The Royal Marsden Hospital Manual of Clinical Nursing Procedures

Third Edition

Also available from Blackwell Science

The Royal Marsden Hospital Manual of Standards of Care

256 pages, illustrated paperback

ISBN 0 632 03386 X

Edited by Joanna M. Luthert and Lorraine Robinson

With the increased need for quality assurance systems, particularly systems to audit nursing and rehabilitative care, this manual will be essential reading and of practical use to a wide range of health care professionals in a variety of settings.

The Royal Marsden Hospital Manual of Standards of Care provides an audit package that can be adapted to be used as part of a quality assurance programme and is the only publication to provide such a complete auditing tool.

The Manual

- makes standards of care practical, attainable and usable
- defines over 40 clinical standards identifying key targets of excellence in clinical care for a variety of health care professionals
- outlines the resources and professional practice necessary to achieve excellence
- describes the expected outcome of such quality care from the perspective of both the health care professional and patients and their families
- demystifies standard writing and measurement

The book has been edited by Joanna Luthert and Lorraine Robinson with contributions from experienced colleagues in a variety of clinical specialties at The Royal Marsden Hospital.

Contents

For further information please contact the Nursing Books Marketing Department on (01865) 206206

The Royal Marsden Hospital Manual of Clinical Nursing Procedures

Third Edition

Edited by

A. Phylip Pritchard

BA, RGN, RMN

Formerly Co-ordinator of European Educational Initiatives,
The Royal Marsden Hospital,
and Executive Secretary,
European Oncology Society

and

Jane Mallett

BSc, MSc, RGN

Research Co-ordinator
The Royal Marsden Hospital

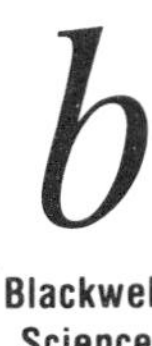

Blackwell
Science

Blackwell Science Ltd
Editorial Offices:
Osney Mead, Oxford OX2 0EL
25 John Street, London WC1N 2BL
23 Ainslie Place, Edinburgh EH3 6AJ
238 Main Street, Cambridge, Massachusetts 02142, USA
54 University Street, Carlton, Victoria 3053, Australia

Other Editorial Offices:
Arnette Blackwell SA
1, rue de Lille
75007 Paris
France

Blackwell Wissenschafts-Verlag GmbH
Kurfürstendamm 57
10707 Berlin
Germany

Blackwell MZV
Feldgasse 13
A-1238 Wien
Austria

First Edition published by Harper and Row Ltd 1984
Second Edition published 1988
Reprinted by HarperCollins 1990
Third Edition published by Blackwell Scientific Publications 1992
Reprinted 1993, 1994 (twice)

Set by Best-set Typesetter Ltd., Hong Kong
Printed and bound in Great Britain by The University Press, Cambridge

DISTRIBUTORS

Marston Book Services Ltd
PO Box 87
Oxford OX2 0DT
(*Orders*: Tel: 01865 791155
Fax: 01865 791927
Telex: 837515)

USA
Blackwell Science, Inc.
238 Main Street
Cambridge, MA 02142
(*Orders*: Tel: 800 759-6102
617 876-7000)

Canada
Times Mirror Professional Publishing Ltd
130 Flaska Drive
Markham, Ontario L6G 1B8
(*Orders*: Tel: 800 268-4178
Fax: 416 470-6739)

Australia
Blackwell Science Pty Ltd
54 University Street
Carlton, Victoria 3053
(*Orders*: Tel: 03 347-5552)

British Library
Cataloguing in Publication Data

The Royal Marsden Hospital manual of clinical nursing.
I. Pritchard, A. Phylip (Albert Phylip)
II. Mallett, Jane
610.73

ISBN 0-632-03387-8

Acknowledgements

Fig. 3.1 is reproduced by kind permission of *Nursing Times* 74(2), 54–5 where the article first appeared: Taylor, L. (1978) An evaluation of handwashing techniques, 1.

Figs 8.1, 8.2, and 8.3 are reproduced with permission from BMJ, publishers.

Fig. 16.12 is taken from Ross & Wilson: *Foundations of Anatomy and Physiology* and is reproduced by kind permission of Churchill Livingstone.

Fig. 28.2 is adapted by kind permission from Fig. 2 Osmosis and Diffusion from *Nursing Times* 22 April 1987.

Fig. 24.1 is reproduced by kind permission of the Backpain Association and is © NBPA: *The Handling of Patients: A Guide for Nurses* 2nd edition.

Fig. 28.2 is reproduced with permission from Professor Teasdale, University of Glasgow.

Fig. 32.1 is reproduced with permission from *Professional Nurse*.

Fig. 46.1 is reproduced by kind permission of Mrs Judy Waterlow, Organiser, Tissue Viability Society Regional Study Days.

Contents

Contributors

Caroline Badger, *BA*, *RGN*, formerly Senior Nurse (Lymphoedema)

Sophia Baty, *RGN*, Sister (Recovery Unit)

Patrick Casey, *RGN*, Clinical Nurse Specialist/ Unit Manager (Genitourinary/Gastrointestinal)

Lisa Coupland, *BSc*, *RGN*, Macmillan Lecturer, Academic Nursing Unit.

Jill David, *MSc*, *RGN*, *HV*, *CERT ED*, *MI BIOL*, formerly Director of Nursing Research

Tonia Dawson, *MSc*, *RGN*, Clinical Nurse Specialist/ Unit Manager (Gynaecology)

Barbara Dicks, *BA*, *RGN*, *RM*, *FETC*, Patient Services Manager

Anne Doherty, *RGN*, formerly Staff Nurse (Operating Theatres)

Shelley Dolan, *BA*, *RGN*, Clinical Nurse Specialist/ Unit Manager (High Dependency Unit)

Lisa Dougherty, *RGN*, *RM*, Clinical Nurse Specialist/ Unit Manager (Intravenous Therapy)

Nuala Durkin, *RGN*, Clinical Nurse Specialist/ Unit Manager (High Dependency Unit)

Sarah Faithfull, *BSc*, *RGN*, Macmillan Lecturer, Academic Nursing Unit

Douglas Guerrero, *BSc*, *RGN*, *NDN*, Clinical Nurse Specialist/Unit Manager (Neuro-Oncology), and formerly Clinical Nurse Specialist (Community Liaison)

Sarah Hart, *RGN*, *FETC*, *Dip Sc*, Clinical Nurse Specialist (Infection Control Radiation Protection)

Pauline Hill, *BA*, *RGN*, *RM*, *HV Cert*, Community Liaison Services Manager

Sian Horn, *RGN*, Sister (High Dependency Unit)

Maureen Hunter, *BSc*, *SRD*, Group Chief Dietitian

Annie Leggett, *RGN*, formerly Clinical Nurse Specialist/Unit Manager (Intravenous Therapy)

Anne Lister, *RGN*, formerly Clinical Nurse Specialist/Unit Manager (Palliative Care Unit)

Jane Mallett, *BSc*, *MSc*, *RGN*, Research Co-ordinator

Marion Morgan, *RGN*, Research Sister (Gynaecology)

Katrina Neal, *RGN*, *FETC*, Clinical Nurse Specialist/ Unit Manager (Palliative Care Unit)

Kate Newlands, *RGN*, *RMN*, Lecturer/Practitioner (Psychological Care)

Cathryn Newton, *BA*, *RGN*, *Dip N*, formerly Senior Nurse (Gastrointestinal/Genitourinary Unit)

Helen Jayne Porter, *RGN*, Clinical Teacher (Leukaemia Unit)

A. Phylip Pritchard *BA*, *RGN*, *RMN*, formerly Co-ordinator of European Educational Initiatives, The Royal Marsden Hospital, and Executive Secretary, European Oncology Nursing Society

Helen Roberts, *RGN*, formerly Senior Nurse (Head and Neck Unit)

Tim Root, *BSc*, *MR PHARMS Soc*, Chief Pharmacist

Miriam Rushton, *MSc*, *RGN*, *Dip N*, *FETC*, formerly Senior Nurse (Gynaecology Unit)

Lena Salter, *BSc, RGN, Dip N, CNT Neurology Certificate*, formerly Senior Nurse, (Neuro-Oncology Unit)

Mave Salter, *BSc, RGN, DN Cert, Cert ED*, Community Liaison Services Manager and formerly Clinical Nurse Specialist/Unit Manager (Gastrointestinal/ Genitourinary Unit)

Valerie Speechley, *RGN, RCNT, Dip N*, formerly Clinical Nurse Specialist (Intravenous Therapy)

Robert Tunmore, *BSc, RGN, RMN*, formerly Clinical Nurse Specialist (Psychological Support)

Kay Wright, *RGN, RCNT, DipN, FETC*, formerly Research Assistant (Nursing Research Unit)

Clare Shaw, *BSc, SRD*, Senior Dietitian

Frances Thurston-Hookway, *RGN*, Clinical Nurse Specialist/Unit Manager (Head and Neck Unit)

Beverley van der Molen, *RGN, FETC*, Clinical Nurse Specialist/Unit Manager (General Oncology)

Foreword

Once again it is my great pleasure to write the foreword to *The Royal Marsden Hospital Manual of Clinical Nursing Procedures*.

This, the third edition, represents a continuation of a successful tradition which dates back to its first publication in 1984. Since that time the nursing profession has developed its scientific and professional base, and the third edition of the manual has sought to reflect this development. A number of new chapters have been added including the Management of Chronic Oedema and Arterial Lines. Other chapters have been thoroughly revised to incorporate up-to-date information and research findings on which a firm base for clinical practice can be founded. As we have emphasized previously, the comments and suggestions of those who use the manual are invaluable in guiding us towards ever improved future editions. We will endeavour to incorporate them into the fourth edition as it begins to take shape.

Robert Tiffany, OBE
Director of Patient Services/
Chief Nursing Officer

PHILOSOPHY FOR NURSING

We believe that the person with cancer should be nursed with full respect for their individuality. The uniqueness of the individual encompasses the physical, emotional, psychosocial and spiritual needs around which the specific contribution of nursing care is planned and given.

We believe that nursing fulfils a central function in co-ordinating the activities of the multidisciplinary team. This role ensures that the individual with cancer receives care that is both responsive to and anticipatory of perceived needs.

We believe that the individual with cancer has a right to be nursed by trained specialist cancer nurses in units designated to treat a specific malignancy or to provide a specialist service.

We believe patients and their families should be encouraged and, where appropriate, instructed to be active participants in setting and achieving realistic health goals.

We believe in facilitating the needs of the individual with cancer to have both conventional and innovative therapies included in their plan of care.

We believe educational opportunities should be available for nurses so that they are better able to act as a resource to patients and their families and provide information to the public about cancer, its prevention and treatment.

We believe in the importance of research and recognize our responsibility to initiate and facilitate this process where appropriate.

We believe in continuous evaluation of standards of care as a basis for the improvement of the quality of nursing practice.

We believe that nurses should manage the provision of nursing care.

We believe that as professionally qualified practitioners, nurses are accountable for their actions.

Acknowledgements

The Royal Marsden Hospital Manual of Clinical Nursing Procedures is the result of a team effort. Some members of the team have changed since the first edition of this work was published in 1984 but the spirit that inspired and drove the original team has remained strong and vital.

We extend our thanks to our contributors for producing procedures that complement and develop the material contained in the previous two editions of the manual and to our medical and paramedical colleagues – notably Lindsey Pegus, Head of the Medical Art Department, and Sue Hall and Peter Walsh also of the Medical Art Department – for their advice and support.

The staff of the libraries of the Royal College of Nursing and the Institute of Cancer Research, in particular Gay Davis, Chief Librarian, have yet again shown that no reference is too obscure to be traced.

To Antoinette Bell, Tina Lisle, Anna Orlowska, David Proudfoot and Carole Merchant we owe a substantial debt for the essential part they played in typing and preparing the manuscripts for publication.

Finally, our thanks to Lisa Field and her colleagues at Blackwell Science Ltd for their help and encouragement.

A. Phylip Pritchard
Jane Mallett

Introduction

The important contribution *The Royal Marsden Hospital Manual of Clinical Nursing Procedures* has made to the process of introducing statements of principle and basing procedures on research findings was quickly recognized by the nursing community (Millar, 1985). The manual now has been adopted in part or in its entirety as the official procedure book by a number of health authorities and remains a source of knowledge which can be used to inform debate on the relationship between nursing theory and practice and the essential nature of nursing procedures and clinical decision making (Crow, Chapman & Roe, 1988).

This edition includes The Royal Marsden Hospital 'Philosophy for nursing'. This philosophy embodies the concept of care practised in the Hospital. The procedures are but one means by which this philosophy is made tangible.

The format of the third edition of *The Royal Marsden Hospital Manual of Clinical Nursing Procedures* remains as for previous editions. Every procedure has two sections: (1) reference material, (2) guidelines. Some procedures also have a third section devoted to nursing care plans.

REFERENCE MATERIAL

The reference material section consists of a short review of the literature and other relevant material. Whenever possible, research findings have been utilized. A list of references and further reading is included at the end to indicate the source of the information and to assist the reader to follow up the topic if more detail is required.

GUIDELINES

The guidelines section provides a list of the equipment needed, followed by a detailed step-by-step account of the procedure and the rationale for the proposed action.

NURSING CARE PLAN

The nursing care plan section gives a list of the problems that may occur, their possible causes and suggestions for their resolution. Items from this sheet can be used on the patient's own nursing care plan.

Procedures have been arranged in alphabetical order although some have been grouped together. The procedures on 'Blood Pressure', 'Respirations' and 'Temperature' will be found under the general heading of 'Observations' (Chapter 29). Correspondingly, many of the procedures associated with wound care (such as care of leg ulcers and pressures ulcers) will be found under the general heading of 'Wound Management' (Chapter 46). Chapter 4, 'Nursing the Infectious or Immunosuppressed Patient', has been expanded considerably and includes new material on infectious diseases that are considered relevant to cancer. Most of the procedures have been rewritten substantially or completely to include the latest research findings. Regrettably, there is still scant literature available on many important clinical nursing activities. If there are still points the reader wants to challenge, then the editors would urge you to let them know. The last word on procedures has yet to be written.

A. Phylip Pritchard
Formerly Co-ordinator of European Educational Initiatives, The Royal Marsden Hospital and Executive Secretary, European Oncology Nursing Society
Jane Mallett
Research Co-ordinator, The Royal Marsden Hospital

References

Crow R. A., Chapman R. G. & Roe B. H. (1988) Nursing procedures and their function as policies for effective practice. *International Journal of Nursing Studies*, 25(3), 217–24.

Millar, A. (1985) The relationship between nursing theory and nursing practice. *Journal of Advanced Nursing*, 10, 417–24.

1

Abdominal Paracentesis

Definition

Abdominal paracentesis is used for the insertion of solutions into, and the withdrawal of fluid from, the peritoneal cavity.

Indications

Abdominal paracentesis is indicated under the following circumstances:

1. To obtain a specimen of fluid for analysis.
2. To relieve pressure when abdominal fluid interferes with respiration or bladder function or is compressing the abdominal viscera and blood vessels.
3. To insert substances such as radioactive gold colloid or cytotoxic drugs (e.g. bleomycin) into the peritoneal cavity; to achieve regression of serosae deposits responsible for fluid formation.

REFERENCE MATERIAL

Abdominal paracentesis is normally performed by a doctor assisted by a nurse. It is an invasive procedure performed at the patient's bedside.

The procedure is most frequently performed for diagnostic purposes. The removal of large amounts of peritoneal fluid is not routine because of the danger of inducing hypovolaemia, hypokalaemia and hyponatraemia. Immediately after removal of large amounts of peritoneal fluid, fluid moves from the vascular space and reaccumulates in the peritoneal cavity so that the problems that occurred before the procedure was performed reappear. In addition, ascitic fluid contains proteins, and body proteins in an already debilitated patient will be further depleted after abdominal paracentesis (Zehner & Hoogstraten, 1985).

Anatomy and physiology

The peritoneum is a semi-permeable serous membrane consisting of two separate layers:

1. Parietal layer: this layer lines the wall of the abdominal cavity.
2. Visceral layer: this layer covers the organs contained within the abdominal cavity (Figure 1.1).

Those organs completely surrounded by peritoneum will be suspended from the posterior abdominal wall by a double fold of the membrane. It is in this way that a mesentery or fold of the peritoneum by which the intestine is attached to the posterior abdominal wall is formed. It is between these two layers that the blood vessels reach the organs, for the abdominal aorta and its branches lie outside the peritoneal cavity (Hinchliff & Montagne, 1988).

The stomach, intestines (except for the duodenum and rectum), liver and spleen are almost completely surrounded by peritoneum. The duodenum, rectum and pancreas are covered only on their anterior surfaces.

The pelvic peritoneum is continuous with that of the rest of the abdominal cavity. It covers the front aspects of the rectum. In the male it passes forwards over the posterior and anterior surfaces of the bladder to become continuous with that on the anterior abdominal wall. In the female it passes from the rectum over the posterior and anterior surfaces of the uterus before reaching the bladder.

Functions of the peritoneum

1. The peritoneum is a serous membrane which enables the abdominal contents to glide over each other without friction.
2. It forms partial or complete cover for the abdominal organs.
3. It forms ligaments and mesenteries which help keep the organs in position.
4. The mesenteries contain fat and act as a store for the body.
5. The mesenteries can move to engulf areas of inflammation and this prevents the spread of infection.

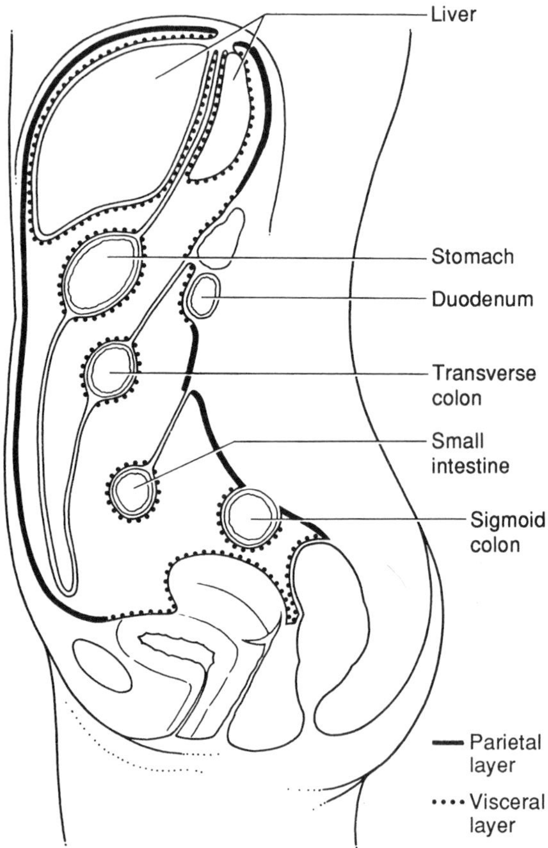

Figure 1.1 Diagram to show peritoneum of female in lateral view.

6. It has the power to absorb fluids and exchange electrolytes.

References and further reading

Alban, C. J. *et al.* (1990) Postoperative chylons ascites: diagnosis and treatment. A series report and literature review. *Archives of Surgery*, 125(2), 270–73.

Hinchliff, S. & Montagne, S. (1988) *Physiology for Nursing Practice*, Ballière Tindall, London.

Kearney, M. (1990) Gynaecological malignancy: Care of the terminally ill. In *Clinical Gynaecological Oncology*, 2nd edn (Ed. by J. H. Shepherd & J. M. Monaghan). Blackwell Scientific Publications, Oxford.

Lentz, S. S. *et al.* (1990) Chylons ascites after whole-abdomen irradiation for gynaecologic malignancy. *International Journal of Radiation, Oncology, Biology and Physics*, 19(2), 435–8.

Marieb, E. N. (1989) *Human Anatomy and Physiology*, The Benjamin/Cummings Publishing Co Inc, Redwood City.

Phipps, W. J. *et al.* (1986) *Medical–Surgical Nursing: Concepts and Clinical Practice*, 3rd edn. C. V. Mosby, St Louis.

Sears, W. G. & Winwood, R. S. (1985) *Anatomy and Physiology for Nurses*, 6th edn. Edward Arnold, London.

Twycross, R. G. & Lack, S. A. (1990) *Therapeutics in Terminal Cancer*, 2nd edn. Churchill Livingstone, Edinburgh.

Wolff, L. (1983) *Fundamental Nursing: the Humanities and the Sciences in Nursing*, 7th edn. J. B. Lippincott, Philadelphia.

Zehner, L. C. & Hoogstraten, B. (1985) Malignant effusions and their management. *Seminars in Oncology Nursing*, 1(4), 259–68.

GUIDELINES: ABDOMINAL PARACENTESIS

Equipment

1. Sterile abdominal paracentesis set containing forceps, blade holder, swabs, towels, suturing equipment, trocar and cannula, rubber tubing to attach to the cannula and guide fluid into the container.
2. Sterile dressing pack.
3. Sterile receiver.
4. Sterile specimen pots.
5. Local anaesthetic.
6. Needles and syringes.
7. Antiseptic solution.
8. Plaster dressing or plastic spray dressing.
9. Large sterile drainage bag or container.
10. Gate clamps.

Procedure

Action	Rationale
1. Explain the procedure to the patient.	To obtain the patient's consent and co-operation.
2. Ask the patient to void bladder.	If the bladder is full there is a chance of it being punctured when the trocar is introduced.
3. Ensure privacy.	
4. The patient should be sitting in Fowler's position or lying in bed.	Normally the pressure in the peritoneal cavity is no greater than atmospheric pressure but, when fluid is present, pressure becomes greater than atmospheric pressure. This position will then aid gravity in the removal of fluid and the fluid will drain of its own accord until the pressure is equalized.
5. The procedure is performed by a doctor:	
(a) The abdomen is prepared aseptically and draped with sterile towels.	To prevent local and/or systemic infection. The peritoneal cavity is normally sterile.
(b) Local anaesthetic is administered	To minimize pain during the procedure and thus ensure maximum co-operation from the patient.
(c) Once the anaesthetic has taken effect the doctor makes an incision approximately halfway between the umbilicus and the symphysis pubic on the midline of the abdomen.	To avoid puncturing the colon.
(d) The trocar and cannula are inserted via the incision and the rubber tubing is attached to the cannula.	
(e) The trocar is removed.	
6. If the cannula is to remain in position, sutures will be inserted and a supportive dry dressing applied and taped firmly in position.	To prevent trauma to the patient. To prevent local and/or systemic infection.
7. A closed drainage system is now attached to the cannula.	A sterile container with a non-return valve is necessary to maintain sterility.
8. Monitor the patient's blood pressure, pulse and respirations and observe drainage. A clamp should be available on the tubing to reduce the flow of fluid if necessary.	To monitor any reaction to the procedure or infection. There may be a major circulatory shift of fluid causing a sudden release of intra-abdominal pressure and possible vasodilation with a consequent fall in blood pressure. While too rapid a removal of fluid can be hazardous, too slow a drainage can also cause hypovolaemia. A rate of 1 litre over 2 hours should not cause problems (Kearney, 1990). However, Kearney (1990) states that the removal of large amounts of ascitic fluid in frail patients can be extremely debilitating, and here a 'partial' paracentesis of 1 to 4 litres may be adequate to relieve symptoms. Twycross and Lack (1990) advise that a tense abdomen should have 2 litres removed immediately followed by 5 to 6 litres over the next 12 hours.

Guidelines: Abdominal paracentesis

Action	Rationale
9. Monitor the patient's fluid balance. Encourage a high-protein and high-calorie diet.	After removal of large amounts of peritoneal fluid, fluid moves from the vascular space and reaccumulates in the peritoneal cavity. Ascitic fluid contains protein in addition to sodium and potassium. Problems of dehydration and electrolyte imbalance may be present.
10. When the cannula is withdrawn, apply a sterile topical swab to the wound.	To maintain asepsis and protect the wound.

NURSING CARE PLAN

Problem	Cause	Suggested action
Patient exhibits shock.	Major circulatory shift of fluid or sudden release of intra-abdominal pressure, vasodilation and subsequent lowering of blood pressure.	Clamp the drainage tube with a gate clamp to prevent further fluid loss. Record the patient's vital signs. Refer to the medical staff for immediate intervention.
Cessation of drainage of ascitic fluid.	Abdomen is empty of ascitic fluid.	Check with the total output of ascitic fluid given on the patient's fluid balance chart. Measure the patient's girth; compare this measurement with the pre-abdominal paracentesis measurement. Suggest to medical staff that the cannula should be removed. Discontinue the drainage system.
	Patient's position is inhibiting drainage.	Change the patient's position, i.e. move the patient upright or onto his/her side to encourage flow by gravity.
	The ascitic fluid has clotted in the drainage system.	'Milk' the tubing. If this is unsuccessful, change the drainage system aseptically.
Signs of local or systemic infection.	Bacterial invasion at site of abdominal paracentesis cannula.	Obtain a swab from the site of the cannula for cultural review. Apply a dry dressing. Refer to the medical staff.
Cannula becomes dislodged.	Ineffective sutures, trauma or infection at the puncture site.	Obtain a swab for culture. Apply a dry dressing. Inform the medical staff.

2

Arterial Lines

Definition
Placement of a catheter into the radial artery.

Reasons for arterial cannulation
Ease of access thereby avoiding the discomfort of frequent punctures of the artery, e.g. blood gases, full blood count, urea and electrolytes. To gain continuous and accurate direct measurement of intra-arterial blood pressure.

Indications
1. During and following major surgery involving prolonged anaesthesia.
2. Patients who are being ventilated mechanically.
3. Patients who require continuous arterial monitoring when rapid alterations in blood pressure are anticipated, e.g. administration of inotropic (e.g. dopamine, adrenaline) and chronotropic (e.g. adrenaline) drugs.
4. Major trauma patients, especially when there is a serious chest injury affecting normal physiology.
5. During inter-hospital transfer of the seriously ill patient.

REFERENCE MATERIAL
Direct haemodyamic monitoring is now performed more frequently than ever before and one particular method, intra-arterial pressure monitoring, is used with increasing frequency in operating theatres, recovery rooms, intensive care units, acute general wards and during inter-hospital transfer of acutely ill patients (Allan, 1984). As a result, the role of the nurse has been extended in line with this increase in the use of invasive techniques. The nurse needs to have an understanding of what is involved when caring for a patient who has an arterial cannula in position.

The most convenient site for arterial cannulation is the right or left radial artery (the cannula should not be positioned close to an adjoining intravenous cannula) and vice versa. The radial artery passes down the radial or lateral side of the forearm to the wrist. Just above the wrist it lies superficially and can be felt in front of the radius, where the radial pulse is palpable. The artery then passes between the first and second metacarpal bones and enters the palm of the hand (Ross & Wilson, 1990).

Intra-arterial cannulation is now an established and essential procedure for the monitoring of arterial blood pressure (Zideman & Morgan, 1981). If the arterial line is used for pressure monitoring, a suitable monitoring system is required to provide a continuous assessment of the patient's intra-arterial pressure, i.e. mean arterial pressure and blood pressure (Allan, 1984). An additional advantage of an indwelling arterial cannula is that repeated sampling for blood gas analysis, etc. can be performed without repeated puncture of the artery (which may be more traumatic than prolonged cannulation) (Hinds, 1987).

Accidental intra-arterial injection of drugs may occur with the presence of an arterial cannula and the multiplicity of venous lines in such patients. In one case Flucloxacillin was accidentally injected and parts of digits became gangrenous, which required amputation and the application of skin grafts. Such a risk can be minimized by clearly labelling the arterial line (Zideman & Morgan, 1981).

Another serious complication is hypovolaemia, due to disconnection. This can be minimized by using Luer locks for all connections and by leaving the site exposed for observation. Ischaemia is rare, however, the signs must be recognized early and the cannula removed promptly (Hinds, 1987). A recent study comparing heparin solution and normal saline for maintenance of arterial patency resulted in catheter survival rate of 86% at 96 hours compared with a rate of 52% after 40 hours with a normal saline solution. This suggests that heparin reduces the frequency of catheter occlusion (Clifton *et al.*, 1991).

References and further reading
Allan, D. (1984) Care of the patient with an arterial

catheter. *Nursing Times*, 14 November, 80(46), 40–41.
Clifton, G. D. *et al.* (1991) Comparison of normal saline and heparin solutions for maintenance of arterial catheter patency. *Heart and Lung*, 20(2), 115–18.
Hinds, C. J. (1987) *Intensive Care*. Baillière Tindall, Gillingham, Kent.
Huddak, C., Gallo, B. M. & Lohr, T. S. (1986) *Critical Care Nursing*, 4th edn. J. B. Lippincott, Philadelphia.
Oh, T. E. (1991) *Intensive Care Manual*, 3rd edn. Butterworths, Sydney, Australia.
Pritchard, A. P. & David, J. A. (1988) *The Royal Marsden Hospital Manual of Clinical Nursing Procedures*, 2nd edn. Harper & Row, London.
Ross, J. S. & Wilson, K. J. (1990) *Anatomy and Physiology and Illness*, 7th edn. Churchill Livingstone, Edinburgh.
Santolla, A. & Weckel, C. (1983) A new closed system for arterial lines. *RN*, June, 46(6), 49–52.
Zideman, D. A. & Morgan, M. (1981) Inadvertent intra-arterial injection of Flucloxacillin. *Anaesthesia*, 36(6), 296–8.

GUIDELINES: SETTING UP AN ARTERIAL LINE

Equipment

1. 600 ml pressure infuser cuff.
2. 500 ml bag of normal saline or prescribed solution.
3. Heparin as prescribed, plus additive label.
4. 22 SWG cannula or other available arterial catheters.
5. Sterile intravenous pack.
6. Gloves.
7. Antiseptic alcoholic cleanser.
8. Semi-occlusive dressing.
9. Syringes – various.
10. Arterial identification label.
11. 1% lignocaine injection.
12. Pressuring monitoring system equipment.

Procedure

Action	Rationale
1. Explain procedure to patient. (*Note*: Most arterial cannulas are inserted when patients are anaesthetized.)	To obtain patient's consent and co-operation.
2. Prepare infusion and additive (heparin 1 unit per ml) as prescribed. Apply additive sticker to front of bag.	To prevent duplication of treatment. To maintain accurate records. To provide a point of reference in the event of any queries.
3. Connect giving set to bag.	
4. Open intravenous controller fully.	
5. Prime the giving set by squeezing the flush device–actuator (see instructions with set). Ensure all three-way tap ports are primed.	
6. Check thoroughly for air bubbles in the circuit.	To prevent an air embolus.
7. Check that all connections are snugly fitted. Do not force because they may crack.	To prevent disconnection.
8. Insert bag of heparinized saline into bottom pressure cuff. Inflate to 300 mm Hg.	This pressure is higher than arterial blood pressure, therefore an automatic flush mode is activated in the system which delivers 3 ml/hr, which maintains patency of circuit, cannula and artery (Allan, 1984).

9. Wash your hands with bactericidal soap and water or bactericidal alcohol hand rub before leaving clinical room.
To reduce the risk of cross-infection.

10. Prepare trolley near the patient as described in Chapter 3, Aseptic Technique.

11. Radial site (or other site chosen by doctor) is prepared aseptically by doctor, shaved if necessary, cleaned with skin cleansing solution and a sterile towel is placed under the arm.
To maintain asepsis.

Note: Before the insertion of a radial artery cannula, circulation to the hand should be evaluated by assessing the circulation of the palmar arch using the Allen test. The Allen test consists of simultaneously compressing both the ulnar and radial arteries for approximately one minute. During this time, the patient rapidly opens and closes the hand to promote exsanguination.

Approximately five seconds after release of the artery (usually the ulnar), the extended hand should blush due to capillary refilling. This reactive hyperaemia indicates adequate circulation in the hand. If blanching occurs, palmer arch circulation is inadequate, and a radial cannula could lead to ischaemia of the hand (Hinds, 1987).

12. Local anaesthetic is administered locally if cannulation is performed while the patient is conscious.
To minimize pain during the procedure and thus ensure maximum co-operation from the patient.

13. Nurse and doctor apply gloves. See Chapter 3, Aseptic Technique, for safe technique and practice guidelines.
To prevent contamination of hands if blood spillage occurs.

14. The nurse holds the patient's arm in suitable position.
To prevent movement and dislodgement of cannula.

15. Cannula is inserted by the doctor.

16. Pressure is applied to radial artery above cannula while infusion is connected.
To prevent blood spillage.

17. Open infusion controller fully

18. Tape the line and cannula securely, and apply semi-occlusive dressing. Clearly label 'arterial' (see Figure 2.1).
Leaving the site exposed allows the observer to recognize immediately any dislodgement or disconnection. Clear labelling prevents accidental injection of drugs.

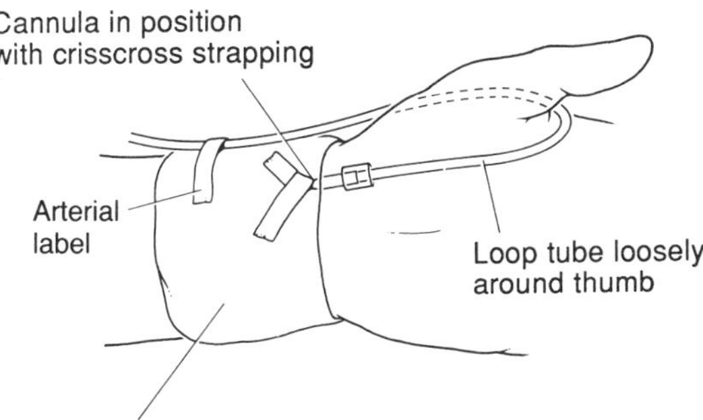

Figure 2.1 Positioning, securing and labelling of the cannula.

Guidelines: Setting up an arterial line

Action	Rationale
19. Inform patient of amount of movement permitted, e.g. arm may be moved gently and fingers may be exercised. Discourage any stress on arm and connections.	To prevent dislodgement.

GUIDELINES: TAKING A BLOOD SAMPLE FROM AN ARTERIAL LINE

This should be carried out by a nurse who is skilled in the procedure. Care must be taken not to introduce air or infection.

Equipment

1. Intravenous sterile dressing pack.
2. Gloves.
3. Appropriate syringes and blood sample bottles.
4. Sterile Luer lock connection.
5. Antiseptic alcoholic cleanser.
6. Bactericidal skin cleanser.

Procedure

Action	Rationale
1. Explain the procedure to the patient.	To obtain the patient's consent and co-operation.
2. Prepare the trolley.	
3. Wash hands with bactericidal soap and water or bactericidal alcohol hand rub before leaving clinical room.	To prevent cross-infection.
4. Check that the three-way tap (Figure 2.2a) is closed to air.	To prevent back-flow of blood and blood spillage.

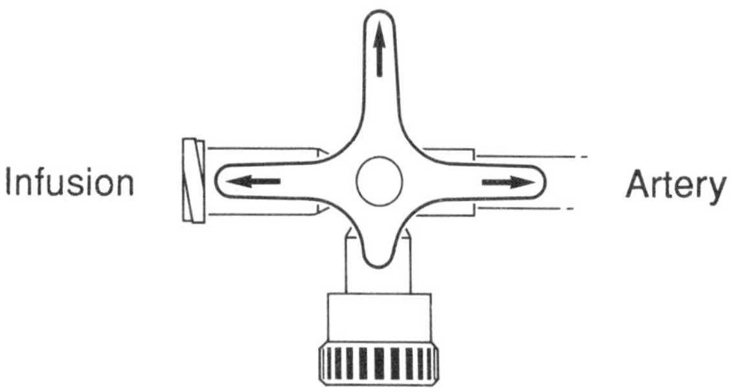

Figure 2.2a Three-way tap closed to port.

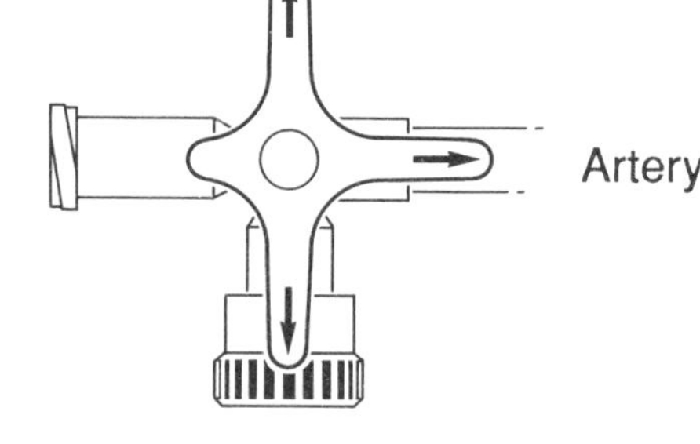

Figure 2.2b Three-way tap turned to artery and port.

Action	Rationale
5. Clean hands with bactericidal alcohol hand rub.	Hands have been contaminated by touching three-way tap.
6. Prepare trolley according to the Guidelines: Aseptic Technique, Chapter 3.	

7. Apply gloves. See Chapter 3 for safe technique and practice guidelines.	To prevent contamination of hand with blood.
8. Remove cap from three-way tap (Figure 2.2a) and clean open port with antiseptic alcoholic cleanser.	To prevent infection.
9. Connect 15 ml syringe to open port.	
10. Turn three-way tap to artery and port (Figure 2.2b).	To prevent contamination of blood sample with heparinized infusion fluid.

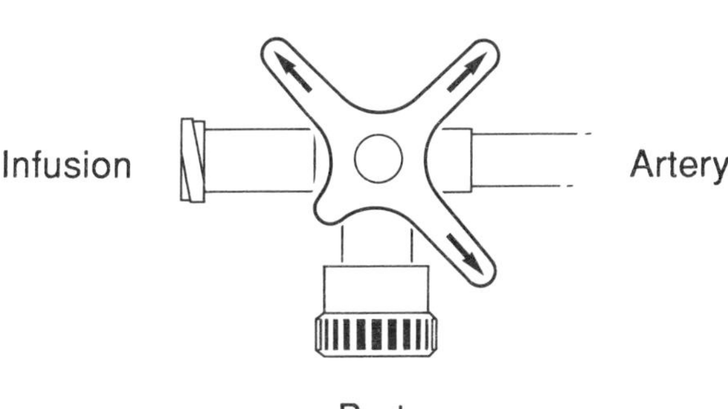

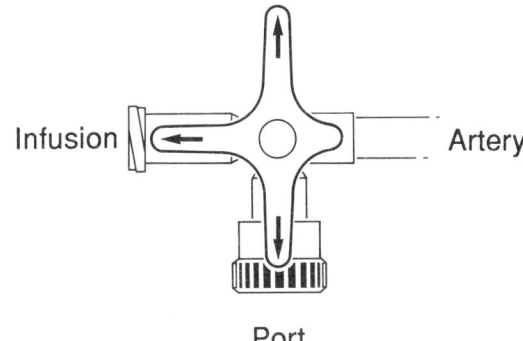

Figure 2.2c Three-way tap turned diagonally to close off infusion, artery and port.

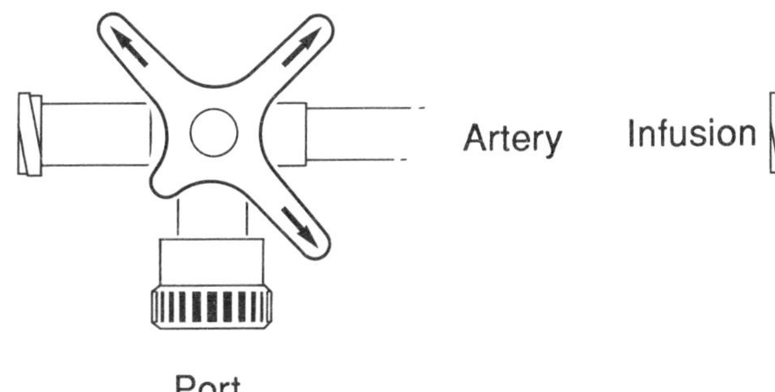

Figure 2.2d Three-way tap turned to infusion and port.

11. Gently withdraw 5 ml of blood or until line is clear of infusion fluid.	To prevent contamination of blood with infusion fluid.
12. Turn three-way tap diagonally to close off infusion, artery and port (Figure 2.2c).	To prevent back-flow of blood from artery, contamination with infusion fluid and blood spillage.
13. Remove syringe.	
14. Connect appropriately sized syringe for sample.	
15. Turn three-way tap to artery and port (Figure 2.2b).	To prevent contamination with infusion fluid.
16. Gently remove amount of blood required.	
17. Turn three-way tap to infusion and artery (Figure 2.2a).	To prevent back flow of blood and blood spillage.
18. Remove syringe.	
19. Turn three-way tap to infusion and port (Figure 2.2d).	To prevent blood clotting in port.
20. Turn three-way tap to infusion and artery (Figure 2.2a). Flush line gently by squeezing actuator (see instructions with set).	To clear blood from line.
21. Clean port with antiseptic.	
22. Apply sterile Luer lock connection and check it is snugly connected.	To prevent haemorrhage or blood spillage.

Guidelines: Taking a blood sample from an arterial line

Action	Rationale
23. Check pressure infuser cuff is inflated to 300 mm Hg.	To prevent back-flow of blood into circuit.
24. Empty blood from syringe into appropriate sample bottle, and immediately label or record blood gas.	

GUIDELINES: REMOVAL OF AN ARTERIAL LINE

Equipment

1. Intravenous sterile dressing pack.
2. Gloves.
3. Hypo-allergenic tape.
4. Antiseptic alcoholic cleanser.
5. Bactericidal skin cleanser.

Procedure

Action	Rationale
1. Explain procedure to patient.	To obtain patient's consent and co-operation.
2. Prepare trolley as described in Chapter 3, Guidelines: Aseptic Technique.	
3. Wash hands with bactericidal soap and water or bactericidal alcohol hand rub before leaving clinical room.	To reduce the risk of cross-infection.
4. Prepare trolley by patient as described in Chapter 3, Guidelines: Aseptic Technique.	
5. Turn three-way tap diagonally (Figure 2.2c).	To prevent back-flow of blood into line.
6. Turn off intravenous controller.	To prevent spillage when removing cannula.
7. Deflate pressure cuff.	Pressure no longer required.
8. Remove semi-occlusive dressing and tape from cannula site.	
9. Clean hands with a bactericidal skin cleanser solution.	
10. Apply gloves. See Chapter 3 for safe technique and practice guidelines.	To prevent contamination of hands with blood.
11. Clean cannula site area with antiseptic alcoholic cleanser.	

12. Place sterile piece of gauze over area and gently remove cannula.

13. Apply pressure to site for a minimum of five minutes or until bleeding stops. — To prevent a haematoma and blood loss.

14. Apply a clean, sterile, dry dressing using a non-touch technique. — To maintain asepsis.

15. Apply strapping.

Following this procedure, check the patient's hand hourly for warmth, colour, swelling and signs of bleeding. Ask the patient to inform staff if feeling faint or if there is oozing from dressing. The medical staff must be informed immediately if the hand or forearm becomes discoloured or swollen, or if the patient complains of pain in the limb.

NURSING CARE PLAN

Problem	**Cause**	**Suggested action**
Haemorrhage.	Luer lock connections are loose or cracked. Blood will be lost from open connection.	Check that Luer locks are fitted securely. Do not force because the locks may crack.
	Blood may ooze around the cannula site.	Place a semi-occlusive dressing over the cannula site and observe hourly.
	Cannula may have become dislodged.	Inform the patient about the amount of movement that is preferred. Take care when moving the patient. Avoid putting stress on the arm and connections. Secure the line well (see Figure 2.1).
Back-flow of blood into the line.	The pressure infusor cuff may not be inflated to the optimal pressure.	Ensure that the pressure infusor cuff is inflated to 300 mm Hg. This pressure is higher than arterial blood pressure and an automatic flush mode is activated in the system which delivers 3 ml/hr. This maintains potency of circuit, cannula and artery (Allan, 1984).
Ischaemia.	A thrombosis may form in the circuit cannula or artery.	Ensure that heparin is added to the saline infusion (Clifton, 1991). Assess limb pulse, colour and temperature hourly. Absent pulses, pallor, cyanosis and coldness denote occlusion. If this occurs medical advice must be sought and the cannula removed promptly (Hinds, 1987).
Erythema or inflammation around the insertion site.	Phlebitis due to sepsis, chemical irritation or mechanical irritation.	Refer to the procedure on pages 258–263.

Nursing care plan

Problem	**Cause**	**Suggested action**
Hypotension, tachycardia, cyanosis, unconsciousness.	Embolism: air particle	Refer to the procedure on pages 104–108.
Arterial spasm.	Forceful flushing or aspiration when withdrawing blood.	Avoid forceful flushing and maintain a slow even pressure when withdrawing blood.
Cerebral vascular accident (CVA).	Large flush volumes can cause back-flow of arterial blood leading to central artery emboli and subsequent CVA (Santolla/Wechel, 1983).	Manual flushing should be kept to a minimum if cerebral vascular accidents are to be prevented.
Gangrene.	Accidental injection of a drug into the artery.	Label the arterial cannula and circuit clearly (see Figure 2.1). In the event of accidental injection of any drug, report the error immediately to medical staff and senior nurse and perform the following: (a) Gently withdraw blood from the three-way tap to try and withdraw the drug. (b) Stop the infusion and wait for instructions from the medical staff. (c) Assess limb pulse, colour and temperature hourly. (d) Complete an accident form.

3

Aseptic Technique

Definition

Aseptic technique is a method used to prevent contamination of wounds and other susceptible sites by organisms that could cause infection. This can be achieved by ensuring that only sterile equipment and fluids are used during invasive medical and nursing procedures.

Indications

An aseptic technique should be implemented during any invasive procedure that bypasses the body's natural defences, e.g. the skin and mucous membranes, or when handling equipment such as intravenous cannulae and urinary catheters that have been used during these procedures.

REFERENCE MATERIAL

The literature shows that a significant number of patients acquire some type of wound infection during their stay in hospital which is directly related to wound contamination at the time of operation (Table 3.1) (Cruse & Foord, 1980).

Sixty per cent of these infections were caused by aerobic Gram-negative bacteria, 30% by Gram-positive bacteria, 3% anaerobic bacteria, while the remaining 7% were attributed to fungi and viruses.

Similarly, urinary tract infections continue to be the most common hospital-acquired infections. The prevalence study in 1980 by the Public Health Laboratory showed that urinary tract infection caused 30.3% of all infections; of the 8.6% of patients catheterized, 21.2% had infections, compared to 2.9% in non-catheterized patients (Meers *et al.*, 1981), illustrating the association between invasive procedure and infection.

Table 3.1 Category of wound and infection rate

Category of wound	*Infection rate (%)*
Clean	1.5
Clean contaminated	7.7
Contaminated	15.2
Dirty	40.0

The diagnosis of infection relies on classic signs of inflammation such as local redness, swelling and pain. These local signs and symptoms can precede a further sequence of events, which can be lymphangitis, lymphadenitis, bacteraemia and septicaemia which, if not promptly recognized and treated, can result in death (Laurence, 1991).

The cost of infection is high, both to the patient and the hospital. The patient may be inconvenienced by a prolonged period of hospitalization, which can cause economic and social hardships to the whole family. The hospital will have increased waiting lists and increased hospital costs. It is essential that when aseptic techniques are used as a method of preventing infection that these procedures are sound in theory and are carried out correctly.

Gwyther (1988) discusses how most teaching occurs on the hospital ward and questions whether this teaching is based on knowledge of the principles of, for example, wound care, or simply on experience.

Principles of asepsis

The risk of infection is increased if the patient is immunocompromised (Hart, 1990) by:

1. Age. Neonates and the elderly are more at risk due to their less efficient immune systems.
2. Underlying disease. For example, those patients with severe debilitating or malignant disease.
3. Prior drug therapy, such as the use of immunosuppresive drugs or the use of broad-spectrum antimicrobials.
4. Patients undergoing surgery or instrumentation.

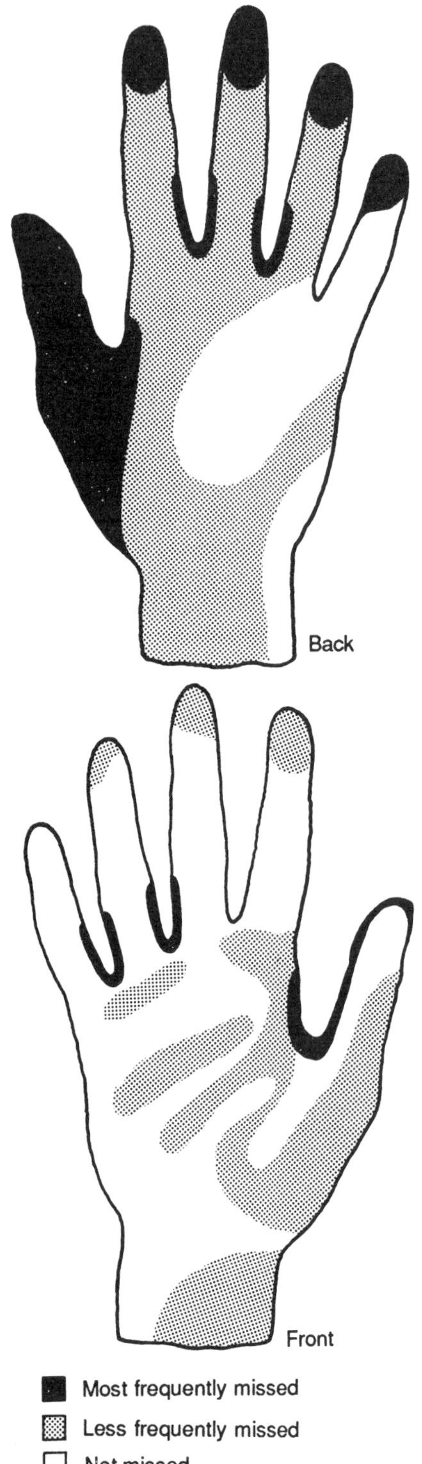

Figure 3.1 Areas most commonly missed following hand washing. (Reproduced by kind permission of *Nursing Times*, where this article first appeared in 1978.)

The following factors must be considered (Trester 1982):

(a) Classic signs and symptoms of infection are often absent.
(b) Untreated infection may disseminate rapidly.
(c) Infections may be caused by non-pathogenic and unusual organisms.
(d) Some antibiotics are less effective in immuno-compromised patients.
(e) Repeated infections may be caused by the same organism.
(f) Superimposed infection is a frequent occurrence requiring nursing care of the highest standard to prevent infection (Gurevich *et al.*, 1986), which includes strict adherence to aseptic techniques.

The most usual means for spread of infection include:

1. Hands of the staff involved.
2. Inanimate objects, e.g. instruments and clothes.
3. Dust particles or droplet nuclei suspended in the atmosphere.

Hand washing

Hand washing is the single most important procedure for preventing nosocomial infection as hands have been shown to be an important route of transmission of infection (Casewell *et al.*, 1977). However, studies have shown that hand washing is rarely carried out in a satisfactory manner (Taylor, 1978a), with the most important factor inhibiting hand washing being busyness (Larson *et al.*, 1982) or inaccessible sinks (Albert *et al.*, 1981). Studies have shown that up to 89% of staff miss some part of the hand surface during hand washing (Taylor, 1978a) (see Figure 3.1).

Taylor (1978b) and Phillips (1989) use Feldman's criteria for handwashing, which include the following:

1. Use soap.
2. Use continuously running water.
3. Position hands to avoid contaminating arms.
4. Avoid splashing clothing or floor.
5. Rub hands together vigorously.
6. Use friction on all surfaces.
7. Rinse hands thoroughly with hand held down to rinse.
8. Dry hands thoroughly.

Paper towels have been shown to be a quick, convenient and reliable method of drying hands, and preferable to roller towel or warm air dryers (Blackmore, 1987). Hand washing should be undertaken after patient contact and before an aseptic technique is performed (Centre for Disease Control, 1986). Dress rings, bracelets, wrist watches and nail varnish must be removed and sleeves rolled up before hand washing.

Transient bacteria can be almost completely removed from the hands by soap and water washing (Lowbury *et al.*, 1974a). Conversely, soap and water do not reduce the number of resident bacteria by any significant amount. Resident skin flora, such as *Staphylococcus aureus*, are removed most effectively by rubbing the hands with a bactericidal alcoholic solution of chlorhexidine. Lowbury *et al.* (1974b) showed that rinsing the hands with alcoholic chlorhexidine 0.5% removed more resident skin flora than did washing the hands with a chlorhexidine 4% detergent wash.

It is suggested that a preparation such as chlorhexidine 4% detergent wash is used for cleaning physically dirty or contaminated hands, while a bactericidal alcoholic hand rub should be used for disinfecting clean hands immediately before carrying out an aseptic technique. A nurse with 'socially clean' hands will not need to wash them during the aseptic procedure, but should use a bactericidal alcoholic hand rub whenever disinfection is required, e.g. after opening the outer wrappers of dressings. This will also remove the need for the nurse to leave the patient during the procedure to wash the hands at a basin, as it is unlikely that nurses' hands will become soiled with blood or body fluids as long as blood and body fluid precautions are adopted at all times (Hart, 1991).

No-touch technique

A no-touch technique is essential to ensure that hands, even though they have been washed, do not contaminate the sterile equipment or the patient. This can be achieved either by the use of forceps or sterile gloves (Lascelles, 1982). However, it must be remembered that gloves can become damaged and allow the passage of bacteria (Rowland *et al.*, 1985), while forceps may damage tissue (David, 1991).

Inanimate objects

All instruments, fluids and materials that come into contact with the wound must be sterile if the risk of contamination is to be reduced. The central sterile supplies department should normally provide all sterile instruments. In the event of supplies being short or in an emergency, it is acceptable to disinfect a clean instrument, such as a pair of scissors, by immersing it completely in alcoholic chlorhexidine 1 in 200 (70%) for five minutes.

Most disinfectants have a limited antimicrobial spectrum and must be used only on clean surfaces or equipment, e.g. instruments, as they may fail to penetrate blood or pus (Ayliffe, 1984). Any equipment that becomes contaminated during a procedure must be discarded. On *no* account should it be returned to the sterile field. Care must also be taken to ensure that equipment and lotions are sterile and that packaging is undamaged before use.

While following aseptic techniques, it is also important to evaluate the whole procedure to ensure the principles are being followed during the whole process; errors such as taking adhesive tape from a contaminated roll (Oldman, 1987) or using dressings left over from a previous dressing (Roberts, 1987) must be avoided.

The dressing trolley

The trolley should be washed every day with detergent and water. It should not need cleaning between dressings unless a surface becomes physically contaminated, since organisms cannot survive on cold, smooth, dry surfaces. The sterile field, usually made of thick waxed paper, will not allow the passage of organisms through it. Trolleys used for aseptic procedures must not be used for any other purpose.

Protective clothing

Protective clothing may be worn for a variety of reasons, including the need to proclaim the identity of the wearer (Sparrow, 1991). Generally, however, protective clothing is worn for the following reasons:

1. Prevent user's clothing becoming contaminated with pathogenic micro-organisms which may subsequently be transferred to other patients in their care.
2. Prevent user's clothing becoming soiled, wet or stained during the course of their duties.
3. Prevent transfer of potentially pathogenic micro-organisms from user to patient.
4. Prevent user acquiring infection from patient.

There is evidence of transfer of organisms from one room to another on clothing (Hambraeus, 1973). An impermeable apron offers better protection than a cotton gown, which allows bacteria and moisture to pass through because of the weave (Mackintosh *et al.*, 1980). It is therefore recommended that a disposable plastic apron, which is impermeable to bacteria, is worn during aseptic procedures. Aprons should be changed after each dressing.

Masks are worn to prevent the dissemination of organisms from the nose and mouth during breathing, talking, sneezing or coughing, and to protect the wearer from inhaling airborne micro-organisms disseminated from infected patients. Studies have shown that not wearing a mask does not alter infection rates (Orr, 1981). However, there may be some justification in wearing masks when giving prolonged close care to major burn patients.

The patient's skin flora is an important source of infection following invasive procedures (Goodinson, 1990). Patient hygiene will reduce this hazard (Mackenzie, 1988). Studies comparing washing with soap or chlorhexidine solution demonstrated a marked decrease in bacteriuria in patients washing with chlorhexidine (Sanderson, 1990).

Studies to establish whether the incidence of infection or prolonged or delayed healing occurred when stitches became wet during bathing, showed that getting stitches wet was not detrimental to wound healing (Noe *et al.*, 1988). Therefore, a patient with, for example, an indwelling intravenous Hickman catheter, while showering with stitches still *in situ* should wear a dressing, and after showering any non-waterproof dressing should be changed immediately (Mitchell, 1984).

Airborne contamination

The spread of infection is most likely to occur in a large, open ward and, ideally, dressings should all be performed in a properly ventilated room. Many dressings, however, are carried out at the patient's bedside. In such cases, ward cleaning should have ceased at least 30 minutes before, and the curtains drawn at least 10 minutes before a dressing is begun. To reduce to a minimum the opportunities for airborne contamination, wounds should be exposed for the shortest time possible and dirty dressings should be placed carefully in a yellow clinical waste bag, preferably plastic, which is sealed before disposal (Lowbury *et al.*, 1981). Clean wounds should be dressed before contaminated wounds. Colostomies and infected wounds should be dressed last of all to minimize environmental contamination and cross-infection.

Air movement should be kept to a minimum during the dressing. This means that adjacent windows should be closed and the movement of personnel within the area discouraged.

References and further reading

Albert, R. K. *et al.*, (1981) Handswashing patterns in medical intensive care units. *New England Journal of Medicine*, 304, 1465–6.

Ayliffe, G. A. J. (1984) *Chemical Disinfection in Hospitals*. Public Health Laboratory Service, London, pp. 7–8.

Blackmore, M. (1987) Hand drying methods. *Nursing Times*, 83(37), 71–4.

Casewell, M. *et al.* (1977) Hands as route of transmission for *klebsiella* species. *British Medical Journal*, 2, 1315–17.

Centre for Disease Control (1986) Guidelines for handwashing and hospital environmental control. *Infection Control*, 7(4), 233–5.

Cruse, P. J. E. & Foord, R. (1980) The epidemiology of wound infection – a 10-year prospective study of 62,939 wounds. *Surgical Clinics of North America*, 60(1), 27–40.

David, J. (1991) Letters. *Wound Management*, 1(2), 15.

Goodinson, S. M. (1990) Keeping the flora out. *The Professional Nurse*, 5(11), 572–5.

Gurevich, I. *et al.* (1986) The compromised host deficit specific infection and the spectrum of prevention. *Cancer Nursing*, 9, 263–75.

Gwyther, J. (1988) Skilled dressing. *Nursing Times*, 84(19), 60–61.

Hambraeus, A. (1973) Transfer of *Staphylococcus aureus* via nurses' uniform. *Journal of Hygiene*, 71, 799–814.

Hart, S. (1990) The immunosuppressed patient in infection control. In *Guidelines for Nursing Care* (Ed. by M. A. Worsley *et al.*), pp. 15–20. Surgikos Ltd.

Hart, S. (1991) Blood and body precautions. *Nursing Standard*, 5(25), 25–8.

Larson, E. *et al.* (1982) Factors influencing handwashing behaviour of patients' care personnel. *American Journal of Infection Control*, 10(3), 93–9.

Lascelles, I. (1982) Wound dressing technique. *Nursing*, 2(8), 217–19.

Laurence, C. (1991) Bacterial infection of wounds. *Wound Management*, 1(1), 13–15.

Lowbury, E. J. *et al.* (1974a) Disinfection of hands: removal of transient organisms. *British Medical Journal*, 2, 230–33.

Lowbury, E. J. *et al.* (1974b) Preoperative disinfection of surgeons' hands: Use of alcoholic solutions and effects of gloves on skin flora. *British Medical Journal*, 4, 369–72.

Lowbury, E. J. *et al.* (1981). *Control of Hospital Infection – A Practical Handbook*, 2nd edn. Chapman & Hall, London.

Mackenzie, I. (1988) Pre-operative skin preparation and surgical outcome. *Journal of Hospital Infection*, Suppl. B., pp. 27–32.

Mackintosh, C. A. *et al.* (1980) The evaluation of fabric in relation to their use as protective garments in nursing and surgery. *Journal of Hygiene*, 85, 393–403.

Meers, P. D. *et al.* (1981) Report on the National Survey of Infection in Hospital 1980. *Journal of Hospital Infection*, 2(Suppl), 1–53.

Mitchell, N. J. (1984) Whole-body disinfection with chlorhexidine in shower bathing more effective than bathing. *Journal of Hospital Infection*, 5, 96–9.

Noe, J. M. *et al.* (1988) Can stitches get wet? *Plastic and Reconstructive Surgery*, 81(1), 82–4.

Oldman, P. M. (1987) An unkind cut. *Nursing Times*, 83(48), 71–4.

Oldman, P. (1991) A sticky situation – microbiological study of adhesive tape used to secure IV cannulae. *The Professional Nurse*, February, 265–9.

Orr, N. W. M. (1981) Is a mask necessary in the operating

theatre? *Annals of the Royal College of Surgeons*, 63, 390–92.

Phillips, C. (1989) Hand hygiene. *Nursing Times*, 85(37), 76–9.

Roberts, J. (1987) Pennywise, pound foolish. *Nursing Times*, 83(37), 68–9.

Rowland, C. *et al.* (1985) In the surgeons' hands. *Nursing Times*, Supplement, 5–7.

Sanderson, P. J. (1990) A comparison of the effect of chlorhexidine antisepsis, soap and antibiotics on bacteriuria, perineal colonization and environmental contamination in spinally injured patients. *Journal of Hospital Infection* 15, 235–43.

Sparrow, S. (1991) An exploration of the role of the nurses' uniform through a period of non-uniform wear on an acute medical ward. *Journal of Advanced Nursing*, 16, 116–22.

Taylor, L. (1978a) An evaluation of handwashing techniques 1. *Nursing Times*, 74(2), 54–5.

Taylor, L. (1978b) An evaluation of handwashing techniques 2. *Nursing Times*, 74(3), 108–10.

Trester, A. (1982) Nursing management of patients receiving cancer chemotherapy. *Cancer Nursing*, 6, 206–10.

GUIDELINES: ASEPTIC TECHNIQUE

Equipment

1. Sterile dressing pack* containing gallipots or an indented plastic tray, low-linting, non-woven swabs and/or medical foam, disposable forceps, gloves, sterile field, disposable bag.
2. Fluids for cleaning and/or irrigation.
3. Hypo-allergenic tape.
4. Appropriate dressing (see Chapter 46, Wound Care).
5. Appropriate hand hygiene preparation.

Any other material will be determined by the nature of the dressing: special features of a dressing should be referred to in the patient's nursing care plan.

Procedure

Action	Rationale
1. Explain the procedure to the patient.	To obtain the patient's consent and co-operation.
2. Wash the trolley with liquid detergent and water. Dry throughly with a paper towel.	To provide a clean working surface.
3. Place all the equipment required for the procedure on the bottom shelf of a clean dressing trolley.	To maintain the top shelf as a clean working surface.
4. Take the patient to the treatment room or screen the bed. Position the patient comfortably so that the area to be dealt with is easily accessible without exposing the patient unduly.	To allow dust and airborne organisms to settle before the sterile field (and in the case of a dressing, the wound) is exposed. Maintain the patient's dignity and comfort.
5. If the procedure is a dressing and the wound is infected or producing copious amounts of exudate, put on a disposable plastic apron.	To reduce the risk of spreading infection.
6. Take the trolley to the treatment room or patient's bedside, disturbing the screens as little as possible.	To minimize airborne contamination.
7. Wash your hands with bactericidal soap and water or a bactericidal alcohol hand rub.	To reduce the risk of wound infection.
8. Check the pack is sterile (i.e., the pack is undamaged, intact and dry. If autoclave tape is	To ensure that only sterile products are used.

Guidelines: Aseptic technique

Action	Rationale
present, check that it has changed colour from beige to beige and brown lines), open the outer cover of the sterile pack and slide the contents onto the top shelf of the trolley.	
9. Open the sterile field using only the corners of the paper.	So that areas of potential contamination are kept to a minimum.
10. Check any other packs for sterility and open, tipping their contents gently onto the centre of the sterile field.	To prepare the equipment and in the case of a wound dressing reduce the amount of time that the wound is uncovered. This reduces the risk of infection and a drop in temperature of the wound.
11. Wash hands with a bactericidal alcohol rub.	Hands may become contaminated by handling outer packets, etc.
12. Using the forceps in the pack, arrange the sterile field with the handles of the instruments in one corner or around the edge of the sterile field. Where appropriate, swab along the 'tear area' of lotion sachet with chlorhexidine gluconate 0.5% and isopropyl alcohol 70%. Tear open sachet and pour lotion into gallipots or an indented plastic tray (see Table 46.3).	The time the patient is exposed is kept to a minimum. To minimize risk of contamination of lotion.
13. If appropriate, put on sterile gloves, touching only the inside wrist end.	To reduce the risk of infection. Gloves provide greater sensitivity than forceps and are less likely to cause trauma to the patient.

Carry out procedure

Action	Rationale
14. Make sure the patient is comfortable.	
15. Dispose of waste in yellow clinical waste bags.	To prevent environmental contamination. Yellow is the recognized colour for clinical waste.
16. If necessary, draw back curtains or, if appropriate, help the patient back to the bed area and ensure the patient is comfortable.	
17. Check that the trolley remains dry and physically clean. If necessary, wash with liquid detergent and water and dry throughly with a paper towel.	To reduce the risk of spreading infection.
18. Wash hands with soap and water.	To reduce the risk of spreading infection.

* **Footnote**: Please note that for some procedures it may be more appropriate to use different types of sterile packs (e.g. intravenous packs). Since usage of these will vary locally reference is generally made to 'sterile dressing pack'.

4

Barrier Nursing: Nursing the Infectious or Immunosuppressed Patient

BARRIER NURSING

Definition

Barrier nursing involves the use of practices aimed at controlling the spread of, and destroying, pathogenic organisms. These practices may require the setting up of mechanical barriers to contain pathogenic organisms within a specified area.

Indication

Barrier nursing is required under the following circumstances:

1. To prevent the spread of infection from patients with communicable diseases (i.e. contagious diseases such as glandular fever, or infectious diseases such as chicken pox).
2. To prevent the spread of infection from patients infected with organisms which are resistant to the usual range of antibiotics; such as methicillin-resistant *Staphylococcus aureus* (MRSA).
3. To protect those patients whose susceptibility to infection is increased (protective isolation or reverse barrier nursing).

REFERENCE MATERIAL

Most precautions against transferring infection demand more effort, take more time and cost more than the comparable procedures in normal circumstances.

For the infected patient the consequences can be considerable and may include the following:

1. Delayed or prevented recovery.
2. Increased pain, discomfort and anxiety.
3. Extended hospitalization, which has implications for the patient, the family and the hospital.
4. Psychological stress as a result of long periods spent in isolation.

Sources of infection

Self-infection (endogenous infection)

Self-infection results when tissue becomes infected from another site in the patient's body. The normal microbial flora of the human body consists largely of the organisms in the alimentary tract, upper respiratory tract and female genital tract and on the skin. This flora may include versatile pathogens (e.g. *Staphylococcus aureus*) that may cause disease in almost any tissue as well as others (e.g. micrococcus species and diphtheroids) which are usually of very low pathogenicity; many organisms exist with capabilities between these extremes.

Cross-infection (exogenous infection)

Cross-infection may be caused by infection from patients, hospital staff or visitors who are suffering from the relevant disease (cases) or who are symptomless carriers. Food and the environment may also be factors in cross-infection.

Routes and reservoirs of infection

A reservior of infection is anywhere where organisms can survive and multiply. For infection to occur there has to be a route of transmission between the reservoir and the susceptible host. Routes of spread include:

Direct contact

Organisms can be transmitted directly to susceptible people by contaminated equipment or by the hands of health care attendants (Casewell *et al.*, 1977). Washing the skin removes harmful organisms quickly. However, studies of hand washing by nurses and others have shown that this procedure is generally not carried out efficiently (Gidley, 1987). The use of disinfectants improves the cleaning process, although no method of chemical disinfection will produce a sterile hand. Soaps and detergent emulsions containing hexachlorophane build a protective barrier in the skin against gram-positive organisms (Mackenzie, 1988). A widely used solution is one containing 4% chlorhexidine. Washing in running water is essential. Basins should be deep enough to contain any splashing water and should be plugless. Taps should not be operated by hand but by elbow, knee or foot as appropriate.

A quick, convenient and effective disinfectant for clean hands, without the use of soap and water, is a hand rub containing 70% isopropyl and a bactericidal agent such as 4% chlorhexidine, with the addition of enough glycerine to prevent excessive drying of the skin.

Hands must be washed after direct patient contact or contact with contaminated material, e.g. toys, bed linen etc., and before contact with susceptible patients (Gidley, 1987), and dried thoroughly using a good quality disposable paper towel (Rowland, 1972). (See Chapter 3, Aseptic Technique.)

Airborne

Organisms can be transmitted in dust or skin scales carried by air. This is likely to occur during procedures such as bed-making when particles may land directly on open wounds or puncture sites (Glenister, 1983). Airborne infection may also occur through droplets. Water from nebulizers or himidifiers may be contaminated by Pseudomonas species (Redding, *et al.*, 1980). Fine droplet spray from ventilation cooling towers or showers contaminated with *Legionella pneumophila* has also been shown to be a hazard (Alderman, 1988).

Food borne

Food poisoning occurs when contaminated foods are ingested, with Salmonella species being one of the most common causes (White, 1986).

Blood borne

Blood, or blood-stained material, is potentially hazardous, transmitting infection through inoculation accidents, existing breaks in the skin, gross contamination of mucous membranes, sexual activity or, prenatally, from mother to baby (Hart, 1991).

Insect borne

Although disease transmitted by biting insects is not a major problem in the United Kingdom, insects such as cockroaches can carry pathogenic organisms on their bodies and in their digestive tracts. This may infect the hospital environment, which includes food and sterile supplies (Burgess, 1979). Storage of supplies in dry, clean, well-ventilated areas is therefore essential.

Types of barrier nursing

1. Protective isolation (see section entitled 'Nursing the immunosuppressed patient', below).
2. Source isolation.

Source isolation

This form of isolation is designed to prevent the spread of pathogenic microrganisms from an infected patient to other patients, hospital personnel and visitors. The need for isolation is determined by the ease with which the disease can be transmitted in hospital and, if it is transmittable, by its severity. As infectious diseases are transmitted by different routes, isolation procedures must, in order to be effective, provide appropriate barriers to the route of transmission. In addition, the procedures imposing these barriers must be adhered to universally by all hospital staff entering the isolation unit.

The decision to isolate a patient will be influenced by the availability of facilities as well as by the physical condition of the area where the isolation is to take place. In determining the most suitable area, a number of criteria need to be met. Among these are the relative cleanliness of the ward, the standard of domestic services support, the microbiological status of the other patients and the anticipated length of the isolation.

Source Isolation may be achieved by:

1. Purpose-built infectious disease wards.
2. Plastic isolators found in high security units and used only for infections such as viral haemorrhage fever (Bowell, 1986).
3. Single rooms on general wards.

Effective barrier nursing practice is achieved most easily by isolating the patient in a single room with the following:

1. An anteroom area for protective clothing.
2. Hand-washing facilities.
3. Toilet facilities.

However, with good technique, an area in the ward away from especially vulnerable patients, can be used. In some instances where cross-infection has occurred, it may be more appropriate to care for these patients together in a small ward with designated staff, so containing the infection to one area, rather than using side rooms on different wards (Duckworth, 1990). Uninfected patients must not be admitted into this area until all the infected patients have been discharged and the area thoroughly cleaned.

General principles of barrier nursing

The main emphasis for successful barrier nursing

procedures is on hand washing and protection of clothes. Several general principles need to be adhered to if effective barrier nursing is to occur. Every effort must be made to ensure that instructions are kept simple and realistic. Regular assessment and evaluation of the situation must take place to ascertain whether barrier nursing continues to remain the most appropriate form of care.

Protective clothing

Gowns or aprons

The wearing of a protective gown or apron is an accepted part of barrier nursing technique to prevent the spread of micro-organisms from one patient to the next on clothing (Hambraeus, 1973).

Disposable plastic aprons are cheap, impermeable to bacteria and water (Babb, 1983), are easy to put on, protect the probable area of maximum contamination and are preferable to cotton gowns, which provide increased cover but are *readily penetrated* by moisture and bacteria (Mackintosh, 1982).

Caps

Although the wearing of disposable caps while nursing infected patients is still practised, hair that is clean and tidy has not been implicated in cross-infection. Therefore, unless heavy contamination or splashing is present, the wearing of caps is not justified (Gaya, 1980).

Masks

Masks are worn to protect the wearer from inhaling airborne micro-organisms. Studies have indicated that masks are generally of little value (Hare, 1982). Masks are sometimes worn when handling patients with viral and bacterial meningitis or those patients with pulmonary tuberculosis who are smear-positive, have a productive cough and are unable to cover their mouth and nose when coughing and sneezing (Joint Tuberculosis Committee of the British Thoracic Society, 1983). If masks are worn, they must be a filter type and fit the face closely.

Overshoes

The floors of hospital wards become easily contaminated by large numbers of bacteria (Ayliffe *et al.*, 1967). However, the wearing of overshoes has little value and there could even be an increased risk of cross-infection by contaminating the hands while putting on overshoes, making it necessary for the hands to be washed after putting on or taking them off (Jone *et al.*, 1988).

If airborne transmission of micro-organisms is a potential risk, a dry dust control mat placed at the patient's door, which is vacuumed daily and washed weekly, will be an effective means of limiting spread of infection by feet and trolley wheels (Meddick, 1977).

Gloves

Clean gloves must be worn when handling blood or body fluids, or cleaning (Hart, 1991), but are not a substitute for hand washing. Therefore, hands must be washed with bactericidal soap and water or bactericidal alcohol hand rub after removing gloves.

Cleaning

Scrupulous daily cleaning of the barrier nursing room is essential. All furniture must be damp-dusted to remove organisms dispersed into the air from bed-making. The floor must be either vacuum-cleaned with a machine fitted with a filter or damp-mopped with hot, soapy water (the mop-head must be laundered daily). Dry dusting or the use of a broom should be forbidden as studies have shown this method of cleaning simply re-disperses the organisms into the air (Ayliffe, 1982). The cleaning equipment must be kept for sole use in this room.

Patient hygiene

The numbers of some micro-organisms on the skin will be reduced by using an antiseptic detergent for skin and hair washing and this has been shown to be effective in eradicating the carriage of MRSA (Duckworth, 1990). The antiseptic should be applied directly to the flannel and rinsed off thoroughly.

Studies comparing standard baths with shower baths showed no overall significant difference between the two bathing techniques. However, one study indicated that shower baths were more effective in disinfecting axillae, and standard baths more efficient in reducing microbes in the perineum (Mitchell, 1984). Assessment and evaluation of the patients must be made to establish which patients will benefit most from a standard bath and which patients, for example, those with indwelling Hickman lines, will benefit from a shower bath.

Waste

Infected rubbish must be disposed of in yellow clinical waste bags. Full bags must be sealed securely within the room before being sent for incineration (Health and Safety Commission, 1982). Sharps must be placed immediately into a sharps disposal box (Department of Health and Social Security, 1983) which, when full, must be sealed and placed in a yellow clinical waste bag before being sent for incineration (Health and Safety Commission, 1982).

Linen
Infected linen must be placed in a polythene bag with red alginate stripe, which is then placed in a red linen bag and sent in a safe manner to the laundry to be 'barrier washed' (Department of Health and Social Security, 1987).

Cutlery, crockery
All crockery must be machine-washed in a dishwasher with a final rinse of 82°C to disinfect it (Collins, 1981). Disposable crockery and cutlery are needed only when gross contamination has occurred or if a dishwasher is not available.

Urine, faeces and vomit
These are to be disposed of immediately down a heat-disinfecting bedpan washer.

Notification of infection
If a patient develops suspicious signs and symptoms or if bacteriological analysis identifies an organism which necessitates barrier nursing, swift communication and action are needed to instigate this. Any problems may be discussed with the microbiologist or infection control nurse.

Informing the patient and visitors
Giving careful explanation to the patient is essential so that he/she can co-operate fully with the restrictions (Wilson-Barnett *et al.*, 1983). The nurse should be sensitive to the psychological implications of being labelled 'infectious' and of being confined in isolation. The patient's visitors must also be informed why the barrier nursing restrictions are necessary. Visitors will generally be allowed into the room at the discretion of the bacteriologist. They must be taught to observe the correct procedures for entering and leaving the room. As children are more susceptible to infection than adults, any visit by a child should be discussed with the appropriate personnel.

Domestic staff
The domestic manager must be informed as soon as barrier nursing is commenced. He or she will then provide the ward domestic with written instructions.

The ward domestic staff must understand clearly why barrier nursing is required and should be instructed on the correct procedure. The nursing staff must check that the ward domestics understand and are following their instructions correctly. If the patient is in a single room, a mop, bucket, cleaning fluid and disposable cloths should be kept solely for this patient's use. If the patient is in a general ward, special care must be taken with the cleaning so that potentially infectious material is not transferred from the area around the infected patient to other patient areas. The infected patient's area must be cleaned last and separately.

Staff allocation
A minimum number of staff should be involved with an infected patient. The nurse concerned with the infected patient should not also attend to other susceptible patients. If barrier nursing is for an infectious disease, it is preferable that only personnel who have already had the disease should attend this patient.

The protection of staff against the risk of infection is one of the main functions of the occupational health department. This department offers an immunization and counselling service.

References and further reading

Alderman, C. (1988) The cooler culprits. *Nursing Standard*, 2(33), 22.

Austin, L. (1988) The Salt Bath Myth. *Nursing Times*, 84(9), 79–83.

Ayliffe, G. A. J. *et al.* (1967) Ward floors and other surfaces as reservoirs of hospital infection. *Journal of Hygiene*, 65, 515–36.

Ayliffe, G. A. J. (1982) Airborne infection in hospital. *Journal of Hospital Infection*, 3, 217–40.

Babb, J. R. *et al.* (1983) Contamination of protective clothing and nurses' uniforms in an isolation ward. *Journal of Hospital Infection*, 4, 149–57.

Bowell, E. (1986) Nursing the isolated patient, Lassa fever. *Nursing Times*, 33, 72–81.

Burgess, N. R. H. (1979) Cockroaches and the hospital environment. *Nursing Times*, 75(11) (Contact), 5–7.

Casewell M. *et al.* (1977) Hands as route of transmission of *Klebsiella* species. *British Medical Journal*, 2, 1315–17.

Collins, B. (1981) Infection and the hospital environment. *Nursing*, 1, Supplement, 1–3.

Department of Health and Social Security (1983) *Containers for the Disposal of Used Needles and Sharp Instruments.* DHSS Specifications TSS/8/330, DHSS, London.

Department of Health and Social Security (1987) *Hospital Laundry Arrangements For Used and Infected Linen*, HC(87) 30. DHSS, London.

Duckworth, G. (1990) Revised guidelines for the control of epidemic methicillin-resistant *Staphylococcus aureus. Journal of Hospital Infection*, 16, 351–77.

Gaya, H. (1980) Questions and answer section. Is it necessary for staff and visitors in an intensive care unit to wear masks, hats, gowns and overshoes? *Journal of Hospital Infection*, 1, 369–71.

Gidley, C. (1987) Now wash your hands. *Nursing Times*, 83(29), 40–42.

Glenister, H. (1983) The passage of infection. *Nursing Mirror*, 12 January, 79, 28–30.

Hambraeus, A. (1973) Transfer of *Staphylococcus aureus* via

nurses' uniform. *Journal of Hygiene*, 71, 799–814.
Hare, R. (1982) To mask or not to mask? *Nursing Times*, 59, 715.
Hart, S. (1991) Blood and body fluid precautions. *Nursing Standard*, 5(25), 25–8.
Health and Safety Commission (1982) *The Safe Disposal of Clinical Waste*. HMSO, London.
Joint Tuberculosis Committee of the British Thoracic Society (1983) Control and prevention of tuberculosis: a code of practice. *British Medical Journal*, 287, 1118–21.
Jones M. *et al.* (1988) Over-estimating overshoes. *Nursing Times*, 84(41), 66–71.
Mackenzie, I. (1988) Pre-operative skin preparation and surgical outcome. *Journal of Hospital Infection II*, Supplement B, 27–32.
Mackintosh, C. A. (1982) A testing time for gowns. *Journal of Hospital Infection*, 3, 5–8.
Meddick, H. M. (1977) Bacterial contamination: control mats; – a comparative study. *Journal of Hygiene*, 79, 133–40.
Mitchell, N. J. (1984) Whole-body disinfection with chlorhexidine in shower bathing more effective than bathing. *Journal of Hospital Infection*, 5, 96–9.
Redding, R. J. *et al.* (1980) *Pseudomonas fluorescens* cross-infection due to contaminated humidifier water. *British Medical Journal*, 26 July, 281, 275.
Rowland A. J. (1972) Transmission of infection through towels. *Community Medicine*, 5 May, 71–2.
White, P. M. B. (1986) Food poisoning in a hospital staff canteen. *Journal of Infection*, 13, 195–8.
Wilson-Barnett, J. *et al.* (1983) Studies evaluating patient teaching implication for practice. *International Journal of Nursing Studies*, 20(1), 33–40.

GUIDELINES: SOURCE ISOLATION

Equipment

1. Isolation suite if possible.
2. All items required to meet the patient's nursing needs during the period of isolation, such as crockery, linen, instruments to assess vital signs, etc.

Procedure

Preparation of the isolation room

Action	Rationale
1. Place a barrier nursing sign outside the door.	To inform anyone intending to enter the room of the situation.
2. List requirements for personnel before entering and after leaving the isolation area.	To decrease entries and exits to the room.
3. Remove all non-essential furniture. The remaining furniture should be easy to clean and should not conceal or retain dirt or moisture either within or around it.	To minimize the risk of furniture harbouring microbial spores or growth colonies.
4. Stock the hand basin with a suitable antibacterial detergent preparation and paper towels for staff use.	Facilities for hand washing within the infected area are essential for effective barrier nursing.
5. Place yellow clinical waste bag in the room on a foot-operated stand. The bag must be sealed with tape before it is removed from the room.	For containing contaminated rubbish within the room. Yellow is the recognized colour for clinical waste.
6. Place a container for 'sharps' in the room.	To contain contaminated 'sharps' within the infected area.
7. When the 'sharps' container is full it must be placed in a yellow clinical waste bag, securely sealed and sent for incineration.	To minimize the risk of leakage from the 'sharps' safe.

Guidelines: Source isolation

Action	Rationale
8. Keep the patient's personal property to a minimum. Advise him/her to wear hospital clothing. All belongings taken into the room should be washable, cleanable or disposable.	The patient's belongings may become contaminated and cannot be taken home unless they are washable or cleanable. Anything else may have to be destroyed.
9. Provide the patient with his/her own thermometer and sphygmomanometer, water jug, glass and tray, and all items necessary for attending to personal hygiene.	Equipment used regularly by the patient should be kept within the infected area to prevent the spread of infection.
10. Keep dressing solutions, creams and lotions, etc. to a minimum and store them within the room.	All partially used materials must be discarded when barrier nursing ends (sterilization is not possible), therefore unnecessary waste should be avoided.
11. Set up a trolley outside the door to hold plastic gowns, aprons, gloves, and bactericidal alcoholic hand rub.	Staff are more likely to use the equipment if it is readily available.

Entering the room

Action	Rationale
1. Collect all equipment needed.	To avoid entering and leaving the infected area unnecessarily.
2. Roll up long sleeves to the elbow.	To protect clothing from contamination.
3. Put on a disposable plastic apron when there is no risk of airborne transmission of organisms or when close contact with the patient is not anticipated.	A plastic apron is inexpensive and adequate to protect clothing from contamination in most situations.
4. Put on a disposable gown for close work, e.g. lifting.	To protect clothing from contamination to shoulders, arms and back. Cotton gowns are an ineffective barrier against bacteria, particularly when wet.
5. Put on a disposable, well-fitting mask if there is a risk of airborne spread, i.e. (a) Smear-positive pulmonary tuberculosis patient with a productive cough. (b) Viral or meningococcus meningitis.	To reduce the risk of inhaling organisms.
6. Safety glasses, visors and goggles should be put on only when blood splashes are expected, e.g. during haemodialysis.	To give protection to the conjunctiva from blood splashes.
7. Put on disposable gloves only if you are intending to deal with blood, excreta or contaminated material.	To reduce the risk of contaminating your hands. Over-use of disposable gloves may ultimately detract from the importance of hand washing.
8. Enter the room, shutting the door.	To reduce the risk of airborne organisms leaving the room.

Attending to the patient

Action	Rationale
1. *Meals.* Meals should be served only on disposable crockery and eaten with disposable cutlery if deemed necessary by the bacteriologist. Disposables and uneaten food should be discarded in the appropriate bag.	Contaminated crockery is a potential disease vector. Cleaning of same may be difficult and time consuming.
2. *Non-disposable crockery.* A personal water jug, glasses and tray should be kept at the bedside. These, and any other non-disposable crockery, should be washed separately from the rest of the ward's utensils, in a dishwasher with a hot disinfecting cycle.	Separation of contaminated crockery reduces the risk of the spread of infection in washing-up water.
3. *Excreta.* Ideally, a toilet should be kept solely for the patient's use. If this is not available, a separate bedpan or urinal and commode should be left in the patient's room. Gloves must be worn by staff when dealing with excreta. Bedpans and urinals should be bagged in the isolation room, emptied and then washed in a bedpan washer, then dried and returned immediately to the patient's room.	To minimize the risk of infection being spread from excreta, e.g. via a toilet seat or a bedpan.
4. *Accidental spills.* Any suspected contaminated fluids must be mopped up immediately and the area cleaned with disinfectant.	Damp areas encourage microbial growth and increase the risk of spread of infection.
5. *Bathing.* An infected patient must be bathed last on the ward. Clean the bath after the previous patient and after the infected patient. If the patient has infected lesions, disinfectant may be added to the bath water. Salt is not a disinfectant and has little antibacterial effect (Austin, 1988).	Leaving the bath dry after disinfection reduces the risk of microbes surviving and infecting others. Bacteria will not grow on clean, dry surfaces.
6. *Dressings.* Aseptic technique must be used for changing all dressings. Waste materials and dirty dressings should be discarded in the appropriate bag. Used lotions, creams, etc. must be kept in the room and not used for other patients.	Aseptic procedure minimizes the risk of cross-infection. Lotions and creams can become easily contaminated.
7. *Linen.* Place linen in a polythene bag with a red alginate stripe, which must be secured tightly before it leaves the room. Just outside the room, place this bag into a red linen bag which must be secured tightly and not used for other patients. These bags should await the laundry collection in a safe area.	Holding dirty linen in a polythene bags with a red alginate stripe confines organisms and allows staff handling the linen to recognize the potential hazard.
8. *Waste.* Yellow clinical waste bags should be kept in the room for disposal of all the patient's rubbish. The bag's top should be sealed by knotting or stapling before it is removed from the room.	Yellow is the international colour for clinical waste.

Guidelines: Source isolation

Leaving the room

Action	Rationale
1. If wearing gloves, remove and discard them in the yellow clinical waste bag. Wash hands again with an appropriate antiseptic solution.	To remove pathogenic organisms acquired during contact with patient before removing gown, so preventing contaminated of uniform.
2. Remove apron and discard it in the appropriate bag. Wash hands again with an appropriate antiseptic solution.	Hands may be contaminated by a dirty gown.
3. Used gowns should not be re-used.	Mistakes are made if gowns have to be re-used, particularly as staff find it hard to distinguish the inside/outside of a gown. If the gown is worn inside out, uniforms can be contaminated.
4. Leave the room, shutting the door behind you.	
5. Rinse hands with a bactericidal alcohol-based hand wash solution.	To remove pathogenic organisms acquired from such items as the door handle.

Cleaning the room

Action	Rationale
1. Domestic staff must understand why barrier nursing is required and should be instructed on the correct procedure.	To reduce the risk of mistakes and to ensure that barrier nursing is maintained.
2. The area where barrier nursing is being carried out must be cleaned last.	To reduce the risk of the transmission of organisms.
3. Separate cleaning equipment must be kept for this area.	Cleaning equipment can easily become infected. Cross-infection may result from shared cleaning equipment.
4. Members of the domestic services staff must wear gloves and plastic aprons.	To reduce the risk of cross-infection.
5. *Floor* (hard surface). This must be washed daily with a disinfectant as appropriate. All excess water must be removed.	Daily cleaning will keep bacterial count reduced. Organisms, especially Gram-negative bacteria, multiply quickly in the presence of moisture.
6. After use, the bucket must be cleaned, dried and stored within the barrier nursing area.	Bacteria will not survive on clean dry surfaces.
7. Ideally, mop heads should be laundered in a hot wash daily, when this is not possible, the mop must be washed, rinsed, all excess water removed and stored with the mop head uppermost to allow for quick drying within the barrier nursing area.	Mop heads become contaminated easily.
8. *Floor* (carpet). An infected patient may have been admitted into a room with a carpet. A vacuum cleaner should be used which is fitted with an efficient filter. After use the dust bag	Vacuum cleaning reduces the dust thus reducing organisms.

Action	Rationale
must be changed and the brush head washed and dried.	
9. On discharge, the carpet must be steam cleaned.	Bacteria can survive in dust trapped in the carpet fibres. The heat of the steam will kill these bacteria.
10. Furniture and fittings should be damp-dusted using a disposable cloth and a detergent solution or a disinfectant if appropriate.	To remove any organisms.
11. The toilet, shower and bathroom area must be cleaned at least once a day using a non-abrasive hypochlorite powder or cream. A disinfectant will only be required if soiling of the area has occurred.	Non-abrasive powders or creams preserve the integrity of the surfaces. These areas recontaminate rapidly after cleaning and routine chemical disinfection is of little value and should be saved for terminal cleaning.

Transporting infected patients outside the barrier nursing area

Action	Rationale
1. Inform the department concerned about the diagnosis.	To allow other departments time to make their own arrangements.
2. Arrange for the patient to have the last appointment of the day.	The department concerned will then be empty of other patients; time can be allowed for special cleaning or disinfecting; hospital corridors, lifts, etc. are usually less busy at this time of day.
3. Any porters involved must be instructed carefully. The trolley or chair should be cleaned after use.	Protection and reassurance of porters are necessary to allay fear and to minimize the risk of the infection being spread to them.
4. It may be necessary for the nurse to escort the patient.	To ensure the necessary precautions are maintained.

Discharging the patient

Action	Rationale
1. Inform the microbiologist when the patient is due for discharge.	The microbiologist will advise on any special precautions.
2. The room should be stripped and aired. All textiles must be changed and curtains sent to the laundry.	Curtains readily become colonized with bacteria.
3. Impervious surfaces, e.g. lockers, stools, blinds and thermometer holders, should be washed with soap and water.	Wiping of surfaces is the most effective way of removing contaminants. Relatively inaccessible places, e.g. ceilings, may be omitted; these are not generally relevant to any infection risk.
4. The floor must be washed and dried thoroughly.	To remove any organisms present.
5. If the room is known to be contaminated with blood or blood-stained excreta from hepatitis B-positive or human immunodeficiency virus (HIV) antibody-positive individuals, a hypochlorite solution should be used.	To remove the source of potential contamination.

6. If the room has been used by a patient with an enteric infection a clean, soluble phenolic should be used.	To remove the source of potential contamination.

ANTIBIOTIC-RESISTANT ORGANISMS

Definition

The term 'antibiotic resistance' denotes a strain of bacteria that is not killed or inhibited by antimicrobial agents to which the species is generally sensitive.

REFERENCE MATERIAL

The importance of antibiotic-resistant organisms cannot to be overemphasized. Patients who are immunocompromised, debilitated or with open wounds are at particular risk and deaths have occurred (Bradley, 1985; Hone *et al.*, 1981). Bacterial resistance to antibiotics may take many years to develop, as in the case of the gonococcus. Strains resistant to penicillin G only appeared after 25 years of use (Sparling *et al.*, 1976). Methicillin-resistant *Staphylococcus aureus* (MRSA), however, was first reported in 1961 (Jevons), only two years after the drug's clinical introduction. MRSA is now increasing with some hospitals reporting its frequenty as high as 20 to 40% of all *Staphylococcus aureus* identified (Ayliffe, 1985).

The widespread and often indiscriminate use of antibiotics for prophylactic and veterinary purposes, as well as the inappropriate selection of antibiotics, are believed to be important factors in the development of resistant forms of bacteria (Swan Joint Committee, 1969; Garrod, 1972). The transmission of genetic material between bacteria by conjugation has been well documented (Jaffe *et al.*, 1980; Mendoza, 1985) and this conjugation accounts in part for the rapid spread of resistance, with mutation, transformation and transduction also being involved (Sande & Mandell, 1980).

The consequences of a patient being infected with a resistant form of bacteria are demanding in terms of increased length of stay, costs of care and treatment (Grazebrook, 1986).

The North East Thames Microbiology Sub-Committee MRSA Working Party (1987) estimated the annual cost to a hospital with a large MRSA infection problem to be £250 000 (Duckworth, 1990).

A recent study from Hong Kong showed that the average cost of antimicrobial therapy per patient with MRSA bacteraemia was £440, compared with £60 for patients with methicillin-sensitive *Staphylococcus aureus* bacteraemia. The extra cost reflected the increased cost of antimicrobials and the longer treatment required (Cheng *et al.*, 1988).

Theoretically, any organism can develop antibiotic resistance. In practice, however, two groups present the major problem: Gram-negative bacteria and *Staphylococcus aureus*.

Gram-negative bacteria

Gram-negative bacteria normally inhabit the gut but cause infections in the urinary tract, respiratory tract and wounds. Outbreaks of resistant forms have been reported (Casewell, 1982; Dance, 1987) which may be the consequence of excessive use of broad-spectrum antibiotics. Pseudomonas species may cause particular problems, being ubiquitous in the hospital environment. This organism can multiply in warm, moist conditions and has been identified in eye drops, soap solutions, lotions and in the tubing used for ventilators and incubators. This is particularly difficult because of the shortage of drugs which are effective against resistant forms of Pseudomonas species.

Gram-negative bacteraemia

Gram-negative bacteraemia is associated with septic shock (Ferguson, 1991), which occurs primarily in debilitated, hospitalized patients who are the group that also develops the resistant form of Gram-negative bacteraemia (Bryant *et al.*, 1971).

The major problem regarding Gram-negative-resistant organisms is that shock progresses before antibiotic sensitivities are known, with increased clinical manifestations which can result in death (Hughes, 1971).

Staphylococcus aureus

Staphylococcus aureus is part of the normal human flora, with large numbers of the organism being found on the skin and mucosa. Colonization or infection by MRSA is therefore more likely to occur in the nose, lesions and sites of abnormal skin, and in indwelling devices such as catheters and tracheostomies (Ayliffe, 1986).

There are many distinguishable strains of MRSA which may or may not be epidemic in character, i.e. epidemic MRSA (EMRSA). Phage typing of the strain to establish strain and epidemiology is important (Richardson *et al.*, 1988) as increased barrier nursing precautions will be required for epidemic strains.

Carriers and infected patients need to be identified and the extent of colonization must be established. Prompt barrier nursing may limit the spread of MRSA (Selkon *et al.*, 1980). Patients transferred from hospitals and countries known to have an MRSA problem should be screened on admission and treated as suspect until the results of screening specimens are known. These restrictions may be minimal, with nursing care involving just good hand washing following patient contact. However, if the patient is obviously ill with, for example, a discharging wound, then this would necessitate barrier nursing (see beginning of Chapter 4).

Contacts of infected patients must be screened to prevent spread. This would include nose swabs, and swabs from skin lesions, catheters and intravenous lines.

If cross-infection occurs it may be necessary to close a ward to new admissions, particularly to surgical or intensive care patients. Once patients have been discharged, the ward must be cleaned thoroughly before patients are readmitted. The use of a phenolic disinfectant for surface disinfection in cross-infection incidences has been advised (Duckworth, 1990).

Screening of staff contacts must include medical, nursing, paramedical and domestic staff. There is no evidence that MRSA poses a risk to healthy staff, but staff may become colonized and could transmit MRSA to other patients. *All* staff in contact with the infected patient should be screened and, if working in a high-dependency unit, may need to be removed from duty if widespread carriage develops. Generally, only nasal carriage occurs, which can be treated with mupirocin ointment, while staff continue at work (Hill *et al.*, 1988).

Agency staff are a particular problem with respect to cross-infection, and may transmit MRSA between hospitals. It is preferable to use a central agency and make it known that staff who have recently worked in an infected hospital will not be employed until negative screening swabs are available (Cookson *et al.*, 1989). Infected patients must be identified clearly and barrier nursing commenced.

Eradication of carriage sites other than the nose is difficult and may often fail. Mupirocin nasal ointment in paraffin base for mucous membranes and mupirocin cream in a miscible macrogol base for non-mucous membrane intact skin has been seen to be most effective (Duckworth, 1990).

The MRSA load on skin can be reduced by twice-weekly hairwashing and daily showering for one week, using an antiseptic detergent such as chlorhexidine povidone iodine or triclosan (Bartzokas *et al.*, 1984). Serious clinical infection should be treated with vancomycin. New agents such as teicoplanin and ciprofloxacin are still being evaluated (Duckworth, 1990).

Relapses may occur, especially in debilitated patients and particularly in sites such as tracheostomies. This means that barrier nursing must be maintained even after three negative cultures have been obtained. The presence of MRSA should be documented in the patient's records in order to alert staff should readmission be necessary (Cookson *et al.*, 1986).

Inter-hospital movement should be restricted to the absolute minimum. If the patient must be transferred to another hospital, the receiving hospital must be informed in plenty of time for the necessary arrangements to be made. The ambulance service should be notified if it is being used to transfer an MRSA patient, mainly to prevent another patient being placed in the same vehicle before it is cleaned. Hand washing by the ambulance service staff and cleaning of local areas of patient contact, i.e. chair or stretcher, is all that is required after transport of an affected patient.

References and further reading

Ayliffe, G. A. J. (1986) Guidelines for the control of epidemic methicillin-resistant *Staphylococcus aureus*, *Journal of Infection*, 7, 193–201.

Bartzokas, C. A. *et al.* (1984) Control and eradication of methicillin-resistant *Staphylococcus aureus* on a surgical unit. *New England Journal of Medicine*, 311, 1422–5.

Bradley, J. M. (1985) Methicillin-resistant *Staphylococcus aureus* in a London hospital. *Lancet*, 1, 1493–5.

Bryant, R. E. *et al.* (1971) Factors affecting mortality of Gram-negative rod bacteraemia. *Archives of International Medicine*, 127, 120.

Casewell, M. W. (1982) The role of multiply resistant coliforms in hospital acquired infection. *Recent Advances in Infection*, 2, 31–50.

Cheng, A. F. *et al.* (1988) Methicillin-resistant *Staphylococcus aureus* bacteraemia in Hong Kong. *Journal of Hospital Infection*, 12, 91–101.

Cookson B. D. *et al.* (1986) A hospital computer system as a tool for infection control. In *Current Perspectives in Health Care Computing* (Ed. by J. Bryant, J. Roberts & P. Windson), pp. 126–31. British Computer Society Health Information, Specialist Group, & *British Journal of Health Care Computing*, London.

Cookson, B. D. *et al.* (1989) Staff carriage of epidemic methicillin-resistant *Staphylococcus aureus*. *Journal of Clinical Microbiology*, 27, 1471–6.

Dance, D. A. B. (1987) A hospital outbreak caused by a chlorhexidine and antibiotic resistant *Proteus mirabilis*. *Journal of Hospital Infection*, 10, 10–16.

Duckworth, G. (1990) Revised guidelines for the control of epidemic methicillin-resistant *Staphylococcus aureus*. *Journal of Hospital Infection*, 16, 351–77.

Ferguson, J. (1991) Septic shock in the critically ill patient. *Surgical Nurse*, 4(2), 21–4.

Garrod, L. P. (1972) Causes of failure in antibiotic treatment. *British Medical Journal*, 4, 473–6.

Grazebrook, J. (1986) Counting the cost of infection. *Nursing Times*, 83(6), 24–6.

Hill, R. L. R. *et al.* (1988) Elimination of nasal carriage of methicillin-resistant *Staphylococcus aureus* with mupirocin during a hospital outbreak. *Journal of Antimicrobial Chemotherapy*, 22, 377–84.

Hone, R. *et al.* (1981) Bacteraemia in Dublin due to gentamicin-resistant *Staphylococcus aureus*, *Journal of Hospital Infection*, 2, 119–25.

Hughes, W. T. (1971) Fatal infections in childhood leukaemia. *American Journal of Diseases in Childhood*, 122, 283–7.

Jaffe, H. W. *et al.* (1980) Identity and interspecific transfer of gentamicin resistant plasmids in *Staphylococcus aureus* and *Staphylococcus epidermidis*, *Journal of Infectious Diseases*, 141, 738.

Jevons, M. P. (1961) Celberin resistant staphylococci. *British Medical Journal*, 1, 124–5.

Mayet, F. (1989) The microbe file. *Nursing Standard*, 3, 57–8.

Mendoza, M. C. (1985) Evidence for the dispersion and evolution of R. plasmids from *Serratia marcescens* in hospital. *Journal of Hospital Infection*, 6, 147–53.

Peters, G. *et al.* (1983) Antibacterial activity of teichomycin – a new glycopeptide antibiotic in comparison to vancomycin. *Journal of Antimicrobial Chemotherapy*, 11, 94–5.

Richardson, J. F. *et al.* (1988) Another strain of methicillin-resistant *Staphylococcus aureus* epidemic in London. *Lancet*, 2, 748–9.

Sande, M. A., and Mandell, G. L. (1980) Chemotherapy of microbial diseases. In *The Pharmacological Basis of Therapeutics* L. S. Goodman *et al.* Macmillan, London.

Selkon, J. B. *et al.* (1980) The role of an isolation unit in the control of hospital infection with multi-resistant *Staphylococcus aureus*. *Journal of Hospital Infection*, 1, 41–6.

Smith, S. M. *et al.* (1989) Ciprofloxacin therapy for methicillin-resistant *Staphylococcus aureus* infection or colonizations. *Antimicrobial Agents and Chemotherapy*, 33, 181–4.

Sparling, F. P. *et al.* (1976) Antibiotic resistance in the gonococcus. In *Microbiology* (Ed. by D. Schlessinger). American Society of Microbiology.

Swan Joint Committee (1969) *Use of Antibiotics in Animal Husbandry and Veterinary Medicine*. HMSO, London.

NURSING THE IMMUNOSUPPRESSED PATIENT

Definition

Immunosuppression is a generalized depression of the immune system, which increases the risk of acquiring an infection. This necessitates protecting immunosuppressed patients from micro-organisms carried in the environment, from health care workers providing care, from visitors and from other patients. Protection can be achieved by protective isolation, previously termed reverse barrier nursing.

Protective isolation provides a safe environment for patients who are susceptible to infection and can be an appropriate form of care for many patients, e.g. burns patients, children with immunodeficiency disease and patients receiving bone marrow transplantation. The aim of protective isolation is to prevent and treat infection until the period of immunosuppression is past.

Indications

Immunosuppression can be caused by many factors including:

1. Primary disease such as leukaemia, lymphoma (Field *et al.*, 1977), acquired immune deficiency syndrome (AIDS) (Centre of Disease Control, 1988), severe combined immunodeficiency disease (SCID) (Hill, 1989).
2. Secondary disease, such as diabetes, which may complicate primary disease (Reeves, 1980).
3. Drugs, in particular, cytotoxic drugs and corticosteroids (Reheis, 1985).
4. Antimicrobial therapy causing changes in the patients' microbial flora (Hahn *et al.*, 1978).
5. Irradiation therapy: the degree of immunosuppression is related directly to the area being treated (Strober *et al.*, 1981).
6. Trauma (Maclean, *et al.*, 1975) and burns (Miller *et al.*, 1979).
7. Age (Leonard, 1986).

The risk of infection will be increased by breaches in the body's natural defence mechanisms, for example:

1. Skin by, for example, indwelling catheters; repeated venepuncture; pressure ulcers (Wade, 1982).
2. Mucous membranes, from oral ulceration.
3. Body cavities by urinary catheters (Meers *et al.*, 1981) or endotracheal tubes.

These risks require nursing care of the highest standards when involved in such procedures to reduce the risk of infection as much as practically possible.

Infection risk is also related to the absolute level or circulating granulocytes (Bodey *et al.*, 1966) with the frequency of infection rising as the granulocytes count drops below 500/μl, with a dramatic increase as the granulocyte count reaches zero (Schimpff *et al.*, 1978).

Granulocytopenia, occurring rapidly, is more likely to be associated with an increased risk of infection than is a slow decline or a stable granulocytopenia (Dale *et al.*, 1979).

Some patients have an increased risk of infection due to a combination of immunosuppressive factors. For example, in the case of a patient with leukaemia who is undergoing bone marrow transplantation and who develops graft-versus-host disease (GVHD), which requires treatment with increased doses of immunosuppressive drug (Armstrong, *et al.*, 1971).

Therefore, the severity and expected length of immunosuppression should be assessed to decide the level of protective isolation which is required (Meyer, 1986). Generally, the greater the state of immunosuppression, the greater the need for protection (Rubin *et al.*, 1990); additionally, more limitation must be placed on the planned nursing care the greater the environmental hazard.

REFERENCE MATERIAL

Protective isolation may be achieved by:

1. Purpose-built units (Borley, 1982).
2. Plastic isolators (Bowell, 1986).
3. Single rooms on a general ward (Nauseef *et al.*, 1981).
4. Shared rooms within a controlled environment on a general ward.

Purpose-built units

A purpose-built unit will include:

1. Filtered air supply.
2. Single rooms with integral toilet, shower, a hatch system for the aseptic transfer of equipment into the room, an entry area for visitors and staff where protective clothing can be donned and hands washed.
3. Facilities to provide pathogen-free food.
4. Gastrointestinal decontamination (Jameson *et al.*, 1971).

These units are expensive to build, maintain and staff. Although evidence shows that this form of protective isolation does reduce infection, it does not affect long-term survival (Levine *et al.*, 1973; Schimpff *et al.*, 1975; Yates *et al.*, 1973) although it may reduce graft-verus-host disease (GVHD) (Storb *et al.*, 1983).

Opinion is also divided as to whether protective isolation causes psychological damage (Kohle, 1979), particularly among paediatric patients (Powazek *et al.*, 1978), necessitating such units to provide psychological support in the form of social workers, play therapists, teachers and psychologists.

Plastic isolators

An isolator consists of a framework erected around a bed from which a PVC tent is suspended. The tent has an air supply attached which keeps the whole apparatus inflated. A positive air pressure is usually maintained within the isolator. In some cases, for example, when nursing patients with Lassa fever, the pressure within the isolator is slightly below atmospheric pressure, which prevents the escape of an infected particles. Although patients may feel a strong sense of containment within the isolator, this system does have the advantage of achieving high standards of bacteriological control, and it can be assembled and dismantled rapidly.

Single rooms and shared rooms in general wards

The decision to isolate a patient will be influenced by the availability of facilities coupled to the general condition of the ward area where the isolation is to take place. In determining the most suitable area, a number of criteria need to be met. Among these are the relative cleanliness of the ward, the standard of domestic services support, the microbiological status of the other patients and the anticipated length of the isolation.

This less vigorous method of protective isolation is unlikely to greatly reduce the acquisition of potential pathogens, as only person-to-person transfer of infection is prevented, since facilities such as clean air and pathogen-free food are not usually available on general wards (Hann *et al.*, 1984).

The prevention of exogenous transmission of infection is important and can be achieved by careful monitoring of the environment to remove items which could predispose to infection, for example, flowers (Taplin *et al.*, 1973). Scrupulous cleaning with special attention to furniture and equipment within the room will also prevent transmission (Crane, 1980).

The limiting of endogenous transmission of infection, which is the major cause of infection in immunosuppressed patients (Schimpff *et al.*, 1970); (Selden *et al.*, 1971), is difficult but good patient hygiene, restriction of invasive devices and procedures are useful.

A thorough and continuing assessment of the patient is essential in order to recognize the first signs of infection (see Chapter 29, Observations). The most common areas of early infection include the lung, pharynx, anorectal area, skin and subcutaneous tissue (Reheis, 1985). Unfortunately, signs and symptoms of infection are often absent (Sickles *et al.*, 1975).

Investigations to establish the cause of infection include chest X-ray, bacteriological and viral culture of blood, urine and sputum, and swabs obtained from any suspicious lesion (see Chapter 36, Specimen Collection).

As progression of infection in the immunosuppressed patient may be rapid and widespread, the earliest sign of infection must be looked for, and appropriate antimicrobial therapy commenced immediately. If an infection is left untreated, fatality rate ranging from 18% to 40% can occur within the first 48 hours (Schimpff, 1977).

Bacterial infections are generally caused by Gram-negative organisms, such as Pseudomonas species, *Escherichia coli* and Klebsiella species, normally found in the gastrointestinal tract. Gram-positive organisms causing infections are commonly *Staphylococcus epidermidis*, which is generally a skin contaminant (Bodey, 1975).

The most common fungal infection is by *Candida albicans*, which is most usually found in the oral cavity, but which may affect the oesophagus, bowel or vagina, and cause systemic infection, pneumonia and septicaemia.

Aspergillus infection, particularly associated with nearby building work has also been seen (see Aspergillosis, p. 47). Viral infections, particularly by Cytomegalovirus and the Herpes virus may occur (see pages 61 and 63, respectively). The main route of infection transmission is by contact transmission from hands and clothes.

Airborne infectious micro-organisms, notably staphylococci, may be inhaled or transferred to the patient via wounds, intravenous cannulae, etc. Patients may also infect themselves directly from their own micro-organisms.

Food is a potential source of infection. Generally, if non-absorbable gut antibiotics are prescribed, pathogen-free food must be provided. Thoroughly cooked foods, canned foods and foods known to be pathogen-free such as cereal, should be served with sterile utensils on sterile trays. If these facilities are unavailable, then the diet should consist only of food that has been well-cooked; foods known to have high bacterial counts should be avoided (Roberts, 1982). This involves eliminating raw fruit and vegetables from the diet (Wright *et al.*, 1976).

Protective isolation can cause increased stress for patients. It is also suggested that nursing on a protective isolation unit, particularly with patients undergoing bone marrow transplantation, increases the stress suffered by nurses themselves (Borley, 1985). This can result in burn-out, producing symptoms such as fatigue, anxiety, depression and poor concentration (Scully, 1980), which can be detrimental to nurses, their colleagues and the patients in their care.

Nursing managers of intensive care units such as protective isolation units need to be aware of this risk and provide support and a treatment plan if burn-out does occur (McElroy, 1982).

The procedure described below (Guidelines: Nursing the neutropenic patient) is intended to protect the patient whose period of neutropenia can reasonably be expected to be measured in days. It does not involve the special precautions of full protective isolation with protection from commensal infection in patients whose neutropenia is likely to be prolonged. Such patients should be nursed in a purpose-built protective isolation unit.

References and further reading

Bodey, C. P. *et al.* (1966) Quantitative relationships between circulating leukocytes and infection in patients with acute leukaemia. *Annals of International Medicine*, 64, 328–40.

Bodey, C. P. (1975) Infections in cancer patients. *Cancer Treatment and Review*, 2, 89–128.

Borley, D. (1982) A protected environment for bone marrow transplantation. *Pictures in Nursing Medical Education*, 156–8.

Borley, D. (1985) Bone marrow patients can plant extra stress on nurses. *Nursing Mirror*, 160(8), 6.

Bowell, E. (1986) Nursing the isolated patient. *Nursing Times*, 33, 72–81.

Centre of Disease Control (CDC) (1988) Revision of CDC surveillance case definition of AIDS. *Morbidity and Mortality Weekly Report*, No. 36, 1–15.

Crane, L. R. (1980) Prevention of infection on the oncology unit. *Nursing Clinics of North America*, 15(4), 843–55.

Dale, D. C. *et al.* (1979) Chronic neutropenia. *Medicine*, 58, 128–44.

Field, R. *et al.* (1977) Infections in patients with malignant lymphoma treated with combination chemotherapy. *Cancer*, 39, 1018–77.

Hahn, D. M. *et al.* (1978) Infection in acute leukaemia patients receiving oral, non-absorbable antibiotics. *Antimicrobial Agents and Chemotherapy*, 13, 958–64.

Hann, I. M. *et al.* (1984) Infection prophylaxis in the patient with bone marrow failure. *Clinics in Haematology*, 13(3), 523–46.

Hill, H. R. (1989) Infections complicating congenital immunodeficiency syndromes. In *Clinical Approaches to*

Infection in the Compromised Host, 2nd edn (Ed. by R. H. Rubin, Lowell & S. Young), pp. 407–32. Plenum Medical Book Co. London.

Jameson, B. *et al.* (1971) Five-year analysis of protective isolation. *Lancet*, 1, 1034–40.

Kohle, K. (1979) Psychological aspects in isolated patients' experience during eight years. *Clinical and Experimental Gnotobiotics*, 7, 45–72.

Leonard, M. (1986) Handling infection. *Nursing Times*, 33, 81–4.

Levine, A. S. *et al.* (1973) Protective environment and prophylactic antibiotics – a prospective controlled study of their utility in the therapy of acute leukaemia. *New England Journal of Medicine*, 288, 477–83.

Maclean, L. D. *et al.* (1975) Host resistance in sepsis and trauma. *Annals of Surgery*, 182, 207–15.

McElroy, A. (1982) Burn-out: a review of the literature with application to cancer nursing. *Cancer Nursing*, June, 3(6), 211–17.

Meers, P. D. *et al.* (1981) Report on the Natural Survey of Infections in Hospitals, 1980. *Journal of Hospital Infection, Supplement*, 2, 1–53.

Meyer, I. D. (1986) Infection in bone marrow transplant recipients. *American Journal of Medicine*, 81, 27–8.

Miller, C. L. *et al.* (1979) Changes in lymphocyte activity after thermal injury. *Journal of Clinical Investigation*, 63, 202–10.

Nauseef, W. M. *et al.* (1981) A study of the value of simple protective isolation in patients with granulocytopenia. *New England Journal of Medicine*, 304(8), 448–53.

Powazek, M. *et al.* (1978) Emotional reaction of children to isolation in a cancer hospital. *Journal of Paediatrics*, 92(5), 834–7.

Reeves, W. G. (1980) Immunology of diabetes and insulin therapy. *Recent Advances in Clinical Immunology*, 2, 183–7.

Reheis, C. E. (1985) Neutropenia causes complications: treatment and resulting nursing care. *Nursing Clinics of North America*, 20(1), 219–25.

Roberts, D. (1982) Factors contributing to outbreaks of food poisoning in England and Wales, 1970–1979. *Journal of Hygiene*, 89, 491.

Rubin, R. H. *et al.* (1990) Therapy, both immunosuppressive and antimicrobial for the transplant patient in the 1990s. In *Organ Transplantation – Current Clinical and Immunological Concepts* (Ed. by L. Brent & R. Sells), pp. 71–89. Baillière Tindall, Eastbourne.

Schimpff, S. C. (1977) Therapy for infection in patients with granulocytopenia. *Medical Clinics of North America*, 61, 1101–18.

Schimpff, S. C. *et al.* (1970) Relationship of colonization with *Pseudomonas aeruginosa* to development of *Pseudomonas bacteraemia* in cancer patients. *Antimicrobials and Chemotherapy*, 10, 240–44.

Schimpff, S. C. *et al.* (1975) Infection prevention in acute non-lymphocytic leukaemia laminar air flow room reverse isolation with oral non-absorbable antibiotic prophylaxis. *Annals of International Medicine*, 82, 351–8.

Schimpff, S. C. *et al.* (1978) Infection prevention in acute leukaemia. *Leukaemia Research*, 2, 231–40.

Scully, R. (1980) Stress in the nurse. *American Journal of Nursing*, May, 80(5), 912–15.

Selden, R. *et al.* (1971) Nosocomial Klebsiella infections. Intestinal colonization as a reservoir. *Annals of International Medicine*, 74, 675–84.

Sickles, E. A. *et al.* (1975) Clinical presentation of infection in granulocytopenia patients. *Archives of International Medicine*, 135, 715–19.

Storb, R. *et al.* (1983) GVHD and survival in patients with asplastic anaemia treated by bone marrow grafts with HLA identifiable siblings. *New England Journal of Medicine*, 308, 302–7.

Strober, S. *et al.* (1981) Immunosuppressive and tolerogenic effect of whole-body total lymphoid regional irradiation. In *Immunosuppressive Therapy* (Ed. by J. R. Salaman). MTP Press, Lancaster.

Strom, T. B. (1990) Immunosuppression in graft rejection. In *Organ Transplantation – Current Clinical and Immunological Concepts* (Ed. by L. Brent & R. Sells) pp. 44–56. Baillière Tindall, Eastbourne.

Taplin, D. *et al.* (1973) Flower vases in hospital as reservoirs of pathogens. *Lancet*, 11, 1279–81.

Wade, J. C. *et al.* (1982) *Staphylococcus epidermidis*, an increasingly but frequently recognised cause of infection in granulocytopenia. *Annals of International Medicine*, 97, 503–8.

Wright, C. *et al.* (1976) *Enterobacteriaceae* and *Pseudomonas aeruginosa* recovered from vegetable salads. *Applied and Environmental Microbiology*, 31(3), 453–4.

Yates, J. W. *et al.* (1973) A controlled study of isolation and endogenous microbial suppression in acute myelocytic leukaemia patients. *Cancer*, 32, 1490–8.

GUIDELINES: NURSING THE NEUTROPENIC PATIENT

Procedure

Preparation of the room and maintenance of general cleanliness

Action	Rationale
1. A single room should be used if possible.	To reduce airborne transfer of micro-organisms.
2. A toilet to be kept for the sole use of the patient.	To reduce the risk of cross-infection.

Guidelines: Nursing the neutropenic patient

Action	Rationale
3. Area to be cleaned meticulously before the patient is admitted.	To reduce the risk of infection.
4. Equipment and supplies to be kept for the sole use of the patient. (This must also include any cleaning equipment used by domestic staff.)	To reduce the risk of cross-infection. Cleaning equipment can easily become colonized with micro-organisms which may cause cross-infection.
5. Surfaces and furniture to be damp dusted daily using disposable cleaning cloths and detergent solution.	Damp dusting and mopping removes micro-organisms without distributing them into the air.
6. Floor to be mopped daily using soap and water.	To reduce the risk of cross-infection.
7. Mop head to be laundered daily.	As above.
8. Bucket and mop handle to be cleaned and dried and stored in the isolation area.	As above.

Nursing procedure

Action	Rationale
1. Hands must be washed thoroughly with bactericidal soap and water or bactericidal alcohol hand rub.	Hands are regarded as the principle source of transfer of micro-organisms. (For further information on aseptic technique see Chapter 3, Aseptic Technique.)
2. A disposable plastic apron should be worn for all nursing procedures.	Staff clothing can easily become contaminated. A disposable plastic apron reduces the risk of transfer of organisms.
3. Door of room to be kept closed. Ideally the air in the room should be under slightly positive pressure. The air flow should be from the room into the corridor.	To reduce the risk of airborne transmission of infection by inhaling organisms from the rest of the ward when entering the protective isolation room.

Visitors

Action	Rationale
1. The patient should be asked to nominate close relatives and friends who may then, after instruction, visit freely. The patient or his or her representative should inform casual acquaintances or non-essential visitors that they should avoid visiting during the period of neutropenia.	The incidence of infection increases in proportion to the number of people visiting. Large numbers of visitors are difficult to screen and educate. Unlimited visiting by close relatives and friends diminishes the sense of isolation that the patient may experience.
2. Any visitor with an infection or who has been in contact with infection should be excluded.	Neutropenic patients are susceptible to infection.
3. Children, unless very close relatives, should be discouraged.	Children are more likely to have been in contact with infectious diseases which can have serious consequences if transmitted to a neutropenic patient.

Diet

Action	Rationale
1. Educate the patient to choose only cooked food from the hospital menu and avoid raw fruit, salads and uncooked vegetables, whether on the menu or brought in by visitors.	Uncooked foods are often heavily colonized by micro-organisms, particularly Gram-negative bacteria.
2. Food brought into the hospital by visitors must be: (a) Obtained from well-known, reliable firms. (b) In undamaged, sealed tins and packets. (c) Within expiry date.	Correctly processed and packaged foods are acceptable as they should not be unacceptably infected.
3. Water should be boiled and allowed to cool in a covered jug.	Tap water is perfectly safe to drink but can become colonized by organisms, particularly Gram-negative organisms found in the plug hole of sinks or overflow outlet when the water is being filled.
4. Bottled concentrated fruit drinks made from whole fruit and containing sugar are invariably pathogen free.	Pathogens do not easily survive or multiply in a high sugar concentrate.
5. Sealed packets of fruit juice (long shelf-life varieties, particularly those rich in vitamins) are suitable. It should be poured directly into a clean jug and drunk the same day.	These juices have been pasteurized and remain pathogen-free until they are opened.

Discharging the patient

Action	Rationale
1. Crowded areas, for example shops, cinemas, pubs and discos, should be avoided.	Although the patient's white cell count is usually high enough for discharge, the patient remains immunocompromised for some time.
2. Pets should not be allowed to lick the patient, and new pets should not be obtained.	Pets are known carriers of infection.
3. Certain foods, for example take-away meals, soft cheese and pâté, should continue to be avoided.	Take-away meals are subject to handling by a large number of individuals and are stored for longer periods, both of which increase the likelihood of contamination.
4. Salads and fruit should be washed carefully, dried and, if possible, peeled.	To remove as many pathogens as possible.
5. Any sign or symptoms of infection should be reported immediately to the patient's general practitioner or to the discharging hospital.	Any infection may continue to have serious consequences if left unlocated.

ACQUIRED IMMUNE DEFICIENCY SYNDROME (AIDS)

Definition

Acquired immune deficiency syndrome (AIDS) is a state of immunosuppression caused by the human immunodeficiency virus 1 (HIV 1) and 2 (HIV 2). As no overall description can be made for AIDS, an internationally agreed case definition has been made (Communicable Disease Centre, 1987) and includes the following:

1. Certain opportunistic infections.
2. Certain cancers.
3. Wasting syndrome.
4. Encephalopathy.

The global programme on AIDS of the World Health Organization (WHO) has developed a clinical, four-part staging system for HIV infection and disease, based on clinical signs and symptoms, and can be used to improve clinical management of patients, and to establish reliable parameters for evaluating drugs and vaccine trials (WHO, 1990).

REFERENCE MATERIAL

The human immunodeficiency virus has been isolated in the blood (Gallo *et al.*, 1984), semen (Zagury *et al.*, 1984), tears and saliva (Fujikawara *et al.*, 1985), breast milk (Thiry *et al.*, 1985), genital secretions of women (Wofsy *et al.*, 1986) and cerebrospinal fluid and the brain (Levy, 1985). In adults, transmission of the virus between individuals most often occurs during sexual activity (male to male (Kingsley *et al.*, 1987); male to female (Padian *et al.*, 1987a), female to male (Padian, 1987b); whereas female to female is rare (Cabane *et al.*, 1984)). Other causes of transmission of virus are by needle sharing in drug abusers (Marmor *et al.*, 1987) and by the administration of contaminated blood and blood products (Peterman, 1987). HIV transmission has been reported rarely by organ transplantation (Communicable Disease Centre, 1987), and following artificial insemination (Steward *et al.*, 1985).

Most infants and children become infected as a result of vertical transmission of HIV from their infected mothers, either during pregnancy, at delivery or during the immediate post-partum period (Sprecher *et al.*, 1986). HIV transmission to newborn infants from infected breast milk has occurred (Lepage *et al.*, 1987), and it has also been recorded as a result of sexual abuse (Rubinstein *et al.*, 1986).

Studies of prolonged social contact with HIV infection have failed to show that transmission has occurred, unless the transmission routes already mentioned are present (Jason *et al.*, 1986), except in one case from a child to a mother who was providing health care (Communicable Disease Centre, 1986).

Transmission of HIV infection to health care workers has occurred following needlestick injuries, contamination of mucous membranes or through breaks in the skin (Department of Health and Social Security, 1990a). The overall risk with a single sharps injury is estimated to be approximately 0.3%, and probably needs to involve a hollow needle, with an inoculation of greater than 0.1 ml of blood (Shanson, 1991).

Trials of prophylactic zidovudine following inoculation accidents involving HIV-antibody-positive blood are in progress (Department of Health and Social Security, 1990b; Henderson *et al.*, 1989). Failure to prevent seroconversion has been seen (Lange, 1990), which emphasizes the need to adopt and promote safe practices at all times (Hart, 1991).

The period immediately following infection with HIV is termed the window period, during which time antibodies to the virus will be produced. This generally occurs within three months of exposure, although longer window periods have been reported (Ranki *et al.*, 1987).

Generally, a negative antibody test six months after a known or expected exposure to HIV 1 will provide a reasonable basis for reassurance, although in a few reported cases detectable antibodies could not be recovered although detected virus was present (Groopman, *et al.*, 1985).

Antibodies to HIV are measured using an enzyme-linked immunosorbent assay (ELISA) (Arpadi *et al.*, 1991). Usually a positive test is retested by ELISA and a confirmatory test is carried out using Western Blot Analysis is undertaken (Schochetman, 1990). (This technique is also called immunoblotting and is used to identify particular antigens in a mixture by separation on polyacrylamide gels blotting onto nitrocellulose, and by labelling with radiolabelled or enzyme-labelled antibodies as probes.)

HIV 1 antigen tests are available and play a major contribution to the serological assessment of HIV infection (Allain, 1986). However, this test has not yet become generally available, as the expense and time involved renders it unsuitable as a screening system.

The Department of Health and Social Security (1985) recommends that no patient should be tested for HIV antibodies without their informed consent, and that counselling should be offered to the patient before and after the test. Miller (1987) discusses the information which should be included in the counselling sessions. Carr and Gee (1986) discuss the significance of positive and negative test results, while Grimshaw (1987) suggests that the time spent on counselling not only provides psychological and emotional support, but is also a good basis for future communication.

Hospitals involved in anonymous HIV antibody screening must ensure that patients are aware of the ongoing research project. No post-test counselling is possible in these circumstances.

Since reporting began in 1982, although the rate of increase in the incidence of AIDS has slowed, the incidence continues to rise. In the final quarter of 1990, an average of 24 new AIDS cases was seen each week. Of 31 European countries for which data are available, the UK has an estimated cumulative AIDS incidence of 72 per million population, which ranks tenth in the order of magnitude of the AIDS pandemic (Communicable Disease Centre, 1991).

AIDS raises many ethical issues (Reisman, 1988). Mindel (1987) discusses the importance of confidentiality when dealing with any antibody-positive patient. This was supported by the United Kingdom Central Council for Nursing, Midwifery and Health Visitors (1986) and the Department of Health and Social Security (1990a) which also states that health care workers dealing with known or suspected seropositive patients or specimens must be made fully aware of the risk.

The Public Health (Infections Diseases) Regulations 1985 make certain provisions to safeguard public health where a person is suffering from AIDS. It is stressed that these provisions are to be used only in exceptional circumstances where transmission of HIV may occur.

Adler (1987) reports that not all infected people go on to develop AIDS, but may develop persistent generalized lymphadenopathy (PGL) or AIDS-related complex (ARC). It is not clear why and when an infected person will develop full-blown AIDS; estimates vary from 15 to 50% or more (Goedert *et al.*, 1987). The 1990 median survival time from the date of diagnosis to death with AIDS disease is estimated to be between 18 and 20 months (Pratt, 1991).

Much research is in progress to identify and evaluate treatments and vaccines for the treatment and prevention of HIV infection. Several drugs have inhibited the action of reverse transcriptase, a viral enzyme which allows HIV to make a deoxyribonucleic acid (DNA) copy of its ribonucleic acid (RNA) genetic material. Zidovudine has been seen to be the most effective drug as yet, by prolonging survival and reducing mortality, but it is expensive and potentially toxic (Richman *et al.*, 1987).

HIV infection alone does not affect a person's ability to continue with regular employment (Department of Employment, 1987) unless injury to the worker could result in blood contaminating the patients' open tissues (UK Health Department, 1991). An incidence of transmission of HIV from a dentist to his patient during a dental procedure has occurred (Communicable Disease Centre, 1990).

AIDS disease is changing all the time. At present, records show a decline in the incidence of Kaposi's sarcoma (Rutherford, *et al.*, 1989) and a reduced mortality from *Pneumocystis carinii* pneumonia (Harris, 1990), but the emergence of new opportunist pathogens (Peters, *et al.*, 1991).

Nurses must keep up to date with improved, earlier diagnosis of AIDS, with better treatments and with the increased use of prophylaxis. They must be ready to adapt to these changes and be prepared and able to provide good care. This process will be achieved only by good education (Armstrong-Esther *et al.*, 1990) and management support.

References and further reading

Adler, M. N. (1987) Range and natural history of infection. *British Medical Journal*, 294, 1145–7.

Allain, J. P. (1986) Serological markers in early stages of human immunodeficiency virus infection in haemophiliacs. *Lancet*, 2, 1233.

Armstrong-Esther, C. *et al.* (1990) The effect of education on nurses' perception of AIDS. *Journal of Advanced Nursing*, 15, 638–51.

Arpadi, S. *et al.* (1991) HIV testing. *Journal of Pediatrics*, 199(1), Part 2, S8–S13.

Cabane, J. *et al.* (1984) AIDS in an apparently risk-free woman. *Lancet*, 2, 105.

Carr, G. & Gee, C. (1986) AIDS and AIDS-related conditions: screening for populations at risk. *Nurse Practitioner*, 11(10), 25–46.

Communicable Disease Centre (CDC) (1986) Apparent transmission of human T-lymphotropic type III/lymphodenopathy associated virus from a child to a mother providing health care. *MMWR*, 35, 76–9.

Communicable Disease Centre (1987) Human immunodeficiency virus infection transmitted from an organ donor screened for HIV antibody. *Morbidity and Mortality Weekly Report*, 36(20), 306–8.

Communicable Disease Centre (1990) Possible transmission of human immunodeficiency virus to a patient during an invasive dental procedure. *Morbidity and Mortality Weekly Report*, 39(29) 489–93.

Communicable Disease Centre (1991) AIDS and HIV 1 Antibody reports. United Kingdom. *Communicable Disease Report*, 1(15), 67–8.

Department of Employment – The Health and Safety Executive (1987) *AIDS and Employment*. DoE, London.

Department of Health and Social Security (1985) *The Public Health (Infectious Diseases) Regulations 1985 (HC(85)17) (LAC(85)10)*. HMSO, London.

Department of Health and Social Security (1990a) *Advisory Committee on Dangerous Pathogens. HIV The Causative Agent of AIDS and Related Conditions. Second Revision of Guidelines HN(90)4*. HMSO, London.

Department of Health and Social Security (1990b) *Guidance for Clinical Health Care Workers. Protection Against Infection with HIVB and Hepatitis Viruses*. HMSO, London.

Fujikawara, L. S. *et al.* (1985) Isolation of human T lymphotropic virus type III from tears of patients with AIDS, *Lancet*, 2, 529–30.

Gallo, R. C. *et al.* (1984) Frequent detection and continuous production of cytopathic retroviruses (HTLV III) from patients with AIDS. *Science*, 224, 497–500.

Goedert, J. J. *et al.* (1987) Effects of T4 counts and co-factors on the incidence of AIDS in homosexual men infected with human immunodeficiency virus. *Journal of the American Medical Association*, 257, 326–30.

Grimshaw, J. (1987) Being HIV antibody positive. *British Medical Journal*, 295, 256–7.

Groopman, J. E. *et al.* (1985) Antibody seronegative human T lymphotropic virus type III (HTLV III) infected patients with acquired immunodeficiency symdrome or related disorders. *Blood*, 66, 742–4.

Harris, J. E. (1990) Improved short-term survival of AIDS patients initially diagnosed with *Pneumocystis carinii* pneumonia 1984 through 1989. *Journal of the American Medical Association*, 263, 397–401.

Hart, S. (1991) Blood and body fluid precautions. *Nursing Standard*, 5, 25–7.

Henderson, D. K. *et al.* (1989) Prophylactic Zidovudine after occupational exposure to the human immunodeficiency virus; an interim analysis. *Journal of Infectious Diseases*, 160, 321–7.

Jason, J. M. *et al.* (1986) HTLV III/LAV antibody and immune status of household contacts and sexual partners of persons with haemophilia. *Journal of the American Medical Association*, 155, 212.

Kingsley, L. A. *et al.* (1987) Risk factors for seroconversion to human immunodeficiency virus among homosexuals. *Lancet*, 1, 345–8.

Lange, J. M. A. (1990) Failure of Zidovudine prophylaxis after accidential exposure to HIV. *New England Journal of Medicine*, 322(19), 1375–7.

Lepage, P. *et al.* (1987) Postnatal transmission of HIV from mother to child. *Lancet*, 2, 400.

Levy, J. A. (1985) Isolation of AIDS-associated retroviruses from cerobrospinal fluid and brain of patients with neurological symptoms. *Lancet*, 2, 586–8.

Marmor, M. *et al.* (1987) Risk factors for infection with human immune-deficiency virus among intravenous drug abusers in New York City. *AIDS*, 1(1), 39–44.

Miller, D. (1987) Counselling. *British Medical Journal*, 294, 1670–4.

Mindel, A. (1987) Management of early HIV infection. *British Medical Journal*, 294, 1145–7.

Padian, N. S. *et al.* (1987a) Male to female transmission of human immunodeficiency virus. *Journal of the American Medical Association*, 258, 788–90.

Padian, N. S. (1987b) Heterosexual transmission of acquired immunodeficiency syndrome. International perspectives and national projections. *Review of Infectious Diseases*, 9, 947–60.

Peterman, T. A. (1987) Transfusion associated acquired immunodeficiency syndrome. *World Journal of Surgery*, 11(1), 36–40.

Peters, B. S. *et al.* (1991) Changing disease pattern in patients with AIDS in a referral centre in the United Kingdom. The changing face of AIDS, *British Medical Journal*, 302, 203–6.

Pratt, R. (1991) AIDS – *A Strategy for Nursing Care*, 3rd edn. Edward Arnold, London.

Ranki, A. *et al.* (1987) Long latency periods precedes overt seroconversion in sexually transmitted human immunodeficiency virus infection. *Lancet*, 2, 589–93.

Reisman, E. C. (1988) Ethical issues confronting nurses. *Nursing Clinics of North America*, 23(4), 789–801.

Richman, D. D. *et al.* (1987) The toxicity of azidothymidine (AZT) in the treatment of patients with AIDS and AIDS-related complex. A double-blind placebo controlled trial. *New England Journal of Medicine*, 317, 192–7.

Rubinstein, A. *et al.* (1986) The epidemiology of paediatric acquired immunodeficiency syndrome. *Clinical Immunology and Immunopathology*, 40, 115–21.

Rutherford, G. W. *et al.* (1989) The epidemiology of AIDS-related Kaposi's sarcoma in San Francisco. *Journal of Infectious Diseases*, 159, 567–71.

Schochetman, G. (1990) Laboratory diagnosis of infection with the AIDS virus. *Lab. Medica*, April/May, 15–24.

Shanson, D. C. (1991) Current surgical controversies over HIV infection. *Journal of Hospital Infection*, 17, 77–81.

Sprecher, S. *et al.* (1986) Vertical transmission of HIV in a 15-week fetus. *Lancet*, 2, 288.

Steward, G. J. *et al.* (1985) Transmission of HTLV III by artificial insemination by donor serum. *Lancet*, 2, 581–4.

Thiry, L. *et al.* (1985) Isolation of AIDS virus from cell-free breast milk of three healthy virus carriers. *Lancet*, 1, 891–2.

UK Health Department (1991) *AIDS-HIV Infected Health Care Workers – Occupational Guidance for Health Care Workers, their Physicians and Employers*. Recommendations of the expert advisory group on AIDS. Copies from Health Publication Unit, Heywood Stores, Lancashire OL10 2PZ.

United Kingdom Central Council for Nursing, Midwifery and Health Visitors (1986) *Confidentiality – An Elaboration of Clause 9 of the Second Edition of the UKCC's Code of Professional Conduct*. UKCC, London.

Wofsy, C. B. *et al.* (1986) Isolation of AIDS associated retrovirus from genital secretions of women with antibodies to the virus. *Lancet*, 1, 527–9.

World Health Organization (WHO) (1990) *WHO Weekly Epidemiology Record*, 20 July, WHO, Geneva.

Zagury, D. *et al.* (1984) HTLV III cells culture from semen in two patients with AIDS, *Science*, 226, 449–51.

HUMAN IMMUNODEFICIENCY VIRUS 2 (HIV2)

Definition

HIV 2 was first recognized in 1986 (Clavel *et al.*, 1986), although evidence that HIV 2 infections were present in many West Africa as far back as 1966 (Karamura *et al.*, 1989) has been disputed (Mohammed *et al.*, 1989). Serological evidence supporting the existence of a second HIV was published in 1985 (Barin *et al.*, 1985). Today, HIV 2 is present in many West African countries and, in some, it is a more common cause of AIDS than HIV 1 (Naucler *et al.*, 1989).

REFERENCE MATERIAL

In the UK, screening of blood donors and people attending genitourinary medicine clinics show that the occurrence of HIV 2 infection is rare. A few HIV 2 infections have been reported in many European countries, and 18 HIV 2 infections have been reported in the United States. Of these, over two-thirds of patients had contact with, or were from, Africa (Evans *et al.*, 1991).

Transmission of HIV 2 follows the same pattern as HIV 1 (Kroegal *et al.*, 1987), although the rate of vertical transmission from mother to child is uncertain, with some studies suggesting that it might be low (Morgan *et al.*, 1990).

Despite the high prevalence of HIV 2 infections in West Africa, there have been many fewer reported AIDS cases compared with East and Central Africa, where HIV 1 predominates, implying HIV 2 is less pathogenic than HIV 1 (Romieu *et al.*, 1990).

The range of opportunistic infections and malignancies and the wasting and dementia associated with progressive HIV 1 infections are also present in HIV 2 disease, although *Pneumocystis carinii* pneumonia (Clavel *et al.*, 1987) and active tuberculosis may be less common in HIV-2-infected people than in those infected with HIV 1. However, this may represent a difference in prevalence of opportunistic pathogens rather than being a direct effect of HIV infection (Kanki, 1989).

In May 1989, the AIDS laboratory diagnostic working group advised combined screening in diagnostic laboratories in the UK (Evans *et al.*, 1991).

Since July 1990, combined anti-HIV 1/HIV 2 testing of all donations of blood was introduced in the UK Blood Transfusion Service. Of the first 250 000 donations, only one HIV-2-infected donor was detected.

Since there is no difference in the method of transmission between HIV 1 and HIV 2, prevention and nursing care are the same.

References and further reading

Barin, F. *et al.* (1985) Serological evidence for virus related to Simian T-lymphotropic retrovirus III in residents of West Africa. *Lancet*, 2, 1387–9.

Clavel, F. *et al.* (1986) Isolation of a new human retrovirus from West African patients with AIDS. *Science*, 233, 343–6.

Clavel, F. *et al.* (1987) Human immunodeficiency virus type 2 infection associated with AIDS in West Africa. *New England Journal of Medicine*, 316, 1180–5.

Evans, B. G. *et al.* (1991) HIV 2 in the United Kingdom. A review. *Communicable Disease Report*, 1(2), R19-R232.

Kanki, P. J. (1989). Clinical significance of HIV 2 infection in West Africa. *AIDS Clin. Rev.*, 95–108.

Karamura, M. *et al.* (1989) HIV 2 in West Africa in 1966. *Lancet*, 1, 385.

Kroegal, C. *et al.* (1987). Routes of HIV 2 transmissions in Western Europe. *Lancet*, 1, 1150.

Mohammed, I. *et al.* (1989) HIV 2 West Africa in 1966. *Lancet*, 1, 385.

Morgan, G. *et al.* (1990) AIDS following mother to child transmission of HIV 2. *AIDS*, 4, 879–82.

Naucler, A. *et al.* (1989) HIV 2-associated AIDS and HIV 2 sero-prevalence in Bissau, Guinea-Bissau. *Journal of AIDS*, 2, 88–93.

Romieu, I. *et al.* (1990) HIV 2 link to AIDS in West Africa, *Journal of AIDS*, 3, 220–30.

GUIDELINES: ACQUIRED IMMUNE DEFICIENCY SYNDROME IN A GENERAL WARD

Procedure

Action	Rationale
1. Staff suffering from eczema should not nurse patients who are HIV antibody positive.	Any break in staff members' skin should be covered with a waterproof dressing to prevent entry of HIV. This would be difficult to accomplish with eczema lesions and would exacerbate the eczema.
2. Immunodeficient-compromised staff, either through illness or therapy, should not nurse patients who are HIV antibody positive.	HIV antibody positive patients who present with generalized infection could put this category of staff at risk.
3. All staff should read and be familiar with government guidelines on AIDS and their own hospital's codes of practice.	To ensure all staff are aware of, and take, the necessary precautions.

Guidelines: Acquired immune deficiency syndrome in a general ward

Action	Rationale
4. Hospital staff should cover any broken skin with a waterproof dressing.	To prevent the entry of infectious material.
5. Accidental inoculations must be avoided at all cost.	Serious inoculation accidents have been seen to be a means of transmission of HIV.
6. In the event of gross contamination of intact skin the affected area must be washed thoroughly with soap under hand hot water. A scrubbing brush must not be used.	Intact skin is a natural barrier against infection. By thorough washing the infectious material can be removed. Scrubbing brushes can cause skin damage which allows infection to enter.
7. Puncture wounds or cuts must be made to bleed freely and washed under hot running water.	To flush out infectious material.
8. A waterproof dressing must be applied and medical advice sought for large wounds.	To prevent further infection.
9. An accident form must be filled in immediately and taken to bacteriology, the occupational health physician or other medical advisor as appropriate.	It is important to have accurate records of all accidents and incidents in order to monitor events.

Low-risk, HIV-positive individuals

Action	Rationale
1. If the patient is not bleeding, incontinent, confused or infected with a contagious disease, he/she may be nursed on an open ward using all the patients' facilities as normal.	HIV cannot be transmitted by social contact.
2. If a low-risk, HIV-positive individual develops an infection, is undergoing invasive procedures or becomes incontinent, nursing care will commence as for high-risk, HIV-positive persons.	Incontinent, bleeding HIV antibody-positive patients have the potential risk of transmitting the HIV virus to others.

High-risk, HIV-positive individuals

Action	Rationale
1. Known or strongly suspected HIV-antibody-positive patients who are bleeding, incontient, infected with a contagious disease or receiving invasive procedures should be nursed in a single room with its own toilet and hand-washing facilities.	To minimize the risk of transmitting infection. HIV can be transmitted via blood and body fluid.

Entering the room

Action	Rationale
1. When the patient is not bleeding, coughing, incontinent or receiving procedures, protective clothing is not required.	Transmission of HIV is not possible from casual social contact.

2. When the patient is incontinent, bleeding or undergoing invasive procedures, disposable well-fitting gloves and a plastic apron are needed. A specification for non-sterile, natural rubber latex examination gloves has been published recently by the Department of Health (Doc. No. TSS/D/300.010, October 1988, Supplies Technology Division, Procurement Directorate). Users should check that their supplier's products conform with this specification.

Transmission of HIV is possible from body fluids.

3. If there is a possibility of airborne contamination, a correctly fitting theatre mask and safety spectacles should be worn.

Transmission of HIV is possible if contaminated material is allowed to contaminate mucous membrane.

Liquid waste

Action	Rationale
1. All liquid waste from AIDS patients must be disposed of in a bedpan washer immediately, taking care to avoid splashing.	To prevent contamination of the environment.
2. Areas without bedpan washers will need to use the slop hopper. Great care must be taken to pour waste slowly and carefully down the hopper to avoid splashing.	To prevent contamination of the environment.

Non-disposable equipment

Action	Rationale
1. Cleaning of non-disposable equipment needs to be performed thoroughly and in a safe manner.	Careless cleaning, immersion, drying, etc. can increase contamination of the environment.
2. Gloves/aprons must be worn, together with masks/eye protection if appropriate.	To prevent self-contamination.
3. Before disinfection, equipment must be cleaned with soap and water, avoiding splashing.	Disinfectants cannot completely penetrate organic matter.
4. The equipment must then be dried carefully.	Wet objects would alter the disinfectant's strength and could inactivate the solution if soap and soiling were still present.
5. If equipment will not be damaged by immersion in freshly activated 2% glutaraldehyde for 30 minutes, this is the method of choice.	Glutaraldehyde's bacteriostatic action is completely effective against the AIDS retrovirus.
6. If the equipment will be damaged by immersion in the glutaraldehyde solution, or is too big to fit into the disinfection container, these items must be first washed thoroughly with soap and water and dried, followed by washing and drying with a hypochlorite 1% solution.	Hypochlorite 1% solution has a non-corrosive action for delicate equipment and is less toxic to staff than glutaraldehyde.
7. If the equipment will be damaged by	70% ethanol is virucidal against most categories of

Guidelines: Acquired immune deficiency syndrome in a general ward

Action	Rationale
glularaldehyde or hypochlorite solution, these items must be first washed thoroughly with soap and water and dried, and immersed in 70% ethanol.	viruses, but does not penetrate organic matter and is inflammable.
8. If the equipment can be autoclaved it must be placed in a central sterile supplies department (CSSD) bag, taped shut with biohazard tape and marked with a biohazard label. The bag must then be taken to CSSD.	Autoclaving is the most effective sterilization method. Correct bagging and transportation of the equipment will prevent contamination of the environment.
9. Expensive, delicate items which have had prolonged, close contact with the patient, i.e. a ventilator, will require ethylene oxide disinfection.	Ethylene oxide disinfection is the second process of choice after autoclaving.
10. Before the ethylene oxide disinfection process, these items must have all their disposable parts, filters, etc. removed and the whole item cleaned completely and thoroughly with hypochlorite 1% solution and dried carefully.	To prevent contamination of the environment.
11. The transportation and ethylene oxide process will take at least one week. Thought must be given beforehand to the use of this equipment for actively bleeding, incontinent patients.	Ethylene oxide disinfection involves lengthy airing of equipment after the process to ensure it is safe to re-use. During this time other patients may be deprived of the item.

Other hospital departments

Action	Rationale
1. It is essential that all request cards for such items as specimens have the biohazard label attached.	To ensure all departments are informed that the sample is potentially dangerous.
2. All specimens must have the biohazard label attached and be double bagged in a specimen polythene biohazard bag with a biohazard label attached to the bag.	To ensure the laboratory is aware of potential risk and that the specimen is correctly contained to prevent cross-infection. (For further information on specimen collection see Chapter 36, Specimen Collection).
3. The specimen should be taken to the laboratory in a washable, covered container.	To prevent contamination of the environment.
4. A nurse should accompany an antibody-positive patient to other departments. If there is not a departmental nurse in the department, the ward nurse should remain with the patient.	To give help and advice.
5. The patient will normally be given the first or last appointment of the day if invasive procedures are planned.	The department will be less crowded and busy, thus allowing time for appropriate precautions to be taken.

Domestic staff

Action	Rationale
1. The room must be prepared and cleaned. (For further information see Guidelines: Source Isolation, above.)	To minimize the risk of cross-infection.
2. A nurse must check the patient's room to establish that it is suitable for the domestic staff to clean.	To ensure the room is not contaminated with blood or body fluids.
3. If contamination of the environment with blood or body fluids occurs it must be treated with a hypochlorite solution containing 10 000 ppm available chlorine.	To prevent cross-infection.

Terminal cleaning of the room

Action	Rationale
1. The room must be cleared of all equipment before it is cleaned.	It is impossible to clean thoroughly if potentially contaminated items are in the room.
2. The carpet must be steamed if contamination by blood or excreta has occurred.	Organisms have been known to survive in carpets. Steam cleaning destroys these.
3. The walls should only be cleaned if contamination is known to have occurred.	HIV does not survive on intact walls.
4. The curtains must be changed if contamination has occurred.	Discretion and assessment need to be used. If the room has only been used for a short time for a patient who has not contaminated the environment, curtains would not need changing.

The patient

Action	Rationale
1. As soon as possible, the probable/known diagnosis must be discussed with the patient and the hospital policy explained.	It is essential that the patient understands fully the reason for these restrictions which, while protecting contacts, also protect the patient from further risks of infection.
2. Psychological support is essential.	Psychological dysfunction is likely and should be recognized and treated early to alleviate and contain the mental distress which an AIDS patient may experience.
3. It if necessary that all nurses caring for antibody-positive patients are familiar with treatment and care procedures.	To ensure appropriate nursing care is delivered.
4. Staff should adopt a non-judgemental approach in their dealings with antibody-positive patients.	It is the responsibility of all health professionals to care for patients and not to pass moral judgements.
5. It may be appropriate to recommend voluntary agencies to antibody-positive patients.	Support groups have knowledge and experience which can help HIV antibody-positive individuals.

Guidelines: Acquired immune deficiency syndrome in a general ward

Visiting

Action	Rationale
1. Visitors should be encouraged.	To prevent isolation.
2. The diagnosis of AIDS is confidential and should not be disclosed.	To maintain confidentiality.

Discharging the patient

Action	Rationale
1. Almost all patients with AIDS will require community services at some time during their illness.	AIDS patients will need to be admitted to hospital for the treatment of clinical illness, but will be encouraged to resume their normal activities when in remission.
2. If an AIDS patient requires community services, the patient must have given consent for HIV antibody-positive diagnosis to be given to the general practitioner and community care personnel.	Confidentiality must not be breached without the patient's consent. However, health care workers such as ambulance men and women and district nurses will need to take precautions if bleeding, incontinence or infections are present.

Disposal of waste in the community

Action	Rationale
1. Excreta, infected fluids and such items as sanitary towels can be discarded into the toilet in the normal manner.	To prevent contamination of the environment.
2. Infected waste such as dressings, gloves and aprons, must be burned or placed in yellow clinical waste bags and the local authority asked to collect them.	Yellow is the international colour for infected waste bags, and they are available on request from the local authority.
3. Sharps must be placed in a sharps box and stored in a safe place when full. They should then be placed in a yellow clinical waste bag and collected by the local health authority.	To prevent inoculation accidents. Yellow is the international colour coding for clinical waste.

Laundry in the community

Action	Rationale
1. Clothes and linen which are heavily soiled or bloodstained should be washed separately by washing machine at 71°C for 25 minutes. Wash as for above in a public launderette.	Heat is effective in destroying the HIV. If the temperature is increased, the duration of the wash may be decreased.

2. If the person is not fit enough, infected linen should be placed in polythene bags with a red alginate stripe and the local authority asked to arrange collection and laundering.

Polythene bags with a red alginate stripe are recognized internationally for infected linen.

Cookery and cutlery

Action	**Rationale**
1. Ideally, crockery and cutlery should be washed in a dishwasher with a final rinse temperature of at least 80°C.	Heat is effective in destroying the HIV.
2. There is no need to keep a separate store of crockery and cutlery.	Crockery and cutlery present no risk of contamination.

Protective clothing in the community

Action	**Rationale**
1. Disposable apron and gloves need be worn only when blood or excreta are being handled.	There is no risk of acquiring infection from casual contact.
2. Disinfectants are required only if blood or excreta spillage has occurred. A strong hypochlorite solution (1 part household bleach to 10 parts water) is recommended.	Unnecessary use of disinfectants is expensive and may be potentially hazardous to staff and the environment.

Visitors in the community

Action	**Rationale**
1. Visitors should be encouraged.	There is no risk of acquiring infection from casual contact.
2. The patient should be encouraged to resume social activities.	Social activities will help to contain any symptoms such as stress and depression.

Prevention of further infection

Action	**Rationale**
1. The patient should be encouraged to stay away from individuals with infections.	AIDS patients are susceptible to infections.
2. If the patient develops any signs and symptoms of ill health, the general practitioner or hospital must be informed immediately.	Early treatment of symptoms will enhance the chances of containing the disease.

(For further details on discharge planning see Chapter 12.)

Death

Action	**Rationale**
1. The body should be laid out as described in the Procedure, Last Offices (Chapter 23). In addition, the nurse should wear gloves and a plastic apron.	To prevent self-contamination.

Guidelines: Acquired immune deficiency syndrome in a general ward

Action	Rationale
2. All orifices must be packed.	The body continues to secrete fluids after death has occurred. Any leakage may contaminate the environment.
3. Any wounds, intravenous sites or skin breakages must be sealed with waterproof dressing.	To prevent leakage of contaminated fluids.
4. All documentation relating to this procedure must have a biohazard label attached.	To alert administration, portering and mortuary staff of the infection risks.
5. Once the body has been laid out and the room made presentable, family and friends may view the body.	Once the body has left the word or home, viewing will be difficult if the funeral director adheres strictly to infectious diseases regulations.
6. The body must be placed in a cadaver bag and sealed securely with biohazard tape.	The cadaver bag will prevent leakage and ensures infectious diseases regulations are complied with.
7. Porters must be given help and support.	There is no infection risk when the body is sealed in a cadaver bag unless the bag becomes torn or damaged in transportation. Gloves and aprons will prevent contamination of the staff handling the body.

Funeral arrangements

Action	Rationale
1. Ideally, the hospital administration should have a list of funeral directors who will attend to an AIDS patient.	It is important that the bereaved relatives and given every help and support to prevent unnecessary distress.

ASPERGILLOSIS

Definition

An infection caused by a fungus of the genus *Aspergillus*, causing inflammatory granulomatous lesions on or in any organ.

REFERENCE MATERIAL

Aspergillus are common saprophytic moulds, easily recognized by their conidiophores, which are swollen ends of hyphae, from which radiate large numbers of sterigmata which end in short chains of spores. Each *Aspergillus* conidiospore releases thousands of spores, which remain suspended in the air for long periods and are viable for many months in dry locations. Over 200 species of *Aspergillus* have been characterized, but less than 20 are reported as being pathogenic to man, the most common species causing allergic and invasive disease being *Aspergillus fumigatus* (Warren *et al.*, 1982). In recent years *Aspergillus flavus* has also emerged as an important pathogen (Bodey *et al.*, 1989).

Aspergillus spores are commonly found in soil, decaying vegetation, spices, potted plants and dried flowers. Cases of allergic and invasive disease have been reported among individuals working in close contact with such substances and who inhale large numbers of *Aspergillus* spores.

Generally, aspergillosis has been associated with building renovation, when large numbers of spores are often liberated into the environment (Arnow *et al.*, 1978). These spores are then inhaled and deposited in the lungs. Ear, cutaneous, sinus and dental infections have also been known to occur.

Normal healthy people rarely develop invasive disease. Aspergillosis is primarily an infection of severely immune-compromised patients. The major predisposing factor of infection includes prolonged neutropenia, chronic administration of steroids, insertion of prosthetic devices and tissue damage due to prior infection or trauma (Khardoni, 1989).

The organism is capable of invasion across all natural barriers, including cartilage and bone, and has a propensity for invading blood vessels, causing thrombosis and infection. The major concern is the potential for severe haemorrhage, which may cause death and which occurs in about 10% of patients.

Generally, infection is chronic, causing symptoms directly related to the site of infection.

Diagnosis is difficult as *Aspergillus* spores are cultured infrequently from the respiratory tract secretions (Weiland, 1983), and there is considerable debate about the significance of isolation as this organism is a common contaminant. Diagnosis generally relies on serological (Trull *et al.*, 1985) or histocytochemical tests (Meyer *et al.*, 1973).

Therapy of invasive aspergillosis has been less than satisfactory, with amphotericin B being the only antifungal agent with established activity against the infection (Pizzo *et al.*, 1982). Newer antifungal agents such as Fluconazole and Itraconazole appear to exhibit good activity against a variety of fungi (Oppo Anaissie, 1992).

Control measures are essential. Air conditioning systems must be functioning and well maintained, and the environment kept scrupulously clean, with emphasis placed on vacuuming, damp dusting and mopping. Instruments, dressings equipment and linen must always be stored properly to prevent contamination by *Aspergillus*. This highlights the importance of removing wound dressings for the shortest period of time possible before dressing changes to prevent contamination of open wounds.

During structural work it is essential to provide and maintain impermeable barriers to ensure that spores from work areas do not enter ventilation systems or get carried to other wards. Ideally, relocation of immune-suppressed patients to unaffected areas is advisable, and thorough cleaning of work areas before the return of patients is essential (Arnow *et al.*, 1978).

Person-to-person spread has not been demonstrated, and therefore barrier nursing is not required. However, careful disposal of sputum, and encouraging patients to cover the mouth and nose when coughing, are necessary precautions.

References and further reading

Arnow, P. M. *et al.* (1978) Pulmonary aspergillosis during hospital renovation. *American Review of Respiratory Disease*, 118, 49–53.

Bodey, G. P. *et al.* (1989) Aspergillosis. *European Journal of Clinical Microbiology and Infectious Disease*, 8(5), 413–37.

Khardoni, N. (1989) Host–parasite interactions in fungal infections. *European Journal of Clinical Microbiology and Infectious Diseases*, 8, 331–52.

Meyer, R. D. *et al.* (1973) Aspergillosis complicating neoplastic disease. *American Journal of Medicine*, 54, 6–54.

Oppo Anaisse E. (1992) Opportunistic mycoses in the immunocompromised host. Experience at a cancer centre and review. *Clinical Infectious Disease*, 14 (suppl II), 543–53.

Pizzo, P. A. *et al.* (1982) Empiric antibiotic and antifungal therapy for cancer patients with prolonged fever and granulocytopenia. *American Journal of Medicine*, 72, 101–11.

Trull, A. *et al.* (1985) IgG enzyme linked immunosorbent essay for diagnosis of invasive aspergillosis: retrospective study over 15 years of transplant recipients. *Journal of Clinical Pathology*, 38, 1045–51.

Warren, R. E. *et al.* (1982) Clinical manifestations and management of aspergillosis in the compromised patient. In *Fungal Infections in the Compromised Patient* (Ed. by D. W. Warnock & M. D. Richardson), pp. 119–53. John Wiley, New York.

Weiland, D. (1983) Aspergillosis in 25 renal transplant patients. *Annals of Surgery*, 198, 622–9.

CRYPTOSPORIDIOSIS

Definition

Cryptosporidium is a protozoan parasite, first isolated in 1907. The only species of the organism known to affect man is *Cryptosporidium parvum*.

Cryptosporidia species were initially considered a cause of severe protracted diarrhoea (Navin *et al.*, 1984) in immunocompromised patients (Wolfson *et al.*, 1985). Cryptosporidium is now being increasingly recognized as the cause of self-limiting enteritis in otherwise healthy people, with sporadic and epidemic cryptosporidiosis most commonly recorded in young children (Holley *et al.*, 1986).

REFERENCE MATERIAL

Cryptosporidium is rarely isolated in people with normal stools (Soave *et al.*, 1986). In Britain, the number of reported cases of crytosporidiosis has been increasing. This may reflect greater public awareness and improved detection methods, rather than a true increase.

The organism infects livestock, particularly calves and lambs, whose faecal matter infects water supplies, which then can infect man (Tzipori, 1983).

Routine water disinfection by chlorination is ineffective in controlling the organism except in small numbers. Contamination of the water supply generally occurs when heavy rains follow drought, causing leakage of effluent or slurry into treated water.

Based on epidemiological evidence, consumption of certain foods (especially undercooked sausages, offal and unpasteurized milk) appears to be a risk factor (Casemore, 1987). Infection can also occur following direct contact with animals, and is easily transmitted from one person to another (Department of Health, 1990) which is probably the main mode of transmission in urban populations. Only a small innoculum of organism appears to be required to cause infection.

The incubation period is between 3 and 11 days, but may be as long as 25 days. Illness usually presents as acute offensive, non-bloody, diarrhoea, sometimes accompanied by fever. Acute illness may last for two to three weeks, with excretion of the organism in faeces for as long as a fortnight after symptoms have cleared. While infection is usually self-limiting in healthy people, it can cause untrackable diarrhoea in immunocompromised people, who will need admission to hospital for care and rehydration. There is no effective antimicrobial agent available to treat this organism.

Strict barrier nursing is required while diarrhoea persists, with segregation from other patients continuing until clear specimen of stool cultures are obtained.

Any sign of cross-infection must be pursued vigorously to prevent further spread. This will include close co-operation with health and local authorities, the appropriate water companies and the outbreak control team with the authority, as recommended by the Department of Health (1990).

The organism is unaffected by chlorine in the concentrations that can be used in the treatment of drinking water, and is inactivated only by being frozen or heated to temperatures of 65 to 85°C for five to ten minutes or by exposure to boiling water. Prevention relies on compliance with safe practices by water companies and health authorities in water treatment processes.

References and further reading

Casemore, D. P. (1987) Cryptosporidiosis PHLS. *Microbiology Digest*, 4, 1–5.

Department of Health (1990) *Report of the Group of Experts on Cryptosporidium in Water Supplies* (Chairman, Sir John Badenock). HMSO, London.

Holley, H. P. *et al.* (1986) Cryptosporidiosis – a common cause of parasitic diarrhoea in otherwise healthy individuals. *Journal of Infectious Diseases*, 153, 365–7.

Navin, T. R. *et al.* (1984) Cryptosporidiosis – clinical, epidemiological and parasitologic review. *Review of Infectious Diseases*, 6, 313–27.

Soave, R. *et al.* (1986) Cryptosporidium and cryptosporidiosis. *Review of Infectious Diseases*, 8, 1012–23.

Tzipori, S. (1983) Cryptosporidiosis in animals and humans. *Microbiological Review*, 47, 84–96.

Wolfson, J. S. *et al.* (1985) Cryptosporidiosis in immunocompetent patients. *New England Journal of Medicine*, 312, 1278–82.

HEPATITIS A

Definition

Hepatitis A is an acute infectious disease caused by the hepatitis A virus (HAV).

REFERENCE MATERIAL

HAV is a small, symmetrical RNA virus (enterovirus type 72) (Melnick, 1982). The virus is unusually stable, resisting heat at 60°C for one hour or 25°C for three months, indefinite cold storage (5°C), acidic conditions (pH3) and non-ionic detergents (Siegl *et al.*, 1984; Sorbey *et al.*, 1988).

HAV is spread predominantly by the faecal–oral route, and viral replication probably occurs in the jejunum before transmission via the portal vein to the liver (Siegl, 1988) and has been associated with the following:

1. Contaminated water, milk and food. Any uncooked foods and drinks could be responsible for infection. However, particular problems are due to contamination at the time of harvesting and packaging of uncooked frozen foods which are then thawed and used (Ramsey *et al.*, 1989).
2. Poor general hygiene and low economic status (Ayoola, 1988).
3. Contact with children in day centres (Hadler *et al.*, 1986) and neonatal intensive care units (Azimi *et al.*, 1986).
4. Foreign travel to countries where HAV is endemic (Skinhof *et al.*, 1981).
5. Blood transfusions (Noble *et al.*, 1984).

The HAV antigen (HAAg) can be detected in stools early in the course of illness. HAAg levels decline rapidly with the onset of symptoms but can remain detectable for up to two weeks after the onset of clinical hepatitis (Coulepis *et al.*, 1980).

Diagnosis of acute HAV infection is usually confirmed serologically, by detecting IgM antibodies to HAAg which appear in serum three to seven weeks after oral inoculation, and may persist for some time, occasionally for more than a year (Lemon *et al.*, 1980). Evidence of past infection and therefore immunity which can persist for life (Lemon, 1985) is obtained by detecting serologically the presence of IgG antibody to HAAg.

HAV usually causes a minor illness in children and young adults, with as few as 5% of cases being symptomatic (Eddleston, 1990). The illness often presents as an upper respiratory infection with the following signs and symptoms: anorexia; malaise; weight loss; pyrexia; diarrhoea and vomiting (Wright *et al.*, 1985); dark urine; and jaundice.

Symptomatic infection is more likely to occur with increasing age, with UK census data for 1979 to 1985 showing a positive correlation between age and death from HAV (Office of Population Censuses and Surveys, 1989). Control and prevention of HAV relies on provision of good sanitation facilities and clean drinking water, and supervision of food handlers. Passive immunization with intramuscular normal pooled immunoglobulin (NHIg) gives protection against clinical hepatitis for about three months in most people. However, it is probable that passive immunization allows HAV infection with greatly attenuating effects which could lead to life-long immunity (Gust *et al.*, 1988). It is advisable before travel in endemic regions; post-exposure prophylaxis is advisable for household contacts during outbreaks of HAV infection (Department of Health, 1988).

References and further reading

Ayoola, E. A. (1988) Viral hepatitis in Africa. In *Viral Hepatitis and Liver Disease* (Ed. by A. J. Zuckerman), pp. 161–9. Alan R. Liss, New York.

Azimi, P. H. *et al.* (1986) Transfusion-acquired hepatitis A in a premature infant with second nosocomial spread in an intensive care nursery. *American Journal of Diseases of Childhood*, 140, 23–7.

Coulepis, A. C. *et al.* (1980) Detection of hepatitis A virus in the faeces of patients with naturally acquired infection. *Journal of Infectious Diseases*, 141, 151–6.

Department of Health (1988) *Immunization Against Infectious Disease.* HMSO, London.

Eddleston, A. (1990) Modern vaccines. Hepatitis. *Lancet*, 335, 1142–5.

Gust, I. D. *et al.* (1988) Prevention and control of hepatitis A. In *Viral Hepatitis and Liver Disease* (Ed. by A. J. Zuckerman), pp. 77–80. Alan R. Liss, New York.

Hadler, S. C. *et al.* (1986) Hepatitis in day care centres. Epidemiology and prevention. *Review of Infectious Diseases*, 8, 548–57.

Lemon, S. M. (1985) Type A viral hepatitis. New developments in an old disease. *New England Journal of Medicine*, 313, 1059–67.

Lemon, S. M. *et al.* (1980) Specific immunoglobulin. A response to hepatitis A virus determined by solid phase radioimmunossay. *Infectious Immunology*, 28, 927–36.

Melnick, J.-L. (1982) Classification of hepatitis A virus as enterovirus type 72 and of hepatitis B virus as hepadnovirus type 1. *Intervirology*, 18, 105–6.

Noble, R. C. *et al.* (1984) Post-transfusion hepatitis A in a neonatal intensive care unit. *Journal of the American Medical Association*, 252, 2711–15.

Office of Population Censuses and Surveys (1989) *Mortality Statistics, Cause, 1979–1985. Series DH2 Nos. 6–12.* HMSO, London.

Ramsey, C. N. *et al.* (1989) Hepatitis A and frozen raspberries. *Lancet*, 1, 43–4.

Siegl, G. *et al.* (1984) Stability of hepatitis A virus. *Intervirology*, 22, 218–26.

Siegl, G. (1988) Virology of hepatitis. In *Viral Hepatitis and Liver Disease* (Ed. by A. J. Zuckerman), pp. 3–7. Alan R. Liss, New York.

Skinhof, P. *et al.* (1981) Travellers' hepatitis: origin and characteristics of cases in Copenhagen, 1976–1978. *Scandinavian Journal of Infectious Diseases*, 13, 1–4.

Sorbey, M. D. *et al.* (1988) Survival and persistence of hepatitis A virus in environmental samples. In *Viral Hepatitis and Liver Disease* (Ed. by A. J. Zuckerman), pp. 121–4. Alan R. Liss, New York.

Wright, R. *et al.* (1985) Acute viral hepatitis. In *Liver and Biliary Disease* (Ed. by R. Wright *et al.*), pp. 677–767. Baillière Tindall, London.

GUIDELINES: HEPATITIS A

Outpatient

Action	Rationale
1. It is not usually necessary to admit the individual to hospital.	Self-limiting disease.
2. Patient education is essential and must include advice on good personal hygiene and careful hand washing.	Limits the spread of the virus. Careful hand washing removes contamination from hands.
3. Separate soap, flannel and towel must be provided.	To minimize the risk of infection being spread via equipment used for hygiene purposes.
4. Meticulous cleaning of bath, wash basin and toilet with a non-abrasive cream cleaner and hot water.	To remove contamination.

Guidelines: Hepatitis A

Action	Rationale
5. Bath and wash basin must be allowed to dry after use.	Viruses will not survive on clean dry surfaces.
6. Soiled bed linen and underclothing should be washed.	To remove contamination.
7. Patient should refrain from intimate kissing and sexual intercourse while symptoms are present.	To prevent cross-infection.
8. Avoid contact with susceptible people, i.e. very young, old or those with debilitating illness.	To reduce the likelihood of infection.
9. Crockery and cutlery must be washed and rinsed in hot water.	Heat destroys the virus.

Inpatient

Action	Rationale
1. Whenever possible, the patient should have medical or surgical treatment postponed under he/she is symptom free.	Medical and surgical treatment will debilitate the patient further and recovery will be slower.
2. Ideally, the patient should be discharged.	Cross-infection is less likely to occur at home among fit, healthy people.
3. A single room with separate toilet should be made available for the patient, although barrier nursing is not necessary.	Although patients are no longer excreting the virus once they have become symptomatic, there are always exceptions.
4. Blood, secretions and excreta (particularly faeces) must be dispesed of immediately in a heat-disinfecting bedpan washer.	To prevent cross-infection.
5. Careful hand washing after patient contact.	To prevent cross-infection.

NON-A NON-B HEPATITIS

Definition

Due to major advances in knowledge concerning hepatitis, hepatitis A, B, C, D and E have been distinguished. There remains the theoretical possibility of hepatitis F and beyond being reported. Until this time, the hepatitis virus non-A non-B (NANB) is the term given to all clinical hepatitis that does not fall into the above-mentioned categories (Editorial, 1990).

REFERENCE MATERIAL

There are no accepted serological tests for NANB. Diagnosis is achieved by excluding infections associated with NANB. These include symptoms associated with hepatitis A, hepatitis B, cytomegalovirus, Epstein–Barr virus, toxic and drug-induced liver injury (including alcoholic liver disease), circulatory abnormalities, shock, sepsis, biliary tract disease and metabolic liver disease (Dienstag, 1983).

Non-A and non-B hepatitis has been shown to occur in patients who have received:

1. Blood transfusions (Dienstag *et al.*, 1977).
2. Clotting factors for coagulation disorders.
3. Haemodialysis.
4. Outbreaks of epidemics in tropical areas (Wong *et al.* 1980).
5. Sporadic cases with no identifiable cause.

Transmission appears to be similar to that of hepatitis B, i.e. principally through blood and blood products. There is an increased incidence in drug addicts due to the sharing of contaminated needles and syringes (Bamber & Thomas, 1983). There is evidence, however, of sporadic cases with no obvious contributory factors (Farrow *et al.*, 1981).

The incubation period is estimated at six to eight weeks followed by clinical features similar to hepatitis

B, although as a rule acute illness tends to be less severe.

Despite its relatively mild, often asymptomatic and anicteric presentation during acute infection, approximately 20% of people infected with NANB will develop cirrhosis and may die from hepatic-related death such as hepatocellular carcinoma (Lefkowitch *et al.*, 1987). Assessment of treatment protocols for chronic NANB hepatitis has been hindered by the lack of viral markers (Ellis, 1990).

Recombinant interferon is showing promising results in the management of NANB hepatitis (Hoofnagle *et al.*, 1986). Generally, treatment involves responding to the signs and symptoms as they occur. Liver transplantation is the treatment of the future for patients with liver failure (Dusheiko, 1990).

It is essential that safe techniques are used at all times when in contact with blood and body fluids. Human immunoglobulin should be given prophylactically following a previous history of needlestick injuries.

References and further reading

Bamber, M. & Thomas, H. C. (1983) Acute type A, B and non-A non-B hepatitis in a hospital population in London clinical and epidemiological features. *Gut*, 24, 561–4.

Dienstag, J. L. (1983) Non-A non-B hepatitis recognition epidemiology and clinical features. *Gastroenterology*, 85, 439–62.

Dienstag, J. L. *et al.* (1977) Non-A non-B post transfusion hepatitis. *Lancet*, 1, 560–2.

Dusheiko, G. M. (1990) Hepatocellular carcinoma associated with chronic viral hepatitis. Aetiology, diagnosis and treatment. *British Medical Bulletin*, 46(2), 492–511.

Editorial (1990) The A to F of viral hepatitis. *Lancet*, 336, 1158–60.

Ellis, M. E. (1990) Non-A non-B hepatitis; quandaries in serological testing and treatment. *Journal of Infection*, 21, 235–40.

Farrow, L. J. *et al.* (1981) Non-A non-B hepatitis in West London. *Lancet*, 1, 982–4.

Hoofnagle, J. H. *et al.* (1986) Treatment of chronic non-A non-B hepatitis with recombinant human alpha interferon. *New England Journal of Medicine*, 315, 1575–8.

Inarson, S. *et al.* (1973) Multiple attacks of hepatitis in drug addicts. *Journal of Infectious Disease*, 12, 165–9.

Lefkowitch, J. H. *et al.* (1987) Liver cell dysplasia and hepatocellular carcinoma in non-A non-B hepatitis. *Arch. Path. Lab. Med.*, III, 170–73.

Wong, O. C. *et al.* (1980) Epidemic and endemic hepatitis in India: evidence for a non-A non-B hepatitis virus aetiology. *Lancet*, 2, 876–8.

GUIDELINES: NON-A NON-B HEPATITIS

The procedure should be as for hepatitis B (see below).

HEPATITIS B

Definition

Hepatitis B is a serious infectious disease caused by the hepatitis B virus (HBV), which produces an inflammatory condition of the liver characterized by jaundice, hepatomegaly, anorexia, abdominal and gastric discomfort, abnormal liver function, clay-coloured stools and dark urine.

REFERENCE MATERIAL

HBV is a 42 nm double-shelled particle, termed initially Dane particles after their discoverer, which represents the intact infectious virion (Dane *et al.*, 1970). Contained within is a 27 nm inner core particle which contains the viral nucleic acid (Hart, 1990).

Epidemiology

HBV may be found in virtually all body secretions and excreta of patients with acute hepatitis B and carriers of the virus. Blood, semen and vaginal fluids are mainly implicated in the transmission of infection, which occurs by:

1. Sexual transmission, both vaginal and anal.
2. Accidental inoculation of blood following a sharps injury, for example, or by drug addicts sharing used needles and syringes (Shattock *et al.*, 1985).
3. Contamination of mucous membranes, eye, nose or mouth.
4. Contamination of non-intact skin.
5. Perinatally at or about the time of birth.
6. Blood transfusion. The frequency of post-transfusion HBV infection has decreased significantly since the exclusion of hepatitis B surface antigen (HBs Ag) seropositive blood donors in Britain (O'Grady *et al.*, 1988), but transfusions abroad are still implicated as sources of infection (Papaevangelou *et al.*, 1984).

This explains why high rates of infection occur in narcotic drug addicts, promiscuous homosexuals and prostitutes. A high prevalence of HBV infection has been reported in areas of the world where socio-economic conditions are poor, and in individuals requiring repeated transfusions of blood or blood products, in institutions for the mentally retarded and in some semi-closed institutions (Follett, 1987).

The number of male homosexuals and intravenous drug abusers developing HBV has decreased, suggesting the concerns about AIDS have influenced safe sex practices among promiscuous individuals and the use of clean needles and syringes among intravenous drug abusers (Polakoff, 1989).

The number of new cases of HBV infection in the United Kingdom is about 1000 reported cases a year. The prevalence of infection in the United Kingdom is not known, but has been suggested to be as low as one in 500 of the general adult population (Department of Health and Social Security, 1988).

Clinical response

HBV infection is clinically extremely variable, with the incubation period varying from four weeks to as long as six months. Approximately 60% of adult cases produce a subclinical infection with only mild symptoms such as fatigue and malaise, which often go unnoticed. Acute infection occurs in about 40% of adults, with spontaneous recovery usually within one month, although prolonged recovery can occur, accompanied by post-viral depression. Only about 5 to 10% of infected people become chronically infected and run the major risk of developing cirrhosis and liver cell cancer (Jacyna *et al.*, 1990). This accounts for less than 1% of deaths due to HBV infection.

The incidence of chronic infection is higher in those in whom there is a relative deficit of T cell function, the young, the aged, those with Down's syndrome, those with malignancy and those receiving immunosuppressive or cytotoxic therapy (Alexander, 1990).

Infectivity

The progress of HBV can be monitored by serological testing. Hepatitis B surface antigen (HBs Ag) is detected in the blood approximately three to four weeks after exposure, with antibodies to hepatitis B core (HBc) antigen (HBc Ag) developing about two weeks after HBs Ag occurs.

Anti-HBc will eventually be replaced by anti-HBs, which is the antibody to HBs Ag, and marks the end of infectivity and the development of immunity to subsequent HBV infection.

The antigen HBe Ag is an internal component of the core of HBs and is an indicator of infectivity; it will be replaced eventually by anti-HBe, which correlates with loss of viral replication (Tedder, 1980). HBV is capable of surviving for at least one week in the environment (Trevelyan, 1991).

Diagnosis

Diagnosis is confirmed by a virological blood test with regular monitoring of antigen status to evaluate progress.

Screening policy for hepatitis B surface antigen

Screening of the entire hospital patient population would be an effective way to identify hepatitis B infection, but this would be costly and time consuming in terms of the benefits derived. It is important, however, to screen patients before their admission to a transplant or renal unit (Tedder, 1980).

In general, the best compromise is to test those patients belonging to groups in which there is a high prevalence of hepatitis B. These include the following people:

1. All new admissions who currently live or were born in countries where there is a high prevalence of hepatitis B, such as the developing countries.
2. Drug addicts.
3. Promiscuous heterosexuals and male homosexuals (i.e. individuals who frequently change sexual partners, particularly those who are prostitutes or male homosexuals).
4. Mentally subnormal patients in institutions.
5. Multiple transfusion patients.
6. All patients acutely or recently jaundiced.

Transmission of HBV in the health care setting

Studies of health care workers who have sustained inoculation accidents involving HBs Ag-positive blood indicates the risk of transmission to be approximately 20%, where the potential source of infection is an HBe Ag-positive patient or carrier (Werner *et al.*, 1982). Most carriers can be classified as low risk where blood contains anti-HBe. The chance of transmission from these patients is approximately 0.1%; overall, the chance of transmission of infection is probably of the order of 5%.

There is no evidence of transmission of HBV by inhalation of droplets, neither has faecal–oral transmission been demonstrated (UK Health Department, 1990). However, one study estimated that up to 94% of HBV infections among health care workers may have been acquired without any inoculation injury (Callender *et al.*, 1982).

Immunization and vaccination

Passive immunization is achieved by hepatitis B

immunoglobulin which is prepared from pooled plasma with a high titre of hepatitis B surface antibody, which confers temporary passive immunity under certain defined conditions, as follows:

1. Administered preferably within 48 hours and no later than seven days following inoculated, ingested or splashed HBs Ag-infected blood. If the blood is HBe Ag positive, a second dose should be given 30 days later (Deinhardt *et al.*, 1985). The Medical Research Council report (1980) describes a low incidence (3%) of subsequent HBV infection when specific HBV immunoglobulin had been given *prophylactically*.
2. Vertical and perinatal spread is the commonest method of spread of HBV world-wide, and accounts, for example, for the very high carrier rate in South East Asia and parts of Africa, (Stevens *et al.*, 1975). Prophylaxis immunoglobulin given as soon as possible after birth reduces by 70% the risk of the baby developing the persistent carrier state. Protection is increased to about 90% when given with active immunization (Zuckerman, 1990).

Active immunization is by hepatitis B vaccine. There are two HBV vaccines available:

1. Human plasma derived from symptomless carriers which has been purified by a combination of ultracentrifugation and biochemical procedures.
2. A genetically engineered vaccine from yeast. Both vaccines are approximately 90% effective, although immune-deficient people respond less well than healthy people. Booster doses can be offered to non-respondents but even then response may be poor. Duration of immunity is not known but it is estimated at three to five years. A booster dose is required when antibody levels fall below 10 mlU/ml (Department of Health and Social Security, 1988).

Indications for immunization include:

1. Personnel including teaching, training and nursing staff directly involved over a period of time in patient care where there is a high prevalence of HBV or where blood and blood products are handled regularly.
2. Laboratory workers.
3. Dentists, dental personnel.
4. Medical and surgical personnel.
5. Health care personnel on secondment to work in areas of the world where there is a high prevalence of HBV.
6. Patients on entry to residential institutions for the mentally handicapped where there is a high prevalence of HBV.
7. Patients treated by maintenance haemodialysis.
8. Sexual contacts of patients with acute HBV or carriers of HBV.
9. Infants born to mothers who are HBs Ag positive.
10. Health care workers who receive an inoculation accident from a needle used on a patient who is HBs Ag positive, either used alone or in combination with hepatitis B immunoglobulin.

Prevention of hepatitis B in health care workers
Safe technique is essential when in contact with blood and body fluids regardless of whether the patient is hepatitis positive or negative. Dienstag and Ryan (1982) have shown that general ward nurses are at no greater risk of acquiring hepatitis B than the general population.

Avoiding inoculation accidents is an essential component of safe techniques. Resheathing needles accounts for 15 to 41% of all needlestick injuries and must not be undertaken (McCormick *et al.*, 1981). Resheathing commonly occurs as a result of trying to ensure safe transit to a disposal sharps bin (Edmond *et al.*, 1990), suggesting that sharps bins should be either attached to trolleys or placed at the bedside (Hart, 1990).

Employment of HBs Ag people
Tedder (1980) discusses the problem of carriers of HBs Ag who want to return to full-time employment, particularly those whose carrier state lasts for many years or possibly for the rest of their lives. Guidelines are available to those individuals working in the health service (Department of Health and Social Security, 1981).

Patient education
The Department of Health and Social Security (1984) recommends that individuals found to be HBs Ag carriers should be educated about the ways in which hepatitis B may spread and the precautions which can be taken to reduce the risk to others. It is stressed that unnecessary restrictions and precautions may cause distress and should be avoided.

Anti-viral therapy

Anti-viral therapy for chronic HBV infection can result in clearance of replicating virus from the liver and prevention of progression to cirrhosis in a substantial proportion of patients (Jacyna *et al.*, 1990). Treatments include:

1. Adenosine arabinoside monophosphate, an inhibitor of HBV replication, is of limited useful-

ness because of neuromuscular toxicity (Bassendine *et al.*, 1981).

2. Acyclovir alone is clinically ineffective but when coupled with interferon has proved useful in eliminating HBV from the liver (Schalm *et al.*, 1986).
3. Alpha-interferon offers up to a 50% chance of long-term inhibition of HBV replication in patients who acquire HBV in adulthood (Caselmann *et al.*, 1989), but is ineffective when HBV is acquired from birth. Trials of interferon and prednisolone are currently under evaluation for this presentation (Perillo *et al.*, 1988).

References and further reading

Alexander, G. J. M. (1990) Immunology of hepatitis B virus infection. *British Medical Bulletin*, 46(2), 354–67.

Bassendine, M. F. *et al.* (1981) Adenine arabinoside therapy in HBs Ag-positive chronic liver disease: a controlled study. *Gastroenterology*, 80, 1016–21.

Callender, M. E. *et al.* (1982) Hepatitis B virus infection in medical and health care personnel. *British Medical Journal*, 284, 423–6.

Caselmann, W. H. *et al.* (1989) Beta and gamma interferons in chronic active hepatitis B: a pilot trial of short-term combination therapy. *Gastroenterology*, 96, 449–55.

Dane, D. S. *et al.* (1970) Virus-like particle in serum of patients with Australian antigen-associated hepatitis. *Lancet*, 1, 695–8.

Deinhardt, F. D. *et al.* (1985) Immunization against hepatitis B. Report on a WHO meeting on viral hepatitis in Europe. *Journal of Medical Virology*, 17, 209–17.

Department of Health and Social Security (1981) *Hepatitis B and NHS Staff (CMO (81)11)*. HMSO, London.

Department of Health and Social Security (1984) *Guidance for Health Service Personnel Dealing with Patients Infected With Hepatitis B Virus, (CMO (84)11, CNO (84)7)*. HMSO, London.

Department of Health and Social Security (1988) *Immunization against infectious diseases*. London Department of Health and Social Security.

Dienstag, J. L. & Ryan, D. M. (1982) Occupational exposure to hepatitis B virus in hospital personnel; infection or immunization. *American Journal of Epidemiology*, 115, 22–9.

Edmond, M. *et al.* (1990) Effects of bedside needle disposal units on needle recapping frequency and needlestick injury. *Canadian Intravenous Nurses Association Journal*, 6(1), 10–11.

Follett, E. (1987) Psychiatric hospitals and the mentally handicapped – a special case. *Royal College of Nursing Wendsly Conference Report*, pp. 7–16.

Hart, S. (1990) Clinical hepatitis B; guidelines for infection control. *Nursing Standard*, 4(45), 24–7.

Jacyna, M. R. *et al.* (1990) Antiviral therapy – hepatitis B. *British Medical Bulletin*, 46(2), 368–82.

McCormick, R. D. *et al.* (1981) Epidemiology of needlestick injuries in hospital personnel. *American Journal of Medicine*, 70, 928–32.

Medical Research Council and Public Health Laboratory Service (1980) The incidence of hepatitis B infection after accidental exposure and anti-HBs immunoglobulin prophylaxis. *Lancet*, 1, 6–8.

O'Grady, J. G. *et al.* (1988) Early indicators of prognosis in acute liver failure and their applications of patients for orthotopic liver transplantation. *Gastroenterology*, 94, A578.

Papaevangelou, G. *et al.* (1984) Etiology of fulminant viral hepatitis in Greece. *Hepatology*, 4, 369–72.

Perillo, R. *et al.* (1988) Prednisalone withdrawal followed by recombinant alpha interferon in the treatment of chronic hepatitis B. *Annals of International Medicine*, 109, 95–100.

Polakoff, S. (1989) *Acute Viral Hepatitis B in Laboratory Reports 1985–1988. Communicable Disease Report 89/92 3–6*. HMSO, London.

Schalm, S. W. *et al.* (1986) Acyclovir enhances the antiviral effect of interferon in chronic hepatitis B. *Lancet*, 2, 358–60.

Shattock, A. C. *et al.* (1985) Increased severity and morbidity of acute hepatitis in drug abusers with simultaneously acquired hepatitis B and hepatitis D infection. *British Medical Journal*, 290, 1377–80.

Stevens, C. F. *et al.* (1975) Vertical transmission of hepatitis B antigen in Taiwan. *New England Journal of Medicine*, 292, 771–4.

Tedder, R. S. (1980) Hepatitis B in hospitals. *British Journal of Hospital Medicine*, 23(3), 266–79.

Trevelyan, J. (1991) Hepatitis B – who is at risk? *Nursing Times*, 87(5), 26–9.

UK Health Department (1990) *Guidance for Clinical Health Care Workers; Protection Against Infection With HIV and Hepatitis Viruses*. HMSO, London.

Werner, B. G. *et al.* (1982) Accidental hepatitis B; surface–antigen-positive inoculations. *Annals of International Medicine*, 97, 367–9.

Zuckerman, A. J. (1990) Immunization against hepatitis B. *British Medical Bulletin*, 46(2), 383–98.

GUIDELINES: HEPATITIS B

Procedure

Action	Rationale
1. The patient may be nursed on an open ward using all the patients' facilities as normal unless	If adequate precautions can be adhered to on an open ward, there is no need to isolate the patient.

Guidelines: Hepatitis B

Action	Rationale
there is a high risk of blood contamination of the ward environment.	
2. The patient must be assessed daily to establish accurately any sites of bleeding. Changes in the patient's condition should be recorded in the care plan.	Sites of bleeding must be identified in order that the appropriate precautions can be taken.
3. An individual container for disposing 'sharps' must be kept by the patient. When half full it must be sealed and put into a yellow clinical waste bag. The bag is then securely sealed, marked 'High Risk' and sent for incineration.	Contaminated 'sharps' are a potential inoculation hazard to others, so particular caution must be taken in handling them. Overloaded 'sharps' containers may cause needles to pierce the walls of the container or even protrude through the top.
4. A personal yellow clinical waste bag should be kept on a regular holder with a lid for the patient's disposable waste. When full this should be securely closed, marked 'High Risk' and sent for incineration.	To confine potentially contaminated material, e.g. bloodstained tissues.
5. The patient's personal hygiene equipment must be kept at the bedside.	To prevent accidental use of equipment by others.
6. Used linen that is not bloodstained is placed in the ward linen bags in the usual way.	Linen free from blood stains is not contaminated and may be dealt with in the normal manner.
7. During venepuncture or other procedures likely to cause bleeding, furniture, bedding and clothing in the adjacent area should be protected with polythene sheeting.	To prevent contamination of the environment with spilled blood.
8. All staff involved with the patient should cover any cuts or grazes on their hands with waterproof dressings.	Broken skin provides a portal of entry for the hepatitis virus in the event of contact with the patient's blood.
9. Routine daily cleaning procedures may be carried out as normal. As part of universal safe technique and practices, domestic staff will be aware of the potential hazard associated with any blood contamination.	Education is necessary so the domestic staff can understand the hazards involved or may over-react to the situation.

Accidental inoculation or spillage of blood

Action	Rationale
1. Any accident involving skin penetration or heavy contamination of abraded skin or mucosal surfaces of staff should be recorded on an accident form and this taken to bacteriology immediately. If the risk of infection from this incident is high, hepatitis B immunoglobulin must be given within 48 hours.	To protect personnel. To comply with legal and/or hospital requirements.
2. Blood spillage onto unbroken skin should be washed off with soap and running water. A	To remove the source of potential contamination.

Guidelines: Hepatitis B

Action	Rationale
scrubbing brush should not be used as this could break the skin. Complete an accident form, as above.	
3. Accidental inoculation sites should be cleaned under running water, encouraged to bleed freely and then sealed. Complete an accident form, as above.	Bleeding helps 'wash' the inoculated virus out of the system.
4. Blood spilled on hard surfaces must be wiped up immediately with paper towels and the area washed well with a solution such as a hypochlorite.	To prevent viral spread. Dried blood remains infectious for several days.
5. Linen stained with blood should be treated as infected linen and placed in a polythene bag with a red alginate stripe before being placed in a red linen bag.	Bloodstained linen is highly infectious. All linen in polythene bags with a red alginate stripe will be washed in a barrier wash at the laundry.

Precautions if bleeding is present

Action	Rationale
1. If serious bleeding is present in the mouth:	
(a) Use disposable crockery and cutlery and discard, with any uneaten food, into the disposal bag at the bedside.	
(b) Keep a personal food tray and water jug at the bedside.	
(c) Disposable mouth-care equipment, sputum pot and tissues should be kept at the bedside.	The sputum may be contaminated with blood from the mouth, therefore precautions must include avoiding contact with the patient's sputum.
2. If haematuria or melaena is present:	Blood present in the urine or faeces makes the patient's excreta a potential source of hepatitis B contamination.
(a) Wear plastic growns and gloves when handling excreta.	
(b) Keep a toilet and handbasin for the patient's sole use, if practicable.	
(c) If a toilet is not available for the paitent's sole use, bedpans or urinals must be used. These should be washed in the usual manner in the bedpan washer and dried carefully. They should then be placed in the appropriate bag, maked 'High Risk', stapled securely and sent to the central sterile supplies department for autoclaving. Disposable bedpans are dealt with in the routine manner.	
3. If the patient has a wound or a break in the skin:	To prevent the spread of the virus from dried or fresh blood. It should be remembered that dried blood can remain infectious for several days.
(a) Cover the area adequately so that there is no seepage.	
(b) Used dressings should be sealed securely in a plastic bag before being disposed of in the appropriate bag.	

(c) All tapes, lotions and creams are kept solely for the patient's use.
(d) The dressing trolley must be cleaned carefully before re-use.
(e) Non-disposable equipment should be emptied and wiped clean, placed in a central sterile supplies department bag, securely stapled shut, marked 'High Risk', and sent to the central sterile supplies department in a safe manner, to be resterilized.

Other hospital departments

Action	Rationale
1. All departments and staff involved with the patient must be made aware of the diagnosis.	To allow them to make their own precautionary arrangements.
2. All request cards to be labelled appropriately.	To alert the receiving department of the diagnosis.
3. All specimens to be labelled appropriately and correctly bagged. (For further information on specimen collection see Chapter 36).	To alert the receiving department of the diagnosis and prevent contamination of the environment.
4. If a patient who is bleeding has to be transported elsewhere, the porter involved should be provided with the following: (a) Disposable gloves and aprons. (b) Disposable trolley sheets or chair covers. (c) Cleaning equipment for the trolley or chair before use by the next patient.	To prevent the contamination of the porter or other patients.

Death of a patient with hepatitis B

Action	Rationale
1. There should be minimal handling of the body.	To reduce the risk of infecting the nursing staff.
2. Nurses should wear disposable plastic aprons and gloves when handling the body.	
3. The body should be totally enclosed in a plastic cadaver bag specifically designed for highly contagious patients.	To reduce the risk of infecting the nursing staff.
4. The mortuary staff should be informed of the diagnosis.	
5. If the relatives want to view the body, they must be supervised.	To prevent contamination.

Discharging the patient

Action	Rationale
1. The majority of precautions can cease.	Discharge normally implies that the risk of cross-infection is no longer present.
2. The patient should be advised not to share	To prevent cross-infection.

Guidelines: Hepatitis B

Action	**Rationale**
razors, toothbrushes or similar personal property likely to be contaminated by blood.	
3. If bleeding occurs, the patient clears up the blood himself/herself and disposes safely of such items as contaminated tissues by burning, flushing down the toilet or sealing in a polythene bag for routine council rubbish collection. If regular persistent blood-stained waste is generated, the health authority must be requested to make special collections.	To prevent cross-infection.
4. If emergency treatment or dental care is required, the patient must inform the health care worker of the fact that he/she has a recent history of hepatitis B infection.	To allow the correct precautions to be taken.

HEPATITIS C VIRUS (HCV)

Definition

Hepatitis C virus (HCV) causes hepatitis which can vary from mild to acute self-limiting infection to chronic infection which can cause chronic liver disease. Recent studies have shown a strong association between HCV and the development of hepatocellular carcinoma (Bruix *et al.*, 1989).

REFERENCE MATERIAL

HCV is an RNA virus and is the major cause of post-transfusion community acquired non-A non-B hepatitis (Bradley *et al.*, 1986). The time required for seroconversion to HCV antibody is extremely variable, with the mean interval from onset of hepatitis to seroconversion being around 15 weeks (range four to 32 weeks). Although approximately one third of seroconversion takes place relatively early in the acute phase of disease, most occur later on in the infection, occasionally up to one year later (Kuo *et al.*, 1989). Diagnosis therefore relies on assaying sequential serum samples for at least six to nine months. Some studies indicate that seroconversion occurs less frequently in acute self-limiting infection compared to chronic infection (Alter *et al.*, 1989).

Transmission in non-transfusion-related cases are as a result of multiple heterosexual partners or sexual or household contact with individuals with a history of hepatitis (Hess *et al.*, 1989). However, intrafamilial transmission has been suggested only on the basis of HCV antibody detection in a family of two patients (Kamitsukasa *et al.*, 1989), making it likely that HCV can be transmitted sexually and via close personal contact, but with low efficiency (Esteban *et al.*, 1989).

Male homosexuals who are HIV antibody positive have shown a significantly higher frequency of HCV antibody than male homosexuals who are negative for HIV antibody (Mortimer *et al.*, 1989). HCV has also been noted to be highly prevalent among haemophiliacs (Noel *et al.*, 1989) and drug addicts (Roggendorf *et al.*, 1989).

The clinical features of hepatitis C are indistinguishable from other viral hepatitis and the illness is likely to go unnoticed in many patients, because of the frequency of asymptomatic or mild disease.

Needle-stick transmission of hepatitis C has been reported once (Vaglia *et al.*, 1990) in a health care worker, suggesting the need for HBV precautions to be implemented for patients infected with HCV. The use of passive prophylaxis with standard immunoglobulins should be considered in post-needlestick inoculation accident management (Sanchez-Quijano *et al.*, 1988).

Recombinant interferon has shown promise in the management of hepatitis C, although much is still unkonwn about this recently discovered virus (Ellis, 1990).

The nursing care is the same as for hepatitis B (see Guidelines: Hepatitis B, above).

References and further reading

Alter, M. J. *et al.* (1989). Detection of antibody to hepatitis C virus in prospectively followed transfusion recipients with acute and chronic non-A non-B hepatitis. *New England Journal of Medicine*, 321, 1494–500.

Bradley, D. W. *et al.* (1986) Etiology and national history of post-transfusion and enterically transmitted non-A non-B hepatitis. *Semin. Liver. Dis.*, 6, 56–66.

Bruix, J. *et al.* (1989) Prevalence of antibodies to hepatitis C virus in Spanish patients with hepatocullular carcinoma and hepatitis cirrhosis. *Lancet*, 2, 1004–6.

Ellis, M. E. (1990) Non-A non-B hepatitis quandaries in serological testing and treatment. *Journal of Infection*, 21, 235–40.
Esteban, J. I. *et al.* (1989) Hepatitis C virus antibodies among risk groups in Spain. *Lancet*, 2, 294–7.
Hess, G. *et al.* (1989) Hepatitis C virus and sexual transmissions. *Lancet*, 2, 987.
Kamitsukasa, H. *et al.* (1989) Intrafamilial transmission of hepatitis C virus. *Lancet*, 1, 987.
Kuo, G. *et al.* (1989) An assay for circulating antibodies to a major etiologic virus of human non-A non-B hepatitis. *Science*, 244, 362–4.
Mortimer, P. P. *et al.* (1989) Hepatitis C virus antibody. *Lancet*, 2, 798.
Noel, L. *et al.* (1989) Antibodies to hepatitis C virus in haemophilia. *Lancet*, 2, 560.
Roggendorf, M. *et al.* (1989) Antibodies to hepatitis C virus. *Lancet*, 2, 324–5.
Sanchez-Quijano, P. *et al.* (1988) Prevention of post-transfusion non-A non-B hepatitis by non-specific immunoglobulin in heart surgery patients. *Lancet*, 1, 1245–9.
Vaglia, A. *et al.* (1990) Needlestick hepatits C virus sero-conversion in a surgeon. *Lancet*, 1, 1315–16.

DELTA HEPATITIS

Definition

Delta hepatitis D virus is a new human pathogen which is always associated with hepatitis B virus (HBV) and causes both fulminant hepatitis and the accelerated progression of pre-existing HBV hepatitis (Monjardino *et al.*, 1990).

REFERENCE MATERIAL

HDV has an RNA genome, is coated in hepatitis B virus surface antigen (HBs Ag), and is dependent in pre-existing or concomitant HBV infection for propagation (Rizzetto, 1983).

Superinfection is frequently associated with 70 to 90% deterioration of the underlying HBV hepatitis, while concomitant infection tends to result in clearance of both HDV and HBV (Rizzetto *et al.*, 1988).

Distribution tends to follow the prevalence of HBV although there are some regions of high HBV endemicity where HDV has not been found, for example the Far East and Southern Africa, suggesting an early HDV dissemination or the possible involvement of additional unknown factors in the spread of infection (Rizzetto *et al.*, 1985).

Diagnosis relies on detection of delta antigens in liver biopsy specimens or serum, or the presence of anti-HDV in serum (Rizzetto *et al.*, 1977).

Presentation, signs and symptoms, treatment and nursing care are as for hepatitis B-positive patients (see Hepatitis B, above).

References

Monjardino, J. P. *et al.* (1990) Delta hepatitis. The disease and the virus, *British Medical Bulletin*, 46, 2, 399–407.
Rizzetto, M. (1983) The delta agent. *Hepatology*, 3, 729–37.
Rizzetto, M. *et al.* (1977) Immunofluorescence detection of a new antigen–antibody system, *Gut*, 18, 997–1003.
Rizzetto, M. *et al.* (1985) Delta hepatitis – present status. *Journal of Hepatology*, 1, 187–93.
Rizzetto, M. *et al.* (1988) Hepatitis delta virus infection – clinical and epidemiological aspects. In *Viral Hepatitis and Liver Disease* (Ed. by A. Zuckerman), pp. 389–94. Alan R. Liss, New York.

HEPATITIS E

Definition

Hepatitis E is the term given for enterically transmitted non-A, non-B, hepatitis, producing a self-limiting disease resembling hepatitis A, although chronic liver disease and persistent viraemia has not been observed.

REFERENCE MATERIAL

Hepatitis E is an RNA virus, which has caused outbreaks of infection involving tens of thousands of cases in developing countries of the world, particularly India and the Indian subcontinent (Wong *et al.*, 1980) with sporadic cases and smaller outbreaks involving hundreds of cases in endemic areas. Cases in western countries are related directly to travel to endemic areas.

Young to middle-aged people are affected primarily, with fatalities of approximately 20% in infected pregnant women (Shrestha *et al.*, 1975).

Hepatitis E is transmitted by faecally contaminated drinking water or by contact with a faecally contaminated environment (Viswanathan, 1957), with a low secondary attack rate occurring among exposed household members. This indicates that person to person transmission is uncommon (Hillis *et al.*, 1973). The incubation period ranges between two and nine weeks, with an average of six weeks.

Diagnosis is made by virological and serological

studies of stool and serum specimens. Very little is known about the virus, but it is considered to be unstable, which may account for the difficulty in producing a clear profile of the virus (Bradley, 1990).

Barrier nursing is not essential for patients with hepatitis E infection. However, much is still to be learned about this virus and prudence dictates a very high standard of nursing care, with particular attention to hand washing after patient contact.

As pregnant women appear to be particularly vulnerable to this virus, it is advisable for infected patients to be provided with a single room and their own toilet facilities if pregnant women are also inpatients on the ward.

References and further reading

Bradley, D. W. (1990) Enterically transmitted non-A non-B hepatitis. *British Medical Bulletin*, 46(2), 442–61.

Hillis, A. *et al.* (1973) An epidemic of infectious hepatitis in the Kathmandu valley. *J. Nepal Med. Assoc.*, 11, 145–51.

Shrestha, S.-M. *et al.* (1975) Viral A hepatitis in pregnancy during Kathmandu epidemic. *J. Nepal Med. Assoc.*, 132, 58–69.

Viswanathan, R. (1957) Infectious hepatitis in Delhi 1955–56. A critical study epidemiology. *Ind. J. Med. Res.* (supplement), 45, 1–30.

Wong, D. C. *et al.* (1980) Epidemic and endemic hepatitis in India: evidence for a non-A non-B hepatitis etiology. *Lancet*, 2, 876–9.

THE HERPES VIRUSES

There are four human herpes viruses which cause infection. These are detected more frequently in immunocompromised people than in immunologically intact individuals (Kedzierski, 1991). The four types are:

1. Cytomegalovirus (CMV).
2. Epstein-Barr virus (EBV).
3. Herpes simplex virus (HSV).
4. Varicella zoster virus (VZV).

CYTOMEGALOVIRUS (CMV)

Definition

Cytomegalovirus produces a severe, often fatal, infection in immunocompromised people.

REFERENCE MATERIAL

CMV is distributed widely throughout the world, mostly among those from the lower socioeconomic groups (Krech *et al.*, 1981), and homosexual males are known to have high rates of CMV seropositivity (Drew *et al.*, 1981). Increased rates of CMV infection can be found in children in group day care and institutions (Pass *et al.*, 1984).

CMV causes asymptomatic infection in the vast majority of individuals. However, serious illness may occur in immunocompromised people and in a small percentage of babies after congenital infection.

CMV infection can be acquired by intrauterine, perinatal (Stagno *et al.*, 1986), intrafamilial and sexual transmission (Handfield *et al.*, 1985) as well as following blood transfusion (Hersman *et al.*, 1982) or transplantation (Peterson *et al.*, 1980).

During primary infection, the virus can be isolated from saliva, tears, urine, breastmilk, blood, semen and cervical secretions (Pomeroy *et al.*, 1987). After initial infection, the virus establishes a latent infection thought to be in the lymphocytes. The latent infection may subsequently reactivate with production of infectious virions. Reactivation is generally controlled by the host's cell-mediated immune response. Hence, CMV infection is common in immunocompromised people (Myers *et al.*, 1986).

Approximately 1% of all babies have congenital CMV infection, and 90 to 95% of these infants are asymptomatic. Some infants with asymptomatic symptoms at birth may have sensorineural hearing loss (Stagno *et al.*, 1977) and others may have mild learning disabilities (Hanshaw *et al.*, 1976). CMV-associated morbidity has been seen in both full-term (Kumar *et al.*, 1984) and pre-term infants (Yeager *et al.*, 1983).

Patients with malignancies, or those receiving chemotherapeutic therapies, transplantation of kidney (Chou, 1986), heart (Hofflin *et al.*, 1987) or bone marrow (Meyers *et al.*, 1988), have a high risk of contracting CMV disease, including CMV pneumonia, hepatitis, pancreatitis, colitis, mononucleosis, retinitis and encephalitis (Rubin, 1979). Diagnosis is obtained by cell culture methods of blood or urine (Stirk, 1987).

Treatment of active CMV infection using acyclovir, vidarabine, ganciclovir and alpha-interferon has been used as therapy in immunosuppressed patients. However, mortality remains high (Meyers *et al.*, 1988).

Prevention relies on decreasing the risk of virus acquisition and reactivation. Therefore, blood products used should either derive from CMV sero-negative donors or be free from viable leucocytes, which can be achieved by irradiating or washing the blood product (Rubin *et al.*, 1979).

Transmission of CMV within the hospital setting from seropositive patients to seronegative patients (Spector, 1983), and staff (Lipscomb *et al.*, 1984) has been seen but is thought to be low. Routine blood and body fluid precautions are essential to maintain these numbers at their low level.

Patients with CMV infection generally do not require barrier nursing as they feel ill and do not mix closely with other patients. Therefore, patient-to-patient transmission is unlikely.

References and further reading

Chou, S. (1986) Acquisition of donor strains of cytomegalovirus by renal transplant recipients. *New England Journal of Medicine*, 314, 1418–23.

Drew, W. L. *et al.* (1981) Prevalence of cytomegalovirus infection in homosexual men. *Journal of Infectious Diseases*, 143, 188.

Handfield, H. N. *et al.* (1985) Cytomegalovirus infection in sex partners – evidence for sexual transmission. *Journal of Infectious Diseases*, 151, 344–8.

Hanshaw, J. B. *et al.* (1976) School failure and deafness after silent congenital cytomegalovirus infection. *New England Journal of Medicine*, 295, 468–70.

Hersman, J. *et al.* (1982) The effect of granulocyte transfusion on the incidence of CMV infection after allogenic marrow transplantation. *Annals of International Medicine*, 96, 149–52.

Hofflin, J. M. *et al.* (1987) Infectious complications in heart transplant recipients receiving cyclosporine and corticesteroids. *Annals of International Medicine*, 106, 209–16.

Krech, U. *et al.* (1981) A collaborative study of cytomegalovirus antibodies in mothers and young children in 19 countries. *Bull. WHO*, 59, 605–10.

Kumar, M. L. *et al.* (1984) Postnatally acquired cytomegalovirus infection in infants of CMV-excreting mothers. *Journal of Paediatrics*, 104, 669.

Lipscomb, J. A. *et al.* (1984) Prevalence of cytomegalovirus antibody in nursing personnel. *Infection Control*, 5(11), 513–18.

Meyers, J. D. *et al.* (1986) Risk factors for cytomegalovirus infection after human marrow transplantation. *Journal of Infectious Diseases*, 153, 478–88.

Meyers, J. D. *et al.* (1988) Infection complicating bone marrow transplantation. In *Clinical Approach to Infection in the Compromised Host* (Ed. by R. H. Rubin & L. S. Young), pp. 525–55. Plenum Medical Books, New York and London.

Pass, R. F. *et al.* (1984) Increased frequency of cytomegalovirus infection in children in group day care. *Paediatrics*, 74, 121–6.

Peterson, P. K. *et al.* (1980) Cytomegalovirus disease in renal allogrant recipients: a prospective study of the clinical features, risk factors and impact on renal transplantation medicine. *Medicine*, 59, 283–300.

Pomeroy, C. *et al.* (1987) Cytomegalovirus epidemiology and infection control. *American Journal of Infection Control*, 15, 107–19.

Rubin, R. H. *et al.* (1979) Summary of workshop on cytomegalovirus infection during organ transplantation. *Journal of Infectious Diseases*, 139, 728–34.

Spector, S. A. (1983) Transmission of cytomegalovirus among infants in hospital documented by restriction-endonuclease-digestion analyses. *Lancet*, 2, 378–81.

Stagno, S. *et al.* (1977) Auditory and visual defects resulting from symptomatic and subclinical congenital cytomegalovirus and toxoplasma infections. *Paediatrics*, 59, 669–78.

Stagno, S. *et al.* (1986) Primary cytomegalovirus infection in pregnancy. *Journal of the American Medical Association*, 256, 1904–8.

Stirk, P. R. *et al.* (1987) The use of monoclonal antibodies for the diagnosis of cytomegalovirus infection by the detection of early antigen fluorescent foci (DEAFFO in cell culture). *Journal of Medical Virology*, 21, 329–37.

Yeager, A. S. *et al.* (1983) Sequelae of maternally derived cytomegalovirus infection in premature infants. *Journal of Paediatrics*, 102, 918.

EPSTEIN-BARR VIRUS

Definition

Epstein-Barr virus (EBV) is a herpes virus which causes infectious mononucleosis.

REFERENCE MATERIAL

EBV primary infection in childhood is usually asymptomatic, although occasional cases have been seen to resemble chronic active hepatitis (Lloyd-Still *et al.*, 1986). In adolescence, approximately 50% of cases are accompanied by fever, malaise, pharyngitis and lymphadenopathy (Hoagland, 1960). In people over 40 years of age, infection can be accompanied by abdominal pain and fever (Horowitz *et al.*, 1983).

EBV can persist in the host and reactivate at a later time, particularly during immunosuppression (Crawford *et al.*, 1981), commonly following transplantation (Strauch *et al.*, 1974) or in people with cancer or leukaemia (Lange *et al.*, 1978). Initially, EBV replication appears to take place in epithelial cells of the nasopharynx (Sixbey, 1984) followed by infection of B lymphocytes. The incubation period between exposure and clinical manifestation in normal people varies from 30 to 50 days.

EBV is found in the saliva (Sixbey *et al.*, 1984) and on the cervix (Sixbey *et al.*, 1986), and can be transmitted by kissing and sexual contact, and rarely by blood transfusion (McMonigal *et al.*, 1983). Diagnosis relies on serological methods that detect the presence of IgG and IgM antibodies to EBV viral capsid antigen (Wielaard *et al.*, 1988).

EBV infection in healthy people is generally self-limiting with spontaneous recovery. Interferon, acyclovir and dihydroxy-2-propoxy-methyl guanine (DHPG) treatment for immunosuppressed patients is being investigated (Hirsch, 1988).

Barrier nursing is not necessary for EBV infection, but the patient should avoid kissing and sexual contact while symptoms persist. The patient's personal hygiene articles must not be shared.

References and further reading

Crawford, D. H. *et al.* (1981) Long-term T cell-mediated immunity to Epstein-Barr virus in renal allograft recipients receiving cyclosporin A. *Lancet*, 1, 10–13.

Hirsch, M. S. (1988) Herpes group virus infections in the compromised host. In *Clinical Approach to Infection in the Compromised Host* (Ed. by R. H. Rubin & L. S. Young), pp. 347–66. Plenum Medical Books, New York and London.

Hoagland, R. J. (1960) The clinical manifestation of infectious mononucleosis. A report of 200 cases. *American Journal of Medical Science*, 240, 55–63.

Horowitz, C. A. *et al.* (1983) Infectious mononucleosis in older patients aged 40 to 72 years. Report of 27 cases including 3 without hyeterophile antibody response. *Medicine*, 62, 256–62.

Lange, B. *et al.* (1978) Longitudinal study of Epstein-Barr virus antibody titre and excretion in paediatric patients with Hodgkin's disease. *International Journal of Cancer*, 22, 521–7.

Lloyd-Still, J. D. *et al.* (1986) The spectrum of Epstein-Barr virus hepatitis in children. *Paediatr. Pathol.*, 5, 337–51.

McMonigal, K. *et al.* (1983) Post-perfusion syndrome due to Epstein-Barr virus. Report of 2 cases and review of the literature. *Transfusion*, 23, 331–5.

Sixbey, J. W. *et al.* (1984) Epstein-Barr virus replication in oropharyngeal epithelial cells. *New England Journal of Medicine*, 310, 1225–30.

Sixbey, J. W. *et al.* (1986) A second site for Epstein-Barr virus shedding the uterine cervix. *Lancet*, 2, 1122–4.

Strauch, J. W. *et al.* (1974) Oropharyngeal excretion of Epstein-Barr virus by renal transplant recipient and other patients treated with immunosuppressive drugs. *Lancet*, 1, 234–7.

Wielaard, F. *et al.* (1988) Development of an antibody-capture IgM enzyme-linked immunosorbent assay for diagnosis of acute Epstein-Barr virus infection. *J. Virol. Meth.*, 21, 105–15.

HERPES SIMPLEX VIRUS (HSV)

Definition

HSV causes infections which have an affinity for the skin and nervous system. It has two presentations.

1. HSV 1 (oral herpes) infections tend to occur in the facial areas.
2. HSV 2 (herpes genitalis) infections are usually limited to the genital region (Corey *et al.*, 1983b).

REFERENCE MATERIAL

Herpes Simplex infections are worldwide in distribution. HSV 1 generally infects children between the ages of two and ten years, and is transmitted primarily by contact with oral secretions. It is chiefly responsible for perioral, ocular and encephalitic infections in adults. HSV 2 is spread by genital contact and generally infects sexually active people. It is the major cause of penile vesicular lesions, cervicovaginitis and proctitis, as well as neonatal disseminated disease (Hirsch, 1988).

Recurrent infection occurs frequently, generally as a result of reactivation of virus, since HSV may become latent within the sensory nerve ganglia, although exogenous reinfection can occur. Recurrences tend to be milder than primary infection.

Immune-deficient people with breaks in natural mucocutaneous barriers are more susceptible to more serious forms of HSV infection. These individuals include organ transplant recipients (Anuras *et al.*, 1976), those with malignancy who are receiving cytotoxic therapy (Faden *et al.*, 1977), the severely malnourished (Becker *et al.*, 1968) and those with congenital or acquired cellular immune defects (Seigal *et al.*, 1981), burns (Foley *et al.*, 1970) or skin disorders (Wheeler *et al.*, 1966).

The HSV infection in immunosuppressed patients includes: chronic, large, ulcerated lesions (Herpes phagenda), which may persist from months to years; eczema herpeticum, a severe cutaneous infection of HSV; diffuse interstitial pneumonitis (Ramsey *et al.*, 1982); and oesophagitis (Nash *et al.*, 1974). Involvement of the liver, adrenals, gastrointestinal tract and central nervous system can also occur.

Transmission of HSV is by direct contact, particularly with oral and/or genital secretions. Prevention involves avoiding contact with infected lesions, and therefore gloves are essential for all health care professionals who come into direct contact with lesions.

The use of condoms to prevent genital spread during sexual intercourse is advisable (Corey *et al.*, 1983a).

Caesarean section for mothers with clinically apparent cervical or genital infection will prevent the baby from acquiring the infection, provided the mother implements good infection control practices when handling the baby (Corey *et al.*, 1983b).

Diagnosis

HSV infections are easily recognizable. Confirmation can be obtained by cytological and histological techniques on vesicle fluids obtained early after the onset of lesions.

Therapy

The majority of infections resolve spontaneously, although acyclovir is the drug of choice for both prophylaxis (Wade, 1984) and therapy (Wade *et al.*, 1982). Intravenous, oral or topical application has been seen to be effective in severe infections.

Nursing care

Barrier nursing is essential for extensive herpes virus infection.

References and further reading

Anuras, S. *et al.* (1976) Fulminant herpes simplex hepatitis in an adult. Report of a case in a renal transplant recipient. *Gastroenterology*, 70, 425–8.

Becker, W. B. *et al.* (1968) Disseminated herpes simplex virus infection, its pathogenesis based on virological and pathological studies in 33 cases. *American Journal of Diseases of Childhood*, 115, 1–8.

Corey, L. *et al.* (1983a) Genital herpes simplex virus infection. Clinical manifestations, course and complications. *Annals of Internal Medicine*, 98, 958–72.

Corey, I. *et al.* (1983b) Genital herpes simplex virus infection. Current concepts in diagnosis, therapy and prevention. *Annals of Internal Medicine*, 98, 973–83.

Faden, H. S. *et al.* (1977) Disseminated herpes virus hominus infection in a child with acute leukaemia. *Journal of Paediatrics*, 90, 951–3.

Foley, F. D. *et al.* (1970) Herpes virus infection in burns patient. *New England Journal of Medicine*, 282, 652–6.

Hirsch, M. S. (1988) Herpes group virus infection in the compromised host. In *Clinical Approach to Infection in the Compromised Host* (Ed. by R. H. Rubin & L. S. Young), pp. 347–66. Plenum Medical Books, New York and London.

Kedzierski, M. (1991) Diseases of the herpes virus. *Nursing Standard*, 5(31), 28–32.

Nash, G. *et al.* (1974) Herpetic oesophagitis – a common cause of oesophagal ulceration. *Human Pathology*, 5, 339–45.

Ramsey, P. G. *et al.* (1982) Herpes simplex virus pneumonia; clinical virologic and pathologic features in 20 patients. *Annals of Internal Medicine*, 97, 813–20.

Seigal, E. P. *et al.* (1981) Severe acquired immunodeficiency in male homosexuals, manifested by chronic perianal ulcerative herpes simplex lesions. *New England Journal of Medicine*, 305, 1439–44.

Wade, J. C. *et al.* (1982) Intravenous acyclovir to treat mucocutaneous *Herpes simplex* virus infection after bone marrow transplantation. A double-blind trial. *Annals of Internal Medicine*, 96(3), 265–9.

Wade, J. C. *et al.* (1984) Oral acyclovir for prevention of *Herpes simplex* virus reactivation after marrow transplantation. *Annals of Internal Medicine*, 100(6), 823–8.

Wheeler, C. E. *et al.* (1966) Eczema herpeticum: primary and recurrent. *Archives of Dermatology*, 93, 162–73.

VARICELLA ZOSTER VIRUS (VZV)

Definition

Initial infection with VZV causes varicella (chicken pox). Following clinical recovery, the virus persists in the latent form in the dorsal root ganglia of nerves; reactivation of the latent VZV causes zoster (shingles).

REFERENCE MATERIAL

The varicella incubation period is 11 to 21 days. The infected individual is infectious for two days before the rash appears and remains so until all the lesions have healed. Initial entry of VZV is unclear, although the respiratory tract, skin or conjunctiva are likely possibilities. Following local replication, the virus will be carried by the bloodstream to other sites. Recovery from varicella in a fit person is usually spontaneous and without sequelae.

In the immunocompromised child, a much more serious presentation occurs. Visceral dissemination and death is not uncommon in children with cancer. When peripheral blood lymphocyte counts are below 500/mm^3, the mortality rate is 7% to 30% (Fieldman *et al.*, 1975). Varicella may be especially severe in transplant recipients, particularly among children who have received bone marrow grafts. The mortality rate for untreated varicella is 35% (Atkinson *et al.*, 1979). Visceral involvement involving the lung usually occurs three to seven days after the onset of skin lesions. Neurological complications occur less commonly and generally present four to eight days after the onset of rash, and often indicate a poor prognosis. The liver is less commonly involved (Hirsch, 1988).

The diagnosis of chicken pox can usually be made from the characteristic pattern of vesicles. Treatment of varicella is normally only necessary for immunosuppressed patients, and involves the use of antiviral agents such as acyclovir, which reduces time of new lesion formation, fever and visceral complications.

Immunosuppressed children without a history of varicella and, in some cases, children with a history of varicella, but who are currently on high-dose chemotherapy, should receive varicella-zoster immunoglobulin (VZIg) when exposed to chicken pox or zoster. To be effective, VZIg must be administered as soon after exposure as possible (Wisnes, 1978), which will give protection for approximately four weeks. Second cases of chicken pox in healthy people are extremely rare. However, among the immunosuppressed, second cases have been seen to occur and are often referred to as atypical disseminated zoster or varicelliform zoster. They do not have dermatomal distribution (Dolin *et al.*, 1978).

Every year, about four in every 1000 people suffer an attack of shingles (Milbourn, 1989). It is still unclear what factors contribute to virus activation, which is more common in those aged over 50 years and during periods of immunosuppression.

Cancer patients are particularly susceptible to zoster, which is more common during advance stage disease and develops more frequently at areas of regionalized tumour and/or localized radiotherapy. Most cases of zoster occur within the first year after diagnosis of cancer.

Patients with AIDS or AIDS-related complex (ARC) appear to be at increased risk of zoster; the incidence of zoster in an HIV antibody-positive person appears to be a sign for the development of AIDS (Melbye *et al.*, 1987).

People who have not been infected with VZV can acquire varicella from individuals infected with varicella or zoster. However, there is little evidence to support the view that in healthy people, zoster can be contracted by exposure to zoster or varicella (Dolin *et al.*, 1978).

Neuralgia often proclaims the onset of zoster and can occur several days before the vesicles appear. The vesicles generally correspond in distribution to one or more sensory nerves. Dissemination of zoster in an immunosuppressed patient generally occurs six to ten days after the onset of localized lesions and is usually limited to cutaneous involvement, with occasional involvement of the central nervous system (CNS), lung, heart or gastrointestinal tract (Jemsek *et al.*, 1983).

The diagnosis of zoster can be made from the typical picture and distribution of the lesions. Confirmation can be obtained from virology culture of vesicle fluid. Treatment involves the use of antiviral agents such as acyclovir, which should begin within 72 hours of lesion formation. Herpetic neuralgia and healing time will be shortened, although scarring may result in severe zoster (Balfour *et al.*, 1983).

Nursing care

Only staff who have had varicella should have contact with patients with varicella or zoster. Barrier nursing is essential (see beginning of Chapter 4).

References and further reading

Atkinson, M. K. *et al.* (1979) Analysis of late infections in 89 long-term survivors of bone marrow transplantation. *Blood*, 53, 720–31.

Balfour, H. H. *et al.* (1983) Acyclovir halts progression of herpes zoster in immune-commpromised patients. *New England Journal of Medicine*, 308, 1448–53.

Dolin, R. *et al.* (1978) Herpes zoster varicella infections in immunosuppressed patients. *Annals of Internal Medicine*, 89, 375–88.

Fieldman, S. *et al.* (1975) Varicella in children with cancer. *Paediatrics*, 56, 388–97.

Hirsch, M. S. (1988) Herpes group virus infection in the compromised host. *Clinical Approach to Infection in the Compromised Host* (Ed. by R. H. Rubin & L. S. Young), pp. 347–66. Plenum Medical Books, New York and London.

Jemsek, J. *et al.* (1983) Herpes zoster-associated encephalitis in immunosuppressed patients. *Annals of Internal Medicine*, 89, 375–88.

Melbye, M. *et al.* (1987) Risk of AIDS after herpes zoster. *Lancet*, 1, 728–31.

Milbourn, S. (1989) Caring for patients with herpes zoster ophthalmicus. *The Professional Nurse*, January, 186–7.

Wisnes, R. (1978) Efficacy of zoster immunoglobulin in prophylaxis of varicella in high-rish patients. *Acta Paediatr. Scand.*, 67, 77–82.

LEGIONNAIRE'S DISEASE

Definition

Legionnaire's disease is an acute bacterial pneumonia caused by infection with *Legionella pneumophilia*.

REFERENCE MATERIAL

In the summer of 1976 an outbreak of pneumonia occurred among about 5000 people who had attended an American Legion convention in Philadelphia. There were 182 cases and 29 deaths. The epidemic aroused enormous public interest. Epidemiological investigations showed that the focus was the lobby of a famous hotel, but the cause remained unidentified for months until a small Gram-negative organism was found, which subsequently became known as *Legionella pneumophilia* (Fraser *et al.*, 1977).

Since 1976 at least 34 additional species, comprising 53 different serogroups, have been isolated from a range of environmental sites including lakes, rivers, soils and man-made water systems such as cooling towers and water distribution systems (Cooper, 1991). The latter two sites have been responsible for numerous outbreaks of Legionnaire's disease, which have occurred mainly during June to October (Center for Disease Control, 1978).

The pattern of infection is unique. The outbreaks are site specific and associated with factors which predispose to infection, including water systems contaminated with the organism. *Legionella pneumophilia* is a thermophile which flourishes at temperatures from 25 to 42°C and can survive a range of temperatures from 5 to 58°C. The most critical temperature is 36°C. Every effort should be made to avoid stagnant water conditions and to store and supply water outside this critical temperature (Harper, 1986).

Legionella is ubiquitous in surface water. It multiplies in warm water, particularly in 'dead ends' and loops in plumbing systems where sludge has formed. This predisposes to proliferation of the organism, providing ideal conditions and the opportunity for the organism to grow and cause infection.

The major route of infection is by aerosal dispersion and inhalation of the bacteria from, for example, shower heads (Alderman, 1988), or more commonly by air conditioning systems where the organism may multiply in the water of cooling towers. Although this water does not come into direct contact with the air, a great deal is lost by evaporation, when droplets containing *Legionella* may be drawn into the air intakes of the building or fall on people passing by.

Virulence is coupled to a susceptible host. The disease tends to affect males, by a factor of 2 or 3 to 1. Those who smoke or consume excess alcohol, people who are already immunocompromised and the elderly are all predisposed to infection (Stout, 1987).

The incubation period is about two to ten days following first exposure. The signs and symptoms include malaise, general aches and headache, diarrhoea and vomiting, followed by high temperature, cough rigors and respiratory distress. Some patients do not develop pneumonia but progress to profound septicaemia with confusion, symptoms of diplopia and mental confusion (Potterton, 1985).

Diagnosis relies on laboratory diagnosis by:

1. Isolation of the causative organism.
2. Demonstration of the presence of the organism, its antigen or its products in the patient's body fluids or tissues (Harrison, 1985).
3. Demonstration of specific antibodies directed against the organism, its antigens or its products (Harrison, 1985).

Coupled to the clinical picture and chest X-ray findings, treatment includes the antibiotic erythromycin (Center for Disease Control, 1978) with supportive therapy for complications as they arise, which may include pulmonary failure, shock and acute renal failure. Person-to-person spread has never been demonstrated and therefore barrier nursing is not required. However, careful disposal of sputum and encouraging patients to cover their mouth and nose when coughing are necessary precautions.

Prevention relies on regular inspection and maintenance of the water system, including planning, installation and commissioning (Finch, 1988).

References and further reading

Alderman, C. (1988) The cooler culprits. *Nursing Standard*, 2(33), 22.

Center for Disease Control (CDC) (1978) Legionnaire's disease, diagnosis and management. *Annals of Internal Medicine*, 88, 363–5.

Cooper, J. (1991) Positive discrimination. *Laboratory Practice*, 40(1), 16–17.

Finch, R. (1988) Minimizing the risk of Legionnaire's disease. *British Medical Journal*, 296, 1343–5.

Fraser, D. W. *et al.* (1977) Legionnaire's disease: description of an epidemic of pneumonia. *New England Journal of Medicine*, 297, 1189–97.

Harper, D. (1986) Legionnaire's disease: prevention better than cure. *Health and Safety at Work*, March, 41–6.

Harrison, T. G. (1985) A nasty family from Philadelphia. *Medical Laboratory World*, September, 19–23.

Potterton, D. (1985) Mystery of the organism. *Nursing Times*, 82(22), 20–21.

Stout, J. E. (1987) Legionnaire's disease acquired within the homes of two patients. *Journal of the American Medical Association*, 257(9), 1215–17.

LISTERIOSIS

Definition

Listeriosis is an infectious disease caused by *Listeria monocytogenes*. Listeria is a Gram-positive bacterium with widespread distribution in the environment, including soil, dust and vegetation (Watkins *et al.*, 1981). It inhabits the gastrointestinal tract of animals and humans, who remain symptomless (Botsen-Moller, 1972).

REFERENCE MATERIAL

The genus Listeria includes many types which are non-pathogenic to man. *Listeria monocytogenes* is recognized as being the cause of listeriosis in man (Lamont *et al.*, 1988).

Growth of this organism is optimal at 37°C but it will survive and multiply at a range of 26°C to 42°C, and is not easily inactivated by environmental influences such as freezing, thawing and strong sunlight (Gray, 1963). Instances of human infection are increasing (McLauchlin, 1988), particularly among immunocompromised people.

The fetus and the newborn are especially prone to infection due to the immaturity of their immune systems. In the United Kingdom, there is about one incidence in every 9700 of perinatal listeriosis births (McLauchlin, 1987). Maternal symptoms are often absent, and neonatal listeriosis presents as meningitis or occasionally as septicaemia (Gill, 1988). Abortion and stillbirths due to listeriosis have been reported (MacNaughton, 1962). Infection in immunocompromised adults varies from a mild, chill-like illness to bacteraemia, septicaemia and meningitis.

Treatment

Ampicillin is usually regarded as the drug of choice (Trautman *et al.*, 1985), often in combination with gentamicin (Azimi *et al.*, 1979). However, even with prompt antibiotic therapy, mortality may be as high as 30% in patients with other serious underlying conditions.

The mode of transmission can be via sexual contact, following localization in both male and female genital tracts (Gray, 1960). However, contaminated food is becoming increasingly important as a vehicle of spread. There are increasing reports of listeria found in raw meat, fruit and vegetables which predispose to contamination of, for example, coleslaw. An outbreak involving coleslaw prepared from contaminated cabbage involved seven adults and 34 newborn babies in Canada (Schlech *et al.*, 1983).

Prevention entails scrupulous preparation of cooked food for immunocompromised people and the avoidance of uncooked foods. Person-to-person transmission during normal contact is unlikely. However, careful disposal of blood fluids and thorough handwashing after contact with the patient is essential.

References and further reading

Azimi, P. H. *et al.* (1979) *Listeria monocytogenes.* Synergistic effects of ampicillin and gentamicin. *American Journal of Clinical Pathology*, 72, 974–7.

Botsen-Moller, J. (1972) Human listeriosis. Diagnostic epidemiological and clinical studies. *Acta. Pathol. Microbiol. Scand.* (suppl.), 229, 1–57.

Gill, P. (1988) Is listeriosis often a food-borne illness? *Journal of Infection*, 17, 1–5.

Gray, M. L. (1960) Genital listeriosis as a cause of repeated abortions. *Lancet*, 2, 315–17.

Gray, M. L. (1963) Epidemiological aspects of listeriosis. *American Journal of Public Health*, 53, 554–63.

Lamont, R. J. *et al.* (1988) *Listeria monocytogenes* and its role in human infection. *Journal of Infection*, 17, 7–28.

MacNaughton, M. C. (1962) *Listeria monocytogenes* in abortion. *Lancet*, 11, 484.

McLauchlin, J. (1987) *Listeria monocytogenes*: recent advances in the taxonomy and epidemiology of listeriosis in humans. *J. Appt. Bacteriol.*, 63, 1–11.

McLauchlin, J. (1988) Listeriosis and food-borne transmission. *Lancet*, 1, 177–8.

Schlech, W. F. *et al.* (1983) Epidemic listeriosis. Evidence of a transmission by food. *New England Journal of Medicine*, 308, 203–6.

Trautman, M. *et al.* (1985) Listeria meningitis: report of 10 cases and review of current therapeutic recommendations. *Journal of Infection*, 10, 107–14.

Watkins, J. *et al.* (1981) Isolation and enumeration of *Listeria monocytogenes* from sewage, sewage study and river water. *J. Appt. Bacteriol.*, 5, 1–9.

PNEUMOCYSTOSIS

Definition

Pneumocystosis is an infection caused by the organism *Pneumocystis carinii.*

REFERENCE MATERIAL

Pneumocystis carinii was first discovered in 1909 and was associated with outbreaks of pneumonia in people subjected to malnutrition and overcrowding (Radman, 1973). The organism has been recognized as being an important cause of pneumonia in the immunocompromised host for over 20 years. Three types of patients have been particularly affected:

1. Patients of all ages receiving immunosuppressive agents for the treatment of cancer and during organ transplantation (Walzer *et al.*, 1973).
2. Children and infants with primary immunodeficiency disorders, particularly severe combined immunodeficiency (SCID) (Gajdusek, 1957).
3. Patients with acquired immune deficiency syndrome (AIDS), particularly in patients whose blood CD_4 T lymphocytes are below 200/mm^3 of

blood (Phair *et al.*, 1990). (CD_4 means an antigenic marker of helper T cells.)

Most epidemiological studies have focused on clusters of cases within hospitals, orphanages or private clinics. All have a common denominator of overcrowding, protein calorie malnutrition, prematurity or immunosuppressive disease, predisposing to *Pneumocystis carinii* pneumonia. These studies give the impression of outbreaks of infection, when no spread has actually occurred; rather the disease probably occurred from reactivation of latent infection triggered by immunosuppression (Dutz, 1970).

Watanable and colleagues (1965) reported a cluster of infection in a family of three. A healthy woman developed fatal *Pneumocystis carinii* pneumonia several days before her husband who had acute lymphatic leukaemia, and who also died. Their seven-year-old daughter had had a typical respiratory disease two months before her parents' illness. Although she recovered, she may have transmitted the disease to her non-immune parents, suggesting that person-to-person or airborne transmission is possible among immunologically naive subjects.

Pneumocystis carinii infections associated with deprivation in children are reported to be slow and insidious in onset, with initial non-specific signs of restlessness, lethargy, poor feeding over a period of weeks, resulting in tachypnoea, severe dyspnoea, use of accessory muscles for breathing, marked cyanosis and exhausting non-productive cough (Perera *et al.*, 1970).

Children and adults with underlying disease such as neoplasm often experience an abrupt onset of illness, with high fever, tachypnoea and cough, which can progress to a fatal outcome even with treatment (Walzer, 1970).

Until recently, diagnosis has relied upon the demonstration of organisms in either open lung or transbronchial biopsy, although considerable controversy surrounds these invasive procedures because of the potential complications of haemorrhage and pneumothorax. Fibreoptic bronchoscopy or bronchial washings are now favoured because of the increase of *Pneumocystis carinii* infection among AIDS patients, where large numbers of organisms are generally present in bronchial secretions, sputum and transtrachial aspirations. Unfortunately, if such specimens yield negative results, open lung biopsy may have to be undertaken expeditiously, before the patient deteriorates further. Survival is related directly to the aggressiveness with which the diagnosis is pursued in the early stages of disease and with the early institution of appropriate therapy (Young, 1984).

Treatment is by pentamidine intramuscularly, daily for 14 days; although longer therapy may be necessary for more recalcitrant infections. Major side-effects can be experienced (Pearson *et al.*, 1985).

Other treatment includes the use of trimethoprim sulphamethoxazole given orally or intravenously. However, the cumulative toxicity from both individual components has made this drug the most toxic of all anti-pneumocystis treatments (Wharton *et al.*, 1986). Oral trimethoprim sulphamethoxazole is generally given prophylactically to severely immunocompromised patients when discharged from hospital. It is continued for the duration of their immunosuppression, and discontinued on improvement of immunological function and/or a decrease in therapeutic immunosuppression.

Aerosolized pentamidine prophylaxis has significantly improved prognosis for patients with AIDS (Miller *et al.*, 1989). However, a real concern has emerged that the use of aerosolized pentamidine has predisposed patients to disseminated disease, which has been reported with increased frequency; for example, *Pneumocystis carinii* thyroiditis (Galland, 1988), otitis media, mastoiditis (Gherman, 1988), choroidopathy (Friedberg *et al.*, 1990), gastrointestinal (Carter *et al.*, 1988), hepatic (Poblete *et al.*, 1989) and splenic disease (Pilon *et al.*, 1987). This indicates that the systemic absorption of aerosolized pentamidine is minimal, allowing *Pneumocystis carinii* to infect extrapulmonary sites. Therefore, patients receiving aerosolized prophylaxis must be monitored carefully for signs of disseminated disease.

Hospitalized patients who develop *Pneumocystis carinii* pneumonia may well be cared for in areas where there are large concentrations of immunosuppressed patients. Due to the reports of clustering of this disease and the difficulty of distinguishing whether this represents person-to-person spread, patients with a productive cough should be placed in a single room until the cough improves. Precautions other than careful hand washing following patient contact are unnecessary.

References and further reading

Carter, T.-R. *et al.* (1988) *Pneumocystis carinii* infection of the small intestine in a patient with acquired immunodeficiency syndrome. *American Journal of Clinical Pathology*, 89, 679–83.

Dutz, W. (1970) *Pneumocystis carinii* pneumonia. *Path. Ann.*, 5, 309.

Friedberg, D.-N. *et al.* (1990) Asymptomatic dissemination *Pneumocystis carinii* infection detected by ophthalmoscopy. *Lancet*, 2, 1256–7.

Gajdusek, D. C. (1957) *Pneumocystis carinii* etiologic agent of interstitial plasma cell pneumonia of young and premature infants. *Paediatrics*, 19, 543.

Galland, J. E. (1988) *Pneumocystis carinii* thyroiditis. *American Journal of Medicine*, 84, 303–6.

Gherman, C. R. (1988) *Pneumocystis carinii* otitis media and mastoiditis as the initial manifestation of the acquired immunodeficiency syndrome. *American Journal of Medicine*, 85, 250–2.

Miller, R. F. *et al.* (1989) Nebulized pentamidine as treatment for *Pneumocystis carinii* pneumonia in the acquired immunodeficiency syndrome. *Thorax*, 44, 565–9.

Pearson, R. D. *et al.* (1985) Pentamidine for the treatment of *Pneumocystis carinii* pneumonia and other protozoan diseases. *Annals of Internal Medicine*, 103, 782–6.

Perera, D. R. *et al.* (1970) *Pneumocystis carinii* pneumonia in a hospital for children. *Journal of the American Medical Association*, 214, 1074–8.

Phair, J. *et al.* (1990) The risk of *Pneumocystis carinii* pneumonia among men infected with human immune deficiency virus type 1. *New England Journal of Medicine*, 322, 161–5.

Pilon, V. A. *et al.* (1987) *Pneumocystis carinii* infection in AIDS. *New England Journal of Medicine*, 316, 1410–11.

Poblete, R. B. *et al.* (1989) *Pneumocystis carinii* hepatitis in the acquired immunodeficiency syndrome. *American Journal of Internal Medicine*, 110, 737–8.

Radman, J. C. (1973) *Pneumocystis carinii* pneumonia in an adopted Vietnamese infant. *Journal of the American Medical Association*, 230, 1561–3.

Walzer, P. D. *et al.* (1973) *Pneumocystis carinii* pneumonia and primary immune deficiency disease in infancy and childhood. *Journal of Paediatrics*, 82, 416–22.

Walzer, P. D. (1970) *Pneumocystis carinii* infection. Review article. *Southern Medical Journal*, 70(11), 1330–33.

Watanable, J. M. *et al.* (1965) *Pneumocystis carinii* pneumonia in a family. *Journal of the American Medical Association*, 193, 113.

Wharton, M. *et al.* (1986) Trimethoprim sulphamethoxazole or pentamidine for *Pneumocystis carinii* pneumonia in the acquired immunodeficiency syndrome. *Annals of Internal Medicine*, 105, 37–44.

Young, L. S. (1984) Clinical aspects of pneumocystosis in man. In *Pneumocystis carinii Pneumonia* (Ed. by L. S. Young), pp. 139–74. Marcel Dekker, New York.

TUBERCULOSIS

Definition

Tuberculosis is a destructive infectious disease caused by *Mycobacterium tuberculosis*, an acid-fast bacillus. It is acid-fast because of a waxy material in the cell wall, which resists simple laboratory staining techniques unless treated with hot carbol fuchsin, which allows impregnation by the dye. This is retained despite attempts to decolourize it with acid or alcohol.

Mycobacteria are distributed widely throughout the world, and only a few species are pathogenic to man, such as *Mycobacterium tuberculosis*, whose main host is man, and *Mycobacterium bovis*, the bovine type of tubercle bacillus, which is pathogenic to man as well as to cattle. This causes characteristically chronic granulamatous lesions, mainly in the lungs, but the glands, bones, joints, brain and meninges and other internal organs may be affected (Alvarez *et al.*, 1984).

Studies have shown that the prevalence of mycobacteria infection is six times greater in patients with cancer than in patients who do not have cancer. Lung cancer was the most common neoplasm in patients with mycobacteria infection (Ortbals, 1978).

There are also three mycobacteria associated with patients who are severely immunocompromised due to human immunodeficiency virus (HIV) infection. These are: *Mycobacterium avium intracellulare*, *M. xenopi* and *M. kansasii*. In the past, these types rarely caused disease in man, but now cause a disease which quickly disseminates to most organs in the body (Young *et al.*, 1986), and they are highly resistant to treatment. However, person-to-person transmission does not appear to occur.

REFERENCE MATERIAL

Between 1982 and 1989, tuberculosis notification for England and Wales fell in total, but geographical distribution figures have changed, with some regions showing small increases in numbers. The increases have been greatest in the North-East and South-East Thames regions for males; and for females in the West Midlands and North-West Thames regions (Watson *et al.*, 1991). The highest notification rates are generally reported from areas with a high proportion of Indian subcontinent ethnic groups (Joint Tuberculosis Committee, 1978).

The number of extra cases of tuberculosis as a result of the HIV pandemic is not clear, but it is unlikely that more than 6% of cases in the United Kingdom develop tuberculosis at any time in the course of their disease (Watson *et al.*, 1991).

Mortality from tuberculosis in England and Wales has declined since recording began in 1913. In recent years, total notification has fallen from 7406 in 1982 to 5432 in 1989, and deaths due to tuberculosis (excluding late effects) have fallen from 564 in 1982 to 443 in 1989 (Office of Population Censuses and Surveys, 1990).

Certain conditions predispose to the development of tuberculosis, including general physical debilitation and lowered resistance due to disease, immunosuppressive drugs and alcoholism. In addition, poor economic status and population groups such as Asians and those with little immunity, such as the very young and elderly are also susceptible (Galbraith, 1981; Joint Tuberculosis Committee, 1978; Joint Tuberculosis Committee of the British Thoracic Society, 1983). The mode of spread for tuberculosis is occasionally by ingestion, for example, by drinking infected milk, but principally by inhalation of small droplets produced by coughing. These droplets are probably the most effective vehicle of spread since they dry rapidly in the air to yield droplet nuclei of less than 5 nm in diameter which, when inhaled, can reach the alveoli. The organism can survive in moist or dried sputum for up to six weeks, but is killed by a few hours' exposure to direct sunlight (Loudon *et al.*, 1969).

Special attention must be given to equipment contaminated with mycobacterium species. Thorough cleaning followed by autoclaving is the sterilization method of choice. As certain equipment such as endoscopes can be damaged by autoclaving, disinfection must be used. A greater resistance by the organism to glutaraldehyde solution has been seen, and so thoroughly pre-cleaned equipment must be totally immersed for 60 minutes in a freshly prepared glutaraldehyde solution (Department of Health and Social Security, 1986).

Diagnosis

A provisional diagnosis can be based on microscopical findings of acid-fast bacilli in sputum, tissue, urine or cerebrospinal fluid, for example. This is termed smear positive. Conformation and species identification by culture may take several weeks and is termed culture positive.

Patients with smear-positive pulmonary disease are infectious, those with smear-negative or non-pulmonary disease are not. Once appropriate combination chemotherapy has commenced (Joint Tuberculosis Committee, 1983), smear-positive people are considered non-infectious after two weeks of treatment (Subcommittee of the Joint Tuberculosis Committee of the British Thoracic Society, 1990).

Treatment

Treatment until the 1960s included bedrest and attention to diet but chemotherapy is now the preferred treatment. It involves the use of combination drugs designed to reduce viable bacteria as rapidly as possible in order to minimize the risk of ineffective treatment in those patients infected by drug-resistant bacteria (Cooke, 1985). Treatment failures generally occur due to poor compliance by the patient and improper supervision (Fox, 1983).

Tuberculosis continues to be a notifiable disease under the revised Public Health Act, 1985. It is the responsibility of the Medical Officer for Environmental Health to follow up all contacts of infected people. This has proved to be a valuable and worthwhile procedure (British Thoracic and Tuberculosis Association, 1978). Generally, hospital staff are followed up by the hospital infection control officer in liaison with the hospital occupational health unit (Thornbury, 1985).

The priorities for tuberculosis control are early detection of cases, examination of contacts, barrier nursing if appropriate and immunization of tubercle-negative people with Bacillus Calmette-Guérin vaccine (BCG). It is recommended that BCG vaccination should be offered routinely in schools to children aged 10 to 14 years. This programme has been shown to be effective in preventing tuberculosis (Sutherland, 1987).

Certain professions, for example, those working in hospitals, prisons, old people's homes and schools, should be screened on employment. This may include a tuberculin test and chest radiography (Jachuck, 1988) for staff who have not received BCG vaccination in the past. It is extremely uncommon for hospital staff to acquire tuberculosis from patients (Capewells *et al.*, 1986). Staff in contact with untreated, smear-positive patients for a week or more should be reported to the occupational health department, and a chest X-ray arranged for six months' time. However, if the employee develops suspicious symptoms such as an unexplained cough lasting longer than three weeks, persistent fever or weight loss, then a full examination must be undertaken.

References and further reading

Alvarez, S. *et al.* (1984) Extrapulmonary tuberculosis revisited. A review of experience at Boston City and other hospitals. *Medicine (Baltimore)*, 63, 25.

Ayliffe, G. A. J. *et al.* (1984) *Chemical Disinfection in Hospital*, p. 3. Public Health Laboratory Service, London.

British Thoracic and Tuberculosis Association (1975) Tuberculosis among immigrants related to length of residence in England and Wales. *British Medical Journal*, 3, 698–9.

British Thoracic and Tuberculosis Association (1978) A study of standardized contact procedure in tuberculosis. *Tubercle*, 59, 245–59.

Capewells, S. *et al.* (1986) Tuberculosis in the NHS – is it a problem? *Thorax*, 41, 708.

Cooke, N. J. (1985) Treatment of tuberculosis. *British Medical Journal*, 291, 497–8.

Department of Health and Social Security (1986) *Safety*

Information Bulletin 28. DHSS, London.

Fox, W. (1983) Compliance of patients and physicians' experience and lessons from tuberculosis. *British Medical Journal*, 298, 101–5.

Galbraith, N. S. (1981) *Changing patterns of infectious disease in the general population of England and Wales*. Infection Control Nurses Associations' Twelfth Annual Symposium, pp. 61–5.

Jachuck, S. J. (1988) Is a pre-employment chest radiograph necessary for NHS employees? *British Medical Journal*, 296, 1187–8.

Joint Tuberculosis Committee (1978) Tuberculosis among immigrants in Britain. *British Medical Journal*, 1, 1038–40.

Joint Tuberculosis Committee of the British Thoracic Society (1983) Control and prevention of tuberculosis – a code of practice. *British Medical Journal*, 287, 1118–21.

Loudon, R. G. *et al.* (1969) Cough frequency and infectivity in patient with pulmonary tuberculosis. *American Review of Respiratory Disease*, 99, 109–111.

Office of Population Censuses and Surveys (1990) *Communicable Disease Statistics, Statistical Tables 1988, Series MB2, No. 15*. HMSO, London.

Ortbals, D. W. (1978) A comparative study of tuberculosis and mycobacterial infection and their associations with malignancy. *American Review of Respiratory Disease*, 117, 39.

Subcommittee of the Joint Tuberculosis Committee of the British Thoracic Society (1990) Control and prevention of tuberculosis in Britain. An updated code of practice. *British Medical Journal*, 300, 995–9.

Sutherland, I. *et al.* (1987) Effectiveness of BCG vaccination in England and Wales in 1983. *Tubercle*, 68, 81–92.

Thornbury, G. (1985) TB or not TB. *Nursing Times*, 81(32), 43–4.

Watson, J. M. *et al.* (1991) Notification of tuberculosis in England and Wales, 1982–1989. *Communicable Disease Report*, 1(2), R13–R16.

Young, L. S. *et al.* (1986) Mycobacterial infection in AIDS patients with the emphasis on the *Mycobacterium* complex. *Review of Infectious Diseases*, 8, 1024–33.

5

Bladder Lavage and Irrigation

Definitions

Lavage
Bladder lavage is the washing out of the bladder with sterile fluid.

Irrigation
Bladder irrigation is the continuous washing out of the bladder with sterile fluid.

Indications
Bladder lavage or irrigation is indicated for the following reasons:

Lavage
1. To clear an obstructed catheter.
2. To remove the potential souces of obstruction, e.g. blood clots or sediment from infection.

Irrigation
1. To prevent the formation and retention of blood clots, e.g. following prostatic surgery.
2. On rare occasions to remove heavily contaminated material from a diseased urinary bladder.

REFERENCE MATERIAL

Solutions used for lavage and irrigation
A number of solutions are available for cleansing the bladder and the selection of a particular solution will depend on its therapeutic properties in relation to the patient's needs. Some studies have suggested that the use of bladder washout regimes to reduce, prevent or treat urinary tract infection (UTI) is ineffective (Dudley & Barriere, 1981; Stickler *et al.*, 1981; Warren *et al.*, 1978). The following conclusions were suggested by these studies:

1. Regular bladder irrigation leads to infection with resistant organisms and may lead to higher rates of infection.
2. Noxythiolin had no bactericidal effect unless in contact with infected urine for two hours.
3. Chlorhexidine was found to lead to the selection of resistant bacterial species.

Elliott *et al.* (1989) therefore called for a reassessment of bladder irrigation methods and the indications for their use. The use of bladder lavage, however, to reduce or prevent catheter obstruction may be beneficial with certain patients (Blannin & Hobden, 1980; Brocklehurst & Brocklehurst, 1978; Ferrie *et al.*, 1979).

Normal saline is the agent most commonly recommended for lavage and irrigation and should be used in every case unless an alternative solution is prescribed. Normal saline is isotonic so it does not affect the body's fluid or electrolyte levels, therefore large volumes may be used as necessary. Three-litre bags of saline are available for irrigation purposes.

Studies of water and saline (Harper & Matz, 1975, 1976) showed them to be the least erosive irrigating solutions when tested in rat bladders. Ferrie *et al.* (1979) and Blannin and Hobden (1980) recommended the use of tap water as a purely mechanical means of flushing out the catheter for patients at home. The use of large volumns of sterile water is not recommended, however, as its absorption through the bladder wall may increase the blood volume to unacceptable levels.

The use of chlorhexidine gluconate as a bladder washout is not recommended unless it is specifically prescribed. The 0.02% solution provided for intravesical use is an effective disinfectant against vegative bacteria, especially Gram-positive organisms. Its activity is reduced, however, by blood and other organic matter (Martindale, 1982) and can cause haematuria and bladder erosion (Harper, 1981).

Traditionally, intermittent bladder washouts using antispetic solutions have been used to try and eradicate urinary tract infections. The research evidence is now conclusive that antiseptic bladder washouts will not prevent or remove urinary tract infections in catheterized patients.

A number of solutions have been recommended for use in specific circumstances but their effectiveness has not been established (Kennedy, 1984). They include citric acid (3.23%) to prevent and dissolve crystallization in the catheter or bladder; mandelic acid (1%) to prevent the growth of urease-producing bacteria by bladder acidification; and citric acid (6%) to dissolve persistent crystallization in the bladder or catheter (Waghorn *et al.*, 1988).

Cytotoxic agents given intravesically

For details on the administration of cytotoxic agents, see Chapter 11, Cytotoxic Drugs, section entitled Guidelines: Intravesical instillation of cytotoxic drugs.

Catheters used for lavage and irrigation

A three-way urinary catheter must be used for irrigation in order that fluid may simultaneously be run into, and drained out from, the bladder. This catheter is passed routinely in theatre when irrigation is required, e.g. after prostatectomy. Occasionally, bladder irrigation is started on the ward. If the patient has an ordinary catheter, this must be replaced with a three-way type (see Figure 5.1).

For bladder lavage it is not necessary to use a three-way catheter. There are three reasons for this:

1. Obstruction is more likely to occur when the drainage lumen is small, as in the three-way type.
2. The catheter may not drain if there is an obstruction. Such an obstruction is most likely to have occurred within the drainage lumen, and lavage via the side-arm is unlikely to have much, if any, effect on the cause of the obstruction.
3. The risk of infection from the recatheterization with a three-way catheter is much greater than the risk of infection from disconnecting a closed drainage system, provided that aseptic techniques are adhered to strictly.

It is recommended, however, that a three-way catheter is passed if frequent intravesical installations of drugs or antiseptic solutions are prescribed and the risk of catheter obstruction is not considered to be very great. In such cases the most important factor is minimizing the risk of introducing infection and

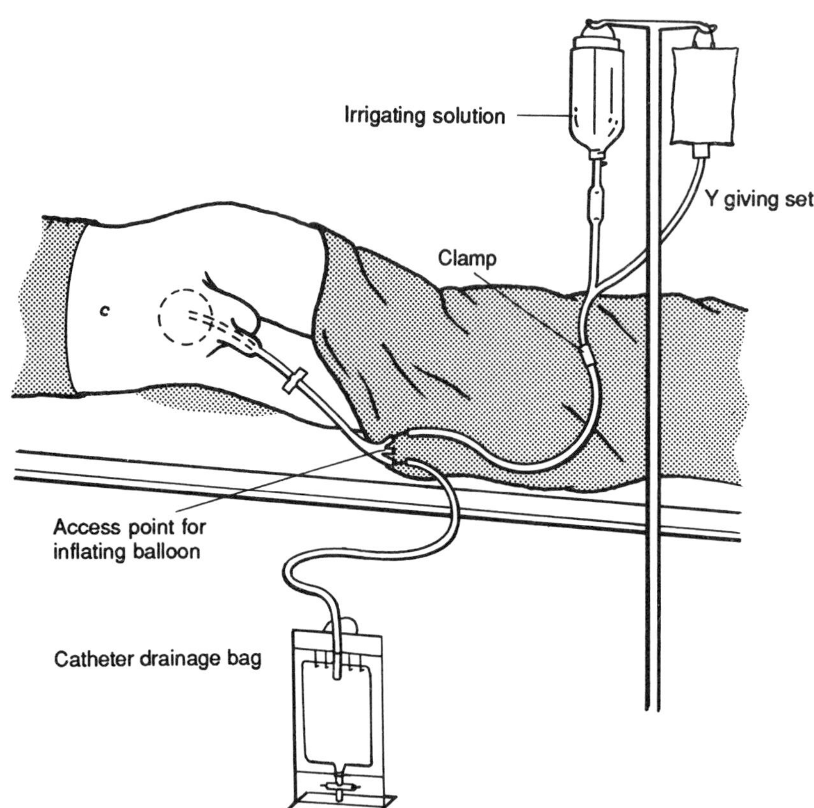

Figure 5.1 Closed urinary drainage system with provision for intermittent or continuous irrigation.

maintaining a closed urinary drainage system, for which the three-way catheter allows.

References and further reading

Blannin J. & Hobden, J. (1980) The catheter of choice. *Nursing Times*, 76, 2092–3.

Brocklehurst, J. C. & Brocklehurst, S. (1978) Management of indwelling catheters. *British Journal of Urology*, 50, 102–5.

Datta, P. K. (1981) The post-prostatectomy patient. *Nursing Times*, 77, 1759–61.

Dudley, M. N. & Barriere, S. L. (1981) Antimicrobial irrigations in the prevention and treatment of catheter-related urinary tract infections. *American Journal of Hospital Pharmacy*, 38, 59–65.

Elliott, T. (1990) Disadvantages of bladder irrigation (in catheterized patients. Brief research report). *Nursing Times*, 86, 52.

Elliott, T. S. *et al.* (1989) Bladder irrigation on irritation? *British Journal of Urology*, 64, 391–4.

Ferrie, B. G. *et al.* (1979) Long-term urethral catheter drainage. *British Medical Journal*, 279, 1046–7.

Gilbert, V. & Gobbi, M. (1989) Bladder irrigation (Principles and methods). *Nursing Times & Nursing Mirror*, 85, 40–2.

Gopal, R. G. & Elliott, T. S. (1988) Bladder irrigation. *Age and Ageing*, 17(6), 373–8.

Harper, W. (1981) An appraisal of 12 solutions used for bladder irrigation or installation. *British Journal of Urology*, 53, 433–8.

Harper, W. & Matz, L. (1975) The effect of chlorhexidine irrigation of the bladder in the rat. *British Journal of Urology*, 47, 539–43.

Harper, W. & Matz, L. (1976) Further studies on effects of irrigating solutions on rat bladders. *British Journal of Urology*, 48, 463–7.

Kennedy, A. (1984) Trial of new bladder washout system. *Nursing Times*, 80, 48–51.

Martindale, W. (1982) *The Extra Pharmacopoeia*, 28th edn. The Pharmaceutical Press, London.

Roe, B. H. (1989) Use of bladder washouts: a study of nurses' recommendations. *Journal of Advanced Nursing*, 14(6) 494–500.

Roe, B. (1990) The basis for sound practice. *Nursing Standard*, 4, 25–7.

Stickler, D. J. *et al.* (1981) Some observations on the activity of three antiseptics used as bladder irrigants in the treatment of UTI in patients with indwelling catheters. *Paraplegia*, 19, 325–33.

Waghorn D. J. *et al.* (1988) Urinary catheters. *British Medical Journal*, 296, 1250.

Warren, J. *et al.* (1978) Antibiotic irrigation and catheter-associated urinary tract infection. *New England Journal of Medicine*, 299, 570–3.

GUIDELINES: BLADDER LAVAGE

Equipment

1. Sterile dressing pack.
2. Bladder syrginge, 60 ml.
3. Sterile jug.
4. Antiseptic solution.
5. Alcohol-based hand wash solution.
6. Clamp.
7. New catheter bag (for Foley-type catheter) or sterile spigot (for three-way catheter).
8. Sterile receiver.
9. Sterile solution for lavage.

Procedure

Action	Rationale
1. Explain the procedure to the patient.	To obtain the patient's consent and co-operation.
2. Screen the bed. Ensure that the patient is in a comfortable position allowing access to the catheter.	For the patient's privacy and to reduce the risk of cross-infection. Curtains are drawn at this stage so that dust and airborne organisms disturbed by the curtains do not settle on the sterile field.
3. Perform the procedure using an aseptic technique.	To prevent infection. (For further information on aseptic technique see Chapter 3.)
4. Draw up solutions using a 60 ml syringe,	It is easier to draw up solutions from vials in the

Guidelines: Bladder lavage

Action	Rationale
preferably with needle adapter. Cap the syringe and place it in a sterile receiver.	clinical area than at the bedside.
5. Take the trolley to the bedside. Open the outer wrappings of packs and put them on the top shelf of the trolley.	
6. Prepare the sterile field. Pour the lavage solution into the sterile jug.	
7. Wash hands with an appropriate antiseptic solution and put on gloves.	To minimize the risk of infection.
8. Clamp the catheter. Place a sterile paper towel under the junction of the catheter and the tubing of the drainage bag and disconnect them.	To prevent leakage when the catheter is disconnected. When the patient has a three-way catheter the drainage bag will not need disconnecting as the washout fluid is injected through the side-arm of the catheter. This should be spigoted off after use and the fluid remaining in the bladder will drain into the catheter bag.
9. Clean gloved hands with an alcohol-based hand wash solution. Clean around the end of the catheter with sterile cotton wool and an antiseptic solution.	To remove surface organisms from gloves and catheter and thus reduce the risk of introducing infection into the catheter.
10. Draw up the irrigating fluid into the bladder syringe and insert the nozzle into the end of the catheter.	
11. Release the clamp on the catheter and gently inject the contents of the syringe into the bladder, trying not to inject air.	Rapid injection of fluid could be uncomfortable for the patient. Large volumes of air in the bladder cause distension and discomfort.
12. Remove the syringe and allow the bladder contents to drain by gravity into a receiver placed on a sterile towel.	
13. Repeat steps 11 and 12 of the procedure until the washout is complete or the returning fluid is clear.	
14. If the fluid does not return naturally, aspirate gently with the syringe.	Gentle suction is sometimes required to remove obstructive material from the catheter.
15. Connect a new catheter bag or sterile spigot if a three-way catheter is in place, and allow the remaining fluid to drain out.	A closed drainage system must be re-established as soon as possible to reduce the risk of bacterial invasion through the catheter.
16. If the solution is to remain in the bladder, the catheter should be clamped when all the fluid has been injected and the clamp released after the desired period.	

Action	Rationale
17. Measure the volume of washout fluid returned and compare it with the volume of fluid injected. Record any discrepancies of volume in the appropriate documents.	To keep an accurate record of urinary output and to observe for catheter obstruction.
18. Make the patient comfortable, remove equipment and clean the trolley.	
19. Wash hands.	To prevent cross-infection.

As an alternative to the use of bladder syringe and irrigating solution, a pre-packed filled reservoir with sterile catheter adaptor called Uro-tainer is now available. Kennedy (1984) found that the use of Uro-tainer compared with traditional saline washout procedure produced a reduced incidence of urinary tract infection.

GUIDELINES: CONTINUOUS BLADDER IRRIGATION

Equipment

1. Sterile dressing pack.
2. Antiseptic solution.
3. Alcohol-based hand wash solution.
4. Clamp.
5. Sterile irrigation fluid.
6. Disposable irrigation set.
7. Infusion stand.
8. Sterile jug.

Procedure

Commencing bladder irrigation

Action	Rationale
1. Explain the procedure to the patient.	To obtain the patient's consent and co-operation.
2. Screen the patient and ensure that he or she is in a comfortable position allowing access to the catheter.	For the patient's privacy and to reduce the risk of cross-infection. Curtains are drawn at this stage so that dust and airborne organisms disturbed by the curtains do not settle on the sterile trolley.
3. Perform the procedure using an aseptic technique.	To prevent infection. (For further information on aseptic technique, see Chapter 3).
4. Open the outer wrappings of the pack and put it on the top shelf of the trolley.	
5. Insert the end of the irrigation giving set into the fluid bag and hang the bag on the infusion stand. Allow fluid to run through the tubing so that air is expelled.	To prime the irrigation set so that it is ready for use. Air is expelled in order to prevent discomfort from air in the patient's bladder.
6. Clamp the catheter.	
7. Prepare the sterile field.	
8. Clean hands with an antiseptic solution. Put on gloves.	To minimize the risk of cross-infection.

Guidelines: Bladder lavage

Action	**Rationale**
9. Place a sterile paper towel under the irrigation inlet of the catheter and remove the spigot.	To prevent leakage of urine through the irrigation arm when the spigot is removed.
10. Discard the spigot.	
11. Clean gloved hands with an alcohol-based hand wash solution. Clean around the end of the irrigation arm with sterile cotton wool and an antiseptic solution.	To remove surface organisms from gloves and catheter and to reduce the risk of introducing infection into the catheter.
12. Attach the irrigation giving set to the irrigation arm of the catheter. Keep the clamp of the irrigation giving set closed.	To prevent over-distension of the bladder, which can occur if fluid is run into the bladder before the drainage tube has been unclamped.
13. Release the clamp on the catheter tube and allow any accumulated urine to drain into the catheter bag. Empty the urine from the catheter bag into a sterile jug.	Urine drainage should be measured before commencing irrigation so that the fluid balance may be monitored more accurately.
14. Discard the gloves.	These will be contaminated, having handled the cathether bag.
15. Set irrigation at the required rate and ensure that fluid is draining into the catheter bag.	To check that the drainage system is patent and to prevent fluid accumulating in the bladder.
16. Make the patient comfortable, remove unnecessary equipment and clean the trolley.	
17. Wash hands.	To prevent cross-infection.

Care of the patient during irrigation

Action	**Rationale**
1. Adjust the rate of infusion according to the degree of haematuria. This will be greatest in the first 12 hours following surgery (average fluid input is 6–9 litres during the first 12 hours, falling to 3–6 litres during the next 12 hours). The aim is to obtain a drainage fluid which is rosè in colour.	To remove blood from the bladder before it clots and to minimize the risk of catheter obstruction and clot retention.
2. Check the volume in the drainage bag frequently when infusion is in progress, e.g. half-hourly or hourly.	To ensure that fluid is draining from the bladder and to detect blockages as soon as possible, also to prevent over-distension of the bladder and patient discomfort. Frequent checking means, in addition, that full catheter bags are noticed and can be emptied before they reach capacity.
3. Using rubber-tipped 'milking' tongs, 'milk' the catheter and drainage tube regularly, as required.	To remove unseen clots from within the drainage system and to maintain an efficient outlet.

(A) Date and time	(B) Volume put up	(C) Volume run in	(D) Total volume	(E) Urine	(F) Urine running total

Figure 5.2 Bladder irrigation recording chart.

4. Record the fluid balance chart accurately. The fluid balance of all patients having bladder irrigation must be monitored.

So that urine output is known and any related problems, e.g. renal dysfunction, may be detected quickly and easily.

BLADDER IRRIGATION RECORDING CHART

The bladder irrigation recording chart (Figure 5.2) is designed to provide an accurate record of the patient's urinary output during the period of irrigation.

Procedure for the use of the chart

Record the time (column A) and the fluid volume in each bag of irrigating solution (column B) as it is put up.

When the irrigating fluid has all run from the first bag into the bladder, record the original volume in the bag in column C. Record the corresponding time in column A. Do not attempt to estimate the fluid volume run in while a bag is in progress as this will cause inaccuracies. If, however, a bag is discontinued, the volume run in can be calculated by measuring the volume left in the bag and deducting this from the original volume. This should be recorded in column C.

The catheter bag should be emptied as often as is necessary, the volume being recorded in column D and the corresponding time in column A. The catheter bag must also be emptied whenever the bag of irrigating fluid is empty, and the volume recorded in column D.

When each bag of fluid has run through, add up the total volume drained by the catheter in column D, and write this in red. Subtract from this the total volume run in (column C) to find the urine output. Write this in column E. Draw a line across the page to indicate that this calculation is complete and continue underneath for the next bag.

NURSING CARE PLAN

Problem	Cause	Suggested action
Fluid retained in the bladder when the catheter is in position.	Fault in drainage apparatus, e.g.:	
	Blocked catheter.	'Milk' the tubing. Wash out the bladder with normal saline.
	Kinked tubing.	Straighten the tubing.
	Overfull drainage bag.	Empty the drainage bag.
	Catheter clamped off.	Unclamp the catheter.
Distended abdomen related to an overfull bladder during the irrigation procedure.	Irrigation fluid is infused at too rapid a rate.	Slow down the infusion rate.
	Fault in drainage apparatus.	Check the patency of the drainage apparatus.
Leakage of fluid from around the catheter.	Catheter slipping out of the bladder.	Insert the catheter further in. Decompress balloon fully to assess the amount of water necessary. Refill balloon until it remains *in situ*, taking care not to over fill beyond safe level (see manufacturer's instructions).
	Catheter too large or unsuitable for the patient's anatomy.	If leakage is profuse or catheter is uncomfortable for the patient, replace the catheter with one of smaller size.
Patient experiences pain during the lavage or irrigation procedure.	Volume of fluid in the bladder is too great for comfort.	Reduce the fluid volume within the bladder.
	Solution is painful to raw areas in the bladder.	Inform the doctor. Administer analgesia as prescribed.
Retention of fluid with or without distended abdomen, with or without pain.	Perforated bladder.	Stop irrigation. Maintain in recovery position. Call medical assistance. Monitor vital signs. Monitor patient for pain, tense abdomen.

6

Bone Marrow Procedures

Definition

Bone marrow procedures involve the removal of bone marrow and other tissue from the iliac crest, sternum or tibia using a special needle. They include the following:

1. Aspiration – the withdrawal of the bone marrow fluid to gain information about the developing cells.
2. Trephine biopsy – the removal of a core of bone including marrow to provide details of the overall marrow architecture whereby abnormal structure can be identified and examined.
3. Harvest – the withdrawal of bone marrow including stem cells for autologous and allogeneic bone marrow transplantation or for cryopreservation.

Indications

Bone marrow procedures are performed by trained medical staff.

Bone marrow aspiration and trephine

Used for:

1. Evaluation of haematopoiesis and establishment of a diagnosis in certain haematological disorders, e.g. anaemia, leukaemia, myeloma and metastatic carcinoma.
2. Monitoring both the course of the patient's disease and the response to therapy.

Bone marrow harvest

Used to provide bone marrow for transplantation or cryopreservation for future use.

Contraindications

This procedure is contraindicated in those patients who are unable to co-operate or who have a coagulation defect such as an increased clotting time, unless it is correctable.

REFERENCE MATERIAL

Bone marrow aspiration was first introduced in Naples in 1909 by Pianese. By 1933 Custer had developed it into a routine technique. It is a quick and relatively simple method of obtaining a marrow specimen and can be performed either in the hospital ward or in an outpatient clinic.

Anatomy and physiology

The bone marrow is the main site for blood cell formation. It contains pluripotent stem cells from which blood cells are derived. In a normal adult the production of cells is dependent on the body's needs.

Bone marrow occupies 85% of the cavities of bones. There are two types of marrow:

1. Red marrow, which is responsible for the production of red and white blood cells and platelets.
2. Yellow marrow. This consists of fat cells, blood vessels, reticulum cells and fibres. As age increases, red marrow is replaced by yellow marrow.

In certain diseases, such as leukaemia, the immature cells of the red marrow may proliferate and replace the yellow marrow. Red marrow is found in the cavities of all the bones during the first years of life. In adults it is found mainly in the flat bones, e.g. skull, vertebrae, clavicles, scapulae, sternum and iliac crests. The preferred sites for marrow procedures, in an adult, are the iliac crests and the sternum (see Figure 6.1). In children the tibia may sometimes be used.

Bone marrow aspirations and biopsies are usually performed under local anaesthesia. The iliac crests are often used for patients requiring frequent marrow aspirations as the use of the right and left crests can be alternated, both anterior and posterior surfaces may be used and there are no vital organs nearby that may be punctured by the procedure. The posterior iliac crest is often preferred as the procedure can then be performed outside the patient's field of vision, often

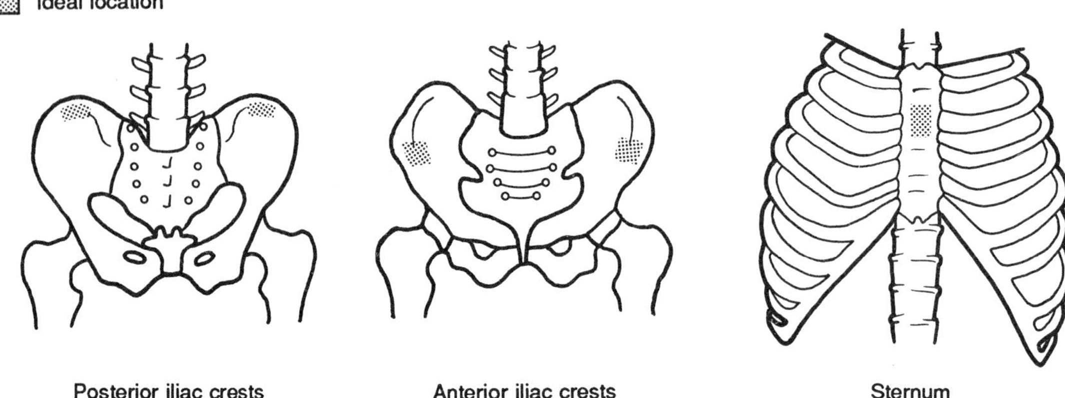

Figure 6.1 Common sites for bone marrow examination, arranged in order of preference. Normally, only aspirations and not biopsies are done on the sternum because of its small size and proximity to vital organs.

reducing his or her anxiety. The actual aspiration of marrow from the bone cavity is painful despite the local anaesthetic which dulls the pain of the passage of the needle through the skin, subcutaneous layer and, to a large extent, the periosteum. To enable the patient to cope with the pain, he/she should be warned about its inevitability beforehand, but it should be emphasized that the pain will be only of short duration. Very anxious patients and children may be prescribed a mild sedative to be given before the procedure begins. In some units the procedure is carried out under a light general anaesthetic.

Bone marrow harvests are performed under a general anaesthetic because:

1. The procedure may last approximately one hour compared to 5 to 15 minutes for an aspiration biopsy.
2. Multiple puncture sites may be used and the patient may be approached from both sides.
3. The procedure can be very painful.

An epidural will be used when the patient is unsuitable for a general anaesthetic.

Complications

Complications are extremely rare but include the following:

1. Cardiac tamponade. This is the compression of the heart produced by the accumulation of blood or fluid in the pericardial sac. It can be caused by the rupture of a blood vessel in the myocardium caused by a penetrating wound such as a bone marrow aspirate.
2. Haemorrhage, which occurs almost exclusively in those patients with thrombocytopenia. It may be avoided by applying adequate pressure to the puncture site for a few minutes following aspiration and by platelet transfusions where indicated.
3. Infection, particularly in the neutropenic patient.
4. Bone fractures, particularly in small children.

References and further reading

Abrahams, P. & Webb, P. (1975) *Clinical Anatomy of Practical Procedures*. Pitman Medical, London.

Bevan, J. (1978) *A Pictorial Handbook of Anatomy and Physiotherapy*. Mitchell Beazley, London.

Booth, J. A. (1983) *Handbook of Investigations*. Harper & Row, London.

Brunner, L. S. & Suddarth, D. S. (1982) *The Lippincott Manual of Medical-Surgical Nursing*, Vol. 2. Harper & Row, London.

Frazer, I. & Gough, K. R. (1968) Bone marrow biopsy. In *Biopsy Procedures in Clinical Medicine* (Ed. by A. E. Read). John Wright, Bristol.

Henke, Y. C. (1990) Physiology of normal bone marrow. *Seminars in Oncology Nursing – Adult Leukaemia*, 6(1), 3–8.

Hoffbrand, A. & Pettit, J. (1985) *Essential Haematology*, 2nd edn. Blackwell Scientific Publications, Oxford.

Keele, C., Neil, E. & Joels, N. (1983) *Samson Wrights Applied Physiology*, 13th edn. Oxford University Press, Oxford.

Markus, S. (1981) Taking the fear out of bone marrow examinations. *Nursing* (US), 11(4), 64–7.

Navarett, D. (1981) Assisting with bone marrow aspiration. In *Mosby's Manual of Clinical Nursing Procedures* (Ed. by J. Hirsch & J. Hancock). C. V. Mosby, St Louis.

Pagnana, K. D. & Pagnana, T. J. (1986) *Diagnostic Testing and Nursing Implications*, 2nd edn. C. V. Mosby, St Louis.

Skydell, B. & Crowder, A. (1975) *Diagnostic Procedures – A Reference for Health Practitioners and a Guide for Patient Counselling*. Little, Brown, Boston.

GUIDELINES: BONE MARROW ASPIRATION

Equipment

1. Antiseptic skin cleansing agent.
2. Sterile dressing pack.
3. Selection of syringes and needles.
4. Local anaesthetic.
5. Marrow aspiration needle and guard, e.g. Salah needle.
6. Microscope slides and coverslips.
7. Specimen bottles (plain and with heparin).
8. Polyurethane semi-permeable dressing or spray.

Procedure

Action	Rationale
1. Explain the procedure to the patient.	To obtain the patient's consent and co-operation.
2. Give medication as ordered, allowing sufficient time for it to have effect.	Usually this is only necessary for very anxious patients.
3. Help the patient into the correct position:	
(a) Supine.	For sternal puncture.
(b) Prone or on side.	For anterior or posterior iliac crest puncture.
4. Continue to observe the patient throughout the procedure. Assist the doctor as required. Reassure the conscious patient. Follow the appropriate procedure if the patient is anaesthetized.	See Chapter 33, Peri-operative Care.
5. Procedure is performed by a doctor:	
(a) Skin is cleansed with antiseptic solution.	To maintain asepsis throughout the procedure and thus minimize the risk of infection.
(b) Local anaesthetic is injected intradermally and through the various layers until the periosteum is infiltrated.	To minimize pain during the procedure. Transitory pain will be felt both as the periosteum is punctured and when the marrow is aspirated.
(c) Once the local anaesthetic has taken effect the doctor inserts the marrow needle, with the guard on, into the anaesthetized area.	The needle guard ensures the correct positioning of the needle in the marrow cavity and diminishes the risk, particularly in the sternal puncture, of inadvertently puncturing vital organs.
(d) If the patient has not been anaesthetized, the doctor warns the patient that he/she will feel a brief episode of sharp pain as the marrow is withdrawn. The needle is advanced into the bone marrow and the required amount of marrow is withdrawn.	To allay anxiety and to ensure the patient's maximum co-operation.
(e) The needle is removed from the puncture site.	
6. Once the doctor has removed the needle, apply pressure over the puncture site using a sterile topical swab until the bleeding stops.	To minimize bruising and to prevent haematoma formation. Prolonged pressure, 5 to 10 minutes, is required if the patient has a low platelet count (thrombocytopenia).
7. Once bleeding stops, cover the site with plaster or a plastic dressing. Ask the patient not to bathe or wash the area for 24 hours.	To provide an airtight seal over the puncture site and to prevent the entry of bacteria.

Guidelines: Bone marrow aspiration

Action	Rationale
8. Make the patient comfortable. He/she may be mobile, as desired, depending on the level of sedation.	Some patients will have this procedure performed in the outpatient department and will be asked to wait in the clinic for a further 30 minutes to ensure that no further bleeding occurs.
9. Remove and dispose of equipment.	To prevent spread of infection.
10. Record necessary information in the appropriate documents and ensure that specimens are sent to the appropriate laboratory department, correctly labelled and with the necessary forms.	

NURSING CARE PLAN

Problem	Cause	Suggested action
Pain experienced over the puncture site for 1 to 2 days following the procedure.	Bruising of the tissues at the time of puncture or haematoma formation due to inadequate pressure ón the puncture site following the procedure.	Administer a mild analgesic as prescribed by the doctor.
Haemorrhage from the puncture site following the procedure.	Low platelet count or inadequate pressure on the puncture site following the procedure.	Ensure that pressure is applied for a minimum of five minutes on the puncture site. Report excessive, uncontrollable bleeding to the appropriate personnel.
Haematoma formation over the puncture site.	Haemorrhage following the procedure.	Administer analgesics as prescribed. If the haematoma is severe, report this to the doctor as aspiration may be required.

7

Bowel Care

GENERAL INTRODUCTION

It should be borne in mind that many patients are too embarrassed to talk about bowel function and will often delay reporting the problem until it has been present for a few days. Generally, complaints will be either that the patient has diarrhoea or is constipated. Both diarrhoea and constipation should be seen as symptoms of some underlying disease or malfunction, and managed accordingly.

The nurse's priority in either case is immediate resolution of the problem and re-education of the patient to avoid such problems in the future. However, it is necessary to assess what the patient means by the terms diarrhoea and constipation as well as to assess the cause.

REFERENCE MATERIAL

Anatomy and physiology

From the ileocaecal sphincter to the anus the colon is approximately 1.5 m in length. Its main function is to eliminate the waste products of digestion by the propulsion of faeces towards the anus. In addition, it produces mucus to lubricate the faecal mass, thus aiding its expulsion. Other functions include the absorption of fluid and electrolytes, the storage of faeces and the synthesis of vitamins B and K by bacterial flora.

Faeces consist of the unabsorbed end products of digestion, bile pigments, cellulose, bacteria, epithelial cells, mucus and some inorganic material. They are normally semi-solid in consistency and contain about 70% water.

The movement of faeces through the colon towards the anus is by peristaltic action. The colon absorbs about two litres of water in 24 hours. If faeces are not expelled they will, therefore, gradually become hard due to dehydration and will be difficult to expel. If there is insufficient roughage (fibre) in the faeces, colonic stasis occurs. This leads to continued water absorption and the faeces will harden still further.

Faeces normally remain in the sigmoid colon until the stimulus to defaecate occurs. This stimulus varies in individuals according to habit. The stimulus can be controlled by conscious effort. After a few minutes the stimulus disappears and does not return for several hours. If these natural reflexes are inhibited on a regular basis they are eventually suppressed and reflex defaecation is inhibited. The result is that the individual becomes severely constipated. In response to the stimulus faeces move into the rectum.

The rectum is very sensitive to rises in pressure, even of 2–3 mm Hg, and distension will cause a perineal sensation with a consequent desire to defaecate. A co-ordinated reflex empties the bowel from mid-transverse colon to the anus. During this phase the diaphragm, abdominal and levator ani muscles contract and the glottis closes. Waves of peristalsis occur in the distal colon and the anal sphincter relaxes, allowing the evacuation of faeces.

Diarrhoea

The cause of diarrhoea needs to be ascertained. Roberts (1987) suggests that *acute* causes of diarrhoea include, for example, the following:

1. Infective agents.
2. Food poisoning.
3. Unwise eating (spices, excessive fruit).
4. Allergy to food constituents.

Chronic causes include:

1. Drugs (e.g. broad-spectrum antibiotics).
2. Gastrectomy.
3. Malabsorption.
4. Systemic illnesses.
5. Diseases of the large colon, including carcinoma, diverticular disease and inflammatory bowel disease, which can affect the small intestine as well.

It must also be remembered that faecal impaction can cause diarrhoea overflow concealing an impacted colon. Continuing episodes of diarrhoea need to be

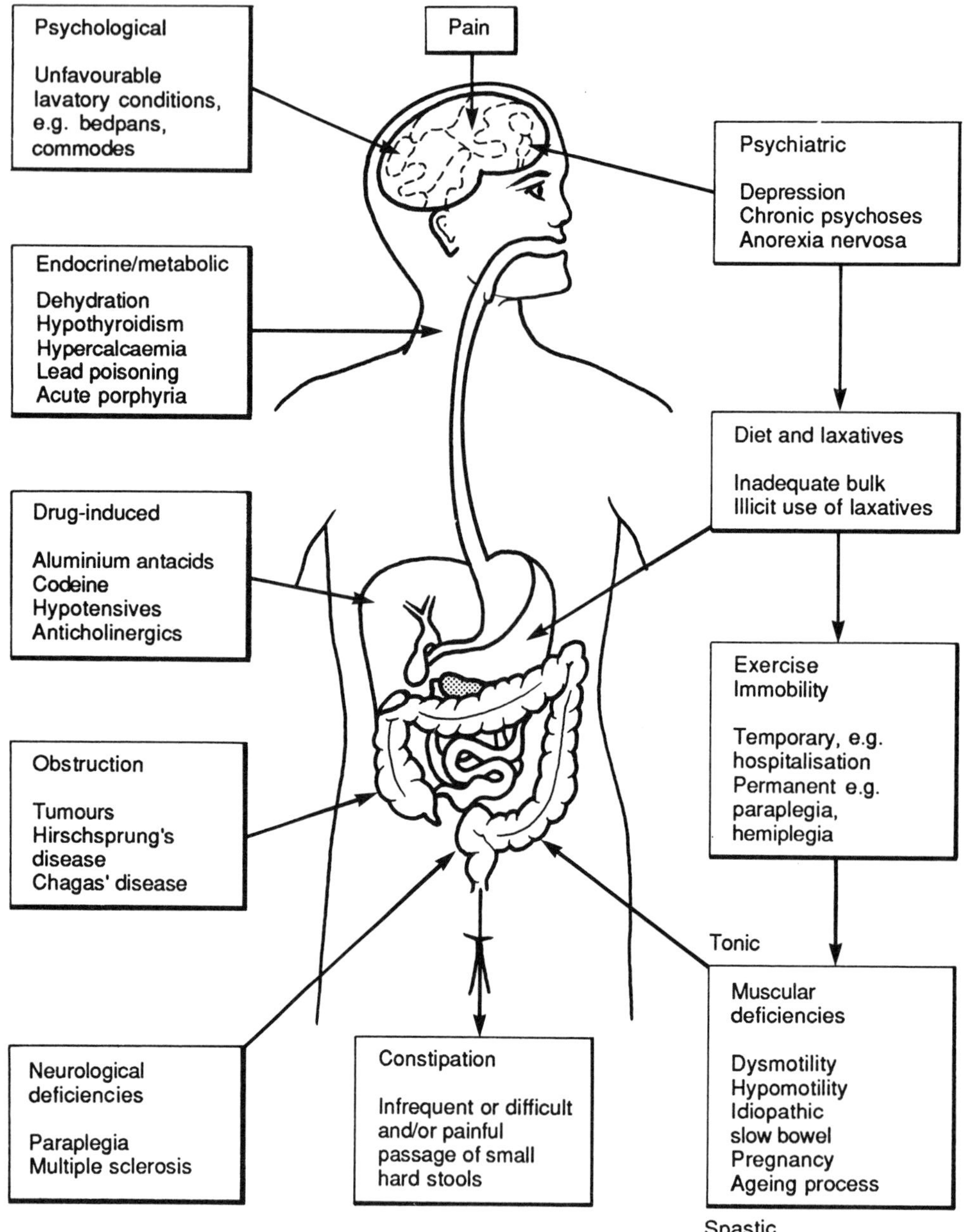

Figure 7.1 Classification of constipation – combined sources.

investigated to rule out inflammatory bowel disease or infection. Mild or severe diarrhoea before or after breakfast can be an indication of irritable bowel disease. In the management of diarrhoea, the nurse can ensure that the patient's diet is altered. Foods having a high fibre content can be avoided and fluid intake can be increased. Such measures as the provision of soft toilet paper, easy access to toilet facilities and a suitable barrier cream to prevent anal excoriation can be implemented and will be much appreciated by the patient. Constipation, however, demands the use of more elaborate nursing skills.

Table 7.1 Types of laxatives

Type of laxative	*Example*	*Brand names and sources*
Bulk producers	Dietary fibre Mucilaginous polysaccharides Methylcellulose	Bran, wholemeal bread, Fybogel, Celevac
Stool softners	Synthetic surface active agents	Dioctyl
Lubricants	Liquid paraffin	Agarol, Petrolager, Milpar
Osmotic agents	Sodium, potassium and magnesium salts	Magnesium sulphate, milk of magnesia, lactulose
Chemical stimulants	Sodium picosulphate, glycerin	Senna, Senokot, bisacodyl, Dulcolax, co-danthrusate, Picolax, glycerol

Constipation

Constipation is a symptom. Its management depends on its cause. Definitions and classifications differ but for most patients it means irregular, infrequent defaecation associated with the passage of hard faeces (see Figure 7.1). The patient usually complains of difficulty in defaecating with accompanying discomfort or pain.

Traditionally, the treatment of constipation has been left to the nurse (Milton-Thompson, 1971). As the patient often presents in hospital with an acute problem of constipation, nurses will need to formulate a short-term plan to evacuate the bowel as completely and as quickly as possible. For this reason enemas, suppositories and laxatives have remained the treatments of choice. Very often little thought is given either to the cause of the problem or to a more long-term plan. Duffin *et al.* (1981) have shown that a total of 3428 enemas were given on the geriatric wards of a district general hospital over a six-month period. There were 1120 admissions in this period, which gave an overall average of three enemas per patient. The same study found that although enemas frequently produced a good bowel evacuation, they also embarrassed the patient and produced symptoms ranging from nausea and abdominal pain to faecal incontinence. Hurst (1970) felt that enemas were probably only of use where there was a mechanical delay between the splenic flexure and anus. Dorgu (1971) felt that the main benefit of enemas was that they acted within minutes of their administration and were useful in acute conditions of impaction before drug therapy could be effective.

Assessment of the problem

The myth of daily bowel evacuation being essential to healthy living has persisted through the centuries. This myth has resulted in laxative abuse becoming one of the commonest type of drug abuse in the Western world.

On the use and abuse of purgatives, Hurst (1970) showed that £10 million was expended in 1921 on patent medicines, the majority of which contained purgatives. In the 1960s, a survey of Londoners showed that over 30% were treating themselves with laxatives (Rutter and Maxwell, 1976).

However, the indications for the use of laxatives are fairly limited. The nurse should always stress the importance of diet and exercise to the patient before recommending other ways of evacuating the bowel.

Defining constipation is undoubtedly a problem while the notion of essential daily evacuations persists. The first objective should be for the nurse to assess what is 'normal' for an individual patient. A bowel action every third day may be quite adequate for some people; for others three times a day will be the norm. This does not mean that the first person is constipated or that the second has diarrhoea.

Many factors may affect normal bowel functioning. Among those pertinent to hospital admission are the following:

1. Change in diet.
2. Lack of exercise.
3. X-ray investigation of the bowel involving the use of barium.
4. The use of drugs, particularly analgesics.

Laxatives are often required to overcome these effects (see Table 7.1).

Weller (1989) defines laxatives as medicine that loosens bowel contents and encourages evacuation. A laxative with a mild or gentle effect is also known as an aperient and one with a strong effect is referred to as a cathartic or a purgative. Purgatives should be used only in exceptional circumstances, i.e. where all other interventions have failed, or when they are prescribed for a specific purpose. Wherever possible the most natural means of bowel evacuation should be employed.

Laxatives alter the natural functioning of the alimentary tract. Often a period of no bowel evacuations follows their use and this usually causes the patient to take more laxatives; thus a cycle of dependence ensues (Mortimer, 1970).

The nurse should always make a rectal examination to establish whether the patient is constipated and to what degree. Wilson and Muir (1975) in their trial on geriatric faecal incontinence found that there was little correlation between a nurse's subjective assessment of whether a patient was constipated and the actual evidence gained from a rectal examination.

The use of the bedpan should always be avoided if possible. If the patient can get out of bed, a commode is preferable as the amount of energy expended is considerably less than that required for balancing on a bedpan. Lewin (1976) quoted from research by an American team investigating the straining forces of bowel evacuation by objective methods. They showed that straining was increased three to six times when a patient uses the bedpan and that its use requires a 50% greater consumption of oxygen than a commode by the bedside.

Manual evacuation of the rectum should be avoided if possible. It is a distressing, often painful and potentially dangerous procedure for the patient. If the procedure proves to be unavoidable, it may be necessary to sedate the patient before carrying it out. It is recommended by Pirrie (1980) that the procedure should be performed only by medical staff.

Laxatives (see Table 7.1)

Stool softeners lower the surface tension of the faeces and allow penetration by water. They act within 24 to 48 hours. Liquid paraffin is a stool softener as well as a lubricant, but its use should be avoided as droplets of oil may be inhaled accidentally, especially by the very young or the elderly, and cause lipoid pneumonia or even pulmonary tumours which may imitate carcinoma (Milton-Thompson, 1971). Repetitive use of liquid paraffin and the mineral oils also interferes with the absorption of fat-soluble vitamins and may increase the risks of alimentary tract malignancies (Janes, 1979).

Osmotic agents retain water in the small bowel and increase the flow of fluid into the colon. This increased volume will cause peristalis and consequent expulsion of faeces. Osmotic agents work within three to six hours. Magnesium salts are contraindicated for patients suffering from chronic renal failure as magnesium poisoning may result (Milton-Thompson, 1971). Sodium-containing laxatives should not be used for patients with cardiac problems or inflammatory bowel disease (Corman *et al.*, 1975).

Chemical stimulants cause irritation of mucosa, nerves or smooth muscle. Most of the stimulants act within two to eight hours. The amount of abdominal cramping produced and the time taken for them to work vary from one drug to another. These drugs can produce electrolyte imbalance, histological changes (melanosis coli) and damage to the mysenteric plexi. Eventually permanent damage affecting motility of the colon can occur, leading the patient to take increasing doses of the drug (Rutter & Maxwell, 1976).

Recently, more favour has been shown towards the bulk laxatives which can be incorporated into the diet, e.g. whole-grain cereals and high-fibre bread. Bulk laxatives work by increasing the mass of the faeces. They do this by attracting water. This in turn promotes peristalsis and reduces the time taken by the faeces to move through the colon. An increased fluid intake is required when bulk laxatives are used, particularly in the elderly, to prevent intestinal obstruction occurring. Another problem initially is that bulk laxatives tend to distend the abdomen, often making the patient feel full and uncomfortable. Sometimes this leads to temporary anorexia. Harris (1980) discussed fully the merits of introducing bran into the diet, especially of the elderly, and the consequent drastic reduction in the number of enemas administered. She also showed that the cost of using bran compared to other laxatives, even other bulk laxatives, was very much lower.

However, more care now needs to be taken in the use of supplementary bran; unprocessed wheat bran, commonly used to increase the fibre in a diet, contains high levels of phytates, which can combine with minerals essential to a healthy diet, such as calcium, iron, copper and zinc. This can lead to a deficit in those people at risk from an inadequate diet, especially the elderly. More use should be made of normal foods which are rich in 'high fibre' content, e.g. cereals, vegetables, especially root vegetables and broad beans, and fruit.

There is evidence indicating that 'dietary fibre' can reduce the levels of postprandial levels of glucose and insulin (Haber *et al.*, 1977; Jenkins *et al.*, 1981). However, the value of this relationship to diabetic patients is unclear. Studies have now shown that there are a number of types and components of 'dietary fibre', which makes this too imprecise a term for health care professionals to use: its closest, more exact description is now 'non-starch polysaccharides'. A more detailed discussion of this area can be found in 'Dietary Reference Values for Food Energy and Nutrients for the United Kingdom' (Department of Health, 1991).

ENEMAS

Definition

An enema is the introduction into the rectum or lower colon of a stream of fluid for the purpose of producing a bowel action or instilling medication.

Indications

Enemas may be prescribed for the following reasons:

1. To clean the lower bowel before surgery; X-ray examination of the bowel using contrast medium; before endoscopy examination or in cases of severe constipation.
2. To introduce medication into the system.
3. To soothe and treat irritated bowel mucosa.
4. To decrease body temperature (due to contact with the proximal vascular system).
5. To stop local haemorrhage.
6. To reduce hyperkalaemia (calcium resonium).
7. To reduce portal systemic encephalopathy (phosphate enema).

Contraindications

Enemas are contraindicated under the following circumstances:

1. In paralytic ileus.
2. In colonic obstruction.
3. Where the administration of tap water or soap and water enemas may cause circulatory overload, water intoxication, mucosal damage and necrosis, hyperkalaemia and cardiac arrhythmias.
4. Where the administration of large amounts of fluid high into the colon may cause perforation and haemorrhage.
5. Following gastrointestinal or gynaecological surgery, where suture lines may be ruptured (unless medical consent has been given).
6. The use of micro-enemas and hypertonic saline enemas in patients with inflammatory or ulcerative conditions of the large colon.

REFERENCE MATERIAL

Types of enemas

Evacuant enemas

An evacuant enema is a solution introduced into the rectum or lower colon with the intention of its being expelled, along with faecal matter and flatus, within a few minutes. The following solutions are used:

1. Phosphate enemas with standard or long rectal tubes in single-dose disposable packs.
2. Dioctyl sodium sulphosuccinate 0.1%, sorbitol 25% in single-dose disposable packs.
3. Sodium citrate 450 mg, sodium alkysulphoacetate 45 mg, sorbic acid 5 mg in single-dose disposable packs.
4. Oxyphenisatin in powder for reconstitution.
5. Tap water.

Enemas containing dioctyl sodium sulphosuccinate lubricate and soften impacted faeces. Phosphate enemas are useful in bowel clearance before X-ray examination and surgery.

Tap water may be dangerous when administered as an enema to a child or to those with poor cardiac function, as excessive absorption could lead to circulatory overload (Milton-Thompson, 1971).

Green soap was formerly very popular as an evacuant enema, especially before childbirth. However, its use has now fallen into disfavour due to numerous adverse reports of mucosal damage, necrosis, extensive sloughing of mucosa, severe haemorrhage, anaphylactic shock and death (Edgell and Johnson, 1973; Lewis, 1965; Pike *et al.*, 1971; Smith, 1967). The limiting factors in soap are alkalis, potash and phenol. In Hirschsprung's disease, deaths following soap enema have occurred when a potassium-based soap was used. Hyperkalaemia resulted, causing cardiac arrhythmias (Lewin, 1976). Soap is probably a simple irritant; the higher the concentration, the greater the mucosal inflammation that results.

Retention enemas

A retention enema is a solution introduced into the rectum or lower colon with the intention of being

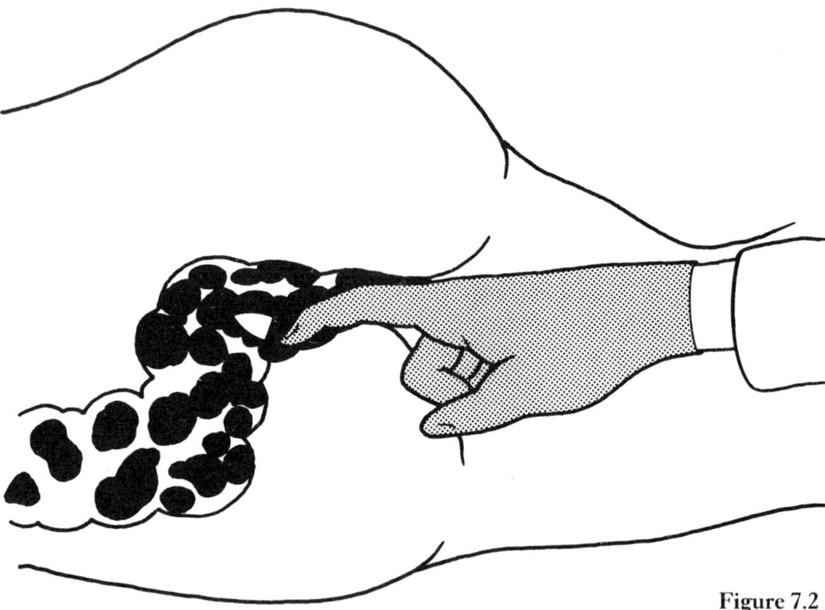

Figure 7.2 Administration of suppositories.

retained for a specified period of time. Three types of retention enema are in common use:

1. Arachis oil (may be obtained in a single-dose disposable pack).
2. Olive oil.
3. Prednisolone.

Enemas containing olive oil will soften and lubricate impacted faeces. Retention enemas given to administer medications will be prescribed by the doctor. The product must be checked with the prescription before its administration.

SUPPOSITORIES

Definition

A suppository is a solid or semi-solid pellet introduced into the anal canal for medicinal purposes.

Indications

The use of suppositories is indicated under the following circumstances:

1. To empty the bowel before certain types of surgery.
2. To empty the bowel to relieve acute constipation or when other treatments for constipation have failed.
3. To empty the bowel before endoscopic examination.
4. To introduce medication into the system.
5. To soothe and treat haemorrhoids or anal puritus.

Contraindications

The use of suppositories is contraindicated when one or more of the following pertain:

1. Chronic constipation, which would require repetitive use.
2. Paralytic ileus.
3. Colonic obstruction.
4. Following gastrointestinal or gynaecological operations, unless on the specific instructions of the doctor.

REFERENCE MATERIAL

Many elderly people find repeated enemas both unpleasant and uncomfortable, and in cases of severe stasis and impaction, whole gut irrigation or colonic lavage may be preferable (Currie, 1979). Hunt (1974) states that the advantages of colonic lavage are that it clears the colon more effectively when visual observation of the interior of the colon is necessary and in cases of disordered action with constipation. However, the disadvantages include the risk of bowel perforation and the inadvertent washing away of the protective mucus which the bowel secretes. Its use is contraindicated in cases of diverticular disease and colitis.

Suppositories may be favoured as they are both easier to adminster (see Figure 7.2) and generally cause the patient less discomfort.

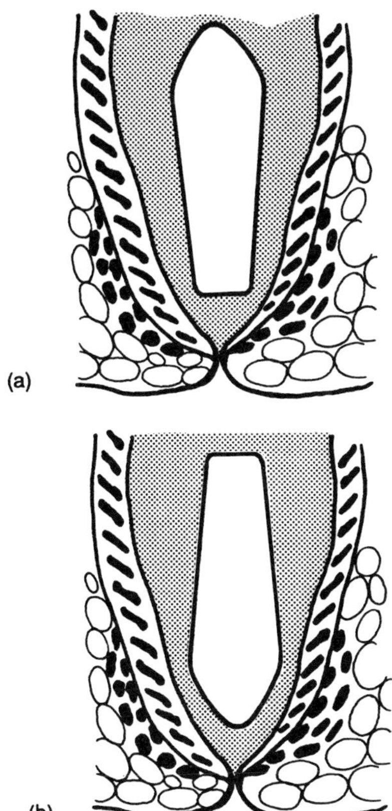

Figure 7.3 (a) A suppository administered in the conventional manner to have a local action and promote defaecation. (b) A suppository administered blunt end forward to minimize local discomfort and maximize systemic therapy.

Administration of suppositories

The use of suppositories dates back to about 460 BC. Hippocrates recommended the use of cylindrical suppostories of honey smeared with ox gall (see Hurst, 1970). Several types are now commonly available.

Lubricant suppositories, e.g. glycerine, should be inserted directly into the faeces and allowed to dissolve to enable softening of the faecal mass (see Figure 7.2). However, stimulant types, such as bisacodyl, must come into contact with the mucus membrane of the rectum if they are to be effective. Other types, such as sodium bicarbonate and anhydrous sodium acid phosphate, exert their influence by releasing carbon dioxide, causing rectal distension when they contact water or mucous membrane.

Walker (1982) has shown that if a suppository is being used to obtain a systemic action it should be inserted blunt end forward to minimize rectal discomfort or irritation and maximize the retention period. It should be inserted in the conventional manner for local action to promote defaecation (Figure 7.3).

RECTAL LAVAGE

Definition

Rectal lavage is the washing out of the rectum using large volumes of non-sterile fluid.

Indications

Rectal lavage is performed for the following purposes:

1. To clear the lower bowel before investigation by barium enema and thus enable good images to be obtained.
2. To assist in clearing the lower bowel before major abdominal surgery and thus decreasing the risk of infection and aiding satisfactory healing.
3. To clear the lower bowel of residual faecal matter following previous surgery, e.g. formation of colostomy.

Contraindications

Rectal lavage is contraindicated in patients who have a history of any one of the following:

1. Severe or prolapsed haemorrhoids.
2. Anal fissure.
3. Inflammatory bowel disease.
4. Large tumour in the rectum or sigmoid colon.
5. Post-radiation proctitis.
6. Internal fistulae.
7. Previous extensive deep X-ray therapy to the pelvis.
8. Recent bowel surgery.
9. Congestive cardiac failure.
10. Impaired renal function.

In points 1 to 8 of the contraindications listed above, the reason for employing caution is because of the damage that could be inflicted by the mechanical aspects of rectal lavage. When the bowel has already been traumatized there is a greater potential risk of causing irritation or, in extreme cases, perforation while inserting the catheter and running large volumes of fluid in and out of the rectum.

With the last two contraindications the potential risk lies with the possibility of large amounts of fluid and/or electrolytes becoming absorbed through the bowel. (Generally speaking, with the amounts and type of fluid used and the relatively short time that it stays in the bowel, this should not present a major problem.)

REFERENCE MATERIAL

Choice of fluid

Several solutions can be used to clear the bowel.

Hypertonic solutions

Hypertonic solutions, e.g. sodium phosphate and sodium acid phosphate in solution, act by drawing water from the intestinal cells by osmosis. This increases the fluid in the faecal mass, causing first distension then contraction and defaecation.

For patients who have a large amount of faecal matter to evacuate, small volumes of these solutions are very effective. Hypertonic solutions should not be given to patients whose capacity to utilize sodium is affected, as some sodium may be absorbed. These solutions are available as commercially prepared enemas but are not suitable for administration in large volumes.

Tap water

Rectal lavage is a procedure that is normally used in combination with other methods of clearing the bowel, e.g. oral aperients and dietary restrictions. In this situation, it can be anticipated that there will be very little residue remaining in the lower bowel. What is needed, therefore, is a simple, non-sterile solution that can be used with relative safety in large volumes to wash out the residual faecal matter. The solution which fulfils these criteria ideally is tap water.

Rectal lavage using tap water is not without risk as large volumes of this hypotonic solution can upset the patient's electrolyte balance. Water is drawn by osmosis into the intestinal cells and water intoxication can result, with symptoms of weakness, sweating, pallor, vomiting, coughing and dizziness. However, this is a relatively rare complication and generally tap water is very well tolerated.

The other advantages of tap water are as follows:

1. It is cheap and easily available.
2. It can be easily warmed to the correct temperature.
3. It is non-irritant to the bowel mucosa.
4. It does not cause excessive peristalsis with resulting cramps and colic.

Caution should be exercised when giving tap water lavage to infants or patients with altered kidneys or cardiac reserve, but otherwise tap water is the solution of choice.

Isotonic saline

An isotonic saline solution can be substituted for patients with compromised electrolyte status. This is prepared by adding two level teaspoons of salt to one litre of plain water. Its effect on the bowel is similar to that of water in that it stimulates peristaltic action by distending the intestinal walls. With isotonic saline, however, there is less danger of electrolyte imbalance.

Choice of catheter

Several manufacturers produce rectal catheters. The criteria for selection should be as follows:

1. The catheter should be of an adequate length. Most are approximately 30 cm long.
2. The lumen should be large enough to allow the free drainage of particulate matter, i.e. a minimum Charrière gauge of 24.
3. The tip of the catheter should be open ended or have large opposed eyelets to minimize the possibility of blockage.
4. The catheter should be made from a soft flexible material; rubber or plastic is suitable.

References and further reading

Booth, S. & Booth, B. (1986) Aperients can be deceptive. *Nursing Times*, 24 September, 82(39), 38–9.

British Medical Association/Pharmaceutical Society of Great Britain (1988) *British National Formulary*. BMA, London.

Clarke, B. (1988) Making sense of enemas. *Nursing Times*, 84(30), 40–4.

Cooper, P. (1976) The treatment of constipation. *Midwife, Health Visitor and Community Nurse*, 12, 165.

Corman, M. *et al.* (1975) Cathartics. *American Journal of Nursing*, 75, 273–9.

Currie, J. E. J. (1979) Whole gut irrigation. *Nursing Times*, 75, 1570–1.

Department of Health (1991) *Report on Health and Social Subjects 41, Dietary Reference Values for Food Energy and Nutrients for the United Kingdom* pp. 61–71. HMSO, London.

Dorgu, R. E. O. (1971) *Bowel Function – Disorders and Management*. Butterworths, London.

Duffin, H. M. *et al.* (1981) Are enemas necessary? *Nursing Times*, 77(45), 1940–1.

Edgell, R. W. & Johnson, W. D. (1973) Postpartum hypotension and erythema: an adverse reaction to soap enema. *American Journal of Obstetrics and Gynecology*, 117, 1146–7.

Haber, G. B. *et al.* (1977) Depletion and disruption of dietary fibre. *Lancet*, 2, 679–82.

Harris, W. (1980) Bran or aperients? *Nursing Times*, 76, 81–3.

Hunt, T. (1974) Colonic irrigation. *Nursing Mirror*, 139(1), 76–7.

Hurst, Sir A. (1970) *Selected Writings of Sir Arthur Hurst (1989–1944)*. Spottiswode, Ballantyne.

Janes, E. (1979) Constipation: keeping a true perspective. *Nursing Mirror*, 149(13), Supplement, p. x.

Jenkins, D. J. A. *et al.* (1981) Glycaemic index of foods: a physiological basis for carbohydrate exchange. *American Journal of Clinical Nutrition*, 34, 362–6.

Lewin, D. (1976) Care of the constipated patient. *Nursing Times*, 72, 444–6.

Lewis, A. E. (1965) Dangers inherent in soap enemas. *Pacific Medicine and Surgery*, 73, 131–3.

Milton-Thompson, G. J. (1971) Constipation. *Nursing Mirror*, 132, 30–3.

Mortimer, P. M. (1970) A worrying problem – constipation. *Health Visitor*, 43, 47–8.

Pike, B. F. *et al.* (1971) Soap colitis. *New England Journal of Medicine*, 285(4), 217–18.

Pirrie, J. (1980) Constipation in the elderly. *Nursing*, 1(17), 753–4.

Roberts, A. (1987) Systems of life, No. 146. *Nursing Times*, 83(5), 47–8.

Rutter, K. & Maxwell, D. (1976) Constipation and laxative abuse. *British Medical Journal*, 2, 997–1000.

Sadler, C. (1988) The power of purgatives. *Community Outlook*, June, 11–12.

Smith, D. (1967) Severe anaphylactic reaction after a soap enema. *British Medical Journal*, 215(4), 215.

Smith, S. (1987) Drugs and the gastrointestinal tract. *Nursing Times*, 83(26), 50–2.

Thompson, M. & Bottomley, H. (1980) Normal and abnormal bowel function. *Nursing*, 1(17), 721–2.

Walker, R. (1982) Suppository insertion. *World Medicine*, 18, 58.

Weller, B. (1989) *Encyclopaedic Dictionary of Nursing and Health Care*, Baillière Tindall, Eastbourne.

Wieck, L. *et al.* (1986) *Illustrated Manual of Nursing Techniques*, 3rd edn. J. B. Lippincott, Philadelphia.

Wilson, A. & Muir, T. (1975) Geriatric faecal incontinence. *Nursing Mirror*, 140(16), 50–2.

GUIDELINES: ADMINISTRATION OF ENEMAS

Equipment

1. Disposable incontinence pad.
2. Disposable gloves.
3. Topical swabs.
4. Lubricating jelly.
5. Rectal tube and funnel (if not using a commercially prepared pack).
6. Solution required or commercially prepared enema.
7. Bath thermometer.

Procedure

Action	**Rationale**
1. Explain the procedure to the patient.	To obtain the patient's consent and co-operation.
2. Ensure privacy.	To avoid unnecessary embarrassment to the patient.
3. Allow patient to empty bladder first if necessary.	A full bladder may cause discomfort during procedure.
4. Ensure that a bedpan, commode or toilet is readily available.	In case the patient feels the need to expel the enema before the procedure is completed.
5. Warm the enema to the required temperature by immersing in a jug of hot water, testing with a bath thermometer. A temperature of 40.5 to 43.3°C is recommended for adults. Oil retention enemas should be warmed to 37.8°C.	Heat is an effective stimulant of the nerve plexi in the intestinal mucosa. An enema temperature of body temperature or just above will not damage the intestinal mucosa. The temperature of the environment, the rate of fluid administration and the length of the tubing will all have an effect on the temperature of the fluid on the rectum.

Guidelines: Administration of enemas

Action	**Rationale**
6. Assist the patient to lie in the required position, i.e. on the left side, with knees well flexed, the upper higher than the lower one, and with the buttocks near the edge of the bed.	This allows ease of passage into the rectum by following the natural anatomy of the colon. In this position gravity will aid the flow of the solution into the colon. Flexing the knees ensures a more comfortable passage of the enema nozzle or rectal tube.
7. Place a disposable incontinence pad beneath the patient's hips and buttocks.	To reduce potential infection caused by soiled linen. To avoid embarrassing the patient if the fluid is ejected prematurely following administration.
8. Wash hands with bactericidal soap and water or bactericidal alcohol hand rub, and put on disposable gloves.	To reduce cross-infection.
9. Place some lubricating jelly on a topical swab and lubricate the nozzle of the enema or the rectal tube.	To prevent trauma to the anal and rectal mucosa by reducing surface friction.
10. Expel excessive air and introduce the nozzle or tube slowly into the anal canal while separating the buttocks.	The introduction of air into the colon causes distention of its walls, resulting in unnecessary discomfort to the patient and increases peristalsis. The slow introduction of the lubricated tube will minimize spasm of the intestinal wall.
(A small amount of air may be introduced if bowel evacuation is desired.)	(Evacuation will be more effectively induced due to the increased peristalsis.)
11. Slowly introduce the tube or nozzle to a depth of 10 to 12.5 cm.	This will bypass the anal canal (2.5 to 4 cm in length) and ensure that the tube or nozzle is in the rectum.
12. If a retention enema is used, introduce the fluid slowly and leave the patient in bed with the foot of the bed elevated by 45° for as long as prescribed.	To avoid increasing peristalsis. The slower the rate at which the fluid is introduced the less pressure is exerted on the intestinal wall. Elevating the foot of the bed aids in retention of the enema by force of gravity.
13. If an evacuant enema is used, introduce the fluid slowly by rolling the pack from the bottom to the top to prevent backflow, until the pack is empty or the solution is completely finished.	The faster the rate of flow of the fluid the greater the pressure on the rectal walls. Distention and irritation of the bowel wall will produce strong peristalsis which is sufficient to empty the lower bowel.
14. If using a funnel and rectal tube, adjust the height of the funnel according to the rate of flow desired.	The forces of gravity will cause the solution to flow from the funnel into the rectum. The greater the elevation of the funnel, the faster the flow of fluid.
15. Clamp the tubing before all the fluid has run in.	To avoid air entering the rectum and causing further discomfort.
16. Slowly withdraw the tube or nozzle.	To avoid reflex emptying of the rectum.
17. Dry the patient's perineal area with a gauze swab.	To promote patient comfort and avoid excoriation and infection.
18. Ask the patient to retain the enema for 10 to 15 minutes before evacuating the bowel.	To enhance the evacuant effect.

19. Ensure that the patient has access to the nurse call system, is near to the bedpan, commode or toilet, and has adequate toilet paper.	
20. Remove and dispose of equipment.	To avoid infection.
21. Wash hands.	
22. Record in the appropriate documents that the enema has been given, its effects on the patient and its results (colour, consistency, content and amount of faeces produced).	To monitor the patient's bowel function.

NURSING CARE PLAN

Problem	Cause	Suggested action
Unable to insert the nozzle of enema pack or rectal tube into the anal canal.	Tube not adequately lubricated.	Apply more lubricating jelly.
	Patient in an incorrect position.	Ask the patient to draw knees up further towards the chest.
	Patient apprehensive and embarrassed about the situation.	Ensure adequate privacy and give frequent explanations to the patient about the procedure.
	Patient unable to relax anal sphincter.	Ask the patient to take deep breaths and 'bear down' as if defaecating.
Unable to advance the tube or nozzle into the anal canal.	Spasm of the canal walls.	Insert the tube or nozzle more slowly, thus minimizing spasm.
Unable to advance the tube or nozzle into the rectum.	Blockage by faeces.	Allow a little solution to flow and then insert the tube further.
	Blockage by tumour.	If resistance is still met, stop the procedure and inform a doctor.
Patient complains of cramping or the desire to evacuate the enema before the end of the procedure.	Distension and irritation of the intestinal wall, which produce a stong peristalsis sufficient to empty the lower bowel.	Temporarily stop the insertion of fluid by clamping the tubing or lowering the funnel until the patient says the feeling has subsided.
Patient unable to open bowels after an evacuant enema and the fluid has not returned.	Reduced neuromuscular response in the bowel wall.	Insert a rectal tube and try to siphon the fluid off. Measure and record the amount. If this is not successful, perform rectal lavage. (For further information, see Rectal Lavage, above.) Measure and record the amount returned.

GUIDELINES: ADMINISTRATION OF SUPPOSITORIES

Equipment

1. Disposable incontinence pad.
2. Disposable gloves.
3. Topical swabs or tissues.
4. Lubricating jelly.
5. Suppository(ies) as required (check the prescription before administering a medicinal suppository, e.g. aminophylline).

Procedure

Action	Rationale
1. Explain the procedure to the patient. If you are administering a medicated suppository, it is best to do so after the patient has emptied his/her bowels.	To obtain the patient's consent and co-operation. To ensure that the active ingredients are not impeded from being absorbed by the rectal mucosa or that the suppository is not expelled before its active ingredients have been released.
2. Ensure privacy.	To avoid unnecessary embarrassment to the patient.
3. Ensure that a bedpan, commode or the toilet is readily available.	In case of premature ejection of the suppositories or rapid bowel evacuation following their administration.
4. Assist the patient to lie in the required position, i.e. on the left side, with the knees flexed, the upper higher than the lower one, with the buttocks near the edge of the bed.	This allows ease of passage of the suppository into the rectum by following the natural anatomy of the colon. Flexing the knees will reduce discomfort as the suppository is passed through the anal sphincter.
5. Place a disposable incontinence pad beneath the patient's hips and buttocks.	To avoid unnecessary soiling of linen, leading to potential infection and embarrassment to the patient if the suppositories are ejected prematurely or there is rapid bowel evacuation following their administration.
6. Wash hands with bactericidal soap and water or bactericidal alcohol hand rub, and put on gloves.	To reduce the risk of cross-infection.
7. Place some lubricating jelly on the topical swab and lubricate the blunt end of the suppository if it is being used to obtain systemic action. Separate the patient's buttocks and insert the suppository blunt end first, advancing it for about 2 to 4 cm. Repeat this procedure if a second suppository is to be inserted.	Lubricating reduces surface friction and thus eases insertion of the suppository and avoids anal mucosal trauma. Research has shown that the suppository is more readily retained if inserted blunt end first. (For further information see Suppositories, above.) The anal canal is approximately 2 to 4 cm long. Inserting the suppository beyond this ensure that it will be retained.
8. Once suppository(ies) has been inserted, clean any excess lubricating jelly from the patient's perineal area.	To ensure the patient's comfort and avoid anal excoriation that may then lead to infection.
9. Ask the patient to retain the suppository(ies) if it is of an evacuant type. If it is medicated, ask the patient to retain the suppository for 20 minutes, or until he/she is no longer able to do so.	This will allow the suppository to melt and release the active ingredients.

10. Remove and dispose of equipment.

To avoid infection.

11. Record that the suppository(ies) have been given, the effect on the patient and the result (amount, colour, consistency and content) in the appropriate documents.

To monitor the patient's bowel function.

GUIDELINES: ADMINISTRATION OF RECTAL LAVAGE

Equipment

1. Rectal lavage pack containing a large funnel, rubber tubing, a straight connector, a one-litre jug and a rectal catheter (Charrière guage 24). (Commercial packs are also available.)
2. Non-sterile topical swabs.
3. Lubricating jelly.
4. Disposable gloves.
5. Disposable incontinence pad.
6. Plastic sheet and draw sheet.
7. Large non-sterile jug.
8. Bucket.
9. Gate clip or clamp.
10. Toilet paper or tissues.
11. Disposable plastic apron.
12. Large disposable bag.
13. Measured volume of warm tap water (37 to 40°C).

Procedure

Action	Rationale
1. Explain the procedure to the patient.	To obtain the patient's consent and co-operation.
2. Prepare the area where the lavage is to be performed, i.e. the patient's bed or a couch in the room where rectal lavage is to take place. Protect the bed or couch with a plastic sheet and draw sheet. Place a disposable incontinence pad on the floor.	To prevent non-disposable equipment becoming contaminated with faecal matter, thus minimizing the risk of cross-infection.
3. Wash hands with bactericidal soap and water or bactericidal alcohol hand rub, and dry hands, clean the trolley and prepare the equipment for the procedure by opening the pack and laying out the contents on the top of the shelf.	Although this is not an aseptic procedure, care must be taken to avoid unnecessary contamination.
4. Attach a large disposable bag to the trolley.	To provide a suitable receptacle for safe disposal of potentially large amounts of contaminated waste.
5. Fill a large non-sterile jug with a measured volume of warm (37 to 40°C) tap water. Check the temperature with a lotion thermometer. Place the filled jug on the lower shelf of the trolley. Put a bucket for receiving effluent by the side of the bed or couch.	As the bowel is not sterile, there is no need to use sterile fluid. A large volume needs to be available for use, up to a maximum of six litres, although the total amount used will vary with each patient and may be much less. If the solution is too warm, the intestinal mucosa may be damaged; if too cold, unnecessary cramping may occur.

Guidelines: Administration of rectal lavage

Action	Rationale
6. Assist the patient to lie in the required position, i.e. on the left side, with the knees well flexed the upper higher than the lower one, and with the buttocks near the edge of the bed. Tilt the foot of the bed slightly upwards if possible.	This position allows ease of access for insertion of the catheter into the rectum, follows the natural anatomy of the colon and aids gravity in promoting the flow of fluid into the sigmoid and descending colon. Tilting the bed also aids the flow.
7. Check that the patient's clothing is tucked out of the way and that both the patient and the bed are adequately protected. Ensure that the patient is as comfortable as possible before continuing with the procedure.	As the procedure can be lengthy and is potentially messy, the patient needs to be as relaxed and well protected as possible to aid successful completion.
8. Wash hands with bactericidal soap and water or bactericidal alcohol hand rub, and put on disposable gloves and a disposable plastic apron.	To reduce cross-infection and for nurse's protection.
9. Connect up the funnel, tubing and rectal catheter, using a straight connector between the latter two items. Fix a gate clamp or clip in position approximately 15 cm from the end of the rectal catheter.	To allow the tubing and the catheter to be primed and filled with fluid, thus preventing the entry of air into the rectum and discomfort to the patient.
10. Using non-sterile topical swab lubricate the last 15 cm of the rectal catheter with a generous amount of lubricating jelly.	To aid insertion and minimize patient discomfort and trauma to the rectal mucosa.
11. Fill a small jug with one litre from the measured volume of warm tap water.	A small jug is more manageable and allows measurement of the amount of fluid used each time.
12. Prime the catheter and the tubing.	
13. Gently insert 7.5 to 10 cm of the catheter into the rectum.	The rectum is approximately 12.5 cm long and the anal canal 2.5 cm. Inserting the catheter 7.5 to 10 cm ensures that the rectum will be adequately filled with the minimum trauma to the patient.
14. Encourage the patient to take deep breaths.	Deep breathing relaxes the anal sphincter.
15. Check that the patient is comfortable.	
16. Fill the funnel with approximately 400 ml of fluid from the jug.	The rectum will hold 200 to 400 ml without causing trauma.
17. Hold the funnel about 30 cm above the rectum, release the clamp and allow the fluid to run into the rectum, holding the catheter in position.	Aqueous solution exerts pressure of 0.225 kg for every 30 cm of elevation. The pressure should not exceed 0.45 kg as this may cause cramping or even rupture of the intestinal wall.
18. Ask the patient to rock gently from side to side.	To ensure efficient lavage of the bowel lumen.
19. Before the funnel is completely empty, invert it over the bucket to allow the lavage fluid and faecal matter to drain out.	To prevent unnecessary amounts of air entering the rectum and causing the patient discomfort.

Action	Rationale
20. Refill the funnel with another measure of fluid, keeping the tubing pinched or clamped and the funnel at patient level until it is filled.	
21. Pepeat the last two procedures until:	
(a) The effluent runs clear. (b) A maximum volume of six litres has been used.	If the bowel is not clear after this volume, other methods need to be employed.
22. Note how much fluid was used during the procedure.	To ensure that not more than six litres are used to reduce the risk of circulatory fluid overload.
23. At the end of the procedure:	
(a) Measure the amount of effluent obtained and compare it with the volume run in.	To ensure that the patient has not absorbed fluid in such a quantity that will carry the risk of fluid overload.
(b) Clear away and dispose of equipment.	To avoid infection.
(c) Ensure that the patient is clean and tidy.	
24. Settle the patient into bed, on an incontinence pad and with a bedpan or commode at hand.	To reduce potential infection caused by soiled linen.

NURSING CARE PLAN

Problem	**Cause**	**Suggested action**
Fluid will not run in freely.	Catheter is pressed against the bowel wall.	Gently manoeuvre the catheter around in the rectum.
	Catheter is blocked with faecal material.	Remove the catheter and unblock. Reinsert and recommence procedure.
	Insufficient gravity flow.	Raise the funnel slightly, but never over 60 cm above the mattress.
Leakage of fluid around the catheter.	Poor positioning of the catheter or displacement following insertion. Poor tone of the anal sphincter muscles.	Check that the catheter is 7 to 10 cm into the rectum. Hold it gently in position. Ask the patient to try and tighten muscles as fluid is run in. Elevate the foot of the bed to aid flow.
Discomfort and/or cramping when the fluid is run in.	Fluid is too cold.	Check the temperature of the fluid and warm it if necessary.
	Pressure of the fluid entering the rectum is too high.	Lower the funnel to stop fluid from running until the spasm passes, but leave the catheter in to relieve distension.
	Extreme tension and anxiety.	When the spasm has passed, gradually raise the funnel and allow fluid to enter very slowly. Encourage deep breathing through the mouth to relax the abdominal muscles and decrease colonic pressures.

Nursing care plan

Problem	**Cause**	**Suggested action**
	Perforation of the rectum.	Stop the procedure immediately. Inform a doctor.
Severe pain accompanied by perspiration, pallor and tachycardia.	Perforation of the gut around the site of a large tumour due to increased peristalsis.	Check the patient's vital signs. Inform a doctor. Do not allow the patient to eat or drink until seen by a doctor.
Blood is returned in the effluent.	Insertion of the catheter has caused internal haemorrhoids to bleed.	Stop the procedure and inform a doctor. Record the appropriate amount of blood that has been passed and observe further bowel motions.
	Trauma to rectal mucosa.	
Large discrepancy between amount of fluid run in and the effluent obtained.	Excessive leakage on to pads during the procedure.	Try to estimate the amount of fluid on pads etc.
	Patient has retained a certain amount of fluid that may be passed later.	Measure carefully all subsequent bowel actions.
	Patient has absorbed the excess fluid.	Check the patient's vital signs. Record further intake and output carefully. Inform a doctor.
Sudden onset of pallor, perspiration, vomiting, coughing and dizziness.	Water intoxication due to absorption of water from the rectum.	Stop the procedure immediately. Inform a doctor. Check the patient's vital signs.

8

Cardiopulmonary Resuscitation

Definition

Cardiac arrest can be defined as the abrupt cessation of cardiac function which is potentially reversible. Respiratory and cardiac arrest may produce similar signs but there is one important difference: cardiac arrest – no arterial pulse; respiratory arrest – arterial pulse is present.

The three main mechanisms of cardiac arrest are:

1. Asystole.
2. Ventricular fibrillation.
3. Electromechanical dissociation.

Indications

Indications of cardiac arrest are as follows:

1. The patient rapidly loses consciousness, becoming pale and cyanosed with absent pulses in major vessels (carotid and femoral arteries).
2. Respiration is slow and stertorous or absent.
3. The pupils become dilated and unresponsive to light.

REFERENCE MATERIAL

Principles

The primary objective of cardiopulmonary resuscitation is to prevent irreversible cerebral damage due to anoxia by restoring effective circulation within four minutes.

Resuscitation is the emergency treatment of any condition in which the brain fails to receive enough oxygen. The basic technique involves a rapid simple assessment of the patient followed by the ABC of resuscitation (Evans, 1990) (see Figure 8.1a–d).

A Assessment and airway control

Check that the patient is conscious by shaking him/her gently and asking, 'Are you all right?' If there is no response, establish and maintain a clear airway.

B Breathing

If the patient is not breathing, commence and maintain artificial ventilation either by expired air method, i.e. mouth to mouth, or use of an airway plus Ambu-bag and face mask. The patient should initially be given two slow expired breaths of air, each sufficient to cause the chest to rise.

C Circulation

If the patient does not have a pulse in a major artery, i.e. carotid or femoral, then circulation must be established by external cardiac massage (Figure 8.2a,b).

If a cardiac arrest is witnessed or monitored, the first intervention should be the pre-cordial thump. This is delivered from about 20 cm above the chest, sharply on the junction between the lower and middle third of the sternum. The pre-cordial thump is of most value in asystole or ventricular tachycardia. A thump can also be effective on rare occasions within a few seconds of the onset of ventricular fibrillation. It carries little risk and takes only a few seconds (Evans, 1990).

Causes

1. *Cardiac*: cardiac causes are due to coronary occlusion, cardiac tamponade, cardiomyopathy and electrocution.
2. *Respiratory*: respiratory causes are due to airway obstruction, i.e. foreign bodies, pulmonary embolism, pneumothorax and drowning.
3. *Cerebral*: cerebral causes are due to depression of respiratory centre due to:
   (a) Head injury with increased intracranial pressure.
   (b) Overdose of depressant drugs.
   (c) Hypothermia.
   (d) Hypertension.
   (e) Lesions of the central nervous system.

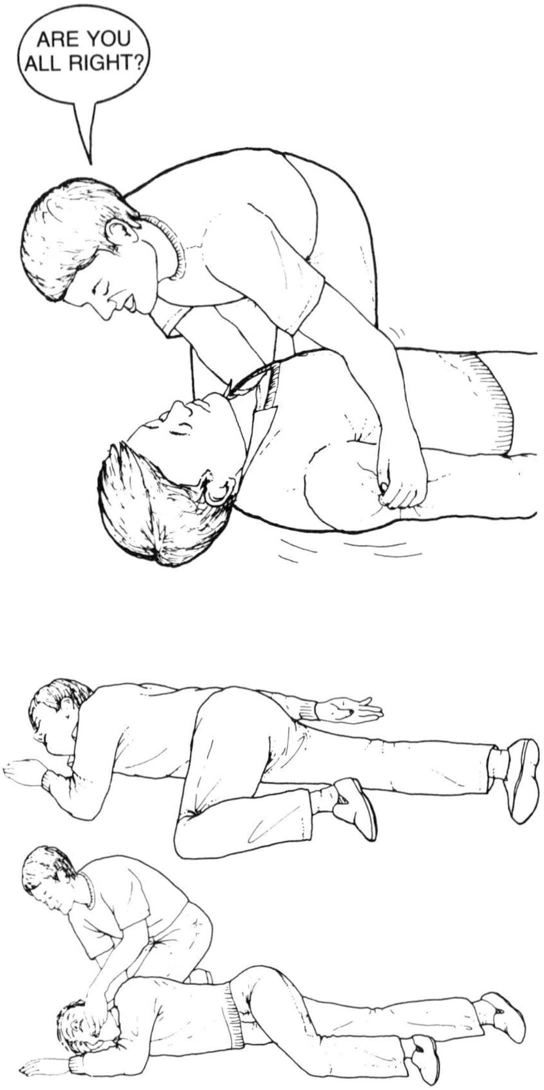

ARE YOU ALL RIGHT?

Recovery position

Figure 8.1 (a) The ABC of resuscitation. Rapid, simple assessment of patient, and placement in the recovery position.

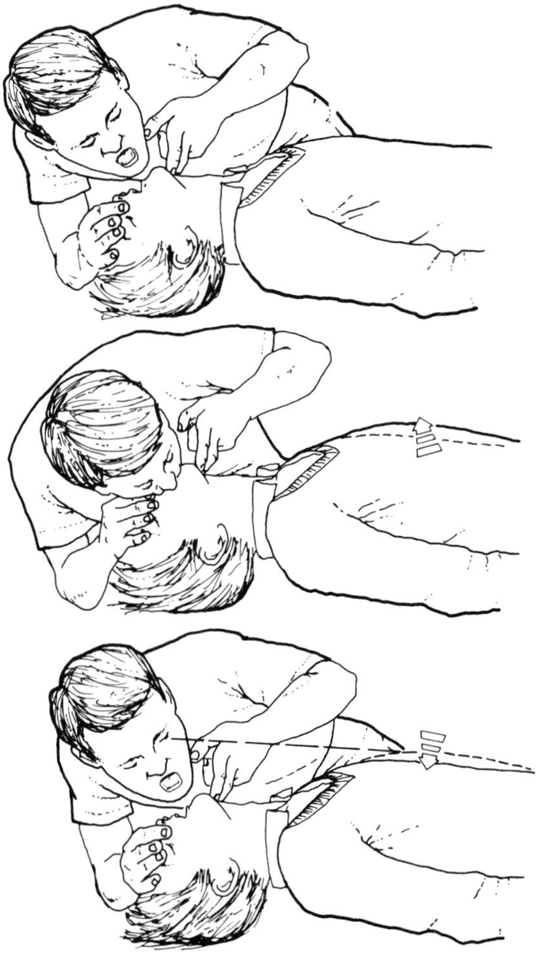

Expired air resuscitation

Figure 8.1 (b) If the patient is not breathing, expired air respiration must be started immediately.

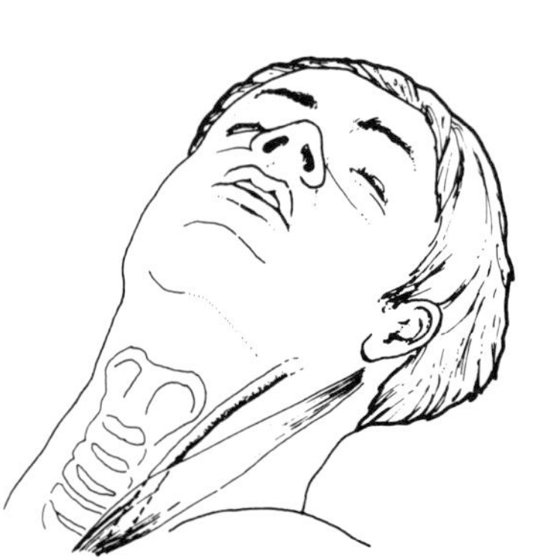

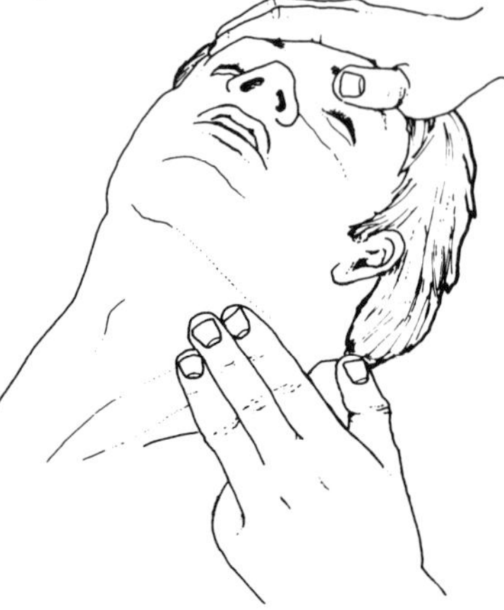

Figure 8.1 (c) If the patient does not have a pulse in a major artery (carotid), or if there is a neck injury, the femoral artery may be felt. Circulation must then be established with compression.

Circulation

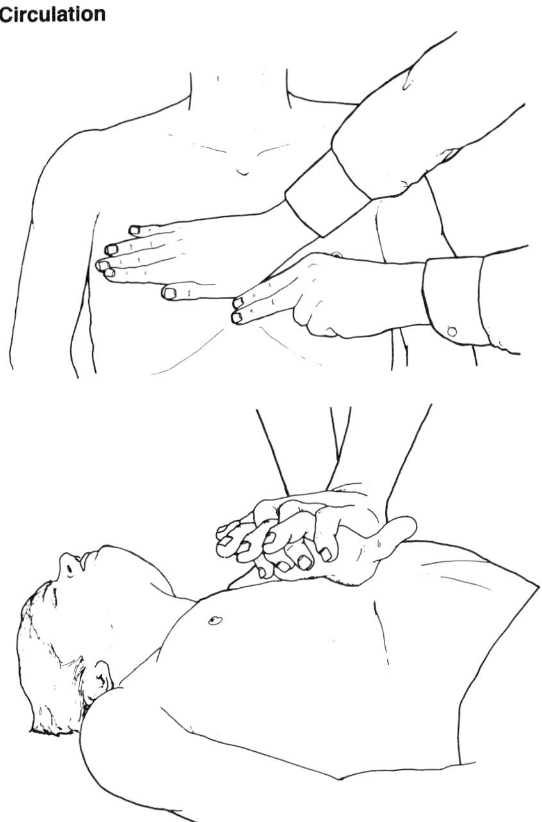

Figure 8.1 (d) Establishing circulation with compression. Note fingers are clear of chest wall. (From *The ABC of Resuscitation*, published by the *British Medical Journal*.).

4. Acid–base balance and electrolyte causes are due to hypo- or hyperkalaemia, acidosis and hypovolaemia caused by severe haemorrhage.

Treatment

Treatment of cardiac arrest is carried out in three stages:

1. Restoration of breathing and circulation.
2. Correction of acid–base balance.
3. Assessment and correction of fluid and electrolyte imbalance.

Drugs

The drugs used in the treatment of cardiac arrest are:

1. Adrenaline 1 mg (10 ml of a 1:10 000 solution) given intravenously. The main purpose of adrenaline is to maintain coronary and cerebral perfusion during a prolonged resuscitation attempt.

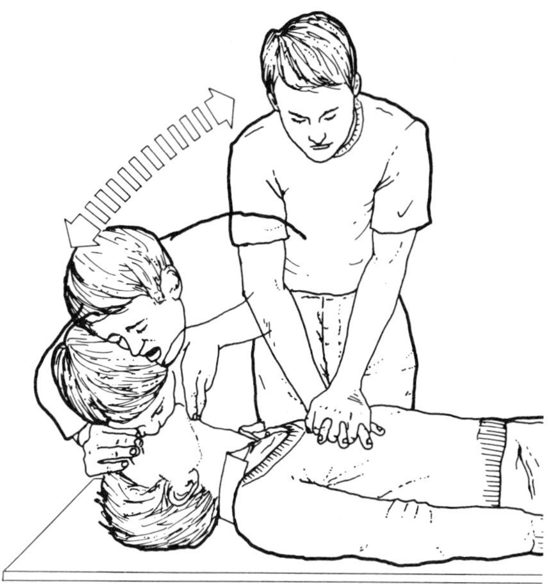

(a) One-rescuer cardiopulmonary resuscitation

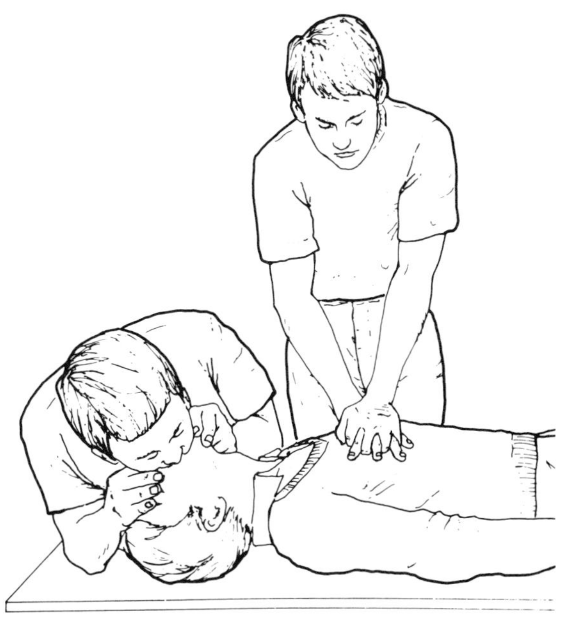

(b) Two-rescuer cardiopulmonary resuscitation

Figure 8.2 Establishing circulation by external cardiac massage. **(a)** When only one rescuer is present, the compression to ventilation ratio is 15:2. **(b)** When two rescuers are present, the compression to ventilation ratio is 5:1. (From *The ABC of Resuscitation*, published by the *British Medical Journal*.)

2. Atropine 2 mg given intravenously. Reduces cardiac vagal tone, increases the rate of discharge of the sinoatrial node and increases the speed of conduction through the atrioventricular node. It is advisable to give atropine for asystole following administration of adrenaline because it blocks all parasympathetic activity.
3. Calcium chloride (10 ml of 10%) is used for the treatment of electromechanical dissociation when the cause is hyperkalaemia, hypocalacaemia, or when calcium antagonist toxicity is present. Calcium has no proven efficacy in asystolic cardiac arrest.
4. Lignocaine 100 mg is given intravenously. The value of lignocaine is its ability to prevent ventricular arrhythmias. It does not facilitate defibrillation. If necessary, the bolus can be repeated, provided that a total of 3 mg/kg is not exceeded. A lignocaine infusion may be commenced if appropriate at a rate of 1 to 3 mg per minute. The side-effects of lignocaine are related to the dosage and size of the patient.
   (a) Early toxic effects are initial stimulation followed by depression of the central nervous system. Early signs appear as sleepiness, dizziness, paraesthesia, blurred or double vision, and sweating.
   (b) More severe signs include hypotension, convulsions and coma.
   (c) At the first signs of toxic effects, the dose should be decreased and it should be stopped altogether if more serious side-effects occur.
5. Sodium bicarbonate 8.4% is now only used in prolonged cardiac arrest or according to blood gas analyses. Potential adverse effects of excessive sodium bicarbonate administration include hypokalaemia, exacerbation of respiratory acidosis and increased affinity of haemoglobin for oxygen. Other adverse effects are increased cardiac irritability and impaired myocardial performance. The usual dose of sodium bicarbonate is 50 mmols (50 ml 8.4%).
6. Bretylium tosylate (400 mg intravenously) is recommended in refractory ventricular fibrillation. It raises the fibrillation threshold, thereby assisting defibrillation. Bretylium achieves its effects relatively slowly, so once this drug is given, chest compressions and defibrillation attempts should continue for a further 20 to 30 minutes. However, this will be appropriate in only a few cases.

The Resuscitation Council of the United Kingdom (Evans, 1990) has issued new guidelines for drug administration and defibrillation sequence. Cardiopulmonary resuscitation should not be interrupted for more than 10 seconds, and should be continued for up to two minutes after each drug is administered. If an intravenous line cannot be established, then double doses of adrenaline or lignocaine may be given via the endotracheal tube, but drug absorption is unpredictable using this method.

Defibrillation

Defibrillation causes a simultaneous depolarization of the myocardium and aims to restore normal rhythm to the heart. This is the immediate treatment for ventricular fibrillation and ventricular tachycardia. Defribillation can be used for a patient who has had a cardiac arrest even if a monitor is not available.

The carrying out of defibrillation by nurses in special units, i.e. coronary care and intensive care, is becoming an accepted practice, provided nurses have received proper training. This also depends on guidelines laid down in hospital policies.

Please see Figure 8.3 for the treatment of electromechanical dissociation, ventricular fibrillation and asystole.

The resuscitation team

Most hospitals now have a designated cardiac arrest team. This usually consists of four or five personnel (Evans, 1990):

1. A duty medical registrar.
2. An anaesthetic registrar.
3. Senior house officer.
4. A porter (and trolley).
5. A senior nurse.

The team will require bleeps, with a speech channel so that the operator can give the exact location of the emergency.

Statistics

Sudden cardiac death most frequently occurs in the first one to two hours after the onset of symptoms due to fatal arrhythmias, usually ventricular fibrillation.

Cozart Rosequist (1987) suggests that if cardiopulmonary resuscitation is initiated quickly and promptly by well-trained lay people or emergency medical personnel, then between 40 and 80% of patients with documented ventricular fibrillation can be resuscitated successfully.

In the United Kingdom, community resuscitation has been slower to improve (Evans, 1990). However, with the advent of a nationwide programme of extended training of ambulance staff in resuscitation, and the introduction of a training programme aimed

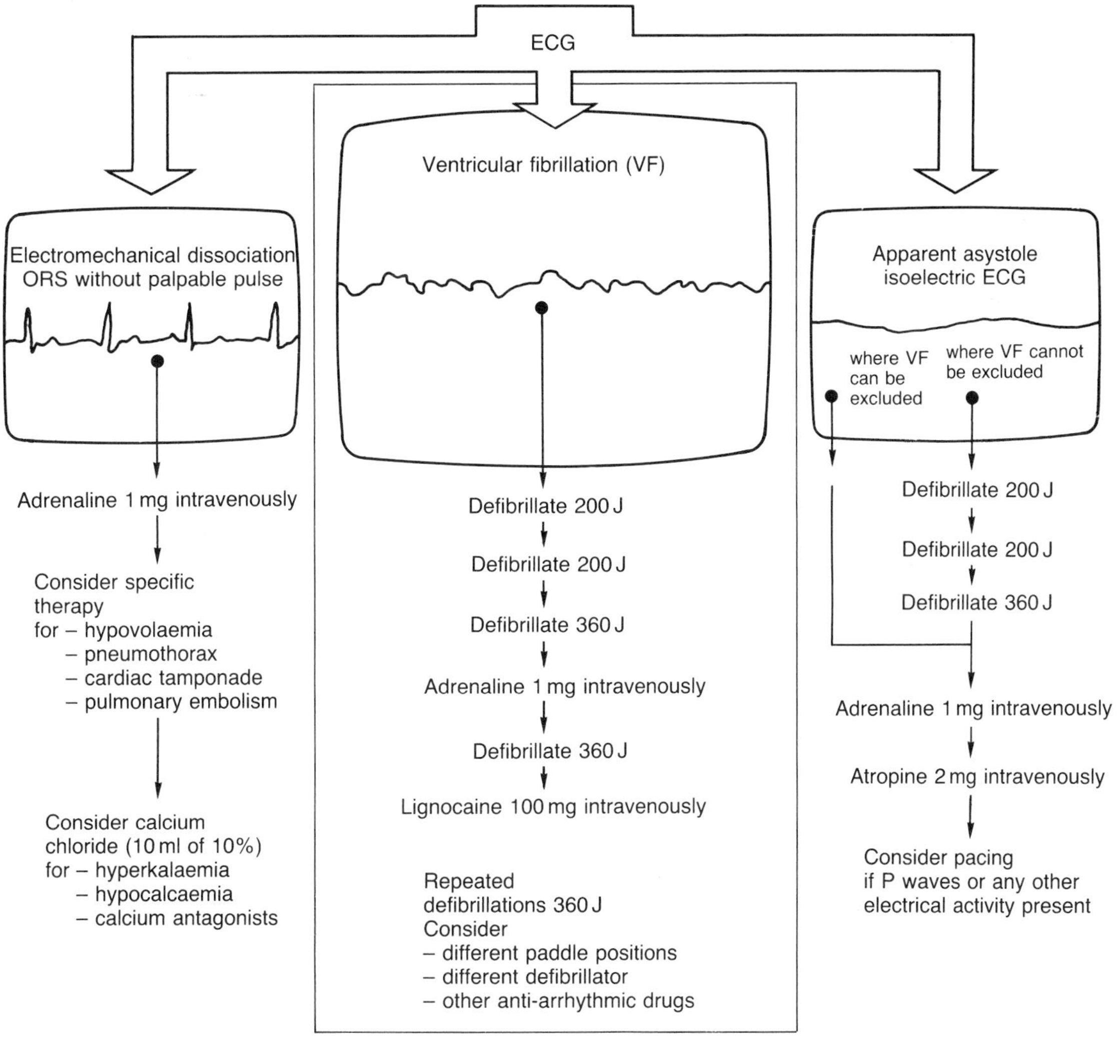

ECG

Electromechanical dissociation
QRS without palpable pulse

Adrenaline 1 mg intravenously
↓
Consider specific therapy
for – hypovolaemia
– pneumothorax
– cardiac tamponade
– pulmonary embolism
↓
Consider calcium chloride (10 ml of 10%)
for – hyperkalaemia
– hypocalcaemia
– calcium antagonists

Ventricular fibrillation (VF)

Defibrillate 200 J
↓
Defibrillate 200 J
↓
Defibrillate 360 J
↓
Adrenaline 1 mg intravenously
↓
Defibrillate 360 J
↓
Lignocaine 100 mg intravenously

Repeated
defibrillations 360 J
Consider
– different paddle positions
– different defibrillator
– other anti-arrhythmic drugs

Apparent asystole
isoelectric ECG

where VF can be excluded → Adrenaline 1 mg intravenously

where VF cannot be excluded
↓
Defibrillate 200 J
↓
Defibrillate 200 J
↓
Defibrillate 360 J
↓
Adrenaline 1 mg intravenously
↓
Atropine 2 mg intravenously
↓
Consider pacing
if P waves or any other
electrical activity present

Continue cardiopulmonary resuscitation for up to 2 minutes after each drug. Do not interrupt CPR for more than 10 seconds, except for defibrillation.
If an intravenous line cannot be established, consider giving double doses of adrenaline, lignocaine or atropine via an endotracheal tube.

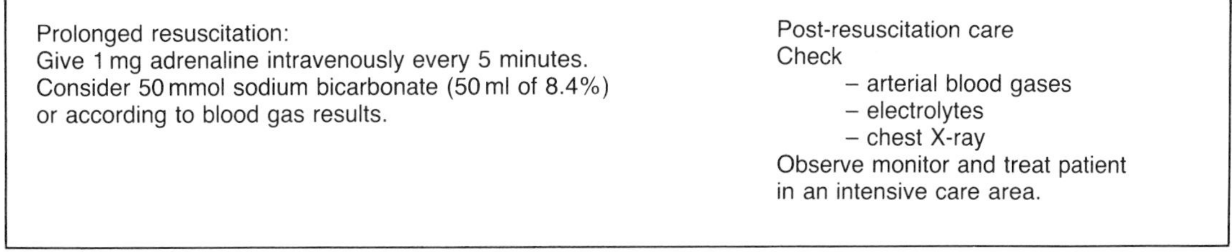

Prolonged resuscitation:
Give 1 mg adrenaline intravenously every 5 minutes.
Consider 50 mmol sodium bicarbonate (50 ml of 8.4%)
or according to blood gas results.

Post-resuscitation care
Check
– arterial blood gases
– electrolytes
– chest X-ray
Observe monitor and treat patient
in an intensive care area.

The Resuscitation Council (UK)

Figure 8.3 Treatment of electromechanical dissociation, ventricular fibrillation and asystole.

at the general public by a few hospitals (Ferguson, 1990), this situation can only improve.

Of equal importance is the fact that hospital staff often do not possess the necessary skills. Wynn (1987) has shown the poor performance by nursing staff in resuscitation. This indicates an obvious need for more training, and a revision of skills.

Ethics

The increase in skills, knowledge, technology and pharmacological support have proved very effective in prolonging quality of life. However, the assessment of patients suitable for resuscitation is controversial. There are many important factors which need to be considered in deciding whether to resuscitate a patient or not:

1. The patient's disease and prognosis.
2. Events leading to cardiopulmonary arrest.
3. The patient's wishes and the wishes of the family or friends.
4. The quality of life of the patient and expected quality after discharge.

The decision on whether or not to resuscitate should involve all personnel in the clinical team. Ideally, this decision should be made before the event. However or whenever these decisions are made, the problems must be discussed openly and freely, so that the medical profession is not accused of prolonging misery because personnel are afraid to make the decision.

Dangers associated with resuscitation

Diseases such as auto-immune deficiency syndrome (AIDS) and hepatitis B have now come into focus with regard to mouth-to-mouth resuscitation. Research into the human immunodeficiency virus (HIV) virus being transmitted during resuscitation is still in its infancy although there is no evidence to date that HIV is transmitted by saliva, and there are airway adjuncts which can be used. Pocket face masks and mouth shields are available commercially, but such devices must not hinder airflow; more importantly, resuscitation should not be delayed until one is at hand.

References and further reading

Andreoti, K. G. *et al.* (1975) *Comprehensive Cardiac Care*, 3rd edn. C. V. Mosby, St Louis.

Bridges, W. & MacLeod Clark, J. (1981) *Communication in Nursing*. HM & M Publishers, London.

Cavanagh, S. J. (1990) Educational aspects of cardiopulmonary resuscitation (CPR) training. *Intensive Care Nursing*, 6(1), 38–40.

Cozart Rosequist, C. (1987) Current standards and guidelines for cardiopulmonary resuscitation and emergency cardiac care. *Heart and Lung Journal of Critical Care (Heart Lung)*, 16(4), 408–18.

Evans, T. R. (1990) *ABC of Resuscitation*, 2nd edn. British Medical Journal Publications, London.

Ferguson, A. (1990) Cardiopulmonary resuscitation . . . a teaching guide. *Nurse Education Today*, 10(1), 50–3.

Lawrence, J. A. (1982) The nurse should consider: critical care ethical issues. *Journal of Advanced Nursing*, 7(3), 223–9.

McPhail, A., Moore, S. *et al.* (1981) One hospital's experience with a 'do not resuscitate' policy. *Canadian Medical Association Journal*, 125, 830–6.

Neatherlin, J. S. & Brillhart, B. (1988) Glasgow Coma Scores in the patient: post-cardiopulmonary resuscitation. *Journal of Neuroscience Nursing*, 20(2), 104–9.

Sloman, M. (1988) Paediatric cardiopulmonary resuscitation. *Nursing Times*, 84(43), 50–2.

Stirba, C. (1988) Cardiopulmonary resuscitation in patients with acquired immunodeficiency syndrome (letter). *Archives of Internal Medicine*, 149(10), 2380.

Voladez L. & Garcia, R. M. (1987) Resusci annie proves safe. *Journal of Continuing Education in Nursing*, 18(5), 160–2.

Wynn, G. (1987) Inability of trained nurses to perform basic life support. *British Medical Journal*, 294(6581), 1198.

GUIDELINES: CARDIOPULMONARY RESUSCITATION

Equipment

All hospital wards and appropriate departments, i.e. computerized axial tomography (CT) scanning department, should have a cardiac arrest trolley or box. A list of the items should be drawn up and checked weekly or immediately after use, by ward staff or designated personnel.

1. Airways (different sizes).
2. Ambu-bag with valve and mask.
3. Oxygen tubing.
4. Tongue forceps.
5. Suction apparatus.
6. Oropharyngeal suction catheters.
7. Laryngoscope with spare bulbs and batteries.

8. Magill's forceps.
9. Endotracheal tubes (different sizes) and introducer.
10. Gauze swabs.
11. Lubricating jelly.
12. 10 ml syringe for use with endotracheal tube.
13. Artery forceps.
14. Endotracheal suction catheter.
15. Bandage or tracheostomy tape.
16. Scissors.
17. Catheter mount with swivel connector.
18. Emergency cardiac drugs (prefilled syringes).
19. Intravenous infusion giving sets.
20. Selection of intravenous cannulae.
21. Strapping.
22. Syringes and needles (various sizes).
23. Alcohol swabs.
24. Intravenous infusion stand.
25. ECG monitor plus adhesive electrodes.
26. Defibrillator with conductive gel pads for defibrillation.

Procedure

Action	Rationale
1. Note time of arrest, if witnessed.	Lack of cerebral perfusion for approximately 3 to 4 minutes can lead to irreversible brain damage.
2. If arrest is witnessed or monitored, give patient pre-cordial thump.	This may restore cardiac rhythm, which will give a cardiac output.
3. Summon help. If a second nurse is available, he/she can call for the cardiac arrest team, bring emergency equipment and screen off the area.	Cardiopulmonary resuscitation is more effective with two rescuers. One is responsible for inflating the lungs, and the other for chest compressions. Continue until medical help arrives.
4. Lie patient flat on firm surface. A King's Fund bed now provides such a surface; failing this, a board may be placed under the mattress, or the patient may be placed on the floor.	Effective external cardiac massage can be performed only on a hard surface.
5. If patient is in bed, remove bed head, and ensure adequate space between back of bed and wall.	To allow easy access to patients' head in order to facilitate intubation.
6. Ensure a clear airway; extend, not hyperextend, the neck (thus lifting the tongue off the posterior wall of the pharynx). This is best achieved by lifting the chin forwards with the finger and thumb of one hand while pressing the forehead backwards with the heel of the other hand. If this fails to establish an airway, there may be obstruction by a foreign body. Try to remove the obstruction if possible.	To establish and maintain airway, thus facilitating ventilation.
Do not remove well-fitted dentures.	They help to create a mouth seal during ventilation.
7. Insert airway, and place mask over patient's mouth and nose, making sure a seal is created.	To ventilate lungs, and avoid escape of air around face mask. It avoids contact with patient's mouth, thus minimizing risk of disease transmission.

Guidelines: Cardiopulmonary resuscitation

Action	Rationale
8. Locate the base of the sternum, then place one hand the width of two fingers above this point over the lower third of the sternum, midline. Ensure that only the heel of the hand is touching the sternum.	To increase and maintain coronary and cerebral blood flow.
Place the other hand on top, straighten the elbows and make sure shoulders are directly over the patient's chest. The sternum should be depressed sharply by 2 to 4 cm. The cardiac compressions should be forceful, and sustained at a rate of 60 to 80 per minute.	Pressure on the lower half of the sternum of sufficient weight will compress the sternum and force blood out of the ventricles and improve blood flow.
9. Compress the Ambu-bag in a rhythmical fashion: the bag should be attached to oxygen source. In order to deliver 100% oxygen, a reservoir may be attached to the Ambu-bag. If, however, oxygen is not immediately available, the Ambu-bag will deliver ambient air.	To ensure a constant and steady supply of oxygen. The brain and heart have a very low tolerance to hypoxia, and any increase in the blood oxygen content will improve the chances of survival of these organs. Room air contains only 21% oxygen.
10. Maintain cardiac compression and ventilation at a ratio of 15:2 for one-rescuer resuscitation, and 5:1 for two-rescuer resuscitation (see Figure 8.2a,b). This rate can be achieved effectively by counting out loud 'one and two' etc. There should be a slight pause to ensure that the delivered breath is sufficient to cause the patient's chest to rise. This must continue until cardiac output returns and the patient has a palpable blood pressure.	To maintain circulation and oxygenation, thus reducing risk of damage to vital organs.
11. When the cardiac arrest team arrives, it will assume responsibility for the arrest.	
12. Attach patient to ECG monitor, apply three electrodes: the negative electrode is applied just under the outer quarter of left shoulder; the ground electrode is applied beneath the right clavicle; and the positive electrode is placed at the fourth right intercostal space, right sternal border (Andreoti *et al.*, 1975).	To obtain adequate ECG signal. Accurate recording of cardiac rhythm will determine the appropriate treatment to be initiated.

Intubation

Action	Rationale
13. Continue to ventilate and oxygenate the patient before intubation.	The risks of cardiac arrhythmias due to hypoxia are decreased.
14. Equipment for intubation should be checked before handing to appropriate medical staff: (a) Suction equipment is operational. (b) The cuff of the endotracheal tube inflates and deflates.	

(c) The endotracheal tube is well lubricated.
(d) That catheter mount with swivel connector are attached.

15. During intubation, the anaesthetist may request cricoid pressure. This involves compressing the oesophegus between the cricoid ring and the sixth cervical vertebra to prevent regurgitation.

Aspiration of stomach contents during intubation can cause a chemical pneumonitis with an increased mortality.

16. Recommence ventilation and oxygenation once intubation is completed.

Intubation should interrupt resuscitation only for a few seconds to prevent the occurrence of cerebral anoxia.

Intravenous lines

Action	**Rationale**
17. Venous access must be established through a large vein as soon as possible.	To administer emergency cardiac drugs and fluid replacement.
18. Asepsis should be maintained throughout.	To prevent local and/or systemic infection.
19. The correct rate of infusion is required.	To ensure maximum drug and/or solution effectiveness.
20. Accurate recording of the administration of solutions infused and drugs added is essential.	For reference in the event of any queries.

Defibrillation

Used to terminate ventricular fibrillation or ventricular tachycardia.

Post-resuscitation care

Complete recovery from cardiac arrest does not happen immediately.

1. Check the patient by assessing breathing, circulation, blood pressure and urine output.
2. Check arterial blood gasses and electrolytes.
3. Monitor patient's cardiac rhythm.
4. Chest X-ray should be taken.
5. Continue oxygen therapy.
6. Assess patient's level of consciousness. This can be done by use of the Glasgow Coma Scale. Although this is intended primarily for head injury, it is clinically relevant. It contains five levels of consciousness:
   (a) Conscious and alert.
   (b) Drowsy but responsive to verbal commands.
   (c) Unconscious but responsive to minimal painful stimuli.
   (d) Unconscious and responsive to deep painful stimuli.
   (e) Unconscious and unresponsive.
7. The patient should be made comfortable and nursed in the appropriate position, i.e. upright or the recovery position. Careful explanation and reassurance is vital at all times, particularly if the patient is conscious and aware. Patients are often subject to strange and uncomfortable sensations due to infusion lines and/or monitoring leads attached to them. These can also leave the patient feeling trapped (Bridges & McCleod Clark, 1981).

The patient should be transferred to a special unit, i.e. coronary care or intensive care.

NURSING CARE PLAN

Problem	Cause	Suggested action
Only one nurse immediately available.	Colleagues in other areas of ward. If an emergency occurs during the night, the second nurse may be having rest break.	Use emergency buzzer to summon help, or shout. Commence resuscitative measures immediately using airway, breathing and circulation (ABC) technique.
Breathing is absent.	Obstructed airway due to the tongue falling onto the posterior pharyngeal wall. Airway obstruction can occasionally be caused by foreign bodies, e.g. food, dentures, etc.	Establish and maintain a clear airway: extend (*not* hyperextend) the neck and lift the chin forward with the finger and thumb of one hand, and press down on the forehead with the other. Check for foreign bodies. If this does not relieve obstruction and patient is still not breathing, commence expired air respiration immediately either by mouth-to-mouth resuscitation or by using an airway or Ambu-bag and mask. For effective ventilation, ensure the mask covers the nose and mouth correctly in order to create an airtight seal.
The patient is a child or infant		Resuscitation should begin at once. An increased rate of compression is necessary (100 to 120 per minute, depending on age). Respirations should be at the rate of 20 to 24 per minute. The adult ratio of two ventilations to 15 compressions can be used in older children. A ratio of five compressions to one ventilation should be used in infants and younger children. Continue resuscitation until help arrives.
Patient has a radioactive source implanted.		See the procedures for iodine-131 (Chapter 22) and sealed radioactive sources (Chapter 35).

9

Central Venous Catheterization

Definition

Placement of an indwelling catheter within the superior or inferior vena cava or right atrium, or a large vein leading to these vessels.

Indications

This procedure is indicated in the following circumstances:

1. To monitor central venous pressure in seriously ill patients.
2. For the administration of large amounts of intravenous fluid or blood, e.g. in cases of shock or major surgery.
3. To provide long-term access for:
   (a) Hydration or electrolyte maintenance.
   (b) Repeated administration of drugs, such as cytotoxic and antibiotic therapy.
   (c) Repeated transfusion of blood or blood products.
   (d) Repeated specimen collection.
4. For total parenteral nutrition.

REFERENCE MATERIAL

The catheter

In the past decade there have been numerous developments in both catheter design and materials, resulting in a greater range of devices. This has had a beneficial effect on patient care due to improvements in insertion techniques and nursing management.

Table 9.1 lists examples of available catheters. This is not intended to be a comprehensive list as recent progress has been rapid, with many new products entering clinical use. Double- and triple-lumen catheters have provided solutions to the problems of multiple access and the inclusion of extra features such as 'on/off' switches has simplified nursing practice.

Insertion of the catheter

The catheter may be inserted at any of the sites shown in Figure 9.1. If the site chosen is the antecubital fossa, a 'long line' will be used as the catheter has to pass a substantial distance through the venous system.

The catheter may be inserted directly into the vein or it may be tunnelled subcutaneously for a short distance prior to entry (see Figure 9.1). Skin tunnelling is usually performed if the catheter is intended to provide long-term access over a number of months, during which the patient may be discharged and readmitted. The purpose of the tunnel is to remove the entry site into the vein from the exit site on the skin, so providing a barrier to infection. Catheters specifically designed for skin tunnelling

Table 9.1 Examples of common catheter materials

Catheter material	*Recommended indwelling life*	*Common site(s) of insertion*	*Capacity for skin tunnelling*
Teflon	5–7 days	Jugular	No
Polyethylene	8–10 days	Jugular Subclavian Antecubital fossa	No
Silicone	Indefinite	Cephalic Axillary Subclavian Antecubital fossa	Yes (may be connected to an implanted port)
Polyurethane II	Indefinite	Subclavian/jugular	No

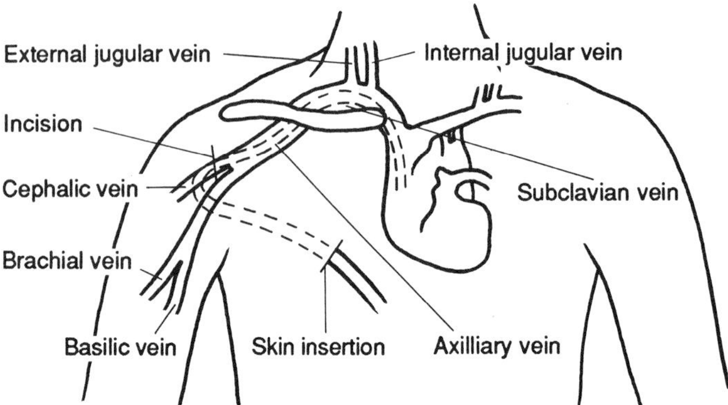

Figure 9.1 The ideal position and site for a long-term indwelling catheter.

frequently have a Dacron cuff sited part way along their length. This cuff is positioned in the subcutaneous tunnel and tissue granulates around it so reinforcing the barrier to invading organisms and providing security. Local site infection can be observed and treated, the incidence of septicaemia is reduced and removal of the catheter due to contamination is not always necessary. An example of this type of catheter is the Hickman.

A recent development aimed at reducing complications due to infections further is an implantable drug delivery system, consisting of a portal attached to a silicone catheter (Figure 9.2). It is usually inserted under general anaesthetic. Among its advantages over conventional central lines or Hickman catheters are that there are fewer risks of sepsis, heparinization is required less frequently and the system is more aesthetically pleasing. It can be used for bolus injections, infusions of drugs, blood products, total parenteral nutrition and blood sampling (Speechley and Davidson, 1989).

The portal is placed under the skin and sutured to the chest wall. The catheter is tunnelled as previously described and the tip rests in a major vein. The reformation of the skin barrier prevents the entry of micro-organisms, and strict aseptic technique should result in a minimal contamination rate.

A variety of catheters and portals are available, the choice of which is dependent on a number of factors. For example, whether the patient is a child or an adult, amount of access necessary etc. The portal is accessed using a special Huber point needle when therapy is required and this may remain in place for up to one week (See Guidelines: Care of Implantable Ports, below).

The hazards associated with the insertion of a central venous catheter are substantial (Table 9.2). For that reason the procedure should be performed in a controlled environment, and the operating theatre or anaesthetic room is preferred. When this is not possible, a quiet environment with a minimum of activity is recommended.

A general anaesthetic may be necessary for some insertions but often the procedure is performed under heavy sedation using local anaesthesia. The doctor inserts the catheter with the nurse assisting. The nurse's responsibilities are:

1. To ensure the patient has been given a full explanation of the procedure and to teach the patient techniques which may be required during

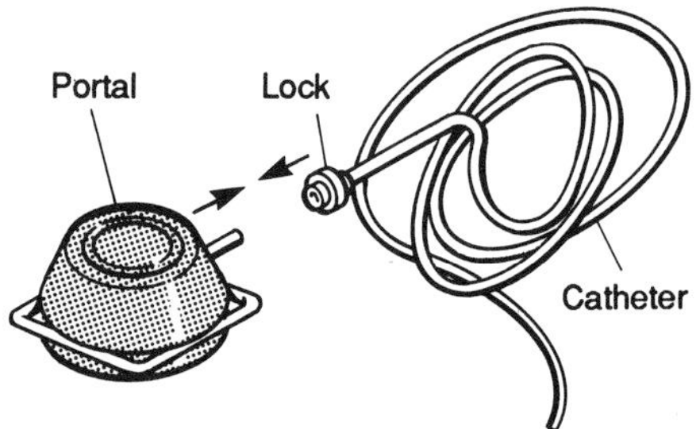

Figure 9.2 Components of a Port-a-Cath implantable delivery system.

Table 9.2 Hazards of catheter insertion

Sepsis	Air embolism	Pneumothorax
Hydrothorax	Haemorrhage	Haemothorax
Brachial plexus injury	Thoracic duct trauma	Misdirection or kinking
Catheter embolism	Thrombosis	Cardiac tamponade
		Cardiac arrhythmias

insertion; for example the Valsalva manoeuvre (see below).
2. To ensure that any specific preoperative instructions have been carried out.
3. To explain the postoperative procedures and the appearance and function of the catheter or device.
4. To assemble the equipment requested.
5. To prepare fluids with which to test the patency of the catheter.
6. To prepare local anaesthesia and dressing materials.
7. To ensure the correct positioning of the patient during insertion, that is, in the supine or Trendelenburg position, with the head down and a roll of towel along the spinal column.
8. To attend to the physical and psychological comfort of the patient during and immediately following the procedure.
9. To ensure that no fluid or medication is infused before the correct position of the catheter is confirmed by X-ray.

Reducing the likelihood of the above complications and preventing distress to the patient may be achieved by careful insertion techniques, strict asepsis, correct positioning and radiological confirmation of the catheter placement. The catheter should be heparinized or normal saline infused slowly, 10 to 20 ml/h, until X-ray results confirm the correct placement of the catheter.

The Valsalva manoeuvre

This may be performed by conscious patients to aid the insertion of the catheter. The patient is placed in the supine or Trendelenburg position which increases venous filling. He/she is asked to breathe in and then try to force the air out with the mouth and nose closed (i.e. against a closed glottis). This increases the intrathoracic pressure so that the return of blood to the heart is reduced momentarily and the veins in the neck region become engorged. A distension of the vein up to 2.5 cm can be achieved in this way.

Principles of catheter care

Prevention of infection

Strict aseptic technique and compliance with recommendations for equipment and dressing changes are essential if microbial contamination is to be prevented. (See Chapter 3, Aseptic Technique.)

Whenever the insertion site is exposed or the closed system is broken, strict aseptic technique should be practised. As blood or body fluids may be present, gloves should be worn to comply with safe technique and practice (see Guidelines: Changing the dressing on a central venous catheter insertion site, below). The insertion site should be checked regularly postoperatively and the dressing renewed if there is haemoserous discharge. There may be local swelling and drainage from the tunnel when a skin-tunnelled catheter has been inserted. A pressure dressing or application of an ice pack may reduce the severity of these problems. The sterile dressing over the insertion site may be renewed weekly. Complaints of soreness, unexpected pyrexia and damaged, wet or soiled dressing are reasons for immediate inspection and renewal. (For further details, see Guidelines: Changing the dressing on a central venous catheter insertion site, below.)

When the dressing is changed, the site should be observed for inflammation and/or discharge and the conditions of the skin noted. Alternatives must be considered in cases where the skin is delicate and a conventional semi-occlusive dressing could traumatize it, for example, in bone marrow transplantation patients and children. For these patients a dry, sterile gauze dressing secured with a minimum of tape may be more suitable. This dressing should be changed daily.

Following the healing of the skin tunnel and removal of the sutures from a Hickman-type catheter at 14 to 21 days, no dressing is necessary unless the patient requests one.

Maintenance of a closed system

If equipment becomes disconnected, air embolism or profuse blood loss may occur, dependent on the condition and position of the patient at the time. Luer locks provide a more secure connection and all equipment should have these fittings, i.e. giving sets, extension sets, injection caps and syringes. Care should be taken to clamp the line firmly when changing equipment, and the switch provided on some catheters must be used. Connections must be double checked and precautions taken to prevent the introduction of air into the system when making additions to, or taking blood from, the central line.

Maintenance of a patent catheter

It is important at all times for the patency of the line to be maintained. Blockage predisposes to damage, injection, inconvenience to patients and disruption to protocols. Occlusion of the catheter is usually the result of clot formation due to:

1. An administration set or mechanical aid being turned off accidentally and left for a prolonged period.

2. Insufficient flushing of the catheter when not in use.
3. Precipitate formation due to inadequate flushing between incompatible medications.

It is therefore important to use an injection technique using positive pressure to ensure fluid is retained in the catheter as this appears to decrease the incidence of clot formation. Patency of the line may also be impaired by kinking of the line. Meticulous intravenous technique will prevent the majority of these problems.

When used for intermittent therapy, the catheter should be flushed after each use with a solution of heparinized saline, containing 10 units/ml. The volume injected must be between 2.5 and 5 ml. Commercial preparations of this strength are available.

Catheters made of polyurethane and silicone are often *in situ* for prolonged periods of time and may not be used frequently, especially if the patient is discharged. In this situation it is recommended that heparinization with the aforementioned solution is performed twice weekly.

If occlusion does occur, gentle aspiration may dislodge the clot and a flush with normal saline may be all that is required to restore patency. Gentle pressure and suction may need to be repeated if the catheter has been left for a long time and a larger thrombus has formed. Silicone catheters expand on pressure and allow fluid around a clot facilitating its dislodgement. Use of heparin solution may also be tried.

The enzymes urokinase and streptokinase have both been used to dissolve thrombi and restore catheter patency. Although effective, these are potentially dangerous substances and their use must be approved by the medical staff and prescribed accordingly.

When using implanted drug delivery systems, the manufacturer's literature should be consulted with reference to heparinization. The most widely stated recommendation is a flush with 500 units of heparin monthly.

Preventing damage of the catheter and performing a repair

Silicone catheters are prone to cracking or splitting if handled incorrectly but fortunately both temporary and permanent repairs can be performed. However, prevention of this occurrence is preferred.

Artery forceps, scissors or sharp-edged clamps should not be used on or near the catheter. A smooth clamp should be placed on the reinforced section of the catheter provided for this purpose. If this is not present, one can be created by placing a tape tab over part of the catheter. A second alternative is to move the clamp up or down the catheter at regular intervals.

Accidents do occur, however, and the nurse must be familiar with the action to be taken. Immediate clamping of the catheter proximal to the fracture or split is essential to prevent blood loss or air embolism. The split area should be covered with an alcohol swab and emergency repair equipment collected, together with sterile gloves to ensure that all manipulations are aseptic. Figure 9.3 illustrates the steps to be followed.

A permanent repair should be performed as soon as possible using the specific kit provided by the manufacturer. This should be done by a member of the medical staff or other designated personnel.

Pyrexia of unknown origin

In the event of the patient developing a persistent pyrexia or tachycardia, contamination of the catheter should be suspected. However, the catheter should not be removed until infection has been confirmed, unless the clinical condition dictates otherwise. The following investigations must be performed:

1. Blood cultures:
   (a) From the catheter.
   (b) From a peripheral vein.
   (c) Swab from entry site.
2. A full blood count.
3. Midstream specimen of urine for microscopy, culture and sensitivity.
4. Chest X-ray.
5. Other tests, e.g. wound swabs, throat swabs, to eliminate other sources of infection, as appropriate.

Septicaemia

If the patient has a suspected septicaemia, antibiotic cover should be initiated but no further action taken with reference to the catheter until positive blood culture results are received and further decisions made by the medical staff concerned. The line should be heparinized and the infusion stopped.

Indications for catheter removal

1. Blood cultures from the line when tested indicate the presence of micro-organisms.
2. A positive wound swab from the entry site.
3. Generalized septicaemia.
4. A leaking or damaged catheter.
5. Blockage.
6. Termination of therapy.

Catheters should not be removed without consultation with medical staff. The device should be removed carefully using aseptic technique, and the tip of the catheter sent for bacteriological examination.

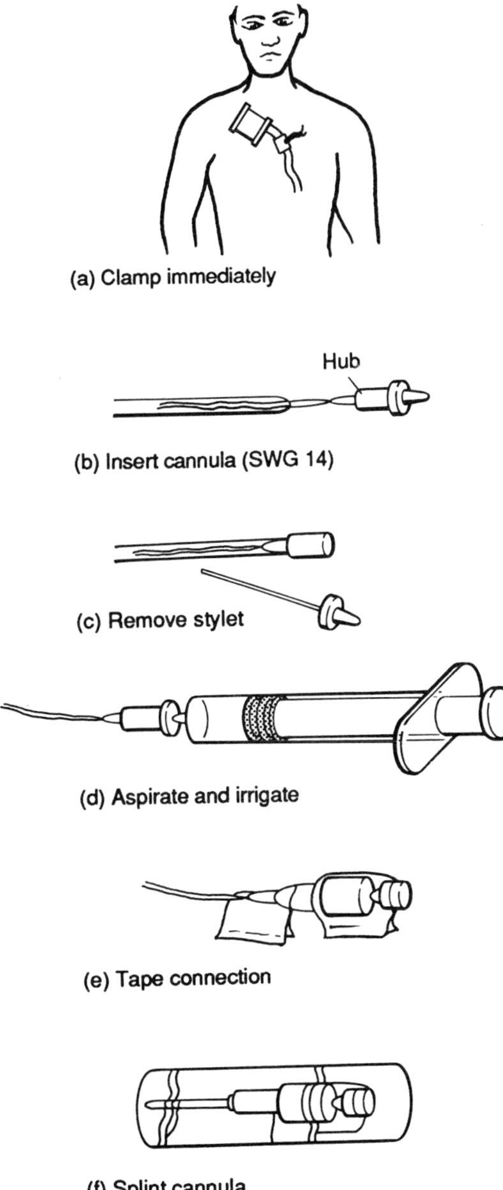

Figure 9.3 Temporary repair of a damaged silicone catheter. (Adapted from Ford, 1986.)

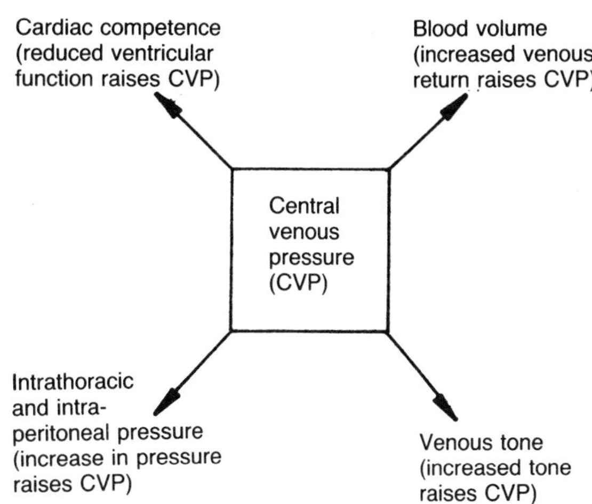

Figure 9.4 Determinants of central venous pressure.

Reading central venous pressure

Central venous pressure (CVP) is the pressure within the superior vena cava or the right atrium. Measurements of CVP reflect the relationship between the circulating blood volume (Figure 9.4), the competence of the heart as a pump and the peripheral vascular resistance.

Purpose of CVP readings

1. To serve as a guide to fluid balance in critically ill patients.
2. To estimate the circulating blood volume.
3. To assist in monitoring circulatory failure.

Measuring CVP

The CVP measurement should be taken from a site in line with the right atrium. Either of the sites indicated in Figure 9.5 may be used, remembering that the sternal angle should be used only with the patient in the supine position, whereas the mid-axilla can be used when the patient is in a variety of other positions. It should be established at the outset which point is to be used, as there is a difference in pressure of about 5 cm of water between them. It is useful to mark the chosen site for future readings and note both the site and the patient's position on the CVP recording chart and also in the patient's care plan. The normal values for CVP readings are: 0 to 5 cm of water at the sternal angle, and 5 to 10 cm of water at the mid-axilla.

Current models of some volumetric infusion pumps have electronic central venous pressure monitoring facilities. These can be accurate, but they are, as yet, no substitute for a manual manometer set which allows greater assessment of patency of line, and accuracy of measurement.

Discharging patients with a central catheter *in situ*

Patients with skin-tunnelled catheters or implanted devices may be discharged home with their line *in situ*. No special instructions are required for implanted

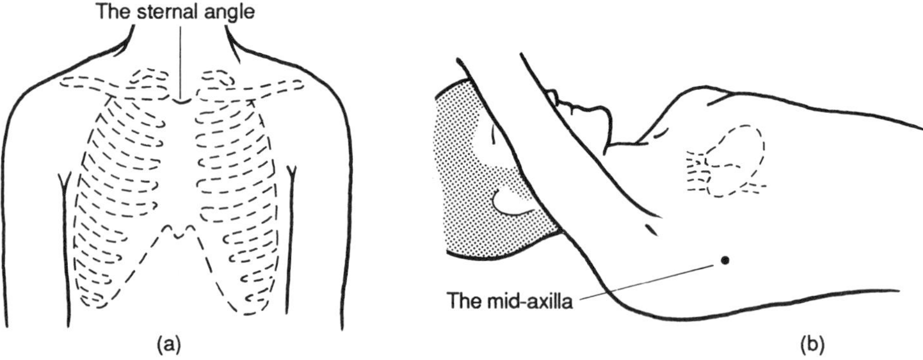

Figure 9.5 Measuring central venous pressure. (a) The sternal angle. (b) The mid-axilla.

ports as the catheter will be heparinized and the needle removed before the patient leaves hospital. Re-heparinization is not necessary for one month.

Patients with Hickman-type catheters must be instructed and supervised in the care of their lines before discharge. Aspects to be covered with the patient, relatives and/or friends include:

1. Care of the exit site.
2. Heparinization techniques.
3. The amount and type of activity permitted.

At the time of discharge the catheter should be well established and the Dacron cuff covered with fibrous tissue, sealing off the catheter insertion site from the skin. In this instance, no dressing is needed unless the patient requests it. If this is so, sterile, low-linting swabs and hypo-allergenic tape may be supplied.

If the individual is discharged before suture removal, the site should be dressed according to hospital policy, and arrangements made for this to be renewed weekly or when the dressing gets wet or soiled. The only other time when a dressing may be required is if the patient participates in water sports. In this instance, the whole catheter and exit site should be covered completely with an occlusive dressing one hour before the activity and removed immediately afterwards. The area should then be dried carefully. Such precautions are not necessary for daily showers or baths, but it must be pointed out to the patient that a separate cloth and towel should always be used to wash and dry the exit site. Similarly, when bathing, the water should not come into contact with the exit site; the site should be cleaned separately with fresh water using low-linting swabs, both to clean and dry.

Before discharge the patient should observe the heparinization technique and perform it with and without supervision. Relatives and friends should be involved in this procedure. Sufficient equipment must be supplied to enable the patient to care for the catheter from the time of discharge until the next outpatient appointment or admission. A kit should be assembled containing the following:

1. Spare Luer lock caps with an injection site.
2. A spare, smooth-edged clamp.
3. A supply of heparinized saline, 50 i.u. in 5 ml.
4. Isopropyl alcohol 70% swabs to clean the injection site on the cap.
5. A supply of sterile 5 ml syringes.
6. 19G needles (white) to draw up the heparinized saline.
7. 25G needles (orange) to inject through the intermittent injection cap.
8. Instruction booklet to provide the patient with a point of reference if in doubt about procedures when at home.
9. A container to store sharps.

The patient's technique and confidence when caring for the catheter should be assessed before discharge and the importance of asepsis during all handling procedures stressed.

There are few restrictions with reference to activity. Modifications of dressing technique to allow the patient to engage in water sports are mentioned above. The psychological impact of an indwelling catheter on body image should not be overlooked, especially when patients are sexually active. Additionally, normal activities may be affected, for example, driving may become uncomfortable due to pressure from a seat belt on the catheter or clamp exit site.

Removal of the catheter

Non-skin tunnelled catheters

If a catheter is not tunnelled through the skin it

may be removed by nursing staff. The nurse must be familiar with the procedure and confident about performing it. Aseptic technique must be adhered to and the site cleaned before removal to prevent a false-positive result when the catheter tip is sent for bacteriological examination. Major vessels usually heal quickly but direct pressure must be applied to the site until cessation of bleeding confirms this. A sterile dressing is applied and should remain in place for at least 24 hours.

Skin-tunnelled catheters

Removal techniques for skin-tunnelled catheters vary but the procedure is normally performed by a doctor due to the risk of the catheter breaking and subsequently resulting in a catheter embolism. This has been reported in a number of studies.

It is recommended that the patient is placed in the same position as for insertion (see above) and that aseptic technique is used throughout. Sedation may be required to relieve anxiety in some patients. The exit site should be cleaned to prevent a false–positive tip culture being obtained. The catheter should be gripped firmly and constant traction applied. It may take a few minutes for the catheter and cuff to become loose before sliding free. Continued steady pressure will remove the complete line. This should be checked immediately after removal before the tip is cut and sent for microbiological examination. The catheter and cuff may be pulled through together, resulting in a slight bleeding from the patient. However, the cuff may remain attached to tissue. This is of no significance and it may be left in place. If the patient or medical staff wish it, the cuff may be surgically excised. Difficulty with removal or a break in the catheter will require surgical intervention. Major vessels usually heal quickly but a dressing may be needed on the exit site for 24 hours (Plumer, 1987).

Note: intravenous management and administration of drugs may be undertaken by means of peripheral or central venous pathways. Only nurses in possession of a certificate of competence, or nurses supervised by a suitably qualified nurse, should perform these procedures.

Total parenteral nutrition

Total parenteral nutrition (TPN) is the direct infusion, into a vein, of solutions containing the essential nutrients in quantities sufficient to meet all the daily needs of the patient.

The decision to administer TPN should be an elective one and should be used only if alternative enteral methods are considered inappropriate or unsatisfactory. Total parenteral nutrition is indicated in any disease or circumstances when the digestive and absorptive functions of the small intestine are seriously impaired (see Table 9.3).

Table 9.3 Indications for total parenteral nutrition (TPN)

Inflammatory bowel disease
Enterocutaneous fistulae
Short bowel syndrome
Severe burns
Bowel obstruction
Infants of very low birth weight
Major abdominal/thoracic surgery

TPN solutions

The basic components of a TPN regime are provided by solutions of:

1. Amino acids (nitrogen source).
2. Glucose (carbohydrate energy source).
3. Fat emulsion (non-carbohydrate energy source).
4. Electrolytes and trace elements.

TPN is usually administered from a single infusion container in which all the requirements for a 24-hour feed are pre-mixed. Such infusions are prepared either by the hospital pharmacy or are purchased. It may be necessary sometimes to exclude fat emulsion from the mixture and to administer it concurrently from separate containers.

To allow for the possible need to vary the constituents of the infusion in response to changes in the patient's nutritional status, TPN solutions should be ordered daily, except on weekends and public holidays, when it is necessary to order and prepare them in advance on Fridays or the last working day before the holiday.

Monitoring of TPN

During TPN, regular observations are required. The following measurements are suggested:

Daily

Sodium mmol/l	Calcium mmol/l
Chloride mmol/l	Potassium mmol/l
Urea mmol/l	Creatinine µmol/l
Glucose mmol/l	
Fluid balance	

Twice weekly

Albumin g/l	Total protein g/l
Magnesium mmol/l	Bicarbonate mmol/l

Table 9.4 An example of a TPN regime for a patient of body weight 60 to 75 kg

Components		*Nutritional composition*	
Vamin 9 glucose	1500 ml	Sodium	97.5 mmol
Glucose 10%	1000 ml	Potassium	72.5 mmol
		Calcium	8.75 mmol
Addiphos	15 ml	Magnesium	3.75 mmol
Potassium chloride 15%	10 ml	Phosphate	37.5 mmol
		Chloride	116 mmol
Addamel	10 ml		
Intralipid 20%	500 ml	Total volume	3045 ml
		Total non-protein calories	2000 kcal
Vitlipid N Adult	10 ml	Total N_2	14.1 g
Solivito N	1 vial	Kcal/N_2 ratio	142:1

Phosphate mmol/l
Bilirubin μmol/l
Aspartate amino transferase (AST) i.u./l
Alkaline phosphatase (ALP) i.u./l
Haemoglobin g/dl
White blood cells × 10^9/l
Packed cell volume %

Delivery of TPN and recommendations for intravenous management

The major hazard associated with delivery of TPN is infection and the following detailed recommendations are designed to prevent this. They reflect the current policy of The Royal Marsden Hospital that was compiled by a multidisciplinary team:

1. Catheter insertion must take place in theatre using full aseptic technique.
2. A skin-tunnelled silicone catheter is the catheter of choice for long-term nutrition.
3. A separate peripheral cannula may be required for insulin infusion via a syringe pump.
4. Peripheral venous access should be assessed before catheter placement; if the veins available are considered inadequate to support the patient for the duration of therapy, a double- or triple-lumen catheter should be inserted.
5. In the event of peripheral access deteriorating during the course of parenteral nutrition, an adaptor for dual access to the nutrition catheter should be used. The adaptor should be streamlined and possess Luer lock fittings.

Dressing of the insertion site

A sterile semi-occlusive transparent dressing will be applied to the insertion site while the patient is in theatre. This should not be touched but the site should be inspected daily. Exceptions to this are:

1. If the site is inflamed, sore or if there is haemoserous discharge.
2. If the dressing is not adequately secured, or torn.

The dressing must be performed in accordance with hospital procedure for the dressing of central venous lines. The entry site is cleaned with 0.4% chlorhexidine in 70% spirit, then an appropriate dressing is applied, e.g. sterile ethylene oxide adhesive surgical dressing. If the site is inflamed, a swab must be sent to the bacteriology department for culture and sensitivity, and the medical staff notified.

Administration sets

Administration sets must be changed every 24 hours, as directed by hospital policy, always using an aseptic technique. Administration sets must have a Luer lock fitting. Infusion containers will be prepared under aseptic conditions in the pharmacy and may be delivered to the ward with administration sets attached. In this instance, the nurse is required to prime the tubing and connect it to the catheter. Before changing the line, the connections should be sprayed with isopropyl 70% and allowed to dry. The line should then be disconnected and the new one attached. All connections should be checked. Existing injection sites on the administration set should never be used for the giving of additional medications. Containers and administration sets should be scheduled for changing in daylight hours, even if this means discarding an incompletely used bag at a time specified on the prescription sheet.

Administration of medications

No additional medications or blood products should be given by means of a parenteral nutrition catheter. It should not be used for central venous pressure (CVP) measurements. The procedure detailed under catheter insertion should be followed, i.e. a peripheral line should be established.

Control of the rate of infusion

Total parenteral nutrition infusions must be closely monitored at all times. An infusion mechanical device (controller or pump) must always be used, especially when TPN is given via a three-litre bag.

No adjustment greater than four drops per minute every 15 minutes should be made to an infusion rate. Never attempt to 'catch up' rapidly if fluid is running slowly. In the event that the patient develops a pyrexia of unknown origin or septicaemia, the same principles outlined above will apply.

Clinical conditions dictating removal of the catheter

Elective

See 'Indications for catheter removal', above.

Termination of therapy

Total parenteral nutrition should not be terminated (except for reasons already stated) until oral or nasogastric feeding is well established. This will be discussed and decided by the medical and surgical staff and dietician. At the end of parenteral nutrition, the catheter need not be removed immediately. It may continue to be used for access or fluids. When the catheter is removed, aseptic technique must be used and the catheter tip sent to bacteriology. A sterile airtight dressing should be placed on the exit site and left in place for at least 24 hours to prevent an air embolism.

Heparinization

Occasionally certain investigations, e.g. computerized tomography, may require the infusion to be discontinued and the catheter heparinized. Simultaneous insulin infusions must also be discontinued. Partly-used infusion containers should never be used again but must be discarded and a fresh one requested from the pharmacy. Problems should be referred to the appropriate member of medical, anaesthetic, pharmacy or nursing staff.

References and further reading

Anderson, M. A. *et al.* (1982) The double-lumen Hickman catheter. *American Journal of Nursing*, 82(2), 272–7.

Bjeletich, J. (1982) Repairing the Hickman catheter. *American Journal of Nursing*, 82(2), 274.

Bjeletich, J. & Hickman, R. O. (1980) The Hickman indwelling catheter. *American Journal of Nursing*, 80(1), 62–5.

Brunner, L. S. & Suddarth, D. S. (1986) *The Lippincott Manual of Nursing Practice*, 4th edn. J. B. Lippincott, Philadelphia.

Davies, J. *et al.* (1978) Disinfection of the skin of the abdomen. *British Journal of Surgery*, 65, 855–8.

Finnegan, S. & Oldfield, K. (1989) When eating is impossible: TPN in maintaining nutritional status. *The Professional Nurse*, March, 4(6), 271–5.

Flannigan, M. (1982) Intravenous feeding. *Nursing Mirror*, 154(16), 44–6; 154(17), 48–52.

Ford, R. (1986) History and organisation of the Seattle-area Hickman catheter committee. *Journal of the Canadian Intravenous Nurses Association*, 2(2), 4–13.

Goodman, M. S. & Wickham, R. (1984) Venous access devices: an overview. *Oncology Nurses Forum*, 11(5), 16–23.

Gyves, J. *et al.* (1982) Totally implanted system for intravenous chemotherapy in patients with cancer. *American Journal of Medicine*, 73, 841–5.

Hinds, C. T. (1988) *Intensive Care*, pp. 32–9. Baillière Tindall, Eastbourne.

Hollingsworth, S. (1987) Getting on line. *Nursing Times*, 83(29), 61–2.

Hurtibise, M. R. *et al.* (1980) Restoring patency of occluded central venous catheters. *Archives of Surgery*, 115, 212–13.

Keohane, P. P. *et al.* (1983) Effects of catheter tunnelling and a nutrition nurse on catheter sepsis during parenteral nutrition. *Lancet*, 2(17), 1388–90.

Lawson, M. *et al.* (1982) The use of urokinase to restore the patency of occluded central venous catheters. *American Journal of IV Therapy and Clinical Nutrition*, 9(9), 29–32.

Mehtar, S. & Taylor, P. (1982) Bacteriological survey of patients undergoing TPN and an IV policy's effects. *British Journal of Intravenous Therapy*, 3(8), 3–11.

Mughal, D. L. (1991) Infected feeding lines. *Care of the Critically Ill*, 6(6), November, 228–32.

Ostrow, L. S. (1981) Air embolism and central venous lines. *American Journal of Nursing*, 81(21), 40–2.

Plumer, A. L. (1987) *Principles and Practices of Intravenous Therapy*, 4th edn. Little, Brown & Co., Boston.

Sellu, D. (1985) Long-term intravenous therapy. *Nursing Times*, 81(21), 40–2.

Speechley, V. & Davidson, T. (1989) Managing an implantable drug delivery system. *The Professional Nurse*, March, 4(6), 284–8.

Thompson, A. *et al.* (1989) Long-term central venous access: the patient's view. *Intensive Therapy and Clinical Monitoring*, May, 10(5), 142–5.

Viall, C. (1990) Daily access of implanted venous port. *Journal of Intravenous Nursing*, 13(5), 294–6.

Wachs, T. (1990) Urokinase administration in paediatric patients with occurred central venous catheters. *Journal of Intravenous Nursing*, 13(2), 100–2.

Woods, S. (1982) Parenteral nutrition. *Nursing*, 2(4), 105–7.

GUIDELINES: READING CENTRAL VENOUS PRESSURE

Equipment

1. Spirit level.
2. Manometer.
3. Central venous pressure (CVP) monitoring intravenous administration set.

Procedure

Action	Rationale
1. Explain the procedure to the patient.	To obtain the patient's consent and co-operation.
2. Ascertain the point of CVP reading, i.e. sternal angle or mid-axilla. If the patient agrees, this point should be marked on the patient and noted in the care plan chart for future reference.	CVP must always be read from the same point because the sternal angle reading is about 5 cm water higher than the mid-axilla reading.
3. Assist the patient to get into a recumbent or semi-recumbent position to a maximum angle of 45°.	The position of the patient must allow the baseline of the manometer to be level with the patient's right atrium. If the patient is upright or is lying on his/her side, the right atrium will not be in line with the sternal angle or the mid-axilla. However, if it is impossible for the patient to be in any other position, the CVP reading may be recorded with the patient sitting up at a 90° angle, but this must be recorded on the observation chart.
4. Position the manometer so that the baseline is level with the right atrium.	To obtain an accurate CVP reading, the baseline and the right atrium must be level.
5. Loosen the securing screw and slide the scale up or down until the baseline figure lies next to the arm of the spirit level (Figure 9.6a) This figure may be 0 but is usually taken as +10 if the CVP reading is more than 2 cm below zero (Figure 9.6b).	Most scales do not extend below 2 cm, therefore the height of the scale must be altered to obtain a reading.

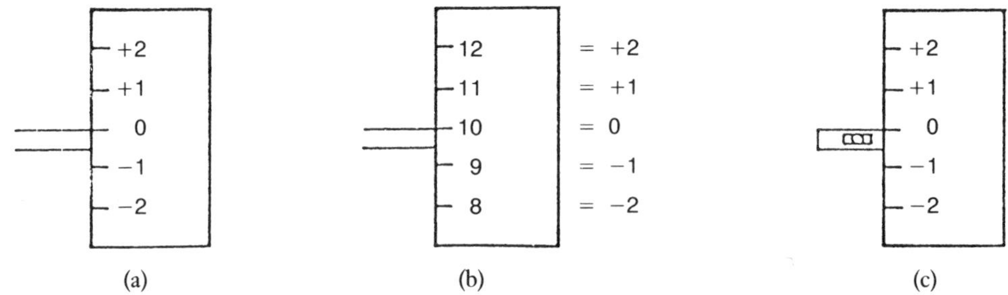

Figure 9.6 (a) and (b) Setting the baseline. (c) Checking the baseline.

Action	Rationale
6. Check that the baseline and right atrium are level by extending the arm of the spirit level to the sternal angle or to the mid-axilla. Move the manometer until the bubble is between the parallel lines of the spirit level (Figure 9.6c).	

7. Flush the line well by allowing the intravenous fluid to run through into the patient.

To ensure the patency of the line and to check for leaks, kinks, blockages, etc.

8. Turn off the three-way tap to the patient (Figure 9.7). Allow the manometer to fill slowly.

To allow the intravenous fluid to run into the manometer. To avoid:
- Bubbles, which cause inaccurate readings.
- Overfilling of, and spillage from, the manometer that would put the patient at risk from infection.

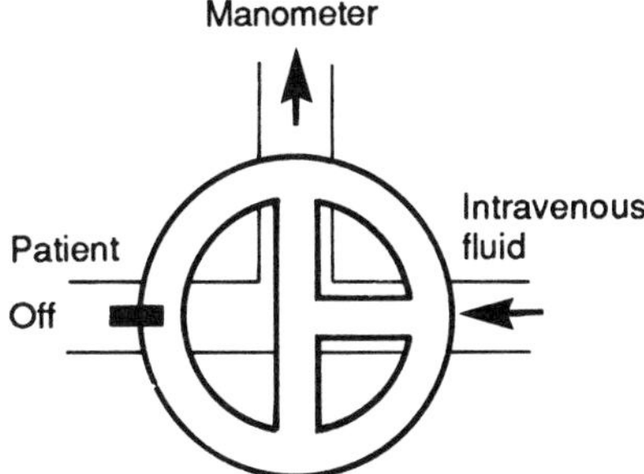

Figure 9.7 Turn off the three-way tap to the patient.

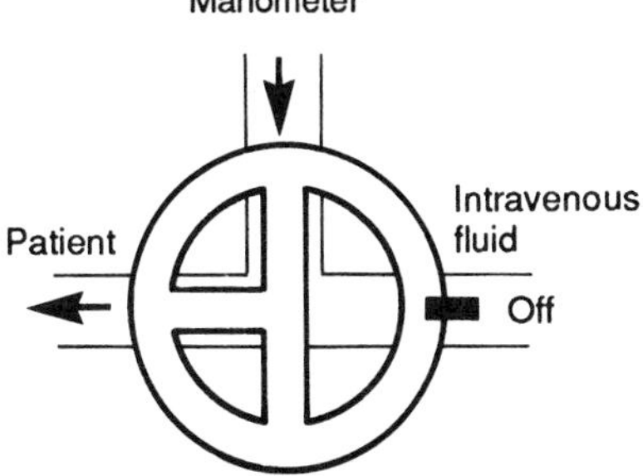

Figure 9.8 Turn off the three-way tap to intravenous fluid.

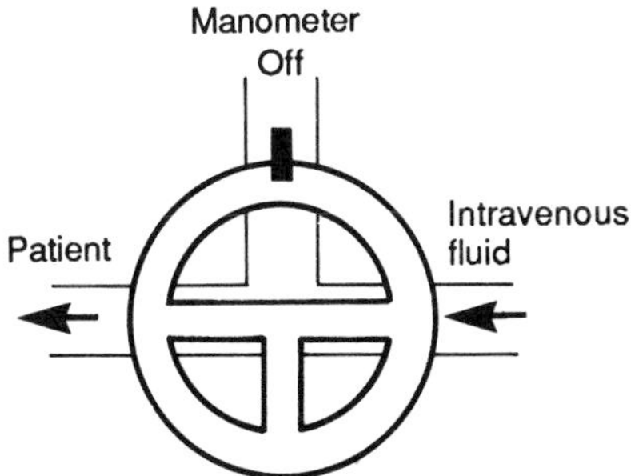

Figure 9.9 Turn off the three-way tap to manometer.

9. Turn off the three-way tap to the intravenous fluid (Figure 9.8)

To allow fluid from the manometer to enter the patient's right atrium.

10. The column of water should fall rapidly.

Indicating patency of the line, resulting in an accurate CVP reading.

11. When the level of fluid in the manometer ceases to drop, and oscillates with the patient's respirations, this is the CVP reading.

The pressure of the column of water in the manometer now equals the pressure in the right atrium.

12. Turn off the three-way tap to the manometer (Figure 9.9).

To restore the intravenous line.

13. Readjust the infusion rate.

14. Record the CVP measurement on the appropriate chart. Compare this measurement with the patient's acceptable CVP limits as stated by the doctor or the anaesthetist.

Acceptable CVP values vary with the patient and his/her overall condition. Deviations from these limits may require urgent medical intervention.

GUIDELINES: CHANGING THE DRESSING ON A CENTRAL VENOUS CATHETER INSERTION SITE

Before commencing the procedure it is important to check whether there is a variation to standard technique for individual patients, e.g. those receiving TPN, children.

Equipment

1. Sterile dressing pack.
2. Clamp for the catheter, if necessary.
3. Alcohol-based hand scrub.
4. Alcohol-based skin cleansing preparation, e.g. chlorhexidine, 0.5% in 70% spirit.
5. Alcohol-based spray, e.g. isopropyl 70% spray (for TPN only).
6. Intravenous administration set and extension set primed with infusion fluid if prescribed or intermittent injection cap.
7. Sterile padded dressing or sterile gauze.
8. Hypo-allergenic tape.
9. Bacteriological swab.

Procedure

Action	Rationale
1. Explain the procedure to the patient.	To obtain the patient's consent and co-operation.
2. Perform the dressing using an aseptic technique.	To prevent infection. (For further information on asepsis, see Chapter 3, Aseptic Technique.)
3. Screen the bed. Assist the patient into supine position, if possible.	To allow dust and airborne organisms to settle before the wound and the sterile field are exposed. To help prevent embolus.
4. Wash hands with bactericidal soap and water or bactericidal alcohol hand rub. Place all equipment required for the dressing on the bottom shelf of a clean dressing trolley.	
5. Prime the giving set, keeping the Luer lock sterile.	So that the infusion is ready for use when the current giving set is discontinued.
6. Take the trolley to the patient's bedside, disturbing the screens as little as possible.	To minimize airborne contamination.
7. Open the outer cover of the sterile dressing pack and slide the contents onto the top shelf of the trolley.	
8. Open the sterile field using the corners of the paper only. Using the forceps in the pack, arrange the sterile field with the handles of the instruments in one corner.	So that areas of potential contamination are kept to a minimum.
9. Attach a yellow clinical waste bag to the side of the trolley below the level of the top shelf.	So that contaminated material is below the level of the sterile field.
10. Open the other sterile packs, tipping their contents gently onto the centre of the sterile field. Pour lotions into gallipots or an indented plastic tray.	

Action	Rationale
11. Wash hands with bactericidal alcohol hand rub.	Hands may have become contaminated by handling the outer packs, etc.
12. Loosen the old dressing gently, touching only the tape, etc securing it.	So that the dressing can be lifted off easily with the forceps.
13. Put on gloves.	To protect the nurse from any contact with patient's blood.
14. Using gloved hands or forceps, remove the old dressing and discard it, together with the forceps into the yellow clinical waste bag.	
15. If the site is red or discharging, take a swab for bacteriogical investigation.	For identification of pathogens. To predict colonization of the site.

Note: routine samples should be taken weekly for all patients and twice-weekly for susceptible patients.

Action	Rationale
16. Clean gloved hands with bactericidal alcohol hand rub.	To minimize the risk of introducing infection.
17. Clean the wound as necessary, working from the inside to the outside of the area and dealing with the cleanest parts of the wound first.	To minimize the risk of infection spread from a 'dirty' to a 'clean' area.
18. Apply dressing, moulding it into place so that there are no folds or creases, or apply dry gauze.	
19. Remove gloves and wash hands with bactericidal soap and water or bactericidal alcohol hand rub.	
20. Discontinue the infusion in progress. Clamp the catheter using a smooth clamp if the catheter is of silicone, or artery forceps over sterile topical swabs if it is of plastic, or move catheter 'on/off' switch to 'off'.	To prevent entry of air or leakage of blood when the catheter is disconnected. Swabs prevent cracking of a plastic catheter by artery forceps.
(If TPN is in progress, spray the ends of the line with isopropyl 70%. Allow to dry.)	(To prevent infection at connection site.)
21. Either (a) put on gloves or (b) clean hands with bactericidal alcohol hand rub.	Where potential spillage of patient's blood or certain drugs may occur, e.g. cytotoxics; to minimize the risk of introducing infection into the catheter after handling unsterile parts of the system.
22. Disconnect the catheter from the old giving set and connect the prepared new set. Check that no air bubbles are present in the system. Unclamp the catheter and continue infusion. Where no clamping of the line is possible, the Valsalva manouvre should be used.	To reduce the risk of air embolism.
23. Tape the extension set into a position comfortable for the patient, and attend to his/her general comfort.	To ensure the patient's comfort and to minimize the risk of accidentally dislodging the catheter.
24. Ensure that the drip rate is satisfactory.	

Guidelines: Changing the dressing on a central venous catheter insertion site

Action	Rationale
25. Alternatively, attach a Luer lock intermittent injection cap and heparinize the catheter, and extension set, if continuous infusion is not required (see Heparinization, below).	To maintain a patent catheter for intermittent use.
26. Fold up the sterile field, place it in the yellow clinical waste bag and seal it before moving the trolley. Draw back the curtains. Dispose of waste in appropriate containers.	To prevent environmental contamination.

GUIDELINES: HEPARINIZATION OF A CENTRAL VENOUS CATHETER

This is a simple procedure which may be performed after each use or twice weekly (or less frequently in some circumstances) when no therapy is necessary.

Equipment

1. Heparinized saline 50 i.u. 5 ml ready prepared in a syringe, with 25G (orange) needle attached, in clinically clean container.
2. Isopropyl alcohol 70% swabs.

Procedure

Action	Rationale
1. Explain the procedure to the patient.	To gain the patient's consent and co-operation.
2. Wash hands thoroughly or use an alcohol-based hand scrub.	To avoid microbiological contamination.
3. Swab the injection cap with 70% alcohol and allow to dry.	To avoid microbiological contamination.
4. Insert the needle, unclamp the catheter and inject contents of the syringe.	To flush the line thoroughly.
5. Clamp the catheter while injecting the final 0.5 ml of solution.	To maintain positive pressure and prevent back-flow of blood into the catheter, and possible clot formation.
6. Remove needle from cap and dispose of equipment safely.	To prevent injury.
7. Follow procedure meticulously.	To ensure the patient is aware of each step, and the need for good hand washing/drying techniques, etc. as he/she may be performing this procedure on discharge.

GUIDELINES: TAKING BLOOD SAMPLES FROM A CENTRAL VENOUS CATHETER

Equipment

1. Sterile dressing pack.
2. Clamp for catheter, if necessary.
3. Alcohol-based hand wash solution.
4. Sterile 10-ml syringe or extra 10-ml blood bottle without heparin.
5. Sterile syringe of appropriate size for sample required
   or
   Vacuum system container holder (shell).
   Vacuum system adaptor.
   Appropriate vacuumed blood bottles.
6. Intermittent injection cap, if necessary.
7. Heparinized saline, as per policy for flushing.

Procedure

Action	**Rationale**
1. Explain the procedure to the patient.	To obtain the patient's consent and co-operation.
2. Perform procedure using an aseptic technique.	To prevent infection. (For further information on asepsis see Chapter 3, Aseptic Technique.)
3. Wash hands with bactericidal soap and water or bactericidal alcohol hand rub.	
4. Prepare a tray or trolley and take it to the bedside. Cleanse hands as above. Open sterile pack and prepare equipment.	
5. If intravenous fluid infusion is in progress, discontinue it.	
6. Clamp the catheter with a smooth clamp if the catheter is of silicone or with artery forceps over sterile topical swabs if it is of plastic, or move catheter 'on/off' switch to 'off'.	To prevent entry of air or leakage of blood via the catheter. Swabs prevent the artery forceps from cracking a plastic catheter.
7. Wash hands with a bactericidal alcohol hand rub. Put on gloves.	To minimize the risk of introducing infection into the catheter.
8. Disconnect the giving set from the catheter and cover the end of the set with the syringe cover or remove the injection cap and discard.	To reduce the risk of contaminating the end of the giving set.
9. For syringe sampling: (a) Attach a 10-ml syringe to the catheter. Release the clamp and withdraw 5 to 10 ml of blood.	
(b) Reclamp the catheter and discard the sample and syringe.	To remove blood, heparin and intravenous fluids from the 'dead space' of the catheter. Samples from this 'dead space' are likely to cause inaccuracies in blood tests.

Guidelines: Taking blood samples from a central venous catheter

Action	Rationale
(c) Attach a new syringe of appropriate size. Release the clamp and withdraw the required amount of blood.	To obtain the sample. To prevent blood loss or air embolism.
(d) Reclamp the catheter and detach the syringe.	
10. For vacuum sampling:	
(a) Attach vacuum container holder and release clamp.	To remove blood, heparin and intravenous fluids from the 'dead space' of the catheter. Samples from this 'dead space' are likely to cause inaccuracies in blood tests.
(b) Attach sample bottles for required specimens.	To obtain sample. It is not necessary to clamp the catheter when changing collection bottles, as the system is not broken.
(c) Reclamp catheter and detach vacuum container holder.	To continue therapy.
11. Reconnect the giving set, unclamp the catheter and recommence infusion or attach new intermittent injection cap, release clamp and heparinize catheter.	To prevent the catheter clotting in between uses.
12. Ensure that blood samples have been placed in the correct containers and agitated as necessary to prevent clotting. Label them with patient's name, number, etc. and send them to the laboratory with the appropriate forms.	To make certain that the specimens, correctly presented and identified, are delivered to the laboratory, enabling the requested tests to be performed and the results returned to the correct patient's records.

Double- or triple-lumen lines are now inserted routinely. Where these lines have different-sized lumens, the largest should be reserved where possible for blood products and blood sampling only.

Difficulty may be encountered when taking blood samples. This is particularly true when the central catheter is made of silicone and has been in place for a period of time. The main cause is that the tip of the soft catheter lays against the wall of the vessel and the suction required to draw blood brings this into close contact, so leading to temporary occlusion.

Measures to try to dislodge the tip include asking the patient to:

1. Cough and breathe deeply.
2. Roll from side to side.
3. Raise his/her arms.
4. Perform the Valsalva manoeuvre, if possible.
5. Increase general activity, e.g. walk up and down stairs.

If these are unsuccessful, irrigation of the catheter with normal saline or a dilute solution of heparin may be helpful. However, it may be necessary to take blood from a peripheral vein (see Chapter 44, Venepuncture).

GUIDELINES: CARE OF IMPLANTABLE PORTS

Placement of a Huber point needle into the implantable port is to be performed by a doctor or by nurses who have been taught and assessed as being competent. The needle will be connected to an extension set and a Luer-lock bung placed at the end of this. The needle and extension set remain in position for seven days and will then be changed, if required, after that time. For general procedures please refer to relevant Guidelines for Intravenous Management, Chapter 21.

Equipment

As for Guidelines: Administration of drugs by direct injection, bolus or push (i.e. items 1–13, p. 255), together with the following:

14. Non-sterile gloves.

Procedure

To give a bolus injection

Action	Rationale
1. Explain the procedure to the patient.	To obtain the patient's consent and co-operation.
2. Perform the procedure using aseptic technique.	To prevent infection.
3. Screen the bed, assist patient into the supine position.	To allow dust and airborne organisms to settle before the sterile field is exposed.
4. Wash hands with bactericidal soap and water or bactericidal alcohol hand rub.	
5. Remove the dressing.	To inspect for any obvious signs of sepsis, inflammation, haematoma, accumulation of serous fluid or movement of needle.
6. Put on gloves.	
7. Using a 10-ml Luer lock syringe, flush the line with normal saline and/or draw back blood (you may not always succeed in drawing back blood). However, if any pressure is experienced when flushing the line, advice should be sought.	Syringes smaller than 10 ml exert too great a pressure on the catheter. To confirm the patency of the line.
8. Inject the drugs as per hospital procedure.	
9. Flush with 10 ml normal saline and heparinize the line using 500 i.u. heparin in at least 5 ml of normal saline.	To maintain patency of catheter.
10. Remove the needle.	

To use for intermittent single injections or infusions

1 to **8** as for bolus injections.

9. Flush with 10 ml normal saline. Heparinize the line with 50 i.u. heparin in 5 ml normal saline.	To maintain patency.

Note: to keep the line patent when accessed, use 50 i.u. of heparin in 5 ml normal saline after use. Only heparinize with 500 i.u. heparin before the removal of the needle or if the catheter will not be used in a 12 hour period.

To commence an infusion or to change giving set

1 to **4** as for bolus injections.

5. Prime a Luer lock giving set.	So infusion is ready to attach.
6. Remove dressing and inspect insertion site as previously described.	To observe for any abnormalities.

Guidelines: Care of implantable ports

Action	Rationale
7. Put on gloves.	
8. Inject at least 10 ml normal saline and draw blood as previously described.	To confirm patency.
9. Clamp extension set with clamp or artery forceps protected with gauze.	To prevent entry of air or leakage of blood when catheter is disconnected; swabs prevent cracking of plastic catheter by forceps.
10. Remove Luer lock bung or old giving set and attach primed giving set.	To commence infusion or change giving set in accordance with hospital policy (24-hour set changes).
11. Unclamp forceps and commence infusion, regulate infusion accordingly.	

Discontinuation of infusion

1 to **4** as for bolus injections.

5. Clamp extension set.	To prevent entry of air or leakage of blood when giving set is disconnected.
6. Disconnect old giving set and replace with Luer lock bung.	
7. Unclamp extension set.	
8. Flush with 10 ml normal saline and heparinize using 500 i.u. heparin in at least 5 ml normal saline.	To maintain patency.

Heparinization of implantable port

It must be heparinized after each use and at monthly intervals between treatments.

Removal of the needle

The needle should be removed if no further treatment is anticpated and/or before discharge.

1 to **6** as for bolus injections.

7. Flush with at least 10 ml normal saline.	To flush the line thoroughly.
8. Heparinize the line using heparin 500 i.u. in 5 ml normal saline.	To maintain patency.
9. Clamp extension set while still maintaining positive pressure (i.e. keep thumb on syringe plunger).	To prevent back-flow of blood and possible clot formation.
10. Press down on portal of implantable port with two fingers.	To support portal.
11. Withdraw the needle using steady traction.	To prevent trauma to the skin.
12. No dressing is required.	

GUIDELINES: REMOVAL OF A NON-SKIN TUNNELLED CENTRAL CATHETER

Equipment

As for Guidelines: Changing the dressing on a central venous catheter insertion site (items 1 to 9, above p 120) plus:

10. Sterile scissors.
11. Small sterile specimen container.
12. Stitch cutter.
13. Additional sterile low-linting gauze swab (a new administration set, etc. is not required).

Procedure

Proceed as for a dressing procedure, steps 1 to 15 (above) then continue as follows:

Action	**Rationale**
16. Clean the insertion site.	To prevent contamination of the catheter on removal, and a false–positive culture result.
17. Discontinue the infusion, if in progress. Clamp the catheter as previously described or move the catheter 'on/off' switch to 'off'.	To prevent entry of air or leakage of blood when the catheter is disconnected.
18. Clean gloved hands with a bactericidal alcohol hand rub.	To minimize the risk of infection after handling unsterile parts of the system.
19. Cut and remove any skin suture securing the catheter.	To facilitate removal.
20. Disconnect the catheter from the remainder of the infusion system.	To ease handling and removal.
21. Ask the patient to perform the Valsalva manoeuvre.	To reduce the risk of air embolus.
22. Cover the insertion site with a thick pad of several sterile topical swabs.	Swabs are used to discourage the entry of organisms into the insertion site and to absorb any leakage of blood.
23. Hold the catheter with one hand near the point of insertion and pull firmly and gently. As the catheter begins to move, press firmly down on the site with the swabs.	Pressure is applied to prevent haemorrhage and to encourage resealing of the vein wall. It also prevents the entry of air into the vein.
Maintain pressure on the swabs for about five minutes after the catheter has been removed.	Continued pressure is necessary to allow time for the puncture in the vein to close.
24. When bleeding has stopped (approximately five minutes), swab site and cover with padded dressing for bacteriological examination.	To detect any infection at exit site.
25. Carefully cut off the tip (approximately 5 cm) of the catheter using sterile scissors and place it in a sterile container for microbiological investigation.	To detect any infection related to the catheter, and thus provide necessary treatment.
26. Fold up the sterile field, place it in the yellow clinical waste bag and seal it before moving the trolley. Dispose of the equipment in the appropriate containers.	To prevent environment contamination.

Guidelines: Removal of a non-skin tunnelled central catheter

Action	Rationale
27. Make the patient comfortable.	

This procedure may be adapted for removal of a skin-tunnelled line.

NURSING CARE PLAN

Problem	Cause	Suggested action
Dyspnoea, chest pain or cyanosis (may be slow in onset).	Hydrothorax, pneumothorax or haemothorax due to insertion technique.	Inform a doctor. Arrange for a chest X-ray. Assist with any immediate treatment and with chest drainage if necessary.
Change in pulse rate and rhythm after insertion of catheter.	Cardiac irritability.	Inform a doctor.
Dyspnoea, chest pain, tachypnoea, disorientation, cyanosis, raised CVP, coma, cardiac arrest.	Air embolism due to air entering circulation during the insertion procedure or via the catheter.	Observe the patient closely. If signs or symptoms develop, clamp the catheter to prevent further air entry. Lay the patient on the left side in Trendelenburg position. Inform a doctor. Give oxygen or external cardiac compression.
Change in pulse rate, rhythm, dyspnoea, cyanosis, cardiac arrest.	Ventricular rupture due to insertion.	Observe patient closely. Inform doctor immediately. Prepare to commence cardiac massage.
Tingling in fingers, shooting pain down arm, paralysis.	Injury to brachial plexus during insertion.	Inform a doctor. Treatment is symptomatic. Physiotherapy may be necessary.
Oedema of the arm on the side of the catheter insertion, may be associated with pain or limb discolouration.	Thoracic duct injury at insertion, resulting in alterations in lymph flow. Thrombosis in major vessel due to irritation by foreign body (catheter).	Inform a doctor. Removal is usually necessary.
Pyrexia, techycardia, rigors indicating systemic infection.	Poor aseptic technique. Careless use and handling of equipment, e.g. stopcocks, over-flooding of manometer.	Culture of the patient's blood is required. Take a swab of the infusion site, employing strict asepsis and minimum handling of the equipment. Administer antimicrobials as prescribed. Observe the patient closely. Removal of line is sometimes indicated.
Unable to draw back blood.	Catheter tip occluded by the vein wall.	Encourage the patient to move arms, or position on the side where catheter is inserted, and ask patient to perform the Valsalva manoeuvre.

	Catheter blocked by blood clots due to: (1) infusion being too slow or switched off; (2) heparinization not having been carried out previously.	Inject 1000 i.u./ml heparin (1 ml) and 1 ml normal saline into the catheter. Clamp and leave for 15 minutes. Attempt to aspirate with a 5- or 10-ml syringe to remove the clots. Irrigate with 5 ml heparinized saline. Repeat if necessary or use other solution, e.g. urokinase. 5000 i.u. in 2 to 5 ml normal saline. Suggested action: inject slowly. Leave for one hour and then attempt to aspirate.
Leakage of fluid onto the dressing.	Loose connection in the system. Cracking of catheter or hub.	Check and tighten connections. Report to the intravenous nursing staff and/or medical staff.
Catheter required for many functions, e.g. blood sampling and extra drug	Limited routes of access available to satisfy the patient's requirements.	Consider multi-lumen catheter before insertion. Simple regimes and methods of administration. Use adaptors and administration sets available for this purpose.
Fluid overload resulting in dyspnoea, oedema, raised pulse rate and blood pressure.	Infusion is too fast. Inaccurate fluid monitoring.	Use flow control devices. Keep accurate records of the patient's fluid balance and weight. Revise the patient's fluid intake regime. Inform a doctor.
Inaccurate CVP readings.	Patient in a position different from that in which the initial reading was taken.	Position should be documented in the patient's records.
	Reference point on the patient not observed.	Zero of the manometer must be level with the patient's right atrium at the point marked on the patient, i.e. mid-axilla or sternal angle.
	Faulty pressure reading technique.	If the CVP reading is outside the limits deemed acceptable for that patient and it is considered to be an accurate reading, recheck it after 15 or 30 minutes and inform a doctor if unchanged.
Elevated CVP.	Increased intrathoracic pressure caused by coughing, increased movement or pain.	Encourage coughing before taking the reading. Ensure that the patient is comfortable and pain free.
	Lower extremities elevated.	Position the patient so that he/she is lying in a supine position.
	Patient having intermittent positive-pressure ventilation.	Read the CVP at the end expiratory level (lowest point of fluctuation). This will always be higher than the 'normal' reading.

Nursing care plan

Problem	**Cause**	**Suggested action**
	Anxiety and/or restlessness.	Verify the cause of the anxiety or restlessness.
	Blood in progress via the CVP line.	Flush the line well with normal saline and read again.
	Shivering and/or muscular spasm, e.g. post-anaesthetic reaction.	Assess the patient's general condition, e.g. pulse, blood pressure, temperature. Check that the patient is warm enough. Inform a doctor.
Low CVP reading.	Leak in the system or equipment adjusted inaccurately.	Check and readjust the system.
	Changing of the patient's position from recumbent to semi-recumbent.	Re-read with the patient in the original position.
Potential pulmonary embolus due to catheter tip embolus. Symptoms include chest pain, cool clammy skin, haemoptysis, tachycardia, hypotension.	Occasionally occurs after the removal of the catheter, especially the skin-tunnelled type.	All skin-tunnelled catheters must be removed by medical staff. Notify a doctor immediately if the patient develops any of the related symptoms.
Bleeding at the insertion site following removal of the catheter.	Opening in the vein wall.	Apply pressure over the site with sterile topical swabs, until bleeding has stopped. Patients prescribed warfarin or heparin will require a longer period of pressure to compensate for the prolonged clotting time. Apply sterile dressing. If bleeding persists, the doctor must be informed.

In addition, the care plan associated with intravenous management (Chapter 13, Drug Administration) may contain useful and relevant information.

10

Continent Urinary Diversions

Definition

A urinary diversion is a surgical procedure to create an alternative method of removing urine from the body when either the bladder or urethra are no longer viable.

The urine leaves the body through an opening on the abdomen created during the operation. This opening is termed a stoma. There are two types of urinary diversion: an ileal conduit urinary diversion (incontinent) and a continent urinary diversion.

The formation of an ileal conduit urinary diversion is an operation involving the construction of a tube of ileum with one end formed into a protruding spout on to the abdomen (called a stoma) and the ureters implanted into the other, as described by Woodhouse (1991). It continually leaks urine (an incontinent stoma) necessitating the wearing of an appliance. (See procedure on stoma care, Chapter 37).

A continent urinary diversion (Figure 10.1) is an operation involving either the preservation of the patient's bladder or the formation of a new bladder called a urinary reservoir, into which the patient's ureters have been implanted. The bladder or urinary reservoir is then connected to the abdomen by a continent urinary stoma created from the appendix, ureter, fallopian tube or small bowel (Figure 10.1). The continent urinary stoma does not leak urine. Instead of wearing an appliance, patients self-catheterize into the continent urinary stoma every three to four hours to empty the urine. These operative techniques were devised by Mitrofanoff (1980) and Kock *et al.* (1987).

Indications for the formation of a continent urinary diversion

1. To expel urine from the body if the ureter, bladder or urethra are no longer viable due to disease.
2. So that urine does not leak continuously, therefore:
   (a) It prevents skin excoriation.
   (b) It improves the individual's body image since it is not necessary to wear an appliance.

REFERENCE MATERIAL

Principles of a continent urinary diversion

Following the formation of an ileal conduit (see Chapter 37, Stoma Care), the patients' perception of their body image and sexuality may be altered, which may affect their ability to form and maintain social and sexual relationships (Delvin & Plant, 1979; Jeffrey *et al.*, 1988; Jones, *et al.*, 1981).

The formation of a continent urinary diversion is an alternative to the formation of an ileal conduit. The opening on the abdomen (stoma), compared to the ileal conduit stoma, is small and flush with the skin. The continent urinary stoma is tunnelled through the muscle of the bladder or reservoir. This prevents urine leaking through the stoma. The size of the continent urinary stoma depends upon the type of material used to create it. The ureter is the smallest (approximately 3.9 mm in diameter), while the small intestine is the largest at 9 to 10 mm in diameter.

The continent urinary diversion involves the patient having two admissions into hospital. The first is to form the continent urinary diversion. Following the operation, a sterile fine-bore tube is left in the continent urinary stoma to keep it patent and allow the urine to drain into a catheter bag. After recovering from the operation, patients are taught how to take care of the tubing, leg bags and night drainage systems. Patients are then discharged home to be readmitted six weeks after the operation to be taught self-catheterization.

Urine drains into the urinary reservoir or bladder through the ureters. Patients self-catheterize into the continent urinary stoma every three or four hours to empty the urine reservoir (Figure 10.2). They go into a toilet, adjust any restrictive clothing and insert a special tube into the continent urinary stoma, pointing

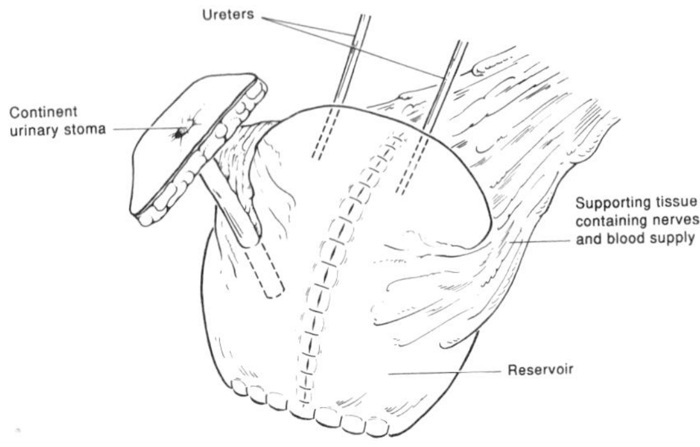

Figure 10.1 Continent urinary diversion.

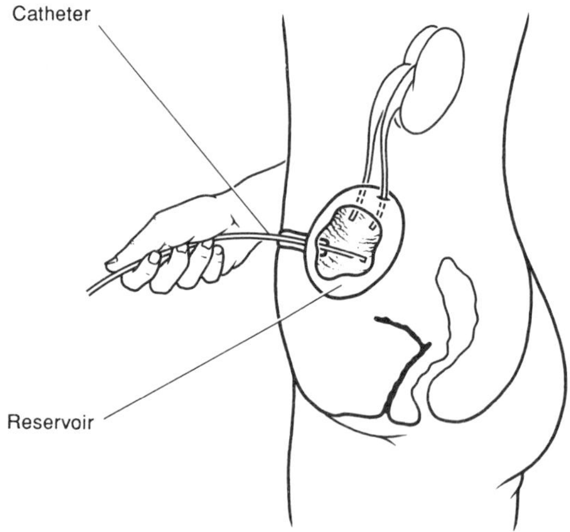

Figure 10.2 Self-catheterization into the continent urinary stoma.

the other end into the toilet. The urine drains out. The tube is then removed, washed with water and replaced in its container (usually a plastic bag, spectacle case or cosmetic bag).

Before each discharge, patients are given verbal and written advice (Horn, 1990), and can contact the hospital 24 hours a day.

Types of continent urinary diversions

There are a number of types of continent urinary diversions. Essentially the principles and the nursing care are the same, with only minor modifications. Two examples are the Mitrofanoff and Kock's pouch (Figures 10.1 and 10.2).

The Mitrofanoff pouch was devised in the late 1970s early 1980s by Paul Mitrofanoff (1980) in France. Initially, it was devised for patients with bladder neck obstruction or incompetence. The bladder was preserved and the appendix was used as the continent urinary stoma. The operation was later modified so that in the absence of an appendix, a piece of ureter or fallopian tube could be used. If the bladder is unviable, the sigmoid colon can be resected and created into a urinary reservoir. Further modifications have been made by Duckett and Snyder (1985; 1986).

The Kock pouch was devised by Kock *et al.* (1987), in Sweden, initially as a continent ileostomy; in the early 1980s it was adapted into a continent urinary diversion. A section of the small bowel is resected and used to create both the reservoir and the continent urinary stoma. The Kock pouch continent urinary stoma is larger then the Mitrofanoff stoma which uses the smaller appendix, ureter or fallopian tube. Skinner and Boyd (1984) have made further modifications.

Indications for the surgical formation of a continent urinary diversion

The indications for the formation of a continent urinary diversion and an ileal conduit are similar. (See Chapter 37, Stoma Care). However, an ileal conduit can be converted into a continent urinary diversion and *vice versa*.

1. Cancer of the bladder, ureters or urethra.
2. Invasive cancer of the cervix or ovary requiring a pelvic exenteration. This is an operation involving a cystectomy, hysterectomy and colectomy.
3. An unviable bladder or urethra following radiotherapy.
4. Congenital urinary tract deformities.
5. Bladder neck obstructions or incompetence.
6. Neuropathic bladder. A condition where the nerve impulses do not reach the bladder.
7. Trauma to the bladder, ureters or urethra.
8. An ileal conduit or ureterostomy can be converted into a continent urinary diversion.

Patient selection

Patients are selected carefully for this type of surgery. Horn (1990) describes how potential patients should have good renal function and a suitable continent urinary stoma. They must be motivated towards self-catheterization and be dexterous. Patients should be physically and psychologically able to undergo major surgery. If they have cancer it should be either curable or controllable and without metastases.

Specific pre-operative preparation

Patients undergo the usual preparation for anaesthesia

Table 10.1 Advantages and disadvantages of an ileal conduit

Advantages	*Disadvantages*
1. Tried and tested technique.	1. Continual urine leakage necessitating the wearing an appliance.
2. Surgery is not as extensive as with a continent urinary diversion.	2. Potential problem of skin excoriation.
3. The skills to care for an ileal conduit are relatively easy to learn.	3. Potential problem of altered body image to patients and others.
4. Lower incidence of postoperative problems.	4. Fear of maintaining or creating new relationships.

Table 10.2 Advantages and disadvantages of a continent urinary diversion

Advantages	*Disadvantages*
1. No need to wear an appliance.	1. Patient must be enthusiastic and motivated towards self-catheterization.
2. Small stoma, 0.5 to 1 cm in diameter.	2. There are problems with the operation technique.
3. No urine leakage.	3. Operation still involves a laparotomy and drain-site scars, which do fade but may cause and altered body image.
4. Improves or maintains body image.	4. Consider whether patient will be able to self-catheterize in five to ten years' time.
5. No skin excoriation.	5. It is a long operation with a high risk of postoperative problems, and requires two hospitalizations.
	6. Lack of familiarity in outside specialist centres.
	7. Long-term problems are unknown.
	8. Surgical and nursing care techniques are modified regularly.
	9. Patients may fear they are being used to test the operation.

(see Chapter 33, Peri-operative Care). Only the specific preparation is discussed here although physical preparation may vary according the individual surgeon's preference.

Pre-operative counselling

Once patients have been selected as suitable candidates, psychological preparation should begin as soon as possible. Boore (1978) and Hayward (1978) have illustrated the importance of pre-operative information and explanation in reducing postoperative physical and psychological stress to the individual following the formation of a stoma (ileal conduit or colostomy). Their research is also applicable to patients receiving continent urinary diversion stomas. This is discussed in Chapter 37, Stoma Care.

Patients should receive a full explanation from the consultant and stoma therapist. This usually takes place in an outpatients clinic, and is reiterated when the patient has been admitted to the ward. The formation of an ileal conduit as well as a continent urinary diversion is discussed with the patient in case the latter is not a viable option. The advantages and disadvantages of both operations should be fully discussed with the patients and their family and friends (Tables 10.1 and 10.2). They should be shown pictures of the continent urinary diversion and ileal conduit stomas, and are encouraged to familiarize themselves with the equipment: pouches, wafers, catheterization tubes and bladder syringes.

Useful aids

1. Information booklets.
2. Samples of equipment.
3. Diagrams.
4. Being visited by patients who have had a continent urinary diversion and an ileal conduit formed (ideally, of similar age, sex and background to the patient).

The effect on diet and bowel movements

Horn (1991) describes in a patient information booklet the effect of evacuating the patient's bowels and intestinal manipulation during the operation, and how the patient can adjust to the temporary effects. Patients should be warned about the necessity to evacuate their bowels of faeces before the operation. The procedure to do this and the surgical manipulation of the bowel during the operation results in the bowel not working for several days after the surgery. When their bowels do start to work again, patients may experience loose, watery stools which will become firmer as the appetite returns.

Horn (1991) describes how the slow return of both a normal appetite and bowel function is a common feature following this type of operation and it can give much anxiety. The patient should be advised to take small, light meals supplemented with nutritious drinks. It may take two or three months before patients return to a completely normal appetite. Once recovered, the patient can eat and drink a normal diet.

Patients are reassured that the new urine reservoir and stoma are completely separate from their normal bowel action. Stools will not pass through the continent urinary stoma.

Bowel preparation

Patients are admitted three days before surgery to commence a regime to evacuate all faecal matter from the intestine. The regime used depends on the surgeon's preference.

Alexander Williams (1980) explains why it is necessary to remove all faecal matter:

1. To prevent hard faecal masses from impacting proximal to an anastomosis.
2. To prevent faeces spilling from the cut ends of the bowel during the operation.
3. To reduce bacterial contamination when the bowel is opened.

However, it is important to know that this faeces-removing procedure can cause the patient to suffer hypovolaemia and electrolyte imbalance. Therefore, it is important that the fluid loss is replaced orally or intravenously.

Sexual dysfunction

Following the formation of a continent urinary diversion possible sexual impairment for both men and women may occur. This is the same as for other stoma patients and is discussed in Chapter 37, Stoma Care.

Pre- and postoperative counselling is given to each patient and partner. Each person's sexual dysfunction is discussed and treated on an individual basis.

Specific postoperative care

Horn (1990) describes the postoperative nursing care given to patients following the formation of a continent urinary diversion. The surgery involves intestinal manipulation, which causes a paralytic ileus. Manipulation of the ureters in a highly vascular area results in a risk of haemorrhage and local oedema, leading to uteric obstruction. This may prevent the urine draining into the urinary reservoir.

Apart from the routine immediate postoperative care (see Chapter 33, Peri-operative Care), nursing care is based on early detection of these problems. Due to the paralytic ileus, patients are unable to eat or drink, and receive total parental nutrition through a cannula in the internal jugular or subclavicular vein. A gastrostomy or nasogastric tube drains any gastric fluid that collects due to gastric stasis. The nasogastric and gastrostomy tubes are removed and parental nutrition is discontinued when the ileus has resolved. A wound drain is inserted into the wound site to prevent haematoma and abscess formation (Figure 10.3).

Ureteric obstruction can be avoided by inserting a small, hollow, plastic tube called a stent into each ureter, which is then passed through the urinary

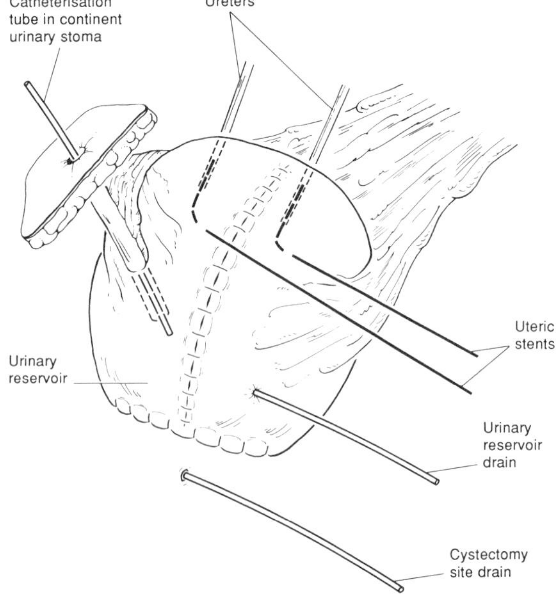

Figure 10.3 Siting of wound drains to prevent haematoma and abscess formation.

reservoir and onto the abdomen, and connected to a urine-measuring apparatus. This allows the urine to drain out and is usually removed ten days post-operatively when local oedema has reduced. A fine-bore nasogastric tube is inserted into the continent urinary stoma to prevent occlusion due to surgical trauma and to allow urine to drain into a measuring device. This remains in position for six weeks (Woodhouse, 1989).

If the urinary reservoir is allowed to fill before the anastomosis can heal it may rupture, and therefore a bladder drain is inserted to drain the urine. It is removed aseptically within seven to ten days. The main postoperative problems are the collection of post-surgery debris and, if a urinary reservoir has been created, the mucus produced by the intestinal lining of the urine reservoir. These can collect and block the bladder drain and continent urinary stoma, which may lead to increased pressure on the anastomosis. Horn (1990) describes how to remove the debris by irrigating the reservoir drain and continent urinary stoma tubing with sterile normal saline twice a day.

Although the debris is eventually removed, the mucus secretion may cause obstruction. Therefore, patients are taught how to flush the reservoir twice a day. At home tap water can be used to flush the continent urinary stoma (Lapides, 1971).

Patient education before first discharge

The stoma therapist visits the patients on the ward to continue the relationship established before the operation, to check on postoperative recovery and to act as a resource for the nursing staff. As patients recover from the operation they are taught the care of the urine drainage systems by the stoma therapist and experienced ward nurses. The care of the urine drainage system then gradually becomes the patient's responsibility rather than the ward nurses'. Before discharge, patients are taught how to flush the continent urinary stoma tubing using tap water (Lapides, 1971), secure the tube in place and attach drainage bags. They are taught how to recognize a urinary tract infection and advised to drink at least two to three litres of fluid daily to prevent it happening. They are also advised to wear a medical aid bracelet, so that if they are found unconscious at any time a doctor or nurse will know how to empty the urine drainage system.

When patients are well enough to be discharged, they are allowed to go home for a few weeks before being readmitted to be taught self-catheterization. Patients are seen by the stoma therapist before discharge and a community nurse is requested to visit the patients after discharge. An explanatory letter and the relevant literature is supplied. Patients are encouraged to seek advice from the ward staff at any time.

Second admission

Patients are readmitted six weeks after the operation to be taught intermittent self-catheterization by the stoma therapist and experienced ward staff, as described by Horn (1990). Before such teaching, a pouchogram is performed. A radio-opaque dye is poured into the urinary reservoir to ascertain the amount of fluid the bladder or urinary reservoir can hold, and to ensure all the anastomoses have healed. The patient is then taught intermittent self-catheterization. See Guidelines: Teaching intermittent self-catheterization, below.

Second discharge advice

Once proficient with intermittent self-catheterization, patients are discharged home with a two- to four-week outpatient clinic appointment to see the surgeon and stoma therapist. The advice now extends to include the following:

1. Emptying the bladder or reservoir every three to four hours, to prevent overdistension of the reservoir.
2. To ensure an undisturbed sleep by reducing the amount of fluid the patient drinks three hours before going to sleep. The patient should catheterize before going to sleep and on waking.
3. To keep a tube available at all times (in suit, car, handbag, at work and at home), in case patient needs to empty the urine.
4. A small amount of mucus may leak from the continent urinary stoma and a piece of gauze can be worn to protect clothing.
5. On discharge, patients are given a supply of nelaton self-catheterization catheters. These are normally used for urethral self-catheterization. Suction catheters should not be used. Various makes of nelaton-type catheter are available on prescription. The hospital will tell the patient how to obtain further supplies.
6. Once the tubing has been taken out of its original sterile packet, it can be used repeatedly for up to seven days providing it is rinsed with tap water between uses and stored in its own container (a plastic bag, cosmetic bag, spectacle case).
7. If the patient finds it difficult to insert the catheter into the stoma, he or she is advised to pause and rest for ten minutes before attempting to insert the catheter again. This is to allow any swelling around the stoma to subside. If it is still difficult, then a warm bath sometimes dilates the stoma. The

patient should then try again, with a size smaller tube. If it is still difficult, the hospital should be contacted.

8. If there trauma during catheterization, such as some spotting of blood, the patient should wait ten minutes and then try again. A doctor should be consulted if the bleeding continues or increases.
9. Patients should be told that it can take a while to become confident with this procedure. However, they can contact the hospital at any time for advice and reassurance.

Long- and short-term problems

Horn (1990) summarized the following problems which were encountered by the surgeons who had performed this technique: septicaemia (due to urine leaking during the operation); breakdown of the anastomosis; perforation or stenosis of the continent urinary stoma; calculi forming on the clips in the anastomosis; swelling due to trauma, which may block the stoma; urine leaking from the stoma which necessitates further surgery. As the formation of a continent urinary diversion is a relatively new surgical technique, it is not known if there are any other short- or long-term problems.

Long-term psychological effects

Boyd *et al.* (1987) carried out a survey comparing the social and sexual affects of ileal conduits versus continent urinary diversions, and the effects on patients who had been converted from a ileal conduit to a continent urinary diversion. The survey revealed that all the patients had adapted to the new skills. However, patients with an ileal conduit had the poorest body image; the most satisfied patients were those who had the conversion performed.

A continent urinary diversion of the type described can offer patients an improved lifestyle, and the nurse has a critical part to play in preparing patients to adapt to it.

Useful addresses

The Urostomy Association
Central Office
'Buckland'
Beaumont Park
Danbury
Essex
CM3 4DE
Tel.: 024541 4294

Impotence Information Centre
PO Box 1130
London
WC1X 9JN

The Royal Marsden Hospital
Fulham Road
London
SW3 6JJ
Tel.: 071–352 8171

Medic-Alert Foundation
17 Bridge Wharf
156 Caledonian Road
London
N1 9UU
Tel.: 071–833 3034

References and further reading

Alexander Williams, J. (1980) Cleaning the gut for colonic surgery. *World Medicine*, 15(10), 18–19.

Blannin, J. P. & Hobden, J. (1980) The catheter of choice. *Nursing Times*, 76, 2092–3.

Boore, J. R. P. (1978) *A Prescription for Recovery: the Effects of Pre-operative Preparation of Surgical Patients on Post-operative Stress, Recovery and Infection*. Royal College of Nursing, London.

Boyd, S. D. *et al.* (1987) Quality of life survey of urinary diversion patients: comparison of ileal conduits versus continent urinary reservoirs. *The Journal of Urology*, 138, 1386–9.

Brocklehurst, J. C. & Brocklehurst, S. (1978) Management of indwelling catheters. *British Journal of Urology*, 50(2), 102–5.

Cummings, J. *et al.* (1987) The choice of suprapubic continent catheterisable urinary stoma. *British Journal of Urology*, 60, 227–30.

Delvin, H. B. & Plant, J. (1979) Sexual function – an aspect of stoma care. *British Journal of Sexual Medicine*, 1, pp. 2, 6, 22, 26, 33–34, 37.

Duckett, J. W. & Snyder, H. M. (1985) Use of the Mitrofanoff principal in urinary reconstruction. *World Journal of Urology*, 3, 191–3.

Duckett, J. W. & Snyder, H. M. (1986) Continent urinary diversion – the Mitrofanoff principal. *The Journal of Urology*, 136, 58–62.

Hayward, J. (1978) *Information – A Prescription Against Pain*. Royal College of Nursing, London.

Horn, S. A. (1990) Nursing patients with a continent urinary diversion. *Nursing Standard*, 4(21), 24–6.

Horn, S. A. (1991) *Continent Urinary Diversions – Your Questions Answered. Patients' Information Booklet*. The Royal Marsden Hospital, London.

Jeffrey, L. *et al.* (1988) The Mitrofanoff principal: an alternative form of continent urinary diversion. *The Journal of Urology*, 140, 1529–31.

Jones, M. A. *et al.* (1981) Life with an ileal conduit: results of a questionnaire – surveys of patients and urological surgeons. *British Journal of Urology*, 52, 21–5.

Kock, N. G. *et al.* (1987) Appliance-free sphincter controlled bladder substitute. *The Journal of Urology*, 138, 1150–4.

Lapides, S. (1971) Clean intermittent self-catheterization in the treatment of urinary tract disease. *Trans-American Association of Genitourinary Surgery*, 63, 92.

Lawson, A. (undated) *Understanding Urostomy*. Squibb Surgicare.

Mitrofanoff, P. (1980) Cystomie continente trans appendiclaire dans le traitment des vessies neurologiques. *Chirurgie Pediatrique*, 21, 297–305.

Skinner, D. G. & Boyd (1984) Techniques of creation of a continent urinary ileal reservoir (Kock pouch) for urinary diversion. *Urological Clinics of North America*, 11(4), 741–9.

Whitfield, H. N. & Hendry, W. F. (1985) *Textbook of Genito-Urinary Surgery*. Churchill Livingstone, Edinburgh. Chapter 101, Pathophysiology of erection and ejaculation (G. S. Brindley); Chapter 102, Investigations and treatment of impotence (J. P. Pryor); Chapter 121, Bladder surgery (W. F. Hendry & H. N. Whitfield).

Woodhouse, C. R. J. (1989) The Mitrofanoff principal for continent urinary diversions. *British Journal of Urology*, 63(1), 53–7.

Woodhouse, C. R. J. (1991) *Longterm Paediatric Urology*. Blackwell Scientific, Oxford.

TEACHING INTERMITTENT SELF-CATHETERIZATION OF A CONTINENT URINARY DIVERSION STOMA

Definition

Intermittent self-catheterization is when patients insert a self-catheterization catheter into the urinary reservoir via the continent urinary stoma using a clean technique. It is performed to evacuate or instill fluids, after which the tube is removed.

Indications

Intermittent self-catheterization may be carried out for the following reasons:

1. To empty the contents of the urinary reservoir every three to four hours. If the reservoir is left too long between emptying it can become overstretched and lose its elasticity.
2. To allow irrigation of the urinary reservoir for the removal of mucus which may occlude the continent urinary stoma.

REFERENCE MATERIAL

The following research has been gathered from urethral self-catheterization. However, the same principles would apply to a continent urinary stoma.

Intermittent self-catheterization is intended to make life easier and not more complicated. Lapides (1971) suggested that this technique can reduce significantly the incidence of urinary tract infection.

Types of tubing used for intermittent self-catheterization

Blannin and Hobden (1980) suggest that the tubing used for intermittent self-catheterization should be: smooth-surfaced and flexible to prevent trauma; sterile so that it will not introduce infection; relatively resistant to the urine's acidity which can cause some materials to disintegrate or become inflexible, resulting in trauma; easily cleaned and stored for repeated use up to seven days. Horn (1990) describes how fine-bore nasogastric tubes and Nelaton catheters may be used. The choice of tubing depends upon the size of the continent urinary stoma: that formed from ureter and fallopian tube may need a size six to ten French gauge Nelaton catheter, while that formed from the appendix and small bowel may need size ten French gauge upwards of a Nelaton catheter (one French gauge = 0.66 mm).

Teaching self-catheterization

Intermittent self-catheterization should be taught in a place that offers privacy, with a good clear light and a full-length mirror (bathroom, toilet or at the patient's bedside) (Horn, 1990). It is a clean and not a sterile procedure. Patients can learn self-catheterization with the aid of a mirror or by touch, and are observed and assisted by a nurse until they are proficient (see Procedure, Guidelines: Self-catheterization, below).

During the day patients are encouraged to drink at least two litres of fluid to prevent any urinary tract infection and to catheterize every three or four hours to prevent the reservoir becoming distended and losing its elasticity. However, patients can reduce their fluid intake during the evening so that they need catheterize only before they go to sleep and again when they get up in the morning. The patient may feel bloated when the urine reservoir is full. Patients whose own bladder has been preserved may get a normal sensation of wanting to pass urine.

If a urinary reservoir has been created it may ooze mucus from its intestinal lining. This is normal, although it may stain the patient's clothing so a small protective dressing is advisable.

GUIDELINES: SELF-CATHETERIZATION

Equipment

1. Tubes for catheterization depending upon the size of the stoma.
2. Catheter-tipped syringe.
3. Tissues.
4. Clean jug or bowl.
5. Non-adherent dressing and skin protective tape to cover stoma if it oozes mucus.

Procedure

Action	Rationale
1. Following explanation of self-catheterization, the patient should collect all the equipment required for the procedure.	To obtain the patient's consent and co-operation. To ensure all the equipment required is easily available.
2. Take the equipment to the toilet, bathroom or screened bed area.	To ensure the patient's privacy.
Ensure there is a good light and a full-length mirror.	To ensure the patient can see the stoma clearly.
3. The equipment should be arranged on a clean surface and within easy reach for the procedure.	To prevent contamination by surface bacteria. So that equipment is easily available.
4. The patient needs to remove any inhibiting clothing.	To ensure the patient can examine the stoma.
5. The patient should wash the hands with soap and water then dry them.	To ensure the hands are clean.
6. The patient should look at the stoma, if necessary with the aid of a hand or full-length mirror.	To look for mucus and swelling around the stoma.
7. The patient should wipe away any mucus with a tissue soaked in warm water and gently pat dry.	To ensure the opening is clear and mucus does not block the catheter during insertion into stoma.
8. Remove the plastic tube from its container. Moisten the tip to be inserted with warm, running water or water-soluble lubricant.	To act as a lubricant preventing internal trauma of the continent urinary stoma, thus allowing the tube to enter the urine reservoir.
9. Ensure the untipped end of the tube is in a receiver, i.e. jug, bowl or toilet.	To ensure the urine goes into a bowl and not onto the patient.
10. The patient can use either a mirror to guide the tube into the opening of the stoma or feel the opening with two fingers slightly apart with the stoma between.	To act as a guide to pass the tube into the continent urinary stoma.
11. Insert the tube gently into the stoma following the pathway inside (usually towards the middle of the abdomen) until urine starts to flow, then insert tube a further 6 cm.	The direction of insertion and the length of catheter inserted depends on the type, size and shape of continent urinary stoma.
12. When all the urine has stopped flowing gently remove the tubing. If urine starts to flow again wait until it stops before removing the tube any further.	To ensure complete emptying of the urinary reservoir.

13. Remove the tube. Hold one end up then the other end.	To allow complete drainage of the tube.
14. Rinse the tubing through with first hot, then cold tap water.	To rinse out any urine. To restore the patency of the tube.
15. Replace the tube in its plastic container.	To keep the tubing clean.
16. Cover the stoma with a non-adherent dressing and secure with skin-protective tape.	To prevent mucus staining the patient's clothing.
17. The patient should wash the hands with soap and water, and then dry them.	To remove any urine on the hands.
18. The patient can then dress, collect equipment and dispose of any soiled dressings.	To prevent cross-infection.

NURSING CARE PLAN

Problem	Cause	Suggested action
Cannot insert the tube into the stoma.	Using too large a tube. Unable to locate opening. Opening occluded, e.g. due to swelling.	Try a smaller sized tube. Use a magnifying mirror to find opening. Rest for 10 minutes to let stoma relax and then reinsert. Have a warm bath which sometimes helps to dilate the opening. If still unable to catheterize, then patient should contact the hospital. Doctor may give subcutaneous injection of steroid to reduce swelling. If the opening remains occluded, a suprapubic catheter may be inserted to allow the swelling to subside and drain the urine from the reservoir. The stoma may need to be dilated by a doctor.
Partial insertion only of tubing is possible.	Tubing kinked. Stricture in the stoma.	Remove tubing and try with fresh tubing of the same size. Or try with a size smaller tubing. If unable to catheterize, contact the hospital.
Patient is easily catheterized but no urine is passed.	Tubing not inserted into reservoir. Tubing kinked.	Insert tubing further. Do not use force. If there is resistance then stop. Contact the hospital.
	Tube blocked with mucus.	Cough. The increased intra-abdominal pressure may dislodge the plug of mucus. Flush the tube while inserted with tap water. Remove tubing, examine for mucus and reinsert once it is clear. Flush the urine reservoir.

Nursing care plan

Problem	**Cause**	**Suggested action**
Stoma leaks urine between catheterizations.	Reservoir not emptied regularly. Mucus plug blocking tubing, preventing complete drainage. Stoma failure.	Catheterise every three to four hours. Flush reservoir at least twice a day. If still leaking inform the hospital. Surgical fashioning of the stoma may be necessary.
Staining of blood during catheterization.	Trauma due to rough technique. Using wrong type of self-catheterization catheter.	Lubricate the tube well with water and insert gently into stoma. Use lubricating jelly. If blood staining continues or increases in amount then inform the hospital. Use nelaton self-catheterization catheter.

11

Cytotoxic Drugs: Handling and Administration

Definition

The term cytotoxic literally translated means 'toxic to cells'. Hence these drugs are those which kill cells (malignant or non-malignant).

REFERENCE MATERIAL

In recent years there has been increasing concern about the occupational hazards associated with the handling of cancer chemotherapeutic agents. On the basis of the evidence available at present, risks to personnel involved in the reconstitution and administration of cytotoxic drugs fall into two categories:

1. The proven local effects caused by direct contact with the skin, eyes and mucous membranes. These include the following:
   (a) Dermatitis.
   (b) Inflammation of mucous membranes.
   (c) Excessive lacrimation.
   (d) Pigmentation.
   (e) Blistering, associated with mustine.
   (f) Other, miscellaneous, allergic reaction.

   These hazards have been recognized for a number of years. Protection using non-absorbent armlets, plastic aprons and gloves and masks (in certain circumstances) for reconstitution, and gloves and aprons for administration are required. Different types of gloves are being used. Wright (1990) says, 'recommendations vary as to which type of glove material (latex, rubber or PVC) provides best protection'. The key issues to consider when selecting gloves are thickness and integrity. Goggles should fully cover the eyes to protect the handler, and meet BS2092C requirements.
2. The potentially harmful short- or long-term systemic effects due to inhalation or ingestion of cytotoxic drugs during preparation. Many of these drugs have been shown to be mutagenic, and several are suspected of being teratogenic and/or carcinogenic when given at the therapeutic levels to animals and humans. With the majority of the compounds there is little or no absorption through intact skin (the exceptions are those which are lipid soluble). Systemic complaints from handlers include:
   (a) Lightheadedness.
   (b) Dizziness.
   (c) Nausea.
   (d) Headache.
   (e) Alopecia.
   (f) Coughing.
   (g) Pruritus.
   (h) General malaise.

The working conditions in which these complaints were experienced were not desirable, i.e. a small, unventilated medicine closet. No formal collection of data was performed and the author readily admits to gathering information on an anecdotal basis, but the data are supported by the literature (Drug Intelligence and Clinical Pharmacy, 1983).

In a number of studies the urine of cytotoxic drug handlers, including that of nurses, has been collected and screened for mutagenic activity using an accepted test (Ames *et al.*, 1975). Although alterations in cell structure have been detected in many of the published works, they appear to be transient and of a low level. It has yet to be demonstrated whether these changes in cell structure are harmful and if this level of mutagenesis can be equated with more serious consequences. Inconclusive or contradictory data, and doubts about the validity of the test, have yet to be quantified.

In summary, localized toxicity due to accidental contact with cytotoxic drugs is well documented and it is therefore only sensible to take precautions to minimize the risks. While long-term hazards remain largely undefined, the suggestion that some compounds may carry the insidious risk of teratogenicity or carcinogenicity is sufficiently strong that the only responsible course of action is that which minimizes exposure. This is best achieved through locally agreed policies based on the available national guidelines. In hospitals where cytotoxic drugs are used frequently, the most satisfactory procedure is for all doses to be prepared in the pharmacy department by trained staff working in a specially equipped area.

Whatever the situation, written guidelines should be available to cover:

1. Preparation of compounds – environment, staff training, staff protection, techniques, equipment.
2. Administration of drugs – staff training, staff protection, technique, equipment.
3. Disposal – of drugs, equipment, waste and excreta.
4. Accidents – spillage and contamination of nurse, doctor or patient.
5. A system for monitoring and recording any effects on hospital staff.

Note: Qualified nursing staff are increasingly given responsibility for the administration of intravenous medication, including cytotoxic drugs. For further information regarding these procedures see Chapter 21, Intravenous Management.

References and further reading

Allwood & Wright (Eds) (1990) *The Cytotoxic Handbook*. Radcliffe Medical Press, Oxford.

Ames, B. N. *et al.* (1975) Methods for detecting carcinogens and mutagens with the salmonella/mammalian microsome mutagenicity test. *Mutation Research*, 31, 347–64.

Anderson, M. *et al.* (1983) Development and operation of a pharmacy-based intravenous cytotoxic reconstitution service. *British Medical Journal*, 286, 32–6.

Anderson, R. *et al.* (1982) Risk of handling injectable antineoplastic agents. *American Journal of Hospital Pharmacy*, 39, 1881–7.

Bauman, B. & Duvall, E. (1980) An unusual accident during the administration of chemotherapy. *Cancer Nursing*, 3(4), 305–6.

Calvert, A. H. (1981) The long-term sequelae of cytotoxic therapy. *Cancer Topics*, 3(7), 77–9.

Colls, B. M. (1985) Safety of handling cytotoxic agents: a cause for concern by pharmaceutical companies. *British Medical Journal*, 291, 318–19.

Cooke, J. *et al.* (1987) Environmental monitoring of personnel who handle cytotoxic drugs. *Pharmaceutical Journal*, 239(6452 suppl. R2).

Crudi, C. B. (1980) A compounding dilemma: I've kept the drug sterile but have I contaminated myself? *National Intravenous Therapy Association*, 3, 77–8.

Darbyshire, P (1986) Handle with care. *Nursing Times*, 82(40), 37–8.

Drug Intelligence and Clinical Pharmacy (1983) 17, 532–7.

Falck, K. *et al.* (1979) Mutagenicity in urine of nurses handling cytotoxic agents. *Lancet*, 1, 1250.

Harris, J. & Dodds, L. (1985) Handling waste from patients receiving cytotoxic drugs. *Pharmaceutical Journal*, 235(6345), 289–91.

Health and Safety Executive (1983) *Precautions for the Safe Handling of Cytotoxic Drugs, Medical Series*. HMSO, London.

HPG Welsh Office (1988) *Policy for the Safe Handling of Cytotoxic Drugs*.

Knowles, R. S. & Virden, J. E. (1980) Handling of injectable antineoplastic agents. *British Medical Journal*, 2, 589–91.

Laidlaw, J. L. *et al.* (1984) Permeability of latex and polyvinyl chloride gloves to 20 antineoplastic drugs. *American Journal of Hospital Pharmacy*, 41, 2018–23.

Nguyen, T. V. *et al.* (1982) Exposure of pharmacy personnel to mutagenic antineoplastic drugs. *Cancer Research*, 42, 4792–6.

Oakley, P. & Reeves, E. (1984) Setting up a reconstitution service. *Pharmaceutical Journal*, 232(6282), 739–40.

Oldcorne, M. A. *et al.* (1987) Letters to the editor. Handling cytotoxic drugs. *The Pharmaceutical Journal*, 18 April, 238, 488.

Oncology Nursing Society (1989) *Staff Practices with Cytotoxics*.

Richardson, M. L. & Bowron, J. M. (1985) The fate of pharmaceutical chemicals in the aquatic environment. *Journal of Pharmaceutical Pharmacology*, 37, 1–12.

Selevan, S. G. (1986) Letter. *New England Journal of Medicine*, 16, 1048–51.

Selevan, S. G. *et al.* (1985) A study of occupational exposure to antineoplastic drugs and fetal loss in nurses. *New England Journal of Medicine*, 19, 1173–8.

Speechley, V. (1982) Better safe than sorry. *Nursing Mirror*, 154(15), 11.

Stokes, M. *et al.* (1987) Permeability of latex and polyvinyl chloride gloves to fluorouracil and methotrexate. *American Journal of Hospital Pharmacy*, 44, 1341–6.

Stuart, M. (1981) Sequence of administering vesicant cytotoxic drugs; Part A. *Oncology Nursing Forum*, 9(1), 53–4.

Thomas, P. H. & Fenton-May, V. (1987) Protection offered by various gloves to carmustine exposure. *The Pharmaceutical Journal*, 20 June, 238, 775–7.

Vennit, S. *et al.* (1983) Monitoring exposure of nursing and pharmacy personnel to cytotoxic drugs: urinary mutation assays and urinary platinum as markers of absorption. *Lancet*, 1, 74–6.

Working Party of the Pharmaceutical Society of Great Britain on the Handling of Cytotoxic Drugs (1983) Guidelines for the handling of cytotoxic drugs. *Pharmaceutical Journal*, 230(6215), 230–1.

Wright, N. P. (1990) Chapter 3, Protective Clothing, *The Cytotoxic Handbook*, Ed. by M. Allwood & P. Wright. Radcliffe Medical Press, Oxford.

GUIDELINES: PROTECTION OF THE ENVIRONMENT

Management of spillage

Action	Rationale
1. Act immediately.	Any spillage may become a health hazard.
2. Collect spillage kit.	It contains all necessary equipment.
3. Put on thick latex or PVC gloves and disposable plastic apron or tabard.	To provide personal protection.
4. If there is visible powder spill, put on a good-quality surgical face mask.	To prevent inhalation of powder.
5. If spillage is on hard floor, put on overshoes.	For protection and to minimize the spread of contamination.
6. Wipe up powder spillage quickly with well-dampened paper towels and dispose of them as 'high-risk' waste.	To prevent dispersal of powder. To protect others and ensure safe disposal by incineration.
7. Mop up liquids which have been spilled on a hard surface with paper towels and dispose of them as 'high risk' waste.	To protect others and ensure safe disposal by incineration.
8. Wash hard surfaces well with copious amounts of cold, soapy water and dry with paper towels.	To remove residual contamination.
9. If spillage is on clothing, remove it as soon as possible and treat as 'soiled linen'.	To decontaminate clothing without hazard to laundry staff.
10. If spillage has penetrated clothing, wash contaminated skin liberally with soap and cold water.	To decontaminate skin and prevent drug absorption.
11. If spillage is on bed linen, change it immediately and treat as 'soiled linen'.	To protect the patient. To protect the laundry staff.
12. Any accident or spillage involving direct skin contact with a cytotoxic drug must be reported to the occupational health department (see Guideline: Protection of nursing staff when handling cytotoxic drugs, below).	To ensure that details of accidental contact are entered in the nurse's health record, and appropriate follow-up initiated.

Disposal of waste

Action	Rationale
1. 'Sharps' should be placed in the special container provided.	To ensure incineration and to prevent laceration and/or inoculation during transit and disposal.
2. Dry waste, intravenous administration sets and other contaminated material should be placed in 'high-risk' waste disposal bags.	To ensure careful handling and disposal by incineration.
3. A small amount (a part dose) of drug solution may be flushed down the main drainage system,	Many water authorities prohibit drug waste disposal in the drainage system. This route of disposal must

Guidelines: Protection of the environment

Action	Rationale
using copious amounts of cold water, only if no alternative means of safe disposal is available.	be used *only* if the waste cannot be safely transported elsewhere for disposal.
4. Re-usable trays and other equipment should be washed with copious amounts of water followed by the usual procedure for disinfection.	To prevent cross-contamination and cross-infection.
5. Unused doses of cytotoxics should be returned, unopened, to the pharmacy.	To enable them to be relabelled and re-issued, stability permitting, or to be destroyed safely.

Disposal of excreta from patients receiving cytotoxic drugs

Few cytotoxic agents are excreted as unchanged drug or active metabolites in urine or faeces. In order to comply with safe technique and practice, gloves should now always be worn, thus minimizing risks to the nursing staff.

GUIDELINES: PROTECTION OF NURSING STAFF WHEN HANDLING CYTOTOXIC DRUGS

Nursing staff should not be involved in routine reconstitution of cytotoxic drugs, as this is the function of the pharmacy unit. However, there may be emergency situations when the nurse is requested to prepare chemotherapy and it is essential that this is performed safely. The following procedure should be used for guidance.

Action	Rationale
1. Reconstitution of cytotoxic drugs should take place in a well-ventilated room. Doors and windows should be closed to prevent draughts.	To prevent any unnecessary airborne exposure from possible powder or droplet aerosol released.
2. While reconstitution is in progress no other activities should be carried out within the area. Movement in and out of that area should be restricted.	As above.
3. The area should contain a sink and running water.	To clean surfaces and/or skin if spillage or contamination occurs.
4. The work surface should be smooth and impermeable.	To enable cleaning of surfaces to be undertaken easily and quickly.
5. Reconstitution should take place in a plastic tray or equivalent.	To enable containment of spillage and ease of cleaning.
6. Nursing staff should receive instruction in the techniques of reconstitution and the reasons for these recommendations.	To ensure staff are safe to practise and are aware of the risks involved.
7. Direct contact with drug solution can be entirely avoided by good technique and the use of thick latex/PVC gloves.	To minimize exposure to handler.
8. All cuts and scratches should be covered.	To prevent infiltration of the skin if damage to gloves occurs.

Action	Rationale
9. Use protective goggles or glasses.	To prevent contact between drugs and the eyes. If the nurse wears glasses these should provide approximately 90% protection.
10. Wash protective goggles after use.	To prevent cross-contamination and/or cross-infection.
11. Use a good quality surgical face mask when reconstituting dry powder, especially if presented in an ampoule, e.g. bleomycin.	To prevent inhalation of any powder released during reconstitution.
12. Put on a disposable plastic apron or tabard.	To provide a barrier between the drug and the handler.
13. Ampoules should be held away from the face and covered with a sterile gauze swab when breaking them.	To prevent contamination of the gloves and skin. To prevent formation of aerosols or liberation of powder.
14. Luer-locking syringes should be used.	To reduce the incidence of accidental disconnection and spillage of drug.
15. A filtered air venting needle is recommended.	To prevent the development of pressure differentials between syringe and vial.
The alternative 'no airway' technique involves a 'push–pull' use of the syringe to add cyclically small quantities of diluent to, and remove air from, the closed vial. This technique is not recommended (see Chapter 13, Drug Administration, under the heading Guidelines: Administration of injections).	In inexperienced hands, the 'no airway' technique results in the danger of contamination. In extreme circumstances the vial and closure may separate, the syringe/needle junction may leak (especially if Luer slip syringes are used) or the vial may explode.
16. The diluent should be introduced slowly down the inside wall of the vial or ampoule.	To ensure that the powder is thoroughly wet before agitation, and is not released into the atmosphere.
17. Needles should be capped before the expulsion of air, or the tip should be covered with a sterile swab or the air should be expelled into the vial or ampoule.	To prevent aerosol formation.
18. Gloves and apron/tabard should continue to be worn during administration as the nurse is still handling the drugs and may become contaminated.	To prevent contamination at a later stage in the procedure.
19. Contamination of the skin, mucous membranes and eyes should be treated promptly. All areas should be washed with copious amounts of tap water or normal saline. Eye wash may be available.	To prevent any local damage to tissue.
20. Accidental infiltration of the skin with a vesicant drug should be treated as an extravasation and the appropriate procedure followed (see Management of extravasation of vesicant drugs, below).	To prevent any local damage to tissue.
21. If erythema and/or other local reaction occurs in any circumstances, contact the occupational	To prevent further damage and/or complications.

Guidelines: Protection of nursing staff when handling cytotoxic drugs

Action	Rationale
health unit or a member of the medical staff so that appropriate treatment may be advised.	
22. It is essential after any accident involving direct contact with a cytotoxic drug, or if any local or systemic symptoms occur after handling such a drug, that the occupational health unit should be contacted.	To assist with recording and monitoring of staff exposure.
23. If pregnancy is suspected or intended, the occupational health unit should be contacted.	To discuss future work patterns and any anxiety that may be felt.

GUIDELINES: INTRAVENOUS ADMINISTRATION OF CYTOTOXIC DRUGS

The most frequently used route for administration of cytotoxic drugs is intravenously. This ensures rapid, reliable delivery of agents to the patients and the tumour site. In addition, many drugs have to be administered into a vein where rapid dilution by the blood can occur, as they are irritant to soft tissue and capable of causing necrosis. These drugs are called 'vesicant agents'. The aim of the procedure for administration of chemotherapy intravenously is to protect both nurse and patient from contamination and also to prevent extravasation of drugs which could result in local tissue damage. An infusion of a cytotoxic vesicant drug may be administered into a verified central line, either with the aid of a mechanical device or by gravity. They should not be administered into a peripheral line by a mechanical pump device, due to the risk of possible extravasation. An infusion by gravity is acceptable only providing that the cannula is observed at all times. The large majority of cytotoxic agents will be delivered to the ward/unit individually packaged for delivery to a named patient, by injection or infusion. If this is not so, specific guidelines should be followed (see 'Guidelines: Protection of nursing staff when handling cytotoxic drugs', above).

Action	Rationale
1. Put on gloves and an apron before commencing the procedure.	To protect the nurse from local contamination of skin or clothing. *Note*: with careful handling technique, this risk is minimal but splashes can occur when changing syringes or infusion containers.
2. Prepare necessary equipment for an aseptic administration procedure, and ensure that this is followed carefully. (For further information on intravenous management, see Chapter 21).	To prevent local and/or systemic infection. Patients are frequently immunosuppressed and at greater risk.
3. Check that all details on the syringe or infusion container are correct when compared with the patient's prescription, before opening the sterile packaging.	To ensure the patient is given the correct drug which has been dispensed for him/her. To prevent wastage.
4. Explain the procedure to the patient.	To obtain the patient's consent and co-operation.
5. Inspect the infusion or injection site, and consult the patient about sensation around the device insertion site.	To detect any phenomena, e.g. phlebitis, which would render the vein unusable.
6. Establish the patency of the vein using normal saline.	To determine whether the vein will accommodate the extra fluid flow and irritant drugs and remain patent.

Action	Rationale
7. Ensure the correct administration rate.	To prevent speed shock. To prevent extra pressure and irritation within the vein.
8. Be aware of the immediate effects of the drug.	To know what to observe during administration. To be prepared to manage any side-effects which occur.
9. Administer drugs in the correct order, i.e. vesicants first.	To ensure that those agents likely to cause tissue damage are given when venous integrity is greatest, i.e. at the beginning. *Note*: because of their irritant nature (approx. pH3 to 3.5) anti-emetics should be given half an hour before chemotherapy administration or at the end of the sequence.
10. Observe the vein throughout.	To detect any problems at the earliest moment.
11. Observe for signs of extravasation, e.g. swelling or leakage at the site of injection. Note the patient's comments about sensation at the site, e.g. pain.	To prevent any unnecessary damage to soft tissue, and to enable the remainder of the drug(s) to be given correctly at another site. To enable prompt treatment to be given, thus minimizing local damage, and possibly preserving venous access for future treatment. (For further information see Management of extravasation of vesicant drugs, below).
12. Flush the line between drugs and after administration.	To prevent drug interaction. To prevent leakage along the path of the cannula or from the puncture site.
13. Be aware of the patient's comfort throughout the procedure.	To minimize trauma to the patient. To involve the patient in treatment and detect any side-effects and/or problems that may then be avoided at the next treatment.
14. Record details of the administration in the appropriate documents.	To prevent any duplication of treatment to provide a point of reference in the event of queries.
15. protect the patient from contact with the drugs by:	
(a) Placing a plastic sheet or small incontinence pad or equivalent under the sterile towel.	To provide a waterproof barrier and protect the skin.
(b) Inserting the needle carefully into the injection site of the giving set, extension set or cannula stopper.	To prevent exiting on the other side and contaminating or inoculating the patient.
(c) Careful removal of the blind hub and changing of needles/syringes, plus care when inserting the administration set into the infusion container or changing bags.	To avoid leakage or splashes and contamination of the nurse or patient.
(d) Securing a good bond between needle and syringe.	To prevent leakage or separation, which may occur due to pressure during administration, resulting in spray and contamination.
(e) Checking the injection site or stopper at the end of the procedure.	To ensure that there is no leakage.
(f) Acting promptly if any contamination is noted and washing the area with cold water or saline.	To prevent any local reaction on skin, mucous membranes, etc.

MANAGEMENT OF EXTRAVASATION OF VESICANT DRUGS

REFERENCE MATERIAL

The treatment of extravasations of chemotherapeutic agents is controversial. The procedure detailed here represents the policy of The Royal Marsden Hospital for the management by nursing staff of extravasion injury, drawn up with the assistance of pharmacy and medical colleagues.

Before administration of cytotoxic drugs the nurse should know which agents are capable of producing tissue necrosis. The following is a list of those in common use:

carmustine (concentrated solution)
dacarbazine (concentrated solution)
dactinomycin
daunorubicin
doxorubicin
epirubicin
mithramycin
mitomycin C
mustine
rubidazone
vinblastine
vincristine
vindesine

If in any doubt, the drug data sheet should be consulted or reference made to a trial protocol. Drugs should not be reconstituted to give solutions that are higher than the manufacturers' recommended concentration, and the method of administration should be checked, e.g. infusion, injection.

A variety of non-cytotoxic agents in frequent use are also capable of causing severe tissue damage if extravasated. They include:

vasoconstrictors, e.g. adrenaline;
antibiotics, e.g. erythromycin;
antivirals, e.g. acyclovir;
electrolytes, e.g. sodium bicarbonate 8.4% injection.

This potential hazard should always be remembered. The actions listed in this procedure may not be appropriate in all these instances. Drug data sheets should always be checked and the pharmacy departments should be consulted if the information is insufficient.

Extravasation should be suspected if:

1. The patient complains of burning, stinging pain or any other acute change at the injection site. This should be distinguished from a feeling of cold which may occur with some drugs.
2. Induration, swelling or leakage at the injection site is observed. There may be redness or 'blistering' with doxorubicin and other red drugs – the 'nettle rash' effect. This is normal.
3. No blood return is obtained. (If found in isolation this should not be regarded as an indication of a non-patent vein.)
4. A resistance is felt on the plunger of the syringe if drugs are given by bolus.
5. There is absence of free flow when administration is by infusion.

Note: One or more of the above may be present. If extravasion is suspected or confirmed, action must be taken immediately.

References and further reading

Oncology Nursing Society (1984) *Cancer Chemotherapy Guidelines and Recommendations for Nursing Education and Practice*. Oncology Nursing Society, Pittsburgh, USA.

Smith, R. (1985a) Extravasation of intravenous fluids. *British Journal of Parenteral Therapy*, 6(2), 30–5/42.

Smith, R. (1985b) Prevention and treatment of extravasation. *British Journal of Parenteral Therapy*, 6(5), 114–20.

Leight, M. D. *et al.* Anthracyclines. In *Cancer Chemotherapy By infusion*. (Ed. by J. Jacob & M. D. Lokich).

Rudolf, R. & Lasson, D. (1987) Etiology and treatment of chemotherapy agent extravasion. *Journal of Clinical Oncology*, 5(7), 1116–26.

GUIDELINES: MANAGEMENT OF EXTRAVASATION

Equipment

To assist the nurse, an extravasation kit should be assembled and should be readily available in each ward/unit. It contains:

1. Instant cold pack × 1.
2. Dexamethasone injection 8 mg in 2 ml × 1.
3. Hydrocortisone cream 1% 15 g tube × 1.
4. 2-ml syringes × 2.
5. 19 G needles × 2 (for drawing up).
6. 25 G needles × 4 (for injection).
7. Alcohol swabs.

8. Documentation slips × 2.
9. Copy of extravasation management procedure.

Procedure

Action	Rationale
1. Explain the procedure to the patient.	To obtain the patient's consent and co-operation.
2. Stop injection *immediately*, leaving the cannula or winged infusion device in place.	To minimize local injury. To allow aspiration of the drug to be attempted.
3. Aspirate any residual drug and blood from the device and suspected infiltration site.	To minimize local injury by removing as much drug as possible. Subsequent damage is related to the volume of the extravasation, in addition to other factors.
4. Remove the cannula or winged infusion device.	To prevent the site from being used as an intravenous route.
5. Apply cold pack or ice instantly.	To localize the area of extravasation, slow cell metabolism and decrease the area of tissue destruction. To reduce local pain.
6. Inform a member of the medical staff.	To enable actions differing from agreed policy to be taken if considered in the best interests of the patient. To notify the doctor of the need to prescribe drugs.
7. Draw up a dexamethasone injection 8 mg in 2 ml and inject 0.1 to 0.2 ml subcutaneously at the points of the compass around the circumference of the area of extravasation. Ensure the whole area is infiltrated.	To reduce local inflammation and improve the survival of tissues, especially those marginally injured.
8. Reapply a long-lasting cold pack or ice for 24 hours.	To localize the steroid effect in the area of extravasation. To reduce local pain and promote patient comfort.
9. Elevate the extremity and/or encourage movement.	To minimize swelling and to prevent adhesion of damaged area to underlying tissue, which could result in restriction of movement.
10. Apply hydrocortisone cream 1% twice daily, and instruct the patient how to do this. Continue as long as erythema persists.	To reduce local inflammation and promote patient comfort.
11. Provide analgesia as required.	To promote patient comfort. To encourage movement of the limb as advised.
12. Document the following details, in duplicate, on the form provided: (a) Patient's name/number. (b) Ward/unit. (c) Date, time. (d) Needle size and type. (e) Venepuncture site (on diagram). (f) Drug sequence. (g) Drug administration technique, i.e. 'bolus', infusion.	To provide an immediate full record of all details of the incident, which may be referred to if necessary. To provide a baseline for future observation and monitoring of patient's condition.

Guidelines: Management of extravasation

Action	Rationale
(h) Approximate amount of the drug extravasated.	
(i) Diameter of erythematous area.	
(j) Appearance of the area.	
(k) Nursing management/action taken/medical officer notified.	
(l) Patient's complaints, comments, statements.	
(m) Signature of the nurse.	
13. Explain to the patient that the site may remain sore for several days.	To reduce anxiety and ensure continued co-operation.
14. Observe the area regularly for erythema, induration, blistering or necrosis. *Inpatients*: monitor daily.	To detect any changes at the earliest possible moment.
15. Request outpatients to observe the area daily and to report immediately any increased discomfort, peeling or blistering of the skin.	To detect any changes as early as possible, and allow for a review of future management. This may include referral to a plastic surgeon.
16. If blistering or tissue breakdown occurs, begin sterile dressing techniques.	To prevent a superimposed infection.
17. If a shallow, clean ulcer develops, consider attempting to heal it using a starch-hydrogel type dressing.	To promote healing and avoid unnecessary surgery. This type of dressing has been observed to have a beneficial effect in some instances.
18. Consider referral for plastic surgery if no healing occurs and the patient's condition permits.	To prevent further pain or other complications as chemically induced ulcers rarely heal spontaneously.

ADMINISTRATION OF CYTOTOXIC DRUGS BY OTHER ROUTES

ORAL ADMINISTRATION

Nurses dispensing tablets or capsules should use a non-touch technique. If tablets have to be counted, this should be done using a triangle, which should be washed and dried after use.

Many tablets are coated and this protects the drug in its inner core. There is no handing risk if these coatings are not broken.

A small number of tablets are compressed powders, but there is no risk where there is no free powder visible. It is important that these tablets are not crushed.

Capsules are free from risk if they have not been opened or have not been either broken or leaked. They should not be crushed or opened.

Any visible spillage should be dealt with as previously directed (see 'Guidelines: Protection of the environment', above).

INTRAMUSCULAR AND SUBCUTANEOUS INJECTION

The local tissue toxicity of many cytotoxic drugs limits the use of this route. Drugs administered in this way are:

1. Methotrexate.
2. Bleomycin.
3. Cytosine arabinoside.
4. L-asparaginase.

Intramuscular and subcutaneous injections are often used for patient convenience, if regular adminstration is required and journeys to the hospital are impractical. Community nurses are responsible for administration and must be supplied with adequate information when the patient is discharged.

Although the volume of drug and diluent handled is less than for the intravenous route, preparation and reconstitution of the agents should be in line with the information listed under Guidelines: Protection of nursing staff when handling cytotoxic drugs, above. The nurse should continue to wear gloves during administration. Spillage and disposal of equipment should be dealt with as previously directed (see 'Guidelines: Protection of the environment', above) and systems of work modified to ensure this is possible.

Recommendations about administration should be followed carefully, e.g. deep intramuscular infection using a Z-track technique to prevent leakage onto the skin; rotation of sites to prevent local irritation developing.

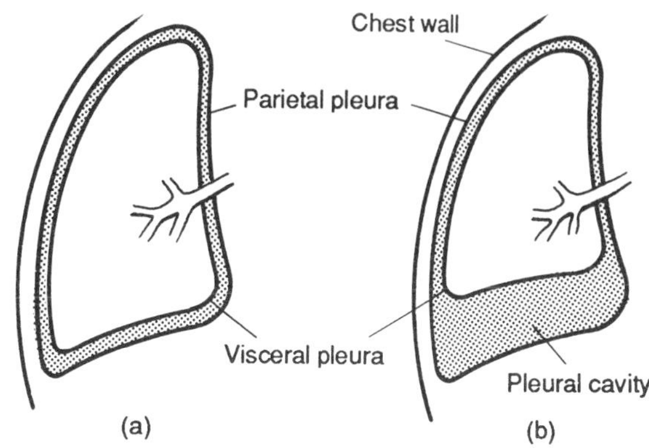

Figure 11.1 Lung anatomy. (a) Normal lung anatomy showing pleura. (b) Lung demonstrating presence of pleural effusion.

INTRAPLEURAL INSTILLATION

Definition

Introduction of cytotoxic drugs, or other substances, into the pleural cavity following drainage of an effusion to prevent or delay a recurrence.

REFERENCE MATERIAL

Pleural effusion is a common complication of malignant disease and may pose a considerable management problem. The most common neoplasms associated with the development of malignant pleural effusions are those of the:

1. Breast.
2. Lung.
3. Gastrointestinal tract.
4. Prostate.
5. Ovary.

The incidence varies, but may be as high as 50% in patients with primary lung or breast carcinoma. Such effusions can be very distressing to the patient, causing progressive discomfort, dyspnoea and death from respiratory insufficiency.

The alteration in normal anatomy due to the pressure of an effusion is illustrated in Figure 11.1. In health less than 5 ml of transudate fluid are present between the visceral and parietal pleurae. This fluid acts as a lubricant and hydraulic seal. Infections and malignancies disrupt this mechanism, often repeatedly. Patients may survive for months or years; therefore, effective palliation is important in maintaining or improving their quality of life.

Several methods have been used to treat pleural effusions, including surgical techniques, such as ablation of the pleural space, radiotherapy and systemic chemotherapy. In addition, instillation of sclerosing agents into the pleural space has been used for 30 years. These agents have included talc, radioactive phosphorus, thiotepa, tetracycline and, more recently, cytotoxic drugs. The drug most frequently instilled is bleomycin.

Cytology may show the presence of tumour cells in effusion fluid but even when these are absent, instillation of drugs may be effective in preventing recurrence due to the inflammatory reaction which obliterates the pleural space.

Improvements in equipment used, for example flexible cannulae or catheters, and lengthening of both the initial drainage period and that following instillation of the drug, have contributed to increased patient comfort and greater effectiveness.

All studies recommend that the patient should be turned regularly following instillation of the drug to ensure its complete distribution over the pleural surfaces. The recommended timing varies and only one paper (Wood, 1981) provides a detailed procedure. The rationale for such turning is based on clinical observation and there is a lack of work comparing patients who were turned with those who were not.

Adequate analgesia and nursing measures must be provided to ensure patient comfort.

References and further reading

Anderson, C. *et al* (1972) The treatment of malignant pleural effusions. *Cancer*, 33, 916–22.

Paladine, W. *et al.* (1976) Intracavity bleomycin in the management of malignant effusions. *Cancer*, 38, 1903–8.

Taylor, L. (1962) A catheter technique for intrapleural adminstration of alkylating agents: a report of ten cases.

American Journal of the Medical Sciences, 244(6), 706–16.

Wallach, H. (1975) Intrapleural tetracycline for malignant pleural effusions. *Chest*, 68, 510–12.

Wood, H. (1981) Developments in the support of patients with malignant pleural effusion. In *Cancer Nursing Update* (Ed. by R. Tiffany) 69–76. Baillière Tindall, London.

GUIDELINES: ADMINISTRATION OF INTRAPLEURAL DRUGS

The procedure and nursing care plans related to intrapleural drainage (see Chapter 20) should be consulted for all aspects of thoracic drainage. The following information covers specific points regarding drug instillation.

Procedure

Instillation of drug

Action	Rationale
1. Explain the procedure to the patient.	To obtain the patient's consent and co-operation.
2. Administer premedication to the patient, if prescribed.	To relax the patient.
3. Prepare the required equipment (see Chapter 13, Drug Administration, under the heading Guidelines: Administration of injections) and cytotoxic drug with protective wear as necessary.	To ensure the procedure goes smoothly without interruption.
4. Assist the doctor with the installation and provide support for the patient.	To increase the efficiency of the procedure and reduce discomfort for the patient.
5. At the end of the procedure clamp the drainage tube and leave for the desired period.	To prevent back-flow of the drug.

Rotation of the patient

Action	Rationale
1. Assess the clinical status of the patient and ability to tolerate the desired rotation.	To prevent undue discomfort the patient may feel and to ensure that the doctor is informed of the patient's inability to comply.
2. Turn the patient in the following rotation: (a) Left side. (b) Supine. (c) Right side. (d) Prone.	To ensure that the drug coats and washes the pleural cavity completely
3. Carry out the rotations as instructed. Examples are as follows: (a) Five minutes in each position, repeated once, equals 40 minutes. (b) Thirty minutes in each position, repeated once, equals four hours. (c) One hour in each position equals four hours.	As above.
4. Observe regularly for patient comfort. Administer analgesic as required.	To keep the patient comfortable and free from pain.

5. Record the patient's respirations, colour and temperature every 15 minutes for one hour, then every hour until stable, then four-hourly, or, as frequently as the patient's condition dictates.	To observe for pyrexia, a common side-effect that may indicate a developing infection or a reaction to chemotherapy. To ensure there is no change in respiratory function following the procedure.

Drainage of thoracotomy tube

Action	Rationale
1. Ensure the patient is in a comfortable position, and is aware of any limitations about movement.	To prevent discomfort or dislodgement of the drainage tube.
2. Unclamp the chest tube.	To allow drainage of the drug instilled.
3. Maintain the underwater seal until a volume of less than 50 ml is drained during 24 hours for 2 consecutive days or for a maximum of 7 days.	To allow complete drainage of the drug instilled, and any additional fluid.
4. Record the colour and amount of fluid drained on the appropriate documents.	To monitor the immediate effectiveness of therapy.

NURSING CARE PLAN

Problem	Cause	Suggested action
Local or systemic effects associated with specific cytotoxic drugs, e.g. rigors due to bleomycin.	Absorption of the drug into circulation in sufficient quantities to cause toxicity.	Be aware that this can occur. Initiate preventive action, e.g. corticosteroid cover to prevent rigors, or observe for a reaction and treat symptomatically.

INTRAVESICAL INSTILLATION

Definition
The instillation of chemotherapeutic agents directly into the bladder, via a urinary catheter.

Indications
This therapy has been shown to be effective in the treatment of superficial papillary carcinoma of the bladder.

REFERENCE MATERIAL
Systemic chemotherapy has repeatedly produced disappointing results in bladder carcinoma although some recent combined modality studies have produced improved response rates. However, instillation of cytotoxic agents into the bladder via a urinary catheter has been used for many years in selected cases with some success.

A high concentration of drug bathes the endothelium. Local toxicity is not a major problem, being mainly confined to burning on urination, and there are minimal general side-effects.

The use of this method of therapy is limited to two clinical situations:

1. Small, multiple, superficial, well-differentiated, non-invasive papillomatous carcinomas.
2. Prophylaxis, to minimize recurrence in patients with a history of multipe tumours known readily to seed locally.

Treatment protocols vary. Contact time with the bladder endothelium is one hour and therapy may be repeated on alternating days for three doses or weekly for varying lengths of time.

In measurable disease, however, response rates are similar with an average of 60% effectiveness. Approximately 30% of patients experience a complete response.

Cytotoxic drugs used are:

1. Thiotepa.
2. Mitomycin C.
3. Doxorubicin.

A paper (Garnick *et al.*, 1987) has questioned the criteria on which efficacy of treatment is based and has suggested that the primary measure of success should be the development or not of invasive bladder carcinoma.

References and further reading

Carter, S. K. & Wasserman, T. H. (1975) The chemotherapy of urologic cancer. *Cancer*, 36, 729–47.

Dorr, R. T. & Fritz, W. L. (1980) *Cancer Chemotherapy Handbook*. Kimpton, London.

Garnick, M. B. *et al.* (1987) A determination of appropriate endpoints in assessing efficacy of intravesical therapies in superficial bladder cancer. *Proceedings of the American Society of Clinical Oncology*, Abstract no. 412.

Manual of Cancer Chemotherapy (1981) *UICC Technical Reports 56*, pp. 223–4.

GUIDELINES: INTRAVESICAL INSTILLATION OF CYTOTOXIC DRUGS

Other relevant procedures are urinary catheterization (see Chapter 43) and bladder lavage and irrigation (see Chapter 5). Details of required procedure and problems which may be encountered are given in these chapters. The following guidelines and care plan deal with specific aspects of chemotherapy administration.

Equipment

1. Urotainer containing prescribed drug in clinically clean tray (delivered from pharmacy reconstitution unit).
2. Sterile, latex gloves.
3. Disposable apron and eye protection.
4. Gate clip or equivalent clamp for catheter.
5. Catheter drainage bag, if catheter is to remain in position.
6. 10- or 20-ml sterile syringe.
7. Small dressing pack, containing sterile field.

Procedure

Action	**Rationale**
1. Explain the procedure to the patient.	To obtain the patient's consent and co-operation.
2. Check the patient's full blood, as instructed by the medical staff, and inform them of any deficit before administration.	Absorption of the drug through the bladder wall may cause some myelosuppression. However, there are differing opinions as to whether regular checks are necessary.
3. Check all the details on the container of cytotoxic drug against the patient's prescription chart.	To minimize the risk of error and comply with legal requirements.
4. Assemble all necessary equipment, including the cytotoxic drug container, and proceed to the patient.	To ensure that the instillation proceeds smoothly and without interruption.
5. Screen the patient's bed/couch.	To ensure privacy during the procedure.
6. Ask the patient to empty bladder.	To enable the instillation of the drug.
7. Ensure the bladder is empty of urine.	To prevent dilution of the drug.
8. Put on an apron/eye protection.	To protect the nurse from contact with the cytotoxic drugs. With correct technique the risk of contamination is minimal, but splashes can occur.
9. If the catheter is already in place, using aseptic technique and sterile latex gloves, proceed to place sterile towel under the end of the catheter, clamp the catheter and disconnect the drainage bag.	To protect the patient from infection. To protect the nurse from drug spillage. To gain access to the catheter. To prevent urine from soiling the bed.

Action	Rationale
10. Remove the cover from the urotainer, connect to the catheter and release the clamp.	To facilitate drug instillation.
11. Gently squeeze the urotainer to administer the cytotoxic agent. Do not use force.	Rapid instillation would be uncomfortable for the patient, especially if the bladder is small or scarred from previous treatment or disease.
13. When the correct volume has been instilled, clamp the catheter.	To prevent drainage of drug from the bladder.
14. (a) If the catheter is to stay in position, connect the catheter to a new drainage bag but do not unclamp it.	To create a closed system, reducing the risk to bacterial contamination, and to retain the drug in the bladder.
(b) If the catheter is to be removed, withdraw the water from the catheter balloon using the sterile syringe and remove the catheter using gentle traction. Dispose of equipment into yellow clinical waste bag and seal.	The catheter may not be required for continued urinary drainage, and may have been inserted to facilitate drug administration, particularly in the outpatient department. The risk of infection is greater if the catheter remains *in situ*.
15. Make the patient comfortable and instruct him/her about changes of position required during the time the drug is *in situ*.	Frequent changes in position ensure the drug bathes all of the bladder mucosa.
16. If the patient is unable to turn himself/herself, nursing assistance must be provided.	As above.
17. Provide outpatients with information about the amount of movement required.	Following outpatient instillation, the journey home is usually sufficient to coat the bladder mucosa.
18. When the drug has been in the bladder for one hour, request the patient to micturate *or* release the clamp on the catheter to allow the drug and urine to drain into the bag.	One hour is the usual time specified for intravesical drugs to ensure the maximum therapeutic effect with minimum toxicity.
19. Advise the patient on fluid intake, suggesting ways in which he or she may increase it in the following 24-hour period. Patients should be aware that their urine may be cloudy.	To provide a good fluid output, washing out the bladder and reducing the likelihood of local irritation or difficulty in urination due to débris from the tumour.
20. Instruct the patient to report any discomfort or inability to pass urine immediately to ward staff or general practitioner/district nurse, or to telephone the hospital if anxious.	To detect any problems at the earliest moment. To reduce anxiety experienced by the patient.

NURSING CARE PLAN

Problem	Cause	Suggested action
No drainage of urine when the catheter is inserted.	Bladder is empty or the catheter is in the wrong place, e.g. in the urethra or in a false track. False tracks may develop after repeated cystoscopy or bladder surgery.	Do not inflate the balloon but tape the catheter to the skin to keep it in position. Check when the patient last micturated. Encourage the patient to drink a few glasses of fluid. Do not give the drug until urine flow is seen or correct positioning of the catheter is established. Inform a

Nursing care plan

Problem	**Cause**	**Suggested action**
		doctor if no urine has drained during the next 30 minutes.
Haematuria.	Trauma of catheterization or loosening of blood clots following cystoscopy by fluid injected into the bladder.	Inform a doctor. Observe the patient for signs of clot retention, shock, haemorrhage or fluid retention. Encourage the patient to drink fluids.
Leakage from around the catheter following administration of the drug.	Catheter slipping out of the bladder or bladder spasm caused by the drug.	Check the position of the catheter. Inform a doctor if leakage persists. Protect the patient's skin by wrapping sterile topical swabs around the catheter. Estimate the volume lost by leakage. Wash contaminated skin thoroughly.
Patient unable to retain the requisite drug volume in the bladder for the time required.	Low bladder capacity; weak sphincter muscles; unstable detrusor muscle causing uncontrolled bladder contractions.	Note actual duration of the drug in the bladder and inform a doctor.
Patient has pain during instillation of the drug or while the drug is in the bladder.	Following resection of mucosa, the bladder can become acutely sensitive to irritants, thus causing painful spasm resulting possible expelling of the cytotoxic agent.	Allow the drug to drain out and/or stop instillation if the pain is severe. Inform a doctor. Administer Entonox if appropriate (see Chapter 15, Entonox Administration) and have analgesics prescribed for subsequent administration.
Patient unable to pass urine after the drug has been *in situ* for the required length of time.	Anxiety; poor bladder tone; prostatism.	Reassure the patient. Encourage the patient to drink fluids.
Urine does not drain from the catheter when the clamp is released.	Catheter wrongly placed. Catheter blocked with clots and/or debris.	Check the position of the catheter. Perform bladder lavage.

INTRA-ARTERIAL CHEMOTHERAPY

Definition

Delivery of a high concentration of cytotoxic drug to the tumour site by catheterization of the artery providing the blood supply to the affected organ.

Drugs may be administered by slow push injection or infusion, the latter being most common. Frequency of administration is determined by the doctor.

REFERENCE MATERIAL

Indications

Intra-arterial chemotherapy has been used to treat a variety of malignancies at a number of different sites during the past 20 years. These include:

Head and neck lesions.
Liver metastases from colorectal cancer.
Sarcomas/melanomas of upper and lower limb (including isolated limb perfusion).
Carcinoma of the stomach.
Carcinoma of the breast.
Carcinoma of the cervix.

Intra-arterial chemotherapy is possible when the regional artery can be easily isolated and catheterized. Confirmation that the artery supplies the desired area can be achieved by installation of yellow fluorescence dye if the tumour site is visible, or contrast medium if an internal organ such as the liver is the target area.

Once the catheter is in place and secured, cytotoxic drugs may be administered by:

1. Injection, using a syringe.
2. Small volume infusion using a syringe pump.
3. Large volume infusion using a volumetric pump.

Other variations on the delivery system include the implantable drug delivery system.

All delivery systems must be under pressure to combat arterial pressure, i.e. 300 mm Hg. The majority of infusion pumps meet this requirement.

The cytotoxic drugs used vary with the histology and site of the tumour. The following have all been used for intra-arterial administration:

actinomycin D	5-FUDR (floxuridine)
BCNU (carmustine)	methotrexate
bleomycin	melphalan
cisplatin	mitomycin C
doxorubicin	vincristine
5-FU (5-fluorouracil)	

A high concentration of drug can be delivered to the primary or secondary tumour mass. A reduction in systemic circulating levels of drugs has been shown to occur in many circumstances resulting in a corresponding reduction in side-effects to the patient, although this is difficult to predict.

Principles of nursing care

Insertion is an operative procedure and consent must be obtained. Adequate explanation to the patient is essential, especially what to expect on return to the ward.

The area: to be shaved or otherwise prepared and the period of fasting should be checked with the doctor.

The catheter is inserted in theatre or in the X-ray department and its position checked at that time. The catheter will be secured and an occlusive dressing applied. This should *not* be touched as it is essential that the catheter is *not* displaced.

A three- or one-way tap is connected to the catheter and it is at this point that all manipulations take place. An extension set should be connected to this at the time of insertion or on return to the ward to prevent unnecessary handling near the skin exit site.

The system will consist of: catheter/tap/extension set/administration set or infusion device.

Certain general rules apply:

1. The dressing must not be touched but should be observed regularly for signs of bleeding. This should be reported immediately to the medical staff, including the radiologist.
2. All procedures or manipulations associated with the pathway must use aseptic technique.
3. All connections must be Luer locking to prevent exsanguination/air embolism or disconnection under pressure.
4. The line must be clamped securely or switched off using the tap *in situ* before any equipment changes.
5. Positive pressure, greater than arterial pressure, must be maintained at all times.
6. When chemotherapy is not being infused, heparinized saline must be used to maintain patency. This should be via a syringe/syringe pump during transfer between wards or departments, or via a syringe pump/infusion pump in the ward. A nurse escort may be necessary for transfers. The concentration of heparin should be 1 unit/ml, i.e.
   1000 i.u./1 litre of fluid
   500 i.u./500 ml of fluid
   50 i.u./50 ml of fluid.
   It should be delivered at the minimum rate sufficient to combat arterial pressure and maintain patency, approximately 5 ml per hour or 10 drops per minute, dependent on the device used. If a special delivery system is used, then manufacturers' instructions should be followed.
7. The patient must be instructed on the amount of mobility allowed. This may vary depending on the site of the catheter. Assistance may be needed to maintain personal hygiene and relieve pressure. Aids may be required to prevent the development of pressure ulcers on all points of contact.
8. The position of the catheter may be checked daily by X-ray, which will be performed on the ward. Fluoroscopy and installation of dye are other methods of confirming position.
9. At the end of treatment, the patency of the arterial line should be maintained using heparinized saline until a decision has been made about removal. Instructions for this and the amount

of heparin to be used should be prescribed in advance to enable the nurse to initiate the procedure when appropriate.

10. Before removal, the tap may be switched off and the catheter allowed to clot. The catheter should be removed by a doctor and firm pressure applied for at least five minutes or until all bleeding has ceased. A dressing should be applied to the site. Pressure dressings are not indicated if bleeding has ceased and can obscure the formation of a haematoma.

Any problems should be referred to the medical staff and the radiologist (Consertino, 1987).

Conclusion

The administration of intra-arterial chemotherapy is an infrequent occurrence but it has been used to achieve significant reductions in tumour size and improved survival. A decrease in systemic circulating levels of drugs and a lessening of side-effects to patients has been shown, although this is variable.

Do not hesitate to contact a radiologist if a problem is suspected as he/she is the expert in catheter placement and management of complications.

References and further reading

Bedford, R. F. (1978) Percutaneous radial artery cannulation. *Surgical News*, no. 4.

Consertino, F. (1987) Chapter 23. *Principles and Practice of Intravenous Therapy*, 4th edn (Ed. by A. Plumer & F. Consertino), pp. 477–504. Little, Brown & Co, Boston, USA.

Dorr, R. T. & Fritz, W. L. (1980) *Cancer Chemotherapy Handbook*. Kimpton, London.

Gilbertson, A. A. (1984) *Intravenous Technique and Therapy*. Heinemann, London.

Plumer, A. L. (1982) *Principles and Practice of Intravenous Therapy*. Little, Brown & Co, Boston, USA.

Taylor, I. (1985) Hepatic arterial infusion of anti-cancer drugs. *Cancer Topics*, 5(5), 50–1.

NURSING CARE PLAN

Problem	Action	Rationale
Haemorrhage.	Observe the dressing at regular intervals. Monitor pulse and blood pressure at least four-hourly.	To prevent blood loss or detect haemorrhage at the earliest possible moment.
	Instruct the patient on the amount of movement permitted and to report any feeling of faintness, or oozing noted on dressing.	
	After removal of the catheter, vital signs and the dressing should be observed every 15 minutes for two hours. Whether the patient should remain on bedrest for 24 hours is dependent on the site that the patient has been catheterized.	
	If bleeding occurs, pressure should be applied immediately and a member of the medical staff contacted.	
Displacement of the catheter.	Do not disturb the dressing placed in the X-ray department.	To prevent displacement or detect it as early as possible, so reducing the likelihood of extravasion of drugs (see Guidelines: Management of extravasation, above).
	Instruct the patient on amount of movement permitted.	
	Check position daily, if requested by the doctor.	

Arterial occlusion.	Check vessel patency daily, if instructed to do so by medical staff. This may be done using a Doppler flowmeter or by manual location of distal pulses. Report any abnormality to the doctor or radiologist.	To prevent this occurring and ensure continued delivery of therapy to the patient.
Infection.	Strict asepsis must be maintained for all procedures and manipulations of the arterial line.	To prevent both localized infection and septicaemia.
	Temperature must be taken every four hours and any pyrexia investigated.	To observe for pyrexia as it may indicate a developing infection.
Exsanguination/air embolism.	Luer-lock connections must be used throughout the pathway. These should be checked at regular intervals, and continuous flow maintained. Care must be taken when changing equipment to prevent blood loss occurring or air entering the line, e.g. shut off tap, firm clamping, if necessary. Care must be taken when injecting medications, as above. The seriousness of an air embolus depends on the siting of the arterial line and whether it is a direct route to the carotid artery and so to the brain.	To prevent a major blood loss progressing to shock. To prevent an air embolus, although this is less likely.
Thrombosis/emboli.	The literature indicates that thrombosis occurs in over 40% of arteries catheterized for over 48 hours. However, this is dependent on the vessel used. Most used for chemotherapy delivery pose no problem and will remain patent for the treatment period. However, a resulting thrombus may embolize causing vascular insufficiency, distal or central embolism. When occlusion occurs due to thrombus formation or spasm, blood flow is usually maintained by collaterals until the vessel recovers. Presence of a pulse and the colour of the area should be checked daily or a Doppler flowmeter may be used.	To detect this problem at the earliest possible moment, so preventing reduced blood flow to the limb or organ.

Nursing care plan

Problem	**Cause**	**Suggested action**
	Any abnormality should be reported to the medical staff and radiologist.	
	The catheter should be removed by the doctor using firm, steady traction, in an attempt to prevent dislodging any thrombus present.	
	The condition of the patient and the limb/area should be observed carefully at the time that vital signs are measured.	
Damage to the artery, arteriovenous fistula, aneurysm formation.	The incidence of these is low and the likelihood of them occurring can be minimized by gentle handling of the catheter and immobilization of the limb/area as soon as appropriate.	To reduce the incidence of these complications, however rare, and to ensure that the medical staff are notified immediately.
Extravasation of drugs/failure of drug to reach target area.	Both of these are very rare but can lead to significant morbidity. The incidence can be reduced by careful placement of the catheter and verification by X-ray or installation of dye.	As above.
	If there is any doubt concerning the placement of the catheter the doctor and radiologist should be notified, as extravasation of the drug may lead to ulceration and necrosis.	
Chemical hepatitis/bilary sclerosis.	The occurrence of these will be evident from elevated liver enzymes. Therefore, monitoring of liver function tests is important. Any elevation is usually transient.	To be aware that this may occur and of the significance.

12

Discharge Planning

Definition

Discharge planning is the plan evolved before a patient is transferred from one environment to another. This process involves the patient, partner, family, friends, and the hospital and community health care teams. An individualized assessment of the patient for future care needs is a continuous process that begins on admission. This enables the formulation of a plan which promotes continuity and co-ordination of health care on discharge from hospital. Discharge planning is an integral part of the continuity of nursing care for patients throughout their hospital stay.

Historical perspective

The discharge of patients from hospital into the community continues to remain an area of concern. Research first conducted in the late 1960s (Hockey, 1968; Noble, 1967) found that little communication between hospital and community nurses actually took place. Skeet (1971) found that of 530 patients interviewed at home after their return from hospital, approximately half had to cope with unmet needs on discharge.

The situation has not improved significantly in the past 30 years. There is considerable evidence that a patient's discharge from hospital is often unplanned, with little attempt made to offer or to arrange the appropriate community services (Altschul, 1984; Armitage, 1985; Jackson, 1990; Jones, 1984; Saddington, 1985).

Inadequate communication networks or a lack of interpersonal co-operation has been identified as contributing to these problems, resulting in the needs of the patient and family being ignored, or inappropriate assistance being engaged. An effective communication process is vital if the patient's home nursing care is to begin without delay (Bowling & Betts, 1984).

Primary responsibility for care-giving rests with the patient's partner, family and friends. The days following discharge can be a period of great vulnerability and anxiety (Waters, 1987). Poor discharge planning and its consequences may result in physiological and psychological problems for both cancer patients and their families (Edstrom & Miller, 1981; Wingate & Lackey, 1989). A lack of information, knowledge and physical care skills can cause psychological distress for patients and families at critical periods following discharge (Oberst & Scott, 1988). In a study conducted by Jackson (1990), none of the family members interviewed were aware of support groups for families. Campbell & Ross (1990) indicated that patients and families were not informed about the availability of aids and equipment, thus leading to stress and difficulty in coping in the home environment.

The chronicity of the cancer disease process, coupled with episodes of acute life-threatening illness necessitates frequent hospital admissions and complex treatment procedures that may have a prolonged effect on the quality of life for patients and their families (Giacquinta, 1977; Sque, 1985). Disruption and distress can be minimized if care is planned and is continuous between hospital and home (Jupp & Simms, 1987). The decision to discharge a patient from hospital depends on many factors other than medical consideration. A multidisciplinary approach is essential to ensure that all available expertise is utilized in planning for discharge.

Collaboration between hospital and community health care professionals is important for continuity in patient care. Community nurses should be involved in the discharge planning process (Guerrero, 1990). Continuity of care occurs only when all health providers make a concerted effort to link their plan of care to the whole plan of care for the patient (Marquez, 1980).

Aims

1. To prepare the patient, partner and family physically and psychologically for transfer home or to an agreed environment.
2. To facilitate a smooth transfer, by ensuring that all

Table 12.1 An assessment of a patient's ability to meet their self-care requisites (Orem, 1980)

Six universal self-care requisites for all healthy individuals:

1. Sufficient intake of air, water, nutrition
2. Satisfactory eliminative functions
3. Activity balanced with rest
4. Time spent alone balanced with time spent with others
5. Prevention of danger to self
6. Being 'normal'

Orem describes two further categories of self-care requisites which arise out of the influence of events on the universal self-care requisites:

1. Developmental self-care requisites
2. Health deviation self-care requisites (Pearson and Vaughan, 1989)

necessary health care facilities are prepared to receive the patient.

3. To promote the highest possible level of independence for the patient, partner and family by encouraging self-care activities.
4. To provide continuity of care between the hospital and the agreed environment by facilitating effective communication.

REFERENCE MATERIAL

Assessment of patients' needs before discharge

Table 12.1 summarizes the assessment factors to be considered before discharge planning. Assessment can be conducted within any relevant model of nursing care. The following assessment outline is based on Orem's self-care model (1980), which attempts to encourage the patient and family or friends to make the best use of their most immediate resource in health care – themselves.

Healthy individuals have sufficient self-care ability to be able to meet their fundamental self care requisites. In Table 12.1 individuals who experience illness or injury are subject to additional demands for self-care. They may be able to meet those needs with nursing assistance or require a nurse to meet those needs for them until they are capable of resuming their own self-care.

First stage of the assessment

Is there a deficit between the individual's self-care requisite and their ability to self-care?

Yes? Nursing intervention required.
No? Nursing intervention not required.

(If patients cannot carry out their self-care requisites *safely or effectively* then nursing will be required.)

Second stage of the assessment

If patients cannot carry out their self-care requisites, then why is there a self-care deficit?

1. Lack of knowledge? This could be related to:
   (a) Physical and psychological needs that are unfamiliar to the patient, family and friends.
   (b) Knowledge of specialist health care activities, e.g. dressing techniques, catheter management, etc.
   (c) Patient's, family's and friends' understanding of illness and treatment.
   (d) Specific aids and equipment that will facilitate health care.
   (e) Community resources available.
2. Lack of skill? This could be related to:
   (a) Techniques of physical and psychological care.
   (b) Ability to learn to manage health care problems.
   (c) Lack of contact with similar health care problems before discharge.
   (d) Inappropriate teaching or experience regarding health care activities before this admission.
3. Lack of motivation? This could be related to:
   (a) Willingness of patient, family and friends to undertake self-care activities.
   (b) Willingness of patient, family and friends to accept help and their ability to assist in care-giving.
   (c) Are the self-care activities culturally and socially acceptable, e.g. self-administration of suppositories, stoma care, etc.?
4. Limited range of behaviour? This could be related to:
   (a) Physical limitations, e.g. effects of disease process and treatment:
   respiration
   eating and drinking
   elimination
   posture
   rest and sleep
   dressing and undressing
   temperature control
   personal hygiene
   protection from danger
   communication
   religion
   work
   recreation
   education (Henderson, 1977).
   (b) Psychological limitations.

(c) Social limitations, e.g. resources within family and friends, occupational and financial resources.
(d) Is the patient safe to engage in self-care activities?

5. Potential for re-establishing self-care in the future.
   (a) Activities which will lead to the patient and family being able to take over self-care activities again.

Conclusion

From the patient's perspective, discharge remains one of the most important events of the hospital stay. The way in which the patient is transferred into the community directly influences the patient's, family's and friends' abilities to cope at home. Therefore, it is essential that discharge planning is considered as an integral part of the nursing process. Assessment, planning, implementation and evaluation of care from the time of hospital admission, up to and including discharge, are essential if care is to be individualized and continuity of care achieved.

References and further reading

Altschul, A. (1984) Safe journey home. *Nursing Times*, 80(41), 18–19.

Armitage, S. (1985) Hospital to home: discharge referrals, who's responsible? *Nursing Times*, 81(8), 26–8.

Bowling, A. & Betts, G. (1984) From hospital to home 2: communication on discharge. *Nursing Times*, 80(30), 44–6.

Campbell, F. & Ross, F. (1990) Aids and equipment. *Journal of District Nursing*, November, 4–10.

Department of Health (1989) *Health Circular HC(89)5. Discharge of Patients from Hospital*. HMSO, London.

Edstrom, S. & Miller, M. (1981) Preparing the family to care for the cancer patient at home: a home care course. *Cancer Nursing*, 5(2), 49–52.

Giacquinta, B. (1977) Helping families to face the crisis of cancer. *American Journal of Nursing*, 77(10), 1585–8.

Guerrero, D. (1990) Working towards a partnership. *Community Outlook*, September 14–18.

Henderson, V. (1977) *Basic Principles of Nursing Care*. International Council of Nurses, Kruger.

Hockey, L. (1968) *Care in the Balance*. Queen's Institute of District Nursing, London.

Jackson, M. F. (1990) Use of community support services by elderly patients discharged from general medical and geriatric medical wards. *Journal of Advanced Nursing*, 15, 167–75.

Jones, I. H. (1984) Cause for complaint 2: lack of communication. *Nursing Times*, 80(32), 51–2.

Jupp, M. & Simms, S. (1987) Going home. *Nursing Times*, 82(33), 40–2.

Marquez, S. (1980) A community homecare co-ordination programme (Chapter 11). *Continuity of Care Between the Hospital and the Community* (Ed. by S. R. Beatty), pp. 147–63. Grune & Stratton, London and New York.

Noble, M. (1967) Communication in the National Health Service – a survey of some published findings. *International Journal of Nursing Studies*, 4, 15–28.

Oberst, M. T. & Scott, D. W. (1988) Post-discharge distress in surgically treated cancer patients and their spouses. *Research in Nursing and Health*, 11, 223–33.

Orem, D. (1980) *Nursing: Concepts of Practice*. McGraw Hill, New York.

Pearson, A. & Vaughan, B. (1989) *Nursing Models for Practice*. Heinemann, Oxford.

Roberts, I. (1975) *Discharge from Hospital*. Royal College of Nursing, London.

Saddington, N. (1985) A communication breakdown. *Nursing Times*, 81(8), 31.

Skeet, M. (1971) *Home from Hospital*. Dan Mason Nursing Research Committee, Macmillan Press, London.

Sque, M. (1985) What's in a name? *Nursing Mirror*, 160, 28–30.

Waters, K. R. (1987) Outcomes of discharge from hospital for elderly patients. *Journal of Advanced Nursing*, 12, 347–55.

Wingate, A. L. & Lackey (1989) A description of the needs of non-institutionalized cancer patients and their primary care givers. *Cancer Nursing*, 12(4), 216–25.

GUIDELINES: DISCHARGE PLANNING

Procedure

Action	Rationale
1. Assess the patient for home care needs and formulate a plan of care to meet the individual physiological, psychological and social needs of patient, family and friends.	To determine as soon as possible after admission potential nursing or social problems.
This must begin on admission and is an ongoing process.	To enable planning to start well in advance of discharge home.
2. Document all relevant social information, communications with community services and	To facilitate planning, co-ordination and communication.

Guidelines: Discharge planning

Action	**Rationale**
plans for discharge. If considerable planning is required, formulate a discharge action plan using a separate problem page in the multidisciplinary care plan.	
3. Ensure that the home address and telephone number of the patient is documented accurately. Document the discharge address if different to the permanent address.	Personal information may not have been updated on previous nursing or medical records. It is crucial that this information is accurate when making referrals to community services.
4. Ensure that the patient is registered with a permanent general practitioner (GP) and with one on a temporary basis if going to a different address on discharge. Check the names, addresses and telephone numbers with the patient and document accurately.	Community nursing services may not wish to accept the patient without medical support. Accurate information is required to establish which district nurse will have responsibility for patient care. It is important for the patient that medical care can be provided at home.
5. Establish whether any statutory community health or Social Services have been involved before the patient's admission. Document names and telephone numbers. Include the health visitor when the patient has children under the age of five years.	To enable contact for exchange of information. Valuable information can be obtained from community services to assist in assessing potential needs on discharge.
Ensure that all services visiting the patient at home are informed of the patient's admission.	To prevent anxiety and wasted time for community services in trying to locate the client.
6. Check whether the patient has dependants, e.g. elderly relatives, children or a disabled or unwell partner. If so, establish who is looking after them and whether they are receiving any services.	Arrangements may need to be made for alternative care or an increase in services.
7. Establish who are the main care-givers and sources of support for the patient and the degree of contact and care they are able to provide, e.g. partner, relatives, friends. Document appropriate names, addresses and telephone numbers and their relationship to the patient.	To assess the support that the patient and carers may require at home so that appropriate services can be mobilized.
Ensure that the next of kin recorded is the person who is willing to accept responsibility for legal and financial affairs.	To ensure information is given to the appropriate people.
8. Establish who else is involved in giving care/support and the type of help given, e.g. local support group, voluntary agency, church.	To establish social network in order to co-ordinate care between voluntary and statutory agencies.
9. Ascertain the type of accommodation the patient is living in, e.g. residential or nursing home, sheltered housing, private or local authority house, flat or bungalow.	To identify early potential housing problems which may entail social work intervention.
Document the names and telephone numbers of	To enable contact to be made to establish that an

Action	Rationale
sheltered housing or officers in charge of homes.	appropriate degree of care and support can continue to be provided.
10. Did the patient experience any functional difficulties before admission, e.g. was he/she able to climb stairs? Is he/she likely to experience difficulties as a result of current problems or treatment?	To establish at an early stage whether an occupational therapy assessment is required.
11. Refer to other hospital personnel as soon as potential need is recognized, e.g. occupational therapist, community liaison nurse, social worker, physiotherapist. Referral as soon as possible after admission is essential – do not wait until treatment is completed and discharge is imminent.	To ensure multidisciplinary planning and co-ordination. Considerable time may be needed to arrange community services.
12. Arrange for the district nurse to make joint home assessment with the occupational therapist where appropriate.	It is valuable for the district nurse to assess the patient in the home before discharge and plan appropriate care and to liaise with occupational therapist regarding equipment.
13. Plan discharge with patient, relatives, friends and all involved hospital and community personnel and set discharge date.	To collate information and co-ordinate planning.
A multidisciplinary meeting is a most helpful forum. Document planned action resulting from meeting.	To ascertain readiness for discharge. To ensure provision of services on discharge.
14. Refer to community nursing services with at least 48 hours' notice of discharge. If a high level of nursing care is required, refer as soon as you have identified that nursing services will be required. Document referrals made with names, telephone numbers and date of referral.	Arrangment made for discharge may depend on availability and level of service which can be provided. Services may be closed temporarily to new referrals. District nurses require time to plan their work.
15. Ascertain whether district nurses are able to carry out necessary clinical procedures, in accordance with their health authority policy, e.g. care of Hickman line, syringe driver.	District nurses may not have been trained in certain procedures or may be unfamiliar with particular equipment.
Consider alternative arrangement if necessary. Give written information or instructions.	
Invite district nurses to visit the ward where appropriate.	
16. Complete the community care referral form. Allow time to complete it fully and accurately. The form should be completed and signed by the same person. Provide a copy for the Macmillan home care nurse, if involved.	The district nurse requires full knowledge of patient's history and nursing requirements. Form may be inaccurate if insufficient time is allowed to complete it.
17. Ensure any essential aids or equipment have been obtained and adaptations made before discharge, e.g. oxygen, commode. Liaise with occupational therapist.	Some equipment may not be available or may take a long time to obtain. The patient may be at risk at home or suffer unnecessary discomfort and distress.

Guidelines: Discharge planning

Action	Rationale
18. Ensure that medical staff have contacted the general practitioner by telephone when medical back-up will be required at home.	Lack of information makes it difficult for the GP to provide the medical care needed.
Ensure that the appropriate community services have been arranged and informed of pending discharge.	To ensure continuity of care.
19. Notify the sheltered housing warden or officer in charge of nursing/residential home, of discharge date.	To ensure preparation of accommodation.
20. Ensure that carers have full information regarding the patient's medical condition and care required. This may require you to initiate a meeting with medical staff.	To prepare carers and to help them to support each other.
21. Teach the patient and carers any necessary skills, allowing sufficient time to practise before discharge.	To enable the patient to be as independent as possible and promote an understanding of self-care techniques.
22. Inform the patient and carers of potential side-effects of treatment and management.	To alleviate anxiety and to promote patient comfort and knowledge.
23. Ensure that the patient and carers have information on other organizations if appropriate, e.g. local support groups, voluntary specialist organizations.	Some patients benefit from the kind of support offered by self-help groups.
24. Reinforce any special instructions with written information or by giving an approved education booklet.	To promote an understanding of disease and treatment.
25. Give patient, family and friends telephone numbers of the community services which will be visiting. Inform them of expected date of first visit or telephone contact. Ensure they have an understanding of service provision and are agreeable to their involvement.	To alleviate anxiety. So that services can be contacted if they do not visit when expected.
26. Ensure that arrangements have been made to provide patient with food at home on discharge and that there will be adequate heating.	To supply immediate needs. Community services may not be able to commence immediately.
27. Ensure that the patient has door key and can gain entrance to their residence. Wherever possible, ensure that someone is at home to receive the patient.	Patient may have left their key with a neighbour. It is helpful for someone to be available to welcome patient and attend to any immediate needs.
28. Book transport if required with 48 hours' notice, using relevant form. Specify if patient needs a stretcher or chair. Ensure that transport is also booked for return clinic appointment if necessary.	Patient may not have private transport facilities and may be too weak to use public transport.

	Action	Rationale
	Cancel transport if discharge date or outpatients department appointment is altered.	
29.	Ensure that all medication, dressings and equipment, e.g. syringes, catheter bags, are ordered for the patient to take home.	Time is needed to obtain items on prescription in the community. To ensure that treatment is continuous and to prevent errors in drug administration.
	Ensure that adequate supplies are given considering availability in the community, according to hospital policy.	
	Ensure that the patient and carers have appropriate knowledge of the route, frequency and side-effects of any drugs and of the use of any equipment given and how to obtain future supplies.	
	Reinforce with written advice.	
30.	Book outpatient clinic appointment and give the patient an appointment card.	To ensure the patient is followed up and to minimize difficulty of attendance.
	If the patient had a previous appointment booked before admission, ensure this appointment is cancelled.	
	If patient requires appointments at different clinics, ensure they are spaced realistically, e.g. not on consecutive days when patient may have a long way to travel.	
31.	Discharge plans should not be altered without consultation with all the hospital personnel who have been involved in the planning, e.g. occupational therapist, social worker, community liaison nurse.	If there is no consultation this causes considerable confusion and stress for the patient, family and friends, and all involved services. It may result in the patient being unsupported at home.
32.	If discharge is cancelled or postponed or if patient dies, ensure that all relevant community services are informed.	To avoid wasted visits and promote good community relations. To avoid distress to relatives.
33.	*Weekend Discharge* Whenever possible, patients who require a high level of district nursing and Social Service support should not be discharged home on a Friday or Saturday. This applies particularly to patients who were previously unknown to community services.	All community services will be operating at a reduced level and emergency medical back-up may be difficult to obtain.
	Note: Assessment and planning for weekend leave is as important as for final discharge.	

13

Drug Administration

REFERENCE MATERIAL

Legislation

The manufacture, supply and use of medicines (and the interactive wound dressings) are controlled by two statutes, the 1968 Medicines Act and the 1971 Misuse of Drugs Act.

The Medicines Act, 1968

This defines 'medicinal products' as substances sold or supplied for administration to humans (or animals) for medicinal purposes. Part 3 of the Act, and regulations and orders made under it, control the manufacture and sale or supply of medicines and for this purpose broadly classifies them into three groups:

1. Prescription-only medicines (POM).
2. Pharmacy medicines (P).
3. General sales list medicines (GSL).

Different requirements apply to the sale, supply and labelling of medicines in each group. In NHS hospitals, adherence to the Act usually means that the purchasing and supply of medicines is supervised by a pharmacist, and that supply or administration to a patient is only on a doctor's prescription.

Sections 9, 10, and 11 of the Act exempt doctors/dentists, pharmacists and nurses, respectively, from many restrictions otherwise imposed by the act on the general public, and thus allow them to supply and use drugs in the practice of their respective professions.

The Misuse of Drugs Act, 1971

This designates and defines as controlled drugs a number of 'dangerous or otherwise harmful' substances. These substances are all also by definition prescription-only medicines under the Medicines Act, 1968.

The controls imposed by the Misuse of Drugs Act are therefore additional to those under the Medicines Act.

The purpose of the 1971 Act is to prevent abuse of controlled drugs, most of which are potentially addictive or habit forming, by prohibiting their manufacture, sale or supply except in accordance with regulations made under the Act. Other regulations govern safe storage, destruction and supply to known addicts.

The level of control to be exercised is related to the potential for abuse or misuse of the substances concerned. Under the current (1985) regulations, controlled drugs are classified into five schedules, each representing a different level of control. The requirements of the Act as they apply to nurses working in a hospital with a pharmacy department are described in Table 13.1. Schedule 2 is the most relevant to everyday nursing practice.

Summary

Hospital wards and departments are authorized to hold a stock of controlled drugs. These are obtained by the use of a special duplicate order form signed by the nurse in charge who is then responsible for them. They should be stored in a locked cupboard used exclusively for this purpose. They may be administered only to a patient in that ward or department when prescribed by a doctor. Appropriate records of their use must be maintained. Completed registers and copies of orders should be kept for two years. Unwanted drugs should normally be destroyed in the pharmacy but may, under some circumstances be disposed of on the ward under the supervision of a pharmacist. An appropriate entry should then be made in the ward register.

Types of medicinal preparations of drugs

Preparations for oral administration

Tablets

These come in a great variety of shapes, sizes, colours and types. The formulation may be very simple and result for instance in a plain, white, uncoated tablet, or complex and designed with specific therapeutic aims. Sugar coatings are used to improve appearances and palatability. In cases where the drug is a gastric irritant or is broken down by gastric acid, an enteric coating may be used. This is designed to allow the tablet to remain intact in the stomach and to pass unchanged into the small bowel where the coating dissolves and hence the drug is released and absorbed. Sustained-release tablets may be formulated in many ways but all with the object of producing a slow continuous rate of drug release as the tablet passes along the alimentary tract. Tablets may also be formulated specifically to dissolve readily ('soluble' or 'effervescent'), to be chewed or to be held under the tongue ('sublingual'). Unscored or coated tablets should not be crushed or broken, nor should most 'slow-release' or 'sustained action' tablets.

Capsules

These consist of a gelatin shell in which is contained the drug powder or granules. They offer a useful method of formulating drugs which are difficult to make into a tablet or are particularly unpalatable. Slow-release capsule formulations also exist. Capsules should not normally be broken or opened.

Lozenges and pastilles

These are designed to be sucked for local treatment of the mouth and throat.

Linctuses, elixirs, syrups

These are usually sweet, syrup-like solutions used to treat coughs or where, in children for instance, a tablet or capsule may be inappropriate.

Mixtures

These are flavoured solutions or suspensions of drugs. It is particularly important the suspensions are thoroughly mixed by shaking before each dose is measured. This ensures that the measured volume always contains the correct amount of drug.

Table 13.1 Summary of the legal requirements for the handling of controlled drugs as they apply to nurses in hospitals with a pharmacy

	Schedule 1	*Schedule 2*	*Schedule 3*	*Schedule 4*	*Schedule 5*
Drugs in schedule	Cannabis + derivatives but excluding nabilone, LSD (lysergic acid diethylamide)	Most opioids in common use including: alfentanye amphetamines cocaine diamorphine methadone morphine papaveretum fentanyl phenoperidine pethidine codeine } dihydrocodeine } pentazocine }	Minor stimulants. Barbiturates (but excluding: hexobarbitone thiopentone methohexitone). diethylpropion buprenorphine injections only	Benzodiazepines	Some preparations containing very low strengths of: cocaine codeine morphine pholcodine and some other opioids
Ordering	Possession and supply permitted only by special licence from the Secretary of State issued (to a doctor only) for scientific or research purposes	A requisition must be signed in duplicate by the nurse in charge. The requisition must be endorsed to indicate that the drugs have been supplied. Copies should be kept for two years	As Schedule 2	No requirement[1]	No requirement[1]
Storage[5]	As Schedule 2	Must be kept in a suitable locked cupboard to which access is restricted	diethylpropion and buprenorphine: as Schedule 2. all other drugs: no requirement	No requirement[1]	No requirement[1]

Table 13.1 *Continued*

	Schedule 1	*Schedule 2*	*Schedule 3*	*Schedule 4*	*Schedule 5*
Record keeping	As Schedule 2	Controlled drugs[3] register must be used	No requirement	No requirement[1]	No requirement[1]
Prescriptions	As Schedule 2	See below for detail of requirements[4]	As Schedule 2 except for phenobarbitone[2]	No requirement[1]	No requirement[1]
Administration to patients	As Schedule 2. Under special licence only	A doctor or dentist or anyone acting on their instructions may administer these drugs to anyone for whom they have been prescribed	As Schedule 2	No requirement[1]	No requirement[1]

[1] 'No requirement' indicates that the Misuse of Drugs Act imposes no legal requirements additional to those imposed by the Medicines Act, 1968.

[2] All references to phenobarbitone should be taken to include all preparations of phenobarbitone and phenobarbitone sodium. Because of its use as an anti-epileptic, phenobarbitone is exempt from the handwriting requirements only of the full prescription requirements (see 4 below).

[3] *Record keeping.*

There is no legal requirement for the nurse in charge or acting in charge of a ward or department to keep a record of Schedule 1 or 2 controlled drugs obtained or supplied. However the Aitken Report recommended that this should be done and in practice a controlled drug register is invariably kept according to the following guidelines:

(a) Each page should be clearly headed to indicate the drug and preparation to which it refers. Records for different classes of drug should be kept on separate pages.
(b) Entries should be made as soon as possible after the relevant transaction has occurred and always within 24 hours.
(c) No cancellations or obliteration of an entry should be made. Corrections should be made by means of a note in the margin or at the foot of the page and this should be signed, dated and cross-referenced to the relevant entry.
(d) All entries should be indelible.
(e) The register should be used for controlled drugs only and for no other purposes.
(f) A completed register should be kept for two years from the date of the last entry.

[4] *Prescription requirements.*

(a) The prescription *must* state:
   (i) The name and address of the patient.
   (ii) The drug, the dose, the form of preparation (e.g. tablet).
   (iii) The total quantity of drug, or the total number of dosage units to be supplied. This quantity must be stated in *words* and *figures*.
   All of the above must be written indelibly in the prescriber's own handwriting and he/she must sign the prescription.
   (iv) The date of the prescription.
   (v) If the prescription is to be dispensed in instalments, the number of instalments and the intervals between them.

   It is illegal to write or dispense a prescription which does not comply with these requirements.
(b) The full handwriting requirements and statement of quantity to be supplied do not apply to prescriptions for hospital inpatients if the controlled drugs concerned are administered from ward or department stocks. They do, however, apply to prescription for drugs 'to take home' or for outpatients.

[5] *Storage and safe custody.*

(a) All controlled drugs should be stored in a suitably secure (usually metal) cupboard which is kept locked and to which access is restricted. This cupboard (which may be within a second outer cupboard) should be used only for the storage of controlled drugs.
(b) The Aitken Report recommends that all controlled drug record entries be checked by two nurses. In conjunction with the pharmacy a procedure should be developed to ensure regular checking of records and reconciliation of receipts and issues.
(c) A programme for regular stock checking should be established and adhered to.

[6] *Destruction.*

Unwanted or unused controlled drugs in Schedule 2 should normally be returned to the pharmacy but may, in some circumstances, be destroyed on the ward under the supervision of a pharmacist.

Rectal and vaginal preparations

Enemas
These are solutions which are instilled into the rectum as laxatives or to obtain other localized therapeutic effects, or for diagnostic purposes.

Suppositories
These are solid wax pellets for rectal administration. They may either melt at body temperature or dissolve or disperse in the mucous secretions of the rectum. They may be used to obtain local effect (e.g. as laxatives) or for systemic therapy. Many drugs, such as the opioids for example, are well absorbed when administered this way. Suppositories sometimes offer a useful alternative to injections for very sick patients unable to take drugs orally.

Pessaries
These are solid pellets for vaginal administration and are usually designed to have a local therapeutic action.

Topical preparations

Creams
These are semi-solid emulsions containing a high proportion of water. When applied they are quickly absorbed into the skin leaving little or no greasy residue. They may be used as a 'base' in which a variety of drugs may be applied for local therapy.

Ointments
These are similar to cream but contain a higher proportion of oil. They are absorbed more slowly into the skin and leave a greasy residue. They have similar uses to creams, and are particularly suitable for dry, scaly lesions.

Injections
Injections are defined by the British Pharmaceutical Codex (BPC) as: 'sterile solutions, suspensions, or emulsions which contain one or more medicaments in a suitable aqueous or non-aqueous vehicle; they are intended to be administered parenterally to produce a localized or systemic, rapid or sustained response'. The parenteral route of administration is often adopted for medicaments which cannot be given orally because of patient intolerance or because of instability, therapeutic inactivity or poor absorption. In an emergency, an injection can provide a rapid and effective response.

Subcutaneous injection
This is given into the highly vascular layer beneath the epidermis, and drugs are absorbed fairly rapidly by this route.

Intradermal injection
This is used mainly for diagnostic tests, e.g. Mantoux.

Intramuscular injection
Many drugs may be administered by this route provided they are not irritant to soft tissues and are sufficiently soluble. Absorption is usually rapid and can produce blood levels comparable to those achieved by intravenous bolus injection. Intramuscular injections should, where possible, be avoided in thrombocytopaenic patients.

Intravenous injection
This type of injection ranges from small volumes for 'bolus' or 'push' administration to large-volume infusions.

Intrathecal injection
This may be used when the drug concerned does not penetrate the blood-brain barrier.

Intra-articular injection
This term refers to the injection of a solution into a joint.

Intra-arterial injection
This special technique allows delivery of a high concentration of drug to the tissues supplied by a particular artery.

Subconjunctival injection
Some drugs may be given by this procedure in ophthalmology.

Inhalations
The term 'inhalation' once referred solely to the inhalation of volatile constituents of such preparations as compound tincture of benzoin. In modern therapeutics two techniques – nebulization and aerosolization – permit the inhalation of a range of drugs with the aim of a localized therapeutic effect.

Nebulization involves the passage of air (or sometimes oxygen) through a solution of the drug concerned to create a fine spray. Some antibiotics and bronchodilators may be given in this way.

Aerosolization involves the use of a solution of drug in an inert diluent. Passing a metred volume of this solution through a valve under pressure allows the delivery to the patient of a measured dose of drug in a very fine spray of controlled particle size. Bronchodilators and steroids are administered commonly in this way. Although a very small total dose of drug is administered, the concentration achieved at the site of action is high. Rapid and effective control of symptoms is achieved but without the side-effects commonly associated with an equivalent systemic (oral or parenteral) dose of the drug(s).

There are now available on the market aerosol and non-aerosol inhaler devices. Each device has its own advantages and disadvantages dependent on the particular situation.

Storage

Certain general principles apply to the storage of medicinal preparations (Department of Health and Social Security, 1988).

Principle	Rationale
1. *Security*: locked cupboards. When not in use drug trolleys should not only be kept locked but should also be secured to a wall and thus immobilized.	To prevent unauthorized access and deter abuse and/or misuse.
2. *Separate storage*: for medicines and non-medicines.	To prevent confusion and hence danger to patients.
Separate storage: for preparations for oral use and those for topical use.	To prevent errors and therefore danger to the patient.
3. *Stability*: no medicinal preparation should be stored where it may be subject to substantial variations in temperature, e.g. not in direct sunlight or over a radiator.	To maintain efficacy of the medicines.
Stability: some preparations require storage under well-defined conditions, e.g. 'below 10°C' or 'store in a refrigerator'.	To maintain efficacy of the medicines.
4. *Labelling*: the wording of labels is chosen carefully to convey clearly all essential information. Printed labels should always be used.	To ensure that the user has all the necessary information.
5. *Containers*: the type of container used may have been chosen for specific reasons.	The design and material of which the container is made may significantly influence the stability of the contents.
Medicinal preparations should never be transferred (in bulk) from one container to another except in the pharmacy.	As above. Inadequate labelling of repackaged medicines is dangerous.
6. *Stock control*: a system of stock rotation must be operated (e.g. 'first in, first out') to ensure that there is no accumulation of 'old' stocks. Regular stock checks should be carried out, if possible by pharmacy staff.	All medicinal preparations, even when stored correctly retain activity only for a limited period of time.

The label on the pack should in most cases give guidance about storage conditions for individual preparations. The term 'a cool place' is normally interpreted as meaning between 1° and 15°C for which a refrigerator will normally suffice. 'Room temperature' allows a range of approximately 15° to 25°C.

If you are in any doubt about the storage requirements for any preparation you should check with a pharmacist, but the following points are noteworthy:

1. Aerosol containers should not be stored in direct sunlight or over radiators – there is a risk of explosion if they are heated.
2. Creams may deteriorate rapidly if subjected to extremes of temperature.
3. Eye drops and ointments may become contaminated with micro-organisms during use, the hence pose a danger to the recipient. Hence, in hospitals, eye preparations should be discarded seven days after they are first opened. For use at home this limit is extended to 28 days.
4. Mixtures may have a relatively short shelf-life. Most antibiotic mixtures require refrigerated storage and even then have a shelf-life of only seven to 14 days. Always check the label for details.
5. Tablets and capsules are relatively stable but are susceptible to moisture unless correctly packed. They should be stored only in the containers in which they were supplied by the pharmacy.
6. Vaccines and similar preparations usually require refrigerated storage and may deteriorate rapidly if exposed to heat.

Administration

The effective and safe administration of drugs to patients demands a partnership between the various health professionals concerned, i.e. doctors, pharmacists and nurses. The nurse is responsible for the correct administration of prescribed drugs to patients in his/her care. To achieve this the nurse must have a sound knowledge of the use, action, usual dose and side-effects of the drugs being administered. Various studies have shown that this is not always the case. Markowitz *et al.* (1981) came to the conclusion that not only nurses but doctors and pharmacists in the survey hospital needed to upgrade their knowledge of the drugs they prescribed or administered. They then went on to suggest that inadequate practitioner knowledge may contribute to the incidence of preventable adverse drug reactions in hospitals. Francis (1980) examined the number of 'hidden', i.e. undeclared, medication errors committed by nurses. In the survey hospital it was found that nurses made ten times more of such errors than they reported.

Observation of the patient receiving medication is important. No drug produces a single effect. The combined effect of two or more drugs taken together may be different from the effects when taken separately. The effectiveness of any drug should be noted and any signs of resistance or dependence reported. Side-effects may vary from slight symptoms to severe reaction and any signs must be brought to the attention of the appropriate personnel.

The nurse must also be aware of the hazards involved in handling drugs, detergents and alcohols. Nurses Action Group (1981) attempts to highlight some hazards and offers advice on how nurses should protect themselves from some of the more common preparations found in hospitals.

Wherever possible, patients should be encouraged to be responsible for storing and administering their own medication. Falconer (1971), in her study, found that patients were able to cope proficiently with the administration of their medication. Even mildly confused patients, who were, initially, judged to be unsuitable for self-medication, were able to become independent after a period of instruction and supervision. Roberts (1978), in her study of self-medication in the elderly, reported that no patient took another's medication. Most patients kept their medicines in handbags or other places of safety. The common factor among those who failed to comply was that of ignoring the tablets altogether. There was no evidence of overdosage.

Injections

Injection is defined as the act of giving medication by use of a syringe and needle.

Newton and Newton (1979) identify eight routes for the use of parental injection:

1. Intra-arterial.
2. Intra-articular.
3. Intracardiac.
4. Intradermal.
5. Intralesional.
6. Intramuscular.
7. Intravenous.
8. Subcutaneous.

Intrathecal routes are employed when the prescribed drug is unable to cross the blood-brain barrier. These authors also include a useful table of the tissues, sites and types of needle used, the amount of medication usually injected and the medications commonly administered via these routes.

Sites of injection

Site selection is predetermined for intra-arterial, intra-articular, intracardiac, intralesional and intrathecal injections. The choice of the remaining sites will normally depend on the desired therapeutic effect and the patient's safety and comfort.

Intradermal

Chosen sites are the ventral forearms and the scapulae. Observation of an inflammatory reaction is a priority, so the best sites are those that are highly pigmented, thinly keratinized and hairless.

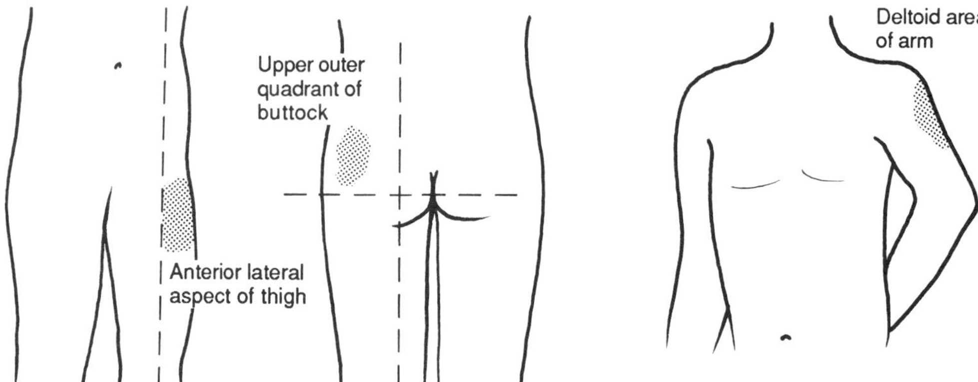

Figure 13.1 Sites for intramuscular injections.

Subcutaneous

Chosen sites are the lateral aspects of the upper arms and thighs, the abdomen in the umbilical region, the back and the lower loins. Slow absorption is a priority so ideal sites are those poorly supplied with sensory nerves. Rotation of these sites decreases the likelihood of irritation and ensures improved absorption.

Intramuscular

Intramuscular injections are given at five sites (see Figure 13.1 for some examples):

1. *Mid-deltoid*: used for the injection of such drugs as narcotics, sedatives, absorbed tetanus toxoid, vaccines, epinephrine in oil and vitamin B_{12}. It has the advantage of being easily accessible whether the patient is standing, sitting or lying down. It is also a better site than the gluteal muscles for small-volume (less than 2 ml), rapid-onset injections. Because the area is small, it limits the number and size of the injections that can be given at this point.
2. *Gluteus medius*: used for deep intramuscular and Z-track injections. The gluteus muscle has the lowest drug absorption rate. The muscle mass is also likely to have atrophied in elderly, non-ambulant and emaciated patients. This site carries with it the danger of the needle hitting the sciatic nerve and the superior gluteal arteries.
3. *Gluteus minimus*: used for antibiotics, anti-emetics, deep intramuscular and Z-track injections in oil, narcotics and sedatives. It is best used when large-volume intramuscular injections are required and for injections in the elderly, non-ambulant and emaciated patient as the site is away from major nerves and vascular structures.
4. *Rectus femoris*: used for anti-emetics, narcotics, sedatives, injections in oil, deep intramuscular and Z-track injections. It is the preferred site for infants and for self-administration of injections.
5. *Vastus lateralis*: used for deep intramuscular and Z-track injections. This site is free from major nerves and blood vessels. It is a large muscle and can accommodate repeated injections.

Skin preparation

McConnell (1982) quotes the two most common solutions for preparing the skin for injection as ethyl alcohol and the iodophors, such as povidone-iodine. If using the iodophors, the nurse must check beforehand that the patient is not allergic to iodine. An iodophor must not be used to prepare the skin for an intradermal injection as the solution discolours the skin and this makes it difficult to assess any expected reaction.

When cleaning the skin, the use of friction together with a circular motion is recommended. The nurse should begin at the centre of the chosen site and progress outwards. The antiseptic must be allowed to dry thoroughly before injection, otherwise the antiseptic may be forced into the tissue with the injection.

Research, however, has questioned the value of skin preparation before injection. Dann (1969) has shown that there is no experimental evidence that skin bacteria are introduced into the deeper tissues by injection, thereby causing infection. Antiseptics in current use cannot act in the time allowed in practice (five seconds on average) and cannot possibly cause complete sterility. Over a period six years, during which time more than 5000 injections were given to unselected patients via all the injection routes, without using any form of skin preparation, no single case of local and/or systemic infection was reported. Only before injections where strict asepsis is needed, as in intrathecal or intra-articular injections, is skin preparation required. Koivistov and Felig (1978) carried out a survey into the need for skin preparation before giving an insulin injection and found that skin preparation did reduce skin bacterial count but was not necessary to prevent infection at the injection site.

Needle bevel

Three categories of needle bevel are available:

1. *Regular*: for all intramuscular and subcutaneous injections.
2. *Intradermal*: for diagnostic injections and other injections into the epidermis.
3. *Short*: rarely used.

Needle size

Lenz (1983) states that when choosing the correct needle length for intramuscular injections it is important to assess the muscle mass of the injection site, the amount of subcutaneous fat and the weight of the patient. Without such an assessment, most injections intended for gluteal muscle are deposited in gluteal fat. The following are suggested by the author as ways of determining the most suitable size of needle to use:

Deltoid and vastus lateralis muscles

The muscle to be used should be grasped between the thumb and forefinger to determine the depth of the muscle mass or the amount of subcutaneous fat at the injection site. One half of the distance between the thumb and forefinger will be the appropriate length of the needle required to penetrate into that muscle.

Gluteal muscles

The layer of fat and skin above the muscle should be gently lifted with the thumb and forefinger for the same reasons as before. Use the patient's weight to calculate the needle length required. Lenz (1983) recommends the following guide:

31.5–40 kg	2.5-cm needle
40.5–90 kg	5–7.5-cm needle
90+ kg	10–15-cm needle

Injections and pain

McConnell (1982) and Newton and Newton (1979) set out, in point form, techniques which may reduce the discomfort experienced by the patient. Kruszewski *et al.* (1979) focus on ways in which positioning can help to minimize pain. Field (1981) attempts to answer the question of what it is like to give an injection, and goes on to explore the meaning and use of language relating to injections, the feelings involved in preparing and administering injections, and the meaning of the patient's response to the nurse.

Intravenous drug administration

The administration of intravenous medications is an area in which the role of the nurse is being increasingly extended. For further information on intravenous drug administration see Chapter 21.

Intra-arterial drug administration

Injection of drugs into an artery is a rare and hazardous procedure. The introduction of the cannula or catheter must be performed with care as the vessel may go into spasm, causing pain and occlusion. This could result in necrosis of an organ or part of a limb. Injection of irritant chemicals increases the risk of spasm and its sequentiae. In patients with some forms of cancer, however, arterial catheterization is occasionally performed when it is desirable to deliver a high concentration of a drug to a tumour mass. The most common procedures are catheterization of the hepatic artery and isolated limb perfusion.

References and further reading

Adamson, L. (1978) Control of medicines in the UK. *Nursing Times*, 74, 973–5.

Bayliss, P. F. C. (1980) *Law on Poisons, Medicines and Related Substances*, 3rd edn. Ravenswood Publications, London.

Central Health Services Council (1958) *Report of Joint Sub-Committee on the Control of Dangerous Drugs and Poisons in Hospitals* (Chairman J. K. Aitken). HMSO, London.

Dale, J. R. & Appelbe, G. E. (1983) *Pharmacy, Law and Ethics*, 3rd edn. The Pharmaceutical Press, London.

Dann, T. C. (1969) Routine skin preparation before injection: an unnecessary procedure. *Lancet*, 2, 96–7.

David, J. A. (1983) *Drug Round Companion*. Blackwell Scientific, Oxford.

Department of Health and Social Security (1988) *Guidelines for the Safe and Secure Handling of Medicines* (The Duthrie Report). HMSO, London.

Dorr, R. & Fritz, W. (1980) *Cancer Chemotherapy Handbook*. Kimpton, London.

Downie, G. *et al.* (1987) *Drug Management for Nurses*. Churchill Livingstone, Edinburgh.

Drugs and Therapeutics Bulletin (1977) Storage and shelf life of drugs: when is it important? *Drugs and Therapeutics Bulletin*. 15(21), 81–3.

Falconer, M. (1971) Self administered medication. *Hospital Administration in Canada*. 13(5), 28–30.

Field, P. A. (1981) A phenomenological look at giving an injection. *Journal of Advanced Nursing*, 6(4), 291–6.

Fink, J. L. (1983) Preventing lawsuits. *Nursing Life*, 3(2), 27–9.

Francis, G. (1980) Nurses' medication 'errors': a new

perspective. *Supervisor Nurse*, 11(8), 11–13.
Hopkins, S. J. (1987) *Drugs and Pharmacology for Nurses*, 9th edn. Churchill Livingstone, Edinburgh.
Koivistov, V. A. & Felig, P. (1978) Is skin preparation necessary before insulin injection? *Lancet*, 1, 1072–3.
Kruszewski, A. Z. *et al.* (1979) Effect of positioning on discomfort from intramuscular injections in the dorsogluteal site. *Nursing Research*, 28(2), 103–5.
Lenz, C. L. (1983) Make your needle selection right to the point. *Nursing (US)*, 13(2), 50–1.
Loebl, S. *et al.* (1980) *The Nurse's Drug Handbook*, 2nd edn. John Wiley, Chichester, pp. 10–22.
Lydiate, P. W. H. (1977) *The Law Relating to the Misuse of Drugs*. Butterworth, London.
McConnell, E. A. (1982) The subtle art of really good injections. *Research Nurse*, 45(2), 25–34.
Markowitz, J. S. *et al.* (1981) Nurses, physicians, and pharmacists: their knowledge of hazards of medication. *Nursing Research*, 30(6), 366–70.
Marks, M. (no date) *Neoplatin Cisplatin: A Nurse's Guide*. Mead Johnson.
Newton, D. W. & Newton, M. (1979) Route, site and technique: three key decisions in giving parenteral injections. *Nursing (US)*, 9(7), 18–25.
Nurses Action Group (1981) Health and safety 3. Beware the drug. *Nursing Mirror*, 152, 22–5.
Pearson, R. M. & Nestor, P. (1977) Drug interactions. *Nursing Mirror*, 145, Suppl. XI.
Roberts, R. (1978) Self medication trial for the elderly. *Nursing Times*, 74(23), 976–7.
Thomas, S. (1979) Practical nursing – medicines: care and administration. *Nursing Mirror*, 148, 28–30.
Wade, A. (1980) *Pharmaceutical Handbook*, 19th edn. The Pharmaceutical Press, London.
Whincup, M. H. (1982) *Legal Rights and Duties in Medical and Nursing Service*, 3rd edn. Ravenswood Publications, London.
Wieck, L. *et al.* (1986) *Illustrated Manual of Nursing Techniques*, 3rd edn. J. B. Lippincott, Philadelphia.

GUIDELINES: ORAL DRUG ADMINISTRATION

Equipment

1. Drug trolley.
2. Jug of water.
3. Tumblers.
4. Graduated medicine containers.
5. Bowl with warm soapy water.
6. Roll of paper towel.
7. Disposable waste bag.
8. Two spoons.

Procedure

Action	Rationale
1. Wash hands with bactericidal soap and water or bactericidal alcohol hand rub.	To prevent cross-infection.
2. Ensure that the drug trolley is prepared before beginning the procedure.	To prevent interruption of the procedure once it has begun.
3. Before administering any prescribed drug, check that it is due and has not been given already. Check that the information contained in the prescription chart is complete, correct and legible.	To protect the patient from harm.
4. Select the required medication and check the expiry date.	Treatment with medication that is outside the expiry date is dangerous. Drugs deteriorate with storage. The expiry date indicates when a particular drug is no longer pharmacologically efficacious.
5. Empty the required dose into a medicine container. Avoid touching the preparation.	To prevent cross-infection. To prevent harm to the nurse.
6. Take the medication and the prescription chart	To prevent error.

Action	Rationale
to the patient. Check the patient's identity and the dose to be given.	
7. Evaluate the patient's knowledge of the medication being offered. If this knowledge appears to be faulty or incorrect, offer an explanation of the use, action, dose and potential side-effects of the drug or drugs involved.	A patient has a right to information about treatment.
8. Administer the drug as prescribed.	
9. Offer a glass of water, if allowed, to facilitate swallowing the medication.	
10. Record the dose given in the prescription chart and in any other place made necessary by legal requirement or hospital policy.	To meet legal requirements and hospital policy.
11. Place the used medicine container and tumbler in the bowl of warm, soapy water.	
12. Administer irritating drugs with meals or snacks.	To minimize their effect on the gastric mucosa.
13. Administer drugs that interfere with foods, or drugs destroyed significant proportions by digestive enzymes, between meals or on an empty stomach.	To prevent interference with the absorption of the drug.
14. Do not break a tablet unless it is scored. Break scored tablets with a file.	Breaking may cause incorrect dosage, gastrointestinal irritation or destruction of a drug in an incompatible pH.
15. Do not interfere with time-release capsules and enteric coated tablets. Ask patients to swallow these whole and not to chew them.	The absorption rate of the drug will be altered.
16. Sublingual tablets must be placed under the tongue and buccal tablets between gum and cheek.	To allow for correct absorption.
17. When administering liquids to babies and young children, or when an accurately measured dose in multiples of 1 ml is needed for an adult, an oral syringe should be used in preference to a medicine spoon or measure.	A syringe is much more accurate than a measure or a 5-ml spoon. Use of a syringe makes administration of the correct dose much easier in an unco-operative child. Special syringes are available for this purpose: (a) They are washable and re-usable; the graduations do not readily rub off. (b) They have a non-Leur fitting to which it is impossible to attach a needle in error.
18. In babies and children especially, correct use of the syringe is very important. The tip should be gently pushed into and towards the side of the mouth. The contents are then *slowly* discharged towards the inside of the cheek, pausing if necessary to allow the liquid to be swallowed.	To prevent injury to the mouth and eliminate the danger of choking the patient.
In difficult children it may help to place the end of the barrel between the teeth!	To get the dose in and to prevent the patient spitting it out.

Guidelines: Oral drug administration

Action	Rationale
Controlled drugs	
1. Select the correct drug from the controlled drug cupboard.	
2. Check the stock against the last entry in the ward record book. (At The Royal Marsden Hospital, a second person is required to check the stock level.)	To comply with hospital policy (Department of Health, 1988).
3. Check the appropriate dose against the prescription sheet.	
4. Return the remaining stock to the cupboard and lock the cupboard.	
5. Enter the date and the patient's name in the ward record book.	
6. Take the prepared dose to the patient, whose identity is checked.	
7. Administer the drug after checking the prescription chart again. Once the drug has been administered, the prescription chart is signed by the nurse responsible for administering the medication.	
8. Complete any documentation required.	

GUIDELINES: ADMINISTRATION OF INJECTIONS

Equipment

1. Clean tray or receiver in which to place drug and equipment.
2. 19G needle(s) to ease reconstitution and drawing up.
3. 21, 23 or 25G needle, size dependent on route of administration.
4. Syringe(s) of appropriate size for amount of drug to be given.
5. Swabs saturated with isopropyl alcohol 70%.
6. Sterile topical swab, if drug is presented in ampoule form.
7. Drug(s) to be administered.
8. Patient's prescription chart, to check dose, route, etc.
9. Recording sheet or book as required by law or hospital policy.
10. Any protective clothing required by hospital policy for specified drugs, such as antibiotics or cytotoxic drugs.

Procedure

Action	Rationale
1. Collect and check all equipment.	To prevent delays and enable full concentration on the procedure.
2. Check that the packaging of all equipment is intact.	To ensure sterility. If the seal is damaged, discard.

3. Wash hands with bactericidal soap and water or bactericidal alcohol hand rub.	To prevent contamination of medication and equipment.
4. Prepare needle(s), syringe(s), etc. on a tray or receiver.	
5. Inspect all equipment.	To check that none is damaged; if so, discard.
6. Consult the patient's prescription sheet, and ascertain the following: (a) Drug. (b) Dose. (c) Date and time of administration. (d) Route and method of administration. (e) Diluent as appropriate. (f) Validity of prescription. (g) Signature of doctor.	To ensure that the patient is given the correct drug in the prescribed dose using the appropriate diluent and by the correct route.
7. Check all details with another nurse if required by hospital policy.	To minimize any risk of error.
8. Select the drug in the appropriate size or dosage and check the expiry date.	To reduce wastage. To prevent an ineffective or toxic compound being administered to the patient.
9. Proceed with the preparation of the drug, using protective clothing if advisable.	

Single-dose ampoule: solution

Action	Rationale
1. Inspect the solution for cloudiness or particulate matter. If this is present, discard and follow hospital guidelines on what action to take, e.g. return drug to pharmacy.	To prevent the patient from receiving an unstable or contaminated drug.
2. Tap the neck of the ampoule gently.	To ensure that all the solution is in the bottom of the ampoule.
3. Cover the neck of the ampoule with a sterile topical swab and snap it open. If there is any difficulty a file may be required.	To aid asepsis. To prevent aerosol formation or contact with the drug which could lead to a sensitivity reaction. To prevent injury to the nurse.
4. Inspect the solution for glass fragments; if present, discard.	To prevent injection of foreign matter into the patient.
5. Withdraw the required amount of solution, tilting the ampoule if necessary.	To avoid drawing in any air.
6. Replace the guard on the needle and tap the syringe to dislodge any air bubbles. Expel air.	To prevent aerosol formation, etc. To ensure that the correct amount of drug is in the syringe.
7. Alternatives to expelling the air with the needle guard in place include the following: (a) Covering the needle tip with sterile topical swab. (b) Using the ampoule or vial to receive any air and/or drug.	

Guidelines: Administration of injections

Action	Rationale
8. Change the needle.	To reduce the risk of infection. To avoid tracking medications through superficial tissues. To ensure that the correct size of needle is used for the injection.

Single-dose ampoule: powder

Action	Rationale
1. Tap the neck of the ampoule gently.	To ensure that any powder lodged here falls to the bottom of the ampoule.
2. Cover the neck of the ampoule with a sterile topical swab and snap it open. If there is any difficulty a file may be required.	To aid asepsis. To prevent contact with the drug which could cause a sensitivity reaction. To prevent injury to the nurse.
3. Add the correct diluent carefully down the wall of the ampoule.	To ensure that the powder is thoroughly wet before agitation and is not released into the atmosphere.
4. Agitate the ampoule and inspect the contents.	To dissolve the drug. To detect any glass fragments or any other particulate matter. If present, continue agitation or discard as appropriate.
5. When the solution is clear withdraw the prescribed amount, tilting the ampoule if necessary.	To avoid drawing in air.
6. Replace the guard on the needle and tap the syringe to dislodge any air bubbles. Expel air.	To prevent aerosol formation, etc. To ensure that the correct amount of drug is in the syringe.
7. Change the needle.	To reduce the risk of infection. To avoid tracking medications though superficial tissues. To ensure that the correct size of needle is used for the injection.

Multidose vial: solution

Action	Rationale
1. Inspect the solution for cloudiness or particulate matter. If this is present, discard. Follow hospital guidelines on what action to take, e.g. return drug to pharmacy.	To prevent patient from receiving an unstable or contaminated drug.
2. Clean the rubber cap with an appropriate antiseptic and let it dry.	To prevent bacterial contamination of the drug.
3. Insert a 19G needle into the cap to vent the bottle (Figure 13.2a).	To prevent pressure differentials which can cause separation of needle and syringe.
4. Withdraw the prescribed amount of solution, and inspect for pieces of rubber which may have 'cored out' of the cap (Figure 13.2b).	To prevent the injection of foreign matter into the patient.

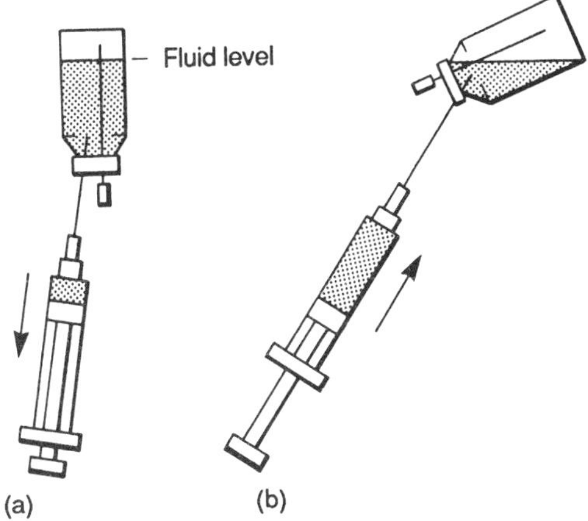

Figure 13.2 (a) To remove reconstituted solution, insert syringe needle and then invert vial. Ensure that tip of second needle is above fluid, and withdraw solution. (b) Remove air from syringe without spraying into the atmosphere by injecting air back into vial.

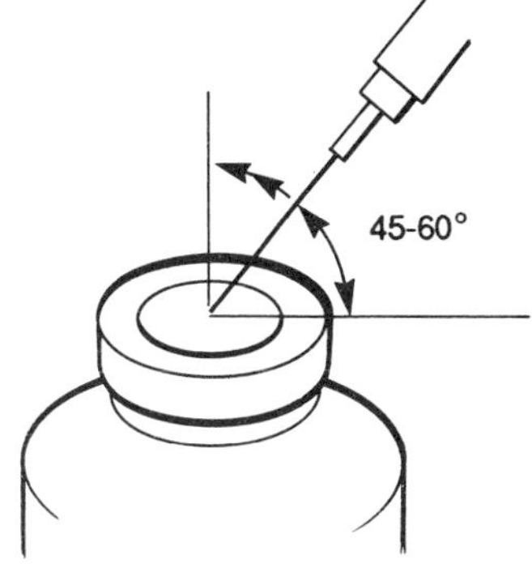

Figure 13.3 Method to minimize coring.

Note: Coring can be minimized by inserting the needle into the cap, bevel up, at an angle of 45° to 60°. Before complete insertion of the needle tip, lift the needle to 90° and proceed (Figure 13.3).

5. Replace the guard on the needle and tap the syringe to dislodge any air bubbles. Expel air.	To prevent aerosol formation. To ensure that the correct amount of drug is in the syringe.
6. Change the needle.	To reduce the risk of infection. To avoid possible trauma to the patient if the needle has barbed. To avoid tracking medications through superficial tissues. To ensure that the correct size of needle is used for the injection.

Multidose vial: powder

Action	Rationale
1. Clean the rubber cap with the chosen antiseptic and let it dry.	To prevent bacterial contamination of the drug.
2. Insert a 19G needle into the cap to vent the bottle (Figure 13.4a).	To prevent pressure differentials, which can cause separation of needle any syringe.
3. Add the correct diluent carefully down the wall of the vial.	To ensure that the powder is thoroughly wet before it is shaken and is not released into the atmosphere.
4. Remove the needle and the syringe.	
5. Place a sterile topical swab over the venting needle (Figure 13.4b).	To prevent contamination of the drug or the atmosphere.

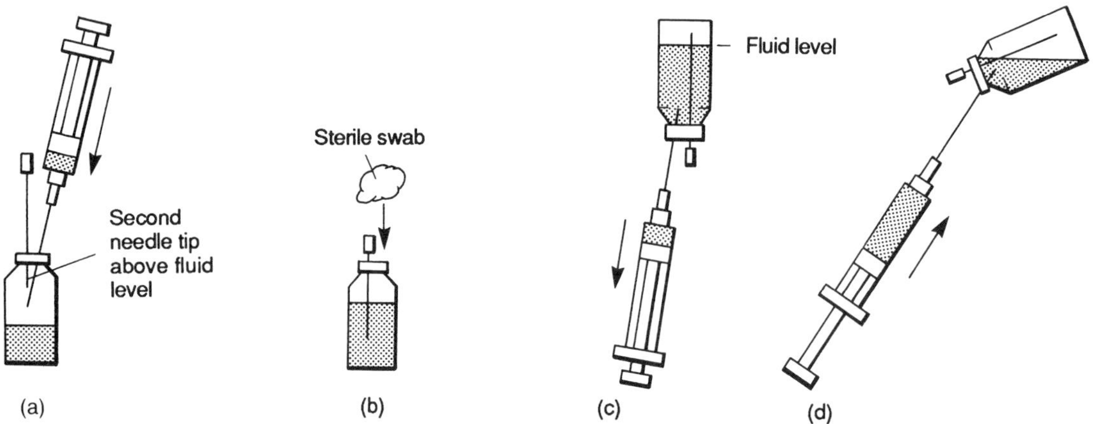

Figure 13.4 Suggested method of vial reconstitution to avoid environmental exposure. (a) When reconstituting vial, insert a second needle to allow air to escape when adding diluent for injection. (b) When shaking the vial to dissolve the powder, push in second needle up to Luer connection and cover with a sterile swab. (c) To remove reconstituted solution, insert syringe needle and then invert vial. Ensuring that tip of second needle is above fluid, withdraw the solution. (d) Remove air from syringe without spraying into the atmosphere by injecting air back into vial.

6. Proceed to the patient.

Note: The nurse may encounter other presentations of drugs for injection, e.g. vials with a transfer needle, and should follow the manufacturer's instructions in these instances.

Subcutaneous injections

Action	**Rationale**
1. Explain the procedure to the patient.	To obtain the patient's consent and co-operation.
2. Assist the patient into the required position.	
3. Expose the chosen site.	
4. Choose the correct needle size.	To minimize the risk of missing the subcutaneous tissue and any ensuing pain.
5. Clean the chosen site with a swab saturated with isopropyl alcohol 70%.	To reduce the number of pathogens introduced into the skin by the needle at the time of insertion. (For further information on this action see 'Skin preparation', above.)
6. Grasp the skin firmly.	To elevate the subcutaneous tissue.
7. Insert the needle into the skin at angle of 45° and release the grasped skin.	Injecting medication into compressed tissue irritates nerve fibres and causes the patient discomfort.
8. Pull back the plunger. If no blood is aspirated, depress the plunger and inject the drug slowly. If blood appears, withdraw the needle completely, replace it and begin again. Explain to the patient what has occurred.	To confirm that the needle is in the correct position. To prevent pain and ensure even distribution of the drug.
9. Withdraw the needle rapidly. Apply pressure to any bleeding point.	To prevent haematoma formation.

Action	Rationale
10. Record in the appropriate documents that the injection has been given.	
11. Ensure that all sharps and non-sharp waste are disposed of safely and in accordance with locally approved procedures. For example, sharps into sharps bin and syringes into yellow clinical waste bag.	To ensure safe disposal and to avoid laceration or other injury to staff.

Intramuscular injections

Action	Rationale
1. Explain the procedure to the patient.	To obtain the patient's consent and co-operation.
2. Assist the patient into the required position.	
3. Expose the chosen site.	
4. Clean the chosen site with a swab saturated with isopropyl alcohol 70%.	To reduce the number of pathogens introduced into the skin by the needle at the time of insertion. (For further information on this action see 'Skin preparation', above.)
5. Stretch the skin around the chosen site.	To facilitate the insertion of the needle and to displace the subcutaneous tissue.
6. Holding the needle at an angle of 90°, quickly plunge it into the skin. Leave a third of the shaft of the needle exposed.	To ensure that the needle penetrates the muscle. To facilitate removal of the needle should it break.
7. Pull back the plunger. If no blood is aspirated, depress the plunger and inject the drug slowly. If blood appears, withdraw the needle completely, replace it and begin again. Explain to the patient what has occurred.	To confirm that the needle is in the correct position. To prevent pain and ensure even distribution of the drug.
8. Withdraw the needle rapidly. Apply pressure to any bleeding point.	To prevent haematoma formation.
9. Record in the appropriate documents that the injection has been given.	
10. Dispose of the equipment in the required fashion.	To ensure safe disposal and to avoid laceration or other injury to staff.

GUIDELINES: ADMINISTRATION OF RECTAL AND VAGINAL PREPARATIONS

Equipment

1. Disposable gloves.
2. Topical swabs.
3. Lubricating jelly.
4. Prescription chart.

Guidelines: Administration of rectal and vaginal preparations

Procedure

Rectal preparations

For further information about the administration of rectal medication see the relevant sections in Chapter 7, Bowel Care.

Vaginal pessaries

Action	Rationale
1. Explain the procedure to the patient.	To obtain the patient's consent and co-operation.
2. Select the appropriate pessary and check it with the prescription chart and another nurse.	To ensure that the correct medication is given to the correct patient at the appropriate time.
3. Assist the patient into the appropriate position, either left lateral with buttocks to the edge of the bed or supine the knees drawn up and legs parted.	To facilitate the correct insertion of the pessary.
4. Wash hands with bactericidal soap and water or bactericidal alcohol hand rub, and put on gloves.	To prevent cross-infection.
5. Apply lubricating jelly to a topical swab and from the swab on to the pessary.	To facilitate insertion of the pessary and ensure the patient's comfort.
6. Insert the pessary along the posterior vaginal wall and into the top of the vagina. *Note*: This procedure is best performed late in the evening when the patient is unlikely to get out of bed.	To ensure that the pessary is retained and that the medication can reach its maximum efficiency.
7. Wipe away any excess lubricating jelly from the patient's vulval and/or perineal area with a topical swab.	To promote patient comfort.
8. Make the patient comfortable and apply a fresh sanitary pad.	To absorb any excess discharge.
9. Record in the appropriate documents that the pessary has been given.	

GUIDELINES: TOPICAL APPLICATIONS OF DRUGS

Equipment

1. Flat wooden spatulae.
2. Sterile topical swabs.
3. Applicators.

Procedure

Action	Rationale
1. Explain the procedure to the patient.	To obtain the patient's consent and co-operation.

Action	Rationale
2. Use aseptic technique if the skin is broken.	To prevent local or systemic infection.
3. Remove semi-solid or stiff preparations from their containers with a flat wooden spatula. Use a different spatula each time if more of the preparation is required.	To prevent cross-infection.
4. If the medication is to be rubbed into the skin, the preparation should be placed on a sterile topical swab. The wearing of gloves may be necessary.	To prevent cross-infection. To protect the nurse.
5. If the preparation causes staining, advise the patient of this.	To ensure that adequate precautions are taken beforehand and to prevent unwanted stains.

GUIDELINES: ADMINISTRATION OF DRUGS IN OTHER FORMS

Procedure

Inhalations

Action	Rationale
1. Seat the patient in an upright position if possible.	To permit full expansion of the diaphragm.
2. Administer only one drug at a time unless specifically instructed to the contrary.	Several drugs used together may cause undesirable reactions or they may inactivate each other.
3. Measure any liquid medication with a syringe.	To ensure the correct dose.
4. Clean any equipment used after use.	To prevent infection.
5. Correct use of inhalers is essential (see manufacturer's information leaflet) and will be achieved only if this is carefully explained and demonstrated to the patient. If further advice is required, contact the hospital pharmacist.	Incorrect use may result in most of the dose remaining in the mouth and/or being expelled almost immediately. This renders treatment ineffective.

Gargles

Action	Rationale
1. Throat irrigations should not be warmer than 49°C.	Any liquid warmer than 49°C will destroy or damage tissue.

Nasal drops

Action	Rationale
1. Have paper tissues available.	To wipe away secretions and/or medication.
2. Clean the patient's nasal passages.	To ensure maximum penetration for the medication.
3. Hyperextend the patient's neck.	To obtain the best position for insertion of the medication.
4. Avoid touching the external nares with the dropper.	To prevent the patient from sneezing.

Guidelines: Administration of drugs in other forms

Action	Rationale
5. Request the patient to maintain his/her position for one or two minutes.	To ensure full absorption of the medication.
6. Each patient should have his/her own medication and dropper.	To prevent cross-infection.

Eye medications

For information on eye care see Chapter 18.

Ear drops

Action	Rationale
1. Ask the patient to lie on his/her side with the ear to be treated uppermost.	To ensure the best position for insertion of the drops.
2. Warm the drops to body temperature if allowed.	To prevent trauma to the patient.
3. Pull the cartilagenous part of the pinna backwards and upwards.	To prepare the auditory meatus for instillation of the drops.
4. Allow the drop(s) to fall in direction of the external canal.	To ensure that the medication reaches the target.
5. Request the patient to remain in this position for one or two minutes.	To allow the medication to reach the eardrum and be absorbed.

SINGLE-NURSE ADMINISTRATION OF DRUGS

Certain nurses may administer drugs by themselves provided it is the policy of the health authority by whom they are employed. Some authorities have policies which require that nurses have received specific training, both in theory and practice, and are in possession of a certificate stating their proficiency in the technique.

It is felt that this will result in greater care being given since that one nurse will be aware that she/he is solely responsible and accountable.

Those nurses who wish or need to have their administration supervised will retain the right to do so until such time as all parties agree that the requested level of proficiency has been achieved.

SELF-ADMINISTRATION OF DRUGS

Definition

Patients are responsible for taking their own prescribed drugs. The self-administration of prescribed drugs should not be confused with self-medication using over-the-counter drugs.

Indications

Ideally self-administration is practised when:

1. There is a safe locked place in which to store drugs.
2. Pharmacy staff are able to dispense the drug individually.
3. The drug regime is not subject to frequent adjustments.

For patients who have psychological or physical problems with taking drugs, the development of an education and training programme for self-administration needs to be undertaken before discharge. This will improve compliance.

REFERENCE MATERIAL

While patient self-medication as a concept is gaining increasing support (Davis, 1989), research has concentrated on the advantages of self-administration for the elderly, mainly because these patients have greater educational needs and frequently take two or more different drugs. Errors in compliance have been shown to increase with the number of drugs having to be taken (Garland, 1979). An increase in compliance has been demonstrated when training and memory aids are given to patients before discharge from hospital (Wandless & Davie, 1977). Such benefits are of equal advantage to other patient groups and are in line with self-care models of nursing. For patients who take drugs long term (for example, endocrine replacement drugs) the removal of their drug-taking responsibility on hospital admission is humiliating, making them immediately dependent on nursing staff. They are also controlled by the timing of drug administration in hospital which may well produce physiological changes in the drug response.

Aids to self-administration are available for those with physical problems such as opening containers, measuring liquids as well as problems with remembering when drugs have to be taken (Williams, 1984).

References and further reading

Brock, A. M. (1979) Self administration of drugs in the elderly. *Nursing Forum*, 18(4), 340–57.

Central Health Services Council (1958) *Report of the Joint Sub-Committee on the Control of Dangerous Drugs and Posions in Hospitals* (Chairman J. K. Aitken). HMSO, London.

David, J. A. (1983) *Drug Round Companion*. Blackwell Scientific Publications, Oxford, Chs 3, 7 and 8.

Davis, S. (1989) A study of patients' drug self-administration patterns in a cancer hospital. In *Cancer Nursing – A Revolution in Care. Proceedings of the Fifth International Conference on Cancer Nursing* (Ed. by A. P. Pritchard), pp. 152–3. Macmillan Press, London.

Department of Health (1988) *Guidelines for the Safe and Secure Handling of Medicines*. Report to the Secretary of State for Social Services by Joint Sub-Committee of the Standing Medical, Nursing, Midwifery and Pharmaceutical Advisory Committees. Chaired by Professor R. B. Duthie, September.

Falconer, M. (1971) Self-administered medication. *Hospital Administration in Canada*. 13(5), 28–30.

Garland, M. H. (1979) Drugs and the elderly. *Nursing Times*, 75, 3–6.

Powys Health Authority (1984) *All Wales Working Party of Review of the Administration of Drugs by Nurses*. Powys Health Authority, Bronllys.

Roberts, R. (1978) Self-medication trial for the elderly. *Nursing Times*, 74(23), 976–7.

Royal College of Nursing (1983) *Drug Administration: A Nursing Responsibility*, 2nd edn. Royal College of Nursing of the United Kingdom, London.

Shannon, M. (1983) Self-medication in the elderly. Nursing Mirror, 157, *Clinical Forum*, Vol. 9, pp. i–iii, vi–viii.

Wandless I. & Davie, J. W. (1977) Can drug compliance in the elderly be improved? *British Medical Journal*, 1, 359–61.

Williams, A. (1984) Medicine management. *Nursing Mirror*, 159(12), Suppl. 1, pp. i–viii.

GUIDELINES: SELF-ADMINISTRATION OF DRUGS

Equipment

1. Individually issued prescribed drugs in suitable containers.
2. Locked drawer or locker for storage.
3. Drug administration record prepared for self-administration.

Procedure

Action	**Rationale**
1. Take a drug history from the patient on admission.	This will record any drugs (prescribed or over-the-counter) being taken, allergies or idiosyncrasies to drugs, problems with self-administration and the patient's current understanding of his/her drugs.
2. Discuss the selection of the patient for self-administration with the charge nurse and pharmacist.	To ensure that the patient is suitable and that the drug can be supplied for self-administration from the pharmacy.
3. Explain self-administration to the patient, making a joint plan for education, storage and recording.	The patient is contracted to self-administer, education can be undertaken and co-operation ensured.
4. Check that drugs are taken correctly.	Checking drugs daily with the patient ensures compliance, offers educational opportunities and enables the nurse to record that drugs have been taken.

Guidelines: Self-Administration of Drugs

Action	Rationale
5. Ensure that new supplies are ordered for the patient, particularly if discharge is anticipated.	To continue administration without problems.
6. Evaluate the patient's capability to self-administer and the effectiveness of drug education.	To allow for a new plan if required and to set long-term goals.

NURSING CARE PLAN

Problem	Cause	Suggested action
Patient unwilling to self-administer.	Anxiety about drugs or present medical condition. Does not see the value of self-administration. Unsure of capabilities.	Discuss the problem, educate the patient and answer questions. Explain how self-administration can establish a routine. Work with the patient gradually giving more responsibility.
Failing memory.	Old age, confusion, anxiety.	Plan memory aids, timing of drug-taking linked to events. Diary or pad to tick off drugs taken. Drugs packed for daily administration.
Physical problems: dexterity, vision, communication.	Arthritis, old age, does not speak English.	Make use of aids (Williams, 1984), an interpreter and the adaptation of practice to meet the individual patient's needs.
Special technique required for administration.	Drug to be given via central line, rectally or vaginally. Drugs to be given by relative (as in the case of children).	Introduce the technique to the patient (relative) and gradually involve in administration. Remain available once competence is achieved.

14

Enteral Tube Feeding and Nutritional Assessment

Definition

Enteral feeding refers to any method of nutrient ingestion via the gastrointestinal tract. Enteral tube feeding includes nasogastric gastrostomy and jejunostomy feeding.

Indications

Enteral tube feeding may be considered in patients who have a functioning gastrointestinal tract but are unable to consume an adequate nutritional intake. Examples of such patients are those:

1. Unable to eat at all, e.g. those with carcinoma of the head and neck area, or oesophagus, post-surgery or radiotherapy to head and neck area, fistula of the oral cavity or oesophagus.
2. Unable to eat sufficient food to meet dietary requirements, e.g. due to difficulties with chewing or swallowing after surgery or radiotherapy, sore mouth, anorexia.

Patients in either group may have increased requirements for nutrients due to an increased metabolic rate, as found in patients with burns, major sepsis, trauma or cancer cachexia.

REFERENCE MATERIAL

Nasogastric feeding is the most commonly used enteral tube feed and is suitable for short-term use. Where long-term feeding is anticipated or if the patient feels that a nasogastric tube is unacceptable for cosmetic reasons, then a gastrostomy or jejunostomy may be more appropriate.

For patients with gastric disease, e.g. pyloric obstruction, or who cannot be endoscoped for the insertion of a fine-bore feeding gastrostomy, then a jejunostomy may be a more suitable feeding route.

Assessment

Before the initiation of enteral tube feeding the patient must be assessed. The purpose of assessment is to identify if the patient is undernourished, the reasons why this may have occurred and to provide baseline data for planning and evaluation of nutritional support. The following methods can be used, preferably not in isolation:

1. Dietary history. This is an important method of assessing nutritional status. A 24-hour recall may be used, as described by Burke (1974), in addition to ascertaining appetite, the presence of any eating difficulties and food preferences. Factors which may influence future food intake, e.g. surgery or radiotherapy, also need to be considered when planning nutritional support, as clinical experience shows these may exert a deleterious effect on appetite.
2. Body weight and weight loss. Accurate weighing scales are necessary for measurement of body weight. Comparison of the patient's weight with charts of ideal body weight for height are not a good indicator of whether the patient is at risk nutritionally, as an apparently normal weight can mask severe muscle wasting. Of greater use is the comparison of current weight with the patient's usual weight (Passmore and Eastwood, 1986). Percentage weight loss is a useful measure of the risk of malnutrition.

   $$\%\text{ weight loss} = \frac{\text{Usual weight} - \text{Actual weight}}{\text{Usual weight}} \times 100$$

   A weight loss of 10% represents malnutrition and a loss of 20%, severe malnutrition. Obesity and oedema may make interpretation of body weight difficult. Both may mask loss of lean body mass and potential malnutrition (Bistrain, 1981)
3. Skinfold thickness measurements can be used to assess stores of body fat. They are rarely used in routine nutritional assessment and are more appropriate for long-term assessments or research purposes. Calipers are used to measure the thickness of subcutaneous fat at four sites, the triceps, biceps, subscapular and supra-iliac. The

measurements can be used to determine the percentage body fat of a person.

4. Clinical examination. General nutritional depletion may be seen on clinical examination. Specific nutritional deficiencies may be identifiable in some patients by a trained observer or clinician, e.g. polyneuropathy, cardiac enlargement and oedema in thiamin deficiency, or swollen, bleeding gums and poor wound healing in vitamin C (ascorbic acid) deficiency.
5. Biochemical investigations. Biochemical tests carried out on blood may give information on the patient's nutritional status. The most commonly used are:
   (a) Serum albumin and total protein. Low levels of plasma proteins often reflect malnutrition. However, changes in plasma albumin may also arise due to physical stress, changes in circulating volume, hepatic and renal function, shock conditions and septicaemia. Additionally, the long half-life of albumin (20 days) makes it an insensitive marker of malnutrition. Prealbumin and retinol binding protein have much shorter half-lives (two days and 10 hours, respectively), and are therefore more sensitive indicators of nutritional depletion (Jensen *et al.*, 1983). However, they are rarely measured routinely.
   (b) Haemoglobin. This is often below haematological reference values in malnourished patients (men, 13.5 to 17.5 g/dl; women, 11.5 to 15.5 g/dl). This can be due to a number of reasons, such as loss of blood from circulation, increased destruction of red blood cells or reduced production of erythrocytes and haemoglobin, e.g. due to dietary deficiency of iron or folate.
   (c) Serum vitamin and mineral levels. These tests are rarely carried out routinely, as they are expensive and often cannot be performed by hospital laboratories.
   (d) Immunological competence:
      (i) Cell-mediated immunity.
      (ii) Total lymphocyte count.

      It should be remembered that other factors may influence immune competence, such as malignancy, zinc deficiency, age and non-specific stress.

If a patient is considered to be malnourished by one or more of the above methods of assessment then a referral to a dietitian should be made immediately.

Calculation of nutritional requirements

Energy requirements may be calculated using equations such as those derived by Schofield (1985), which take into account height, weight, age, sex and injury. However, an easier method is to use body weight and allowances based on the patient's clinical condition (Table 14.1).

Nitrogen (or protein) requirements can be calculated in a similar way. If additional nitrogen is being given in situations where losses are increased, e.g. due to trauma, gastrointestinal losses or major sepsis, then additional energy intake is required to assist in promoting a positive nitrogen balance.

Types of enteral feeding tubes

1. Nasogastric/nasoduodenal. Fine-bore feeding tubes should be used whenever possible as these are more comfortable for the patient than wide-bore tubes. They are less likely to interfere with swallowing or cause oesophageal irritation (Passmore & Eastwood 1986). Polyurethane or silicone tubes are preferable to PVC as they withstand gastric acid and can stay in position longer than the 10–14-day lifespan of the PVC tube. Nasogastric tubes may have a tungsten-weighted tip or be unweighted. A wire introducer is provided with many of the tubes to aid intubation if necessary. The weighted tip of a tube may facilitate the passage of the tube towards the soft palate and pharynx after insertion into the nasal passage.

Table 14.1 Guidelines for estimation of patient's protein and energy requirements

	Normal	*Intermediate (moderate infection postoperative patients); most cancer patients)*	*Severly hypermetabolic (multiple injuries, severe infection, severe burns)*
Energy per kg body weight	30 kcal	35–40 kcal	40–60 kcal
Nitrogen per kg body weight	0.16 g	0.2–0.3 g	0.3–0.5 g
Protein per kg body weight	1 g	1.3–1.9 g	1.9–3.1 g

2. Gastrostomy. Percutaneous endoscopically guided gastrostomy (PEG) tubes are the gastrostomy tube of choice. They are made from polyurethane or silicone and are therefore suitable for long-term feeding. A flange or inflated balloon holds the tube in position. The use of conventional balloon urinary catheters is now outdated, particularly as these are at risk of allowing gastric acid to leak at the tube entry site. Clinical trials have shown that complications with PEG gastrostomy tubes, such as leakage, are rare (Ruppin & Lux, 1986).
3. Jejunostomy. Fine-bore feeding jejunostomy tubes may be placed with the use of a 'jejunostomy kit' consisting of a needle-fine catheter necessary for the insertion of a feeding jejunostomy. The use of needles and an introducer wire allow a fine-bore polyurethane catheter to be inserted into a loop of jejunum. Alternatively, some gastrostomy tubes allow the passage of a fine-bore tube into the jejunum.

Enteral feeding equipment

The administration of enteral feeds may be via gravity drip or pump assisted. There are many enteral feeding pumps available which vary in their range of flow rate from 1 ml to 300 ml per hour. The following systems are used for gravity-drip feeding:

1. Plastic bottles into which the feed is decanted before connection to a gravity-giving set.
2. PVC bag into which the feed is decanted. The giving set may be an integral part of the bag and some bags may have a rigid neck to assist filling.
3. Glass bottle containing feed which is attached directly to the giving set. This gives less flexibility in choice of feed or additional liquids than the plastic bottle or bag.

Enteral feeds

Commercially prepared feeds should be used for nasogastric, gastrostomy or jejunostomy feeding. Available as liquid or powder, they have the advantage of being of known composition and are sterile when packaged.

1. Whole protein/polymeric feeds contain protein, hydrolysed fat and carbohydrate and so require digestion. These may provide 1 kcal/ml or 1.5 kcal/ml (see manufacturer's specifications). As the energy density of the feed increases so does the osmolarity. Hyperosmolar feeds tend to draw water into the lumen of the gut and can contribute to diarrhoea if given too rapidly. The majority of feeds are low residue although some contain dietary fibre.
2. Medium chain triglyceride (MCT) containing feeds. In some whole protein feeds a proportion of the fat or long-chain triglycerides may be replaced with medium-chain triglycerides. The feed often has a lower osmolarity, and is therefore less likely to draw fluid from the plasma into the gut lumen due to the ability of MCT to be absorbed directly into the lymphatic system. These feeds are suitable for patients with mildly impaired gastrointestinal function (Colin-Jones, 1985).
3. Chemically defined/elemental feeds. These contain free amino acids, short-chain peptides or a combination of both as the nitrogen source. They are often low in fat or may contain some fat as MCT. Glucose polymers provide the main energy source. These feeds require little or no digestion and are suitable for those patients with impaired gastrointestinal function (O'Morain *et al.*, 1984). They are hyperosmolar and low in residue.

Up to date information on the exact composition of enteral feeds can be obtained from the manufacturers.

References and further reading

Bistrain, B. (1981) Assessment of protein energy malnutrition in surgical patients. In *Nutrition and the Surgical Patient* (Ed. by G. L. Hill), pp. 39–54. Churchill Livingstone, Edinburgh.

Burke, B. S. (1974) The dietary history as a tool in research. *Journal of the American Dietetic Association*, 23, 1041–6.

Colin-Jones, D. G. (1985) Sorting out inflammatory bowel disease. *Update*, 17–26.

Elwyn, D. H. (1980) Nutritional requirements of adult surgical patients. *Critical Care Medicine*, 8, 9–20.

Grant, A. & Todd, E. (1982) *Enteral and Parenteral Nutrition*. Blackwell Scientific Publications, Oxford.

Jensen, T. G. *et al.* (1983) *Nutritional Assessment – A Manual for Practitioners*. Prentice-Hall, London.

O'Morain, C. *et al.* (1984) Elemental diet as a primary treatment of acute Crohn's disease: a controlled trial. *British Medical Journal*, 288, 1859–62.

Passmore, R. & Eastwood, M. A. (1986) Chapter 52, pp. 491–501. In *Human Nutrition and Dietetics* 8th edition (Ed. by Davidson & Passmore). Churchill Livingstone, Edinburgh.

Ruppin, H. & Lux, G. (1986) Percutaneous endoscopic gastrostomy in patients with head and neck cancer. *Endoscopy*, 18, 149–52.

Schofield, W. N. (1985) Predicting basal metabolic rate. New standards and review of previous work. *Human Nutrition and Clinical Nutrition*, 39C, Suppl. 15, 41.

GUIDELINES: NASOGASTRIC INTUBATION WITH TUBES USING AN INTRODUCER

Equipment

1. Clinically clean tray.
2. Fine-bore nasogastric tube.
3. Introducer for tube.
4. Sterile receiver.
5. Sterile water.
6. Hypo-allergenic tape.
7. Adhesive patch if available.
8. Glass of water.
9. Lubricating jelly.

Procedure

Action	Rationale
1. Explain the procedure to the patient.	To obtain the patient's consent and co-operation.
2. Arrange a signal by which the patient can communicate if he/she wants the nurse to stop, e.g. by raising his /her hand.	The patient is often less frightened if he/she feels able to have some control over the procedure.
3. Assist the patient to sit in a semi-upright position in the bed or chair. Support the patient's head with pillows *Note*: The head should not be tilted backwards or forwards.	To allow for easy passage of the tube. This position enables easy swallowing and ensures that the epiglottis is not obstructing the oesophagus.
4. Select the appropriate distance mark on the tube by measuring the distance on the tube from the patient's ear lobe to the bridge of the nose plus the distance from the bridge of the nose to the bottom of the xiphisternum.	To ensure that the appropriate length of tube is passed into the stomach.
5. Wash hands with bactericidal soap and water or bactericidal alcohol hand rub, and assemble the equipment required.	To minimize cross infection.
6. Inject 10 ml sterile water down the tube before inserting introducer. Lubricate proximal end of tube with jelly.	Contact with water activates coating inside tube and on the tip. This lubricates the tube assisting its passage through the nasopharynx and allowing easy withdrawal of the introducer.
7. Check that the nostrils are patent by asking the patient to sniff with one nostril closed. Repeat with the other nostril.	To identify any obstructions liable to prevent intubation.
8. Insert the rounded end of the tube into the clearest nostril and slide it backwards and inwards along the floor of the nose to the nasopharynx. If any obstruction is felt, withdraw the tube and try again in a slightly different direction or use the other nostril.	To facilitate the passage of the tube by following the natural anatomy of the nose.
9. As the tube passes down into the nasopharynx, ask the patient to start swallowing and sipping water.	To focus the patient's attention on something other than the tube. A swallowing action closes the glottis, enabling the tube to pass into the oesophagus.

Action	Rationale
10. Advance the tube through the pharynx, as the patient swallows until the predetermined mark has been reached. If the patient shows signs of distress, e.g. gasping or cyanosis, remove the tube immediately.	
11. Remove the introducer by using gentle traction. If it is difficult to remove, then remove the tube as well.	If the introducer sticks in the tube, it may be indicative that the tube is in the bronchus.
12. Check the position of the tube to confirm that it is in the stomach by:	
(a) Introducing 2 to 5 ml of air into the stomach via the tube and check for bubbling using a stethoscope placed over the epigastrium, and	Air can be detected by a 'whooshing' sound when entering the stomach.
(b) Taking an X-ray of chest and upper abdomen.	Radio-opaque tube shows up on the X-ray.
13. Secure the tube to the nostril with hypo-allergenic tape and to the cheek with an adhesive patch (if available).	To main the tube in place. To ensure patient comfort. Feeding via the tube must not begin until the correct position of the tube has been confirmed by X-ray.

GUIDELINES: NASOGASTRIC INTUBATION WITH TUBES WITHOUT USING AN INTRODUCER E.G. A RYLE'S TUBE

Equipment

1. Clinically clean tray.
2. Nasogastric tube that has been stored in a deep freeze for at least half an hour before the procedure is to begin, to ensure a rigid tube that will allow for easy passage.
3. Topical gauze.
4. Lubricating jelly.
5. Hypo-allergenic tape.
6. 20 ml syringe.
7. Blue litmus paper.
8. Receiver.
9. Spigot.
10. Glass of water.
11. Stethoscope.

Procedure

Action	**Rationale**
1. Explain the procedure to the patient.	To obtain the patient's consent and co-operation.
2. Arrange a signal by which the patient can communicate if he/she wants the nurse to stop, e.g. by raising his/her hand.	The patient is often less frightened if he/she feels able to have some control over the procedure.
3. Assist the patient to sit in a semi-upright position in the bed or chair. Support the patient's head with pillows.	To allow for easy passage of the tube. This position enables easy swallowing and ensures that the epiglottis is not obstructing the oesophagus.

Guidelines: Nasogastric intubation with tubes without using an introducer

Action	Rationale
4. Mark the distance which the tube is to be passed by measuring the distance on the tube from the patient's ear lobe to the bridge of the nose plus the distance from the bridge of the nose to the bottom of the xiphisternum.	To indicate the length of tube required for entry into the stomach.
5. Wash hands with bactericidal soap and water or bactericidal alcohol hand rub, and assemble the equipment required.	To minimize cross infection.
6. Check the patient's nostrils are patent by asking him/her to sniff with one nostril close. Repeat with the other nostril.	To identify any obstructions liable to prevent intubation.
7. Lubricate about 15 to 20 cm of the tube with a thin coat of lubricating jelly that has been placed on a topical swab.	To reduce the friction between the mucous membranes and the tube.
8. Insert the proximal end of the tube into the clearest nostril and slide it backwards and inwards along the floor of the nose to the nasopharynx. If an obstruction is felt, withdraw the tube and try again in a slightly different direction or use the other nostril.	To facilitate the passage of the tube by following the natural anatomy of the nose.
9. As the tube passes down into the nasopharynx, ask the patient to start swallowing and sipping water.	To focus the patient's attention on something other than the tube. The swallowing action closes the glottis, enabling the tube to pass into the oesophagus.
10. Advance the tube through the pharynx as the patient swallows until the tape-marked tube reaches the point of entry into the external nares. If the patient shows signs of distress, e.g. gasping or cyanosis, remove the tube immediately.	Distress may indicate that the tube is in the bronchus.
11. Ascertain whether the tube is in the stomach by:	
(a) Aspirating the contents of the stomach with a syringe. The aspirate should turn blue litumus paper red.	The acid nature of the stomach contents verifies the position of the tube.
(b) Placing a stethoscope over the epigastrium and injecting 2 to 3 ml of air into the tube.	Air can be detected by a 'whooshing' sound when entering the stomach.
12. Tape the tube to the patient's nose and secure the distal end in a suitable position. Spigot the tube.	To maintain the tube in place. To ensure patient comfort.

GUIDELINES: ADMINISTRATION OF AN ENTERAL FEED

Suitable for nasogastric, gastrostomy or jejunostomy feeding.

The administration of a feed should be discussed with a dietitian to ensure patient requirements are met.

Two methods are available:

1. Intermittent or cyclical feeding: a small quantity of feed (200 to 500 ml) is given over a limited period of time using either a syringe or a reservoir and giving set. For the latter, gravity drip or pump-assisted feeding can be used. This process is repeated at different times throughout the day until the correct amount of feed has been administered. This method of feeding allows the patient more control over the regime and more freedom of movement.
2. Continuous feeding: the total volume of feed required by the patient is given over a 16 to 24-hour period (or a proportion of feed may be given continuously overnight). Pump-assisted feeding is usually used in these cases, as the feed is administered much more slowly than in intermittent feeding. This method is suitable for patients experiencing problems with tolerance of feed or for whom the intermittent method is unsuitable. It is often the method of choice for jejunostomy feeding. However, it often reduces the mobility of patients and they may feel restricted. The method of administering the feed and feed type should be decided for each individual patient on their own merit.

Equipment

1. Prescribed feed.*
2. Reservoir* and airway.**
3. Giving set.
4. 2 and 10 ml syringes.
5. 10 ml water in a syringe.
6. Clean jug.
7. Suitable stand for holding reservoir.

* These may come as one unit
** This may be an integral part of the giving set

Procedure

Intermittent feeding

Action	Rationale
1. Explain the procedure to the patient.	To obtain the patient's consent and co-operation.
2. Wash hands with bactericidal soap and water or bactericidal alcohol hand rub.	To minimize cross-infection.
3. Take the feed and necessary equipment to the patient's bedside. If the patient is capable of doing so, he/she should assist in the procedure.	To encourage feelings of independence.
4. Remove the cap of the reservoir, and pour the prescribed feed into it. (This step may be omitted if a prepacked bottled feed is used.)	
5. Replace the cap and insert the giving set. Close the airway. Hang the reservoir on the stand beside the patient. Run the feed through to the end of the tubing. Clamp the tubing firmly.	To prevent the feed escaping from the reservoir via the airway. Running the feed through the tubing removes excess solution and any air bubbles from the system, and prevents them from reaching the patient's stomach.
6. Connect the giving set to the nasogastric tube using an appropriate connector if required.	

Guidelines: Administration of an enteral feed

Action	Rationale
7. Open the airway and set the flow of feed at the prescribed rate using the roller clamp. Pumps are available commercially for administering feeds at a constant rate, approximately 200 to 250 ml/hour.	The rate of feed must be regulated to meet the patient's need. If possible, the patient should control own feeding rate.
8. Return periodically to check the patient's comfort and the rate of flow of the feed.	The rate of flow of the feed may alter suddenly, especially if the patient is mobile.
9. On completion of a feed, disconnect the giving set from the distal end of the nasogastric tube and flush the tube with 10 ml of water.	To remove particles of feed likely to block the tube.
10. Discard or clean and sterilize equipment according to manufacturer's instructions and hospital policy.	Washing with detergent removes any feed left in the equipment. Thorough rinsing is required to prevent inactivation of sterilizing agent by the detergent.

After completing step 10, the procedure begins again at step 1 after the patient has rested for a period of time, usually approximately two hours.

Continuous feeding

Following the above procedure for intermittent feeding and repeat continuously. In step 7, the feed rate will be much slower according to the length of time the continuous feed is to run for.

Note: with both the continuous and intermittent methods of feeding, the giving set and reservoir must be discarded after 24 hours.

NURSING CARE PLAN

Problem	Cause	Suggested action
Abdominal distension, nausea or diarrhoea.	Feed given too rapidly.	Reduce the rate of feed. Administer any medication prescribed for nausea or diarrhoea. If this fails, consider other causes for nausea and diarrhoea.
	Malabsorption due to enzyme depletion, villous atrophy following periods of starvation or inadequate nutrition.	Dilute the feed or decrease the rate of feed. Inform the dietitian and medical team or nutrition team.
	Hyperosmolar feeds.	As above.
	Lactose intolerance, especially in patients of African and Asian origin or severely debilitated patients.	Use a lactose-free feed.
	Contaminated feed and/or equipment.	Obtain a stool for bacteriological investigation. Take swabs from the equipment and any solutions used.

Nursing care plan

Problem	Cause	Suggested action
Weight gain is unsatisfactory and/or urea output high.	Inadequate nutrition for patient's needs.	Inform the dietitian or nutrition team.
Dehydration.	Inadequate water intake to meet patient's needs.	Offer fluids. Inform the dietitian or nutrition team.

APPENDIX: SUGGESTED MANAGEMENT OF AN ENTERAL FEEDING REGIMEN

Suitable for nasogastric, gastrostomy or jejunostomy feeding.

The management of the enteral feed should be discussed with a dietitian to ensure that the patient's requirements are met.

Starting the regimen

This will vary depending on the following:
1. Nutritional requirements of patient.
2. Condition of the patient, e.g. has the patient been starved before starting the regimen?
3. Type of feed being used.

Action	Rationale
1. Gradual build up, over four to five days, of volume and rate of feed to meet nutritional requirements.	Gradual increase in regime allows the gastrointestinal tract to adjust to a liquid diet, thus reducing the risk of intolerance.

Timing of the feed

Action	Rationale
Either	
1. A continuous drip feed over 24 hours.	Patients may find this restricting but it has the advantage of allowing a large volume of feed to be dripped in slowly over a long period of time, thus giving a high level of nutrition while keeping the osmotic load low.
or	
2. Four or five feeds daily. Timing determined by convenience to patient and staff. (See 'Guidelines: Administration of an enteral feed', above.)	Patients may prefer intermittent feeds given throughout the day.

Duration of the feed

Action	Rationale
1. The number of feeds and the drip rate should be decided based upon the patient's requirements, condition and personal preference, by the dietitian, medical team, nursing staff and patient.	Feed should be given according to individual patient's needs and preferences.

Appendix: Suggested management of an enteral feeding regime

Monitoring the patient

	Action	Rationale
1. Fluid balance.	Measure daily input and output. Observe for thirst, lethargy.	To monitor state of hydration.
2. Weight.	Weigh twice weekly (in same clothing and at same time of day).	To monitor weight changes which may be associated with a tube-feeding regimen.
3. Urine.	Daily urine analysis for glucose during first week of feeding. If glucose detected, notify dietitian and medical team and check blood sugar using glucose-sensitive strip.	To ensure that the glucose levels remains within normal limits.
4. Bowels.	Check daily, by observation or by asking the patient about the frequency and nature of stools.	To detect and combat diarrhoea or constipation related to tube feeding.
5. Haematological investigations.	Test for urea and electrolytes and glucose levels once or twice weekly.	To monitor the patient's state of hydration and glucose levels. Nitrogen balance may be of value in some patients, with heavy nitrogen losses in fistula or major sepsis.

15

Entonox Administration

Definition

Entonox is a gaseous mixture of 50% oxygen and 50% nitrous oxide which acts as an analgesic agent when inhaled. The mixture remains stable at temperatures of above −6°C.

The Entonox cylinder is coloured blue and has white segments on the shoulder. The apparatus consists of the cylinder, the Bodok seal, inhalation tubing and the handpiece. Either a mask or a mouthpiece may be used (Figure 15.1).

Indications

The use of Entonox is indicated before or during a number of painful procedures:

1. Changing packs, drains and dressings.
2. Removal of sutures from sensitive areas, e.g. the vulva.
3. Re-dressing burns, where an occlusive or open technique is not used.
4. Invasive procedures such as catheterization and sigmoidoscopy.
5. Childbirth.
6. Removal of radioactive intracavity gynaecological applicators.
7. Following myocardial infarction (Entonox provides safe analgesia as well as supplementary oxygen).
8. Altering the position of a patient who is in pain.
9. Manual evacuation of the bowel to relieve constipation.
10. Traumatic injuries.
11. Applying orthopaedic traction.
12. Physiotherapy procedures, particularly postoperatively.

Contraindications

Its use is contraindicated in the following cases and situations:

1. Maxillofacial injuries, as the patient may not be able to hold the mask tightly to the face or to use the mouthpiece adequately.
2. Head injuries with impairment of consciousness.
3. Heavily sedated patients.
4. Intoxicated patients.
5. Pneumothorax, as it will increase the problem.
6. The 'bends', as nitrous oxide escapes into the bloodstream and increases the size of the nitrogen bubbles in the tissues.
7. Laryngectomy patients, as they will be unable to use the apparatus.
8. Administration over continuous periods of longer than 48 to 72 hours as leucopenia may occur.
9. Temperatures below −6°C as separation of the gases occurs.

REFERENCE MATERIAL

The relief of pain for patients undergoing painful procedures is often not met adequately. The reasons for this are varied and range from the inability of professional personnel to measure adequately how much pain a patient is suffering, to the difficulty of judging at the outset how painful a procedure will prove to be for a patient. Nurses are able to administer analgesics only if the doctor has specifically prescribed their use. Many procedures can only be assessed as painful once their performance has begun. At this stage it is difficult either to wait for a doctor to prescribe analgesics or to wait for a prescribed analgesic to take effect. In these situations an analgesic that could be prescribed and administered by nurses, would take rapid effect, would be equally rapidly excreted from the body and would have few side-effects is the ideal (Diggory, 1979). Entonox meets all these criteria. See Table 15.1 for a comparison between opiates and Entonox.

Principle of administration

Entonox is designed for self-administration by the patient. The apparatus works as a demand unit, i.e. gas can be obtained only by the patient inhaling and producing a negative pressure. When the patient exhales, the gas flow stops. The patient must hold the mask firmly over the face to produce an airtight fit

Table 15.1 Comparison of opiates and Entonox

Opiates	*Entonox*
1. Usually have to be given by injection – an added discomfort for the patient. There is also the risk of local or systemic infection.	Inhaled, i.e. a painless procedure.
2. May take up to one hour to become effective.	Rapid onset, i.e. $1\frac{1}{2}$ to 2 minutes.
3. Effects that last for approximately one hour or more.	Effects wear off rapidly, i.e. in approximately 2 to 5 minutes.
4. Need to be prescribed by a doctor.	Can be prescribed by an appropriately qualified trained nurse or physiotherapist.
5. Side-effects include respiratory and cardiovascular depression, emesis, drowsiness and thus an inability to co-operate.	Side-effects are few and self-limiting as the gas is self-administered. Recovery from side-effects such as drowsiness and amnesia is rapid.
6. Tend to decrease peripheral circulation in patients suffering from shock due to their effect on the cardiovascular system.	The extra oxygen in Entonox increases peripheral circulation oxygenation in patients suffering from shock.

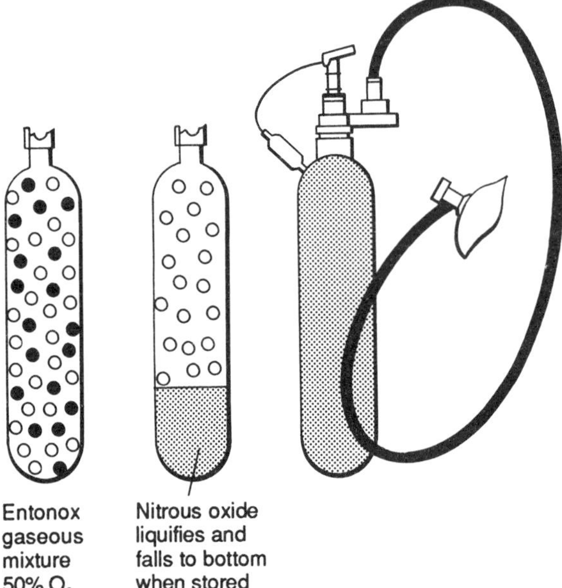
Entonox gaseous mixture 50% O_2 50% N_2O
Nitrous oxide liquifies and falls to bottom when stored below -6°C

Figure 15.1 Entonox cylinder. The apparatus consists of the cylinder, the Bodok seal, inhalation tubing and the handpiece. Either a mask or a mouthpiece may be used.

before the gas will flow. Expired gases escape by the expiratory valve on the handpiece. Alternatively, a mouthpiece can be used. It is essential to adhere to this method of self-administration as it is impossible for patients to overdose themselves because if they become drowsy they will relax their grip on the hand set and the gas flow will cease when no negative pressure is applied.

A smaller dose than normal of an opiate may be given to augment the effects of Entonox (Entonox, 1975). This should be given in sufficient time to take effect before the procedure begins.

Entonox has an oxygen content two and a half times that of air and is, therefore, a good way of giving extra oxygen as well as providing analgesia.

Personnel qualified to teach and supervise the use of Entonox

Only those staff who have been trained and supervised in the use of Entonox should be allowed to train and supervise patients. Usually these will be:

1. Registered general nurses or certified midwives.
2. Physiotherapists.

References and further reading

Diggory, G. (1979) Entonox and its role in nursing care. *Nursing*, April, pp. 28–31.

Entonox (1975) Abstracted proceedings of the symposium on Entonox organized by the Department of Anaesthesia, St Bartholomew's Hospital, London.

Msi, J. (1981) The use of Entonox for the relief of pain experienced by cancer patients. In *Cancer Nursing Update* (Ed. by R. Tiffany). Baillière Tindall, London.

Toulson, S. (1990) More than a lot of hot air. *Nursing*, 4(2), 23–6.

Audiovisual aids

Entonox in Hospitals, BOC's Audio Visual Services, 42 Upper Richmond Road, West London SW14 8DD.

GUIDELINES: ENTONOX ADMINISTRATION

Equipment

1. Entonox cylinder and head.
2. Face mask or mouthpiece.

Procedure

Action	Rationale
1. Check to see if there is gas in the Entonox cylinder by turning the tap in an anticlockwise direction.	
2. Examine the gauge to determine how much gas is in the cylinder.	To ensure an adequate supply of gas throughout the procedure.
3. Ensure that the patient is in as comfortable a position as possible.	
4. Demonstrate how to use the apparatus by holding the mask tightly to your face and breathing in and out regularly and deeply. A hissing sound will indicate that the gas is being inhaled.	To ensure that the patient understands what to do before any painful procedure commences. To reassure the patient of the non-toxic effects of the gas. To provide a correct role model.
5. Allow the patient to practise using the apparatus.	To enable the patient to adopt the correct technique and observe the analgesic effect of the gas before the procedure commences.
6. Encourage the patient to breathe gas in and out for at least two minutes before commencing any painful procedure.	To allow sufficient time for an adequate circulatory level of nitrous oxide to provide analgesia. (When the patient inhales, gas enters first the lungs then the pulmonary and systemic circulations. It takes one to two minutes to build up reasonable concentrations of nitrous oxide in the brain.)
7. During the procedure keep encouraging the patient to breathe in and out regularly and deeply.	To maintain adequate circulatory levels, thus providing adequate analgesia.
8. At the end of the procedure observe the patient until the effects of the gas have worn off.	Some patients may feel a transient drowsiness or giddiness and should be discouraged from getting out of bed until these effects have worn off. It is rare for the patient to experience transient amnesia.
9. Turn off the Entonox supply from the cylinder by turning the tap in a clockwise direction. The gauge should then read 'Empty'.	To avoid potential seepage of gas from the apparatus.
10. Depress the diaphragm under the valve to express residual gas.	
11. Wash the face mask, expiratory valve and handpiece in a neutral detergent.	To minimize the risk of cross-infection.

NURSING CARE PLAN

Problem	Cause	Suggested action
Patient not experiencing adequate analgesic effect.	Entonox cylinder empty. Apparatus not properly connected.	Check before procedure commences.
	Patient not inhaling deeply enough.	Encourage the patient to breathe in until a hissing noise can be heard from the cylinder.
	Patient inhaling pure oxygen, i.e. cylinder has been stored below −6°C and nitrous oxide has liquified and settled at the bottom of the cylinder. (All cylinders should be stored horizontally at a temperature of 10°C or above for 24 hours before use.)	Initially safe, but later the patient may inhale pure nitrous oxide and be asphyxiated. Discontinue the procedure. Ensure adequate warming of the cylinder and inversion of the cylinder to remix the gases adequately.
	Not enough time has been allowed for nitrous oxide to exert its analgesic effect.	Allow at least two minutes of Entonox use before commencing the procedure.
Patient experiences generalized muscle rigidity.	Hyperventilation during inhalation.	Discontinue Entonox and allow the patient to recover. Explain the procedure again, stressing deep and regular inspiration. Try a mouthpiece instead of a mask.
Patient unable to tolerate a mask.	Smell of rubber, feeling of claustrophobia.	Try a mouthpiece.
Patient feels nauseated, drowsy or giddy.	Effect of nitrous oxide accumulation.	Discontinue Entonox administration – the effect will then rapidly disappear.
Patient afraid to use Entonox.	Associates gases with previous hospital procedures, e.g. anaesthesia before surgery.	Demonstrate use and thus its non-toxic effects.

16

Epidural Analgesia

Definition

This is the administration of analgesics and anti-inflammatory drugs into the epidural space. Analgesic drugs may be divided into two categories:

1. Local anaesthetics, which provide a conduction block for sensory stimuli.
2. Opiates which act within the central nervous system by attaching to specific opiate receptors in the substantia gelatinosa and the thalamus.

Both groups of drug provide excellent analgesia and each has its own specific side-effects:

1. Local anaesthetics. The main side-effects are related to sympathetic and motor neuronal blockade. Sympathetic blockade may result in hypotension, due to vascular dilatation, requiring treatment with volume expanders and/or vasoconstrictors such as ephedrine. Motor blockade will result in temporary paralysis of muscle groups supplied by the affected segments.
2. Opiates. The main side-effect is that of respiratory depression, which may require treatment with intravenous naloxone and oxygen therapy. A further minor, though significant, side-effect can be pruritis, requiring treatment with antihistamine and calamine.

A side-effect common to both classes of analgesics is urinary retention which may require catheterization.

Indications

1. Provision of analgesia during labour.
2. As an alternative to general anaesthesia, e.g. in severe respiratory disease or for patients with malignant hyperthermia.
3. As a supplement to general anaesthesia.
4. Provision of postoperative analgesia.
5. Provision of analgesia resulting from trauma, e.g. fractured ribs, which may result in respiratory failure due to pain on breathing.
6. Management of chronic intractable pain, e.g. from bone metastases.
7. To relieve muscle spasm and pain resulting from lumbar cord pressure due to disc protrusion or local oedema and inflammation.

Contraindications

These may be absolute or relative

Absolute:

1. Patients with coagulation defects, which may result in epidural haematoma formation and spinal cord compression, e.g. iatrogenic (anticoagulated patient) or congenital (haemophiliacs).
2. Local sepsis at the site of proposed epidural injection; the result might be meningitis or epidural abscess formation.
3. Proven allergy to the intended drug.
4. Unstable spinal fracture.
5. Patient refusal to consent to the procedure.

Relative:

1. Unstable cardiovascular system.
2. Spinal deformity.
3. Raised intracranial pressure (a risk of coning if a dural tap occurs).
4. Certain neurological conditions (though this may be because of fear of litigation, rather than for good medical reasons).

REFERENCE MATERIAL

Anatomy of the epidural space

The epidural space lies between the spinal dura and ligamentum flavum. Its average diameter is 0.5 cm, and is widest in the midline posteriorly in the lumbar region. The contents of the epidural space include a rich venous plexus, spinal arterioles, lymphatics and extradural fat.

Spinal nerves traverse the epidural space laterally. There are 31 pairs of spinal nerves of varying size. The two main groups of nerve fibres are:

1. Myelinated – myelin is a thin, fatty sheath which insulates the fibres, preventing impulses being

transmitted to adjacent fibres. Myelin also protects fibres and speeds of impulses.
2. Unmyelinated – delicate fibres, more susceptible to hypoxia and toxins than myelinated fibres.

The spinal nerves are composed of a posterior and anterior root, which join to form a spinal nerve:

1. Posterior root – transmits ascending sensory impulses from the periphery to the spinal cord.
2. Anterior root – transmits descending motor impulses from the spinal cord to the periphery by means of its corresponding spinal nerve.

Principal insertion technique

1. The patient is positioned either in the left or right lateral position, with the knees curled into the abdomen and the chin into the chest (the 'fetal' position), or seated on the edge of the trolley with the feet on a stool and bent forward onto a pillow placed across the knees.
2. Full asepsis is observed, i.e. the operator is scrubbed, gowned and gloved.
3. The skin is prepared with an alcoholic solution (chlorhexidine or betadine).
4. The site of injection is isolated with a fenestrated towel.
5. Local anaesthetic is injected at the site of epidural injection.
6. The skin is punctured at the site with an appropriate needle, and the 16 gauge Tuohy needle is inserted as far as the ligamentum flavum. This is identified by applying pressure on the plunger of a glass syringe filled with air or saline, which meets with resistance while the needle tip lies within the ligamentum flavum. Needle and syringe are then advanced with a constant pressure being applied to the syringe plunger, which will suddenly plunge 'home' when the tip of the Tuohy needle enters the epidural space, i.e. loss of resistance technique.
7. The epidural catheter is then passed by means of the Tuohy needle into the epidural space, the needle is withdrawn and the catheter length adjusted so that there are approximately four or five centimetres left in the space.
8. The catheter is aspirated to exclude accidental insertion into an epidural vein.
9. The catheter is taped into position.

Common solutions used

1. Local anaesthetics – either plain or with adrenaline 1:200 000:
   (a) Lignocaine 0.5 to 2%: rapid onset, short duration (one to two hours).

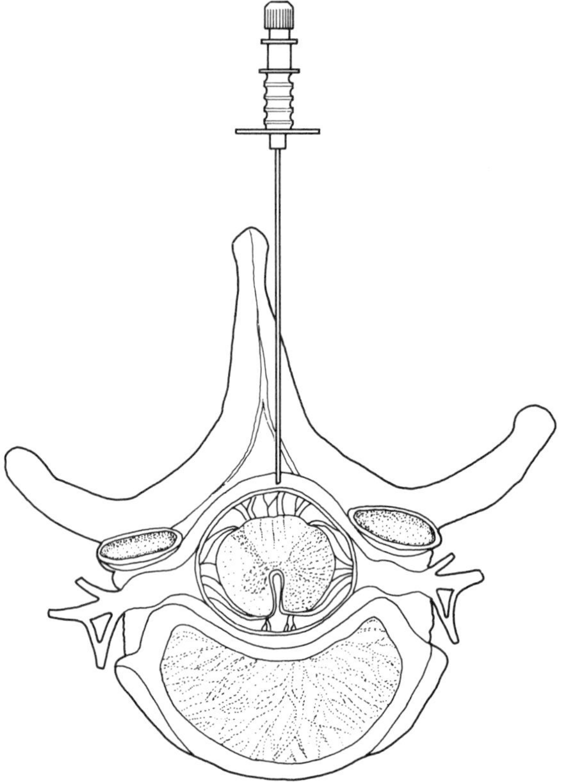

Figure 16.1 Diagram showing positioning of Tuohy needle. (*Source*: Regional Anaesthesia (American Society of Regional Anaesthesia)).

   (b) Bupivacaine: slower onset of action, but longer duration (two to eight hours).
   (c) Others: amethocaine hydrochloride, prilocaine.
2. Opiates: Diamorphine, morphine and fentanyl are the most commonly used opiates.

Spread of local anaesthetic solutions

Spread of local anaesthetic solutions is influenced by the following:

1. Volume injected.
2. Age of patient.
3. Force of injection.
4. Level of catheter.
5. Drug concentration.

Mode of injection

1. Bolus injections.
2. Continuous infusions.
3. Combined infusion/bolus method, i.e. back-

ground infusion with boluses as required if analgesia inadequate.

Methods of administration

1. Bolus administered by nurse or doctor, when required.
2. Patient-controlled administration using a microprocessor-controlled infusion device.

Complications of epidural analgesia

1. Paraplegia is a rare occurrence. It may be caused by cord infarction.
2. Intraocular haemorrhage has been reported after rapid injection of 30 ml of fluid. This is thought to raise cerebrospinal fluid pressure with resultant intraocular bleeding.
3. Backache has been produced occasionally from local irritation caused by the needle or catheter.
4. Extradural abscess may take up to 16 days to develop. Extradural abscess or haematoma should be drained on diagnosis otherwise paraplegia may result (Pritchard & David, 1988).

References and further reading

Adam, S. (1985) Epidural anaesthesia. *Nursing Mirror*, 160(10), 38–41.

Atkinson, R. S. *et al.* (1982) *A Synopsis of Anaesthesia*, 9th edn. John Wright, Bristol.

Bibbings, J. (1984) Epidural analgesia. *Nursing Times*, 80(35), 53–5.

Brown, E. (1990) Narcotics via the epidural route (Part I). *Nursing Standard*, 4(38), 24–39; Part II, *Nursing Standard*, 4(39), 37–9.

de Boek, R. *et al.* (1990) *Patient-Controlled Analgesia*, The Royal Marsden Hospital (Patient Information Series) (unpublished), London.

Morgan, M. (1989) The rational use of intrathecal and extradural opioids. *British Journal of Anaesthetists*, 63, 165–8.

Owen, H. *et al.* (1988) The development and clinical use of patient-controlled analgesia. *Anaesthetic Intensive Care*, 16, 437–47.

Pritchard, A. P. & David, J. (1988) *The Royal Marsden Hospital Manual of Clinical Nursing Procedures*, 2nd edn. Harper & Row, London.

Sheargold, L. (1986) Epidural and spinal anaesthetics. *Nursing Times*, 82(27), 44–5.

The Royal College of Surgeons of England & The College of Anaesthetists (1990) *Report of the Working Party on Pain After Surgery*, pp. 15–17.

Ward, M. E. (1978) Epidural analgesia. *Nursing*, (May) No. 2, 78–81.

Yarde, A. (1989) Epidural analgesia. *The Professional Nurse*, September, Vol. 4, Part 12, 608–13.

GUIDELINES: EPIDURAL ANALGESIA

Note: patients undergoing epidural analgesia should always have venous access or an intravenous infusion in situ before the procedure.

Equipment

1. Antiseptic skin cleansing agent.
2. Local anaesthetic.
3. Selection of needles and syringes.
4. Sterile dressing pack.
5. Face mask.
6. Tuohy needle or assorted gauge lumbar puncture needles.
7. Epidural catheter.
8. Bacterial filter.
9. Waterproof dressing and plastic adhesive dressing to tape catheter securely.

Procedure

Action	Rationale
1. Explain the procedure to patient.	To obtain the patient's consent and co-operation.
2. Assist the patient into the required position: (a) Lying: Position pillow under patient's head. Firm surface.	To ensure maximum widening of the intervertebral spaces, providing easier access to the epidural space.

Guidelines: Epidural analgesia

Action	**Rationale**
On side with knee drawn up to the abdomen and clasped by the hands. Support the patient in this position.	To prevent sudden movement.
(b) Sitting: Patient sits on firm surface with arms resting on a table, and with the head resting on the arms.	Allows proper identification of the spinal processes and therefore invertebral spaces.
3. Support, encourage and observe the patient throughout the procedure.	
4. Assist the doctor as required. The doctor will proceed as follows:	
(a) Clean the skin with alcohol-based solution (chlorhexidine) or povidone–iodine solution.	To maintain asepsis.
(b) Identify the area to be punctured and inject the skin and subcutaneous layers with local anaesthetic.	
(c) Introduce Tuohy or spinal needles usually between third and fourth lumbar vertebrae.	
(d) Ensure epidural space has been entered.	To prevent anaesthesia being given directly into spinal cord or intravenously by means of the dural veins.
(e) Inject test dose of drug (may be performed).	To ensure the position of the needle.
(f) Thread epidural catheter through barrel of Tuohy needle.	To facilitate intermittent topping-up of anaesthesia and to allow greater control.
(g) Attach the bacterial filter.	To prevent injection of contaminants into epidural space.
(h) Apply dressing and tape to the catheter insertion site.	To prevent the catheter being dislodged.
(i) Inject solution into epidural space via catheter.	To provide anaesthesia.
5. Position the patient according to the doctor's instructions, tilting if appropriate.	To ensure spread of solution to provide optimum effect.
6. Take vital signs observations: blood pressure and respirations every five minutes for 30 minutes, and then 15 minutes for next 90 minutes. Take pulse every 15 minutes for two hours, or more frequently if the patient's condition dictates.	To monitor for signs of hypotension and respiratory depression.
7. Make the patient comfortable. Usually the patient is nursed flat for the first three to six hours, then slowly elevated into a sitting position. Bedclothes should not constrict the feet.	To prevent the development of footdrop.

GUIDELINES: TOPPING UP EPIDURAL ANALGESIA

Usually performed by the doctor. Local anaesthetic agents *or* opioids may be given by nursing staff as part of an extended role, according to local policy. This should follow an agreed period of education and supervised practice.

Equipment

1. Antiseptic cleaning agent.
2. Syringes and needles.
3. Drug as prescribed.
4. Water or saline for injection as necessary.
5. Patient's prescription chart.
6. Sterile hub/bung.

Procedure

Action	Rationale
1. Wash hands with bactericidal soap and water or bactericidal alcohol hand rub.	To prevent cross-infection.
2. Check the drug to be administered and diluents, according to policy.	To ensure the correct drug, amount and concentration is administered to the correct patient.
3. Draw up the drug.	
4. Clean the access portal of the bacterial filter.	To prevent the introduction of contaminants and micro-organisms into the epidural space.
5. Inject drug as prescribed.	
6. Make the patient comfortable.	
7. Monitor vital signs, blood pressure and respirations every five minutes for 30 minutes, then every 15 minutes for 90 minutes. Take pulse every 15 minutes for two hours or more frequently if the patient's condition dictates.	To monitor signs of hypotension and respiratory depression.
8. Dispose of the equipment appropriately.	

GUIDELINES: REMOVAL OF AN EPIDURAL CATHETER

Equipment

1. Dressing pack.
2. Skin cleansing agent, i.e. normal saline.
3. Spray dressing (moisture vapour permeable), i.e. op-site.
4. Occlusive dressing.

Procedure

Action	Rationale
1. Wash hands with bactericidal soap and water or bactericidal alcohol hand rub.	To minimize cross-infection.
2. Open dressing pack.	
3. Remove tape and dressing from catheter insertion site.	
4. Gently, in one swift movement, remove catheter. Check that it is removed intact by observing marks along the barrel.	To ensure the catheter is removed intact.

Guidelines: Removal of an epidural catheter

Action	***Rationale***
5. Spray dressing (moisture vapour permeable), i.e. op-site with povidone–iodine and op-site spray.	As prophylaxis against infection along the catheter tract.
6. Apply an occlusive dressing and leave *in situ* for 24 hours.	To prevent inadvertent access of micro-organisms along the tract.

The epidural tip may be sent for culture and sensitivity if infection is suspected, or according to local policy.

NURSING CARE PLAN

Problem	**Cause**	**Suggested action**
Rapid fall in blood pressure.	Sympathetic blockade producing hypotension.	Turn off infusion pump if in progress. If systolic blood pressure falls below 85 mm Hg: Summon duty anaesthetist or doctor. Tilt the patient's head down unless contraindicated. Give oxygen 4 litres/minute via a mask. To prevent hypoxia caused by reduced cardiac output. Open fully intravenous infusion unless contraindicated e.g. congestive heart failure. To increase circulatory volume and blood pressure. Prepare 15 to 30 mg of ephedrine for intravenous injection, which may be required by the doctor. Ephedrine increases heart rate and cardiac output and produces vasoconstriction by direct and indirect action on the sympathetic nervous system.
Respiratory depression.	Opiate analgesia.	Call for medical assistance. Turn off infusion pump or patient-controlled analgesia (PCA) pump if in progress. Prepare naloxone 0.4 mg intravenously. If prescribed, give dose according to criteria, i.e. respiratory rate <8/minute. Dosage counteracts respiratory depression and might also reverse the analgesic effect. If no improvement, administer second dose. A further 0.4 mg naloxone intravenously can be given 5 to 10 minutes after first.

		Prepare emergency equipment to support respiration. The patient's respiratory rate pattern and depth should be observed at all times. Continuous display of oxygen saturation and monitors are available. Access to blood gas machines should be available. Observe pupil constriction.
Total spinal anaesthesia.		Prepare emergency equipment to support respiration. Call for medical assistance. Turn patient into the supine position. Ventilate the lungs. Elevate the legs. Prepare emergency drugs. Open intravenous infusion. Prepare equipment for intubation.
Total central neurological blockade: 1. Marked hypotension. 2. Apnoea. 3. Dilated pupils. 4. Loss of consciousness.		Call for medical assistance and begin emergency procedures.
Toxicity due to injected drug: 1. Disorientation. 2. Twitching. 3. Convulsions. 4. Apnoea.		Call for medical assistance and institute emergency procedures.
Nausea or vomiting.	Side-effect of opiates. Due to stimulation of the vomiting centre in the brain stem and stimulation of the chemoreceptor zone in the fourth ventricle of the brain.	Administer antiemetics as prescribed. Inform an anaesthetist.
Headache.	May be caused by accidental dural puncture.	Administer systemic analgesia Lie patient flat. Oral and intravenous fluids may be increased to encourage cerebrospinal fluid formation.
Pruritis. Especially of the face and/or neck.	Following administration of opiates histamine release.	Inform anaesthetist. Administer antihistamine as prescribed. Keep patient cool. Use calamine lotion.
Urinary retention.	Due to parasympathetic block at the sacral level of the spinal cord.	Inform anaesthetist. Catheterize as required. The majority of patients on an intensive therapy unit or high

Nursing care plan

Problem	**Cause**	**Suggested action**
		dependency unit are usually catheterized.
Infection.		Check temperature four-hourly. Check catheter entry site for inflammation or exudate. Remove epidural cannula if appropriate.

Assess pain regularly using a visual analogue scale or pain chart if appropriate. Observe the patient's movements and facial expressions. Discuss insufficient or ineffective analgesia with the anaesthetist.

PATIENT-CONTROLLED ANALGESIA AND INFUSIONS

Patient-controlled analgesia (PCA) is a technique developed over 20 years ago which allows patients to administer their own analgesia. The PCA syringe pump can deliver an opioid analgesic, e.g. diamorphine, in three different ways:

1. By pressing a button, the patient can deliver a programmed *bolus dose* as required. A *lockout period* is set so that the syringe pump will not respond to further pressing of the button for the set amount of time. This allows time for each dose to work before patients can give themselves another bolus. This mechanism prevents the occurrence of overdosage.
2. A continuous *background infusion* can be delivered by the pump just as by any continuous syringe driver.
3. A combination of *background infusion* and *bolus dose* can be used.

For patient safety, all patients receiving epidural analgesia should be nursed on a high dependency unit by skilled staff with appropriate equipment.

Continuous monitoring and observation is essential

Facilities for resuscitation should be readily available for all of these patients. The patient should be the *only* person who operates the patient-controlled analgesia pump. Inappropriate pressing of the button by nursing staff or doctors may lead to oversedation and respiratory arrest.

Patient-controlled analgesia may not be suitable for all patients and it is important that every patient is assessed carefully by the nursing and medical staff.

The use of pain charts is advocated in most units. Patients can be assessed 30 minutes after commencing therapy, then at designated times according to local policy.

Continuous in-service training of staff is essential in order to detect rare cases of equipment malfunction and to minimize error.

Continuous infusions

An increasing number of units are using a combination of one or more drugs as a continuous infusion. Drugs used vary according to the anaesthetist. A variety of opiates may be used, e.g. diamorphine, fentanyl.

In most cases, a 30 cc or 60 cc syringe containing the selected drug is run at a rate prescribed by the anaesthetic team. The rate can be increased or decreased as necessary.

The syringe pump should be monitored and marked hourly to ensure that the correct dose is given and that the pump is working accurately.

The most important, and potentially fatal, complication of spinal opiates is respiratory depression, which may be considerably delayed many hours after these infusions commence.

All patients must be observed constantly and their respiratory rate, depth and pattern recorded. The use of pulse oximeters to continually display oxygen saturation is now employed in most units. Blood gasses may need to be taken and oxygen therapy administered if appropriate.

17

External Compression and Support in the Management of Chronic Oedema

Definition

'Support can be thought of as sub-bandage (sub-hosiery) pressure achieved by the body tissue pushing the bandage outwards . . . Compression, on the other hand, is where the forces within a bandage (or hose) cause pressure to be exerted beneath it' (Collyer, 1990). 'Support may be defined as the retention and control of tissue without the application of compression . . . Compression implies the deliberate application of pressure' (Thomas, 1990).

Indications

Graduated external compression is the mainstay of conservative physical treatment of chronic oedema. It is important for several reasons:

1. It ensures that fluid in the limb flows upwards towards the root of the limb.
2. It limits the formation of lymph in the tissues.
3. It supports the tissues of the swollen limb and helps to maintain a normal shape to the limb.
4. It provides muscles in the affected limb with a firm wall against which to work, thus maximizing the effect of the muscle pump (Leduc *et al.*, 1990; Olszewski and Engeset, 1990).

In the cancer setting, external support is used in situations where significant reduction of swelling is unlikely (such as obstructive oedema due to advanced cancer), since should the limb reduce under a support bandage, the bandage will become loose and fall off.

Bandages are used in the following situations:

1. To reduce large limbs.
2. To restore normal shape to a limb that is distorted.
3. To provide support and alleviate discomfort in the palliative treatment of gross oedema.
4. To protect fragile or damaged skin on oedematous limbs.
5. To resolve lymphorrhoea (leakage of lymph through the skin).

Hosiery is used:

1. To contain the drained tissues of a reduced limb and maintain reduced limb size.
2. To reduce mild, pitting oedema.
3. To prevent oedema accumulating in situations where lymph drainage is known to be compromised.
4. To provide support and alleviate discomfort in the palliative treatment of mild to moderate oedema.

Contraindications for compression

1. Arterial disease in the arm or leg.
2. Acute deep vein thrombosis in the leg.

REFERENCE MATERIAL

Chronic oedema (or lymphoedema) is defined as 'tissue swelling due to a failure of lymph drainage' (Mortimer, 1990). Lymph drainage commonly fails in cancer patients as a result of damage to lymph nodes from surgery and/or radiotherapy, or from the obstructive effects of local tumour. A study carried out at the Royal Marsden Hospital (Kissen *et al.*, 1986) found an incidence of lymphoedema of 25% in 200 patients following treatment for breast cancer. The incidence rose to 38% in patients who had received both surgery and radiotherapy to the axilla.

The incidence of leg oedema following treatment for abdominal and pelvic tumours is not known, nor is the incidence in patients with soft tissue sarcoma or melanoma. However, lymphoedema is not uncommon in these patients.

Lymphoedema can affect any part of the body including the head, but it most commonly affects the limbs (Mortimer, 1990). The high protein concentration of lymphoedema causes skin and tissue changes in the oedematous limb, leading to the characteristic deepened skin folds, distorted limb shape and hyperkeratosis associated with longstanding lymphoedema. There is an increased risk of infection in the affected limb (fungal infections, cellulitis) and recurrent acute inflammatory episodes are common (Mortimer, 1990).

Chronic venous disease of the lower limbs, commonly seen in the elderly, can result in oedema usually affecting the lower legs. This oedema often has a lymphatic component (Prasad *et al.*, 1990). The increased load on the lymphatic system from the outpouring of fluid from incompetent veins leads to lymphatic failure. Dependency or gravitational oedema is another problem commonly seen in the immobile, elderly patient. It arises from a lack of propulsion to venous blood flow and lymph flow.

There is no cure for lymphoedema but it is possible to reduce the size of the swollen limb and, in the patient free of active cancer, to control the swelling in the long term (Badger & Twycross, 1988). For patients with recurrent or advanced cancer, treatment can be modified with the aim of palliating the symptoms associated with oedema (Badger, 1987).

Types of compression and support

There are two main forms of external compression, compression bandages and elastic hosiery. Each has a distinct function and each is used at a specific stage of treatment.

In the active treatment of severe or complicated lymphoedema, bandages are generally the first-line approach. High compression bandages (25 to 35 mm Hg at the ankle) are used. Crepe bandages do not fall into the this category. Bandages are applied using a multi-layer technique over layers of padding and foam, and are left in place for 24 hours a day (Badger & Twycross, 1988). They are re-applied once every 24 hours, thus ensuring that a high level of pressure is maintained.

In the palliative setting, where the aim is simply to provide support, lower levels of pressure are used and bandages may be left in place for longer periods (two to three days). Though bulky, the bandages should always feel comfortable to the patient and should not prevent the patient from moving all of the bandaged joints.

Normal use of the bandaged limb should be encouraged as much as possible to stimulate the drainage of lymph. Bandages should never result in trauma to the skin, nor should they result in constricted blood flow. Patients must be advised to report any symptoms of pain, tingling or numbness in the limb.

Elastic hosiery is available in a wide range of off-the-shelf sizes and designs. Ready-made stockings come in three compression classes:

1. Class 1: 20 to 30 mm Hg at the ankle.
2. Class 2: 30 to 40 mm Hg at the ankle.
3. Class 3: 40 to 50 mm Hg at the ankle.

Lymphoedema usually calls for the use of class 3 stockings, while classes 1 and 2 are more appropriate for mixed lympho-venous oedema or dependency oedema where the swelling is usually soft and pitting in nature. Classes 1 and 2 stockings are available on general prescription, while class 3 hosiery has to be obtained through a hospital appliance department. Elastic sleeves, like class 3 stockings, are not available on general prescriptions and must also be obtained through the hospital appliance department. These, too, come in a range of sizes and designs but are limited to one compression class (between 30 and 40 mm Hg). Anti-embolism stockings are designed to improve blood flow in the lower limbs and are inappropriate for the treatment of oedema, but shaped, elasticated surgical tubular stockinette may be used in situations where class 1 hose is called for. Hosiery is used to maintain improvement in limb size following bandaging. Ideally, it should be applied before the patient gets out of bed in the morning or, if this is not feasible, as soon after rising as possible. At night, when the limb is in a horizontal position, there is no need for the patient to wear hosiery and the stocking or sleeve is removed. An elastic sleeve or stocking should always feel comfortable and supportive. It should not cause pain or trauma and, while it should be firm-fitting, it should not constrict the limb. Hosiery may also be used as the initial treatment for mild, uncomplicated oedema, or to provide support in the palliative treatment of oedema.

Assessment

A full and careful assessment will highlight the patient's main problems and any co-existing complications. This information is then used to set realistic treatment goals and to determine the initial treatment approach. Assessment should establish:

1. The cause and type of oedema (lymphoedema, venous oedema).
2. The degree and extent of the swelling.
3. The duration of the swelling.
4. Any distortion in limb shape.
5. The condition of the skin.
6. The degree of mobility in the limb.
7. Any obstruction to blood flow.
8. Symptoms and causes of pain.
9. Neurological impairment.

References and further reading

Badger, C. M. A. (1987) Lymphoedema: Management of patients with advanced cancer. *Professional Nurse*, 2(4), 200–2.

Badger, C. M. A. & Regnard, C. F. B. (1989) Oedema in advanced disease: a flow diagram. *Palliative Medicine*, 3, 213–15.
Badger, C. M. A. & Twycross, R. G. (1988) *The Management of Lymphoedema – Guidelines*. Sobell Study Centre, Oxford.
Collyer, G. J. (1990) *Classification of extensible bandages*. Unpublished.
Foldi, M. (1983) Lymphology today. *Angiology*, February, 84–90.
Foldi, E. *et al.* (1985) Conservative treatment of lymphoedema of the limbs. *Angiology*, 36, 171–80.
Kissen, M. W. *et al.* (1986) Risk of lymphoedema following the treatment of breast cancer. *British Journal of Surgery*, 73, 580–4.
Leduc, O. *et al.* (1990) Bandages: scintigraphic demonstration of its efficacy on colloidal protein reabsorbtion during muscle activity. In *Progress in Lymphology – X11: Excerpta Medica* (Ed. by M. Nishi, S. Uchino & S. Yabuki), pp. 421–3. Elsevier, Tokyo.
Mortimer, P. S. (1990) Investigation and management of lymphoedema. *Vascular Medicine Review*, 1, 1–20.
Olszewski, W. L. & Engeset, A. (1990) Peripheral lymph dynamics. *Progress in Lymphology – X11, Excerpta Medica* (Ed. by M. Nishi, S. Uchino & S. Yabuki), pp. 213–14. Elsevier, Tokyo.
Prasad, A. *et al.* (1990) Leg ulcers and oedema: a study exploring the prevalence, aetiology and possible significance of oedema in venous ulcers. *Phlebology*, 5, 181–7.
Stillwell, G. K. (1973) The law of Laplace: some clinical applications. *Mayo Clinic Proceedings*, December, 48, 863–9.
Stillwell, G. K. (1977) Management of arm oedema. In *Breast Cancer Management: Early and Late* (Ed. by B. A. Stoll). Royal Free Hospital, London.
Thomas, S. (1990) Bandages and bandaging: the science behind the art. *CARE Science and Practice*, 8(2), 56–60.
Thomas, S. (1990) Bandages and bandaging. *Nursing Standard, Special Supplement 8*, 4(39), 4–6.

GUIDELINES: STANDARD MULTI-LAYER COMPRESSION BANDAGING

The bandages used should be strong compression bandages (crepe bandages are not suitable). Light retention bandages are used to bandage digits and to hold foam padding in place. The swollen limb should be clean and well moisturized with a bland cream (e.g. E45) before being bandaged. Pressure must be applied in a graduated profile, i.e. highest over the hand or foot, and gradually reducing as the limb is bandaged upwards, to ensure that fluid is encouraged to drain towards the root of the limb. The degree of pressure is influenced by:

1. The circumference of the limb – pressure will be highest over a small circumference and lowest over a large circumference (Laplace's law (Stillwell, 1973)).
2. The amount of tension placed on the bandage.
3. The amount of bandage overlap.
4. The number of bandage layers (Thomas, 1990).

Thus, on a normally shaped limb, maintaining the same amount of bandage tension and the same amount of bandage overlap all the way up the limb will result in a natural graduation of pressure due to the gradual increase in the size of the limb from ankle to groin, or wrist to axilla. In cases where swelling has distorted the shape of the limb, additional padding is used to create a suitable profile on which to bandage, and adjustments may be needed in bandage tension and bandage overlap. Very large limbs may also require extra layers of bandage to be used in order to ensure that sufficient pressure is applied (Badger & Twycross, 1988).

Equipment for bandaging an arm

1. Stockinette.
2. Light retention bandages, 6 cm and 10 cm.
3. Padding, 6 cm roll.
4. Foam.
5. Strong compression bandages, 6 cm and 8 cm.
6. Tape.
7. Scissors.

Procedure

Action	Rationale
1. Explain the procedure to the patient.	To gain the patient's co-operation and consent.

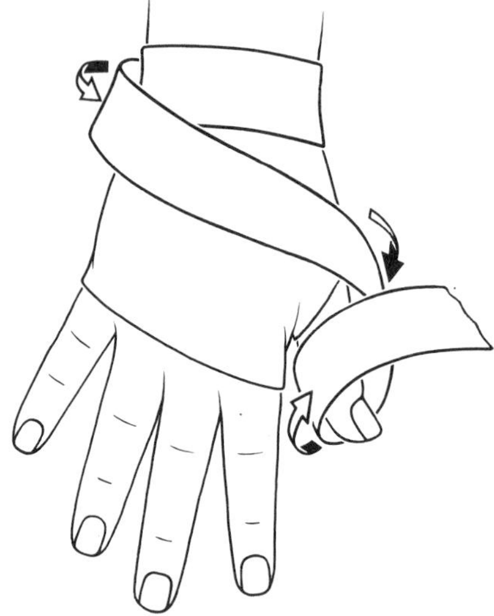

Figure 17.1 Bandaging swollen fingers.

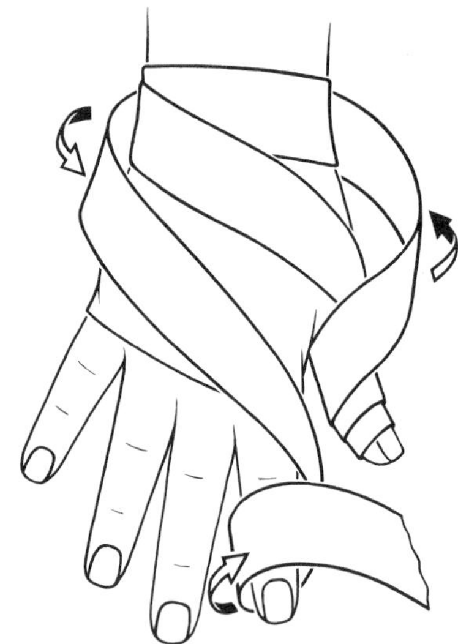

Figure 17.2 The bandage is taken under the wrist, back over the hand, to the index finger.

Guidelines: Standard multi-layer compression bandaging

Action	Rationale
2. If possible, the patient should be seated in a chair. The nurse should be positioned in front of the patient.	To ensure the comfort of both the patient and nurse.
3. Cut a length of stockinette long enough to fit the patient's arm. Cut a small hole for the thumb and slip over the patient's arm.	To protect the skin from chafing.
4. If the fingers are swollen or have a tendency to swell, they must be bandaged (Figure 17.1). Anchor the bandage loosely at the wrist and bring across the back of the hand to the thumb. Bandage around the thumb from the tip downwards (start at the level of the nail bed). Do not pull the bandage tight but go gently and firmly. Take the bandage under the wrist and back over the back of the hand to the index finger (Figure 17.2). Again, bandage from the nail bed down to the webs of the finger. Repeat the same procedure for all fingers. Finish by tucking in the end of the bandage (Figure 17.3).	To reduce or prevent swelling.
5. Check the colour and temperature of the tips of the fingers.	To ensure that the blood supply is not compromised.
6. Check that the patient can move the fingers and make a fist.	To check that the bandage is not too tight.

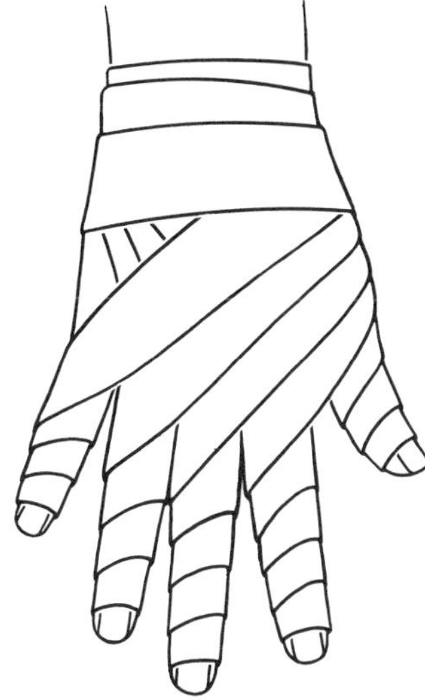

Figure 17.3 The finished bandage.

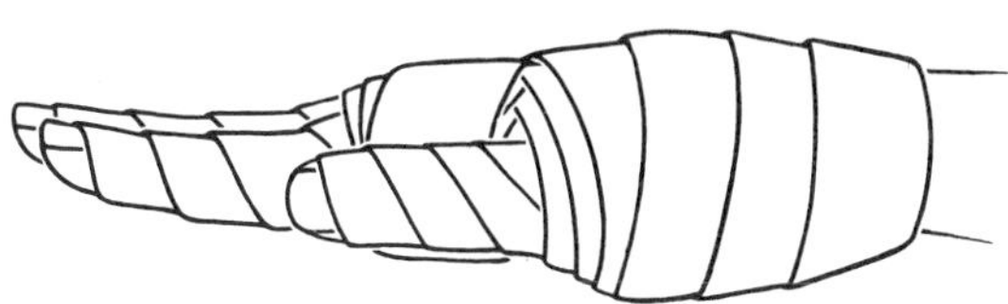

Figure 17.4 The palm and back of the hand are padded out.

7. Using the roll of padding, cover the hand in a figure of eight, padding out the palm and back of the hand (Figure 17.4).	Padding out the hand ensures even pressure distribution.
8. Cut foam to fit the length of the arm from the wrist to axilla ensure that the width is sufficient to encircle the arm with a small overlap.	To protect the elbow joint and provide a smooth, even profile on which to bandage.
9. Wrap the foam around the arm, securing with a light retention bandage. Finish by tucking in the end of the bandage (Figure 17.5).	
10. Take a 6 cm compression bandage and start by anchoring it loosely at the wrist. Bandage the hand firmly in a figure of eight until all of the hand is covered (Figure 17.6). Continue the rest of the bandage up the forearm in a spiral, covering half of the bandage with each turn. Keep the bandage as smooth as possible.	To avoid constriction at the wrist.
11. Take an 8 or 10 cm bandage and, starting at the wrist, bandage in a spiral, still covering half of the bandage with each turn, up to the top of the arm (Figure 17.7).	Two layers are used on the forearm to ensure that pressure is highest distally.
12. Secure the end of the bandage with tape.	
13. Once again, check the colour of the finger tips and check that the patient can move all joints.	To check that the blood flow is not compromised.
14. Remind the patient to use the limb as normally as possible and to report any feelings of discomfort, tingling or numbness.	To ensure good lymph flow.

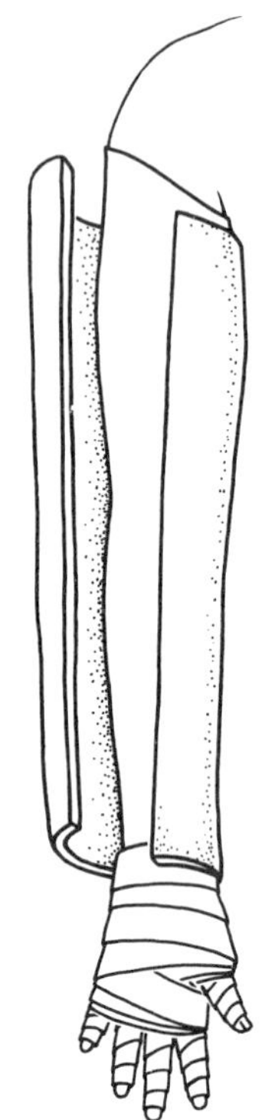

Figure 17.5 Foam is wrapped around the arm, secured with a light retention bandage.

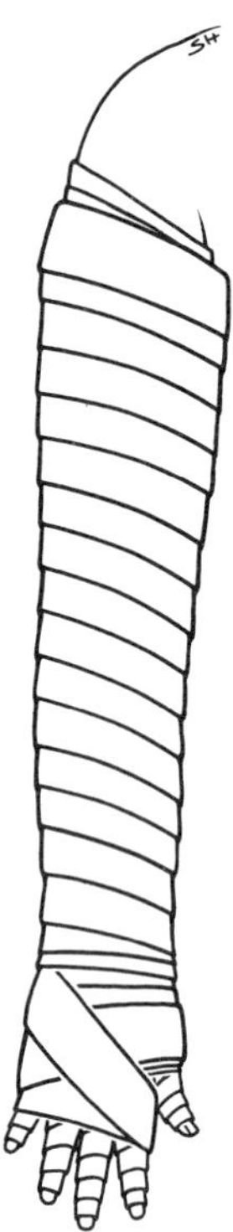

Figure 17.7 Starting at the wrist, an 8 cm or 10 cm bandage is used to cover to the top of the arm, in a spiral fashion.

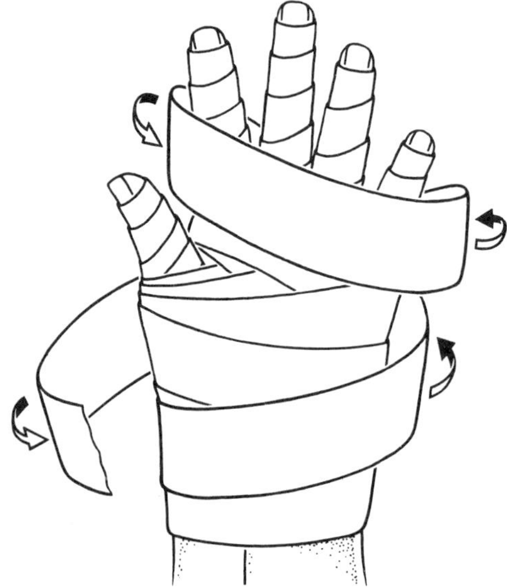

Figure 17.6 The hand is bandaged firmly in a figure of eight using a 6 cm compression bandage.

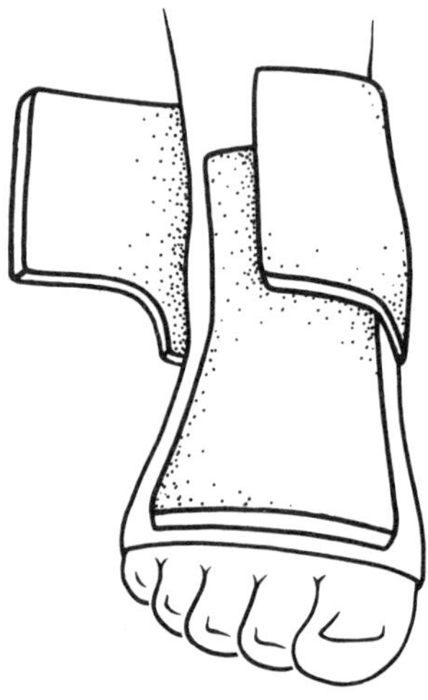

Figure 17.8 Foam is used to cover the dorsum of the foot and around the ankle.

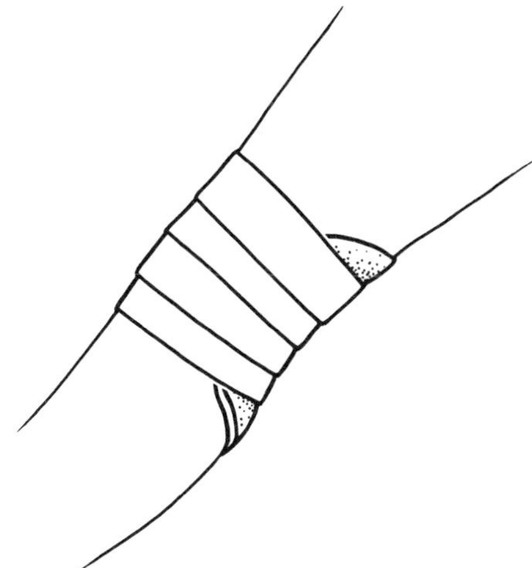

Figure 17.9 A foam pad is bandaged into position behind the knee.

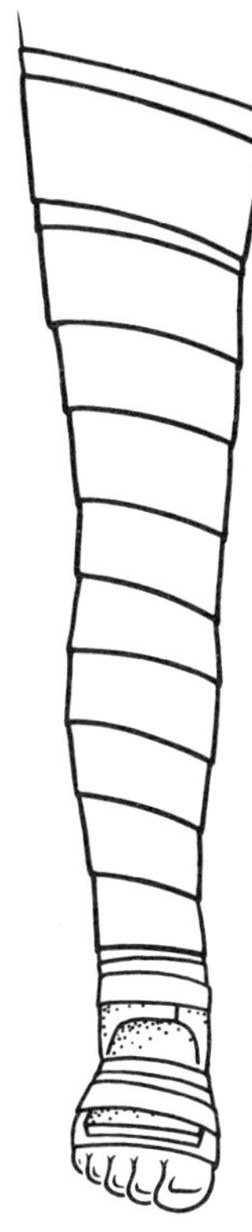

Figure 17.10 Rolls of padding are applied firmly in a spiral up the leg, starting at the ankle.

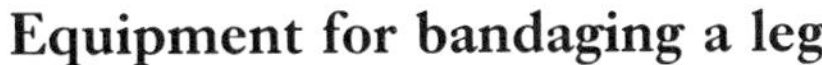

Equipment for bandaging a leg

1. Stockinette.
2. Light retention bandages, 10 cm or 12 cm.
3. Padding, 10 cm and 20 cm.
4. Foam.
5. Strong compression bandages, 8 cm, 10 cm and 12 cm.
6. Tape.
7. Scissors.

Procedure

Action	Rationale
1. Explain the procedure to the patient.	To gain the patient's co-operation and consent.
2. If possible, the patient should be seated upright on a bed or treatment couch. Raise the bed or couch to a comfortable height.	To ensure the comfort of both the patient and nurse.
3. Cut a length of stockinette long enough to fit the patient's leg. Slip over the leg.	To protect the skin from chafing.
4. Cut the foam into pads to fit over the dorsum of the foot, around the ankle (Figure 17.8) and behind the knee (Figure 17.9).	To protect bony prominences and joint flexures.
5. Secure the pads firmly in place with light retention bandages.	
6. Using a 10 cm roll of padding, apply firmly in a spiral up the leg, starting at the ankle. Use the 20 cm padding over the thigh (Figure 17.10).	To protect the skin and create a smooth profile on which to bandage.

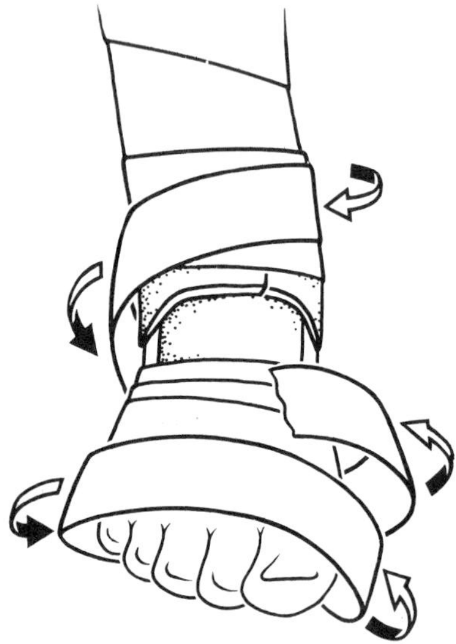

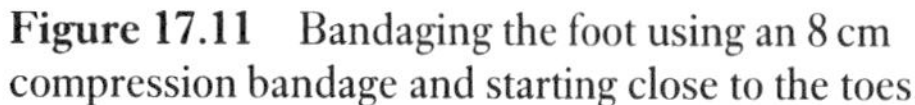

Figure 17.11 Bandaging the foot using an 8 cm compression bandage and starting close to the toes.

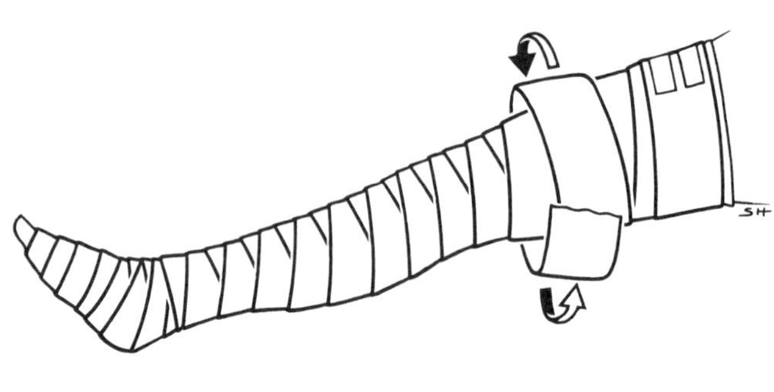

Figure 17.12 Applying a second layer of bandage, from ankle to thigh.

Action	**Rationale**
7. Take an 8 cm compression bandage and start by anchoring it loosely at the ankle. Bandage the foot, starting as close as possible to the toes (Figure 17.11). Use a spiral over the instep, covering half of the bandage with each turn, and use a figure of eight over the heel and ankle.	To avoid constriction at the ankle.
Bandage firmly and do not leave any gaps.	Fluid will accumulate in any unbandaged areas.
8. Using a 10 cm bandage, continue from where the first bandage finished, using a spiral up the leg and covering half of the bandage with each turn. Remember to bandage firmly. Use the widest bandage over the thigh. Secure the end of the last bandage with tape.	
9. Apply a second layer of bandage, from ankle to thigh, using a figure of eight. Secure the end with tape (Figure 17.12).	
10. Check the colour and temperature of the patient's toes. It may be difficult for the patient to flex the knee at first but this should get easier as the bandages loosen slightly.	To check that the blood flow is not compromised.
11. Remind the patient to use the limb as normally as possible and to report any feelings of discomfort, tingling or numbness.	To ensure good lymph flow.

GUIDELINES: THE APPLICATION OF ELASTIC HOSIERY AND ELASTICATED SURGICAL TUBULAR STOCKINETTE

The application of hosiery is made easier by applying any necessary moisturizing creams at night-time, rather than in the morning just before putting on a sleeve or stocking. A very light layer of talcum powder applied to hot, sticky skin will also ease application. If this is the first time a patient has worn compression hosiery, explain that the feeling of pressure may seem strange for the first few hours but that it should not cause pain.

Procedure for applying hosiery to the leg

Action	Rationale
1. Explain the procedure to the patient.	To obtain the patient's co-operation and consent.
2. If possible, position the patient seated upright on a bed or couch and raise the height to a comfortable level.	To ensure the comfort of both the patient and nurse.
3. Turn the stocking inside-out to the heel.	
4. Pull the foot of the stocking over the patient's foot.	
5. Turn the top of the stocking back over the foot and up the leg.	
6. Ask the patient to keep the leg straight and if possible to push against the nurse.	This makes it easier to ease the stocking up.
7. Starting at the foot, gradually ease the stocking over the heel and up the leg a bit at a time.	
Do not pull from the top. Remember that since it is the material of the stocking that provides the pressure, it must be distributed evenly to ensure an even distribution of pressure.	This will cause the stocking top to become overstretched and will lead to an uneven distribution of the stocking material.
8. Once the stocking is in place, check that there are no creases or wrinkles, particularly around the joints.	Wrinkles cause chafing of the skin and constricting bands of pressure.
9. Check that the patient finds the stocking comfortable and ask that any feelings of pain, tingling or numbness be reported.	
10. To remove the stocking, simply peel off the limb from the top downwards. Do not roll it down.	Rolling the stocking can result in tight bands of material forming, which are difficult to move.

Procedure for applying hosiery to the arm

Action	Rationale
1. Explain the procedure to the patient.	To ensure the patient's co-operation and consent.
2. The patient may be seated or standing.	

Guidelines: the application of elastic hosiery and elasticated surgical tubular stockinette

Action	Rationale
3. Turn the sleeve inside-out to the wrist. Pull over the patient's hand. *Note*: If the handpiece is separate from the sleeve, always put the handpiece on before the sleeve.	To avoid increasing swelling in the hand.
4. Turn the top of the sleeve back over the hand and up the arm.	
5. Ask the patient to grip something stable, such as a towel rail or the back of a chair.	This steadies the arm and gives the patient something to pull against.
6. Working from the hand or wrist, gradually ease the sleeve up the arm. Do not pull up from the top. Remember that since it is the material that provides the pressure, it must be evenly distributed to ensure an even distribution of pressure.	This will cause the top to become overstretched and will result in an uneven distribution of pressure.
7. Once the sleeve is in place, check that there are no creases or wrinkles, particularly around the joints.	Wrinkles and creases cause chafing of the skin and constricting bands of pressure.
8. Check that the patient finds the sleeve comfortable and ask that any signs of pain, tingling or numbness be reported.	
9. To remove the sleeve simply peel off the limb from the top. Do not roll it down.	Rolling the sleeve down can lead to tight bands of material forming which are difficult to move.

18

Eye Care

Indications

Eye care may be necessary under the following circumstances:

1. To relieve pain and discomfort.
2. To prevent infection.
3. To prevent any further injury to the eye.

REFERENCE MATERIAL

Patients should be encouraged after instruction to carry out for themselves many of the procedures involved in eye care. However, the nurse is often involved in caring for the postoperative, very ill or unconscious patient. Infection can easily be transmitted, by careless technique, from one eye to another. In some cases this can lead to loss of sight (Burton, 1989).

Anatomy and physiology

The eyeball is protected from injury by the bony cavity of the orbit, the conjunctiva, the lacrimal apparatus, the eyebrows and the eyelashes.

The eyeball itself has three layers (Figure 18.1):

1. The outermost, composed of the cornea and sclera.
2. The middle, composed of the choroid, ciliary body and iris (uveal tract).
3. The innermost, composed of the retina, macula lutea (yellow spot) and fovea centralis.

The function of the outer coat is protective. The middle layer is vascular and pigmented, while the innermost layer contains the light-sensitive nerve endings concerned with vision, i.e. the rods and cones.

The blood vessels of the retina are seen readily with an ophthalmoscope. Abnormal changes in these vessels can be indicative of both generalized diseases, such as diabetes and hypertension, and diseases of the eye itself (Tortora and Anagnostakos, 1987).

The optic nerve (cranial II) has two tracts which cross over at the optic chiasma. Each tract supplies the opposite side of the body. These tracts enter the eyeball to the side of the macula lutea. This area is known as the optic disc and is an area of no vision (blind spot) (Figure 18.2).

An additional blind spot or scotoma may be indicative of a brain tumour. In 90% of pituitary tumours there is a defect in the field of vision (Tortora and Anagnostakos, 1987).

The inside of the eyeball is divided by the lens into an anterior and posterior chamber. The anterior chamber is filled with a clear, watery fluid called the aqueous humour and the posterior chamber by a jelly-like substance called the vitreous humour which gives the eyeball its shape (Figure 18.3).

The aqueous humour is secreted into the posterior chamber by choroid plexuses of the ciliary processes of the ciliary bodies behind the iris. This fluid then permeates the posterior chamber and passes through between the iris and the lens, through the pupil, into the anterior chamber. From the anterior chamber the aqueous humour, which is produced continually, is drained off into the scleral venous sinus (canal of Schlemm) and then into the blood. The intraocular

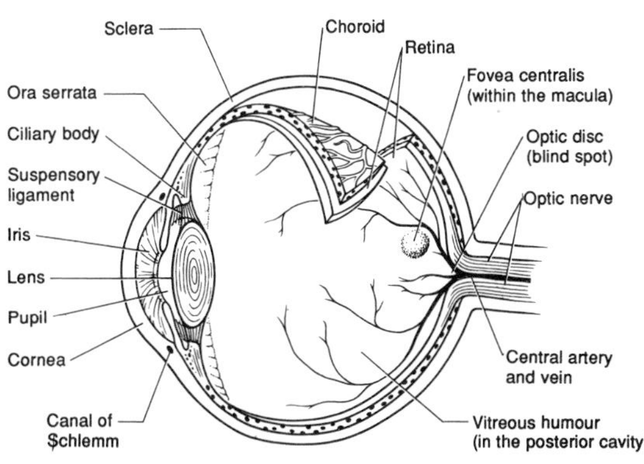

Figure 18.1 Internal structure of the eye (sagittal section). (From Marieb (1989), with kind permission.)

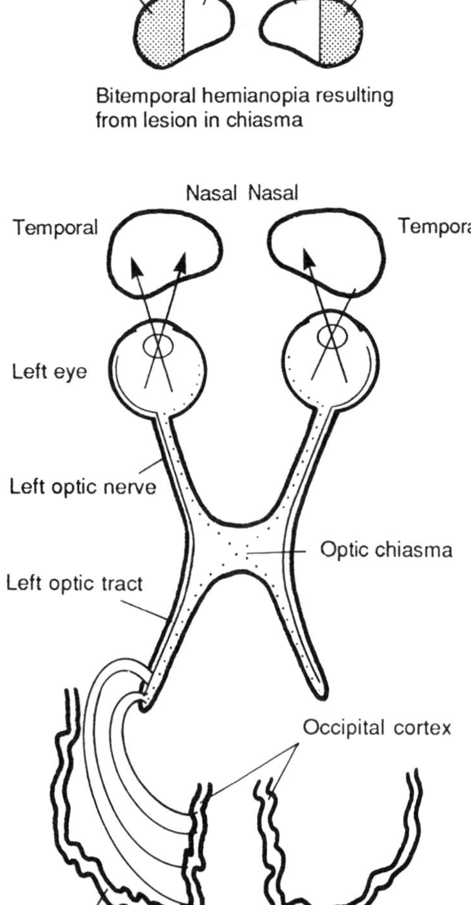

Figure 18.2 Visual pathways and visual fields.

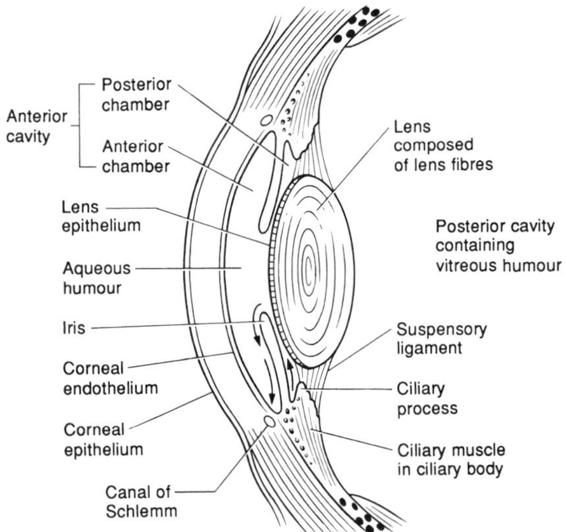

Figure 18.3 Structures seen in a transverse section through the anterior portion of the eye. The anterior cavity in front of the lens is incompletely divided into the anterior chamber (anterior to the iris) and the posterior chamber (behind the iris), which are continuous through the pupil. Aqueous humour, which fills the cavity, is formed by the ciliary processes and reabsorbed into the venous blood by the canal of Schlemm. The arrows indicate the circulation pathway. (From Marieb (1989), with kind permission.)

pressure is produced mainly by the aqueous humour, which together with the vitreous humour helps to counteract the pull of the extrinsic eye muscles and maintain the shape of the eyeball. Glaucoma is a disease which can cause degeneration of the retina and blindness due to the excessive intraocular pressure. The aqueous humour also acts as the principal link between the cardiovascular system, the lens and the cornea (Marieb, 1989).

The tears are produced in the lacrimal gland (Figure 18.4). Their function is to wash over the eyeball, removing any foreign substances and providing antisepsis by the action of the enzyme lysozyme. Lysozymes can rupture the cell walls of some bacteria and cause their lysis or death (e.g. Gram-negative bacteria). The tears drain through the lacrimal puncti into the nasolacrimal duct. In health, the surface of the eye should always be slightly moist. The cornea has no blood vessels and is dependant on tears and aqueous humour for its nourishment (Marieb, 1989).

General principles of eye care

Aseptic technique is necessary only in certain circumstances, for example, when the eye is damaged or following ophthalmic surgery. The positions of the patient and the nurse in relation to the light source are vital in order for the procedure to be carried out safely and efficiently.

Position of the patient

Where possible, the patient should be lying down with the head tilted backwards and the chin pointing upwards. This enables ease of access to the eyes and is a good position for patient comfort and ease of compliance.

Position of the light source

A good light source before commencing eye procedures is necessary in order to be able to assess carefully the state of the eyes and to avoid damaging their delicate structures during the procedure. The

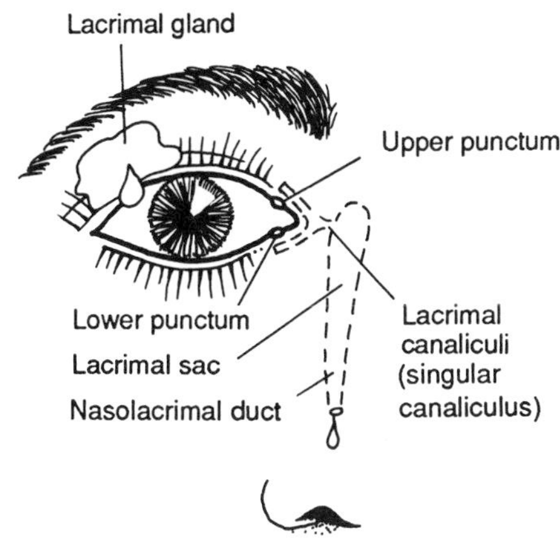

Figure 18.4 Lacrimal apparatus.

light should be above and behind the nurse or to the side. Light should never be allowed to shine directly into the patient's eyes as this will be painful to the patient.

Instillation of drops

Most types of drops are instilled into the outer rim of the lower fornix as the conjunctiva is less sensitive than the cornea, and the outer rim avoids loss of the drops into the nasolacrimal passage. Exceptions to this are as follows:

1. *Drugs used to lubricate the cornea*: these should be directed into the lower fornix. Oil-based drops produce less corneal reaction than aqueous ones as they do not feel as cold to the cornea when administered.
2. *Anaesthetic drops*: the first drop should be instilled into the conjunctiva and then directly onto the cornea one drop at a time until the patient is no longer able to feel the drops.
3. *Drops used to treat the nasal passages*: these should be instilled at the punctal end of the eye.

The number of drops used depends on the type of solution used and its purpose. Usually, one drop only is ordered and will be sufficient if it is instilled in the correct manner. The exceptions to the 'one drop' rule are:

1. Oil-based solutions: these are used for lubricating the eyeball, one drop being instilled and repeated as required.
2. Anaesthetic drops: it is usual to instil two or three drops at a time at intervals, until the drop cannot be felt on the eye.

The dropper should be held as close to the eye as possible without touching either the lids or the cornea, i.e. at approximately 2.5 cm. This will avoid corneal damage and the risk of infection. If the drop falls from too great a height it is difficult to control and will also be uncomfortable for the patient.

There are a variety of droppers and bottles available, including pipettes, pipettes incorporated into the eyedrop bottle, plastic bottles and single-dose packs. Pipettes are easy to use but need drying and sterilizing between doses. Plastic bottles can be squeezed and so avoid the need for a pipette and are cheaper than glass bottles with a dropper. Ideally, single-dose containers should be used if they do not prove to be too expensive for routine use.

Eye irrigation

The most common use of eye irrigation is for the removal of caustic substances from the eye, e.g. domestic cleaning agents or (in the hospital setting) medications, particularly cytotoxic material. This should be done as soon as possible to minimize damage. The procedure is also used as a pre-operative preparation or to remove infected material. The lotion most commonly used is normal saline. In an emergency tap water may be used.

Care of the insensitive eye

Any interference with the sensory nerve supply to the eye, such as unconsciousness, will cause the eye reflex to become insensitive. The blink reflex is often lost, the eye's surface becomes dry and the cornea may be damaged. Corneal ulcers, infection, scarring and loss of vision may be the end result. When the patient has lost these protective reflexes measures, the nurse must institute measures to replace them. The surface of the eye should be kept clean and moist by gentle swabbing of the eye with sterile saline and the instillation of artificial tears where necessary.

If there is no blink reflex the eyelids should be kept closed by the use of non-allergenic tape or by the

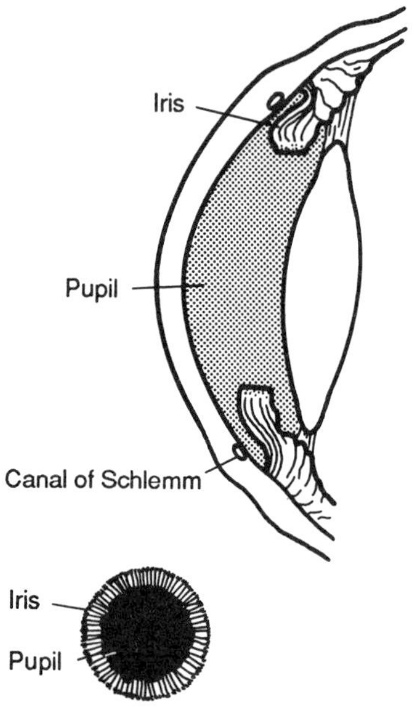

Figure 18.5 Effect of mydriatics.

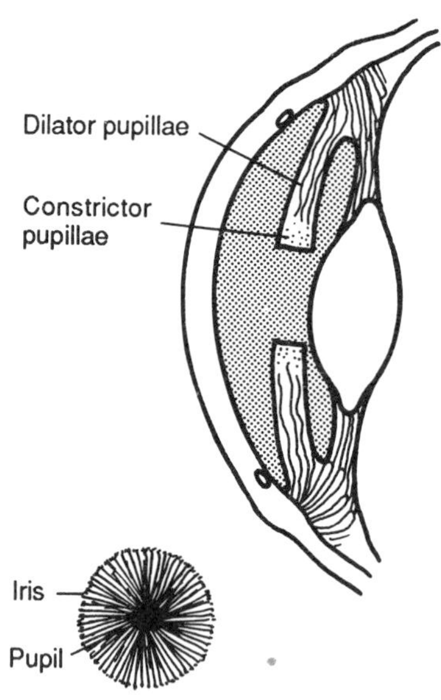

Figure 18.6 Effect of miotics.

application of new water–gel preparations. If the eyes become infected the relevant medication should be applied.

With each of these measures care must be taken not to spread infection between the eyes. Any alteration to the appearance of the eye must be reported to the doctor.

Eye medications

Drugs may be given either systemically or topically to exert an effect on the eye. However, if given systemically the prescribing doctor needs to take account of the physiological barrier and the blood–aqueous barrier which exists within the eye and which is selective in allowing drugs to pass into the intraocular fluids. Permeability of this barrier may be altered in inflammatory conditions and following paracentesis.

Drugs applied locally meet some resistance at the tear film. The cornea allows the passage of water but not of drugs. This resistance may alter where there are corneal epithelial changes. Wetting agents may be employed to alter corneal permeability.

Many drugs will produce similar effects on a diseased or a healthy eye. Drugs for use in the eye are usually classified according to their action:

Mydriatics and cycloplegics

These drugs produce their effects by paralysing the ciliary muscle, by stimulating the dilator muscle of the pupil or by a combination of both (Figure 18.5). They are used mainly for diagnostic purposes and most have an anticholinergic action (Burton, 1989). The most commonly used preparations are cyclopentolate 1% and tropicamide 1%.

Miotics

These drugs produce their effects by constriciting the pupil and contracting the ciliary muscle (Figure 18.6). Miotics help in the drainage of aqueous humour and are used primarily in the treatment of glaucoma.

Local anaesthetics

These render the eye and the inner surfaces of the lids insensitive. They are used before minor surgery, removal of foreign bodies and tonometry. Cocaine is less used now as some patients develop an idiosyncrasy to it and may suddenly collapse after its use. Its effects do not wear off for at least half an hour after administration.

Anti-inflammatories

These may be steroids, antihistamines or pyrazole

derivatives, such as oxyphenabutazone 10%. The most commonly used preparations are dexamethasone, prednisolone and betamethasone.

Corticosteroid eye drops should be used with caution as they can cause a serious rise in intraocular pressure in a small percentage of people (especially if they have a history of glaucoma) (Burton, 1989).

Antibiotics

Antibiotics can be used in the active treatment of infection and as prophylactics both pre- and post-operatively, following removal of a foreign body or following an injury. Antibiotic preparations in common use are framycetin 0.5%, neomycin 0.5% and chloramphenicol 0.5%.

Artificial tears

Where tear deficiency exists due to disease processes, treatment with radiation or reduction of the blink reflex, artificial lubricants such as methyl cellulose or hypromellose may be used.

Toxic effects of common systemic drugs on the eye

As the eye may be the first place to show signs of systemic disease, so some systemic drugs may now show their toxic effects in the eye. These effects range from pruritis, irritation, redness, excess tear formation with overflow (epiphora), photophobia and blapharo-conjunctivitis, to disturbance of vision. Particular effects of specific drugs are listed below:

1. *Methotrexate and related antimetabolites*: these drugs can affect the Meibomian glands, causing blepharoconjunctivitis, and produce photophobia, epiphora, periorbital oedema and conjunctival hyperaemia.
2. *5-Fluorouracil (5-FU)*: 5-FU can cause canalicular fibrosis and oculomotor disturbances (probably secondary to a local neurotoxicity affecting the brainstem).
3. *Antihistamines*: these drugs decrease tear production and may lead to 'dry eye', especially in patients with Sjogren's syndrome or ocular pemphigus, in patients who wear contact lenses and in the elderly.
4. *Tamoxifen*: this drug can cause subepithelial, whirl-like, corneal deposits and retinal lesions.
5. *Indomethacin*: this can cause corneal deposits and retinal pigmentary toxicity.
6. *Oral contraceptives*: these can stimulate corneal steeping and intolerance to contact lenses.
7. *Atropine, scopalamine and belladonna-like substances*: such drugs cause mydriasis and cycloplegia.
8. *Corticosteroids*: prolonged use of corticosteroids produces posterior subcapsular cataracts.
9. *Chloramphenicol*: chloramphenicol treatment can lead to optic neuritis.
10. *Ethambutol*: this drug can cause damage to the optic nerve.
11. *Rifampicin*: stains soft contact lenses.
12. *Digoxin*: in overdose results in blurred vision and yellow/green vision.
13. *Oxygen*: in neonates, high concentrations for a long period can cause retrolental fibroplasia (Burton, 1989).

References and further reading

Bryant, W. M. (1981) Common toxic effects of systemic drugs on the eye. *Occupational Health Nursing*, 29, 15–17.

Chilman, A. M. & Thomas, M. (1987) *Understanding Nursing Care*, 3rd edn. Churchill Livingstone, Edinburgh.

Darling, V. H. & Thorpe, M. R. (1981) *Ophthalmic Nursing*, 2nd edn. Baillière Tindall, London.

Garland, P. (1975) *Ophthalmic Nursing*, 6th edn. Faber & Faber, London.

Marieb, E. N. (1989) *Human Anatomy and Physiology*. Benjamin Cummings, California.

Percy, E. & Smith W. A. M. (1973) *Ophthalmology (Ophthalmic Techniques)*. William Heinemann Medical Books, London.

Phillips, M. (1982) Ophthalmic preparations. *Nursing Mirror*, 155, 69–71.

Rooke, F. C. E. *et al.* (1980) *Ophthalmic Nursing – Its Practice and Management*. Churchill Livingstone, Edinburgh.

Smith, J. & Nachazel, D. P. (1980) *Ophthalmologic Nursing*, Little, Brown, Boston.

Tortora, G. J. & Anagnostakos, N. P. (1987) *Principles of Anatomy & Physiology*, 5th edn. Harper & Row, London, pp. 373–85.

Wilson, P. (1976) *Modern Ophthalmic Nursing*. Edward Arnold, London.

GUIDELINES: EYE SWABBING

Equipment

1. Sterile dressing pack.
2. Sterile water.

Procedure

Guidelines: Eye swabbing

Action	**Rationale**
1. Explain the procedure to the patient.	To obtain the patient's consent and co-operation.
2. Assist the patient into the correct position: (a) Head well supported and tilted back. (b) Preferably the patient should be in bed or lying on a couch.	The patient needs to be discouraged from flinching or making unexpected movements and so should be in the most comfortable position possible at the start of the procedure.
3. Ensure an adequate light source, taking care not to dazzle the patient.	To enable maximum observation of the eyes without causing the patient harm or discomfort.
4. Wash hands thoroughly using bactericidal soap and water or bactericidal alcohol hand rub, then dry hands.	Use a non-touch technique where the patient has a damaged eye or has just had an operation on the eye. Infection can lead to loss of an eye.
5. Always treat the uninfected or uninflamed eye first.	To avoid cross-infection.
6. Always bathe lids with the eyes closed first.	To avoid damage to the cornea.
7. Using a slightly moistened lint square or wool swab, ask the patient to look up and swab the lower lid from the nasal corner outwards.	If the swab is too wet the solution will run down the patient's cheek. This increases the risk of cross-infection and causes the patient discomfort. Swabbing from the nasal corner outwards avoids the risk of swabbing discharge into the lacrymal punctum, or even across the bridge of the nose into other eye.
8. Ensure that the edge of the swab is not above the lid margin.	To avoid touching the sensitive cornea.
9. Using a new swab each time, repeat the procedure until all the discharge has been removed.	To avoid infection.
10. Swab the upper lid by slightly everting the lid margin and asking the patient to look down. Swab from the nasal corner outwards and use a new swab each time until all discharge has been removed.	To effectively remove any foreign material from eye. To reduce the risk of infection.
11. Once both eyelids have been cleansed and dried, make the patient comfortable.	
12. Remove and dispose of equipment.	
13. Wash hands.	To reduce the risk of cross-infection.

14. Record the procedure in the appropriate documents.	To monitor trends and fluctuations.

Note: For information about obtaining an eye swab for pathological investigations, see the appropriate section in Chapter 36, Specimen Collection.

GUIDELINES: INSTILLATION OF EYE DROPS

Equipment

1. Sterile dressing pack.
2. Sterile water.
3. Appropriate eye drops. (Any preparation must be checked against the doctor's prescription.)
4. Cotton wool.

Procedure

Action	**Rationale**
1. Explain the procedure to the patient.	To obtain the patient's consent and co-operation.
2. If there is any discharge, proceed as for eye swabbing.	To remove any infected material and thus ensure adequate absorption of the drops.
3. Check the following:	
(a) Prescription against bottle label.	To ensure that appropriate drops are instilled.
(b) For which eye the drops are prescribed.	To avoid cross-infection and instillation of the drug into the wrong eye.
(c) Expiry date on bottle.	To ensure that medication has not expired.
4. Assist the patient into the correct position, i.e. head well supported and tilted back.	To ensure that drops are instilled beneath the lower lid into the fornix and to avoid excess solution running down the patient's cheek.
5. Wash hands thoroughly using bactericidal soap and water or bactericidal alcohol hand rub, and dry them.	Asepsis is essential, particularly when the patient has a damaged eye or has just had an operation on the eye. Infection can lead to loss of an eye.
6. Place a wet cotton wool swab on the lower lid against the lid margin.	To absorb any excess solution which may be irritating to the surrounding skin.
7. Ask the patient to look up immediately before instilling the drop.	This opens the eye and allows the drop to be instilled into the outer side of the lower fornix. If done too soon the patient may blink as the drop is instilled.
8. Ask the patient to close the eye. Keep the wet wool swab on the lower lid.	To ensure absorption of the fluid and to avoid excess running down the cheek.
9. Make the patient comfortable.	
10. Remove and dispose of equipment.	
11. Wash hands with soap and water.	To avoid cross-infection.
12. Record the procedure in the appropriate documents.	To monitor trends and fluctuations.

GUIDELINES: INSTILLATION OF EYE OINTMENT

Equipment

1. Sterile dressing pack.
2. Sterile water.
3. Appropriate eye ointment. (Any preparation must be checked against the doctor's prescription.)

Procedure

Guidelines: Instillation of eye ointment

Action	Rationale
1. Explain the procedure to the patient.	To obtain the patient's consent and co-operation.
2. If there is any discharge, and to remove any previous application of ointment, proceed as for eye swabbing.	To remove any infected material and previous ointment to allow for absorption of ointment.
3. Check the following:	
(a) Prescription against tube of ointment.	To ensure that appropriate ointment applied.
(b) For which eye the ointment is prescribed.	To avoid cross-infection and administration of an inappropriate treatment.
(c) Expiry date on tube.	To ensure that medication has not expired.
4. Wash hands thoroughly using bactericidal soap and water or bactericidal alcohol hand rub.	To avoid infection.
5. Place a wet wool swab on the lower lid against the lid margin.	To absorb excess ointment which may be irritating to the surrounding skin.
6. Slightly evert the lower lid by pulling on the wool swab. Ask the patient to look up immediately before applying the cream.	To allow the application to be made inside the lower lid into the lower fornix.
7. Apply the ointment by gently squeezing the tube and, with the nozzle 2.5 cm above the lower lid, drawing a line along the inner edge of the lower lid from the nasal corner outward.	To avoid possible contamination and trauma.
8. Ask the patient to close the eye and remove excess ointment with a new wet wool swab.	To avoid excess ointment irritating the surrounding skin.
9. Warn the patient that, when the eye is opened, vision will be a little blurred for a few minutes.	
10. Make the patient comfortable.	
11. Remove and dispose of equipment.	
12. Wash hands with soap and water.	To avoid infection.
13. Record the procedure in the appropriate documents.	To monitor trends and fluctuations.

GUIDELINES: EYE IRRIGATION

Equipment

1. Sterile dressing pack.
2. Irrigation fluid (usually sterile normal saline but, in an emergency, tap water may be used).
3. Receiver.
4. Towel.
5. Plastic cape.
6. Irrigating flask.
7. Hot water in a bowl to warm irrigating fluid to tepid temperature.
8. Anaesthetic drops.

Procedure

Action	Rationale
1. Explain the procedure to the patient.	To gain the patient's consent and co-operation.
2. Instil anaesthetic drops if required.	To avoid any discomfort.
3. Prepare the irrigation fluid to the appropriate temperature.	Tepid fluid will be more comfortable for the patient. The solution should be poured across the inner aspect of the nurse's wrist to test the temperature.
4. Assist the patient into the appropriate position: (a) Head comfortably supported with chin almost horizontal. (b) Head inclined to the side of the eye to be treated.	To avoid the solution running either over the cheek into the eye or out of the eye and down the side of the nose.
5. Wash hands using bactericidal soap and water or bactericidal alcohol hand rub, and dry.	To avoid infection.
6. Remove any discharge from the eye by swabbing.	To prevent washing the discharge down the lacrimal duct or across the cheek.
7. Ask the patient to hold the receiver against the cheek below the eye being tested.	To collect irrigation fluid as it runs away from the eye.
8. Position the towel and plastic cape.	To protect the patient's clothing.
9. Hold the patient's eyelids apart, using your first and second fingers, against the orbital ridge.	The patient will be unable to hold the eye open once irrigation commences.
10. Do not press on the eyeball.	To avoid causing the patient discomfort or pain.
11. Warn the patient that the flow of solution is going to start and pour a little onto the cheek first.	
12. Direct the flow of the fluid from the nasal corner outwards.	To wash away from the lacrimal punctum.
13. Ask the patient to look up, down and to either side while irrigating.	To ensure that the whole area is washed.
14. Evert lids while irrigating.	To ensure complete removal of any foreign body.

Guidelines: Eye irrigation

Action	Rationale
15. Keep the flow of irrigation fluid constant.	To ensure swift removal of any foreign body.
16. When the eye has been thoroughly irrigated, ask the patient to close the eyes and use a new swab to dry the lids.	
17. Take the receiver from the patient and dry the cheek.	If the receiver is removed first, solution may run down the patient's neck.
18. Make the patient comfortable.	
19. Remove and dispose of equipment.	
20. Wash hands with soap and water.	To avoid infection.
21. Record the procedure in the appropriate documents.	To monitor trends and fluctuations.

19

Gastric Lavage

Definition

Gastric lavage is the irrigation or washing out of the stomach with repeated flushing of an appropriate fluid. It is used to obtain a specimen of gastric contents and to remove poisons or other harmful substances, that were swallowed deliberately or accidentally, thus preventing further absorption.

Indications

Gastric lavage may be used under the following circumstances:

1. If the patient is seen within four hours of ingesting poisons or harmful substances.
2. If the patient is unconscious and the time of ingestion is not known.
3. In all cases of salicylate poisoning within 12 hours of ingestion.
4. For gastrointestinal haemorrhage (Evans, 1981).
5. Before surgery in patients with pyloric obstruction.

REFERENCE MATERIAL

The reliability of gastric lavage is debatable, advice on its use is conflicting, and its value is questionable (Burstom, 1970; Goth & Vesell, 1984; Matthew, 1971; Stoddart, 1975). Blake *et al.* (1978) attempted to identify those factors that influenced the decision to perform gastric lavage in 236 cases of deliberate self-poisoning seen over a period of six months in one hospital. Of patients seen within four hours of ingesting the poison, 87% had a lavage performed irrespective of the number of tablets and the nature of the drug taken. Overall, 77% had a gastric lavage. Most of the late lavages were carried out for salicylate ingestion. The authors concluded that given the changing pattern of drugs used for attempted self-poisoning, at least 50% of patients were subjected to gastric lavage unnecessarily.

Gastric lavage is generally carried out by medical staff assisted by nurses. Registered general nurses in specialized units, mainly accident and emergency departments, may carry out the procedure without medical involvement after initial assessment.

Gastric lavage versus induced emesis

Research has not shown clearly which of these two methods is most effective at removing the gastric contents in cases of drug overdose. Commonly, ipecacuanha is used in children, while gastric lavage tends to be used in adults. However, one method cannot be applied to the exclusion of the other in all cases.

Ipecacuanha is a centrally acting drug, its site of action being the chemotrigger zone in the medulla oblongata. It also has an irritant effect on the lining of the stomach. It can take up to 20 minutes to produce an effect: if this fact is not appreciated, repeated doses may be given before the first dose has had time to work. This may result in protracted vomiting. However, if after 20 minutes no emesis has occurred, a further dose can be given. It is recommended by the manufacturing company that a glass of water is taken following a dose of ipecacuanha.

Ipecacuanha should not be given if: corrosive or petroleum distillate agents have been taken, or medications which could cause a rapid onset of symptoms (especially fitting), or agents that depress the central nervous system.

Induced emesis should be used only when the patient is alert and when the development of lethargy and coma are unlikely. Unless the patient is awake, the cough reflex may be depressed and this may result in the patient inhaling the vomitus. When a drug with strong antiemetic properties has been ingested, e.g. chlorpromazine, induced emesis will have little or no effect, and gastric lavage may become the method of choice.

Gastric lavage is contraindicated when a caustic or corrosive substance has been ingested because of the possibility of perforating the oesophagus when passing the tube. It is also contraindicated when strychnine has been ingested since stimulation while passing the tube into the stomach may precipitate convulsions.

Careful assessment needs to be made of comatose and especially drowsy patients. A gastric lavage should not be performed if they do not have a strong enough cough reflex or if the airway cannot be protected by a cuffed endotracheal tube. In patients brought to a hospital's emergency department several hours (four hours is quoted in the literature) after the ingestion of drugs, gastric lavage is held to be of little value in that after such a period of time very little if any of the drug will remain in the stomach. Any drug that does remain may then be washed into the small intestines by the procedure. Gastric lavage within six hours is quoted by Evans (1981) as valuable in methanol poisoning. Drugs such as aspirin and glutethimide remain in the small intestines for long periods and act as a reservoir for continued absorption. Gastric lavage is useful at any time within 12 hours of ingestion in these cases.

Gastric lavage tubes

Cosgriff (1978) gives a brief, illustrated summary of some of the tubes used for gastric lavage in the United States of America. The tube of choice in the United Kingdom appears to be the 30 gauge Jacques stomach tube (Evans, 1981; Matthew, 1971). This wide-bore tube enables tablets, food with adherent tablet particles and virtually all the contents of the stomach to be evacuated through it.

Further information

For more specific information on the ingestion of poisons, and whenever there is any doubt about the management of such patients, the Poisons Information Centres should be contacted:

Poisons Information Services:

1. Belfast (0232 240503).
2. Birmingham (021-554 3801).
3. Cardiff (0222 709901).
4. Dublin (0001 379964 *or* 0001 379966).
5. Edinburgh (031-229 2477; 031-228 2441 – Viewdata, a service whereby information on drugs can be assessed via a computer. It is free to NHS hospitals, which have to provide their own computer systems).
6. Leeds (0532 430715 *or* 0532 432799).
7. London (071-635 9191 *or* 071-955 5095).
8. Newcastle (091-232 5131).

References and further reading

Arena, J. (1974) *Poisoning: Toxicology, Symptoms, Treatment*, 3rd edn. Charles C. Thomas, Springfield, Ill.

Beckett, A. & Rowland, M. (1965) Urinary excretion kinetics of amphetamine in man. *Journal of Pharmacy and Pharmacology*, 17, 628.

Bell, D. S. (1969) Dangers of treatment of status espilepticus with diazepam. *British Medical Journal*, 1, 159.

Blake, D. R. *et al.* (1978) Is there excessive use of gastric lavage in the treatment of self-poisoning? *Lancet*, 2, 1362–4.

Budassi, S. A. & Barber, J. M. (1985) *Emergency Nursing: Principles and Practice*. C. V. Mosby, St Louis.

Burstom, G. R. (1970) *Self-poisoning*. Lloyd-Luke, London.

Chazan, J. & Cohen, J. (1969) Clinical spectrum of glutethimide intoxication. *Journal of the American Medical Association*, 208, 837.

Cosgriff, J. H. (1978) *An Atlas of Diagnostic and Therapeutic Procedures for Emergency Personnel*. J. B. Lippincott, Phildelphia.

Cosgriff, J. H. *et al.* (1984) *The Practice of Emergency Nursing*, 2nd edn. J. B. Lippincott, Philadelphia.

Danel, V. *et al.* (1988) Activated charcoal, emesis and gastric lavage in aspirin overdose (study). *British Medical Journal*, 296, 1507.

Eaves, D. (1988) Making sense of gastric lavage. *Nursing Times and Nursing Mirror*, 84(20), 52–3.

Evans, R. (1981) *Emergency Medicine*. Butterworth, London.

Goth, A. & Vesell (1984) *Medical Pharmacology: Principles and Concepts*, 11th edn. C. V. Mosby, St Louis.

Matthew, H. (1971) Acute poisoning: some myths and misconceptions. *British Medical Journal*, 1, 521.

Stoddart, J. C. (1975) *Intensive Therapy*. Blackwell Scientific Publications, Oxford.

GUIDELINES: GASTRIC LAVAGE

Equipment

1. Clean gastric tube with connector.
2. Connecting tubing.
3. Lubricating jelly.
4. Tape.
5. Syringe (50 ml).
6. Receiver.
7. Litmus paper.
8. Mouth gag.
9. Funnel.

10. Jug.
11. Tepid water or prescribed irrigation fluid.
12. Plastic sheet.
13. Disposable paper sheets.
14. Disposable plastic aprons.
15. Disposable plastic gloves.
16. Bucket.
17. Suction equipment.
18. Emergency resuscitation equipment.

Procedure

Action	Rationale
1. Explain the procedure to the patient whenever possible.	To obtain the patient's consent and co-operation. (The efficacy of explanations is questionable, however, on the basis that an adult who has ingested a toxic substance deliberately is unlikely to want to co-operate with agents whose aim is to prevent suicidal gestures. Tact must be employed in these circumstances.)
2. Unconscious patients must be intubated.	To maintain a clear airway.
3. Place the patient on a firm surface, lying in the left lateral position, with the head down (Figure 19.1). (A standard emergency department trolley should be available ideally.)	To maintain a clear airway.
4. Remove any prostheses from the buccal cavity. Remove débris and/or vomitus from the buccal cavity with suction.	To maintain a clear airway.
5. Have emergency resuscitation equipment available.	Strong vagal stimulation can induce cardiac dysrhythmias and cardiopulmonary arrest.
6. Place a disposable sheet under the patient's head and a plastic sheet over the floor.	To protect nurse and patient should vomiting occur.

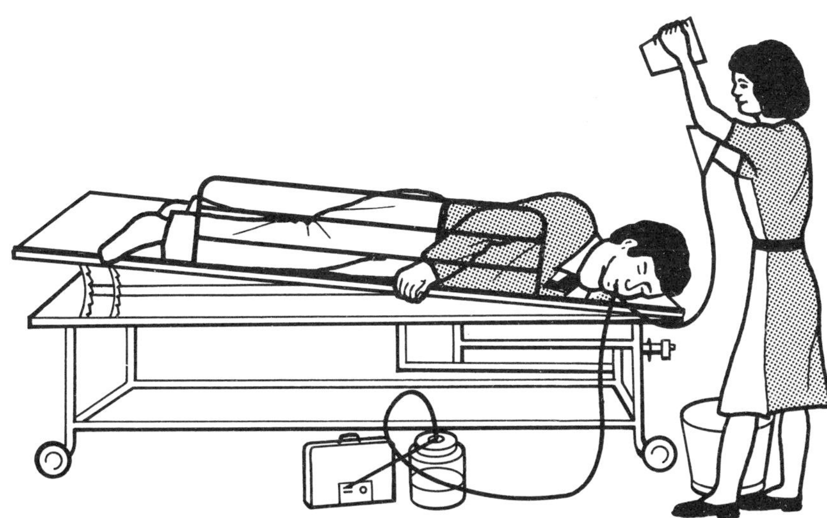

Figure 19.1 Gastric lavage.

Guidelines: Gastric lavage

Action	**Rationale**
7. Lubricate the tube with lubricating jelly.	To facilitate passage of the tube.
8. If the patient is able to co-operate ask him/her to sit up and swallow sips of water.	Swallowing will cause the epiglottis to close and prevent accidental passage of the tube into trachea.
9. Secure the tube with tape once inserted.	To prevent dislodgement of the tube.
10. Either aspirate the tube before lavage begins and test the aspirate with litmus paper, or listen with a stethoscope over the stomach as air is introduced into the tube via a syringe.	To ensure that the tube is in the stomach.
11. Retain a specimen of aspirate in a labelled specimen bottle.	For analysis.
12. Instil, via a funnel, water or the prescribed irrigation fluid, in volumes of 100 to 500 ml.	Approximately 500 ml of fluid are necessary to flatten out the rugae of the stomach so that the fluid may reach all parts of the mucous membrane.
13. Any fluid instilled must be tepid.	To prevent a sudden lowering of body temperature and possible shock.
14. Hold the funnel below the level of the patient. Once the required amount of fluid has been poured into the funnel, raise it gradually until the fluid empties into the stomach. Do not allow the contents of the funnel to empty.	To control the rate at which the fluid is instilled. A siphoning action is needed to return the contents of the stomach.
15. Lower the funnel and observe all the contents as they return from the stomach. Empty the contents into a bucket. If blood returns, stop the procedure and inform the medical staff. Otherwise lavage until the returning fluid is clear.	
16. Once lavage is completed, pinch the tube off and remove the tube quickly. Have suction at hand.	Gagging and possible vomiting may occur when the tube is removed. As the tube reaches the pharynx, any fluid left may escape and infiltrate into the lungs.
17. Check buccal cavity for signs of trauma. Provide oral hygiene facilities as required.	To maintain a clean, moist mouth. To prevent the accumulation of oral secretions. To prevent the development of mouth infections.
18. Explain to patient that procedure is completed and ensure patient comfort.	

20

Intrapleural Drainage

Definition

Intrapleural drainage is an underwater-seal system of drainage that prevents the entry of air into the pleural space, thus avoiding pneumothorax.

Indications

1. To remove matter from the pleural space or thoracic cavity:
   (a) Solids, e.g. fibrin or clotted blood.
   (b) Liquids, e.g. serous fluids, blood, pus, chyle or gastric juice.
   (c) Gas, e.g. air from the lungs, trachea or oesophagus.
2. To allow the lung to re-expand following surgery (Oh, 1989).

REFERENCE MATERIAL

Anatomy and physiology

The pleura is a thin sheet of tissue covering the undersurface of the ribs, diaphragm and the structures of the mediastinum. It continues over the surface of both lungs, thus forming a space known as the pleural space. The layer in contact with the surface of the lungs is known as the visceral pleura; that in contact with the thoracic wall, the parietal pleura. These two membranes are continuous with each other but are separated by a thin serous fluid that allows the pleurae to slide smoothly over each other during respiration. In health the pleural space is a potential space only. This space has a negative pressure normally. The elastic tissues of the lungs and the chest wall continually pull in opposite directions, the lungs tending to recoil inwards and the chest wall outwards. As these opposing forces attempt to pull the visceral and parietal pleurae apart, they create a negative pressure in the pleural space. Pressures in the pleural space are approximately 8 mm water during inspiration and 2 mm water on expiration. A negative pressure of 54 mm water can be measured during forced inspiration; during expiration, e.g. coughing, a positive pressure of approximately 68 mm water develops (Marieb, 1989).

Any opening of the thoracic cavity results in a loss of negative pressure and the lungs collapse. Collections of fluids or materials can also cause the lung to collapse as these substances are incompressible and restrict expansion of the lungs and inhibit cardiopulmonary function.

When a tube is inserted to remove air it is normally inserted fairly high in the intrapleural space, usually through the second anterior intercostal space, as air will rise. If a tube is inserted to remove liquid or debris, it is usually inserted fairly low through the sixth or seventh intercostal space to achieve satisfactory drainage (Hinds, 1987). If more than one tube is inserted, e.g. following intrathoracic surgery, to remove air and fluid or debris the higher tube, known as the apical drain, is used to remove air, and the lower tube, known as the basal drain, is used to remove liquid and debris.

Types of chest drain

Any system must be capable of removing whatever collects in the pleural space more rapidly than it accumulates (Figure 20.1).

Single bottle water-seal system

In this system the end of the drainage tube from the patient's chest is covered by a layer of water that permits drainage and prevents lung collapse by stopping atmospheric air entering the pleural space. Drainage depends on gravity, the mechanics of respiration and, if necessary, suction by the addition of a controlled vacuum. The tube from the patient should extend approximately 2.5 cm below the level of the water in the container (Figure 20.2).

Two-bottle water-seal system

This system consists of the same water seal chamber with the addition of a manometer bottle. Effective

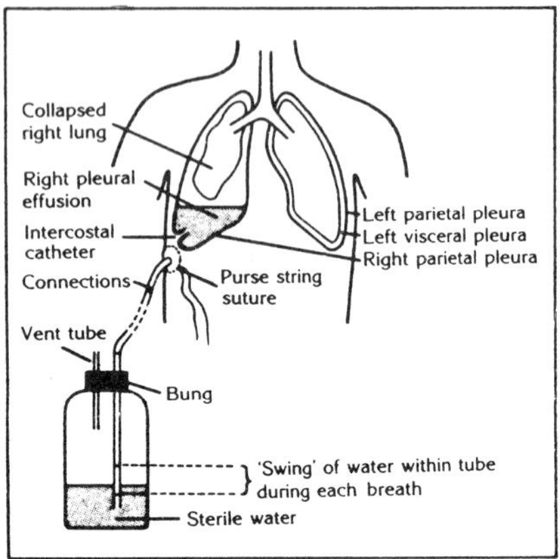

Figure 20.1 Drainage of a right pleural effusion using an intercostal catheter attached to an underwater seal. (From Munford (1986); reproduced with permission from *The Professional Nurse.*)

drainage depends on gravity and the amount of suction added as controlled by the manometer bottle.

Three-bottle water-seal system

The initial chamber in this system collects the drainage, so that the fluid in the water-seal chamber stays constant as drainage accumulates. This has an advantage over the single and two-bottle systems in that as the chest drainage collects in the water-seal chamber, the resistance to flow from the pleural space is increased therefore there is more resistance to elastic recoil of the lung. When the fluid in the water-seal chamber equals the amount of fluid in the manometer bottle, any effective suction is cancelled. In this system drainage depends on gravity and the amount of suction added, as controlled by the manometer. The suction system maintains a negative pressure throughout the closed drainage system. The manometer bottle regulates the amount of vacuum in the system (Figure 20.2).

The argyle 'double-seal' system

This system consists of four chambers and is portable. The second chamber is the collection chamber and is divided into three subchambers. The next chamber is the water-seal chamber. It is essentially U-shaped. The last chamber is the suction control chamber. Again this is U-shaped. The extra chamber in an Argyle unit is also a water-seal chamber. The patient's air passes through the third chamber into the suction source. If, however, the passage into the suction source is obstructed accidentally, the patient's air will pass instead through the first chamber into the atmosphere. The first chamber provides a safety vent for the patient's air (Figure 20.3).

Use of pump or suction apparatus

If there is no response to any of the above methods of drainage, external suction apparatus can be applied. Suction at approximately 15 to 20 cm water pressure can be used via a pump such as the Roberts' pump.

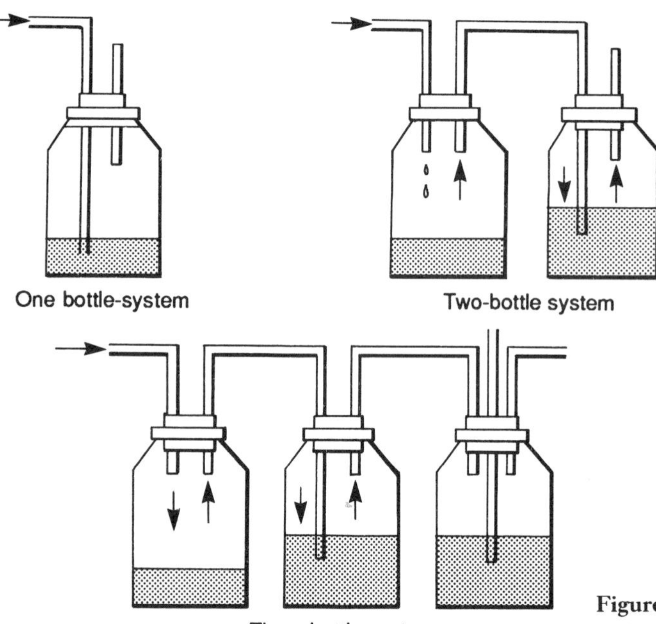

Figure 20.2 One-, two- and three-bottle chest drainage systems.

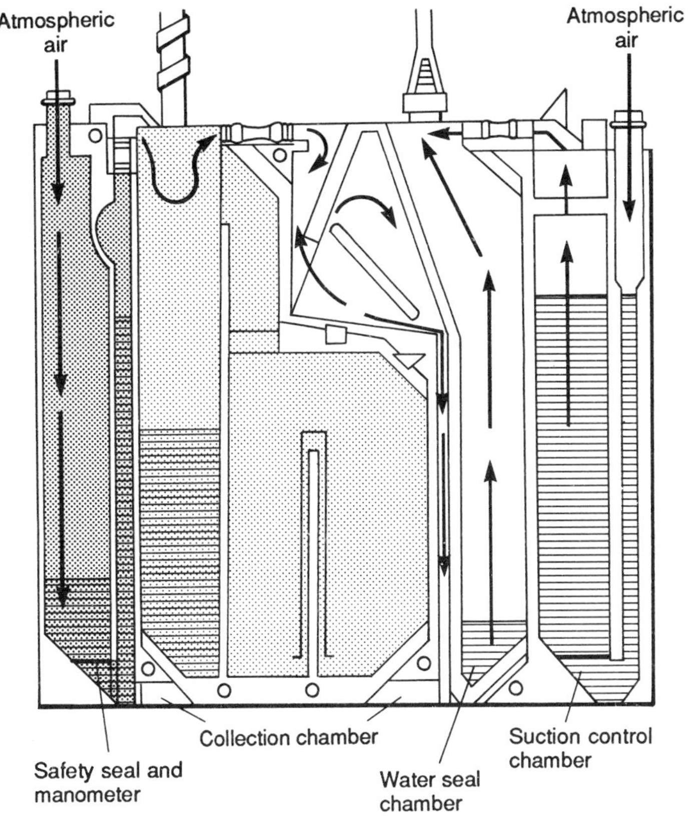

Figure 20.3 Argyle double-seal system.

The efficacy of added suction has still to be confirmed (Mumford, 1986).

References and further reading

Brunner, L. S. & Suddarth, D. S. (1986) *The Lippincott Manual of Nursing Practice*, 4th edn. J. B. Lipincott, Philadelphia.

Cohen, S. & Stack, M. (1980) Programmed instruction: how to work with chest tubes. *American Journal of Nursing*, 80, 685–712.

Erickson, R. (1981) Chest tubes: they're really not that complicated. *Nursing* (US), 11(5), 34–43.

Erickson, R. (1981) Solving chest tube problems. *Nursing* (US), 11(6), 62–8.

Hinds, C. J. (1987) *A Concise Textbook of Intensive Care*. Baillière Tindall, London, pp. 164–5, 235.

Marieb, E. N. (1989) *Human Anatomy and Physiology*. Benjamin Cummings, California.

Mumford, S. P. (1986) Draining the pleural cavity. *The Professional Nurse*, 1(9), 240–2.

GUIDELINES: MANAGEMENT OF UNDER WATER-SEAL DRAINAGE

Equipment

1. Sterile chest drainage bottle.
2. Sterile disposable tubing.
3. Drainage bottle holder, if available.
4. Suction pump, if required.
5. Two pairs of large artery forceps (tips covered with rubber).

Procedure

Action	**Rationale**
1. Attach the intrapleural drain to the drainage tube.	Water-seal drainage provides for the escape of air, fluid and débris into a drainage bottle. The water

Guidelines: Management of under water-seal drainage

Action	**Rationale**
Note: This should lead to the long tube whose end is under water seal.	acts as a seal and keeps the air from being drawn back into the pleural space.
2. Ensure that drainage tubing is 2.5 cm below the water level (Figure 20.4).	If the tube is not deep enough under the water level, there is a danger of it emerging above the water line if the bottle is moved. If the tube is too deep, a higher intrapleural pressure is required to expel air.
3. The other, shorter tube, is:	
(a) Left open to the atmosphere.	To allow gas to escape.
(b) Attached to a controlled suction apparatus.	Although drainage of liquids and/or débris relies on gravity and the mechanics of respiration, additional controlled suction may be necessary to accelerate the process.
4. Establish the original level of fluid by: (a) Marking with a piece of tape. (b) Filling to a preset amount. *Note*: All bottles used should, preferably, be calibrated.	This provides a baseline for measurement of fluid drainage.
5. When recording fluid drainage:	
(a) Note the date and time. (b) Mark hourly or daily increments, or more frequently if there is excessive drainage, by taping the level on the drainage bottles. *Note*: When using tape specify whether the upper, mid or lower border of the tape is the level to be measured at (Figure 20.5).	This marking will show the amount of fluid loss and how fast fluid is collecting in the drainage bottle. If the fluid is blood, it serves as a basis for retransfusion or reoperation, if following surgery. Inaccuracies of 100 to 200 ml can occur if the incorrect border is used.
6. Secure tubing to the bed clothes by the use of tape and safety pins.	This will prevent kinking, looping or pressure on the tubing which may cause reflux of fluid into the pleural space or impede drainage, causing blocking of the intrapleural drain by débris.
7. Ensure that artery clamps are in close proximity to patient, i.e. taped to the wall, clamped to the bed clothes or on the bedside locker.	In the event of accidental disconnection of the drainage tubing from the intrapleural drain, the artery clamps should be applied immediately to the

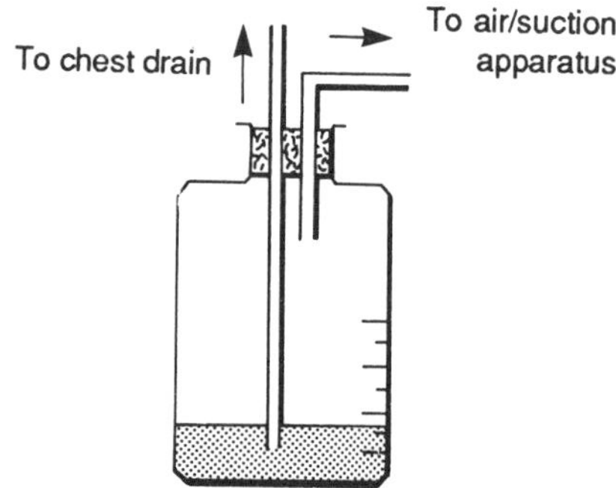

Figure 20.4 Underwater-seal drainage.

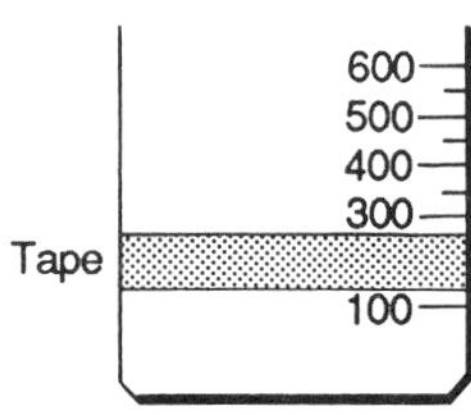

Figure 20.5 Specify whether the upper, mid- or lower level of the tape is to be measured.

	intrapleural drain to prevent entry of air (on inspiration) into the pleural space – leading to pneumothorax. When moving the patient, the drainage tubing is more likely to become disconnected, therefore the artery clamps should be readily available. There may be medical orders to apply the clamps, at set intervals, to delay drainage; e.g. following instillation of drugs or radioactive substances it is normal to clamp the tubing for 24 hours.
8. Ensure that the patient is sitting in a comfortable position which allows optimum drainage. Encourage the patient to change position frequently. This may be enhanced by adequate pain control, using drugs which do not depress respiration.	Correct poisitioning aids drainage by gravity and by ensuring that the patient breathes freely, to promote gaseous exchange. Changing position also promotes better drainage as well as avoiding discomfort and pressure sores.
9. Ask the physiotherapist to help encourage the patient with mobility, chest and arm exercises.	To promote drainage and avoid the complications of pressure sores and stiffness of the arm on the side of drain insertion.
10. Ensure patency of tubing by 'milking' tubing towards the drainage bottle, if necessary. Take care not to disconnect tubing while executing this manoeuvre. *Note*: This is only necessary if draining fluid.	'Milking' the tubing prevents it from becoming clogged with clots or fibrin. Constant attention to maintaining the patency of the tube will facilitate prompt expansion of the lung and minimize complications.
11. Ensure that there is fluctuation (swinging) of the fluid level in the drainage tube under water seal.	Fluctuation of the water level in the tube shows that there is effective communication between the pleural cavity and the drainage bottle, provides a valuable indication of the patency of the drainage system, and is a gauge of intrapleural pressure.
12. Ensure that the drainage bottle remains at floor level, except when the patient is being helped to move. The drainage bottle should never be raised above the level of the intrapleural drain.	To prevent back-flow of fluid and débris into the pleural space.
13. Caution visitors and ancillary staff against handling any part of the system or displacing the drainage bottle.	To prevent backflow and to guard against accidental disconnection of the tubing which would allow air entry.

GUIDELINES: CHANGING DRAINAGE TUBING AND BOTTLES

Equipment

1. Sterile drainage bottle.
2. Sterile water.
3. Two pairs of artery clamps (tips covered with rubber).
4. Suitable antiseptic solution, e.g. chlorhexidine.
5. Sterile tubing.

Procedure

Action	Rationale
1. Explain the procedure to the patient.	To gain the patient's consent and co-operation.

Guidelines: Changing drainage tubing and bottles

Action	Rationale
2. Wash hands with bactericidal soap and water or bactericidal alcohol hand rub.	To minimize the risk of infection.
3. Prepare drainage bottle by putting in a set amount (enough to cover the end of the long arm of the drainage tubing) of sterile water and taking note of that level. Mark this level with tape. If tubing is to be changed, attach clean tubing to the prepared drainage bottle.	To provide an underwater seal. Enough water should be in the bottle to ensure maintenance of the seal. Too much water creates pressure and reduces the capacity of the bottle for drainage. It is essential to note the amount of water added to the bottle for accurate measurement of drainage.
4. Take the equipment to the bedside.	
5. Clamp the intrapleural drain using both artery clamps, before changing the bottle for tubing.	To avoid tension pneumothorax occurring when the water seal is broken.
6. Clean hands with a suitable solution, e.g. bactericidal hand rub.	To minimize the risk of infection.
7. Remove the bung with the drainage tubing from the underwater-seal bottle and replace it in the clean bottle. Ensure that there is an airtight connection between the bung and bottle. If tubing is being changed, the bung will already be in place in the sterile bottle.	To prevent air entry and reduce the risk of infection.
8. Take the clamps off the intrapleural drainage tube.	To re-establish drainage.
9. Ensure that there is fluctuation (swinging) of the fluid level in the drainage tube under water seal.	To establish communication between pleural cavity and the drainage bottle.
10. Make the patient comfortable.	
11. Remove equipment.	
12. Record in appropriate documentation the amount of drainage, deducting the amount of water originally in the bottle.	For accurate recording of the amount of drainage.
13. Empty and clean the bottle and return it to the central sterile supplies department.	

Note: if an underwater-seal drain is established to drain air from the pleural space, there is probably no need to change either connection tubing or bottle. However, if fluid and débris are drained the bottle may need changing frequently (at least daily), depending on the amount drained. The tubing need be changed only if there is a copious amount of débris and there is a danger of it becoming blocked. Changing the tubing or the bottle breaks the closed system and provides a potential portal of entry for bacteria.

GUIDELINES: REMOVAL OF AN INTRAPLEURAL DRAIN

Equipment

1. Sterile dressing pack.
2. Cleansing lotion.
3. Surgical gloves.
4. Stitch cutter.
5. Collodion lotion.
6. Adhesive tape, waterproof.
7. Plaster remover.

Procedure

This procedure is usually carried out by a member of the medical staff, preferably the doctor who inserted the drain. However, it may be performed by a qualified nurse if he/she has been instructed and supervised in the removal of intrapleural drains.

Action		**Rationale**
Doctor/First nurse	*Assisting nurse*	
1. Explain the procedure to patient and allow the patient to practise the procedure beforehand.	Wash hands with bactericidal soap and water or bactericidal alcohol hand rub.	To obtain the patient's consent and co-operation. Speed and accuracy are essential in this procedure so all equipment must be at hand.
2. Establish patient is not allergic to tape or collodion.		To avoid allergic reactions.
3. Wash hands with bactericidal soap and water or bactericidal alcohol hand rub.		To minimize the risk of infection.
4. Prepare equipment using strict aseptic technique.	Assist in preparation of equipment without causing contamination.	
5. Remove the old dressing.		
6. Cut the knot from the purse-string suture.		Allows mobility of the suture.
7. Cut the suture holding the drain in place.	Hold the drain in place.	To prevent the drain falling out.
8. Tie the purse-string suture lightly to skin level.		To enable rapid tightening of the suture when the drain is removed.
9. Instruct the patient to breathe in to the maximum and to hold the breath. This manoeuvre should have been practised beforehand.		To minimize the risk of tension pneumothorax occurring as the drain is removed. Prior preparation of the patient ensures full co-operation.
	Steadily pull out the drain.	If the drain is pulled out too quickly, tension pneumothorax

Guidelines: Removal of an intrapleural drain

Action		**Rationale**
		may occur through further rupture of the pleura.
10. As the drain leaves the skin, tighten the purse-string suture and tie a firm double-knot. Speed is essential. Cut the end to 1.25 cm.		The purse-string suture must be tightened immediately the drain leaves the chest to avoid tension pneumothorax.
11. Place gauze with collodion over the suture.	Strap the gauze firmly in place.	To provide a tight seal.
12. Tell the patient that he/she may exhale and relax.		
	Remove any débris from the site of the wound and ensure that the patient is comfortable.	
	Clear equipment away.	
	Wash hands with soap and water.	To prevent cross-infection.
	Measure fluid drained.	
	Empty and clean the drainage bottles and send them to the central sterile supplies department.	
	Record the amount of drainage in appropriate documents.	To provide an accurate record.

NURSING CARE PLAN

Problem	**Cause**	**Suggested action**
Lack of drainage.	Kinking, looping or pressure on the tubing may cause reflux of fluid into the intrapleural space or may impede drainage, causing blocking of the intrapleural drain.	Check the system and straighten tubing as required. Secure the tubing to prevent a recurrence of the problem.
No fluctuation of fluid in tubing from the underwater seal.	Re-expansion of the lung.	Ask medical staff if the drain may be removed following chest X-ray. The purpose of the drain has been fulfilled. Keeping the drain in any longer than necessary may lead to hazards from infection or air re-entry.

	Tubing is obstructed by blood clots or fibrin.	'Milk' the tubing towards the drainage bottle to try to dislodge the obstruction and re-establish patency.
	Tubing is looped or kinked.	Straighten tubing as required. Secure the tubing to prevent a recurrence.
	Failure of the suction apparatus.	Disconnect the suction apparatus and ensure drain is patent.
Constant bubbling of fluid in the drainage bottle.	An air leak in the system.	Clamp the intrapleural drain, momentarily, close to the chest wall and establish whether there is a leak in the rest of the system. Clamping the tubing shows whether the leak is below the level of the clamp. However, if the clamp is left on for too long, and the leak is at thoracic level, i.e. air is entering the pleura, this will increase the patient's pneumothorax. Inform medical staff as leaking and trapping of air in the pleural space can result in tension pneumothorax.
Patient shows signs of rapid, shallow breathing, cyanosis, pressure in the chest, subscutaneous emphysema or haemorrhage.	Tension pneumothorax; mediastinal shift; postoperative haemorrhage; severe incisional pain; pulmonary embolus or cardiac tamponade.	Observe, record and report any of these signs to a doctor immediately.
Incisional pain.		Provide adequate analgesia, as prescribed, to reduce the patient's discomfort and to enable deep-breathing exercises to be performed and mobilization to ensure adequate drainage and to avoid complications.
Accidental disconnection of the drainage tubing from the intrapleural drain.		Apply an artery clamp to the drain immediately in order to avoid air entering the pleural space. Re-establish the connection as soon as possible in order to re-establish drainage. If necessary, use a clean, sterile drainage tube; tubing may have been contaminated when it became disconnected. Report to the doctor, who may wish to X-ray. Record the incident in the relevant records. The patient may have been upset by the incident and will need reassurance.

Nursing care plan

Problem	**Cause**	**Suggested action**
Patient needs to be moved to another area, e.g. X-ray department.		Place the drainage bottle below the level of the intrapleural drain, as close to the floor as possible, in order to prevent reflux of fluid into the pleural space. Do not clamp the drain unless the doctor has ordered it; this may obstruct drainage and allow clot formation if fluid is being drained. Ensure clamps are readily available in case of accidental disconnection *en route*.
Intrapleural drain falls out.		Pull the purse-string suture immediately to close the wound. Cover the wound with an occlusive sterile dressing. Inform a doctor. The objective is to minimize the amount of air entering the pleural space. The drain will probably need reinserting. Reassure the patient with appropriate explanations.

21

Intravenous Management

DRUG ADMINISTRATION

REFERENCE MATERIAL

The involvement of nursing staff in the administration of intravenous drugs was formally recognized in the mid-1970s following the publication of the Breckenridge Report (Department of Health and Social Security, 1976). A working party had been established in 1974 under the chairmanship of Professor Breckenridge as a result of the increasing use of the intravenous route for drug administration. There was concern that hazards such as microbial contamination and drug incompatibilities were not fully appreciated and that the staff participating were not adequately trained in the procedures used.

The terms of reference of the working party were as follows:

1. To identify and investigate the problems associated with this form of intravenous therapy.
2. To consider the responsibilities of the various parties involved.
3. To consider modification of nurse training to ensure safe practice.
4. To produce guidelines for the three main professions, i.e. doctor, pharmacists and nurses.
5. To assess the value of various aids, e.g. charts for reference.

The working party received evidence from a number of sources and considered pharmaceutical data. In 1976 the findings were published by the Department of Health and Social Security. The report proposed a rational approach to intravenous drug administration, established guidelines for documentation and outlined the responsibilities of health authorities and health professionals. The responsibility of medical staff was to ensure that the drug was administered by the most effective and safest route and that the instructions to facilitate this were clearly written.

An intravenous additive service provided by pharmacists was favoured. In situations where this was not practical, pharmacists were to act as an information source for other personnel. It was accepted that nursing staff could undertake the addition and administration of intravenous drugs. The nurse, however, should be qualified (i.e. should be a registered general nurse or an enrolled nurse) and have undergone a period of training and assessment in both the theoretical knowledge and practical procedures involved in such drug administration. He/she should be issued with a certificate of competence and fully understand the legal implications of undertaking such an extension of the role of the nurse.

In all intravenous therapy the nurse's responsibility continued to include the following:

1. Checking the infusion fluid and container for any obvious faults or contamination.
2. Ensuring the administration of the prescribed fluid to the correct patient.
3. Observing whether the intravenous line remains patent.
4. Inspecting the site of insertion and reporting abnormalities.
5. Controlling the rate of flow as prescribed.
6. Monitoring the condition of the patient and reporting any changes.
7. Maintaining appropriate records.

Permitted methods of intravenous drug administration by nurses were identified:

1. Continuously, or intermittently, by addition to an intravenous infusion in a bottle, bag or burette. This method may include the use of a variety of equipment, e.g. a small-volume syringe pump or a Y administration set.
2. Intermittently by injection into the latex rubber section of an intravenous administration set.
3. Intermittently by injection into a cannula or winged infusion device. The device's patency may be maintained by:

(a) Injecting heparinized saline.
(b) Injecting saline.
(c) Placing a stylet in the cannula.

4. Intermittently by injection via a three-way tap or stopcock. This method is not advised, however, due to the increased risk of contamination associated with these devices. Streamlined adaptors are now available and are preferred.

Additional guidelines

Certain guidelines were also issued in 1976 about general intravenous management related to the area of nursing involvement. These included the following:

1. The infusion container should not hang for more than 24 hours. This was reduced to eight hours in the case of blood or blood products.
2. The administration set must be changed every 24 hours. More recent research indicates that a 48 to 72-hour set change is not associated with an increase in infection (Department of Health and Social Security, 1973; Goodison, 1990a,b,c; Maki *et al.*, 1987). It is desirable to record the time and date when this is due.
3. The site of the infusion should be inspected at least daily for complications such as infiltration or inflammation.
4. The sterile dressing covering the insertion site must be changed daily, at the time of inspection or whenever it touched, e.g. at the time of administration of an intravenous injection.

Further recommendations in the light of recent research have shown that it is desirable that a closed system of infusion is maintained wherever possible, with as few connections or stopcocks as is necessary for its purpose (Speechley, 1986). This reduces the risk of extrinsic bacterial contamination, especially if three-way taps or their equivalent are excluded. The dead space in this equipment has been identified as a reservoir for micro-organisms which may be released into the circulation (Weinbaum, 1987).

The majority of sepsis is cannula related, and both infective and non-infective complications have been shown to increase substantially after the device has been in position for 48 hours (Maki, 1977). Routine resiting is, therefore, advised if at all possible. Although nurses are not normally responsible for this duty, they may be able to remind the doctor when this time has elapsed.

In order for the insertion site to be readily available for inspection, it may be necessary for the nurse to assume responsibility for taping the cannula in place as well as dressing the insertion site. Non-sterile tape should not cover the site, the equivalent of an open wound, and a method must be devised so that the site remains visible and the cannula is stable. The procedure illustrated in Figure 21.1 is recommended.

The purpose of all recommendations is to reduce the complications associated with intravenous therapy. Competent, informed management and adherence to basic principles will ensure this.

Removal of the intravenous device or cannula should be an aseptic procedure. The cannula must be taken out gently in order to prevent damage to the vein and pressure should be applied immediately. This pressure should be firm and not involve any rubbing movement. A haematoma will occur if the needle is carelessly removed, causing discomfort and a focus for infection. Pressure should be applied until bleeding has stopped, then a light sterile dressing applied.

Drugs are used for three basic purposes:

1. Diagnostic purposes, e.g. assessment of liver function or diagnosis of myasthenia gravis.
2. Prophylaxis, e.g. heparin to prevent thrombosis or antibiotics to prevent infection.
3. Therapeutic purposes, e.g. replacement of fluids or vitamins, supportive purposes (to enable other treatments, such as anaesthesia), palliation of pain and cure (as in the case of antibiotics).

Drugs administered intravenously also fall within the above-mentioned categories.

Advantages of using the intravenous route

1. An immediate therapeutic effect is achieved due to rapid delivery of the drug to its target site.
2. Total absorption allows precise dose calculation and more reliable treatment.
3. The rate of administration can be controlled and the therapeutic effect maintained or modified as required.
4. Pain and irritation caused by some substances when given intramuscularly or subcutaneously are avoided.
5. Intravenous administration is suitable for drugs which cannot be absorbed by any other route due to large molecular size and irritation to, or instability in, the gastrointestinal tract.

Disadvantages of using the intravenous route

1. There is an inability to recall the drug and reverse the action of it. This may lead to increased toxicity or a sensitivity reaction.
2. Insufficient control of administration may lead to speed shock. This is characterized by a flushed

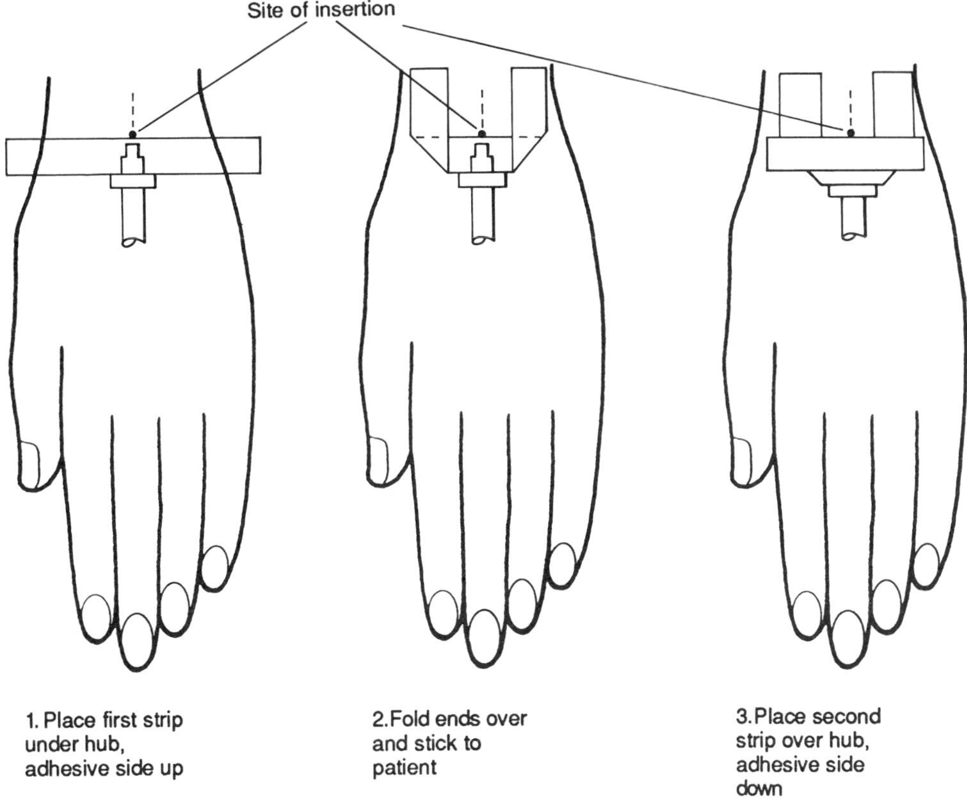
Site of insertion
1. Place first strip under hub, adhesive side up
2. Fold ends over and stick to patient
3. Place second strip over hub, adhesive side down

Figure 21.1 Site of insertion.

face, headache, congestion, tightness in the chest, etc.

3. Additional complications may occur, such as the following:
   (a) Microbial contamination through a point of access into the circulation for a period of time.
   (b) Vascular irritation, e.g. chemical phlebitis.
   (c) Drug incompatibilities and interactions if multiple additives are prescribed.

Principles to be applied throughout preparation and administration

Asepsis

Aseptic technique must be adhered to throughout all intravenous procedures to prevent extrinsic bacterial contamination. The nurse must employ good hand washing and drying techniques or use an alcohol-based skin cleanser as an alternative. Injection sites or bungs should be cleaned using an alcohol-based antiseptic, allowing time for it to dry. A non-touch technique should be employed when changing infusion bags or bottles and these procedures should be completed as quickly as possible. If asepsis is not maintained, local infection, septic phlebitis or septicaemia may result. Any indication of infection, e.g. redness at the insertion site of the device or pyrexia, requires removal of the cannula and further investigation.

Inspection of fluids, drugs, equipment and their packaging must be undertaken to detect any points where contamination may have occurred during manufacture and/or transport. This intrinsic contamination may be detected as cloudiness, discoloration or the presence of particles.

Sterility will ensure that the patient does not receive an injection or infusion of microbes.

Safety

All details of the prescription and all calculations must be checked carefully in accordance with hospital policy in order to ensure safe preparation and administration of the drug(s). The nurse must also check the compatibility of the drug with the diluent or infusion fluid. The nurse should be aware of the types of incompatibilities, and the factors which could influence them. These include pH, concentration, time, temperature, light and the brand of the drug. If insufficient information is available, a reference book must also be checked and constant monitoring of both the mixture and the patient is important. The preferred method and rate of intravenous administration must be determined.

Drugs should never be added to the following: blood; blood products, i.e. plasma or platelet concentrate; mannitol solutions; sodium bicarbonate solution. Only specially prepared additives should be used with fat emulsions or amino acid preparations.

Accurate labelling of additives and records of administration are essential.

Any protective clothing which is advised should be worn.

Comfort

Both the physical and psychological comfort of the patient must be considered. By maintaining high standards throughout, the patient's physical comfort should be assured. Comprehensive explanation of the practical aspects of the procedure together with balanced information about the effects of treatment will contribute to reducing anxiety.

Methods of administering intravenous drugs

Three methods are recommended: continuous infusion, intermittent infusion and intermittent injection.

Continuous infusion

Continuous infusion may be defined as the administration of a large volume of fluid, i.e. 250 to 1000 ml, over a number of hours that may be repeated over a period of days. An exception of this may be a small-volume infusion (e.g. of heparin) delivered continously via a syringe pump.

A continuous infusion may be used when:

1. The drugs to be administered must be highly diluted.
2. A maintenance of steady blood levels of the drug is required.

Pre-prepared infusion fluids with additives such as those containing potassium chloride should be used whenever possible. Only one addition should be made to each bottle or bag of fluid after the compatibility has been ascertained. The additive and fluid must be mixed well to prevent a layering effect which can occur with some drugs. The danger is that a bolus injection of the drug may be delivered. To safeguard this, any additions should be made to the infusion fluid before the fluid is hung on the infusion stand. The infusion container should be labelled clearly after the addition has been made. Constant monitoring of the infusion fluid mixture and the patient should occur.

Intermittent infusion

Intermittent infusion is the administration of a small-volume infusion, i.e. 50 to 250 ml, over a period of between 20 minutes and two hours. This may be given as a specific dose at one time or at repeated intervals during 24 hours.

An intermittent infusion may be used when:

1. A peak plasma level is required therapeutically.
2. The pharmacology of the drug dictates this specific dilution.
3. The drug is not stable for the time required to administer a large-volume infusion.
4. The patient does not require or cannot tolerate large volumes of fluid.

Delivery of the drug by intermittent infusion may utilize a system such as a Y set, if the simultaneous infusion is of a compatible fluid, or a burette set with a chamber capacity of 100 or 150 ml. A small-volume infusion may also be connected to a heparinized cannula if no fluids are required between doses.

All the points considered when preparing for a continuous infusion should be taken into account here, e.g. pre-prepared fluids, single additions, adequate mixing, labelling and monitoring.

Calculations of accurate rate of administration (continuous or intermittent)

The rate of administration of a continuous or intermittent infusion may be calculated from the following equation:

$$\frac{\text{No. millilitres to be infused}}{\text{No. hours over which infusion is to be delivered}} \times \frac{\text{No. drops per millilitre}}{\text{60 minutes}} = \text{No. drops to be delivered per minute}$$

In this equation, 60 is a factor for the conversion of the number of hours to the number of minutes; the number of drops per millilitre is dependent on the administration set used and the viscosity of the infusion fluid. For example, crystalloid fluid administered via a solution set is delivered at the rate of 20 drops/ml; the rate of packed red cells given via a blood set will be calculated at 15 drops/ml.

Direct intermittent injection

Direct intermittent injection is a procedure for the introduction of a small volume of drug(s) into the cannula or the injection site of the administration set using a needle and syringe. This may take a few seconds or a number of minutes.

A direct injection may be used when:

1. A maximum concentration of the drug is required to vital organs. This is a 'bolus' injection which is given rapidly over seconds, as in an emergency.
2. The drug cannot be diluted due to pharmacological or therapeutic reasons. This is given as a controlled 'push' injection over a few minutes. Rapid administration could result in toxic levels and an anaphylactic-type reaction. Manufacturers' recommendations of rates of administration (i.e. millilitres or milligrams per minute) should be adhered to. In the absence of such recommendations, administration should proceed slowly.
3. A peak blood level is required and cannot be achieved by small-volume infusion.

Delivery of the drug by direct injection may be via the cannula through a resealable latex bung, extension set or via the injection site of an administration set. Whatever method is chosen, the same procedure should be followed. This includes the following:

1. Removal of any bandage or dressing present to inspect the insertion of the cannula.
2. Confirmation of the patency of the vein and its ability to accept an extra flow of fluid or irritant chemical.

Administration into the injection site of a fast-running drip may be advised if the infusion progress is compatible. Alternatively, a stop–start procedure may be employed if there is doubt about venous integrity. If the infusion fluid is incompatible with the drug, the line may be switched off and a syringe of normal saline used as a flush.

In some centres a heparin lock may be utilized. This means maintaining the patency of the cannula using a weak solution of heparin. A plug with a resealable injection cap is inserted into the end of the intravenous device. Sufficient heparin to fill the 'dead space' and of a concentration to prevent fibrin formation is injected. The cannula can then be left for a number of hours before reheparinization is required. The time is dependent on the strength of heparin used. After every use, reheparinization is required.

The advantage of using a heparin lock are as follows:

1. It reduces the risk of circulatory overload.
2. It reduces the risk of vascular irritation.
3. It decreases the risk of bacterial contamination as it eliminates a continuous intravenous pathway.
4. It increases patient comfort and mobility.
5. It may reduce the cost of intravenous equipment.

Some centres are now using normal saline flush to maintain the patency of cannulae. This could have the advantage of being cheaper than heparanized saline. An alternative method of maintaining patency is the use of a stylet which can be inserted into certain cannulae.

If a number of drugs are being administered, normal saline must be used to flush in between each to prevent interactions. This fluid should also be repeated at the end of the administration.

The insertion site of the device should be observed throughout for swelling or redness. Patients must be consulted constantly about any pain or discomfort they may be experiencing. Problems that arise during administration will involve the vein. Patency throughout should not be assumed. Early detection of extravasation of any drug, especially in concentrated form, is essential to meet the aims of therapy.

These aims can be summarized as the effective delivery of treatment without discomfort or tissue damage to the patient and without compromising venous access, especially if long-term therapy is proposed.

Summary

The nurse is responsible for administering intravenous drugs safely by the methods listed. In order to do this he/she requires a thorough knowledge of the principles and their application, and a responsible attitude which ensures that intravenous medications are not given without full knowledge of immediate and late effects, toxicities and nursing implications.

Knowledge of equipment and techniques for combining multiple additives is also essential.

Only by investigating these topics can the nurse develop into a confident and safe practitioner.

References and further reading

Band, J. & Maki, D. (1979) Safety of changing intravenous delivery systems at longer than 24-hour intervals. *Annals of Internal Medicine*, 90, 173–8.

British Intravenous Therapy Association (1987) *Guidelines for the Preparation of Nurses for Intravenous Drug Administration and Associated Intravenous Therapy*.

British Medical Association/Pharmaceutical Society of Great Britain (1988) *British National Formulary*. BMA, London.

Buxton, A. *et al.* (1979) Contamination of intravenous infusion fluid: effects of changing administration sets. *Annals of Internal Medicine*, 90, 764–8.

Cyganski, J. *et al.* (1987) The case for the heparin flush. *American Journal of Nursing* 87, 796–7.

Department of Health and Social Security (1973) *Medicines Commission Report on Prevention of Microbial Contamination of Medicinal Products*. HMSO, London.

Department of Health and Social Security (1976) *Health Services Development, Addition of Drugs to Intravenous Fluids, HC(76)9 (Breckenridge Report)*. HMSO, London.

Dunn, D. & Lenihan, S. (1987) The case for the saline flush. *American Journal of Nursing*, 87(6), 798–9.

Goodison, S. M. (1990a) The risks of IV therapy. *The Professional Nurse*, February, 235.

Goodison, S. M. (1990b) Keeping the flora out. *The Professional Nurse*, August, 572.

Goodison, S. M. (1990c) Good practice insures minimum risk factors. *The Professional Nurse*, December, 175.

Hook, M. (1990) Heparian vs normal saline. Letters to the Editor, *Journal of Intravenous Nursing*, 13(3), 150–1.

Josephson, A. *et al.* (1985) The relationship between intravenous fluid contamination and the frequency of tubing replacement. *Infection Control*, 9, 367–70.

Maki, D. (1977) A semi-quantative culture method for identifying intravenous catheter-related infections. *New England Journal of Medicine*, 296, 1305–6.

Maki, D. *et al.* (1987) Prospective study replacing administration sets for intravenous therapy, at 48 to 72 hour intervals. *Journal of the American Medical Association*, 258(13), 1777–81.

Nystrom, B. *et al.* (1983) Bacteraemia in surgical patients with intravenous devices: a European multicentre incidence study. *Journal of Hospital Infection*, 4, 338–49.

Parish, P. (1982) Benefits to risks of IV therapies. *British Journal of Intravenous Therapy*, 3(6), 10–19.

Peters, J. *et al.* (1984) Peripheral venous cannulation: reducing the risks. *British Journal of Parenteral Therapy*, 5(2), 56–68.

Plumer, A. L. (1987) *Principles and Practice of Intravenous Therapy*, 4th edn. Little Brown & Co, Boston, USA.

Sager, D. & Bomar, S. (1980) *Intravenous Medications*. J. B. Lippincott, Philadelphia.

Sager, D. & Bomar, S. (1983) *Quick Reference to Intravenous Drugs*. J. B. Lippincott, Philadelphia.

Smith, R. (1985a) Extravasation of intravenous fluids. *British Journal of Parenteral Therapy* 6(2), 30–5.

Smith, R. (1985b) Prevention and treatment of extravasation. *British Journal of Parenteral Therapy*, 6(5), 114–19.

Speechley, V. (1984) The nurse's role in intravenous management. *Nursing Times*, 2 May, 31–2.

Speechley, V. (1986) Intravenous therapy: peripheral/central lines. *Nursing*, 3(3), 95–100.

Speechley, V. & Toovey, J. (1987) Factsheets: problems in IV therapy 1, 2, 3. *The Professional Nurse*, 2(8), 240–2; 2(12), 413; 3(3), 90–1.

Weinbaum, D. L. (1987) Nosocomial bacterias. In *Infection Control in Intensive Care* (Ed. by B. F. Faser), pp. 39–58. Churchill Livingstone, New York.

GUIDELINES: ADMINISTRATION OF DRUGS BY CONTINUOUS INFUSION

This procedure may be carried out by the infusion of drugs from a bag, bottle or burette.

Equipment

1. Clinically clean receiver or tray containing the prepared drug to be administered.
2. Patient's prescription chart.
3. Recording sheet or book as required by law or hospital policy.
4. Protective clothing as required by hospital policy for specific drugs.
5. Container of appropriate intravenous infusion fluid.
6. Swab saturated with isopropyl alcohol 70%.
7. Drug additive label.

Procedure

Action	**Rationale**
1. Explain the procedure to the patient.	To obtain the patient's consent and co-operation.
2. Inspect the infusion.	To check it is running satisfactorily and if the patient is experiencing any discomfort at the site of insertion.
3. Wash hands with bactericidal soap and water or bactericidal alcohol hand rub, and assemble the necessary equipment.	
4. Prepare the drug for injection described in the procedure.	

5. Check the name, strength and volume of intravenous fluid against the prescription chart.

To ensure that the correct type and quantity of fluid are administered.

6. Check the expiry date of the fluid.

To prevent an ineffective or toxic compound being administered to the patient.

7. Check that the packaging is intact.

To maintain asepsis.

8. Inspect the container and contents in a good light for cracks, punctures, air bubbles, discolouration, haziness and crystalline or particulate matter.

To maintain asepsis. To prevent any toxic or foreign matter being infused into the patient.

9. Check the identity and amount of drug to be added. Consider:
(a) Compatibility of fluid and additive.
(b) Stability of mixture over the prescription time.
(c) Any special directions for dilution, e.g. pH, optimum concentration, etc.
(d) Sensitivity to external factors such as light.
(e) Any anticipated allergic reaction.
If any doubts exist about the listed points, consult the pharmacist or appropriate reference works.

To minimize any risk of error. To ensure safe and effective administration of the drug. To enable anticipation of toxicities and the nursing implications of these.

10. Any additions must be made immediately before use.

To prevent any possible microbial growth or degradation.

11. Wash hands thoroughly using bactericidal soap and water or bactericidal alcohol hand rub.

To maintain asepsis.

12. Expose the injection site on the container by removing any seal present.

13. Clean the site with the swab and allow it to dry.

To maintain asepsis.

14. Inject the drug using a new sterile needle into the bag, bottle or burette. A 23 or 25G needle should be used.

To enable resealing of the latex or rubber injection site.

15. If the addition is made into a burette at the bedside:
(a) Avoid contamination of the needle and inlet port.
(b) Check that the correct quantity of fluid is in the chamber.
(c) Switch the infusion off briefly so that a bolus injection is not given.

To maintain asepsis and prevent incompatibility, etc.

16. Invert the container a number of times, especially if adding to a flexible infusion bag.

To ensure adequate mixing of the drug.

17. Check again for haziness, discolouration, etc. This can occur even if the mixture is theoretically compatible, thus making vigilance essential.

To detect any incompatibility or degradation.

18. Complete the drug additive label and fix it on the bag, bottle or burette. Complete the

To maintain accurate records. To provide a point of reference in the event of any queries. To prevent any

Guidelines: Administration of drugs by continuous infusion

Action	Rationale
patient's recording chart and other hospital and/or legally required documents.	duplication of treatment.
19. Place the container in a clinically clean receptacle. Wash hands and proceed to the patient.	To maintain aspesis.
20. Check again that the infusion is running well and that the contents of the previous container have been delivered.	To confirm that the vein and/or cannula remain patent. To ensure that the preceding prescription has been administered.
21. Switch off the infusion and hang the new container quickly using a non-touch technique.	To achieve a safe and aseptic change-over.
22. Restart the infusion and adjust the rate of flow as prescribed.	To deliver the mixture accurately.
23. If the addition is made into a burette, the infusion can be restarted immediately following mixing and recording and the infusion rate adjusted accordingly.	
24. Ask the patient if any abnormal sensations, etc. are experienced.	To ascertain whether there are any problems. If so, investigate.
25. Discard waste, making sure that it is placed in the correct containers, e.g. 'sharps' into a designated receptacle.	To ensure safe disposal and avoid injury to staff. To prevent re-use of equipment.

GUIDELINES: ADMINISTRATION OF DRUGS BY INTERMITTENT INFUSION

This procedure is carried out via a heparinized cannula or when patency is maintained by a stylet.

Equipment

Equipment for this procedure is as described for the previous procedure (i.e. items 1–7), together with the following:

8. Intravenous administration set.
9. Intravenous infusion stand.
10. Clean dressing trolley.
11. Clinically clean receiver or tray.
12. Sterile needles and syringes.
13. Normal saline 0.9%, 20 ml for injection.
14. Flushing solution, in accordance with hospital policy, plus sterile bung or sterile stylet.
15. Alcohol-based lotion for cleaning injection site.
16. Alcohol-based hand wash solution.
17. Sterile dressing pack.
18. Hypo-allergenic tape.
19. Gloves.

Procedure

Action	Rationale
1. Explain the procedure to the patient.	To obtain the patient's consent and co-operation.

Action	Rationale
2. Prepare the intravenous infusion and additive as described for the previous procedure (i.e. items 2–11).	
3. Prime the intravenous administration set with infusion fluid mixture and hang it on the infusion stand.	
4. Draw up 10 ml of normal saline 0.9% for injection in two separate syringes, using an aseptic technique.	
5. Draw up flushing solution, as required by hospital policy, and check.	
6. Place the syringes in a clinically clean receiver or tray on the bottom shelf of the dressing trolley.	
7. Collect the other equipment and place it on the bottom shelf of the dressing trolley.	
8. Place a sterile dressing pack on the top of the trolley.	
9. Check that all necessary equipment is present.	To prevent delays and interruption of the procedure.
10. Wash hands thoroughly using bactericidal soap and water or bactericidal alcohol hand rub before leaving the clinical room.	To maintain asepsis.
11. Proceed to the patient.	
12. Open the sterile dressing pack.	To maintain asepsis.
13. Add lotion for cleaning the skin to the gallipot in order to wet the cotton wool balls.	
14. Wash hands with bactericidal soap and water or with a bactericidal alcohol-based hand wash solution.	To maintain asepsis.
15. Remove the patient's bandage and dressing.	To observe the insertion site.
16. Inspect the insertion site of the cannula.	To detect any signs of inflammation, infiltration, etc. If present, take appropriate action.
17. Wash hands as above (see point 14).	To maintain asepsis.
18. Put on gloves.	To comply with safe technique and practice.
19. Place a sterile towel under the patient's arm.	To create a sterile field.
20. Remove the injection bung or stylet from the cannula while applying digital pressure at the point in the vein where the cannula tip rests. This may be achieved easier using a sterile cotton wool ball.	To prevent blood spillage.
21. Inject gently 10 ml of normal saline 0.9% for injection.	To confirm the patency of the cannula.

Guidelines: Administration of drugs by intermittent infusion

Action	**Rationale**
22. If no resistance is met, no pain or discomfort is felt by the patient, no swelling is evident, no leakage occurs around the cannula and there is a good back-flow of blood on aspiration, it can be assumed that the cannula is patent.	
23. Connect to the infusion.	To commence treatment.
24. Open the control valve.	To check free flow.
25. Check the insertion site and ask the patient if he/she is comfortable.	To confirm that the vein can accommodate the extra fluid flow and that the patient experiences no pain, etc.
26. Adjust the flow rate as prescribed.	To ensure that the correct speed of administration is established.
27. Tape the administration set in a way that places no strain on the cannula.	To reduce the risk of mechanical phlebitis or infiltration.
28. Cover the cannula with a sterile topical swab and tape it in place.	To maintain asepsis.
29. Remove gloves.	
30. If the infusion is to be completed within 40 minutes, bandaging is unnecessary and the patient may be instructed to keep the arm resting on the sterile field.	
31. Cover the dressing trolley and equipment with a sterile towel and leave by the bedside.	To maintain asepsis.
32. Return at frequent intervals.	To check the flow rate, the patient's comfort and for signs of infiltration.
33. If the infusion is to be in progress for longer than 40 minutes, a bandage should be applied. The equipment may be cleared away and reassembled at the end of the infusion.	To provide support and to promote patient comfort.
34. When the infusion is complete, wash hands using bactericidal soap and water or bactericidal alcohol hand rub, and recheck that all the equipment required is present.	To maintain asepsis and ensure that the procedure runs smoothly.
35. Stop the infusion when all the fluid has been delivered.	To ensure that all of the prescribed mixture has been delivered.
36. Wash hands with bactericidal soap and water or bactericidal alcohol hand rub.	To maintain asepsis.
37. Put on gloves.	To comply with safe technique and practice.
38. Disconnect the infusion set and flush the	To flush any remaining irritating solution away from

Action	Rationale
cannula with 10 ml of normal saline 0.9% for injection. (A 'minibag' may be used to flush the drug through the tubing but the cost implications of this should be considered before this is adopted routinely.)	the cannula.
39. Insert a new sterile bung.	To maintain the patency of the cannula for future use.
40. Flushing must follow.	
41. Clean the injection site of the bung with a swab saturated with isopropyl alcohol 70%.	To maintain asepsis.
42. Administer flush, as prescribed (using a 23 or 25G needle) using the positive pressure technique.	To maintain the patency of the cannula and enable reseal of the latex injection site.
43. Cover the insertion site and cannula with a new sterile topical swab. Tape it in place.	To maintain asepsis.
44. Apply a bandage.	To provide support and increase the patient's comfort.
45. Ensure that the patient is comfortable.	
46. Discard waste, placing it in the correct containers, e.g. 'sharps' into a designated container.	To ensure safe disposal and avoid injury to staff. To prevent re-use of equipment.
47. Remove gloves.	

GUIDELINES: ADMINISTRATION OF DRUGS BY DIRECT INJECTION, BOLUS OR PUSH

This procedure may be carried out via any one of the following:

1. The injection site of an intravenous administration set.
2. An adaptor or injectable plug into a cannula or winged infusion device (patency may be maintained by stylet or by heparinization).
3. An extension set, multiple adaptor or stopcock (one-, two- or three-way).

Equipment

1. Clinically clean receiver or tray containing the prepared drug(s) to be administered.
2. Patient's prescription chart.
3. Recording sheet or book as required by law or hospital policy.
4. Protective clothing as required by hospital policy or specific drugs.
5. Clean dressing trolley.
6. Clinically clean receiver or tray.
7. Sterile needles and syringes.
8. Normal saline 0.9%, 20 ml for injection.
9. Flushing solution, in accordance with hospital policy, or a sterile intravenous stylet.
10. Alcohol-based lotion for cleaning injection site.
11. Sterile dressing pack.
12. Hypo-allergenic tape.
13. Sharps container.

Guidelines: Administration of drugs by direct injection, bolus or push

Procedure

Action	Rationale
1. Explain the procedure to the patient.	To obtain the patient's consent and co-operation.
2. Check any infusion in progress.	To see if it is running satisfactorily, and that the patient is not experiencing any discomfort at the site of insertion.
3. Wash hands with bactericidal soap and water or bactericidal alcohol hand rub, and assemble necessary equipment.	
4. Prepare the drug for injection as per procedure described earlier.	
5. Prepare a 20-ml syringe of normal saline 0.9% for injection, as described, using aseptic technique.	
6. Draw up flushing solution, as required by hospital policy, and check.	
7. Place syringes in a clinically clean receptacle on the bottom shelf of the dressing trolley, along with the receptacle containing any drug(s) to be administered.	
8. Collect the other equipment and place it on the bottom of the trolley.	
9. Place a sterile dressing pack on top of the trolley.	
10. Check that all necessary equipment is present.	To prevent delays and interruption of the procedure.
11. Wash hands thoroughly (see point 3, above).	To maintain asepsis.
12. Proceed to the patient.	
13. Open the sterile dressing pack. Add lotion to wet the low-linting swab.	
14. Wash hands with bactericidal soap and water or with bactericidal alcohol hand rub.	To reduce the risk of infection.
15. Remove the bandage and dressing.	To observe the insertion site.
16. Inspect the insertion site of the cannula.	To detect any signs of inflammation, infiltration, etc. If present, take appropriate action.
17. Observe the infusion, if in progress, to confirm that it is running as desired. If the infusion is normal saline 0.9% with no additives, confirmation of patency and flushing with a separate syringe of normal saline are not necessary.	

18. Wash hands or clean them with an alcohol-based hand wash solution.

To maintain asepsis.

19. Place a sterile towel under the patient's arm.

To create a sterile field.

20. Clean the injection site with a swab saturated with 70% is opropyl alcohol. Wait until alcohol evaporates.

To reduce the number of pathogens introduced into the skin by the needle at the time of the insertion. Reduces pain on insertion which may be caused by introducing alcohol.

21. Switch off the infusion or close the fluid path of a tap or stopcock.

To prevent excessive pressure within the vein. To prevent contact with an incompatible infusion fluid. To allow the nurse to concentrate on the site of insertion and injection.

22. Inject normal saline 0.9% gently.

To confirm patency of the vein. To prevent contact with an incompatible infusion fluid.

23. Use a sterile 23 or 25G needle if the injection is made through a resealable latex site.

To enable resealing of the site at the end of the injection.

24. Change syringes and inject the drug smoothly in the direction of flow at the specified rate.

To prevent excessive pressure within the vein. To prevent speed shock.

25. Observe the insertion site of the cannula throughout.

To detect any complications at an early stage, e.g. extravasation or local allergic reaction.

26. Blood return and/or 'flashback' must be checked frequently throughout the injection.

To confirm that the device is correctly placed and that the vein remains patent.

27. Consult the patient during the injection about any discomfort, etc.

To detect any complications at an early stage, and ensure patient comfort.

28. If more than one drug is to be administered, flush with normal saline between administrations by restarting the infusion or changing syringes.

To prevent drug interactions.

29. At the end of the injection, flush with normal saline by restarting the infusion or changing syringes.

To flush any remaining irritant solution away from the cannula site.

30. Instructions in the manufacturers' literature may specifically recommend that the drug is given into the injection site of an infusion that is running rapidly.

To increase dilution and reduce venous irritation.

31. Check that the infusion fluid in progress and the drug are compatible. If not, change the fluid.

To prevent drug interaction.

32. Open the control clamp of the giving set fully. Inject the drug at a speed sufficient to slow but not stop the infusion.

To prevent a back-flow of drug up the tubing.

33. Observe the insertion site of the cannula carefully.

To detect any complications at an early stage. Extra pressure within the vein caused by both fluid flow and injection of the may cause rupture.

34. After the final flush of normal saline adjust the

Guidelines: Administration of drugs by direct injection, bolus or push

Action	Rationale
infusion rate as prescribed or open the fluid path of the tap or stopcock or maintain the patency of the cannula by using flushing solution or an intravenous stylet.	
35. Cover the insertion site with new sterile topical dressing and tape it in place.	To continue accurate delivery of therapy.
36. Apply a bandage.	To maintain asepsis.
37. Make sure that the patient is comfortable.	To provide support and increase the patient's comfort.
38. Record the administration on appropriate sheets.	To maintain accurate records, provide a point of reference in the event of any queries and prevent any duplication of treatment.
39. Once injection has been administered, place all used syringes with needle unsheathed directly into 'sharps' container. Other waste should be placed into the appropriate plastic bags.	To avoid needle stick injury.

NURSING CARE PLAN

The problems associated with injection and infusion of intravenous fluids and drugs fall into two categories:

1. Local venous complications associated with the cannula insertion site.
2. Systemic problems which affect the whole patient, exerting effects on vital organs and their functions.

The nurse must observe regularly the insertion site, the infusion and the patient to detect any complications at the earliest possible moment and to prevent progression to more serious conditions. Early detection also includes paying attention to the patient's comments. The patient's symptoms and physical signs both constitute reasons for a resiting of the cannula or discontinuation of the infusion. Signs and symptoms are used as problem headings.

Problem	Possible causes	Preventive nursing measures	Suggested action
Infusion slows or stops.	Change in position of the following:		
	(a) Patient.	Check the height of the fluid container if the patient is active, as all infusions run by gravity.	Adjust the height accordingly.
	(b) Limb.	Tape, bandage or splint the limb if infusion is sited at a point of flexion.	Move the arm or hand until infusion starts again.
		Instruct the patient on the amount of movement permitted. Continued movement could result in mechanical phlebitis.	Retape, bandage or splint the limb again carefully in the desired position.
	(c) Administration set.	Check for kinks and/or compression if the patient is active or restless.	Correct accordingly.

(d) Cannula.	Tape the cannula firmly to prevent movement. It may come into contact with the vein wall or a valve. Infusions sited in small veins are prone to this problem.	Remove the bandage and dressing and manoeuvre the cannula gently until the infusion starts again. Retape carefully.
Technical problems:		
(a) No air inlet in the rigid container.	Ensure that the container is vented.	Vent if necessary.
(b) Empty container.	Check fluid levels regularly.	Replace the fluid container before it runs dry.
(c) Venous spasm due to chemical irritation or coldness.	Dilute drugs as recommended. Remove solutions from the refrigerator a short time before use.	Apply a warm compress to soothe and dilate the vein, increase blood flow and dilute the infusion mixture.
(d) Injury to the vein.	Detect any injury early as it is likely to progress and cause more serious conditions (see below).	Stop the infusion and request a resiting of the cannula.
(e) Occlusion of the cannula due to fibrin formation.	Maintain a continuous, regular fluid flow or ensure that patency is maintained by heparinization or by placement of a stylet. Instruct the patient to keep limb at waist level or below if ambulant.	Attempt to flush the cannula gently using a 1 ml syringe of normal saline. If resistance is met, stop and request a resiting of the cannula.
(f) The cannula has become displaced either completely or partially, i.e. it has 'tissued'.	Tape the cannula and the giving set so that no stress is placed on them. Instruct the patient on the amount of movement permitted.	Confirm that infiltration has occurred by (i) inspecting the site for leakage, swelling, etc.; (ii) testing the temperature of the skin – it will be cooler if infiltration has occurred; (iii) comparing the size of the limb with the opposite one; (iv) applying a tourniquet above the cannula site or lower the infusion below the height of the limb. If the vein is patent, blood will flow back into the giving set. Once infiltration has been confirmed, stop the infusion and request a resiting of the cannula. If the infusion is allowed to progress, discomfort and tissue damage will result. Apply cold or warm compresses to provide

Nursing care plan

Problem	Possible causes	Preventive nursing measures	Suggested action
			symptomatic relief. Reassure the patient by explaining what is happening.
Erythema or inflammation around the insertion site.	Phlebitis due to:		
	(a) Sepsis.	Adhere to aseptic techniques when performing all intravenous procedures.	Stop the infusion and request a resiting of the cannula. Follow hospital policy about sending equipment for bacterial analysis. Clean the area and apply a sterile dressing. Check regularly.
	(b) Chemical irritation.	Dilute drugs according to instructions. Check compatibilities carefully to reduce the risk of particulate formation. Be aware of the factors involved, e.g. pH.	Stop the infusion and request a resiting of the cannula. If the infusion is allowed to progress, tissue damage and severe pain will result. Apply cold or warm compresses to provide symptomatic relief. Encourage movement of the limb. Reassure the patient by explaining what is happening.
	(c) Mechanical irritation.	Tape, bandage or splint the limb if the infusion is sited at a point of flexion. Use an extension set to minimize direct handling if cannula sited in awkward position. Instruct the patient on the amount of movement permitted.	Stop the infusion and request a resiting of the cannula. Although inflammation of this type progresses more slowly, it will cause discomfort. Provide symptomatic relief as above. Encourage movement and reassure the patient by explaining what is happening. Failure to detect and act when phlebitis is at an early stage, for whatever reason, will result in painful and incapacitating thrombophlebitis. Dislodgement of a thrombus could cause a pulmonary embolus.
	Infection with or without discharge.	Adhere to aseptic techniques when	Stop the infusion and request a resiting of the

		performing all intravenous procedures. Observe all recommendations for equipment changes, etc.	cannula. Follow hospital policy about sending equipment for bacterial analysis. Clean the area and apply a sterile dressing. Check regularly. Observe the patient for signs of systemic infection.
	Cellulitis due to: (a) Sepsis. (b) Non-specific sterile inflammation.	As above.	As above. Due to the nature of the connective tissue any infection or inflammation spreads quickly, especially if the limb is oedematous.
	Local allergic reaction.	Ask if the patient has any allergies before administration of any drugs or fluids, including sensitivities to topical solutions. Check whether the particular medication is commonly associated with local or venous flushing.	Observe the patient for systemic reaction. Treat the local area symptomatically. Reassure the patient.
Local oedema.	During infusion: (a) Infiltration. (b) Phlebitis.	Tape the cannula and giving set so that no stress is placed on the cannula. Use an extension set. Instruct the patient on the amount of movement permitted. Check regularly for swelling, e.g. tightness of bandages or a wedding ring.	Stop the infusion and request a resiting of the cannula before proceeding. Apply cold or warm compresses to provide symptomatic relief. Reassure the patient by explaining what is happening.
	During injection: (a) Extravasation of medication.	Observe the patient carefully throughout drug administration.	Stop the injection immediately extravasation is suspected. Act in accordance with hospital policy. Some drugs may cause inflammation and supportive, symptomatic relief will be required. Others may have the potential to cause necrosis of tissue and further action may be necessary.
Oedema of the limb.	Infiltration.	Tape the cannula and giving set so that no stress is placed on the cannula. Use an	Stop the infusion and request a resiting of the cannula. Provide symptomatic relief and

Nursing care plan

Problem	**Possible causes**	**Preventive nursing measures**	**Suggested action**
		extension set. Instruct the patient on the amount of movement permitted. Check regularly for swelling, as above.	support. Reassure the patient.
	Circulatory overload.	Administer infusion fluids at the prescribed rate and do not make sudden alterations of flow. Be aware of the patient's renal and cardiac status. Monitor intake and output routinely.	Slow the infusion. Monitor vital signs for increase in blood pressure and respirations. Place the patient in an upright position and keep him/her warm to promote peripheral circulation and relieve stress on the central veins. Reassure the patient. Notify a doctor immediately.
Pain at the insertion site.	All of the previous listed conditions may be accompanied by soreness or pain.	As previously listed.	Provide local symptomatic relief as required. Administer systemic analgesia, as prescribed, if necessary.
Pyrexia, rigors, tachycardia.	Septicaemia.	Adhere to aseptic techniques when performing all intravenous procedures. Inspect all equipment, infusion fluids, etc., before use. Observe recommendations for additives, equipment changes and general management. Avoid hazardous equipment, e.g. stopcocks.	Notify a doctor immediately. Follow hospital policy about sending equipment for bacterial analysis.
Decrease in blood pressure, tachycardia, cyanosis, unconsciousness.	Embolism: (a) Air.	Check the containers and change before they run dry, especially bottles. Clear all air from tubing before commencing infusion. Check all connections regularly and make sure they are secure.	Turn the patient onto left side and lower the head of the bed to prevent air from entering the pulmonary artery. Notify a doctor immediately. Reassure the patient by explaining what is happening.
	(b) Particle.	Check all infusion fluids before and after any additions have been made. Check drug compatibility and	As above, but also change the container and giving set. Replace with new equipment and normal saline 0.9%

		stability. Observe the solution throughout the infusion for precipitate formation.	infusion from a different batch. Follow hospital policy about sending contaminated fluid and equipment for bacterial analysis.
Itching, rash, shortness of breath.	Allergic reaction due to sensitivity to an intravenous fluid, additive or drug.	Ask the patient if he/she has any allergies *before* administration of any drugs or fluids. Check whether the particular medication is commonly associated with any allergic reactions and observe the patient more closely.	Stop drug infusion or injection and maintain the patency of the intravenous line using normal saline 0.9%. Notify a doctor immediately. Reassure the patient.
Flushed face, headache, congestion of the chest, possibly progressing to loss of consciousness.	Speed shock due to too rapid administration of drugs.	Administer drugs and infusion at the correct rate. Check the flow rate frequently. Use mechanical aids if the delivery rate is crucial.	As above.

FLOW CONTROL

Definition

The delivery of intravenous fluids and medications at an appropriate rate and in a constant, accurate manner, to achieve the desired therapeutic response and to prevent complications. The nurse has a responsibility to determine the correct rate in individual circumstances and to maintain that rate throughout the infusion.

Indications

The following should be considered when a decision on flow control is to be made.

Complications associated with over-infusion include:

1. Fluid overload with accompanying electrolyte imbalance.
2. Metabolic disturbances during parenteral nutrition, mainly related to serum glucose levels.
3. Toxic concentrations of medications, which may result in a shock-like syndrome ('speed shock').
4. Air embolism, due to containers running dry before expected.
5. An increase in venous complications, e.g. chemical phlebitis, caused by reduced dilution of irritant substances.

Complications associated with under-infusion include:

1. Dehydration.
2. Metabolic disturbances, as above.
3. A delayed response to medications.
4. Occlusion of a cannula/catheter due to slow cessation of flow.

Delivery of fluids and medications should be constant over a period with no major adjustments to 'catch up' Small alterations are permissible.

REFERENCE MATERIAL

Factors affecting infusion rates

Fluid and container

The type of fluid, viscosity and the temperature at which it is delivered affect the rate of flow. The amount of fluid within the container exerts a pressure which falls as delivery continues. Therefore, adjustments in height may be required. The optimum height of the container above the patient is 0.9 m and consequently changes in the patient's position may mean further adjustment.

Flow control clamps

The roller clamps used to control fluid flow may slip, loosen or distort the tubing causing a phenomenon known as 'cold flow'. Any marked tension or stretching of the tubing, due to movement by the patient, can render the clamp ineffective.

Cannula/catheter/intravenous line

The flow rate may be affected by any of the following:

1. The condition and size of the vein.
2. The gauge of the cannula/catheter.
3. The position of the device within the vein.
4. The site of the intravenous device, e.g. it may be positional.
5. Kinking or compression of the cannula/catheter.
6. Occlusion of the cannula/catheter due to clot formation.

The drop calibration of the administration set limits flow rate and when slower delivery is required microdrip sets should be used.

The tubing of the administration set may become pinched or kinked causing variations in the set rate.

Inclusion of other in-line devices, e.g. filters, may also affect the flow.

The patient

Patients occasionally tamper with the control clamp or other parts of the delivery system, e.g. adjusting the height of the infusion container, thereby making flow unreliable.

Complications associated with flow control

At-risk groups include:

1. Infants and young children.
2. The elderly.
3. Patients with compromised cardiovascular status.
4. Patients with impairment or failure of organs, e.g. kidneys.
5. Patients with major sepsis.
6. Patients suffering from shock, whatever the cause.
7. Postoperative or post-trauma patients.
8. Stressed patients, whose endocrine homeostatic controls may be affected.
9. Patients receiving multiple medications, whose clinical status may change rapidly.

Fluid/electrolyte imbalance

The most common disorder of fluid and electrolyte balance is circulatory overload, that is isotonic fluid expansion. It is caused by infusion of excessive quantities of isotonic fluids such as normal saline 0.9%. No flow of fluid from the extracellular to the intracellular compartment occurs and, therefore, the extracellular volume increases.

Due to electrolyte concentration, no extra water is available to enable the kidneys selectively to excrete and restore the balance. Early clinical manifestations of this condition are:

1. Weight gain.
2. An increase in fluid intake over output.
3. A high pulse pressure.
4. Raised central venous pressure measurements.
5. An increased peripheral hand vein emptying time (normally three to five seconds).
6. Peripheral oedema.
7. Hoarseness.

Progression will lead to dyspnoea and cyanosis, due to pulmonary oedema, and neck vein engorgement.

The nurse needs to recognize the condition early so that fluid can be withheld until excesses have been excreted. Careful monitoring should continue to prevent isotonic contraction occurring.

If a patient is receiving large quantities of electrolyte free water, such as glucose 5% in water, to replace losses from gastric suction, vomit, diarrhoea, diuresis or insensible loss, hypotonic expansion may develop. This involves both extracellular and intracellular compartments.

This condition is more frequently seen in the early postoperative period and in the elderly patient. Signs which differentiate hypotonic from isotonic expansion are:

1. The pulse and blood pressure usually remain normal.
2. Intracranial pressure is raised causing headache, nausea, vomiting, muscle twitching and confusion.
3. Tibial oedema is present.

Fluids will be withheld and careful correction of electrolyte balance undertaken.

Metabolic disturbance

Metabolic disturbances are related to total parenteral nutrition and most commonly to glucose intolerance. This may result in either a hyper- or hypoglycaemic state. Signs of hypoglycaemia include weakness, headache, thirst and a cold clammy skin. Hyperglycaemia will lead rapidly to coma.

Disturbances in fat metabolism may occur if too rapid infusion takes place. These are most likely in patients with disordered liver function, major infections or other conditions which create stress.

Accurate control of flow rates of all feeding solutions is essential and the *maximum* recommended adjustment of flow is four drops per minute every 15 minutes.

Administration of drugs

Rapid, uncontrolled administration of drugs will result in toxic concentrations reaching vital organs. Toxicity may be manifested by an exaggeration of the usual pharmacological actions of the drug or by signs and symptoms specific for that drug or class of drugs. The most extreme toxic response which can occur if a drug is given at a dose or rate exceeding that recommended, is the lethal response.

Signs of speed shock include:

1. Flushed face.
2. Headache.
3. Congestion of the chest.
4. Tachycardia, fall in blood pressure.
5. Syncope.
6. Shock.
7. Cardiovascular collapse.

Administration must be slowed down or discontinued, and the medical staff notified (see Nursing care plan, above, final entry).

Paediatric intravenous therapy

Paediatrics is an area where extra care is required. The heart and circulatory system are smaller, therefore fluid and electrolyte imbalance and circulatory overload can occur more rapidly. Maintenance of flow is usually achieved by the use of special sets and regular monitoring of intake and output is performed.

For example:

Intake

1. An hourly record of the amount and type of fluid.
2. A running total of the amount administered.
3. Regular checks of the infusion device and the rate of flow.
4. Recording the volume of diluent used in drug reconstitution.
5. Checking the electrolyte content of drug presentations, especially sodium and potassium.
6. Consideration of additional water needs due to a faster metabolic rate, and a greater loss in urine due to immature renal function.

Output

1. Careful recording all output, including weighing nappies.
2. Recording any other drainage, e.g. from a wound site.
3. Adjustments to allow for insensible loss via a greater surface area.

Other observations include weight and general condition and behaviour, e.g. tachycardia, raised blood pressure and respirations, oedema, headache, abdominal cramps.

Dose calculations of medications should be checked carefully as micrograms are frequently used, and amounts often include a decimal point.

Total parenteral nutrition in children requires extra careful delivery and monitoring.

Summary

Careful calculation and control of flow rates are essential as delivery of fluids and medications may be critical due to any of the factors mentioned above. There are many infusion control devices available to assist the nurse in this task, ranging from the simple to the complex. A knowledge of these systems and of their application is necessary to ensure appropriate choices are made.

References and further reading

Auty, B. (1989) Choice of instrumentation for controlled IV infusion. *Intensive Therapy & Clinical Monitoring*, 10(4), 117–22.

British Medical Association/Pharmaceutical Society of Great Britain (1987) *British National Formulary No. 14.* BMA, London.

Department of Health and Society Security (1984) *Health Equipment Information Evaluation Issue No. 125.* HMSO, London.

Department of Health and Society Security (1985) *Health Equipment Information Evaluation Issue No. 135/147.* HMSO, London.

Department of Health and Society Security (1986) *Health Equipment Information Evaluation Issue No. 157.* HMSO, London.

Department of Health and Society Security (1987) *Health Equipment Information Evaluation Issue No. 175.* HMSO, London.

Department of Health and Society Security (1989) *Health Equipment Information Evaluation Issue No. 193.* HMSO, London.

Department of Health and Society Security (1990) *Health Equipment Information Evaluation Issue No. 198.* HMSO, London.

Hudek, K. (1986) Compliance in intravenous therapy. *Journal of Canadian Intravenous Nurses Association*, 2(3), 7–8.

Leggett, A. (1990) Intravenous infusion pumps. *Nursing Standard*, 4 April, 4(28), 24–6.

Leggett, A. (1990) Looking at infusion devices. *Nursing Standard*, 18 April, 4(30), 29–31.

Luken, J. & Middleton, J. (1990) Intravenous infusion controllers. *Nursing Standard*, 11 April, 4(29), 30–2.

Miller, J. (1989) Intravenous therapy in fluid and electrolyte imbalance. *The Professional Nurse*, February, p. 237.

Plumer, A. L. (1987) *Principles and Practice of Intravenous Therapy*, 4th edn. Little, Brown & Co, Boston, USA.

Sager, D. & Bomar, S. (1980) *Intravenous Medications.* J. B.

Lippincott, Philadelphia.
Sepion, B. (1990) Intravenous care for children. *Paediatric Nursing*. April, 14–16.
Wittig, P. & Semmler-Bertanzi, D. J. (1983) Pumps and controllers: a nurse's assessment guide. *American Journal of Nursing*, 7, 1023–5.

GUIDELINES: CHOICE OF AN INFUSION CONTROL SYSTEM

Common available choices

1. Gravity drip, including measured volume sets.
2. Drip rate controller.
3. Volumetric controllers.
4. Volumetric pump.
5. Syringe pump/ambulatory pump.

Simple gravity drip

Advantages	**Disadvantages**
Low cost.	Infusion pressure limited by height of fluid container.
Familiar to all staff.	Requires frequent observation and adjustment.
Minimal risk of extravascular infusion.	Variability of drop size influences accuracy of flow rate. Inclusion of a burette chamber increases accuracy as delivery in millitres/hour.
Infusion of air is unlikely.	Infusion rates limited especially with viscous fluids and small cannula or catheters.
	Arterial infusion impossible.

Indications for use

1. Delivery of fluids without additives on the majority of peripheral lines.
2. Delivery of fluids without additives on some central venous lines.
3. Administration of fluids containing a small amount or low concentration of medication, e.g. 20 mmol KCl/litre, in the above circumstances.
4. Administration of drugs where adverse effects are not anticipated if the infusion rate varies slightly.
5. When the patient's condition does not give cause for concern and no complications are predicted.
6. In situations where the rate of infusion is too great to be controlled by the devices available, e.g. 500 ml/hr.

Comments

Many infusions are controlled adequately using the above method. Increased accuracy can be achieved by use of a burette set.

Over recent years, mechanical infusion devices have been used increasingly to ensure greater accuracy than the simple gravity drip can offer. To meet the increase in demand, manufacturers have produced a number of new products, ranging from the basic to the advanced. It is important to consider the following points before purchasing new devices.

1. The most *appropriate* device to deliver safe care to patients.
2. Accuracy of device.
3. Device that is easy to use ('user friendly').
4. Standardizing of equipment (where possible).
5. Cost and running cost of device.

A controller is a mechanical device that operates by gravity rather than positive pressure. There are a variety of different controllers available ranging from the drops/minute set, to volumetric, non-designated, or designated giving sets, to basic alarm systems and even more complex sets.

Drip rate controllers

Advantages	**Disadvantages**
Automatic control eliminates the frequent adjustment required by the simple gravity drop.	Infusion pressure limited by height of fluid container.
Conventional low-cost administration sets usually used (some devices require disposable rate clip to be attached to non-designated giving sets).	Variability of drop size makes accurate determination of flow rate difficult.
Minimal risk of extravascular infusion.	Infusion rates limited especially with viscous fluids and small cannulae.
Infusion of air unlikely.	Not suitable for blood transfusion.
Alarms available.	Arterial infusion impossible.
May be used on central lines.	

Indications for use
As for simple gravity drip (see above).

Comments
The maximum rate at which this device can deliver is 500 ml/hr.

Mechanical infusion pumps

The mechanical infusion pump is a device that delivers fluid or medication by pressure in spite of variable resistence. There are a variety of different pumps available, ranging from the basic to the more advanced, non-designated or designated giving sets. Volumetric pumps have now superseded the drops/minute devices.

In recent years, the occlusion alarm has increasingly become an important factor in device selection. The occlusion alarm will sound when increased pressure is detected by the device. There are now a number of different pumps on the market with varying occlusion alarm pressures.

The standard volumetric pump will often have a set occlusion of 499 mm/hr, whereas a more advanced pump device allows the user to alter the occlusion alarm to suit the situation, or has the occlusion alarm set at a lower level.

A lower occlusion alarm has a number of advantages:

1. An increase in pressure will be detected at an early stage.
2. Less bolus on correction of occlusion.
3. Less time where patient is not receiving fluid or drug.

No device can detect extravasation; however, where an early detection of an occlusion is identified, extravasation might be avoided.

In some devices the occlusion alarm can sound at a low setting initially, and can then be moved to a higher occlusion pressure if the alarm is over-ridden by the user.

Consideration of running costs must be made when purchasing a device, as these may exceed the cost of the device within a short time if designated giving sets are used. Thus a number of volumetric pumps have recently been introduced which do not require designated giving sets, and this has substantial implications for costing. It must be remembered, however, that quality of care must always be the most important factor when considering device selection.

Volumetric pump

Advantages	**Disadvantages**
Accurate control of rate in ml/hr.	Generally higher volumetric instrument cost.

Guidelines: Choice of an infusion control system

Advantages	**Disadvantages**
Accurate control of volume infused.	Where special designated administration sets are required, higher cost will be incurred (cost of disposables may soon exceed instrument cost if used frequently).
Pressure maintains rate in spite of variable resistance.	Pressure may produce extensive extravascular infusion.
Wide choice of infusion rates.	
Wide range of features provided, e.g. central venous pressure (CVP) monitoring.	
Variable pressure setting capacity.	More complicated device.
Alarms available, including protection against air embolism usually provided.	

Indications for use

Advanced volumetric pump

1. Central lines:
   (a) When infusion of drugs of fluids is critical, e.g. high-dependency situations where drugs are used which affect cardiovascular, respiratory or central nervous system.
   (b) Where other features provided by the device are required, e.g. central venous pressure monitoring.
2. Arterial lines.
3. Peripheral lines (where correct use of variable pressure facility is used):
   (a) An infusion sited in lower limb.
   (b) An infusion sited in a precarious vein – regular flow under pressure may prolong the life of the line.
4. Paediatrics.

Standard volumetric pump

Central lines
When higher occlusion alarm will not compromise safe delivery of intravenous fluid. When infusion of fluids and drugs are not critical, e.g. total parenteral nutrition, or chemotherapy.

Comments
The standard volumetric pump is used on peripheral lines in many areas. However, with the varied device selection that is now offered, it is more appropriate to use either a controller device or advanced volumetric pump device (used correctly), thus further reducing the risk of high pressure in the vein.

Syringe/ambulatory pump

The syringe pump usually accommodates either 60 ml syringe or a variety of sizes up to 60 ml. The device delivers in ml/hr. It is used in situations where patients are immobile, e.g. high-dependency situations, or for short-term therapy, i.e. one hour or less.

The ambulatory pump can be divided into two types:

1. Syringe driver.
2. Reservoir pump.

The syringe driver takes a variety of different sized syringes, ranging from 2 to 20 ml. The syringe driver is small, battery fed and is appropriate for an ambulatory patient, when non-critical drug delivery is being administered. Over a number of years, syringe drivers have been used for intravenous delivery. Due to their basic design they should be used with caution on intravenous lines. All syringe drivers must have a clip on the device to prevent possible negative pressure drawing the fluid or medication at an uncontrolled rate into the patient. The volume is delivered in mm/hr or mm/24 hr. (See Chapter 38, Syringe Drivers, for further details.)

The reservoir pump is being used increasingly for patients receiving continuous therapy lasting from an hour or hours, to a number of days. These devices have the added advantage of being able to accommodate a higher volume, e.g. up to 65 ml. The reservoir is encased in the device, leading to greater safety. However, these disposable devices are more expensive, as with some portable infusion systems, where a completely new system is used each time.

Patient-controlled analgesic pumps are also available in both syringe pumps and reservoir pumps.

Syringe pump/driver/reservoir

Advantages	**Disadvantages**
Accurate control of volumetric rate.	Unsuitable for large volumes.
Accurate control of volume infused.	Pressure may produce extravascular infusion.
Particularly suited for small volumes and low infusion rates.	Comprehensive alarm systems not always provided.
Pressure maintains rate in spite of variable resistance.	
Infusion of air unlikely.	
Some alarms are available.	
Some pumps are portable (battery/mains powered).	
Arterial infusion is possible.	
Generally cheaper than volumetric pumps, with low-cost disposables (with exception of reservoir pumps).	

Indications for use
Delivery of small-volume continuous infusions, e.g. insulin, heparin, analgesia, chemotherapy.

Comments
When using a syringe pump/driver on a peripheral line, it must be regularly checked to detect any extravasation at the earliest moment.

PROBLEM SOLVING

Problems are listed under general headings. The action to be taken to prevent or correct these may vary depending on the make or model of the equipment. Therefore, the most important point of reference is the manufacturer's instruction sheet or booklet, which should be read carefully before use.

Occasional malfunctions, including false alarms

Although machines provide a valuable aid to patient care, they do not replace the need for good nursing assessment and intervention. They should be checked frequently to ensure the device is functioning correctly, the flow rate is maintained and that no infiltration has occurred, if attached to a peripheral line.

Infection

Strict aseptic technique should be maintained when setting up or changing the pump/controller administration

Problem solving

set. Connections must be secure, preferably Luer locks when fluid is delivered under pressure. All components of the system should be changed every 24 hours, as per hospital policy.

Air embolism

Administration sets should be primed carefully and all air eliminated. Connections must be secure, preferably Luer locks when fluid is delivered under pressure. Pumps with a peristaltic action can pump air if it enters the tubing below the drip chamber.

Flow rate inaccuracies

These may occur due to:

1. Variability of drop size.
2. Air trapped in the cassette chamber of volumetric sets.
3. A malposition of the drop sensor – drops may be missed or splashes counted as drops.
4. Tilting or dirt on the drip chamber may affect the sensor.

Occlusion

Occlusion of the tubing or kinking can cause alarms. Tubing should be looped and taped to prevent this. If maximum pressure is reached by a pump, connections may repture and if a catheter becomes occluded the pressure may cause it to split with serious consequences for the patient. A peripheral insertion site should be checked frequently for infiltration.

Crushing of the tubing

Crushing of the tubing of the administration set may occur resulting in malfunction. Tubing should be repositioned every few hours to prevent this if using a peristaltic mechanism. A movement of 5 to 7.5 cm forward or backward is sufficient.

Opaque fluids

Fluids such as blood and fat emulsions may not be detected by some drop sensors. Manufacturers' information should be checked. Most models can pump blood without causing haemolysis but again refer to the literature.

The alarm

An alarm should always be turned on, and taken notice of, to be of value. It may be silenced while the problem is being assessed but should not be turned off permanently. The delivery system should be checked and the device reset. Only after a thorough assessment should malfunction be assumed to be the cause.

Dislodgement of the tubing or cassette

The patient may accidentally or deliberately dislodge the tubing or casette or manipulate flow rate setting. Adequate explanation may prevent this but restraint may be necessary in confused or restless patients.

Electrical or mechanical malfunction

Electrical or mechanical malfunction may occur due to inadequate cleaning or inexperienced handling. All equipment requires regular servicing, but simple measures – such as ensuring the drop sensor is clean and moves freely – can result in trouble-free usage.

22

Iodine-131 Treatment Protocol

Definition

Radioactive iodine-131 is a beta-gamma emitter with a half-life of eight days, and is used mainly in the form of iodide solution (an unsealed source). The beta radiation gives a high, local dose in iodine-concentrating tissue. The gamma component is useful for external measurement and scanning.

Indications

1. *Iodide*
   Thyroid tissue selectively concentrates iodide and this enables iodine-131 to be used in the diagnosis and treatment of thyroid disorders:
   (a) For thyrotoxicosis, treatment doses usually between 75 and 400 megabecquerel (MBq) (Table 22.1) activity of iodine-131 can be given, usually on an outpatient basis.
   (b) For well differentiated thyroid cancers (papillary and follicular), and metastases that function similarly to the thyroid tissue. Treatment is usually on an inpatient basis because of the higher activities involved.
   Iodine-131 is normally administered as a solution taken orally by the patient, although occasionally it may be given in the form of capsules. It can also be administered intravenously.
2. *Meta-iodobenzylguanidine (MIBG)*
   This is used to treat patients with neural crest tumours such as neuroblastomas in children and phaeochromocytomas in adults. MIBG stimulates noradrenaline and is localized, therefore, by receptive sympathetic nervous tissue. MIBG is administered as an intravenous infusion over 30 to 60 minutes. Care of patients receiving MIBG follows the same guidelines as for patients receiving iodine-131 for thyroid cancers, particularly where it relates to radiation protection. Treatment doses are based on dosimetry calculations and are typically 7 to 12 gigabecquerel (GBq).

Table 22.1

A Becquerel is the Système International (SI) unit of activity and is 1 disintegration per second

K (Kilo) = 1×10^3

M (Mega) = 1×10^6 e.g. megabecquerel (MBq)

G (Giga) = 1×10^9

REFERENCE MATERIAL

Treatment programme for carcinoma of the thyroid

Surgical removal of the thyroid

Normal thyroid tissue usually concentrates iodine more efficiently than malignant tissue, and some malignant tissues concentrate iodine-131 only after removal of normal tissue. It is recommended, therefore, that a surgical near-total thyroidectomy is performed before administration of iodine-131.

Iodine-131 treatment

Following thyroidectomy an ablation dose of, typically, 3 GBq of iodine-131 is administered to ablate remnants of thyroid tissue. Further treatments of 5.5 GBq may be necessary to destroy deposits in local lymph nodes and distant metastases.

Principles of protection policies

Iodine-131 is excreted rapidly in patients who have had a thyroidectomy via all body fluids, in particular, the urine (see Figure 22.1). In those patients who have not undergone thyroidectomy, excretion is rapid initially, slowing as the iodine-131 is bound by the thyroid tissue. Consequently, great care must be taken with all body fluids, especially during the first few days.

The precautions to be observed must be available to

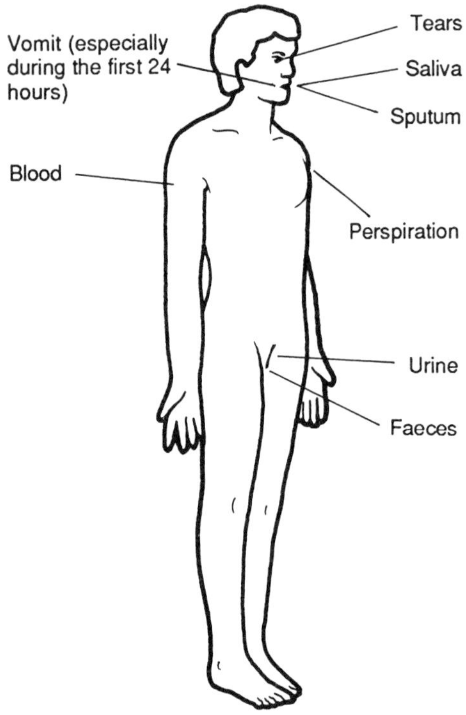

Figure 22.1 The patient's body fluids will be highly radioactive, especially during the first few days after administration of iodine-131.

hospital personnel as a written system of work. Nurses must follow the procedures as set out during the period when controlled area restrictions apply. This, and careful planning of work, will ensure radiation exposure is minimized, compatible with good nursing care.

The principles of distance, shielding and time limitation must be observed to minimize radiation exposure.

The following radiation protection policies and nursing guidelines are written to conform with the *Ionizing Radiations Regulations, 1985 and 1988* and associated guidance notes. They are applicable to The Royal Marsden Hospital, where dedicated single-bed treatment rooms with en suite toilet and bathing facilities are available.

Further precautions may be necessary when these conditions are not met. The advice of the radiation protection advisor must then be sought.

Controlled area
The entrance to the controlled area must be marked with a warning sign. Information is displayed to indicate the following:

1. The radioactive material and activity administered.
2. The nursing time allowed per day:
   (a) Essential nursing procedures only should be carried out and unnecessary time must not be spent in close proximity to the patient while the sign is displayed.
   (b) The time given is such that a nurse remaining at a distance of approximately 60 cm from the patient for the time indicated each day would, after five consecutive days, receive the maximum permissible dose for the working week.

Appropriate barriers, i.e. lead shields, should be placed at the entrance to the controlled area to:

1. Prevent inadvertent entry by unauthorized personnel.
2. Minimize radiation exposure to visitors and staff.

Patients treated with iodine-131 should be confined to their rooms, except for special medical or nursing procedures, when they must be accompanied by suitably trained staff.

Film badges
Film badges should be worn at all times when on duty.

Contamination control
With iodine-131 in an unsealed form, it is important to guard against contamination both of personnel and the hospital environment by the correct use of protective gloves, gowns and overshoes. The application of cosmetics, eating, drinking or smoking while there is any possibility that the hands are contaminated is prohibited.

In the event of any incident involving radioactive material, the physics department must be advised immediately, even if the incident occurs outside normal working hours.

Preparation of the iodine-131 therapy room

Equipment
Equipment should be kept to a minimum. It must be checked to ensure that it is in working order, as maintenance staff will only be allowed into the room in exceptional circumstances.

Bed linen and disposable items (gloves, aprons, overshoes, cutlery and crockery) should be kept in a utility room or ante-room along with the patient's treatment chart and a radiation monitor.

Personal items
Nurses should be sensitive to the psychological implications for patients of being labelled 'radioactive' and confined in isolation. Although patients may want to bring some personal belongings with them, they should be advised to keep these to a minimum, as items may become contaminated and need to be left in an appropriate place in hospital for a while after the patient's discharge.

Protective floor covering
Plastic-backed absorbent paper, kept in place by adhesive tape, is used to retain accidental urine spills or splashes on the floor immediately surrounding the toilet. Each patient is assessed to decide if further floor covering is necessary, e.g. catheterized patients will require floor covering below a catheter bag.

Cleaning of an iodine-131 treatment room

During occupancy of the treatment room by the patient, cleaning of the room is kept to a minimum and should be supervised by the physics staff. After the patient is discharged, monitoring and any necessary decontamination of the room will be arranged by the physics department, which will inform the relevant personnel when this has been completed. Only then may the room be entered and thoroughly cleaned.

Preparation of the patient

Consent

Patients are required to sign a consent form agreeing to treatment with iodine-131, iodide or MIBG, following a full explanation from the treating clinician. This is to comply with legal requirments and local hospital policy. Consent is usually obtained in the outpatient clinic before ordering the radioactive material.

Before admission

Thyroid treatments

Twenty-one days before admission:
Patients taking tetraiodothyronine (T4) (thyroxine) must stop taking this medication.

Ten days before admission:
Patients taking triiodothyronine (T3) must stop taking this medication.

Three days before admission:
Occasionally, to enhance the uptake of iodine-131, three daily injections of thyroid-stimulating hormone are administered.

MIBG

To prevent the uptake of any free iodine-131, the thyroid gland is blocked by giving patients oral iodine three days before and three weeks post-administration of MIBG.

As MIBG simulates noradrenaline, there are some drugs that act as antagonists, e.g. phenothiazines, and these are contraindicated during treatment.

On admission

Before the administration of iodine-131, any symptoms of diarrhoea or constipation must be remedied. Diarrhoea could result in contamination of the treatment area. Constipation not only inhibits the elimination of radioactivity but could also obscure radiological investigations, e.g. scanning.

Patients and relatives should be educated about the principles of radiation protection and the procedures with which the patient has to comply while in isolation. It is important to identify potential anxieties before the administration of iodine-131 while the nurse is able to reassure the patient and is unconstrained by time limits.

The patient must also agree to stay in hospital until the physics department advises that the level of radioactivity permits discharge.

Discharge of the patient

A patient should not be discharged from hospital until the activity of iodine-131 retained has fallen below recommended levels. This level will depend on several factors, including:

1. Mode of transport on leaving hospital.
2. Journey time involved.
3. Personal circumstances, i.e. young children or pregnant women at home.

Patients will be assessed individually for radiation clearance by the physics department before discharge, and the results will be given to the treating clinician. Advice will be given to patients on issues such as return to work and visits to public places. Patients who are discharged with more than 150 MBq of iodine-131 retained will be given appropriate information in the form of an instruction card carrying details of precautions to be taken. This card must be signed by the treating clinician.

It must be emphasized that this card is to be carried and the instructions followed until the latest date shown so that, for instance, staff would be alerted should the patient be readmitted to hospital. Additional verbal instructions may be necessary.

Regulations

Ionizing Radiations Regulations (1985) HMSO, London.

Ionizing Radiations (Protection of Persons Undergoing Medical Examination or Treatment), Regulations (1988) HMSO, London.

References and further reading

International Commission on Radiological Protection Publication 57: Radiological Protection of the Worker in Medicine and Dentistry, 1990, Pergamon Press, Oxford.

National Council for Radiation Protection (NCRP) Report 105 (1989) *Radiation Protection for Medical and Allied Health Personnel*. NCRP.

National Radiological Protection Board (NRPB) (1988) *Guidance Notes For the Protection of Persons Against Ionizing Radiations Arising from Medical Use*. HMSO, London.

Mould, R. F. (1985) *Radiation Protection in Hospitals*. Adam Hilger, Bristol and Boston.

Tiffany, R. (Ed.) (1988) *Oncology for Nurses and Health Care Professionals, Volumes 1 and 2*. George Allen & Unwin, London.

Walter, J. (1977) *Cancer and Radiotherapy*. Churchill Livingstone, Edinburgh.

GUIDELINES: NURSING THE PATIENT BEFORE THE ADMINISTRATION OF IODINE-131

Action	Rationale
1. The patient is to be fasted for two hours before and after administration of an iodine-131 dose. Offer a light diet for the remainder of the day.	To reduce the risk of nausea and/or vomiting.
2. Administer a prophylactic antiemetic 30 minutes before scheduled administration of the dose.	To prevent vomiting.
3. Check that the preparation of the room and the patient is complete. Ensure that any surplus items have been removed.	To prevent contamination of extraneous equipment.
4. Apply a wristband showing the radiation warning symbol to the patient's wrist.	To identify the patient as radioactive.
5. Place the radiation warning sign at the entrance to the therapy room.	To identify the room as a controlled area.

GUIDELINES: NURSING THE PATIENT RECEIVING IODINE-131 THYROID TREATMENT

Action	Rationale
1. Assist the patient to remove dentures/bridges.	To prevent radioactive material being trapped behind dental plates.
2. The patient drinks the iodine-131 through a straw, physically directed by an authorized physicist in the presence of the clinician directing treatment.	Drinking through a straw reduces the amount of radioactive material left around the mouth. To meet current regulations.
3. Offer the patient a drink of water to rinse out the mouth. (This must be swallowed.) Assist the patient to replace dentures.	To remove any iodine-131 from inside the mouth.

GUIDELINES: NURSING THE PATIENT RECEIVING IODINE-131 MIBG TREATMENT

Action	Rationale
1. Apply a vital signs monitor with a variable time setting mode to the patient that will be visible to staff from outside the room	Following the administration of MIBG, a transient rise in blood pressure and pulse may occur.
2. Check that the patient has been cannulated, and commence prescribed intravenous fluids three hours before iodine-131 MIBG administration.	Iodine-131 MIBG is administered intravenously through a three-way tap attached to the giving set.
3. Set up iodine-131 MIBG infusion and give over 30 to 60 minutes.	To minimize transient rise in blood pressure and pulse.
4. Monitor blood pressure and pulse: (a) Every five minutes during infusion. (b) Every ten minutes for the first 45 minutes post-infusion; (c) Hourly for four hours. (d) Four-hourly or more frequently if required.	To detect and monitor any change.
5. Continue intravenous hydration for 24 hours post-infusion and simultaneously encourage oral fluids.	To increase the urinary output and elimination of radioactivity from the bladder.

GUIDELINES: NURSING THE PATIENT AFTER ADMINISTRATION OF IODINE-131

Entering the room

Action	Rationale
1. Put on disposable gloves.	To prevent contamination of the hands.
2. Put on disposable overshoes.	To prevent spread of contamination outside the treatment area.
3. Put on a suitable protective gown: (a) Long-sleeve cotton gown, e.g. for lifting patient. (b) Disposable water-repellent gown, e.g. for dealing with vomit or incontinence.	 To protect against low levels of contamination, e.g. from the patient's skin. To protect against high levels of contamination.
4. Plan work before entering the controlled area and then work quickly and efficiently, keeping within the time allowance stated.	To minimize radiation exposure, as consistent with good nursing care.
5. Use disposable crockery and cutlery only, to present meals to patients.	China crockery and cutlery may become contaminated.

Maintaining patient comfort and hygiene

Action	Rationale
1. Encourage the patient to bathe/shower frequently, at least once a day.	To reduce any radioactive perspiration on the skin.

Guidelines: Nursing the patient after administration of iodine-131

Action	Rationale
2. Encourage the patient to wash the hands thoroughly after each possible contact with bodily fluids, e.g. cleaning teeth, going to the toilet, etc.	To remove radioactivity from the hands.
3. The patient should remove and clean regularly any dentures under running water.	To remove radioactive saliva from around dentures.
4. The patient should remove and rinse regularly any contact lenses in their usual cleaning fluid.	To remove any radioactive tears from lenses.
5. Encourage a good fluid intake of between two and three litres per day.	To increase the urinary output and elimination of radioactivity from the bladder.
6. Ensure that the patient has own personal toilet facilities and flushes the toilet twice after use.	To reduce contamination of others and of the environment. Urine of patients treated with iodine-131 is initially extremely radioactive.
7. Bedbound patients should be catheterized before the dose is given. Empty the catheter bag every four to six hours, or more frequently if necessary.	Catheterization reduces the nursing time spent with the patient. Frequent emptying of the bag reduces the radiation level in the room.
8. If the patient requires a bedpan or urinal, this item must be kept solely for this patient's use. The bedpan or urinal must be handled carefully with gloved hands and the contents disposed of in the toilet, which is flushed twice. The bedpan or urinal may be washed in the bedpan washer. It should be sealed in a plastic bag for the journey to and from the sluice.	To reduce contamination of the environment and of other patients and staff.
9. If leakage occurs from injection sites, wound sites etc., the nurse should contact the medical staff and the physics department immediately. Any contact with the dressing should be done with long-handled forceps.	It must be remembered that all body fluids are potentially radioactive.
10. Gloves and a protective gown must be worn whenever handling soiled bed linen.	To prevent contamination.
11. All soiled linen must be deposited in a special container provided for this purpose.	Soiled linen must be monitored for contamination before going to the laundry.

Visitors

Action	Rationale
1. Visiting time is limited as advised by the physicist during the first day following administration of iodine-131 or iodine-131 MIBG.	The patient is extremely radioactive during this period.
2. On subsequent days visiting is unlimited, providing visitors remain outside the room behind the lead screen.	To minimize the exposure of visitors to radiation.

Action	Rationale
3. Physical contact with the patient or bed linen is not allowed.	To prevent contamination of visitors.
4. Children under 16 years of age and pregnant women should be discouraged from visiting.	Radiation exposure of children and the unborn must be kept as low as practicable.

On leaving the room

Action	Rationale
1. Remove overshoes, taking care not to touch the shoes worn underneath.	These are removed first to prevent the spread of contamination.
2. Remove the plastic apron, by holding the front of apron and breaking the neck and waist ties.	
3. Remove gloves by peeling them off the hands, taking care not to touch the outside surfaces with bare hands, and discard them in the bin provided.	To prevent transfer of contamination from the gloves' outer surfaces to the hands.
4. Wash hands thoroughly using soap and water.	To remove any contamination.
5. Use the radiation monitor each time after entering the room and monitor for contamination of the hands, feet and clothing. If contamination has occurred, inform the physics department immediately and follow the decontamination procedure (see page 278).	To ensure that the nurse is not contaminated.
6. Use the thyroid monitor to monitor thyroid uptake after each shift.	To check for thyroid and lung uptake.

GUIDELINES: EMERGENCY PROCEDURES

In an emergency, the safety and medical care of the patient must take precedence over any potential radiation hazards to staff. Written radiation safety instructions must be available in all radiation areas where an emergency may arise. These instructions must contain a detailed description of how to manage a patient in the event of a medical emergency and the action required in other emergency situations such as fire. The course of action in an emergency procedure depends on local circumstances and the nature of the emergency.

An incident occurring within the first 24 hours of iodine-131 being administered is obviously a greater hazard than a similar incident on the day of discharge.

Incontinence and/or vomiting

Action	Rationale
1. Inform the physics department immediately. Put on gloves and a gown. Remove the patient from the contaminated area.	So that the physics department can advise on radiation protection as soon as possible.
2. If physics department staff are not immediately available, use a radiation monitor to assess the extent of the spillage.	To define extent of contamination and determine what further measures need to be taken.

Guidelines: Emergency procedures

Action	**Rationale**
3. Put some absorbent material on top of all the radioactive wet area.	To absorb contamination.
4. Leave the area until physics department staff arrive. Polythene sheets may be placed over all of the contaminated area.	To prevent spread of contamination.

Contamination of bare hands

Action	**Rationale**
1. Wash hands in warm soapy water, paying special attention to the areas around the fingernails, between the fingers and on the outer edges of the hands. Continue washing until contamination is below the permissible limits indicated by local monitoring protocols.	To remove radioactive material from any areas where it might be trapped. Hot water should not be used as it may increase skin absorption.
2. If a wound is produced in a contamination accident, wash thoroughly under running water, opening the edges of the cut. This should be continued until physics department staff can demonstrate that no residual radioactivity remains in the wound.	To stimulate bleeding and permit thorough flushing of the cut.

Death

Action	**Rationale**
1. Inform the physics department immediately.	So that the physics department staff can begin making the necessary arrangements for removal of the body to the mortuary.
2. Two nurses wearing gloves, plastic aprons, gowns and overshoes should perform last offices. All orifices must be packed carefully. Any vomit, blood, faeces or urine must be cleaned from the body.	To avoid contamination with body fluids. Minimal handling of the body reduces the risk of contamination.
3. The body should be totally enclosed in a plastic cadaver bag.	To avoid contamination of the porters and the mortuary staff.
4. Transfer of the body should be arranged with the physics department.	The physics department will supervise the transfer of the body.

Cardiac arrest

Action	**Rationale**
1. The switchboard must be told to inform the physics department as soon as possible after alerting the emergency resuscitation team.	So that the physics department can advise on radiation protection as soon as possible.

2. Do not use mouth-to-mouth resuscitation. All areas must be supplied with an Ambu bag for this purpose.	Mouth-to-mouth contact could result in contamination of the resuscitator.
3. Overshoes, gloves and gowns must be put on as soon as it is practicably possible.	To minimize personal contamination.
4. All emergency equipment must be monitored and decontaminated as necessary before being returned to general use.	To prevent contaminated equipment leaving the controlled area.

Fire

Action	Rationale
1. Every effort should be made to contact the physics department without compromising the patient's safety.	To help in the evacuation of the patients treated with iodine-131.
2. Following evacuation, patients treated with iodine-131 should be kept at a safe distance from other patients and staff.	To minimize exposure of others to radiation.

23

Last Offices

When a person dies, a number of procedures are carried out under the generic term 'postmortem care'. As nursing students, we learned to wash the body carefully, protect orifices and pad certain areas to prevent bruising. The rationale for these actions was generally presented as 'showing respect for the deceased'. Respect is not the only reason for these procedures: there is a scientific rationale for them.

(Pennington, 1978)

REFERENCE MATERIAL

'Death with dignity' receives much coverage both in the literature and, more locally, within institutions where the patient's demise is often the termination of a bonding that has developed between nurse and patient. It is the performance of respectful last offices that concludes the care given. Today, the United Kingdom is a multicultural, multireligious, multiracial society and nurses should equip themselves with the knowledge of the legal requirements for the care of the dead and a basic understanding of religious and cultural rituals associated with death. The respectful and correct procedure of last offices is so integral to the holistic care of the patient that disregard for them is essentially disregard for the patient. The bibliography listed below should be utilized to develop greater understanding but the nurse should, where possible and appropriate, discover what is required in order to respect the faith.

References and further reading

Ayrton, W. A. (1982) Last offices in cases of notifiable disease. *Nursing Times*, 78, 35; *Journal of Infection Control Nursing, Suppl. 16.*

Berkovits, B. (1990) Multicultural care: a Jewish perspective on nursing. *Nursing Standard*, 4(28), 32–4.

Buckles, A. (1985) Last offices: precautions for dealing with a patient with a known infection. *Nursing Times*, 81(10); *Journal of Infection Control Nursing, Suppl. 12.*

Department of Social Security (1990) *What To Do After A Death*. Department of Social Security, London.

Green, J. (1991) Death with dignity. Meeting the Spiritual Needs of Patients in a Multi-cultural Society. *Nursing Times Publication*. Macmillan Magazines Ltd, London.

Green, J. (1989) Death with dignity – funerals abroad. Part 7. *Nursing Times & Nursing Mirror*, 85(11), 63.

Henley, A. (1982) *Caring for Muslims and Their Families: Religious Aspects of Care*. DHSS/King Edward's Hospital Fund for London, London.

Henley, A. (1983) *Caring for Hindus and Their Families: Religious Aspects of Care*. DHSS/King Edward's Hospital Fund for London, London.

Henley, A. (1983) *Caring for Sikhs and Their Families: Religious Aspects of Care*. DHSS/King Edward's Hospital Fund for London, London.

Lally, M. M. (1978) Last rites and funeral customs of minority groups. *Midwife, Health Visitor & Community Nurse*, 14(7), 224–5.

McGilloway, O. & Myco, F. (eds) (1985) *Nursing and Spiritual Care*. Harper & Row, London.

McGuiness, S. (1986) Coping with death: death rites – initiatives introduced to help nurses in accident and emergency departments cope with patients who die suddenly. *Nursing Times & Nursing Mirror*, 82(12), 28–31.

Mascar, J. (ed) (1962) *Bhagavad Gita*. Penguin, Harmondsworth.

Neuberger, J. (1978) *Caring for Dying People of Different Faiths*. Austen Cornish Publishers, in association with the Lisa Sainsbury Foundation, London.

Olivant, P. (1986) Coping with death: last offices . . . steps nurses should take to help bereaved relatives. *Nursing Times*, 82(12), 32–3.

Pennington, E. A. (1978) Postmortem care: more than ritual. *American Journal of Nursing*, 78, 846–7.

Royal College of Nursing of the United Kingdom. (1981) *Verification of Death and Performances of Last Offices. Typescript B5/pn.* Royal College of Nursing, London.

Sambhi, S. P. & Cole, W. O. (1990) Caring for Sikh patients. *Palliative Medicine*, 4, 229–33.

Sampson, C. (1982) *The Neglected Ethic: Religious and Cultural Factors in the Care of Patients*. McGraw-Hill, New York.

Sharma, D. L. (1990) Hindu attitudes toward suffering, dying and death. *Palliative Medicine*, 4, 235–8.

Storr, E. (1986) The cost of dying – practical details the relatives have to face. *Geriatric Medicine*, 16(16), 40–4.

Thomas, C. H. (1971) Last offices – a reassessment. *Nursing Mirror*, 132(15), 30.

Weymont, G. (1982) The Howie Report. *Nursing Times*, 78(35); *Journal of Infection Control Nursing, Suppl. 16.*

Which? (1987) *What To Do When Someone Dies*. Hodder, London.

Williams, A. (1982) *Procedures Following Deaths in Hospitals*. Institute of Health Services Administrators. London.

Useful addresses

Buddhist Society, 58 Eccleston Square, London SW1 (Tel. 071-834 5858).

Hindu Society, Unit 43, 95 Tooting High Street, London SW17 (Tel. 081-672 1543).

Hospital Chaplaincies Committee, Church House, Deans Yard, Westminster, London, SW1 (Tel. 071-222 9011).

Islamic Cultural Centre, London Central Mosque, 146 Park Road, London NW8 (Tel. 071 724 3362).

Sexton's Office of United Synagogue Burial Society, Woburn House, Upper Woburn Place, London, WC1 (Tel. 071-837 7891).

The Sikh Missionary Society, 10 Featherstone Road, Southall, Middlesex UB2 5AA (Tel. 081 574 1902).

GUIDELINES: LAST OFFICES

Equipment

1. Bowl, soap, disposable towel.
2. Razor, comb, scissors.
3. Foamsticks for oral toilet.
4. Receiver.
5. Identification labels.
6. Any documents required by law or hospital policy, for example, notification of death cards.
7. Plastic or paper shroud or patient's personal clothing.
8. Mortuary sheet (or cadaver bag, if appropriate).
9. Tape or Sellotape.
10. Sterile dressing pack.
11. Bandages.
12. Valuables or property book.
13. Plastic bag for waste.

Procedure

Action	**Rationale**
1. Inform the appropriate medical staff.	A registered medical practitioner who has attended the deceased person during the last illness is required to give a medical certificate of the cause of death. The certificate requires the doctor to state the last date on which he/she saw the deceased alive and whether or not he/she has seen the body after death.
2. Inform the appropriate senior nurse.	Necessary if relatives are not in the hospital at the time of death and need to be informed. Courtesy for administrative purposes.
3. Lay the patient on his/her back. Close his/her eyelids. Remove any pillows. Support the jaw by placing a pillow on the chest underneath the jaw. Remove any mechanical aids, such as syringe drivers, heel pads, etc. Straighten the limbs.	For the patient's dignity, as *rigor mortis* occurs four to six hours after death.
4. Drain the bladder by pressing on the lower abdomen. Pack orifices if fluid secretion continues or may be anticipated. Wear gloves and plastic apron.	Leaking orifices pose a health hazard to staff coming into contact with the body.
5. Remove dressings, drainage tubes etc., unless	If a postmortem is required, because, for example,

Guidelines: Last offices

Action	Rationale
otherwise instructed. A small suture may be required to prevent leakage. If tubes are required to be left in position, they may be cut and spigotted. Cover them with an appropriate dressing and secure with adhesive tape.	the patient dies within 24 hours of surgery or the cause of death is unclear or suspicious.
6. Wash the patient, unless requested not to for religious reasons. Clean nails, nostrils, ears and mouth. Replace any dentures. Shave normally clean-shaven male patients.	For aesthetic and hygienic reasons.
7. Re-dress any wounds, secure dressings with tape or a loose bandage.	Clean dressings are reapplied to contain further leakage from wound sites.
8. Remove all jewellery, in the presence of another nurse, unless requested to do otherwise.	To meet with legal requirements and relatives' wishes.
9. Put a shroud or personal clothing on the body unless requested to do otherwise.	For aesthetic reasons, particularly if relatives want to view the body.
10. Label one wrist and one ankle with an identification label. Complete any documents such as notification of death cards. Copies of such cards are usually required (refer to hospital policy for details). Tape one securely to shroud.	To ensure correct and easy identification of the body in the mortuary.
11. Wrap the body in a mortuary sheet, ensuring that the face and feet are covered and that all limbs are held securely in position.	To avoid possible damage to the body during transfer and to prevent distress to colleagues, e.g. portering staff.
12. Secure the sheet with tape.	Pins, although providing more security, are contraindicated. If they open, they pose a potential health hazard to staff since bacterial fermentation occurs consequent to decomposition of the body.
If necessary, or according to hospital policy, place body in plastic cadaver bag.	Leakage of fluid, whether infection is present or not, poses a health hazard to all those who come into contact with the deceased patient.
13. If required, tape the second notification of death card to the outside of the sheet (or cadaver bag).	For ease of identification of the body in the mortuary.
14. Request the portering staff to remove the body.	Decomposition occurs rapidly particularly in hot weather and in overheated rooms, and may create a bacterial hazard for those handling the body. Autolysis and growth of bacteria are delayed if the body is cooled.
Screen off the appropriate area.	Avoid causing unnecessary distress to other patients and relatives.
15. Check the patient's property with a second nurse. List the property in the valuables or property book. Lock the property in a safe place.	To ensure that all property can be accounted for.

16. Amend appropriate nursing documentation.	To record patient's demise.
17. Transfer property, patient records etc. to the appropriate administrative department.	The administrative department cannot begin to process the formalities such as the death certificate or the collection of property by the next-of-kin until the required documents are in its possession.

NURSING CARE PLAN

Problem	**Suggested action**
Death occurring within 24 hours of an operation.	All tubes and/or drains must be left in position. Spigot any cannulae or catheters. Treat stomas as open wounds. Leave any endotracheal or tracheostomy tubes in place. Postmortem examination will be required to establish the cause of death. Any tubes, drains, etc. may have been a major contributing factor to the death.
Unexpected death.	As above. Postmortem examination of the body will be required to establish the cause of death.
Unknown cause of death.	As above.
Patient brought in dead.	As above, unless patient seen by a medical practitioner within 14 days before death.
Patient with leaking wounds/orifices with or without infection present.	Follow procedures outlined in section on hepatitis B (Chapter 4).
Patient with hepatitis B or who is HIV positive.	For further information see the procedures in the sections on hepatitis B and AIDS (Chapter 4).
Patient who dies after receiving systemic radioactive iodine.	For further information, see the procedure on iodine-131 (Chapter 22).
Patient who dies after insertion of gold grains or colloidal radioactive solution. Patient who dies after insertion of caesium needles or applicators or irridium wires or hair pins.	Inform the physics department as well as appropriate medical staff. Once a doctor has verified death, the sources are removed and placed in a lead container. A Geiger count is used to check that all sources have been removed. This reduces the radiation risk when completing the last offices procedures. Record the time and date of removal of the sources.
Relatives not present at the time of the patient's death.	Inform the relatives as soon as possible of the death. Consider also that they may want to view the body before last offices are completed.
Relatives or next-of-kin not contactable by telephone or by the general practitioner.	If within United Kingdom, local police will go to next-of-kin's house. If abroad, the British Embassy will assist.
Relatives want to see the body after removal from the ward.	Inform the mortuary staff in order to allow time for them to prepare the body. The body will normally be placed in the hospital's chapel of rest. As required, religious artefacts should be removed

Nursing care plan

Problem	**Suggested action**
	from or placed in the non-denominational chapel of rest. The nurse should check that all is ready before accompanying the relatives into the chapel. The relatives may want to be alone with the deceased, but the nurse should wait outside the chapel in order that support may be provided should the relatives become distressed. After the relatives have left, the nurse should contact the portering service, who will return the body to the mortuary.
Relatives want the body to be placed in the hospital's chapel of rest.	The environment of the mortuary may cause great distress to the relatives. A sympathetic and understanding attitude to immense grief may help to alleviate some anxieties and if they wish to view the body (see above).

GUIDELINES: REQUIREMENTS FOR PEOPLE OF DIFFERENT RELIGIOUS FAITHS

Buddhism

1. A Buddhist may request a Buddhist monk (bhikku) or nun (sister) to be present. There are different schools with varying observances. Ascertain to which school the patient is affiliated.
2. At death, inform the Buddhist priest as soon as possible. This may be done by relatives. The body should not be moved for at least one hour after informing the priest as prayers will need to be said. The body is also wrapped in an unmarked sheet.
3. Check all details with the family for there are many different types of Buddhism and each form may vary in its local practices.

Hinduism

1. Inform the Hindu priest (Brahmin). If the priest is unavailable, read from the *Bhagavad Gita* (1962; Chapters 2, 8 and 15; Ed. by Mascar, J.) before or during the last offices. There may be a request to place the body on the floor and to burn incense.
2. The family will usually remain with the patient. The eldest son should be present. Relatives, of the same sex as the deceased, wash the body. Nursing staff may do this if the relatives prefer.
3. Postmortems are not usually carried out since they are regarded as disrespectful to the deceased.

Islam

1. Family members stay with the dying patient and perform all rites and ceremonies. If possible, the patient should face Mecca (south-east).
2. The body should be left untouched. If Moslems are present, they will perform their own procedures. Disposable gloves should be worn if the deceased has to be touched. The eyes may be closed and the body straightened. The head should be turned towards the right shoulder and covered with a plain sheet. The body should not be washed and will normally be taken home or to a mosque as soon as possible where it will be washed by another Moslem of the same sex. A wife may wash her husband but a husband may not wash his wife.
3. Moslems are buried, never cremated, preferably within 24 hours of death.
4. Postmortems are only allowed if required by law. Organ donation is only permitted if absolutely necessary.

Judaism

1. The family will contact their own community leader if they have one; otherwise, the hospital chaplaincy will advise. Prayers are recited by those present.
2. Eight minutes are required to elapse before the body is moved.

3. Usually close relatives will straighten the body but it is permitted for nursing staff to perform any procedure for the preservation of dignity and honour. Therefore they may:
   (a) Close the eyes.
   (b) Tie up the jaw.
   (c) Put the arms and hands straight and by the side of the body.
   (d) Any tubes or instruments may be removed.
   (e) The patient must not be washed. A plain shroud may be put on. (The body is washed by a nominated group – the Holy Assembly – who perform ritual purification.)
4. Watchers stay with the body until burial (normally within 24 hours of death). A non-denominational room set aside for this purpose is appreciated where the body may be placed on the floor with feet towards the door. A lighted candle is placed near the head.
5. It is not possible for funerals to take place over the Sabbath (from sunset Friday to sunset Saturday).
6. Postmortems are permitted only if required by law.

Sikhism

1. Family and friends are normally present.
2. The family may want to be responsible for carrying out the last office. If requested by the family, close the eyes, straighten the body and wrap it in a plain sheet.
3. The family will wash and dress the body.
4. Cremation will take place as soon as possible, preferably within 24 hours of death.
5. Postmortems are permitted only if required by law.
6. Organ donation for transplants is not permitted.

24

Lifting

The aim of successful lifting is to achieve the required results with minimal effort by the lifter and minimal discomfort to the patient. By fully assessing every situation in which it is necessary to lift, both patient and staff can be protected from injury.

REFERENCE MATERIAL

Potential hazards of lifting

When a patient has to be lifted, both he/she and the nurses involved are potentially at risk of injury. The patient may experience discomfort or pain due to being held or lifted in an unsuitable fashion. For example, dragging a patient up the bed causes friction against the sheets and may cause or exacerbate a sore area. Being lifted physically by others can be an unpleasant or even a frightening experience, particularly if the patient has not had the manoeuvre explained beforehand.

The occupational hazard of back pain is well known. It is estimated that 185 000 nurses (43% of the National Health Service's total nursing population of England and Wales) suffer back pain at least once a year (Nursing Practice Research Unit, 1980). Of these episodes of back pain, 44% occur while the nurse is on duty and 84% of them are attributed directly to moving or supporting a patient. Thus one out of every six nurses is likely to suffer back pain while on duty as a result of moving of lifting a patient.

As well as the personal suffering and inconvenience caused by back pain among nurses, sick leave reduces the staffing levels and patient care may be correspondingly affected. It is estimated that 764 000 nurse working days per year are lost in the National Health Service due to back pain. Stubbs *et al.* (1983, 1984) offer a comprehensive account of back pain in the nursing profession.

It is, therefore, of the utmost importance that nurses are aware of the principles of safe lifting and can employ techniques that reduce the hazard of lifting both to their patients and to themselves. Lifting a patient demands considerable effort but the lifter will be at far less risk of strain if he/she uses skill rather than strength (Gonnet & Kryzwon, 1991; McCall, 1991).

Biomechanics of lifting

The spine is capable of bearing large compression forces but is vulnerable to damage from shearing forces along the surface of the discs as well as torsional and twisting forces (Figure 24.1). Structural damage to the cartilaginous structures may occur as the result not only of one bad lifting experience, but also from continual poor posture or repeated lifting of comparatively light objects in an incorrect manner.

If the trunk is nearly erect, most of the weight of the upper body and the lifted load is directly down through the vertebral column, stabilizing it and causing some compression of the discs. If, however, the trunk is horizontal, these weights produce a shearing force, rather than compression, on the discs.

The erector spinae muscles which provide some of the tension support of the spine during lifting are able to exert greater force lifting a given weight when the spine is in the upright rather than flexed position.

It is not only safer but also more mechanically efficient to lift with a straight back, using the strong thigh and hip muscles to provide the lifting force. When lifting, therefore, the hips and knees should be bent as the quadriceps muscles can be employed to gain vertical movement with minimum reliance on the erector spinae muscles.

The stress on the spine during lifting can be reduced by standing as close as possible to the patient. A large distance of separation will increase the force on the spine and, therefore, increase stress. For the same reasons twisting and jerking should be avoided during lifting.

Factors affecting spinal stress during lifting

By using a pressure-sensitive radio pill it is possible to measure intra-abdominal pressure (IAP) during lifting procedures. Intra-abdominal pressure may be used as

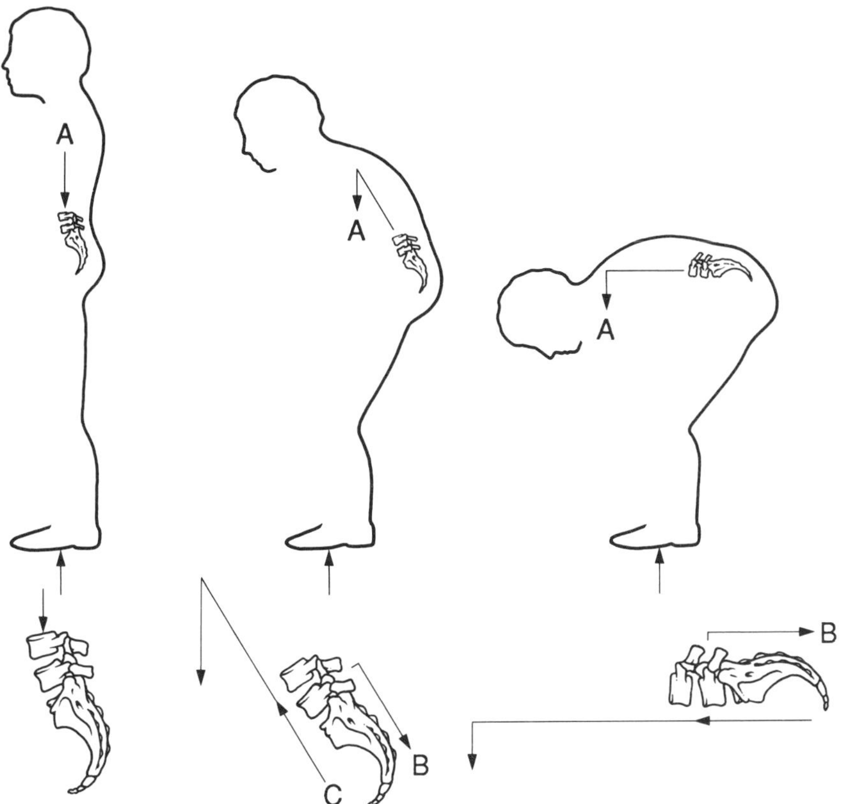

Figure 24.1 Biomechanics of lifting (Back Pain Association and The Royal College of Nursing (1987), with permission). A = weight of upper part of body; B = tension in back muscles; C = equal and opposite reaction to compressing disc.

an index of spinal stress as research has shown a close correlation between the magnitude of the IAP, the size of the load and the forces acting on the spinal mechanism (Davis, 1981).

The load

Studies have shown that the nurse's IAP increases when heavier patients are lifted (Hyde, 1980). Confused, unco-operative or paralysed patients produce higher pressures than others, usually because they make the lift unpredictable or impossible to carry out in a pre-arranged fashion. Patient behaviour as well as weight therefore contribute to the potential hazard of lifting. Many patients, however, can assist the nurses when being lifted, e.g. by digging their heels into the bed.

The lifting technique

The stress experienced by the spine when lifting is largely affected by the technique used. However skilful the lifter may become, he/she must always recognize his/her limitations and get further assistance when necessary.

The lifts most frequently used by nurses are now listed.

The shoulder (Australian) lift (Figure 24.2a)

If a hoist is not available then this is the lift of choice, although it is not suitable for patients with rib or shoulder injuries. It is particularly valuable when lifting heavy patients as using the shoulders gives the lifter a mechanical advantage.

The patient sits forward and both nurses stand level with the patient's hips. The foot nearer the head of the bed points in the direction of the lift and the knees and hips are bent, keeping the back straight and the head up.

The nurses press their near shoulder against the chest wall under the axillae and, if possible, the patient rests his/her arms on the nurses' backs. One nurse grasps the other's forearm well up under the patient's thighs. The lift is then accomplished by pressing the free hand on the bed, straightening the hips and knees and transferring weight on to the forward leg.

This technique may be used for lifting the patient up and down the bed, or from the bed to the chair or commode, for example.

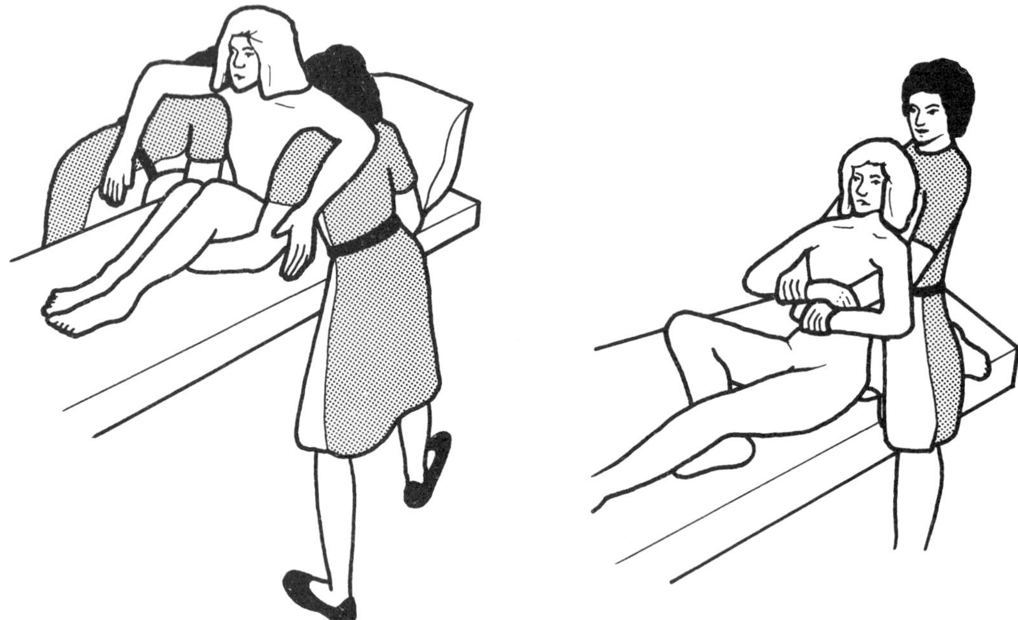

Figure 24.2 (a) Shoulder Australian lift. (b) Through arm lift (second nurse not shown).

The orthodox lift
This lift in which two nurses hold each other's hands under the patient involves excessive stooping and twisting for its successful completion. *It is now not recommended as a safe manual lift* (Back Pain Association, 1987).

The through arm lift (Figure 24.2b)
The nurse stands behind the patient, who is in the sitting position, and places his/her arms under the patient's axillae. The nurse then grips the patient's forearms as near to the wrists as possible by placing his/her hands between the patient's chest and upper arms. The patient is asked to grip one of his/her wrists firmly.

The other nurse faces the patient and puts his/her arms under the patient's thighs from opposite sides so that the nurse can grab his/her wrist. The lift is performed by the nurses extending their hips and knees while keeping their backs straight.

This lift does put unequal strain on the nurses and the one who lifts the upper part of the patient experiences higher spinal stress. However, it is a useful procedure, for example, moving a severely disabled patient from chair to bed. It may also be used to lift a patient from the floor and in this situation one nurse stops the patient's feet from slipping, while the other lifts with a through arm grip.

In comparing these lifting techniques, the shoulder lift has been shown to produce significantly lower intra-abdominal pressures (IAPs), and therefore less spinal stress than the other two manoeuvres. The reason for the higher IAPs of the other lifts as compared to the shoulder lift is an outcome of the initial stooped or semi-stooped starting position. The shoulder lift is, therefore, recommended whenever practically possible.

The through arm lift may also be carried out with two nurses one on either side of the patient. The patient is 'parcelled up' more effectively by holding him/her forward in a sitting position with the through arm grip. The nurses place one knee on the bed and face the foot of the bed. With their free hands they grasp the handling sling placed under the patient's thighs and lift the patient back towards them, sitting back on their heels as they do so.

Equipment

Patients should be encouraged to move themselves whenever possible or to assist nurses to move them by using monkey poles, blocks or other suitable equipment. It has been noted, however, that nurses often do not use lifting aids because they do not know about them or how to use them (Royal College of Nursing, 1990).

References and further reading

Back Pain Association (1987) *The Handling of Patients: A Guide for Nurses*, 2nd ed. Back Pain Association in collaboration with the Royal College of Nursing of the United Kingdom, London.

Davis, P. R. (1981) The use of intra-abdominal pressure in evaluating stresses on the lumbar spine. *Spine*, 6(1), 90–2.

Gonnet, L. & Kryzwon, A. (1991) Preventing back pain through education. *Nursing Standard*, 5(24), 25–7.

Hyde, N. J. (1980) *A comparative analysis of a lifting method commonly used by nurses versus a recommended method of lifting patients, using pressure-sensitive radio pill methodology*. BSc thesis, Leeds Polytechnic.

McCall, J. (1991) Watch your back. *Nursing Standard*, 5(24), 50–1.

Nursing Practice Research Unit (1980) *Prevention of Back Pain in Nursing*, Proceedings of the Conference held at Northwick Park Hospital, 26 September 1980, Nursing Practice Research Unit.

Rodgers, S. (1985) Shouldering the load. *Nursing Times*, 81(3), 24–6.

Royal College of Nursing (1990) Equipment to save your back. *Nursing Standard*, 4(34), 26–8.

Sorenson, K. C. & Luckan, J. (1979) *Basic Nursing – A Psychophysiological Approach*. W.B. Saunders, London.

Stubbs, D. A. *et al.* (1983) Back pain in the nursing profession – Part I. Epidemiology and pilot methodology. *Ergonomics*, 26, 755–65.

Stubbs, D. A. *et al.* (1984) *Patients Handling and Back Pain in Nurses: Main Study*, Report no. JR 125/120). DHSS, London.

Swaffield, L. (1985) Out of court, out of mind. *Nursing Times*, 91(3), 27–8.

GUIDELINES: LIFTING

Procedure

Action	Rationale
1. Assess the patient and the environment to establish what help or aids will be required for the lift.	To ensure that the patient is well enough to be lifted and that all necessary help and equipment can be acquired before disturbing the patient.
2. Decide how the patient is to be lifted and ensure that the other nurse(s) and the patient understand what they are going to do.	So that those involved in the lift can co-operate and co-ordinate their movements and any problems can be taken into account beforehand.
3. Prepare the area. Move equipment into a suitable position, put brakes on the bed and move any unnecessary equipment out of the way. Screen the area if necessary.	The environment must allow safe lifting and reduce the need for the nurse to twist or be impeded in his/her movements.
4. Adopt a suitable stance for the proposed lift as described and illustrated in the reference section, above.	To ensure the lift is carried out correctly.
5. Stand as close as possible to the patient.	To reduce the spinal stress.
6. Lift the patient into the desired position. One nurse acts as leader and co-ordinates the moment of lifting.	So that effort is exerted simultaneously by those involved and unequal strain does not fall on any one person.
7. Check that the lift was comfortable for the patient and nurses, and note any points which could be improved on for future use.	

Note: if something goes wrong when lifting and patient appears to be falling, it is safest to let the patient fall in a controlled fashion, i.e. by allowing the patient to slide gently to the floor or the bed. The nurse should make the patient comfortable and get assistance to lift again.

25

Liver Biopsy

Definition

Liver biopsy is the removal of a small piece of liver tissue by percutaneous puncture using a special needle.

Indications

Liver biopsy is a procedure performed by trained medical staff to establish a diagnosis in certain liver diseases, e.g. cirrhosis, carcinoma (primary or secondary), amyloidosis, miliary tuberculosis.

Contraindications

Liver biopsy is contraindicated in patients who:

1. Are confused or unco-operative.
2. Have a prolonged clotting time.
3. Have an increased bleeding time.
4. Have severe purpura.
5. Have a coagulation defect.
6. Are severely jaundiced.
7. Are under the age of three years.
8. Have a right lower lobe pneumonia or pleuritis.

REFERENCE MATERIAL

Needle biopsy of the liver was first used by Ehrlich in 1883. For varying reasons it fell out of favour as a diagnostic method until reintroduced in 1939 by Iversen and Roholm. It is now a widely practised technique for the diagnosis of certain liver diseases (see Figures 25.1 and 25.2). It has the advantage of being performed at the patient's bedside. No general anesthetic is required and the patient suffers significantly less pain than with open biopsy.

Anatomy and physiology

The liver is the largest organ in the body, weighing about 1.5 kg. It is highly vascular, is situated to the right upper side of the abdomen below the diaphragm and extends vertically for 15–18 cm. Laterally it measures about 20–30 cm and its anterior posterior measurement is about 10–13 cm. The lower surface is covered with peritoneum. The liver has two lobes: a large right lobe, under which the gall bladder lies and a smaller left lobe. The hepatic flexure of the colon lies underneath the liver.

The functions of the liver include:

1. Storage of glycogen, fat, proteins, vitamins A and B_{12}, and blood.
2. Synthesis of plasma proteins, fibrinogen, prothrombin and heparin.
3. Bile secretion.
4. Formation and destruction of red cells.
5. Detoxification.
6. Metabolism of carbohydrates, fats and protein (Keele *et al.*, 1983).

Investigations before biopsy

1. Blood is taken for:
   (a) Bleeding, clotting and prothrombin times.
   (b) Platelet count.
   (c) Grouping and, if necessary, cross-matching.
2. A plain abdominal X-ray is taken to ensure avoidance of colonic puncture if the patient has a small liver.

Physical preparation of the patient

Fasting

Fasting is required as for preoperative cases.

Sedation

For very anxious patients a mild tranquillizer may be ordered by the doctor.

Complications

Haemorrhage

Haemorrhage may occur as a result of inadvertent puncture of an intra- or extrahepatic blood vessel. Signs of this will appear within four hours of the

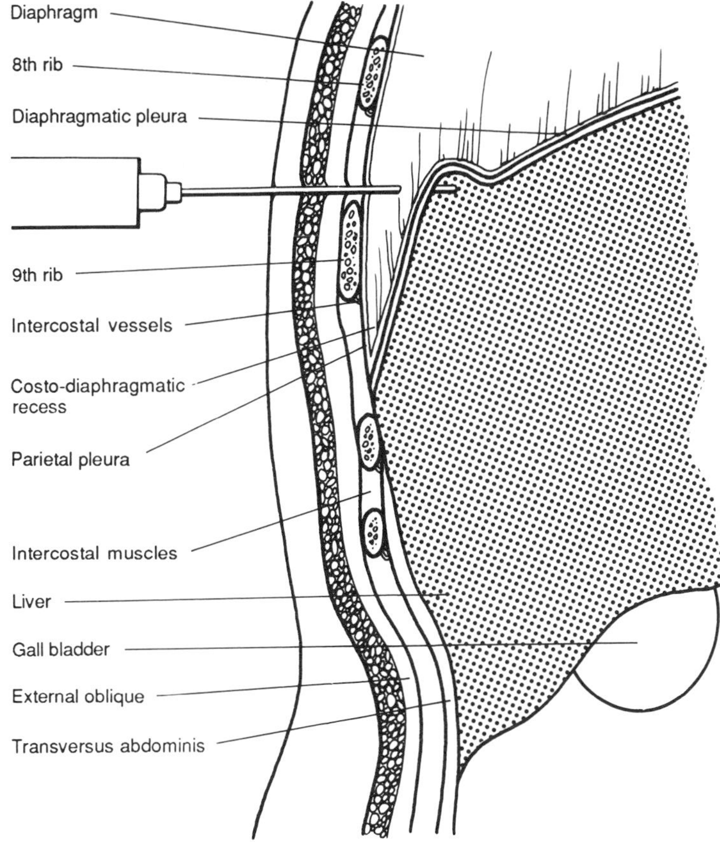

Figure 25.1 Longitudinal section showing liver biopsy from the front.

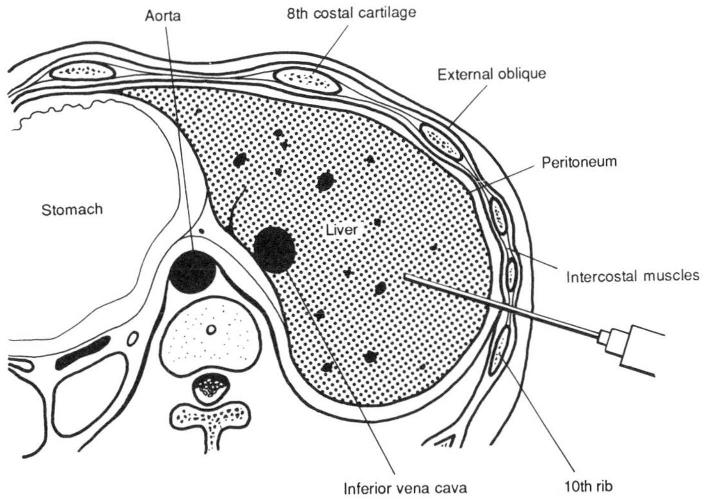

Figure 25.2 Transverse section showing liver biopsy from above.

biopsy. (Loss of 5 to 10 ml of blood from the liver surface is normal following needle biopsy.)

Peritonitis

Peritonitis may be caused by inadvertent puncture of the bile duct, resulting in bile leaking into the peritoneal cavity.

Pneumothorax

Pneumothorax may result from inadvertent puncture of the pleura.

Mortality rate

Scott *et al.* (1991) cite a mortality rate of less than 0.01%, and a morbidity rate of less than 0.1% in patients with normal coagulation.

References and further reading

Abrahams, P. and Webb, P. (1975) *Clinical Anatomy of Practical Procedures*. Pitman Medical, London.

Booth, J. A. (1983) *Handbook of Investigations*. Harper & Row, London.

Deeley, T. J. (1974) *Needle Biopsy*. Butterworth, London.

Keele, C. A. *et al.* (1983) *Samson Wright's Applied Physiology*. Oxford Medical Publications, Oxford.

Kilday, D. (1981) Assisting with liver biopsy. In *Mosby's Manual of Clinical Nursing Procedures* (Ed. by J. Hirsch & I. Hancock). C. V. Mosby, St Louis.

Pagnana, K. D. & Pagnana, T. J. (1982) *Diagnostic Testing and Nursing Implications*. C. V. Mosby, St Louis.

Read, A. E. (1968) Needle biopsy of the liver. In *Biopsy Procedures in Clinical Medicine* (Ed. by A. E. Read). John Wright and Sons, Bristol.

Scott, D. A. *et al.* (1991) Delayed subcapsular hematoma after percutaneous liver biopsy as a manifestation of warfarin toxicity. *American Journal of Gastroenterology*, 86(4), 503–5.

Skydell, B. & Crowder, A. (1975) *Diagnostic Procedures – A Reference for Health Practitioners and a Guide for Patient Counselling*. Little, Brown & Co. Boston.

Zamcheck, N. & Klausenstock, O. (1953) The risk of needle biopsy. *New England Journal of Medicine*, 249, 1062–9.

GUIDELINES: LIVER BIOPSY

Equipment

1. Antiseptic skin cleansing agent.
2. Syringes and needles.
3. Local anaesthetic.
4. Sterile normal saline.
5. Disposable scalpel.
6. Plaster dressing or plastic dressing spray.
7. Hypo-allergenic tape.
8. Liver biopsy needle, usually a Menghini or disposable Trucut needle.
9. Sterile dressing pack.
10. Sterile gloves.
11. Normal saline.

Procedure

Action	Rationale
1. Explain the procedure to the patient.	To obtain the patient's consent and co-operation.
2. Demonstrate holding the breath on expiration and observe the patient practising the manoeuvre.	To minimize the risk of accidental puncture of lung tissue when the biopsy needle is inserted into the liver, the patient will be asked to hold his/her breath on expiration.
3. Administer a sedative at an appropriate time, if ordered.	To reduce the patient's anxiety.
4. Assist the patient to lie in supine position with the right side as close to the edge of the bed as possible, the left side may be supported by a pillow. The right hand should be placed beneath the head and the head turned to the left.	To allow the doctor ease of access to the eighth or ninth intercostal space.

Action	Rationale
5. Continue to observe and reassure the patient throughout the procedure.	
6. Assist the doctor as required. The doctor will:	
(a) Clean the appropriate area with an antiseptic solution.	To maintain asepsis throughout the procedure and thus diminish the risk of infection.
(b) Give a local anaesthetic intradermally and in successive layers down to the pleura.	To minimize pain during the procedure and ensure maximum co-operation of the patient. (No further pain should be felt once the local anaesthetic has been introduced.)
(c) Make a small incision in the skin over the area to be punctured.	To allow ease of introduction of the borer (part of the biopsy set).
(d) Flush the biopsy apparatus with saline to check for patency of the needle. Some saline will be left in the syringe barrel.	To flush out the piece of liver obtained at biopsy, which will be in the core of the needle.
(e) Introduce the needle through the diaphragm and inject a little of the saline.	To remove any pieces of tissue caught in the needle during its introduction.
(f) Ask the patient to breathe in and out fully several times. The patient will then be asked to breathe out and hold the breath. The biopsy needle is then rapidly inserted and withdrawn from the liver.	At this stage there is minimal risk of puncturing lung tissue as the biopsy is obtained. Delay increases the risk of a liver tear.
7. Once the doctor has indicated that the biopsy has been obtained, cover the puncture site with a sterile topical swab and apply pressure for five minutes.	To prevent infection and stop bleeding.
8. Once bleeding is minimal or has ceased, apply a small dry dressing and secure with hypo-allergenic tape. (A plastic dressing spray may be used over the puncture site.)	
9. Make the patient comfortable and position onto right side for the next one to two hours.	To compress the liver capsule against the chest wall and prevent haemorrhage.
10. Observe the patient, monitoring in particular: (a) Pulse rate. (b) Blood pressure. (c) Respiration rate. (d) Pain – local or referred shoulder pain. (e) Abdominal tenderness and/or rigidity. (f) Leakage from the wound site. (g) Haematoma formation. (h) Skin colour. (i) Restlessness. (j) Abdominal swelling. Observations may be decreased or increased according to the patient's condition, but should be monitored every 15 to 30 minutes for the first one to two hours.	To monitor any complications that may occur as a result of the procedure.
11. Remove and dispose of equipment as appropriate.	To prevent spread of infection.
12. Food and fluids may be recommenced when observations are stable.	To allow adequate time for assessment of potential complications before reintroducing diet.
13. Record necessary information in the	

Guidelines: Liver biopsy

Action	Rationale
appropriate documents and ensure that the specimen obtained is sent to the appropriate laboratory with any necessary forms and labelling.	

NURSING CARE PLAN

Problem	Cause	Suggested action
Patient restless and perspiring with a low blood pressure and fast pulse rate.	Haemorrhage from biopsy site due to either a tear in the liver or inadvertent puncture of a blood vessel.	Ensure that the patient lies on his/her right side to produce pressure over puncture site for one to two hours. Record the patient's pulse and blood pressure every 15 to 30 minutes for the first one to two hours and increase or decrease the frequency as the patient's condition allows. Call a doctor if there is any alteration in observations as the patient may require blood transfusion, analgesia and sedation.
Patient complains of severe pain which may be accompanied by signs of shock and collapse, with abdominal tenderness and rigidity.	Leakage of bile into the peritoneal cavity from an accidentally perforated bile duct.	Record the patient's pulse and blood pressure every 15 to 30 minutes for the first one to two hours and increase or decrease the frequency as the patient's condition allows. Call a doctor if there is any alteration in observations as the patient may require a laparotomy to rectify biliary duct puncture.
Patient complains of dyspnoea.	Pneumothorax due to a puncture of the lung tissue caused by the patient inhaling as the biopsy needle is introduced into the liver.	Record the patient's respiration rate every 15 to 20 minutes for the first one to two hours and increase or decrease the frequency as the patient's condition allows. Call a doctor if there is any change in observations as the patient may require intrapleural drainage and oxygen therapy.

26

Lumbar Puncture

Definition

Lumbar puncture is the withdrawal of cerebrospinal fluid by the insertion of a special needle into the lumbar subarachnoid space for diagnostic or therapeutic purposes.

Indications

Lumbar puncture is indicated for the following purposes:

1. Diagnostic purposes.
2. Introducing contrast media for radiological examination.
3. Introducing chemotherapeutic agents, e.g. antibiotics or cytotoxics.

Contraindications

This procedure is contraindicated in the following cases:

1. *Raised intracranial pressure.* The procedure could lead to herniation of the brainstem (coning).
2. *Suspected cord compression.*
3. *Local infection.* Meningitis is a rare complication of lumbar puncture. If skin infection is present, examination should be delayed until the problem is resolved.
4. *Unco-operative patients.* Lumbar puncture is a potentially hazardous procedure which requires maximum patient co-operation.
5. *Severe degenerative spinal joint disease.* In such cases difficulty will be experienced both in positioning the patient and in access between the vertebra.

REFERENCE MATERIAL

Anatomy and physiology

The spinal cord lies within the spinal column (Figure 26.1). It is encased and protected by the vertebrae and extends from the base of the brain to below the second lumbar vertebra where it continues as a fine thread – the filum terminale – which is attached internally to the coccyx. Like the brain, the spinal cord is completely surrounded by three membranes known as the meninges. They are the dura, the arachnoid and the pia maters.

The dura and arachnoid are separated by a potential space called the subdural space. The arachnoid and pia maters are separated by the subarachnoid space which contains the cerebrospinal fluid (CSF). The cerebrospinal fluid is fairly narrow until the first lumbar vertebra, when it widens as the spinal cord terminates. Below the first lumbar vertebra the subarachnoid space contains cerebrospinal fluid, the filum terminale and the cauda equinae (the anterior and posterior roots of the lumbar and sacral nerves). This area is used to obtain specimens of cerebrospinal fluid by lumbar puncture as there is no danger of damage to the spinal cord (Figure 26.2).

The cerebrospinal fluid is secreted by the choroid plexus which is situated in the ventricles of the brain. The fluid is clear, colourless and slightly alkaline, with a specific gravity of 1005. It consists of:

1. Water.
2. Mineral salts.
3. Glucose.
4. Protein – 20 to 30 mg per 100 ml (Keele *et al.*, 1983).
5. Creatinine.
6. Urea.

It is reabsorbed into blood capillaries via the arachnoid villi and is returned to the circulating blood.

The functions of cerebrospinal fluid are to:

1. Act as a shock absorber.
2. Carry nutrients to the brain.
3. Remove metabolites from the brain.
4. Support and protect the brain and spinal cord.
5. Keep the brain and spinal cord moist.

Investigations

Depending on the investigations required, about 5 to

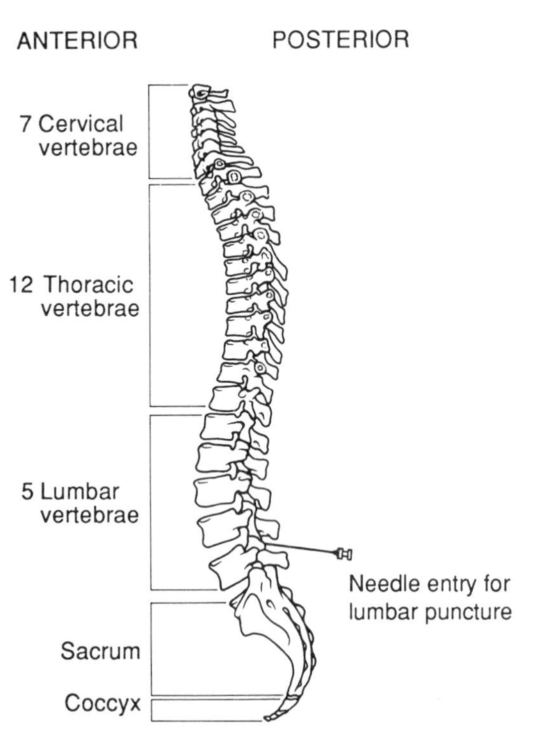

Figure 26.1 Lateral view of the spinal column and vertebrae, showing the needle entry site for lumbar puncture.

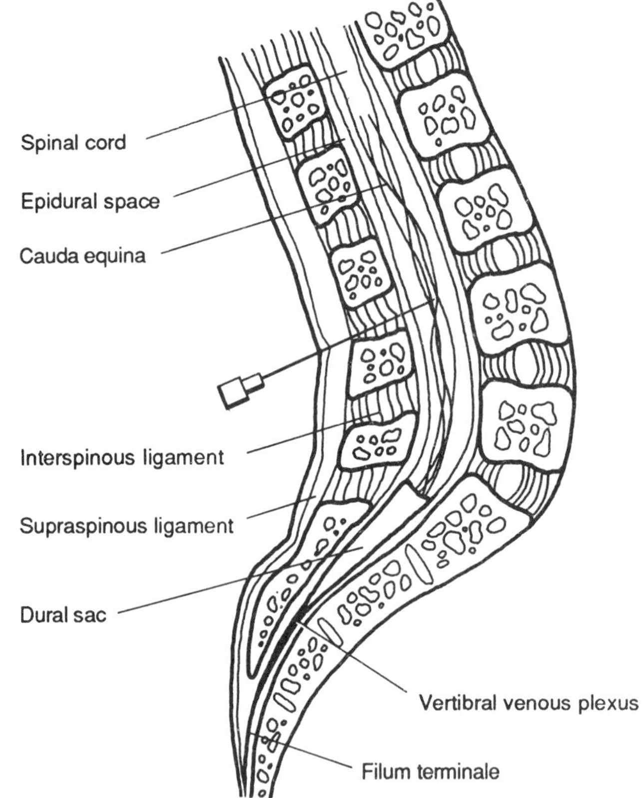

Figure 26.2 Lumbar puncture. Saggital section through lumbosacral spine.

10 ml of cerebrospinal fluid is removed for laboratory analysis.

Pressure

The pressure of the cerebrospinal fluid is investigated at the time of lumbar puncture, using a manometer. Queckenstedt's test may also be performed. The latter consists of applying pressure to the jugular vein. When normal, there is a sharp rise in pressure followed by a fall as the pressure is released. Blockage of the spinal canal will result in a sluggish rise and fall or absence of response. Queckenstedt's manoeuvre is a potentially hazardous procedure if both jugular veins are compressed at the same time. Temporal lobe or brainstem herniation may occur. Normal cerebrospinal fluid pressure is approximately 60 to 180 mm H_2O.

Colour

The fluid should be clear and colourless. The first 3 to 4 ml may be blood-stained due to local trauma at the time of insertion of the lumbar needle. In this case the blood will usually clot. The fluid clears as the procedure continues. However, if blood-staining is due to subarachnoid haemorrhage, no clotting will occur and all samples will be blood-stained.

Blood

There should not be any blood in the samples. The presence of blood indicates either a traumatic puncture or subarachnoid haemorrhage.

Blood cells

There should be no blood cells, except for a few lymphocytes, in the sample. The presence of polymorphonuclear leucocytes is indicative of meningitis or cerebral abscess. Monocytes would indicated viral or tubercular meningitis or encephalitis.

Culture and sensitivity

The presence of microorganisms would indicate meningitis or cerebral abscess. By isolating the specific organism the appropriate antibiotic therapy may be commenced.

Serology for syphilis
If other tests are positive, the appropriate antibiotic therapy may be commenced.

Protein
The total amount of the protein in the cerebrospinal fluid should be 15.45 mg/dl (= 154.5 μg/ml). Proteins are large molecules which do not readily cross the blood–brain barrier. There is normally more albumin (approximately 80% of total protein) than globulin (approximately 12 to 20% of total protein) in cerebrospinal fluid as albumens are smaller molecules. Raised globulin levels are indicative of multiple sclerosis, neurosyphilis, degenative cord or brain disease. Raised protein levels may indicate meningitis, encephalitis, myelitis or the presence of a tumour.

Cytology
Central nervous system tumours tend to shed cells into the cerebrospinal fluid, where they float freely. Examination of these cells after lumbar puncture will determine whether the tumour is benign or malignant.

Instillation of chemotherapy

Lumbar puncture may be used as a means of introducing drugs into the central nervous system which do not cross the blood–brain barrier. Antibiotics may be instilled to treat specific infections such as bacterial meningitis; cytotoxics may be instilled to treat for malignant diseases such as leukaemia and to prevent recurrence in the central nervous system when the patient is in remission.

Complications

1. Infection.
2. Haemorrhage/bruising.
3. Transtentorial or tonsillar herniation (if Queckenstedt's test is carried out in the presence of raised CSF pressure).
4. Headache.
5. Backache.
6. Leakage from puncture site.

References and further reading

Abrahms, P. & Webb, P. (1975) *Clinical Anatomy of Practical Procedures*. Pitman Medical, London.
Booth, J. A. (1983) *Handbook of Investigations*. Harper & Row, London.
Brunner, L. S. & Suddarth, D. S. (1982) *The Lippincott Manual of Medical-Surgical Nursing*. Harper & Row, London, Vol. 3.
Clough, C. & Pearce, J. M. S. (1980) Lumbar puncture. *British Medical Journal*, 280, 297–9.
Keele, C. A. *et al.* (1983) *Samson Wright's Applied Physiology*. Oxford Medical Publications, Oxford.
Pagana, K. D. & Pagana, T. J. (1986) *Diagnostic Testing and Nursing Implications*, 2nd edn. C. V. Mosby, St Louis.
Skydell, B. & Crowder, A. S. (1975) *Diagnostic Procedures – A Reference for Health Practitioners and a Guide for Patient Counselling*. Little, Brown & Co, Boston.
Vannini, V. & Pogliani, G. (1980) *The New Atlas of the Human Body*. Corgi, London.

GUIDELINES: LUMBAR PUNCTURE

Equipment

1. Antiseptic skin-cleansing agent.
2. Selection of needles and syringes.
3. Local anaesthetic.
4. Sterile gloves.
5. Sterile dressing pack.
6. Lumbar puncture needles of assorted sizes.
7. Disposable manometer.
8. Three sterile specimen bottles. (These should be labelled 1, 2 and 3. The first specimen, which may be blood-stained due to needle trauma, should go into bottle 1. This will assist the laboratory to differentiate between blood due to procedure trauma and that due to subarachnoid haemorrhage.)
9. Plaster dressing or plastic dressing spray.

Procedure

Action	Rationale
1. Explain the procedure to the patient.	To obtain patient's consent and co-operation.
2. Assist the patient into the required position:	

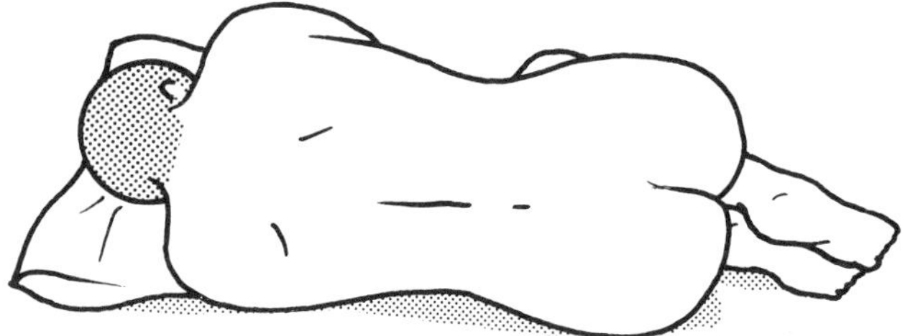

Figure 26.3 Position for lumbar puncture. Head is flexed onto chest and knees are drawn up.

Guidelines: Lumbar puncture

Action	**Rationale**
(a) Lying (Figure 26.3): (i) One pillow under the patient's head. (ii) Firm surface. (iii) On side with knees drawn up to the abdomen and clasped by the hands.	To ensure maximum widening of the intervertebral spaces and thus easier access to the subarachnoid space.
(iv) Support patient in this position by holding him/her behind the knees and neck.	To avoid sudden movement by the patient which would produce bloodstained fluid.
(b) Sitting: (i) Patient straddles a straight-backed chair so that his/her back is facing the doctor. (ii) Patient folds arms on the back of the chair and rests head on them.	This position may be used for those patients unable to maintain the lying position. It allows more accurate identification of the spinous processes and thus the intervertebral spaces.
3. Continue to support, encourage and observe the patient throughout the procedure.	To monitor any physical or psychological changes.
4. Assist the doctor as required. The doctor will proceed as follows:	
(a) Clean the skin with the antiseptic cleansing agent.	To maintain asepsis throughout the procedure.
(b) Identify the area to be punctured and infiltrate the skin and subcutaneous layers with local anasthetic.	
(c) Introduce a spinal puncture needle between the third and fourth or fourth and fifth lumbar vertebrae and into the subarachnoid space.	This is below the level of the spinal cord but still within the subarachnoid space.
(d) Ensure that the subarachnoid space has been entered and attach the manometer to the spinal needle, if required.	To obtain a cerebrospinal fluid pressure reading (normal pressure is 60 to 180 mm H_2O).
(e) Decide whether Queckenstedt's manoeuvre may be performed (Figure 26.4).	To check for obstruction to cerebrospinal fluid flow in the spinal column. (Usually obstruction is caused by a tumour.)
(f) The appropriate specimens of cerebrospinal fluid about 10 ml in total) are obtained for analysis.	
(g) Once all specimens have been obtained and the appropriate pressure measurements made, the spinal needle is withdrawn.	
5. When the needle is withdrawn, apply pressure	To maintain asepsis and to stop blood and

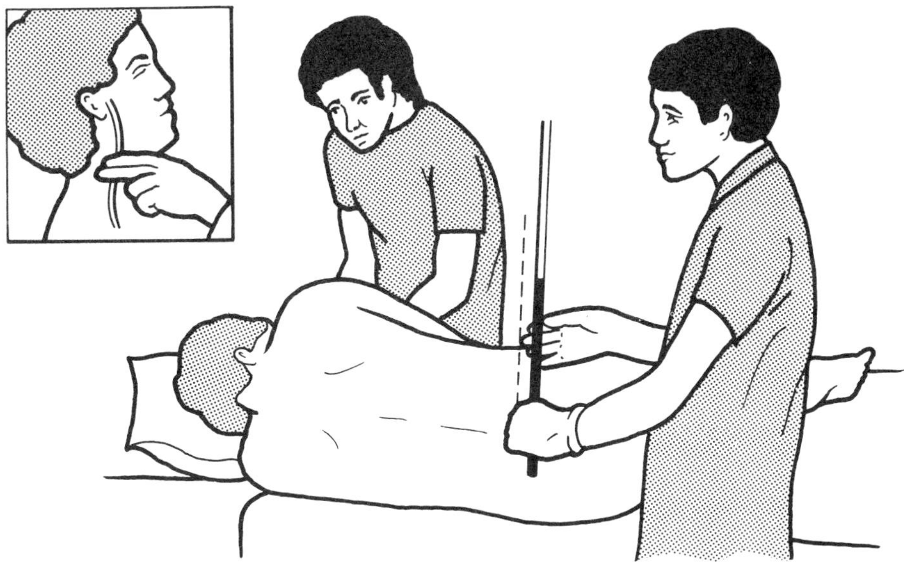

Figure 26.4 Queckenstedt's manoeuvre.

Action	Rationale
over the lumbar puncture site using a sterile topical swab.	cerebrospinal fluid flow.
6. When all leakage from the puncture site has ceased, apply a plaster dressing or plastic dressing spray.	To prevent secondary infection.
7. Make the patient comfortable. He/she should lie flat or the head should be tilted slightly downwards for a period of up to 24 hours (according to the doctor's instructions).	To avoid headache and decrease the possibility of brainstem herniation (coning) due to a reduction in cerebrospinal fluid pressure.
8. Observe patient for the next 24 hours for the following:	
(a) Leakage from the puncture site.	There may be a small amount of bloodstained oozing. The presence of clear fluid should be reported immediately to the doctor, especially if accompanied by fluctuation of other observations, as it may be a cerebrospinal fluid leak.
(b) Headache.	Not unusual following lumbar puncture. Usually relieved by lying flat and, if ordered by the doctor, a mild analgesic.
(c) Backache.	As above.
(d) Neurological observations/vital signs.	These may indicate signs of a change in intracranial pressure. (For further information on neurological observations and the vital signs, see Chapter 28).
9. Encourage a fluid intake of two to three litres in 24 hours.	To replace lost fluid and assist the patient to micturate, which may be difficult due to the supine position.
10. Remove equipment and dispose of as appropriate.	To prevent the spread of infection.

Guidelines: Lumbar puncture

Action	Rationale
11. Record the procedure in the appropriate documents.	
12. Ensure that specimens are labelled appropriately and sent with the correct forms to the laboratory.	

NURSING CARE PLAN

Problem	Cause	Suggested action
Pain down one leg during the procedure.	A dorsal nerve root may have been touched by the spinal needle.	Inform the doctor, who will probably move the needle. Reassure the patient.
Headache following procedure (may persist for up to a week).	Removal of the sample of cerebrospinal fluid.	Reassure the patient that it is a transient symptom. Ensure that he/she lies flat for the specified period of time. Encourage a high fluid intake to replace fluid lost during the procedure. Administer an analgesic as ordered. If the headache is severe and increasing, inform a doctor – there is a possibility of rising intracranial pressure.
Backache following procedure.	(a) Removal of the sample of cerebrospinal fluid. (b) Position required for puncture.	Reassure the patient that it is usually a transient symptom. Ensure that he/she lies flat for the appropriate period of time. Administer an analgesic as ordered.
Fluctuation of neurological observations, i.e. level of consciousness, pulse, respirations, blood pressure or pupillary reaction.	Herniation (coning) of the brainstem due to the decrease of intracranial pressure. (Raised intracranial pressure is a contraindication to lumbar puncture.)	Observe the patient every 30 minutes for the first two hours for signs of alteration in intracranial pressure. The frequency may be increased or decreased to four-hourly as the patient's condition allows. Report any fluctuations in these observations to a doctor immediately.
Leakage from the puncture site.	(a) Resolution of bleeding. (b) Leakage of cerebrospinal fluid.	(a) No further action required. (b) Report immediately to a doctor, especially if accompanied by fluctuation in neurological observations.

27

Mouth Care

Definition

Oral hygiene is performed to prevent a build up of plaque and debris which, if left, could lead to infection.

Indications

1. To achieve and maintain oral hygiene.
2. To prevent plaque build up, dental decay and infections.
3. To keep oral mucosa moist.
4. To promote patient comfort.

These aims are interrelated, as healthy oral tissues are dependent on the mouth remaining clean, moist and free from infection (Trenter & Creason, 1986). The only effective way to achieve this is to ensure that the patient is hydrated adequately and that the correct equipment, solutions and mouth cleaning methods are used.

Patients most at risk of developing mouth problems are those who become unable to maintain good oral hygiene themselves. Predisposing factors to poor oral health are:

1. The inability to take adequate fluids.
2. Poor nutritional status.
3. Insufficient saliva production leading to dry mouth, collection of debris and possible infection.
4. Major intervention altering oral status – surgery, radiotherapy or chemotherapy.
5. Lack of knowledge or motivation towards maintaining correct oral hygiene (Trenter & Creason, 1986).

REFERENCE MATERIAL

Agents used for mouth care

The choice of agents used for mouth care is determined by the individual needs of the patient together with a detailed nursing assessment of the oral cavity. The most commonly used agents are evaluated below.

Saline

This solution is made up as required by dissolving table salt in water. An isotonic solution is recommended for mouth care, i.e. 4.5 g of salt to 500 ml of water (4.5 g of salt are equivalent to one level teaspoonful). Stronger solutions may be irritating to the mucosa and will be unpleasant to the taste. Sterile sachets of normal saline are available for immunosuppressed patients. No damaging effects are known at concentrations that are isotonic or below and the solution is cheap and easy to use. Normal saline is ineffective for removing hardened mucus, debris or crusts. However, the effectiveness of saline compared to water requires further evaluation.

Sodium bicarbonate

This solution is prepared as required by dissolving approximately 1 g sodium bicarbonate in 100 ml of warm water (1% w/v). It has a good cleaning effect and is suitable for making the mucus less viscid (*The Pharmaceutical Codex*, 1979) and loosening debris. If the solution is made too concentrated, it will taste unpleasant and may damage the mucosa. It is recommended that sodium bicarbonate is used in mouth care only when tenacious mucous is present. However, there is evidence to support the view that it is not suitable for removing longstanding or hardened debris from the tongue and surrounding tissues (Hallett, 1984).

Hydrogen peroxide

This mouthwash solution is made up immediately before use by diluting the preparation in the strength advised by the hospital pharmacist. Hydrogen peroxide is broken down into water and oxygen on contact with the enzyme catalase present in blood and tissues. The vigorous release of oxygen bubbles during this reaction acts as a mechanical cleaning agent and is useful, therefore, for loosening necrotic ulcers, crusting and debris (Crosby, 1989). This may also result in the breakdown of new tissue in fresh granulation surfaces. The increased oxygen concentration created by the reaction does inhibit the growth of anaerobic organisms but the foaming effect within the mouth is potentially dangerous if the cough reflex is impaired in any way. Suction should be available if this is the case. Hydrogen peroxide may act as an irritant to the tongue and buccal mucosa, especially where stomatitis is present. It is advisable, therefore, to clean the mouth after its use with warm water or normal saline.

Chlorhexidine
An aqueous solution of chlorhexidine 0.1 to 0.2% is sometimes prescribed as a mouthwash. It has a disinfectant action on Gram-positive and Gram-negative bacteria, and is useful in preventing the accumulation of plaque and the development of gingivitis when brushing is contraindicated. It does, however, have an unpleasant taste. An alcoholic solution of chlorhexidine may be used for soaking dentures in patients with oral infections of Candida species (Crosby, 1989).

If patients are unable to use a mouthwash, a chlorhexidine gel may be applied directly to teeth and gums. Chlorhexidine may stain teeth if used over long periods.

Benzydamine mouth wash
This solution consists of 0.15% benzydamine hydrochloride. It contains a topical anaesthetic and has anti-inflammatory and anti-microbial properties. It is useful for patients who have a sore oral cavity. The patient may rinse or gargle with 15 ml (diluted with half a cup of water, if preferred by the patient) every one-and-a-half to three hours as required (Data Sheet Compendium, 1991–92).

Moist-air swabs
A moist air swab is a stick with a contoured cotton wool end which is impregnated with the following minerals to make it moist: potassium chloride; sodium chloride; calcium chloride; magnesium chloride; and sodium phosphate.

These swabs are useful for cleaning all intra-oral surfaces. However, the taste of the swab is not very pleasant and so it is suitable only for those patients who can tolerate the taste or who have no sense of taste. They may be less irritating to oral tissues than pink foam sticks.

Stannous fluoride gel (0.4%)
This helps to prevent and arrest tooth decay, especially radiation caries, demineralization and decalcification. After normal cleaning, a small amount of gel is placed on a dry toothbrush and brushed onto all tooth surfaces for one minute. The patient can expectorate excess liquid in the mouth, but must not rinse the mouth, or eat or drink anything for at least 30 minutes following procedure in order to let it work (Forrest, 1987).

Sodium fluoride daily rinse (0.05%)
One to two teaspoonfuls (5 to 10 ml) can be placed in the mouth for one minute, and then the liquid can be expectorated, but the mouth must not be rinsed. No diet or fluids can be taken for at least 30 minutes following the procedure in order to let it work (Myers & Mitchell, 1988).

Commercially available mouthwashes
Some commercially available mouthwashes are acidic in nature and may have a high alcohol content that patients with an impaired oral mucosa may find painful.

Synthetic saliva
This product was designed for use by astronauts unable to produce saliva in a low-gravity environment. The constituents resemble those of natural saliva and may be used as often as required for dry mouths without any detrimental effect. This is particularly useful for patients with impaired saliva production (Duxbury *et al.*, 1989).

Vaseline
Vaseline may be used sparingly on the lips to create an occlusive oil film that prevents the loss of moisture by evaporation. A water-soluble lubricating agent, such as petroleum jelly, is preferably for intra-oral use.

Equipment used in mouth care

The most commonly used instruments in mouth care are evaluated below.

Foam sticks
Foam sticks are useful for cleaning oral mucosa but will not remove debris between or from the surface of the teeth. They are easy to use and there is little risk of mechanical trauma from them. The stick should be rotated gently over the mucosa so that all of the foam surface is utilized.

Toothbrushes
Research indicates that a toothbrush is the best way of cleaning teeth as the fine hairs loosen the debris trapped between the teeth and remove plaque from the tooth surface: 'The present evidence in favour of the use of a toothbrush for the care of teeth is so

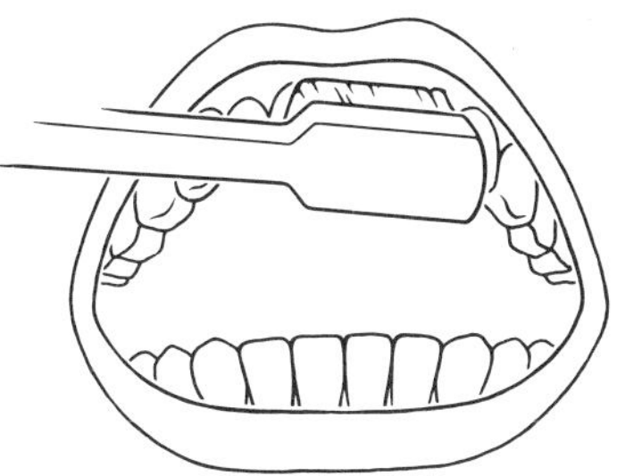
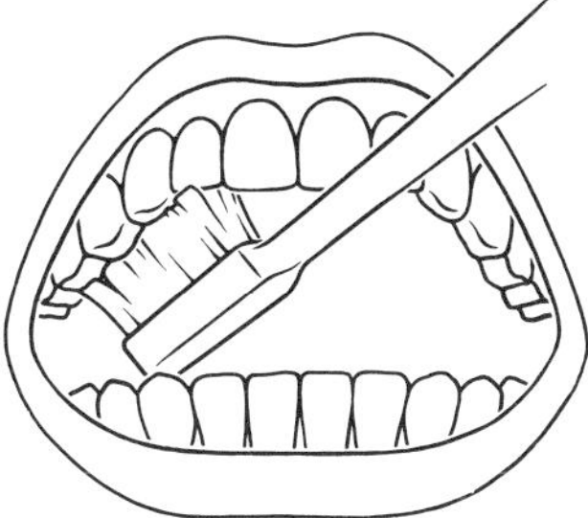
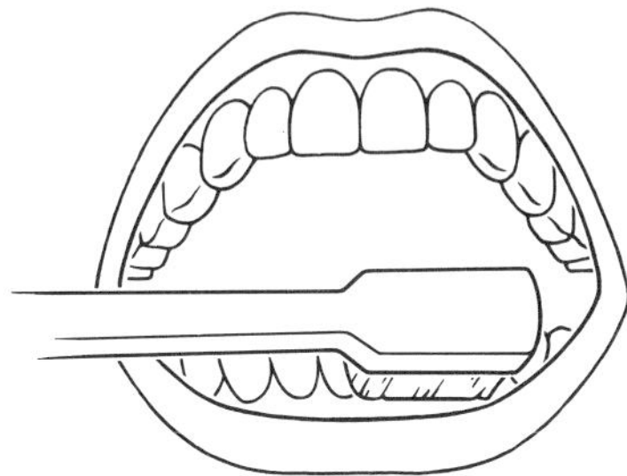

Figure 27.1 The 'Bass' method of toothbrushing using a small-headed toothbrush.

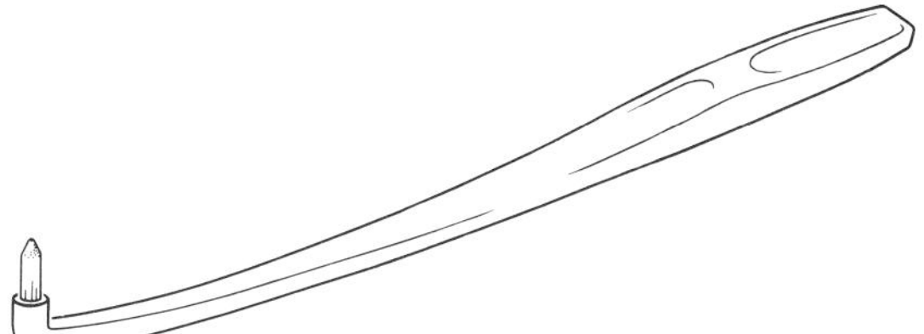
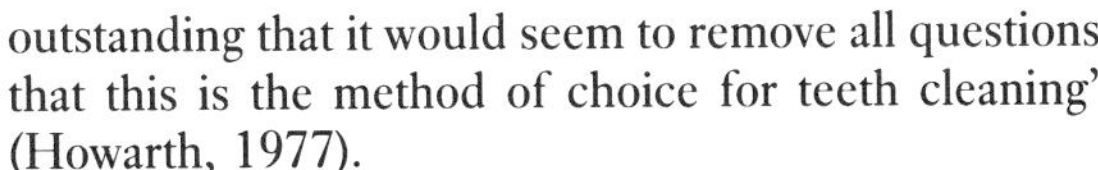

Figure 27.2 Interspace brush.

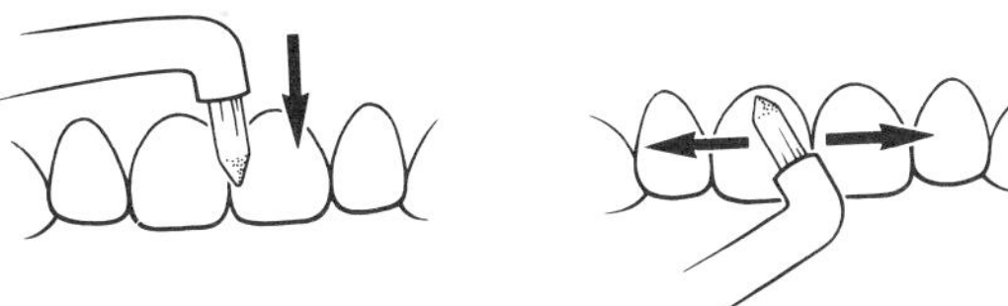

Figure 27.3 The tip of the brush is placed into the gingival margin and follows the contour of the teeth.

outstanding that it would seem to remove all questions that this is the method of choice for teeth cleaning' (Howarth, 1977).

Most patients are familiar with toothbrushing and it would seem sensible for this practice to be encouraged. Brushing the teeth, gums and oral tissues with a toothbrush not only removes debris and keeps the mouth fresh and clean but also stimulates tissue blood flow, thus promoting good oral health.

A small toothbrush with soft bristles that the patient can keep throughout the hospital stay is recommended. Using an automatic toothbrush may be easier for patients who are unable to use an ordinary toothbrush correctly. The type with an oscillating movement is favoured as those with a purely rotational movement may damage the gums. Teeth should be brushed with firm individual strokes so that any loosened debris is directed away from the gums. The toothbrush should be rinsed and dried after use.

Small-headed toothbrush

This is the best way of removing plaque and debris from the teeth. One of the main areas plaque collects is in the gingival crevice. The 'Bass' method of toothbrushing is the most effective way of removing it from this area. The toothbrush is placed on the gingival margin at an angle of 45°. With a very small vibratory movement, the bristles of the brush will go subgingivally and collect the plaque (Figure 27.1).

Interspace brush

This consists of a single tufted brush with a pointed tip (Figure 27.2). Useful for patients with trismus (limited mouth opening). It will not clean interdentally, but will help to remove debris lodged between the teeth and in the gingival crevice. The tip of the brush is placed into the gingival margin and, with a small vibratory movement, the brush follows the contour of the teeth (Figure 27.3).

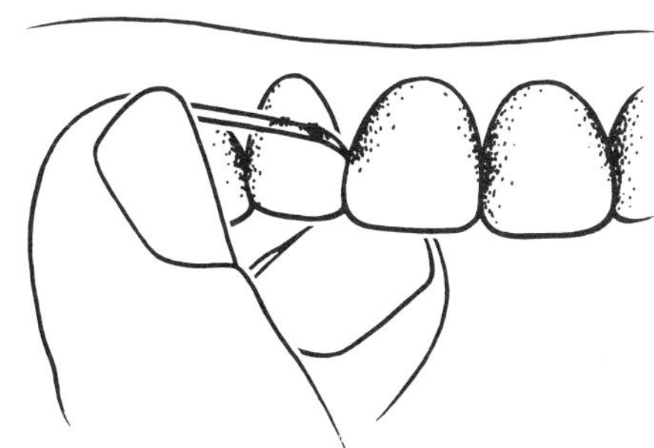

Figure 27.4 Interdental cleansing.

Interdental cleansing

This could involve the use of dental floss or tape, wood sticks and special brushes which will help to remove plaque and increase patient comfort (Figure 27.4).

Frequency of mouth care

The frequency of mouthcare depends entirely on

patient assessment and varies with the particular circumstances of the individual. Dental decay will not take place until plaque and debris have been in place for 24 hours or more. Brushing the teeth after each meal should minimize this risk. Certain factors act as stressors to the state or the oral mucosa. These include the following:

1. Mouth breathing.
2. Continuous oxygen therapy.
3. Intermittent suction.
4. No oral intake.

After experiencing all of the above for only one hour, a healthy young adult developed dryness of the lips and mouth, and colour changes in the oral mucosa (DeWalt & Haines, 1969). It is reasonable to expect more rapid changes in a more debilitated individual. Normally, the saliva lubricates and cleans the mouth and reduces the need for frequent mouth care. For patients who complain of a dry mouth, saliva production may be stimulated by the use of chewing gum or an artificial saliva preparation. Patients with poor appetites should be offered mouth care before and after a meal as a dirty mouth may inhibit the appetite.

References and further reading

Bersan, I. G. & Carl, W. (1983) Oral care for cancer patients. *American Journal of Nursing*, 83, 533–6.

British National Formulary (1991) No. 21, p. 360.

Bruya, M. A. & Madeira, N. P. (1975) Stomatitis after chemotherapy. *American Journal of Nursing*, 75, 1349–52.

Campbell, D. G. (1980) Prevention of infection in extended care facilities. *Nursing Clinics of North America*, 15, 857–68.

Crosby, C. (1989) Method in mouth care. *Nursing Times*, 30 August, 85(35), 38–41.

Daeffler, R. (1980) Oral hygiene measures for patients with cancer I–II. *Cancer Nursing*, 3, 347–56, 427–32.

Daeffler, R. (1981) Oral hygiene measures for patients with cancer III. *Cancer Nursing*, 4, 29–35.

Data Sheet Compendium (1991–92) 3M Health Care Limited, p. 858.

DeWalt, E. M. & Haines, A. K. (1969) The effects of specific stressors on healthy oral mucosa. *Nursing Research*, 18(1), 22–7.

Duxbury, A. J. *et al.* (1989) A double-blind cross-over trial of a mucin-containing artificial saliva. *Oral Medicine*. 25 February, 115–20.

Forrest, J. O. (1987) Stannous fluoride gel in preventative practice. *Dental Practice*. 5 March.

Gibbons, D. E. (1983) Mouth care procedures, *Nursing Times*, 79, 30.

Hallett, N. (1984) Mouth care, *Nursing Times*, 159, 31–3.

Harris, M. D. (1980) Tools for mouth care. *Nursing Times*, 76(8), 340–2,

Hilton, D. (1980) Oral hygiene and infection. *Nursing Times*, 76, 1270–2.

Howarth, H. (1977) Mouth care procedures for the very ill. *Nursing Times*, 73, 354–5.

Imperial Chemical Industries PLC, Pharmaceutical Division, Alderley Park, Macclesfield, Cheshire, England, June 1981.

Katz, S. (1982) The use of fluoride and chlohexidine for the prevention of radiation caries. *Journal of the American Dental Association*, 104(2), 164–70.

Lane, B. & Forgay, M. (1981) Upgrading your oral hygiene protocol for the patient with cancer. *Canadian Nurse*, 77, 27–9.

Lewis, L. A. (1984) Developing a research-based curriculum: an exercise in relation to oral care. *Nurse Education Today*, 3, 143–4.

Macmillan, K. (1981) New goals for oral hygiene. *Cancer Nursing*, 77, 40–2.

Munday, P. & Geilbier, S. (1984) Provision of dental health education in nurse training. *Nurse Education Today*, 3, 124–5.

Myers, R. E. & Mitchell, L. D. (1988) Fluoride for the head and neck radiation patient. *Military Medicine*, 153(8), 411.

Ostchega, Y. (1980) Preventing and treating cancer chemotherapy's oral complications. *Nursing* (US), 10(8), 47–52.

Riker, Z. M. *ABPI Data Sheet Compendium* 1990–1.

Schwiger, T. L. *et al.* (1980) Oral assessment – how to do it. *American Journal of Nursing*, 80, 654–7.

The Pharmaceutical Codex (1979) 11th edn.

Todd, B. (1982) Drugs and the elderly – dry mouth causes and cures. *Geriatric Nursing*, 3(2), 22–3.

Trenter, P. & Creason, N. S. (1986) Nurse-administered oral hygiene: is there a scientific basis? *Journal of Advanced Nursing*, 11, 323–31.

Trowbridge, T. E. & Carl, W. (1975) Oral care of the patient having head and neck irradiation. *American Journal of Nursing*, 75, 921–2.

GUIDELINES: MOUTH CARE

Equipment

1. Clinically clean tray.
2. Plastic cups.
3. Mouthwash or clean solutions.
4. Appropriate equipment for cleaning.
5. Clean receiver or bowl.
6. Paper tissues.

7. Wooden spatula.
8. Small-headed, soft toothbrush.
9. Toothpaste.
10. Disposable gloves.
11. Denture pot.

All the above items may be left on the patient's locker when appropriate, and should be cleaned, renewed or replenished daily.

12. Small torch.

Procedure

Action	**Rationale**
1. Explain the procedure to the patient.	To obtain the patient's consent and co-operation.
2. Wash hands with bactericidal soap and water or with bactericidal alcohol hand rub and dry with paper towel.	To reduce the risk of cross-infection.
3. Prepare solutions required.	Solutions must always be prepared immediately before use to maximize their efficacy and minimize the risk of microbial contamination.
4. Remove the patient's dentures if necessary, using paper tissues or topical swabs, and place them in a denture pot.	Removal of dentures is necessary for cleaning of underlying tissues. A tissue or topical swab provides a firmer grip of the dentures and prevents contact with patient's saliva.
5. Inspect the patient's mouth with the aid of a torch and spatula.	The mouth is examined for changes in condition with respect to moisture, cleanliness, infected or bleeding areas, ulcers, etc.
6. Using a small toothbrush and toothpaste, brush the patient's natural teeth, gums and tongue.	To remove adherent materials from the teeth, tongue and gum surfaces. Brushing stimulates gingival tissues to maintain tone and prevent circulatory stasis.
7. Brush the inner and outer aspects of the teeth with firm, individual strokes directed outwards from the gums.	Brushing loosens and removes debris trapped on and between the teeth and gums. This reduces growth medium for pathogenic organisms and minimizes the risk of plaque formulation and dental caries. Foam sticks are ineffective for this.
8. Give a beaker of water or mouthwash to the patient. Encourage patient to rinse the mouth vigorously then void contents into a receiver. Paper tissues should be to hand.	Rinsing removes loosened debris and toothpaste and makes the mouth taste fresher. The glycerine content of toothpaste will have a drying effect if left in the mouth.
9. If the patient is unable to rinse and void, use a rinsed toothbrush to clean the teeth and moistened foam sticks to wipe the gums and oral mucosa. Foam sticks should be used with a rotating action so that most of the surface is utilized.	
10. Apply artificial saliva to the tongue if appropriate and/or suitable lubricant to dry lips.	To increase the patient's feeling of comfort and wellbeing.

Guidelines: Mouth care

Action	Rationale
11. Clean the patient's dentures on all surfaces with a denture brush or toothbrush. Rinse them well and return them to the patient.	Cleaning dentures removes accumulated food debris which could be broken down by salivary enzymes to products which irritate and cause inflammation of the adjacent mucosal tissue. Some commercial denture cleaners may have an abrasive effect on the denture surface. This then attracts plaque and encourages bacterial growth.
12. Dentures should be soaked in chlorhexidine for ten minutes if oral Candida species are present.	Soaking in chlorhexidine reduces the risk of reinfecting the mouth with infected dentures.
13. Discard remaining mouthwash solutions.	To prevent the risk of contamination.
14. Wash hands with soap and water or alcohol hand rub and dry with paper towel.	To reduce the risk of cross-infection.

NURSING CARE PLAN

Problem	Cause	Suggested action
Dry mouth.	Inadequate hydration.	Monitor the fluid balance and increase the fluid intake where necessary.
	Impaired production of saliva, e.g. as a consequence of radiotherapy.	Apply artificial saliva to the oral cavity as required. Give the patient ice cubes to suck.
	Presence of specific stressors, e.g. mouth breathing, oxygen therapy, no oral intake, intermittent oral suction.	Inspect the mouth frequently, e.g. half-hourly. Swab mucosa with water.
Dry lips.	As above.	Smear a thin layer of appropriate lubricant.
Thick mucus.	Postoperative closure of a tracheostomy. Radiotherapy. Poor swallowing mechanism.	Use sodium bicarbonate solution in the mouth care procedure. Rinse the mouth afterwards with water or saline.
Patient unable to tolerate toothbrush.	Pain, e.g. postoperatively; stomatitis.	Use foam sticks or moist air swab to clean the patient's gums and mucosa. Saline is advisable. For severe pain use an anaesthetic mouth spray or mouthwash before giving mouth care.

Toothbrush inappropriate or ineffective.	Infected stomatitis. Accumulation of dried mucus, blood or debris.	Take a swab of any new lesions for culture before giving mouth care. Use a cleaning agent, e.g. chlorhexidine for swabbing or rinsing around the mouth.
Patient at risk of developing systemic or widespread infection from oral invasion of pathogens.	Immunosuppressive or neutropenic states.	Use sterile water and/or sterile saline for mouthwashing and dilution of agents.

28

Neurological Observations

Definition

Neurological observations relate to the evaluation of the integrity of an individual's nervous system by obtaining specific information about it.

Indications

Neurological observations are required to monitor and evaluate changes in the nervous system by indicating trends, thus aiding diagnosis and treatment, which in turn may affect prognosis and rehabilitation (Abelson, 1982; Jennett & Teasdale, 1984).

The frequency of neurological observations will depend upon the patient's condition and the rapidity with which changes are occurring or expected to occur.

REFERENCE MATERIAL

The main emphasis is on observing five critical areas:

1. Level of consciousness.
2. Pupillary activity.
3. Motor function.
4. Sensory function.
5. Vital signs.

Level of consciousness

Level of consciousness is the single most important indicator of a patient's brain function (derived from Abelson (1982), Allen (1986) & Nikas (1982)). It ranges, on a continuum, from alert wakefulness to deep coma with no apparent responsiveness. Categories of impaired consciousness include the following:

1. *Full consciousness*: the patient is aware of self and environment and this is reflected in the ability of the patient to be aroused, perceive internal or external stimuli and respond appropriately on a cognitive or motor level. Responses may be altered by focal sensory and/or motor deficits.
2. *Lethargy/drowsiness*: the patient is inactive and indifferent, responds slowly or unpurposefully to stimuli and may not respond verbally. The patient may be described as drowsy but rousable (Abelson, 1982).
3. *Coma*: the patient has total absence of awareness of self and environment. Response to arousal from painful stimulus may be absent.

Specific diseases and injuries can impair level of consciousness since they may depress or destroy the reticular activating system (RAS) (Figure 28.1).

Arousability

This depends on the integrity of the RAS. This core of nucleii extend from the brain stem to the thalamic nucleii in the cerebral hemispheres. Thus cognitive ability depends on the ability of the cerebral cortex to permit reciprocal stimulation and conscious behaviour.

Awareness

This requires an intact cerebral cortex to interpret sensory input and respond accordingly. This is the content of consciousness (Nikas, 1982; Scherer, 1986).

Levels of consciousness may vary and are dependent on the location and extent of any neurological damage. Previous and/or co-existing problems should be heeded when noting levels of consciousness, e.g. deafness.

Assessment of level of consciousness

This involves three phases:

1. Eye opening.
2. Evaluation of verbal responses.
3. Evaluation of motor response.

There is no universally accepted method for recording neurological assessment. The Glasgow Coma Scale has been found to be reliable and easy to use to measure conscious level, since it gives an instant graphic representation of the conscious state. It

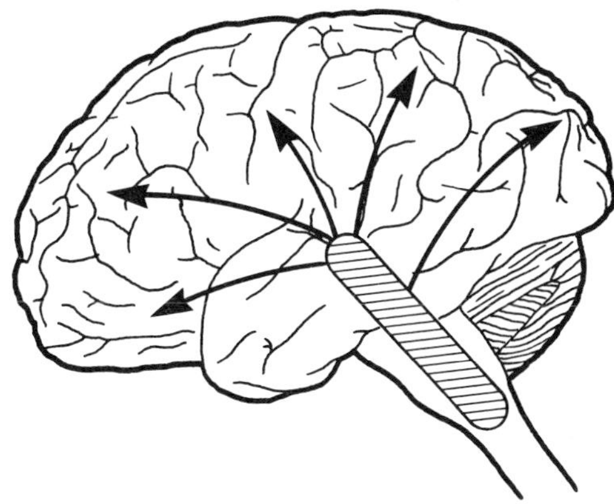

Figure 28.1 Reticular activating system. (From Allen, 1986; reproduced with permission from *The Professional Nurse.*)

Table 28.1 The Glasgow Coma Scale (taken from Sherman, 1990)

1. *Eye opening:*
   - Score 4. Spontaneously
   - 3. In response to voice
   - 2. In response to pain
   - 1. No response

2. *Best verbal response:*
   - Score 5. Orientated
   - 4. Confused
   - 3. Inappropriate speech
   - 2. Incomprehensible speech
   - 1. No response

3. *Best motor response:*
   - Score 6. Obeys commands
   - 5. Localizes pain
   - 4. Flexes and withdraws from pain
   - 3. Assumes flexor posturing in response to pain
   - 2. Assumes extensor posturing in response to pain
   - 1. No response

Lowest score could be 3; highest score, 15.

avoids making divisions between consciousness and unconsciousness, which are times on a continuum (Jennett and Teasdale, 1984) (Figure 28.2).

The Glasgow Coma Scale gives an objective measure of level of consciousness and eliminates the need for potentially ambiguous terms such as 'obtunded'. Possible scores range from 3 to 15 (Sherman, 1990) (Table 28.1). The score (according to Allen, 1984) is of little practical use and was developed as a statistical research tool. It is not used universally.

Eye opening

This indicates that the arousal mechanism in the brain is active. Eye opening may be: spontaneous; to speech, e.g. spoken name; to painful stimulus; none at all.

It must be remembered that swollen or permanently closed eyes (e.g. after tarsorrhaphy) will not open and do not necessarily indicate a falling conscious level.

Evaluation of verbal response

This may be:

1. Orientated; the patient is aware of self and environment.
2. Confused; the patient's responses to questions are incorrect and patient is unaware of self or environment.
3. Incomprehensible; the patient may moan and groan without recognizable words.
4. None; the patient does not speak or make sounds at all.

The absence of speech may not always indicate a falling level of consciousness. The patient may not speak English, may have a tracheostomy or may be dysphasic.

Evaluation of motor response

This is the best response from the patient; it is important and should be recorded. The patient should be asked to obey commands, e.g. 'squeeze my hands' (both sides). The nurse should note power in the hands. If movement is spontaneous, the nurse should note which limbs move, and how, e.g. purposefully or not.

Response to painful stimulus (pressure on nail bed with a pencil) may be:

1. Localized; the patient moves the other hand to the site of the stimulus.
2. Flexor; the patient's limb flexes away from pain.
3. Extensor; the patient's limb extends from pain.
4. Flaccid – no motor response at all.

Use of the terms 'decerebrate' and 'decorticate' should be avoided as they carry anatomical implications (Abelson, 1982; Scherer, 1986).

Painful stimuli

Painful stimuli should be employed only if the patient does not respond to firm, clear commands. Use the least amount of pressure to elicit a response.

THE ROYAL MARSDEN HOSPITAL

NEUROLOGICAL OBSERVATION CHART

NAME

RECORD No.

			DATE / TIME
COMA SCALE	Eyes open	Spontaneously	Eyes closed by swelling = C
		To speech	
		To pain	
		None	
	Best verbal response	Orientated	Endotracheal tube or tracheostomy = T
		Confused	
		Inappropriate Words	
		Incomprehensible Sounds	
		None	
	Best motor response	Obey commands	Usually record the best arm response Muscle relaxant = M
		Localise pain	
		Flexion to pain	
		Extension to pain	
		None	
• 1		240	
		230	40
• 2		220	39
		210	38
• 3		200	37 Temperature °C •
		190	36
		180	35
• 4		170	34

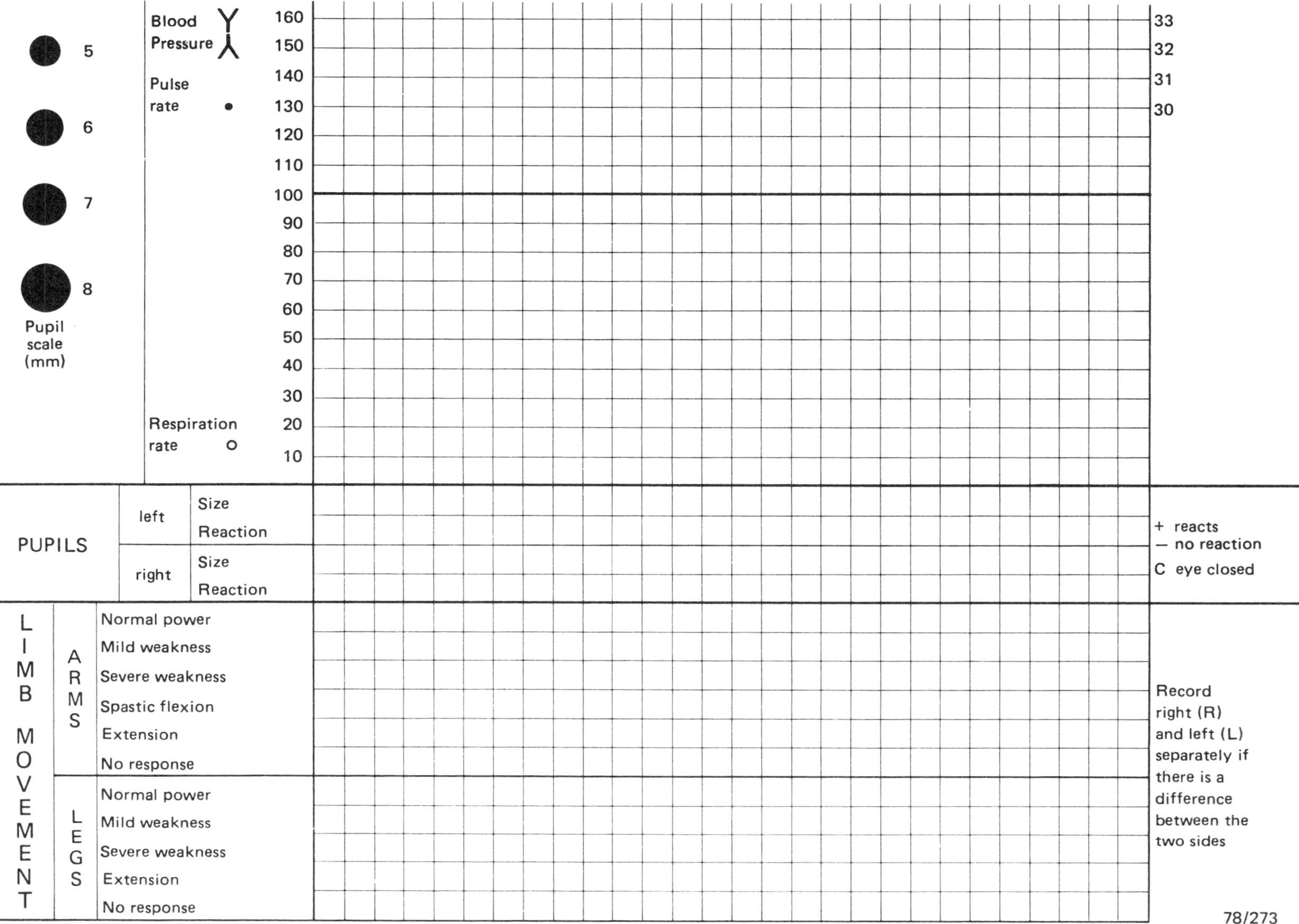

Figure 28.2 Glasgow Coma Scale. (Reproduced with permission of Institute of Neurological Sciences, The Southern General Hospital, Glasgow.)

(For suggested methods see below.) As the ability to localize pain is lost, various responses may be observed when painful stimuli are applied (Hudak *et al.*, 1982).

Painful stimuli can be applied in the following ways (Vernberg *et al.*, 1983):

1. Apply blunt pressure with an object, such as a pencil or pen to the fingernail at the point where it enters the skin of the finger.
2. Press in a circular motion between the fifth and sixth intercostal space over the border of the sternum.
3. Pinch the muscles at the side of the neck (trapezius muscle).
4. Apply pressure (with knuckles) in a circular motion over the sternum (sternal rub).

Note: take care not to mark or bruise the patient's skin. Do not stick pins into the patient (Nikas, 1982).

Pupillary activity

Careful examination of the reactions of the pupils to light is an important part of neurological assessment. Note the size, shape, equality and reaction to light (both direct and consensual responses). Check the position of the eyes. Are they deviated upwards or downwards? Are both eyes looking in the same direction or are they disconjugate (Stolarik, 1985)? Impaired pupillary accommodation signifies that the midbrain itself may be suffering from pressure exerted by a swelling mass in the brain (or inside the cranium). (Pupillary constriction and dilation are controlled by cranial nerve III (oculomotor). Any changes may indicate pressure on this nerve, or brain stem damage) (Figure 28.3).

Motor function

Damage to any part of the motor nervous system can affect the ability to move. Motor function assessment involves an evaluation of the following:

1. Muscle strength.
2. Muscle tone.
3. Muscle co-ordination.
4. Reflexes.
5. Abnormal movements.

Muscle strength

This involves testing the patient's muscle strength against one's own muscle resistance and then against the pull of gravity.

Muscle tone

This involves flexing and extending the patient's limbs on both sides and nothing how well such movements are resisted. Increased resistance would denote increased muscle tone and *vice versa*.

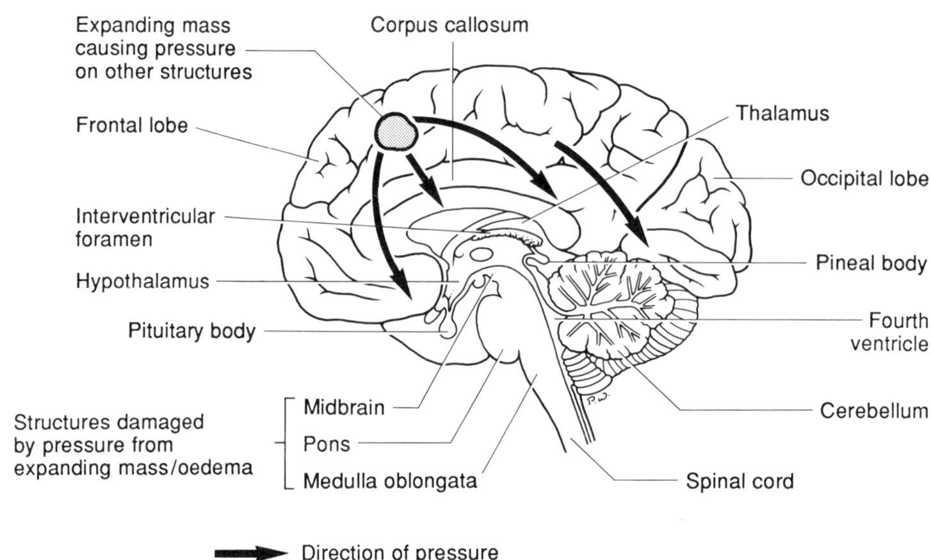

Figure 28.3 Diagrammatic representation of pressure from expanding mass and/or cerebral oedema.

Muscle co-ordination

Any disease or injury that involves the cerebellum or basal ganglia will affect co-ordination. Assessment of hand and arm and leg co-ordination can be achieved by testing the rapidity and rhythm of alternating movements and of point-to-point movements. Nikas (1982) and Hudak *et al.* (1982) describe cerebellar function tests in detail.

Reflexes

Among the most important reflexes are: blink; gag and swallow; oculocephalic; and plantar.

1. *Blink*: is a protective reflex and can be affected by the Vth nerve (trigeminal) and the VIIth nerve (facial) involvement (Hudak *et al.*, 1982).
2. *Gag and swallow*: also protective reflexes. Involvement of the IXth nerve (glosso-pharyngeal) and Xth nerve (vagus) may impair these reflexes (Hudak *et al.*, 1982).
3. *Oculocephalic*: this reflex is an ocular movement that occurs only in patients with a severely decreased level of consciousness. When the reflex is present, the patient's eyes will move in the opposite direction from the side to which the head is turned. If the reflex is impaired, the eyes may not move at all, or only one eye may move (Hudak *et al.*, 1982; Scherer, 1986).
4. *Plantar*: this reflex helps to locate the site of the lesion (Nikas, 1982).

Abnormal movements

When carrying out neurological observations, any abnormal movements such as seizures, tics and tremors must be noted.

Sensory functions

Constant sensory input enables an individual to alter responses and behaviour to suit the environment. When disease or injury damages the sensory pathways, the sensory responses are always affected. Any assessment of sensory function should include an evaluation of the following:

1. Central and peripheral vision.
2. Hearing and ability to understand verbal communication.
3. Superficial sensations (light touch, pain) and deep sensations (muscle and joint pain, muscle and joint position) (Hudak *et al.*, 1982).

Vital signs

It is recommended that assessments of vital signs should be made in the following order:

1. Respirations.
2. Temperature.
3. Blood pressure.
4. Pulse.

Respirations

Of these four vital signs, respiratory patterns give the clearest indication of how the brain is functioning since respirations are controlled by different areas of the brain. Any disease or injury that affects these areas may produce respiratory changes. The rate, character

Table 28.2 Abnormal respiratory patterns

Type	*Pattern*	*Significance*
Cheyne-Stokes	Rhythmic waxing and waning of both rate and depth of respirations, alternating regularly with briefer periods of apnoea	May indicate deep cerebral or cerebellar lesions, usually bilateral; may occur with upper brainstem involvement
Central neurogenic hyperventilation	Sustained, regular, rapid respirations, with forced inspiration and expiration	May indicate a lesion of the low midbrain or upper pons areas of the brainstem
Apnoeustic	Prolonged inspiration with a pause at full inspiration; there may also be expiratory pauses	May indicate a lesion of the low pons or upper medulla, or hypoglycaemia, or drug-induced respiratory depression
Cluster breathing	Clusters of irregular respirations alternating with longer periods of apnoea	May indicate a lesion of low pons or upper medulla
Ataxic breathing	A completely irregular pattern with random deep and shallow respirations; irregular pauses may also appear	May indicate a lesion of the medulla

and pattern of a patient's respiration must be noted. Abnormal respiratory patterns are listed in Table 28.2.

Temperature

Damage to the hypothalamus, the temperature-regulating centre, may result in grossly fluctuating temperatures (Nikas, 1982).

Blood pressure and pulse

Observations of blood pressure and pulse will provide evidence of increased intracranial pressure. Hypertension and bradycardia need to be monitored closely. Abnormalities of blood pressure and pulse usually occur late, after the patient's level of consciousness has begun to deteriorate.

General points

The initial assessment of a patient should include a history (taken from relatives or friends if appropriate) including noting changes in: mood, intellect, memory and personality, since these may be indicators of a longstanding problem, e.g. brain tumour (Barker, 1990).

Visual acuity

May be tested using Snellen charts or newspaper prints, with and without glasses if worn.

Visual fields

Plotting may indicate a lesion in the retina, optic nerve, optic tract, temporal lobe, parietal lobe or occipital lobe. Nikas (1982) and Hudak (1982) discuss visual field defects in detail.

References and further reading

Abelson, N. M. (1982) Observation of the neurosurgical patient. *Curiatonis*, 5(3), 32–7.

Allen, D. (1984) Glasgow Coma Scale. *Nursing Mirror*, 158(2), 32.

Allen, D. (1986) Nursing the unconscious patient. *The Professional Nurse*, 2(1), 15–17.

Barker, E. (1990) Brain tumour frightening diagnosis, nursing challenge. *Registered Nurse*, 53(9), 46–56.

Barr, M. L. & Kiernan, J. A. (1983) *The Human Nervous System*, 4th edn. Harper and Rowe, Phil.

Hinkle, J. L. (1986) Treating traumatic coma. *American Journal of Nursing*, 86(5), 550–6.

Hudak, C. M. *et al.* (1982) Nervous system (B. Fuller) pp. 321–34; Pathophysiology of CNS, pp. 335–48; Management modalities, pp. 349–78; Assessment skills, pp. 379–89. In *Critical Care Nursing*, 3rd edn. Lippincot, N.J.

Jennett, B. & Teasdale (1984) *An Introduction to Neurosurgery*, 4th edn, pp. 23–9. William Heinemann Medical Books, London.

Netter, F. H. (1975) *IHL Printing of CIBA Collection of Medical Illustrations, Volume 1, Nervous System*, pp. 58–9, CIBA, Summit, N.J.

Nikas, D. (Ed.) (1982) *The Critically Ill Neurosurgical Patient.* Churchill Livingstone, New York, Edinburgh, London and Melbourne, pp. 1–27, 77–80, 100–3.

Scherer, P. (1986) The logic of coma. *American Journal of Nursing*, pp. 542–9.

Sherman, D. W. (1990) Managing an acute head injury. *Nursing*, April, 20(4), 47–51.

Stolarik, A. (1985) What the comatose patient can tell you. *Registered Nurse*, April, 48(4), 26–33.

Tortora, G. J. & Anagnostakos (1987) *Principles of Anatomy and Physiology*, 5th edn. Harper Collins, London, pp. 579–83.

Vernberg, K. *et al.* (1983) The Glasgow Coma Scale: How do you rate? *Nurse Educator*, 8(3), pp. 33–7.

GUIDELINES: NEUROLOGICAL OBSERVATIONS AND ASSESSMENT

Note: The following describes a full neurological assessment. It may be inappropriate, unnecessary or impossible for the nurse to carry out all of the procedures every time the patient is observed.

Equipment

1. Pencil torch.
2. Thermometer.
3. Sphygmomanometer.
4. Tongue depressor.
5. Cotton wool balls.
6. Patella hammer.
7. Sterile needle.
8. Two test tubes.

Procedure

Action	**Rationale**
1. Inform the patient, whether conscious or not,	Sense of hearing is frequently unimpaired even in

Action	Rationale
and explain the observations.	unconscious patients. To ensure, as far as is possible, that the patient consents to and understands the procedure.
2. Talk to the patient. Note whether he/she is alert and is giving full attention or whether he/she is restless or lethargic and drowsy. Ask the patient who he/she is, the correct day, month and year, where he/she is, and to give details about family.	To establish whether the patient's level of consciousness is deteriorating. If the patient is becoming disorientated, changes will occur in this order: (a) Disorientation as to time. (b) Disorientation as to place. (c) Disorientation as to person.
3. Ask the patient to squeeze and release your fingers (include both sides of the body) and then to stick out the tongue.	To evaluate motor responses.
4. If the patient does not respond, apply painful stimuli. Suggested methods have been discussed earlier.	Responses grow less purposeful as the patient's level of consciousness deteriorates. As the condition worsens, the patient may no longer localize pain and respond to it in a purposeful way (Vernberg *et al.*, 1983).
5. Record, precisely, the findings. Write exactly what stimulus was used, where it was applied, how much pressure was needed to elicit a response, and how the patient responded.	Vague terms can be easily misinterpreted. Record the patient's best response (Allen, 1984).
6. Hold the eyelids open and note the size, shape and equality of the pupils.	To assess the size, shape and equality of the pupils as an indication of brain damage. Normal pupils are spherical, usually at mid-position and have a diameter ranging from 1.5 to 6 mm (Nikas, 1982).
7. Darken the room, if necessary.	To enable a better view of the eye.
8. Hold each eyelid open in turn. Move torch towards the patient from the side. Shine it directly into the eye. This should cause the pupil to constrict promptly.	To assess the reaction of the pupils to light. A normal reaction indicates no lesions in the area of the brainstem regulating pupil constriction.
9. Hold both eyelids open but shine the light into one eye only. The pupil into which the light is not shone should also constrict.	To assess consensual light reflex. Prompt constriction indicates intact connections between the brainstem areas regulating pupil constriction (Scherer, 1986).
10. Record unusual eye movements.	To assess cranial nerve damage.
11. Extend your hands and ask the patient to squeeze your fingers as hard as possible. Compare grip and strength.	To test grip.
12. Ask the patient to close the eyes and hold the arms straight out in front, with palms upwards, for 20 to 30 seconds. The weaker limb will 'fall away'.	To show weakness in limbs.
13. Stand in front of the patient and extend your hands. Ask the patient to push and pull against your hands. Ask the patient to lie on his/her back in bed. Place the patient's leg with knee flexed and foot resting on the bed. Instruct the	To test arm strength. If one arm drifts downwards or turns inwards, it may indicate hemipharesis. To test flexion and extension strength in the patient's extremities by having patient push and pull against your resistance.

Guidelines: Neurological observations and assessment

Action	Rationale
patient to keep the foot down as you attempt to extend the leg. Flex the knee and place your hand in the flexion. Instruct the patient to straighten the leg while you offer resistance. *Note*: if a patient cannot follow the instruction due to a language barrier or unconsciousness, observe spontaneous movements and note how strong they appear. Then, if necessary, apply painful stimuli.	
14. Flex and extend all the patient's limbs. Note how well the movements are resisted.	To test muscle tone.
15. Ask the patient to pat the thigh as fast as possible. Note whether the movements seen slow or clumsy. Ask the patient to turn the hand over and back several times in succession. Evaluate co-ordination. Ask the patient to touch the back of the fingers with the thumb in sequence rapidly.	To assess hand and arm co-ordination. The dominant hand should perform better.
16. Extend one of your hands towards the patient. Ask the patient to touch your index finger, then his/her nose, several times in succession. Repeat the test with the patient's eyes closed.	To assess hand and arm co-ordination.
17. Ask the patient to place a heel on the opposite knee and slide it down the shin to the foot. Check each leg separately.	To assess leg co-ordination.
18. Ask the patient to look up or hold the eyelid open. With your hand, approach the eye unexpectedly or touch the eyelashes.	To test the blink reflex.
19. Ask the patient to open the mouth, and hold down the tongue with a tongue depressor. Touch the back of the pharynx, on each side, with a cotton wool swab.	To test the gag reflex.
20. Ask the patient to lie to his/her back in bed. Place your hand under the knee, raise and flex it. Tap the patellar tendon. Note whether the leg responds.	To assess the deep tendon reflex.
21. Stroke the lateral aspect of the sole of the patient's foot. If the response is abnormal (Babinski's response), the big toe will dorsiflex and the remaining toes will fan out.	To assess for upper motor neurone lesion.
22. Ask the patient to read something aloud. Check each eye separately. If vision is so poor that the patient is unable to read, ask the patient to count your upraised fingers or distinguish light from dark.	To test the visual acuity.
23. Occlude the ear with a cotton wool swab. Stand a short way from the patient. Whisper	To test hearing and comprehension.

Action	Rationale
numbers into the open ear. Ask for feedback. Repeat for both ears.	
24. Ask the patient to close the eyes. Using the point of a sterile needle, stroke the skin. Use the blunt end occasionally. Ask patient to tell you what is felt. See if the patient can distinguish between sharp and dull sensations.	To test superficial sensations to pain.
25. Ask the patient to close the eyes. Fill two test tubes with water: one warm, one cold. Touch the patient's skin with each test tube and ask patient to distinguish between them.	To test superficial sensations to temperature.
26. Stroke a cotton wool swab lightly over the patient's skin. Ask the patient to say what he/she feels.	To test superficial sensations to touch.
27. Ask the patient to close the eyes. Hold the tip of one of the patient's fingers between your thumb and index finger. Move it up and down and ask the patient to say in which direction it is moving. Repeat with the other hand. For the legs, hold the big toe.	To test proprioception. (Netter, 1975; Tortora & Anagnostakos, 1987). *Definition of proprioception*: the receipt of information from muscles and tendons to the labyrinth that enables the brain to determine movements and the position of the body.
28. Note the rate, character and pattern of the patient's respirations.	Respirations are controlled by different areas of the brain. When disease or injury affects these areas, respiratory changes may occur.
29. Take and record the patient's temperature at specified intervals.	Damage to the hypothalamus, the temperature-regulating centre in the brain, will be reflected in grossly abnormal temperatures.
30. Take and record the patient's blood pressure and pulse at specified intervals.	To monitor signs of increased intracranial pressure. Hypertension and bradycardia usually occur late, after the patient's level of consciousness has begun to deteriorate. Call for medical assistance as soon as it is evident that there is a deterioration in the patient's level of consciousness (Scherer, 1986; Tortora & Anagnostakos, 1987).

NURSING CARE PLAN

Category	**Frequency**	**Rationale**
All patients diagnosed as suffering from neurological or neurosurgical conditions.	At least four-hourly. affected by the patient's condition.	To monitor the condition of the patient so that any necessary action can be instigated.
Unconscious patients (including ventilated and anaesthetized patients).	Frequency indicated by patient's condition.	To monitor the condition closely and to detect trends so that appropriate action may be taken.

29

Observations

PULSE

Definition

The pulse is a pressure wave of blood caused by the alternating expansion and recoil of elastic arteries during each cardiac cycle.

Indications

The pulse is taken for the following reasons:

1. To determine the individual's pulse on admission as a base for comparing future measurements.
2. To monitor fluctuations in pulse.
3. To gather information on the heart rate, pattern of beats (rhythm) and amplitude (strength) of pulse.

REFERENCE MATERIAL

The arterial pulse rate reflects the heart rate and is influenced by activity, postural changes and emotion (Marieb, 1989). Each time the heart beats, it propels blood through the arteries. This pumping action of the heart causes the walls of the arteries to expand and distend. The effect can be felt with the fingers as a wave-like sensation felt as the pulse (Timby, 1989). The pulse can be felt in any arteries lying close to the body surface (Figure 29.1) by lightly compressing the artery against firm tissue and by recording the number of beats (Timby, 1989).

The pulse is palpated to note the following:

1. Rate.
2. Rhythm.
3. Amplitude.

Rate

The normal pulse rate varies in different client groups as age related changes affect the pulse rate, the approximate range is illustrated in Table 29.1 (Timby, 1989).

The pulse may vary depending on the posture of an individual. For example, the pulse of a healthy man may be around 66 beats per minute when he is lying down; this increases to 70 when sitting up, and 80 when he stands suddenly (Marieb, 1989).

The rate of the pulse of an individual with a healthy heart tends to be relatively constant. However, when blood volume drops suddenly or when the heart has been weakened by disease, the stroke volume declines and cardiac output is maintained only by increasing the rate of heart beat.

Cardiac output is the amount of blood pumped out by each heart ventricle in one minute, while the stroke volume is the amount of blood pumped out by a ventricle with each contraction. The relationship between these and the heart rate is expressed in the following equation:

Cardiac output = heart rate × stroke volume.

The heart rate and hence pulse rate are influenced by various factors acting through neural, chemical and physically induced homeostatic mechanisms (Figure 29.2):

1. Neural changes in heart rate are caused by the activation of the sympathetic nervous system which increases heart rate, while parasympathetic activation decreases heart rate (Ganong, 1987).
2. Chemical regulation of the heart is affected by hormones (adrenaline and thyroxine) and electrolytes (sodium, potassium and calcium) (Ganong, 1987). Imbalances of electrolytes may excite or depress heart muscle, posing a danger to health (Brunner & Suddarth, 1989).
3. Physical factors that influence heart rate are age, sex, exercise and body temperature (Marieb, 1989).

Tachycardia is defined as an abnormally fast heart rate, over 100 beats per minute in adults, which may result from a raised body temperature, stress, certain drugs or heart disease (Marieb, 1989).

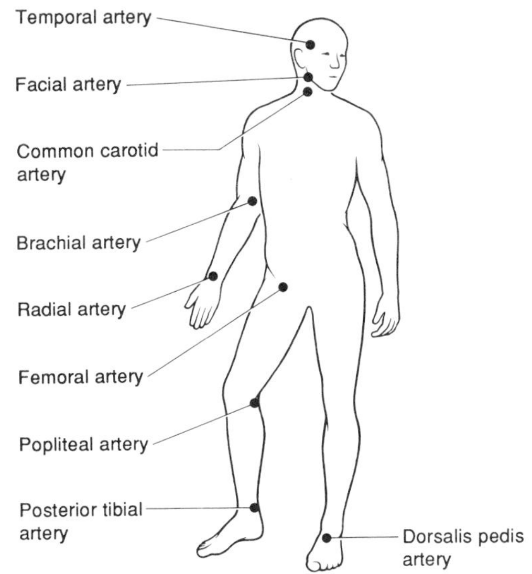

Figure 29.1 The pulse can be felt in arteries lying close to the body surface.

Bradycardia is a heart rate slower than 60 beats per minute. It may be the result of a low body temperature, certain drugs or parasympathetic nervous system activation. It is also found in fit athletes when physical and cardiovascular conditioning occurs. This results in hypertrophy of the heart with an increase in its stroke volume. These heart changes result in a lower resting heart rate but with the same cardiac output (Marieb, 1989). If persistent bradycardia occurs in an individual as a result of ill health, this may result in inadequate blood circulation to body tissues.

Table 29.1 Normal pulse rates per minute at various ages

Age	*Approximate range*	*Average*
Newborn	120–160	140
1–12 months	80–140	120
12 mths–2 years	80–130	110
2 years–6 years	75–120	100
6 years–12 years	75–110	95
Adolescent	60–100	80
Adult	60–100	80

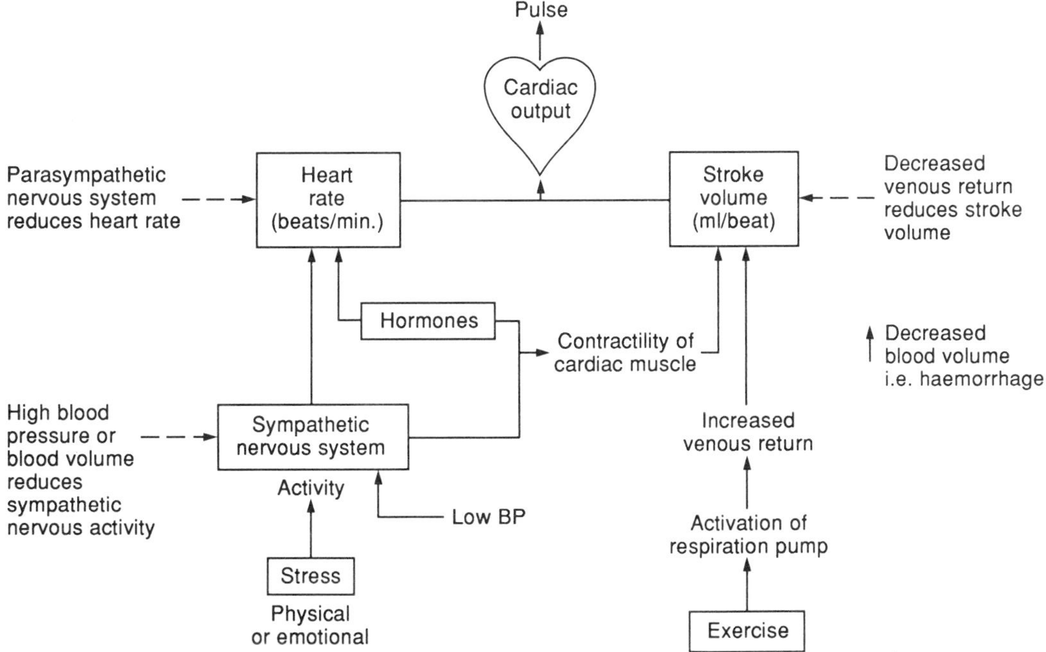

Figure 29.2 Factors affecting cardiac output and pulse.

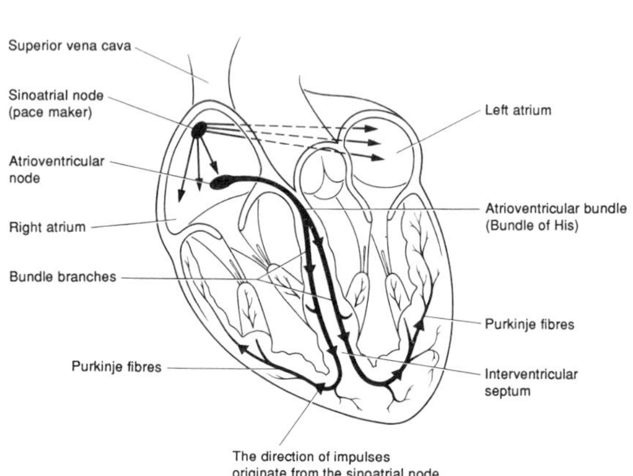

Figure 29.3 Intrinsic conduction system of the heart.

Bradycardia is a sign of brain oedema after head trauma or surgery (Hickey, 1986).

Rhythm

The pulse rhythm is the sequence of beats. In health, these are regular. The co-ordinated action of the muscles of the heart in producing a regular heart rhythm is due to the ability of cardiac muscle to contract inherently without nervous control (Marieb, 1989). The co-ordinated action of the muscles in the heart results from two physiological factors:

1. Gap junctions in the cardiac muscles which form interconnections between adjacent cardiac muscles and allow transmission of nervous impulses from cell to cell (Marieb, 1989).
2. Specialized nerve-like cardiac cells that form the nodal system. These initiate and distribute impulses throughout the heart, so that the heart beats as one unit (Marieb, 1989). These are the sinoatrial node, atrioventricular node, atrioventricular bundle and the Purkinje fibres.

The sinoatrial node is the pacemaker, initiating each wave of contraction, this sets the rhythm for the heart as a whole (Figure 29.3). Its characteristic rhythm is called *sinus rhythm*.

Defects in the conduction system of the heart can cause irregular heart rhythms, or arrhythmias, resulting in unco-ordinated contraction of the heart.

Fibrillation is a condition of rapid and irregular contractions. A fibrillating heart is ineffective as a pump (Marieb, 1989). *Atrial fibrillation* is a disruption of rhythm in the atrial areas of the heart occurring at extremely rapid and unco-ordinated intervals. The rapid impulses result in the ventricles not being able to respond to every atrial beat and, therefore, the ventricles contract irregularly. The cause of this condition is usually due to ischaemic heart disease (Brunner & Suddarth, 1989).

Ventricular fibrillation is an irregular heart rhythm characterized by chaotic contraction of the ventricles at very rapid rates. Ventricular fibrillation can cause death in minutes if it is not reversed rapidly. The frequent cause of this condition is often myocardial infarction, electrical shock, acidosis and electrolyte disturbances (Brunner & Suddarth, 1989).

Amplitude

Amplitude is a reflection of pulse strength and the elasticity of the arterial wall. The flexibility of the artery of the young adult feels very different from the hard artery of the patient suffering from arteriosclerosis. A full, throbbing pulse may indicate such conditions as complete heart block, anaemia or heart failure. Anxiety, alcohol or exercise may produce the same result (Brunner & Suddarth, 1989).

Assessing gross pulse irregularity

Paradoxical pulse is a pulse that markedly decreases in size during inspiration (Brunner & Suddarth, 1989). On inspiration, more blood is pooled in the lungs and so decreases the return to the left side of the heart; this affects the consequent stroke volume. A paradoxical pulse is usually regarded as normal, although in conjunction with such features as hypotension and dyspnoea, it may indicate cardiac tamponade.

When there is a gross pulse irregularity, it may be useful to use a stethoscope to assess the apical heart beat. This is done by placing the bell of the stethoscope over the apex of the heart and counting the beats for 60 seconds. A second nurse should record the radial pulse at the same time. The deficit between the two should be noted using, for example, different colours on the patient's chart to indicate the apex and radial rates.

Conditions where a patient's pulse may need careful monitoring are described below:

1. Postoperative and critically ill patients require monitoring of the pulse to assess for cardiovascular stability. The patient's pulse should be recorded pre-operatively in order to be able to make comparisons. Hypovalaemic shock post surgery from the loss of plasma or whole blood results in a decrease in circulatory blood volume. The resulting acceleration in heart rate causes a tachycardia that can be felt in the pulse. A large volume deficit

of 1800 ml to 2500 ml results in a thready as well as a tachycardic pulse (Brunner & Suddarth, 1989).
2. Blood transfusions require the careful monitoring of the pulse as an incompatible blood transfusion may lead to a rise in pulse rate (Cluroe, 1989).
3. Patients receiving intravenous infusions require the monitoring of pulse to observe for bacteraemia. Contamination of equipment or solutions may cause a sudden rise in pulse rate (Brunner & Suddarth, 1989).
4. Patients with local, systemic infections or neutropenia require monitoring of their pulse to detect septicaemic shock. This is characterized by a decrease in the circulatory blood volume with a resulting rise in pulse rate (Brunner & Suddarth, 1989).
5. Patients with cardiovascular conditions require monitoring of the pulse to evaluate the condition of the patient and the effectiveness of the medication.

References and further reading

Birdsall, C. (1985) How do you interpret pulses? *American Journal of Nursing*, 85(7), 785–6.

Brunner, L. S. & Suddarth, D. S. (1989) *The Lippincott Manual of Medical-Surgical Nursing, Volume 2*. Harper & Row, London.

Cluroe, S. (1989) Blood transfusions. *Nursing*, 3(40), 8–11.

Ganong, W. F. (1987) *Review of Medical Physiology*, 13 edn. Appelton & Lange, Norwalk, Connecticut.

Jarvis, C. M. (1980) Vital signs: a preview of problems. In *Assessing Vital Functions Accurately*, Intermed Communications,

Hickey, J. V. (1986) *The Clinical Practice of Neurological and Neurosurgical Nursing*, 2nd edn. J. B. Lippincott, Philadelphia.

Marieb, E. M. (1989) *Human Anatomy and Physiology*. Benjamin Cummings, California.

Timby, B. (1989) *Clinical Nursing Procedure*. J. B. Lippincott, Philadelphia.

Wieck, L. *et al.* (1986) *Illustrated Manual of Nursing Techniques*, 3rd edn. J. B. Lippincott, Philadelphia.

GUIDELINES: PULSE

Procedure

Action	**Rationale**
1. Explain the procedure to the patient.	To obtain the patient's consent and co-operation.
2. Measure where possible the pulse under the same conditions each time. Ensure that the patient is comfortable.	To ensure continuity and consistency in recording. To ensure that the patient is comfortable.
3. Press gently against the peripheral artery being used to record the pulse.	The radial artery is usually used as it is often the most readily accessible.
4. Place the second or third fingers along the appropriate artery and press gently.	The fingertips are sensitive to touch. The thumb and forefinger have pulses of their own that may be mistaken for the patient's pulse.
5. The pulse should be counted for 60 seconds.	Sufficient time is required to detect irregularities or other defects.
6. Record the pulse rate.	To monitor differences and detect trends, any irregularities should be brought to the attention of the appropriate personnel.

Note: in children under two years of age, the pulse should not be taken in this way; the rapid pulse rate and small area for palpation can lead to inaccurate data. The heart rate should be assessed by utilizing a stethoscope and listening to the apical heart beat (Brunner & Suddarth, 1989).

BLOOD PRESSURE

Definition

Blood pressure may be defined as the force exerted by blood against the walls of the vessels in which it is contained. Differences in blood pressure between different areas of the circulation provide the driving force that keeps the blood moving through the body (Marieb, 1989). Blood pressure is usually expressed in terms of millimetres of mercury (mm Hg).

Indications

Blood pressure is measured for one of two reasons:

1. To determine the patient's blood pressure on admission as a base for comparing future measurements.
2. To monitor fluctuations in blood pressure.

REFERENCE MATERIAL

Blood flow is defined as the volume of blood flowing through a vessel at a given time from the heart. Blood flow is equivalent to cardiac output. Resistance to the cardiac output is opposite to flow and is a measure of the friction the blood encounters as it passes through the differently sized vessels (Marieb, 1989). There are three important sources of resistance: blood viscosity, vessel length and vessel diameter (Figure 29.4).

Viscosity is the internal resistance to flow and may be thought of as the 'stickiness' of a fluid. Blood is more viscous than water due to the elements of plasma proteins and cells that form its constituent parts, and consequently blood moves more slowly. The longer the vessel length, the greater the resistance encountered. The relationship between vessel length and viscosity is often constant; however, blood vessel diameter changes frequently and is an important factor in altering peripheral resistance. Increased peripheral resistance occurs by altering the fluid flow. In a small blood vessel more of the fluid is in contact with the vessel walls which results in increased friction. Arterioles are the major determinants of peripheral resistance because they are small diameter blood vessels which can expand in response to neural and chemical controls (Ganong, 1987).

Normal blood pressure is maintained by neural, chemical and renal controls. The neural controls operate via reflex arcs (Marieb, 1989) derived from stretch receptors found in the wall of the proximal arterial tree, especially in the region of the aortic arch and carotid sinuses. When arterial pressure rises, there is increased stimulation of these nerve endings. The increased number of impulses along

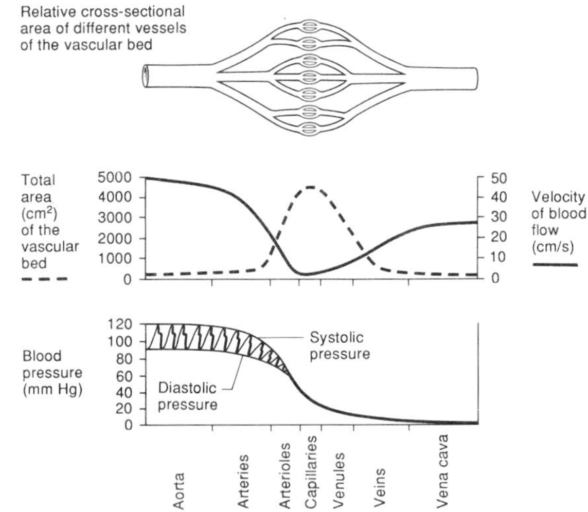

Figure 29.4 Effect of vessel length and diameter on blood pressure and blood flow.

the vagus and glossopharyngeal nerves leads to reflex vagal slowing of the heart and reflex release of vasoconstrictor tone in the peripheral blood vessels. The resulting fall in cardiac output and the reduction of peripheral resistance tend to restore the blood pressure to the normal value. A fall in the arterial pressure decreases the stimulation of the arterial stretch receptors. The reflex tachycardia and vasoconstriction that ensue tend to raise the blood pressure to its normal value forming a continuous homeostatic process (Ganong, 1987). When the oxygen content of the blood drops sharply, chemoreceptors in the aortic arch transmit impulses to the vasomotor centre and reflex constriction occurs. The rise in blood pressure that follows helps to increase blood return to the heart and lungs (Marieb, 1989). Renal regulation provides a major long-term mechanism of influencing blood pressure. When there is a fall in arterial pressure this results in chemical changes which lead to the release of the enzyme renin. Renin triggers a series of enzymatic reactions that result in the formation of angiotensin, a powerful vasoconstrictor chemical. Angiotensin also stimulates the adrenal cortex to release aldosterone, a hormone that increases renal reabsorption of sodium. The sodium, in turn, increases the volume of water reabsorbed by the kidneys; such retention of fluid and vasoconstriction of blood vessels raises arterial pressure.

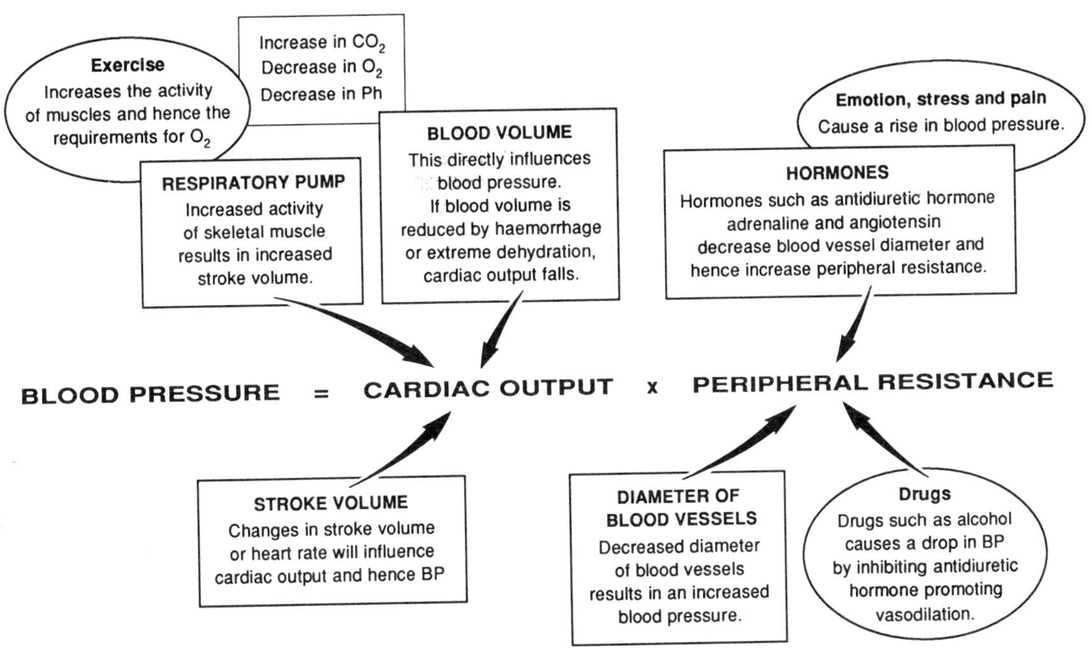

Figure 29.5 Factors affecting changes in blood pressure.

Blood pressure varies not only from moment to moment but also in the distribution between various organs and areas of the body. It is lowest in neonates and increases with age, weight gain, with stress and anxiety (Brunner & Suddarth, 1989). Shock, myocardial infarction and haemorrhage are factors which cause a fall in blood pressure as they reduce cardiac output and peripheral vessel resistance or they diminish venous return after fluid loss (Figure 29.5).

Normal blood pressure

Normal blood pressure generally ranges from 100/60 to 140/90 mm Hg. Blood pressure can fluctuate within a wide range and still be normal. Table 29.2 provides a guide for average normal and upper limits of normal blood pressure measurements for people of various ages.

Table 29.2 Average and upper limits of blood pressure according to age (Timby, 1989)

Age	*Average normal blood pressure*	*Upper limits of normal blood pressure*
1 year	95/65	Undetermined
6–9 years	100/65	119/79
10–13 years	110/65	124/84
14–17 years	120/80	134/89
18+ years	120/80	139/89

Systolic pressure

The systolic pressure is the maximum pressure of the blood against the wall of the vessel following ventricular contraction and is taken as an indication of the integrity of the heart, arteries and arterioles (Marieb, 1989).

Diastolic pressure

The diastolic pressure is the minimum pressure of the blood against the wall of the vessel following closure of the aortic valve and is taken as a direct indication of blood vessel resistance (Marieb, 1989).

Hypotension or low blood pressure is generally defined in adults as a systolic blood pressure below 100 mm Hg (Marieb, 1989). In many cases, hypotension simply reflects individual variations; however, it may indicate orthostatic hypotension, i.e. postural changes that result in a lack of normal reflex response leading to a low blood pressure.

Hypertension is defined as an elevation of systolic blood pressure. This may be a temporary response to fever, physical exertion or stress. Persistent hypertension is a common disease and approximately 30% of people over the age of 50 years are hypertensive (Marieb, 1989). Persistent hypertension is diagnosed in an individual when the average of three or more blood pressure readings taken at rest, several days apart, exceeds the upper limits illustrated in Table 29.2.

Mean arterial pressure

The mean arterial pressure is the average pressure required to push blood through the circulatory system. This can be determined electronically or mathematically as well as by using an intra-arterial catheter (see Chapter 2) and mercury manometer, e.g.

(mathematically)
mean arterial pressure
$= \frac{1}{3}$ systolic pressure + $\frac{2}{3}$ diastolic pressure

A blood pressure of 130/85 mm Hg gives a mean arterial pressure of 100 mg Hg.

Factors affecting blood pressure

The main factors that regulate blood pressure by altering peripheral resistance and blood volume are shown in Figure 29.5.

Methods of recording and equipment

There are two main methods for recording the blood pressure: direct and indirect.

Direct methods are more accurate than indirect methods. The ideal method of measuring blood pressure involves the insertion of a minute pressure transducer unit into an artery for transmission of a waveform or digital display on a monitor. The most commonly used techniques involve placing a cannula in an artery and attaching a pressure-sensitive device to the external end (see Chapter 2).

The *indirect* method is the auscultatory method. This procedure is used to measure blood pressure in the brachial artery of the arm.

The sphygmomanometer

The sphygmomanometer (see Figure 29.6) consists of a compression bag enclosed in an unyielding cuff, and inflating bulb, pump or other device by which the pressure is increased, a manometer from which the applied pressure is read, and a control valve to deflate the system.

Manometer

Mercury sphygmomanometers are reliable, on the whole, and easily maintained. Care should be taken to avoid loss of mercury. Substantial errors may occur if the manometer is not kept vertical during the measurement. The air vent at the top of the manometer must be kept patent. Aneroid sphygmomanometers are generally less accurate than mercury ones (Campbell *et al.*, 1990).

Cuff

The cuff is an inelastic cloth that encircles the arm and encloses the inflatable rubber bladder. It is secured around the arm or leg by wrapping its tapering end to the encircling material, by Velcro surfaces or by hooks.

Croft & Cruikshank (1990) in studying adults found that in terms of precision there is no basis for using two different cuff sizes. Readings from large cuffs came close to intra-arterial pressures in large arms and were also accurate for small arms. They recommend the use of large cuffs only.

Inflatable bladder

A bladder that is too short and/or too narrow will give falsely high pressures. The British Hypertension Society recommended in 1986 that the bladder length should be 80% of the arm circumference and the width at least 40%.

Control valve, pump and rubber tubing

The control valve is a common source of error. It should allow the passage of air without excessive pressure needing to be applied on the pump. When the valve is closed it should hold the mercury at a constant level and, when released, it should allow a controlled fall in the level of mercury. The rubber tubing should be long (approximately 80 cm) and with airtight connections that can easily be separated.

Campbell *et al.* (1990), in reviewing the methods for sphygmomanometer inaccuracies, found that errors in technique and equipment malfunction accounted for differences in readings of more than 15 mm Hg.

It is essential that the sphygmomanometer be kept in good working order. Conceicao *et al.* (1976) and North (1979) have shown that as many as 50% of the sphygmomanometers used in the hospitals they studied were inaccurate.

The stethoscope

Using the stethoscope it is possible to identify a series of five phases as blood pressure falls from the systolic to the diastolic. These phases are known as Korotkoff's sounds (Figure 29.7).

When the cuff pressure has fallen to just below the systolic pressure, a clear but often faint tapping sound suddenly appears in phase with each cardiac contraction. The tapping sound is produced by the transient

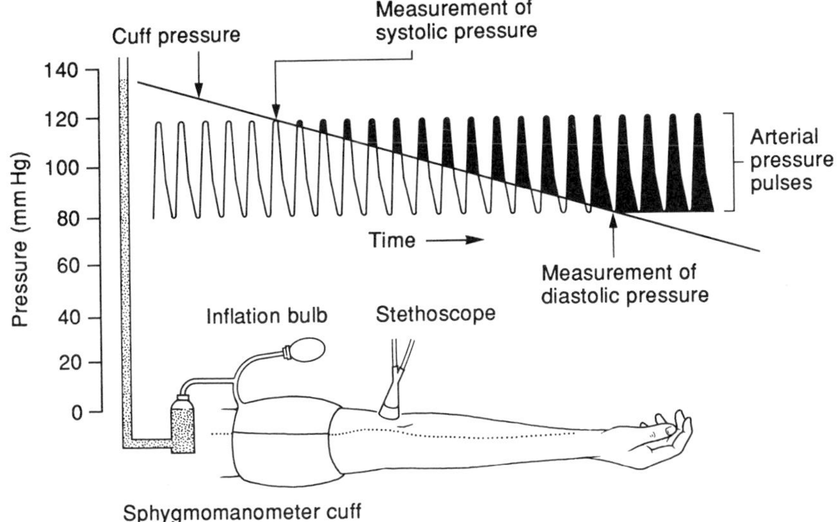

Figure 29.6 Using a sphygmomanometer.

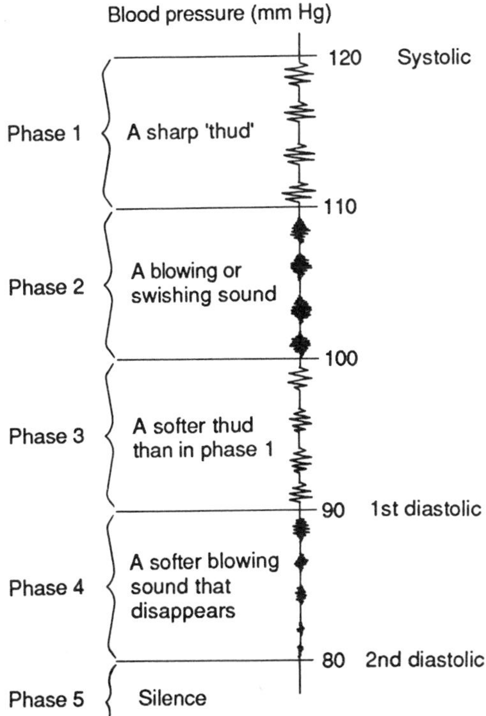

Figure 29.7 Korotkoff's sounds.

and turbulent blood flowing through the brachial artery during the peak of each systole.

As the pressure in the cuff is reduced further, the sound becomes louder, but when the artery is no longer constricted and the blood flows freely, the sounds become muffled and then can no longer be heard. The diastolic pressure is usually defined as the cuff pressure at which 'muffling' and not disappearance occurs. However, if there is an obvious difference between these, both values are reported (Figure 29.7) (Brunner & Suddarth, 1989).

The stethoscope's bell should be placed lightly over the brachial artery (Frohlich *et al.*, 1988). The bell is designed to amplify low frequency sounds such as Korotkoff's sounds (Hill & Grim, 1991). Excessive pressure on the stethoscope's bell may partially occlude the brachial artery and delay the occurrence of Korotkoff's sounds.

Korotkoff's sounds form five phases:

1. The appearance of faint, clear tapping sounds which gradually increase in intensity.
2. The softening of sounds, which may become swishing.
3. The return of sharper sounds which become crisper but never fully regain the intensity of the phase 1 sounds.

4. The distinct muffling sound which become soft and blowing.
5. The point at which all sound ceases.

Additional Information

Much recent research has focused on the faulty techniques employed when blood pressures are taken (Campbell *et al.*, 1990). Blood pressure readings are altered by various factors that influence the patient, the techniques used and the accuracy of the sphygmomanometer. The variability of any readings can be reduced by an improved technique and by several readings (Campbell *et al.*, 1990). Maxwell (1982) and the British Hypertension Society (1986) have shown that the number of patients diagnosed as hypertensive may be grossly over-estimated due to the use of cuffs that were too small. Thompson (1981) discussed, analysed and evaluated the methodology of blood pressure recording. Poor technique and observer bias as potential sources of error were also examined. He concluded that many nurses are often trained inadequately in blood pressure measurement and that, with increasing reliance on the nurse for recording vital signs, more attention needs to be paid to this area.

Variations in the procedure and frequency of taking blood pressure may be required in different patient groups with differing conditions. With a child it is important that the correctly sized cuff is used and that the average of repeated measurements is recorded. Low diastolic pressures are common in children and thus the pressure at muffling (Korotkoff phase 4.) may be difficult to determine. Hill & Grim (1991) suggest recording the onset of muffling sounds as well as that of no sounds (Korotkoff phase 5.) and record it as, for example, 96/54/46 mm Hg. Low diastolic pressures are common in elderly patients who may have atherosclerosis, and in patients with an increased cardiac output, i.e. as a result of pregnancy, exercise and hypothyroidism. These patients may need to have their blood pressure recorded in a similar way to those of children.

In pregnancy, changes in blood pressure may indicate pregnancy-induced hypertension. An increase of 30 mm Hg or more systolic pressure and 15 mm Hg diastolic pressure over the previous readings may be indicative of this condition (Ferris, 1990).

Patients with lines or shunts in their arms may preclude arm measurements of blood pressure; however, the blood pressure may be measured in the leg or forearm. For this procedure the patient lies prone and a thigh or large cuff is applied to the lower third of the thigh. The cuff is wrapped securely with its lower edge above the knee and its bladder centred over the posterior popliteal artery. The stethoscope bell should be applied on the artery below the cuff. Systolic blood pressure is normally 20 to 30 mm Hg higher in the leg than in the arm. The right-sized cuff should be used for obtaining the blood pressure using the forearm, and the bladder should be centred over the radial artery below the elbow, and the cuff wrapped in a similar manner to the normal procedure. The stethoscope bell should be positioned over the radial artery about 2.5 cm above the wrist. Forearm blood pressure measurements may vary significantly from an upper arm measurement, and therefore it is important to document cuff size and location (Hill & Grim, 1991).

Conditions where a patient's blood pressure may need careful monitoring are described below:

1. Hypertension is never diagnosed on a single blood pressure reading. The blood pressure is monitored to evaluate the condition of the patient and the effectiveness of medication (Marieb, 1989).
2. Postoperative and critically ill patients require monitoring of blood pressure to assess for cardiovascular stability. The patient's blood pressure should be recorded pre-operatively in order to make significant comparisons. The reduction in cardiac diastole post surgery may result in a lessened coronary perfusion and therefore a reduced cardiac output and vasoconstriction. Report immediately a falling systolic pressure as this may be an indication of hypovolaemic shock (Brunner & Suddarth, 1989). Haemorrhage may be primary at the time of operation or intermediary in the first few hours after surgery. The blood pressure returns to the patient's normal levels and causes loosening of poorly tied vessels and the flushing out of clots. The resulting blood loss causes a decrease in cardiac output and hypotension. Secondary haemorrhage can occur some time after surgery and is due to infection, this also results in a fall in blood pressure (Brunner & Suddarth, 1989).
3. Blood transfusions require careful monitoring of the blood pressure for several reasons. An incompatible blood transfusion may lead to agglutination and a resulting fall in the blood pressure. Circulatory overload may lead to a rise in blood pressure, while the infusion of large quantities of blood may alter clotting factors and result in bleeding, causing a fall in blood pressure (Cluroe, 1989).
4. Patients receiving intravenous infusions require blood pressure monitoring to observe for circula-

tory overload (this occurs more frequently in elderly patients). The resulting increase in blood volume causes a rise in blood pressure (Brunner & Suddarth, 1989).

5. Patients with local, systemic infections or neutropenia require monitoring of their blood pressure in order to detect septicaemic shock. This is characterized by a change in the capillary epithelium, permitting loss of blood and plasma through capillary walls into surrounding tissues. The decrease in the circulating volume of blood results in impaired tissue perfusion culminating in cellular hypoxia (Ganong, 1989).

References and further reading

Brunner, L. S. & Suddarth, D. S. (1989) *The Lippincott Manual of Medical-Surgical Nursing, Volume 2*. Harper & Row, London.

Campbell, N. R. *et al.* (1990) Accurate, reproducible measurement of blood pressure. *Can. Med. Assoc. J.*, 143(1), 19–24.

Cluroe, S. (1989) Blood transfusions. *Nursing*, 3(40), 8–11.

Conceicao, S. *et al.* (1976) Defects in sphygmanometers. *British Medical Journal*, 2, 886–8.

Croft, P. R. & Cruikshank, J. K. (1990) Blood pressure measurement in adults: large cuffs for all. *Journal of Epidemiology and Community Health*, 44, 107–73.

Ferris, T. F. (1990) Hypertension in pregnancy. *The Kidney*, 23(1), 1–5.

Frohlich, E. D. *et al.* (1988) Recommendations for human blood pressure determination by sphygmomanometers. Report of a special task force appointed by the steering committee, American Heart Association. *Hypertension*, 11, 210a–21a.

Ganong, W. F. (1987) *Review of Medical Physiology*, 13 edn. Appelton & Lange, Norwalk, Connecticut.

Hill, M. N. & Grim, C. M. (1991) How to take a precise blood pressure. *American Journal of Nursing*, 91(2), 38–42.

Jamieson, M. (1990) The measurement of blood pressure, sitting or supine, once or twice? *Journal of Hypertension*, 8, 635–40.

Jarvis, C. M. (1980) Vital signs: a preview of problems. In *Assessing Vital Functions Accurately*, Intermed Communications,

Kilgour, D. & Speedie, G. (1985) Taking the pressure off. *Nursing Mirror*, 160(9), 39–40.

Londe, S. & Klitzner, T. (1984) Auscultatory blood pressure measurement: effect of pressure on the head of stethoscope. *West J. Med.*, 141(2), 193–5.

Marieb, E. M. (1989) *Human Anatomy and Physiology*. Benjamin Cummings, California.

Maxwell, M. H. (1982) Error in blood pressure measurement due to incorrect cuff size in obese patients. *Lancet*, 2, 33–6.

North, L. W. (1979) Accuracy of sphygmomanometers. *Association of Operating Room Nurses Journal*, 30, 996–1000.

Petrie, J. C. *et al.* (1986) Recommendations on blood pressure measurement. *British Medical Journal*, 293, 611–5.

Padfield, D. *et al.* (1990) Problems in the measurement of blood pressure. *Journal of Human Hypertension*, 4(Suppl. 2), 3–7.

Rebenson-Piano, M. *et al.* (1987) An examination of the differences that occur between direct and indirect blood pressure measurement. *Heart and Lung*, 16(3), 285–94.

Thompson, D. R. (1981) Recording patients' blood pressure: a review. *Journal of Advanced Nursing*, 6(4), 283–90.

Timby, B. (1989) *Clinical Nursing Procedure*. J. B. Lippincott, Philadelphia.

Webster, J. *et al.* (1984) Influence of arm position on measurement of blood pressure. *British Medical Journal*, 288, 1574–5.

Wells, D. (1990) A case for accuracy – monitoring blood pressure. *The Professional Nurse*, 6(1), 30–2.

GUIDELINES: BLOOD PRESSURE

Equipment

1. Sphygmomanometer.
2. Stethoscope.

Procedure

Action	Rationale
1. Explain to the patient that blood pressure is to be taken.	To obtain the patient's consent and co-operation.
2. Measure where possible the blood pressure under the same conditions each time.	To ensure continuity and consistency in recording.
3. Ensure that the patient is in the desired position:	To obtain an accurate reading. Measurement made

Guidelines: Blood pressure

Action	Rationale
lying, standing or sitting. Also ensure that the sphygmomanometer is positioned at heart level, with the palm of the hand facing upwards, regardless of whether the patient is standing or sitting (Frohlich *et al.*, 1988).	with the arm dangling by the hip have been 11 to 12 mm Hg higher than those made with the arm supported and the cuff at heart level. Measurements with the arm raised can be falsely high (Webster *et al.*, 1984).
4. Use a large cuff size (Croft & Cruikshank 1990)	To obtain the correct reading.
5. Apply the cuff of the sphygmomanometer snugly around the arm, 2.5 cm above the anticubital fosa (Timby, 1989). If the patient is sitting or standing, the blood pressure cuff must be placed at the level of the patient's heart. If the patient is supine, rest arm next to patient on a flat surface with the cuff in line with the midaxillar (Hill & Grim, 1991).	Measurement made with the cuff in the wrong position may give false results. For every cm that the cuff sits above or below the heart level, the blood pressure varies by 0.8 mm Hg (Hill & Grim, 1991).
6. Inflate cuff until radial pulse can no longer be felt. This provides an estimation of systolic pressure. Deflate the cuff completely and wait 15 to 30 seconds before continuing to measure (Hill & Grim, 1991).	A low systolic pressure may be reported in patients who have an auscultatory gap. This is when Korotkoff's sounds disappear shortly after what corresponds to the systolic pressure is heard, and resuming well above what corresponds to the diastolic pressure. About 5% of the population have an auscultatory gap and it is commonest in those with hypertension (Hill & Grim, 1991). This error can be avoided if the systolic pressure is first estimated by palpitation.
7. The cuff is then inflated to a pressure 30 mm Hg higher than the estimated systolic pressure (Timby, 1989).	Pressure exerted by the inflated cuff prevents blood from flowing through the artery.
8. Place the bell of the stethoscope over the brachial artery.	Apply just enough pressure on the stethoscope to keep it in its place over the brachial artery. Excessive pressure can distort sounds or make them persist for longer than normal (Londe & Klitzner, 1984).
9. Deflate the cuff at 2 to 3 mm Hg per second.	At a slower rate of deflation, venous congestion and arm pain can develop, resulting in a falsely low reading. At faster rates of deflation the mercury may fall too quickly, resulting in an imprecise reading (Hill & Grim, 1991).
10. Record the systolic and diastolic pressures and compare the present reading with previous readings. It may be necessary to record both phases 4 and 5 of Korotkoff's sounds if they are indistinct. Any irregularities should be brought to the attention of the appropriate personnel.	The average of two or more blood pressure readings are often taken to represent a patient's normal blood pressure. Taking more than one measurement reduces the influence of anxiety and may provide a more accurate record (Hill & Grim, 1991).
11. Remove the equipment and clean after use.	To prevent the spread of infection.

RESPIRATIONS

Definition

The function of the respiratory system is to supply the body with oxygen and remove carbon dioxide. This is achieved by the diffusion of gases between the air in the alveoli of the lungs and the blood in the alveolar capillaries (Marieb, 1989).

Indications

The respiration rate is evaluated:

1. To determine the per minute rate on admission as a base for comparing future measurements.
2. To monitor fluctuations in respiration.
3. To evaluate the patient's response to medications or treatments that affect the respiratory system.

REFERENCE MATERIAL

The body cells require a continuous supply of oxygen to carry out their vital functions and this is provided by respiration (Marieb, 1989).

To accomplish respiration, four distinct events must occur:

1. Ventilation is where air is moved into and out of the lungs so that gas in the air sacs is replenished.
2. Gaseous exchange between the blood and the alveoli.
3. Oxygen and carbon dioxide are transported to and from the lungs by the cardiovascular system. This is called respiratory transportation.
4. Internal respiration is the cellular respiration that occurs in the cell where oxygen is utilized and carbon dioxide produced.

Ventilation

Ventilation results from pressure changes transmitted from the thoracic cavity to the lungs (Figure 29.8). Inspiration is initiated by contraction of the diaphragm and external intercostal muscles. This results in the rib cage rising up, and the thrusting forward of the sternum. The ribs also swing outwards expanding their diameter and hence the volume of the thorax (Marieb, 1989). Because the lungs adhere tightly to the thoracic wall, attached by the layers of parietal and visceral pleura, this increases the intrapulmonary volume (Marieb, 1989). Gases travel from an area of high pressure to areas of low pressure. The increased intrapulmonary volume results in a negative pressure of 1 to 3 mm Hg less than the atmospheric pressure (Marieb, 1989). The resulting pressure gradient causes air to rush into the lungs (Figure 29.9).

Expiration is largely passive, occurring as the inspiratory muscles relax, the lungs recoil as a result of their elastic properties (Marieb, 1989). When intrapulmonary pressure exceeds atmospheric pressure this compresses the microscopic air sacs (alveoli) and an expiration of gases occurs.

Disease that effects the pleura of the individual may influence ventilation. Pleurisy, inflammation of the pleura where secretion of pleural fluid declines, causes a stabbing pain with each inspiration. Alternatively an excessive increase in pleural secretions may hinder breathing (Marieb, 1989). Air in the pleural space results in lung collapse (atelectasis). This affects the intrapulmonary pressure and hence ventilation. A chest wound or rupture of the visceral pleural may allow air to enter the pleural space from the respiratory tract. The presence of air in the intrapleural space is referred to as a pneumothorax.

The degree to which the lungs stretch and fill during inspiration and return to normal during expiration is due to the compliance and elasticity of lung tissue.

Lung compliance depends on the elasticity of lung tissue and the flexibility of the thorax (Marieb, 1989). When this is impaired expiration becomes an active process, requiring the use of energy. Emphysema is an example of a disease that influences the elasticity of the lung walls (Marieb, 1989). In emphysema the lungs become progressively less elastic and more fibrous which hinders both inspiration and expiration. The increased muscular activity results in greater energy required to breath.

Compliance is diminished by any factor that:

1. Reduces the natural resilience of the lungs.
2. Blocks the bronchi or respiratory passageways.
3. Impairs the flexibility of the thoracic cage.

Friction in the air passage ways causes resistance and affects ventilation (Ganong, 1987). Normally, airway resistance is reduced so that minimal opposition to airflow occurs. However, any factor that amplifies airway resistance such as the presence of mucus, tumour or infected material in the airways demands that breathing movements become more strenuous (Marieb, 1989).

Respiratory volumes and capacity tests

The amount of air that is breathed varies depending on the condition of inspiration and expiration. Information about an patient's respiratory status can be gained by measuring various lung capacities, which consist of the sum of different respiratory volumes.

The respiratory volumes shown in Figure 29.10 represent normal values for a healthy 20-year-old male weighing about 70 kg (Marieb, 1989).

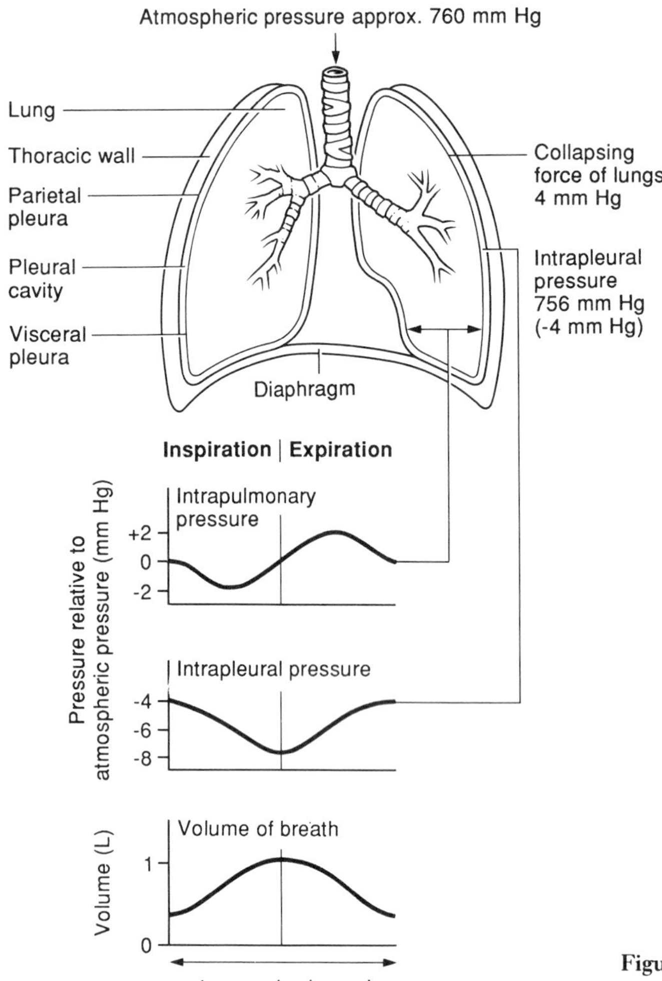

Figure 29.8 Ventilation occurs due to pressure changes transmitted from the thoracic cavity to the lungs.

Tidal volume (TV)

The tidal volume is the amount of air inhaled or exhaled with each breath under resting conditions (about 500 ml).

Inspiratory reserve volume (IRV)

The amount of air that can be inhaled forcibly after a normal tidal value inhalation (about 3100 ml).

Expiratory reserve volume (ERV)

The expiratory reserve volume is the maximum amount that can be exhaled forcibly after a normal tidal value exhalation (about 1200 ml).

Residual volume (RV)

The residual volume is the amount of air remaining in the lungs after a forced expiration (about 1200 ml).

Respiratory capacities

These values are measured for diagnostic purposes. They consist of two or more respiratory lung volumes.

Total lung capacity (TLC)

The total long capacity is the amount of air in the lungs at the end of a maximum inspiration.

TLC = TV + IRV + ERV + RV (6000 ml).

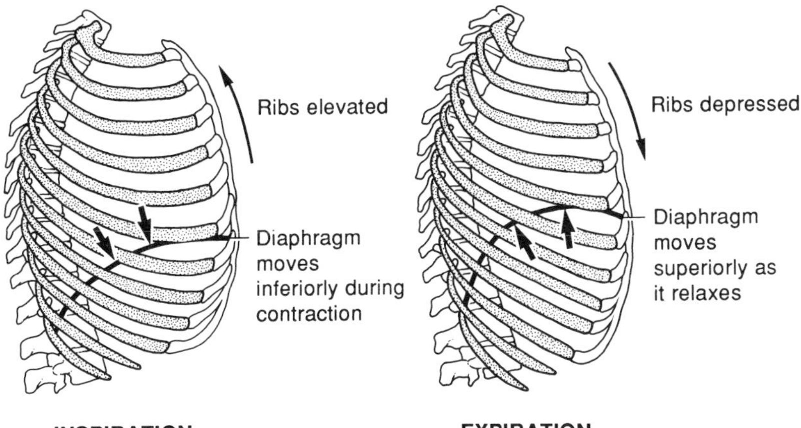

Figure 29.9 Changes in thoracic volume during breathing.

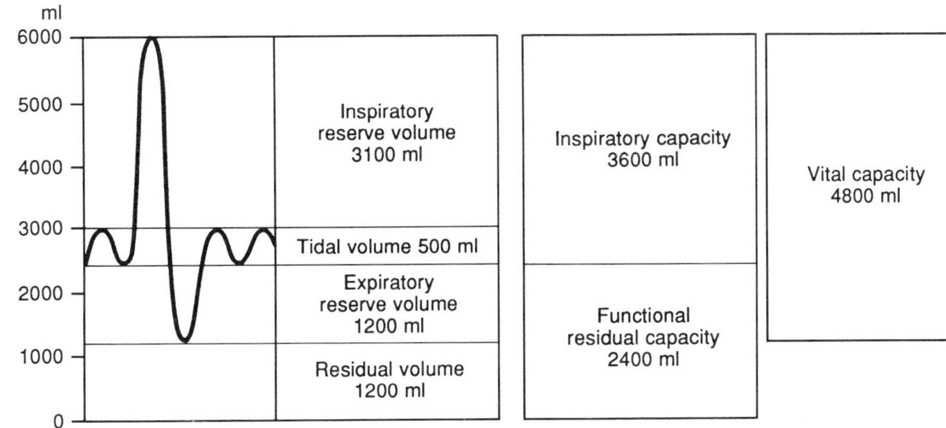

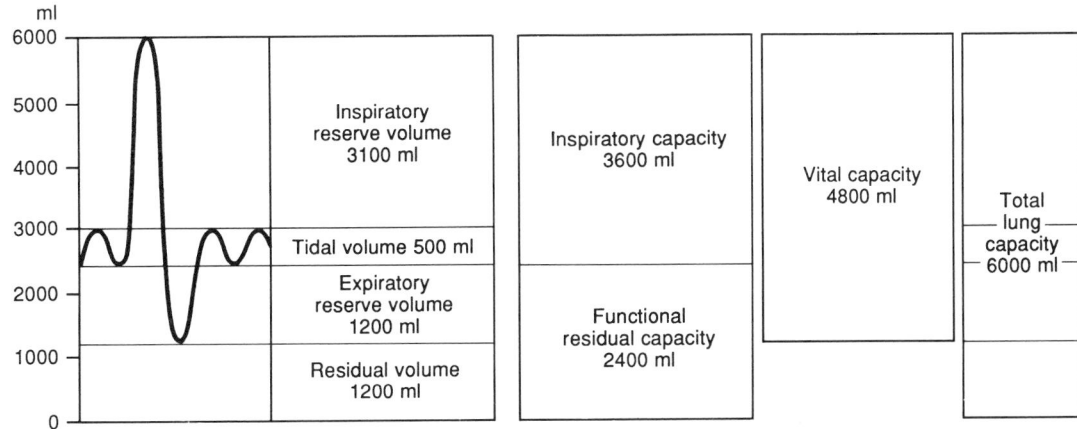

Figure 29.10 Respiratory volumes and capacities.

Vital capacity (VC)
The vital capacity is the maximum amount of air that can be expired after a maximum inspiration.

VC = TV + IRV + ERV (4800 ml)

Inspiratory capacity (IC)
The inspiratory capacity is the maximum amount of air that can be inspired after a normal expiration.

IC = TV + IVR (3600 ml).

Functional residual capacity (FRC)
This describes the amount of air remaining in the lungs after a normal tidal volume expiration.

FRC = ERV + RV (2400 ml).

Dead space
Some of the inspired air fills the respiratory passageways and does not contribute to gaseous exchange. This is termed the anatomical dead space.

Gaseous exchange

Oxygen in the inspired air enters while carbon dioxide leaves the blood in the lungs in the process of ventilation. These gases move in opposite directions in the alveoli by the mechanism of diffusion (Marieb, 1989). Adjacent to the alveoli is a dense vascular network. Oxygen moves into the alveolar capillaries and carbon dioxide moves out (Figure 29.11). This process is called gaseous exchange. Factors influencing this process include the partial pressure gradients, the

TRANSPORT AND EXCHANGE OF CARBON DIOXIDE AND OXYGEN

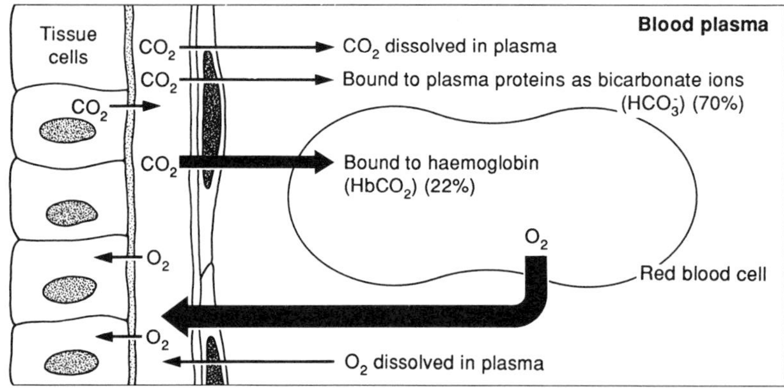

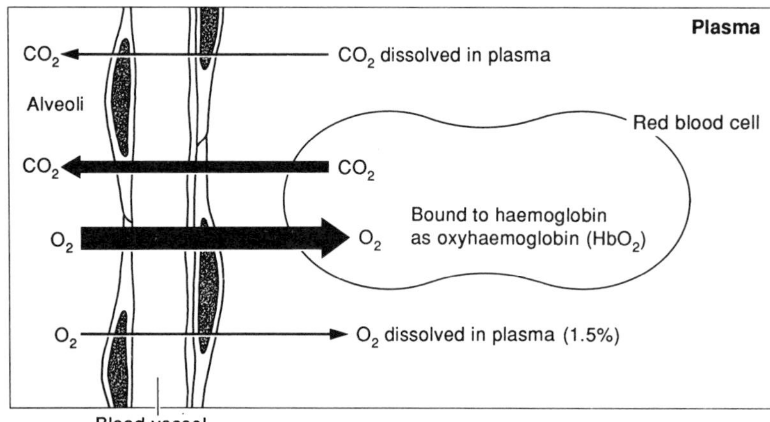

Figure 29.11 Gaseous exchange.

thickness of the respiratory membrane and the surface area available.

The gaseous composition of the atmosphere and alveoli are demonstrated in Table 29.3. The atmosphere consists almost entirely of oxygen and nitrogen, the alveoli contain more carbon dioxide and water vapour and considerably less oxygen. These different figures reflect the following processes:

1. Gaseous exchange in the lungs.
2. Humidification of air by the respiratory passageways.
3. The mixing of alveolar gas that occurs with each breath.

Respiratory transportation

Oxygen is carried in the blood in two ways, bound to the haemoglobin within the red blood cells and dissolved in plasma. Haemoglobin carries 98.5% of the oxygen from the lungs and the tissues. The amount of oxygen bound to haemoglobin depends on several factors:

Table 29.3 Composition of gas in the atmosphere and alveoli

	Atmosphere inspired	*Alveoli*
Oxygen	20.9%	13.7%
Carbon dioxide	0.04%	5.2%
Nitrogen	78.6%	74.9%
Water	0.46%	6.2%

1. The partial pressure of oxygen (PO_2) and the partial pressure of carbon dioxide (PCO_2) in the blood. The gradient of partial pressure influences the rates of diffusion, the oxygen gradient being steeper than that of carbon dioxide. Carbon dioxide is transported from the tissue primarily as bicarbonate ions in the plasma (70%), whereas only small amounts are transported by haemoglobin in the red blood cells (22%).
2. The blood pH influences the affinity of haemoglobin for oxygen: as the pH decreases, as in acidosis, the amount of oxygen unloaded in the tissues increases.
3. As body temperature rises above normal levels, the affinity of haemoglobin for oxygen declines, and therefore oxygen unloading is enhanced. This effect is seen in localized temperature changes such as inflammation.

Diseases that reduce the oxygen-carrying ability of the blood whatever the cause are termed anaemia. This is characterized by oxygen blood levels that are inadequate to support normal metabolism (Marieb, 1989). Common causes of anaemia include:

1. Insufficient number of red cells, including destruction of red cells, haemorrhage and bone marrow failure.
2. Decreases in haemoglobin content, including iron deficiency anaemia and pernicious anaemia.
3. Abnormal haemoglobin, including thalassaemia and sickle cell anaemia (Marieb, 1989).

Internal respiration

Internal respiration is the exchange of gases that occurs within the tissues between the capillaries and the cells. Carbon dioxide enters the blood and oxygen moves into the cells (see Figure 29.11).

Hypoxia is the result of an inadequate amount of oxygen delivered to body tissues. The blue coloration of tissues and mucosal membranes is termed cyanosis.

Control of respiration

Respiratory centre

The respiratory centre generates the basic pattern of breathing. It is located in the brain and is made up of groups of nerve cells in the reticular formation of the medulla oblongata. Regular impulses are sent by these cells to the motor neurones in the anterior horn of the spinal cord which supply the intercostal muscles and the diaphragm (Ganong, 1987). When the motor neurones are stimulated, the muscles contract and inspiration occurs. When the neurones are inhibited, the muscles relax and expiration follows.

Although the respiratory centre generates the basic rhythm, the depth and rate of breathing can be altered in response to the body's changing needs. The most important factors are those of nervous and chemical control (Figure 29.12).

Nervous control

Lung tissue is stretched on inspiration and this stimulates afferent fibres in the vagus nerve. These impulses cause inspiration to cease and expiration occurs. Emotion, pain and anxiety also cause an increased respiratory rate (Marieb, 1989).

Chemical control

An increase in the amount of carbon dioxide in the blood supplying the respiratory centre stimulates the respiratory centre and breathing becomes faster and deeper.

During exercise, carbon dioxide is produced in the muscles by the oxidation of carbohydrate. The amount of carbon dioxide in the blood increases and this stimulates the respiratory centre, producing an increase in depth and rate of respiration. More oxygen is made available in the alveoli for the blood to transport to the muscles, at the same time eliminating more carbon dioxide.

Any substance which, like carbon dioxide, lowers the pH of the blood will stimulate the respiratory centre. Figure 29.12 illustrates the factors influencing the rate and depth of breathing.

Patients with respiratory disease, e.g. emphysema and chronic bronchitis, who maintain high levels of carbon dioxide, will have arterial oxygen levels below 60 mm Hg. This is termed the 'hypoxic drive'. This chronic elevation of the partial pressure of carbon dioxide results in the chemoreceptors becoming unresponsive to this chemical stimulus. The change in respiratory drive results in respiration being stimulated by decreases in oxygen levels rather than that of carbon dioxide (Marieb, 1989). This may be detrimental to the patient's respiration if oxygen is administered therapeutically at high levels (see Chapter 30).

Lung defence mechanisms

The upper airway is designed to warm, humidify and filter inspired air. The nasal passages absorb noxious gases and trap inhaled particles. Smaller particles are removed by the cough reflex.

Observation of respiration

Respirations in an individual should be observed for rate, depth and pattern of breathing.

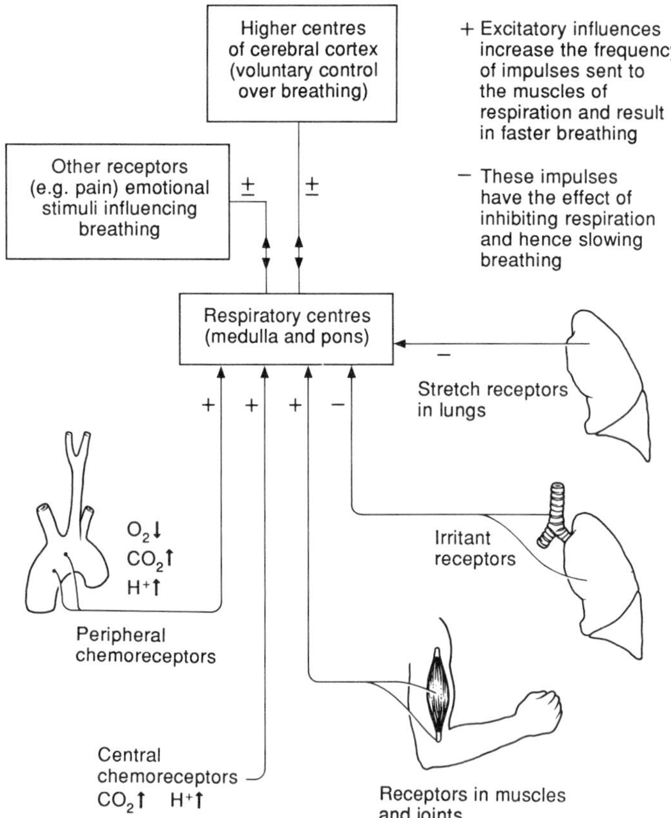

Figure 29.12 Control of respiration.

Table 29.4 Respiratory rates (Timby, 1989)

Age	*Average range/minute*
Newborn	30–80
Early childhood	20–40
Late childhood	15–25
Adulthood – male	14–18
Adulthood – female	16–20

Rate

Rate and depth determine the type of respiration. The normal rate at rest is approximately 14 to 18 breaths per minute in adults and is faster in infants and children (Table 29.4). The ratio of pulse rate to respiration rate is approximately 5:1.

Changes in the rate of ventilation may be defined as follows: *Tachypnoea* is an increased respiratory rate, seen in fever, for example, as the body tries to rid itself of excess heat. Respirations increase by about seven breaths a minute for every 1°C rise in temperature above normal. They also increase with pneumonia, other obstructive airway diseases, respiratory insufficiency and lesions in the pons of the brainstem (Brunner & Suddarth, 1989).

Bradypnoea is a decreased but regular respiratory rate, such as that caused by the depression of the respiratory centre in the medulla by opiate narcotics, or by a brain tumour.

Depth

The depth of respiration is the volume of air moving in and out with each respiration. This tidal volume is normally about 500 ml in an adult and should be constant with each breath. A spirometer is used to measure the precise amount (see respiratory capacities). Normal, relaxed breathing is effortless, automatic, regular and almost silent.

Dyspnoea is undue breathlessness and an awareness

of discomfort with breathing. There are several types of dyspnoea:

1. Exertional dyspnoea is shortness of breath on exercise and is seen with heart failure.
2. Orthopnoea is a shortness of breath on lying down which is relieved by the patient sitting upright. This is often caused by left ventricular failure of the heart.
3. Paroxysmal, nocturnal dyspnoea is a sudden breathlessness that occurs at night when the patient is lying down and is often caused by pulmonary oedema and left ventricular failure (Brunner & Suddarth, 1989).

Pattern

Changes in the pattern of respiration are often found in disorders of the respiratory control centre (Brunner & Suddarth, 1989). Examples of changes in respiratory pattern follow:

Hyperventilation is an increase in both the rate and depth of respiration. This follows extreme exertion, fear and anxiety, fever, hepatic coma, midbrain lesions of the brainstem, and acid–base imbalance such as diabetic ketoacidosis (Kussmaul's respiration) or salicylate overdose (in both of these situations the body compensates for the metabolic acidosis by increased respiration), as well as an alteration in blood gas concentration (either increased carbon dioxide or decreased oxygen). The breathing pattern is normally regular and consists of inspiration, pause, longer expiration and another pause. But this may be altered by some defects and diseases. In adults, more than 20 breaths per minute is considered moderate, more than 30 is severe.

Apnoeustic respiration is a pattern of prolonged, gasping inspiration, followed by extremely short, inefficient expiration, seen in lesions of the pons in the midbrain.

Cheyne-Stokes respiration is periodic breathing, characterized by a gradual increase in depth of respiration followed by a decrease in respiration, resulting in apnoea (Brunner & Suddarth, 1989).

Biot's respiration is an interrupted breathing pattern, like Cheyne-Stokes respiration, except that each breath is of the same depth. It may be seen with spiral meningitis or other central nervous system conditions.

Conditions where a patient's respirations may need careful monitoring are described below:

1. Patients with conditions that effect respiration, such as those described in the text, require monitoring of respiration to evaluate their condition and the effectiveness of medication.
2. Postoperative and critically ill patients require monitoring of respiration. The patient's respiration should be recorded pre-operatively in order to make significant comparisons. The breathing is observed to assess for the return to normal respiratory function.
3. Patients receiving oxygen inhalation therapy or receiving artificial respiration require monitoring of breathing to assess respiratory function (see Chapter 30).

References and further reading

Bell, G. H. *et al.* (1980) *Textbook of Physiology and Biochemistry*, 10th edn. Churchill Livingstone, Edinburgh.

Boylan, A. & Brown, P. (1985) Respirations. *Nursing Times*, 81, 35–8.

Brunner, L. S. & Suddarth, D. S. (1989) *The Lippincott Manual of Medical Surgical Nursing*, Vol. 2. Harper & Row, London.

Ganong, W. F. (1987) *Review of Medical Physiology*, 13th edn. Appelton & Lange, New York.

Glennister, T. W. A. & Ross, R. W. (1980) *Anatomy and Physiology for Nurses*, 3rd edn. William Heinemann Medical Books, London.

Jarvis, C. M. (1980) Vital signs: a preview of problems. In *Assessing Vital Functions Accurately*, Intermed Communications,

Roberts, A. (1980) Systems and signs. Respiration 1, 2. *Nursing Times*, 76, *Systems of Life*, Nos. 71, 72, p. 8.

Rokosky, J. S. (1981) Assessment of the individual with altered respiratory function. *Nursing Clinics of North America*, 16(2), 195–9.

Marieb, E. M. (1989) *Human Anatomy and Physiology*. Benjamin Cummings, California.

Timby, B. (1989) *Clinical Nursing Procedure*. J. B. Lippincott, Philadelphia.

TEMPERATURE

Definition

Body temperature represents the balance between heat gain and heat loss.

Indications

Measurement of body temperature is carried out for two reasons:

1. To determine the patient's temperature on admission as a base for comparing future measurements.
2. To monitor fluctuations in temperature.

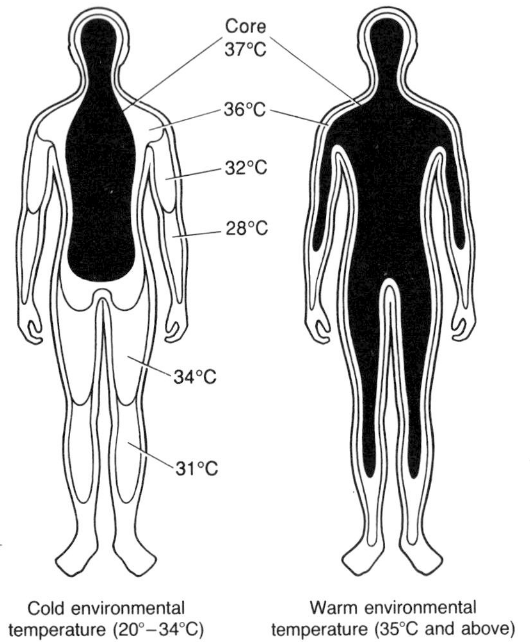

Figure 29.13 Body core and skin temperatures.

REFERENCE MATERIAL

All tissues produce heat as a result of cell metabolism, and this is increased by exercise and activity (Marieb, 1989). Body temperature is usually maintained between 36°C and 37.5°C regardless of the environmental temperature (Sims-Williams, 1976). Man is described as homoiothermic, that is, having a core temperature that remains constant in spite of environmental changes. The body core generally has the highest temperature while the skin is the coolest (Figure 29.13). Core temperature reflects the heat of arterial blood and represents the balance between the heat generated by body tissues in metabolic activity and that lost through various mechanisms.

A relative constant temperature is maintained by homeostasis, which is a constant process of heat gain and heat loss. The body requires stability of its temperature to produce an optimum environment for biochemical and enzyme reactions to maintain cellular function. A body temperature above or below this normal range affects total body function (Boore *et al.*, 1987). A temperature above 41°C can cause convulsions and a temperature of 43°C is unsustainable for life.

The hypothalamus within the brain acts as the body's thermostat, controlling the body's temperature by various physiological mechanisms (Figure 29.14). Heat is gained through metabolic activity of the body, especially of the muscles and liver. Heat loss is achieved through the skin by the processes of radiation, convection, conduction and evaporation.

There are various factors that cause fluctuations of temperature:

1. The body's circadian rhythms cause daily fluctuations. The body temperature is higher in the evening than in the morning (Brown, 1990). Minor and Waterhouse (1981) in a research study recorded a difference of 0.5 to 1.5°C between morning and evening measurements.
2. Ovulation results in a fluctuation of temperature.
3. Exercise and eating cause an elevation in temperature (Boylan & Brown, 1985).
4. Extremes of age affect a person's response to environmental change. The young or elderly are unable to maintain an efficient equilibrium. Thermoregulation is inadequate in the newborn and especially in low birth weight babies. In old people there is an increased sensitivity to cold, and a lower body temperature generally (Howell, 1972).

Hypothermia is where body temperature drops and mechanisms to increase heat production are ineffective. This causes a decline in the metabolic rate and a resulting decrease in all bodily functions (Boore *et al.*, 1987). Hypothermia can be classified according to the severity and the length of time of the condition. Hypothermia is recognized at temperature recordings of below 35°C (Sims-Williams, 1976).

Pyrexia is defined as a significant rise in body temperature. *Fever* caused by pyrexia is the result of the internal thermostat resetting to higher levels. This resetting of the thermostat results from the action of pyrogens in the thermoregulatory centre of the hypothalamus. The endogenous pyrogens involved are released mainly from leucocytes as a result of cell damage (Hensel, 1981). The exact mechanisms of their influence on the hypothalamus are not understood but it has been suggested that prostaglandins, chemicals produced in inflammatory responses, are involved (Boore *et al.*, 1987).

Rigor is a condition that results from the rapid rise in body temperature. In a rigor, shivering is marked and the patient complains of feeling cold. The temperature quickly rises as a result of the normal physiological response to cold. This results in the following physiological changes:

1. Thermoreceptors in the skin are stimulated resulting in vasoconstriction. This decreases heat loss through conduction and convection.

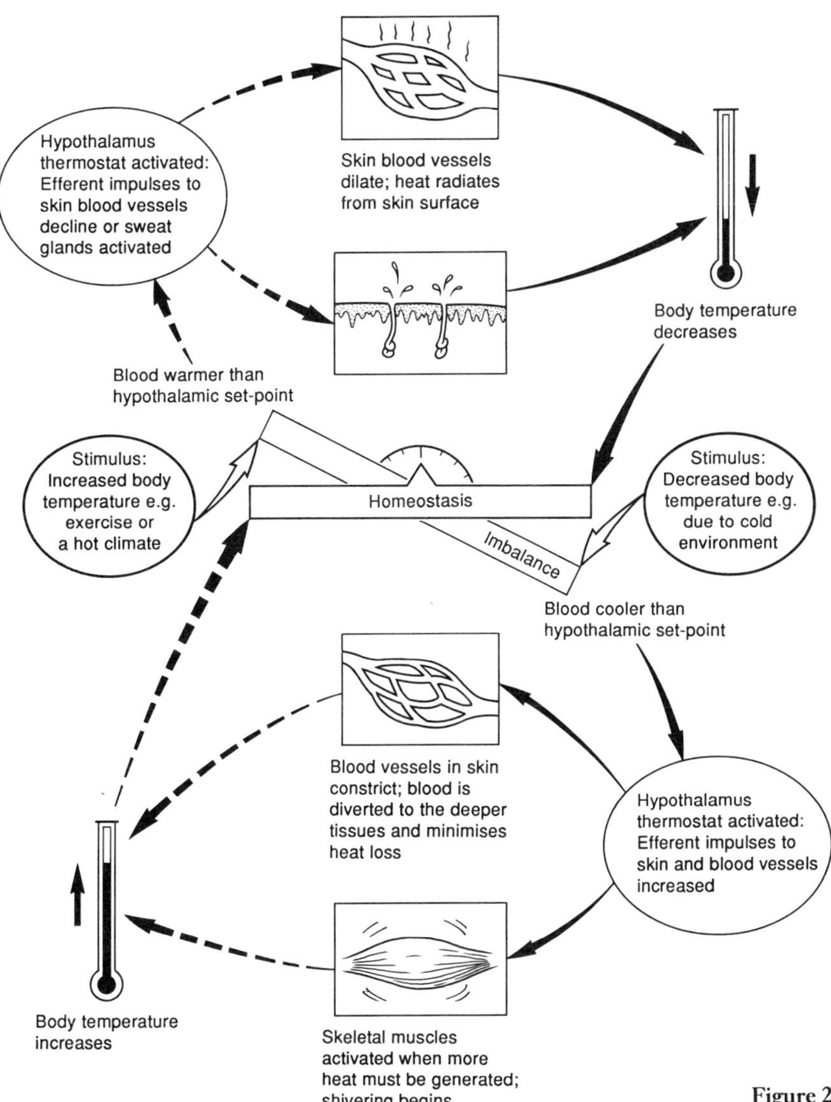

Figure 29.14 Body temperature control.

2. Sweat gland activity is reduced to minimize evaporation.
3. Shivering occurs, muscles contract and relax out of sequence with each other, thus generating heat.
4. The body increases catecholamine and thyroxine levels, elevating the metabolic rate in an attempt to increase temperature (Boore *et al.*, 1987).

All of these changes contribute to a rise in metabolism with an increase in carbon dioxide excretion and the need for oxygen. This leads to an increased respiratory rate. When the body temperature reaches its new 'set-point' the patient no longer complains of feeling cold, shivering ceases and sweating commences. High temperatures may also be the result of heat exhaustion or heat stroke from hot environmental conditions or the loss of the normal body mechanisms for heat loss. Heat exhaustion occurs predominantly in individuals as a result of sodium depletion. Heat stroke may develop from heat exhaustion but, more commonly, appears to develop rapidly in those exposed to high temperatures who are not yet acclimatized to heat (Boore *et al.*, 1987).

There are several grades of pyrexia, and these are described in Table 29.5.

There are different methods for lowering body

Table 29.5 Grades of pyrexia

Low-grade pyrexia	Normal to 38°C	Indicative of an inflammatory response due to a mild infection, allergy, disturbance of body tissue by trauma, surgery, malignancy or thrombosis
Moderate to high-grade pyrexia	38 to 40°C	This may be caused by wound, respiratory or urinary tract infections
Hyperpyrexia	40°C and above	A pyrexia in this range may arise because of bacteraemia, damage to the hypothalamus or high environmental temperatures

temperature. Antipyretics such as the drugs like aspirin can cause a marked fall in temperature (Vane, 1978). It is thought that these drugs inhibit the inflammatory action of prostaglandins, affecting the hypothalamus by temporarily resetting the thermostat to normal levels. Treatment with aspirin is effective for approximately two hours.

Fanning is of benefit for moderate to high pyrexias. Fanning is not recommended while the patient's temperature is still rising as this will only make the patient feel colder and increase shivering (Krikler, 1990).

Recordings of body temperature are an index of biological function and are a valuable indicator of a patient's health.

Temperature recording site

Oral

The most common site for measuring body temperature is the oral method (Brown, 1990). This is measured in the sublingual pocket of tissue at the base of the tongue. This area is in close proximity to the thermoreceptors which respond rapidly to changes in the core temperature, hence changes in core temperatures are reflected quickly here (Blainey, 1974).

Oral temperatures are affected by the temperatures of ingested foods and fluids and by the muscular activity of chewing. Smoking will also affect the thermometer reading. It is recommended that the nurse waits 15 minutes following any of these activities before inserting the thermometer to allow the temperature to return to baseline level (Kozier & Erb, 1982).

It is important that the thermometer is placed in the sublingual pocket and not in the area under the front of the tongue as there may be a temperature difference of up to 1.7°C between these areas. This temperature difference is due to the sublingual pockets being more protected from the air currents which cool the frontal areas (Neff *et al.*, 1989). Oxygen therapy has been shown not to affect the oral temperature reading (Hasler & Cohen, 1982; Lim-Levy, 1982).

Rectal

The rectal temperature is often higher than the oral temperature because this site is more sheltered from the external environment. However, this does not necessarily imply an increase in accuracy as the rectum is far from the central circulation and is inferior to the oral site in reflecting changes in temperature in the vital central organs. The presence of soft stool may separate the thermometer from the bowel wall and give a false reading, especially if the central temperature is changing rapidly. In infants this method is not recommended as it provides a risk of rectal ulceration or perforation.

A rectal thermometer should be inserted at least 4 cm in an adult to obtain the most accurate reading.

Axilla

The axilla is considered less desirable than the other sites since it is not close to major vessels, and skin surface temperatures vary more with changes in temperature of the environment. It is a convenient site for patients who are unsuitable for, or who cannot tolerate, oral thermometers, e.g. after general anaesthetic or those patients with mouth injuries.

To take an axillary temperature reading the thermometer should be placed in the centre of the armpit, with the patient's arm firmly against the side of the chest. It is important that the same arm is used for each measurement as there is often a variation in temperature between left and right (Howell, 1972).

Whichever route is used for temperature measurement, it is important that this is then used consistently, as switching between sites can produce a record that is misleading or difficult to interpret. The assumption that the rectal temperature is about 0.5°C higher, and axillary recordings 0.5°C lower, than oral temperatures is not supported by research findings (Boore *et al.*, 1987).

Time for recording temperatures

The average person experiences circadian rhythms which make their highest body temperature occur in the late afternoon or early evening, i.e. between 4 p.m. and 8 p.m. The most sensitive time for detecting pyrexias appears to be between 7 p.m. and

8 p.m. (Angerami, 1980). This should be considered when interpreting variations in four-hourly or six-hourly observations, and when taking once-daily temperatures.

The time required to record an accurate temperature has been the subject of much research. Nichols *et al.* (1972) have studied this area extensively and suggest that, with a glass thermometer, oral or axillary temperatures should be taken for one to 12 minutes, and rectal temperatures for one to nine minutes. The commonly used three-minute timing led to marked inaccuracy. It was recommended that the thermometer should be left in position for seven to eight minutes in the mouth, nine minutes in the axilla or two minutes in the rectum. The use of the appropriate timings was found to give 90% accuracy for recording the patient's temperature. Takacs and Valenti (1981) observed nurses' temperature-taking practice and found that the timing of thermometer placement varied from 42 seconds to 9.5 minutes, and that this time was determined by the other nursing tasks being carried out. Electronic thermometers take only approximately 30 seconds to record temperatures accurately (Boore *et al.*, 1987).

Types of thermometer

A variety of thermometers, are now available, from clinical glass thermometers with oral or rectal bulbs to the electronic sensor thermometer. The glass thermometer is the most extensively used. Moorat (1976) compared the cost-effectiveness of the different methods of taking temperatures. He used three types of thermometer, the heat-sensitive strip, the glass thermometer and the electronic sensor thermometer. The electronic thermometer proved to be the most cost-effective, reducing costs by 300%. This was largely because of the amount of time saved. Stronge (1980) costed the difference between the use of a glass thermometer (using a two-minute placement) with that of the electronic sensor, and found that the electronic thermometer saved a substantial amount of time and was therefore more cost-effective.

Conditions where a patient's temperature requires careful monitoring are described below:

1. Patients with conditions that affect basal metabolic rate, such as disorders of the thyroid gland require monitoring of body temperature. Hypothyroidism is a condition where an inadequate secretion of hormones from the thyroid gland results in a slowing of physical and metabolic activity, thus the individual has a decrease in body temperature. Hyperthyroidism is excessive activity of the thyroid gland; a hypermetabolic condition results, with an increase in all metabolic processes. The patient complains of a low heat tolerance. Thyrotoxic crisis is a sudden increase in thyroid hormones and can cause a hyperpyrexia (Brunner & Suddarth, 1989).
2. Postoperative and critically ill patients require monitoring of temperature. The patient's temperature should be observed pre-operatively in order to make any significant comparisons. In the post-operative period the nurse should observe the patient for hyperthermia or hypothermia as a reaction to the surgical procedures (Brunner & Suddarth, 1989).
3. Patients with a susceptibility to infection, for example; those with a low white blood cell count (less than 1000 cells/mm^3), or those undergoing radiotherapy, chemotherapy or steroid treatment will require a more frequent observation of temperature. The fluctuation in temperature is influenced by the body's response to pyrogens. Immunocompromised patients are less able to respond to infection. Bacteraemia means a bacterial invasion of the blood stream. Septic shock is a circulatory collapse as a result of severe infection. Pyrexia may be absent in those who are immunosupressed or in the elderly.
4. Patients with a systemic or local infection require monitoring of temperature to assess development or regression of infection.
5. Patients receiving a blood transfusion require careful monitoring of temperature for incompatible blood reactions. Reaction to a blood transfusion is most likely to occur in the early stages and a rise in the patient's temperature is indicative of a reaction. Cluroe (1989) suggests frequent recordings of temperature in the first 15 minutes of a blood transfusion as well as general observation of the patient. Pyrexia can occur throughout a blood transfusion, and results from a reaction to recipient antibodies. This may be as little as one to one-and-a-half hours after the start of blood transfusion (Cluroe, 1989).

References and further reading

Abbey, J. C. *et al.* (1978) How long is that thermometer accurate? *American Journal of Nursing*, 78, 1375–6.

Angerami, E. L. S. (1980) Epidemiological study of body temperature in patients in a teaching hospital. *International Journal of Nursing Studies*, 17, 91–9.

Blainey, C. G. (1974) Site selection in taking body temperatures. *American Journal of Nursing*, 74, 1859–61.

Boore, J. *et al.* (1987) Disturbances of temperature control. In *Nursing the Physically Ill Adult. A Textbook of Medical–Surgical Nursing*. Churchill Livingstone, Edinburgh.

Boylan, A. & Brown, P. (1985) Temperature. *Nursing Times*, 81(16), 36–40.

Brown, S. (1990) Temperature taking – getting it right. *Nursing Standard*, 5(12), 4–5.

Campbell, K. (1983) Taking temperature. *Nursing Times*, 79(32), 63–5.

Cluroe, S. (1989) Blood transfusions. *Nursing*, 3(40), 8–11.

Davies, S. P. *et al.* (1986) A comparison of mercury and digital clinical thermometers. *Journal of Advanced Nursing*, 11(5), 273–4.

Erikson, R. (1980) Oral temperature differences in relation to thermometer and technique. *Nursing Research*, 29(3), 157–64.

Gooch, J. (1986) Taking temperature. *The Professional Nurse*, 1(10), 273–4.

Hasler, M. & Cohen, J. (1982) The effect of oxygen administration on oral temperature assessment. *Nursing Research*, 31, 265–8.

Hensel, H. (1981) *Thermoreception and Temperature Regulation*. Academic Press, London.

Howell, T. (1972) Axillary temperature in aged women. *Age and Ageing*, 1, 250–4.

Kozier, B. & Erb, G. (1982) *Foundations of Nursing: Concepts and Procedures*. Addison Wesley, London.

Krikler, S. (1990) Pyrexia: what to do about temperatures. *Nursing Standard*, 4(25), 37–8.

Litsky, B. Y. (1976) A study of temperature-taking systems. *Supervisor Nurse*, 7(5), 48–53.

Lim-Levy, F. (1982) The effect of oxygen inhalation on oral temperature. *Nursing Research*, 31, 150–2.

Marieb, E. M. (1989) *Human Anatomy and Physiology*. Benjamin Cummings, California.

Minor, D. G. & Waterhouse, J. M. (1981) *Circadian Rhythms and the Human*. Wright, Bristol.

Moorat, D. S. (1976) The cost of taking temperatures. *Nursing Times*, 72(20), 767–70.

Neff, J. *et al.* (1989) Effect of respiratory rate, respiratory depth, and open versus closed mouth breathing on sublingual temperature. *Research in Nursing & Health*, 12, 195–202.

Nichols, G. A. *et al.* (1972) Time analysis of afebrile and febrile temperature readings. *Nursing Research*, 21, 463–4.

Samples, J. F. *et al.* (1985) Circadian rhythms: basis for screening fever. *Nursing Research*, 34(6), 377–9.

Sims-Williams, A. (1976) Temperature-taking with glass thermometers: a review. *Journal of Advanced Nursing*, 1(6), 481–93.

Stronge, J. L. (1980) Electronic thermometers: a costly rise in efficiency? *Nursing Mirror*, 151(8).

Takacs, K. & Valenti, W. (1981) Temperature measurement in a clinical setting. *Nursing Research*, 31(6), 368–70.

Vane, J. R. (1978) In *Pharmacology of the Hypothalamus* (Ed. by Cox *et al.*). Macmillan, London.

GUIDELINES: TEMPERATURE

Equipment

1. Electronic thermometer and oral probe.
2. Disposable probe covers.

Procedure

Action	Rationale
1. Explain the procedure to the patient.	To obtain patient's consent and co-operation.
2. Remove the probe from the stored position in the thermometer and check that the reading is 34°C.	If the readout does not register the machine is faulty and should not be used.
3. Push the probe firmly into the probe cover.	The probe cover protects the tip of the probe and is necessary for the functioning of the instrument.
4. Ask the patient to open the mouth and insert the probe under the tongue into the 'heat pocket' at the posterior base of the tongue.	The highest oral temperature reading is at the posterior base of the tongue, which is least affected by environmental conditions.
5. Ask the patient to close the mouth.	To increase the patient's comfort and to keep the probe in place.
6. Hold the thermometer in place until an audible tone is heard and the machine signals the correct temperature.	Tissue contact must be maintained for an accurate reading to be obtained.

7. If figures on the display stop rising without an audible tone, tissue contact has been lost. Regain tissue contact and continue.	The probe must be supported outside the mouth as its top-heavy shape tends to move the sensitive tip out of the heat pocket.
8. Remove the probe from the patient's mouth when signalled by the machine and note the temperature displayed.	An audible tone indicates that the reading is complete.
9. Discard the probe cover into a waste bag by pressing the probe from the thumb.	Probe covers are for single use only. The discard mechanism prevents transfer of the patient's saliva to the nurse's hands.
10. Return the probe to its storage position in the thermometer, cancelling the temperature reading.	The probe is best protected from damage in this storage position.

30

Oxygen Therapy

Definition

Oxygen therapy is the administration of supplementary oxygen when tissue oxygenation is impaired. Oxygen is essential to allow aerobic metabolism to produce energy from the intake of food.

If tissue oxygenation becomes inadequate, anaerobic metabolism will lead to lactic acidosis and cell death (Oh, 1989).

Indications

There are many indications for oxygen therapy. The major ones are listed below:

1. Acute respiratory failure, this can be subdivided into two groups, i.e. with or without carbon dioxide retention:
   (a) With carbon dioxide retention – the most common causes are chronic bronchitis, chest injuries, e.g. flail segment and rupture of the diaphragm, unconscious drug overdose, post-operative hypoxaemia and the neuromuscular diseases.
   (b) Without carbon dioxide retention – the most common causes are asthma, infective conditions, e.g. pneumonia and legionella, pulmonary oedema and pulmonary embolism (Oh, 1989).
2. Acute myocardial infarction.
3. Cardiac failure.
4. Shock, particularly haemorrhagic, bacteraemic and cardiogenic.
5. For a hypermetabolic state induced, for example, by major sepsis, trauma or burns.
6. States where there is a reduced ability to transport oxygen, e.g. anaemia.
7. Inability to utilize the oxygen carried, as in cyanide poisoning (Foss, 1990).
8. During cardiorespiratory resuscitation.

REFERENCE MATERIAL

Physiology (see also Chapter 29)

Tissue oxygenation is reliant on the following factors:

1. The oxygen cascade.
2. Association and disociation of haemoglobin and oxygen.
3. Cardiac output (Oh, 1989).

An understanding of these factors and their interaction is essential in understanding the physiology of oxygen transport and transfer in the body.

The movement of oxygen from the alveoli in the lungs to the pulmonary blood is effected rapidly due to the pressure gradient that exists. The partial pressure of oxygen (PO_2) in the alveoli is 13.7 kilo Pascal (kPa) (103 mm Hg) as compared to 5.3 kPa (40 mm Hg) in the pulmonary capillaries. This allows a swift exchange of oxygen through diffusion. Similarly, oxygen is easily given up by the arterial blood to the tissues, again because of the steep pressure gradient. The partial pressure of arterial blood is 13.3 kPa (100 mm Hg) and that of the tissues 2.7 kPa (20 mm Hg) (Marieb, 1989). Table 30.1 and Figure 30.1 show the various pressure gradients in the oxygen cascade.

Oxygen is carried in the blood in the following two ways: dissolved in plasma; and bound to the haemoglobin within the red blood cells. Only about 1.5% of oxygen is carried in the plasma as oxygen is poorly soluble in water. Therefore, 98.5% of

Table 30.1 Oxygen cascade. Pressure gradients for oxygen transfer from inspired gas to tissue cells

	mmHg	*(kPa)*
Inspired air	150	(20.0)
Alveolar	103	(13.7)
Arterial	100	(13.3)
Capillary	51	(6.8)
Tissue	20	(2.7)
Mitochondrial	1–20	(0.13–1.3)

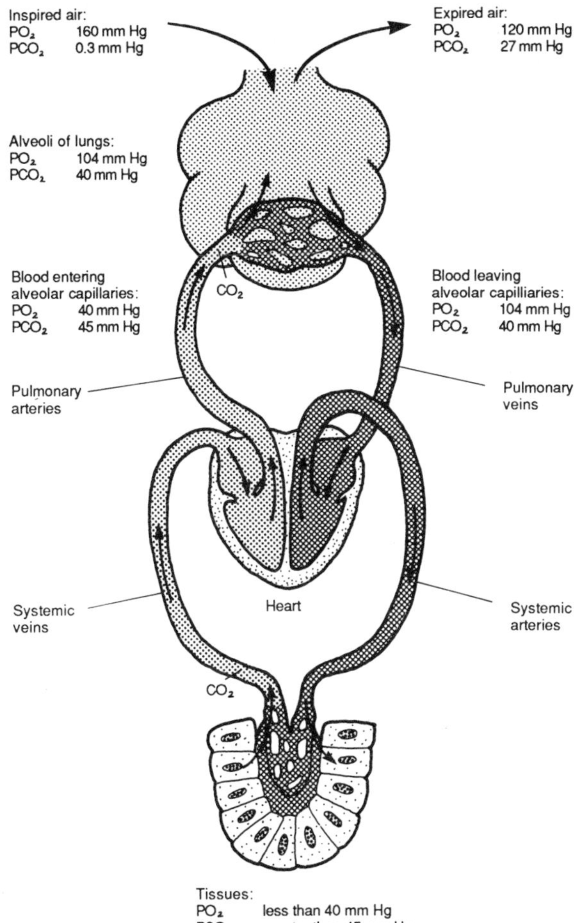

Figure 30.1 Partial pressure gradients promoting gas movements in the body. Gradients promoting oxygen and carbon dioxide exchanges across the respiratory membrane in the lungs (external respiration) are shown in the top part of the figure. Gradients promoting gas movements across systemic capillary membranes in the body tissues (internal respiration) are indicated in the bottom part of the figure. (From Marieb (1989), with permission.)

oxygen is transported around the body in a loose chemical alliance with haemoglobin (Marieb, 1989). Haemoglobin is made up of four polypeptide chains, each of which is bound to a heme group that contains iron. The iron groups bind to oxygen, and therefore each molecule of haemoglobin can combine with four molecules of oxygen. A haemoglobin molecule is said to be fully saturated with oxygen when all four heme groups are attached to oxygen. When less than four are so attached, the haemoglobin is said to be partially saturated (Marieb, 1989).

The action of the four polypeptide molecules and their relationship to oxygen is interlinked so that when one molecule has taken up a molecule of oxygen, the others are facilitated to do the same. The same is also true for the opposite action when the heme molecules unload their oxygen molecules to the tissues (Marieb, 1989).

The timing of haemoglobin uptake and release of oxygen is affected by the following factors:

1. The partial pressure of oxygen (PO_2).
2. Temperature.
3. Blood pH.
4. Partial pressure of carbon dioxide (PCO_2) (Marieb, 1989).

The oxygen dissociation curve

This curve illustrates the factors affecting tissue oxygenation (Figures 30.2, 30.3 and 30.4).

Haemoglobin and oxygenation

The extent of oxygen binding to haemoglobin depends on the PO_2 of the blood, but the relationship is not precisely linear (see Figure 30.2). The slope is steeply progressive between 1.5 kPa and 7 kPa (10 to 50 mm Hg) and then plateaus out between 9 and

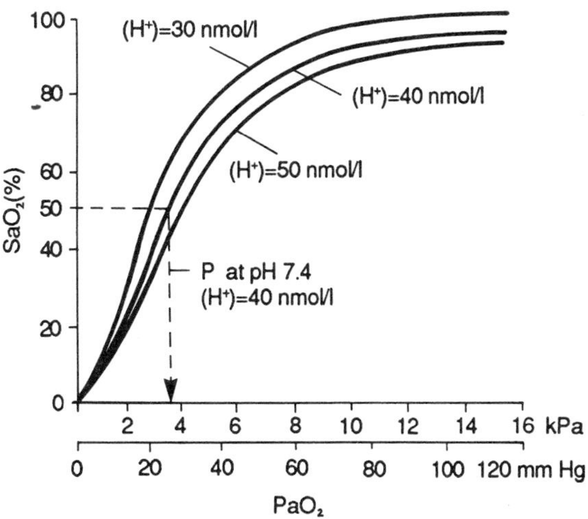

Figure 30.2 Oxygen dissociation curve. Normal curve at 40 nmol/l (H^+), and shifts to left and right. (P_{50} = tension at 50% saturation.) (From Marieb (1989), with permission.)

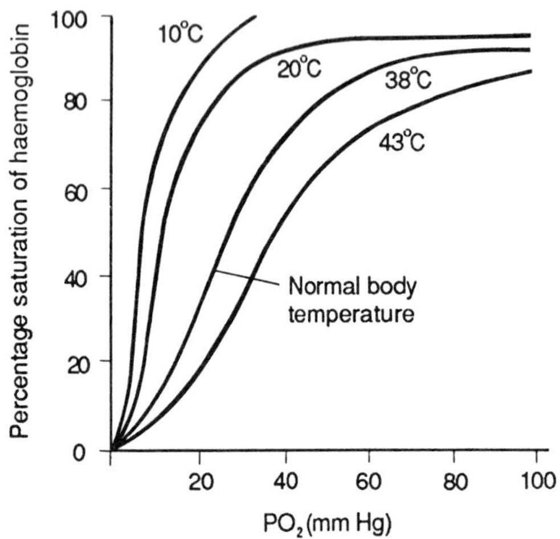

Figure 30.3 Effect of temperature on the oxygen–haemoglobin dissociation curve. Oxygen unloading is accelerated under conditions of increased temperature, resulting in a shift to the right of the dissociation curve. (From Marieb (1989), with permission.)

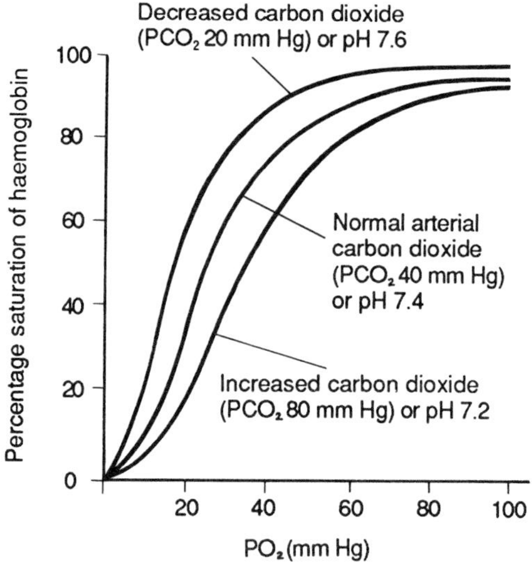

Figure 30.4 Effect of PCO_2 and blood pH on the oxygen–haemoglobin dissociation curve. Oxygen unloading is accelerated under conditions of increased PCO_2 and/or decreased pH, resulting in a shift to the right of the dissociation curve. (From Marieb (1989), with permission.)

13.5 kPa (70 to 100 mm Hg). This is important for oxygen therapy because it illustrates that haemoglobin is almost completely saturated at 9 kPa (70 mm Hg) and therefore further increases in the partial pressure of oxygen will cause only a slight rise in oxygen binding.

The most rapid uptake and delivery of oxygen to and from haemoglobin occurs during the steep portion of the curve (Marieb, 1989).

Haemoglobin, temperature and oxygen

As body temperature rises the affinity of haemoglobin for oxygen is reduced and less oxygen is bound while more oxygen is unloaded (Marieb, 1989) (Figure 30.3).

Haemoglobin, pH and oxygen

As the pH of the blood declines (acidosis) the affinity of haemoglobin for oxygen decreases and more oxygen will be unloaded to the tissues. This is known as the Bohr effect. The same effect occurs when the partial pressure of carbon dioxide rises as this will also lead to a fall in blood pH and acidosis (Marieb, 1989) (Figure 30.4)

Generally, a shift in the oxygen dissociation curve to the right will favour unloading of oxygen to the tissues, and a shift to the left will favour reduced tissue oxygenation (Oh, 1989).

Cardiac output

The final factor influencing tissue oxygenation is the cardiac output. When this is severely reduced, for example in shock states, there will be a severely reduced amount of oxygen available to the tissues. (Edwards, 1988).

Oxygen consumption

At rest the normal oxygen consumption is approximately 200 to 250 millilitres per minute (ml/min). As the available oxygen per minute in a normal man is about 700 ml, this means there is an oxygen reserve of 450 to 500 ml/min. Factors which increase the above consumption of oxygen include fever, sepsis, shivering, restlessness and increased metabolism (Oh, 1989). It is difficult to say at which absolute level oxygen therapy is necessary as each situation should be judged by the requirements for oxygen and the availability of oxygen. Therefore, all of the above information needs to be taken into account together with the measurement of the arterial blood gases.

Generally, additional oxygen will be required when the PaO_2 has fallen to 8 kPa (60 mm Hg) or less (Oh, 1989). Oxygen saturation level at the tissues is also useful and can be measured using a pulse oximeter, which works by emitting narrow shafts of red and infra-red light through the tissue of a finger, toe or earlobe. Different amounts of light rays are absorbed by the arterial blood depending on its saturation with oxygen. The final oxygen saturation (SaO_2) is then calculated by computer (Ehrhardt and Graham, 1990).

Hazards of oxygen therapy

Carbon dioxide narcosis

Carbon dioxide is the chemical that most directly influences respiration by its direct effect on the efficiency of alveolar ventilation. The normal partial pressure of carbon dioxide in the blood is 4 to 5.5 kPa (30 to 40 mm Hg). When this level rises, the pH of the cerebrospinal fluid drops which in turn causes excitation of the central chemoreceptors, and hyperventilation occurs (Marieb, 1989).

In people who always retain carbon dioxide, and are therefore usually hypercapnic because of chronic pulmonary disease such as chronic bronchitis, the chemoreceptors are no longer sensitive to a raised level of carbon dioxide. In these cases the falling PO_2 becomes the principle respiratory stimulus (the hypoxic drive) (Marieb, 1989). Therefore, if a high level of supplementary oxygen was delivered to such patients, severe respiratory depression would ensue and ultimately unconsciousness and death.

Oxygen toxicity

Pulmonary toxicity following prolonged higher percentages of oxygen therapy is recognized clinically, but there is still much to be learnt about the condition. The pattern is one of decreasing lung compliance as a result of a sequelae of haemorrhagic interstitial and intra-alveolar oedema, leading ultimately to fibrosis (Oh, 1990).

It is thought that where possible, long periods (that is 24 hours or more) of oxygen therapy above 50% should be avoided, although clinically it seems that there is much variance in the response of individual patients (Higgins, 1990).

Retrolental fibroplasia

This is a disease affecting premature babies that weigh under 1200 g (about 28 weeks' gestation) if they are exposed to high concentrations of oxygen. It appears that the oxygen stimulates immature blood vessels in the eye to vasoconstrict and obliterate, which results in neovascularization, accompanied by haemorrhage, fibrosis and then retinal detachment and blindness (Oh, 1990).

General considerations

1. Oxygen is an odourless, tasteless, colourless, transparent gas that is slightly heavier than air.
2. Oxygen supports combustion, therefore there is always a danger of fire when oxygen is being used. The following safety measures should be remembered:
   (a) Oil or grease around oxygen connections should be avoided.
   (b) Alcohol, ether and other inflammatory liquids should be used with caution in the vicinity of oxygen.
   (c) No electrical device must be used in or near an oxygen tent.
   (d) Oxygen cylinders should be kept secure in an upright position and away from heat.
   (e) There must be no smoking in the vicinity of oxygen.
   (f) A fire extinguisher should be readily available.

Equipment necessary to administer oxygen therapy

Any oxygen delivery system will include these basic components:

1. Oxygen supply, either from a piped supply or a portable cylinder. All medical gas cylinders have to conform to a standardized colour-coding: oxygen cylinders are black with a white shoulder and are labelled 'Oxygen' or 'O_2'.
2. A reduction gauge – to reduce the pressure to that of atmospheric pressure.
3. Flowmeter – a device which controls the flow of oxygen in litres per minute.
4. Tubing – disposable tubing of varying diameter and length.
5. Mechanism for delivery – a mask or nasal cannulae.
6. Humidifier – to warm and moisten the oxygen before administration (Allan, 1989).

Methods of administration

Simple semi-rigid plastic masks (Figure 30.5)

These are low-flow masks which entrain the air from the atmosphere and therefore are able to deliver a variable oxygen percentage (anything from 21 to 60%) (Allan, 1990). Large discrepancies between the delivered fractional inspired oxygen (FiO_2) and the actual amount received by the patient will occur with increased rate and depth of respiration (Oh, 1989).

Nasal cannuli catheter (Figure 30.6)

These provide an alternative to a mask but again there are great discrepancies between the delivered FiO_2 and the actual oxygen percentage received by the patient. When used at low flow rates, for example two litres per minute, they are well tolerated and afford

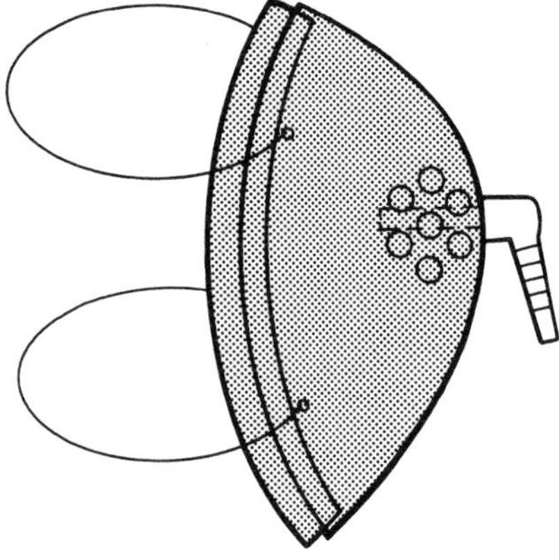

Figure 30.5 Semi-rigid plastic mask.

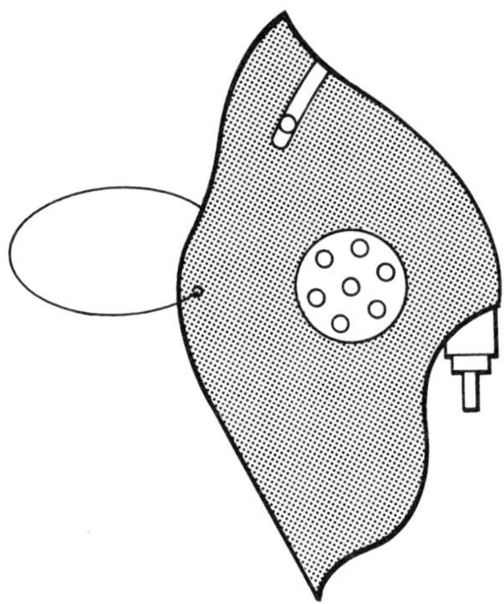

Figure 30.7 High-flow mask.

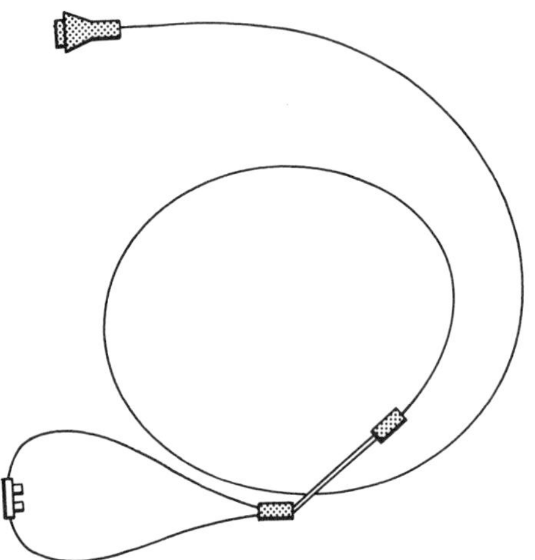

Figure 30.6 Nasal cannula.

the patient more freedom than a mask. At high flow rates, above eight litres per minute, they may cause discomfort and dryness of the nasal mucosa. Nasal cannuli cannot be attached satisfactorily to an external humidification device (Allan, 1989).

Fixed performance masks or high-flow masks (Venturi-type masks) (Figure 30.7)
With these masks it is possible to achieve an unvarying mixture of gases and a known concentration of oxygen using the high air flow oxygen enrichment principle. These masks derive their name from the Venturi barrel in which a relatively low flow rate of oxygen is forced through a narrow jet. There are side holes in the barrel and this jet causes the air to be drawn in at a high rate. As the mixture of gas created is at a flow rate above that of inspiration, the mixture will be constant (Foss, 1990). There are many Venturi-type masks available but the larger-capacity masks are the most accurate and therefore the safest when a known concentration of oxygen is required or when efficient elimination of carbon dioxide is essential, for example, to provide oxygen therapy for the patient with chronic respiratory disease (Allan, 1990).

T-piece circuit
This is a simple, large-bore, non-rebreathing circuit which is attached directly to an endotracheal or tracheostomy tube. Humidified oxygen is delivered through one part of the T, and expired gases leave through the other part. This device may be used as part of the weaning process when a patient has been ventilated previously by a mechanical ventilator (Oh, 1989).

Paediatric circuits
A child's compliance with oxygen masks or cannuli may be limited, requiring other devices to be used. Some examples of these are listed below:

1. *Headbox or hood.*
   Oxygen can be delivered to infants and small children using a headbox or hood. The clear plastic box is fitted carefully over the child's head, encasing the head and neck. It is essential to monitor the oxygen concentration near the face to enable an accurate assessment of FiO_2 (Oh, 1989).
2. *Oxygen tent/cot.*
   An oxygen tent can be used to supply oxygen therapy to larger children. The child is placed in a

clear plastic tent which fits over the bed. The humidified oxygen supply is then directed into the tent. The advantages with the oxygen tent are that the child has freedom from any device over the face, and high degrees of humidity can be reached which may be especially useful in obstructive conditions e.g. croup (Allan, 1990). The main disadvantage is the difficulty in maintaining a constant oxygen concentration (Oh, 1989).

Tracheostomy mask

These perform in a similar way to the simple semi-rigid plastic face mask, outlined above. The mask is placed over the tracheostomy tube or stoma, and the patient will receive less oxygen than is delivered as it will be diluted by room air (Oh, 1989).

Mechanical ventilation

This is indicated when there is reversible acute respiratory failure. The decision to use mechanical ventilation will be made after an assessment of respiratory mechanics, oxygenation and ventilation (Oh, 1989). There are a wide range of ventilators available and they all have slight differences of application but fall into two major groups:

1. Positive pressure ventilators – these are the most widely used for the acute treatment of adults and children.
2. Negative pressure ventilators – these are used much more rarely (usually for patients with chronic neurological problems such as poliomyelitis and some forms of muscular dystrophy). (Hinds, 1988). (For a detailed outline of oxygen therapy using mechanical ventilation, see Hinds, 1988; Oh, 1989.)

Hyperbaric oxygen therapy

This form of treatment is now used mainly in the treatment of skin lesions and soft tissue injury and has also been used more recently for the patient with multiple sclerosis (Bolton, 1981). The therapy is designed to administer 100% oxygen at a range of pressures greater than atmospheric pressure.

Hyperbaric therapy can be used topically or systemically depending on the patient's need, and the treatment is usually intermittent over a period of weeks or months (Oh, 1989).

Humidification

Humidity is the amount of water vapour present in a gaseous environment (Oh, 1989). For the purpose of clinical application, humidity is usually divided into absolute and relative humidity. Absolute humidity is a measurement of the total mass of water in a specified volume of gas at a known temperature. Relative humidity is the ratio (expressed as a percentage) of the mass of water in a given volume of gas (as above) with the mass of water required to saturate the same volume of gas at a given temperature (Oh, 1989).

Normally, the air travelling through the airways is warmed, moistened and filtered by the columnar mucus-secreting epithelial cells of the nasopharynx (Foss, 1990). The air entering the trachea will have a relative humidity of about 90% and a temperature between 32° and 36°C. The humidification and warming process then continues down the airways so that at the alveoli it is fully saturated at 37°C (Oh, 1990).

The humidification pathway is necessary to compensate for the normal loss of water from the respiratory tract (about 250 ml under resting conditions) (Oh, 1990). If the humidification apparatus is impaired due to disease such as upper respiratory tract infection or dehydration, alternative methods of humidification may need to be considered (Allan, 1989).

Oxygen therapy will compound these problems because the added gas will cause further dehydration of the mucous membranes and pulmonary secretions, making it more difficult for the patient to expectorate (Foss, 1990). External humidification is essential when oxygen therapy is being delivered to a patient whose physiological humidification has been bypassed by an endotracheal or tracheostomy tube (Oh, 1989).

Methods of humidification

There are many devices that can be used to supply humidification, the best of these will fulfil the following requirements:

1. The inspired gas must be delivered to the trachea at a room temperature of 32° to 36°C and should have a water content of 33 to 43 g/m^3 (Oh, 1989).
2. The set temperature should remain constant; humidification and temperature should not be affected by large ranges of flow.
3. The device should have a safety and alarm system to guard against overheating, overhydration and electric shocks.
4. It is important that the appliance should not increase resistance or affect the compliance to respiration.
5. It is essential that whichever device is selected, wide-bore tubing (elephant tubing) must be used.

Devices for humidification

1. *Condensers.* These are also known as heat and moisture exchangers or 'Swedish nose'. They

perform the function of the nasopharynx, retaining the heat and water from expired gas through condensation and returning them to the inspired gas. A new range of disposable condensers are now widely used to humidify oxygen delivered through an endotracheal or tracheostomy tube, but heated humidifiers may still be preferred for long-term use (Oh, 1989).

2. *Cold water bubble humidifier*. This device delivers partially humidified oxygen that is about 50% relative humidity. Its use is not advised as it is so inefficient (Oh, 1989).
3. *Water bath humidifiers*. With these devices, inspired gas is forced over or through a heated reservoir of water. To achieve an adequate humidity for the patient, the water bath must reach temperatures of 45° to 60°C. The gas will then cool as it moves down the breathing circuit to the patient, and a relative humidity of 100% will be reached. Hot water bath humidifiers are therefore very efficient and useful in the care of the immobile patient, particularly in an intensive therapy unit. However, they have four main disadvantages:
   (a) Danger of overheating and causing damage to the trachea.
   (b) Their efficiency can alter with changes in gas flow rate, surface area and the water temperature.
   (c) Condensation and collection of water in the oxygen delivery tubes.
   (d) The possibility of microcontamination of stagnant water.
4. *Aerosol generators*. These devices are not governed by temperature, but provide micro-droplets of water suspended in the gas (Oh, 1989). The gas provided through aerosol devices can be very highly saturated with water, especially when ultrasonic nebulizers are used. There are three main types of aerosol humidifier:
   (a) Gas-drive nebulizer.
   (b) Mechanical (spinning disc) nebulizer.
   (c) Ultrasonic nebulizer.

References and further reading

Allan, D. (1988) Making sense of oxygen delivery. *Nursing Times*, 83(18), 40–2.

Bolton, M. E. (1981) Hyperbolic Oxygen Therapy. *American Journal of Nursing*, 1981, 81, pp. 1199–201.

Edwards, D. (1988) Principles of oxygen transport. *Care of the Critically Ill*, 4(5), 13–16.

Ehrhardt, B. S. & Graham, M. (1990) Making sense of oxygen delivery. *Nursing* (US), March, 50–4.

Foss, M. A. (1990) Oxygen therapy. *The Professional Nurse*, January, 180–90.

Higgins, J. (1990) Pulmonary oxygen toxicity. *Physiotherapy*, October, 76(10), 588–92.

Hinds, C. J. (1988) *Intensive Care. A Concise Textbook.* Baillière Tindall, London.

Marieb, E. N. (1989) *Human Anatomy and Physiology*. Benjamin Cummings Publishing, USA.

Oh, T. E. (1989) *Intensive Care Manual.* Butterworths, Australia.

31

Pain Assessment

Definition

Pain is not a simple sensation but a complex phenomenon having both a cognitive (physical) and an affective (emotional) component. Because pain is subjective the favoured definition for use in clinical practice, proposed originally by McCaffery (1968), is: 'Pain is whatever the experiencing person says it is, existing whenever the experiencing person says it does.' The aim of pain assessment, therefore, is to identify *all* the factors – physical and non-physical – which affect the patient's perception of pain.

REFERENCE MATERIAL

Melzack and Dennis (1980) have distinguished three forms of pain:

1. Phasic pain.
2. Acute pain.
3. Chronic pain.

Phasic pain

This is pain of short duration which occurs at the onset of injury.

Acute pain

This is provoked by tissue damage which comprises both phasic pain and a tonic stage which persists for variable periods of time until healing takes place. The distinguishing characteristics of acute pain are that:

1. It subsides as healing takes place, i.e. it has a predictable end.
2. It is of brief duration, at least less than six months.

Chronic pain

This is pain which persists beyond the period of time required for healing. Although distinct affective states appear to be associated with acute and chronic pain, chronic pain has the greatest potential for impact on the psychological wellbeing of the patient. Physical, psychological and social problems become more complex. Therefore, while the principle of assessing the non-physical as well as the physical components of pain is applicable to all forms of pain, it is essential in the case of chronic pain. Therefore, it is intended that pain assessment be seen for the purpose of this procedure in the context of the management of chronic pain.

Factors affecting pain assessment

Patients with chronic, particularly cancer-related, pain rarely present with this one symptom. For example, approximately two-thirds of advanced cancer patients will also complain of anorexia, one half will have a symptomatic dry mouth and constipation, and one-third will suffer nausea, vomiting, insomnia, dyspnoea, cough or oedema (Hanks, 1983). It will be clear from those figures that pain assessment cannot be seen in isolation; identification of all related symptoms is of equal importance as they will contribute to a lowered pain threshold (the least stimulus intensity at which a person perceives pain) and impaired pain tolerance (the greatest stimulus intensity causing pain that a person is prepared to tolerate).

Furthermore, cancer pain is often multifocal. Less than 20% of advanced cancer patients will have a single site of pain, and approximately 50% of patients will have three or more individual pains (Twycross and Fairfield, 1982).

A diagnosis of cancer does not necessarily mean that the malignant process is the cause of the pain. Pain in cancer may be:

1. Caused by the cancer itself.
2. Caused by treatment.
3. Associated with debilitating disease, such as a pressure ulcer.
4. Unrelated to either the disease or the treatment, such as headache.

The cause of *each* pain should therefore be identified carefully; many pains unrelated to the cancer will respond to specific treatment. If the pain is due to the cancer, then it is important to determine the precise

The Royal Marsden Hospital

Pain Assessment Chart

Surname: *Hospital no.*

First name: *Date*:

Initial Assessment

Patient's own description of the pain(s):

What helps relieve the pain?

What makes the pain worse?

Do you have pain

1 *At night*? Yes/No (comment if required).

2 *At rest*? Yes/No (comment if required).

3 *On movement*? Yes/No (comment if required).

Pain sites

Please draw on the body outlines below to show where you feel pain. Label each site of pain with a letter A.B.C. etc.

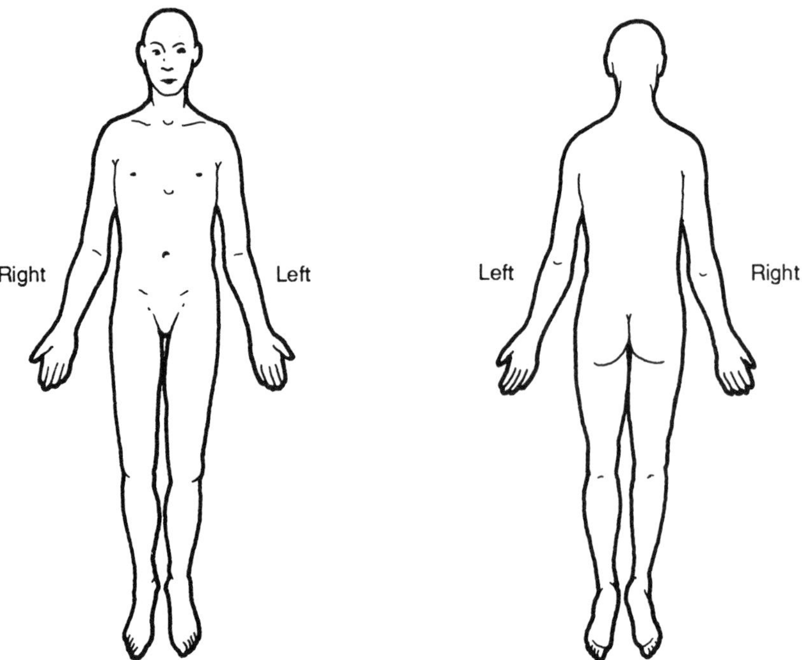

Figure 31.1 The Royal Marsden Hospital Pain Assessment Chart.

Pain Assessment Chart

Continuation no: ________

Key to pain intensity:

0 = no pain
1 = mild pain
2 = moderate pain
3 = severe pain
4 = very severe pain
5 = intolerable/overwhelming pain
s = sleeping

It may be easier to determine the intensity of pain by looking at the pain scale below.

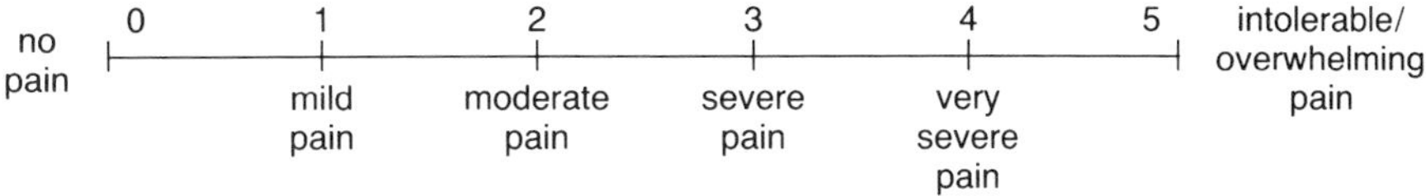

Date	Times	Pain sites								Analgesia name, route & dose	Patient activity and comments
		A	B	C	D	E	F	G	H		

Figure 31.1 Continued

Table 31.1 Factors affecting pain sensitivity

Sensitivity increased:
Discomfort
Insomnia
Fatigue
Anxiety
Fear
Anger
Sadness
Depression
Boredom
Sensitivity lowered:
Relief of symptoms
Sleep
Rest
Sympathy
Understanding
Companionship
Diversional activity
Reduction in anxiety
Elevation of mood

mechanism of pain because treatment will vary accordingly.

The perception of painful stimuli will always be modulated by the emotional response to that perception. Changes in mood may alter considerably the experience of pain. Pain assessment needs to acknowledge this fact, and particular attention must be paid to factors which will modulate pain sensitivity (Table 31.1).

Need for assessment tools

Accurate pain assessment is a prerequisite of effective control and is an essential component of nursing care. In the assessment process, the nurse gathers information from the patient that allows an understanding of the patient's experience and its effect on the patient's life. The information obtained guides the nurse in planning and evaluating strategies for care. Pain is rarely static; therefore its assessment is not a one-time process but is ongoing.

Objective pain assessment is difficult to achieve. For example, the tendency suggested by both research and clinical practice is for the patient not to report any pain or to do so inadequately or inaccurately, minimizing the pain experience (McCaffery, 1983; McCaffery & Beeber, 1989). Hunt *et al.* (1977) found that nurses tended to overestimate the pain relief obtained from analgesia and underestimate the level of the patient's pain.

Pain charts have been considered as useful tools for assisting nurses to assess pain and plan nursing care. Raiman (1986) found that the use of a chart improved communication between staff and patients. Walker *et al.* (1987) found that the specific advantages of using a chart lie in promoting greater objectivity in both the initial assessment of pain and its monitoring. It was also found that the involvement of many patients in their pain management helped to increase their confidence in it.

Introduction to the use of assessment tools

There are numerous methods of assessing pain, and the published literature indicates that pain assessment charts can be used successfully to assess and monitor pain (McCaffery & Beeber, 1989). Some degree of caution, however, must be exercised in their use. The nurse must be careful to select the tool which is most appropriate for a particular type of pain experience. For example, it would not be appropriate to use a pain assessment chart which had been designed for use with patients with chronic pain, to assess postoperative pain. Furthermore, pain charts should not be used totally indiscriminately. Walker *et al.* (1987) found that charts appeared to have little value in cases of unresolved or intractable pain.

The Royal Marsden Hospital Pain Assessment Chart

A study was carried out at The Royal Marsden Hospital in order to design a chart for use with patients with chronic cancer pain and to evaluate its effectiveness (Walker *et al.*, 1987). The study indicated that the chart (Figure 31.1) was a valuable tool for pain assessment in 98% of cases. The following guidelines are written with reference to The Royal Marsden Hospital pain chart, but it is recognized that nurses may modify the chart to meet the needs of their own particular branch of nursing.

References and further reading

Dicks, B. (1990) Programmed instruction, cancer pain. *Cancer Nursing*, 13(4), 256–61.

Hanks, G. W. (1983) Management of symptoms in advanced cancer. *Update*, 26, 1691–702.

Hoskin, P. J. & Dicks, B. (1988) *Symptom Control in Oncology for Nurses and Health Care Professionals: Volume 2*, 2nd edn (Ed. by R. Tiffany, P. Webb). Harper & Row, London.

Hunt, J. M. *et al.* (1977) Patients with protracted pain; a survey conducted at the London Hospital. *Journal of Medical Ethics*, 3(2), 61–73.

McCaffery, M. (1968) *Nursing practice theories related to cognition, bodily pain, and man-environment interactions*. University of California, Los Angeles.

McCaffery, M. (1983) *Nursing the Patient in Pain*. Harper & Row, London.

McCaffery, M. & Beeber, A. (1989) *Pain, Clinical Manual for Nursing Practice.* Mosby, USA.
Melzac, R. & Dennis, S. G. (1980) Phylogenetic evolution of pain expression in animals. In *Pain and Society* (Ed. by H. W. Kosterlitz & L. Y. Teranius). Chomie, New York.
Raiman, J. (1986) Pain relief – a two way process. *Nursing Times*, 82(15), 24–8.
Twycross, R. G. & Fairfield, S. (1982) Pain in far advanced cancer. *Pain*, 14, 303–10.
Walker, V. S. *et al.* (1987) Pain assessment charts in the management of chronic cancer pain. *Palliative Medicine*, 1, 111–16.
World Health Organization (1990) *Cancer Pain Relief and Palliative Care.* WHO, Geneva.

GUIDELINES: INITIAL ASSESSMENT

Action	Rationale
1. Explain the purpose of using the chart to the patient.	To obtain the patient's consent and co-operation.
2. Where appropriate, encourage the patient to complete the pain chart himself/herself.	To encourage patient participation.
3. Where the nurse completes chart, record the patient's *own* description of his/her pain.	To reduce the risk of misrepresentation.
4. (a) Record any factors which influence the intensity of the pain, e.g. activities or interventions which reduce or increase the pain such as distractions or a heat pad. (b) Record whether or not the patient is pain free at night, at rest or on movement.	Ascertaining how and when the patient experiences pain enables the nurse to plan realistic goals. For example, relieving the patient's pain during the night and while he/she is at rest is usually easier to achieve than relief from pain on movement.

GUIDELINES: PAIN SITES

Action	Rationale
1. Encourage the patient, where appropriate, to identify pain himself/herself.	The body outline (Figure 31.1) is ideally a vehicle for the patient to describe own pain experience.
2. Index each site (A to H) (see Figure 31.1) in whatever way seems most appropriate, e.g. shading or colouring of areas or arrows to indicate shooting pains.	This enables individual pain sites to be located.

GUIDELINES: MONITORING PAIN INTENSITY

Action	Rationale
1. Give each pain site a numerical value according to the key to pain intensity or the pain scale and note time recorded.	To indicate the intensity of the pain at each site.
2. Record any analgesia given and note route and dose.	To monitor efficacy of prescribed analgesia.

3. Record any significant activities which are likely to influence the patient's pain.	Extra pharmacological or non-pharmacological interventions might be indicated.

Note: Fixed times for reviewing the pain have been omitted intentionally to allow for flexibility. It is suggested that, initially, the patient's pain be reviewed every four hours. When a patient's level of pain has stabilized, recordings may be made less frequently, e.g. 12-hourly or daily. The chart should be discontinued if a patient's pain becomes totally controlled.

32

Peritoneal Dialysis

Definition

Peritoneal dialysis is a procedure used for patients with inadequate renal function to rid the body of waste products, such as urea, using the peritoneum as a dialysing membrane (Bloe, 1990).

Indications

Peritoneal dialysis is indicated for the following:

1. To aid in the removal of toxic substances and metabolic waste.
2. To assist in regulating fluid and electrolyte balance.
3. To remove excessive body fluid.
4. To control blood pressure (Bloe, 1990).

Choice of dialysis method

Peritoneal dialysis may be selected over haemodialysis for the following reasons:

1. Widespread availability.
2. Technical simplicity.
3. Where haemodialysis is contraindicated because of circulatory or coagulation problems (Oh, 1989).

REFERENCE MATERIAL

In 1926 Rosenak, basing his work on that of Ganter, conceived the possibility of using the peritoneum of humans as a dialysing membrane (Blumenkrantz & Roberts, 1979). The use of peritoneal dialysis reached a peak in 1959 with the introduction of commercial dialysis solutions and tubing. In the 1960s advances in peritoneal dialysis were being made by Tenckhoff (Warren, 1989), and long-term access now became a reality. At this time the technique of haemodialysis was introduced and the two treatments are now used widely (Warren, 1989).

Anatomy and physiology

The peritoneum is the largest serous membrane of the body. In adults it has a surface area of approximately $2.2\,m^2$. It is a closed unit consisting of two parts:

1. The parietal peritoneum that lines the inside of the abdominal wall.
2. The visceral peritoneum that is reflected over the viscera.

The space between the two parts is the peritoneal cavity. This cavity is normally a potential space containing only a small amount of serous fluid. The serous fluid lubricates the viscera and allows them to move freely upon one another and the parietal peritoneum (Marieb, 1989).

The visceral peritoneum (consists of five layers of fibrous and elastic connective tissue and a sixth layer called the mesothelium. Blood and lymphatic capillaries are found only in the deepest layer of tissue in adults. A substance that passes from the bloodstream into the peritoneal cavity must pass through the capillary endothelium, the mesothelium and the five layers of the visceral peritoneum. The mesothelium represents the major barrier to mass transfer for most substances (Marieb, 1989).

Diffusion and osmosis are the physical processes involved in the exchange of substances across the peritoneal membrane (Figure 32.1). Diffusion is the force acting on gaseous, solid or liquid molecules to spread them from a region of high concentration to a region of lower concentration. Osmosis is the passage of a solvent through a semipermeable membrane that separates solutions of different concentrations. The force that causes this movement of solvents is osmotic pressure and this varies directly with the concentration of the solution. As the solvent moves across the membrane, it tends to pull certain amounts of solute with it. This is known as the solvent drag effect. Solvent drag enhances the efficiency of peritoneal dialysis. Equilibration is the achievement of equalization of solute and solvent concentrations on both sides of the membrane. As equilibration is achieved, dialysis ceases and solvents and solutes can be absorbed back into the bloodstream. For peritoneal dialysis to achieve maximum effectiveness, fresh

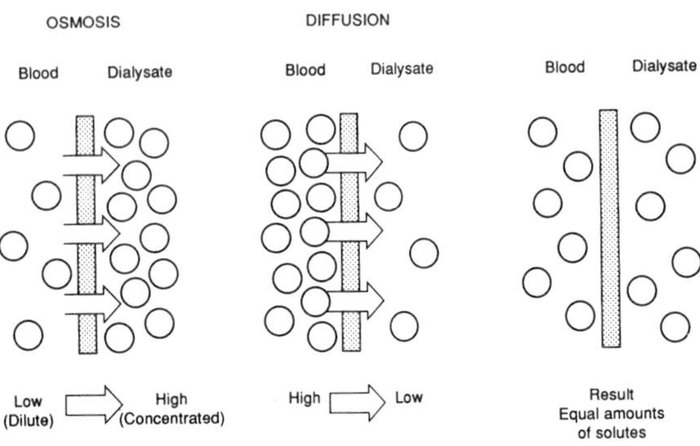

Figure 32.1 The process of osmosis and diffusion. (From 1987, *Nursing Times*, 22 April, p. 41; with permission.)

solutions must be instilled at the point of equilibration to prevent reabsorption of water and uraemic toxins (Smith, 1980).

Solution concentrations

The osmotic pressure of dextrose is utilized in peritoneal dialysis to remove water and solids from the patient. The composition of most commercially available peritoneal dialysis solutions fall into the following three groups:

1. The solution's electrolyte composition approximates normal extracellular fluid, i.e. its potassium concentration is 4 mmol/l and its glucose concentration is 1.3 to 1.5%.
2. As solution 1, but contains no potassium.
3. Hypertonic solution with a glucose concentration of 6.3% and the same potassium concentration as solution 1.

The choice of dialysate solution will depend on the primary aim of dialysis and the patient's baseline plasma electrolyte levels (Bloe, 1990).

Dialysis cycle

Normally, a cycle consists of three stages (Figure 32.2).

Stage 1 (inflow)

The dialysis solution at body temperature is infused into the peritoneal cavity to initiate the dialysis. The fluid infuses by gravity and its rate can be controlled

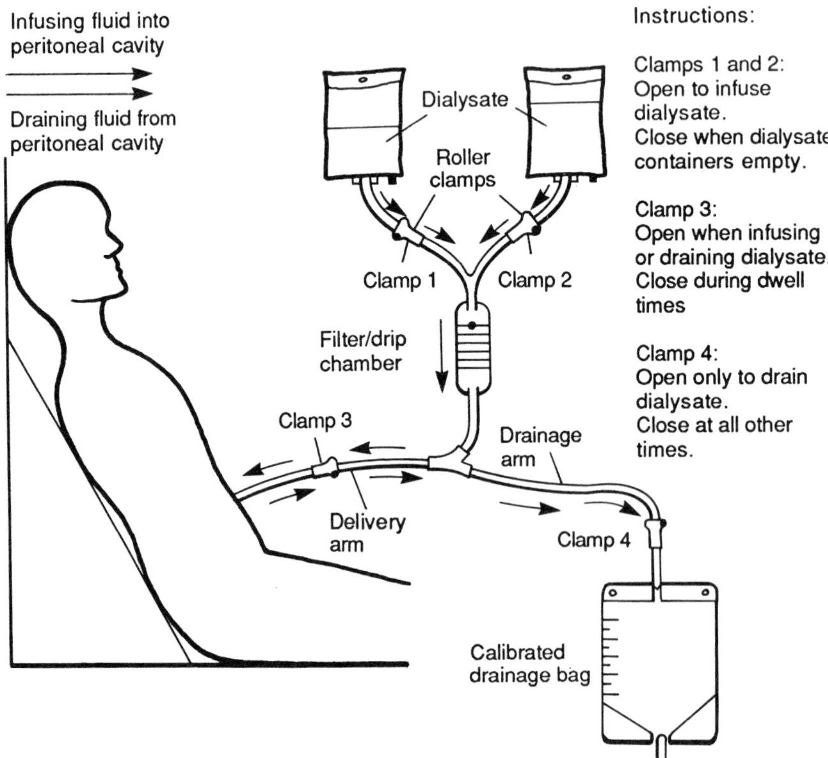

Figure 32.2 Using the Y-type administration set. (From Bloe (1990) Peritoneal dialysis. *The Professional Nurse*, April, 5(7), 345–9; with permission.)

by raising or lowering the container in relation to the patient's abdomen or by releasing or compressing the occluding clamp on the tubing.

Stage 2 (dwell time)
The dwell time is the time that the fluid remains in the peritoneal cavity to allow for equilibration. Different dwell times may be established to remove substances of differing molecular weights. The dwell time is relevant to the type of solute and the amount of solute removed.

Stage 3 (drainage)
The drainage stage is that of emptying the equilibrated solution from the peritoneal cavity to complete dialysis or to prepare for the infusion of fresh solution. Drainage is also dependent on gravity.

Types of peritoneal dialysis

Intermittent
For peritoneal dialysis used in the acute situation, a manual system is usually used to effect a quick and gentle dialysis (Figure 32.3). Optimal dialysis is achieved with short dialysis cycles of about one hour each, with a dwell time of 30 minutes and drainage time of 20 minutes. Specific numbers of exchanges are prescribed and dialysis is then discontinued temporarily, with initiation recurring as uraemia increases (Bloe, 1990).

Continuous ambulatory peritoneal dialysis (CAPD)
CAPD technique was first introduced in 1975. It is a closed, continuous system of peritoneal dialysis and allows the patient the independence of a life free from dialysis machines. The regime practised is usually four exchanges per day with the last staying in the peritoneal cavity overnight. Many devices have been developed to assist patients in their own homes to cope with the treatment while remaining free from the danger of infection and peritonitis (Warren, 1989).

Clear outlines of CAPD can be found in Ainge (1981), Arenz (1982), Sorrels (1981), Stansfield (1985), and Zappacosta & Perras (1984).

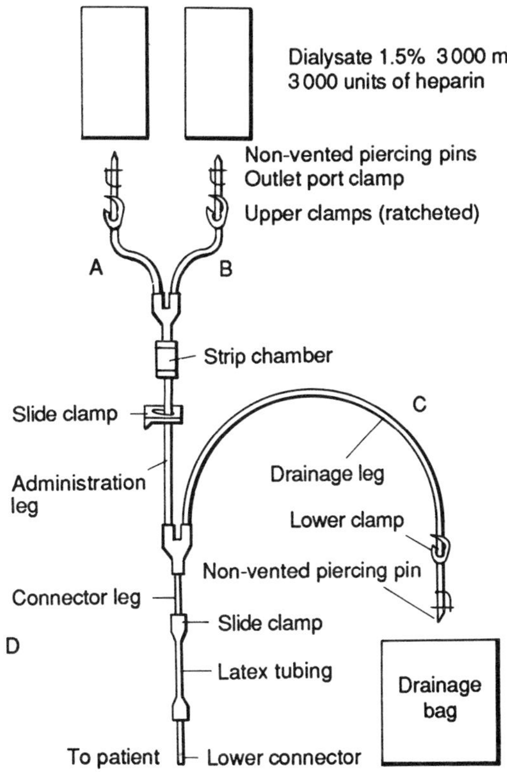

Figure 32.3 Peritoneal dialysis system set-up (courtesy of Abbott Renal Care). (From Prowant *et al.* (1988) Peritoneal dialysis: catheter exit site care. *ANNA Journal*, 15(4), 219–40; with permission.)

References and further reading

Ainge, T. M. (1981) Continuous ambulatory peritoneal dialysis. *Nursing Times*, 77, 1636–8.

Arenz, R. (1982) Continuous ambulatory peritoneal dialysis. *Association of Operating Room Nurses Journal*, 35(5), 946, 948, 950, 952, 954.

Bloe, C. G. (1990) Peritoneal dialysis. *The Professional Nurse*, April, 5(7), 345–9.

Blumenkrantz, M. J. & Roberts, M. (1979) Progress in peritoneal dialysis: an historical prospective. *Contrib. Nephrology*, 17, 101–10.

Brunner, L. S. & Suddarth, D. S. (1982) *The Lippincott Manual of Medical–Surgical Nursing, Vol. 3.* Harper & Row, London, pp. 253–8.

Marieb, E. N. (1989) *Human Anatomy and Physiology*, Benjamin Cummings, California.

Nursing (US) (1982) Fear of floating to a renal unit: nurses' guide to peritoneal dialysis complications. *Nursing*, 12, 42–3.

Oh, T. E. (1989) *Intensive Care Manual*, Butterworth, London.

Smith, K. (1980) *Fluids and Electrolytes: A Conceptual Approach*. Churchill Livingstone, Edinburgh.

Sorrels, A. J. (1981) Peritoneal dialysis: a rediscovery. *Nursing Clinics of North America*, 16(3), 515–29.

Stansfield, G. (1985) Coping with CAPD. *Nursing Mirror*, 161(14), 28–9.

Warren, H. (1989) Changes in peritoneal dialysis nursing. *ANNA Journal*, 16(3), 237–41.

Zappacosta, A. & Perras, S. (1984) *CAPD*. J. B. Lippincott, Philadelphia.

GUIDELINES: PERITONEAL DIALYSIS

Equipment

1. Dialysis Y type administration set and drainage bag.
2. Sterile peritoneal set containing forceps, blade and holder, topical swabs, towels, suturing equipment.
3. Sterile gown, gloves.
4. Peritoneal catheter stylet or trocar and drainage bag.
5. Local anaesthetic – 1 to 2% lignocaine hydrochloride.
6. Syringe, needle.
7. Skin antiseptic.
8. Supplementary drugs as prescribed.
9. Peritoneal dialysis fluid, as prescribed, warmed to 37°C.

Procedure

Action	Rationale
1. Explain the procedure to the patient. An acutely ill patient may be confused and restless but every effort should be made to inform patient of what is about to happen.	To obtain the patient's consent and co-operation. Some hospitals require a patient to sign a consent form before the procedure can be carried out.
2. Ask the patient to micturate and defaecate before the procedure begins.	To avoid perforation of the bladder and/or rectum when the trocar is introduced into the peritoneum.
3. Record the patient's vital signs before the procedure begins.	To assess physical/psychological state and to monitor changes.
4. Weigh the patient before the procedure begins and then daily.	To assess hydration and to monitor any fluid losses.
5. Assist the patient to lie in the semi-recumbent position.	To ensure that the patient is in the best position for the procedure's requirements.
6. Continue to observe and reassure the patient throughout the procedure.	To assess and monitor any physical/psychological changes.
7. Assist the doctor as required.	To facilitate a smooth and effective procedure for the patient.

Insertion of catheter

Action	Rationale
1. Using aseptic technique, the doctor prepares the abdomen surgically and injects the skin and subcutaneous tissues with a local anaesthetic.	To prevent the possibility of contamination and infection. To minimize the pain of the incision.
2. A small incision is made in the abdominal wall 3 to 5 cm below the umbilicus. The trocar is inserted through the incision. The patient is asked to raise the head from the pillow after the trocar is introduced.	This tightens the abdominal muscles and permits easier penetration of the trocar without danger of injury to the internal organs.
3. When the peritoneum is punctured, the trocar is directed to the left side of the pelvis. The stylet is removed and the catheter is inserted through the trocar and gently manoeuvred into position.	To prevent the omentum from adhering to the catheter or occluding its opening.

4. Once the trocar is removed, the skin may be sutured and a sterile dressing placed around the catheter.

To prevent the loss of the catheter in the abdomen. To prevent leakage of peritoneal fluid onto the surrounding skin.

5. The tubing is flushed with the dialysis fluid.

To prevent air from entering the peritoneal cavity.

Preparation of dialysis fluid

Action	Rationale
1. Wash hands with bactericidal soap and water or bactericidal alcohol hand rub. Proceed using aseptic technique.	To reduce risk of infection.
2. The dialysis fluid should have been warmed to body temperature (37°C).	For the patient's comfort. To prevent abdominal pain. Heating causes dilation of the peritoneal vessels and increases clearance of urea. Cold fluid would decrease rate of removal of large molecular solutes and can cause abdominal cramp pain.
3. Add any drugs, e.g. heparin, to the dialysis fluid if prescribed.	Heparin prevents fibrin clots from occluding the catheter.
4. Attach the dialysis fluid to the giving set via Luer lock connections.	
5. Attach the catheter connector to the giving set.	
6. Allow the dialysis fluid to flow freely into the peritoneal cavity. (This normally takes from five to ten minutes.)	To ascertain whether the catheter is in the required position. The flow should be steady and brisk. If not, the tip of the catheter may be buried in the omentum or it may have been occluded by a blood clot.
7. Allow fluid to remain in the peritoneal cavity for the prescribed time. Prepare the next exchange while the first container of fluid is in the peritoneal cavity.	The fluid must remain in the peritoneal cavity for the prescribed dwell time so that potassium, urea and other waste products may be removed. The solution is most effective over the first five to ten minutes when the concentration gradient is at its greatest.
8. Unclamp the drainage tube. Drainage time will vary with each patient but, on average, should be completed in ten minutes.	To rid the body of the required products. The abdomen is drained by a siphon effect through the closed system. Drainage is normally straw coloured.
9. Clamp off the drainage tube when outflow ceases and begin infusing the next exchange, again using aseptic technique.	To enable the next cycle to begin. To prevent local and/or systemic infection.
10. Record the following: (a) Time of commencement and completion of each exchange and the start and finish of the drainage stage (b) Amount of fluid infused and recovered (c) Fluid balance after each complete exchange (d) Any medication added to the dialysis fluid.	To detect and monitor trends and fluctuations.
11. Take and record the vital signs: (a) Blood pressure and pulse every 15 minutes during the first exchange and hourly	Hypotension may be indicative of excessive fluid loss due to the glucose concentration of the dialysis

Guidelines: Peritoneal dialysis

Action	Rationale
thereafter, depending on the patient's condition.	fluid. Changes in pulse may indicate impending shock or overhydration.
(b) Temperature every four hours, or more frequently if condition demands.	To monitor for any signs of infection. Infection is more likely to become evident after dialysis has been discontinued.
12. Record fluid balance accurately.	To prevent complications such as circulatory overload and hypertension that may occur if most of the fluid is not recovered during the drainage stage. The fluid balance should be about even or show slight fluid loss, unless the reason for treatment was to remove excess fluid.
13. Dialysis is usually continued until blood chemistry levels are satisfactory.	The duration of dialysis is related to the severity of the condition and the size and weight of the patient. The usual time is about 12 to 36 hours, giving between 24 to 28 exchanges.
14. Ensure that the patient is comfortable during dialysis by attending to pressure area care and altering the patient's position as required. Assist the patient to sit in a chair for short periods as the condition allows.	The period of dialysis is lengthy and often exhausts the patient.
15. Send a daily specimen of peritoneal fluid for microscopy and culture.	To monitor for any infections, etc.

NURSING CARE PLAN

Problem	Cause	Suggested action
Peritonitis, indicated by fever, persistent abdominal pain and cramping, abdominal fullness, abdominal rigidity, slow dialysis drainage, cloudy and offensive smelling drainage, swelling and tenderness around the catheter and increased white blood cell count.	Poor aseptic technique during catheter insertion or dialysis.	If peritonitis is suspected, notify the doctor immediately. Send a peritoneal fluid sample to the laboratory for fluid analysis, culture and sensitivity testing, Gram staining and cell count. Antibiotics may be prescribed by the doctor either locally or systemically in severe cases. Monitor vital signs; careful pain control is required.
Infection at the site of entry, indicated by redness, swelling, rigidity, tenderness and purulent drainage around the catheter.	Poor aseptic technique during catheter insertion or dialysis, or incomplete healing around the site of entry.	Notify a doctor. Obtain a specimen of the drainage fluid and send it to the laboratory. Antibiotics and pain control may be prescribed as above. Monitor vital signs.
Subcutaneous tunnel infection with cuffed catheter indicated by	Poor aseptic technique during catheter insertion or dialysis, or	Notify a doctor. Antibiotics may be prescribed as above. Monitor

redness, rigidity and tenderness over subcutaneous tunnel.	incomplete healing in subcutaneous tunnel.	vital signs.
Perforation of the bladder or the bowel, indicated by signs and symptoms of peritonitis, bright yellow dialysis fluid drainage (if bladder is perforated) or faeces in drainage (if bowel is perforated).	Catheter inserted when the patient had a full bladder or bowel.	If perforation is suspected, notify a doctor immediately. Monitor vital signs. Only minimal oral fluids should be given.
Bleeding through the catheter.	Minor trauma to the abdomen or minor trauma to the subcutaneous tunnel (with a cuffed catheter) or perforation of a major abdominal blood vessel during surgery.	Bleeding usually stops spontaneously. If it does not, notify the doctor, who may order blood transfusions. One-litre hourly dialysis exchanges may be ordered until the drainage fluid is clear.
Dialysis fluid leaking around the catheter.	Excessive instillation of dialysis fluid or incomplete healing. Incomplete healing around the cuff of the catheter. Catheter obstruction. Catheter dislodged or positioned improperly.	Instil less dialysis fluid at exchanges. Drain the patient's abdomen completely during outflow. Use small volumes of dialysis fluid in exchanges through a new catheter. Also, drain the patient's abdomen completely during outflow. Irrigate the catheter with sterile normal saline solution. Inform a doctor, who will replace the catheter or revise its position surgically.
Kinking of the cuffed catheter.	Subcutaneous tunnel too short or scarring in the subcutaneous tunnel.	Inform a doctor, who will remove the catheter and implant a new one.
Lower back pain.	Pressure and weight of dialysis fluid in the abdomen (particularly so in continuous ambulatory peritoneal dialysis (CAPD) patients).	Doctor may order analgesics. Exercises to strengthen the patient's muscles and improve posture may also be ordered.
Abdominal or rectal pain (with possible referred pain in shoulder).	Improperly positioned catheter tip causing irritation.	Catheter position to be revised surgically.
	Dialysis fluid accumulating under the diaphragm. Dialysis fluid not at 37°C. With two litres of 6.36% solution, severe shoulder pain can occur.	Drain the abdomen completely during outflow. Ensure that the fluid is infused at the correct temperature. If hypertonic dialysis fluid is used, only one container should be used per cycle.
	If air enters the peritoneal cavity, pain may occur.	Maintain a closed system.
Paralytic ileus indicated by sharp	Catheter manipulated excessively	Notify the doctor immediately as

Nursing care plan

Problem	**Cause**	**Suggested action**
pain in abdomen, constipation, abdominal distension, nausea and vomiting, and diarrhoea.	during insertion.	signs and symptoms may indicate peritonitis. A nasogastric tube to suction the stomach may be ordered. Cholinergic medication, such as neostigmine, may be prescribed. Administer fluids and electrolytes as prescribed. If general condition allows, encourage patient to walk, unless advised otherwise by the doctor. Prepare the patient for surgery, as advised by the doctor. The condition may disappear spontaneously after 12 hours.
Cramping.	Dialysis fluid warmer or cooler than 37°C.	Adjust the temperature of the dialysis fluid to 37°C before infusion.
	Too rapid infusion or drainage.	Decrease the infusion or drainage rate to a regime the patient can tolerate.
	Pressure from excess dialysis fluid in the abdomen.	Infuse less dialysis fluid at exchanges to a total volume that the patient can tolerate.
	Chemical irritation.	Use a dialysis fluid with a dextrose concentration lower than 7%.
	Air in the abdomen.	Clamp off the dialysis tubing before the dialysis fluid empties completely into the abdomen.
Excessive fluid loss.	Use of dialysis fluid with too great a dextrose concentration for the patient or inadequate sodium intake or inadequate fluid intake.	Monitor the patient's weight and blood pressure. Ensure that the patient is receiving dialysis fluid with the correct dextrose concentration. The doctor may prescribe a reduced dextrose concentration.
Fluid overload.	Use of dialysis fluid with an osmotic pressure that is too low for the patient or excessive sodium intake or excessive fluid intake.	Monitor the patient's weight and blood pressure. The doctor will order a reduced fluid and sodium intake. The doctor may also order increased use of dialysis fluid with a 4.25% dextrose concentration.
Metabolic disturbance usually affects plasma levels of glucose, potassium or sodium.	Continued use of inappropriate dialysate fluid.	Monitor relevant plasma levels pre- and post-dialysis. If patient has pre-existing diabetic mellitus or insulin deficiency, insulin dosage should be titrated carefully.

Respiratory difficulties.	Pressure from the fluid in the peritoneal cavity and upward displacement of the diaphragm or 'splinting' of the diaphragm, resulting in shallow breathing.	Elevate the head of the bed. Encourage breathing exercises and coughing. Involve the physiotherapist.

33

Peri-Operative Care

Definition

Peri-operative care is the preparation and assessment, physical and psychological, of a patient before surgery.

Peri-operative objectives

Physical

1. To minimize postoperative complications, e.g. by teaching the patient deep-breathing exercises and the relevance after surgery to wellbeing.
2. To assess the physical condition of the patient so that potential problems can be anticipated and prevented.
3. To ensure that the patient is in an optimum physical condition before surgery.

Psychological

1. To ensure that the patient fully understands the nature of the surgery to be undergone.
2. To teach the patient what to expect postoperatively, e.g. about any drains, catheters and so on that may be necessary afterwards.
3. To assess areas of anxiety that the patient may have and discuss them, using nursing interventions if appropriate.

REFERENCE MATERIAL

Patient education and postoperative pain

Much research and discussion has been devoted to the subject of postoperative pain and the ways in which pre-operative patient education can influence the pain experience. Since pain and anaesthesia are often the patient's greatest fears (Carnevali, 1966) it is necessary to address this cause of anxiety in the pre-operative period.

Reducing patient anxiety by giving pre-operative information has been shown to reduce postoperative pain (Haywood, 1975). It also results in the patient requiring less analgesia. The reduction of anxiety and promoting postoperative recovery can be achieved in several ways. The fragmentation of nursing care could account for some patient anxiety (Copp, 1988), and pre-operative visiting by nurses from theatres is being undertaken in many hospitals. It has been found that this can 'help the patient to manage his anxiety, not least by providing a continuity of care in collaboration with other members of the surgical teams' (Leonard & Kalideen, 1985). Copp (1988) also found that teaching patients recovery exercises decreased their feelings of helplessness and, therefore, reduced anxiety, and that the use of cognitive coping methods is an effective way of reducing anxiety.

Further research (Balfour, 1989) has shown that 'patients continue to suffer unrelieved pain following abdomen surgery' and that 'nurses continue to under-administer prescribed analgesics'. Postoperative analgesia is often administered on a *pro re nata* (as required) basis so that patients request it when they are in pain. One strategy is to use methods to maintain a constant drug concentration in the blood via a continuous infusion. This often reduces side-effects, such as nausea, while providing good analgesic cover. Use of patient-controlled analgesia (PCA) gives the patient a sense of autonomy which may decrease anxiety, and which will in turn influence the patient's pain perception (Carr, 1989).

Skin preparation

Before surgery the patient is required to have a bath or shower. The aim of a pre-operative bath or shower is to reduce the risk of postoperative wound infection.

Research into the use of antiseptic preparations to be used in the pre-operative bath or shower is contradictory. Wells *et al.* (1983) found a single bath using chlorhexidine did not reduce postoperative infections in patients undergoing open heart surgery. This is supported by Leigh *et al.* (1983), who found that a single chlorhexidine bath eliminated the skin carriage of *Staphylococcus aureus* but did not reduce postoperative wound infection rates.

Hayek *et al.* (1987) studied the effects of two pre-operative baths comparing the use of chlorhexidine against ordinary soap and a placebo. The findings indicated that the two pre-operative chlorhexidine showers reduced the postoperative infection rate in 'clean' surgery. In the clean group, chlothexidine use reduced the incidence of *Staphylococcus* by 50%; in the clean/contaminated surgery group there was some reduction of staphylococcal infections. Although chlorhexidine caused a reduction of overall infection in the contaminated wounds, it was not statistically significant.

Shaving is also a common pre-operative procedure. Studies suggest that there is a direct relationship between wound infection and hair removal, with the lowest wound infection rates obtained in cases where no hair was removed and the highest infection rate occurring when a razor was used (Alexander *et al.*, 1983; Willford, 1983).

One alternative method is to use a depilatory cream, which has demonstrated lower postoperative infection rates when the absence of hair from the operation site is required (*Lancet*, 1983). Winfield (1986) found that although depilatory cream is more expensive than shaving, it can save nursing time as most patients can apply the cream themselves. Similarly, although skin irritation can occur (in 9% of cases), it compares favourably with skin irritation from razors (13%), including grazes and small cuts.

Pre-operative fasting

Any patient presenting for anaesthesia may have undigested food in the stomach. For elective surgery the patient is usually 'nil by mouth' for long enough to allow the stomach to empty. Research by Thomas (1987) has revealed that patients often did not know why they were fasting, and that they were often deprived of food and drink for longer than the recommended time of six hours. Patients on an afternoon theatre list were less likely to be starved for as long as those on the morning list, who were frequently starved from midnight.

Stomach-emptying on average takes six hours for solid food and four hours for fluids (Carrie & Simpson, 1988). However, gastric emptying may be delayed by anxiety or the action of some drugs, e.g. opiates. Atropine and hyoscine are sometimes prescribed as part of the patient's premedication, primarily to reduce saliva production. However, they also have a blocking action on the parasympathetic nervous system, which reduces motility of the digestive tract and therefore reduces the likelihood of vomiting (Green, 1986).

Antiembolic stockings

Deep vein thrombosis, if it occurs, is usually diagnosed three to 14 days postoperatively. The incidence is highest in middle-aged and elderly patients, those on prolonged bedrest, and after major surgery of the lower abdomen, pelvis or hip joints. Patients with a history of coronary artery disease are also at risk (Carrie & Simpson, 1988). Once high-risk patients have been identified, prophylactic treatment can begin.

One such treatment is the use of antiembolic stockings (Allen *et al.*, 1983) which should be fitted from ankle to midthigh. These stockings work by promoting venous flow and reducing stasis. They increase the velocity of flow, not only in the legs, but also in the pelvic veins and inferior vena cava (Drinkwater, 1989).

During surgery the use of heel supports which reduce the pressure on the calves on the operating table will also encourage venous return. The use of intermittent calf compression air boots which promote venous flow during surgery have also been reported to be effective. Good pain control will encourage patients to mobilize early and carry out postoperative exercises, which are also important in preventing serious postoperative complications.

References and further reading

Alexander *et al.* (1983) The influence of hair removal methods on wound infections. *Archives of Surgery*, 118, 347–52.

Allen *et al.* (1983) The use of graduated compression stockings in the prevention of deep vein thrombosis. *British Journal of Surgery*, 10, 172–4.

Balfour, S. E. (1989) Will I be in pain? Patient and nurse attitudes to pain after abdominal surgery. *The Professional Nurse*, 1(5), 28–33.

Biley, F. C. (1989) Nurse perception of stress in pre-operative surgical patients. *Journal of Advanced Nursing*, 14, 575–81.

Brown, S. A. (1983) Venous thrombosis: another complication of cancer (care plan). *Oncology Nurse Forum*, 10(2), 41–7.

Carnevali, D. L. (1966) Pre-operative anxiety. *American Journal of Nursing*, 66(7), 1536–8.

Carr, F. (1989) Waking up to post-operative pain. *Nursing Times*, 85(3), 38–9.

Carrie, L. E. S. & Simpson, P. J. (1988) *Understanding Anaesthesia*. William Heinemann, London.

Clarke, J. (1983) The effectiveness of surgical skin preparations. *Nursing Times*, *Theatre Nursing Supplement*, 28 September, 79(39), 8–17.

Copp, G. (1988) Intra-operative information and pre-operative visiting. *Surgical Nurse*, 1(2), 27–8.

Davis, P. S. (1988) Changing nursing practice for more effective control of post-operative pain through a staff-initiated educational programme. *Nurse Education Today*, 8, 325–31.

Drinkwater, K. (1989) Management of deep vein thrombosis.

Surgical Nurse, 2(1), 24–6.

Gooch, J. (1989) Who should manage pain – patient or nurse? *The Professional Nurse*, 4(6), 295–6.

Green, J. H. (1986) *Basic Clinical Physiology*, 3rd edn. Oxford University Press, Oxford.

Hayek, L. J. *et al.* (1987) A placebo-controlled trial of the effect of pre-operative baths or showers with chlorhexidine detergent on postoperative wound infection rates. *Journal of Hospital Infection*, 10(2), 165–72.

Hayward, J. (1975) *Information: A Prescription Against Pain*. Royal College of Nursing (Research Series), London.

Johnson, A. (1989) Preparing for elective surgery. *Nursing Standard*, 3(23), 22–4.

Lancet (1983) Pre-operative depilation. *Lancet*, 1(8337), 1311.

Leigh, D. A. *et al.* (1983) Total body bathing with 'Hibiscrub' (chlorhexidine) in surgical patients. A controlled trial. *Journal of Hospital Infection*, 4(3), 229–35.

Leonard, M. D. & Kalideen, P. (1985) 'So you're going to have an operation.' *National Association of Theatre Nurses News*, 22(2), 12–21.

Lore, C. (1990) Deep vein thrombosis: threat to recovery. Part 1, *Nursing Times*, 86(5), 40–3.

McConnell, E. A. (1990) *Clinical Do's and Don'ts: applying* antiembolism stockings (pictoral, protocol). *Nursing*, 20(10), 92.

Thomas, A. E. (1987) Pre-operative fasting – a question of routine? *Nursing Times*, 83(49), 46–7.

Wells, F. C. *et al.*. (1983) Wound infection in cardiothoracic surgery. *Lancet* 1, 1209–10.

Willford, P. S. (1983) Hair removal – shave, preps, depilation, and other pre-operative considerations. Are they really necessary? *Journal of Operating Room Research Institute*, 3(3), 26–8.

Winfield, V. (1986) Too close a shave? *Nursing Times, Journal of Infection Control Nursing*, 82(10), 64–8.

GUIDELINES: PERI-OPERATIVE CARE

Equipment

1 Theatre gown.
2 Labelled denture container if necessary.
3 Hypo-allergenic tape to cover wedding rings.
4 Any equipment and documents required by law and hospital policy if a pre-medication has been prescribed.

Procedure

Action	Rationale
1. Ensure the patient is wearing an identification bracelet with the correct information.	To ensure correct identification and prevent possible problems.
2. Assess the pre-operative education received by the patient and ensure that it is complete and understood.	To ensure that the patient understands the nature and outcome of the surgery and reduce anxiety and possible post-operative complications.
3. Record the patient's pulse, blood pressure, respirations, temperature and weight.	To provide data for comparison postoperatively. The weight is recorded so that the anaesthetist can calculate the dose of drugs to be used.
4. Check that the patient has undergone relevant procedures, e.g. X-ray, ECG, blood tests and that these results are included with the patient's notes.	To ensure all relevant information is available to the nurses, anaesthetists and surgeons. Absence of results may delay or cause cancellation of an operation.
5. Instruct the patient on showering or bathing. Ensure hair removal has been completed *if* required by the surgeon.	To minimize risk of postoperative wound infection.
6. Assist the patient to change into a theatre gown.	
7. Long hair should be held back with, for example, a non-metallic tie.	

Action	Rationale
8. Ensure that patients undergoing major surgery or abdominal/pelvic surgery, the elderly frail or bedbound patients or those with a previous history of emboli or other high-risk factors have antiembolic stockings applied correctly. The use of intermittent calf compression boots should be considered.	To reduce the risk of postoperative deep vein thrombosis or pulmonary emboli.
9. Complete the pre-operative check list by asking the patient and checking records and notes before giving any pre-medication.	*Note*: questioning pre-medicated patients is not a reliable source of checking information as the patient may be drowsy and/or disorientated.
(a) Check when patient last had food or drink and ensure that it was at least six hours before.	To reduce the risk of regurgitation and inhalation of stomach contents on induction of anaesthetic.
(b) Check whether patient micturated before pre-medication.	To prevent urinary incontinence and embarrassment. To allow better access to abdominal cavity for abdomen or pelvic surgery if a catheter is not to be used.
(c) Note whether the patient has dental crowns, bridge work or loose teeth.	The anaesthetist needs to be informed to prevent accidental damage. Loose teeth or a dental prosthesis could be inhaled by the patient when an endotracheal tube is inserted.
(d) Ensure prostheses, dentures and contact lenses are removed.	To prevent trauma to the patient.
(e) Spectacles may be retained until the patient is in the anaesthetic room. Hearing aids may be retained until the patient has been anaesthetized. (These may be left in position if a local anaesthetic is being used.) Any prosthesis should then be labelled clearly and retained in the recovery room.	To reduce anxiety and enable the patient to understand any procedures carried out.
(f) All jewellery (apart from wedding ring), cosmetics, nail varnish and clothing, other than the theatre gown, are to be removed.	Metal jewellery may be accidentally lost or may be cause of harm to patient, e.g. – diathermy burns. Facial cosmetics can make the patient's colour difficult to assess. Nail varnish makes the use of the pulse oximeter, used to monitor the patient's pulse and oxygen saturation levels, impossible and masks peripheral cyanosis.
10. Valuables should be placed in the hospital's custody and recorded according to the hospital policy.	To prevent loss of valuables.
11. Check the consent form is correctly completed, signed and dated.	To comply with legal requirements and hospital policy.
12. Check the operation site is marked correctly.	To ensure the patient undergoes the correct surgery for which he/she has consented.
13. Check that the patient has undergone pre-anaesthetic assessment by the anaesthetist.	To ensure that the patient can be given the most suitable anaesthetic.
14. Give the pre-medication, if prescribed, in accordance with the anaesthetist's instructions and conforming to legal requirements and hospital policy.	Different drugs may be prescribed to complement the anaesthetic to be given, e.g. temazepam to reduce patient anxiety by inducing sleep and relaxation.

Guidelines: Peri-operative care

Action	Rationale
15. Advise the patient to remain in bed once the pre-medication has been given and to use the nurse call system if assistance is needed.	To prevent accidental patient injury as the pre-medication may make the patient drowsy and disorientated.
16. Ensure the patient is supported fully on the canvas, especially the head, when transferred from the ward bed to the trolley.	To prevent injury to the neck, etc. during transfer from the ward to the operating theatre.
17. Ensure that all relevant information, e.g. X-rays, notes, blood results, accompany the patient to the operating theatre.	To prevent delays which can increase the patient's anxiety, and to ensure that the anaesthetist and surgeon have all the information they require for the safe treatment of the patient.
18. The patient should be accompanied to the theatre by a ward nurse who remains until the patient is anaesthetized.	To reduce the patient's anxiety.
19. The ward nurse should give a full handover to the anaesthetic nurse or operating department assistant on arrival of the patient to the anaesthetic room.	To ensure the patient has the correct operation. To ensure continuity of care by exchanging all relevant information.

INTRA-OPERATIVE CARE

Definition

Intra-operative care is the physical and psychological care given to the patient in the anaesthetic room and theatre until transferral to the recovery room.

Objectives

1. To ensure that the patient fully understands what is happening at all times in order to minimize anxiety.
2. To ensure that the patient has the surgery for which the consent form was signed.
3. To ensure patient safety at all times and minimize postoperative complications by:
   (a) Giving the required care for the unconscious patient.
   (b) Ensuring no injury is sustained from hazards associated with the use of swabs, needles, instruments, diathermy and power tools.
   (c) Minimizing postoperative problems associated with patient positioning, such as nerve or tissue damage.
   (d) Maintaining asepsis during surgical procedures to reduce the risk of postoperative wound infection in accordance with hospital policies on infection control.

REFERENCE MATERIAL

Diathermy

Diathermy is used routinely during many operations to control haemorrhage by cauterizing blood vessels or cutting or fulgerizing body tissues. Diathermy is potentially hazardous to the patient if used incorrectly. It is important that all theatre nurses know how to test and use all diathermy equipment in their department to prevent patient injury (3M, 1986; Theatre Safeguards, 1988).

The main risk when using diathermy is of thermo-electrical burns. The most common cause is incorrect application of the patient plate or a break in the connecting lead (Moakes, 1991). If this occurs when using an isolated diathermy machine then the current output will stop. However, if a grounded diathermy machine is used then the electrical current will find an alternative route back to the diathermy machine (Wainwright, 1988). If the patient is in contact with any metal, e.g. on the operating table (3M, 1986, p. 4), then loss of plate contact using a grounded unit could result in a serious burn.

Other causes of burns include skin preparation solutions or other liquids pooling around the plate site. With alcohol-based skin preparations especially, the skin should be allowed to dry before diathermy is used, as the alcohol can ignite (Wainwright, 1988). If the patient's position is changed during the operation the patient plate should be rechecked to ensure that it is still in contact and that the connecting clamp or lead is not causing pressure in the new position.

Use of diathermy and the plate position should be noted on the nursing care plan, and the patient's skin condition should be checked postoperatively.

Patient positioning

The position of the patient on the operating table must be such as to facilitate access to the operation site(s) by the surgeon, taking into account the patient's airway, monitoring equipment or intravenous lines. Nor should it compromise the patient's circulation, respiratory system or nerves (*American Operating Room Nursing*, 1990). Pre-operative assessment will identify patients with particular needs which may be influenced by factors such as weight, nutritional state, age, skin condition and pre-existing disease. All these factors may indicate the need for extra precautions during positioning. Consideration by and the co-operation of all theatre personnel can help prevent many of the pre-operative complications related to intra-operative positioning.

All equipment that may be needed to support the patient during surgery, e.g. the table, arm supports, lithotomy poles and securing straps, should be checked to ensure that they are in working order, clean and free from sharp edges. Metal parts that may come into contact with the patient should be covered as there is an increased risk of burns if diathermy is used (Wainwright, 1988). Padding should be placed at the patient's elbows and heels, and pillows positioned between the legs if the patient is lying in a lateral position. Special consideration should also be given to areas such as the back of the head and ears. The use of a warm air mattress on the operating table can also help to reduce pressure on vulnerable areas such as the hips or sacrum, as well as reducing the risk of hypothermia.

When a patient is transferred between the trolley or bed and operating table, adequate personnel should be present to ensure patient and staff safety (*American Operating Room Nursing Journal*, 1990). If poles and a canvas are to be used then the integrity of the canvas must be assured, also that the patient's head is fully supported by the canvas (Theatre Safeguards, 1988).

All movements of the limbs of the unconscious patient should take into account the anatomy and natural planes of movement of that limb to avoid stretching and pressure on the related nerve planes (Theatre Safeguards, 1988). Hyperabduction of the arm when placed on a board, for example, could stretch the brachial plexus causing some postoperative loss of sensation and reduced movement of the forearm, wrist and fingers. The ulnar and radial nerves may be affected by direct pressure as a result of insufficient padding on arm supports or lack of care when inserting poles into the canvas and hitting the elbows.

Pre-existing conditions such as backache or sciatica can be exacerbated, particularly if the patient is in the lithotomy position as the sciatic nerve can be compressed against the poles (Underwood & Jameson, 1990). Most postoperative palsies are due to improper positioning of the patient on the operating table (Nightingale, 1985).

References and further reading

American Operating Room Nursing Journal (1990) Proposed recommended practices; positioning the surgical patient. *AORN Journal*, 51(1), 216–22.

Gillette, M. K. & Cansico, C. C. (1989) Intra-operative tissue injury, major causes and preventative measures (study). *American Operating Room Nursing Journal*, 50(1), July, 66–8.

Joint Memorandum by Medical Defence Union and Royal College of Nursing (1978) *Safeguards Against Failure to Remove Swabs and Instruments From Patients*.

Lamp (cover story) (1990) There's more in the wash than dirty linen! *Lamp*, 47(3), 12.

3M (1986) *Safety in Diathermy*. 3M Health Care Ltd.

Moakes, E. (1991) Electrosurgical unit safety. *American Operating Room Nursing Journal*, 53(3), 744–52.

Nightingale, K. (1985) Hazards to patients during surgery. *National Association of Theatre Nurses News*, January, 13–16.

Theatre Safeguards (1988) MDU, RCN, NATN.

Underwood, M. J. & Jameson J. (1990) Preventing nerve injuries. *Technic*, 83, 11–13.

Wainwright, D. (1988) Diathermy – How safe is it? *National Association of Theatre Nurses News*, 25(1), 7–8.

GUIDELINES: INTRA-OPERATIVE CARE

Action	**Rationale**
1. Greet the patient by name. Confirm with the ward nurse that it is the correct patient for the scheduled operation.	To make the patient feel welcome. To ensure that the patient is safeguarded against problems related to misidentity.

Guidelines: Intra-operative care

Action	Rationale
2. Identify the patient by checking the name bracelet and number against the patient's notes and the operating list.	To question the pre-medicated patient can be unreliable (Theatre Safeguards, 1988).
3. Examine the pre-operative checklist (Figure 33.1).	To ensure that all of the listed measures have been completed and that any additional information has been recorded.
4. Check that the blood results, X-rays, ect. are present in the patient's notes.	To ensure that all of the required results are available for the medical team's use.
5. Maintain a calm, quiet environment and explain all the procedures to patient.	To reduce anxiety and enhance the smooth induction of anaesthesia.
6. When the patient is anaesthetized ensure that the eyes are closed and hypo-allergenic tape is applied.	To prevent corneal damage due to drying or accidental abrasion.
7. Ensure that there are adequate staff to transfer the patient to the operating table. Ensure the brakes on the trolley and operating table have been applied. Ensure the patient's head and limbs are supported when transferring to the operating table.	To ensure that the patient receives no injury during the transfer.
8. Check with anaesthetist before moving patient.	To ensure airway is protected.
9. Ensure all limbs are supported and secure on the table. Ensure adequate padding and cushioning of bony prominences. The patient's position will be dictated by the nature of the surgery but must take into account the requirements of the anaesthetist and the physical, psychological and social needs of the patient.	If the patient is unconscious and unable to maintain a safe environment, support is necessary to prevent injury. The patient is especially at risk from damage due to pressure and stretching, so measures to maintain the skin's integrity are vital. Nerve damage due to compression or stretching must be prevented.
10. Ensure the patient is well covered by the gown or blanket. These items should only be removed immediately before surgery.	To maintain the patient's dignity. To help prevent a reduction in body temperature or accidental hypothermia.
11. Use a warm air mattress on the operating table. Ensure all fluids used are warmed if possible.	To help maintain the patient's body temperature and prevent postoperative complications due to hypothermia.
12. Ensure all the equipment to be used is checked and in working order before the operating list commences, including suction, the anaesthetic machine, medical gases, monitoring equipment, diathermy and operating table.	To prevent accidental injury due to faulty equipment and to ensure all equipment necessary to the patient's treatment is present.
13. Ensure diathermy patient plate is attached securely in accordance with the manufacturer's instructions and hospital policy.	To ensure that no injury is sustained from the use of diathermy during surgery.
14. Follow hospital policy for the checking of	To ensure that swabs, needles and instruments are

swabs, needles and instruments.	accounted for at the end of the operation (Joint Memorandum MDU and RCN, 1978).
15. Follow hospital policy for the disposal of sharps and clinical waste.	To prevent risk of injury to the patient and staff.
16. Ensure the surgeon is informed that the number of swabs, needles and instruments is correct.	It is the responsibility of the nurse and surgeon to check that nothing is accidentally left inside the patient on completion of surgery.
17. The scrub nurse accompanies the patient with the anaesthetist to the recovery area. A handover is given that includes:	To ensure continuity of care of the patient.
(a) What procedure was performed.	To ensure that the recovery nurse has all the information required to assess the patient's recovery needs.
(b) The presence, position and nature of any drains, infusions or intravenous or arterial lines.	
(c) Information including allergies or pre-existing medical conditions, such as diabetes mellitus.	To assist the recovery nurse in the assessment of postoperative problems with which the patient may present.
(d) The patient's cardiovascular state and pattern of anaesthesia used.	
(e) Specific instructions from the anaesthetist for postoperative care.	
(f) Information about any anxieties of the patient expressed before surgery such as a fear of not waking after anaesthesia or fear about coping with pain.	To ensure appropriate action can be taken as the patient regains consciousness and to enable an assessment of the efficacy of nursing interventions used.
(g) All information is to be recorded on the theatre nursing care plan.	To provide a written record of nursing intervention for use by recovery staff and ward nursing staff.

POST-ANAESTHETIC RECOVERY

Definition

Post-anaesthetic recovery involves the short-term critical care required by patients during their immediate postoperative period until they are stable, conscious and orientated.

Indication

All patients undergoing surgery and anaesthesia.

REFERENCE MATERIAL

The post-anaesthetic recovery room is an area within the operating department that is specifically designed, equipped and staffed for the support, monitoring and assessment of patients through the reversing stages of anaesthesia.

The recovery period is potentially hazardous. 'About 20% of the deaths associated with anaesthesia occur during the first 30 minutes after operation', and 'almost half the deaths occurring in the immediate postoperative period are due to inadequate nursing' (Atkinson *et al.*, 1982). While the majority of patients can be expected to achieve an uneventful recovery, they are vulnerable to many complications, notably respiratory and circulatory ones. One in 5.5 patients develop one or more complications during their time in the recovery room (Farman, 1978). Continuous individual nursing is required until patients are able to maintain their own airway (Association of Anaesthetists of Great Britain and Ireland, 1985). Obstruction of the upper airway is the commonest respiratory complication in the immediate postoperative period. Close observation and appropriate action can prevent the sequence of respiratory obstruction resulting in hypoxia leading to cardiac arrest (Campbell & Spence, 1990).

Guedels' classification of general anaesthesia

Guedel first published his systemization of the signs of inhalation anaesthesia, based on the description of patients under open-drop ether anaesthesia in 1920.

THE ROYAL MARSDEN HOSPITAL

Date ....Patient Name ....Hospital No. ....

Consultant .... Ward ....

PRE-OPERATIVE ASSESSMENT
(Relevant information to include potential medical/physical and communication problems e.g. Diabetes, Blindness/Deafness, Language differences etc.)

T.P.R. B/P

ALLERGIES:

PRE-OPERATIVE CHECKLIST

	YES/NO	INITIAL
SECTION A – To be checked by observing/asking patient		
Identiband present and correct	....	....
Time food or drink last taken	....	....
Urine passed prior to pre-medication	....	....
Dental crowns /bridge work / loose teeth	....	....
Dentures removed (with patient)	....	....
Hearing Aid (with patient)	....	....
Contact lenses removed	....	....

Patient correctly prepared for theatre –		
e.g. shaved if necessary	....	....
Jewellery removed (rings taped)	....	....
Cosmetic and clothing removed	....	....
Valuables placed in hospital custody	....	....

SECTION B – To be checked from nursing/medical notes

Consent to anaesthetic/operation form signed	....	....
Operation site marked if appropriate	....	....
Patient has undergone pre-anaesthetic examination	....	....
Pre-medication given at	(time).....................	....
Case notes accompany patient –	....	....
X-rays accompany patient –	....	....

TIME IN ANAESTHETIC ROOM ....SIGNATURE WARD NURSE ....

SIGNATURE OF CHECKING ODA / NURSE ....

Figure 33.1 The Royal Marsden Hospital theatre care document.

DOCUMENTATION OF CARE

TIME IN THEATRE. . . . .

TEMP (18 - 21C) YES/NO
HUMIDITY (30% - 50%) YES/NO
EQUIPMENT CHECKED YES/NO

PATIENT CARE
identification / consent YES/NO

POSITION OF PATIENT: Supine Prone Lateral Lithotomy Trendelenburg

Other (please specify) ....

Apparatus used for safe positioning of patient:

Arm supports Heel support Gamgee Arm Boards Head Ring

Other (please specify) ....

Hot air mattress Yes/No TED Stockings/Venous stimulators

Position of Diathermy Plate ....

Catheter (size/type/balloon size) ....

Skin preparation Iodine – Aqueous / Alcoholic

Chlorhexidine – Aqueous / Alcoholic

Other (please specify) ....

Throat pack ....

Tourniquet times on......................off ....

SURGEON(S) ....

SCRUB PERSON(S) .... CIRCULATING PERSON(S) ....

....

ANAESTHETIST .... ODA/NURSE ....
LA / GA

PROCEDURE PERFORMED ....

....

Swab / Needle / Instrument Count ....

Condition of patient's skin at end of surgery ....

Diathermy site checked (Initial) ....

Skin Closure : Sutures (Interrupted / Continuous) – Type ....

Staples Other (please specify) ....

Drains : Vacuum Silicone Yeates / Corrugated Other (specify) ....

Dressings: .... Packs vaginal / nasal ....

Specimens – Histology (Formalin / Fresh / Frozen Section) Microbiology Cytology

Signature of Scrub Person ....

Figure 33.1 Continued

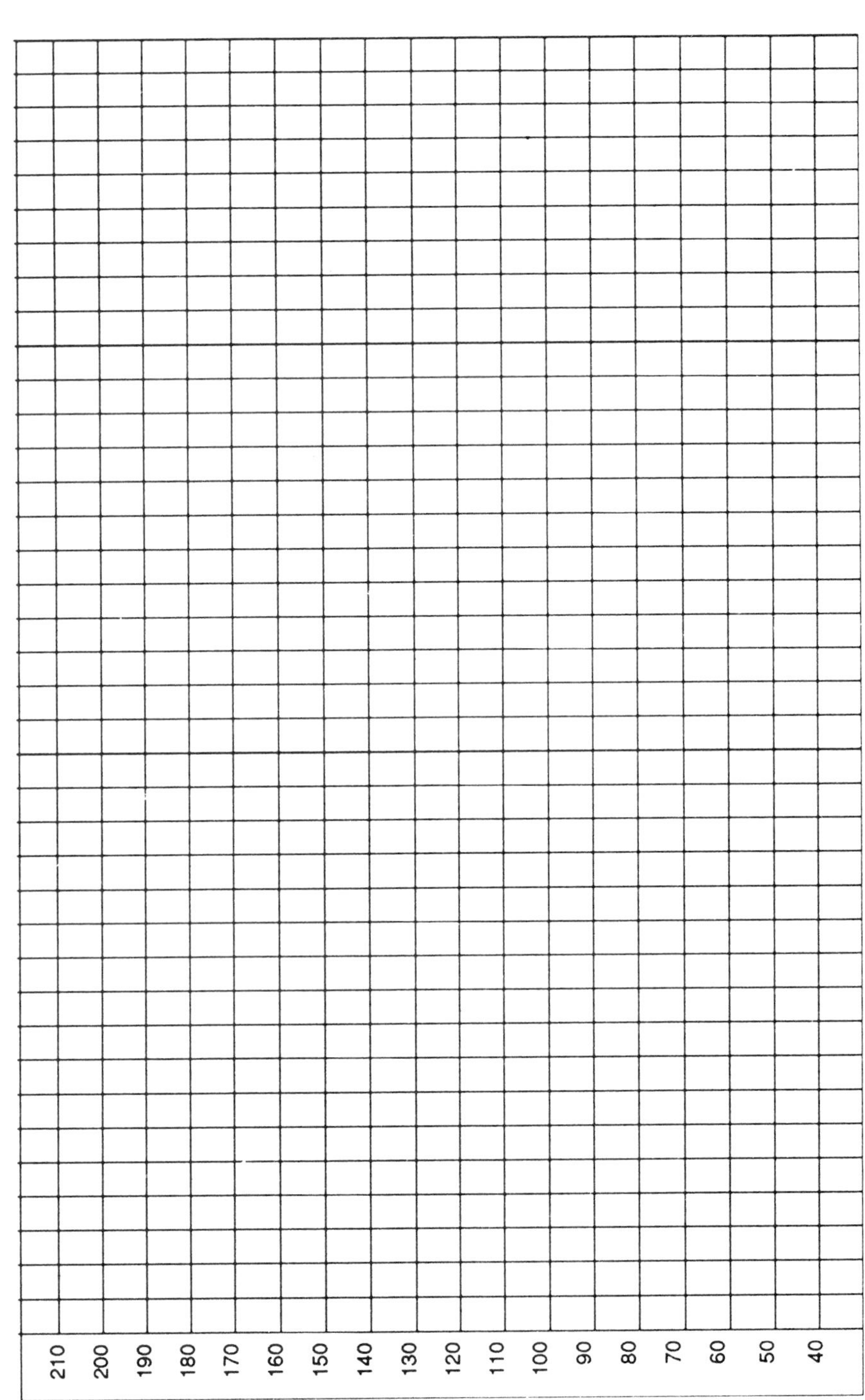
THEATRE RECOVERY
TIME IN ....
210
200
190
180
170
160
150
140
130
120
110
100
90
80
70
60
50
40
PULSE AND BLOOD PRESSURE

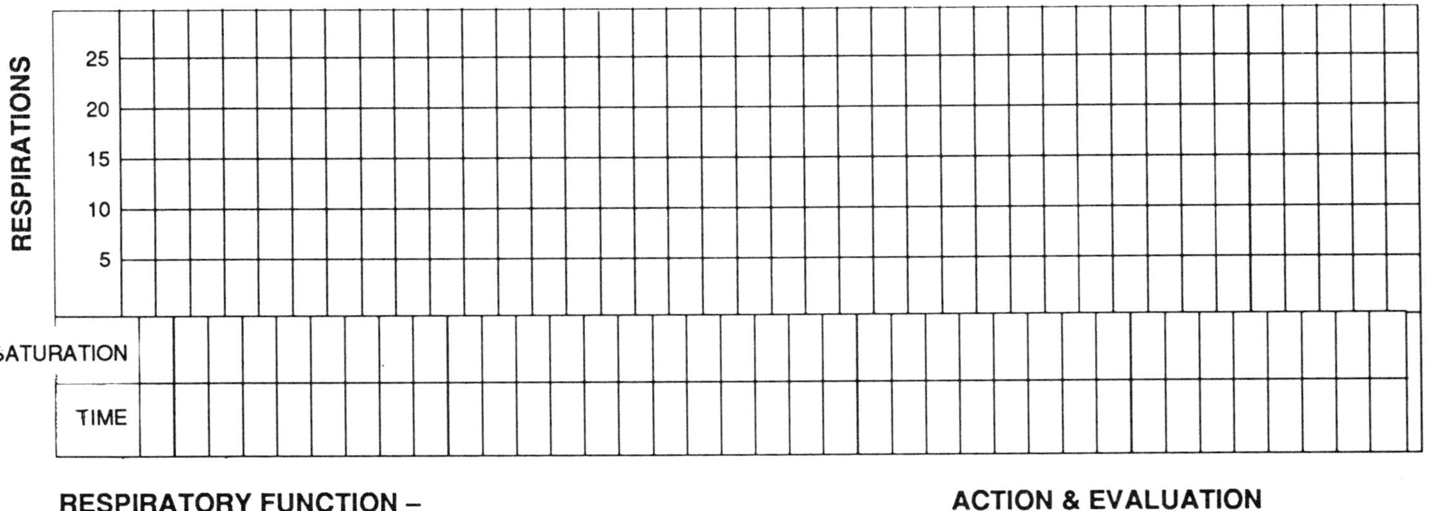

RESPIRATORY FUNCTION –

ACTION & EVALUATION

AIRWAY – observe, assess and ensure patency

BREATHING – record respiratory rate, observe chest movement

Give O_2 as prescribed

Record O_2 saturation

Figure 33.1 Continued

CARDIOVASCULAR FUNCTION	**ACTION & EVALUATION**
Record Pulse & Blood Pressure	
Observe skin/ mucosa for temperature and perfusion	
Observe wound sites, dressings and drains	
LEVEL OF CONSCIOUSNESS Observe responsiveness, orientation & mobility	
FLUID BALANCE Observe and record all input/drainage from IVIs, catheters, NG tubes etc.	

MEDICATION
Record all drugs given, time of administration and effect

COMMENTS AND INSTRUCTIONS SPECIFIC TO PATIENT

....

SIGNATURE OF RECOVERY NURSE

Figure 33.1 Continued

Current practice does not depend on the use of a single agent administered in this way and the effects of opiates and muscle relaxants will affect the signs of the stages of anaesthesia as formulated in his classification. However, the system can still be used as a framework within which to assess the progress of post-anaesthetic recovery as long as other factors influencing the return of consciousness are taken into consideration (Table 33.1).

Assessment for discharge

The length of any patient's stay in the recovery room is dependent on the patient's condition and the rate at which that patient returns to a physical, mental and emotional state where he or she can be left unattended between routine observations.

Minimum criteria for discharge are:

1. The patient is conscious and orientated and all protective reflexes have returned to normal.
2. Respiratory function is adequate and good oxygenation is being maintained.
3. Pulse and blood pressure are within normal pre-operative limits on consecutive observation.
4. There is no persistent or excessive bleeding from wound or drainage sites.
5. Patients with urinary catheters have passed adequate amounts of urine (more than 0.5 ml/kg/hr) (Eltringham *et al.*, 1989).
6. Satisfactory analgesia has been provided for the patient, prescribed by the anaesthetist.

Table 33.1 Guedel's classification of general anaesthesia (Guedel, 1937; Lunn, 1982)

Classification	
Stage I	Analgesia or the stage of disorientation from induction of anaesthesia to loss of consciousness
Stage II	Excitement: reflexes remain and coughing, vomiting and struggling may occur, respiration can be irregular with breath holding
Stage III	Surgical anaesthesia, divided into four planes:
	Plane I – eyelid reflex lost, swallowing reflex disappears, marked eyeball movement but loss of conjunctival reflex
	Plane II – eyeball movement ceases, laryngeal reflex lost although inflammation of the upper respiratory tract increases reflex irritability, corneal reflex disappears, secretion of tears increases, respiration automatic and regular, movement and deep breathing as a response to skin stimulation disappears
	Plane III – diaphragmatic respiration, progressive intercostal paralysis, pupils dilated and light reflex abolished. The laryngeal reflex lost in plane II can still be initiated by stimuli arising in the anus or cervix
	Plane IV – complete intercostal paralysis to diaphragmatic paralysis
Stage IV	Medullary paralysis with respiratory arrest and vasomotor collapse as a result of anaesthetic overdose

Wherever possible, a prior knowledge of patients gained from pre-operative contact is of great value in assessing their return to a normal state. It also has the advantage of helping their orientation to time and place, as familiarity generates a degree of security and confidence.

Local and regional anaesthesia

Patients having surgical procedures performed under local or spinal anaesthesia, whether intra- or extra- (epi-) dural, will require a period of postoperative observation, although the priorities of their care will be geared towards different considerations.

Layout of equipment

While a greater part of the nursing procedures carried out in the recovery room will of necessity be of a routine and repetitive nature, the reason for their performance is for the detection of potential as well as actual complications and the initiation of appropriate intervention. The need for speed, efficiency and economy of movement is essential when time becomes a critical factor in the ultimate safety of the patient. Thus the basic equipment for monitoring, airway maintenance and assisted ventilation must be available at the patient's head in each recovery bay. Theatre equipment must be arranged for ease of access and always be clean and in full working order. Further support equipment should be available centrally, whenever possible being stored on trolleys for ease of transportation.

Summary

Post-anaesthetic care can best be described and understood as a series of many nursing procedures performed in sequence and simultaneously on patients who are in an artificially induced and traumatized condition. These patients will display varying degrees of responsiveness and physical and emotional states. It is important to establish a rapport with each individual to prevent the feeling of 'conveyor-belt processing' and gain the patient's confidence and co-operation. It is also necessary to understand that when emerging from the final stage of anaesthesia, some patients can behave in an emotional and disinhibited fashion, at variance with their normal behaviour (Lambrechts & Parkhouse, 1961). These displays are always transient and fortunately patients seldom have any recollection of them. While most patients can be expected to achieve an uneventful recovery, the duration and extent of surgery and anaesthesia are indicators of the pattern of recovery from the procedure and it can be judged to be uneventful only from hindsight. Physical and psychological recovery can be unpredictable at times.

References and further reading

Andrewes, S. J. (1979) The recovery room as a nursing service. *Journal of the Royal Society of Medicine*, 72, 275–7.

Atkinson, R. S. *et al.* (1982) *A Synopsis of Anaesthesia*, 9th edn. John Wright, Bristol.

Asbury, A. J. (1981) Problems of the immediate post-anaesthesia period. *British Journal of Hospital Medicine*, 25, 159–63.

Association of Anaesthetists of Great Britain and Ireland (1985) *Post-Anaesthetic Recovery Facilities – Working Party Recommendations*.

Bales, R. (1988) Hypothermia, a postoperative problem that's easy to miss. *Registered Nurse*, 51(4), 42–3.

Bowers Feldman, M. E. (1988) Inadvertent hypothermia, a threat to homeostasis in the postanaesthetic patient. *Journal of Postanaesthetic Nurse*, 3(2), 82–7.

Campbell, D. & Spence, A. A. (1990) *Norris and Campbell's Anaesthetics, Resuscitation and Intensive Care*, 7th edn. Churchill Livingstone, Edinburgh.

Crayne, H. E. *et al.* (1988) Thermoresuscitation for post-operative hypothermia using reflective blankets. *American Operating Room Nursing Journal*, 47(1), 222–3, 226–7.

Eltringham, R. (1979) Complications in the recovery room. *Journal of the Royal Society of Medicine*, 72, 278–80.

Eltringham, R. *et al.* (1989) Post-*Anaesthetic Recovery: A Practical Approach*, 2nd edn. Springer-Verlag, Berlin.

Fallaccaro, M. *et al.* (1986) Inadvertent hypothermia – etiology, effects and preparation. 44(1), 54–61.

Farman, J. V. (1978) The work of the recovery room. *British Journal of Hospital Medicine*, 19, 606–16.

Farman, J. V. (1979) Do we need recovery rooms? *Journal of the Royal Society of Medicine*, 72, 270–2.

Guedel, A. E. (1937) *Inhalation Anaesthesia, A Fundamental Guide*. Macmillan, New York.

Hudson, R. B. S. (1979) Pattern of work in the recovery room. *Journal of the Royal Society of Medicine*, 72, 273–5.

Lambrechts, W. & Parkhouse, J. (1961) *British Journal of Anaesthesia*, 33, 397.

Levinson B. W. (1965) *British Journal of Anaesthesia*, 37, 544.

Lunn, J. N. (1982) *Lecture Notes on Anaesthetics*, 2nd edn. Blackwell Scientific Publications, Oxford.

Mallett, J. (1989) Talking patients round. *Nursing Times*, 85(38), 37–9.

White H. E. *et al.* (1987) Body temperature in elderly surgical patients. *Research Nurse Health*, 10(5), 317–21.

GUIDELINES: POST-ANAESTHETIC RECOVERY

Equipment

1. Theatre trolley, which must incorporate the following features:
   (a) Oxygen supply.
   (b) Trendelenburg tilt mechanism.
   (c) Adjustable cot sides.
   (d) Adjustable back rest.
   (e) Brakes.
   (f) Radio translucency.
2. Basic equipment required for each patient:
   (a) Oxygen supply, preferably wall mounted with tubing, facemasks and Venturi masks, a T-piece system and full range of oropharyngeal and nasopharyngeal airways.
   (b) Suction – regulatable with tubing, Yankauer's suckers and range of suction catheters.

   Note: spare oxygen cylinders with flowmeters and an electrically powered portable suction machine should always be available in case of pipeline failure.

   (c) Sphygmomanometer and stethoscope. Automatic blood pressure recorders are a valuable means of saving time and of minimizing disturbance to patients, especially those in pain or disorientated, and leaving the nurse's hands free to attend to other needs. However, such equipment can be nonfunctioning in certain cases, e.g. shivering or profoundly bradycardic patients, and is subject to electrical and mechanical failure.
   (d) Pulse oximeter, whenever possible.
   (e) Miscellaneous items: receivers, tissues, disposable gloves, sharps container and waste receptacle.
3. Essential equipment centrally available for respiratory and cardiovascular support:

Guidelines: Post-anaesthetic recovery

(a) Self-inflating resuscitator bag, e.g. Ambu bag and/or Mapleson C circuit with facemask.
(b) Full intubation equipment: laryngoscopes with spare bulbs and batteries, range of endotracheal tubes, bougies and Magill's forceps, syringe and catheter mount.
(c) Anaesthetic machine and ventilator.
(d) Wright respirometer.
(e) Cricothyroid puncture set.
(f) Range of tracheostomy tubes and tracheal dilator.
(g) Intravenous infusion sets and cannulae, range of intravenous fluids.
(h) Central venous cannulae and manometer.
(i) Emergency drug box – contents in accordance with current hospital policy
(j) Defibrillator.

4. Standard equipment for routine nursing procedures.

Procedure

The following recommended actions are not necessarily listed in order of priority. Many will be carried out simultaneously and much will depend on the patient's condition, surgery and level of consciousness. All actions must be accompanied by commentary and explanation regardless of the apparent responsiveness as the sense of hearing returns before the patient's ability to respond (Lambrechts & Parkhouse, 1961; Levinson, 1965).

Action	Rationale
1. Assess the patency of the airway by feeling for movement of expired air.	To determine the presence of any respiratory depression or neuromuscular blockade. Observe chest and abdominal movement, respiratory rate, depth and pattern.
(a) Listen for inspiration and expiration. Apply suction if indicated. Observe any use of accessory muscles of respiration and check for tracheal tug.	To ensure absence of material in the airway, i.e. blood, mucus, vomitus. To ascertain absence of laryngeal spasm.
(b) If indicated, support the chin with the neck extended.	In the unconscious patient the tongue is liable to fall back and obstruct the airway and protective reflexes are absent.
(c) Apply a facemask and administer oxygen at the rate prescribed by the anaesthetist. If an endotracheal tube or laryngeal mask is in position, check whether the cuff or mask is inflated and administer oxygen by means of a T-piece system.	To maintain adequate oxygenation.
(d) Observe skin colour and temperature. Check the colour of lips and conjunctiva, then peripheral colour and perfusion.	Central cyanosis indicates impaired gaseous exchange between the alveoli and pulmonary capillaries. Peripheral cyanosis indicates low cardiac output.
2. Feel the pulse. The patient's position will probably mean that the head, carotid, facial or temporal arteries will offer the easiest access. Note the rate, rhythm and volume and record.	To assess cardiovascular function and establish a postoperative baseline for future observations.
3. Obtain full information about anaesthetic technique, potential problems and the patient's general medical condition.	To plan subsequent treatment.
4. Obtain full information about the surgical procedure and any drains, packs, blood loss and specific postoperative instructions.	To ensure treatment is based on informed observation.

Note: the information gained from points 3 and 4 will be recorded on the anaesthetic chart and the nursing care document (Figure 33.1), but an initial verbal handover will ensure that there is no delay in providing care that may be needed before all relevant information can be gathered from documentation.

5. Take and record blood pressure on reception and at a minimum of five-minute intervals. Record the pulse and respiratory rate at the same interval unless patient's condition dictates otherwise.

To enable any fluctuations or gross abnormalities in observations to be established quickly. Accurate records are of medico-legal importance in the event of an enquiry.

6. Hypothermia. Check the temperature of the patient, especially those who are high risk of hypothermia, e.g. the elderly, children, those who have undergone long surgery or where large amounts of blood or fluid replacement therapy has been used. Check patients who are shivering, restless, confused or with respiratory depression (hypothermia interferes with the effective reversal of muscle relaxants: Bowers Feldman, 1988). Use 'space' (reflective) blankets and warm blankets to warm the patient.

More than 90% of patients undergoing surgery experience some degree of postoperative hypothermia (Fallaccaro *et al.*, 1986; White *et al.*, 1987).
The symptoms of hypothermia can mimic those of other postoperative complications, which may result in inappropriate treatment. Some of the symptoms, such as shivering, put an increased demand on cardiopulmonary systems as oxygen consumption is increased (Bowers Feldman, 1988). Other complications such as arrhythmias or myocardial infarct can result (Bales, 1988), and the longer the duration of the postoperative hypothermia, the greater the patient mortality (Crayne *et al.*, 1988).

7. Check wound site(s) and observe dressings and any drains. Note and record drainage.

To be aware of any changes or bleeding and take appropriate action, e.g. inform the surgeon.

8. Ensure any intravenous infusions are running at the prescribed rate. Check the prescription chart for any medications prescribed for administration during the immediate postoperative period.

To ensure correct treatment given.

9. Remain with the patient at all times. Assess level of consciousness during reversing stages of anaesthesia, observing for returning reflexes, i.e. swallowing, tear secretion and eyelash and lid reflexes and response to stimuli – both physical (*not* painful) and verbal (do not shout).

To ascertain progress towards normal function.

10. Orientate the patient to time and place as frequently as is necessary.

To alleviate anxiety, provide reassurance, gain the patient's confidence and co-operation. Pre-medication and anaesthesia can induce a degree of amnesia and disorientation.

11. Suction of the upper airway is indicated if gurgling sounds are present on respiration and if blood secretions or vomitus are evident or suspected, and the patient is unable to swallow or cough either at all or adequately. Suction must be applied with care to avoid damage to mucosal surfaces and further irritation or initiation of a gag reflex or laryngeal spasm.

Foreign matter can obstruct the airway or cause laryngeal spasm in light planes of anaesthesia. It can also be inhaled when protective laryngeal reflexes are absent. Vagal stimulation can induce bradycardia in susceptible patients (Atkinson *et al.*, 1982, p. 819).

12. Endotracheal suction is performed following the same procedure as that for suction of tracheostomy tubes. (For further information see the procedure on mouth care, Chapter 27).

To maintain the patency of the tube and remove secretions.

Guidelines: Post-anaesthetic recovery

13. Give mouth care. (For further information, see 'Guidelines: Mouth care', Chapter 27.)	Pre-operative fasting, drying gases and manipulation of lips, etc. leave mucosa vulnerable, sore and foul tasting.
14. After regional and/or spinal anaesthesia, assess the return of sensation and mobility of limbs. Check that the limbs are anatomically aligned.	To prevent inadvertent injury following sensory loss.

NURSING CARE PLAN

Note: no observation of cardiovascular function is informative when taken in isolation. Full assessment must be made of respiratory function in conjunction with observations of pulse, blood pressure, emotional state and significant medical history.

Problem	**Cause**	**Suggested action**
Airway obstruction.	Tongue occluding the airway.	Support chin forward from the angle of the jaw. If necessary insert a Guedel airway. Use a nasopharyngeal airway if the teeth are clenched or crowned.
	Foreign material, blood, secretions, vomitus.	Apply suction. Always check for the presence of throat pack.
	Laryngeal spasm	Increase the rate of oxygen. Assist ventilation with an Ambu bag and facemask. If there is no improvement inform anaesthetist and have intubation equipment ready. Offer the patient reassurance.
Hypoventilation.	Respiratory depression from opiates, inhalations, agents, barbiturates.	Inform the anaesthetist and have available naloxone (opiate antagonist and doxampram (respiratory stimulant) *Note*: if naxolone is given it can reverse the analgesic effects of opiates and has a duration of action of only 20 to 30 minutes. The patient must be observed for signs of returning hypoventilation.
	Decreased respiratory drive from a low partial pressure of carbon dioxide ($PaCO_2$), loss of hypoxic drive in patients with chronic pulmonary disease.	With chronic pulmonary disease, give oxygen using a Venturi mask with graded low concentrations (Atkinson *et al.*, 1982).
	Neuromuscular blockade from continued action of non-depolarising muscle relaxants, potentiation of relaxants caused by electrolyte imbalance,	Inform the anaesthetist, have available neostigmine and glycopyrolate, or atropine potassium chloride and 10% calcium chloride.

	imparied excretion with renal or liver disease.	Often the degree of blockade is mild and will wear off in minutes without treatment, but it is extremely frightening and patients will need continuous reassurance that their condition is not unnoticed and is resolving and that they will not be left alone.
Hypotension.	Hypovolaemia.	Take central venous pressure (CVP) readings if catheter is in place. Give oxygen. Lower the head of the trolley unless contraindicated, e.g. hiatus hernia, gross obesity. Check the record of anaesthetic agents used which might cause hypotension, e.g. enflurane, halothane, beta-blockers, nitroprusside, opiates, droperidol, sympathetic blockade following spinal anaesthesia. Check the peripheral perfusion. If the CVP is low increase intravenous infusion unless contraindicated, e.g. congestive cardiac failure. Check drains and dressings for visible bleeding and haematomata. Inform the anaesthetist or surgeon.
Hypertension.	Pain, carbon dioxide retention.	Treat pain with prescribed analgesia. Pain from certain operation sites can also be alleviated by a changing the patient's position.
	Distended bladder.	Offer a bedpan or urinal.
	Some anaesthetic drugs.	Check the prescription chart for those patients on regular antihypertensive therapy. If the situation is not resolved inform the anaesthetist.
Bradycardia.	Very fit patient, opiates, reversal agents, beta-blockers, pain, vagal stimulation, hypoxaemia from respiratory depression.	Check the prescription chart and anaesthetic sheet. Connect the patient to the ECG monitor to exclude heart block. Inform the anaesthetist.
Tachycardia	Pain, hypovolaemia, some anaesthetic drugs, septicaemia, fear, fluid overload.	Provide analgesia. Check the anaesthetic chart. Connect the patient to the ECG monitor to exclude ventricular tachycardia.
Pain.	Surgical trauma, worsened by fear, anxiety and restlessness.	Provide prescribed analgesia and assess its efficacy. Reassure and orientate the patients who

Nursing care plan

Problem	**Cause**	**Suggested action**
		can be unaware that surgery has been performed, in which case their pain is more frightening. Try positional changes where feasible, e.g. experience has shown that after breast surgery some relief can be obtained from raising the back support by 20 to 40 degrees; patients with abdominal or gynaecological surgery can be more comfortable lying on their side; elevate limbs to reduce swelling where appropriate. Unless significant relief is obtained, inform the anaesthetist.
Nausea and vomiting.	Opiates, hypotension, abdominal surgery, pain; some patients are prone to vomiting.	Offer antiemetics if the patient is conscious. Encourage slow, regular breathing. If the patient is unconscious, turn onto the side, tip the head down and suck out pharynx, give oxygen. *Note*: have wire-cutters available if the jaws are wired.
Hypothermia.	Depression of the heat-regulating centre, vasodilatation, following abdominal surgery, large infusions of blood and fluids.	Use extra blankets or a 'space blanket'. Monitor the patient's temperature.
Shivering.	Some inhalational anaesthetics, especially halothane, hypothermia.	Give oxygen, reassure the patient and take patient's temperature.
Hyperthermia.	Infection, blood transfusion reaction. Malignant hyperpyrexia.	Give oxygen, use a fan or tepid sponging if this is warranted. Medical assessment of antibiotic therapy. Malignant hyperpyrexia is a medical emergency and a malignant hyperpyrexia pack with the necessary drugs should be readily available.
Oliguria.	Mechanical obstruction of catheter, e.g. clots, kinking. Inadequate renal perfusion, e.g. hypotension, systolic pressures under 60 mm Hg, hypovolaemia, dehydration. Renal damage, e.g. from blood transfusion, infection, drugs, surgical damage to the ureters.	Check the patency of the catheter. Take blood pressure and CVP if available. Increase intravenous fluids. Inform the anaesthetist. Refer to the anaesthetist or surgeon.

After discharge from the recovery room to the ward, the nursing care given during the postoperative period is directed towards the prevention of those potential complications resulting from surgery and anaesthesia which might be anticipated to develop over a longer period of time.

Consideration of the psychological and emotional aspects of recovery will of necessity be altered by the changed state of consciousness, awareness and knowledge of patients and their differing responses to surgery, diagnosis and treatment.

Potential respiratory complications

Action	Rationale
1. Observe respirations, noting rate and depth and any presence dyspnoea or orthopnoea. (a) Observe chest movement for equal, bilateral expansion. (b) Observe colour and perfusion. (c) Position the patient to facilitate optimum lung expansion and reinforce preoperative teaching of deep-breathing exercises and coughing.	Respiratory function postoperatively can be influenced by a number of factors: increased bronchial secretions from inhalation anaesthesia; decreased respiratory effort from opiate medication; pain or anticipation of pain from surgical wounds; surgical trauma to the phrenic nerve; pneumothorax as a result of surgical or anaesthetic procedures. All factors limiting the adequate expansion of the lung and the ejection of bronchial secretions will encourage the development of atelectasis and consolidation of the affected lung tissue.
2. Change position of patients on bedrest every two to three hours.	
3. Provide adequate prescribed analgesia.	
4. Record temperature and pulse. If sputum produced observe nature and quantity for culture.	If infection follows there may be a rise in temperature, pulse and respiratory rate.

Potential circulatory problems

Deep venous thrombosis and pulmonary embolus

Action	Rationale
1. Encourage early mobilization where patient's condition allows. For patient's on bedrest, encourage deep breathing and exercises of the leg – flexion/extension and rotation of the ankles.	Patients are at increased risk of developing deep venous thrombosis as a result of muscular inactivity, postoperative respiratory and circulatory depression, abdominal and pelvic surgery, prolonged pressure on calves from lithotomy poles, etc., increased production of thromboplastin as a result of surgical trauma, pre-existing coronary artery disease.
2. Where worn, ensure that antiembolic stockings are of the correct size, fit smoothly and do not constrict at the knees.	
3. Advise against crossing of legs or ankles.	
4. Record temperature.	
5. Report any complaints of calf of thigh pain to medical staff.	
6. Observe for any dyspnoea, chest pain or signs of shock.	

Nursing care plan

Haemorrhage

Action	Rationale
1. Observe dressings, drains and wound sites; and quantity and nature of drainage. Observe pulse, blood pressure respirations and colour.	Early haemorrhage may occur as the patient's blood pressure rises. Record postoperatively re-establishing blood flow or blood as a result of the slipping of a ligature or the dislodging of a clot.
2. Observe wound for redness, tenderness and increased temperature.	Secondary haemorrhage may occur after a period of days as a result of infection and sloughing.

Potential fluid and electrolyte imbalance and malnutrition

Action	Rationale
1. Maintain accurate records of intravenous infusions, oral fluids, wound and stoma drainage, nasogastric drainage, vomitus, urine and urological irrigation.	Pre-operative fasting and dehydration, increased secretion of antidiuretic hormone, blood loss and paralytic ileus all contribute to potential fluid and electrolyte imbalance. Vomiting and stasis of intestinal fluid may lead to potassium depletion.
2. Observe nature and quantity of all drainage, aspirate, faeces, etc.	
3. Give prescribed antiemetics if nausea or vomiting occur.	
4. Observe state of mouth for coating, furring and dryness.	
5. Encourage oral fluids as soon the patient is able to take them unless the nature of the surgery contraindicates this.	
6. Encourage early resumption of diet.	Return to an adequate nutritional state is necessary for wound healing; it is particularly important that diabetic patients should return to their preoperative insulin/diet regime to avoid increased risk of metabolic disturbance.

Potential problem of pain

Action	Rationale
1. Observe the patient, noting physiological signs indicative of pain, e.g. sweating, tachycardia, hypotension, pallor or flushed appearance.	Some postoperative pain is common for 24 to 48 hours but may persist for longer depending on the nature and extent of the surgery and the patient's psychological response.
2. Note restlessness, immobility and facial expressions.	Continuous severe pain can cause restlessness, anxiety, insomnia and anorexia, and may thus interfere with recovery by impeding deep breathing, mobilization and nutrition.

3. Listen to the patient and ascertain the location and nature of the pain.

Communication skills are necessary for the effective assessment and alleviation of pain as there may be multiple contributory factors, both physical and emotional in origin.

4. Administer prescribed analgesia and observe effect.

5. Try changing position of patient. Give attention, information and reassurance; assist with relaxation exercises.

34

Scalp Cooling

Definition

Scalp cooling is a method of reducing scalp temperature and causing constriction of blood vessels, thus decreasing the amount of drug that can pass into the hair follicles and to reduce cellular uptake of drug.

Indications

The effectiveness of scalp cooling has been demonstrated satisfactorily only with doxorubicin and epirubicin (Dean *et al.*, 1979; Middleton *et al.*, 1982; Robinson, 1987). However, patients receiving other cytotoxic drugs (vindesine and vincristine), which may cause alopecia, have undergone the procedure. The data collected are insufficient for evaluation at the time of writing. It is not performed routinely and the consultant's permission must be obtained as there is a risk of protecting scalp micrometastases, especially where there is the possibility of circulating cancer cells, e.g. in cases of leukaemia and lymphoma (Witman *et al.*, 1981).

REFERENCE MATERIAL

Doxorubicin is one of the most active cytotoxic agents currently used in cancer chemotherapy. It belongs to the anthracycline antibiotic group of drugs and has a wide spectrum of activity (Benjamin, 1975; Benjamin *et al.*, 1974). Unfortunately, administration of doxorubicin is associated with alopecia in approximately 90% of cases, and this is often total. Hair loss is distressing for the patient and may lead to refusal to accept treatment.

Initial research into methods to prevent hair loss using a scalp tourniquet (Maxwell, 1980) or crushed ice (Dean *et al.*, 1979) was carried out in the United States of America. Promising results led to follow-up research at The Royal Marsden Hospital (Hunt *et al.*, 1982). The method, using a home-made cap (see Guidelines, below), differed on a number of points to previous work, and the results regarding prevention of total hair loss were considerably better. The success rate in the research project was 85% and this has been maintained in everyday practice (David & Speechley, 1987).

Further work (Guy *et al.*, 1982; Symonds & McCormick, 1986) has been carried out to find a system that allowed precise temperature control. The thermocirculator allows coolant to be pumped between two layers of a plastic cap, while another method was produced using a vortex refrigeration tube to provide cold air to the scalp. The success of these methods varies in the prevention of hair loss.

Two factors affect the amount of hair loss experienced by the patient:

1. Involvement of the liver with metastatic disease leads to elevated plasma levels of doxorubicin for a longer period. Extension of the cooling period does not seem to improve results (Satterwhite & Zimm, 1984).
2. Inadequate cooling because of exceptionally thick hair may lead to partial loss. It has been demonstrated that maximum cooling occurs 20 minutes after the cap has been placed in position. The weight of the cap (as well as the temperature) is a factor, as this ensures that the contact is maintained over the complete scalp (Hunt *et al.*, 1982). Success does not appear to be dose dependent as was first thought (David & Speechley, 1987).

Patients should be selected carefully for scalp cooling and should be well motivated to undertake the procedure. Patients must consent when they have been fully informed about the nature and length of the procedure, and know that they may discontinue the procedure at any time if they find it too traumatic, physically or psychologically (Tierney, 1987), or if any hair loss occurs.

Research shows that scalp cooling can be more distressing than originally thought (Tierney *et al.*, 1989), and work is now being carried out into how patients feel about the procedure and if it is worthwhile. Patients have reported adverse effects during and following treatment such as headaches, claustrophobia and 'ice phobias' (Tierney *et al.*, 1989).

It is important to ensure that if a patient refuses scalp cooling or fails to retain hair, adequate time is spent helping the patient to adapt to the hair loss physically, psychologically and socially. These can be achieved by ensuring that the patient sees the surgical appliance officer as soon as possible, in order to obtain a wig that can be matched to the style and colour of the patient's natural hair. Advice can be given on hair care and various ideas of hats, turbans and so on, and reinforced with a hair care information booklet.

References and further reading

Anderson, J. *et al.* (1981) Prevention of doxorubicin-induced alopecia by scalp cooling in patients with advanced breast cancer. *British Medical Journal*, 282, 423–4

Benjamin, R. S. (1975) A practical approach to Adriamycin toxicology. *Cancer Chemotherapy Reports*, 6, 319–27.

Benjamin, R. S. *et al.* (1974) Adriamycin chemotherapy – efficacy, safety and pharmacologic basis of an intermittent, single, high-dosage schedule. *Cancer*, 33, 19–27.

Cline, B. W. (1984) Prevention of chemotherapy-induced alopecia; a review of the literature. *Cancer Nursing*, June, 221–8

David, J. A. & Speechley, V. (1987) Scalp cooling to prevent alopecia. *Nursing Times*, 83(32), 36–7.

Dean, J. C. *et al.* (1979) Prevention of doxorubicin-induced hair loss with scalp hypothermia. *New England Journal of Medicine*, 301, 1427–9.

Edelstyn, G. A. *et al.* (1977) Doxorubicin-induced hair loss and possible modification by scalp cooling. *Lancet*, 2, 253–4.

Guy, R. *et al.* (1982) Scalp cooling by Thermocirculator. *Lancet*, 24 April, 937–8.

Hayward, J. L. (1977) Assessment of response to therapy in advanced breast cancer. *British Journal of Cancer*, 35, 292–8.

Hunt, J. *et al.* (1982) Scalp hypothermia to prevent Adriamycin-induced hair loss. *Cancer Nursing*, 5(1), 25–31.

Keller, J. F. & Blausey, L. A. (1988) Nursing issues and management in chemotherapy-induced alopecia. *Oncology Nursing Forum*, 15(5), 603–7.

Maxwell, M. B. (1980) Scalp tourniquets for chemotherapy-induced alopecia. *American Journal of Nursing*, 5, 900–2.

Middleton, J. *et al.* (1982) Prevention of doxorubicin-induced alopecia by scalp hypothermia: relation to degree of cooling. *British Medical Journal*, 284, 1674.

Middleton, J. *et al.* (1985) Failure of scalp hypothermia to prevent hair loss when cyclophosphamide is added to doxorubicin and vincristine. *Cancer Treatment Reports*, 69(4), 373–5.

Robinson, M. H. (1987) Effectiveness of scalp cooling in reducing alopecia caused by epirubicin treatment of advanced breast cancer. *Cancer Treatment Reports*, 71, 913–4.

Satterwhite, B. & Zimm, S. (1984) The use of scalp hypothermia in the prevention of doxorubicin-induced hair loss. *Cancer*, 54, 34–7.

Symonds, R. P. & McCormick, C. V. (1986) Adriamycin alopecia prevented by cold air scalp cooling. *American Journal of Clinical Oncology*, 9(5), 454–7.

Tierney, A. J. (1987) Preventing chemotherapy-induced alopecia in cancer patients: is scalp cooling worthwhile? *Journal of Advanced Nursing*, 12, 303–10.

Tierney, A. J. *et al.* (1989) *A Study to Inform Nursing Support of Patients Coping with Chemotherapy for Breast Cancer.* Report prepared for the Scottish Home and Health Department.

Wagner, L. & Bye, M. G. (1979) Body image and patients experiencing alopecia as a result of cancer chemotherapy. *Cancer Nursing*, 2, 365–9.

Witman, G. *et al.* (1981) Misuse of scalp hypothermia. *Cancer Treatment Reports*, 65(5–6), 507–8.

GUIDELINES: SCALP COOLING

Equipment

1. A scalp cooling cap:
   (a) Commercial make.
   (b) Home-made from eight hot/cold packs. These must be taped together and moulded around a wig stand. When bandaged in position, the cap is placed in a deep freeze (temperature approximately −18°C) for 24 hours.
   (c) Rubber cap with tubing for thermocirculator machine.
2. Ear protection – gauze, cotton wool pads.
3. Bottle of hair conditioner.
4. Two crepe bandages (10 and 15 cm wide).
5. Two towels.
6. Comfortable chair (recliner) or bed.
7. Extra pillows and blankets as required.

Guidelines: Scalp cooling

Procedure

Action	Rationale
1. Before beginning, it is important to explain the procedure fully to the patient. The patient should understand that the scalp cooling can be discontinued at any time and that it will not jeopardize the chemotherapy.	To obtain the patient's co-operation and consent.
2. If both machine and gel-pack method are available, the patient should be offered the choice, and told the advantages and disadvantages of each method. (a) Gel-pack method. *Advantages*: shorter procedure. *Disadvantages*: heavy and cold when placed initially on head. (b) Thermocirculator method. *Advantages*: cap placed on head first and then cooling allowed to occur gradually over 30 minutes. *Disadvantage* longer procedure.	To allow an informed choice to be made by the patient.
3. Check the cap has been in the deep freeze for 24 hours (gel-pack). Ensure the machine is switched on and set at the correct temperature (machine).	To ensure the cap is cold enough to be effective. To ensure coolant in pump can reach its correct temperature of −5°C.
4. Wet patient's hair thoroughly (gel-pack). Comb conditioner through the patient's hair (machine only).	To aid conduction of coldness and to aid with fitting of cap.
5. Place the ear protection in position.	To prevent cold injury.
6. Soak one crepe bandage in cold water and use it to bandage the patient's head tightly. The bandage should be applied evenly and should provide a thin layer over the scalp (gel-pack only).	To aid conduction of coldness. To compress the hair and prevent any air being trapped between the cap and scalp.
7. Place the cap on the patient's head making sure it fits closely and covers the whole hairline.	To ensure cooling over the head, including all the hair roots.
8. Add supplementary packs if necessary (gel-pack only).	
9. Bandage the cap in place.	To maintain even and close contact of the cap to the scalp and provide some insulation of the cold.
10. Switch the pump on (machine only).	To commence the flow of coolant around the cap and machine.
11. Add pillows etc. as required.	To provide support for the patient's head and neck and to reduce the weight of the gel-pack cap (approximately 2 to 3 kg).

12. Place a dry towel around the patient's shoulders.	To catch any water as the gel-pack cap defrosts.
13. Offer the patient the use of a blanket.	To prevent any chilling.
14. Leave the patient for at least 15 minutes before injection of the drug (gel-pack). Leave the patient for at least 30 minutes (machine).	To obtain initial cooling of the scalp.
15. Administer the drug by intravenous injection.	
16. Leave the patient for a further 45 minutes (both methods).	To maintain cooling until the plasma levels of drug have fallen (Hunt *et al.*, 1982).
17. When sufficient time has elapsed, remove the cap and bandages carefully.	To prevent damage to the scalp and hair.
18. Encourage the patient to rest, if desired.	To prevent faintness due to the weight being lifted off.
19. Towel the patient's hair dry. (gel-pack). Rinse the conditioner from the patient's hair (machine). Allow the patient to style it gently.	To prevent damage to the hair. To ensure that the patient is comfortable and has a chance to rearrange hair before leaving hospital.
20. Ensure the patient is given a hair care information booklet in order to care for hair correctly between treatments.	To reinforce verbal information given during procedure.

NURSING CARE PLAN

Problem	**Cause**	**Suggested action**
Inadequate cooling: (a) Gel pack cap (−20°C). (b) Machine cap (−5°C).	Poorly fitting cap. Incorrect temperature.	Follow the procedure carefully. Check that the cap is as cold as possible. Ensure the cap size is correct and that the hair roots are covered. If the patient has very thick hair, use the heaviest cap available.
Excess cooling.	Thin hair.	Use extra layers of bandages between the cap and scalp. If it is still painful then discontinue the procedure.
Complaints of headache.	Weight and coldness of cap.	Provide support and blankets as required.
Distressed patient.	Claustrophobia.	Support and reassure the patient. If necessary remove the cap.
	Ice phobia.	Be aware of this possible problem, encourage the patient to discuss feelings.

Nursing care plan

Problem	Cause	Suggested action
Hair loss.	Scalp cooling was not successful.	Offer the patient the opportunity to discontinue the scalp cooling. Make arrangements for the patient to see the appliance officer and obtain a wig. Discuss care of hair and scalp and give information booklet.

35

Sealed Radioactive Sources

Definition

Sealed sources are radioactive isotopes used for therapy which are permanently and completely enclosed in a metal casing.

Most radioactive isotopes used as sealed sources for brachytherapy emit both beta (β) and gamma (γ) radiation. Brachytherapy is where there is a very short distance between the radiation source and the tumour. It is either intracavitary, where radioisotope sources are placed in pre-existing body cavities, such as the uterine cavity or vagina, or interstitial, where radioisotope sources are inserted directly into the tissues in tubes or needles (Lambert & Blake, 1992).

The radiation useful in treating malignant disease includes X-rays, produced artificially by electron bombardment of a metal target, and gamma rays, a natural emission in the nuclear decay of radioisotopes. They are sometimes referred to as 'photon' radiation. Beta particles are also capable of ionization; these are distinguishable from electromagnetic radiation by their ability to carry an electrical charge (either positive or negative). Beta particles result when a neutron within the nucleus disintegrates to form a proton and an electron. The electron is ejected from the nucleus, producing beta radiation (Holmes, 1988).

Indications

Permanent or temporary insertions of small, sealed sources are used to deliver very high doses of radiation into tumours or tumour-bearing tissue while giving rapidly diminishing doses to adjacent structures. This will limit the damage caused to normal tissue. A specific dose of radiation will be received by the cancer. This is delivered continuously over a period of hours or days. Small sealed sources inserted into the body may take the form of:

1. *Intracavitary applicators*: sources that are placed against tissue and usually held in place by packing.
2. *Interstitial implants*: sources that are inserted directly into the tumour-bearing tissue.

(*Note*: surface applicators or moulds: sources are applied directly to superficial cancers.)

REFERENCE MATERIAL

Measures of radiation

Radiation kills by causing ionization within living cells. The sensitive 'target' appears to be deoxyribonucleic acid (DNA) in the nucleus of the cell. The ionizing radiation thus passes through the cells and tissues, and the dose of radiation received is measured in terms of the energy absorbed. The unit of absorbed dose, the 'rad' (radiation absorbed dose), has now been replaced by the 'Gray', which equals 100 rads.

100 centigray (cGy) = 1 Gray (Gy)
1000 milligray (mGy) = 1 Gray
1 million microgray (μGy) = 1 Gray

The exposure of radiation to a patient is described by the term 'dose equivalents'. When the absorbed dose is measured in grays, the dose equivalent is in 'sieverts'. For instance, for staff over 18 who are not pregnant, wearing a monitoring badge to monitor exposure to radiation, the maximum permissable dose equivalent is 50 millisieverts (0.05 Sievert) per year (Department of Health and Social Security, 1985).

Radioactive isotopes used as sealed sources

Caesium-137

Caesium-137 is a radioisotope that can be used in the form of implants or in applicators.

The half-life of caesium-137 is 30 years and it has largely replaced radium as a source in brachytherapy.

Oral implants

Caesium-137 may be used in a needle-like implant that can be positioned directly into the tissue surrounding the tumour. This is a fairly common treatment for early lesions of the cheek, lip and anterior two-thirds of the tongue. If bone involvement is suspected, e.g. in the mandible, alternative treatment will be given.

Gynaecological applicators

Caesium-137 may be used in applicators. The commonest malignancies treated by use of radioactive applicators are tumours of the female genital tract. Intracavity applicators are used which deliver a high dose to the region of the cervix, the paracervical tissue, the upper part of the vagina and the uterine body.

Iridium-192

Iridium-192 is a radioisotope which can be used in the form of pins or wires as in interstitial therapy.

The half-life of iridium-192 is 74.2 days. It is an ideal choice because of the low energy of its gamma emission, which simplifies radiation protection, and because in the form of a platinum–iridium alloy it can be drawn into thin flexible wires. The wires consist of an active platinum–iridium alloy core encased in a sheath of platinum, 10 cm thick, which screens out the beta radiation from the iridium-192.

Modern afterloading techniques reduce the radiation exposure to the radiotherapist and other staff involved.

Iridium-192 implants are used under the following circumstances:

1. As a primary treatment for small primary lesions, especially tongue or breast lesions.
2. As a 'boost' dose after external radiotherapy for larger primary tumours or where nodes are also involved.
3. To treat recurrence.

Gold-198

Gold-198 is used as an interstitial source of radiation in the form of gold grains.

The half-life of the gold-198 radioisotope is 2.76 days. Gamma and beta rays are emitted. The gamma rays are of relatively low energy and the beta rays are filtered out by the platinum casing around the gold. Gold-198 grains are used primarily in the treatment of tumours of the lung, breast, bladder neck, prostate and nodes.

When a patient is selected for interstitial or intracavitary therapy the medical staff assess the size of the tumour. The physics department is responsible for ordering the source and co-ordinating with the radiotherapists.

Intraoral implants

Caesium-137 needles

The sources (see Figure 35.1) are inserted in theatre under a general anaesthetic. They are inserted individually in a predetermined pattern so that the implant covers the whole growth with a safety margin of at least 1 cm. Each needle is positioned by pushers so that its eye, through which silk is threaded, is just visible beneath the mucosal surface. Each silk is then stitched to the tongue with a single suture. When all the needles have been inserted, the silks are counted and gathered together. They are threaded through a piece of rubber to prevent friction and trauma to the mouth. The silks are strapped to the cheek to prevent any needle being swallowed should it work loose. Small beads are attached to the ends of the threads to facilitate counting the needles. X-rays are always taken to check the positions of the needles and to enable estimation of the dose distribution.

Iridium-192 hair pins and single pins

These types of implants are usually used intraorally (Figure 35.2). They are slotted into tissue using steel

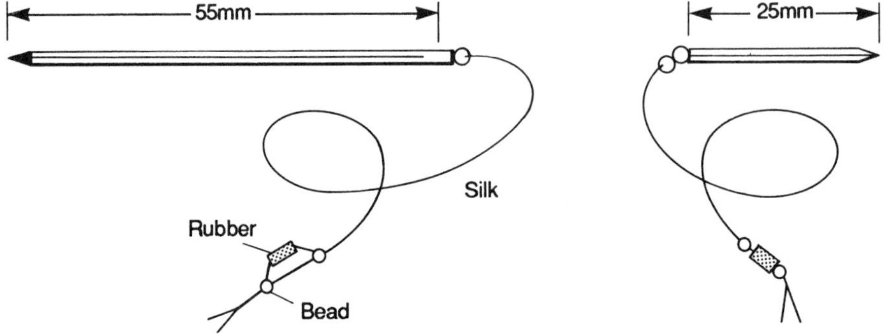

Figure 35.1 Caesium-137 needles.

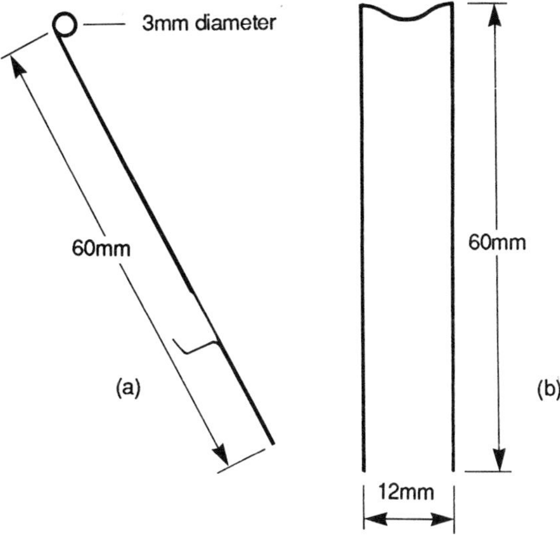

Figure 35.2 Iridium pins. (a) Iridium single pin. (b) Iridium-192 hair pin.

guides to obtain accurate alignment. Radiological examination is used to check the position of the guides before the iridium is inserted. The pins are held in place by sutures.

The staff of the physics department are normally responsible for calculating how long a radioactive implant is to stay in place. This is usually about six days, depending on the size of the tumour. Removal is carried out in theatre by the radiotherapist.

Breast or perineal implants

Iridium-192 wires

These are usually used for breast lesions or lesions of the vulva or perineum (Figure 35.3). Polythene cannulae are inserted under a general anaesthetic. In the case of breast lesions, both ends of each tube protrude through the skin. Correct alignment is established often with the aid of a perspex template which fits over the breast. In the case of vulval or perineal insertions only one end of the tube protrudes. For these, alignment of the sources may be achieved by using a perspex template and vaginal obtivator.

The iridium wire source is afterloaded usually on the ward and the wires are held in the cannulae with crimped lead washers.

The radiotherapist is responsible for calculating how long a radioactive implant should stay in place. This is usually for three to six days, depending on the size of the tumour. Removal of the implant is usually carried out on the ward by the radiotherapist.

Gold-198 grains

Gold-198 grains are 2.5 mm long and 0.5 mm in diameter, made of gold encased in platinum. Fourteen gold-198 grains are contained in an aluminium magazine which fits into the barrel of the implantation gun (Figure 35.4). An injector needle is attached to the gun which is inserted into the tissue that is to be irradiated. The patient requires a general anaesthetic for the insertion.

Gold grains have the following advantages over more classical methods of wires and pin in the irradiation of comparatively inaccessible tumours:

1. Placing gold-198 grains is easier than placing needles or pins.
2. Gold-198 grains do not need any fixing sutures.
3. They are a permanent insertion, therefore the closure of any surgical wound can be immediate.

The disadvantage of this method is that higher numbers of gold-198 grains are required, which means that more precautions must be taken in order to achieve a regular geometrical arrangement to ensure satisfactory distribution of the dose. This can

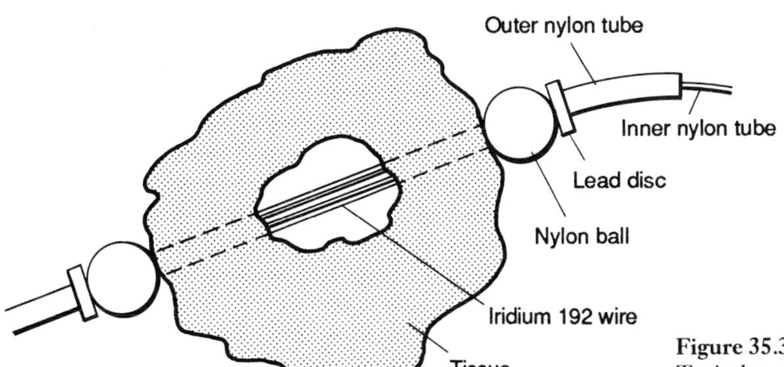

Figure 35.3 Iridium-192 wire in polythene cannula. Typical assembly in tissue.

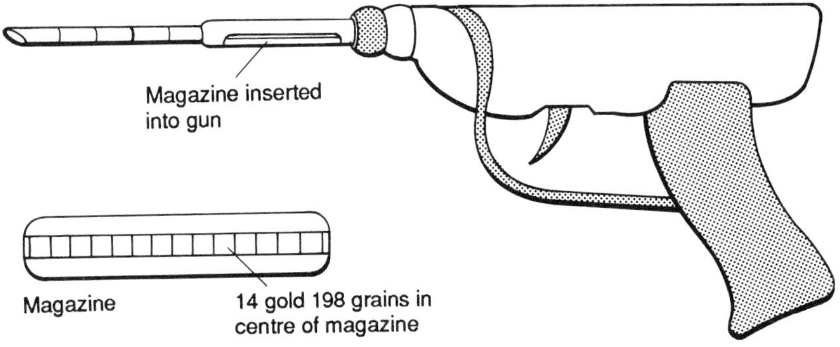

Figure 35.4 Gold grain gun.

increase the length of time the doctors, nursing staff and other personnel present are exposed to irradiation.

Intracavitary applicators

The applicators are inserted under a general anaesthetic, and the position of the applicator is checked by X-ray before the patient returns to the ward. A urinary catheter is also inserted in theatre to reduce the risk of the sources becoming dislodged by the patient when micturating.

Types of applicator

There are several different types of applicator available and choice is usually determined by the site of the tumour, the anatomy of the patient and the preference of the treatment centre. The most commonly used types of applicator are described below (see Figure 35.5).

Stockholm applicator

This is used for carcinoma of the body of the uterus or cervix. Usually a uterine tube and two vaginal packets are inserted. Occasionally, if the vaginal vault is small, one packet is omitted or replaced by a vaginal tube. The radioactive material is held in place with a flavine-soaked gauze pack. It is usually left in place for 22 hours. Tubes and packets have strings attached for removal and colour-coded beads indicate which should be removed first.

Modified Stockholm applicator

This is used for carcinoma of the body of the uterus and cervix. It consists of a uterine tube and a square box which connect together by a point and a hole. The vagina is then packed with gauze saturated with proflavine. They are usually left in place for 20 hours. The box should be removed first. The uterine tube is plain.

Fletcher applicator

This is used for carcinoma of the corpus or cervix, but the patient needs to have a fairly capacious vaginal vault. Hollow applicators, a uterine tube and two vaginal ovoids are inserted in theatre and loaded with the radioactive sources later, on the ward, by the radiotherapist. The apparatus is held in place with a flavine pack. Long ends project through the vulva so that afterloading can be done. These insertions are usually left in place for 60 to 72 hours. No strings are needed as the apparatus itself projects from the vulva.

Curietron afterloading applicator

This is used for carcinoma of the corpus or cervix, but patients need to have a fairly capacious and symmetrical vault. Hollow metal applicators, consisting of two vaginal ovoids and a uterine tube, are inserted in the theatre and are loaded with radioactive 'Curietron' sources later, on the ward, by the radiotherapist. The apparatus is held in place with approximately 90 cm of ribbon gauze flavine pack. The long ends of the applicators project through the vulva so that afterloading can be carried out. The patient may need to be nursed with a sorbo pad or pillow under the dorsal area to keep the projecting ends off the bed.

These insertions last 60 to 72 hours. Patients usually have two insertions but may sometimes be given a single pre-operative insertion or a single insertion following external inrradiation.

Heyman's capsules

These are used for carcinoma of the corpus where there is enlargement of the uterus and expanded uterine cavity. They consist of small metal capsules, each of which contains a small, radioactive source. As many capsules as possible are placed into the uterus. Usually two vaginal packets are used as well. They are held in place by a flavine gauze pack and are left in for about 12 to 18 hours. Each capsule has a flexible wire

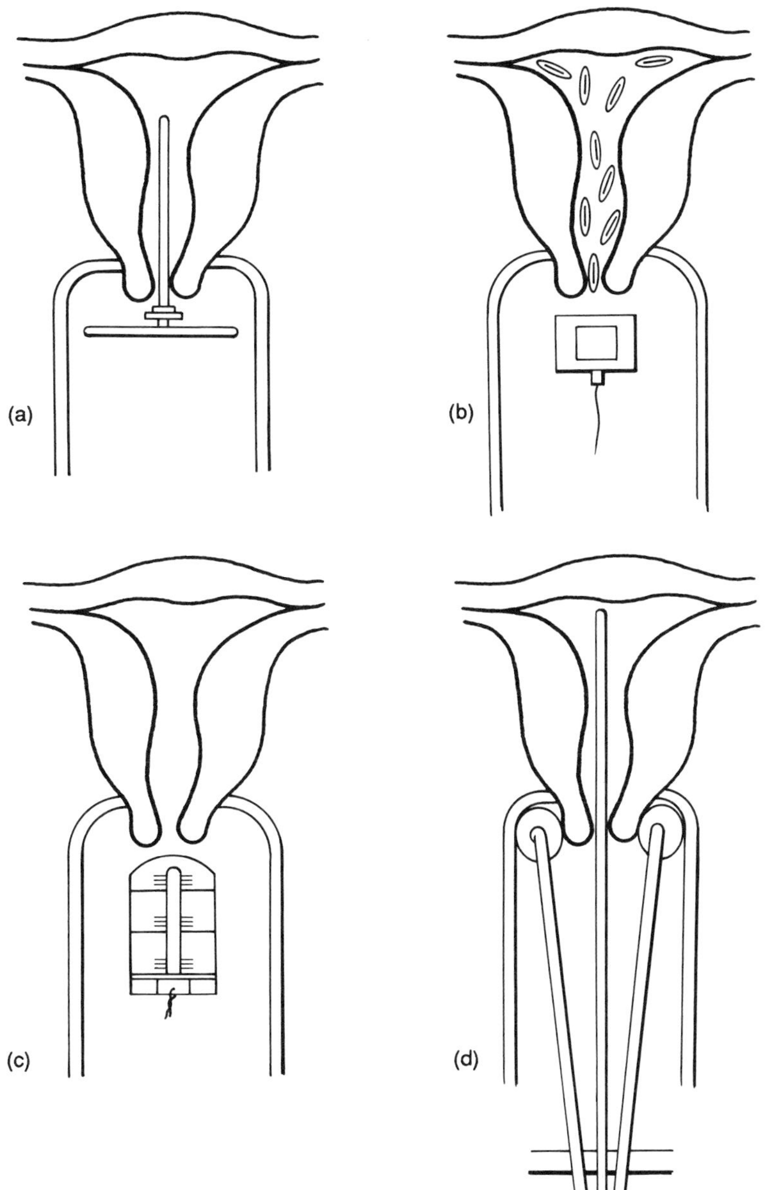

Figure 35.5 Gynaecological caesium applicators. (a) Modified Stockholm applicator. (b) Heyman's capsules and packet. (c) Dobbie applicator. (d) Fletcher applicator.

attached, strapped to the thigh, for removal, and a numbered tag to indicate the order of removal.

Dobbie applicator

This is used to irradiate the whole vagina. A perspex cylindrical applicator, with radioactive sources in the centre, is inserted into the vagina and sutured in place to the vulva. It is usually left in for about 18 hours. Strings are attached to the applicator for removal.

Modified Dobbie applicator

This is a polyacetal cylindrical applicator with a long hollow through the middle. A uterine tube is loaded and slipped into the long hollow. The applicator is inserted into the vagina and sutured in place. It is usually left in position for about 18 hours, but this will depend on the rectal dose of radiation. Strings are attached to aid removal.

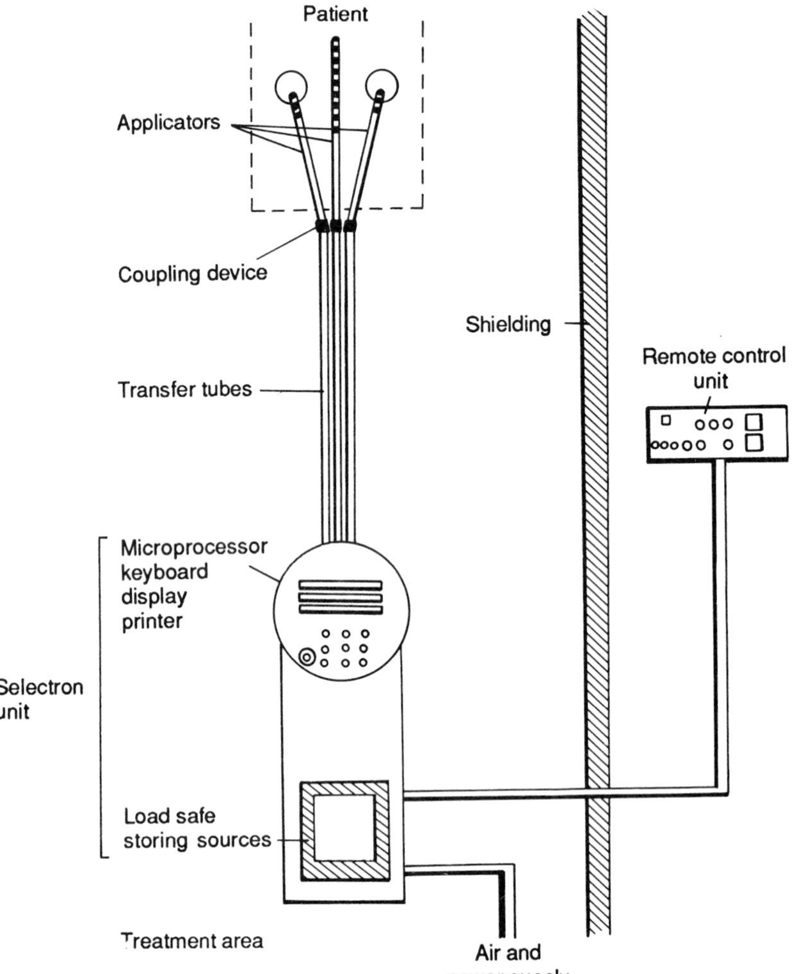

Figure 35.6 Selectron unit.

THE LOW DOSE RATE SELECTRON

Definition

The selectron is a remote-controlled afterloading system and has been designed to deliver intracavitary radiotherapy to patients without exposing hospital personnel to radiation.

Indication

It is gradually replacing conventional intracavitary radium and caesium applicators and other manual and mechanical afterloading techniques.

REFERENCE MATERIAL

The selectron unit comprises of a lead-shielded safe containing caesium-137 sources in the form of small spherical pellets, a microprocessor, keyboard, display unit and printer (Figure 35.6). Leading from the selectron unit are between three and six flexible plastic transfer tubes corresponding to numbered

France

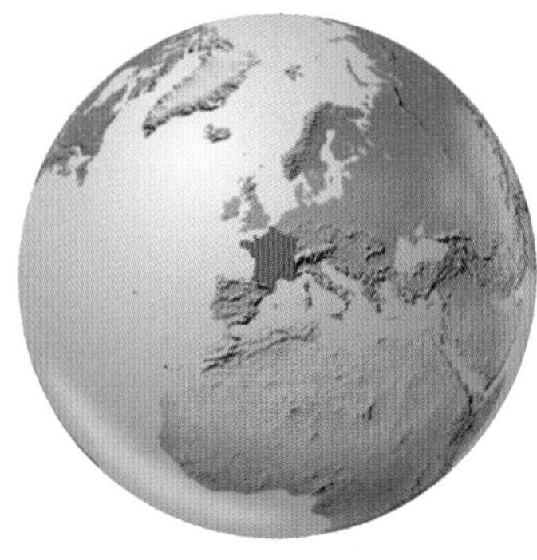

France shares its long eastern border with Italy, Switzerland, Germany, Luxembourg, and Belgium. Spain is to the south. The south of France lies on the Mediterranean Sea coast, and the Atlantic Ocean is to the west.

THE LARGEST COUNTRY in western Europe is France – a land of green, open spaces dotted with picturesque towns and small cities. Its many fine old country palaces, or châteaux, are reminders of France's long history. But it is a modern nation too, with flourishing industries. France is also one of the leading countries in the European Union (EU), the organization that promotes political and economic union between the member states. Northern France has cool, wet weather. The south, with its Mediterranean coast, is drier and warmer. Rolling hills rise from the coasts and valleys, providing good farmland. The rugged hills of the Massif Central occupy the middle of the country. The mountains of the Pyrenees and the Alps line the southwest and eastern borders. France also includes the Mediterranean island of Corsica, and some islands thousands of kilometres away in the Pacific Ocean and the Caribbean Sea. A democratically elected government and president rule France from Paris.

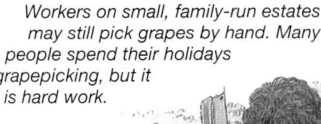

Workers on small, family-run estates may still pick grapes by hand. Many people spend their holidays grapepicking, but it is hard work.

Even the smaller winemakers now use some modern equipment, such as stainless-steel fermentation vats.

Winemaking

France produces about a fifth of the world's wine. Many famous wines are named after French regions, such as Champagne and Bordeaux. Most French wine comes from co-operatives – local groups of farms that share wine-producing and bottling facilities. Some wine, however, is still made on the small estates attached to the old châteaux. The grapes are picked in the early autumn. Pressing the grapes extracts the juice, which then ferments (reacts with yeast) in large vats to produce the alcohol and the delicious taste of the wine. Only when this process is complete can the wine be bottled.

The Louvre, in Paris, is one of the world's most famous art galleries. The glass pyramid was added in 1989.

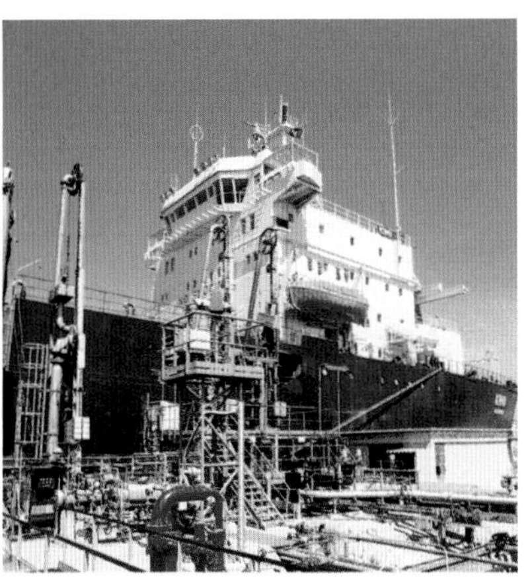

MARSEILLES
France's biggest seaport is Marseilles, on the Mediterranean coast. The warm climate of southern France makes possible the lively, outdoor lifestyle of the city. There is a long history of trade with the rest of the Mediterranean. Marseilles has a large Arab population, mainly from North Africa.

Paris

People have lived on the river Seine where Paris now stands since ancient times. Paris is the capital of France. France has a population of more than 60 million; one fifth live in and around Paris. It is one of Europe's great cities, with wide, tree-lined streets called boulevards, and many famous monuments and museums. The city of today was largely replanned and rebuilt during the 19th century.

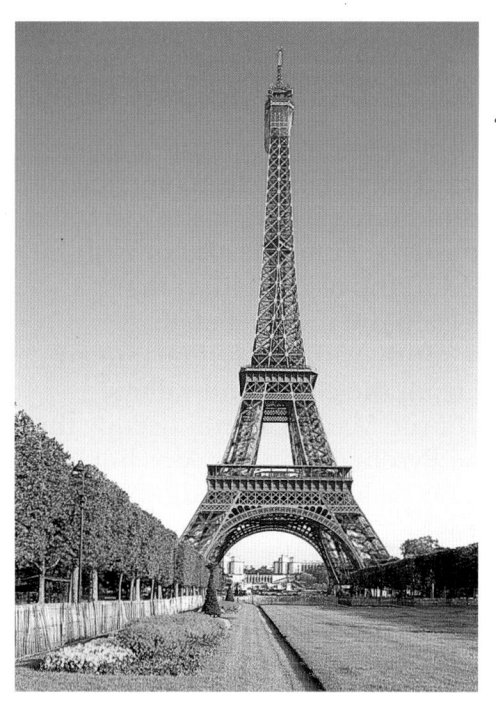

EIFFEL TOWER

Built to impress visitors to the Paris Exhibition of 1889, the Eiffel Tower was originally meant to be a temporary structure. It was designed by the French engineer Alexandre-Gustave Eiffel. Eiffel was internationally famous for his bridge and aqueduct designs. The tower is built of steel girders weighing 7,000 tonnes (7,700 US tons), and 2.5 million rivets hold it together. It reaches a height of 322 m (1,050 ft) and up until the erection of the Empire State Building in New York in 1931, it was the tallest building in the world. Visitors can reach its various levels by lift or by climbing hundreds of steps.

When it was first built in the 19th century, the Eiffel Tower was fiercely criticized. It has now become the symbol of Paris and a much loved feature of the city.

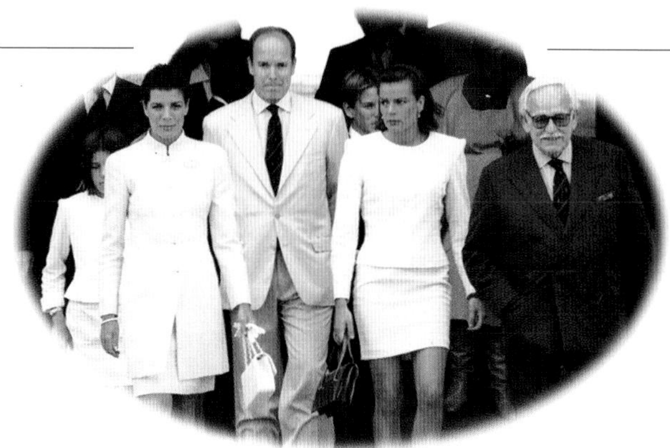

Monaco

A tiny country on the Côte d'Azur, Monaco lies in southeastern France. The heart of the country is the sophisticated city of Monte Carlo, famous for its casinos and motor racing Grand Prix. Monaco is an independent principality, ruled for much of its history by the Grimaldi family (above). Only a small part of the population is originally from Monaco; more than half the people are citizens of France. They are drawn by the lenient tax laws and high standard of living, and earn more per capita than any other country in the world.

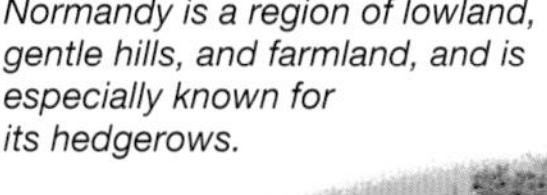

Normandy is a region of lowland, gentle hills, and farmland, and is especially known for its hedgerows.

NORMANDY

The region of Normandy lies between Paris and the English Channel. Normandy is a farming area, known throughout France for its dairy products and its apples. By grazing their cattle in the orchards, many local farmers get double use from the land. They sell the apples as dessert fruit, or turn them into cider and a delicious apple brandy called calvados. Cream from the Normandy cattle makes some of France's most famous cheeses, including Brie and Camembert.

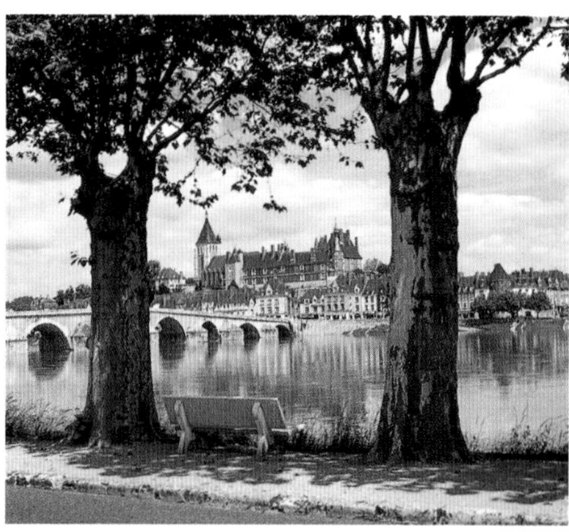

Loire river

The valley of the Loire river is famous for its beautiful castles, called châteaux, such as this one at Gien. Kings, nobles, or wealthy landowners built the châteaux as their homes. They often chose a site on high ground and surrounded the château with a moat, which made it easy to defend the château from attackers. The Loire valley is also an important wine-producing area.

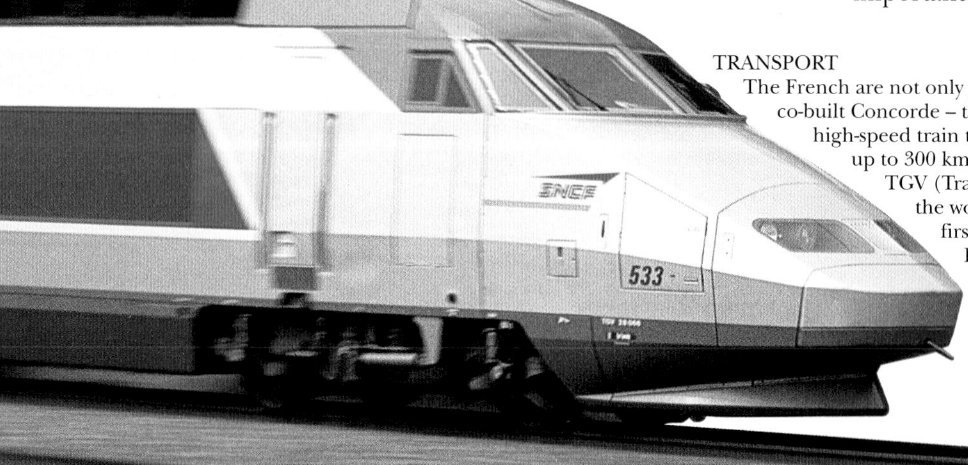

TGV design has evolved over the years. This train has a sharp aerodynamic nose to increase its speed.

TRANSPORT

The French are not only pioneers of aviation – they co-built Concorde – they also lead the world in high-speed train technology. With speeds of up to 300 km/h (185 mph) the French TGV (Trains à Grande Vitesse) is the world's fastest train. The first TGV line, from Paris to Lyon, was opened in 1983. TGV lines have since been built to Belgium, Italy, and Spain. The Channel Tunnel links France to the United Kingdom.

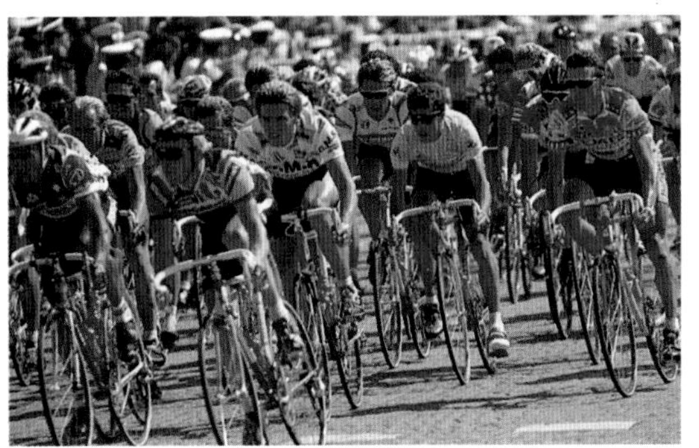

TOUR DE FRANCE
Cycling is an enormously popular pastime in France. The world's most famous cycling race is the Tour de France (Tour of France), which takes place every summer. The route follows public roads, covering about 3,500 km (2,200 miles), primarily in France and Belgium, but briefly in four other countries. The race takes place over 26 days, and the world's best cyclists take part.

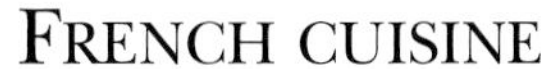

French cuisine

French cooks are considered among the best in the world. There are numerous good restaurants, even in quite small towns, and the quality of ordinary daily food is very high. Food specialists who take great pride in their work produce outstanding cooked meats, pastries, and bread, including the famous stick-shaped baguette. French cheeses, such as Camembert, are eaten all over the world.

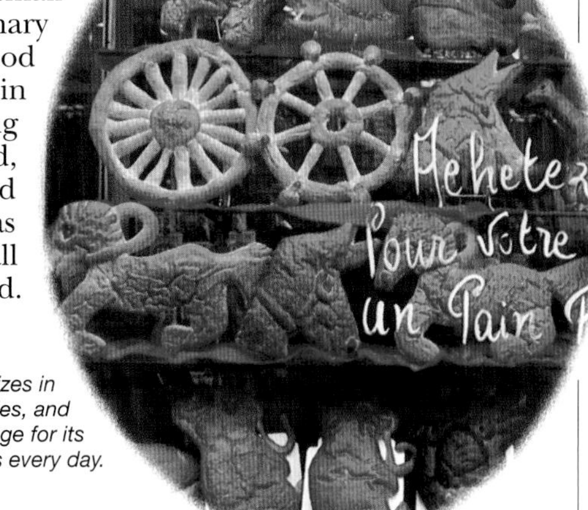

A patisserie specializes in sweet, delicious pastries, and produces a wide range for its customers every day.

The town square is the traditional spot for games such as boules or petanque, French versions of bowling.

In fine weather, café owners put tables and chairs out on the pavements so their customers can eat and drink in the open air.

Country towns

Much of France consists of open country where most working people earn a living from farming. One in every five French people lives and works in the countryside. The farming communities spread out around small market towns, which provide markets, banks, restaurants, and shops and supermarkets. Each town contains a *mairie,* the offices of the local government administration. The *mairie* often overlooks the central square, where people meet to talk and perhaps enjoy a game of *boules.*

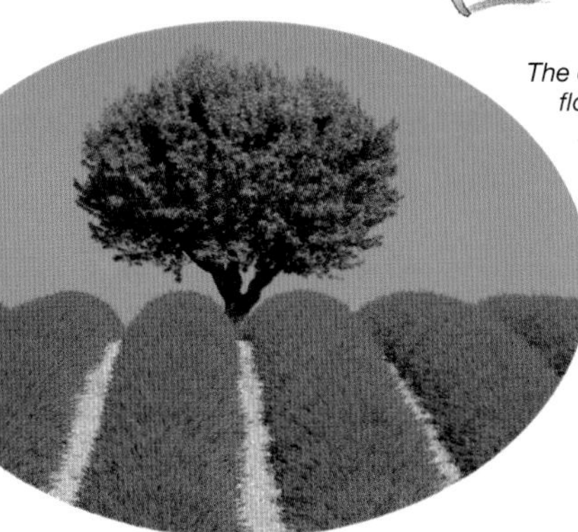

The extract of scented flowers, such as lavender, is a major ingredient in perfume.

PERFUME AND FASHION
Two of France's best-known industries are the manufacture of perfume and haute couture, or high fashion. Many of the most famous and most expensive brands of perfume are French. French designers dominated fashion for most of the last century. The Paris collections, shown in the spring of each year, are the most important of the international fashion shows and are attended by designers from all over the world. They set the trends which the rest of the world will follow.

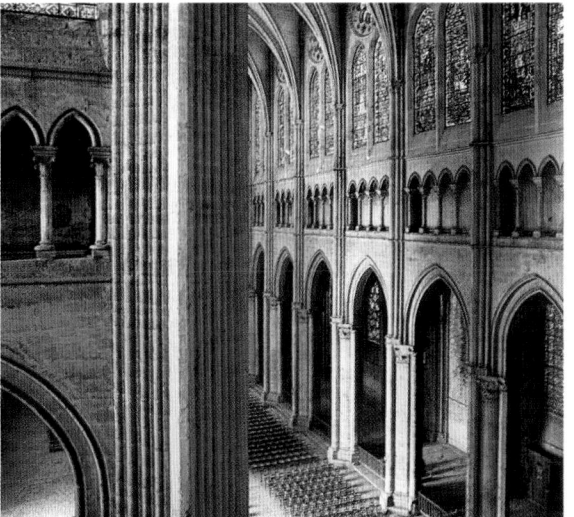

The 176 luminous stained-glass windows of Chartres Cathedral (right) attest to the talents of Chartres craftsmen.

CHARTRES
France is a mainly Roman Catholic country. There are churches in every village, and cathedrals in the cities. The cathedral of Chartres, in northern France, was completed in 1260. It is famous not only for its fine architecture but also for its magnificent stained-glass windows. There are 176 windows, covering a total area of 2,600 sq m (28,000 sq ft), the equivalent of 10 tennis courts.

Find out more

Churches and cathedrals
Europe
France, history of
French revolution
Normans

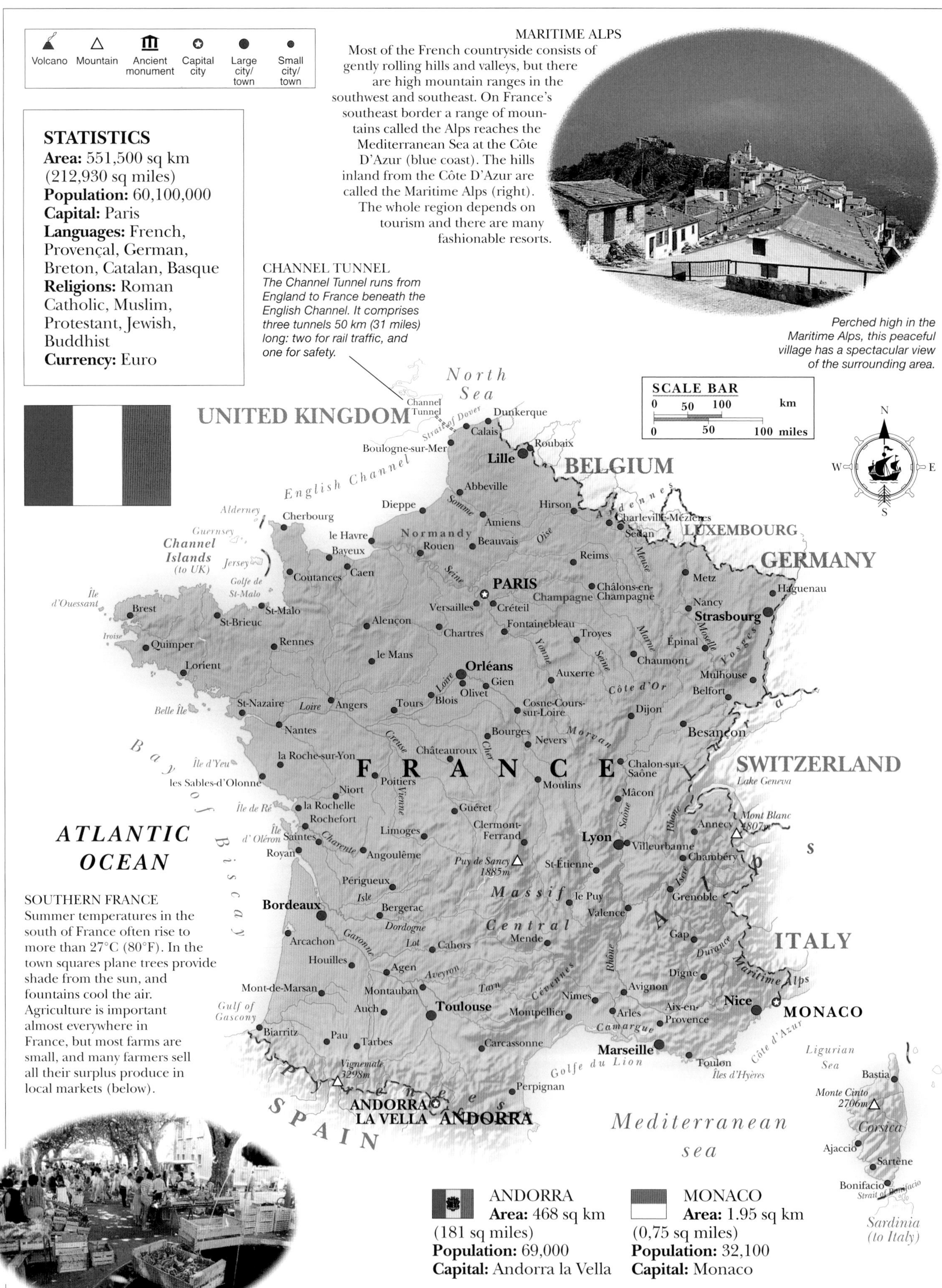

STATISTICS

Area: 551,500 sq km (212,930 sq miles)
Population: 60,100,000
Capital: Paris
Languages: French, Provençal, German, Breton, Catalan, Basque
Religions: Roman Catholic, Muslim, Protestant, Jewish, Buddhist
Currency: Euro

MARITIME ALPS

Most of the French countryside consists of gently rolling hills and valleys, but there are high mountain ranges in the southwest and southeast. On France's southeast border a range of mountains called the Alps reaches the Mediterranean Sea at the Côte D'Azur (blue coast). The hills inland from the Côte D'Azur are called the Maritime Alps (right). The whole region depends on tourism and there are many fashionable resorts.

Perched high in the Maritime Alps, this peaceful village has a spectacular view of the surrounding area.

CHANNEL TUNNEL

The Channel Tunnel runs from England to France beneath the English Channel. It comprises three tunnels 50 km (31 miles) long: two for rail traffic, and one for safety.

SOUTHERN FRANCE

Summer temperatures in the south of France often rise to more than 27°C (80°F). In the town squares plane trees provide shade from the sun, and fountains cool the air. Agriculture is important almost everywhere in France, but most farms are small, and many farmers sell all their surplus produce in local markets (below).

ANDORRA
Area: 468 sq km (181 sq miles)
Population: 69,000
Capital: Andorra la Vella

MONACO
Area: 1.95 sq km (0,75 sq miles)
Population: 32,100
Capital: Monaco

HISTORY OF
FRANCE

THE AREA OF EUROPE that we call France took its name from a tribe of warriors who conquered the region more than 1,000 years ago. The Franks ruled much of Europe for more than four centuries and were the first people to dominate all of France after the Roman Empire collapsed in A.D. 476. Frankish power was strongest under Charlemagne at the start of the ninth century, but ended in 895 when Vikings from Scandinavia settled in northern France. These Northmen, or Normans, as they became known, invaded England in 1066, establishing a link between these lands that was to last for 500 years. The English at one time dominated France, but by 1453 were driven out of everywhere except Calais. Over the next 300 years, the French kings gained immense power and set a pattern for other European royal families of the time. However, the monarchy became increasingly unpopular with the common people, and in 1789 King Louis XVI was overthrown in a revolution that shocked and inspired people all over the world. The French people abolished royal rule and instead chose to govern themselves. They set up the first of a series of republics that have made France one of the most powerful countries in the western Europe.

CARNAC
The ancient Stone Age inhabitants of France were highly developed. More than 7,500 years ago they built many long straight rows of standing stones at Carnac in Brittany. These stones were probably used in religious ceremonies.

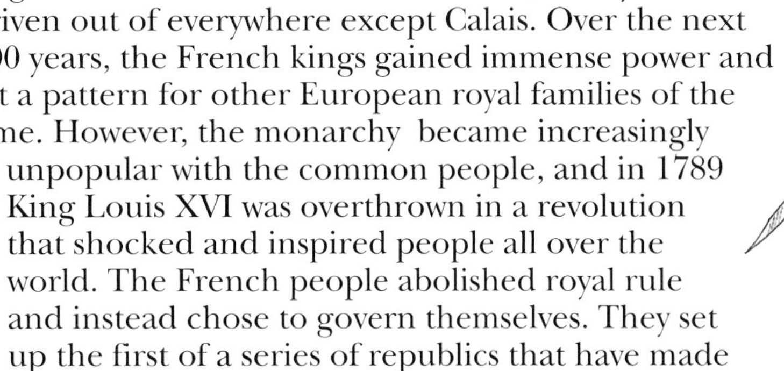

FRANKISH SOLDIERS
When the Roman Empire withdrew from Gaul (ancient France), different invading armies colonized parts of the region. Only when the fearsome Frankish warriors swept through Europe was France united again.

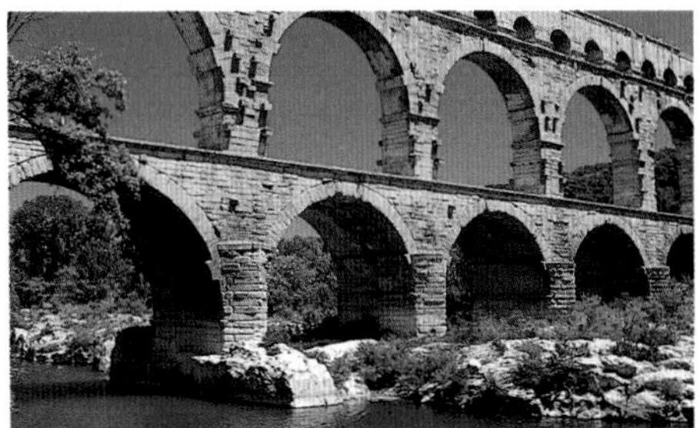

ROMAN ENGINEERING
The Romans occupied Gaul from 58 B.C. to A.D. 486. They constructed many roads and towns, which they supplied with running water from canals. To carry the canals across valleys they built aqueducts, such as this one crossing the River Gard.

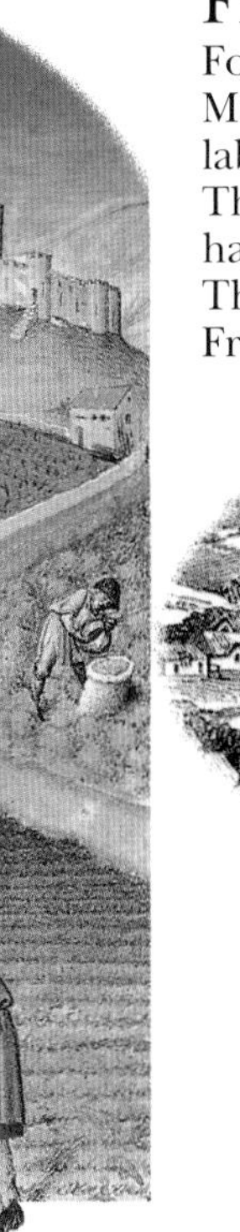

Landowners built huge fortresses with the great wealth they made from the feudal system.The château, or castle, was at the centre of the system.

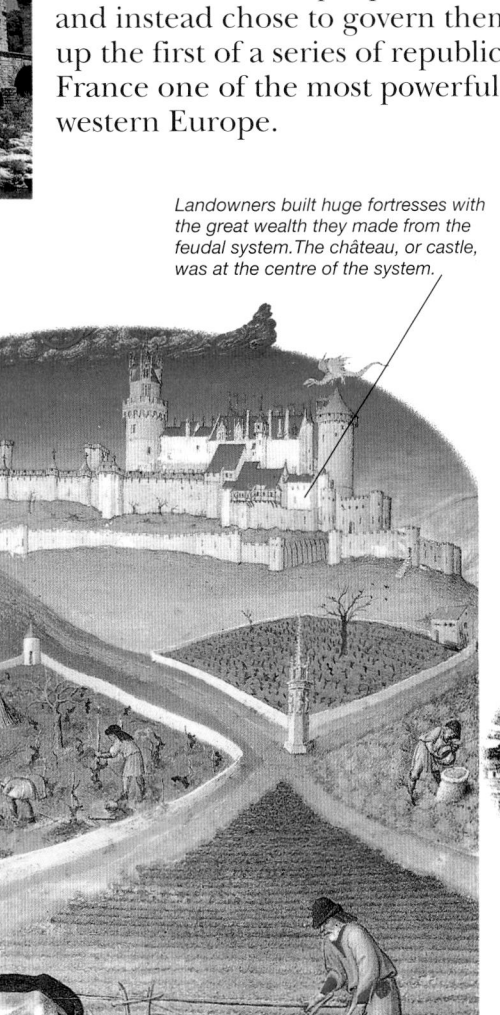

Peasants worked hard on the owner's land, and in return were allowed to grow their own food.

The peasants worked the land with ploughs drawn by oxen.

FEUDAL FRANCE

For almost 1,000 years, during the Middle Ages, French peasants laboured under the feudal system. They had no land of their own and had to work for the local landowners. The system was finally abolished by the French Revolution.

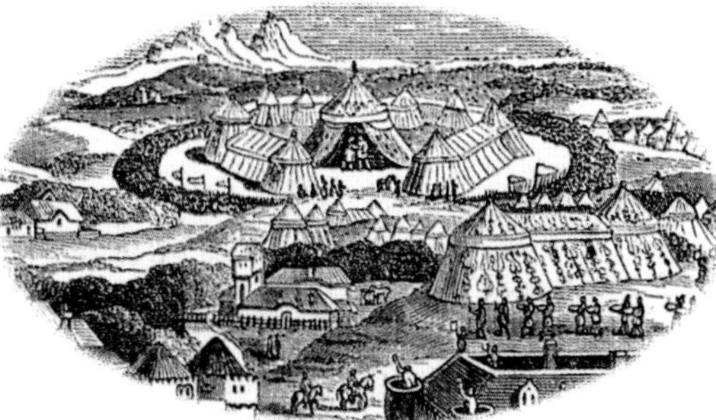

FIELD OF THE CLOTH OF GOLD
By the 16th century, France was a major power in Europe. In 1520, the French king Francis I met Henry VIII of England at a lavish ceremony to sign a peace treaty between the two countries. The place where they met was later called the Field of the Cloth of Gold.

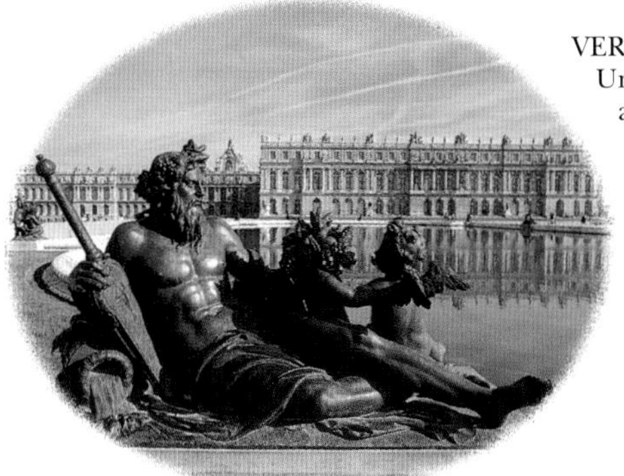

VERSAILLES
Under King Louis XIV and his successors in the 18th century, the arts and crafts in France were among the finest in Europe. Louis built a magnificent palace at Versailles, outside Paris. Ornate sculptures and fountains filled the grounds.

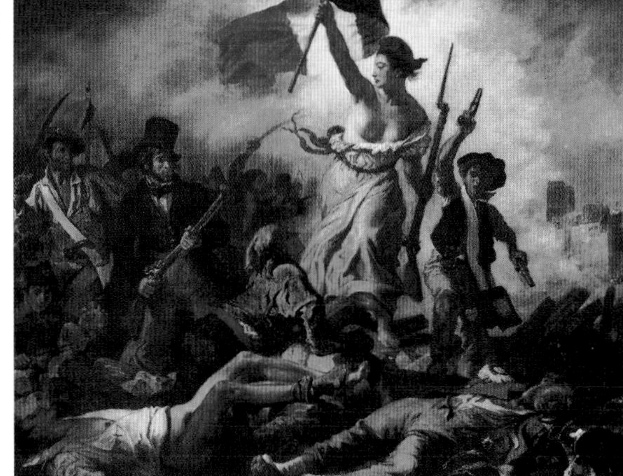

JEAN JACQUES ROUSSEAU
A philosopher and a writer, Rousseau (1712-78) greatly influenced 18th-century French thinking. He criticized society, thinking that it made people evil. His ideas directly influenced the development of the 1789 French Revolution.

REVOLUTIONS
France has a strong tradition of revolution by the people against absolute domination by a king. In the July revolution of 1830, the people rose up against Charles X, who tried to rule with the total power of Louis XIV. This uprising is shown in a patriotic painting by Eugene Delacroix (above).

Paris

The French capital has always been at the centre of the country's politics. In 1871 the city rebelled against the terms the government had accepted to end a war against Prussia. The Parisians barricaded the streets and set up a commune to run the city. The government savagely crushed the rebellion, killing 17,000 people. After the commune the architect Baron Haussmann (1809-91) made the streets of Paris wider to make the setting up of barricades impossible.

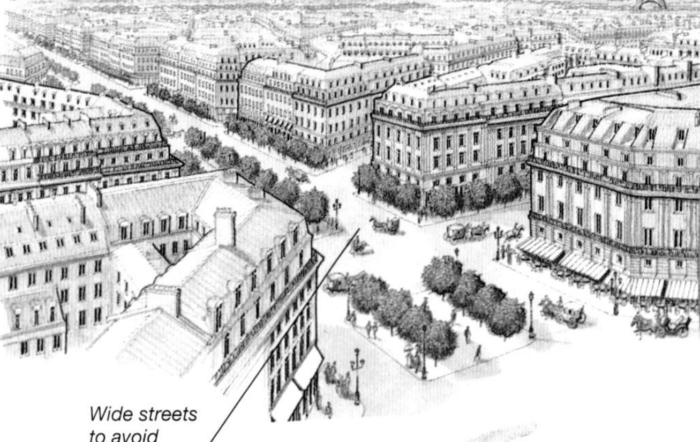

The engineer Alexandre Gustave Eiffel (1832-1923) built his famous Eiffel Tower to celebrate the 100th anniversary of the French Revolution.

Wide streets to avoid barricading

HISTORY OF FRANCE

5700 B.C. Carnac constructed.

58 B.C.-A.D. 486 Roman occupation.

500 Franks settle in country.

768-814 Charlemagne rules Frankish empire.

895 Vikings begin to raid France.

1337-1453 Hundred Years' War against England.

1431 Joan of Arc is burned to death by the English.

1515-47 Reign of Francis I.

1562-98 Wars of Religion between Catholics and Protestants.

1643-1715 Reign of Louis XIV.

1789 Outbreak of French Revolution.

1792 France becomes a republic.

1799 Napoleon seizes power.

1815 Defeat of Napoleon at Waterloo; king restored.

1830 July Revolution throws out king.

1848 Second Republic set up.

1852 Napoleon III sets up Second Empire.

1870-71 Prussia defeats France in Franco-Prussian War. Leads to Third Republic.

1914-18 World War I. France at war with Germany.

1940 Germany invades France.

1944 France liberated from Germany.

1954-62 War with Algeria.

1957 France and other western European nations set up the European Community.

1958-69 Charles De Gaulle is president.

1981 France elects its first socialist president, François Mitterand; he served until 1995.

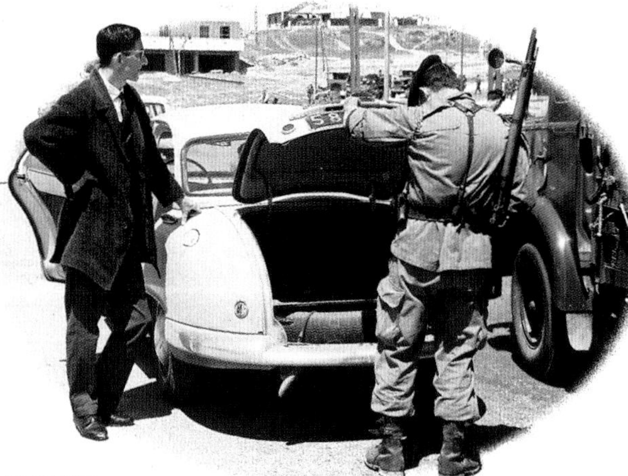

ALGERIA
The French had colonies in North Africa, including Algeria. During the 1950s many colonies gained independence, but France wanted to keep Algeria, home to almost a million French settlers. Discontent and bad living conditions led the Algerians to revolt, and a war followed. French troops occupied Algeria (above). In 1962, after much fighting, France finally granted Algeria independence.

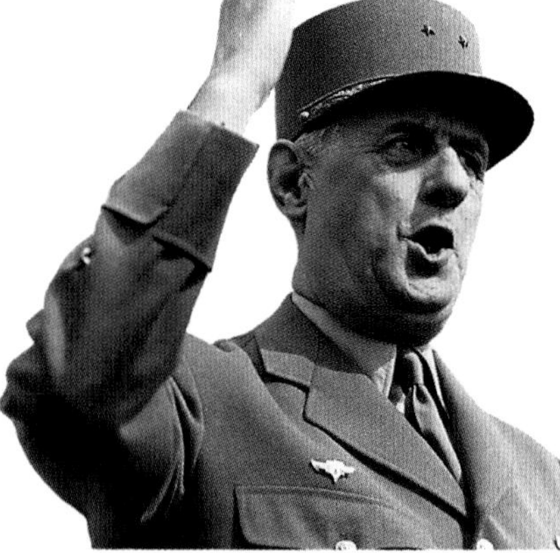

CHARLES DE GAULLE
During World War II, De Gaulle (1890-1970) was leader of the Free French. He became president of France in 1958. As president he led France through difficult times during which Algeria became independent. De Gaulle retired in 1969.

Find out more
FRANCE
FRENCH REVOLUTION
JOAN OF ARC
LOUIS XIV
NAPOLEON BONAPARTE

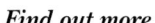

FRENCH REVOLUTION

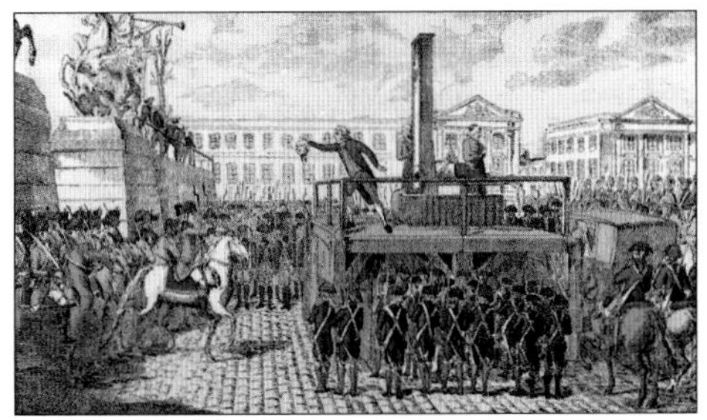

THE EXECUTION OF LOUIS XVI
"Because the country must live, Louis must die." With those words, the king of France was killed on the guillotine on 21 January 1793.

"LIBERTY! EQUALITY! FRATERNITY!" This slogan echoed through France in 1789 as the hungry French people united to overthrow the rich noblemen who ruled the country. The Revolution put ordinary people in control of France and gave hope to oppressed people all over the world. The Revolution started when the bankrupt king Louis XVI summoned the French parliament for the first time since 1614. Instead of helping him raise taxes, they siezed power. In Paris, a crowd stormed the Bastille prison, the symbol of royal authority. The king had to support the Revolution, but in 1792 France became a republic, and Louis was executed. Counterrevolution broke out in parts of France in 1793, which led to a Reign of Terror that undid many of the benefits of the revolution. In 1799 a military takeover put Napoleon in power and ended the Revolution.

THE REVOLUTION

May 1789 Estates General (parliament) meets at Versailles.

July 1789 Paris crowd storms Bastille prison.

Aug 1789 Declaration of the Rights of Man.

June 1790 Nobility is abolished.

June 1791 Louis XVI tries to flee from Paris.

Aug 1792 King Louis imprisoned.

Sept 1792 Monarchy abolished and France becomes a republic.

Mar 1793 Counter-revolution in Vendée region.

Sept 1793 Start of Reign of Terror.

July 1794 Terror ends when Robespierre is overthrown.

Nov 1795 A new republic, the Directory, takes power.

Nov 1799 Napoleon Bonaparte overthrows Directory and assumes power.

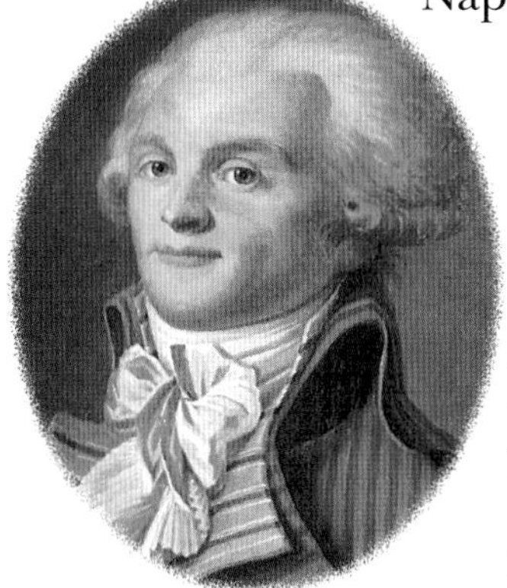

MAXIMILIEN ROBESPIERRE
When 35-year-old lawyer Robespierre came to power in 1793, he took severe measures to safeguard the Revolution. He presided over the Reign of Terror but was himself executed in 1794.

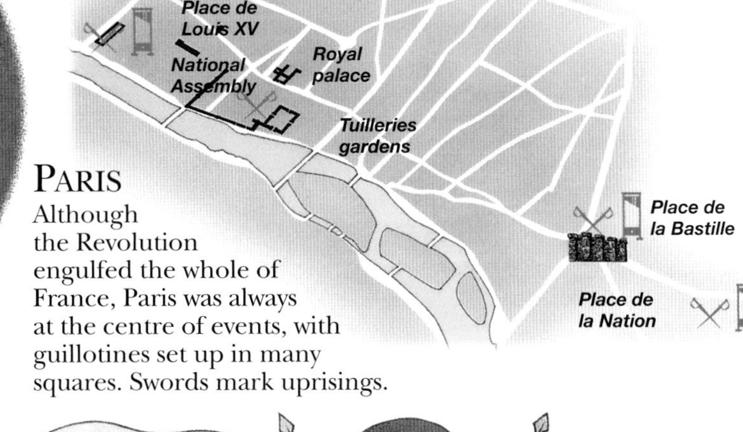

PARIS

Although the Revolution engulfed the whole of France, Paris was always at the centre of events, with guillotines set up in many squares. Swords mark uprisings.

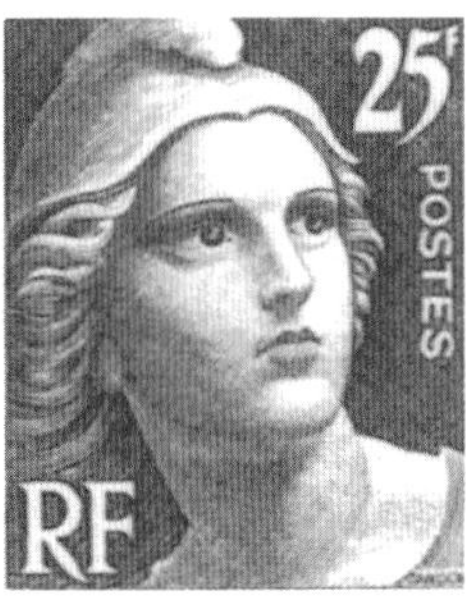

MARIANNE
The new revolutionary calendar started from the day the king was overthrown. Marianne – a symbolic but imaginary revolutionary woman shown here on a stamp – illustrated the first month.

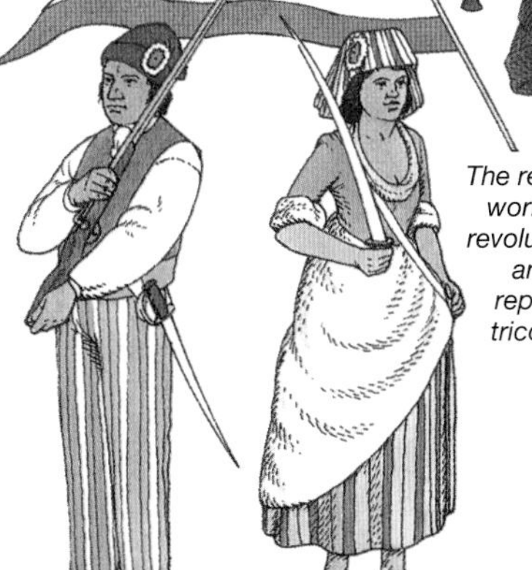

The red bonnet worn by the revolutionaries, and the republican tricolor flag

SANS-CULOTTES

The well-dressed aristocrats sneered at the revolutionaries and called them sans-culottes, or people without trousers. The revolutionaries adopted this name as their own. Their simple clothes came to symbolize the new way of life in revolutionary France.

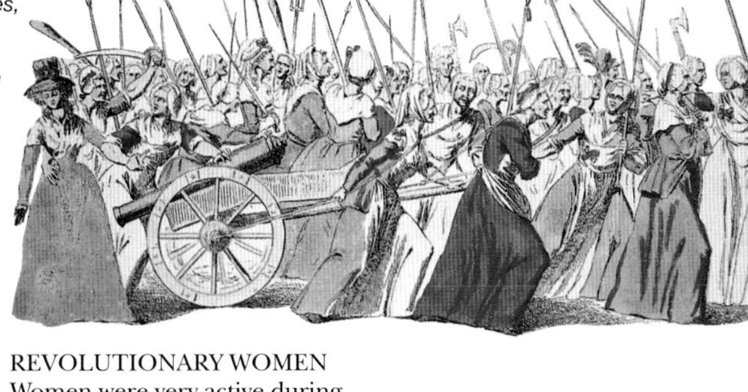

REVOLUTIONARY WOMEN
Women were very active during the Revolution and led many of the marches. But women were never allowed to vote or to participate in the government, and the Rights of Man (the revolutionary charter of human rights) did not apply to them.

Find out more

FRANCE, HISTORY OF
NAPOLEON BONAPARTE
NAPOLEONIC WARS

FROGS AND OTHER AMPHIBIANS

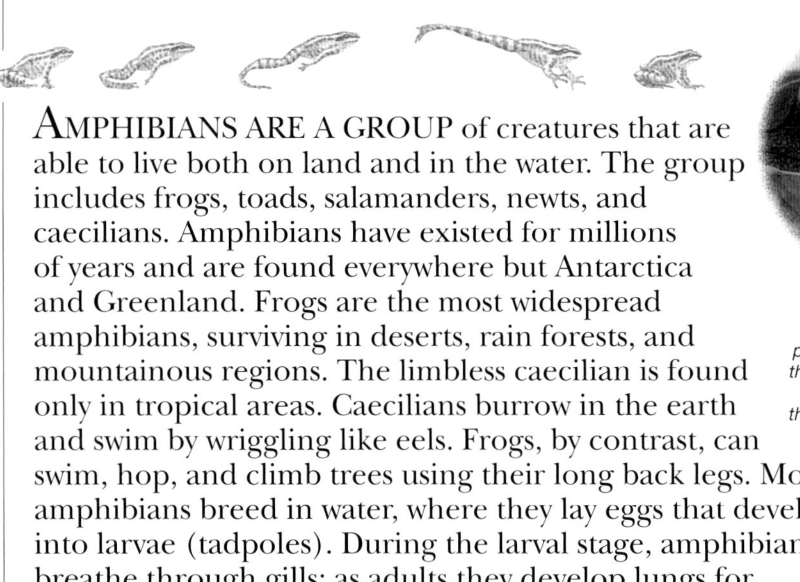

AMPHIBIANS ARE A GROUP of creatures that are able to live both on land and in the water. The group includes frogs, toads, salamanders, newts, and caecilians. Amphibians have existed for millions of years and are found everywhere but Antarctica and Greenland. Frogs are the most widespread amphibians, surviving in deserts, rain forests, and mountainous regions. The limbless caecilian is found only in tropical areas. Caecilians burrow in the earth and swim by wriggling like eels. Frogs, by contrast, can swim, hop, and climb trees using their long back legs. Most amphibians breed in water, where they lay eggs that develop into larvae (tadpoles). During the larval stage, amphibians breathe through gills; as adults they develop lungs for breathing on land. Several kinds of frogs and salamanders are brightly coloured, and some have glands in the skin that produce toxins (poisons) to ward off predators.

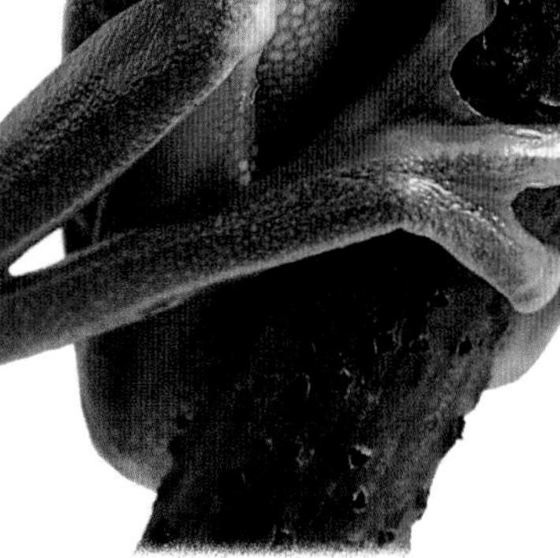

Frogs rely on their eyes to watch for prey. They also use their eyes to judge distances when they are leaping.

Front legs act as shock absorbers when the frog lands.

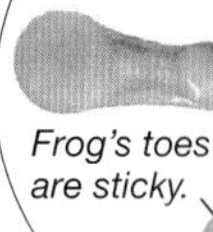

Frog's toes are sticky.

AMPHIBIANS
Some amphibians lay spawn (eggs) in water; others lay eggs out of water, on leaves, or in holes underground. The frog spawn you see in a pond hatches into limbless tadpoles. As the tadpoles grow in the water, they develop limbs. They gradually change into frogs and climb onto the land. This process is called metamorphosis.

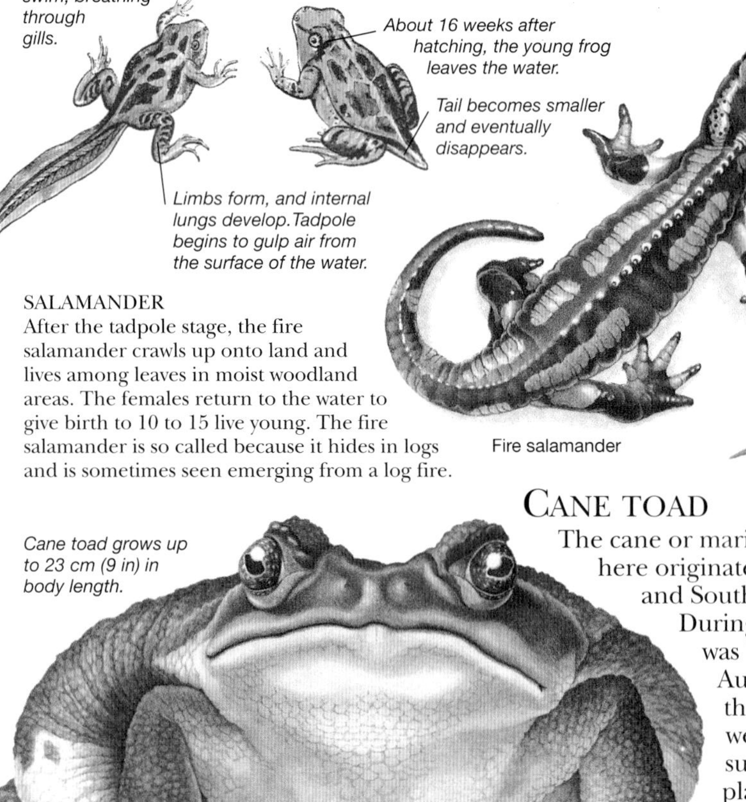

After hatching from its egg, the tadpole starts to swim, breathing through gills.

About 16 weeks after hatching, the young frog leaves the water.

Tail becomes smaller and eventually disappears.

Limbs form, and internal lungs develop. Tadpole begins to gulp air from the surface of the water.

RED-EYED TREE FROG

Tree frogs often have longer, leaner bodies than frogs that live mainly in water. A frog's long back legs can kick powerfully for swimming and leaping away from predators. The red-eyed tree frog shown above has sticky discs on its toes that give a good grip on leaves and bark. Today, red-eyed tree frogs are in danger of extinction.

SALAMANDER
After the tadpole stage, the fire salamander crawls up onto land and lives among leaves in moist woodland areas. The females return to the water to give birth to 10 to 15 live young. The fire salamander is so called because it hides in logs and is sometimes seen emerging from a log fire.

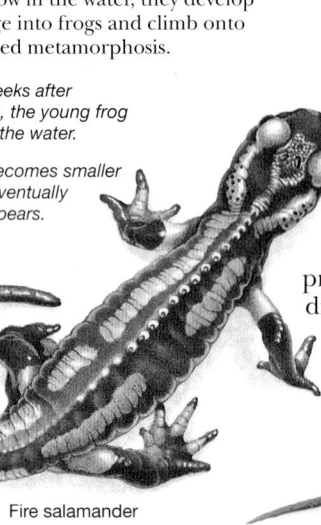

Fire salamander

Mandarin newt

CANE TOAD

The cane or marine toad shown here originated in Central and South America. During the 1930s it was brought to Australia to eat the beetles that were pests in sugar cane plantations. Today the cane toad itself is regarded as a pest.

Cane toad grows up to 23 cm (9 in) in body length.

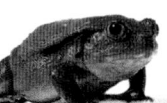

NEWT
Salamanders and their relatives, the newts, resemble lizards in shape. In the breeding season newts often become brighter in colour, and may be red, yellow, or orange, such as the mandarin newt shown here. These colours warn predators that the glands in the skin produce horrible-tasting or poisonous fluids.

Asian leaf frog

Tomato frog

Find out more

ANIMALS
AUSTRALIAN WILDLIFE
CONSERVATION
and endangered species

FRUITS AND SEEDS

ALL FLOWERING PLANTS, from tiny duckweeds to mighty oaks, develop from seeds. Each seed contains an embryo (a young plant) plus a store of food for the embryo's growth. A fruit is the seed container; it protects the developing seeds until they are dispersed by animals, the wind, water, or the plant itself. Fruits include lemons, melons, cherries, and tomatoes. The hard little stones or pips inside are the seeds. Many fruits, such as oranges and black-currants, are an important source of food. They contain large amounts of vitamin C, necessary for good health. People have cultivated fruits for centuries; today, fruit growers produce millions of tonnes of fruit every year. Strangely enough, some foods that we call vegetables, such as cucumber, are in fact fruits, bursting with tiny seeds. So too are spices such as whole chillis and peppercorns. Yet rhubarb, which is often cooked as a fruit, is really the pink stem of a leaf.

Seeds (pips)

Core

There are more than 1,000 varieties of cultivated apples.

APPLE

The apple's flesh, which is what we eat, grows from the receptacle of the flower, so it is a false fruit. The apple core is formed from the ovary, and the pips inside are the seeds. Pears, quinces, and hawthorn berries are formed in the same way; they are also known as pomes.

TRUE AND FALSE FRUITS

Fruits have different names, depending on which part of the flower develops into the main part of the fruit. Fruits are usually described as either true or false fruits. A true fruit develops from the female parts of the flower. A false fruit is one that includes some other part of the flower, such as the receptacle, or flower base.

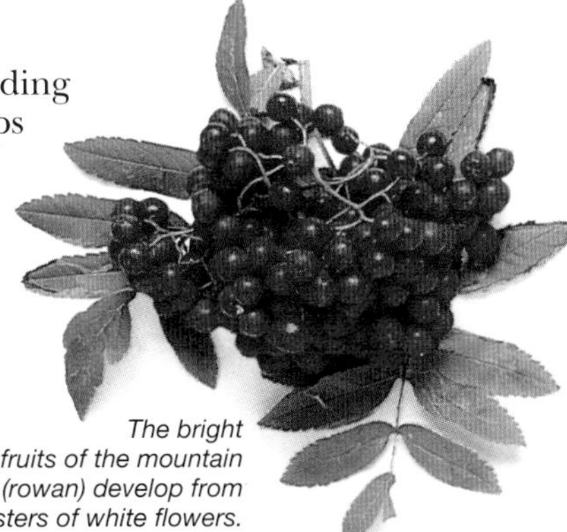

The bright red fruits of the mountain ash (rowan) develop from clusters of white flowers.

GRAPE

Berries are juicy, succulent true fruits with pips inside. They include grapevine berries, which we call grapes. About 5,000 kinds of grapes are used to make wine, or are dried into currants and raisins for cakes and biscuits. Other berries include gooseberries, tomatoes, and bananas. Citrus fruits, such as oranges, lemons, and grapefruits, are also berries.

Runner bean pod

Pea

Pea pod

PEA LEGUME

Legumes are dry, non-juicy fruits. Their seeds are contained in a long outer casing called a pod. Pods are found on pea and bean plants, as well as sweet peas and laburnums. We eat the fruits of pea and bean plants.

POPPY CAPSULE

Capsules are hard, dry fruits found on poppies, violets, snapdragons, and the horse chestnut tree. The poppy capsule is like a saltshaker. The tiny seeds fall through holes at the top when the wind blows.

PLUM DRUPE

Drupes are juicy, succulent true fruits like berries. Unlike berries, however, drupes do not have pips. Instead, they have a hard stone which contains the seed. Plums, cherries, and apricots are all drupes. A blackberry is a collection of drupes.

Cherry

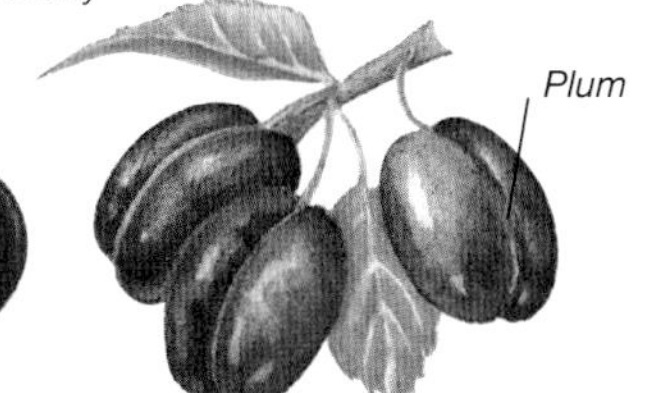

NUT

A nut is a dry, hard-cased fruit such as an acorn or hazelnut, with only one seed inside. Most hard, woody fruits or seeds are called nuts, but the fruit of the walnut is actually a drupe, and the Brazil nut is really a seed.

Walnut fruit (drupe)

Walnut "nut" is the seed.

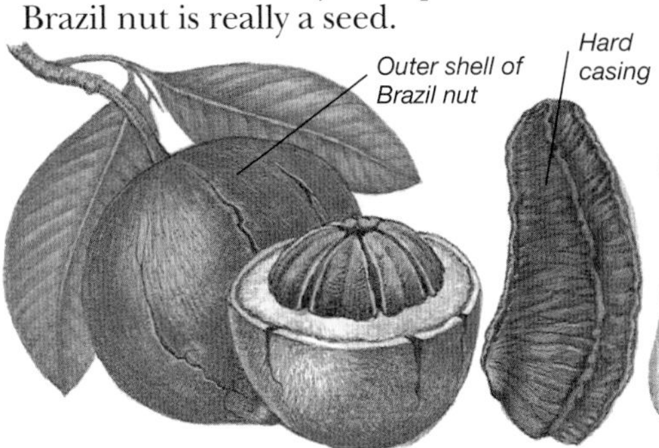

Hard casing

Brazil "nuts" are the seeds of a South American tree. The seeds grow in melon-sized fruit pods.

Brazil nut (seed) that we eat

Seed cases

Seed head

Seeds

Sunflower seeds are used in margarine, animal food, and as a snack.

SUNFLOWER

The sunflower grows about 2.5 m (8 ft) high. After fertilization, the large flower ripens to form a plate-sized seed head. Sunflower seeds contain large amounts of vitamins and edible oil.

Germination

Seeds need warmth, moisture, and air in order to germinate (grow). The seeds of certain tropical plants start to germinate within a few days; the seeds of most other plants remain dormant, or asleep, until conditions are right. Many tree and shrub seeds must pass through a cold winter before they can begin to grow.

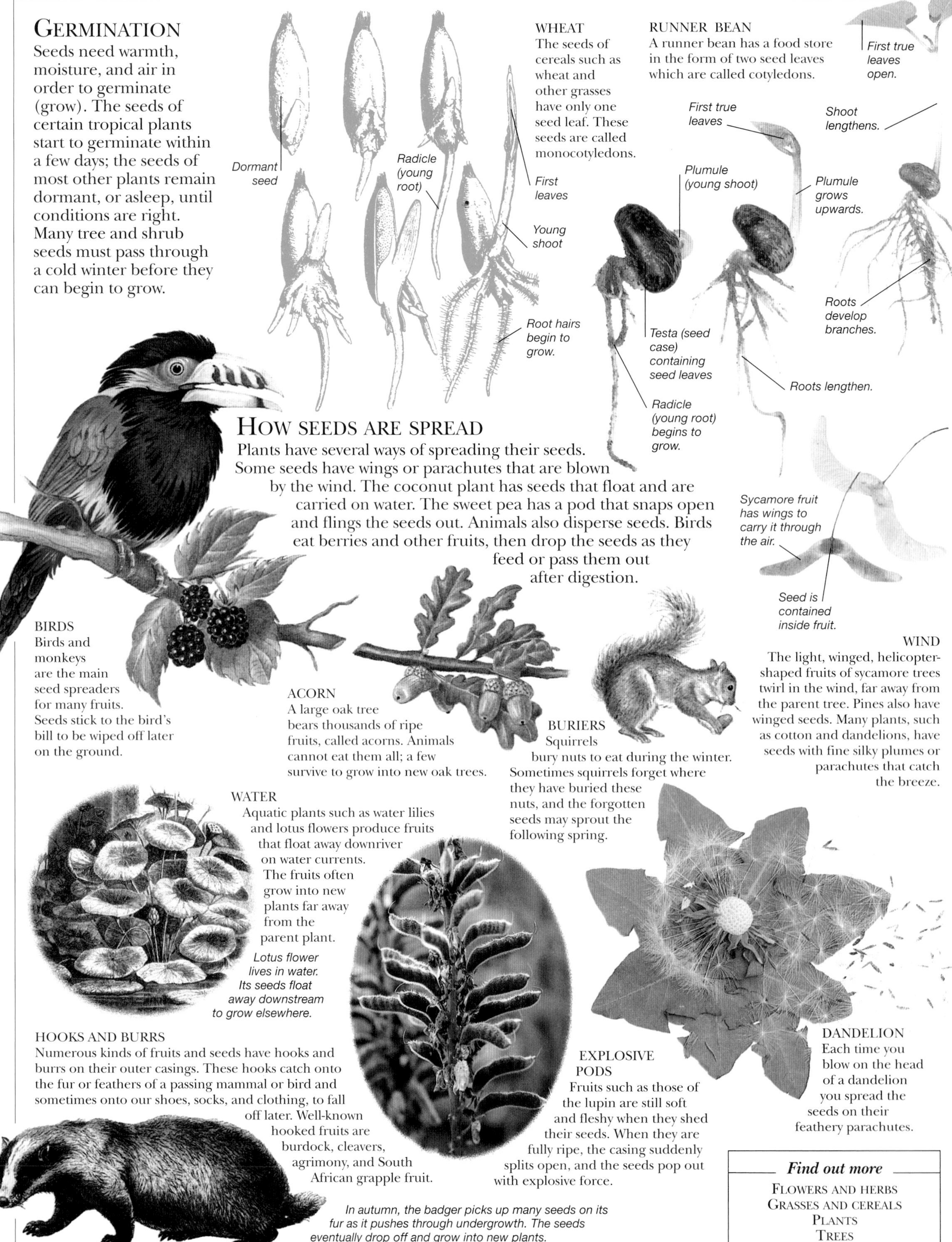

WHEAT
The seeds of cereals such as wheat and other grasses have only one seed leaf. These seeds are called monocotyledons.

RUNNER BEAN
A runner bean has a food store in the form of two seed leaves which are called cotyledons.

How seeds are spread

Plants have several ways of spreading their seeds. Some seeds have wings or parachutes that are blown by the wind. The coconut plant has seeds that float and are carried on water. The sweet pea has a pod that snaps open and flings the seeds out. Animals also disperse seeds. Birds eat berries and other fruits, then drop the seeds as they feed or pass them out after digestion.

BIRDS
Birds and monkeys are the main seed spreaders for many fruits. Seeds stick to the bird's bill to be wiped off later on the ground.

ACORN
A large oak tree bears thousands of ripe fruits, called acorns. Animals cannot eat them all; a few survive to grow into new oak trees.

BURIERS
Squirrels bury nuts to eat during the winter. Sometimes squirrels forget where they have buried these nuts, and the forgotten seeds may sprout the following spring.

WIND
The light, winged, helicopter-shaped fruits of sycamore trees twirl in the wind, far away from the parent tree. Pines also have winged seeds. Many plants, such as cotton and dandelions, have seeds with fine silky plumes or parachutes that catch the breeze.

WATER
Aquatic plants such as water lilies and lotus flowers produce fruits that float away downriver on water currents. The fruits often grow into new plants far away from the parent plant.

Lotus flower lives in water. Its seeds float away downstream to grow elsewhere.

HOOKS AND BURRS
Numerous kinds of fruits and seeds have hooks and burrs on their outer casings. These hooks catch onto the fur or feathers of a passing mammal or bird and sometimes onto our shoes, socks, and clothing, to fall off later. Well-known hooked fruits are burdock, cleavers, agrimony, and South African grapple fruit.

EXPLOSIVE PODS
Fruits such as those of the lupin are still soft and fleshy when they shed their seeds. When they are fully ripe, the casing suddenly splits open, and the seeds pop out with explosive force.

DANDELION
Each time you blow on the head of a dandelion you spread the seeds on their feathery parachutes.

In autumn, the badger picks up many seeds on its fur as it pushes through undergrowth. The seeds eventually drop off and grow into new plants.

Find out more
FLOWERS AND HERBS
GRASSES AND CEREALS
PLANTS
TREES

FURNITURE

WHEN WE SIT DOWN to work or eat, when we lie down to sleep, furniture supports our bodies comfortably. When we carry out tasks in the office, school, or kitchen, furniture has surfaces at just the right height so that we do not bend or stretch. And furniture organizes all our belongings close at hand yet out of sight. We take for granted our chairs, beds, tables, and cabinets because we use them every day. But until the 19th century furniture was handmade, and few families could afford very much. Most homes had a table but only simple stools or benches to sit on. People stored their few clothes and possessions in a chest and slept on mattresses on the floor. Today most furniture is made in factories. Much of it is very practical, with easy-to-clean surfaces at convenient heights. But there are other styles, too, to fit in with any interior. Reproduction furniture, for example, imitates the styles of the past, with rich upholstery and carved wood.

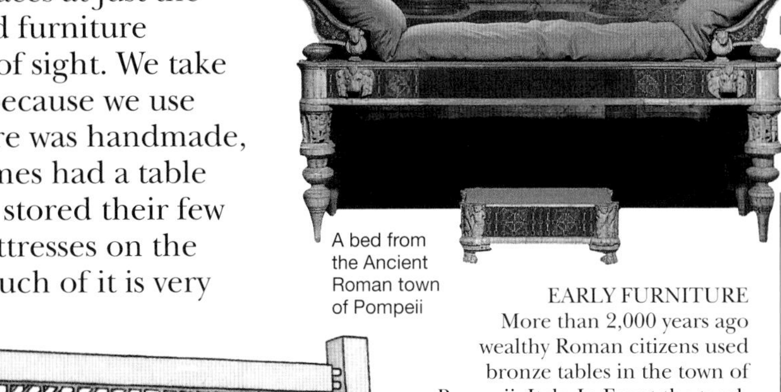

A bed from the Ancient Roman town of Pompeii

EARLY FURNITURE
More than 2,000 years ago wealthy Roman citizens used bronze tables in the town of Pompeii, Italy. In Egypt the tomb of Tutankhamun contained exquisite furniture that was buried with the boy king 3,500 years ago.

The woven rush back holds the sitter upright.

The covering material is attractive and hardwearing.

The chair frame of jointed wood supports the upholstery.

Padding is thick and even for comfort.

Horsehair was once the traditional material for padding; most furniture makers now use plastic foam.

Sturdy material such as hessian covers the springs and distributes the sitter's weight.

Coiled steel springs make the chair soft to sit on.

The upholsterer stretches cotton webbing across the frame.

ANTIQUES
When carpenters such as Englishman Thomas Chippendale (1718-79) were making furniture by hand, many of the objects they crafted were both beautiful and easy to use. Today these items of furniture are called antiques. Some are valuable and highly prized.

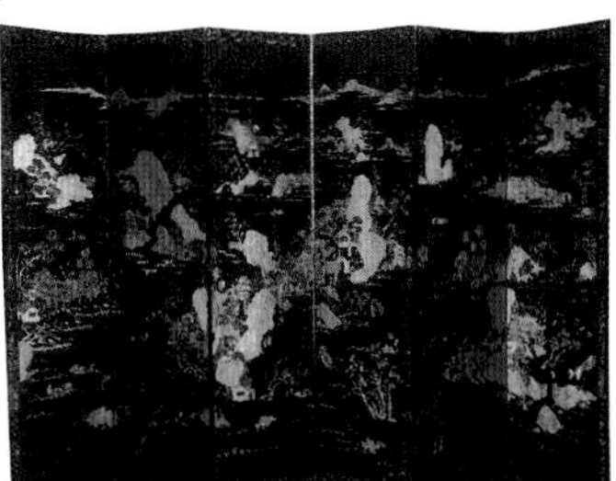

Antique screen from Japan

MOVABLE FURNITURE
European and North American families do not move into new homes often, so their furniture is made to stay in one place. But nomadic people carry their homes with them, so big chairs and tables are not practical. For example, the Bedouin of the Middle East furnish their desert tents with easy-to-pack rugs, cushions, and bedrolls.

South American Indians invented the hammock as a bed they could carry easily.

UPHOLSTERY

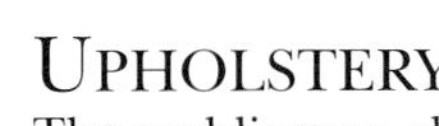

The padding on chairs and sofas is called upholstery. It stops the hard frame of the furniture from digging into your body. Many different materials are needed to make a comfortable seat, because upholstery must be firm in some places to provide support and prevent backache, but soft and yielding elsewhere for comfort.

TYPES OF FURNITURE
Furniture designs have evolved to suit their role. For example, kitchen cabinets have solid doors to hide pots and pans, but the doors of china cabinets are glass to display attractive crockery.

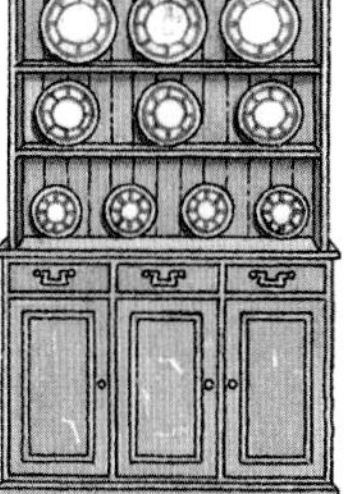

Drawers in the cupboard store cutlery and keep it clean. The upper part shows off the best china.

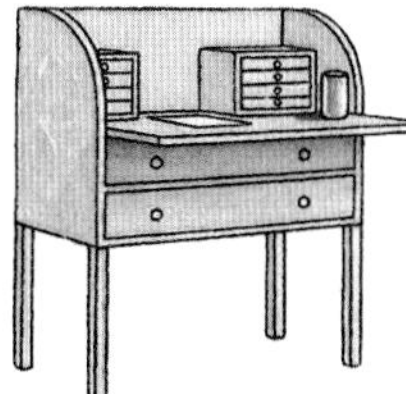

A well-designed desk is a miniature office. The locking drawers hide precious documents, and compartments keep stationery clean.

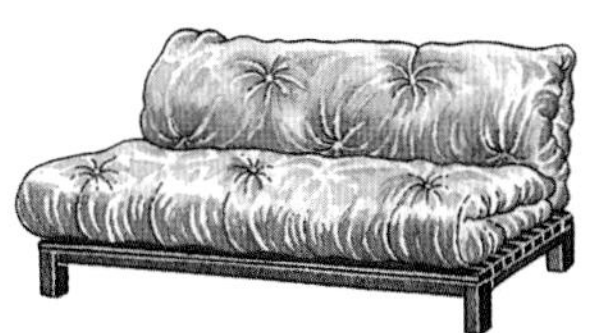

The cotton-filled futon is a sofa which folds out to make a bed. It originated in Japan as a way to save space in small homes.

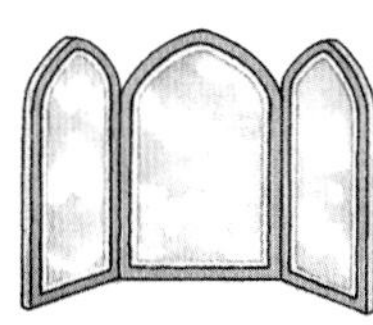

Glassmakers first made mirrors in the 16th century. The three hinged panels enable the user to see his or her face from the side.

Find out more
DESIGN
EGYPT, ANCIENT
HOUSES

GAMES

SKIPPING in the schoolyard and playing world championship chess have one thing in common – they are both games. Some games are similar to organized sports and, like sports, games provide pleasure, relaxation, excitement, and a challenge. There are thousands of different games. Some, such as chess, have the same rules everywhere. But others vary from place to place; for example, there are many variations on the rules of the card game poker. Many games share the same playing equipment: dice are similar all over the world, but players use dice in a huge range of games. Not all games require special equipment: you can make the playing pieces for some games in a few minutes from string, toothpicks, sticks, or stones. Some games make you think, others call for physical skills, and some require both. You can play some games by yourself, some need two to play, while others are fun only when played in a group.

DICE
Throwing dice, usually in pairs, adds chance and luck to a game. In many board games, such as Monopoly, the number of spots facing up when the dice come to rest determines the number of squares or sections players may move along. Standard dice have spots from one to six. Variations include poker dice, which have faces similar to playing cards.

COMPUTER GAMES
To operate computer games, players use buttons, a keyboard, or levers called joysticks. People play against the computer or against each other.

SKIPPING
Players usually chant traditional songs when skipping. With a long enough rope, several players can skip together.

TAG
In tag, the player chosen to be "it" tries to catch the other players.

HOPSCOTCH
Most hopscotch games have 9 to 12 numbered squares. Hopscotch calls for good balance when hopping between squares.

PIGGY IN THE MIDDLE
Two players throw a ball to each other. The "piggy" in the middle tries to intercept or catch it.

PLAYGROUND GAMES

Around any playground you will see a variety of games taking place. Some, such as skipping, occupy a small corner and people wait their turn. Others, such as tag, need more space.

SUITS
A pack of playing cards has four suits or groups, each with thirteen similar cards. The four suits are, from left to right, hearts, clubs, diamonds, and spades.

BOARD GAMES

People first marked out boards to play games 4,000 years ago. Board games such as chess and draughts originally represented the field of battle, in which the players captured enemy soldiers. In backgammon, players take their pieces through enemy territory. Many modern board games imitate common aspects of life, such as buying and selling property, as in Monopoly.

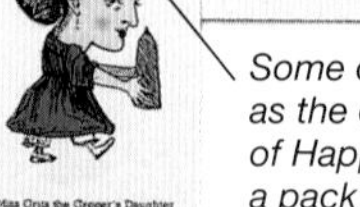
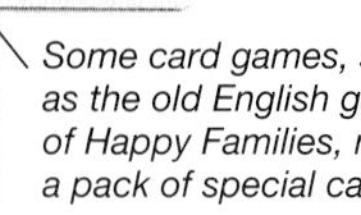
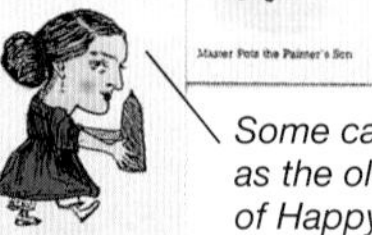
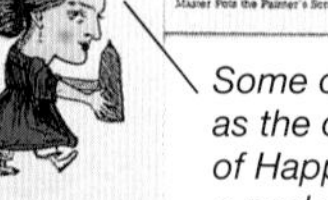
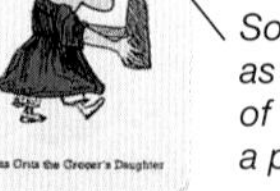
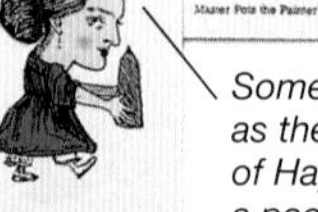
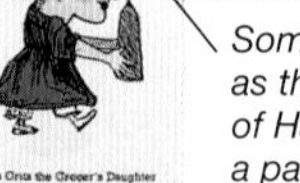

Some card games, such as the old English game of Happy Families, require a pack of special cards.

Cards in suits are numbered from one, or ace, to ten, and there are three "royal" cards: jack, queen, and king.

CARD GAMES
A standard set of cards is called a pack or deck. With its 52 cards you can play countless games of skill or chance. The game of bridge requires good concentration and an excellent memory. But you can learn to play snap in a few seconds, and all you need are quick reflexes.

PACHISI
A variation of backgammon, pachisi is an ancient royal game of India. Two or four players throw dice and try to get their counters to the inner centre of the board.

Find out more
PUZZLES
SPORTS
TOYS

GAS

BURNING GAS TO MAKE HEAT is a quick and easy way to warm the home and to cook. Gas is also used in industry, both for heat and as a raw material. Most of the gas we use for fuel is natural gas. It is extracted from deposits buried deep underground or under the seabed. Gas for burning can also be made by processing coal to produce coal gas. These fuel gases are not the only kinds of gas: there are many others with different uses. For instance, the air we breathe is made up of several gases mixed together.

FORMATION OF NATURAL GAS
The natural gas we use today is millions of years old. It was formed from the remains of prehistoric plants that lived on land and in the sea. New gas deposits are still being created.

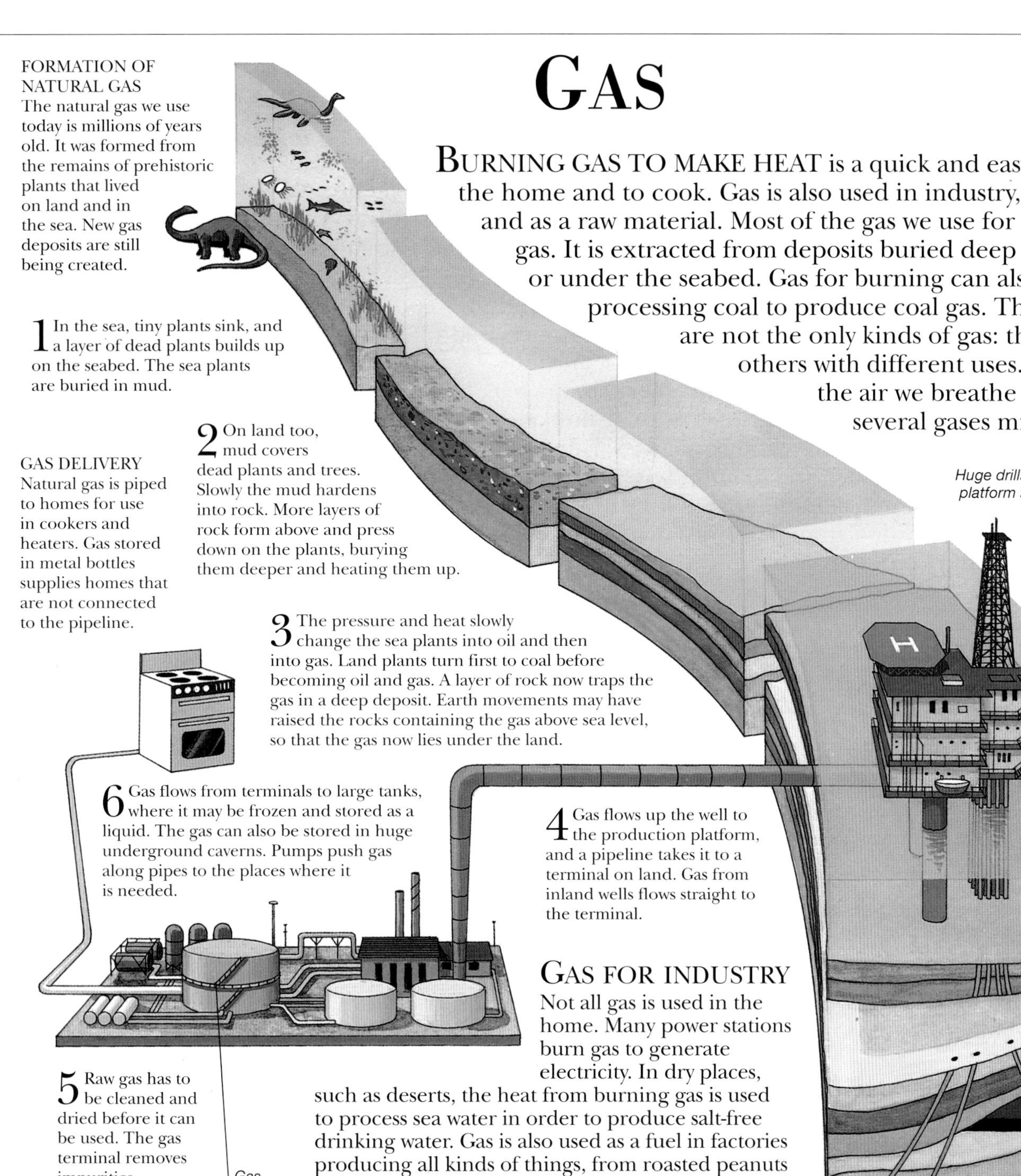

Huge drills on a production platform sink wells to reach gas deposits, which lie as deep as 6 km (4 miles) below the seabed.
Gas storage tank
Gas deposit
Oil deposit
A gas layer often forms above a layer of oil.
The pressure of the gas helps force the oil up wells to the production platform.

1 In the sea, tiny plants sink, and a layer of dead plants builds up on the seabed. The sea plants are buried in mud.

2 On land too, mud covers dead plants and trees. Slowly the mud hardens into rock. More layers of rock form above and press down on the plants, burying them deeper and heating them up.

3 The pressure and heat slowly change the sea plants into oil and then into gas. Land plants turn first to coal before becoming oil and gas. A layer of rock now traps the gas in a deep deposit. Earth movements may have raised the rocks containing the gas above sea level, so that the gas now lies under the land.

4 Gas flows up the well to the production platform, and a pipeline takes it to a terminal on land. Gas from inland wells flows straight to the terminal.

5 Raw gas has to be cleaned and dried before it can be used. The gas terminal removes impurities and water.

6 Gas flows from terminals to large tanks, where it may be frozen and stored as a liquid. The gas can also be stored in huge underground caverns. Pumps push gas along pipes to the places where it is needed.

GAS DELIVERY
Natural gas is piped to homes for use in cookers and heaters. Gas stored in metal bottles supplies homes that are not connected to the pipeline.

GAS FOR INDUSTRY

Not all gas is used in the home. Many power stations burn gas to generate electricity. In dry places, such as deserts, the heat from burning gas is used to process sea water in order to produce salt-free drinking water. Gas is also used as a fuel in factories producing all kinds of things, from roasted peanuts to cars. Chemicals made from gas are vital ingredients in the manufacture of plastics, fertilizers, paints, synthetic fibre, and many other products.

USEFUL GASES

Gas wells produce several different sorts of gas. Methane is the main component, but other fuel gases, called propane and butane, also come from gas deposits. The gas terminal stores these gases in metal cylinders for use in houses where the gas pipe does not reach. Gas deposits are also a source of helium. Helium is used to fill balloons because it is very light and does not burn. Air is another source of useful gases. Carbon dioxide, the gas that makes the bubbles in fizzy drinks, comes from air. Air also contains a little neon gas. Some advertising signs are glass tubes filled with neon. The gas glows when electricity passes through it.

Neon sign

Helium gas balloons

Find out more
AIR
COAL
HEAT
OIL
OXYGEN

GEMS AND JEWELLERY

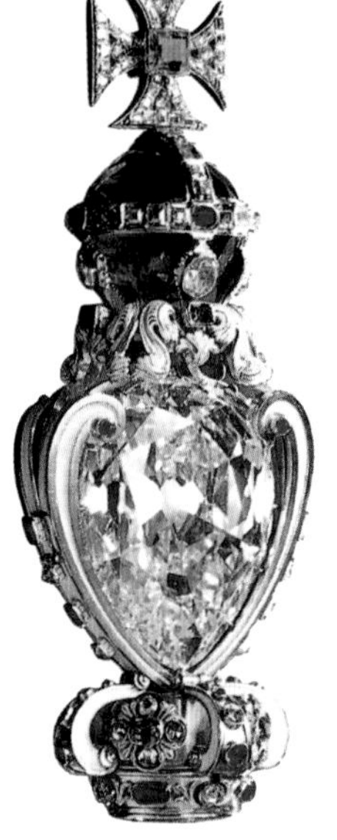

CROWN JEWELS
Priceless gems line the British crown jewels. The Royal Sceptre (above) contains the world's largest cut diamond, the 106 g (3.7 oz) Star of Africa.

A RING MOUNTED with beautiful gems, such as diamonds, seems to flash with fire as it catches the light. Yet the gems were once dull stones buried in rock. Their beauty is the work of gem cutters who shape the gems, and jewellers who mount them in settings of gold, silver, and other precious metals. Sometimes people wear gems, such as sapphires and diamonds, for good luck. Gems are stones used to make jewellery. They are either precious stones, such as rubies and emeralds, or semiprecious stones, such as opal and jade.

Gems also have industrial uses: rubies are used in lasers, and diamond-tipped drills dig through rock in the search for oil. Most gems are hard; diamond, for instance, is the hardest material in the world.

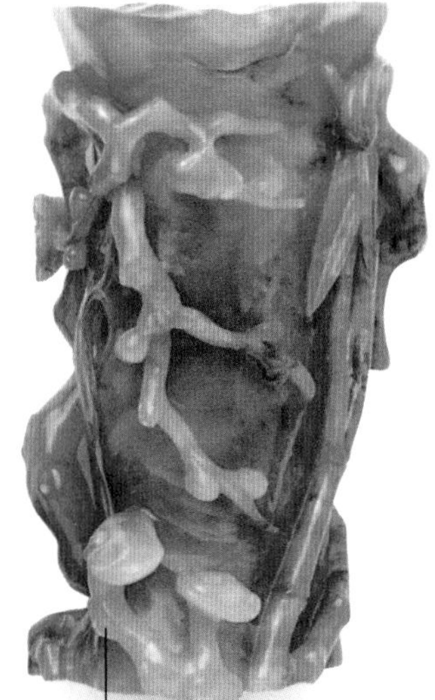

Jade is a hard gem made up of many tiny crystals.

Polished blue sapphire

This ruby crystal, called the Edwardes Ruby, is famous for its size and quality.

Cut ruby

SAPPHIRE AND RUBY
The crystals of coloured minerals make valuable gems. Sapphires and rubies are varieties of a mineral called corundum. The presence of iron and titanium turns corundum blue, to produce sapphires; chromium produces red rubies.

PRECIOUS STONES

Gems such as diamonds come from transparent minerals found in rocks. In their pure form, these minerals are colourless. But metals and other impurities in the minerals produce colour. The metal chromium turns the colourless mineral beryl green, producing emerald, a precious stone. Gemstones are often found in river beds. They are long-lasting and remain in the bed after running water has worn away the surrounding rock.

Vein of opal embedded in sedimentary rock

Polished white opal

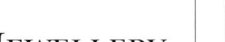

OPAL
Beautiful patterns of rainbow-like colours glisten inside opals. These gems consist mainly of silica, the same mineral found in sand. Opals do not need facets; instead, tiny spheres of silica within opal reflect and scatter light, producing colours from milky white to black, the most highly prized opal.

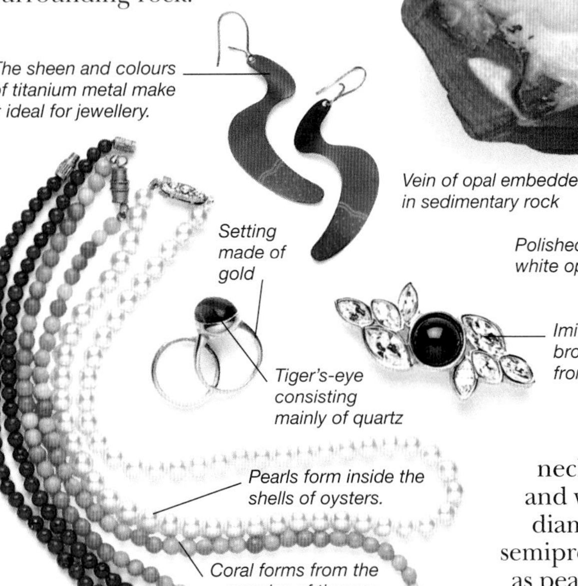

The sheen and colours of titanium metal make it ideal for jewellery.

Setting made of gold

Tiger's-eye consisting mainly of quartz

Imitation diamond brooch made from cut glass

Pearls form inside the shells of oysters.

Coral forms from the remains of tiny sea creatures.

Lapis lazuli jewellery has been known of for more than 6,000 years.

JEWELLERY

Rings, brooches, bracelets, earrings, and necklaces are worn as jewellery by both men and women. Fine pieces are made from gold, diamonds, and other precious materials. But semiprecious stones and organic materials such as pearls and amber also make lovely jewellery. So do inexpensive materials such as shells, coral, wood, and plastic. Some jewellery contains imitation gems made of cheap materials, such as glass, instead of precious stones.

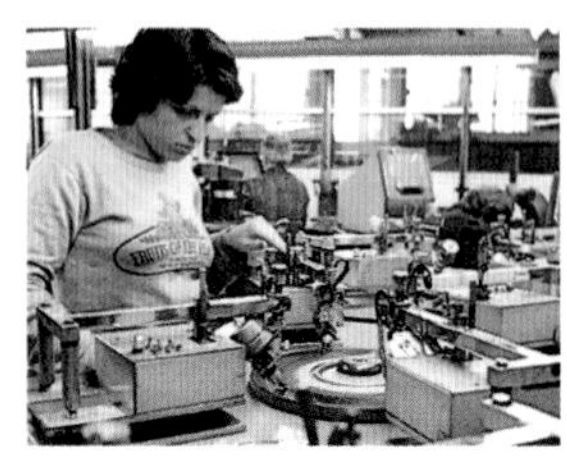

CUTTING GEMS

A gem sparkles because it has many-angled sides, or facets, that reflect light striking and entering the gem. Gem cutters split gemstones and then carve and polish the pieces to form the facets. There are several different kinds of cuts, some with complex patterns of facets.

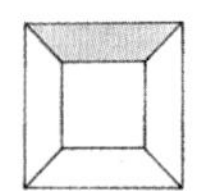

Table cut

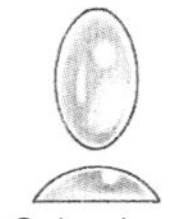

Cabochon

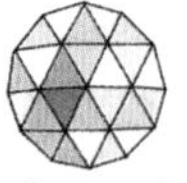

Rose cut

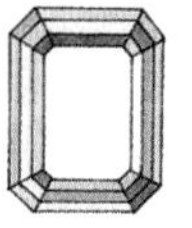

Step cut

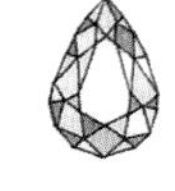

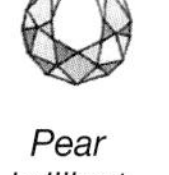

Pear brilliant

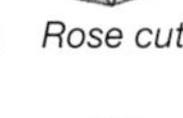

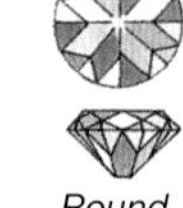

Round brilliant

Find out more

CORALS, anemones, and jellyfish
METALS
ROCKS AND MINERALS
SHELLS AND SHELLFISH

GENETICS

THE SCIENCE OF GENETICS has officially existed ever since the word "gene" was coined in 1909 by the Danish botanist Wilhelm Johannsen (1857-1927). He invented the term to describe the "particles" of inheritance that pass characteristics from one generation of plant or animal to the next. The field of genetics developed over the course of the 20th century, and produced important discoveries about how genes work. Scientists showed that genes are made up of lengths of deoxyribonucleic acid (DNA), which are connected together to make chromosomes. Genes contain the instructions by which plant and animal cells are built. Genes are passed from both parents to their children through sexual reproduction. By this process, called heredity, inheritable characteristics are passed from one generation to the next.

Each "rung" is a pair of chemicals called bases.

The sides of the "ladder" are made up of phosphate and sugar molecules.

The DNA molecule looks something like a twisted ladder in this model. In real life it is a chain of tens of thousands of atoms.

DNA

Deoxyribonucleic acid is the full name of DNA. It is the molecule that holds the genetic code within genes. Its structure is a double helix, with chemical bonds that attach one side of the helix to the other, rather like the rungs on a ladder. Each "rung" is made up of a pair of chemicals selected from a choice of four chemicals, so the way in which genetic information is coded is actually very simple.

HEREDITY

When a plant or animal is created, it inherits a combination of genetic information from both of its parents. Heredity is the passing of characteristics from parents to children. It means that a baby shares characteristics from each of its parents, but it also ensures that each baby is usually different from its brothers and sisters.

Children resemble their parents but are not identical to them.

Blue eye

Some of the traits controlled by genes can be easily seen. The genes in this girl's cells make her eyes blue, her hair straight, and her skin fair.

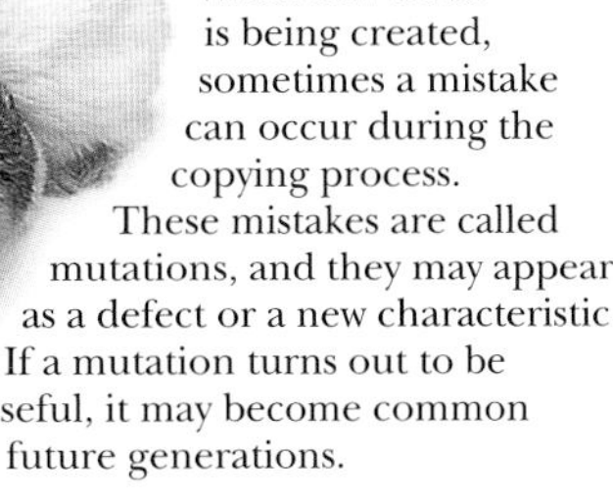

Albino hamster has white fur and red eyes.

Hamster with normal colouring

MUTATION

When new DNA is being created, sometimes a mistake can occur during the copying process. These mistakes are called mutations, and they may appear as a defect or a new characteristic. If a mutation turns out to be useful, it may become common in future generations.

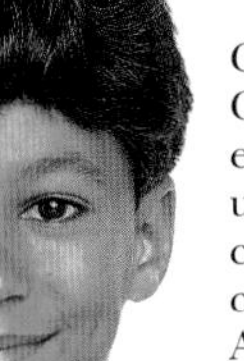

Wavy hair

The genes in this boy's cells make his eyes brown, his hair wavy, and his skin dark.

GENES

Chromosomes become extremely long when they are untangled. This is because a chromosome consists of a tightly coiled, long string of segments. A single segment is called a gene. A gene is a part of a chromosome that is responsible for a particular trait, such as eye colour. Genes vary in length depending on how much code they need to contain the information required for a trait.

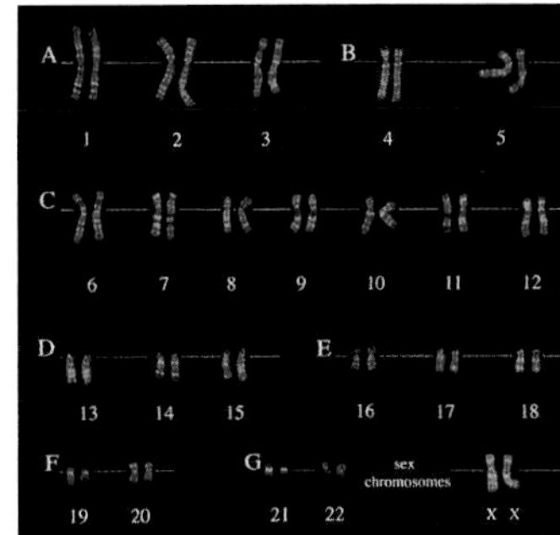

The sex chromosomes determine whether a cell is male or female. Males contain an XY pair, while females contain an XX pair.

CHROMOSOMES

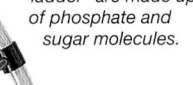

The nucleus of a living cell contains a number of pairs of chromosomes. They are rather like filing cabinets that store all of the genetic information of the plant or animal. Chromosomes are arranged in pairs that separate in the course of reproduction and in the creation of new cells.

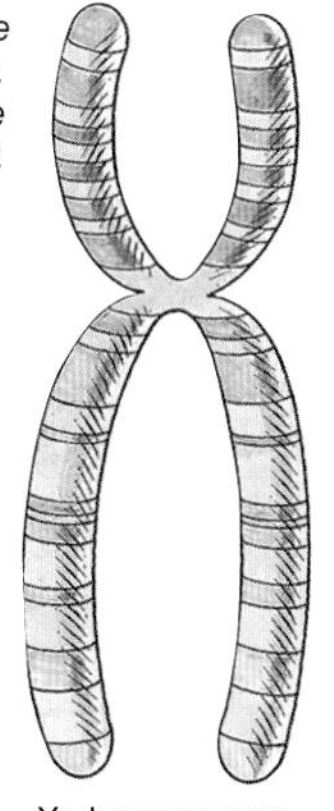

X chromosome

Mendel

Gregor Mendel (1822-84), Austrian scientist, discovered the laws of heredity through experiments with pea plants. In 1866, he showed that features in a plant, such as the production of a smooth or a wrinkled pea, are determined by the genetic information given to the plant by its parents. He called this information "particles", some 43 years before the word "gene" was invented by the Danish scientist Wilhelm Johannsen (1857-1927).

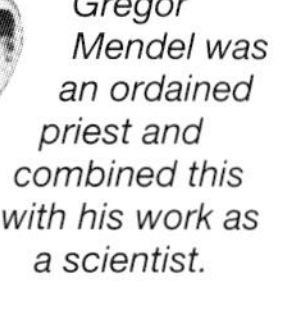

Gregor Mendel was an ordained priest and combined this with his work as a scientist.

PATTERNS OF INHERITANCE

Different forms of the same gene are called alleles, and they can be dominant or recessive. Dominant alleles always show up, even if the information they carry comes from only one parent. Recessive means that a certain feature might not be seen in a plant or animal even though it is carrying the right alleles. Recessiveness is sometimes linked to gender.

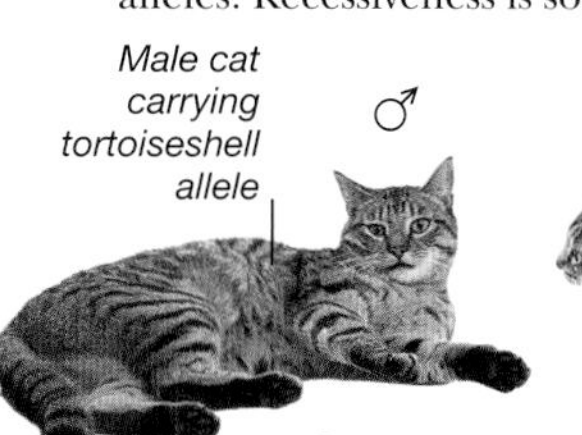

Male cat carrying tortoiseshell allele

Female tortoiseshell cat

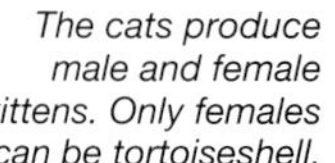

The cats produce male and female kittens. Only females can be tortoiseshell.

The second kitten, who carries two tortoiseshell alleles, does not have a tortoiseshell coat because he is male.

Only one kitten is tortoiseshell like her mother, because she carries two alleles and is female.

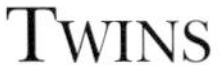

Twins

If a fertilized human embryo splits in two it will develop into identical twins. Each twin shares the same genetic information. In fact, they are not entirely identical because each foetus develops in a slightly different way after the original split. Therefore identical twins can appear to be remarkably similar yet have quite different personalities. Non-identical twins develop from two separate embryos.

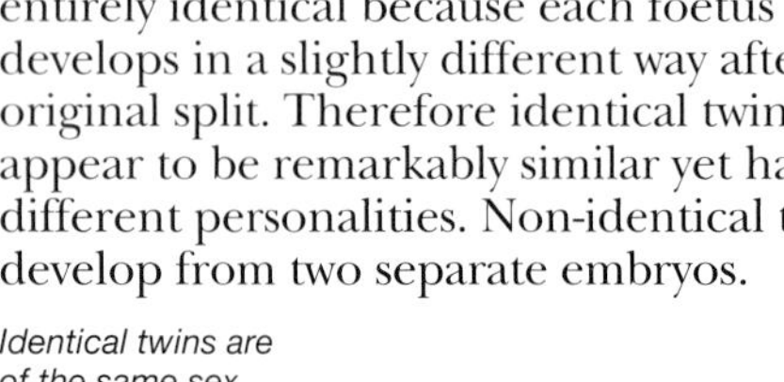

Identical twins are of the same sex because they come from a single embryo.

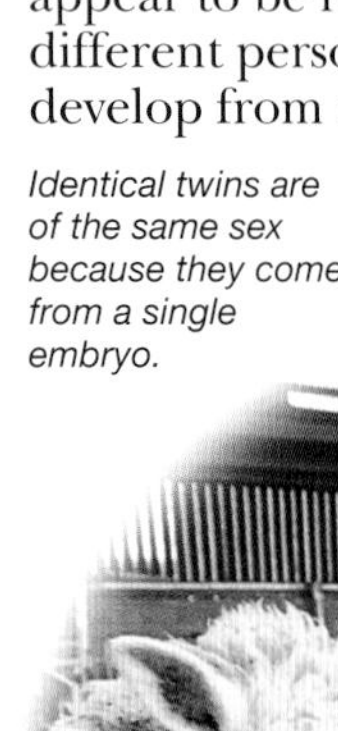

The world's media took a great interest in Dolly, the first large mammal to be cloned.

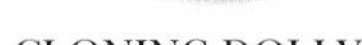

CLONING DOLLY

Clones are one or more identical organisms that share identical genes but unlike twins are not produced by natural reproduction. For many years, scientists have been interested in cloning identical copies of animals and plants. In 1997, scientists successfully cloned a sheep, known as Dolly. The experiment led to a worldwide debate about the ethics of cloning.

GENETICS

1858 Darwin publishes his theory of evolution.

1866 Mendel discovers laws of heredity.

1905 X and Y sex chromosomes discovered.

1918 Forty-eight chromosomes discovered in all human cells.

1927 Genetic mutation in fruit flies created using x-rays.

1950 DNA and RNA discovered.

1953 Watson, Crick, and Wilkins discover the double helix of DNA.

1967 DNA synthesized.

1976 Artificial gene created.

1981 First gene transplant at Ohio University, USA.

1984 Embryonic clone produced.

1985 Genetic fingerprinting introduced.

1997 Dolly the sheep cloned.

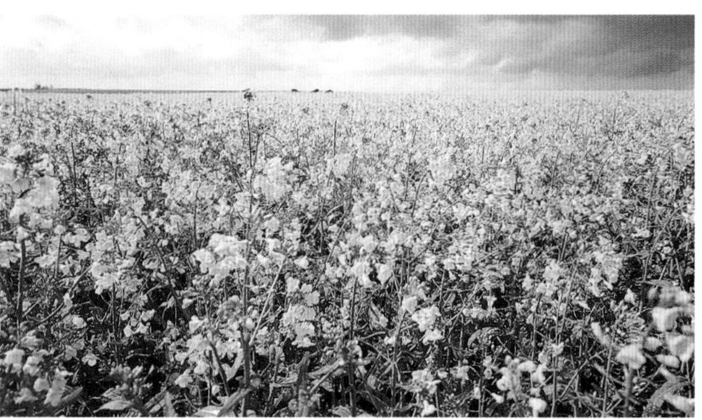

GM foods

The plants and animals that produce GM (genetically modified) foods have had their genes changed by scientists. In theory, genetic modification is just a way of speeding up the process of selection by breeding, which is already done in the natural way. There is much to be learnt before we can be sure that genetic modification is a safe thing to do.

Find out more

Atoms and molecules
Radioactivity
Reproduction

GEOLOGY

OUR EARTH CHANGES all the time. Mountains rise and wear away. Continents move, causing oceans to widen and narrow. These changes are slow. It would take a million years to notice much difference. Other changes, such as when an earthquake shakes the land or a volcano erupts, are sudden. Geology is the study of how the Earth changes, how it was formed, and the rocks that it is made of.

Clues to the Earth's history are hidden in its rocks. Geologists survey (map out) the land and dig down to the rocks in the Earth's crust. The age and nature of the rocks and fossils (remains of prehistoric plants and animals) help geologists understand the workings of the Earth. Geologists also help discover valuable deposits of coal, oil, and other useful minerals. They study the land before a large structure such as a dam is built, to make sure that the land can support the great weight. Geologists also warn people about possible disasters. Using special instruments, they detect the movement of rocks and try to predict volcanic eruptions and earthquakes.

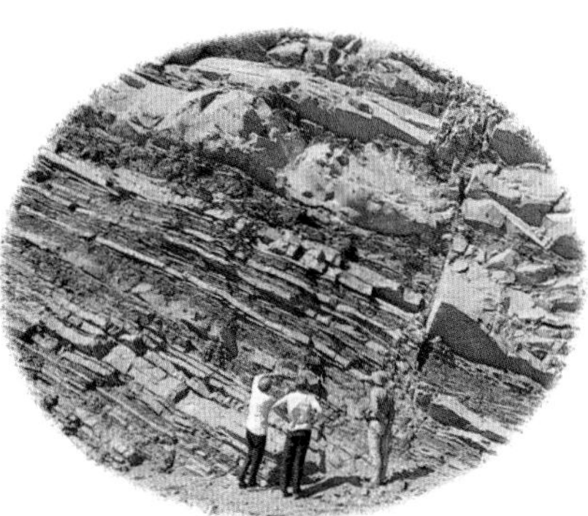

GEOLOGISTS AT WORK
Rocks at the Earth's surface reveal their past to the expert eyes of geologists. For example, huge cracks in layers of rock show that powerful forces once squeezed the rocks.

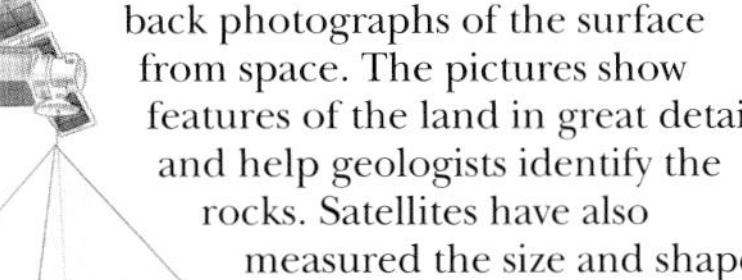

SATELLITE MAPPING
Satellites circle the Earth and send back photographs of the surface from space. The pictures show features of the land in great detail and help geologists identify the rocks. Satellites have also measured the size and shape of the Earth.

Studying the rocks in the ocean floor can reveal the slow movements of the Earth's crust.

AERIAL SURVEYS
Aeroplanes carry special cameras that produce three-dimensional views of the land below, and instruments that measure the strength of the Earth's magnetism and gravity.

SEISMIC TESTS
Special trucks strike the ground with huge hammers, producing shock waves, called seismic waves, which bounce off the layers of rock below. Computers use these waves to draw pictures of the layers of rock within the Earth.

RADIOACTIVE DATING
Rocks contain substances which decay over millions of years, giving off tiny amounts of nuclear radiation. By a process called radioactive dating, which measures this radioactivity, geologists can find out how old the rocks are.

DRILLING
Rigs bore shafts as deep as 3,000 m (10,000 ft) below the ground and bring up samples of the rock layers beneath.

SANDSTONE
The top and youngest layer of rock is sandstone. It sometimes forms from desert sands. The criss-cross pattern shows how the wind blew sand to form the rock.

SHALE
A layer of shale rock shows that the land must have been beneath shallow water. Mud from a nearby river built up and compacted, forming shale.

BASALT
Lava from a volcano formed this layer of basalt. The land rose from the sea, and a volcano erupted nearby to cover the rock below with lava.

LIMESTONE
The lowest and oldest layer contains fossils of tiny creatures, showing that 100 million years ago, during the time of the dinosaurs, the region was under the sea.

ROCK SAMPLE
The layers of rock in this sample (above) come from deep underground.

THE HISTORY OF GEOLOGY

The Ancient Greeks and Hindus were the first peoples to study and date the rocks of the Earth. During the late 18th century, the Scottish scientist James Hutton became the first European geologist to realize that the Earth is millions of years old and that it changes constantly. But his ideas were not accepted until after his death. In 1912, Alfred Wegener, a German meteorologist, proposed that the continents move. But it was more than 50 years before his idea was found to be true.

In 1795 James Hutton founded the modern science of geology with his book The Theory of the Earth.

EXAMINING THE EARTH

The Earth's crust is made of layer upon layer of different kinds of rock which have been laid down over millions of years. The topmost layers usually formed most recently and the lowest layers are the oldest. By uncovering these layers of rock, geologists can trace back the history of the Earth.

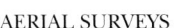

Find out more
COAL
CONTINENTS
EARTH
EARTHQUAKES
FOSSILS
GAS
OIL
ROCKS AND MINERALS

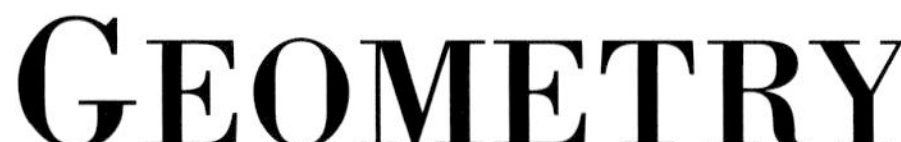

GEOMETRY

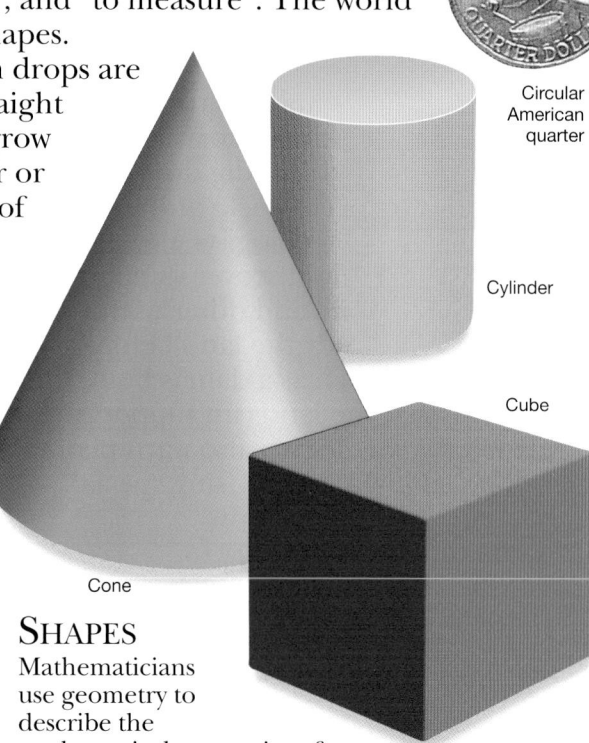

Seven-sided twenty-pence piece

Circular American quarter

THALES
The Ancient Greek philosopher and scientist Thales (c. 624-c. 547 B.C.) visited Egypt and Babylon where he studied local methods of astronomy and land-surveying. He developed the first theories about geometry based on his studies. He is also said to have predicted the solar eclipse of 585 B.C.

THE STUDY OF SHAPES, POINTS, LINES, curves, surfaces, and angles is called geometry. It takes its name from two Greek words meaning "Earth", and "to measure". The world around us is full of geometrical shapes. Liquids have flat surfaces and rain drops are perfect spheres. Objects fall in straight lines and spin in circles. Crystals grow into prisms with square, triangular or hexagonal sections. A knowledge of geometry helps us to understand these shapes. Geometry also has many practical everyday uses. Architects use geometry to construct buildings that will not fall down. Engineers need geometry to build safe roads and bridges. Pilots and sailors use geometrical principles when plotting routes. The principles of geometry were first discovered and written down by Ancient Greek scholars, but we still use them today.

Cylinder

Cube

Cone

SHAPES

Mathematicians use geometry to describe the mathematical properties of shapes. They use terms such as lengths, angles, areas, and volumes to describe the relationships between sides, corners, and surfaces. Shapes may be two-dimensional, such as circles, triangles, rectangles, and polygons. Or they may be three-dimensional, such as cones, cylinders, and cubes.

The diagram above shows that the shell uses a sequence of curves within squares. These decrease in size by a particular percentage each time, so creating the shell's spiral.

NATURAL GEOMETRY

Many things in nature possess geometric properties. An Italian mathematician, Leonardo Fibonacci (c. 1170-c. 1250), noticed that objects such as snail shells have shapes that use geometric sequences of measurements to form complicated curves such as spirals.

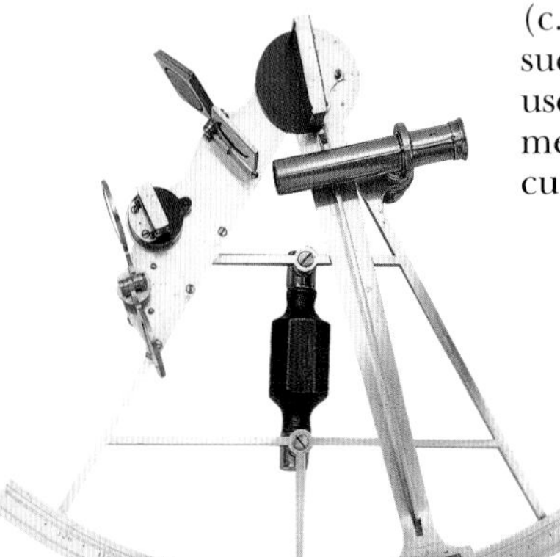

SEXTANT
The sextant was invented in the 1730s for navigating on board ship. By measuring the angle between a particular star and the horizon, the sextant uses the geometry of triangles to calculate the ship's position.

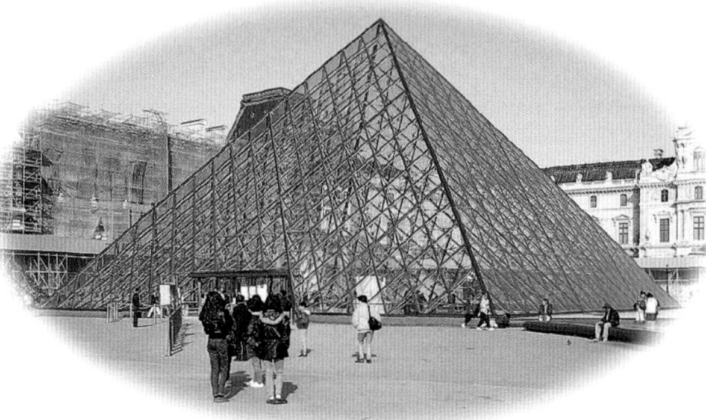

GEOMETRY IN USE
Many everyday activities make use of geometry, including architecture and engineering. For example, the famous glass pyramid at the Louvre in Paris, France, is triangular, and is made up from hundreds of smaller triangles. The entire structure is a combination of two- and three-dimensional geometric shapes.

ANGLES
Geometry is concerned with angles, or the amount by which a line or object turns in relation to a given point. Angles are formed by lines meeting at points, and are measured in degrees (°). A right angle is at 90° to a straight line. An obtuse angle is greater than 90°, and an acute angle is less than 90°.

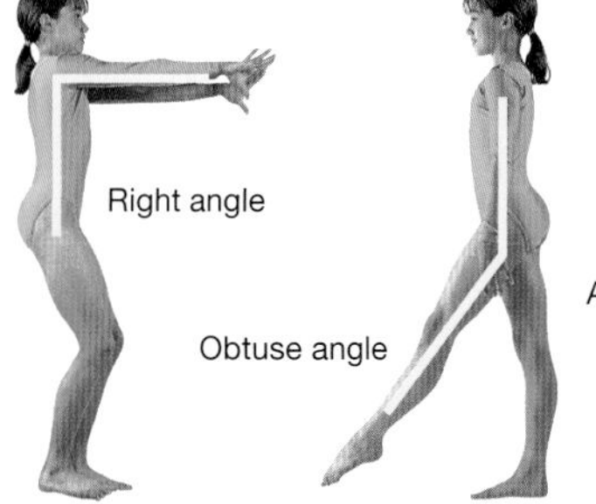

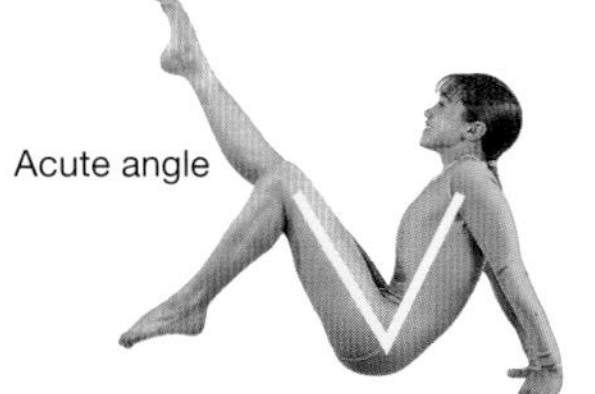

Find out more
ARCHITECTURE
GREECE, ANCIENT
MATHEMATICS
NAVIGATION

GERMANY

GERMANY OCCUPIES A CENTRAL position in northern Europe, and its 82.5 million people play a central role in the economy, way of life, and traditions of Europe. Germany is an old country, and its borders have changed often over the centuries. For much of the second half of the 20th century, Germany consisted of two separate nations: West Germany (the Federal Republic of Germany) and East Germany (the German Democratic Republic). In 1990 they became one nation and the Berlin Wall was removed. Germany is a rich and fertile land, and its farms are among the world's most productive. The landscape rises gently from the sandy coasts and islands on the North Sea and Baltic Sea. Flat plains dominate the northern part of the country, and in the south there are forests and the soaring Alps. The region's cool, rainy weather helps agriculture. Farms produce livestock and dairy products, cereals, potatoes, sugar beet, fruits, and vegetables. Most people, however, live in and around the towns where Germany's energetic industries are based.

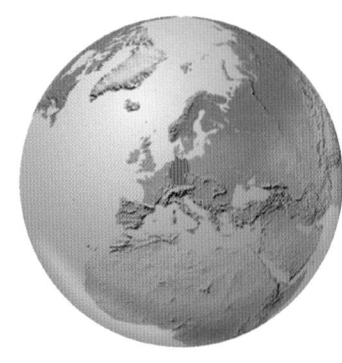

Germany lies at the heart of Europe. From the flat plains of the north to the snow-capped peaks of the Bavarian Alps, the landscape is varied.

Sausage sellers specialize in various kinds of wurst and often sell their wares from tiny stalls or vans.

Beer gardens attached to bars and pubs are popular in warm weather.

WURST AND BEER

Germany produces some excellent wine and is also famous for its beer. Germans often drink beer with the traditional snack of a sausage (or wurst) and a bread roll, accompanied by a large dollop of mild mustard. There are numerous kinds of wurst, and every region has its speciality. Frankfurters, a type of wurst, originally came from Frankfurt.

The Brandenburg Gate stands on the line that once divided East and West Berlin.

BERLIN

Reinstated as the capital of all Germany in 1990, Berlin grew up on the banks of the River Spree. Canals also link Berlin to the Elbe and Oder rivers. Berlin was devastated in World War II. In 1949 the city was split between the two states of East and West Germany. For many years a wall separated the people in the eastern and western sectors, and the two parts of the city still look very different. New buildings have made western Berlin look like any other modern European city. Eastern Berlin still suffers poor infrastructure and buildings.

Leitz camera factory

INDUSTRY

There is a wide range of industries in Germany that produce electrical goods, computers, tools, textiles, and medicines. Coal mines in the central Ruhr region produce large quantities of brown coal, or lignite, to fuel the factories. Western Germany is famous for high-quality precision goods, such as BMW cars and Leitz cameras.

Bavaria

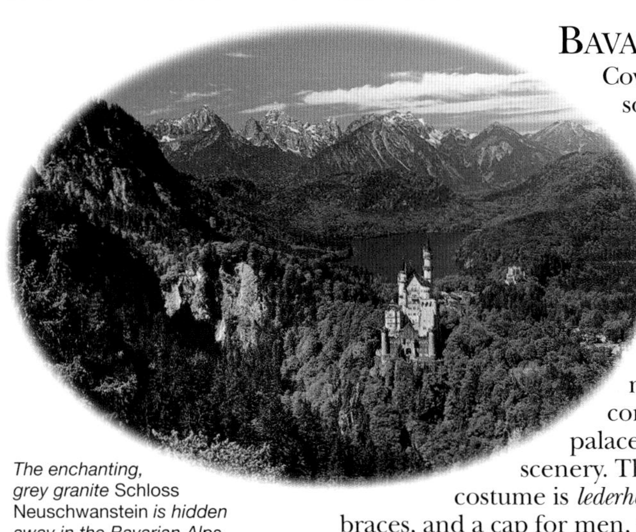

The enchanting, grey granite Schloss Neuschwanstein *is hidden away in the Bavarian Alps.*

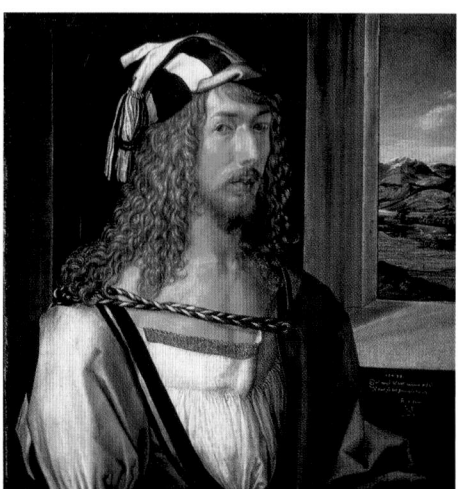

Covering the entire southeastern part of the country, Bavaria is the largest state in Germany. Most of the region is cloaked by forests and farms. In the south, the Bavarian Alps form a natural border with Austria. Bavaria is a magnet to tourists, who come to see its fairy-tale palaces (left) and spectacular scenery. The region's traditional costume is *lederhosen* (leather shorts), braces, and a cap for men, and *dirndlkleider* (a full-length dress with puffed sleeves) for women.

DÜRER
Born in Nuremberg, Albrecht Dürer (1471-1528), is famous for his paintings and engravings. He produced his first self-portrait at the age of 13, and painted himself at intervals throughout his life. He produced this self-portrait (above) when he was 26. At the age of 15 Dürer was apprenticed to Michael Wolgemut, Nuremberg's chief painter and book illustrator. He was inspired by the painters of the Italian Renaissance and resolved to depict people and things in realistic detail. In 1512, Dürer became court painter to the Emperor Maximilian, and gained international fame.

SEMPER OPERA HOUSE
The architect Gottfried Semper (1803-79) built his first opera house, the Royal Theatre, on Theaterplatz square in Dresden, in the years 1838-1841. Almost 30 years later it burnt to the ground and the opera was forced to move to temporary premises. Public pressure persuaded Semper to create a second opera house between 1871 and 1878. The new building (right) followed the style of the Italian High Renaissance. Following its destruction during an air raid in the Second World War, it was rebuilt in its original form between 1977 and 1985. Its exquisite acoustics and opulent interior decoration make it a model for opera houses throughout the world.

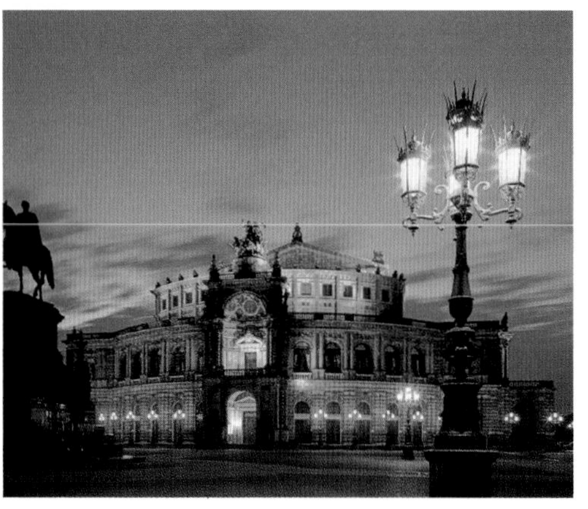

DRESDEN
The city of Dresden in eastern Germany was once the capital of a historic German state called Saxony. Although there are still some beautiful buildings in Dresden, including the former royal palace (below), most of the city's fine architecture was destroyed by Allied bombing in World War II (1939-45). Dresden has now been completely rebuilt, and many of the buildings restored.

Dresden was once admired as the "Florence on the Elbe".

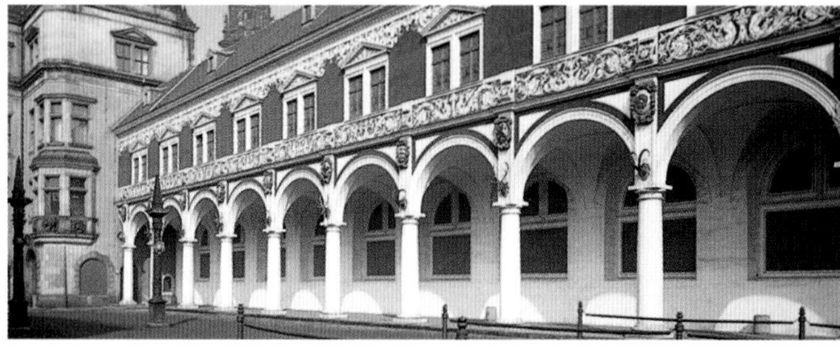

Brothers Grimm

Jakob (1785-1863) and Wilhelm (1786-1859) Grimm were born in Hanau, near Frankfurt. Devoted to each other, the brothers went to the same school and university, and lived together until Wilhelm's death. The Grimm brothers are famous for their collections of German folktales, which include the well-known tales of *Cinderella, Hänsel and Gretel, Rapunzel, Snow White and the Seven Dwarfs, Sleeping Beauty* and *Little Red Riding Hood.* The brothers did not create these stories themselves, but gathered them together from the accounts of country folk, and old books. Most of the stories date back hundreds of years.

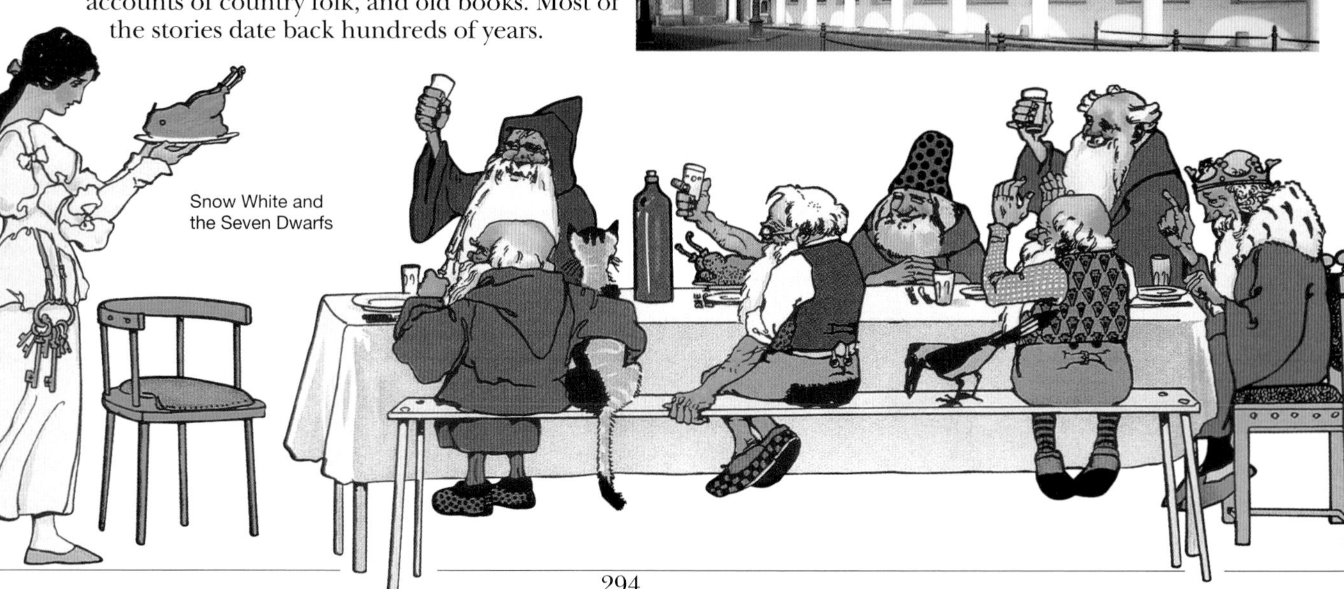

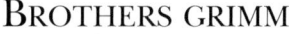

Snow White and the Seven Dwarfs

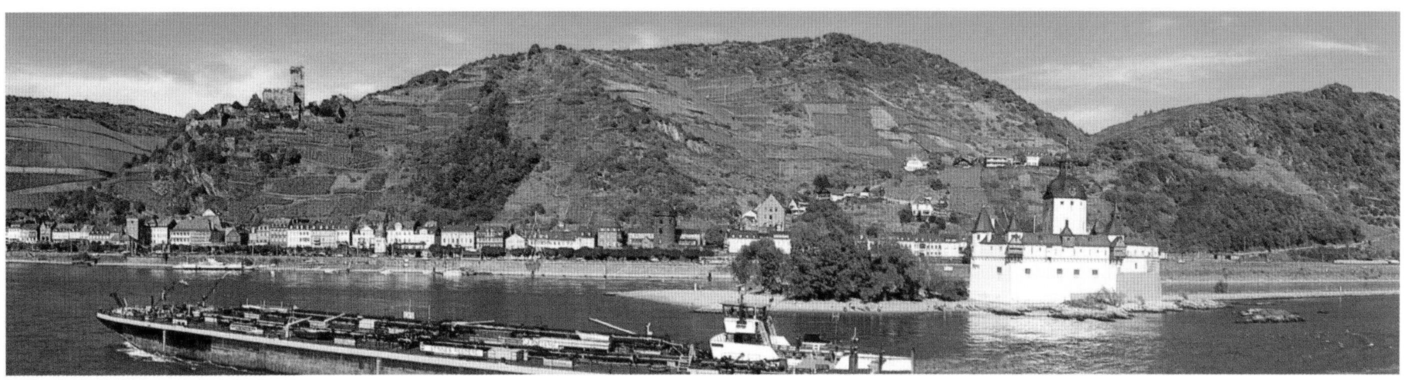

RIVER RHINE
The Rhine is the longest river in Germany. It begins in Switzerland and later forms the German border with France. Then it cuts through the western part of Germany towards the Netherlands and the sea. Large river barges can sail up the Rhine as far as Basle, Switzerland. Vineyards on the steep banks of the southern part of the river produce much of Germany's famous white wine.

SPORTING ACHIEVEMENT
Germany has produced some excellent sports people over the last few decades. Sporting stars include Boris Becker, Steffi Graf, and Michael Stich in tennis, Michael Schumacher in motor racing, and Katja Seizinger in skiing. The German government encourages sports, mainly because it promotes good health. Prizewinning athletes also bring great honour to their country.

The joining of East and West Germany brought together some of the world's finest athletes. When the two countries were rivals, East German competitors were aided by excellent sports facilities, and special privileges gave them time to train. They won many more events than West German counterparts.

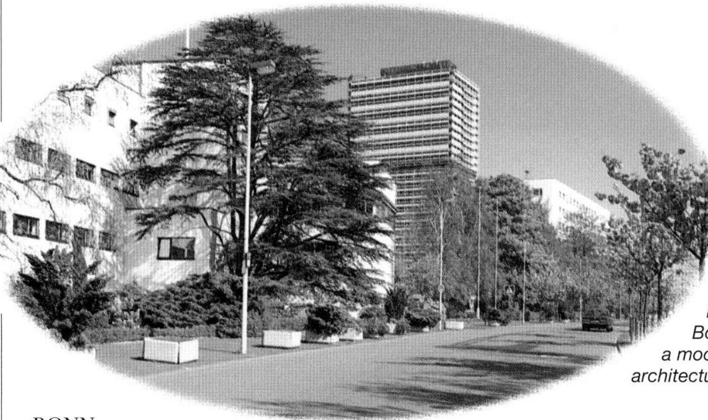

The buildings in parts of Bonn have a modern architectural style.

BONN
Between 1949 and 1990, Bonn was the capital of West Germany. Bonn, an ancient city, stands on the River Rhine on the site of a Roman camp. It is an old university town with many beautiful buildings in traditional German style. Bonn was the birthplace of composer Ludwig van Beethoven (1770-1827).

RUHR VALLEY

Much of Germany's heavy industry is concentrated in the valley of the Ruhr river. Huge coal seams provide the valley with a rich source of power, and factories in the region produce iron, steel, and chemicals. The Ruhr Valley is Germany's most densely populated area.

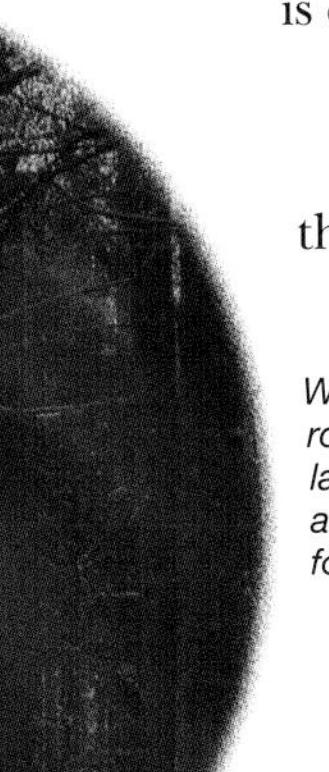

Wild boar still roam in the larger forests and are hunted for their meat.

FORESTS
Great forests cover many of the hills and mountains of the central and southern regions of Germany. These forests are prized for their beauty and for their valuable timber, which is used widely in industry. The most famous forests include the Thüringer Wald, the forests of the Harz Mountains in central Germany, and the Schwarzwald, or Black Forest, in southwest Germany.

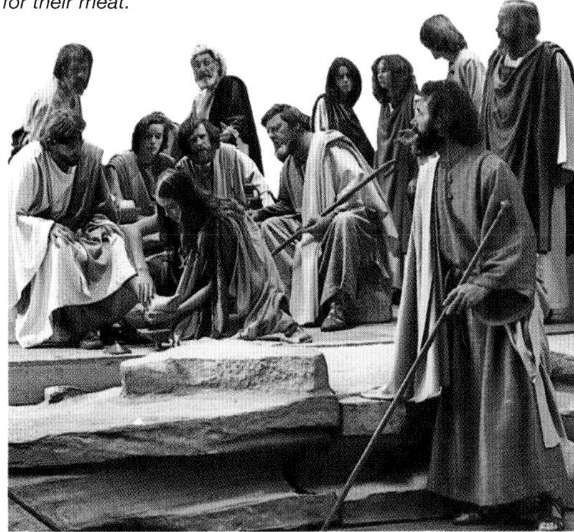

OBERAMMERGAU
Once every 10 years an extraordinary event takes place in this small town in the Bavarian Alps in southern Germany. The inhabitants of Oberammergau get together to perform a passion play, which tells the story of Christ's crucifixion. The villagers first performed the play in 1634 in an effort to stop the plague. They have maintained the custom ever since. It is now a major tourist attraction, and thousands of visitors from Germany and abroad attend.

Find out more
EUROPE
GERMANY, HISTORY OF

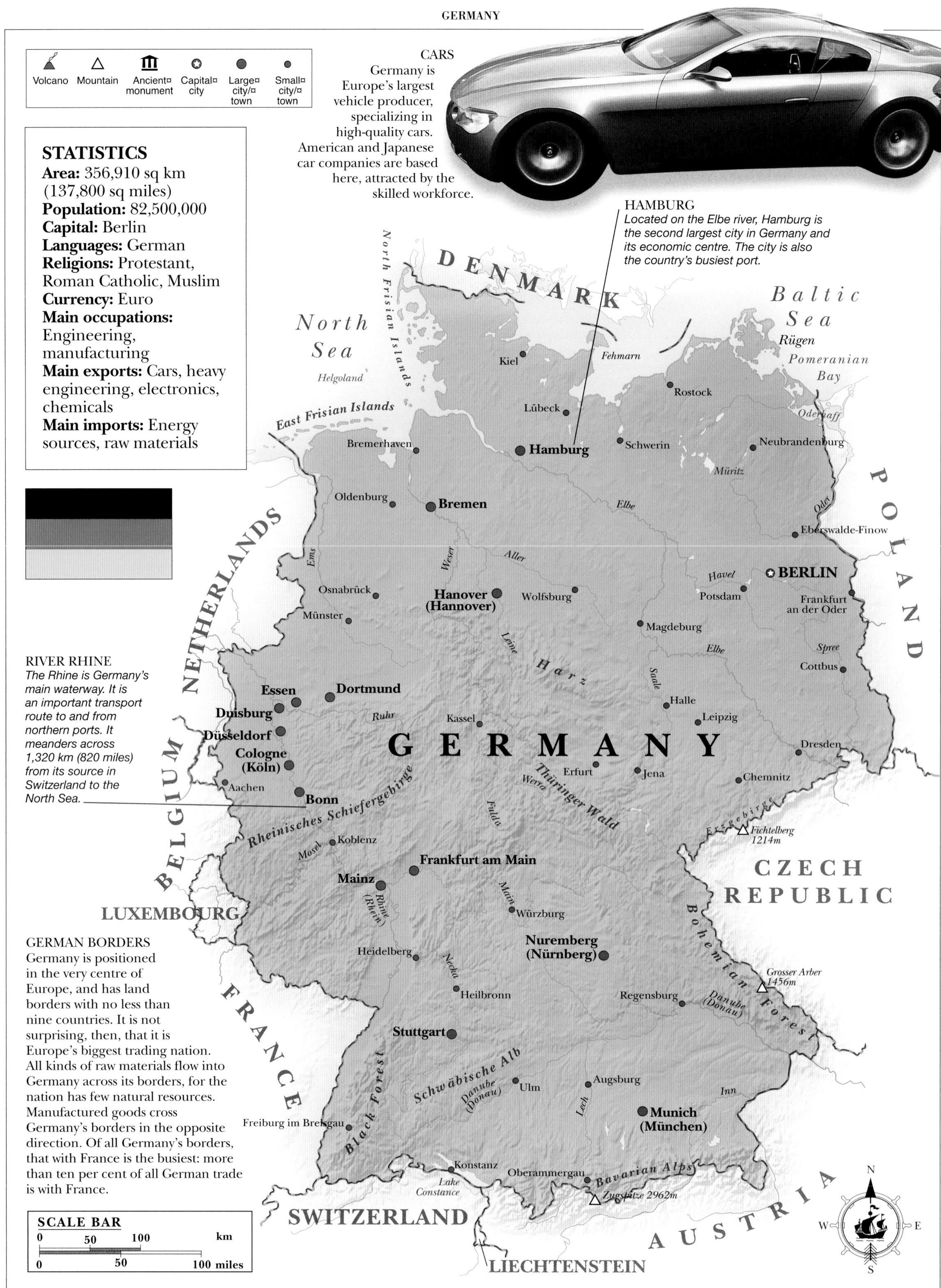

CARS
Germany is Europe's largest vehicle producer, specializing in high-quality cars. American and Japanese car companies are based here, attracted by the skilled workforce.

STATISTICS
Area: 356,910 sq km (137,800 sq miles)
Population: 82,500,000
Capital: Berlin
Languages: German
Religions: Protestant, Roman Catholic, Muslim
Currency: Euro
Main occupations: Engineering, manufacturing
Main exports: Cars, heavy engineering, electronics, chemicals
Main imports: Energy sources, raw materials

HAMBURG
Located on the Elbe river, Hamburg is the second largest city in Germany and its economic centre. The city is also the country's busiest port.

RIVER RHINE
The Rhine is Germany's main waterway. It is an important transport route to and from northern ports. It meanders across 1,320 km (820 miles) from its source in Switzerland to the North Sea.

GERMAN BORDERS
Germany is positioned in the very centre of Europe, and has land borders with no less than nine countries. It is not surprising, then, that it is Europe's biggest trading nation. All kinds of raw materials flow into Germany across its borders, for the nation has few natural resources. Manufactured goods cross Germany's borders in the opposite direction. Of all Germany's borders, that with France is the busiest: more than ten per cent of all German trade is with France.

HISTORY OF

GERMANY

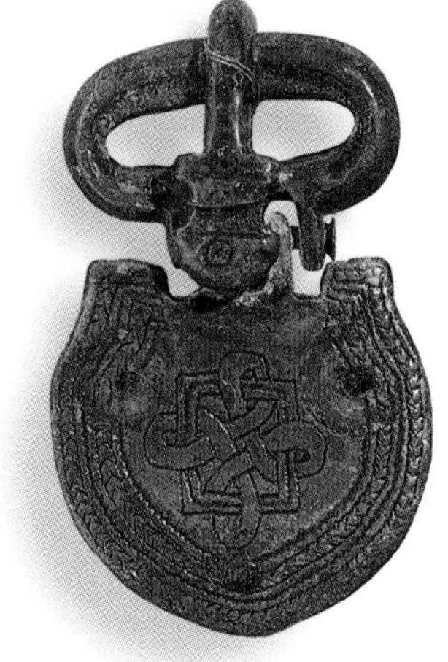

FRANKISH KINGDOM
During the 3rd century the Franks, one of many warlike tribes in Germany, settled along the River Rhine. By the 800s the West Franks ruled what is now France, and the East Franks governed Germany. The Franks were skilled metalworkers, as shown by the bronze buckle and belt fitting above.

FOR MOST OF ITS HISTORY, the land of Germany has consisted of many small independent states, each with its own ruler and set of laws. Over the years there have been many attempts to unite these states into one country. In the 800s Charlemagne, emperor of the Franks, ruled most of Germany and what is now France. His successors tried to maintain this union by setting up the Holy Roman Empire. This empire consisted of Germany and surrounding areas, but Germany was united only in name, for the different states fiercely protected their independence. During the 1500s the Reformation, a movement to reform the Church, divided Germany into Protestant and Catholic states. Prussia emerged as the strongest state, challenging the dominance of the Austrian Hapsburg family. In 1871, the various states of Germany became one country under Prussian rule. But after Germany was defeated in World War II (1939-45), the country was divided again into two separate states – Communist East Germany (German Democratic Republic) and non-Communist West Germany (Federal Republic of Germany). In 1990, East and West Germany were once again united into one country.

PEASANTS' WAR

In 1524, the German peasants rose against their lords. They demanded better social and economic conditions, including the right to elect their clergy and to hunt and fish. They were encouraged by the teachings of Martin Luther (1483-1546), who wanted to reform the Church. But Luther supported the lords, who crushed the revolt without mercy a year after it had begun.

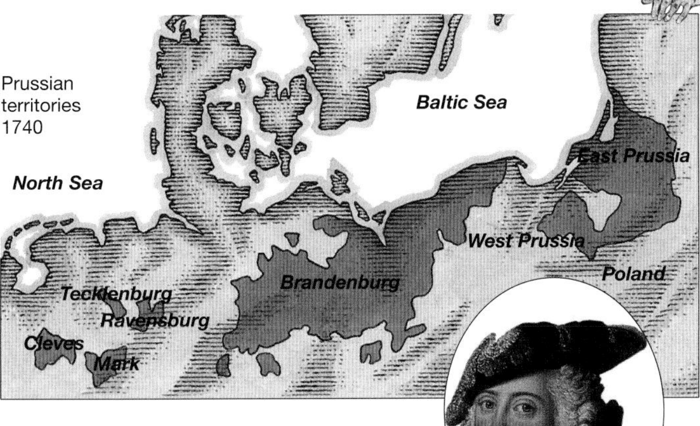

PRUSSIA
Following the Thirty Years' religious war, which destroyed Germany, there was no central power, until Prussia began its rise to power. Prussia was originally a small state in what is now northern Poland. It slowly grew in size until, under the leadership of King Frederick the Great (reigned 1740-86), it became the most powerful state in Germany.

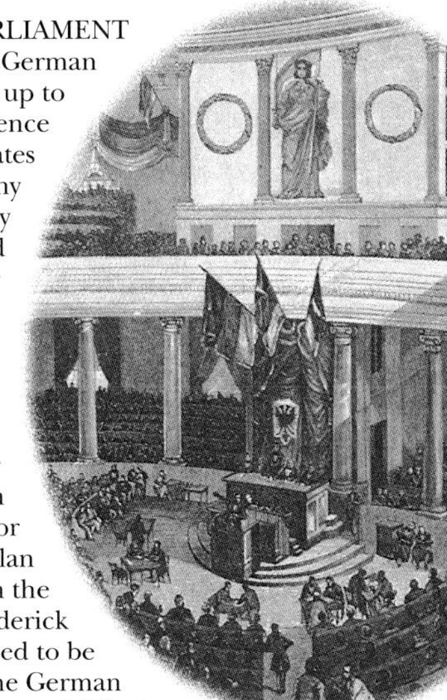

FRANKFURT PARLIAMENT
In 1815, a German Confederation was set up to protect the independence of the 39 separate states that existed in Germany at the time. But Germany was less advanced and prosperous than other European countries. Many people were dissatisfied and wanted unity. In 1848, a group of politicians set up a parliament (law-making group) to meet in Frankfurt to prepare for German unity. The plan failed in 1849 when the Prussian king, Frederick William IV, refused to be emperor. Soon the German Confederation was re-established.

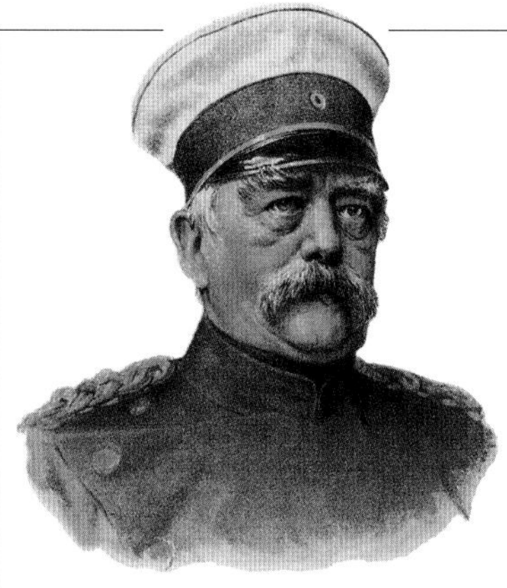

OTTO VON BISMARCK
In 1871, statesman Otto von Bismarck (1815-98), chancellor of Prussia, united Germany under Prussian leadership. Bismarck built the new republic of Germany into a great power. He was famous for his political skill.

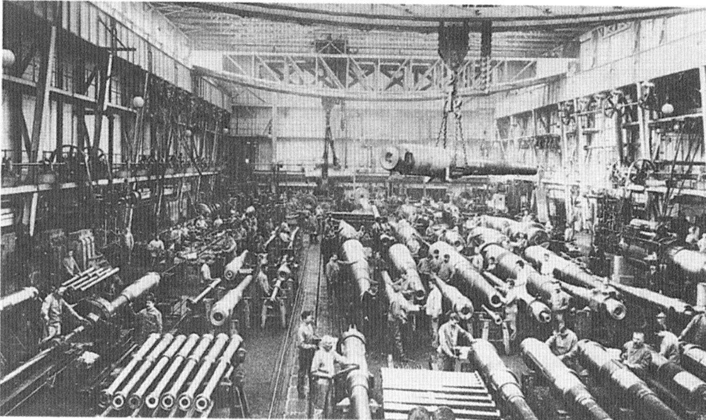

KRUPPS FACTORY
Arms manufacturers, such as Krupps (above), founded in 1811, helped create a powerful German army for the new united Germany.

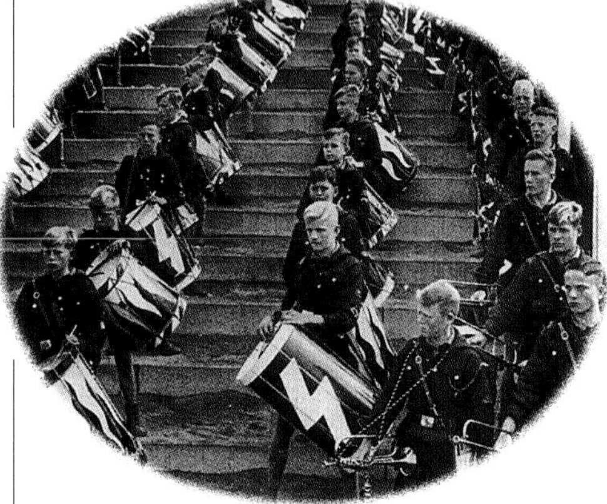

HITLER YOUTH MOVEMENT
In 1933, Adolf Hitler and the Nazis came to power. The Nazis (National Socialist German Workers' Party) believed in strong national government and restricted personal freedom. They organized all sections of society to support the Nazi party. Every young person between the ages of 10 and 18 had to join the Hitler Youth Movement, which became the only youth group allowed to exist under German law.

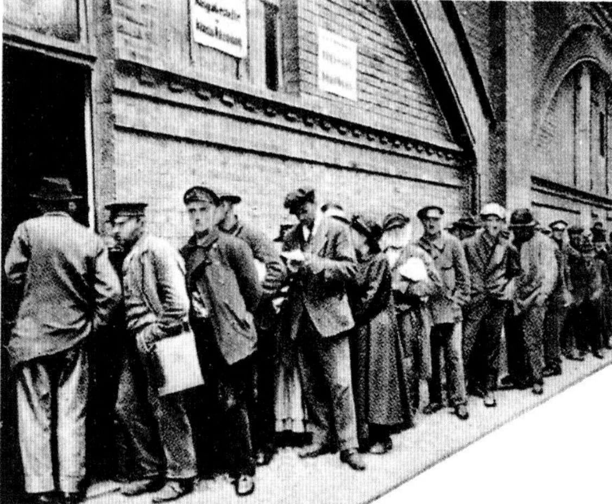

DEPRESSION
The German economy was hit badly by the peace settlements after World War I (1914-18). By 1931, the country, like the rest of the world, was in an economic slump. Thousands of people were out of work and had to line up for food. In desperation, many supported extreme political parties, such as the Nazis, which they hoped would help them out of their poverty.

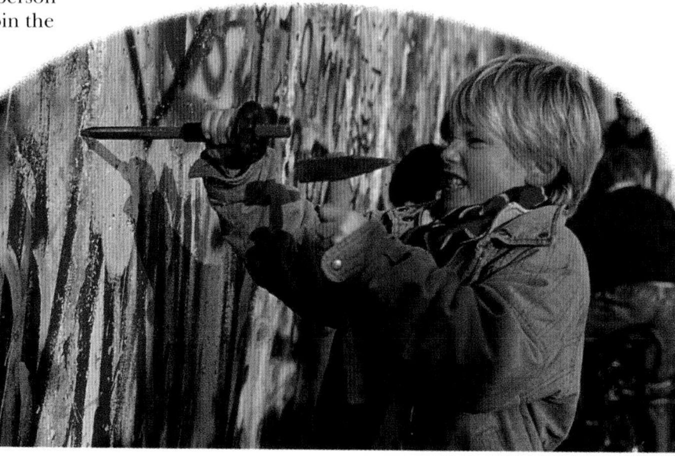

UNITED GERMANY
In 1961 the Communists built a big wall of concrete and barbed wire in Berlin, the former German capital, dividing it into East and West Berlin. This was to block the escape route into West Germany where living and working conditions were much better. In 1989, the people of Berlin demolished the wall, and the following year, East and West Germany were united.

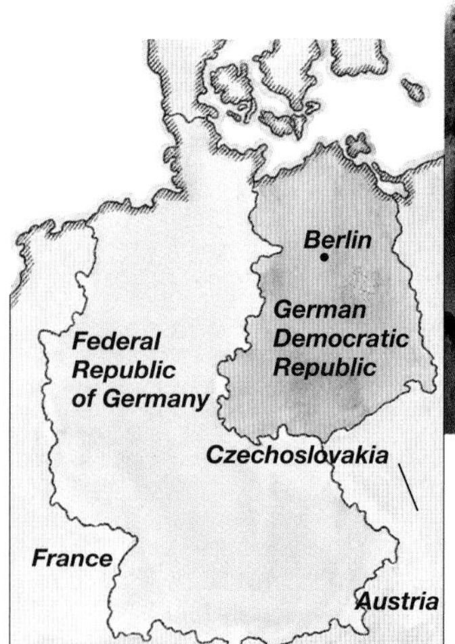

DIVIDED GERMANY
After losing World War II, Germany was divided into two: the Federal Republic of Germany (non-Communist) in the West, and the German Democratic Republic (Communist) in the East.

GERMANY

200s Franks settle along the River Rhine.

c. 800 Charlemagne creates a huge Frankish kingdom in western Europe, uniting Germany for the first time.

843 East Franks form the first all-German kingdom.

962 King Otto I is crowned the first Holy Roman Emperor; the empire consists of a loose grouping of German states.

1300s Austrian Hapsburg family begins to dominate Germany.

1517 Martin Luther begins Reformation in Wittenberg.

1524-25 Peasants' War

1555 Religious conflict following the Reformation ends at the Peace of Augsburg.

1740-86 Prussia emerges as the most powerful German state.

1815 German Confederation is established.

1848-49 Frankfurt Parliament attempts to unify Germany.

1862 Otto von Bismarck becomes chancellor of Prussia.

1914-18 Germany and Austria fight Russia, France, and Britain in World War I.

1919 Treaty of Versailles imposes harsh peace terms on Germany, which becomes a republic.

1933 Nazi party takes power.

1939-45 Germany invades rest of Europe during World War II.

1945 Russian, American, and British troops defeat Hitler and occupy Germany.

1949 Germany is divided into two states, Communist East Germany and non-Communist West Germany.

1961 Berlin Wall divides city.

1989 People of Berlin demolish Berlin Wall.

1990 East and West Germany unite to form one state.

Find out more
Charlemagne
Germany
Holocaust
Reformation
World war II

GLACIERS
AND ICECAPS

SNOW FALLING on the world's tallest mountain peaks never melts. The temperature rarely rises above freezing, and fresh falls of snow press down on those below, turning them to ice. A thick cover of ice, called an icecap or ice sheet, builds up, or snow collects in hollows. Ice flows down from the hollows in rivers of ice called glaciers. They move very slowly, usually less than 1 m (3.3 ft) a day, down towards the lower slopes. There it is usually warmer, and the glaciers melt. However, in the Arctic and the Antarctic, glaciers do not melt. Instead they flow down to the sea and break up into icebergs or form a floating ice shelf. A huge icecap covered much of North America and Europe a million years ago during the last Ice Age. When the weather became warmer, about 10,000 years ago, some ice melted, and the ice sheet shrank. Ice sheets now exist only in Greenland and Antarctica.

GLACIERS
Glaciers often join together, just as small rivers meet to form bigger rivers. The ice may be more than 1 km (0.5 mile) deep.

ICECAP
Icecaps cover vast areas. When the thickness of the ice reaches about 60 m (200 ft) its enormous weight sets it moving.

VALLEY GLACIER
The ice fills a valley, moving faster at the centre than at the sides of the glacier. Cracks called crevasses open in the surface.

MORAINE
The glacier acts like a huge conveyor belt, carrying broken rocks, called moraines, down from the mountaintop. The moving ice also plucks stones and boulders from the base and sides of the valley. This material is carried along within the glacier, and is called englacial moraine.

CIRQUES
The hollow where the ice collects to start the glacier is called a cirque or corrie.

Streams of water form as the glacier melts.

Rocks in the melting ice build up a wall called a terminal moraine.

SHAPING THE LANDSCAPE
Glaciers slowly grind away even the hardest rock and reveal a changed landscape when they retreat. Deep valleys and lakes, together with rivers and waterfalls, now exist where there were none before.

Waterfall

A river flows down the centre of the valley.

Deep U-shaped valley carved out by the glacier

Lake formed behind moraines

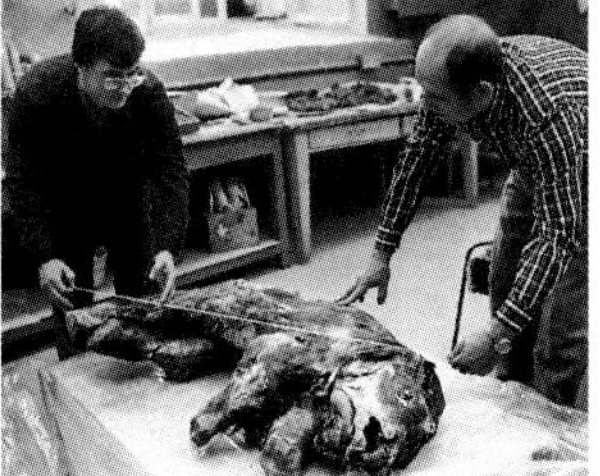

FROZEN MAMMOTHS
In the Russian Federation, ice and frozen soil have preserved huge hairy elephants, called mammoths, just as if they were in a deep freeze. The last mammoths lived in North America, Europe, and Asia during the Ice Age.

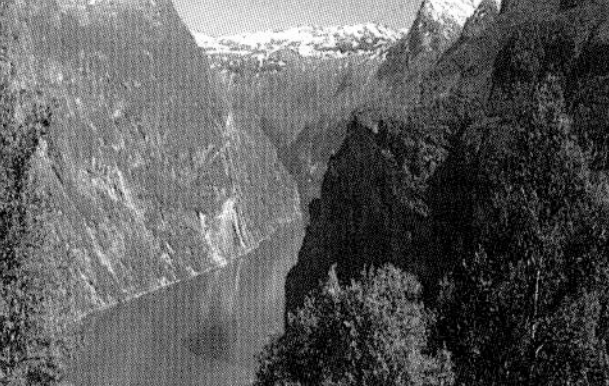

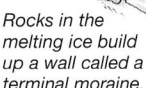

FJORDS
The sea rose at the end of the Ice Age, drowning valleys formed by glaciers. These deep, steep-sided inlets are called fjords. The coast of Norway has many fjords.

ICEBERGS
Huge pieces of floating ice are called icebergs. Nine tenths of the ice floats below the water, so icebergs are a danger to ships. In 1912 the ocean liner *Titanic* sank after colliding with an iceberg.

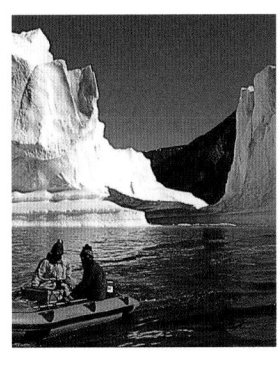

ICE AGE
A deep ice sheet covered about a third of the world's land during the last Ice Age. Ice extended as far south as St. Louis, Missouri, and London. There had been ice ages before the last one, and there could be more in the future.

Find out more
ANTARCTICA
ARCTIC
MOUNTAINS
POLAR WILDLIFE
RAIN AND SNOW

Glass and Ceramics

Sticky clay and dry sand are more familiar on the end of a spade than on the dinner table. Yet these are the basic ingredients in the manufacture of the pottery plates we eat from, and the jars and bottles in which we buy preserved food and drink. Glass and ceramic materials share some useful qualities: they resist the flow of heat and electricity, and they have a hard, non-reactive surface. But they are different in other ways: light passes through glass but not ceramics, and ceramics stay strong when they are heated. In their most basic forms glass and ceramic objects are brittle, but special additives and manufacturing methods make both materials much tougher.

Glass and ceramics are ancient materials. The Egyptians made decorative glass beads more than 5,000 years ago, and pottery is even older.

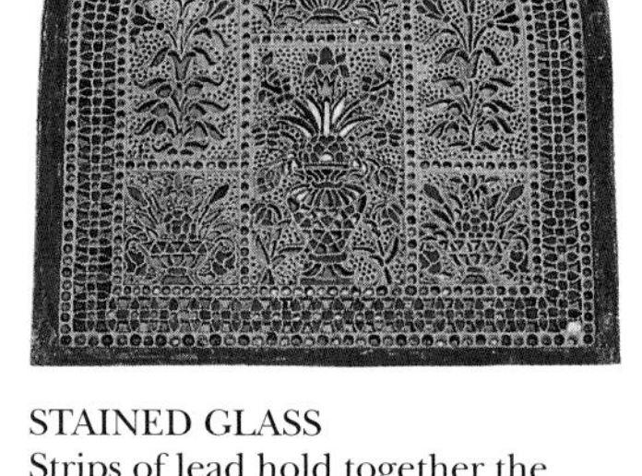

STAINED GLASS
Strips of lead hold together the many pieces of coloured glass in the stained glass windows that decorate homes, churches, and temples.

Glass

Containers of clear glass protect their contents and display them to good advantage. Lenses are specially shaped pieces of glass that bend and concentrate light. But not all glass is functional; some glassware is simply decorative.

Glass bottle for holding medicines

Glass bottle for holding ink

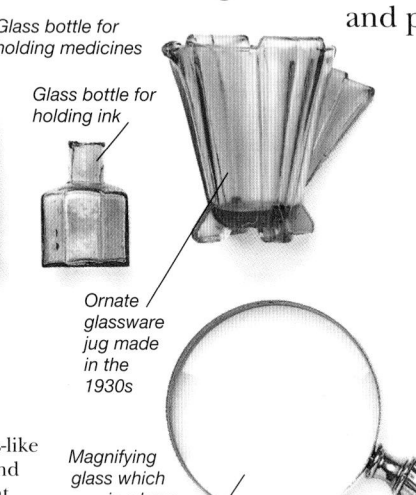

Ornate glassware jug made in the 1930s

Magnifying glass which is a large convex lens.

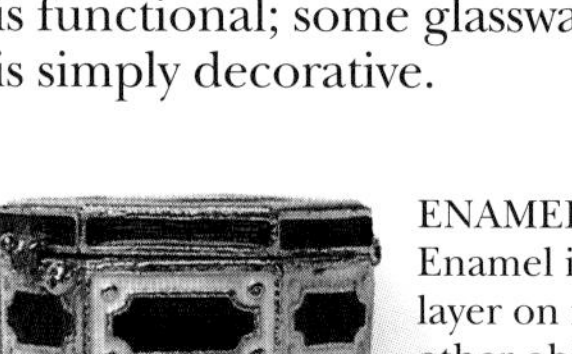

ENAMEL
Enamel is a glass-like layer on metal and other objects that protects them from damage and corrosion. Coloured enamel gives ornaments a beautiful appearance.

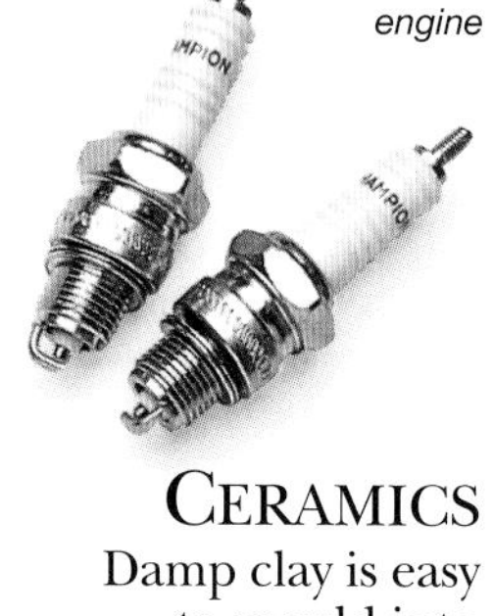

Spark plug for car engine

Ceramics

Damp clay is easy to mould into pottery and tiles; heat sets the shape permanently. Ceramics resist heat and electricity, so they are ideal for insulating objects that get hot, such as spark plugs.

Ceramic tile

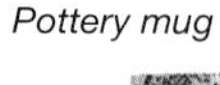

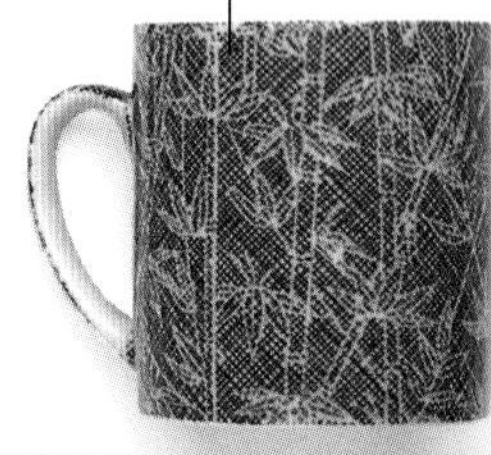

Pottery mug

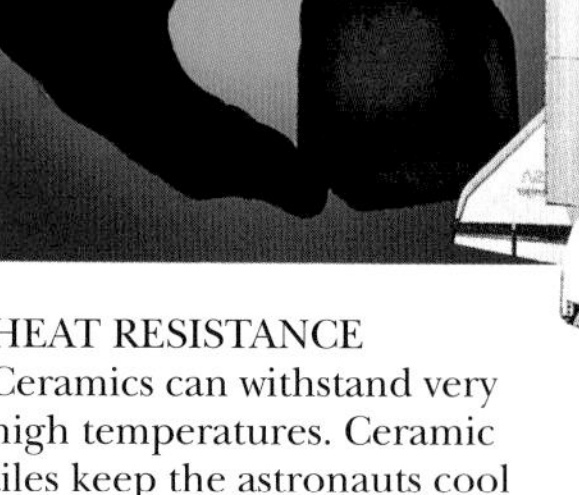

HEAT RESISTANCE
Ceramics can withstand very high temperatures. Ceramic tiles keep the astronauts cool even when the space shuttle glows red from the intense heat of re-entry.

Making glass

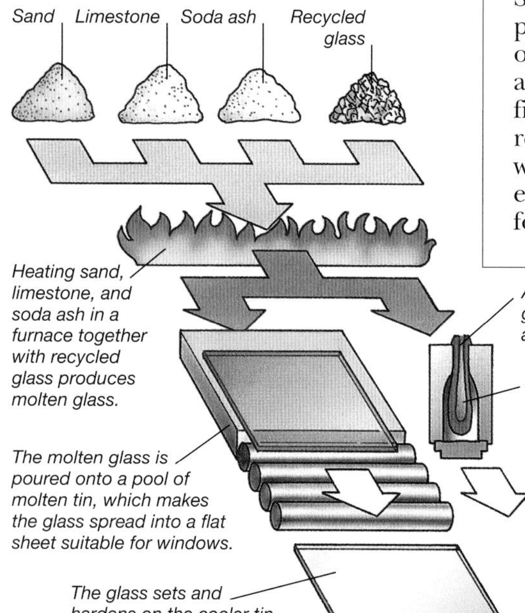
Sand
Limestone
Soda ash
Recycled glass
Heating sand, limestone, and soda ash in a furnace together with recycled glass produces molten glass.
The molten glass is poured onto a pool of molten tin, which makes the glass spread into a flat sheet suitable for windows.
The glass sets and hardens on the cooler tin.
A lump of hot, soft glass is placed in a bottle-shaped mould.
Blowing air into the mould makes the glass inflate into a bubble, which expands to form the bottle.
The glass then cools and sets hard.

Fibreglass

Strengthening plastic with fibres of glass produces a material called fibreglass or glass-reinforced plastic, which is tough enough to be used for car bodies.

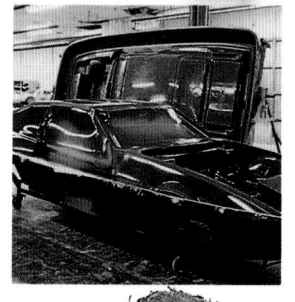

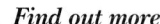

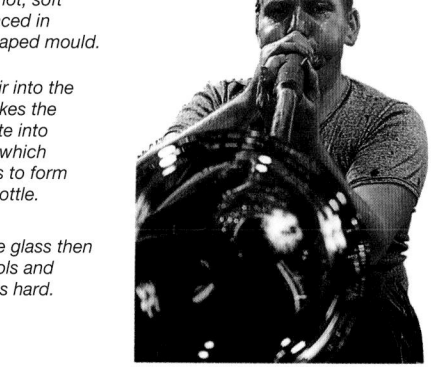

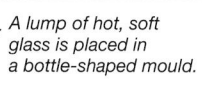

GLASS BLOWING
The breath of the glass blower inflates soft glass on the end of a tube into a bubble. Skilful shaping makes the bubble into fine glassware as it cools.

Find out more
Churches and cathedrals
Light
Plastics
Pottery

GOVERNMENT AND POLITICS

THE ADMINISTRATION OF A COUNTRY'S affairs is undertaken by a government whose policies direct decision making. Governments have many roles: they decide how money raised through taxes will be divided among the different public services, such as health, education, welfare, and defence. They also maintain the police for the safety of society and the armed forces for the defence of the nation. As a result of differing cultural and political traditions, government and policies vary from country to country. There are, however, three main types of government: republican, monarchical, and dictatorial. Most countries are republics, with people voting in an election to choose their government and head of state. In a monarchy, the head of the royal family is the head of state. Countries in which a single ruler has seized absolute power – often through a military takeover – are known as dictatorships.

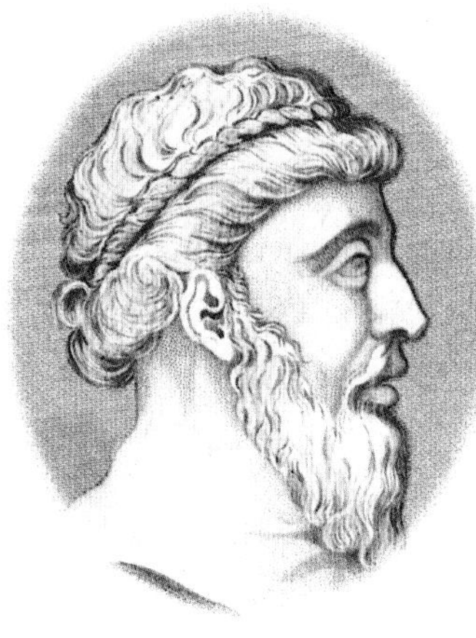

PLATO
More than 2,000 years ago the Greek philosopher Plato wrote the first book about governments and how they rule people – what we today call politics. His book, *The Republic,* set out ideas for democracy, a Greek word meaning "government by the people".

MONARCHY
In a monarchy a king or queen rules the country. Few modern monarchs have real political power, but four centuries ago, European monarchs made the laws and collected taxes.

PARLIAMENT

Many Western nations are democracies – they hold elections, in which the people vote for, or select, the next government from a range of political parties. Some countries, such as Britain and the Netherlands, have a parliamentary democracy. Elected politicians from different parties sit in parliament with the government and discuss the best way to run the country. The government is usually from the political party with the greatest number of votes in the election, and the leader of this party becomes leader of the government and the country.

Parliament buildings in The Hague, Netherlands

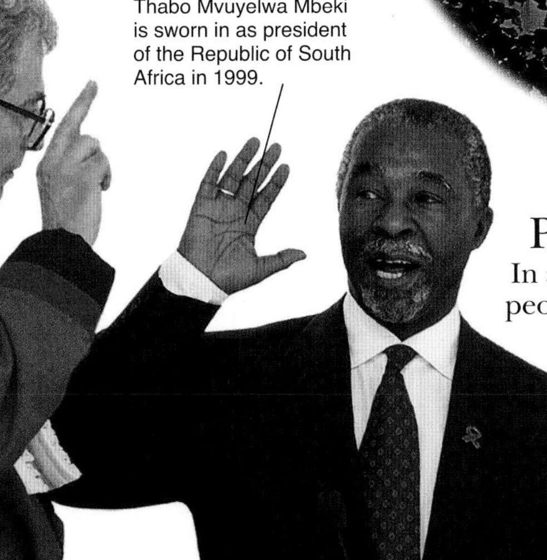

Thabo Mvuyelwa Mbeki is sworn in as president of the Republic of South Africa in 1999.

PRESIDENCY

In a republic, such as South Africa, the people vote for their head of state. In this case, the president holds real political power, and is responsible for the administration of the country and for its foreign policy. In France, power is divided between the president and the prime minister. In some countries, such as India, the president is more of a symbolic figurehead, who takes on a ceremonial role, rather like that of some monarchs.

ANARCHISM
Not everyone believes in governments. Anarchists prefer a society without central control. The 19th-century picture below shows a bomb placed at a Paris opera house by French anti-government protestors.

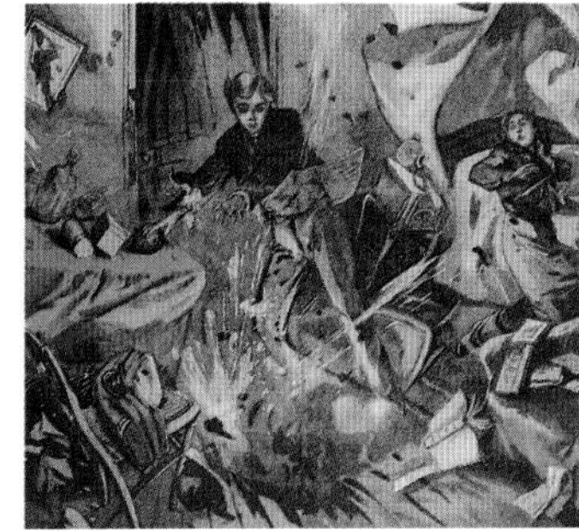

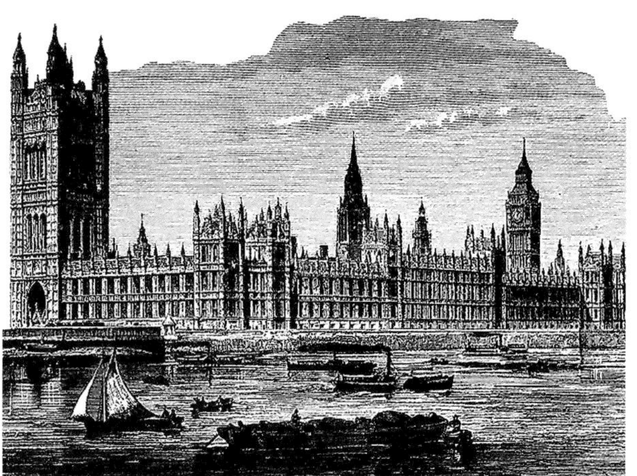

HOUSE OF LORDS

The House of Lords can amend or reject government legislation. It used to contain only hereditary peers, that is men who inherited titles such as earl from their fathers, as well as bishops and law lords. Many people thought this system undemocratic, so, in 1999, all but 92 hereditary peers were removed, leaving only peers chosen for life.

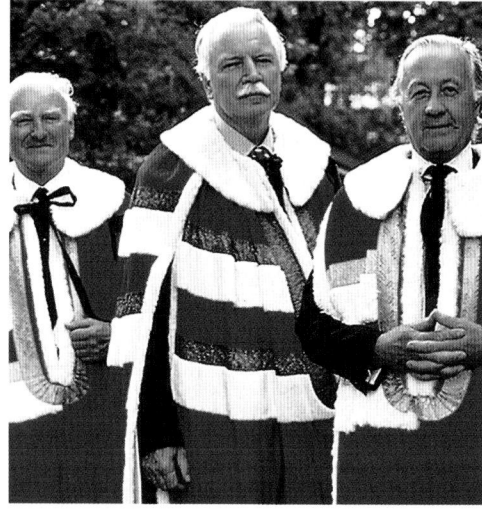

Westminster

There are three Houses of Parliament at Westminster: the House of Commons, the House of Lords, and the Crown in parliament – the monarch. Laws can be proposed in either the Commons or the Lords, but all three houses must give assent to a bill (a proposed law) before it becomes an Act of Parliament, or law.

BRITISH MONARCHY

The monarchy once had great power but now plays a ceremonial role. The monarch has the right to be consulted about government policy, can chose a new prime minister, and can call a general election, although in practice she or he only acts on the advice of the prime minister.

Elizabeth II, current monarch of the UK

Government

The government runs the country. It proposes new laws to parliament, and takes decisions on every aspect of our daily lives. The British government consists of 20 or so ministers who sit in the Cabinet, plus another 90 or so junior ministers. The head is the prime minister, who always sits in the House of Commons and is usually the leader of the largest political party. Other ministers can sit in the Commons or the Lords.

CIVIL SERVICE

The civil service is the bureaucracy, or administrative machine, that carries out the instructions of the government once a law is passed. Civil servants collect taxes and duties, distribute benefits, and run the many government departments.

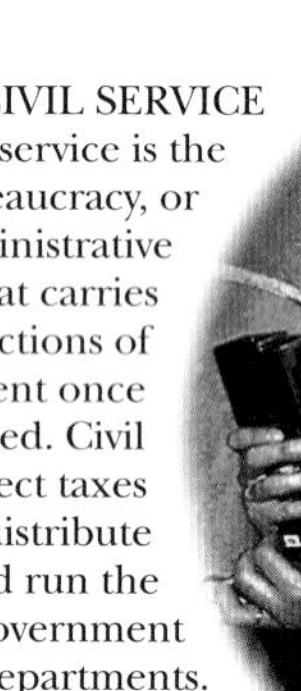

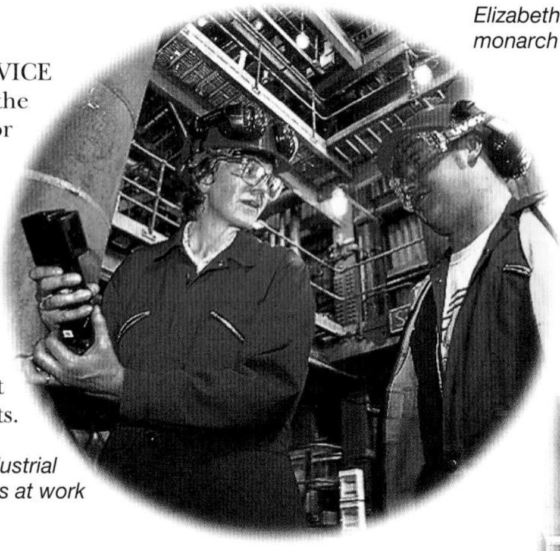

Government industrial chemists at work

THE SPEAKER

The Speaker of the House of Commons controls debates and keeps order in the Commons. She or he is a member of parliament (MP) and is elected at the start of each new session, once a year. Once elected, the speaker becomes neutral and may not cast a vote.

Betty Boothroyd MP, Speaker of the House of Commons from 1992 to 2000

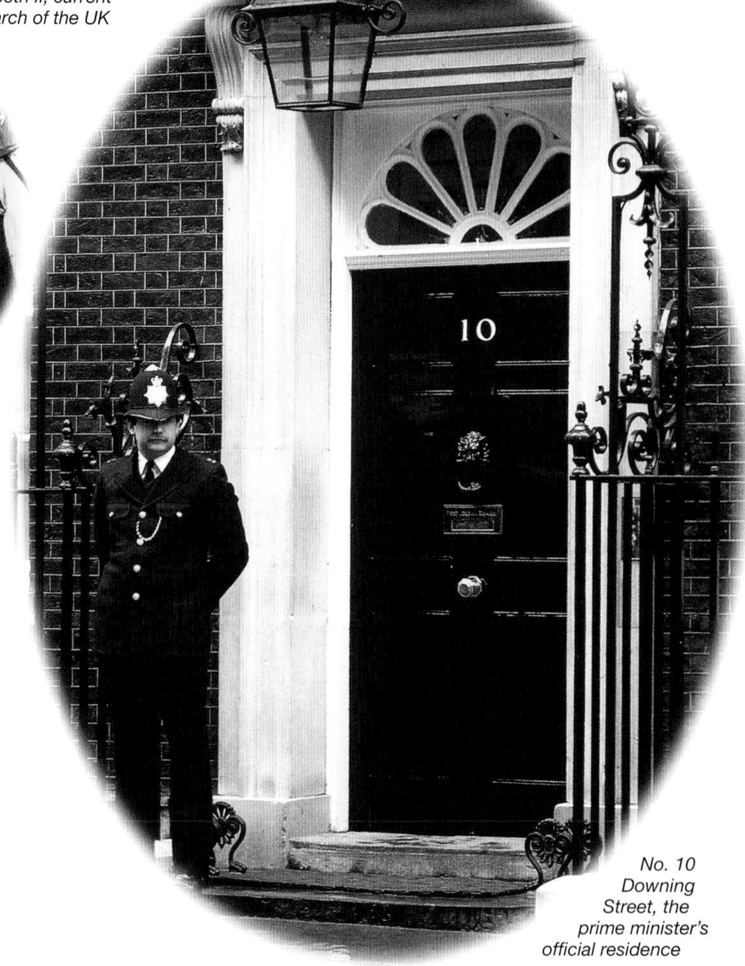

No. 10 Downing Street, the prime minister's official residence

Political parties

Political parties are organizations formed to represent particular views in government or local councils. Britain has three main parties: the Labour, Conservative, and Liberal Democrat Parties. Since 1945, the government has always been either Labour or Conservative. Nationalist parties support independence for their own areas. Politicians who do not belong to a political party are called independents.

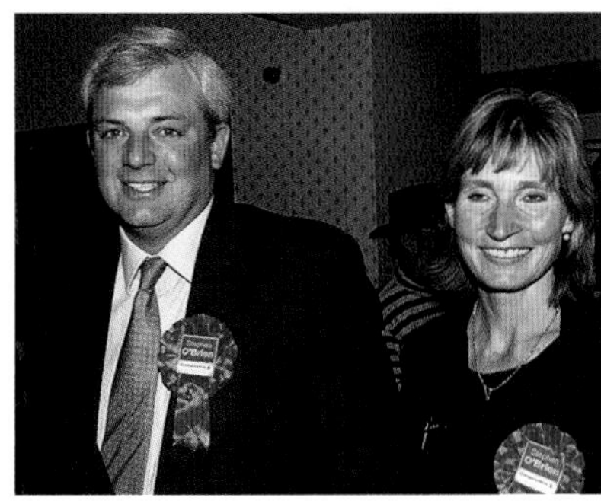

VOTING SYSTEMS

Most British elections are held under the first-past-the-post system, in which the person who gains the biggest number of votes wins. Other elections are based on proportional representation. In this system, w inning places are shared out according to the number of votes cast for each candidate.

PRESSURE GROUPS

People form pressure groups to obtain action or change in a particular cause. Some groups, such as the environmental organization Greenpeace, campaign on a range of issues, often taking direct action such as confronting whaling ships. Others are concerned with local causes, such as stopping a hospital closure, or individual cases, such as freeing a wrongly convicted person in jail. Pressure groups can be very effective in achieving their demands or getting politicians to change their minds.

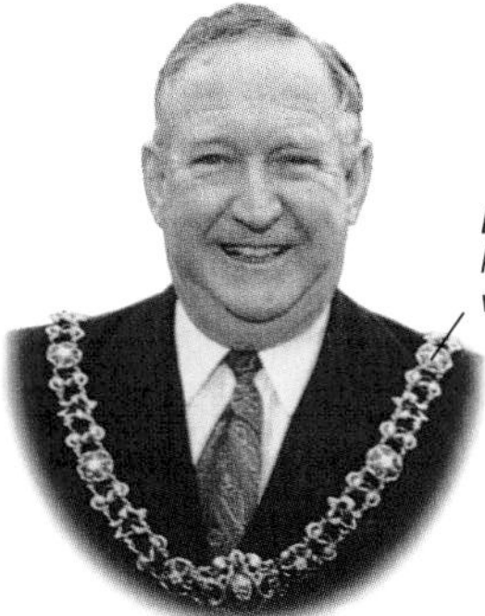

Local governments are led by a mayor who wears a chain of office.

LOCAL GOVERNMENT

Every British city and town has its own city or district council. In rural areas, county and district councils share power. Local government looks after education, housing, social services, the environment, and public health, and carries out national government's orders.

Devolution

Until recently, parliament in London was the only law-making body in the country. In 1999, parliament agreed to devolve (hand down) power to parliaments in Scotland and Wales, giving them limited powers to make their own laws. Similar attempts to devolve power to Northern Ireland have not been as successful because local politicians cannot agree on the best way to work together.

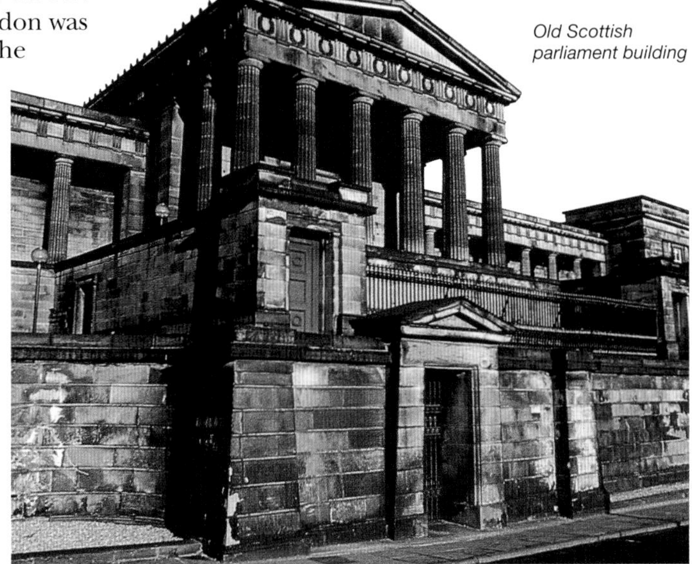

Old Scottish parliament building

BRITISH GOVERNMENT

1265 Representatives from each county and town summoned to parliament, the first time "commoners" attend.

1300s Commons and Lords become separate Houses of Parliament.

1376 First speaker elected.

1642 English Civil War between King and parliament.

1688 Glorious Revolution: monarch cannot pass laws without parliament's consent.

1707 English and Scottish parliaments united.

1832 Property-owning men gain vote.

1835 Town councils set up.

1853 Modern civil service begins.

1867 Working-class men in towns gain the vote.

1872 Secret voting introduced to stop bribery of voters.

1911 Payment for MPs.

1911 Power of House of Lords reduced; House of Commons is supreme.

1918 Women aged 30 gain the vote.

1928 Every adult aged 21 has the vote.

1958 Life Peers first sit in the House of Lords.

1969 Voting age reduced to 18.

1999 Scottish parliament and Welsh Assembly meet for the first time.

1999 House of Lords reformed, only 92 hereditary peers remain.

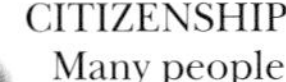

CITIZENSHIP

Many people know little about the government and politics of Britain because they did not learn much about them at school. In 2002, a new subject, citizenship, became part of the national curriculum. Every child learns how the government works and how they can influence and take part in decisions through voting in elections.

Tony Blair and the citizens of the future

Find out more

Democracy
English civil war
Law

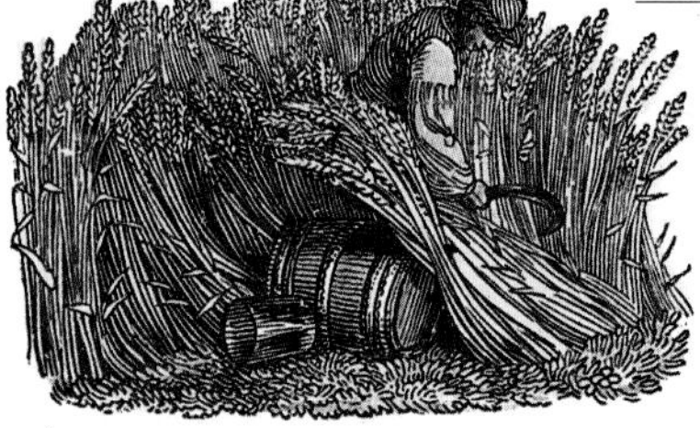

Grasses and Cereals

Harvesting cereal grain by hand is slow, hard work. A modern combine harvester can do the work of up to 100 farm hands.

THERE ARE MORE THAN 10,000 different kinds of grasses throughout the world. They include garden lawns, fields of barley, towering bamboos, and the African grasslands, where huge ostriches graze. Grasses are slender, flowering plants, with stiff stems and long narrow leaves called blades. Their many small roots are matted together. The flowers are feathery tufts without petals at the top of the stem. Grasses are pollinated by the wind, and seeds develop from the flowers in the same way as other flowering plants. Inside each seed is a grain, a rich food store for the plant, and also for us. Grasses are the major source of food for humans. We eat cereal grains in the form of bread, biscuits, and cakes, and also feed them to animals. Wheat and barley were two of the first plants cultivated (grown) by humans, about 10,000 years ago. Today wheat, rice, and corn are among the world's most important food crops.

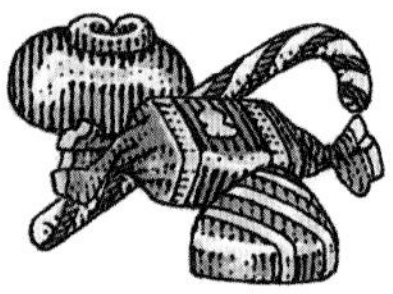

SUGAR CANE
Sugar cane plants grow up to 4.5 m (15 ft) high. At harvest time, the cane is cut off close to the ground and stripped of its leaves, then brought to a sugar mill. In the sugar mill the cane is shredded and then squeezed, and the syrup is turned into sugar for cooking and making sweets.

Oats

Wheat

Single rye grass flower

Stamen (male part)

Rye

Barley

Millet

Rice

Cereals

The ripe seeds of cereals such as oats, wheat, barley, rye, and corn are farmed to make breakfast cereals and other kinds of food. The stems are woven into baskets and turned into straw for animal bedding and thatching on houses. The leaves and stalks are put into a tower or a pit called a silo, where they are kept soft and damp. In time they turn into silage, or animal fodder.

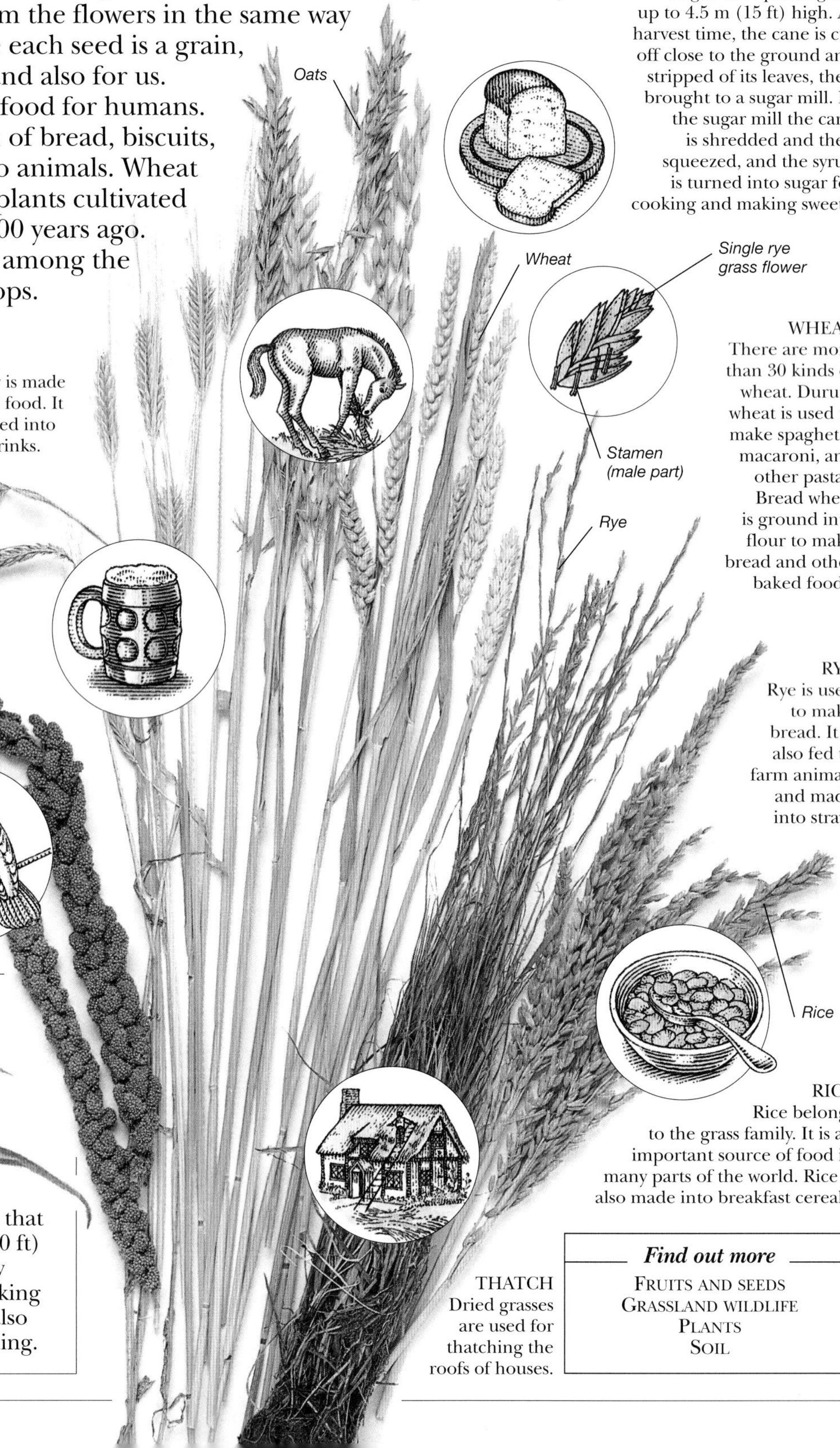

BARLEY
Most barley is made into animal food. It is also brewed into alcoholic drinks.

MILLET
Millet seeds are made into flat breads and porridges. Millet is also common in birdseed and animal fodder.

WHEAT
There are more than 30 kinds of wheat. Durum wheat is used to make spaghetti, macaroni, and other pastas. Bread wheat is ground into flour to make bread and other baked foods.

RYE
Rye is used to make bread. It is also fed to farm animals and made into straw.

RICE
Rice belongs to the grass family. It is an important source of food in many parts of the world. Rice is also made into breakfast cereals.

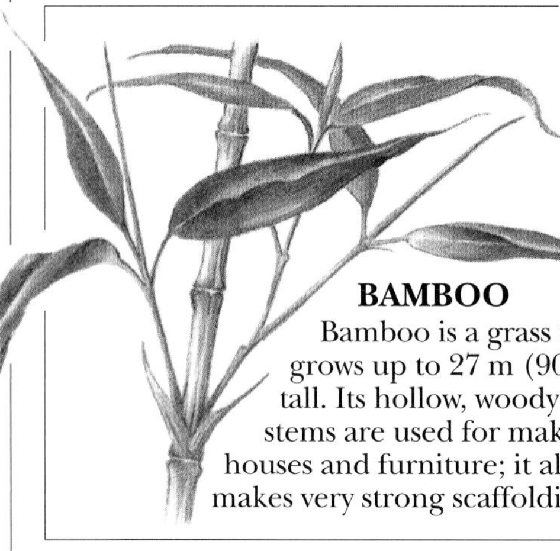

BAMBOO
Bamboo is a grass that grows up to 27 m (90 ft) tall. Its hollow, woody stems are used for making houses and furniture; it also makes very strong scaffolding.

THATCH
Dried grasses are used for thatching the roofs of houses.

Find out more
FRUITS AND SEEDS
GRASSLAND WILDLIFE
PLANTS
SOIL

GRASSHOPPERS AND CRICKETS

THE CHIRPING OF A GRASSHOPPER or a cricket is one of nature's most recognizable sounds. The sound is made by a male to attract a female or to warn off rival males. The insect produces the sound by rubbing together the ridged veins on the front wings, or by rubbing part of the back leg against the wing vein. Grasshoppers and crickets belong to the insect group called Orthoptera – a group that also includes katydids and locusts. There are more than 20,000 kinds of grasshoppers and crickets, living in all but the coldest regions. Grasshoppers are herbivores (plant eaters), feeding on leaves and stems, and crickets are omnivores (plant and meat eaters). A few of these creatures live underground and eat roots or digest nutrients in the soil. Most crickets and katydids have long antennae, sometimes longer than their bodies. Grasshoppers and locusts have much shorter antennae. All these insects have long back legs adapted for leaping. A large grasshopper can jump over a metre in one leap.

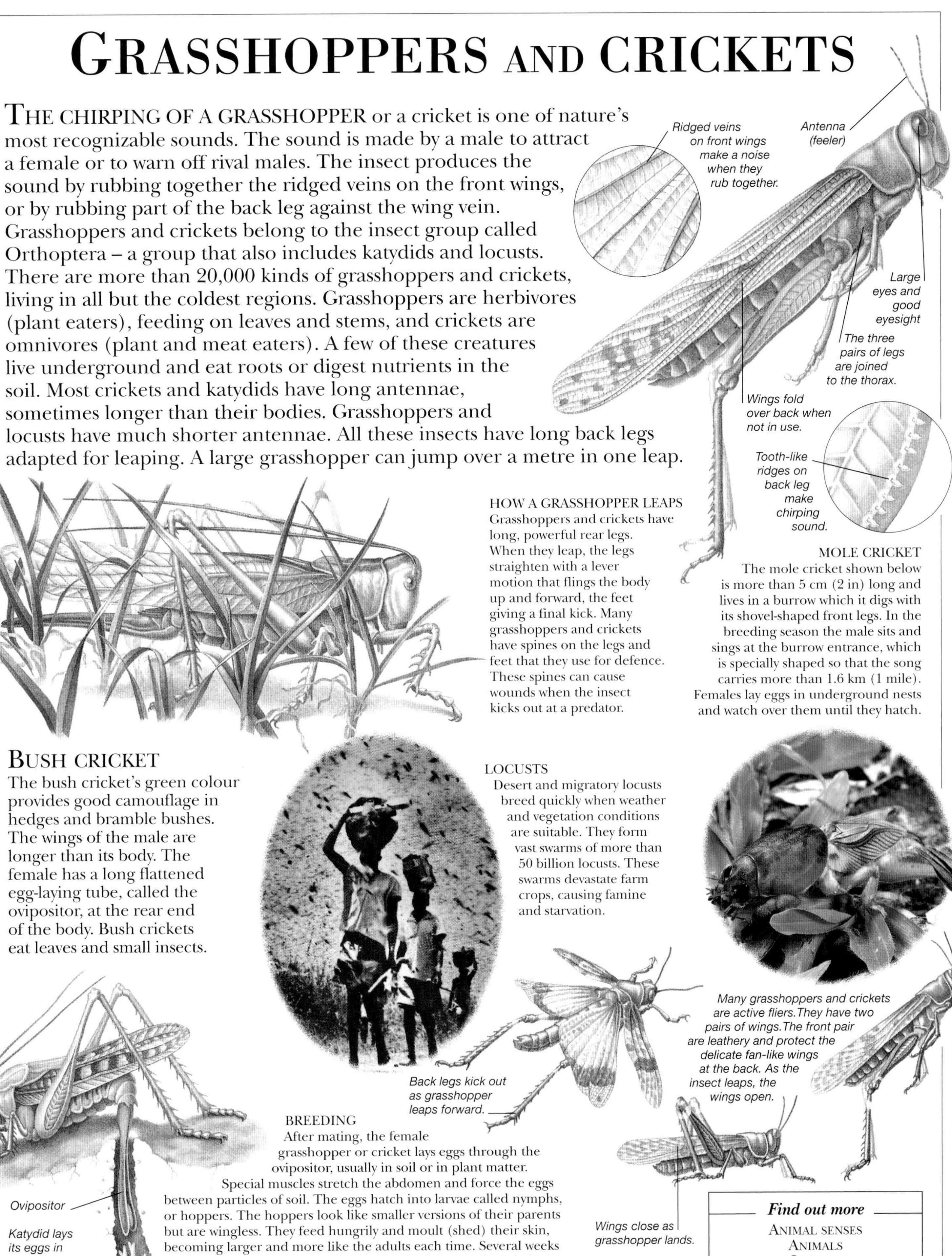

Ridged veins on front wings make a noise when they rub together.
Antenna (feeler)
Large eyes and good eyesight
The three pairs of legs are joined to the thorax.
Wings fold over back when not in use.
Tooth-like ridges on back leg make chirping sound.
Back legs kick out as grasshopper leaps forward.
Many grasshoppers and crickets are active fliers. They have two pairs of wings. The front pair are leathery and protect the delicate fan-like wings at the back. As the insect leaps, the wings open.
Wings close as grasshopper lands.
Ovipositor
Katydid lays its eggs in the soil.

HOW A GRASSHOPPER LEAPS

Grasshoppers and crickets have long, powerful rear legs. When they leap, the legs straighten with a lever motion that flings the body up and forward, the feet giving a final kick. Many grasshoppers and crickets have spines on the legs and feet that they use for defence. These spines can cause wounds when the insect kicks out at a predator.

MOLE CRICKET

The mole cricket shown below is more than 5 cm (2 in) long and lives in a burrow which it digs with its shovel-shaped front legs. In the breeding season the male sits and sings at the burrow entrance, which is specially shaped so that the song carries more than 1.6 km (1 mile). Females lay eggs in underground nests and watch over them until they hatch.

BUSH CRICKET

The bush cricket's green colour provides good camouflage in hedges and bramble bushes. The wings of the male are longer than its body. The female has a long flattened egg-laying tube, called the ovipositor, at the rear end of the body. Bush crickets eat leaves and small insects.

LOCUSTS

Desert and migratory locusts breed quickly when weather and vegetation conditions are suitable. They form vast swarms of more than 50 billion locusts. These swarms devastate farm crops, causing famine and starvation.

BREEDING

After mating, the female grasshopper or cricket lays eggs through the ovipositor, usually in soil or in plant matter. Special muscles stretch the abdomen and force the eggs between particles of soil. The eggs hatch into larvae called nymphs, or hoppers. The hoppers look like smaller versions of their parents but are wingless. They feed hungrily and moult (shed) their skin, becoming larger and more like the adults each time. Several weeks or months later, after about five moults, the hoppers shed their skin again and become full-sized winged adults.

Find out more

ANIMAL SENSES
ANIMALS
INSECTS

GRASSLAND WILDLIFE

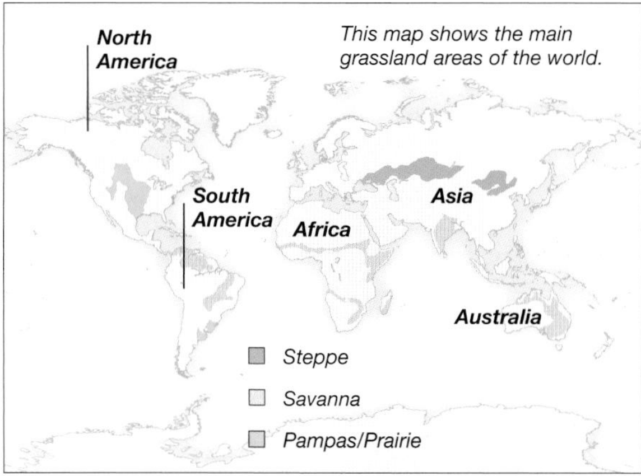

GRASSLAND AREAS
The main grassland areas in the world are the Asian steppes, African savannas and grasslands, North American prairies, and South American pampas, which blend into tropical Amazonian savanna. There are also tropical grasslands in parts of India and across Australia.

VAST AREAS OF AFRICA, the Americas, Asia, and Australia consist of grasslands – areas too dry for forests but not too dry for grasses. Grasses themselves are flowering plants that can grow again quickly after animals eat them. Grasses also recover quickly if fire sweeps across the plains in the hot, dry season. The fire burns only the upper parts of the grass, so the roots and stems are not damaged. Grasslands provide a home for many different animals; each survives by feeding on a different part of the grass plants. Zebras, for example, eat the coarse, older grass, while wildebeest (gnu) graze on new shoots. Thomson's gazelles nibble close to the ground. Grasshoppers, ants, and termites shelter among the grass stems and roots; these insects, in turn, are food for larger animals such as anteaters and armadillos. The lack of trees in grassland areas means that small animals and certain birds have to dig burrows for shelter and for breeding. Each type of grassland has burrowing rodents; prairie dogs and pocket gophers live in North America, susliks in Asia, ground squirrels in Africa, and vizcachas and tuco-tucos in South America.

Thistles grow in grassy areas throughout the world. Their prickles protect them against grazing animals. The flowers are often purple, and form fluffy white seed heads.

SOUTH AMERICAN PAMPAS

The largest mammals on the South American pampas are the pampas deer, guanaco, and rodents such as the viscacha, which burrows for shelter and safety. A fast-running bird called the rhea also lives on the South American pampas, feeding on grasses and other plants.

VISCACHA
The viscacha is related to the guinea pig. A male viscacha weighs about 8 kg (17 lb), almost twice the size of the female. Viscachas dig a system of burrows with their front feet and pile up sticks and stones near the various entrances. They eat mainly plant leaves and stems.

BURROWING OWL
The burrowing owl lives on the South American pampas. It often makes its nest in an empty burrow taken over from a viscacha. Burrowing owls eat grasshoppers, insects, small mammals, birds, lizards, and snakes.

GIANT ANTEATER

With large claws on its second and third fingers, the giant anteater can easily rip a hole in an ants' nest or a termite mound as it searches for food. The giant anteater uses its long, sticky tongue to lick up the ants and termites. Its tongue measures about 60 cm (24 in) in length.

Tail protects anteater's body as it sleeps in a shallow hole, listening for predators such as pumas.

PAMPAS GRASS
The white, fluffy seed heads of pampas grass are a familiar sight in parks and gardens. Wild pampas grass covers huge areas of Argentina, in South America. Pampas leaves have tiny teeth, like miniature saws, that easily cut human skin.

JACKAL
Golden jackals eat whatever they can find on the African savanna, including fruits, small mammals, eggs, birds, and the carcasses (dead bodies) of larger animals such as zebras.

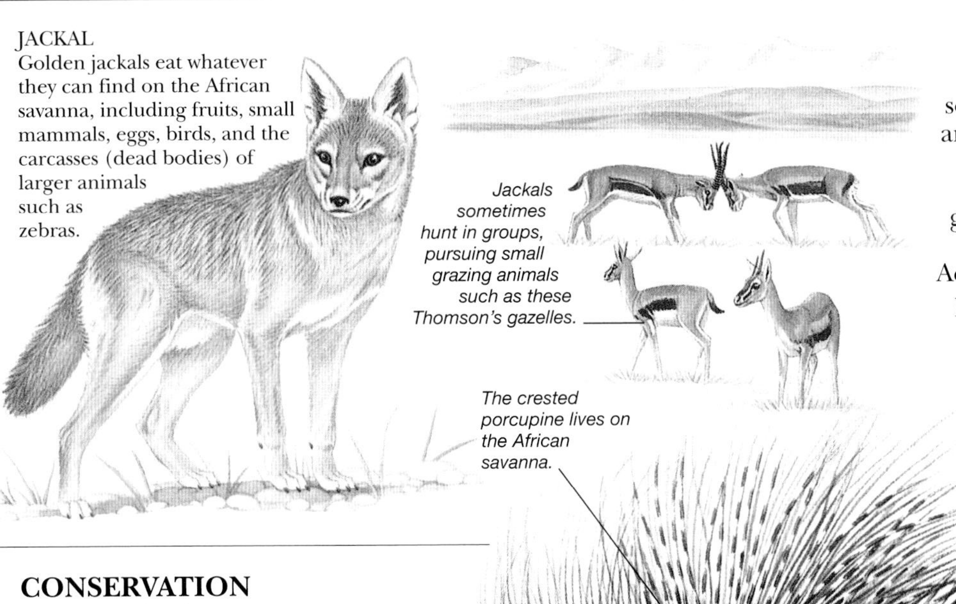

Jackals sometimes hunt in groups, pursuing small grazing animals such as these Thomson's gazelles.

Savanna

The huge grassland areas of eastern and southern Africa are called savannas. These areas are home to the world's largest herds of grazing animals, including zebra, wildebeest, and hartebeest. Many large grazers wander from one area to the next, following the rains to find fresh pasture. Acacia and baobab trees dot the landscape, providing shade for resting lions, ambush cover for leopards, and sleeping places for baboons.

THOMSON'S GAZELLE
These swift-moving mammals live on the grassy plains of Africa in herds of up to 30 animals. They all have horns, but those of the male are larger than those of the female. Thomson's gazelles are often the prey of other grassland animals, such as the cheetah and the jackal.

CONSERVATION

Many grassland areas are now used as farmland, and the natural wildlife is being squeezed into smaller areas. As a result, these areas become overgrazed and barren. Grassland animals are also threatened by human hunters. In the past the Asian saiga antelope was killed for its horns. Today it is protected by law, but it is still seriously endangered with only 50,000 left in the wild.

A newborn saiga antelope is fluffy and has no horns.

The crested porcupine lives on the African savanna.

CRESTED PORCUPINE
The crested porcupine has sharp spines on its back for protection. It warns enemies to stay away by rattling the hollow quills on its tail. If an intruder ignores these warnings, the porcupine runs backwards into the enemy, and the quills come away and stick into the intruder's flesh.

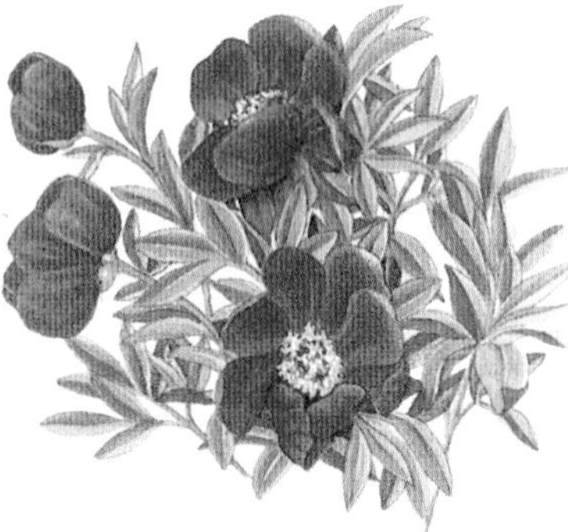

Wild peonies are found in many grassy habitats around the world. Many garden peony plants came originally from the hardy wild peonies that grow in grassland areas.

Steppe

The vast plains of Asia are called steppes. In the western part of Asia the rainfall is more than 25 cm (10 in) each year, and grasses and other plants grow well. Towards the eastern part of Asia there is less than 6 cm (2.5 in) of rainfall yearly, and the grasses fade away into the harsh Gobi Desert. Saiga antelopes, red deer, and roe deer graze on the rolling plains.

GRASS SNAKE
The grass snake lives on riverbanks and in marshes, mainly in Europe and Asia. Grass snakes are good swimmers.

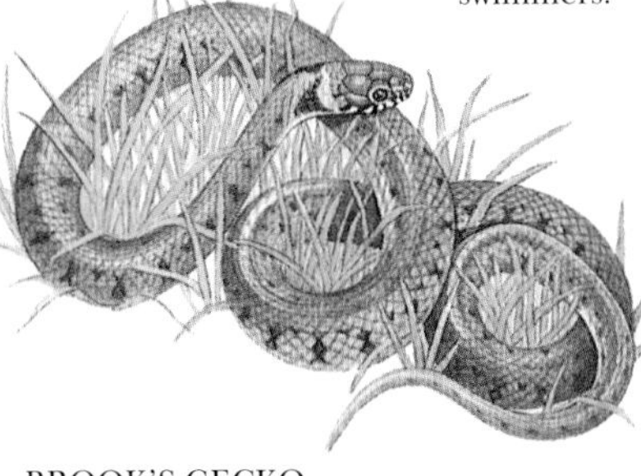

PALLAS'S CAT
This long-furred cat lives in mountains, high steppes, and open country across central Asia. At night it hunts for hares, birds, and mice.

Total body length of about 60 cm (24 in)

Strong, agile, stout body with short legs

Soft, thick fur to keep out the cold winds

BROOK'S GECKO
Sharp claws and sticky toe pads enable the gecko to climb well over smooth rocks, along crevices, and in cracks. The Brook's gecko is active at night, catching insects, and hides by day under rocks or in an empty termite or ant nest.

PALLAS'S SANDGROUSE
The mottled plumage (feathers) of Pallas's sandgrouse gives it excellent camouflage among the brownish grasses and stones of the Asian steppe. It needs little water and can survive on very dry, tough seeds and other plant parts.

Find out more
AFRICAN WILDLIFE
HORSES, ASSES, AND ZEBRAS
LIONS, TIGERS, and other big cats
LIZARDS

GRAVITY

FALLING
Earth's gravity makes falling objects accelerate (speed up). Their speed does not depend on how heavy they are: a light object falls as fast as a heavy object unless air slows it down. The Italian scientist Galileo Galilei (1564-1642) noticed this about 400 years ago.

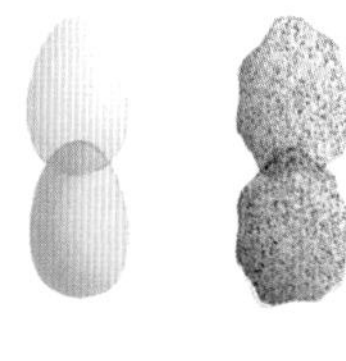

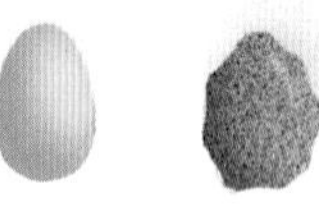

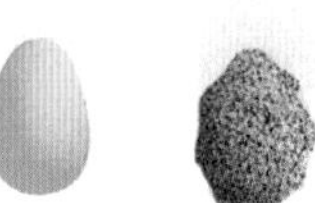

A heavy rock weighs much more than an egg of the same size. However, both objects fall at the same rate and hit the ground at the same time.

THE EARTH MOVES around the sun, travelling about 50 times faster than a rifle bullet. A strong force holds the Earth in this orbit. This is the force of gravity; without it, the Earth would shoot off into space like a stone from a catapult. Everything possesses gravity; it is a force that attracts all objects to each other. However, the strength of the force depends on how much mass is in an object, so gravity is only strong in huge objects such as planets. Although you cannot feel it, the force of gravity is also pulling on you. The Earth's gravity holds you to the surface of the Earth, no matter where you are. This is because gravity always pulls towards the centre of the Earth. Sometimes you can see or feel the effects of gravity. For example, the effort you feel when you climb up a flight of stairs is because you are fighting against the force of gravity.

MASS AND WEIGHT
An object's mass is the amount of material it contains. Mass stays the same wherever the object is in the universe. The weight of an object is the force of gravity pulling on it. Weight can change. Because the moon is smaller than the Earth, its gravity is weaker, about one sixth as strong as Earth's. Therefore, an astronaut on the moon weighs only one sixth of her weight on Earth, but her mass remains the same.

MOON AND EARTH
Gravity keeps the moon moving in its orbit around the Earth. The moon's gravity has effects on the Earth, too. When the moon is directly over the sea, its gravity pulls the sea water towards it, which produces a high tide; low tide follows when the Earth rotates away again.

Objects fall in the opposite direction on the other side of the Earth.

The force of gravity gets weaker as you go further from the centre of the Earth. On top of a high mountain, gravity is slightly weaker than at sea level; so objects weigh fractionally less.

When you drop a ball, it falls because gravity is pulling it towards the centre of the Earth.

Gravity pulls all objects down towards the centre of the Earth.

EARTH'S GRAVITY

People on the opposite side of the Earth are upside down in relation to you. But they do not fall off into space. They are held on to the surface of the Earth just as you are. This is because the force of gravity pulls everything towards the centre of the Earth. Down is always the direction of the Earth's centre.

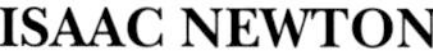

ISAAC NEWTON

British scientist Isaac Newton (1642-1727) was the first person to understand the force of gravity. In 1666, after watching an apple fall to the ground, he wondered whether the force of gravity that makes things fall also holds the moon in its orbit around the Earth. This was a daring idea, and it took Newton many years to prove it to be true. He declared his law of gravity to be a universal law – a law that is true throughout the universe.

CENTRE OF GRAVITY
It is best to carry a large, unwieldy object such as a ladder by holding it above its centre. The weight of the ladder balances at the centre, which is called its centre of gravity or centre of mass. An object with a large or heavy base has a low centre of gravity. This stops it from falling over easily.

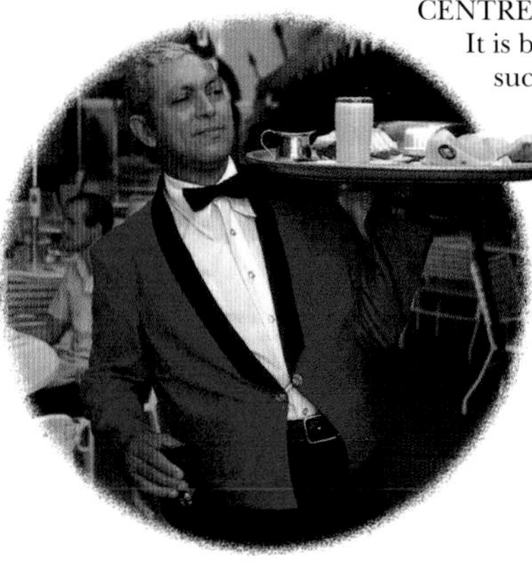

Objects such as a loaded tray balance if supported directly beneath their centre of gravity.

Find out more

ASTRONAUTS
PHYSICS
PLANETS
SCIENCE, HISTORY OF
UNIVERSE
WEIGHTS AND MEASURES

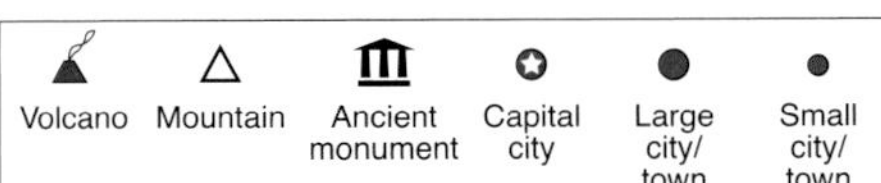

GREECE

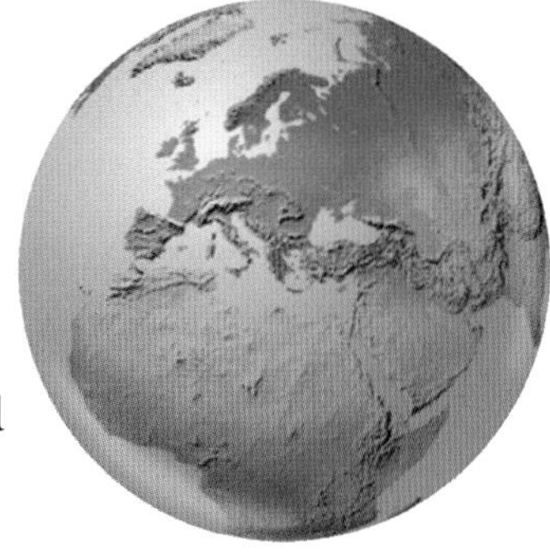

Lying at the eastern end of the Mediterranean, Greece is surrounded by the Mediterranean, Aegean, and Ionian Seas. It consists of a mainland, the Peloponnese peninsula, and over 2,000 islands.

STATISTICS
Area: 131,990 sq km (50,961 sq miles)
Population: 11,000,000
Capital: Athens
Languages: Greek, Turkish, Macedonian, Albanian
Religions: Greek Orthodox, Muslim
Currency: Euro

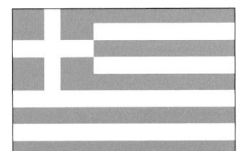

GREECE IS A LAND of wild mountains, remote valleys, and scattered islands. Most people make their living by farming; olives can grow on the dry hillsides, hardy sheep and goats thrive in the rugged landscape. Greece is the world's third largest producer of olive oil, and also exports citrus fruits, grapes, and tomatoes. With one of the largest merchant fleets in the world, Greece is a seafaring nation – people and goods travel by boat. In recent years, tourism has transformed the Greek economy. Millions of visitors are attracted to Greece by its landscape, and by its rich history as the birthplace of democracy in the 5th century B.C.

THE GREEK ISLANDS

The Greek mainland is surrounded by many islands. Ships and ferries unite these scattered communities. In summer, the islands, with their warm climate, fishing villages, and beautiful beaches, are major tourist centres, attracting over nine million visitors. In winter, the small islands are deserted by summer residents, who return to the mainland.

ORTHODOX PRIESTS
The Eastern Orthodox Church was founded in Constantinople (Istanbul) in the 4th century A.D. The Greek Orthodox Church became independent in 1850 and is the official religion of Greece, with more than 10 million faithful. Distinctively dressed priests are a common sight.

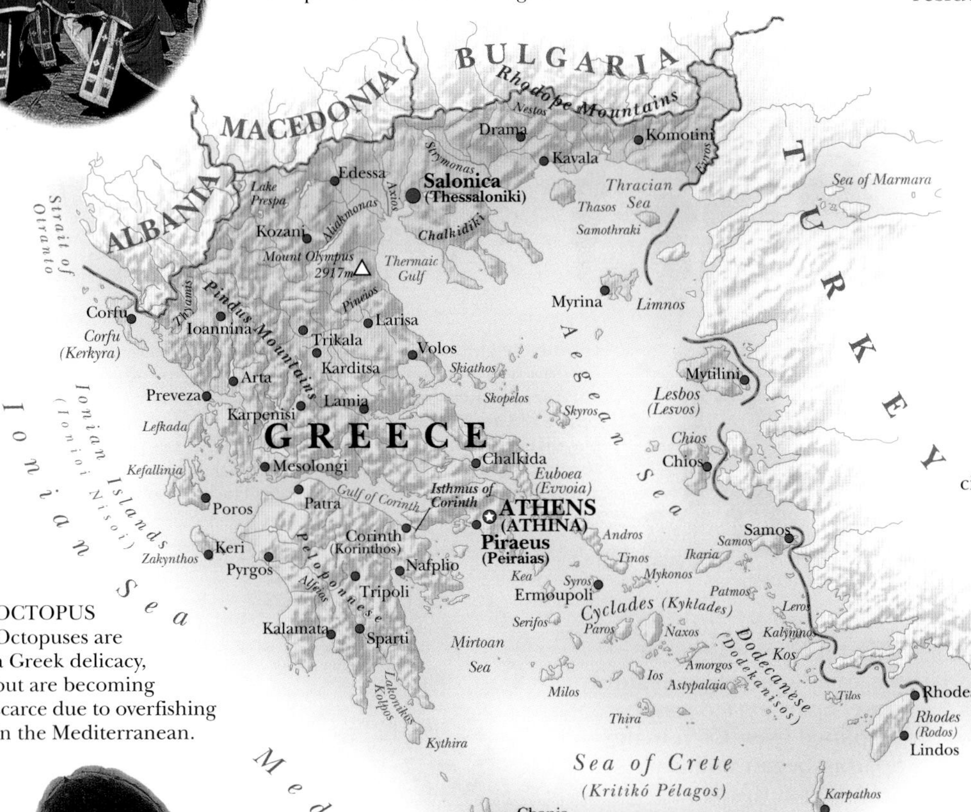

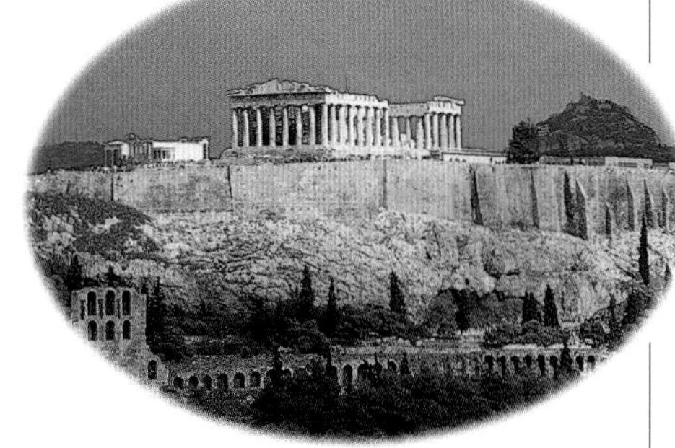

ATHENS
The ancient city of Athens, the cultural centre of Greece in the 5th century B.C., is generally believed to be the birthplace of western civilization. The fortified acropolis (above) rises 100 m (328 ft) above the city. It is crowned by the Parthenon temple, dedicated to the city's patron goddess Athena, and built in 432 B.C. Today, this busy modern city is a major commercial, shipping and tourist centre, and seat of the Greek government.

OCTOPUS
Octopuses are a Greek delicacy, but are becoming scarce due to overfishing in the Mediterranean.

SCALE BAR
0 50 100 km
0 50 100 miles

N
W E
S

Find out more

ARCHAEOLOGY
CHRISTIANITY
DEMOCRACY
GREECE, ANCIENT

ANCIENT
GREECE

MANY WESTERN WORDS, monuments, ideas, and sources of entertainment have their roots in the world of Ancient Greece. About 2,500 years ago, the Greeks set up a society that became the most influential in the world. Greek architects designed a style of building that is copied to this day. Greek thinkers asked searching questions about life that are still discussed. Modern theatre is founded on the Ancient Greek plays that were performed under the skies thousands of years ago. And the Greeks set up the world's first democracy (government by the people) in Athens. However, only free men born in Athens were actually allowed to have a say in government. Ancient Greek society went through many phases, with a "golden age" between around 600 and 300 B.C. Arts and culture flourished at that time. The Macedonians, under Philip of Macedon, finally conquered the civilization, but it continued under Philip's son Alexander, who spread Greek culture and thinking throughout the Middle East and North Africa.

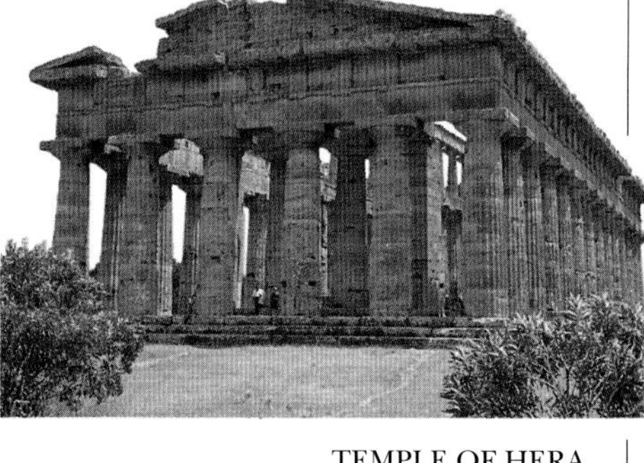

TEMPLE OF HERA
The Greeks built temples to worship their many gods. This temple at Paestum, Italy, was built to honour the goddess Hera, who was the protector of women and marriage.

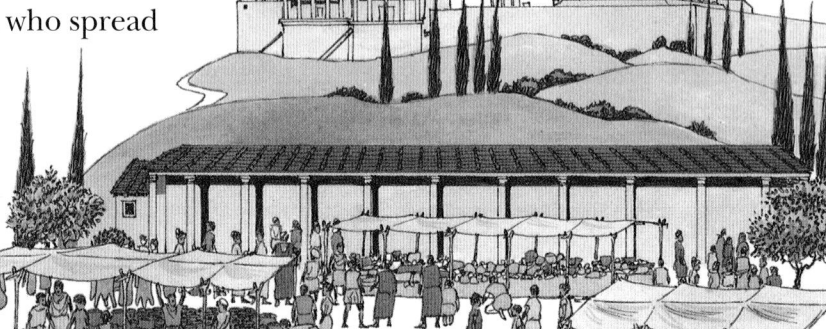

PERICLES
As leader of Athens, Pericles (c.490-429 B.C.) carried out a programme to beautify the city. This included the building of the Parthenon, a temple to the goddess Athena.

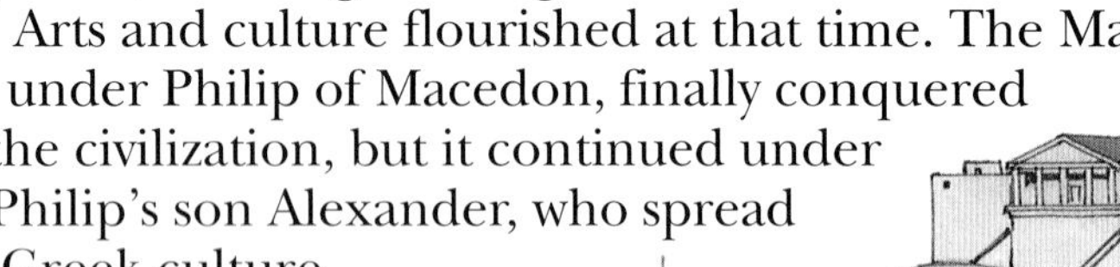

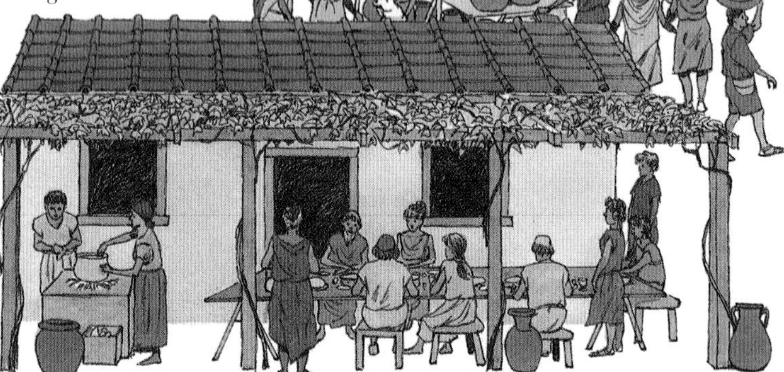

There were many busy markets in Athens, where people came to buy and sell their goods.

ATHENS
During the golden age, the Greek world consisted of independent, self-governing cities, known as city-states. With its own superb port at Piraeus, Athens was the most important city-state. It became the centre of Greek civilization and culture, attracting many famous playwrights and thinkers, such as Socrates. Athens practised the system of *demokratia* (democracy). People gathered together in the agora (marketplace) to shop and talk. The acropolis (high city) towered above Athens.

SPARTA

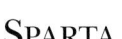

The second major city-state of Greece, Sparta, revolved around warfare. Spartans led tough, disciplined lives. Each male Spartan began military training at the age of seven and remained a soldier until 60. Women kept very fit by running and wrestling. The fierce Spartan hoplites (foot soldiers) were feared throughout the Greek world.

Spartan hoplites

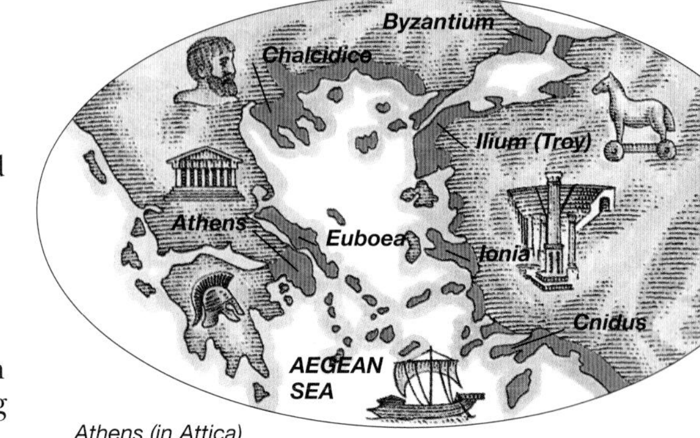

Athens (in Attica) and dependent states (shown in pink), c. 450 B.C.

GREEK WORLD
The Greek world consisted of many city-states and their colonies, spread throughout the Mediterranean region.

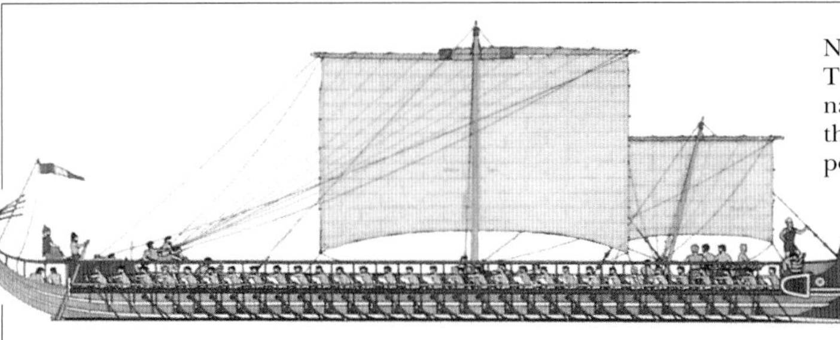

Modern reconstruction of a Greek trireme

NAVY
The Athenians possessed a powerful navy, consisting of a fleet of more than 200 triremes – warships powered by a square sail and rowed by 170 men seated in three ranks. The battle tactic involved rowing furiously and ramming the enemy's ship. In 480 B.C., during wars against the Persians, the Athenian navy crushed the Persian fleet at the sea battle of Salamis.

The main actors performed on the proskenion (stage).

All the actors were men, even those playing women's roles. They wore painted masks to hide their faces.

The audience bought stone tokens, which were like tickets, and sat in a semi-circle of tiered seats set into the hillside.

The chorus commented on the action of the play in song and dance.

The circular space in front of the stage was called the orchestra.

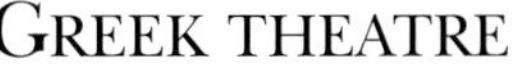

Greek Theatre

Drama was born in Athens. It began as singing and acting as part of a religious festival to honour the god Dionysus. The audience watched a series of plays; at the end of the festival, prizes were given for the best play and best actor. From these beginnings, playwrights such as Sophocles and Aristophanes started to write tragedies and comedies. Tragedies involved dreadful suffering; comedies featured slapstick humour and rude jokes.

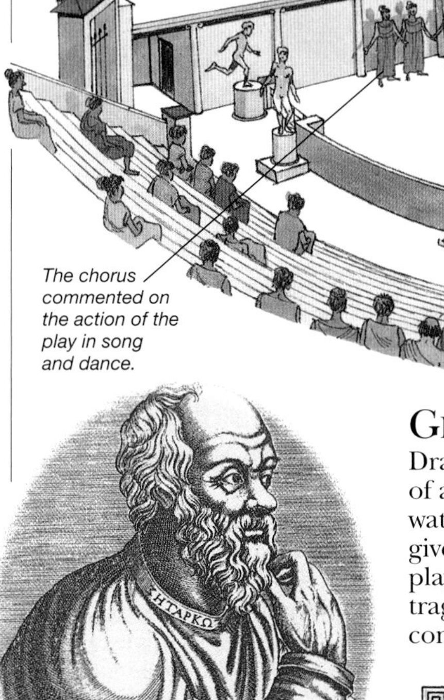

THINKERS
Great thinkers from Athens dominated Greek learning and culture during the 5th and 4th centuries B.C. Socrates (469-399 B.C.; above) was one of the most famous. He discussed the meaning and conduct of life. He also questioned people cleverly, often proving that their ideas were wrong. Socrates wrote no books himself, but one of his followers, Plato (427-347 B.C.), made him the subject of many of his books.

VASE PAINTING

Painted scenes on Greek pottery give us clear clues about daily life in Ancient Greece. The paintings often show a touching scene, such as a warrior bidding his family farewell as he goes off to war. They also show the many gods that the Greeks worshipped.

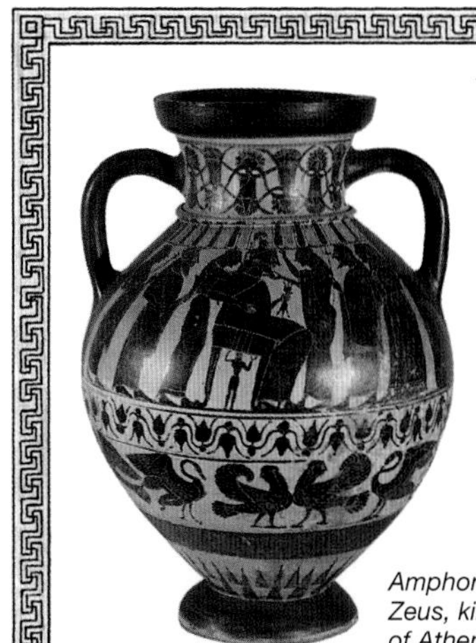

Amphora (vase) from Attica shows Zeus, king of the gods, at the birth of Athena, his daughter.

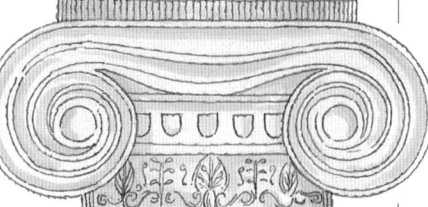

ANCIENT GREECE

1500 B.C. Minoan civilization (on island of Crete) at its height.

c. 1400 Mycenaean civilization, centred in great palaces on the Greek mainland, dominates Greece.

c. 1250 Probable date of the Trojan Wars between Mycenaeans and the city of Troy.

c. 1000 Greek-speaking peoples arrive in Greece and establish the first city-states.

776 First Olympic Games held at Olympia, Greece.

750s First Greek colonies founded.

c. 505 Democracy is established in Athens.

400s Golden age of Greek theatre.

490-479 Persian Wars; Greek states unite to defeat Persians.

490 Greeks defeat Persians at Marathon.

480 Greeks destroy the Persian fleet at the Battle of Salamis.

479 Final defeat of Persians at Plataea.

461-429 Pericles rules in Athens; Parthenon built.

431-404 Peloponnesian War between Athens and Sparta leads to Spartan domination of Greece.

359 Philip becomes king of Macedonia.

338 Philip of Macedonia conquers Greece.

336-323 Alexander the Great, son of Philip, sets up Greek empire in Middle East.

Find out more

Alexander the Great
Architecture
Democracy
Minoans
Sculpture
Theatre

GUNPOWDER PLOT

IN THE LATE 1500s AND EARLY 1600s, Roman Catholics in England, urged on by the Catholic rulers of Spain, constantly schemed to replace England's Protestant rulers with Catholics. In 1605, a small group of Catholics hatched a plot to blow up James I and his government when the king opened a new session of parliament. The so-called Gunpowder Plot was due to take place on 5 November, but it failed because one of the conspirators warned his brother-in-law, Lord Mounteagle, not to attend parliament on that day. Mounteagle warned the government, and the cellars under parliament were searched. There, the king's soldiers found a young conspirator, Guy Fawkes, with 20 barrels of gunpowder. He was arrested, tortured, tried, and executed. The other plotters fled, but were later caught and were also executed.

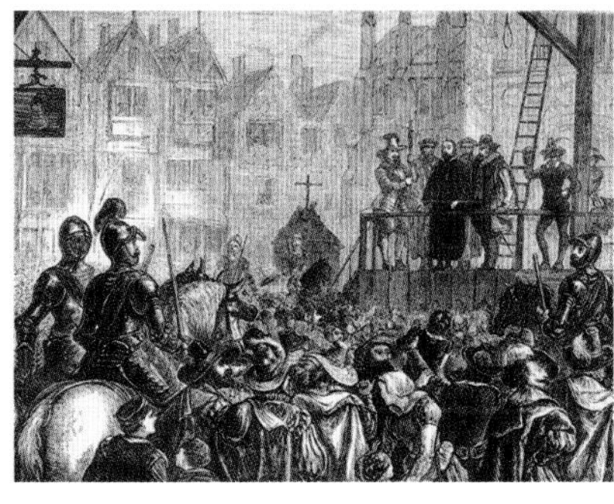

RELIGIOUS INTOLERANCE
Anti-Catholic feeling was common in England and Scotland. Protestants distrusted Roman Catholics because they feared the political power of the pope. After the Plot, fear of Catholics intensifed, and the conspirators were executed.

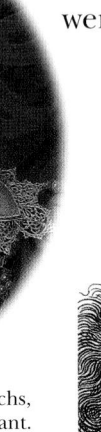

JAMES I
The first of the Stuart monarchs, James I was a staunch Protestant. He came to the throne in 1603, after the death of Elizabeth I. During Elizabeth's reign, Catholics had been persecuted. Mass was forbidden and Catholics could not hold high office. There were many Catholic plots. James I also distrusted Catholics. He angered them by refusing to reverse anti-Catholic laws.

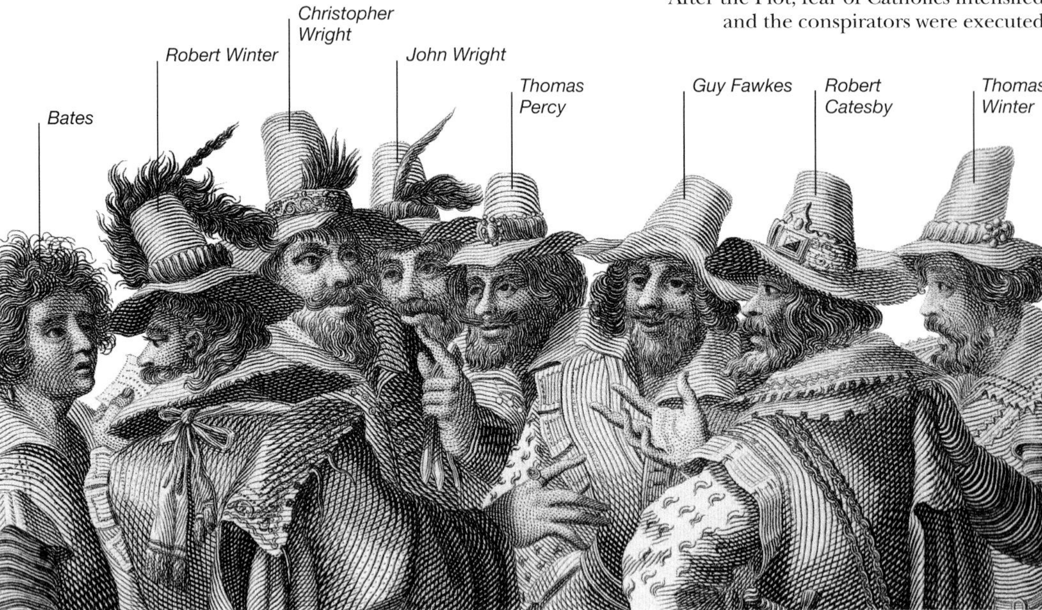

THE CONSPIRACY

The leader of the Gunpowder Plot was Robert Catesby (1573-1605), a wealthy Roman Catholic. He recruited 12 other conspirators, including Guy Fawkes, who was chosen to light the fuse, and blow up the Houses of Parliament. The conspirators hoped that their actions would encourage a rebellion, which would lead to England becoming a Catholic nation. Thomas Tresham, one of the conspirators, gave the plot away.

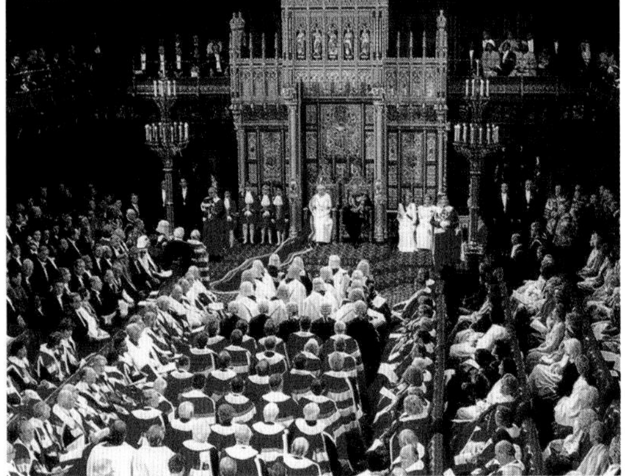

The House of Lords as the Queen formally opens parliament

STATE OPENING
Today, the British monarch still opens each session of parliament. There is a formal opening ceremony, at which the Queen reads out the government's programme for the year. It is the only day on which the Queen wears her crown, the symbol of her authority.

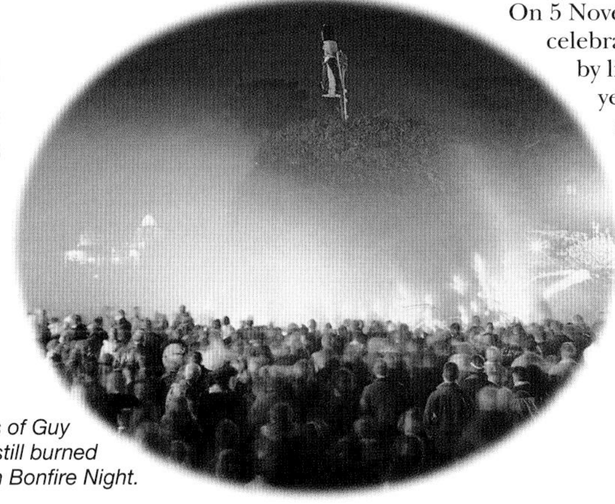

Models of Guy Fawkes are still burned on Bonfire Night.

BONFIRE NIGHT
On 5 November 1605, supporters of the king celebrated the failure of the Gunpowder Plot by lighting bonfires. Ever since then, every year on 5 November, people in Britain remember the Gunpowder Plot. They build bonfires and let off fireworks. Children make dummy "guys" and ask people for a "penny for the guy". In some towns elaborate bonfire processions still take place.

Find out more
ELIZABETH I
HENRY VIII
GOVERNMENT AND POLITICS
STUARTS

GUNS

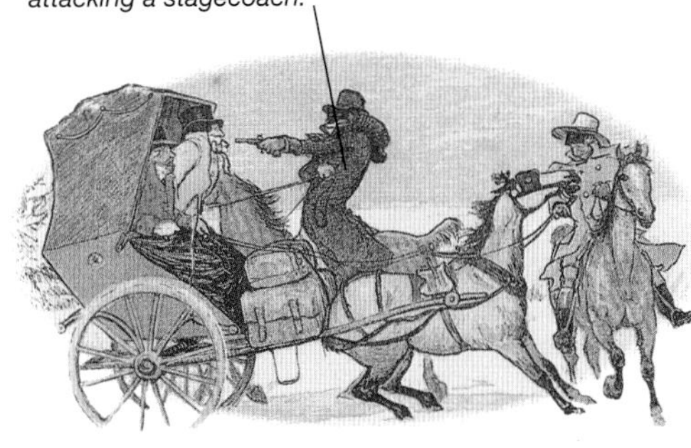

Eighteenth-century highwaymen, armed with early pistols, attacking a stagecoach.

THE FIRST GUNS, called cannons, appeared during the early 14th century. They consisted of a thick metal tube which was closed at one end and was packed with gunpowder. Lighting the fuse caused the gunpowder to explode, blasting a steel ball out of the end of the tube. In the 16th century, pistols were invented to be used as concealed weapons and for personal protection. However, they were useless at a range of more than 9 m (30 ft), and once fired had to be laboriously reloaded. Modern guns range from large, powerful artillery weapons to small, light pistols. Sophisticated engineering has given guns great accuracy and power, and many guns can be fired several times without reloading. However, even the most modern guns work on the same basic principle as the early cannon.

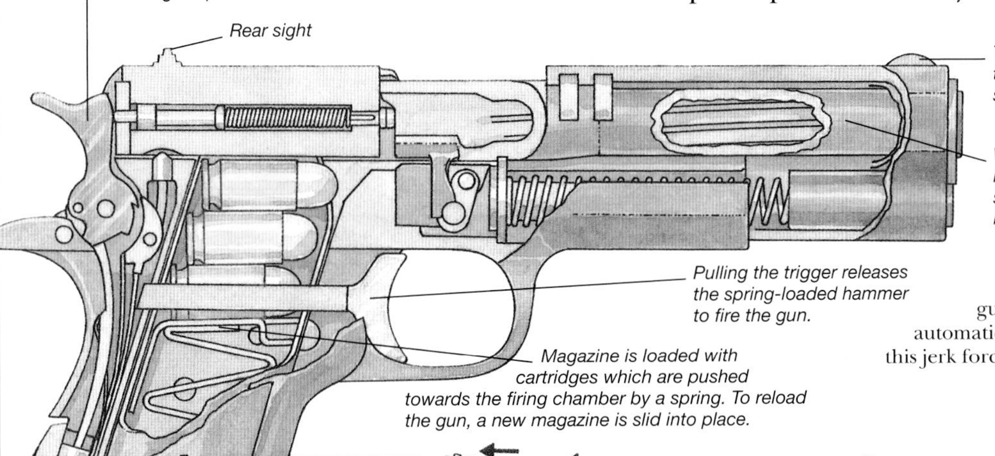

Hammer drives firing pin into the back of the cartridge, making the charge explode.

Rear sight

To aim the pistol, the front and rear sights are lined up.

When the gun is fired, bullet shoots along barrel.

Pulling the trigger releases the spring-loaded hammer to fire the gun.

Magazine is loaded with cartridges which are pushed towards the firing chamber by a spring. To reload the gun, a new magazine is slid into place.

AUTOMATIC PISTOL
The pistol is loaded with cartridges, each of which contains a lead bullet and a small charge of explosive. When the hammer of the gun strikes the charge it explodes, producing gases that expand violently. The force of the expanding gases pushes the bullet along the barrel. The gun recoils, or jerks backwards, when it is fired. In automatic or self-loading weapons such as machine guns, this jerk forces another cartridge into place, ready for firing.

Pulling trigger makes firing pin strike the cartridge, detonating its explosive charge.

Recoil pushes back slide which ejects spent cartridge case; the next cartridge springs into firing chamber.

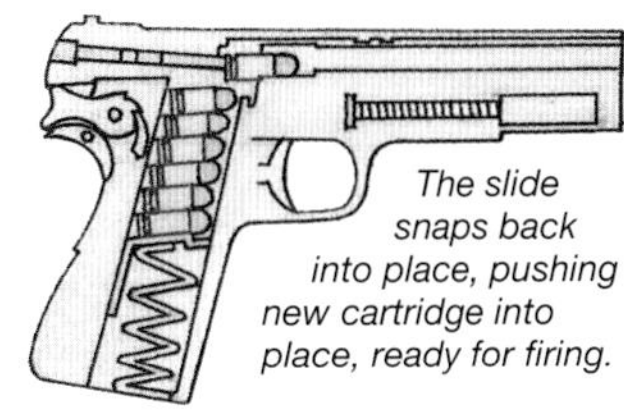

The slide snaps back into place, pushing new cartridge into place, ready for firing.

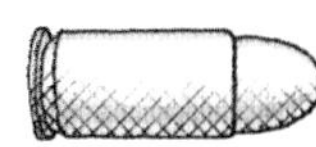

BULLETS
When a bullet is fired, its casing remains behind. The force of the explosion ejects the spent cartridge case through a slot in the barrel.

ARTILLERY

Heavy guns, or artillery, are used to bombard enemy positions. They fire shells – hollow bullet-shaped cylinders packed with high explosive – over distances of more than 32 km (20 miles). The latest artillery weapons are guided by computers and laser rangefinders, and their shells are equipped with special homing devices so that they can hit their targets with great accuracy.

Pakistani soldiers aiming a light artillery weapon high up in the Himalayas.

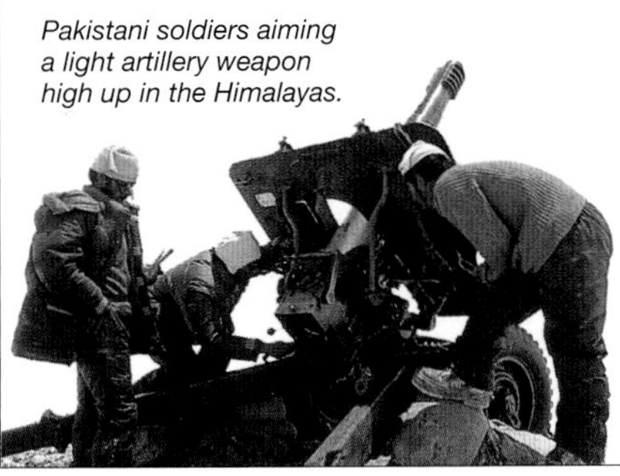

KINDS OF GUN

There are four main types of hand-held gun: pistols for personal protection, rifles for accurate firing over long distances, submachine guns which produce a spray of bullets, and shotguns which fire a mass of lead fragments for sport shooting.

REVOLVER
Revolvers have a rotating drum with six chambers, allowing six shots to be fired without reloading.

RIFLE
A rifle is a long-barrelled gun that is fired from the shoulder. Inside the barrel is a spiral of grooves which make the bullet spin as it is fired. The flight of a spinning bullet is very stable, which makes the rifle a very accurate weapon. A rifle bullet can travel at about 3,500 km/h (2,200 mph).

SUBMACHINE GUN
With one squeeze of the trigger, a submachine gun can fire several bullets in quick succession. It is small and light so that a soldier can carry it easily into battle.

MACHINE GUN
A machine gun is often mounted onto a jeep or armoured vehicle because it is too heavy to hold. It is fed with bullets fixed on a long belt and can fire about 600 rounds per minute.

Find out more
ARMIES
TANKS
WEAPONS

GYMNASTICS

TO SUCCEED, GYMNASTS must be strong, flexible, brave, and graceful. Most people, however, can do some gymnastics. Children, for instance, learn to do handstands and cartwheels at school, and these simple activities are the basis for all gymnastic moves. Gymnastics, as a form of acrobatic exercise, dates back to Ancient Greece. Today, it is an increasingly popular spectator sport. There are two main types: rhythmic gymnastics and artistic gymnastics, performed on apparatus such as the horse or vault. There are eight competitive events. Both men and women do floor exercises, and the vault. Men compete on bars, horse, and rings. Women compete on the beam and asymmetric bars. Judges award points out of ten. Many champions are teenagers.

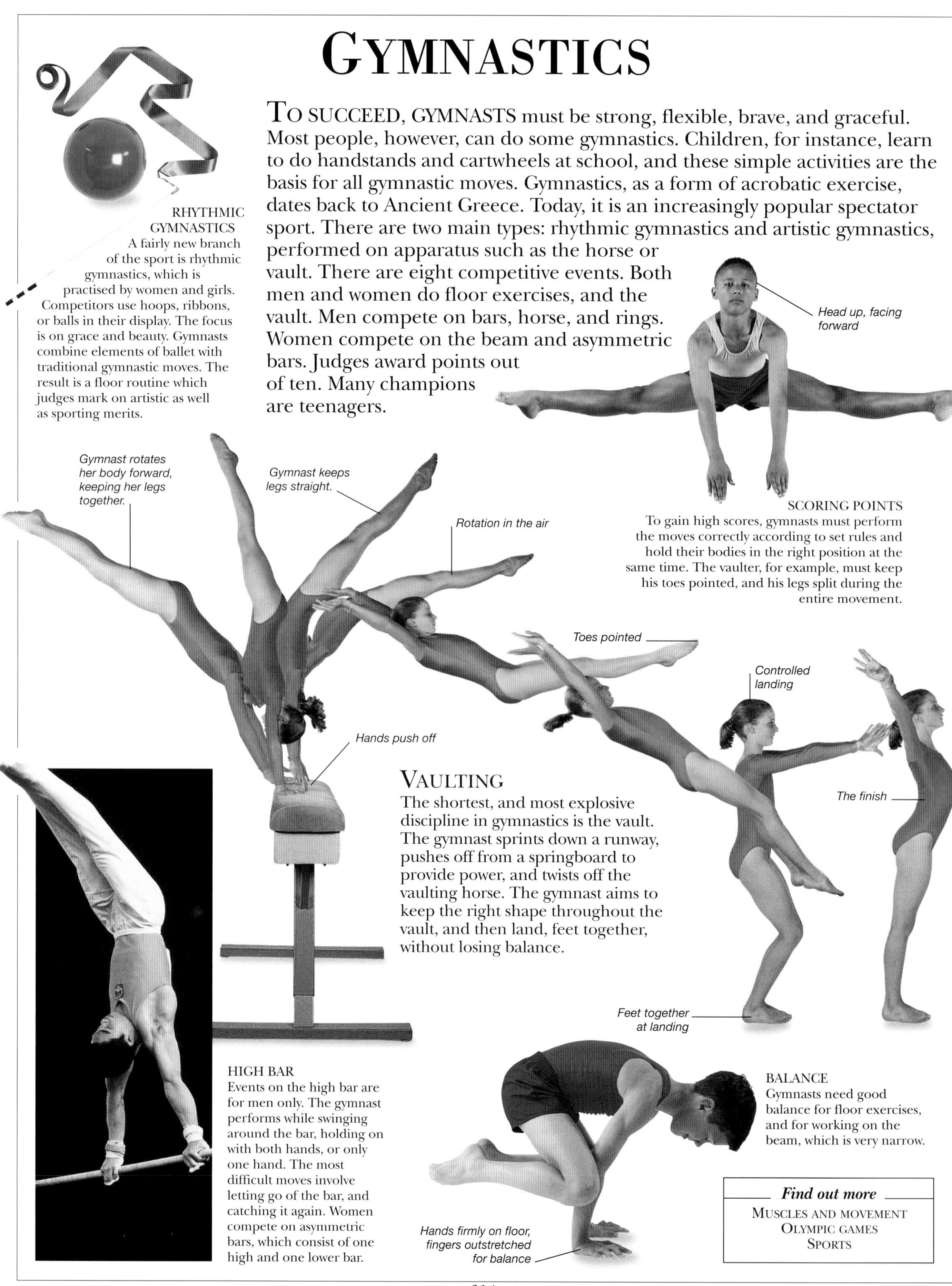

Head up, facing forward
Gymnast rotates her body forward, keeping her legs together.
Gymnast keeps legs straight.
Rotation in the air
Toes pointed
Controlled landing
Hands push off
The finish
Feet together at landing
Hands firmly on floor, fingers outstretched for balance

RHYTHMIC GYMNASTICS
A fairly new branch of the sport is rhythmic gymnastics, which is practised by women and girls. Competitors use hoops, ribbons, or balls in their display. The focus is on grace and beauty. Gymnasts combine elements of ballet with traditional gymnastic moves. The result is a floor routine which judges mark on artistic as well as sporting merits.

SCORING POINTS
To gain high scores, gymnasts must perform the moves correctly according to set rules and hold their bodies in the right position at the same time. The vaulter, for example, must keep his toes pointed, and his legs split during the entire movement.

VAULTING

The shortest, and most explosive discipline in gymnastics is the vault. The gymnast sprints down a runway, pushes off from a springboard to provide power, and twists off the vaulting horse. The gymnast aims to keep the right shape throughout the vault, and then land, feet together, without losing balance.

HIGH BAR
Events on the high bar are for men only. The gymnast performs while swinging around the bar, holding on with both hands, or only one hand. The most difficult moves involve letting go of the bar, and catching it again. Women compete on asymmetric bars, which consist of one high and one lower bar.

BALANCE
Gymnasts need good balance for floor exercises, and for working on the beam, which is very narrow.

Find out more

MUSCLES AND MOVEMENT
OLYMPIC GAMES
SPORTS

HAPSBURGS

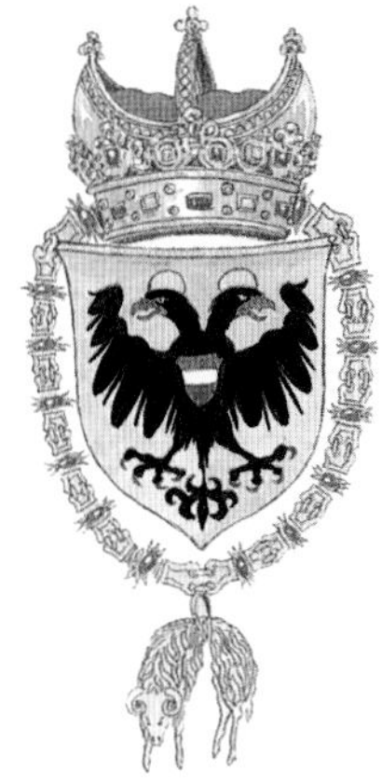

FAMILY CREST
The crest of the Hapsburg family was the black double-headed eagle. It appeared on all their flags and banners.

DURING THE 900s a family named Hapsburg owned some land in France and Switzerland. From this they rose to dominate European history for more than 1,000 years. The name Hapsburg comes from one of the family's first castles, the Habichtsburg, in Switzerland. Through a series of wars, inheritances, and careful marriages, the family acquired more and more land. By the 1500s it owned most of southern and central Europe and much land in the Americas. The Hapsburg possessions became so big that in 1556 the Hapsburg emperor, Charles V, split the land between members of his family. Philip II governed one half from Madrid, Spain, while Ferdinand of Austria governed the other half from Vienna, Austria. The Spanish Hapsburgs died out in 1700, but the Austrian Hapsburgs continued to expand their empire. In the 19th century, however, their power began to weaken because the empire contained so many different peoples. When it collapsed after World War I (1914-18), four new nations emerged: Austria, Czechoslovakia, Hungary, and Yugoslavia.

CHARLES V
Under Charles V, who reigned as Holy Roman Emperor from 1519 to 1556, the Hapsburgs reached the height of their power. Charles V ruled a vast empire shown in pink on the map above.

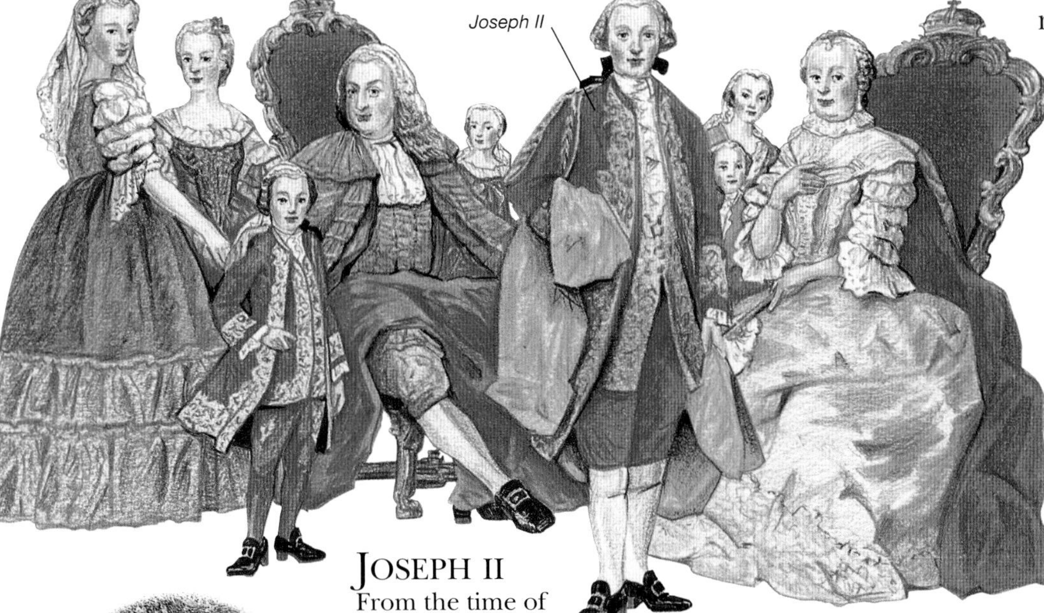

JOSEPH II
From the time of Rudolf I onwards, the Hapsburg family extended its power throughout Europe. Joseph II, son of Maria Theresa, was appalled by the living conditions of his poorer subjects. He began reforms that included freeing serfs and abolishing privileges.

HAPSBURGS

1273 Rudolf I becomes the Holy Roman Emperor.

1282 Albert I becomes first Hapsburg ruler of Austria.

1438 Albert II becomes Holy Roman Emperor.

1519 Charles V becomes Holy Roman Emperor.

1526 Ferdinand, brother of Charles, acquires Bohemia.

1556 Charles V splits Hapsburg lands in half.

1700 Charles II, last Spanish Hapsburg monarch, dies.

1740-1780 Maria Theresa increases Hapsburg power in Europe.

1781 Joseph II, son of Maria Theresa, introduces major reforms and frees serfs.

1867 Austrian empire is split between two monarchs: Austrian and Hungarian.

1918 Charles I, last Hapsburg emperor, gives up throne.

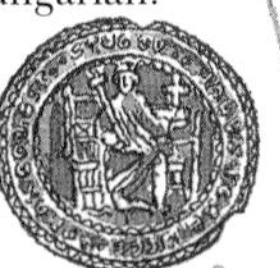

MARIA THERESA
In 1740, Maria Theresa came to the Austrian throne. She was only 23 and her empire was bankrupt. Over the next 40 years, she pulled Austria back from poverty and restored Hapsburg power in Europe.

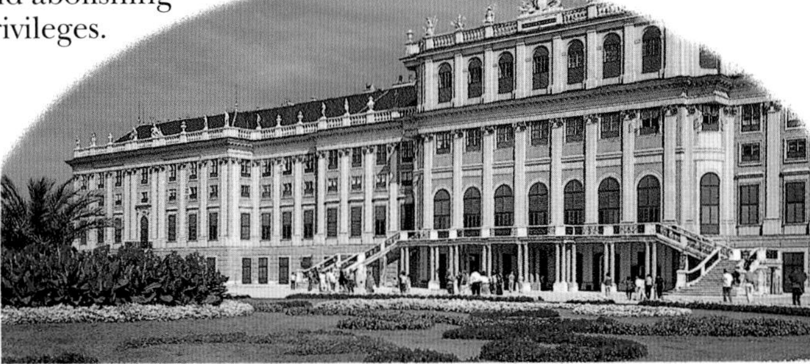

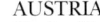

AUSTRIA
Under Maria Theresa, Austria became the leading artistic centre of Europe. Austria was home to the composers Franz Joseph Haydn and Wolfgang Amadeus Mozart. Artists and architects came from all over Europe to work on great palaces such as the Schönbrunn in Vienna (above).

Find out more
AUSTRIA
CHARLEMAGNE
EUROPE, HISTORY OF
GERMANY, HISTORY OF
SPAIN, HISTORY OF

HEALTH AND FITNESS

Regular, vigorous exercise helps prevent heart disease.

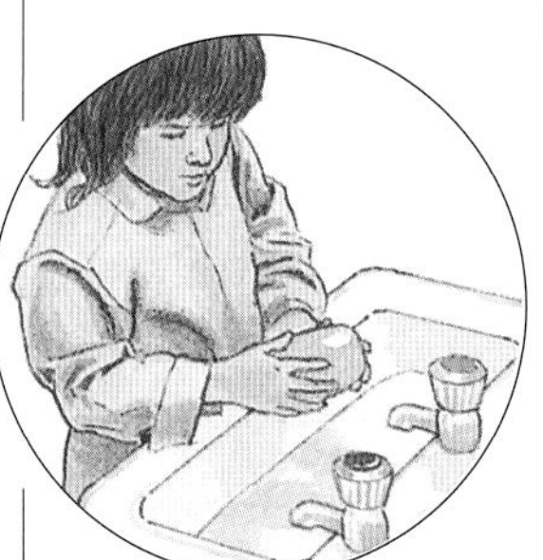

Better hygiene and a more balanced diet could eliminate much ill health in developed nations.

ARE YOU HEALTHY? Before answering, think about what you understand by "health". It doesn't just mean freedom from disease. Health is a measure of how sound and vigorous both your body and mind are. A truly healthy person has a sense of physical and mental well-being. Our health is precious and easily damaged. But there is much we can do to maintain it. Eating well, exercising, and getting enough sleep all help keep us healthy. Standards of health and health hazards are different from place to place. In some parts of the world many people have serious health problems because they are poor, hungry, and without clean drinking water. In other places stress at work, lack of exercise, and too much food bring their own health problems, such as heart disease. People also damage their health through the use of alcohol, tobacco, and dangerous drugs.

KEEPING HEALTHY

Food plays a large part in health. A healthy diet includes fresh fruit and vegetables, meat, fish, bread, eggs, and milk, but not too many fatty, salty, or sugary foods. Exercise keeps the heart strong and prevents us from gaining too much weight.

IMMUNIZATION

Good health includes preventing disease. Immunization, sometimes called inoculation or vaccination, involves injecting the body with a vaccine. This is a tiny dose of the infecting agent of the disease, which has been specially treated to render it safe. The vaccination provides immunity, or protection, against the disease. It is now possible to immunize against diphtheria, polio, tetanus, measles, mumps, rubella, tuberculosis, meningitis, and lots of others. Immunization has completely eliminated one disease, that is smallpox.

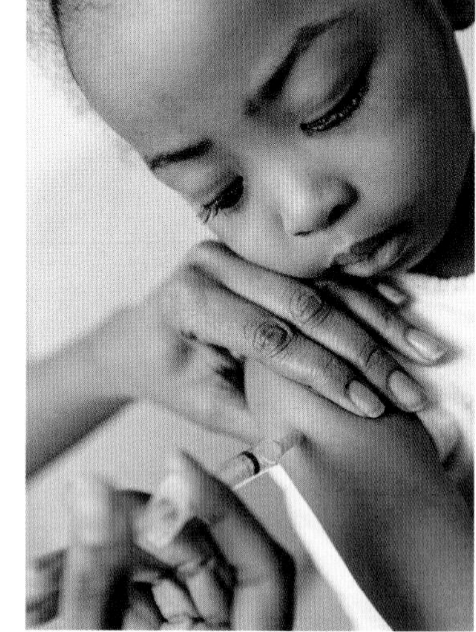

A doctor or nurse usually gives immunizations by injection.

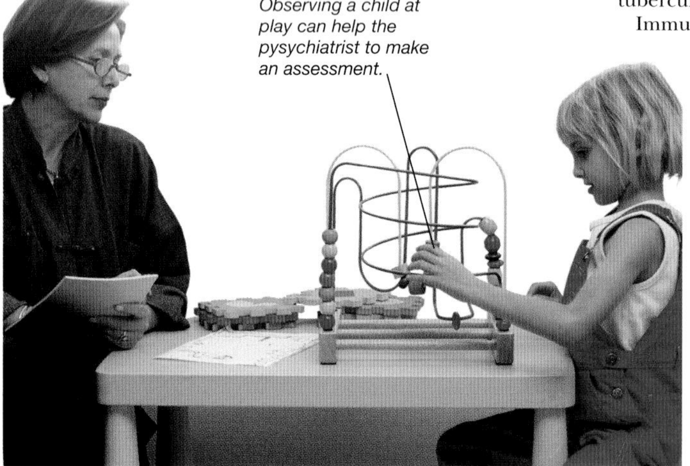

Observing a child at play can help the pysychiatrist to make an assessment.

MENTAL HEALTH

A healthy mind is just as important as a healthy body. Stress, drug abuse, physical disease, and family problems such as divorce can all damage mental health. Specialist doctors who treat mental health problems are called psychiatrists. Other sources of help include drug therapy, counselling, and self-help groups.

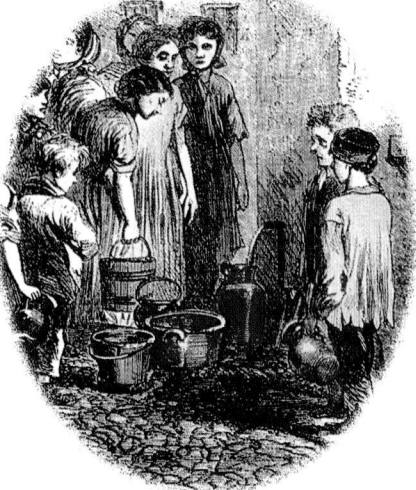

HEALTH CHECKUPS

Through routine medical checkups, doctors can detect health problems such as cancer at the early stages, when treatment is most effective. Checkups can also reveal hereditary health problems – diseases that pass from parents to children.

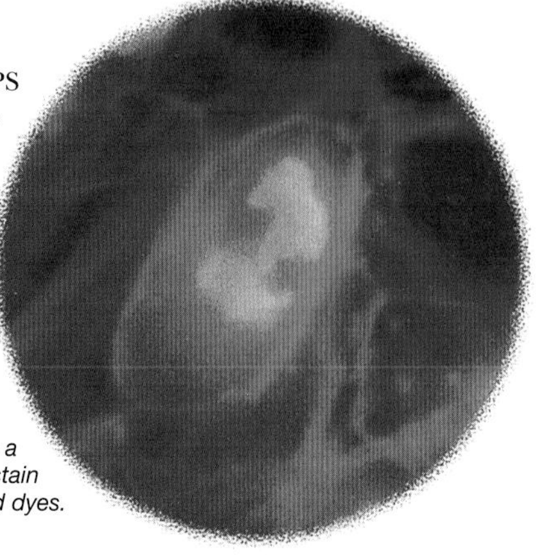

To reveal cancer cells on a microscope slide, technicians stain the tissue sample with coloured dyes.

PUBLIC HEALTH

Dirty conditions and lack of hygiene can affect health. If not controlled, insanitary conditions can spread throughout cities and affect large populations. The Great Plague of London in 1665 was caused by poor hygiene. During the 1840s, pioneers of public health in Europe worked to introduce clean water supplies and good sewage systems. Institutions such as the World Health Organization, have been set up to monitor public health internationally.

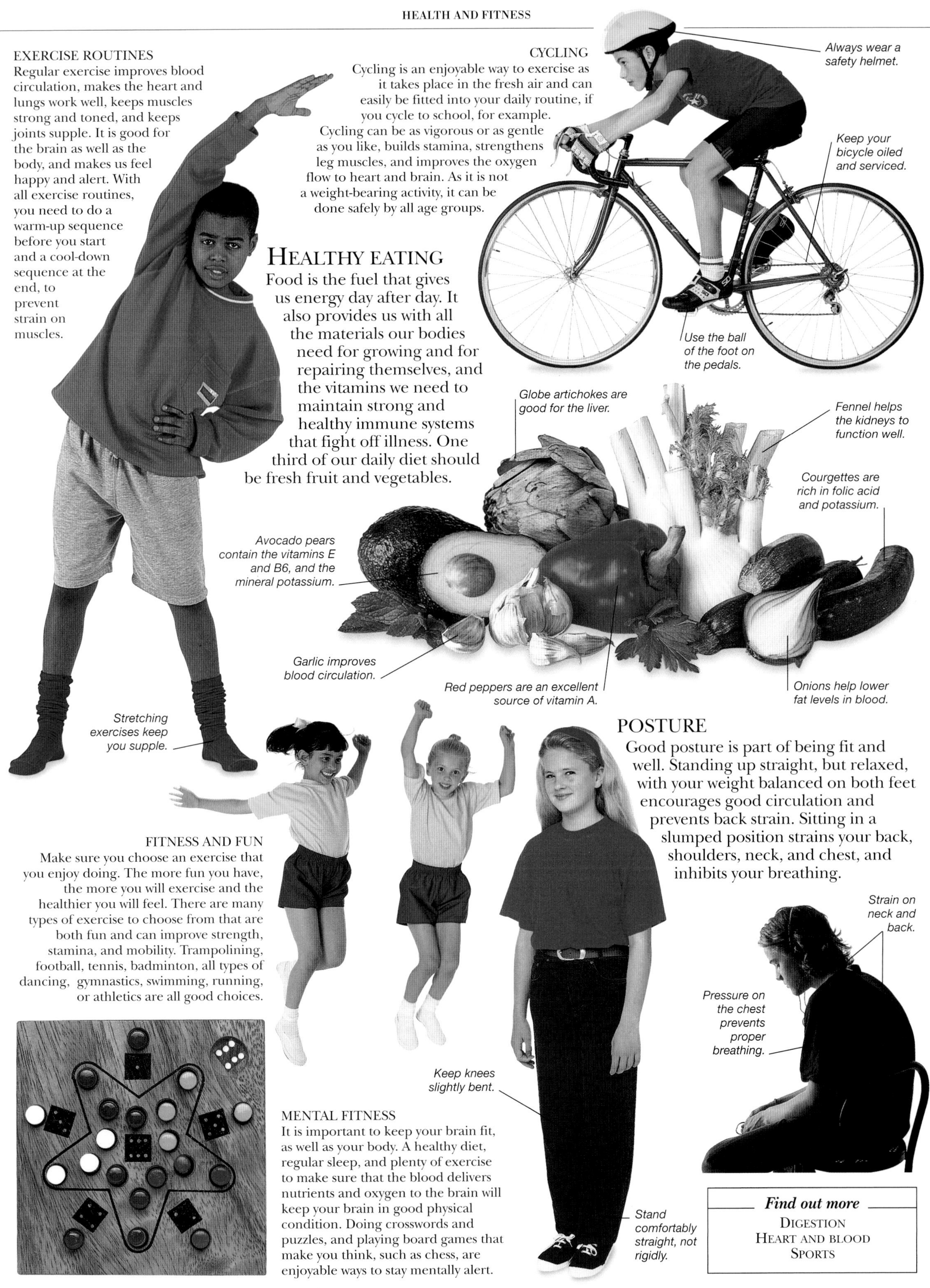

Always wear a safety helmet.
Keep your bicycle oiled and serviced.
Use the ball of the foot on the pedals.
Globe artichokes are good for the liver.
Fennel helps the kidneys to function well.
Courgettes are rich in folic acid and potassium.
Avocado pears contain the vitamins E and B6, and the mineral potassium.
Garlic improves blood circulation.
Red peppers are an excellent source of vitamin A.
Onions help lower fat levels in blood.
Stretching exercises keep you supple.
Strain on neck and back.
Pressure on the chest prevents proper breathing.
Keep knees slightly bent.
Stand comfortably straight, not rigidly.

EXERCISE ROUTINES

Regular exercise improves blood circulation, makes the heart and lungs work well, keeps muscles strong and toned, and keeps joints supple. It is good for the brain as well as the body, and makes us feel happy and alert. With all exercise routines, you need to do a warm-up sequence before you start and a cool-down sequence at the end, to prevent strain on muscles.

CYCLING

Cycling is an enjoyable way to exercise as it takes place in the fresh air and can easily be fitted into your daily routine, if you cycle to school, for example. Cycling can be as vigorous or as gentle as you like, builds stamina, strengthens leg muscles, and improves the oxygen flow to heart and brain. As it is not a weight-bearing activity, it can be done safely by all age groups.

HEALTHY EATING

Food is the fuel that gives us energy day after day. It also provides us with all the materials our bodies need for growing and for repairing themselves, and the vitamins we need to maintain strong and healthy immune systems that fight off illness. One third of our daily diet should be fresh fruit and vegetables.

POSTURE

Good posture is part of being fit and well. Standing up straight, but relaxed, with your weight balanced on both feet encourages good circulation and prevents back strain. Sitting in a slumped position strains your back, shoulders, neck, and chest, and inhibits your breathing.

FITNESS AND FUN

Make sure you choose an exercise that you enjoy doing. The more fun you have, the more you will exercise and the healthier you will feel. There are many types of exercise to choose from that are both fun and can improve strength, stamina, and mobility. Trampolining, football, tennis, badminton, all types of dancing, gymnastics, swimming, running, or athletics are all good choices.

MENTAL FITNESS

It is important to keep your brain fit, as well as your body. A healthy diet, regular sleep, and plenty of exercise to make sure that the blood delivers nutrients and oxygen to the brain will keep your brain in good physical condition. Doing crosswords and puzzles, and playing board games that make you think, such as chess, are enjoyable ways to stay mentally alert.

Find out more

DIGESTION
HEART AND BLOOD
SPORTS

HEART AND BLOOD

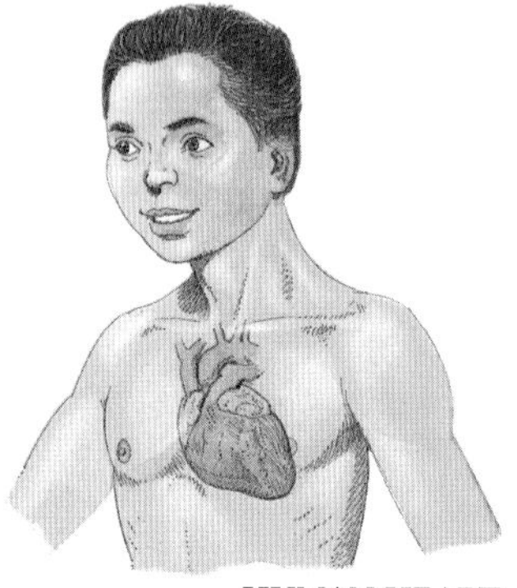

HUMAN HEART
The heart is protected by the rib cage. An adult's heart is the size of a clenched fist and weighs about 300 g (9 oz).

OUR BODIES CONTAIN about 4.5 litres (8 pints) of blood. Throughout life the organ inside the chest, the heart, pumps blood to every part of the body, keeping us alive. The heart is such a powerful pump that it takes only about a minute for each blood cell to travel all the way around the body and back to the heart. Travelling along tubes called blood vessels, blood carries oxygen and nourishment from digested food to every part of the body. Blood also carries away harmful waste products such as carbon dioxide. Blood consists of red and white blood cells, platelets, and a watery liquid called plasma. A drop of blood the size of a pinhead contains about five million cells. About once every second the muscular walls of the heart contract, squeezing blood out of the heart and into blood vessels called arteries. The arteries divide many times until they form a network of tiny blood vessels called capillaries. The capillaries gradually join up again to form veins, which carry the blood back to the heart, where it is sent to the lungs for fresh oxygen.

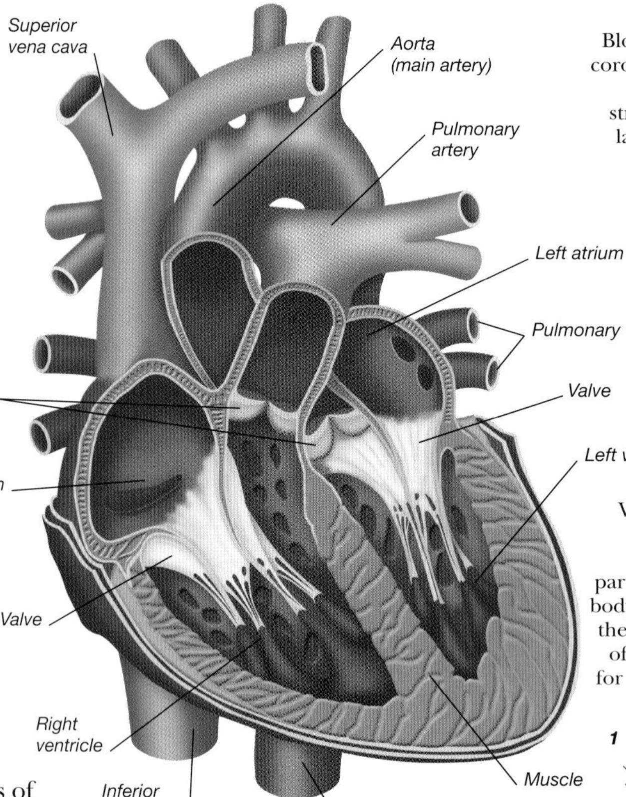

INSIDE THE HEART

The heart has four chambers, two on each side. The upper chamber is called the atrium. Blood from the veins flows into the right atrium, and then into the lower chamber, called the ventricle. The thick, muscular walls of the left ventricle force the blood out into the arteries. The heart consists of two pumps, working side by side. The left pump sends blood full of oxygen (oxygenated) around the body. As the blood passes its oxygen to various parts of the body, it becomes stale (deoxygenated) and returns to the heart through the right pump. The right pump sends it to the lungs for fresh oxygen, then back through the left pump again to be sent around the body once more.

ARTERIES
Blood reaches the heart muscle through coronary arteries. The two main coronary arteries are about as wide as drinking straws. Arteries have thick walls in three layers – a tough outer layer, a muscular middle layer, and a smooth lining.

CAPILLARIES
The tiny blood vessels that carry blood between the smallest arteries (arterioles) and the smallest veins (venules) are called capillaries. Capillaries allow oxygen and nutrients to pass through their walls to all the body cells.

VEINS
Veins carry deoxygenated blood (blue-coloured blood which contains little oxygen) back to the heart from other parts of the body. The largest veins in the body are the two venae cavae, which carry the deoxygenated blood to the right side of the heart, to be pumped to the lungs for oxygen. Veins are thinner, less elastic, and less muscular than arteries.

HEARTBEAT
On average, an adult's heart beats 60 to 70 times each minute, and this rises to more than 150 beats after strenuous activity. Each heartbeat has two main phases. The phase when the heart muscle is fully contracted, squeezing out blood, is called systole. The phase when the heart relaxes and refills with blood is called diastole.

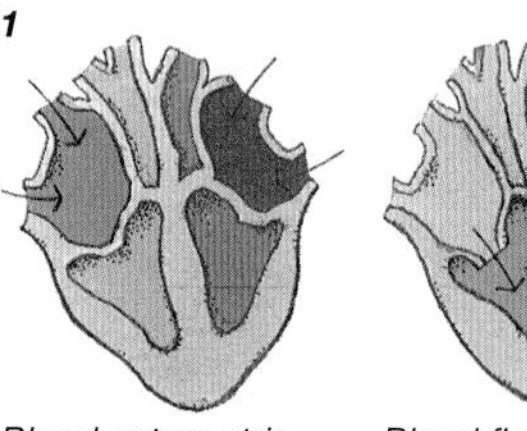

1 Blood enters atria (upper chambers).

2 Blood flows through to ventricles (lower chambers).

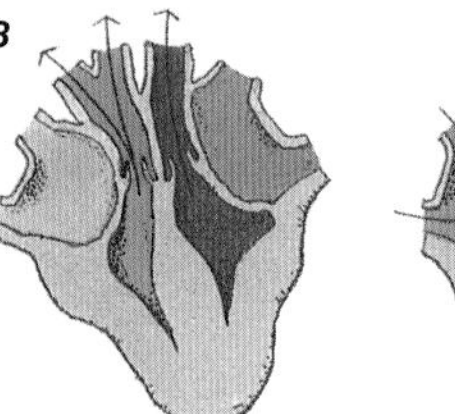

3 Ventricles contract to pump blood into arteries.

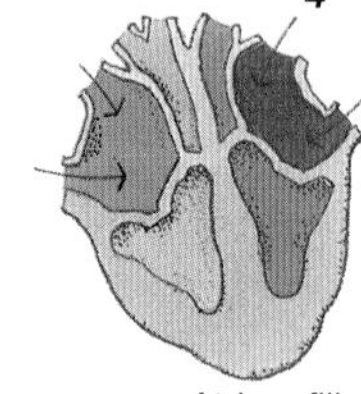

4 Atria refill with blood.

BLOOD CELLS
There are three types of blood cells. Red blood cells carry oxygen from the lungs to the rest of the body. White blood cells protect the body against illness and fight infection. Platelets, which are the smallest type of blood cell, help the blood to clot. All blood cells are produced in the bone marrow inside the bones.

White cell
Red cell
Platelets

HOW BLOOD CLOTS
When you cut yourself and blood flows out of the wound, platelets in the blood stick together and a fine meshwork of fibres forms. This meshwork traps more blood cells and forms a clot to seal the wound.

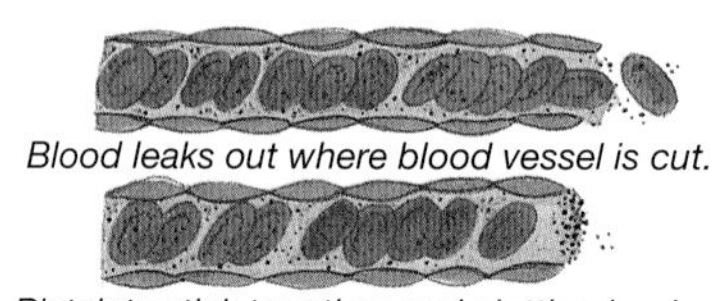

Blood leaks out where blood vessel is cut.

Platelets stick together, and clotting begins.

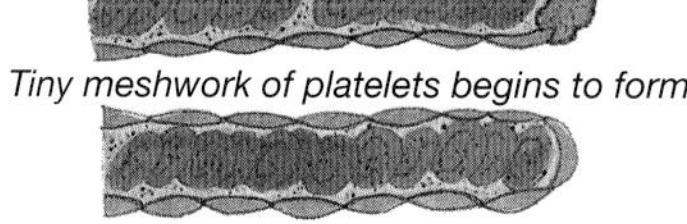

Tiny meshwork of platelets begins to form.

Blood clot forms, sealing the cut.

Find out more

BRAIN AND NERVES
HUMAN BODY
LUNGS AND BREATHING
MUSCLES AND MOVEMENT

HEAT

White-hot steel

STAND IN THE SUNSHINE: you feel warm. Go for a fast run: you will get hot. The warmth of sunshine comes from heat generated in the centre of the sun. Your body also produces heat all the time, and this heat keeps you alive. Heat is important to us in many ways. The sun's heat causes the weather, making winds blow and rain fall. The Earth's interior contains great heat, which causes volcanoes to erupt and earthquakes to shake the ground. Engines in cars, aircraft, and other forms of transport use the heat from burning fuel to produce movement. Power stations change heat into electricity which comes to our homes. Heat is a form of energy. Everything, even the coldest object, contains heat – a cold object simply has less heat than a hot object. All things are made of tiny particles called molecules. Heat energy comes from the vibrating movement of molecules. Hot objects have fast-moving molecules; molecules in colder objects move more slowly.

A solid, such as the ice on this window pane, has rows of molecules that vibrate back and forth. The molecules are locked together, so solids are often hard and cannot be squashed.

SOLIDS, LIQUIDS, AND GASES
A substance can be a solid, a liquid, or a gas, depending on how hot it is. Changing the temperature changes the substance from one state to another. For instance, liquid water becomes a solid – ice – when it is cold and a gas – steam – when it is hot.

A gas, such as steam, has molecules that move about freely so that the gas spreads out to fill its container.

A liquid, such as water, has molecules that are close together. The molecules can move around more easily than in a solid, so a liquid can flow.

A process called convection spreads heat through gases and liquids. For example, hot air above a heater rises. Cold air flows in to take its place, becomes hot, and rises. In this way, a circular current of air moves around a room, carrying heat with it.

Warm rising air

Convection heater

Cool incoming air

BOILING POINT
At a temperature called the boiling point, a liquid changes into a gas. Below the boiling point the gas changes back to a liquid again. The boiling point of water is 100°C (212°F).

MELTING POINT
Heating a solid makes it melt into liquid. This happens only at a certain temperature, which is called the melting point. Below this temperature, the liquid freezes to a solid again. The melting point of ice is 0°C (32°F).

All objects give out heat rays that travel through air and space. The heating element of an oven cooks food with heat rays. The transmission (movement) of heat by heat rays is called radiation. It is not the same as nuclear radiation.

Heat travels through solid objects by a process called conduction. Metal conducts heat well. For instance, a metal spoon in a cup of coffee gets hot quickly. Other substances, such as wood and plastic, do not conduct heat well. They are called insulators and are used to make items such as saucepan handles.

A liquid slowly changes into a gas at a temperature lower than its boiling point. This is called evaporation. The steam from this hot cup of coffee is evaporated water.

HEAT ENERGY

Heat is just one of many forms of energy. Sources of heat change one type of energy into heat energy. A burning fire, for example, changes chemical energy in its fuel into heat energy. Electric heaters change electrical energy into heat.

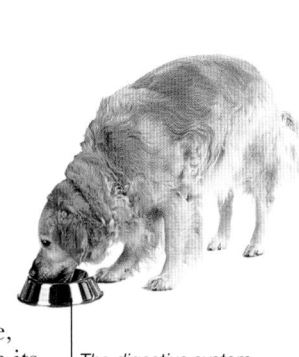

The digestive system of an animal or a person changes chemical energy from food into heat energy inside the body.

INFRA-RED RAYS

Heat rays are also called infra-red rays. They are invisible rays very similar to red light rays, which is why the rays are called infra-red. All objects give out these rays, and hot objects produce stronger infra-red rays than cold objects. Some electric heaters have curved reflectors that send heat rays forward just as a mirror reflects light rays.

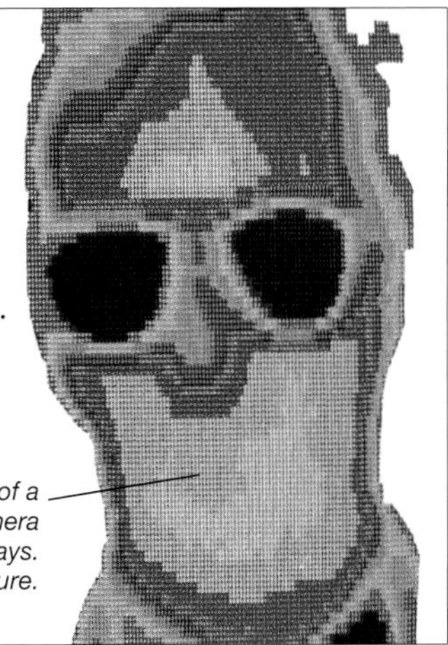

This is a thermogram (heat picture) of a person's face. It was taken by a special camera that uses infra-red rays instead of light rays. The hottest parts are yellow in the picture.

Temperature

Temperature is a measure of how hot an object is. A hot object has a higher temperature than a cold object. When objects are extremely cold, they have negative temperatures: a minus sign indicates how many degrees the temperature is below zero on the temperature scale.

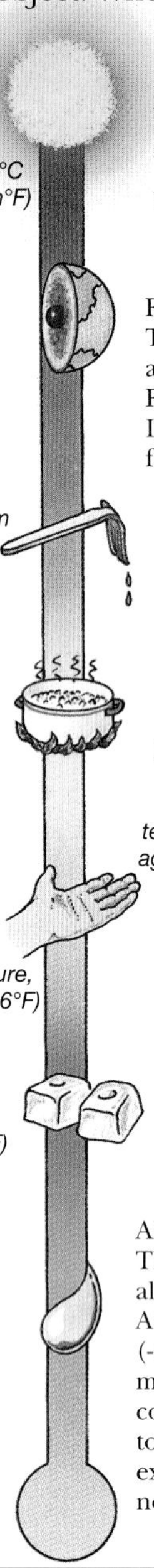

Centre of the Sun, about 15 million°C (27 million°F)

Centre of the Earth, about 4,500°C (8,100°F)

Aluminium melts, 660°C (1,220°F)

Water boils, 100°C (212°F)

Normal body temperature, 37°C (98.6°F)

Water freezes, 0°C (32°F)

Oxygen becomes liquid, -218°C (-360°F)

Absolute zero, -273°C (-460°F)

Fahrenheit

Temperatures marked with an "F" are recorded using the Fahrenheit scale of temperature. In the Fahrenheit scale, water freezes at 32°F and boils at 212°F. A few countries, including the United States, use the Fahrenheit scale.

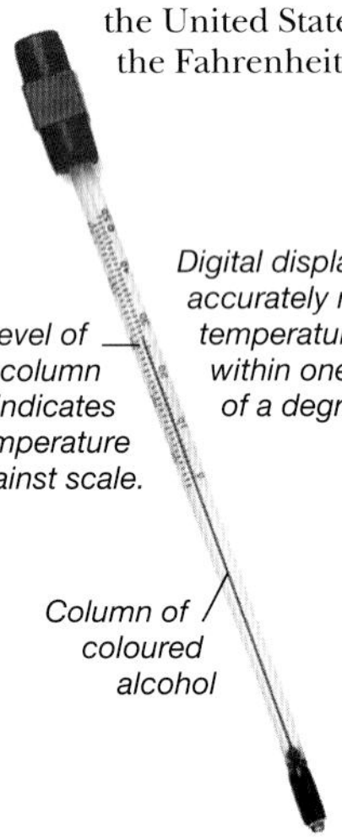

Level of column indicates temperature against scale.

Column of coloured alcohol

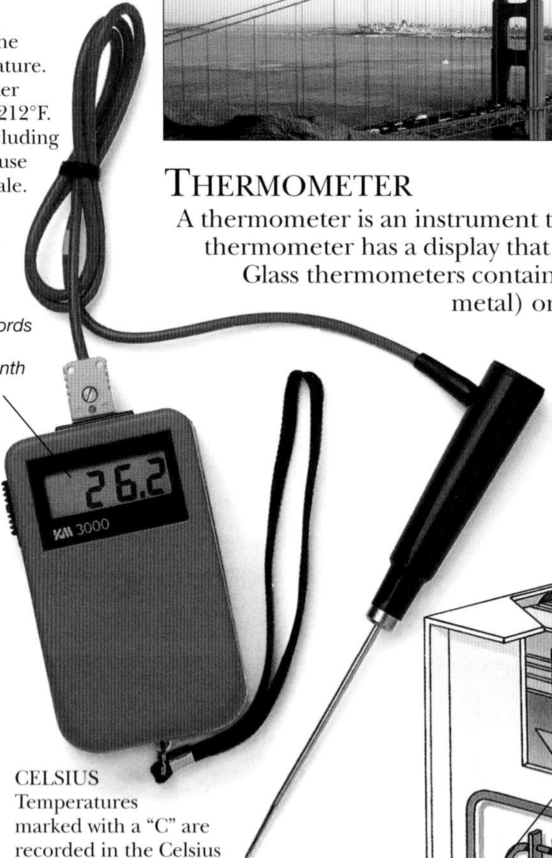

Digital display accurately records temperature within one tenth of a degree.

Absolute zero

The lowest temperature of all is called absolute zero. At absolute zero, -273°C (-460°F), molecules stop moving. Scientists have cooled substances almost to absolute zero, but the exact temperature can never be reached.

Celsius

Temperatures marked with a "C" are recorded in the Celsius (also called Centigrade) scale of temperature. In this scale, water freezes at 0°C and boils at 100°C. Scientists and most countries of the world use the Celsius scale.

Expansion and contraction

Most things expand (get slightly larger) when they get hot. They contract (shrink) again when they cool. This happens because the molecules inside an object make larger, more rapid vibrations as the object heats up. The molecules therefore take up more space, causing the object to expand. The Golden Gate bridge in San Francisco expands by up to 0.9 m (3 feet) in the summer months because of the hotter weather.

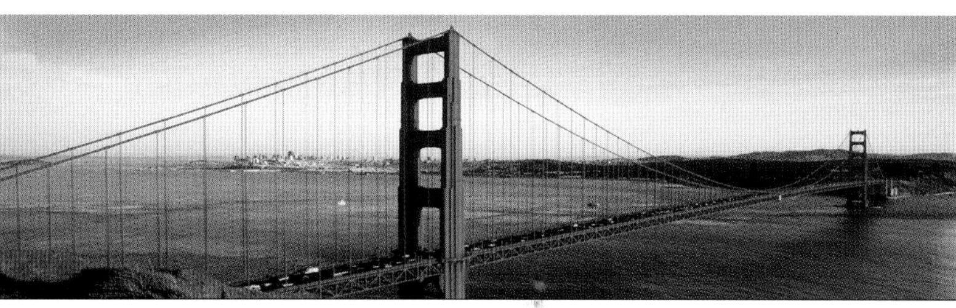

Thermometer

A thermometer is an instrument that measures temperature. A digital thermometer has a display that shows the temperature in numbers. Glass thermometers contain a thin column of mercury (a liquid metal) or coloured alcohol that expands and rises in the thermometer as the temperature increases.

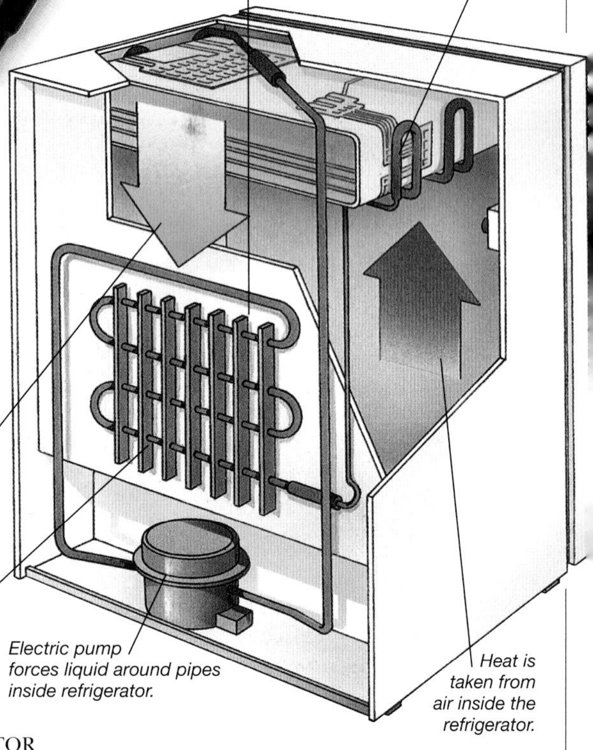

When vapour condenses back into a liquid, it gives out heat to the air around the condenser.

Liquid changes to vapour in evaporator by taking heat from inside the refrigerator and cooling it.

Surrounding cool air outside the refrigerator removes heat.

Vapour changes back to liquid in condenser, and continues its cycle around the refrigerator.

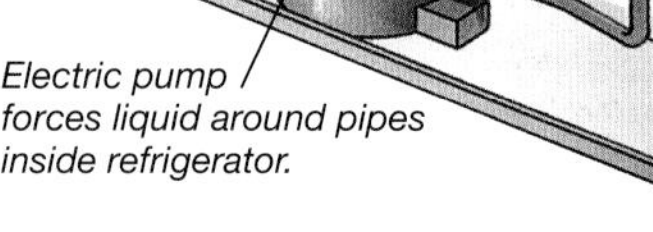

Electric pump forces liquid around pipes inside refrigerator.

Heat is taken from air inside the refrigerator.

Refrigerator

When liquids evaporate (change into a gas), they take heat from their surroundings. In a refrigerator, a liquid circulates, going through a cycle of evaporation and condensation (changing back into a liquid again). As the liquid evaporates, it takes heat from the food in the refrigerator.

Sweating and shivering

Your body usually has a steady temperature of 37°C (98.6°F). It automatically keeps you from getting too hot or too cold. Sweating cools you down if you get too hot. Shivering helps to warm you up when you get too cold. Hairs on your skin stand up when your body gets cold and help to trap a layer of air around the skin, which stops heat loss.

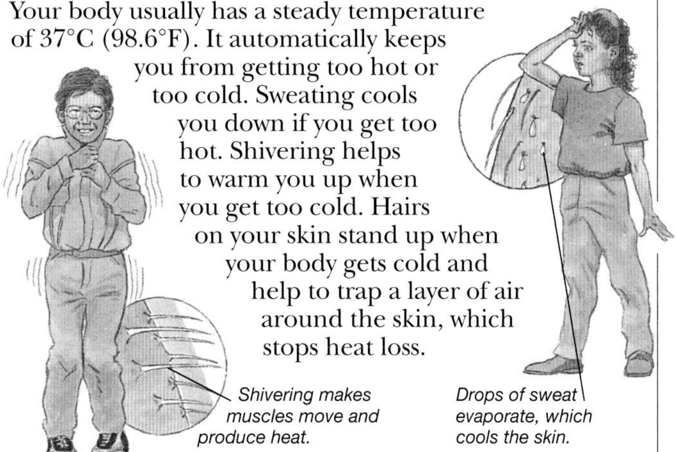

Shivering makes muscles move and produce heat.

Drops of sweat evaporate, which cools the skin.

Find out more

Atoms and molecules
Earth
Engines
Fire
Stars
Sun
Volcanoes

HEDGEHOGS

MOLES, AND SHREWS

Despite having short legs a hedgehog can move surprisingly fast.

NIGHT-TIME IS WHEN hedgehogs, moles, and shrews are most active. These small mammals are well adapted to living in the dark. Their eyesight and hearing are poor, but their sense of smell is keen, and their sensitive whiskers enable them to feel their way in the dark. Hedgehogs measure about 23 cm (9 in) in length, with a short tail, a long snout, and stiff needle-like spines covering the top of the body. Most hedgehogs rest in burrows during the day and emerge at night to hunt for insects and earthworms. The common European mole spends most of its life underground. Its soft, velvety fur lies flat and smooth in any direction, which enables the mole to move around easily in the earth. The mole uses its curved front feet and long claws for digging tunnels in search of insects. Shrews are also suited to dark conditions. They look like mice but are smaller, with a longer nose and tiny eyes. Most shrews live on land; the water shrew has adapted to life in rivers and streams where it hunts for fish and tadpoles. Hedgehogs, moles, and shrews all belong to a large animal group called insectivores (insect eaters).

When alarmed, the hedgehog rolls itself into a ball.The legs and face are gradually hidden.

The hedgehog usually peeps out to check that the danger has passed, before rolling over onto its front.

HIBERNATION
During winter, hedgehogs roll up into a ball and hibernate until spring arrives.

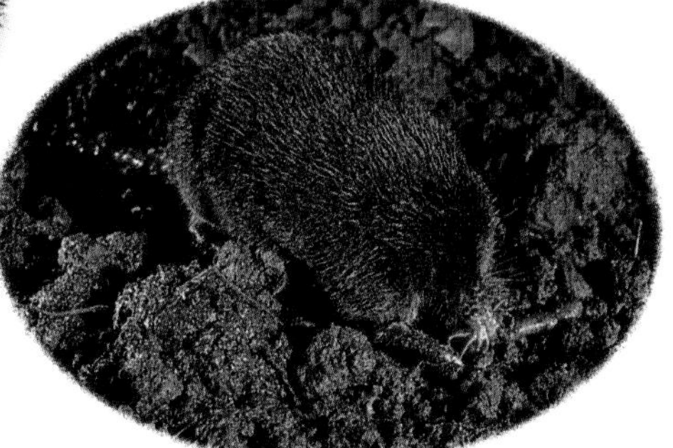

EUROPEAN HEDGEHOG

When it senses danger, the European hedgehog rolls itself into a ball. It tucks its head and feet into the centre of the ball, and a ring of muscles around the lower part of its body tightens like a drawstring on a purse. Hedgehogs have about 5,000 spines; when danger threatens, the spines stick straight out.

STAR-NOSED MOLE
The star-nosed mole shown here has an unusual nose which is very sensitive to touch and vibrations. The mole's nose helps it find worms and beetles in the darkness.

MOLE

There are about 35 different kinds of moles, found throughout the world. Like other moles, the European mole shown here lives mainly underground, digging new tunnels daily, each about 5 cm (2 in) wide. The mole patrols the tunnels regularly in search of worms and insects that have fallen through the walls.

SHREW
The smallest shrews measure just 5 to 8 cm (2 to 3 in) in length from nose to tail. Their tiny bodies lose heat so rapidly that in order to survive, shrews have to eat their own weight in food every day.

MOLEHILL
A molehill is made from the excess soil that the mole pushes out of the way as it digs. The large burrow shown here is where the mole rests and raises its young.

Moles have broad front paws with strong claws that work like shovels as they dig tunnels in the earth.

European hedgehog

American short-tailed shrew

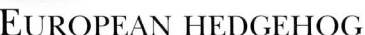

Mole's larder is stocked with worms and other creatures that have been bitten and wounded to keep them from escaping.

The central chamber of the breeding nest is lined with grass and leaves in the breeding season. A female mole gives birth to about four young each spring.

Shrews are active both day and night, searching for food, and rest only a few minutes every now and then.

Find out more

ANIMALS
MAMMALS
NESTS AND BURROWS

HELICOPTERS

OF ALL FLYING machines, the helicopter is the most versatile. It can fly forwards, backwards, or sideways. It can go straight up and down, and even hover in the air without moving. Because helicopters can take off vertically, they do not need to use airport runways and can fly almost anywhere. They can rescue people from mountains, fly to oil rigs out at sea, and even land on the roofs of skyscrapers. Helicopters come in many shapes and sizes. Some are designed to carry only one person; others are powerful enough to lift a truck. All helicopters have one or two large rotors. The rotor blades are shaped like long, thin wings. When they spin around, they lift the helicopter up and drive it through the air.

Gas turbine engine (one of three)

Rotor blades, made of ultra-strong plastics

Cockpit with automatic flight control system

ALL-PURPOSE HELICOPTER

The EH101 can transport 30 passengers or troops, carry 16 stretcher patients as an air ambulance, or lift a load of more than 6 tonnes (5.9 tons). It flies at 280 km/h (170 mph).

Radar dome contains radar antenna.

Mission control console, equipped with radar screens and computers

Helicopter body, made of light metal alloys and strong plastics

Tail plane and fins keep the helicopter stable as it flies.

Tail rotor steers the helicopter and keeps it from spinning around.

Wheels fold into pods on sides of helicopter.

Crewman lowered down to life raft

Life raft contains survivors from shipwreck.

TAKING OFF

The rotor blades produce a lifting force which supports the helicopter.

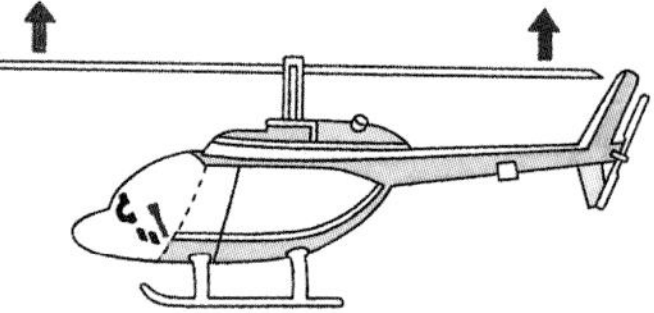

The "collective pitch" stick adjusts the rotors so the helicopter can go up, hover, or go down.

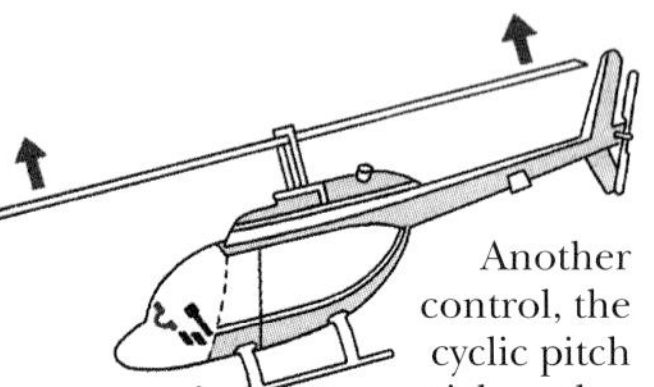

Another control, the cyclic pitch stick, makes the main rotor tilt so that it can pull the helicopter in any direction – backwards, forwards, or sideways.

The tail rotor keeps the helicopter from spinning around. Pedals control the tail rotor so the helicopter can be turned to face any direction.

DEVELOPMENT

The Italian artist and scientist Leonardo da Vinci sketched a simple helicopter about 500 years ago, but it was never built. It was not until 1907 that a helicopter carried a person. It was built by a French mechanic named Paul Cornu.

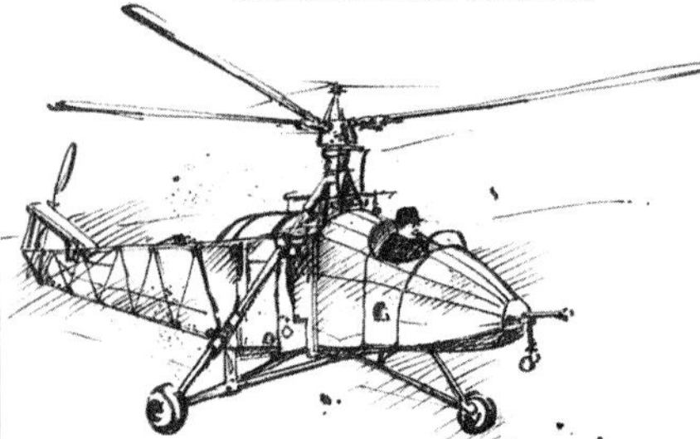

Igor Sikorsky, a Russian-American, built the VS-300 in 1939. It was the first single-rotor helicopter, and it set the style for machines to come.

TWIN-ROTOR HELICOPTER

Large helicopters, such as this Boeing Chinook, may be twin-rotor machines. They have two main rotors that spin in opposite directions, and no tail rotor. The largest helicopter in the world is the Russian Mil Mi 12. It has twin rotors and is powered by four gas turbine engines.

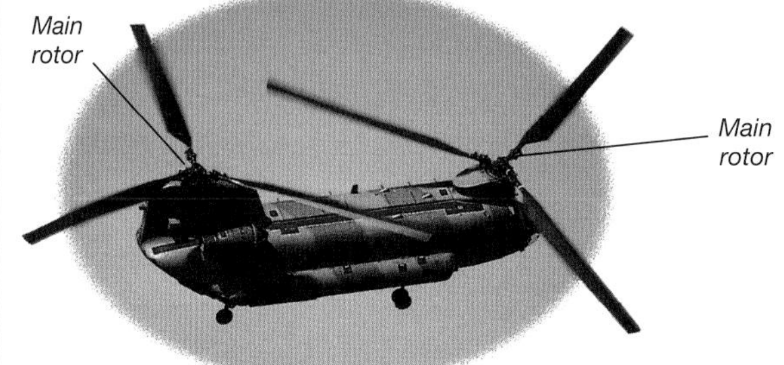

Find out more

AIRCRAFT
ARMIES
MILITARY AIRCRAFT
PLASTICS

HENRY VIII

THE SON OF HENRY VII, Henry VIII was the second of the Tudor monarchs, and probably the most famous king of England. Strong-willed, pleasure-loving, unpredictable, and obstinate, he inspired both admiration and fear. Henry wanted England to be a great power in Renaissance Europe, and used the money his father had amassed to establish Britain as a great naval force and to fight wars all over Europe. Resenting the power of the pope, who would not grant him a divorce from his first wife, Henry passed the Act of Supremacy in 1534. This set up the Church of England as a separate institution to the Catholic Church, and made the monarch its supreme head. Henry married six times, trying to produce a male heir.

1491 Born at Greenwich.

1509 Becomes king and marries Catherine of Aragon.

1533 Marries Anne Boleyn.

1535 Suppresses the monasteries.

1536 Anne Boleyn beheaded. Henry marries Jane Seymour.

1537 Son Edward born. Queen Jane dies.

1540 Henry marries Anne of Cleves; the marriage is annulled. Then marries Catherine Howard.

1542 Catherine is executed for treason.

1543 Henry marries Catherine Parr.

1547 Dies; buried at Whitehall.

WAR AND PEACE

Henry sought glory through war with France. He strengthened the navy and had many powerful new ships built. At the Battle of the Spurs (1513), he led his army to victory, then in 1520 he organized a peace treaty between France and England at the ceremony of the Field of the Cloth of Gold. In 1544 he again made war with France. England captured Boulogne and France agreed to pay the king the sum of 2,000,000 crowns.

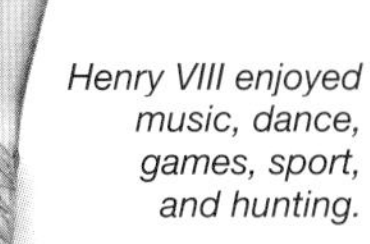

Henry VIII enjoyed music, dance, games, sport, and hunting.

THOMAS CRANMER

Henry had many advisors. Those who disagreed with him were usually executed, but Thomas Cranmer (1499-1556), who supported Henry's marriage to Anne Boleyn, was made Archbishop of Canterbury in 1533.

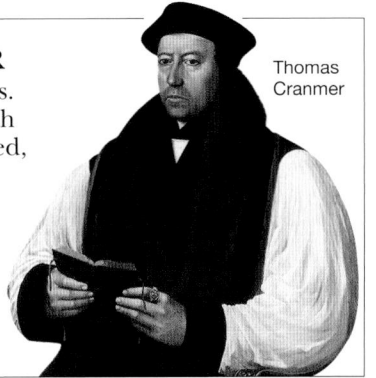

Thomas Cranmer

THE SIX WIVES

Henry's first wife was Catherine of Aragon, mother of Mary I. Because no male heir was born, the king divorced Catherine and married Anne Boleyn, mother of Elizabeth I. For this, he was excommunicated by the pope. After Anne, Henry had four more wives: Jane Seymour, mother of King Edward VI; Anne of Cleves; Catherine Howard; and Catherine Parr, who outlived the king.

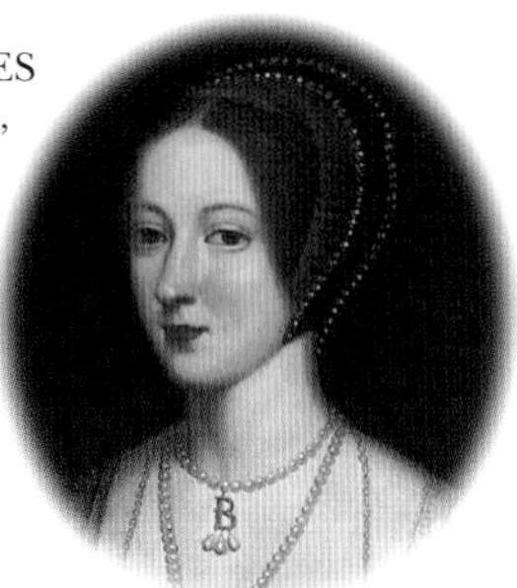

Anne Boleyn

THE ENGLISH REFORMATION

In 1534, Henry abolished the authority of the pope in England and founded the Church of England. This was the beginning of the English Reformation. Monasteries were closed and the king acquired their wealth and lands. The buildings fell into ruin or were destroyed.

Kirkstall Abbey, Yorkshire, destroyed in the Reformation.

HAMPTON COURT

During Henry's reign, great houses were built by rich landowners and the king's courtiers, while many people lived in poverty. Henry himself oversaw the final building stages of Hampton Court, the largest house in England, begun by Cardinal Wolsey and built in brick, like many Tudor houses.

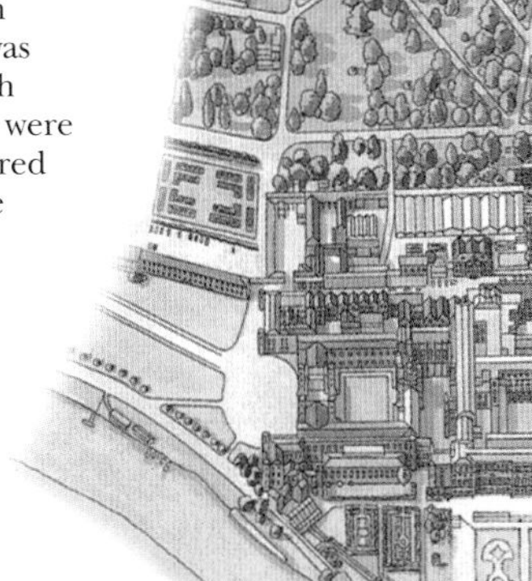

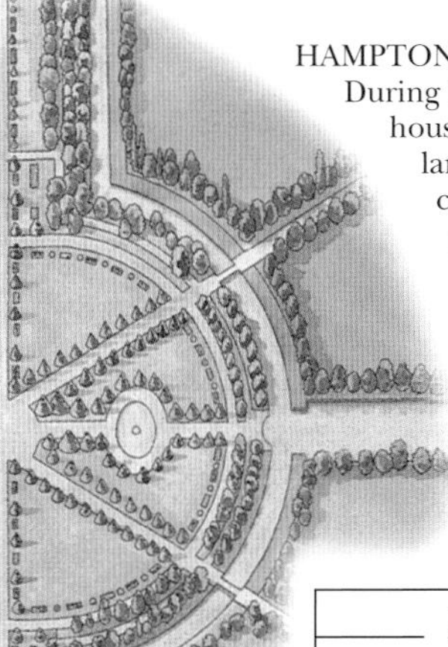

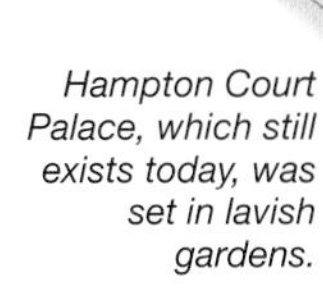

Hampton Court Palace, which still exists today, was set in lavish gardens.

Find out more

MONASTERIES
REFORMATION
RENAISSANCE
TUDORS

HIBERNATION

MANY WARM-BLOODED ANIMALS need extra energy in order to stay warm in the cold winter months, but the source of that energy – food – is scarce in winter. Some animals survive winter by migrating to a warmer place; others, such as bats and hedgehogs, hibernate in a safe and unexposed place such as a nest, burrow, or cave. In true hibernation, the body processes slow down almost to a standstill – the heartbeat occurs only every now and then, and the animal takes only a few breaths per minute. The body temperature falls to only a few degrees above the outside temperature – as low as 0°C (32°F) in a hamster. If the outside temperature drops below zero, chemical reactions in the animal's body switch on to keep it from freezing to death. A hibernating animal feasts on extra food in the autumn so it can build up reserves of fat in its body and survive the winter months without food.

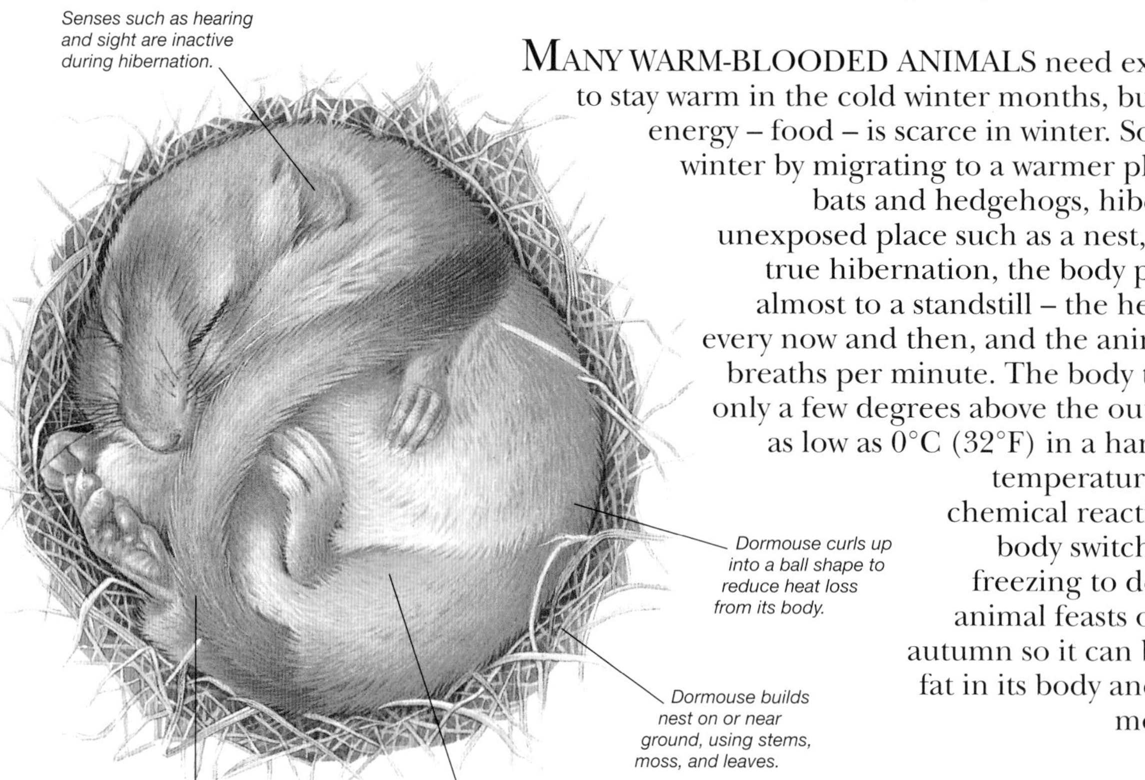

Senses such as hearing and sight are inactive during hibernation.
Dormouse curls up into a ball shape to reduce heat loss from its body.
Dormouse builds nest on or near ground, using stems, moss, and leaves.
Furry tail wraps around face for protection and insulation.
Up to half of body weight is lost during hibernation.

DORMOUSE

One of the best-known hibernators is the dormouse. In autumn it feeds eagerly to build up stores of body fat, then settles into a winter nest among tree roots or in dense undergrowth. Its heart slows to only one beat every few minutes, and its breathing slows down. Its body temperature also drops to a few degrees above the surroundings.

BLACK BEAR

The winter sleep of bears, skunks, and chipmunks is not as deep as the true hibernation of bats and mice. The American black bear's heartbeat slows but the body temperature drops by only a few degrees. This means that the bear can rouse itself from its sleep quite rapidly during a spell of slightly warmer weather. Although it wakes up, the bear does not eat and continues to live off its body fat until the spring. Some female bears give birth during the winter months.

TORPOR

To save energy, some small, warm-blooded animals such as bats and hummingbirds allow their bodies to cool and their heartbeat and breathing to slow down for part of the day or night. This is called torpor. Large animals such as bears do not become torpid because they would need too much energy to warm up again afterwards. Bats often huddle together as they hang upside down to prevent too much heat loss. When the cold season comes, bats fly to a special cave or tree called a hibernaculum, where they begin true hibernation.

AESTIVATION

Many desert animals sleep during the hot, dry season to survive the intense heat. This is called aestivation – the opposite of hibernation. Desert creatures which aestivate include lizards, frogs, insects, and snails. Before aestivation begins, snails seal their shell openings with a film of mucus that hardens in the heat.

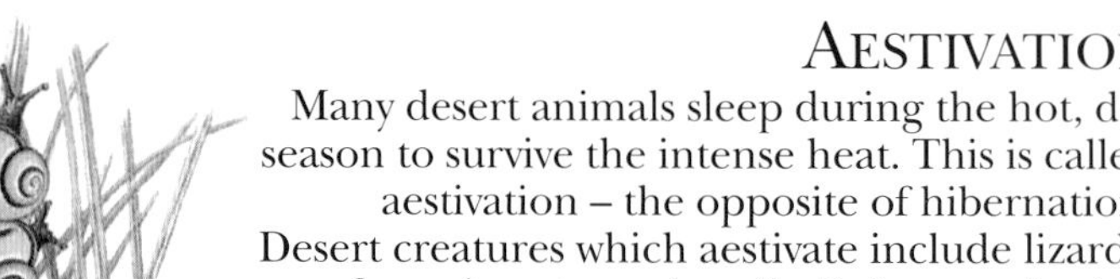

Snails cluster on grass stems to aestivate, away from predators on the ground.

Find out more

BATS
BEARS AND PANDAS
MICE, RATS, AND SQUIRRELS
MIGRATION, ANIMAL
SNAILS AND SLUGS

HINDUISM

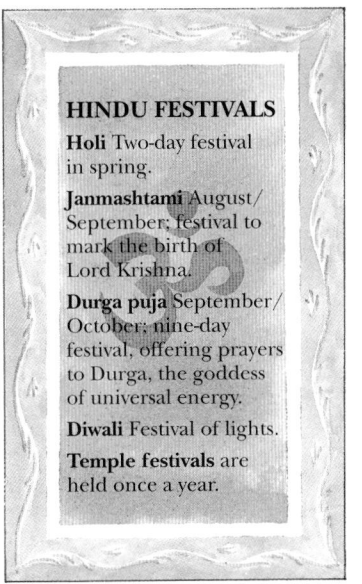

HINDU FESTIVALS

Holi Two-day festival in spring.

Janmashtami August/ September; festival to mark the birth of Lord Krishna.

Durga puja September/ October; nine-day festival, offering prayers to Durga, the goddess of universal energy.

Diwali Festival of lights.

Temple festivals are held once a year.

MORE THAN 5,000 YEARS ago Hinduism, one of the world's oldest religions, began in India. Hinduism has no single founder but grew gradually from early beliefs. Today there are many different Hindu groups or sects. They may worship the same Hindu gods, but they do not all share the same religious beliefs. Nevertheless, most Hindus believe that people have a soul which does not die with them. Instead the soul moves out from a dying body and enters the new one being born. People who live good lives are reincarnated, or born again, in a higher state. Bad deeds can lead to rebirth as animal or an insect. It is possible to escape from the cycle of death and rebirth through Karma, that is, good deeds that bring an individual to the state of Moksha (liberation). Hindus are born into castes, or groups, which give them their rank in society. Rules restrict how people of different castes may mix and marry. Today, there are about 900 million Hindus in the world. They live mainly in India and East Africa.

GODS

There are three primary gods – Vishnu, Brahma, and Shiva – created by the energy of the universe. For the purpose of worship, however, a Hindu may choose any one of the gods as his deity. Vishnu, the preserver, appears in ten different incarnations (forms). Two of the most popular are Rama and Krishna. Stories of the gods and their battles against evil are told in ancient Indian scriptures (writings) such as the Mahabharata.

More gentle than the fierce Shiva, Vishnu comes to restore order and peace to the world.

The four heads of Brahma, the creator, looking in all four directions, show that he has knowledge of all things.

Shiva, the destroyer, rules over the death and life of everything in the world. It is thought that when Shiva dances, he destroys all life.

MARRIAGE

Family life and marriage are very important to Hindus. Parents are often involved in their children's choice of partner. Women are required to be dutiful and obedient to their fathers and husbands. A wedding ceremony is accompanied by music and feasting. The bride and groom exchange colourful garlands of flowers and make solemn promises to each other before a priest.

TEMPLES

In southern and central India there are large temples that contain ornate carvings and statues of the many Hindu gods. Priests look after the temples. They bathe the idols every day, and decorate them with ornaments. Visitors come to pray and bring offerings of flowers and food. After the food has been blessed, it is shared by the worshippers or given to the poor.

Find out more

FESTIVALS
INDIA
RELIGIONS

HOLOCAUST

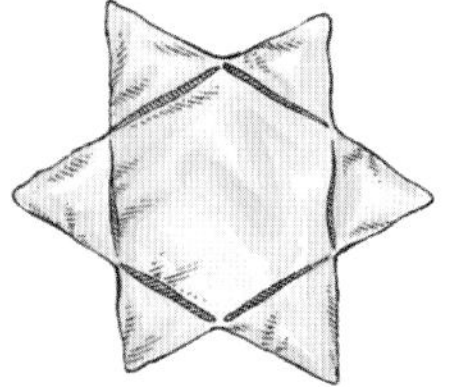

YELLOW STAR
After 1941, Jews over the age of six in German-occupied Europe had to sew a yellow star, the Star of David, onto their clothes. This made it easier to identify them. Jews also wore yellow stars in the camps.

IN 1933, ADOLF HITLER'S NAZI PARTY came to power in Germany. The Nazis were deeply anti-Semitic (prejudiced against Jews) and began to attack German Jews. At first they rounded up Jews and sent them to labour or concentration camps, together with other people the Nazis did not like, such as gypsies, homosexuals, communists, and others. Jews in German-occupied Europe were forced into ghettos (closed-off areas of a city) or shot. In 1942, the Nazis decided to kill all European Jews in an act of genocide (the deliberate extermination of an entire people). No-one knows how many were murdered in death camps such as Auschwitz and Treblinka, but more than six million Jews lost their lives before the end of World War II. This terrible event in human history is called the Holocaust.

Oscar Schindler

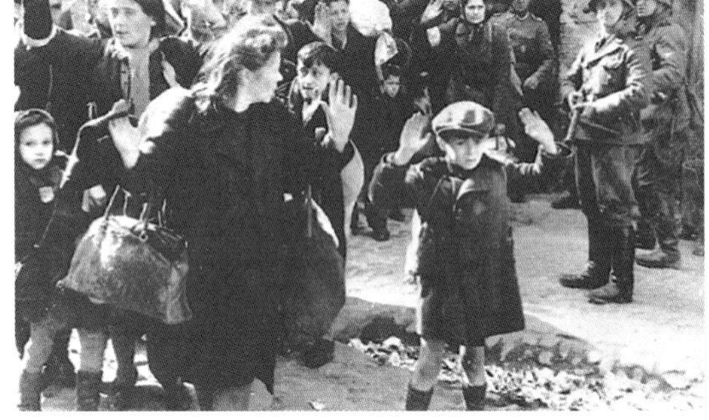

GHETTOS

In Warsaw and other East European cities occupied by the Germans after 1939, Jews were herded into ghettos. These ghettos were isolated from the rest of the city and their inhabitants denied proper food or medical care. In 1943, the Germans attacked the Warsaw ghetto in order to kill everyone inside. The Jews fought back, but by 1945 only about 100 of the original 500,000 inhabitants were still alive.

RESISTANCE
Many Jews resisted the Nazis, by attacking German forces and supplies. Both the Hungarian and Italian governments, although German allies, refused to hand over their Jews, while the Swedish diplomat Raoul Wallenberg helped many Jews escape to Sweden in 1944. Most famously, German businessman Oscar Schindler saved about 1,200 Jews from death, by giving them essential war work in his munitions factory.

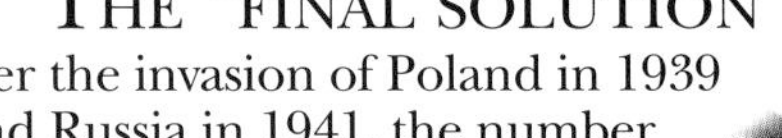

THE "FINAL SOLUTION"

After the invasion of Poland in 1939 and Russia in 1941, the number of Jews under German rule increased. At a conference at Wannsee, Berlin in 1942, the Nazis decided on what they called the "Final Solution": to kill all Jews in specially built extermination camps. These included Auschwitz and Treblinka in Poland, and Belsen, Dachau, and Buchenwald in Germany.

Gates to Auschwitz

COMMEMORATION
After the war, the United Nations tried to repay the Jews for their suffering by creating a Jewish homeland – Israel – in Palestine in 1948. Holocaust museums have been opened in Berlin and elsewhere. Many countries have an official Holocaust commemoration day on 27 January – the anniversary of the liberation of Auschwitz, the first camp to be freed.

THE HOLOCAUST

1933 Hitler's Nazi Party takes power in Germany.

1935 Nuremberg Laws forbid marriage between Jews and non-Jews.

1937 Jewish businesses confiscated.

1938 The Night of Broken Glass (9-10 November); synagogues, shops and homes destroyed.

1942 "Final Solution" begins.

1943 Jews in the Warsaw ghetto wiped out.

1945 Concentration camps liberated.

1948 Israel founded.

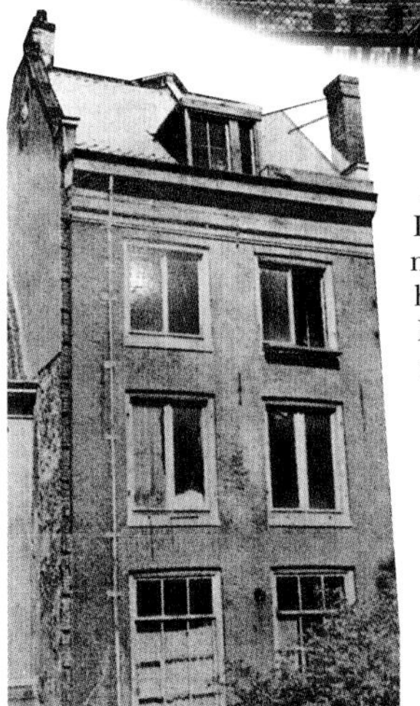

ANNE FRANK
In order to escape the Nazis, many European Jews went into hiding. Thirteen-year-old Anne Frank and her family hid for two years in the back attic of a house in Amsterdam, Holland. In 1944, they were betrayed and sent to a concentration camp, where Anne died of typhus in 1945, aged 16. While in hiding, Anne kept a diary of daily events and her hopes for the future. Published in 1947, her diary was translated into more than 50 languages.

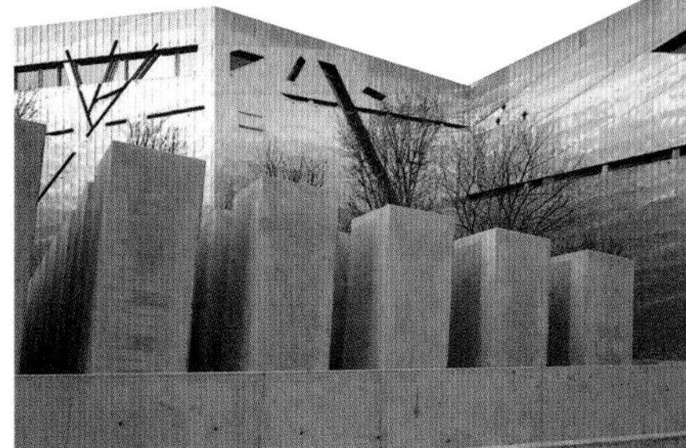

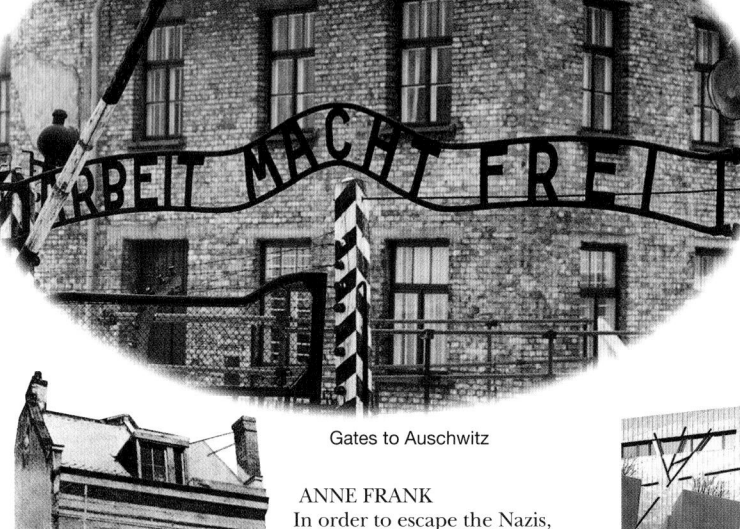

Jewish Museum, Berlin

Find out more
ISRAEL
JUDAISM
WORLD WAR II

Horse-riding

Horses and humans have teamed up for more than 2,000 years, and horses were an essential means of transport for many centuries. Riding for sport and leisure developed in the 17th century and is still enjoyed today. Horse-riding is a wonderful pastime, particularly for young people, and there are many competitive events. These range from polo, and eventing, through to cross-country competitions. Riding is fun, but it also takes skill, practice, and even some courage, especially for jumping. Riders sit on a saddle and put their feet in stirrups, which hang from the saddle. They hold reins attached to a bit in the horse's delicate mouth. The rider controls the horse, urging it into a walk, trot, canter, or turn, using gentle pressure from legs, hands, and body. Riders wear special clothing, including helmets.

STIRRUPS
Around 300 B.C., tribes in Central Asia developed a stirrup to hold a rider's feet. Stirrups made it easier to fight in the saddle. Modern stirrups are usually made of steel.

Rider presses with inside leg to encourage pony to turn.

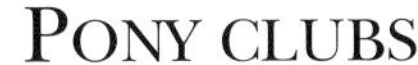

Pony clubs

Many young riders who want to compete in horse events join pony clubs. These organize sporting events and games, which improve riding skills. Pony clubs also teach young riders how to look after their horse and its tack (saddle, bridle, and other equipment), and organize riding camps.

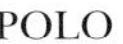

POLO
In this fast and exciting game, two teams, each consisting of four riders, compete against each other on a large field. Players use a mallet to hit a wooden ball through the goal. The team that scores the most goals wins. Polo ponies have to be very agile, and players use their legs to guide them. The game is fast and ponies become tired quickly. Players may change ponies several times during a game.

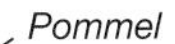

Pommel

SADDLES
The saddle is an important piece of horse-riding equipment. It provides a comfortable seat for the rider, and helps to protect the horse's spine. A strap, called a girth, runs under the horse's body to keep the saddle in place. The Western saddle has a horn-shaped pommel and wide stirrups.

Western saddle

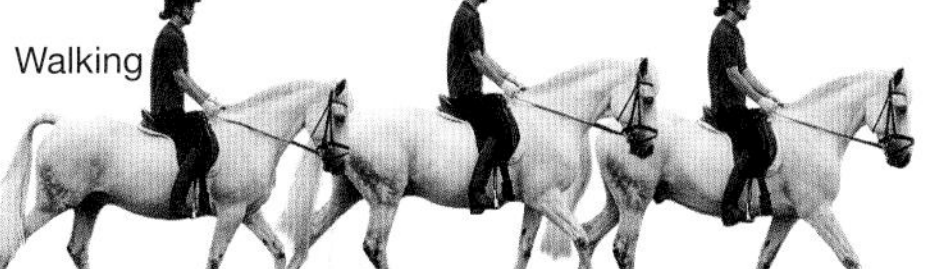

Walking

Trotting

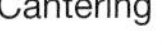

Cantering

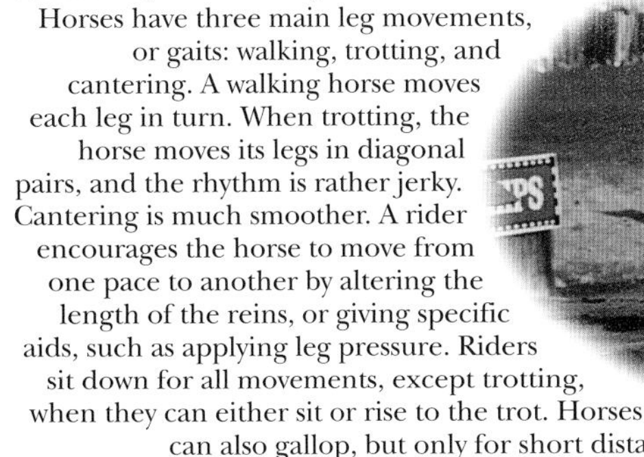

WALKING, TROTTING, AND CANTERING
Horses have three main leg movements, or gaits: walking, trotting, and cantering. A walking horse moves each leg in turn. When trotting, the horse moves its legs in diagonal pairs, and the rhythm is rather jerky. Cantering is much smoother. A rider encourages the horse to move from one pace to another by altering the length of the reins, or giving specific aids, such as applying leg pressure. Riders sit down for all movements, except trotting, when they can either sit or rise to the trot. Horses can also gallop, but only for short distances.

EVENTING
Eventing can last for one, two, or three days, and tests a horse's and rider's agility and endurance. Activities include dressage, which tests obedience, and a gruelling cross-country race. Showjumping, over high fences and tricky water jumps, is the final event.

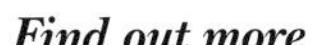

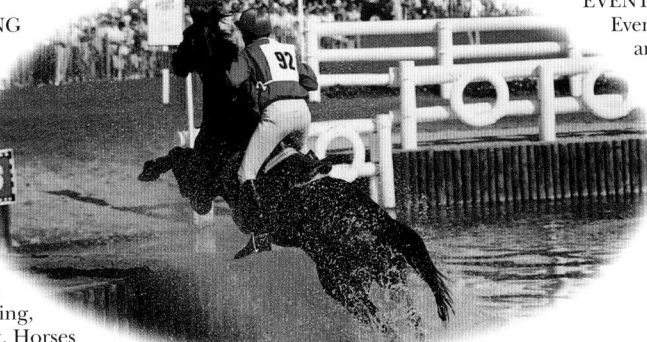

Find out more

Horses, zebras and asses
Olympic games
Sports

HORSES
ZEBRAS, AND ASSES

FOR THREE THOUSAND YEARS before trains and cars were invented, horses were a fast, efficient method of transport. These swift, graceful creatures are easy for humans to train. Today there are more than 75 million domestic (tame) horses, and they are divided into more than 100 different breeds. Horses, asses, and zebras belong to the equid family, a group that includes donkeys and mules. Equids are long-legged mammals with hoofed feet, flowing tails, and a mane on the upper part of the neck. They can run or gallop with great speed. A keen sense of smell, good eyesight, and sharp hearing mean that they are always alert and ready to flee from danger. Horses, asses, and zebras are grazing animals that feed almost entirely on grasses, which they crop with their sharp front teeth.

TEETH
Experts can tell the age of a horse by the number, angle, and size of its teeth, and the way the teeth have worn down with use. Most adult horses have between 40 and 42 teeth.

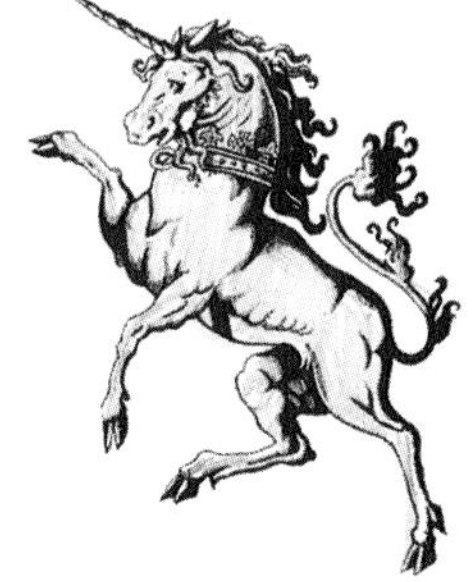

UNICORN
The unicorn is an imaginary horselike creature. It often appears in legends and folktales as a symbol of purity.

Poll
Forelock
Large ears can swivel to detect which direction a sound comes from.
Eyes are on the side of the head for good all-round vision.
Mane covers upper neck.
Withers
Back
Flank
Croup
Dock
Muzzle
Long jaws and strong cheek muscles for chewing grass
Neck
Chest
Elbow
Knee
Horse uses long, coarse hairs of tail as a fly-whisk and as a social signal.
Cannon
Fetlock
Pastern
Hoof

Today's domestic horse
Hyracotherium

THE FIRST HORSES
Hyracotherium, one of the first horses, lived in woodland areas more than 50 million years ago. It was only 60 cm (2 ft) high. Through evolution, horses gradually became larger and began to live in more open grassland areas.

HOOVES
Horses walk on the tips of their toes. On each foot is a strong, hard hoof made of bone. There is a pad on the sole of the hoof called the frog. The frog acts like a shock absorber when the horse runs. People also put metal horseshoes on a horse's hooves to protect them on hard roads and rough ground.

Heel
Frog
Sole
Horseshoe
Bones

ADULTS AND YOUNG
An adult male horse is called a stallion; an adult female is a mare. Young males are called colts; young females are fillies.

HORSES AND HUMANS

Domestic horses are trained to do many jobs, from pulling carts to carrying soldiers into battle. Many sports and leisure activities involve horses, such as show jumping, polo, rodeo, flat racing, and steeplechasing. Champion horses are worth millions of pounds, and the first prize at a famous horse race may be thousands of pounds.

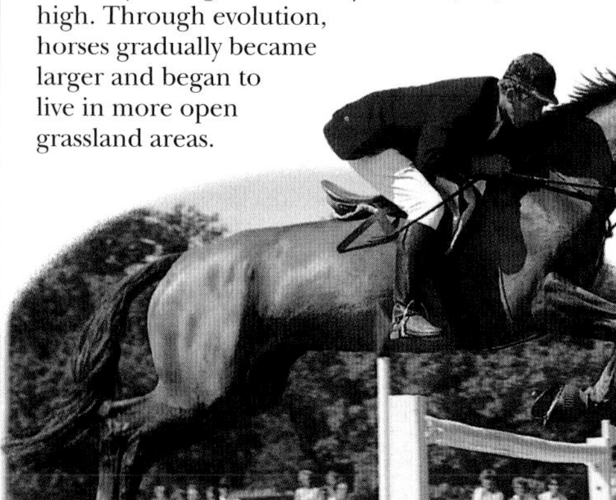

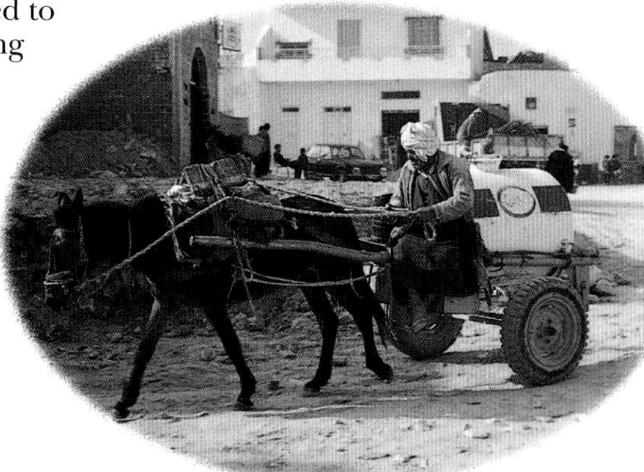

In some countries horses and mules are still used instead of cars. They are also used on farms to till fields, fertilize the crops, and pull produce to market.

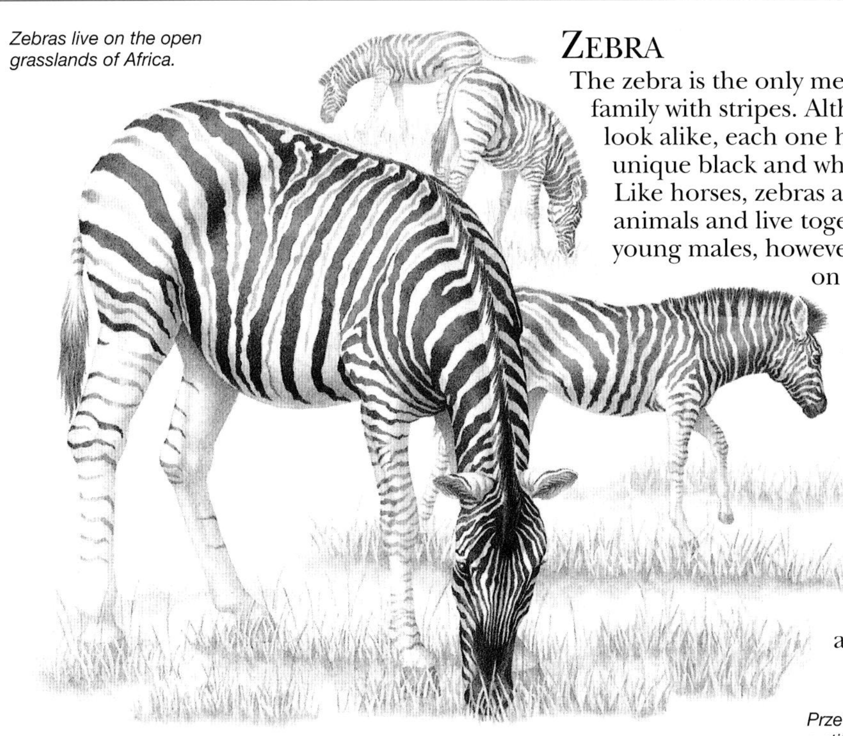

Zebras live on the open grasslands of Africa.

Zebra

The zebra is the only member of the horse family with stripes. Although zebras look alike, each one has its own unique black and white markings. Like horses, zebras are social animals and live together in herds; young males, however, often live on their own until they are mature. As they become adults, male zebras battle with other males to collect a group, or harem, of females to breed with. A zebra can run at about 65 km/h (40 mph) to escape from a predator such as a lion.

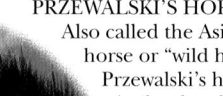

DONKEY
A donkey is a domesticated ass. Donkeys, together with horses and asses, have been hauling loads for people for thousands of years. They are often called beasts of burden. Another beast of burden, the mule, is the offspring of a female horse and a male donkey.

Ass

There are two kinds of wild ass – the African ass and the Asian ass. The African ass lives in dry, rocky areas of North Africa; the Asian ass is found in Asia. Asses need very little water and survive in the wild by eating tough, spiky grasses. Like other members of the horse family, the female ass has one young at a time, called a foal. The foal can walk a few minutes after birth.

A wild ass and a smaller domesticated ass

Przewalski's horse has a stiff upright mane.

PRZEWALSKI'S HORSE
Also called the Asian horse or "wild horse", Przewalski's horse is closely related to the domestic horse. Herds of these horses once lived on the high plains of Mongolia, in northern Asia. Today there are only a few hundred left in zoos and wildlife parks around the world, although there have been attempts to introduce them back into the wild in Mongolia.

GALLOPING
Horses move at a walk, trot, canter, or gallop, in increasing order of speed. When a horse gallops, all its hooves are off the ground for a split second during each stride. The fastest race horses can gallop at more than 65 km/h (40 mph) over a short distance.

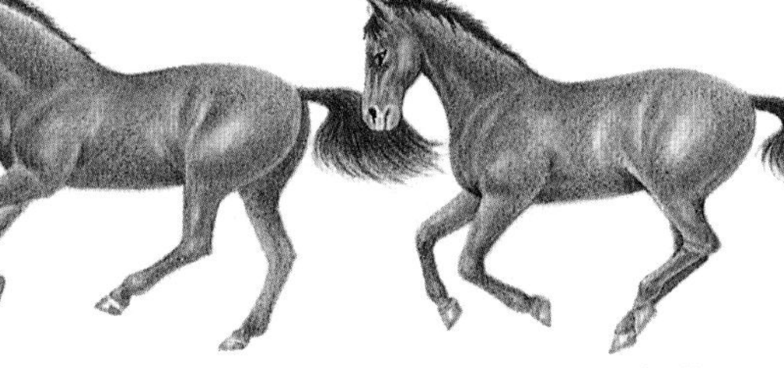

All four hooves lift off the ground in mid-gallop.

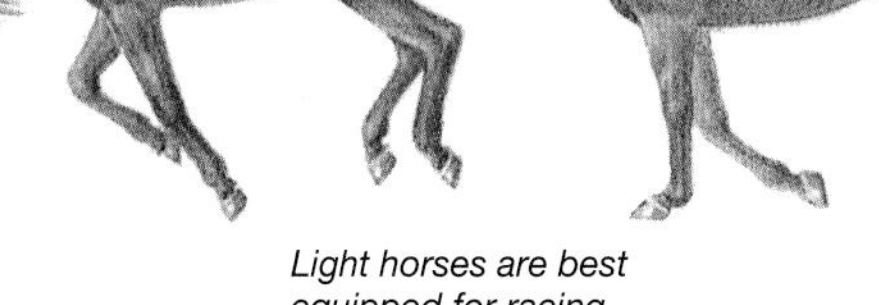

Light horses are best equipped for racing.

HOW WE MEASURE HORSES

Horses are measured in hands from the ground to the withers (the highest point of the shoulder). One hand equals 10 cm (4 in). Shire horses are the largest and Shetland ponies are among the smallest horses.

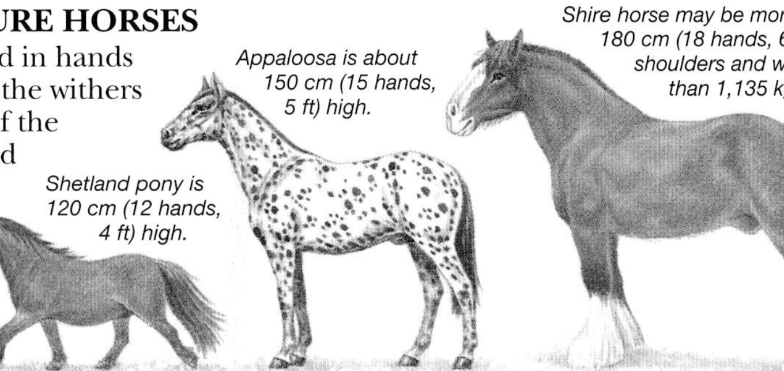

Shetland pony is 120 cm (12 hands, 4 ft) high.

Appaloosa is about 150 cm (15 hands, 5 ft) high.

Shire horse may be more than 180 cm (18 hands, 6 ft) at the shoulders and weigh more than 1,135 kg (2,500 lb).

TYPES OF HORSES
There are three main kinds of horses – draught horses such as Shires; light horses such as Arabian horses; and ponies such as Shetland ponies. Draught horses pull ploughs, and light horses take part in races.

Find out more

ANIMALS
HORSE-RIDING
MAMMALS
TRANSPORT, HISTORY OF

Hospitals

A MACHINE THAT CAN make sick people well sounds like an inventor's dream, but it already exists – it is a hospital. Like a machine, a hospital is a well-run unit that contains all the equipment and facilities needed to treat every kind of illness. But unlike a machine, a hospital is a human place staffed by doctors, nurses, and operating staff, all of them trained to make patients well. Hospitals are needed because there are some disorders that physicians cannot treat in the home or the doctor's office. Someone needing surgery, for instance, usually has to spend a day or more in the hospital. Other people may visit the hospital for a short time during the day, perhaps to see a skin specialist, or for medical tests such as x-rays. In this way, hospitals also provide facilities for diagnosing illness, and care for people who, though not ill, need medical attention, such as women giving birth.

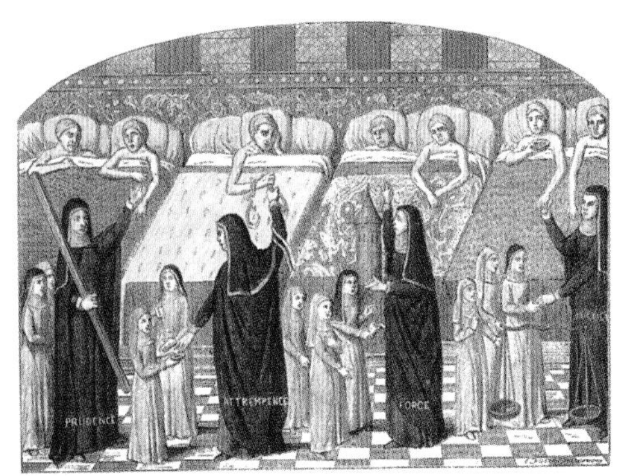

EARLY HOSPITALS
Until the 19th century, hospitals were unhealthy, crowded places where the poor were treated. People with dangerous infectious diseases were also taken to hospitals to prevent them from infecting others.

General hospitals

Some hospitals treat only certain patients, such as those with mental illnesses, but general hospitals treat patients suffering from all kinds of problems. Most towns and cities have a general hospital. General hospitals contain medical wards, surgical wards for people having operations, maternity wards for women having babies, and children's wards. They also have intensive care units, casualty departments, and operating rooms.

ACCIDENTS AND EMERGENCIES
People who are injured or suddenly taken very ill may be rushed by ambulance to the casualty department.

A powerful lamp lights the area where the surgeon operates.

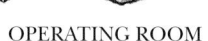

OPERATING ROOM
Surgeons carry out operations in specially equipped rooms where everything is kept very clean to prevent infection.

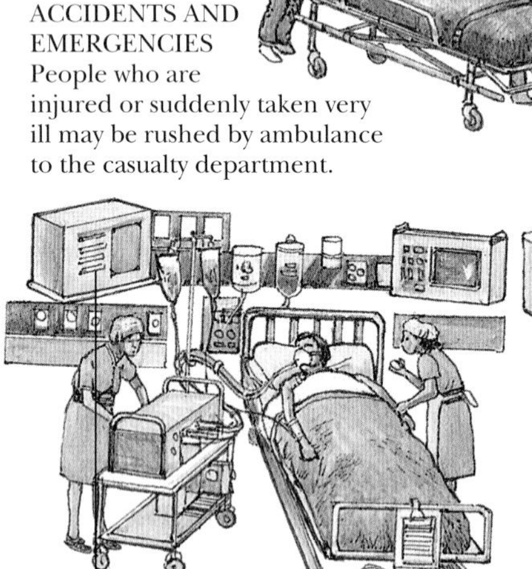

In the intensive care unit the staff uses electronic monitoring devices to keep constant track of the condition of seriously ill patients.

Nurses carefully monitor the medication that each patient receives.

WARDS
Some patients stay in a ward – a room with several beds. Hospital departments, such as surgery, are also called wards.

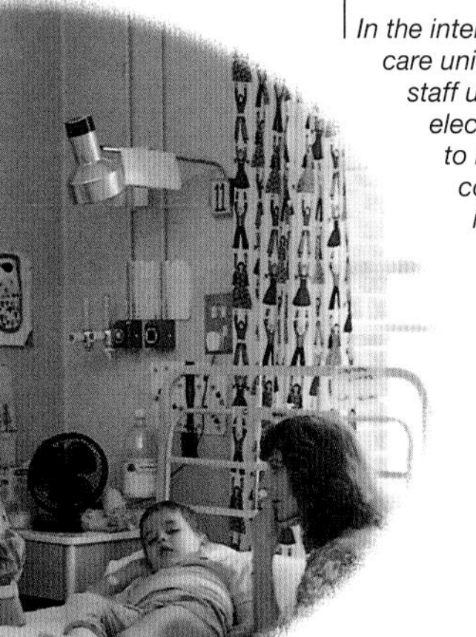

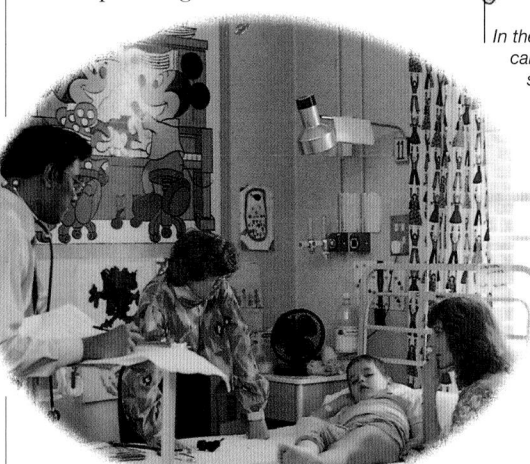

Children's hospitals

Some cities have special hospitals that are only for children. Nurses and doctors who work in children's hospitals are specially trained to care for babies and children. Parents can usually stay with their children throughout the day and, if necessary, can sleep in the hospital at night.

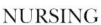

NURSING
A nurse is a man or a woman who is trained to care for the ill and injured. Nurses check the condition of their patients, give them medication, and keep them as comfortable as possible.

Find out more

Doctors
Medicine
Medicine, history of
X-rays

Houses

Learning the art of building enabled our ancestors to escape from the dark caves in which they sheltered from the weather and from hungry beasts. Building houses as they went, these first settlers moved to parts of the world where there was no natural shelter. Even in the icy wastes of the Arctic, the Eskimo people learned to use ice to build domed igloos. Most houses, though, consist of walls and a roof, built in a huge variety of styles. Local materials dictate the kind of house that rises in a particular place, but climate is important too. For instance, houses in the mountains of the Alps have steep roofs to shed the heavy layers of snow that fall in the winter. Modern houses are often complex structures, hiding in their walls networks of pipes and cables that supply water and energy and carry away waste. But in central Turkey, some people live in caves like those that provided the first shelter in prehistoric times.

MOBILE HOMES
The horse-drawn caravan which took fairground workers from place to place was the forerunner of today's mobile home.

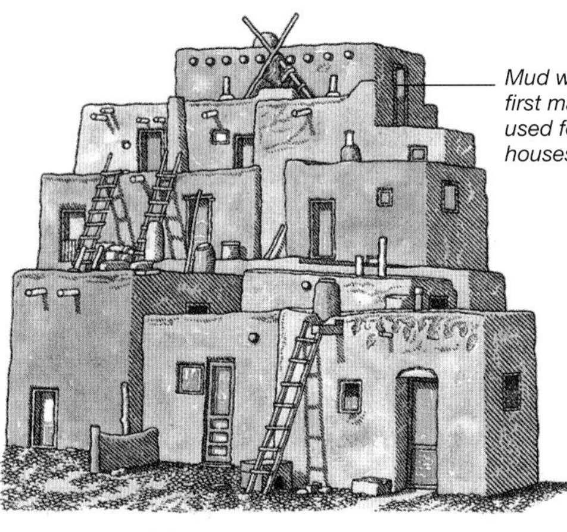

Mud was one of the first materials to be used for building houses.

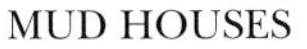

MUD HOUSES
The people of New Mexico traditionally use dried mud to build houses. Because there is little rain, the mud stays hard, and building and repairs are quick and easy. Thick walls and small windows keep out the sun's fierce heat and retain warmth at night.

HOUSEBOATS
A floating house solves the problem of finding a place to live in an overcrowded city where there is no more room to build. The houseboats are usually permanently moored.

This kind of houseboat is found in Hong Kong.

WOODEN HOUSES
American pioneers built their houses with wood, the best building material at hand. Wooden houses are well suited to cold, forested regions, not only because wood is plentiful but also because it is a good insulator and keeps out the cold.

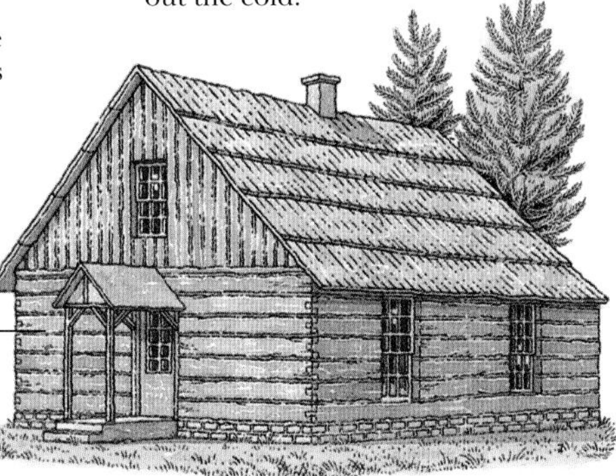

The earliest wooden houses were crude log cabins. The walls and roof of this house are made of sawed timber.

FLATS
City and town flats house hundreds of families on small plots of land, where there is room for just a few low-rise homes. The tallest buildings are made of strong materials such as steel and concrete.

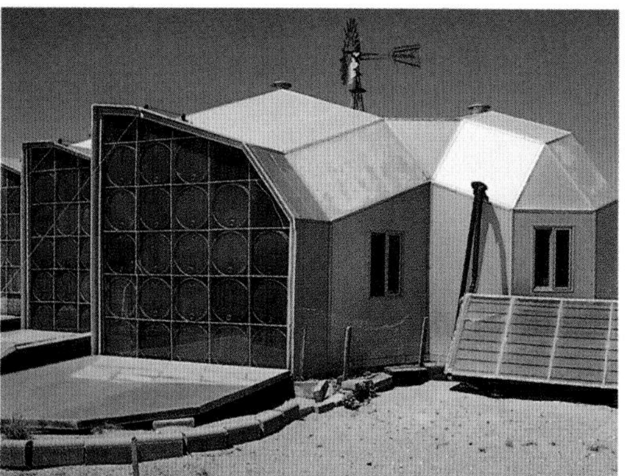

HOUSE OF THE FUTURE
The newest building techniques aim to conserve energy. In the future, people may live in better-insulated homes that need little fuel. The wind will generate electricity, the sun's rays will heat water, and computers will control the windows and heating system.

SHANTYTOWN
Many cities are ringed with shantytowns because people crowd in to the city to seek work but can find nowhere affordable to live. Some build their own homes with any materials they can find. Others remain homeless, sleeping on the streets.

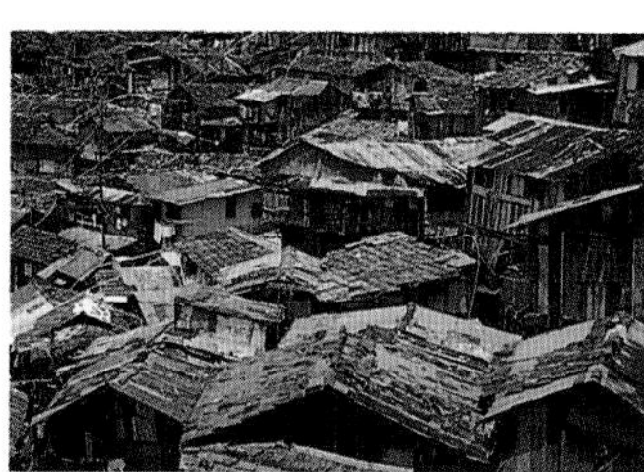

Find out more
Architecture
Building
Furniture
Inuits

Human body

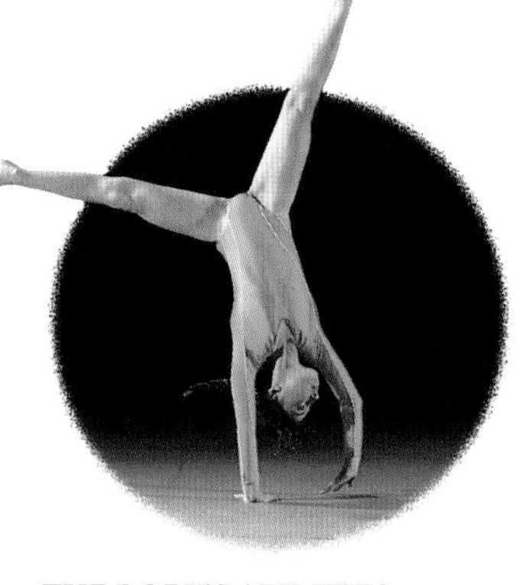

THE BODY'S ABILITIES
The human body is capable of amazing feats of balance and co-ordination. Many animals can run faster or jump higher, but our bodies are very adaptable. An extremely complex brain controls the body and gives us the intelligence to use our physical abilities to the best advantage.

FROM THE MOMENT we are born to the moment we die, our bodies do not stop working for a second. The human body is a complex collection of more than 50,000 million living units called cells. There are about 200 different types of cells, including nerve cells, called neurons, and specialized cells called gland cells. Glands produce substances such as hormones and enzymes, which they release into the body for different purposes. Each type of cell in the body does a particular job. Cells that do similar jobs are grouped together to form tissues, such as muscle tissue and nerve tissue. Tissues, in turn, are grouped together to form organs, which are the main separate parts of the body. The lungs, heart, liver, and kidneys are some of the main organs. The organs work together as systems, and each system carries out one major function. For example, the heart, blood vessels, and blood form the circulatory system, which carries oxygen and nutrients around the body and carries away waste products. All the different systems work together, controlled by the brain. The entire body is a living marvel of design.

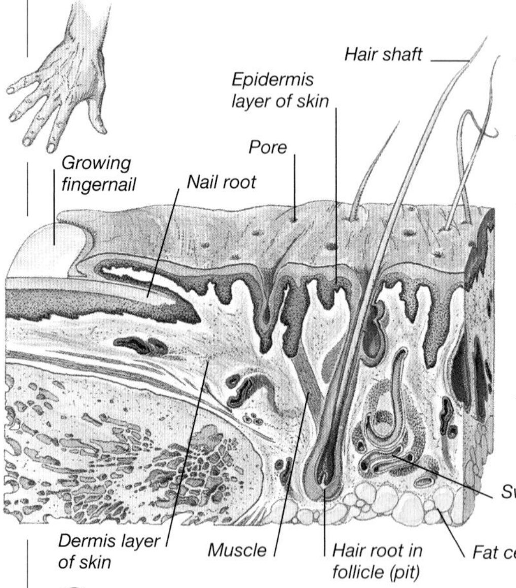

SKIN
The body is covered by skin. Skin is flexible and helps protect the body. It keeps water and harmful bacteria out, and keeps body fluids in. Skin is also wear-resistant because it continually renews itself. The base of the upper layer, or epidermis, divides constantly to make new cells. The new cells move upwards as if on a conveyor belt, to replace cells that are worn out.

Cell

Every second, millions of cells die and millions more replace them. An average cell measures about 0.025 mm (one thousandth of an inch) across, but there are many different kinds of cells in the body, each shaped for a certain job. Nerve cells are long and thin. Like wires, the nerves conduct (carry) electrical nerve signals. Red blood cells are doughnut-shaped and contain chemicals that carry oxygen around the body. Epithelial cells on body surfaces, such as the lining of the mouth, are broad and flat and fit together like paving stones.

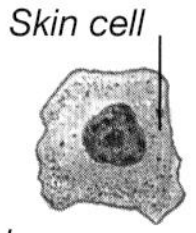

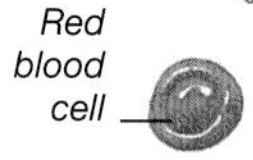

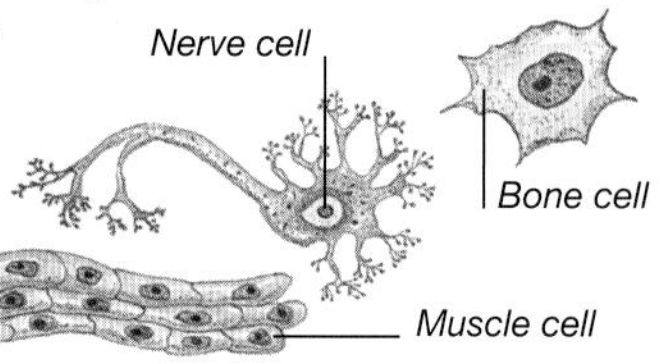

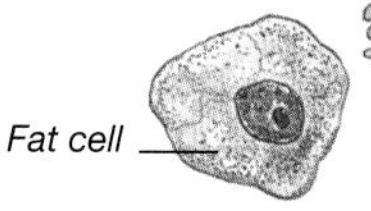

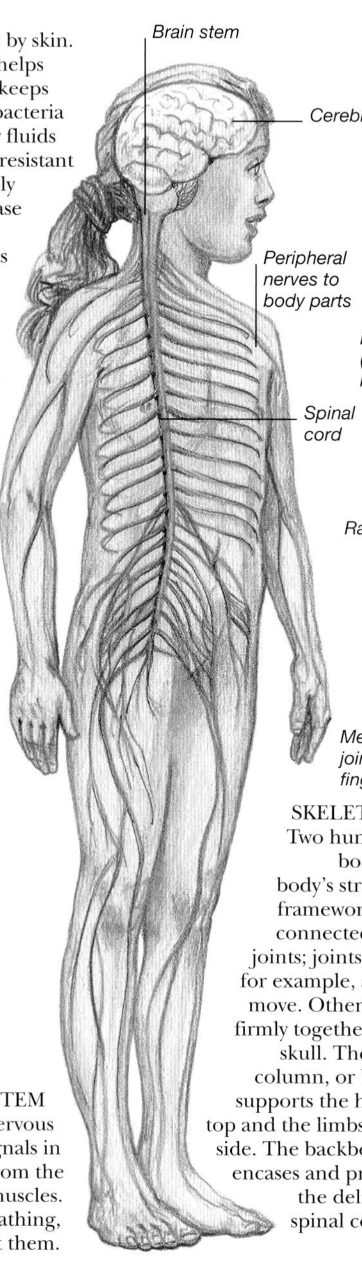

NERVOUS SYSTEM
The brain and the nerves make up the nervous system. Nerves spread from the brain to all body parts, carrying signals in the form of tiny electrical impulses. The signals bring information from the sense organs to the brain and take instructions from the brain to the muscles. The brain controls many processes automatically, such as breathing, heartbeat, and digestion, without our having to think about them.

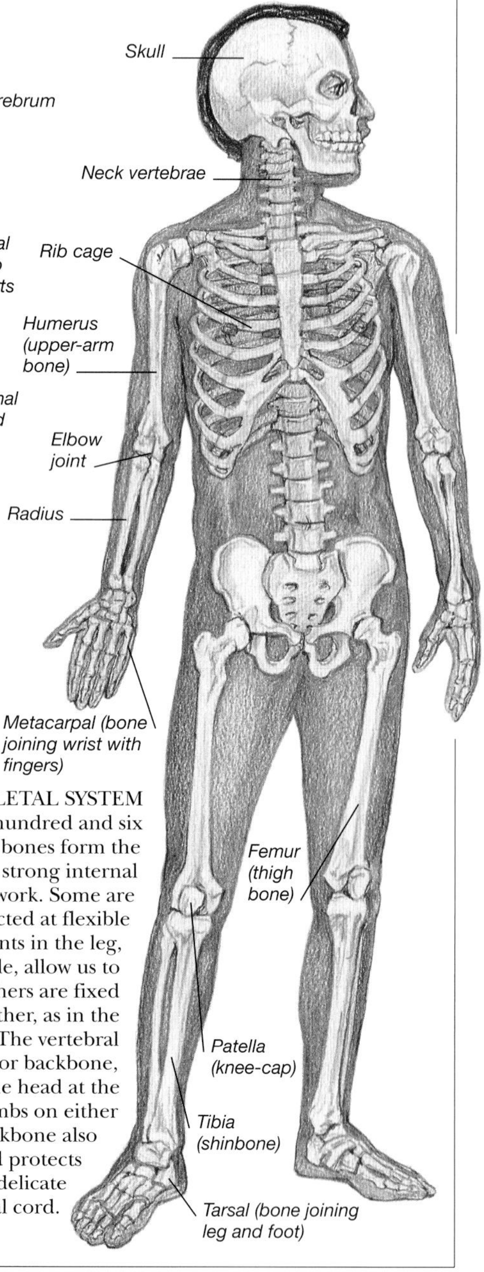

SKELETAL SYSTEM
Two hundred and six bones form the body's strong internal framework. Some are connected at flexible joints; joints in the leg, for example, allow us to move. Others are fixed firmly together, as in the skull. The vertebral column, or backbone, supports the head at the top and the limbs on either side. The backbone also encases and protects the delicate spinal cord.

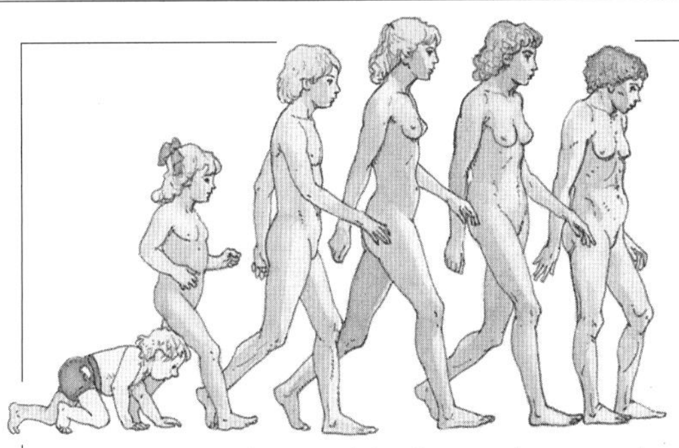

There are several stages of development in everyone's lifetime – from birth through childhood, adolescence, and adulthood, to old age.

GROWTH AND DEVELOPMENT

As the human body grows, it develops many skills. Babies learn to smile, sit up, crawl, walk, and talk. Learning continues at school. On average, the peak of physical abilities is reached at about 18 to 25 years of age. Later, more changes occur with age. The skin becomes wrinkled and less elastic, the joints are less flexible, bones become more brittle, muscles are less powerful, and there is some loss of height and greying of hair.

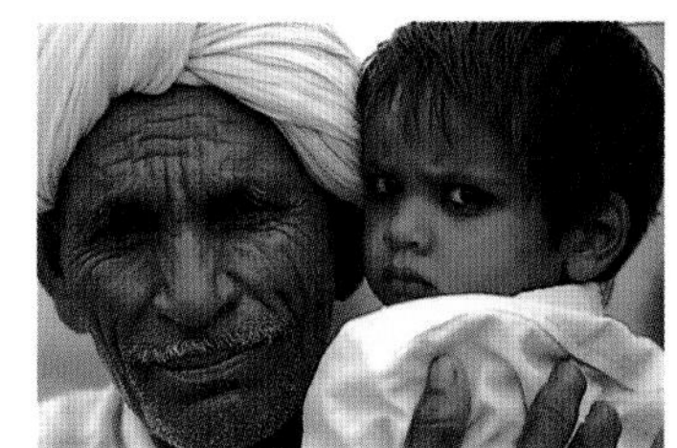

In many older people, decrease in physical strength is offset by the wisdom and knowledge gained from a lifetime of experience.

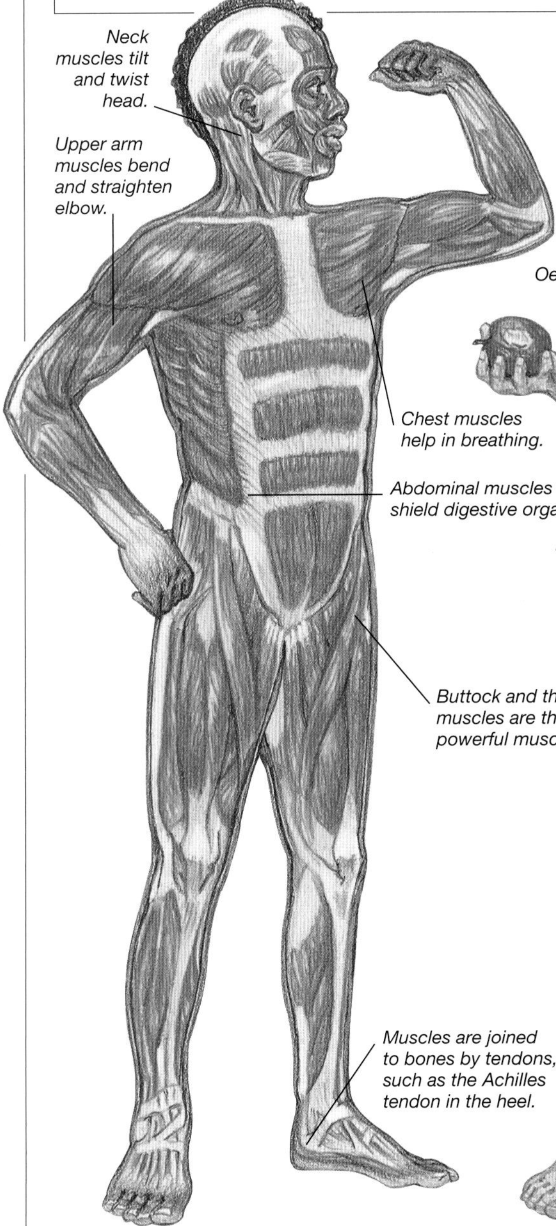

Neck muscles tilt and twist head.

Upper arm muscles bend and straighten elbow.

Chest muscles help in breathing.

Abdominal muscles shield digestive organs.

Buttock and thigh muscles are the most powerful muscles.

Muscles are joined to bones by tendons, such as the Achilles tendon in the heel.

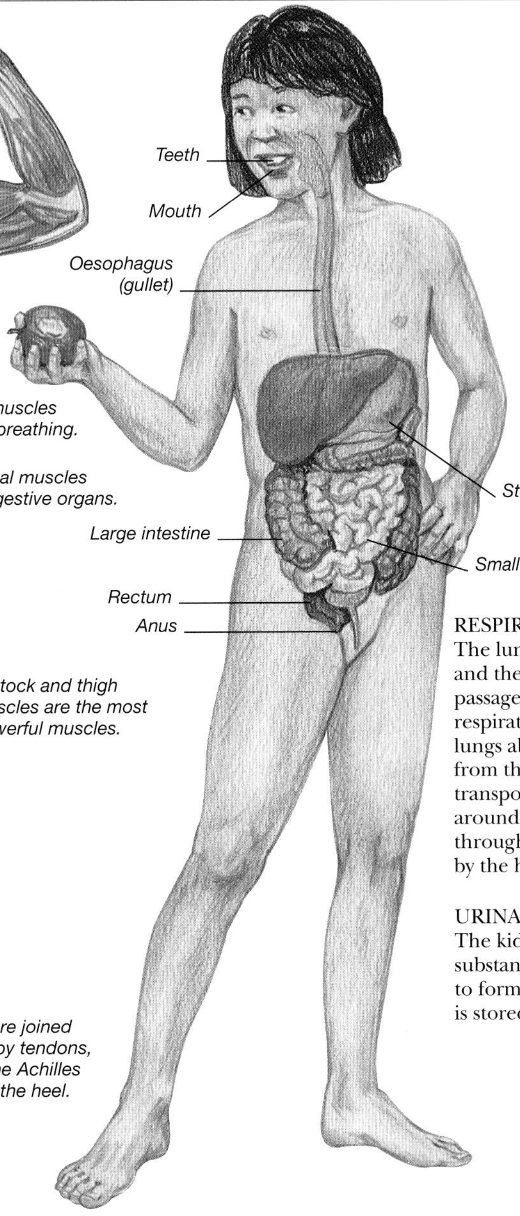

MUSCULAR SYSTEM

There are about 650 muscles in the body. Some, such as the arm muscles, can be controlled at will, to pull on the bones of the skeleton and move the body. Others, such as the muscles of the heart and intestine, work automatically.

Teeth

Mouth

Oesophagus (gullet)

Stomach

Large intestine

Small intestine

Rectum

Anus

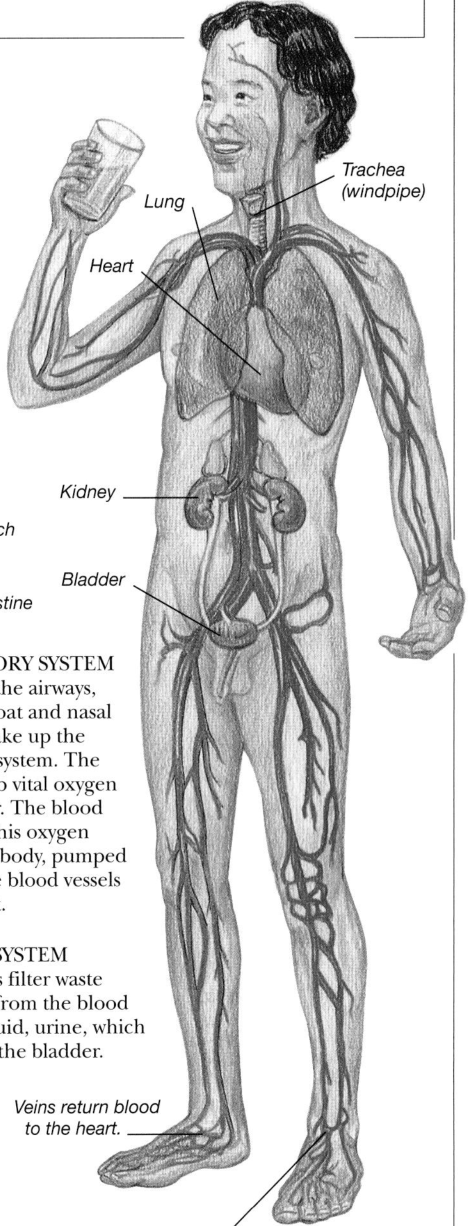

DIGESTIVE SYSTEM

The mouth, oesophagus, stomach, and intestines are part of the digestive system. These organs work together to break down food into particles that are small enough to pass through the lining of the intestine and into the blood. The mouth and teeth chop and chew food, and the stomach churns it with powerful digestive chemicals. The liver is the main organ for converting absorbed nutrients into forms more suitable for use by the various organs. The large intestine deals with wastes and leftover food.

Lung

Trachea (windpipe)

Heart

Kidney

Bladder

RESPIRATORY SYSTEM

The lungs, the airways, and the throat and nasal passages make up the respiratory system. The lungs absorb vital oxygen from the air. The blood transports this oxygen around the body, pumped through the blood vessels by the heart.

URINARY SYSTEM

The kidneys filter waste substances from the blood to form a fluid, urine, which is stored in the bladder.

Veins return blood to the heart.

Arteries carry blood from the heart.

Find out more

BRAIN AND NERVES
EARS
EYES
HEART AND BLOOD
LUNGS AND BREATHING
REPRODUCTION
SKELETONS
TEETH

HUMAN RIGHTS

MOST OF US BELIEVE that we have the right to be treated fairly and equally within society, regardless of our race, sex, religion, or social group. This equal treatment includes the right to vote, to work, and to be educated. When these rights are protected by law, they are called legal or human rights. In some countries, they are spelled out in the constitution. However, through history, many groups, including African-Americans, black South Africans, Native Americans, and women, have not been considered equal to others, and have had few, if any, civil or human rights. This kind of targetted mistreatment is called discrimination. In the 20th century, many different groups, including blacks, homosexuals, women, and people with disabilities, fought long and sometimes bitter campaigns to achieve their rights and obtain equal treatment within society.

NELSON MANDELA
In 1948, the South African government introduced apartheid, under which the black majority had no civil rights. The African National Congress (ANC), headed by Nelson Mandela (b.1918), led a long fight against apartheid. It was finally repealed in 1991.

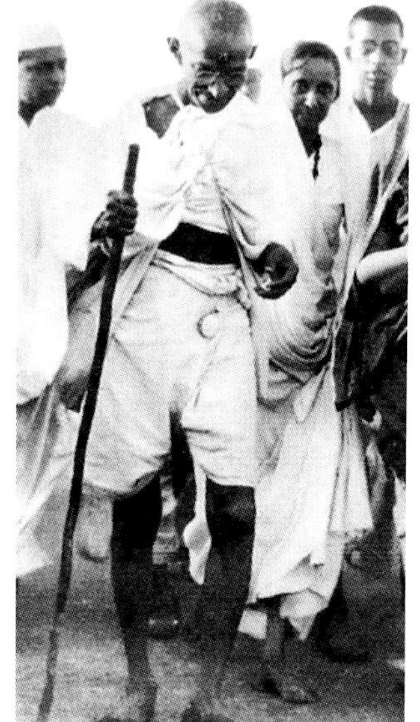

MOHANDAS GANDHI
Human rights activists – those who fight for civil rights – use peaceful methods. They unite and mobilize people. In 1915, Mohandas Gandhi (1869-1948) began to lead the struggle against British rule in India. Using non-violent civil disobedience, Gandhi's fasts and marches led to India's independence from British rule in 1947.

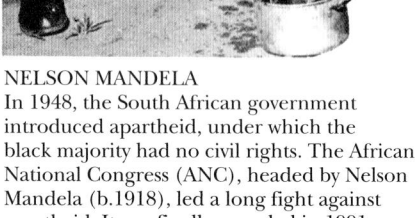

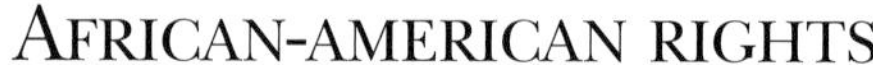

AFRICAN-AMERICAN RIGHTS

Under the American Constitution, African-Americans are guaranteed full citizenship, including the right to vote. But in the 1890s, laws passed in the southern States removed these rights, reducing African-Americans to second-class citizens, and introducing racial segregation (separation). Under the leadership of Martin Luther King, Jr. (1929-68), a civil rights movement emerged. It used non-violent methods, such as sit-ins (see left), where African-Americans peacefully occupied segregated public places. Finally Congress passed the Civil Rights Act in 1964 and the Voting Rights Act in 1965. These laws outlawed discrimination on the grounds of race, colour, or religion in schooling, voting, and employment.

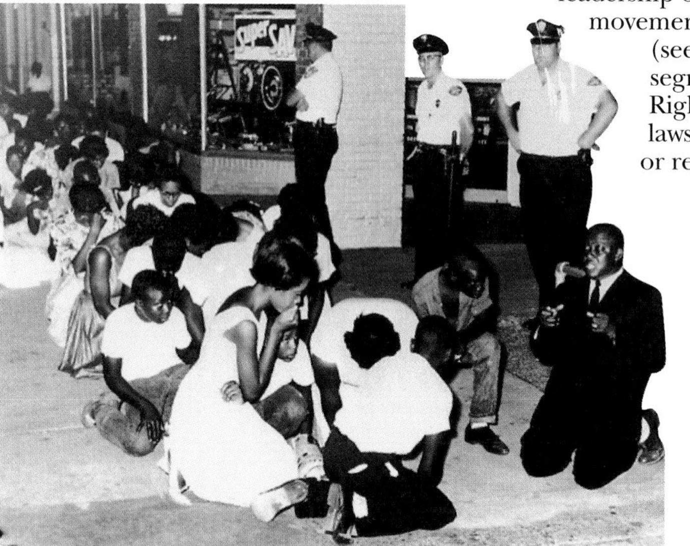

AMNESTY INTERNATIONAL

A worldwide human rights organization, Amnesty International was founded in 1961 following a legal appeal by a British lawyer, Peter Benenson, after he read about two Portuguese students who were imprisoned for raising their glasses in a toast to freedom. Amnesty works to obtain prompt and fair trials for all prisoners, to end torture and executions, and to secure the release of people imprisoned solely for their political or religious beliefs and who have not used or advocated violence. The organization has more than one million members and has its headquarters in London. In 1977, Amnesty International was awarded the Nobel Peace Prize for its work.

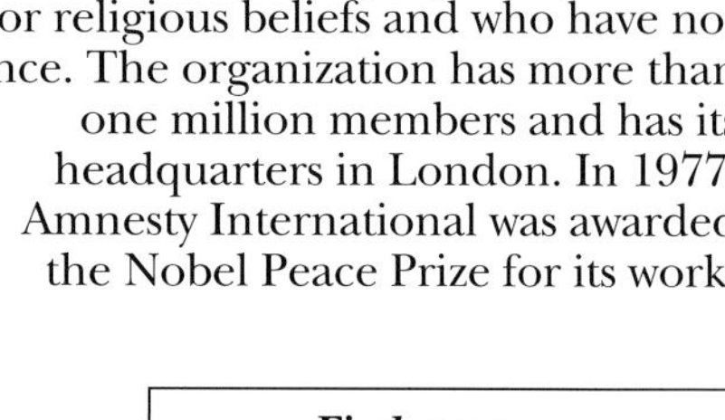

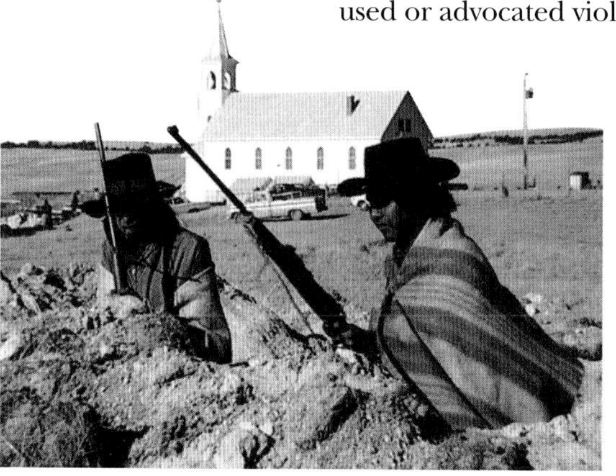

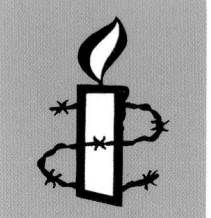

AMERICAN INDIAN MOVEMENT
Since the 1960s, Native Americans have become more forceful in demanding equal rights. In 1968, the American Indian Movement (AIM) formed to fight for civil rights and improved conditions on reservations. A militant organization, AIM conducted a number of high-profile protests. In 1973, they occupied Wounded Knee in South Dakota, the site of a massacre of Sioux people in 1890. Federal marshals surrounded the protestors, and a siege began in which two AIM members were killed. Since then, some Native Americans have won land rights, but discrimination still continues today.

Find out more

AFRICA, HISTORY OF
KING, MARTIN LUTHER
LAW
MANDELA, NELSON
NATIVE AMERICANS
SLAVERY
TUBMAN, HARRIET

Hundred Years War

In 1337, THE ENGLISH KING EDWARD III, whose mother was French, landed in Normandy, laid claim to the French crown, and began what historians call the Hundred Years War. To the people who fought it, it was more like a series of small wars separated by truces. It lasted through the reigns of five English and five French kings. Edward III failed to gain the French crown, and died in 1377. His heir, Richard II, took little interest in the war, but Henry V, who came to the throne in 1413, wanted to fight for the French crown and started the conflict again. Before 1420, the English won most of the battles, including Créçy (1346), Poitiers (1356), and Agincourt (1415), but by 1453, France had taken back all England's French lands, except Calais, which England lost in 1558.

Normandy
Brittany
Paris
Burgundy
Aquitaine
Gascony

ENGLAND AND FRANCE
Through royal marriages, the English already held large areas in the north and west of France. At the Treaty of Troyes in 1420, Henry V claimed almost half of what is now France, including Paris.

English troops kept the sun behind them so that it shone directly into the eyes of the French soldiers.

French troops had to attack uphill.

Welsh and English archers fired faster than French cross-bow men.

French cavalry bogged down in the mud.

Battle of Creçy

On 26 August 1346, Edward III's 8,000 troops were trapped at Créçy, but clever tactics and the skill of the English archers defeated a French army of 20,000. Edward's 16-year-old son, known as the Black Prince because of the black armour he wore, commanded his own troops in the battle.

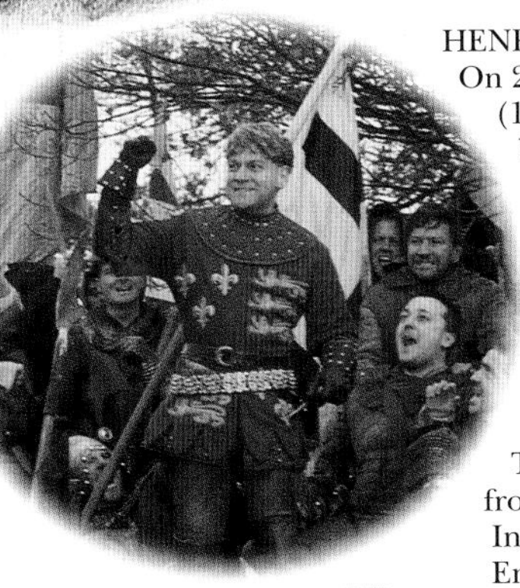

HENRY V AND AGINCOURT
On 25 October 1415, Henry V (1387-1422) led his troops into battle at Agincourt. An English army of only 13,000 archers, pikemen, and cavalry defeated a French force of 50,000. Shakespeare described this English victory in *Henry V.*

Archers practise with their longbows.

ENGLISH LONGBOW
The longbow was normally made from yew, and the arrows were ash. In the 14th and 15th centuries, all English men were required by law to practise archery after church on Sundays, to be ready for war.

HUNDRED YEARS WAR

1338 Edward III of England claims French crown.

1346 Battle of Créçy.

1347 English capture Calais.

1356 Battle of Poitiers.

1415 Henry V declares war on Charles VI of France.

1415 Siege of Harfleur.

1415 Battle of Agincourt.

1419 English capture Normandy.

1420 Treaty of Troyes. Henry V marries King of France's daughter and claims French throne.

1428-29 Siege of Orléans.

1430 Joan of Arc taken.

1450 French reconquer Normandy.

1453 Battle of Castillon.

1453 Fall of Bordeaux ends war.

Find out more
France, history of
Joan of Arc
Knights and heraldry
United kingdom, history of
Weapons

INCAS

IN THE 12TH CENTURY, a tribe of Native Americans moved down from the Andes mountains in South America to settle in the fertile Cuzco valley. By the end of the 15th century they had conquered a huge territory of 1,140,000 sq km (440,000 sq miles) containing more than 10 million people. The Incas won this land with their powerful army and then controlled it with a remarkable system of communications. Inca engineers built a network of paved roads that crisscrossed the empire. Relays of imperial messengers ran along these roads (there were no horses or wheeled vehicles), travelling 250 km (150 miles) a day as they took messages to and from the capital city of Cuzco. At the head of the empire was the chief Inca, who was worshipped as a god and held absolute power over all his subjects. But in 1525 the chief Inca, Huayna Capac, died, and civil war broke out between two rivals for his throne. In 1532 a small force of Spanish soldiers arrived in the country and found it in disarray. They quickly overwhelmed the Incan army, and by 1533 the Inca empire was completely under Spanish rule.

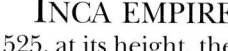

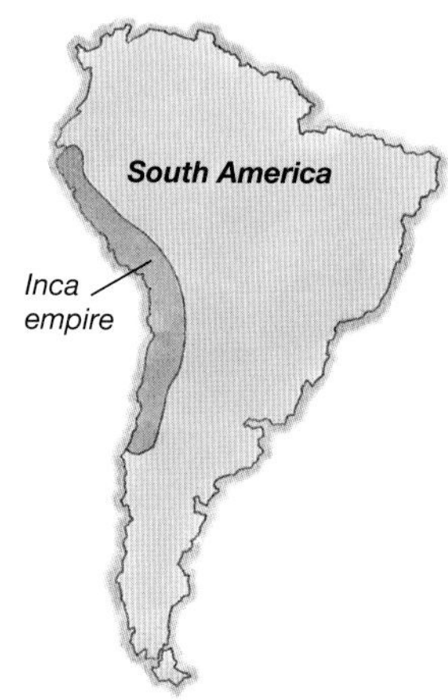

INCA EMPIRE

In 1525, at its height, the Inca empire stretched for more than 3,200 km (2,000 miles) along the Pacific coast of South America, ruling over much of present-day Ecuador, Peru, Bolivia, and Chile.

MACHU PICCHU

Covering an area of 13 sq km (5 sq miles), the fortress city of Machu Picchu was built on a series of terraces carved into the side of a mountain more than 2,280 m (7,500 ft) above sea level.

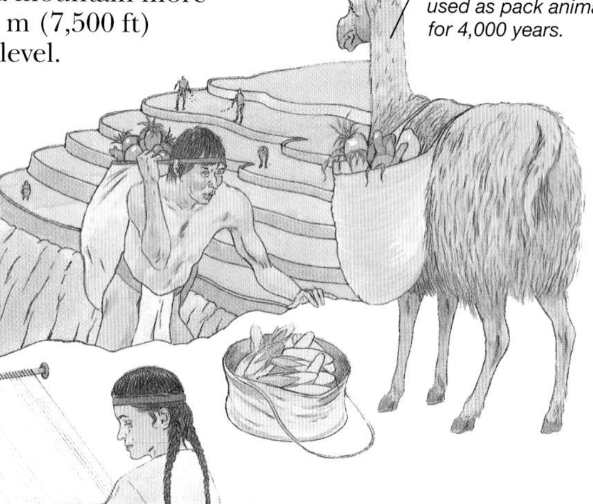

Llamas have been used as pack animals for 4,000 years.

An Inca woman weaving an elaborately designed piece of cloth.

TERRACE FARMING

The Incas were expert at farming every available piece of fertile land in their mountainous empire. They built terraces along the steep hillsides and watered them with mountain streams so that crops could be grown and animals kept to feed all the people who lived in the cities.

WEAVING

The Incas wove lengths of beautiful, colourful cloth with elaborate patterns. The wool they used came from the mountain animals – llamas, alpacas, and vicunas – that the Incas kept on their farms. Many of their designs depicted jaguars and pumas.

QUIPU

The Incas did not read or write. Instead, they used quipus – lengths of knotted string – to record every aspect of their daily life. Historic events, laws, gold reserves, population statistics, and other items of information were all stored accurately in this way.

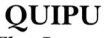

Colour of string, number of knots, and length of string indicated what was recorded on the quipu.

The Incas were expert goldsmiths and often placed gold figurines (right) in their graves. Much of the Incan gold was melted down by Spanish invaders.

Find out more

CAMELS AND LLAMAS
CONQUISTADORS
SOUTH AMERICA, history of

INDIA
AND SUBCONTINENT

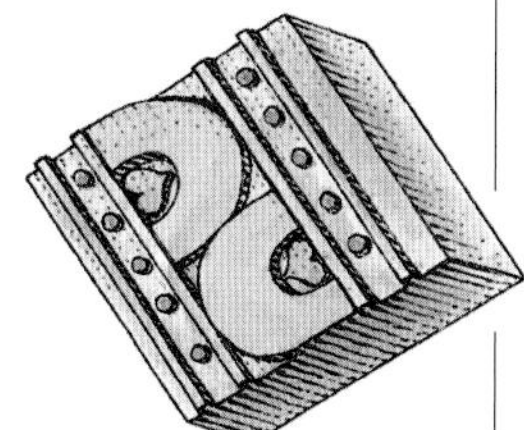

PRINTING BLOCKS
Traditional wooden printing blocks are still used in the production of colourful textiles.

A TRAVELLER IN INDIA would need to speak more than 1,000 languages to understand conversations in every part of the country. Hindi and English are the two official languages, and 14 other languages are spoken nationwide. Many people, however, speak a local language of their own. The majority of Indians are Hindu in religion, but there are many Muslims, Sikhs, Christians, and Buddhists. Geographically, the country is very varied too. The north is mountainous, and in the centre the River Ganges waters a rich plain of productive farmland. In the south a hot and fertile coastal region surrounds a dry inland plateau. With a population of more than 1,000 million, India is the second most populated country in the world (China is the first). About 70 per cent of the people live in small, often very poor villages, and work on the land. The rest live in big cities where some work in modern factories and offices. Recent advances in farming have made the land more productive, and after many years of famine, India can now feed itself.

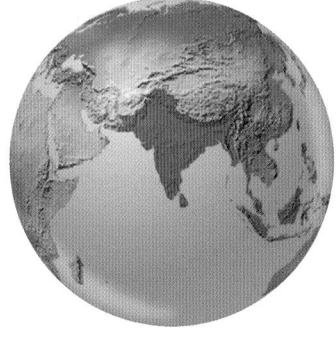

India, Pakistan, Nepal, Bhutan, Bangladesh, and Sri Lanka occupy the Indian subcontinent. China is to the north, and to the east lie the jungles of Southeast Asia. The Indian Ocean washes the southern shores; the mountains and deserts of Iran and Afghanistan enclose the subcontinent on the west.

TEA

In 1824, tea plants were discovered in the hills along the frontier between Burma and the Indian state of Assam. The British first introduced tea culture to India in 1836 and Sri Lanka in 1867, and today most of the world's tea comes from the Indian subcontinent. The low tea bushes grow well on the sheltered, well-drained foothills of the Himalayas. Only the leaves near the tip of the plant are picked; they are then dried, rolled, and heated to produce the final product. Tea also grows in southern India and Sri Lanka.

Picking tea is laborious and often painful work. Most tea pickers are women. They spend long days picking the crop by hand.

KARAKORAM MOUNTAINS

A high mountain range separates the Indian subcontinent from China to the north. Most of the range is part of the Himalayas. At its western end, the Himalayas continue as the Karakoram range, which forms Pakistan's northern border. Few people have their homes in these mountainous regions. Nevertheless, the mountains have a great influence on people living thousands of kilometres away. Most of the rivers that irrigate the fertile plains of the Indian subcontinent begin in the Himalayas.

TEXTILES
The production of textiles, carpets, and clothing is one of the major industries in India. Millions of people work at spinning, weaving, and finishing a wide range of cotton and other goods, often printed with designs that have been in use for centuries. Many of these products are exported. There are large factories, but some people also work in their own homes.

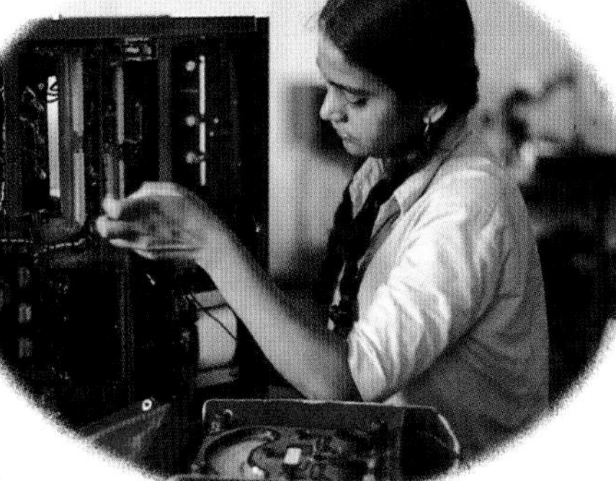

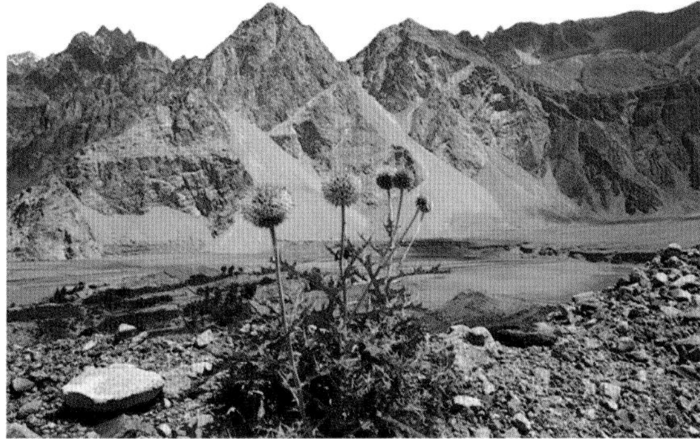

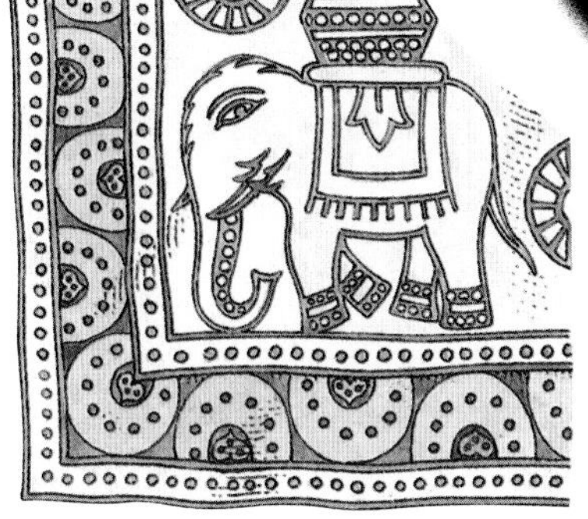

MODERN INDIA
India is one of the most industrial countries in Asia, with a wide range of engineering, electronic, and manufacturing industries. Its railway system is one of the world's biggest. However, traditional costumes and ways of life coexist with modern industries.

PAKISTAN

Pakistan was formed in 1947, when the end of British rule in India led to the creation of two separate states; the predominantly Hindu India, and the predominantly Muslim Pakistan. Pakistan originally included what is now Bangladesh, then known as East Pakistan. Bangladesh became independent in 1971 after a revolt against rule from West Pakistan (present-day Pakistan). India and Pakistan are in bitter conflict over the area at Pakistan's northeastern border known as Kashmir; both India and Pakistan consider the region to be a part of their country. Pakistan's other major concern at present is overpopulation; the country's resources are relatively small in comparison to the size of its population.

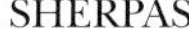

SHERPAS

The Sherpa people (right) of Nepal are famed for their mountaineering skills. They often act as guides for trekkers and tourists on expeditions in the Nepalese Himalayas.

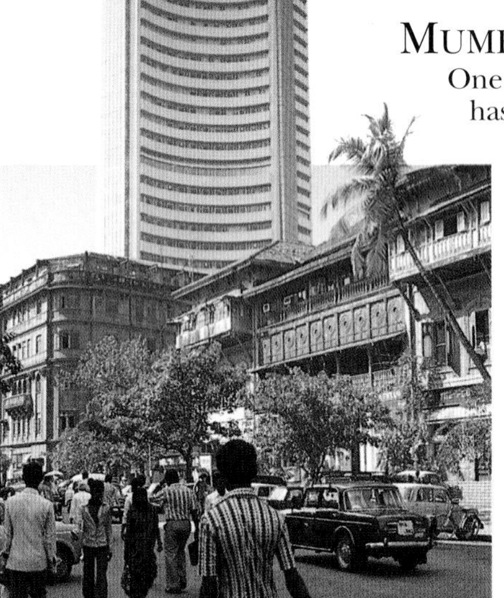

Expansion of Mumbai is confined by its island location, therefore the city has one of the highest population densities in the world.

MUMBAI

One of India's largest cities is Mumbai, which has a population of more than 10 million. The city is the capital of the western state of Maharashtra, and is a major port for western commerce. Mumbai is built on an island, and has a superb natural harbour to the east. Cotton is grown nearby, and Mumbai is the largest cotton textile centre in the country. One half of the people living in Mumbai work in the textile industry.

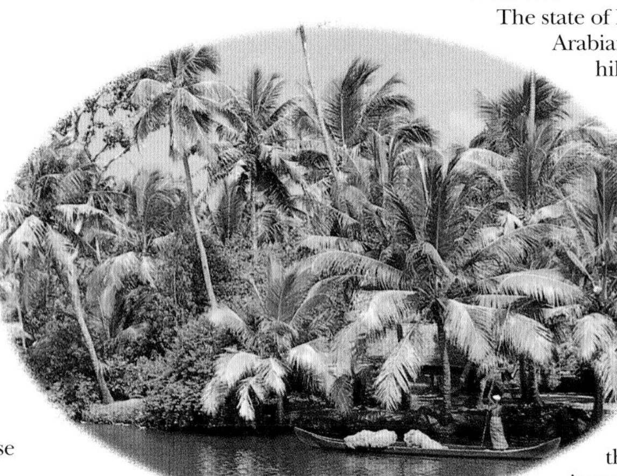

KERALA

The state of Kerala in southwest India borders the Arabian Sea. The eastern part of the state is hilly, but much of the land area is a flat plain. Kerala is one of the most densely-populated states in India. Fishing is important for the local economy. Near the coast, the people of Kerala grow crops of cashew nuts, coconuts, and rice, and there are tea, rubber, coffee, and pepper plantations to the east. Although the government has encouraged modern farming techniques, traditional methods of agriculture and transport are common, such as the canoe in the picture (left). Forestry is also important in Kerala. In the mountains there are forests of teak, ebony, and rosewood, as well as a wide variety of wildlife.

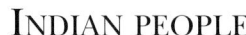

BHUTAN

Most people in Bhutan are descendants of Tibetans who migrated to the area centuries ago. Like their neighbours, they are predominantly Buddhist, and look on the Dalai Lama as their spiritual leader. The dense forests and high mountains that cover the country are home to many animals native to the Indian subcontinent, such as tigers (left), monkeys and elephants. In an effort to protect Bhutan's culture and natural environment the government of Bhutan does not allow many tourists to enter the country.

INDIAN PEOPLE

India has one of the most diverse populations in the world. Throughout history, one race after another has settled in India, each bringing its own culture, customs, and languages. The races often intermarried, but not all aspects of society became mixed and diluted: many groups clung to their traditions. For instance, there is no one Indian language, and people in different parts of the country often have their own unique local language.

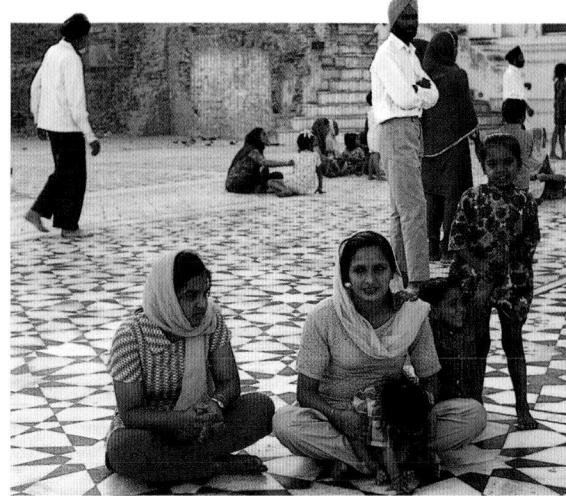

BOLLYWOOD

The Indian film industry produces even more films than Hollywood, in the United States. About 800 full-length feature films are shot each year, mainly in Mumbai, nicknamed "Bollywood". Chennai (Madras) is also a centre of the film industry.

A still from a film by Indian film director, Satyajit Ray. His work is shown and admired worldwide.

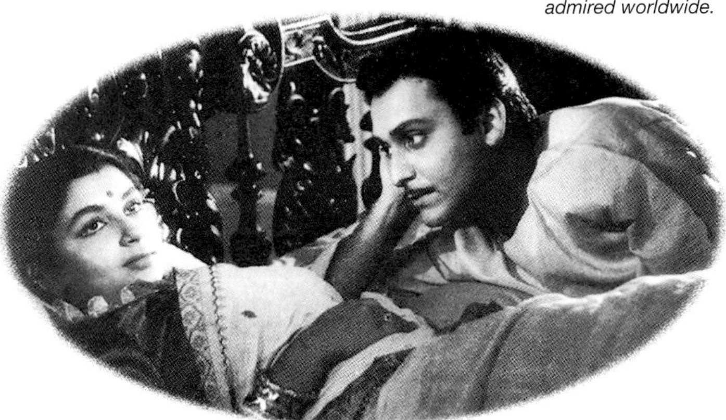

MUSIC

Traditional Indian music is very complex, with a wide range of rhythms. Melodies are based on ragas – a fixed series of notes the performer must play as a basis for improvising or making up the tune. In recent years, bhangra, a new music combining traditional Indian music from the province of Punjab with western rock music, has become popular among young people.

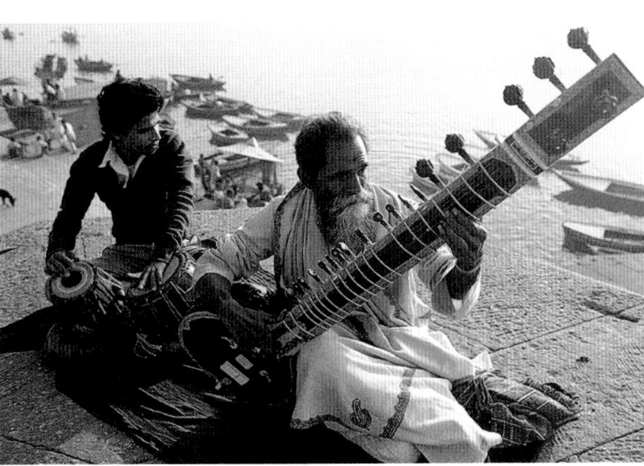

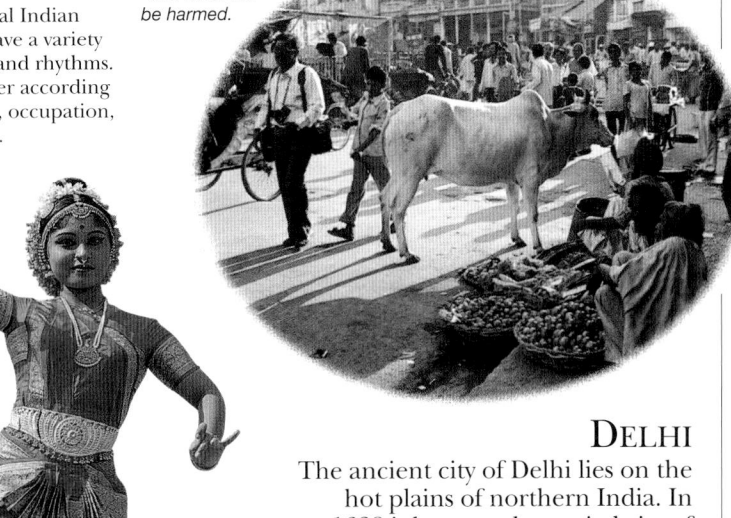

The Taj Mahal is built of the finest white marble and is a supreme example of Islamic architecture.

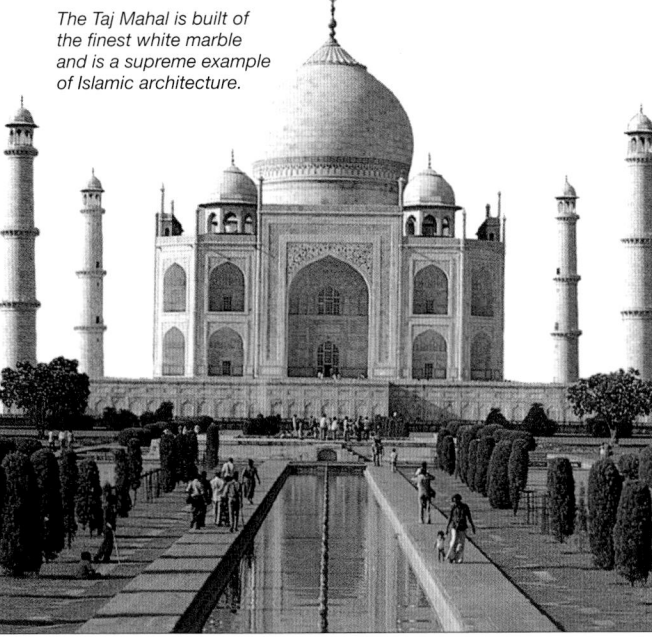

SACRED WATERS

From its source in the Himalayas, the Ganges river (below) flows eastward across India, then turns south. The river's 2,510-km (1,560-mile) course takes it through Bangladesh to reach the sea in the Bay of Bengal. Hindus consider the river to be sacred. They believe that bathing in its waters washes away sins, and cures illness. Indians rely on the waters of the Ganges for the irrigation of agricultural land.

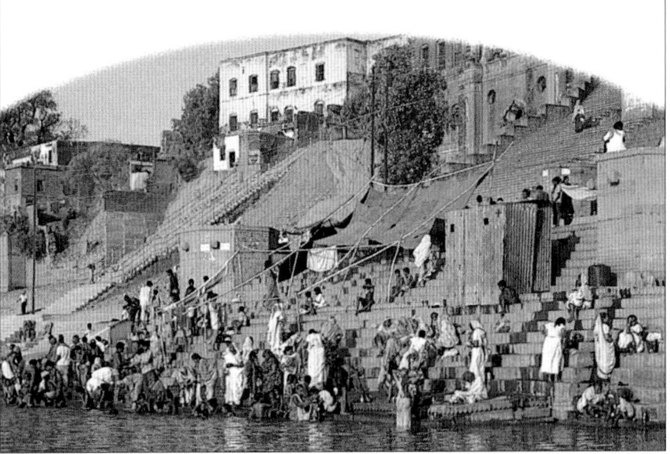

DANCE

Traditional Indian dances have a variety of forms and rhythms. They differ according to region, occupation, and caste.

Cows are sacred to Hindus in India and must not be harmed.

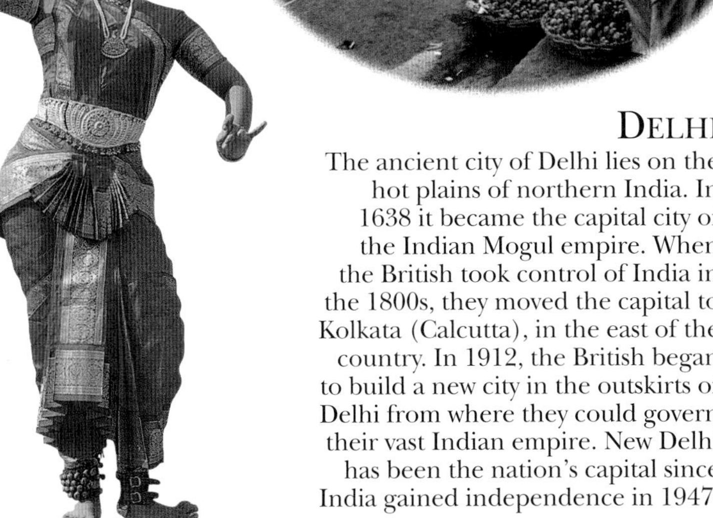

DELHI

The ancient city of Delhi lies on the hot plains of northern India. In 1638 it became the capital city of the Indian Mogul empire. When the British took control of India in the 1800s, they moved the capital to Kolkata (Calcutta), in the east of the country. In 1912, the British began to build a new city in the outskirts of Delhi from where they could govern their vast Indian empire. New Delhi has been the nation's capital since India gained independence in 1947.

TAJ MAHAL

The Taj Mahal (left), at Agra in northern India, was built in 1631 by Shah Jahan, the Mogul emperor of India. It was constructed as a tomb and memorial for his beloved wife, Mumtaz Mahal. She was the mother of 14 children. The Taj Mahal is built of white marble and inlaid with semi-precious stones.

Find out more

ASIA
BUDDHISM
DANCE
HINDUISM
INDIA, HISTORY OF
SOUTHEAST ASIA, HISTORY OF

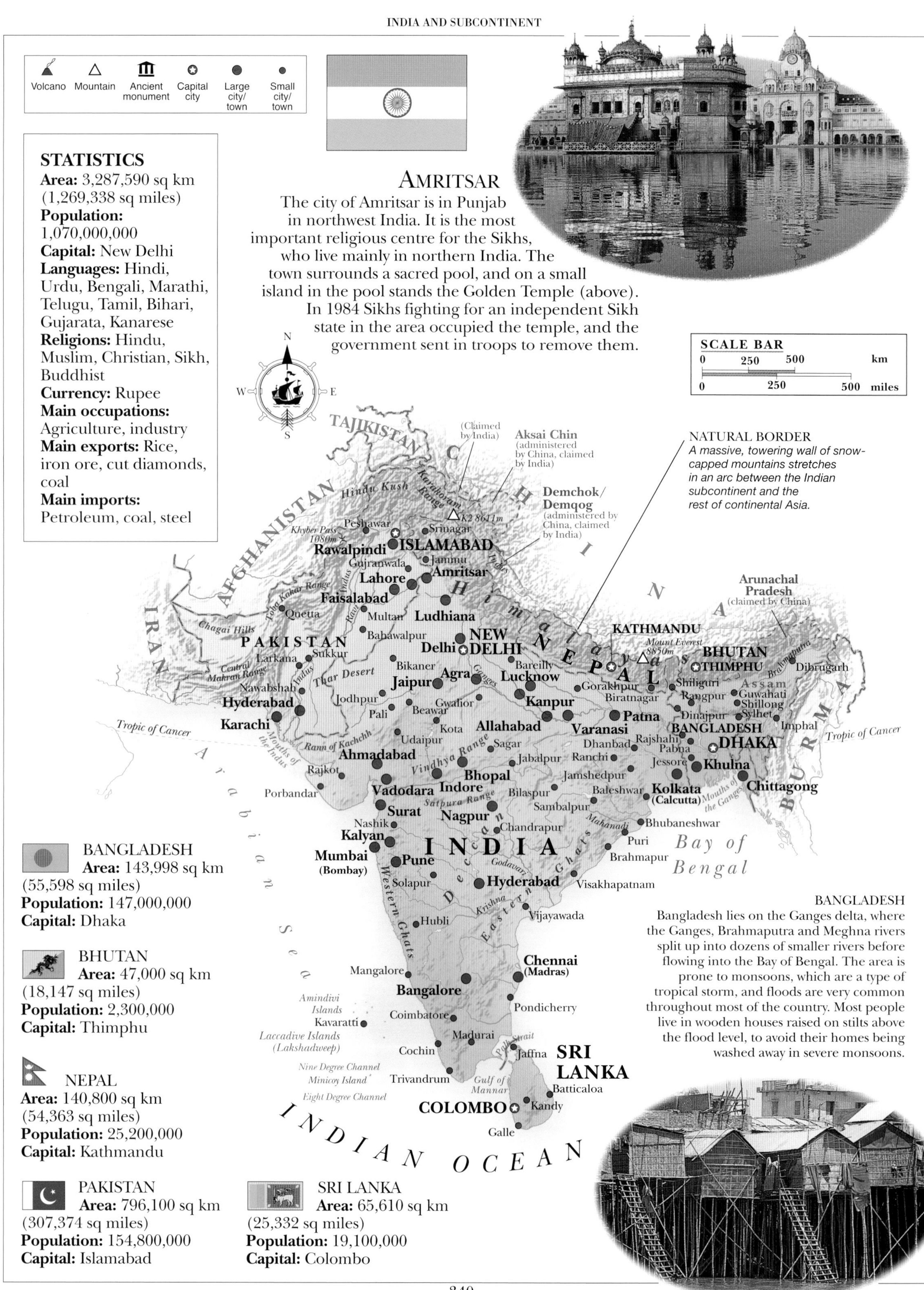

STATISTICS

Area: 3,287,590 sq km (1,269,338 sq miles)
Population: 1,070,000,000
Capital: New Delhi
Languages: Hindi, Urdu, Bengali, Marathi, Telugu, Tamil, Bihari, Gujarata, Kanarese
Religions: Hindu, Muslim, Christian, Sikh, Buddhist
Currency: Rupee
Main occupations: Agriculture, industry
Main exports: Rice, iron ore, cut diamonds, coal
Main imports: Petroleum, coal, steel

AMRITSAR

The city of Amritsar is in Punjab in northwest India. It is the most important religious centre for the Sikhs, who live mainly in northern India. The town surrounds a sacred pool, and on a small island in the pool stands the Golden Temple (above). In 1984 Sikhs fighting for an independent Sikh state in the area occupied the temple, and the government sent in troops to remove them.

BANGLADESH
Bangladesh lies on the Ganges delta, where the Ganges, Brahmaputra and Meghna rivers split up into dozens of smaller rivers before flowing into the Bay of Bengal. The area is prone to monsoons, which are a type of tropical storm, and floods are very common throughout most of the country. Most people live in wooden houses raised on stilts above the flood level, to avoid their homes being washed away in severe monsoons.

BANGLADESH
Area: 143,998 sq km (55,598 sq miles)
Population: 147,000,000
Capital: Dhaka

BHUTAN
Area: 47,000 sq km (18,147 sq miles)
Population: 2,300,000
Capital: Thimphu

NEPAL
Area: 140,800 sq km (54,363 sq miles)
Population: 25,200,000
Capital: Kathmandu

PAKISTAN
Area: 796,100 sq km (307,374 sq miles)
Population: 154,800,000
Capital: Islamabad

SRI LANKA
Area: 65,610 sq km (25,332 sq miles)
Population: 19,100,000
Capital: Colombo

HISTORY OF

INDIA

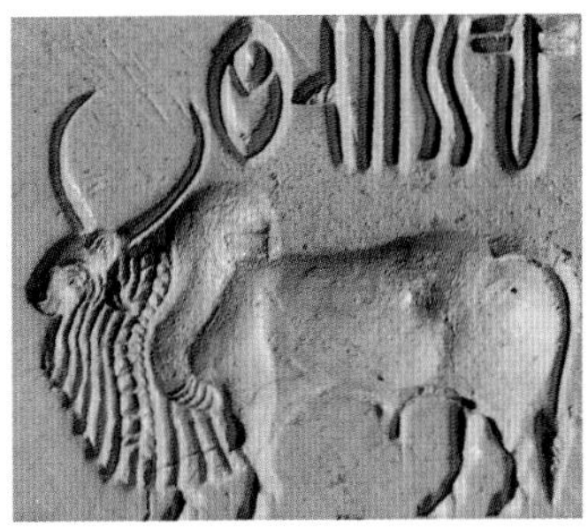

INDUS VALLEY CIVILIZATION
The peoples of the Indus Valley used the water from the River Indus to enrich their soil. They built Mohenjo-Daro and Harappa, the world's first cities. Craftsworkers created elegant and beautiful figures of people, animals, and gods, such as this seal in the form of a bull.

NEARLY 5,000 YEARS AGO, a civilization grew up around the Indus River in southern Asia. The peoples of this region built the world's first cities. Since that time India has been the birthplace of two great religions, Hinduism and Buddhism. Over the centuries, India has had many rulers and has been invaded many times. The first invaders were the Aryans, from the northwest. At the time, India consisted of several city-states, often in conflict. The Maurya dynasty, or ruling family, finally emerged around 322 B.C., and under one of its emperors Asoka, India entered a period of peace. The Gupta dynasty came next, followed by the Moguls, who created a splendid civilization. But differences between various religious groups of Muslims, Sikhs, and Hindus weakened India. Between the 17th and 18th centuries, the British East India Company took control of much of the country; a century later the British government took over India. Many Indian people wanted independence. In 1947 India gained freedom from Britain, but was plunged into conflict between Muslims and Hindus. British and Indian leaders divided the country into two nations: India and Pakistan.

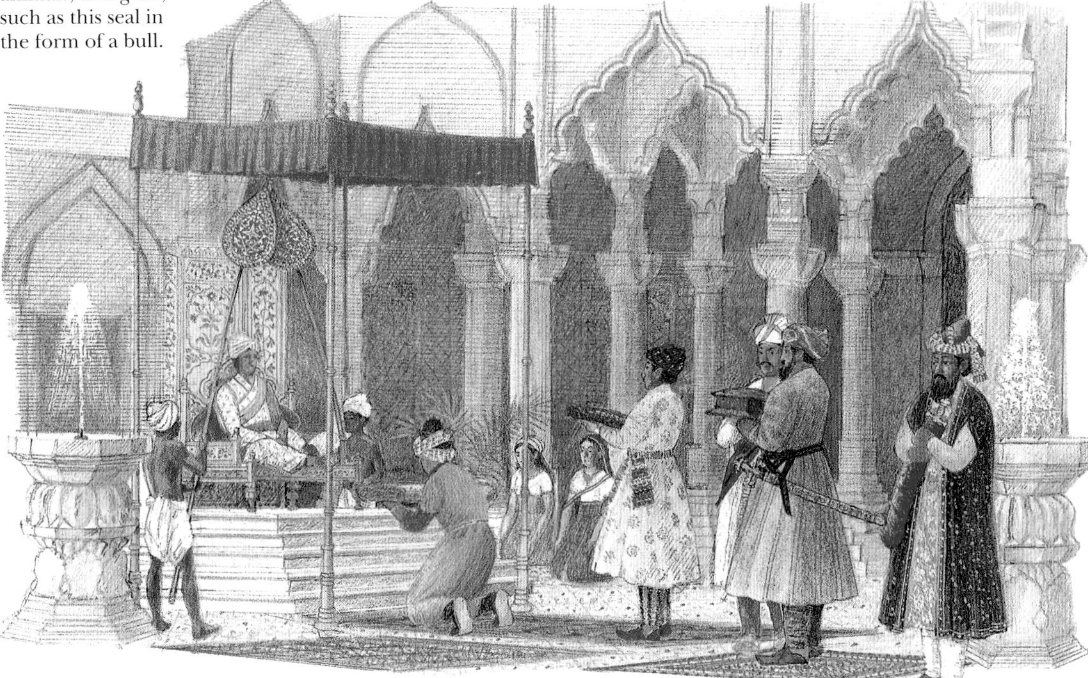

GUPTA EMPIRE
A family of wealthy land owners, the Guptas, founded their empire in A.D. 320, under Chandra Gupta I. Within a century the empire covered much of northern and eastern India. A golden age of cultural life began. The Guptas devised the decimal system of counting and writing numbers that we still use today. The empire collapsed in the seventh century after tribes invaded from Central Asia.

EAST INDIA COMPANY
In 1600, the British founded the East India Company to trade with India. By 1765, the company was governing parts of India itself, but in 1858 the British government took over. The company ceased to exist in 1873. The drawing on the right shows an Englishman travelling by Indian elephant.

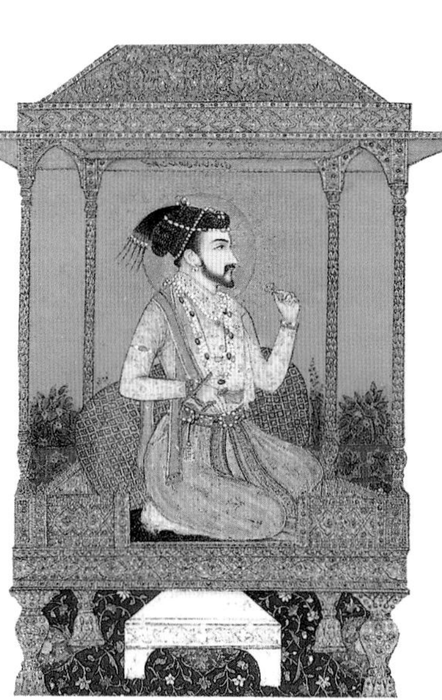

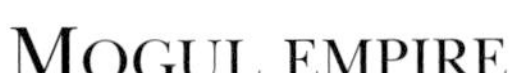

MOGUL EMPIRE

In 1526, Babur, the Mogul ruler arrived from central Asia and established his rule on an administratively weak India. The Moguls were Muslims, and they built some of the most magnificent mosques (Muslim places of worship) and palaces in the world. In 1858, Mogul empire collapsed and the British took control of almost all the landmass.

British Raj

From the early 16th century, Portugal, France, Britain, and the Netherlands all tried to take control of India. The British were the most successful. By the mid-1800s, they ruled the entire Indian subcontinent. In 1876 the British queen, Victoria, became empress of India. The government of India was called the British Raj (from an Indian word meaning "rule"). The Raj employed a civil service to administer the country from the capital city of New Delhi, which was completed in 1931.

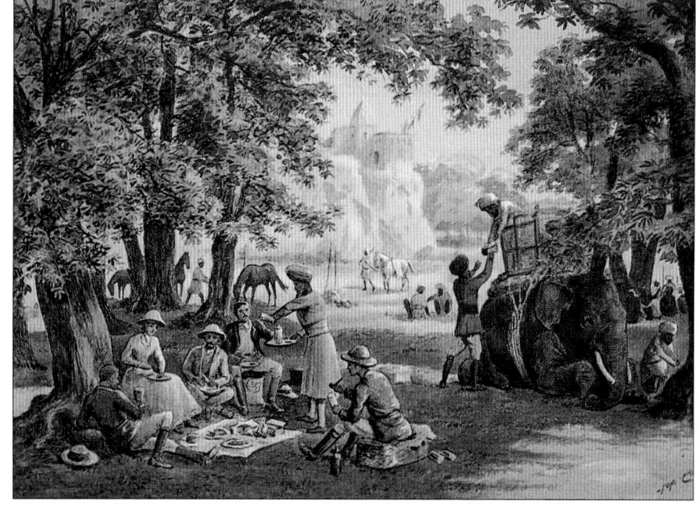

Mohandas Gandhi

The leader of the movement for Indian independence from British rule was Mohandas Gandhi (1869-1948). Called the Mahatma, meaning "great soul", Gandhi attempted to unite all of India's different religions and peoples. He stressed the importance of *satyagraha*, or non-violent resistance to British rule.

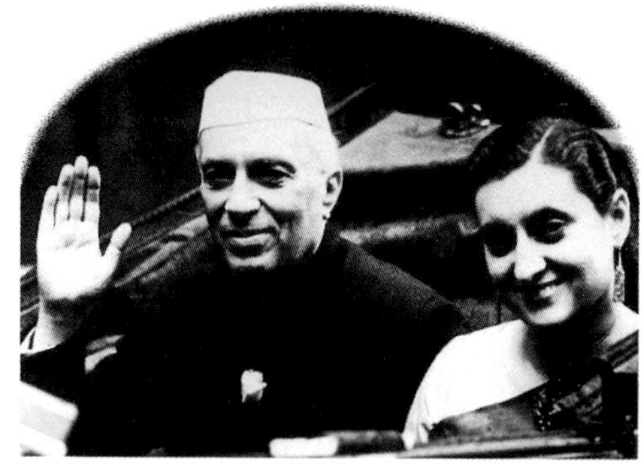

NEHRU FAMILY
The first prime minister of India was Jawaharlal Nehru (1889-1964; above). Two years after his death, his daughter, Indira Gandhi (right), became prime minister. She remained India's leader almost continuously until she was assassinated in 1984, when her son Rajiv succeeded her. In 1989, he lost majority in the Parliament; in 1991 he too was assassinated.

PAKISTAN AND BANGLADESH

When the British ruled the country most Indians were Hindus, but there were Muslims also. There was much conflict between Hindus and Muslims. In 1947 when India achieved independence, the British partitioned (divided) India.

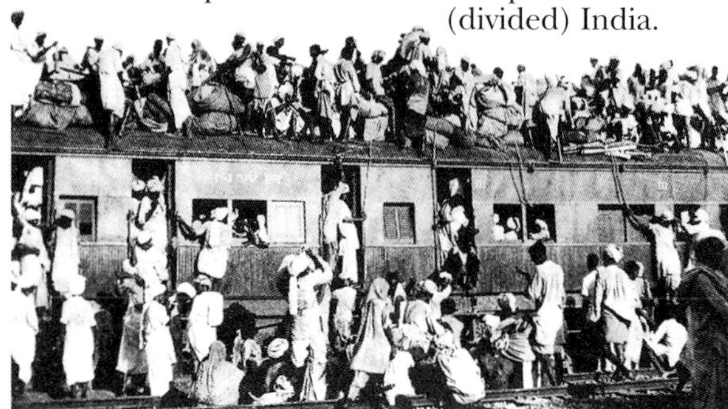

A train from Pakistan carries terrified Hindu refugees.

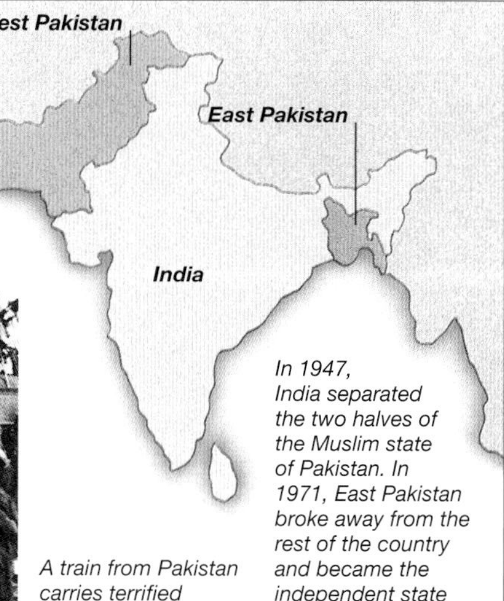

In 1947, India separated the two halves of the Muslim state of Pakistan. In 1971, East Pakistan broke away from the rest of the country and became the independent state of Bangladesh.

INDIA

c. 2500 B.C. Indus Valley civilization sets up cities.

c. 1500 B.C. Aryan invaders destroy Indus Valley civilization and introduce Hinduism.

c. A.D. 320-c.550 Gupta dynasty rules country.

500s Huns from central Asia overthrow Guptas.

700s Arab traders arrive in India; Turks introduce Muslim religion of Islam.

900s Muslim invasion.

1206-1526 The Delhi Sultanate (first Muslim kingdom) rules most of the country.

1526 Babur unites India with Mogul Empire.

1877 Queen Victoria is empress of India.

1885 Indian National Congress formed to campaign for Indian independence.

1947 British India divided into independent India and Pakistan. More than 500,000 people killed during partition.

1948 Hindu fanatic assassinates Mohandas Gandhi.

1956, 1961 India takes over remaining French and Portuguese colonies in India.

1962 Border dispute with China leads to war.

1964 Death of Prime Minister Nehru.

1965 War between India and Pakistan over province of Kashmir.

1966 Indira Gandhi becomes prime minister.

1971 Bangladesh achieves independence.

1984 Indira Gandhi assassinated.

1991 Rajiv Gandhi assassinated.

1998 India, Pakistan explode nuclear devices.

Find out more

BUDDHISM
HINDUISM
INDIA
INDUS VALLEY CIVILIZATION
SOUTHEAST ASIA, HISTORY OF

INDIAN OCEAN

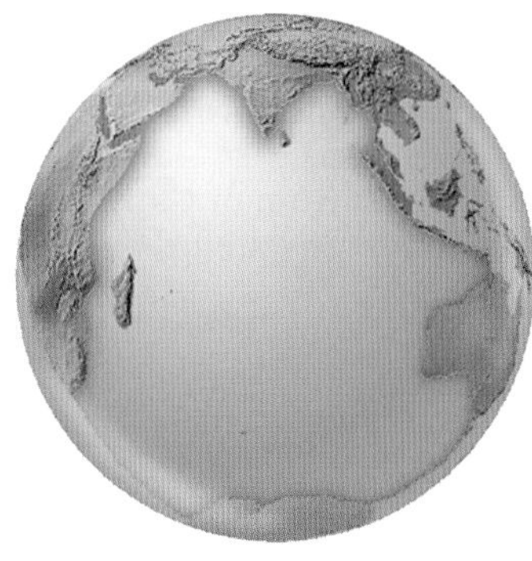

The Indian Ocean is bounded by Africa to the west, India and Australia to the east, and Asia to the north. In the south, it merges with the Antarctic Ocean. In the north, the Suez Canal gives access, via the Red Sea, to the Mediterranean.

MORE THAN 1,000 MILLION PEOPLE live in the countries that fringe the Indian Ocean, and on some of the 5,000 islands that are scattered across its surface. The world's third-largest ocean provides a major link between Europe and Asia. The monsoon winds, which bring heavy rainfall to many of the countries surrounding the ocean, also have an impact on the currents, which reverse direction completely between March and August. Early navigators used the winds and currents to carry them from Arabia to southern India and Indonesia, bringing Islamic religion and culture with them. Malays and Indonesians took the journey westwards, settling in Madagascar. Most of the islands of the Indian Ocean are small and uninhabited. However, many tourists are drawn to their beautiful palm-fringed beaches, and in some places tourism is beginning to supplement traditional ways of life based on fishing and farming.

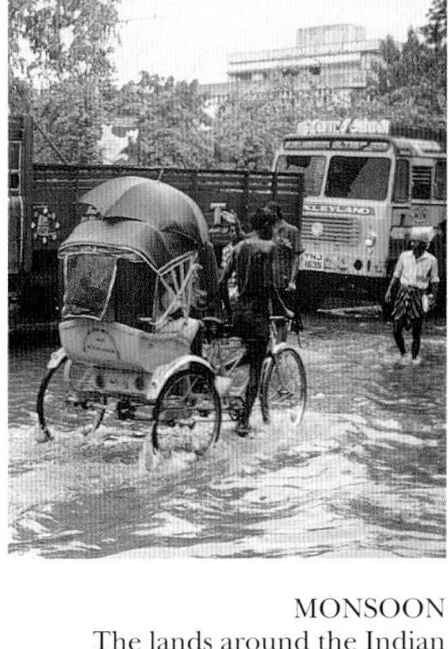

MONSOON
The lands around the Indian Ocean are dependent on monsoon rainfall. Monsoons are seasonal winds, blowing from the southwest in summer and northeast in winter, that bring torrential downpours. Very heavy monsoon rains swell rivers, causing disastrous flooding often accompanied by diseases such as cholera. The Bay of Bengal is especially vulnerable to flooding.

STILT FISHERMEN

There are less areas of shallow seas, where fish breed, in the Indian Ocean than in the Pacific or the Atlantic. Large-scale fishing, using trawlers and factory ships, has therefore not developed in the region. Most fishing takes place on a local basis, near island coastlines. Tuna is the most valuable catch. In Sri Lanka, fishermen – precariously perched on stilts – use poles and lines to catch their fish.

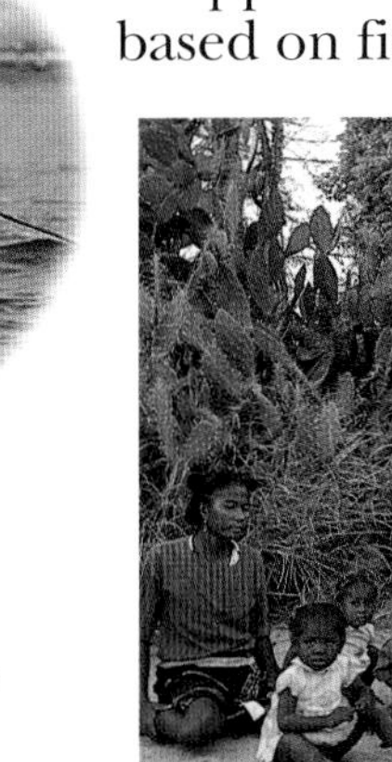

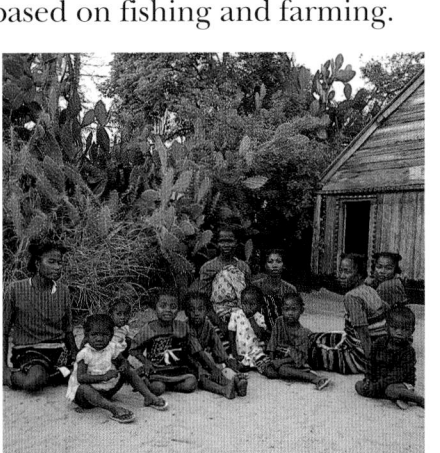

MADAGASCAN VILLAGE
Most Madagascans are descended from Malays and Indonesians, who crossed the Indian Ocean in the 7th century A.D. These villagers come from the southeastern coast. The east coast is densely populated and poor. Most of Madagascar's ruling class come from the central plateau.

SEYCHELLES

The island republic of the Seychelles consists of 40 scattered mountainous islands. These are surrounded by over 70 coral islands, which are low-lying and sparsely populated. The main islands are outstandingly beautiful; their hillsides blanketed with tropical vegetation, fringed by silvery-white beaches. Temperatures are constant throughout the year, reaching a daytime high of 30° C (86° F). The Seychelles attract year-round visitors from the northern hemisphere.

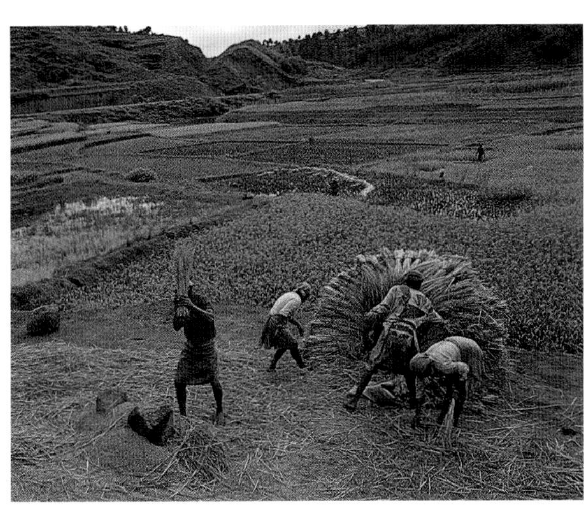

MADAGASCAR

The world's fourth-largest island lies off Africa's eastern coast. Most of the population is concentrated in the narrow strip of fertile land along the east coast, which has a humid, tropical climate. Farming dominates the economy. Rice and cassava are the main crops, while coffee and vanilla are grown for export. Poultry, sheep, pigs, and goats are all kept on a small scale. The government's attempts to modernize livestock farming have not been successful.

Find out more

AFRICA
ASIA
CORALS
OCEANS AND SEAS
SOUTHEAST ASIA

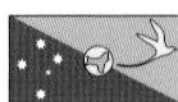

CHRISTMAS ISLAND
Area: 134.6 sq km (52 sq miles)
Status: Australian external territory
Claimed: 1958
Population: 1,300
Capital: Flying Fish Cove

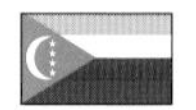

COMOROS
Area: 2,230 sq km (861 sq miles)
Population: 768,000
Capital: Moroni
Languages: Arabic, Comoran, French
Religions: Muslim, Roman Catholic
Currency: Comoros franc

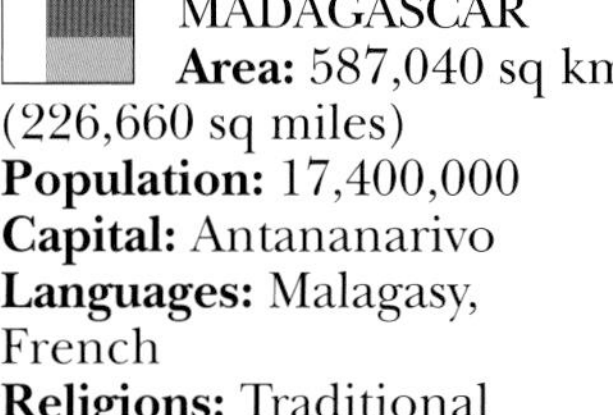

MADAGASCAR
Area: 587,040 sq km (226,660 sq miles)
Population: 17,400,000
Capital: Antananarivo
Languages: Malagasy, French
Religions: Traditional beliefs, Christian, Muslim
Currency: Malagasy franc

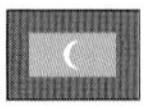

MALDIVES
Area: 300 sq km (116 sq miles)
Population: 318,000
Capital: Male'
Languages: Dhivehi (Maldavian)
Religions: Sunni Muslim
Currency: Rufiyaa

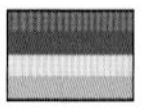

MAURITIUS
Area: 2,400 sq km (927 sq miles)
Population: 1,200,000
Capital: Port Louis
Languages: English, French, French Creole
Religions: Hindu, Roman Catholic
Currency: Mauritian rupee

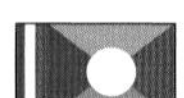

REUNION
Area: 2,517 sq km (972 sq miles)
Status: French overseas department
Claimed: 1649
Population: 777,000
Capital: Saint-Denis

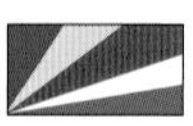

SEYCHELLES
Area: 455 sq km (176 sq miles)
Population: 80,500
Capital: Victoria
Languages: English, French, French Creole
Religions: Roman Catholic
Currency: Seychelles rupee

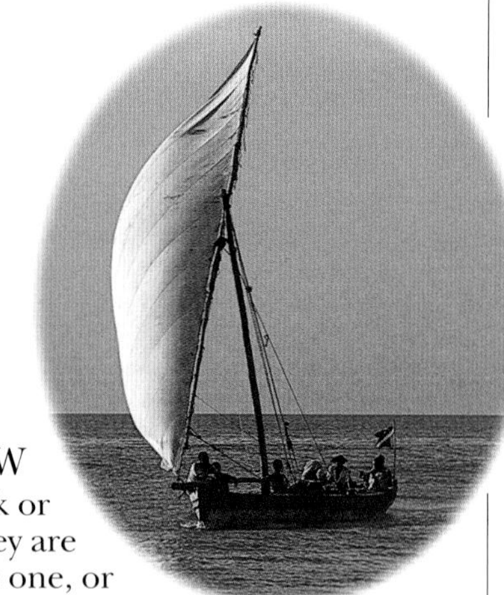

ARAB DHOW

Dhows are Arab trading boats made of teak or coconut planks, sewn together with twine. They are lateen-rigged, which means that they have one, or sometimes two, triangular sails. Dhows are fast and manoeuvrable. They were a vital tool in the Arab exploration of the Indian Ocean from the 8th century A.D. Using the monsoon winds, Arab merchants soon gained control of Indian Ocean trade and spread Islam as far as Indonesia.

Volcano | Mountain | Ancient monument | Capital city | Large city/town | Small city/town

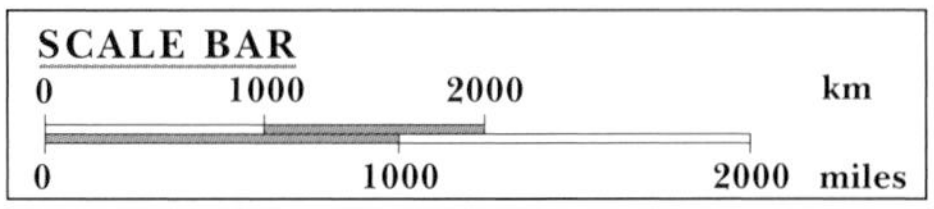

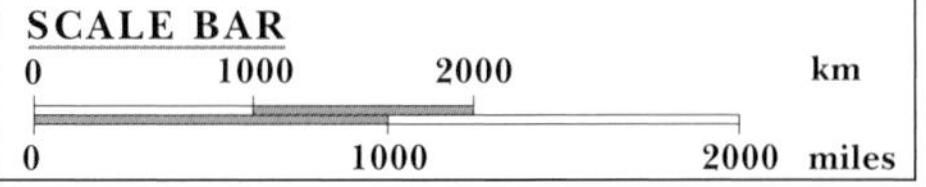

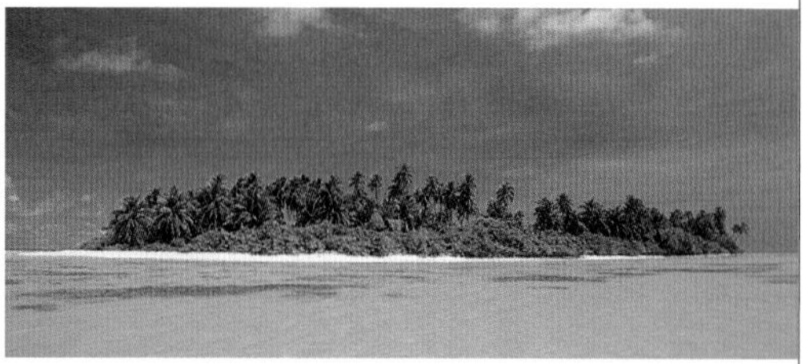

THE MALDIVES
The Maldives consist of 1,800 low-lying coral islands, which form the crowns of ancient submerged volcanoes. None of the islands are higher than 1.8 m (6 ft), and all but 20 have fewer than 1,000 inhabitants. Rising sea levels, caused by global warming, threaten to submerge the islands.

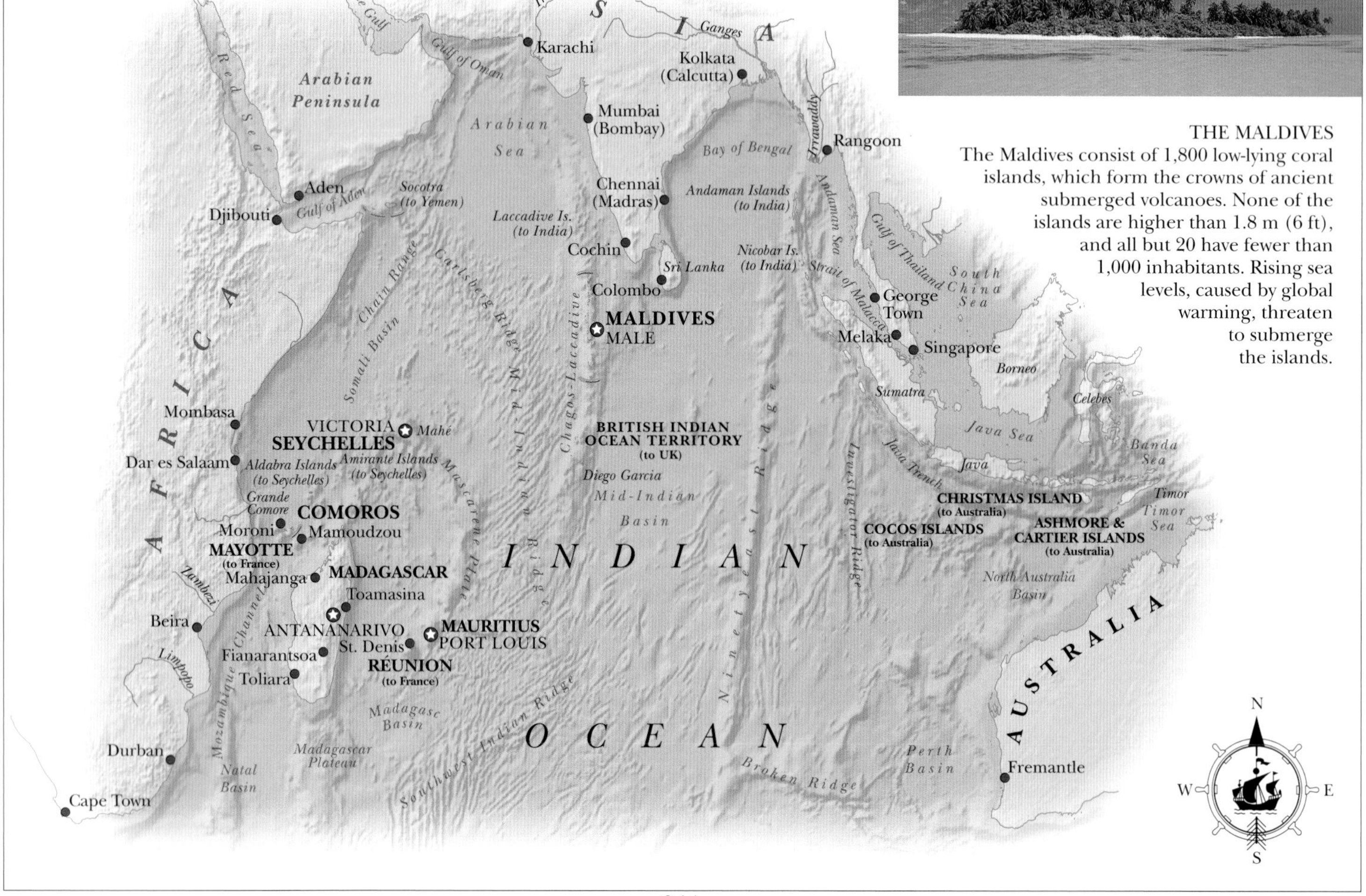

INDUSTRIAL REVOLUTION

THE WORLD WE LIVE IN TODAY, with its factories and huge cities, began less than 300 years ago in Britain, then spread to Europe and the United States. Beginning in about 1760, great changes took place that altered people's lives and methods of work forever, changes that are known today as the Industrial Revolution. Machines powered by water and, later, steam were invented to produce cloth and other goods more quickly. It took many workers to run these big machines, so poor people moved from the country into the new industrial towns to be near the factories. There were more jobs and higher wages in the cities, but life was often miserable. Although the Factory Act in 1833 banned young children in Britain from working in factories, there were no laws to control how long people worked each day, or to make sure the machines were safe.

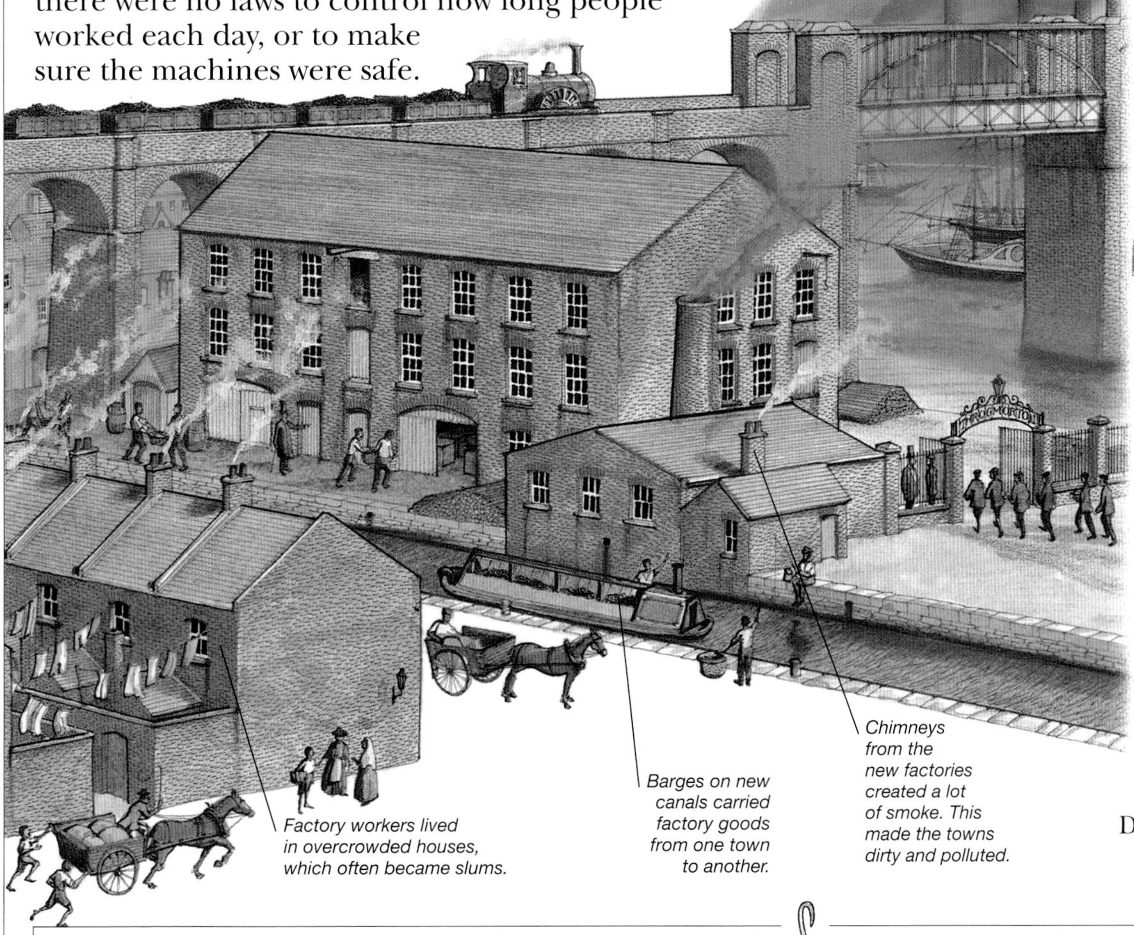

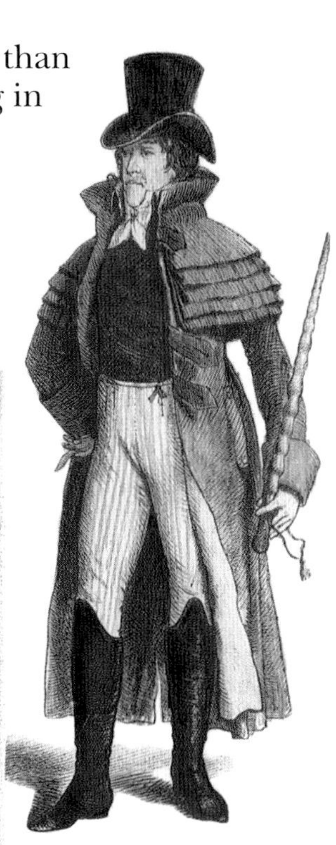

Factory workers lived in overcrowded houses, which often became slums.

Barges on new canals carried factory goods from one town to another.

Chimneys from the new factories created a lot of smoke. This made the towns dirty and polluted.

FACTORY OWNERS
Robert Owen (1771-1858) was a generous British factory owner who tried to improve working conditions. Many other owners grew rich by demanding long hours of work for low wages.

NEW TOWNS

Factory towns were built as fast and as cheaply as possible. Large families were crowded into tiny houses, and the water supply was often polluted. Diseases spread rapidly, and many people died young.

NEW TECHNOLOGY

Stronger metals were needed to make machines, so cast iron and steel were developed. Steam to drive the new engines was made by burning coal to boil water. Coal mines were driven deep into the ground. Cotton cloth was the first product to be made completely by machine. The new goods were produced in large numbers so they were cheap to buy.

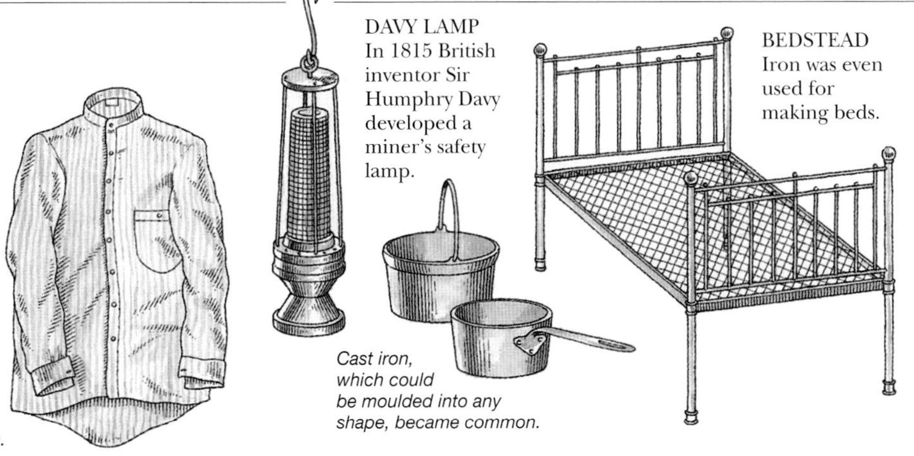

Cotton replaced wool as the main material for making clothes.

DAVY LAMP
In 1815 British inventor Sir Humphry Davy developed a miner's safety lamp.

Cast iron, which could be moulded into any shape, became common.

BEDSTEAD
Iron was even used for making beds.

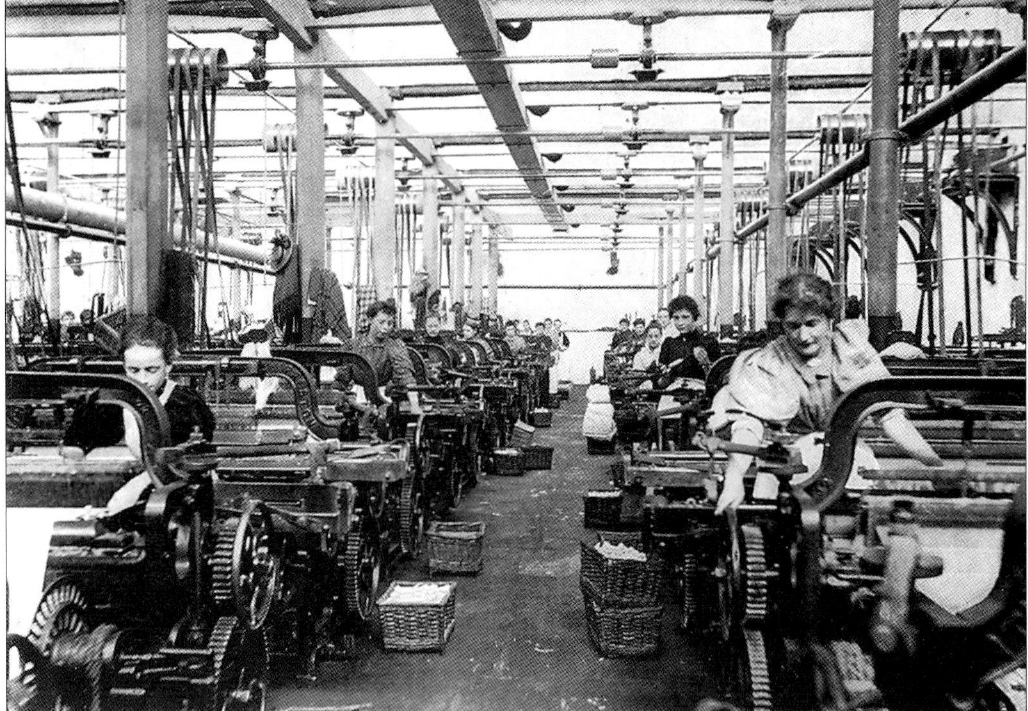

MILLS

The first factories were water-driven cotton mills which produced cloth. They were noisy, dangerous places to work in. Mill owners employed many women and children because they could pay them lower wages than men.

STEAM HAMMER
Unlike humans, steam-powered machines could work tirelessly, turning out vast quantities of goods. This steam hammer, invented in 1839, could hammer iron forgings with tremendous power and great accuracy.

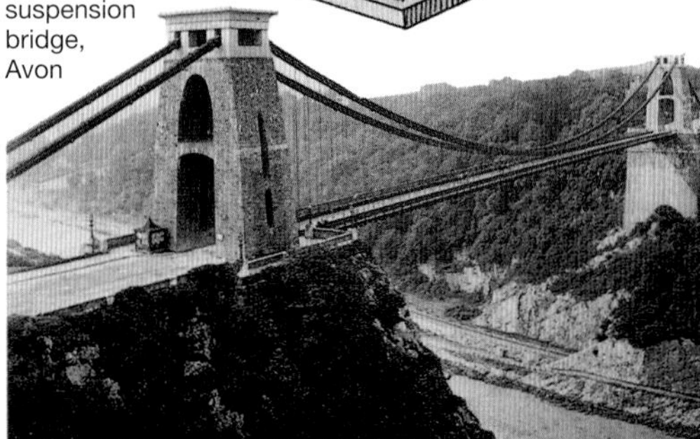

The Clifton suspension bridge, Avon

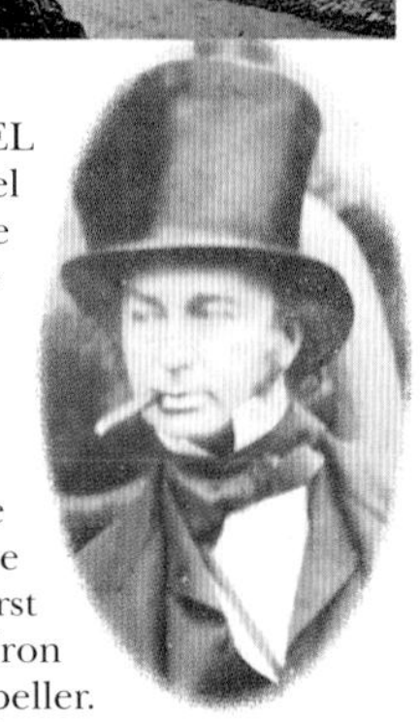

BRUNEL
Isambard Kingdom Brunel (1806-59) was probably the greatest engineer of the Industrial Revolution. His most famous bridge was the Clifton suspension bridge across the Avon Gorge. He also designed and built the Great Western Railway and the *Great Britain*, which was the first large steamship with an iron hull and a screw propeller.

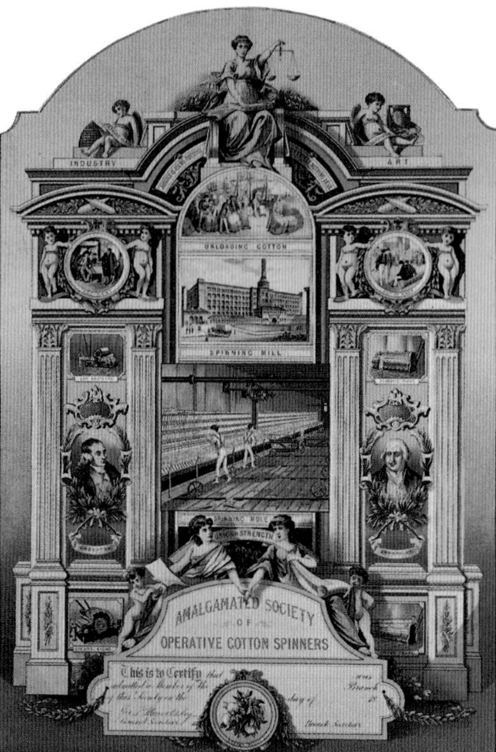

CO-OPS AND UNIONS

Working people fought to improve their conditions. Some set up labour unions to fight for shorter hours and better pay. Others created co-op stores to provide wholesome food at reasonable prices. These stores later grew into a co-operative movement.

INDUSTRIAL REVOLUTION

1708 Englishman Abraham Darby invents coke-smelting of iron.

1733 John Kay, England, develops "flying shuttle", which mechanizes weaving.

1760 Start of Industrial Revolution, Britain.

1765 James Hargreaves, England, invents "spinning jenny". It increases output of spun cotton. Scotsman James Watt develops steam engine, which is used to drive machinery in cotton industry.

1769 Richard Arkwright's water frame used to spin strong thread. Speeds up production; early beginning of Factory Age, England.

1779 English weaver Samuel Crompton develops spinning "mule", which spins many threads at once.

1784 Henry Cort, England, develops puddling furnace and rolling mill. Produces high quality iron.

1789 First steam-powered spinning loom, England. Speeds up textile production.

1793 Eli Whitney's cotton gin mechanizes cotton production, United States.

1804 Englishman Richard Trevithick builds first railway locomotive.

1825 First public railway from Stockton to Darlington, England.

1828 Development of hot-blast smelting furnace, England.

1842 Mines Act, Britain, bans women and children from working underground.

1851 Great Exhibition, London, displays new industrial products and techniques.

1856 Bessemer converter developed in England. Changes pig iron into steel.

1870 Industrialization established in Britain, Germany, and United States.

Find out more

FACTORIES
FARMING
SCIENCE, HISTORY OF
TEXTILES
TRADE AND INDUSTRY
VICTORIANS

INDUS VALLEY CIVILIZATION

ABOUT 4,500 YEARS AGO, one of the greatest ancient civilizations developed along the banks of the Indus River in the western Punjab. The Indus Valley people occupied a huge area, bigger than Ancient Egypt and Sumer together. Many of them lived in villages, farming the valley's fertile soil. But the civilization centered on the two large cities, Harappa and Mohenjo-daro. These cities were carefully planned, with streets running in straight lines, similar to a modern American town. With their courtyard houses and walled citadels, they were the most impressive cities of their time. But floods often damaged the walls, and the buildings needed repairing regularly. It was probably a combination of water damage and poor harvests that led to the decline of the civilization. After 1800 B.C. the Indus Valley civilization came to an end.

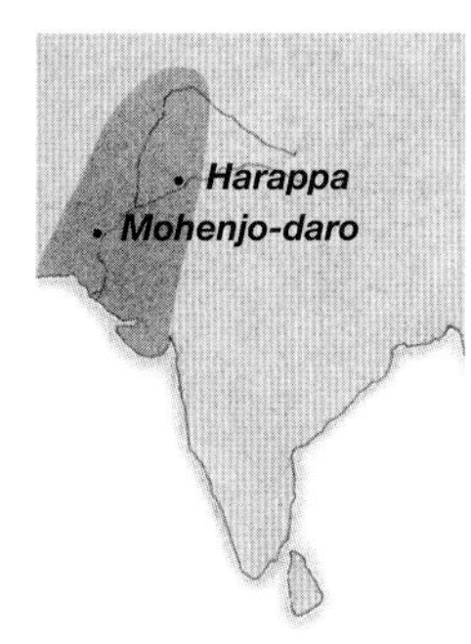

INDUS VALLEY
The Indus River flows through eastern Pakistan. The Indus people lived in a broad strip of land on either side of the river.

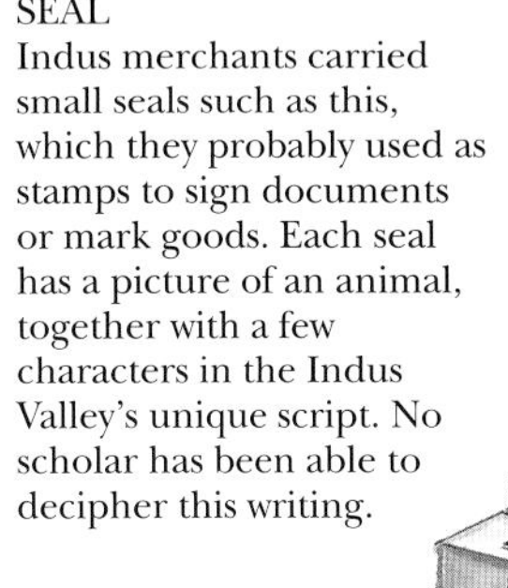

SEAL
Indus merchants carried small seals such as this, which they probably used as stamps to sign documents or mark goods. Each seal has a picture of an animal, together with a few characters in the Indus Valley's unique script. No scholar has been able to decipher this writing.

Citadel area contained large buildings, such as the great bath and granary, protected by a strong wall.

Most houses had two stories and a central courtyard.

Straight main streets show that city was carefully planned.

MOHENJO-DARO

Flat-roofed, mud-brick houses lined the straight streets of Mohenjo-daro. Each house had several rooms, with small windows to keep out the hot sun. A courtyard provided a shaded space for working. Most houses also had a bathroom, with a toilet that drained out into sewers beneath the streets. The city also contained a great bathhouse, which may have been used for religious purposes. Historians think that Mohenjo-daro and Harappa each had about 40,000 inhabitants.

INDUS GODS

Many houses in Mohenjo-daro and Harappa contained small pottery statues of a female figure with a head-dress and jewellery. She was probably a mother goddess. Indus Valley people may have worshipped her at home, hoping that she would bring them good harvests, and a plentiful food supply.

WHEELED TOYS
The children of the Indus Valley played with pottery toys such as this wheeled ox-cart. It is probably a model of similar, full-size carts that were used to take corn to the city's great granary. Archaeologists have also found dice, marbles, and small wheeled animals.

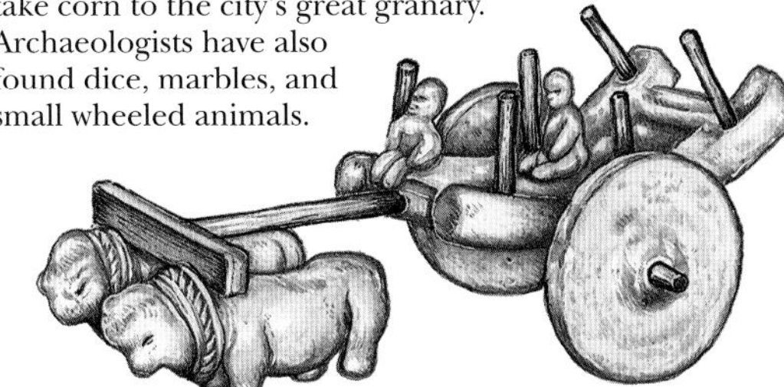

Find out more
CITIES
INDIA, HISTORY OF
RELIGIONS
WHEELS

INFORMATION TECHNOLOGY

THE TERM "INFORMATION TECHNOLOGY", or IT for short, is used to describe technologies that handle, store, process, and transmit, or pass on, information. When people talk about IT, they usually mean the use of computers to store and pass on information, but radio, television, telephones, fax machines, and DVDs are also examples of information technology. Information technology in some form has existed since humans developed pictures and writing, while later inventions such as printing made information more widely available. But modern information technology is based on electronics; vast amounts of information, including pictures and sounds, can be stored as electric signals and transmitted anywhere in the world. Information technology is used in every part of our lives from schools and hospitals, to shopping. Its impact has been enormous, making the world truly a "global village".

An early dial telephone

Camera

EARLY IT
The telephone and the camera were the information technology tools of the 19th century. They had a great impact on society. With the telephone, people could talk to each other all around the world. Using the camera, they could make a record of their lives and families.

USING INFORMATION TECHNOLOGY

To use information technology, you need access to hardware and software. Hardware means the actual machinery, namely computers. Software refers to the programs or applications inside the computer, which actually run it. Programs range from word processing to multimedia and games. They are constantly being updated.

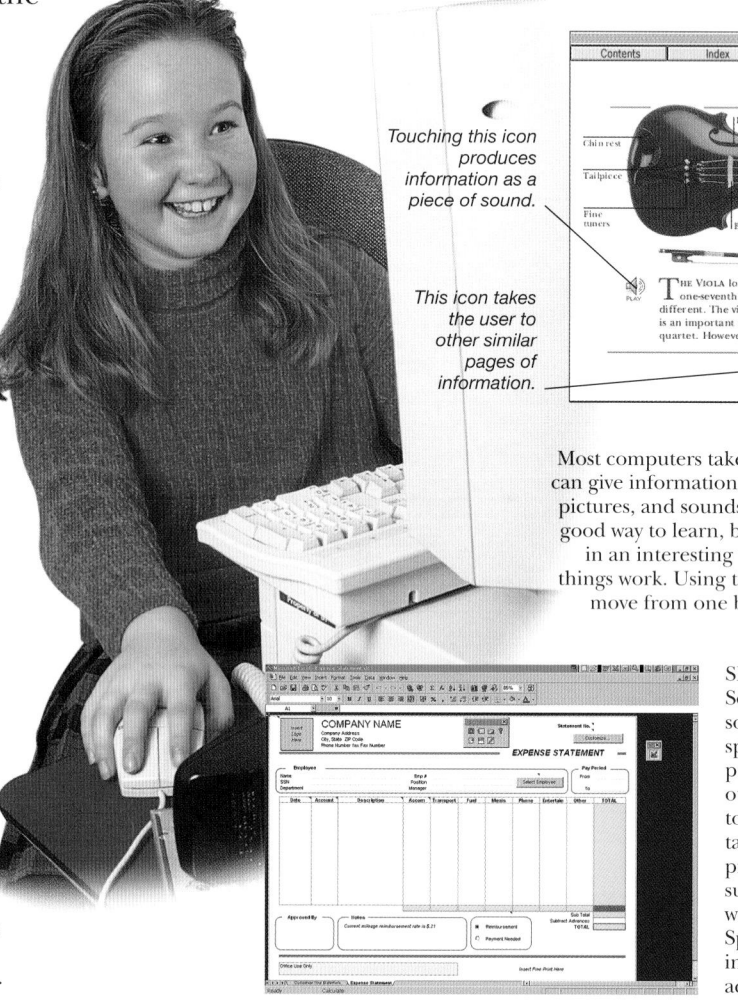

Musical Instruments
Contents | Index | Back | Next | Random

Viola

Chin rest, Tailpiece, Fine tuners, F-hole, Bridge, Strings, Neck, Tuning pegs, Belly, Scroll, Bow

THE VIOLA looks very similar to a violin, but it is about one-seventh larger and its proportions are slightly different. The viola produces a warm, mellow tone, and it is an important member of the orchestra and string quartet. However, viola solos are not often heard.

Touching this icon produces information as a piece of sound.

This icon takes the user to other similar pages of information.

MULTIMEDIA
Most computers take compact discs (CDs), which can give information in multimedia form – words, pictures, and sounds. Multimedia programs are a good way to learn, because they give information in an interesting way and allow you to see how things work. Using the computer mouse, you can move from one bit of information to another.

DESKTOP PUBLISHING
Software programs known as desktop publishing (DTP) enable words and pictures to be moved around on screen. DTP is used in publishing, but it also means people can write and design fan magazines, posters, and newsletters in their own homes.

COMPANY NAME
EXPENSE STATEMENT

SPREADSHEETS
Some computers contain software programs called spreadsheets. A spreadsheet program stores figures or other information that needs to be shown in the form of tables or charts. The program can do calcuations, such as adding up, or working out percentages. Spreadsheets have many uses, including working out accounts or progress charts.

EARLY ELECTRONICS

The use of electronics in information technology has a long history. Materials and designs used for early technology may look dated, but the the early inventions served the same purpose as today's modern examples.

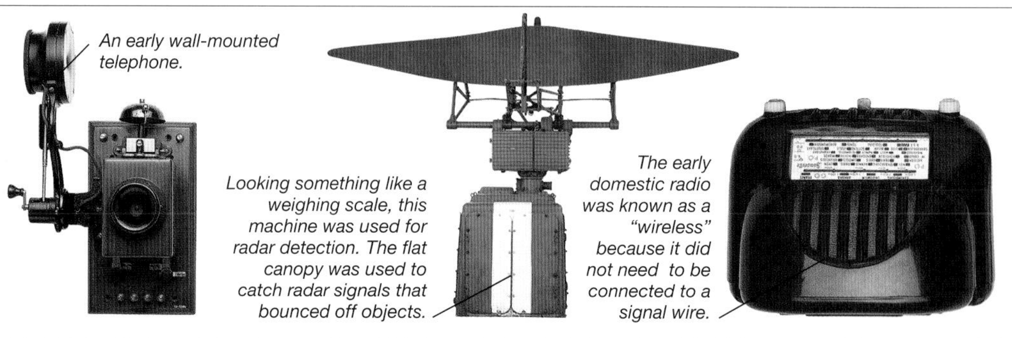

An early wall-mounted telephone.

Looking something like a weighing scale, this machine was used for radar detection. The flat canopy was used to catch radar signals that bounced off objects.

The early domestic radio was known as a "wireless" because it did not need to be connected to a signal wire.

OFFICE COMMUNICATION

In the early 20th century, a new kind of work place came into being – the office. Early offices contained manual typewriters and telephones. These were followed by machines powered by electricity, such as electric typewriters and photocopiers. Today, the modern office is absolutely computerized, and relies completely on the latest information technology, from computers and e-mail to fax machines and picture scanners.

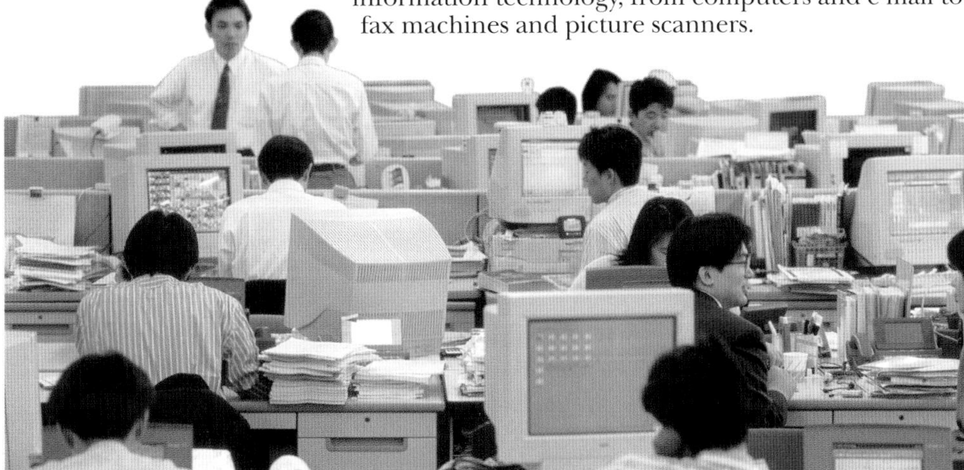

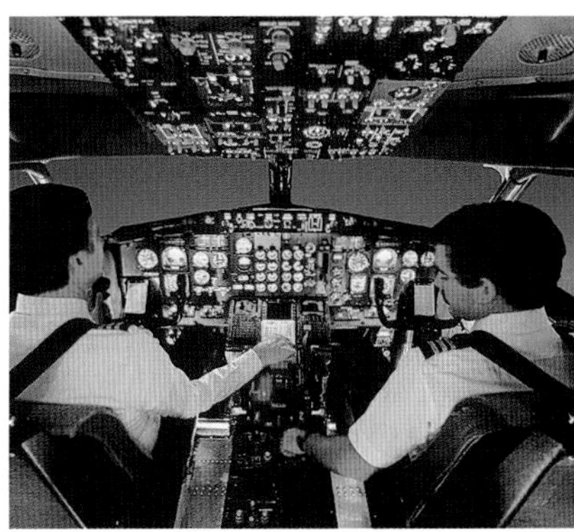

TRANSPORT
Information technology is important in transport, and is used to control airplanes, large ships, and even some cars. The cockpit of an aircraft in particular has become very sophisticated. The information supplied by the technology to the pilots is so accurate that pilots do not need to look out of the aircraft to fly safely, but can rely on the technology.

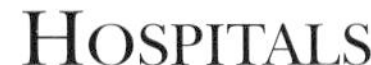

HOSPITALS

Information technology is very useful in hospitals, and medicine generally, and it is now possible to diagnose and treat many illnesses without physically looking inside the body. Scanning devices enable a doctor to monitor the development of an unborn baby on screen, checking on progress and identifying any problems at an early stage.

On-line shoppers can browse through pictures of items for sale displayed in virtual shops.

ON-LINE SHOPPING
E-commerce – buying and selling over the Internet – is a recent development, and many people now shop on-line. To do so, you must pay with a credit card. Fraud is a risk, but special programs can check credit card numbers.

By using the image displayed on a monitor screen, the doctor can show a woman how her baby is developing inside her.

The scanning device is held in the doctor's hand and moved over the woman's stomach, where it collects information that is shown on screen.

DISABILITY

Information technology has brought major advantages for people with disability. This is because the technology can be designed to make the most of each person's physical abilities. For example, word-activated processors are available for blind people, who can both receive and send sound messages. People with physical disabilities can communicate via e-mail, or access information through the Internet, without leaving home.

Find out more
COMPUTERS
ELECTRONICS
INTERNET
TECHNOLOGY

INSECTS

THE EARTH IS CRAWLING with insects; in fact, they make up the largest group of animals. There are at least one million different species, including beetles, butterflies, ants, and bees. Insects first appeared on Earth more than 500 million years ago and are found in almost every kind of habitat, from cold mountains to tropical rain forests. Although all insects have six legs and a body covered by a hard exoskeleton (outer skeleton), they vary enormously in size and shape. The goliath beetle weighs more than 100 gm (3.5 oz); the tiny fairyfly is almost invisible to the human eye. Some insects cause problems for humans. Flies spread disease, and weevils and locusts eat farm crops. Parasites such as ticks and lice live and feed on farm animals and sometimes on humans, too. But insects are a vital part of nature. They pollinate flowers and are an important source of food for many birds, bats, and reptiles. Certain insects are also very useful to humans – without bees, for example, there would be no honey.

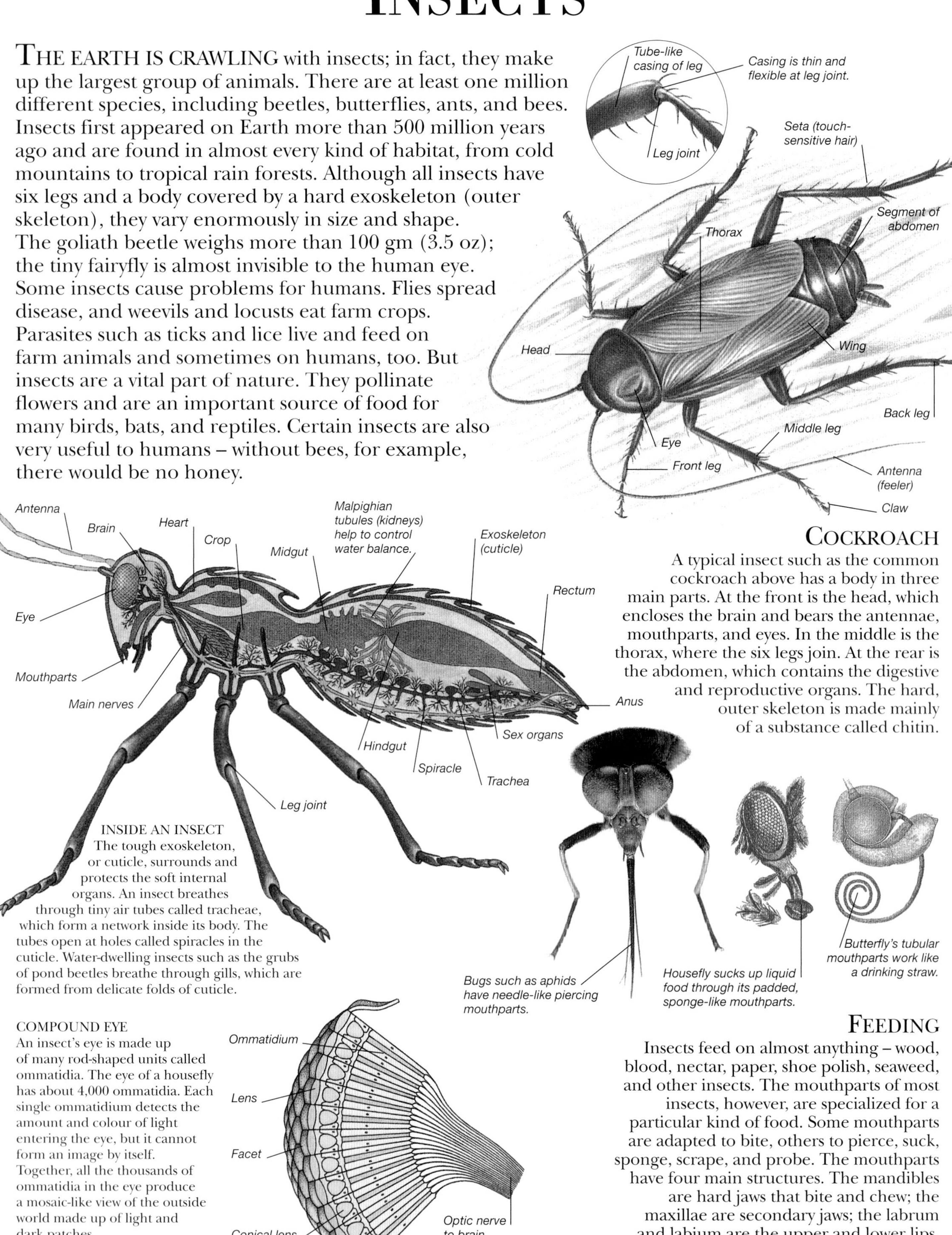

COCKROACH

A typical insect such as the common cockroach above has a body in three main parts. At the front is the head, which encloses the brain and bears the antennae, mouthparts, and eyes. In the middle is the thorax, where the six legs join. At the rear is the abdomen, which contains the digestive and reproductive organs. The hard, outer skeleton is made mainly of a substance called chitin.

INSIDE AN INSECT

The tough exoskeleton, or cuticle, surrounds and protects the soft internal organs. An insect breathes through tiny air tubes called tracheae, which form a network inside its body. The tubes open at holes called spiracles in the cuticle. Water-dwelling insects such as the grubs of pond beetles breathe through gills, which are formed from delicate folds of cuticle.

COMPOUND EYE

An insect's eye is made up of many rod-shaped units called ommatidia. The eye of a housefly has about 4,000 ommatidia. Each single ommatidium detects the amount and colour of light entering the eye, but it cannot form an image by itself. Together, all the thousands of ommatidia in the eye produce a mosaic-like view of the outside world made up of light and dark patches.

FEEDING

Insects feed on almost anything – wood, blood, nectar, paper, shoe polish, seaweed, and other insects. The mouthparts of most insects, however, are specialized for a particular kind of food. Some mouthparts are adapted to bite, others to pierce, suck, sponge, scrape, and probe. The mouthparts have four main structures. The mandibles are hard jaws that bite and chew; the maxillae are secondary jaws; the labrum and labium are the upper and lower lips.

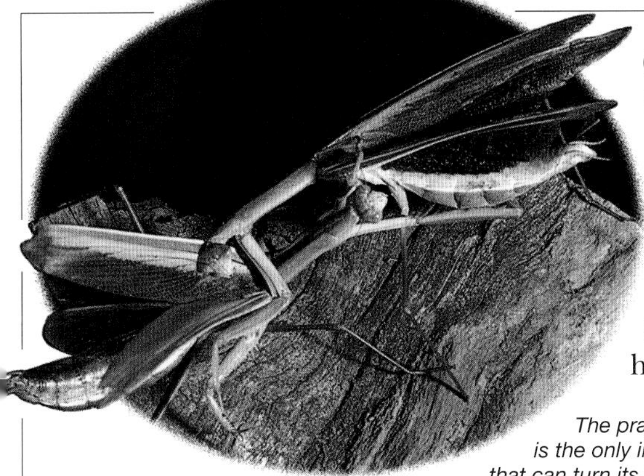

COURTSHIP

Some insects, such as the praying mantises shown here, have complicated courtship behaviour. After mating, the female mantis often grasps and eats the male mantis; the nutrients in the body of the male help the eggs to develop.

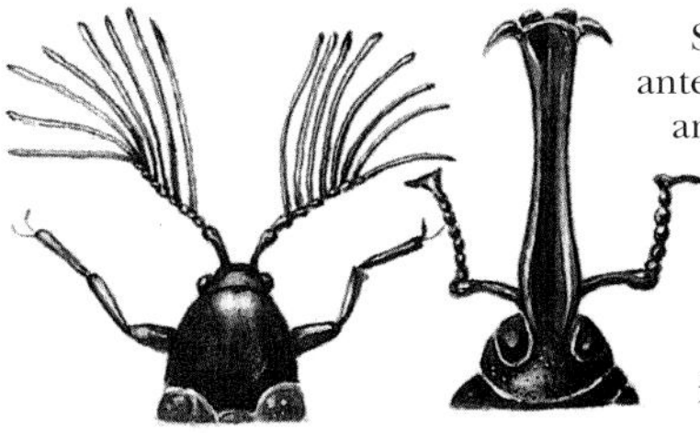

The praying mantis is the only insect that can turn its head to look directly behind.

ANTENNAE

Sense organs called antennae detect smells and vibrations in the air and in solid objects. Often, the male has larger, more branched antennae than the female. These help detect the scent that she releases into the air at mating time. Near the antennae there are often several tiny single-lens eyes called ocelli.

Indian beetle has antler-like antennae.

Weevil has elbow-jointed antennae.

METAMORPHOSIS

Most insects hatch from eggs. Some insects, such as the butterfly, hatch into a larva or caterpillar, which feeds voraciously and moults (sheds its skin) several times. It then forms a chrysalis and pupates, finally emerging as a mature adult butterfly. These great changes in form are known as complete metamorphosis. Other insects, such as grasshoppers, hatch into nymphs, which look like small versions of the parent but without proper wings. They moult in order to grow and finally become adult after the final moult when they have wings. This is called incomplete metamorphosis.

Female damselfly lays eggs on stem of reed.

Emerging nymph climbs up reed stem.

Adult emerges from nymph skin.

Young nymph (larva)

Older nymph (larva) develops wings.

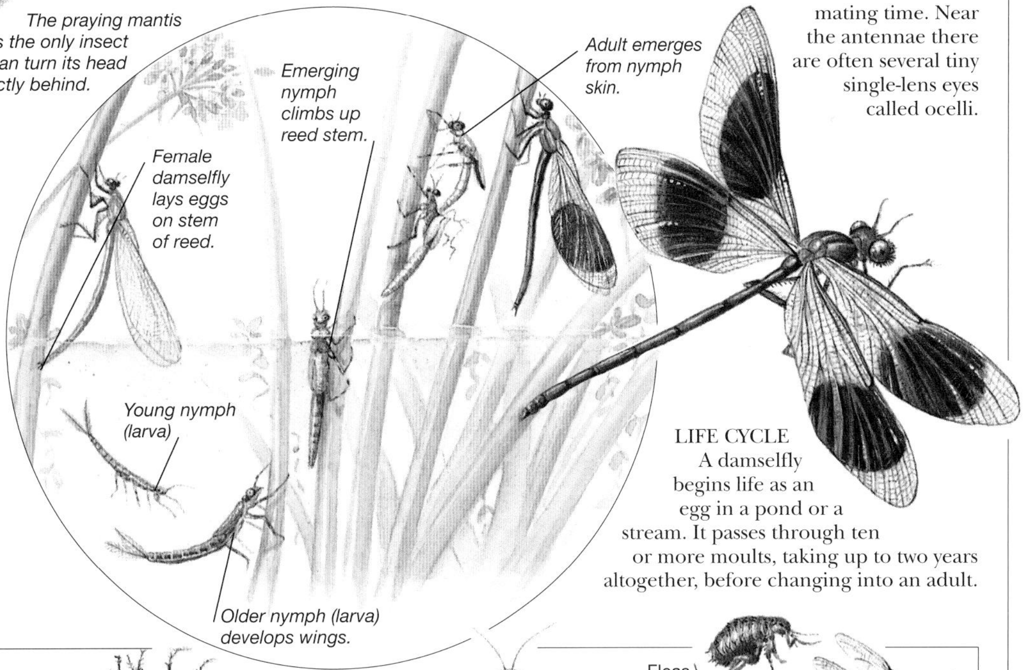

LIFE CYCLE

A damselfly begins life as an egg in a pond or a stream. It passes through ten or more moults, taking up to two years altogether, before changing into an adult.

TYPES OF INSECTS

There are about 20 main groups of insects. Beetles and weevils form the largest single group of insects, which contains more than 300,000 species known to entomologists (scientists who study insects). Most insects have wings at some stage during their life cycle; bristletails, silverfish, and firebrats do not. Fleas are also wingless; their wings have disappeared during the course of evolution.

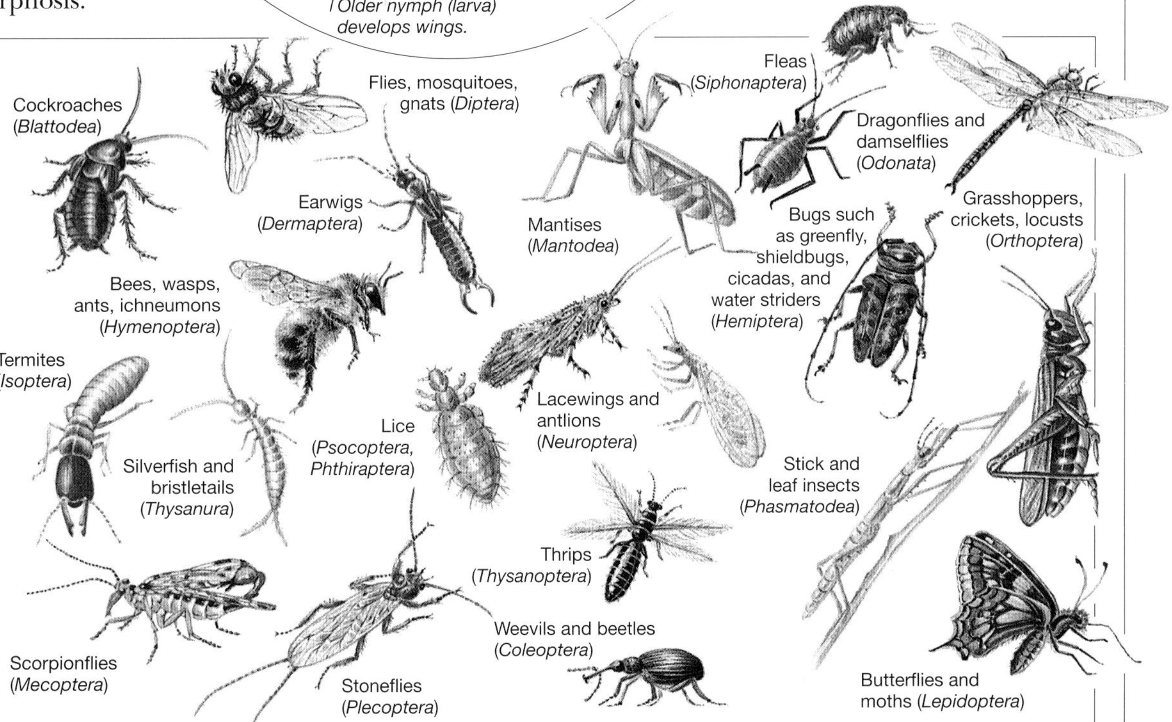

Cockroaches (*Blattodea*)

Flies, mosquitoes, gnats (*Diptera*)

Fleas (*Siphonaptera*)

Dragonflies and damselflies (*Odonata*)

Earwigs (*Dermaptera*)

Mantises (*Mantodea*)

Bugs such as greenfly, shieldbugs, cicadas, and water striders (*Hemiptera*)

Grasshoppers, crickets, locusts (*Orthoptera*)

Bees, wasps, ants, ichneumons (*Hymenoptera*)

Termites (*Isoptera*)

Lice (*Psocoptera, Phthiraptera*)

Lacewings and antlions (*Neuroptera*)

Silverfish and bristletails (*Thysanura*)

Stick and leaf insects (*Phasmatodea*)

Thrips (*Thysanoptera*)

Weevils and beetles (*Coleoptera*)

Scorpionflies (*Mecoptera*)

Stoneflies (*Plecoptera*)

Butterflies and moths (*Lepidoptera*)

FLEA

A flea can leap more than 30 cm (12 in) up into the air, which is similar to a person jumping 245 m (800 ft), or a 70-storey building, or St. Paul's Cathedral in London, England.

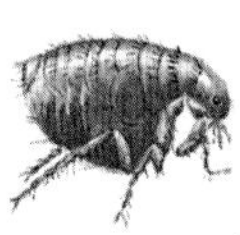

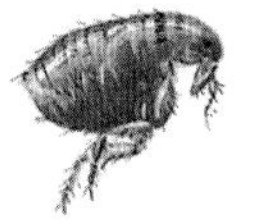

Legs kick down for extra acceleration.

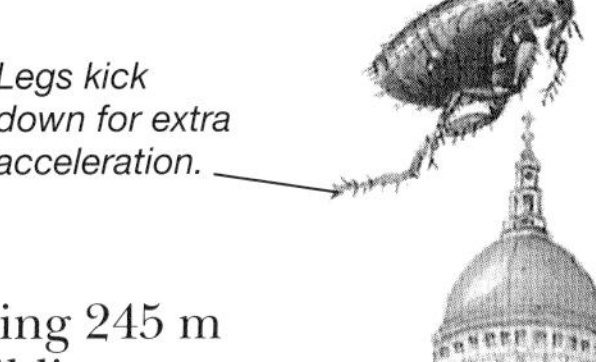

St. Paul's Cathedral

Like other insects, fleas have powerful muscles, and the elastic springiness of the cuticle helps the legs to rebound quickly during movement.

Find out more

ANTS AND TERMITES
BEETLES
BUTTERFLIES AND MOTHS
FLIES AND MOSQUITOES
GRASSHOPPERS and crickets

INTERNET

FOR CENTURIES THE MOST IMPORTANT way of passing on knowledge was through books, but when the Internet (short for international network) was established, it gave people a way of sending and receiving information through personal computers. Words, pictures, music, videos, and any other type of data that can be turned into digital form are all sent from computer to computer, as electronic signals travelling over telephone, radio, or satellite links. The Internet was first set up in 1969 by the US Defense Department, but in 1994 it became open to everybody. We now use the Internet to search for information, send and receive e-mail messages, share photos, buy and sell goods, play games, listen to music, and watch movies and TV.

INFORMATION
The Internet is like a vast library of electronic books. No one knows exactly how many pages there are. Search engines cover nearly 10 billion – but the number grows by millions more every day.

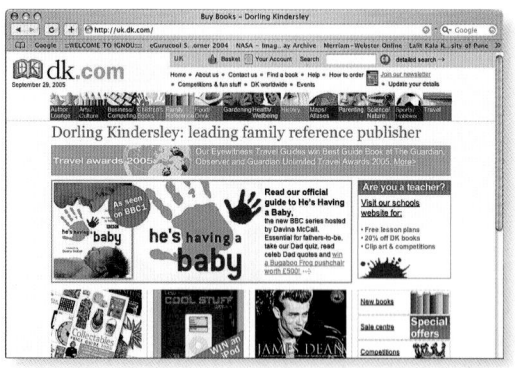

A page from the Dorling Kindersley web site: web pages are regularly updated.

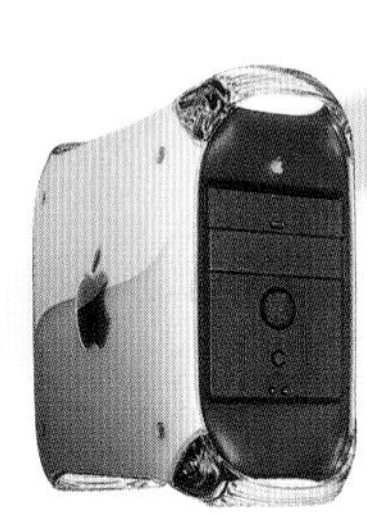

Electronic mail can send a letter halfway round the world in seconds.

Information can be sent all over the world via global satellite links.

The Internet uses the telephone system to link computers with each other.

WORLD WIDE WEB

Most information on the Internet is given in the form of "web pages". These are electronically linked to form "web sites" stored on the World Wide Web (WWW). Web site information is released through "web servers" (very large computers). To link up with the web, you send a request from your computer to a web server.

SURFING THE NET

Looking for information on the Internet is called "surfing". Using a search engine (a kind of electronic catalogue), you type in one or more keywords describing what you are looking for. The search engine matches your keywords against its huge index of the web and produces a list of sites likely to contain what you want. Usually, the most popular and relevant sites are listed first.

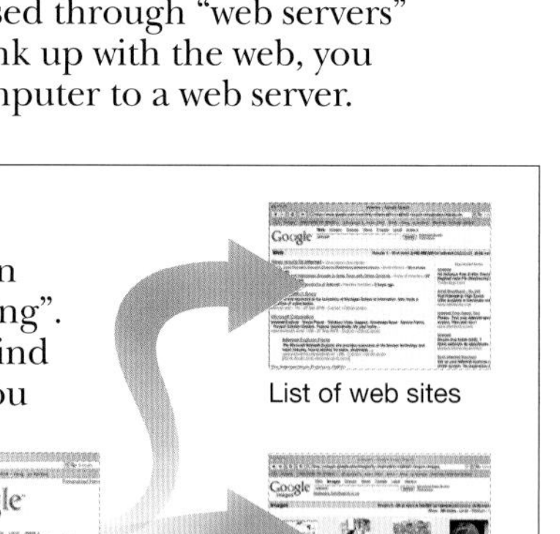

Search engine

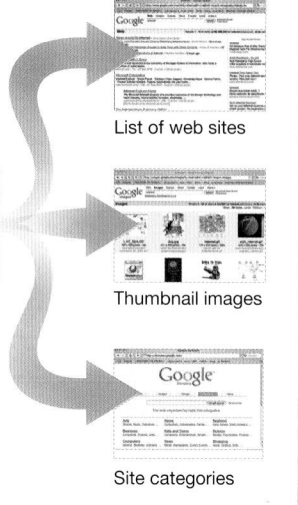

List of web sites

Thumbnail images

Site categories

E-MAIL

Any Internet user can send a message directly to another by electronic mail or e-mail. You need your own e-mail address and a computer with a modem so it can connect to the Internet. A modem translates messages into electronic data that can be sent from one computer to another and displayed on screen.

You can use the Internet to send an e-mail message around the world as easily as making a local telephone call.

Find out more
COMPUTERS
INFORMATION TECHNOLOGY
TELEPHONES
SATELLITES

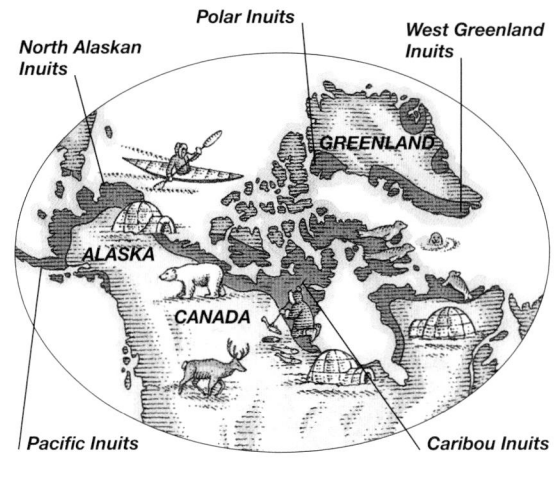

INUITS

THE FROZEN ARCTIC was one of the last regions of the world to be inhabited by humans. The Inuit (Eskimo) people, who originally came from Asia, settled in the Arctic about 4,000 years ago. A Native American tribe named them *Eskimo*, which means "eaters of raw meat"; but the newcomers called themselves *Inuit*, which simply means "real men". Inuits were nomadic. They moved about in family groups, hunting animals such as seals and caribou. Inuit families survived the bitter cold of winter by digging shelters into the ground. They made roofs for the shelters from driftwood or whalebone, with a covering of turf. For clothes, they used double layers of caribou or polar bear fur. Today, most Inuits live in small settlements or towns, but they are proud of their culture. They preserve it in language, art, and song, and hunting is still an essential part of Inuit life.

Polar Inuits
West Greenland Inuits
North Alaskan Inuits
GREENLAND
ALASKA
CANADA
Pacific Inuits
Caribou Inuits

INUIT COMMUNITIES
Inuits live in Siberia in the Russian Federation, in Alaska, Canada, and Greenland. There are many different groups, each named after the area in which they live. The Polar Inuits of Greenland live the furthest north of all the world's peoples.

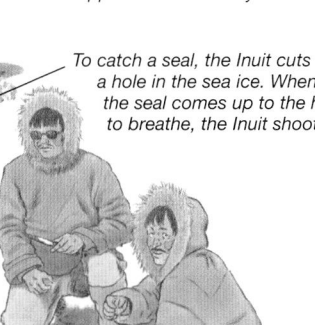

Today, Inuits hunt on snowmobiles instead of sledges.

A hunting trip takes many days, and supplies are carried by snowmobile.

To catch a seal, the Inuit cuts a hole in the sea ice. When the seal comes up to the hole to breathe, the Inuit shoots it.

HUNTING
Inuits hunt for food to eat, and furs to sell. They do not hunt animals for sport. They respect foxes, caribou, seal, walrus, and other Arctic wildlife, and their hunting does not threaten the long-term survival of these animal species. Hunting takes patience and skill, and some Inuits travel 5,000 km (3,000 miles) a year on hunting trips. When they are hunting away from home in winter, they build temporary shelters, called igloos, from blocks of snow.

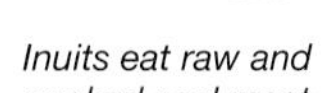

Inuits eat raw and cooked seal meat.

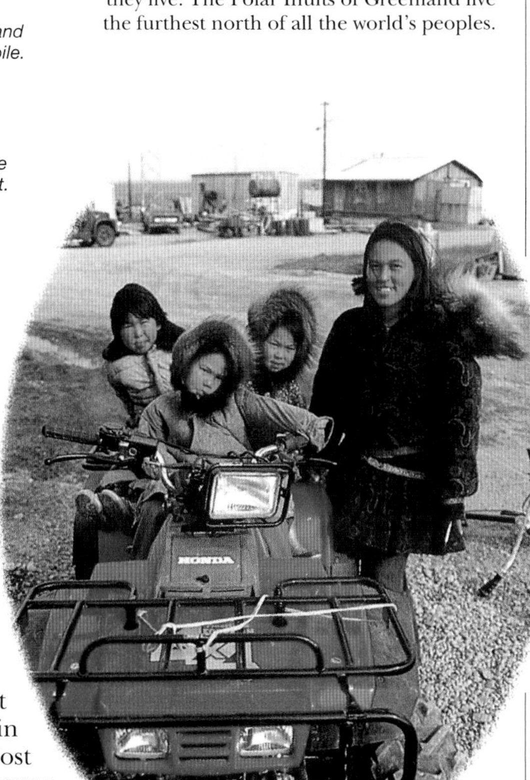

INUIT ART
During the long winter months there is little daylight in the Arctic, so the hours of hunting are limited. In the past, skilled Inuit carvers used the time to work wood, bone, soapstone (soft rock), and walrus tusks. They created beautiful statues of animals, people, and especially favoured hunting scenes. Today, museums and collectors eagerly seek good Inuit carvings.

Inuit artists use their skills to decorate everyday tools, such as this arrow straightener.

INUIT LIFE
There are about 25,000 Inuits in North America. Most live in wooden houses equipped like a typical North American home. Some Inuits are still full-time hunters; most others work in many different businesses and industries.

A team of 10 to 15 husky dogs pull the traditional Inuit sledge. With an expert driver at the reins, a dog team can travel 80 km (50 miles) in a day.

Find out more
ANTARCTICA
ARCTIC
CANADA
POLAR EXPLORATION
POLAR WILDLIFE

IRAN

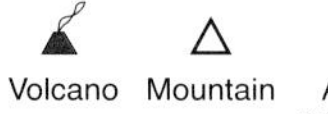

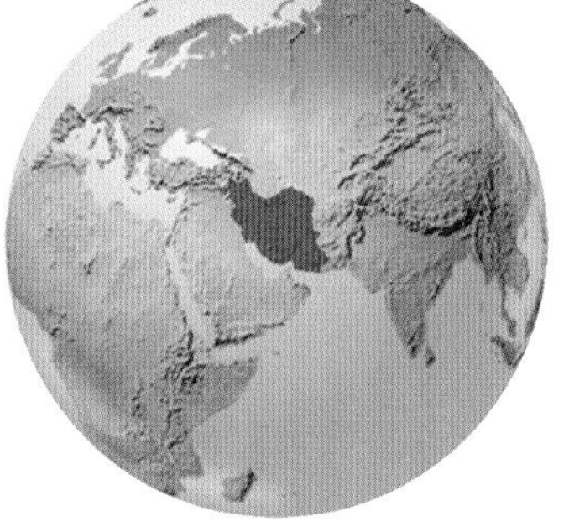

Iran lies at the heart of Asia, bordered by the Caspian Sea in the north, and The Gulf and Gulf of Oman to the south. The Elburz Mountains and Zagros Mountains enclose the central plateau, a land of barren, rocky deserts.

A LAND OF RUGGED MOUNTAINS and harsh deserts, Iran was ruled for many centuries by the shah, or king. In the 1979 revolution, the shah was overthrown and Iran became an Islamic republic, ruled according to strict Islamic laws. Between 1980 and 1988, border disputes led to a devastating war between Iran and its western neighbour, Iraq. The cost of the prolonged war has strained the economy. Although Iran has very substantial oil reserves, it has very few other industries. Eggs from sturgeon caught in the Caspian Sea are used to make caviar, an expensive delicacy, which is exported. Fine, hand-made carpets are also an important source of income for villagers, who grow wheat, barley, and rice and herd sheep. Iran's strict Islamic laws have discouraged tourists, although the country has a great wealth of historic buildings and magnificent mosques.

STATISTICS
Area: 1,648,000 sq km (636,293 sq miles)
Population: 68,900,000
Capital: Tehran
Languages: Farsi (Persian), Azerbaijani, Gilaki, Mazenderani, Kurdish, Baluchi, Arabic, Turkmen
Religions: Shi'ite Muslim, Sunni Muslim
Currency: Iranian rial

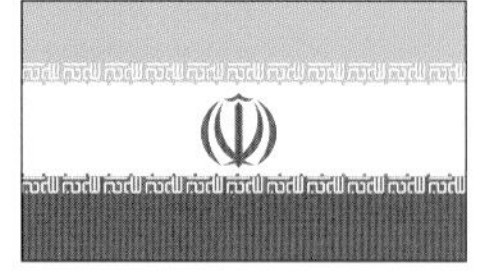

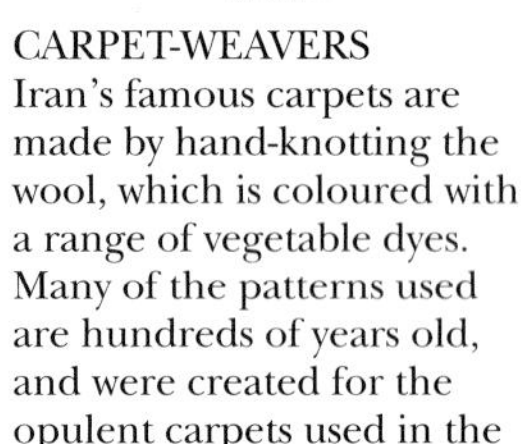

CARPET-WEAVERS
Iran's famous carpets are made by hand-knotting the wool, which is coloured with a range of vegetable dyes. Many of the patterns used are hundreds of years old, and were created for the opulent carpets used in the royal palaces and mosques. Each region prides itself on its carpets, specializing in unique designs and colour combinations.

CASPIAN SEA
The Caspian is a salt lake that lies between Europe and Asia. It sits 28m (92 ft) below sea level.

THE KURDS

The Kurds are an ethnically and linguistically distinctive group, who live in Iran, Iraq, and Turkey. They were once sheep- and goat-herding nomads in the Iranian highlands, although in recent years they have turned to farming and village life. There are about 25 million Kurds, the largest group of stateless people in the world. In Iran, they are pressured to become part of mainstream society, and they are severely discriminated against in Turkey.

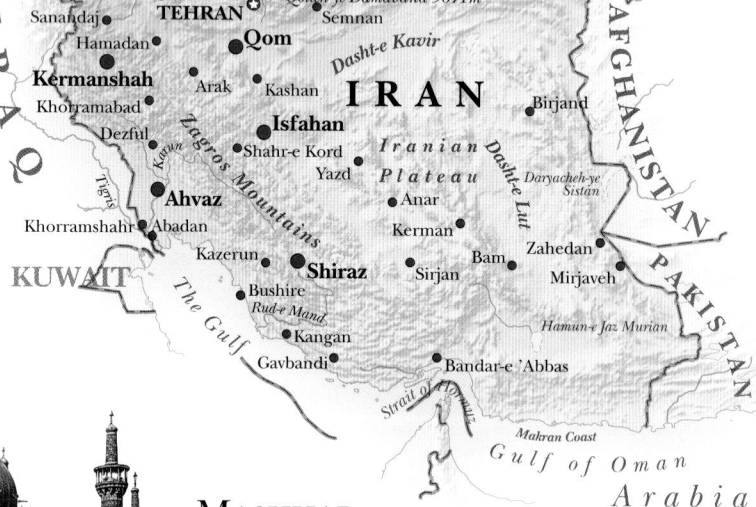

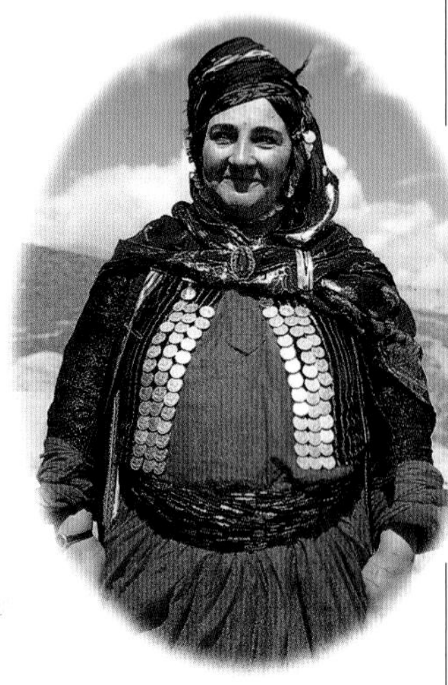

MASHHAD

Most Iranians belong to the minority Shi'ah branch of Islam, and Mashhad is their main shrine, the place where the Shi'ah leader Riza (770–819) was martyred. Iran has a religious government that imposes severe restrictions on the people. Women must wear the chador, a dress covering all but the face and hands, and behaviour is closely monitored.

SCALE BAR
0 100 200 300 km
0 100 200 300 miles

Find out more
ASIA
EARTHQUAKES
ISLAM
PERSIANS, ANCIENT

IRELAND

OFF THE NORTHWEST COAST of Europe lies one of the most beautiful islands in the world. For centuries, writers and singers have praised the lush countryside and wild mountains of Ireland. Despite its beauty, Ireland is not a rich country and has few natural resources. It has no coal, no iron ore or vast reserves of oil. Nevertheless, Ireland's influence has been far-reaching, for the country is rich in its people and their distinctive Gaelic culture. Few corners of the world lack an Irish community whose members keep alive the memory and customs of their homeland. In 1973, Ireland (Eire) joined the European Economic Community (now the European Union). Until then, its powerful neighbour and former ruler, the United Kingdom, had always dominated the country's economy. As a member of the Union, Eire is becoming more prosperous and economically independent of the United Kingdom. New high-tech industries are replacing traditional agriculture and textiles as the main sources of employment.

Ireland is the smaller of the two main British Isles. The other – Britain – is to the east, and the Atlantic Ocean is to the west. Ireland is divided into Ireland (Eire), which is independent, and the province of Northern Ireland, which is part of the United Kingdom.

Blocks of peat – carbon-rich soil consisting of decomposed plant life – are dug up from the marshy countryside and left to dry before being used as fuel.

DUBLIN

The capital city of Ireland is Dublin. It lies on the Liffey river not far from the Irish Sea. The Vikings founded Dublin in the 9th century, and the city has many historic buildings and beautiful town squares.

The Ha'penny Bridge, which spans the Liffey river, is accepted as the symbol of Dublin. Opened in 1816, its name comes from the fee once charged to use it.

COUNTRYSIDE

Wet west winds blow across Ireland from the Atlantic Ocean, soaking parts of the country with more than 200 cm (80 in) of rain each year. This makes the farmland very productive; about 16 per cent of the people work in farming and food processing industries.

GEOGRAPHY

Mountains to the south, west, and north surround Ireland's large, central plain. The plain is marshy in places, and there are many lakes, called loughs. Lough Neagh (right) in Northern Ireland, the biggest lake in the British Isles, is famous for its wildfowl and salmon.

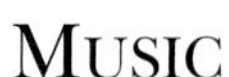

MUSIC

Ireland has a strong musical tradition. Irish rock and classical artists are well known internationally. The Corrs, U2, and Boyzone are all very successful Irish bands. Traditional Irish music and dancing is also very important to Ireland's cultural heritage.

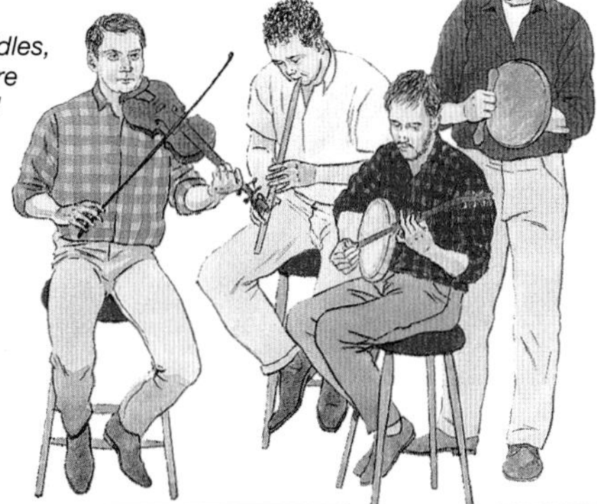

Pipes, fiddles, and banjos are all used in traditional Irish music.

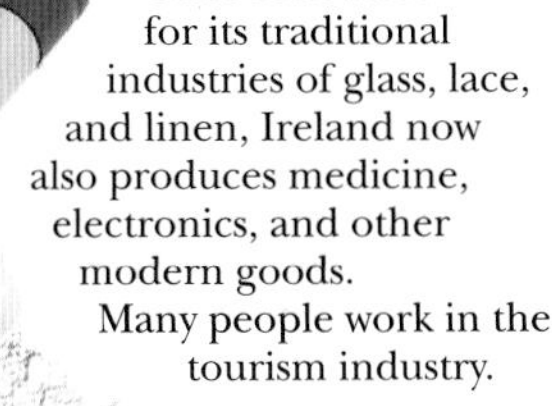

INDUSTRY

Once renowned for its traditional industries of glass, lace, and linen, Ireland now also produces medicine, electronics, and other modern goods. Many people work in the tourism industry.

Find out more

CELTS
EUROPE
IRELAND, HISTORY OF
UNITED KINGDOM
UNITED KINGDOM, HISTORY OF
VIKINGS

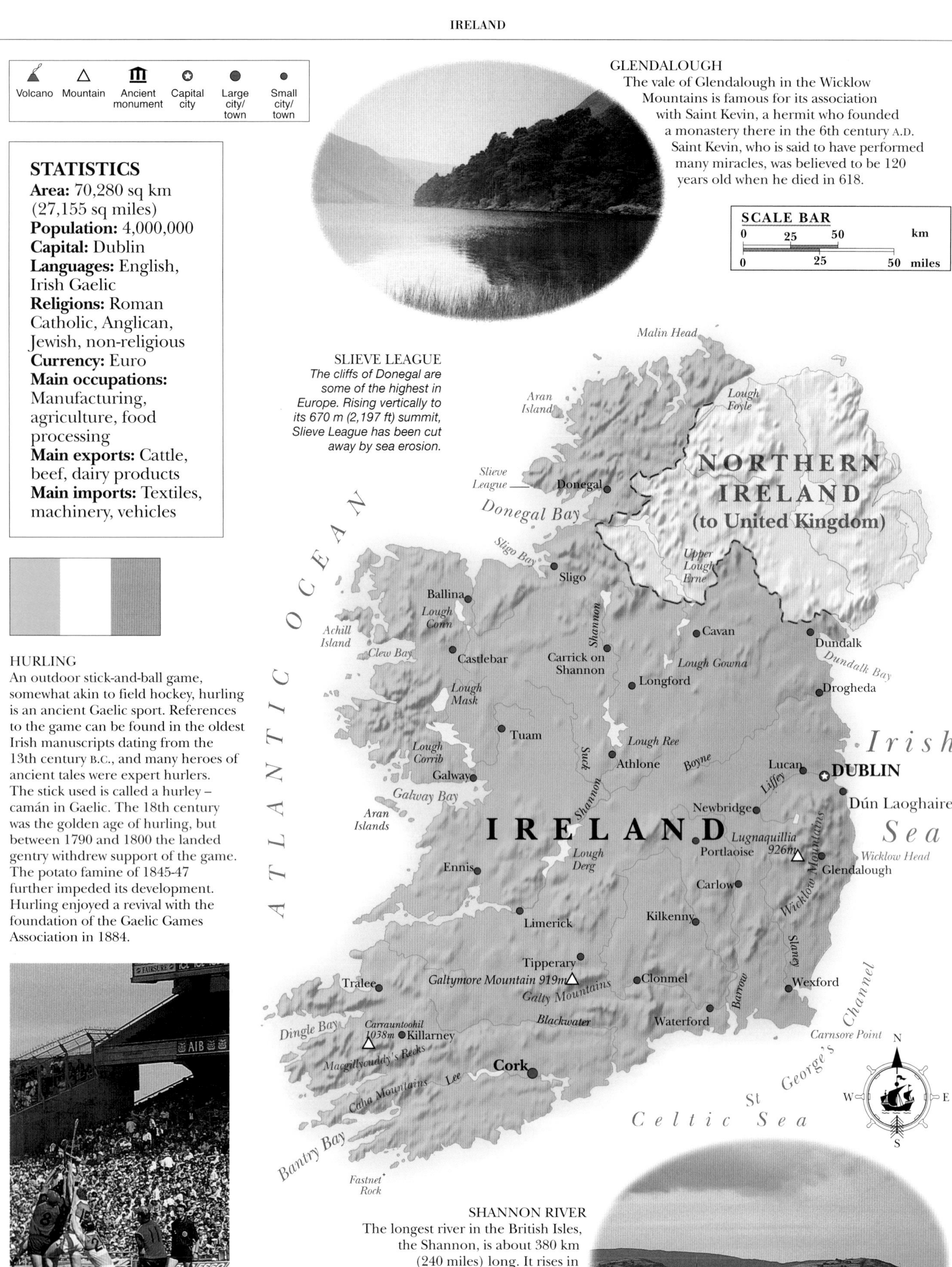

GLENDALOUGH
The vale of Glendalough in the Wicklow Mountains is famous for its association with Saint Kevin, a hermit who founded a monastery there in the 6th century A.D. Saint Kevin, who is said to have performed many miracles, was believed to be 120 years old when he died in 618.

STATISTICS

Area: 70,280 sq km (27,155 sq miles)
Population: 4,000,000
Capital: Dublin
Languages: English, Irish Gaelic
Religions: Roman Catholic, Anglican, Jewish, non-religious
Currency: Euro
Main occupations: Manufacturing, agriculture, food processing
Main exports: Cattle, beef, dairy products
Main imports: Textiles, machinery, vehicles

SLIEVE LEAGUE
The cliffs of Donegal are some of the highest in Europe. Rising vertically to its 670 m (2,197 ft) summit, Slieve League has been cut away by sea erosion.

HURLING
An outdoor stick-and-ball game, somewhat akin to field hockey, hurling is an ancient Gaelic sport. References to the game can be found in the oldest Irish manuscripts dating from the 13th century B.C., and many heroes of ancient tales were expert hurlers. The stick used is called a hurley – camán in Gaelic. The 18th century was the golden age of hurling, but between 1790 and 1800 the landed gentry withdrew support of the game. The potato famine of 1845-47 further impeded its development. Hurling enjoyed a revival with the foundation of the Gaelic Games Association in 1884.

SHANNON RIVER
The longest river in the British Isles, the Shannon, is about 380 km (240 miles) long. It rises in northwest Ireland, and flows into the sea just west of Limerick. As it winds its way down the country, the river passes through numerous lakes, the largest of which is Lough Derg.

HISTORY OF

IRELAND

THE FIRST STONE AGE hunters arrived in Ireland from Europe. The Celts followed and divided Ireland into small kingdoms. The Celtic age produced fantastic legends and wonderful stories of gods, battles, and heroes. In A.D. 432, St. Patrick brought Christianity to the land, and became Ireland's patron saint. A golden age followed during which Irish Christians studied, painted, and wrote literature. Ireland became the cultural centre of Europe. In 795, Viking raiders shattered this peace. They built settlements, including Dublin, the capital. During the 12th century the Normans gained control of most of Ireland. Monarchs Henry VIII, Elizabeth I, and James VI all used the planting of Protestant English and Scottish people on lands seized from the Irish as a way of increasing the number of subjects loyal to the British crown. This worked especially well in areas of Ulster, which accounts for much of today's conflicts in Northern Ireland.

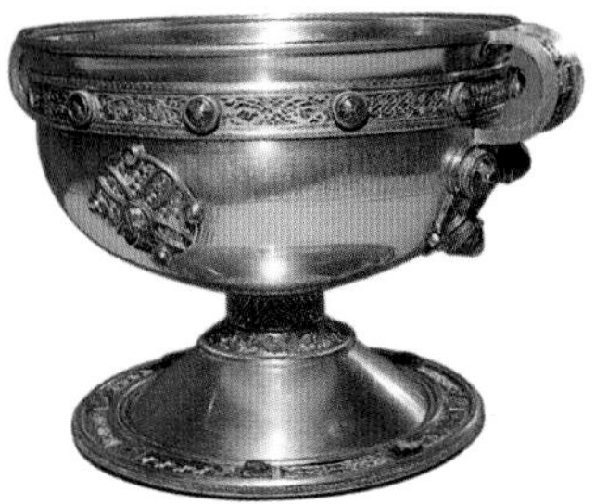

ARDAGH CHALICE
During its golden age, Irish craftsworkers made many magnificent treasures. The silver Ardagh chalice, one of the most famous, is decorated with bronze and gold.

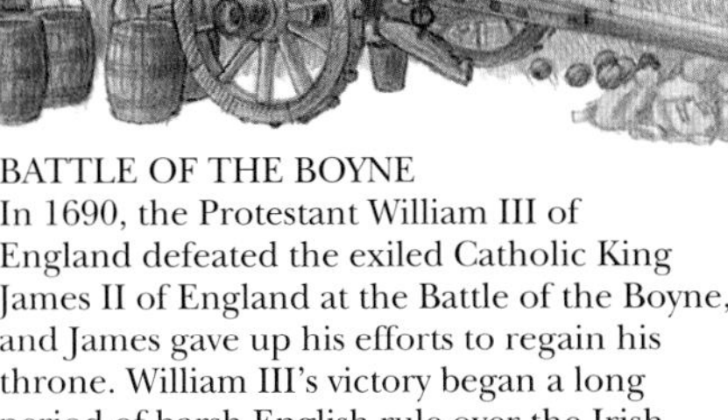

BATTLE OF THE BOYNE
In 1690, the Protestant William III of England defeated the exiled Catholic King James II of England at the Battle of the Boyne, and James gave up his efforts to regain his throne. William III's victory began a long period of harsh English rule over the Irish Catholics. This was called the Penal Law.

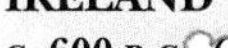

IRELAND

c. 600 B.C. Celts invade Ireland.

A.D. 795 Vikings raid Ireland.

1014 King Brian Boru defeats the Vikings at Clontarf.

1170 Normans land in Ireland.

1641 Rebellion by the Irish against English government.

1690 Battle of the Boyne followed by Protestant domination.

1798 United Irishmen rebellion is defeated.

1845-49 Potato famine. Population falls by three million.

1916 Easter Rebellion.

1919-23 War of Independence. Six counties of Ulster remain with the UK. Anglo-Irish treaty causes civil war in the south.

1973 Ireland joins the EC.

1997 Belfast-born Mary McAleese succeeds Mary Robinson as Ireland's president.

POTATO FAMINE
In the 1800s, most Irish people lived on small holdings and were very poor. They ate mainly potatoes. The crop failed many times, but 1845 and 1848 were the worst years. More than 750,000 people starved and thousands emigrated.

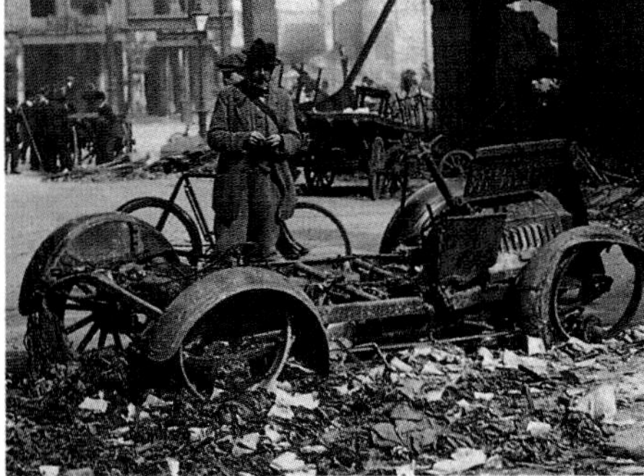

EASTER REBELLION

On Easter Monday in 1916, Irish Republicans, impatient with the delay in implementing Home Rule, rose up in armed revolt. The British army crushed the rebellion and executed 15 of the rebels. The dead rebels became heroes, and support for the Republican cause grew.

THE TROUBLES
In 1922, the Irish Free State (South) was created. In Northern Ireland the Protestant majority ran the government. In 1968 Catholic marches for civil rights were suppressed, and years of mistrust sparked off new violence. The British army was called in to keep peace but conflict developed with their arrival. People from all sides of the community still seek a peaceful solution.

Find out more

ENGLISH CIVIL WAR
IRELAND
NORTHERN IRELAND
UNITED KINGDOM, HISTORY OF

IRON AGE

IRON AGE

4000 B.C. First iron objects, made from meteoric iron, appear in the Middle East.

c. 1500 B.C. People in the Middle East find out how to extract (smelt) iron from iron ore and how to work it by heating and hammering (wrought iron). The Hittites dominate the trade.

1000 B.C. Iron Age begins in the Middle East and Greece. Iron- working also develops in India.

c. 800 B.C. Use of iron spreads across Europe. Celts become expert workers in iron.

c. 400 B.C. Chinese discover how to make cast-iron objects by melting iron ore and pouring it into moulds.

A.D. 1760 Industrial revolution leads to a renewed use of iron. Also leads to great advances in ironworking techniques.

IN SEVERAL EARLY LANGUAGES the word for iron meant "metal from the sky". This was probably because the first iron used to make tools and weapons came from meteorites which fell to Earth from space. Ironworking probably began in the Middle East some 6,000 years ago. At first, people hammered iron while it was cold. Later they learned how to smelt iron – heat the iron ore so they could extract the iron and work with it properly. Unlike bronze, which early people also used, iron did not melt. Instead it was reduced to a spongy mass which people hammered and reheated until it was the right shape. Special furnaces were needed to reach the right temperature. The Hittites, who lived in what is now Turkey, were the first people we know of who traded in iron. But it was not until around 1000 B.C. that knowledge of smelting spread and the Iron Age truly began. In western Europe, the Celts were one of the first peoples to make and use iron.

This razor is around 2,500 years old and would have been as sharp as a modern razor.

HILL FORT
The Celts fortified hill tops with ditches and ramparts. These forts were places of refuge in wartime; they were also administrative and trading centres, and enclosures for livestock.

Iron horseshoe

Heating iron ore in a furnace

Hammering the iron into shape

IRONWORKING

Early furnaces were shallow stone hearths which people filled with iron ore and charcoal. Bellows helped raise the temperature to about 1,200°C (2,192°F), hot enough to make the iron workable. The Celts used deeper furnaces in which the iron collected at the bottom and impurities, called slag, gathered at the top.

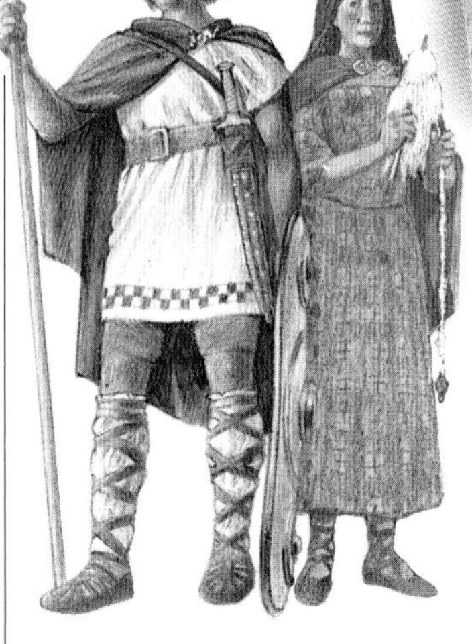

Spring

Iron pin

Brooch made of glass discs

CLOTHING
The Celts loved decoration. Celtic clothes were woollen, often with checked patterns. Richer men and women wore heavy twisted neckbands called torcs in gold or bronze, and cloaks fastened with ornate brooches.

TOOLS
People made useful tools from iron such as a saw with a serrated edge (far left) and tongs (left); the tongs were used to hold metal while beating it into shape.

WEAPONS
Iron weapons were greatly superior to bronze ones. They had much sharper edges and, thus, were more effective. This dagger has a handle shaped like a human figure.

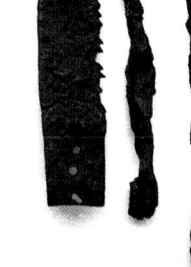

Find out more

BRONZE AGE
CELTS
INDUSTRIAL REVOLUTION
IRON AND STEEL

IRON AND STEEL

HUGE STRUCTURES such as oil tankers and bridges, and tiny objects such as nuts and bolts are made from steel. The world produces more than 800 million tonnes (787 million tons) of steel every year; it is the most widely used of all metals. Steel is made from iron, one of the most common metals in the Earth's crust, and carbon, which comes from coal. Iron has many uses, which include making car engine parts and magnets. Our bodies need iron to work properly. A healthy diet must include foods such as green vegetables, which contain iron. Pieces of iron fall to Earth in meteorites from space. But most iron comes from iron ore in rock. Heating the ore with coke (from coal) produces iron. The Hittites of Turkey perfected iron smelting about 1500 B.C. This was the beginning of the Iron Age, during which iron gained widespread use for making weapons and tools.

Iron and steel were once used to make weapons and armour, such as this 16th-century helmet.

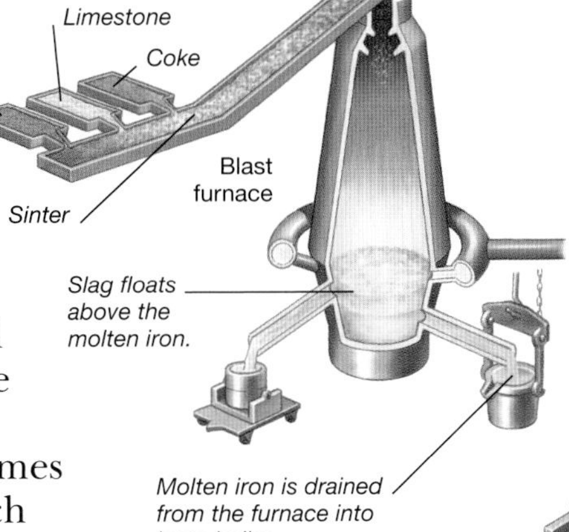

RAW MATERIALS
Iron-making starts with iron ore, coke (a form of carbon from coal), and limestone. They are mixed and treated to make lumps called sinter.

BLAST FURNACE
Slag floats above the molten iron.
Molten iron is drained from the furnace into large ladles.
The ingredients enter the top of the blast furnace and move down inside. A blast of very hot air flows up the furnace. The heat produces molten iron from the ore and coke. Limestone removes impurities which form a layer called slag.

Oxygen is blown through pipe onto surface of pig iron.

After blowing with oxygen, the converter tilts to discharge molten steel.

Molten steel from converter

Continuous casting

The molten steel may be cast into large blocks called ingots.

MAKING IRON AND STEEL

Making metals by heating their ores is called smelting. Huge factories smelt iron ore by heating it with coke to produce iron, which is rich in carbon. Removing most of the carbon produces steel. Steels of different quality are made by adding metals, such as nickel.

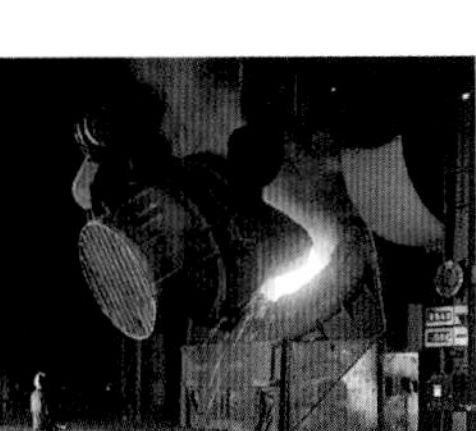

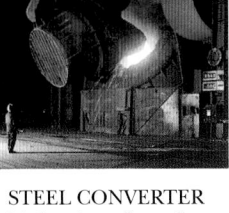

STEEL CONVERTER
Molten iron from the blast furnace is poured into a steel converter where hot air or oxygen is blown over it. The heat burns up most of the carbon from the iron, leaving molten steel. Steel from old cars and other waste can be recycled by adding it to the converter.

Casting uses molten steel from the converter.

Forging

Rolling

CONTINUOUS CASTING
Molten steel from the converter sets as it cools and is held in shape by rollers. The long slab is then cut up into lengths and rolled into steel products.

RUST
Iron and steel objects get rusty when they are left outside in damp conditions. Moist air causes rust. It changes iron into iron oxide, a red-brown compound of iron and oxygen. Rusting weakens the metal so that it crumbles away.

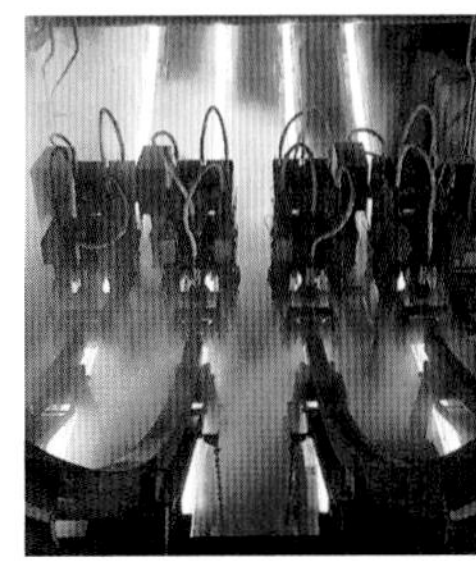

SHAPING STEEL
Passing a hot slab between rollers presses the soft steel into plates or sheets. A forge presses the steel into more complex shapes. Casting uses a mould, in which molten steel cools and sets into shape.

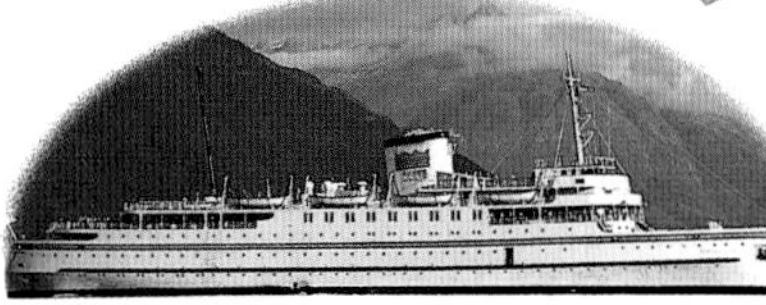

USES OF STEEL

Different kinds of steel are made by varying the amount of carbon and other metals in it. Low-carbon steel goes into car bodies; stronger medium-carbon steel is used for making ships and steel beams that support structures. High-carbon steel is very strong but difficult to shape, and is used for springs and rails that get much wear. Steel containing tungsten metal resists heat and is used in jet engines.

STAINLESS STEEL
Adding the metals chromium and nickel produces stainless steel, which does not rust. Cutlery and saucepans are often made of stainless steel. This metal is also used to make equipment that must be kept very clean in places such as hospitals and dairies.

Find out more
COAL
INDUSTRIAL REVOLUTION
IRON AGE
METALS

ISLAM

IN THE 7TH CENTURY, the prophet Muhammad founded a religion in Arabia that was to become a powerful force in the world. The religion came to be known as Islam and its followers are called Muslims (or Moslems). Muslims believe that many prophets or teachers have been sent by God, including Moses and Jesus Christ, but Muhammad was the last of them. Like Christians and Jews, Muslims believe in one God, Allah.

Islam means "submission to the will of God", and Muslims commit themselves to absolute obedience to Allah.

Islamic life is based on a set of rules called the five pillars of Islam. Muslims believe that by following these rules, they will reach heaven. There is also a strict code of social behaviour, and alcohol and gambling are forbidden. Some Muslim women wear clothes that cover their bodies completely.

Today there are around 1,300 million Muslims living mainly in the Middle East, Asia, and Africa. Islam is a rapidly growing faith. Its popularity has been increased by Islamic fundamentalists – extremely religious people who call for a return to strict, traditional Islamic values.

KORAN
The sacred book of Islam is the Koran. Muslims believe the Koran is the direct word of God as revealed to his messenger, Muhammad.

ISLAMIC FESTIVALS

Day of Hijrah First day of Islamic year.

Ramadan Month-long fast.

Eid ul-Fitr Feast to mark the end of Ramadan.

Lailat ul-Qadr Revelation of Koran to Muhammad.

Meelad ul-Nabi Muhammad's birthday.

Lailut ul-Isra Death of Muhammad.

MOSQUES

The Muslim place of worship is the mosque. Before entering, Muslims remove their shoes and wash. The faithful kneel to pray, with their heads touching the floor. At prayer time Muslims face the mihrab, an empty recess which faces the direction of Mecca. Although they must attend the mosque on Fridays, at other times Muslims pray wherever they are.

MINARETS
Five times a day muezzins, or criers, stand at the top of tall towers called minarets to call fellow Muslims to prayer.

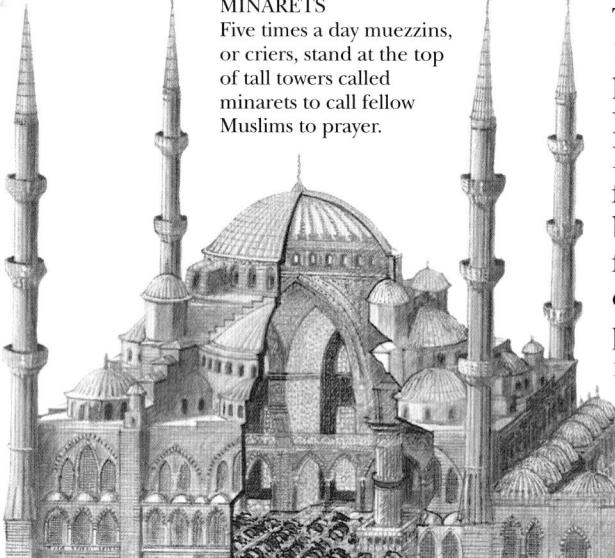

BLUE MOSQUE
The first mosques were very simple, but some later buildings such as the Blue Mosque at Istanbul, Turkey (right), are magnificent examples of Islamic art. Islam forbids realistic images of humans or other living things, so the tiled walls are decorated with intricate designs and beautiful calligraphy.

Before kneeling in prayer in the mosque, Muslims wash their faces, hands, and feet.

لا إله إلا الله محمد رسول الله

MUHAMMAD
The shahada is the Islamic declaration of faith. "None is to be worshipped save Allah: Muhammad is his prophet."

MECCA

The birthplace of Muhammad is Mecca, Saudi Arabia, and every Muslim tries to visit the holy city at least once in a lifetime. The Kaaba, the sacred shrine, is the central point of this pilgrimage. Inside the Kaaba is a black stone which dates from ancient times.

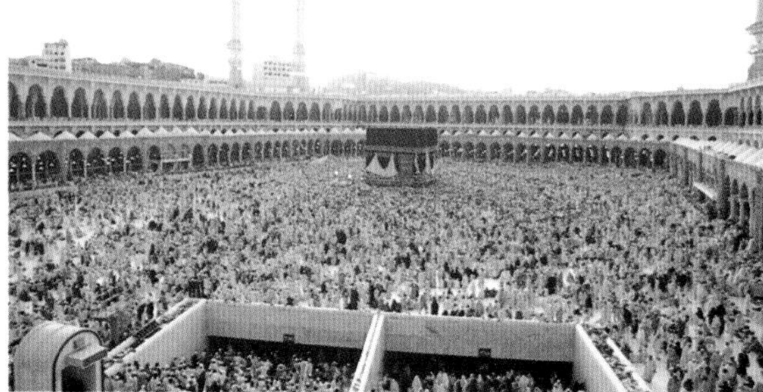

Muslim pilgrims must walk seven times around the Kaaba.

Find out more
CRUSADES
FESTIVALS
MUHAMMAD
RELIGIONS

ISRAEL

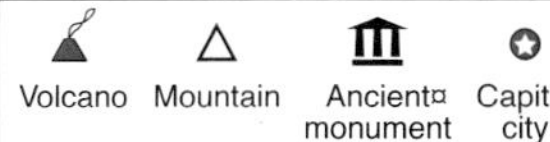

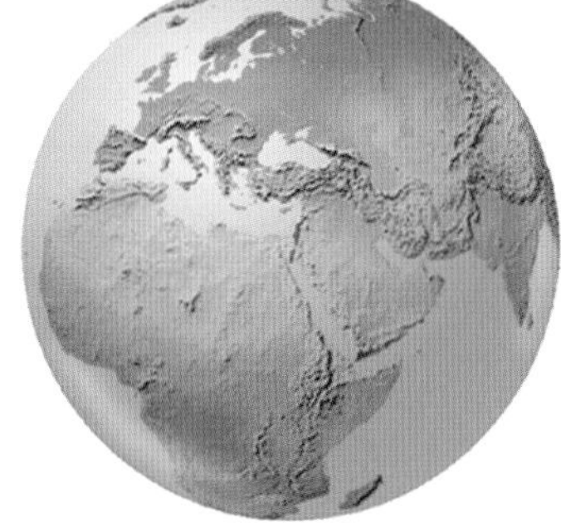

Israel lies at the eastern end of the Mediterranean Sea. Lebanon lies to the north, Syria and Jordan to the east, and Egypt to the southwest.

THE MODERN STATE OF ISRAEL has existed only since 1948. It was created on the sites where there had been Jewish settlements in earlier times. Jews from all over the world flocked to the new state, especially the survivors of Nazi anti-semitism. They revived the ancient language of Hebrew as the national language of Israel. But there have been many problems. The region had previously been the land of Palestine, and many Arab Palestinians had to leave when the country became Israel. However, others have remained, and today they make up about 15 per cent of Israel's 6.4 million population. Israel has also fought wars with neighbouring Arab countries to secure its borders. It still occupies some territory gained in these wars, causing continual Palestinian unrest. Israel is now a wealthy country. The Israelis have developed many modern industries and converted large areas of desert into farmland.

STATISTICS
Area: 20,700 sq km (7,992 sq miles)
Population: 6,400,000
Capital: Jerusalem
Languages: Hebrew, Arabic, Yiddish, German, Russian, Polish, Romanian, Persian
Religions: Jewish, Muslim, Christian, Druze
Currency: New Israeli shekel
Main occupations: Agriculture, manufacturing, finance
Main exports: Potash, bromine, salt, wine, citrus fruits
Main imports: Water

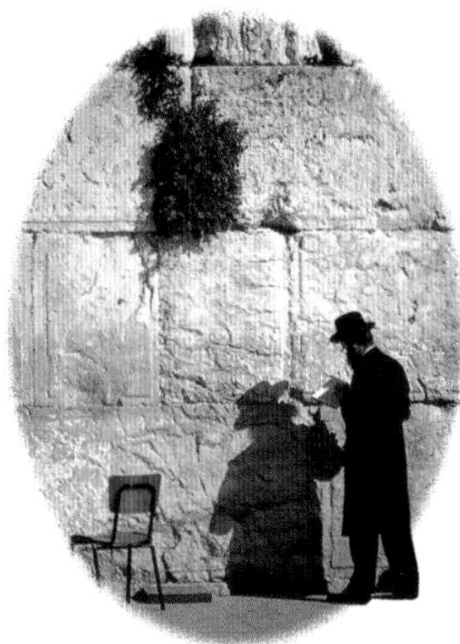

WAILING WALL
Israel occupies much of the "Holy Land" described in the Bible. The land is sacred, not only to Jews but also to Christians and Muslims. The Wailing Wall in Jerusalem is the most sacred Jewish monument. It is all that remains of a temple built by King Herod 2,000 years ago. Visitors gave the wall its name when they heard the sad sound of devout Jews mourning the destruction of the temple.

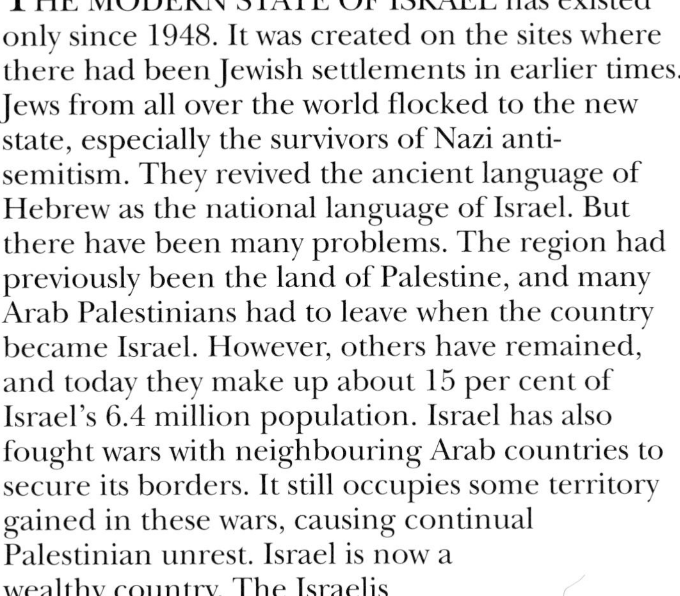

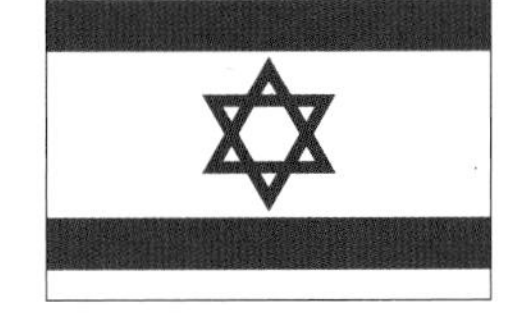

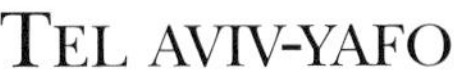

TEL AVIV-YAFO

The main commercial and industrial centre of Israel is Tel Aviv-Yafo, the country's second largest city. It was once two separate towns, but Tel Aviv grew rapidly and absorbed its neighbour, the ancient port of Yafo.

DEAD SEA
The world's saltiest sea, the Dead Sea, is also the lowest area of water on Earth; it is 400 m (1,312 ft) below the level of the Mediterranean Sea. The River Jordan flows into this hot, barren place. The water evaporates in the heat of the sun, but the salt in the water is left behind. Over the centuries the salt has become very concentrated.

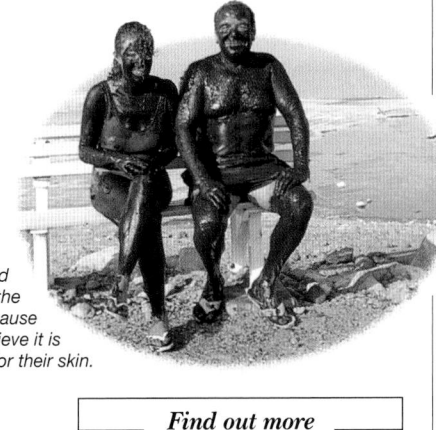

Visitors to Dead Sea resorts bathe in mud because they believe it is good for their skin.

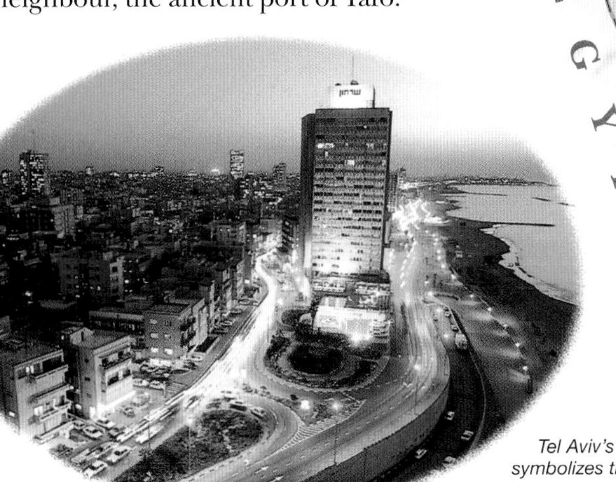

Tel Aviv's centre symbolizes the modern, prosperous face of Israel.

SCALE BAR
0 25 50 km
0 25 50 miles

Find out more
CHRISTIANITY
CRUSADES
ISLAM
JUDAISM
MIDDLE EAST

ITALY

Italy is in southern Europe and forms part of the northern coast of the Mediterranean Sea. It shares borders with France, Switzerland, Austria, and Slovenia.

SHAPED LIKE A BOOT, complete with heel and toe, Italy juts out far into the Mediterranean Sea from southern Europe. Between the country's east and west coasts rise the Apennine Mountains, which divide Italy into two along its length. Northern Italy is green and fertile, stretching from the snow-capped Alps to the middle of the country. It includes farmlands in the great flat valley of the Po River, and large industrial towns such as Turin and Milan. Factories in the north produce cars, textiles, clothes, and electrical goods. These products have helped make Italy one of the most prosperous countries in Europe. Southern Italy, by contrast, is dry and rocky. There is less farming and industry, and the people are poorer. Sicily and Sardinia, the two largest islands of the Mediterranean, are also part of Italy.

Rome, the capital, lies at the centre of the nation. It is the home of Italy's democratic government and also the Vatican, the headquarters of the Roman Catholic Church.

Many Italian farmhouses are old and picturesque; the machinery is usually modern.

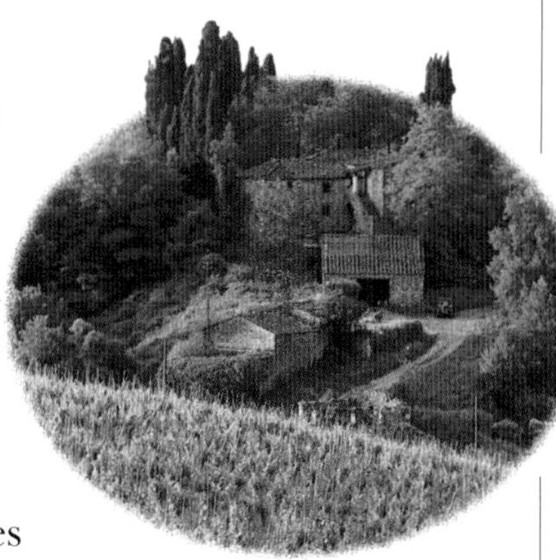

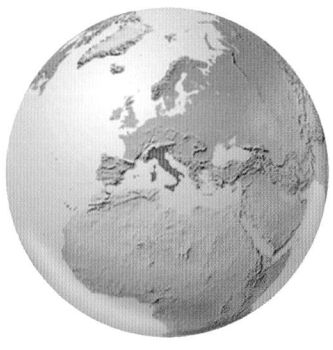

AGRICULTURE
Italian farmers use modern machinery to grow food for Italy's 57.4 million people, and for exporting. Italy is famous for its olives and olive oil, tomatoes, wine, pasta, cheese, fruit, and meat products, such as salami and ham. Italy also grows large quantities of grain, particularly wheat, as well as rice, potatoes, and sunflowers, which are used to make cooking oil. Almost one-third of Italians live in rural areas, many in old farmhouses.

ROME
A walk through Rome is like a walk through history. Since the city was first built, more than 2,500 years ago, each new generation has added something. Today, modern city life goes on around Ancient Roman arenas, 15th-century churches, and 17th-century palaces. Like many of Italy's historic towns, Rome attracts thousands of tourists every year.

PASTA
There are at least 200 shapes of pasta, including ravioli, spaghetti, and macaroni. Pasta is a type of dough made from durum wheat flour, which is rich in gluten, a kind of protein. Served with a tasty sauce, it is Italy's favorite dish. Marco Polo is said to have brought the recipe for pasta from China to Italy.

VENICE

Venice is one of the world's oldest cultural and tourist cities. From the late medieval period, it became Europe's greatest seaport, serving as the continent's commercial and cultural link to Asia. Like several other Italian towns, Venice boasts many magnificent buildings from the past. Its ornate marbled and frescoed palaces, towers, and domes attract thousands of tourists every year. The city was built on about 120 small islands, in a lagoon which remains permanently flooded. A causeway over 4 km (2.5 miles) long connects Venice with mainland Italy. Cars are not allowed in the old city, and people travel by boat on more than 170 canals. The traditional boat, called a gondola (above), is still a common form of transport.

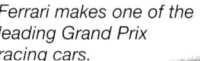

Ferrari makes one of the leading Grand Prix racing cars.

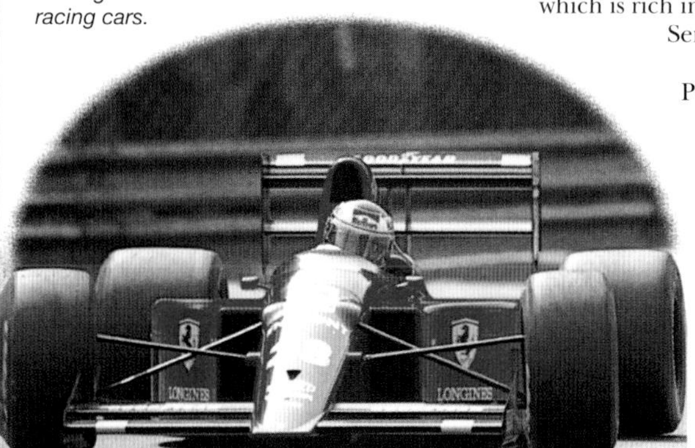

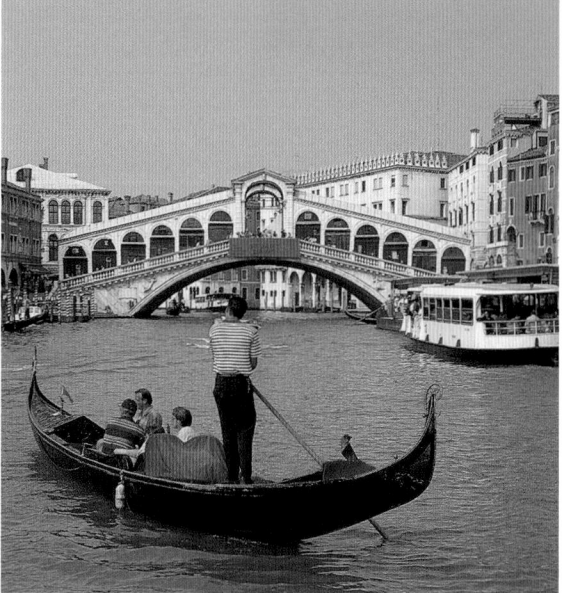

CARS
The Italian motor industry produces some of Europe's finest cars. Manufacturers such as Alfa Romeo, Ferrari, and Lamborghini have always had a reputation for speed and stylish design.

The fairytale fortress of Rocca Tower, perched high on a rocky outcrop, overlooks San Marino.

San Marino

San Marino is the third-smallest independent state in Europe, after Monaco and the Vatican City. It is about 14 km (9 miles) long and 8 km (5 miles) wide, and is situated mostly on the slopes of Monte Titano on the Adriatic coast. Tourism provides a great source of income to the country, as do the frequent issues of its own postage stamps. The Sammarinese, as the inhabitants of San Marino are called, are ruled by two capitani reggenti ("captains regent") who are elected every six months. San Marino has had a treaty of friendship with Italy since 1862.

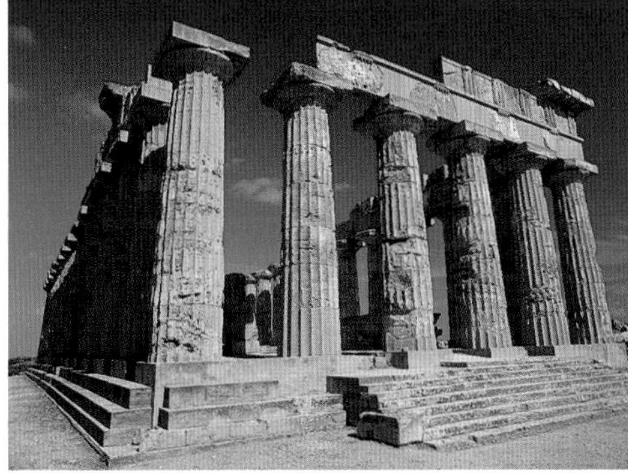

The Doric Temple (right) in the Valley of the Temples, Sicily, was built during the period 460-450 B.C.

SICILY

Sicily is the largest island in the Mediterranean Sea. It belongs to Italy, from which it is separated by the Strait of Messina. The island's highest point is Mount Etna, an active volcano which reaches a height of 3,332 m (10,930 ft). Farming and tourism are the primary sources of income. Increasing numbers of tourists are attracted by the island's beautiful beaches and ancient ruins.

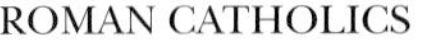

ROMAN CATHOLICS

More than half of all Christians are Roman Catholics. They follow the leadership of the Pope in the Vatican and, together with other Christians, believe in three beings in one God: the Creator and Father; Jesus Christ as God become man; and the Holy Spirit. More than 80 per cent of Italians are Roman Catholic.

Mary, the virgin mother of Christ, is regarded by Roman Catholics as the highest of all human beings.

St. Peter's Basilica, Vatican City, Rome, is the world's largest Christian church. Shaped like a cross, it is nearly 210 m (700 ft) long and extends to about 137 m (450 ft) at its widest point.

Vatican City

Vatican City is a walled city in Rome, and the headquarters of the Catholic Church. It is the official residence of the Pope, and the smallest independent state in the world, with an area of 0.44 sq km (0.17 sq miles). The Vatican has its own flag, national anthem, stamps, and coins, as well as a newspaper and radio station. St. Peter's Basilica, which overlooks a grand piazza (left), dominates the city.

SARDINIA

Sardinia is an island 175 km (109 miles) off mainland Italy, in the Mediterranean Sea. It is a self-governing political region of Italy with its own president and elected regional assembly. The central Italian government, however, controls education, justice, communications such as railways and postal services, defence, and national taxation.

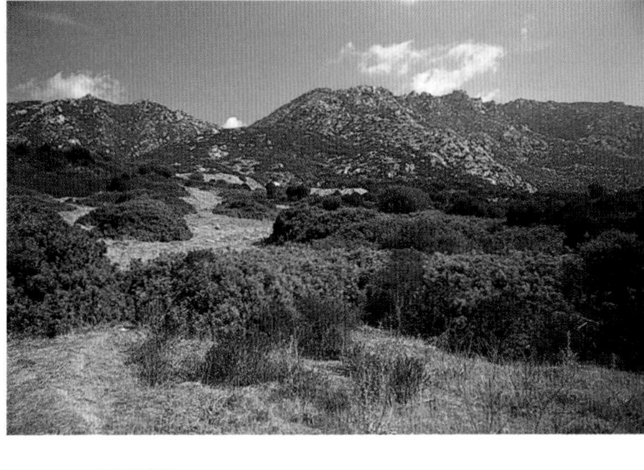

This is the southernmost reach of the Gennargentu Mountains, Sardinia.

MALTA

Malta is a small country in the Mediterranean Sea just south of Sicily. Since ancient times, it has been a vital naval base because of its position on trade routes to the East. Romans, Arabs, French, Turks, Spanish, and British have all colonized or fought over the island. Malta finally gained independence from Britain in 1964, joining the EU in 2004. Tourism is a major source of the country's income.

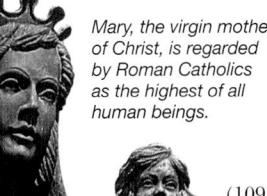

Find out more

Europe
Italy, history of
Renaissance
Roman empire

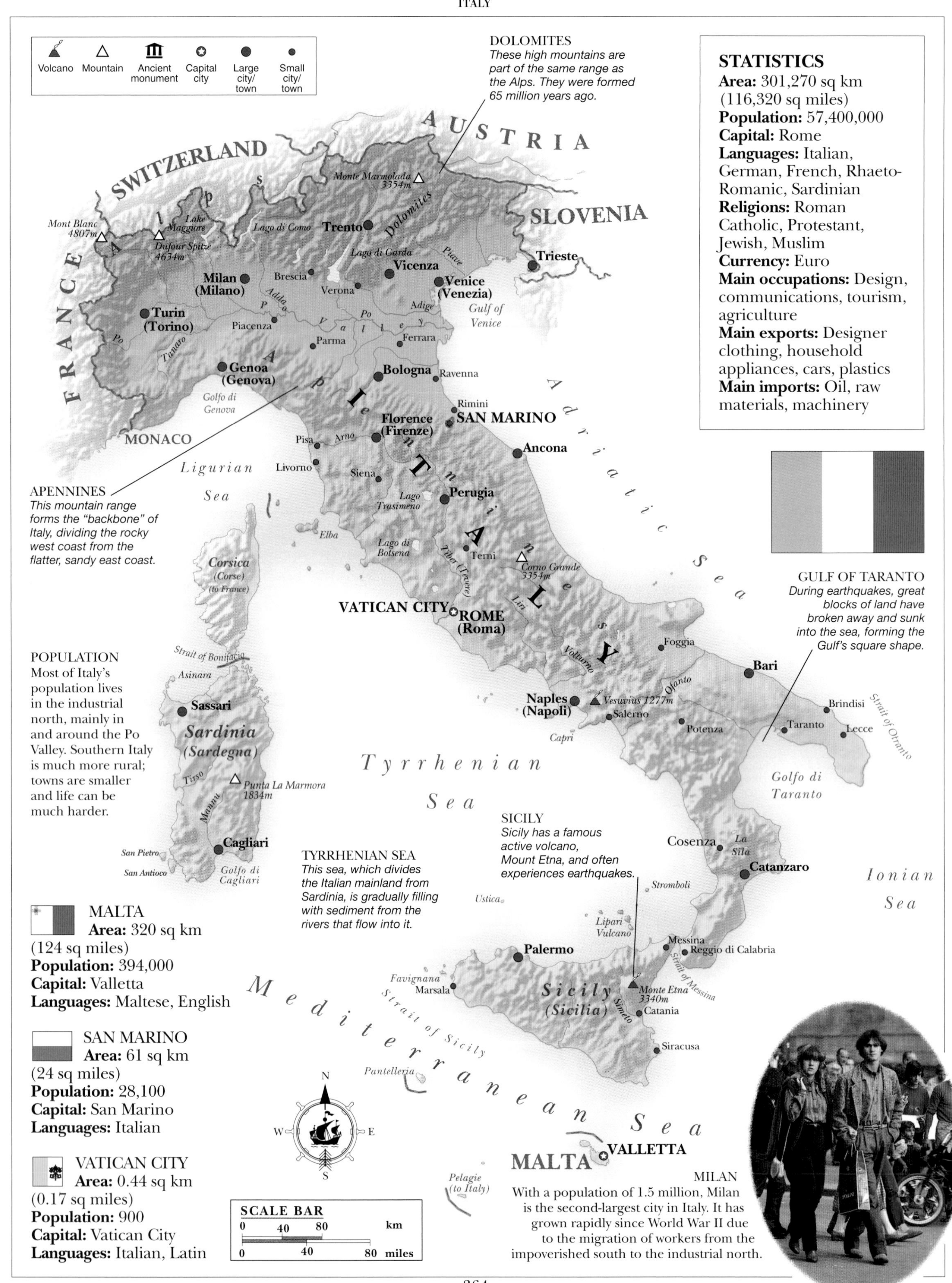

STATISTICS
Area: 301,270 sq km (116,320 sq miles)
Population: 57,400,000
Capital: Rome
Languages: Italian, German, French, Rhaeto-Romanic, Sardinian
Religions: Roman Catholic, Protestant, Jewish, Muslim
Currency: Euro
Main occupations: Design, communications, tourism, agriculture
Main exports: Designer clothing, household appliances, cars, plastics
Main imports: Oil, raw materials, machinery

POPULATION
Most of Italy's population lives in the industrial north, mainly in and around the Po Valley. Southern Italy is much more rural; towns are smaller and life can be much harder.

MALTA
Area: 320 sq km (124 sq miles)
Population: 394,000
Capital: Valletta
Languages: Maltese, English

SAN MARINO
Area: 61 sq km (24 sq miles)
Population: 28,100
Capital: San Marino
Languages: Italian

VATICAN CITY
Area: 0.44 sq km (0.17 sq miles)
Population: 900
Capital: Vatican City
Languages: Italian, Latin

MILAN
With a population of 1.5 million, Milan is the second-largest city in Italy. It has grown rapidly since World War II due to the migration of workers from the impoverished south to the industrial north.

HISTORY OF ITALY

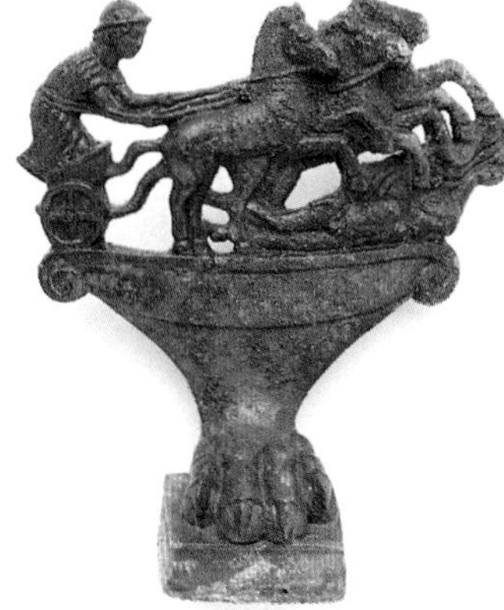

ETRUSCANS
The Etruscans lived in an area of western Italy called Etruria in about 800 B.C. They were great traders, farmers, artists, and engineers and built a civilization of small city-states. The Romans eventually conquered the Etruscans but adopted many of their customs, including gladiatorial fights and chariot racing. Above is a sculpture of an Etruscan chariot running over a fallen man.

FOR 500 YEARS Italy was at the centre of the powerful Roman Empire. In 476 the empire fell. Various tribes conquered Italy and divided it between them. The Italian popes became prominent in both religion and politics and managed to drive out the strongest tribe, the Lombards. During the 1300s, independent "city-states" developed from cities that had grown rich through industry, trade, and banking. These city-states became very powerful, and their wealthy rulers propagated Renaissance arts during the 15th century. For a time, Italian ideas and styles dominated the whole of Europe. But the city-states, weakened by constant squabbling and wars among themselves, were taken over by the Hapsburg family of Austria and Spain. In 1796 Napoleon invaded Italy, and a movement for unification of the various city-states grew. This unification was achieved in 1861. But Italy never regained her former power in Europe. Dictator Benito Mussolini (1883-1945) involved Italy disastrously in World War II. Since then, Italy has become a leading European country.

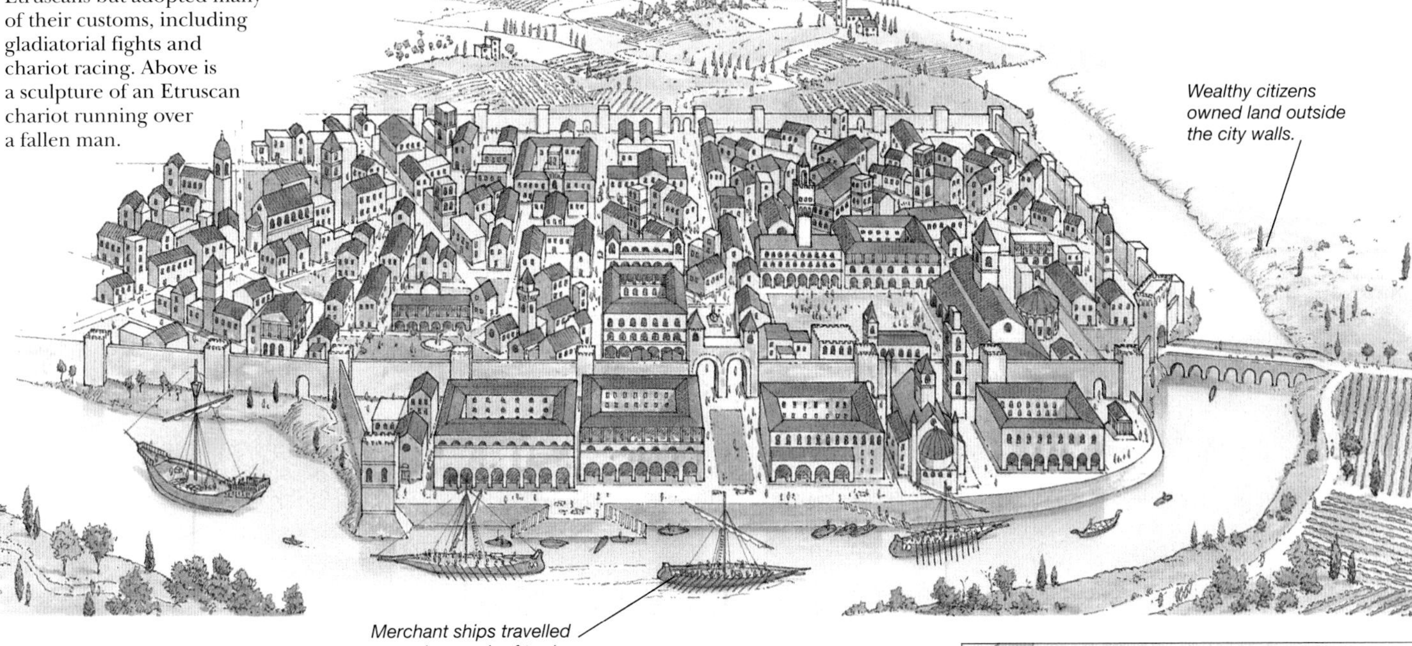

CITY-STATES
During the Renaissance (a flourishing of arts and learning), Italian city-states such as Venice and Florence were important centres of learning. In Florence, a famous Medici family came to power in 1434 and ruled for almost 300 years. Many other city-states were ruled by princes elected by rich citizens who owned huge estates outside the city walls. The estates produced food for the craftworkers and scholars who lived in the city. Most city-states were near the sea, making it easy for Italian merchants to travel to distant countries in search of trade.

DOGE'S BARGE
Venice, the most powerful Italian city-state, was built on a lagoon and crisscrossed by canals. Its huge fleet of ships enabled it to set up a rich empire in the eastern Mediterranean. Each year the ruler of Venice, called the doge, went to sea in his magnificent barge and gave thanks for this wealth by "marrying" the sea with a golden ring. The doge lived in the doge's palace, shown right.

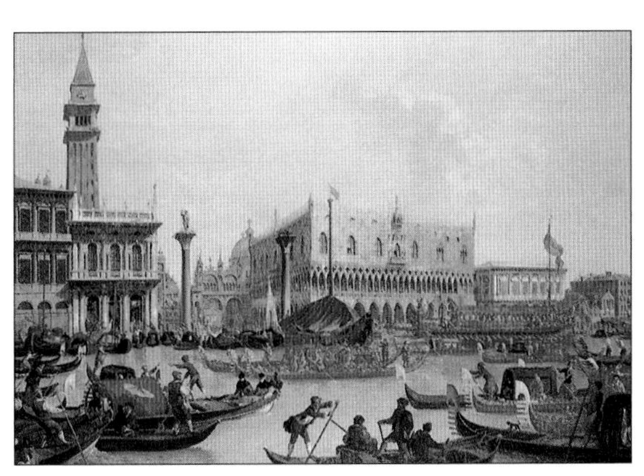

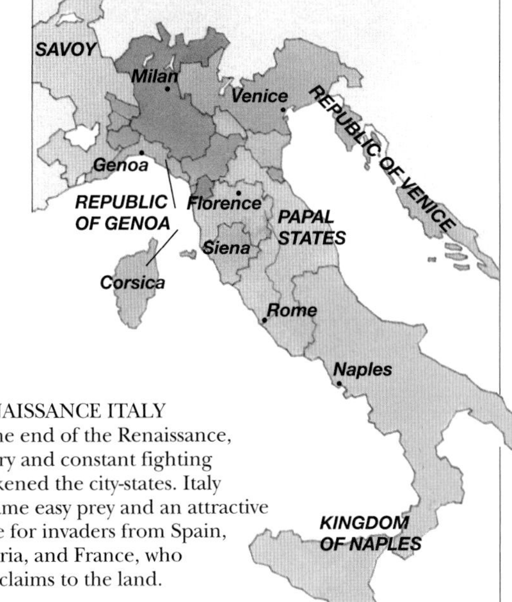

RENAISSANCE ITALY
At the end of the Renaissance, rivalry and constant fighting weakened the city-states. Italy became easy prey and an attractive prize for invaders from Spain, Austria, and France, who laid claims to the land.

Garibaldi

In 1860, Giuseppe Garibaldi (1807-82) became an Italian hero. He led a small army of 1,000 volunteer soldiers, called red shirts, to free Sicily from the rule of the king of Naples, so that the island of Sicily could become part of a new united Italy.

MUSSOLINI

In 1922, Benito Mussolini (below) became premier of Italy. Two years later he was dictator, leading a new movement called fascism, under which the government controlled everything in the country. Mussolini's vast building projects created jobs, but his secret police silenced his opponents. Mussolini, who was also called Il Duce (the leader), wanted to make Italy great, but he became unpopular when his armies were defeated in World War II.

Benito Mussolini making a speech

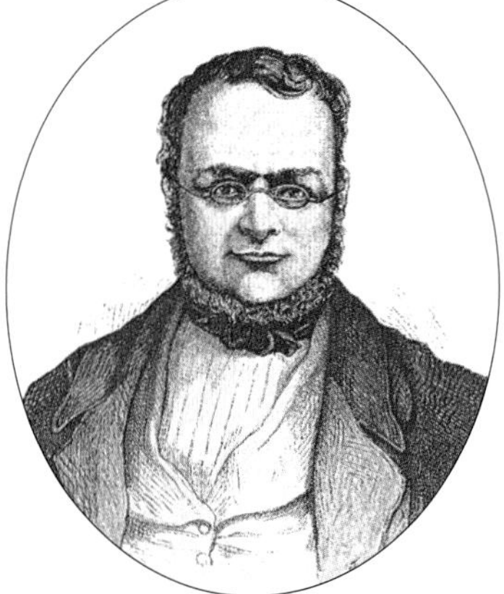

Cavour

Camillo di Cavour (1810-61), prime minister of Piedmont city-state, was a brilliant statesman who dreamed of a united Italy. He led the movement to unite all the Italian states into one country.

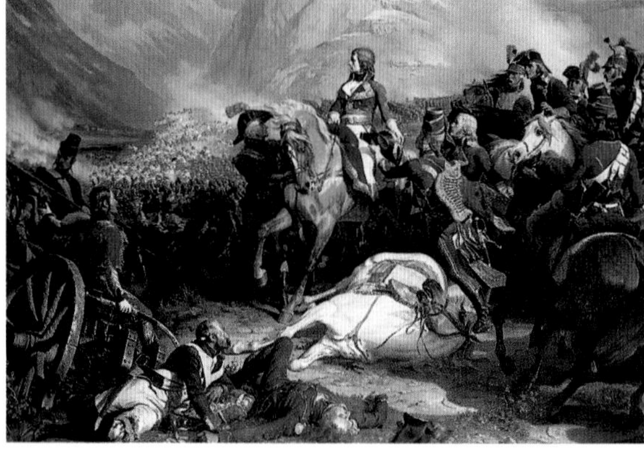

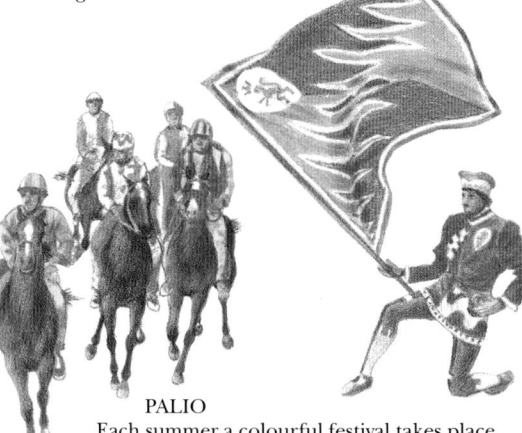

NAPOLEON

Napoleon Bonaparte (above, on horseback) invaded Italy and defeated the Austrian Hapsburgs, who ruled it at the time. He destroyed the old system of many different governments and introduced a single system with the same laws. For the first time since the days of Ancient Rome, Italians from different regions were ruled in the same way. Many began to dream of a united Italy, free from foreign rulers.

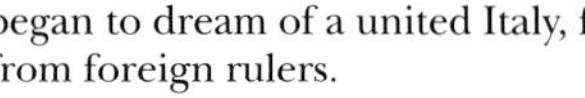

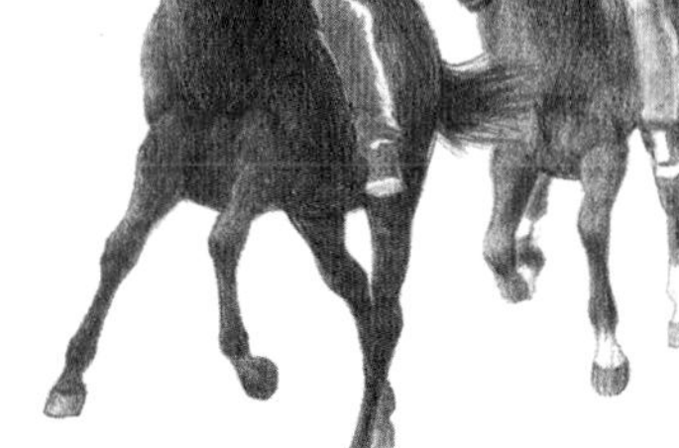

PALIO

Each summer a colourful festival takes place in the ancient Etruscan city of Siena, northern Italy. This pageant, called the Palio, celebrates the power of the city-state, and comes to a climax with a horse race staged in the main square of the city. The race is fast and dangerous. Each *contrada* (city district) is represented by a colourful flag and symbol, and competes fiercely for the honour of winning.

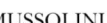

ITALY

509 B.C. Romans drive out Etruscans and establish the Roman republic.

A.D. 476 German barbarians depose last Roman emperor, Romulus Augustulus. Invading German tribes break up empire.

c. 1300 Renaissance begins in Italy.

1796 Napoleon Bonaparte invades and seizes Italy.

1815 Napoleon defeated at Waterloo. Representatives from Austria, Great Britain, Prussia, and Russia (the victorious nations) meet at the Congress of Vienna. Most of Italy is returned to its old rulers.

1858 Cavour, prime minister of the kingdom of Piedmont, makes a treaty with Napoleon III of France to defend the kingdom from the Austrians.

1859 Combined French and Piedmontese army defeats Austrians.

1861 All of Italy, except Venice, San Marino, and the city of Rome, join to become the kingdom of Italy. Victor Emmanuel II, king of Piedmont, becomes king of Italy.

1871 Rome becomes capital of Italy, but the Pope's territory of Vatican City remains an independent state.

1915 Italy joins World War I, fighting with the Allies (Britain, France, Russia, and the United States).

1922 Benito Mussolini becomes premier of Italy.

1940 Italy joins World War II, fighting for the Germans.

1943 Italy surrenders to Allies.

1945 Italian resistance fighters kill Mussolini.

1946 Italy becomes a republic.

1949 Italy joins North Atlantic Treaty Organization (NATO) with 11 other Western countries, to protect against Soviet expansion.

1957 Italy joins the E.E.C.

Find out more

ITALY
NAPOLEON BONAPARTE
NAPOLEONIC WARS
RENAISSANCE
ROMAN EMPIRE

JAPAN

THE TOPS OF A SUBMERGED mountain chain form the islands of Japan. About three-quarters of the country is too steep to farm or build on. Japan has a population of 128 million, most of whom live in valleys and on the narrow coastal plain. Japan is a leading industrial nation, but its success is fairly recent: until 1853 the country was closed to foreigners and the government refused to import modern machines. More recently, Japanese companies have been very successful in exporting their own goods, so Japan sells more than it buys and has become very wealthy. Western influence is strong, but the Japanese are very proud of their traditional culture and religion. They continue to practise old customs while developing more modern technology. Most people follow both the Buddhist and Shinto religions. The head of state is an emperor, but the government is democratic. In the past the country was ruled by noblemen and samurai, professional soldiers who had a strict code of honour. Although the samurai have long been disbanded, their code still influences everyday life.

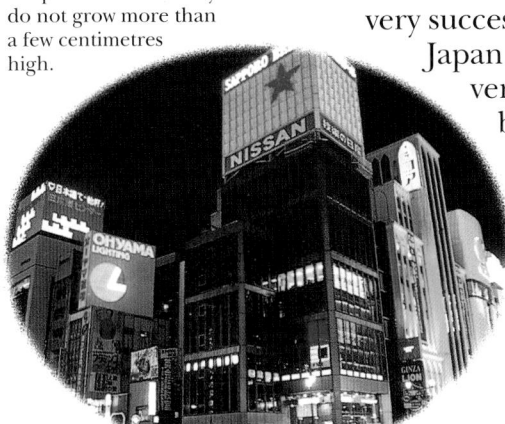

BONSAI
Japanese bonsai trees are pruned so that they do not grow more than a few centimetres high.

Japan is located in the Pacific Ocean, off the east coast of Asia. North and South Korea are to the west, and the Russian Federation to the north. There are four main islands, covering almost 370,000 sq km (144 sq miles).

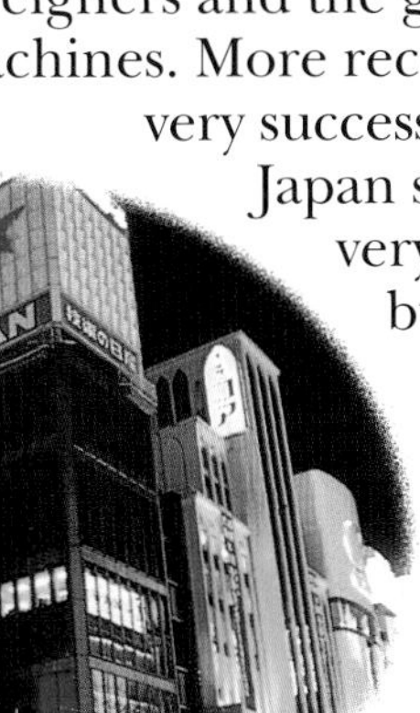

TOKYO

The largest city in Japan is the capital, Tokyo. More than 20 million people live in the city and suburbs, and the whole area is extremely overcrowded. Fumes from cars and industry are a major problem, but effective measures are being taken to reduce pollution.

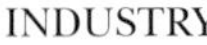

INDUSTRY
Although Japan has few raw materials such as metal ores or coal, Japanese industry is among the most successful in the world. The country's main resource is its workforce. Japanese workers are very loyal to their companies, and workers take their holidays together, exercise together, and sing the company song daily. Managers are equally devoted to the company and pride themselves on their cooperation with the workers. New technology and techniques are introduced quickly and help boost prosperity.

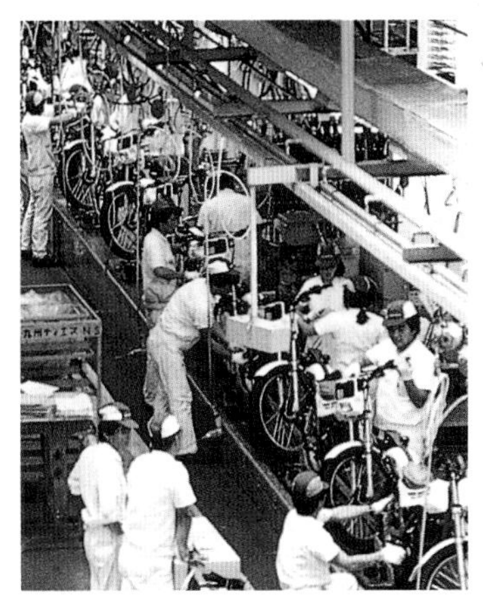

SUSHI
Traditional Japanese food consists mainly of fish and rice. Often the fish is eaten raw or lightly cooked in dishes called sushi.

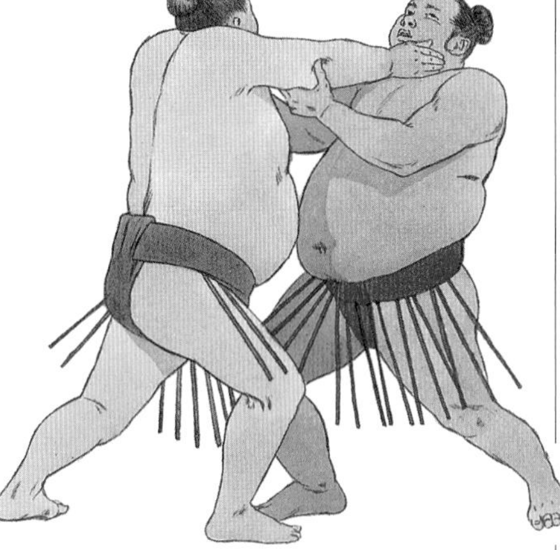

SUMO WRESTLING
The national sport of Japan is sumo wrestling. It attracts large crowds and is shown on television. The two contestants try to push each other out of a small ring. Success depends on strength and weight, so sumo wrestlers go to schools where they train and follow a special diet. Successful wrestlers may become extremely rich and famous. The sport is traditional and follows an elaborate pattern controlled by officials in decorative costume.

BULLET TRAIN
Japan has more than 25,000 km (16,000 miles) of railway. The most famous train is the Shinkansen, or bullet train, which runs from Tokyo to Fukuoka. The train covers the 1,176 km (731 miles) in less than six hours at an average speed of 195 km/h (122 mph) per hour.

Mount Fuji, a 3,776 m (12,388 ft) tall volcano is sacred to the Japanese.

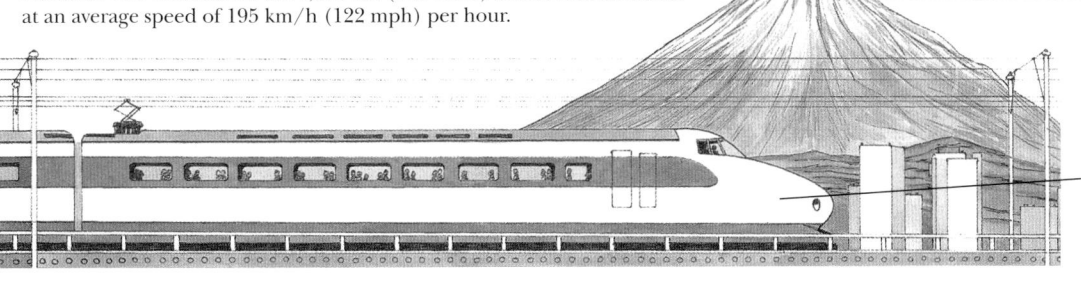

Japanese people travel more by train than travellers in any other country.

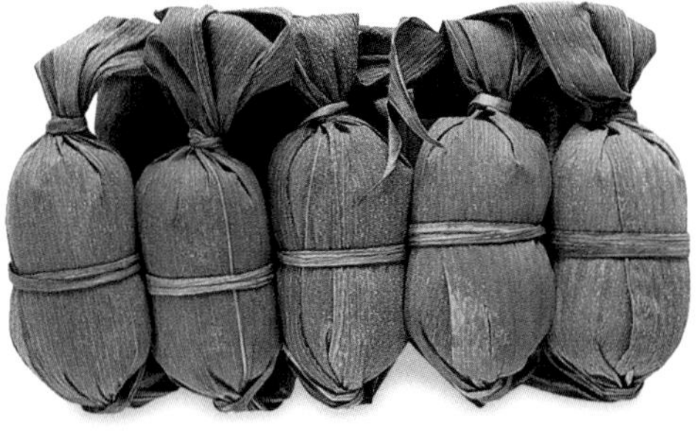

RICE CAKES
Rice cakes called *chimaki* are traditionally eaten throughout Japan. The rice cakes are cone-shaped and wrapped in a bamboo leaf. A similar snack, called *sasadango*, is also eaten in some areas of northern Japan.

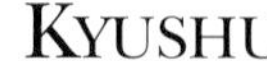

KYUSHU

The southernmost island of Japan, Kyushu, is mountainous; the highest point is a volcano, Mount Aso. Kyushu is the most densely populated of the Japanese islands, and is linked to Honshu island by a railway tunnel under the Shimonoseki Strait.

VEHICLE INDUSTRY

Japanese vehicle manufacturers became world leaders in the 1980s thanks to their stylish designs, new technology and efficient production methods. Today, motor vehicles are the country's biggest export. Japanese vehicle manufacturers have also opened a number of factories in Europe and the USA.

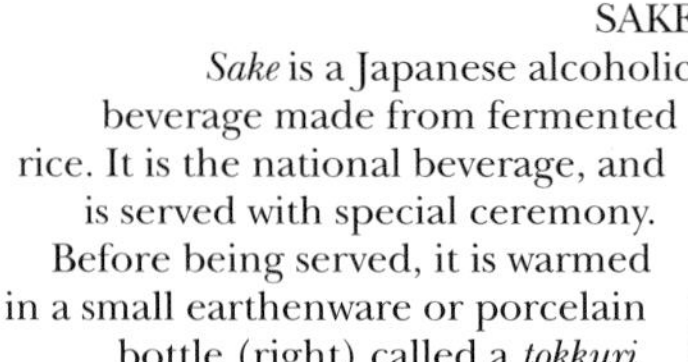

SAKE
Sake is a Japanese alcoholic beverage made from fermented rice. It is the national beverage, and is served with special ceremony. Before being served, it is warmed in a small earthenware or porcelain bottle (right) called a *tokkuri*.

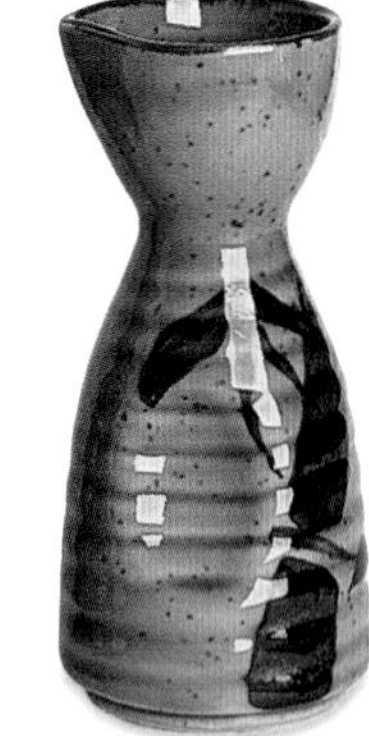

This Kawasaki ZZ-R1100 has a top speed of 282 km/h (175 mph).

ZEN GARDEN

Rock gardens, designed to represent the universe in miniature, are found in Zen Buddhist monasteries in Japan. These gardens are not literal representations of a landscape, but they give the impression of water and land. Sand or gravel symbolizes water, while rocks represent land. The Zen garden has no plants, trees or water, only raked gravel or sand, and rock groupings. These "dry gardens" were introduced by Buddhist monks in the 1300s.

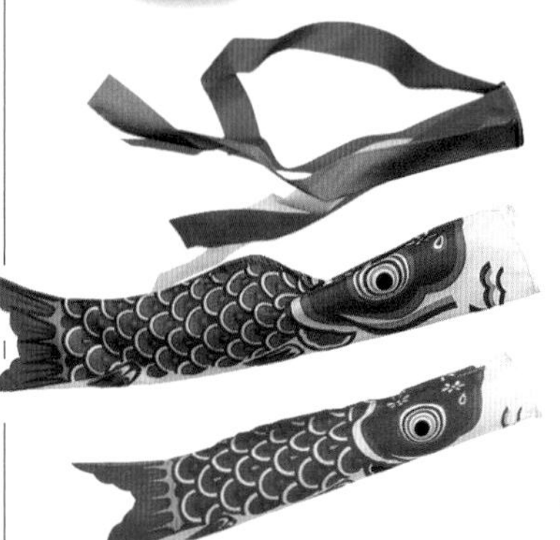

KITES
Carp kites are flown on the fifth day of May to celebrate *Kodomono-hi* or children's day. The carp is a strong robust fish, renowned for its energy and determination, as it must swim upstream against the current, often jumping high out of the water. The carp therefore provides a good example to Japanese boys in particular, who must overcome obstacles and be successful. A group of carp kites represent a family and the largest kite symbolizes the father.

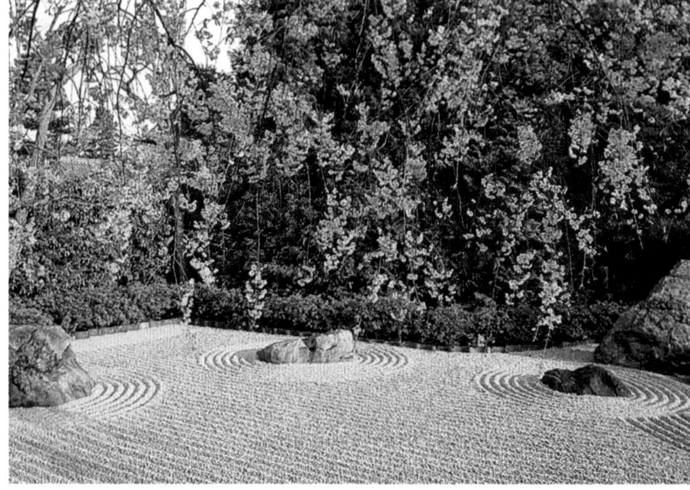

Zen Buddhists believe that performing simple tasks such as raking pebbles in a Zen garden can bring enlightenment to the mind.

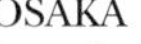

OSAKA
Japan's third-largest city is Osaka, on the south coast of the island of Honshu. Osaka is a major industrial centre, with steel, chemical, and electrical industries. It is also one of the oldest cities in Japan, and has many Buddhist and Shinto temples. Osaka is the site of an impressive castle built in the 16th century by the shogun (warlord) Toyomoti Hideyoshi, who once ruled Japan. In 1970 Osaka was the host city for the World's Fair.

Find out more
ASIA
DEMOCRACY
EARTHQUAKES
JAPAN, HISTORY OF
WEAPONS

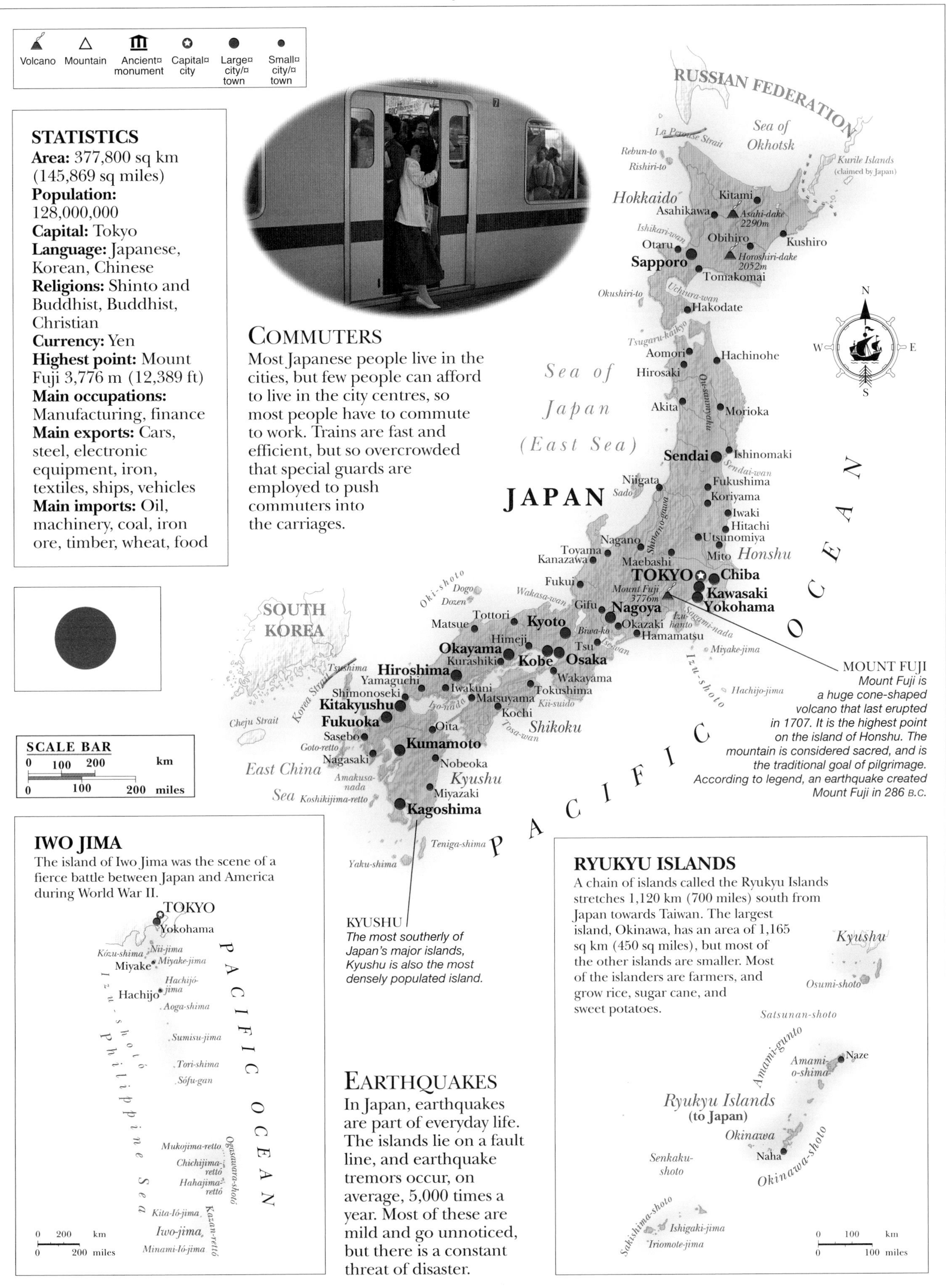

STATISTICS

Area: 377,800 sq km (145,869 sq miles)
Population: 128,000,000
Capital: Tokyo
Language: Japanese, Korean, Chinese
Religions: Shinto and Buddhist, Buddhist, Christian
Currency: Yen
Highest point: Mount Fuji 3,776 m (12,389 ft)
Main occupations: Manufacturing, finance
Main exports: Cars, steel, electronic equipment, iron, textiles, ships, vehicles
Main imports: Oil, machinery, coal, iron ore, timber, wheat, food

COMMUTERS

Most Japanese people live in the cities, but few people can afford to live in the city centres, so most people have to commute to work. Trains are fast and efficient, but so overcrowded that special guards are employed to push commuters into the carriages.

MOUNT FUJI
Mount Fuji is a huge cone-shaped volcano that last erupted in 1707. It is the highest point on the island of Honshu. The mountain is considered sacred, and is the traditional goal of pilgrimage. According to legend, an earthquake created Mount Fuji in 286 B.C.

KYUSHU
The most southerly of Japan's major islands, Kyushu is also the most densely populated island.

IWO JIMA

The island of Iwo Jima was the scene of a fierce battle between Japan and America during World War II.

RYUKYU ISLANDS

A chain of islands called the Ryukyu Islands stretches 1,120 km (700 miles) south from Japan towards Taiwan. The largest island, Okinawa, has an area of 1,165 sq km (450 sq miles), but most of the other islands are smaller. Most of the islanders are farmers, and grow rice, sugar cane, and sweet potatoes.

EARTHQUAKES

In Japan, earthquakes are part of everyday life. The islands lie on a fault line, and earthquake tremors occur, on average, 5,000 times a year. Most of these are mild and go unnoticed, but there is a constant threat of disaster.

HISTORY OF JAPAN

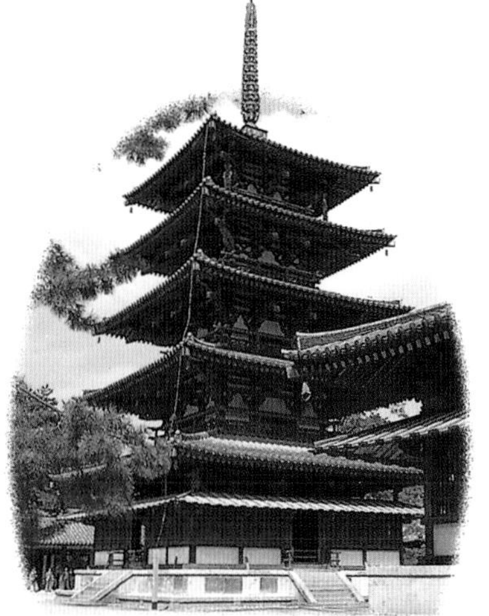

NARA
Nara, the first capital city of Japan, was the political and religious centre of the country. It was the site of the Buddhist Horyuji Temple (above).

THE GROUP OF ISLANDS THAT IS JAPAN remained isolated from the rest of the world until quite recently. During the 6th century A.D., Japan absorbed ideas from its neighbour, China. It also adopted China's Buddhist religion and the Chinese system of imperial rule. But 200 years later, Chinese influence declined, and the imperial system broke down. Until the 1860s, powerful families, and then shoguns (military generals), ruled Japan in the name of the emperor. People rarely invaded Japan successfully. The Mongols tried and failed in the 13th century. During the 16th century, European traders were also unsuccessful. But in 1868, Japan began to look towards the West. Within 50 years it had built up a strong, modern economy and a large empire. All this was destroyed during World War II (1939-45). However, Japan has recovered and is once again rich.

TEA CEREMONY
After the 14th century, the ritual ceremony of drinking tea became very popular in Japan. The ceremony was based on the Zen Buddhist principles of self-discipline and meditation, and was very popular among the war-like shoguns and samurai.

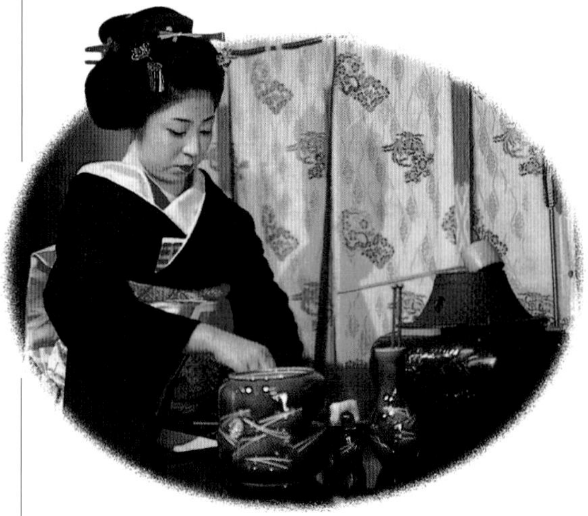

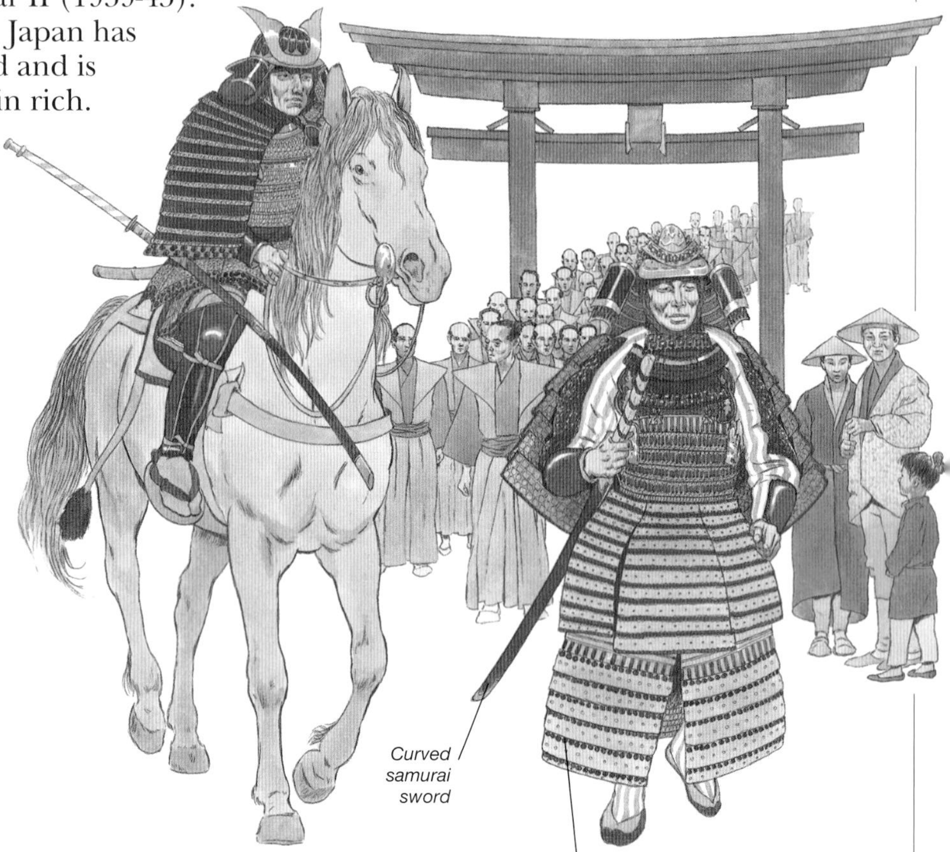

Curved samurai sword

Special suit of armour which a samurai could get into quickly from the side or from below

THE TALE OF GENJI

In the early 11th century a Japanese woman named Murasaki Shikibu wrote one of the world's first novels. More than 600,000 words long, *The Tale of Genji* describes the adventures of a young prince and his travels in search of love and education. The novel was written in Japanese at a time when the official language of the country was Chinese: only commoners and women were allowed to speak Japanese.

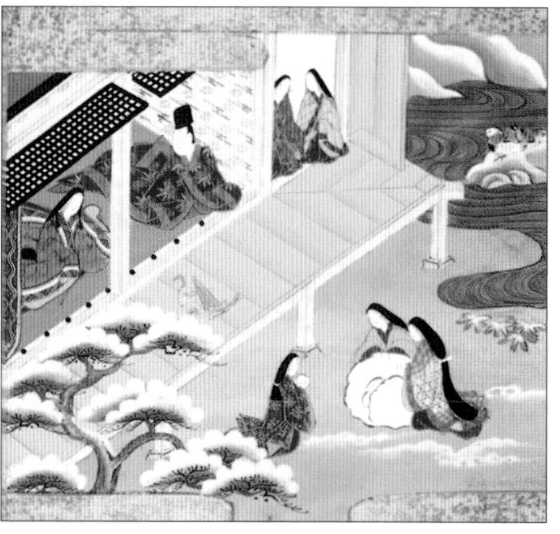

SHOGUNATE

The shogunate was a hereditary military dictatorship. During shogun rule, an aristocratic class of knights called the samurai gained considerable power. These warriors protected the lands of the daimyo (local lords) and followed a code of honour known as the Bushido – "the way of the warrior". Samurai warriors committed hara kiri (suicide) if they lost their honour.

A.D. 400s Yamato clan unites Japan.

794 Capital city of Kyoto founded.

1192 Minamoto Yoritomo becomes first shogun.

1281 "Divine wind" saves Japan from Mongols.

1338-1573 Civil wars.

1542 Portuguese sailors visit Japan.

1549 St. Francis Xavier introduces Christianity to Japan.

1592, 1597 Japan invades Korea.

1639 Almost all Europeans leave.

1853 U.S. Navy forces Japan to trade with the West.

1868 Meiji restoration returns power to emperor.

1868 Tokyo becomes national capital.

1889 Constitutional government.

1904-5 Russo-Japanese War.

1910 Japan takes control of Korea.

1914-18 Japan fights Germany in World War I.

1937-45 Japan invades China, Southeast Asia; bombs Pearl Harbor in 1941, bringing United States into World War II.

1945 U.S. drops first atomic bombs on Hiroshima and Nagasaki; Japanese surrender.

1989 Hirohito dies.

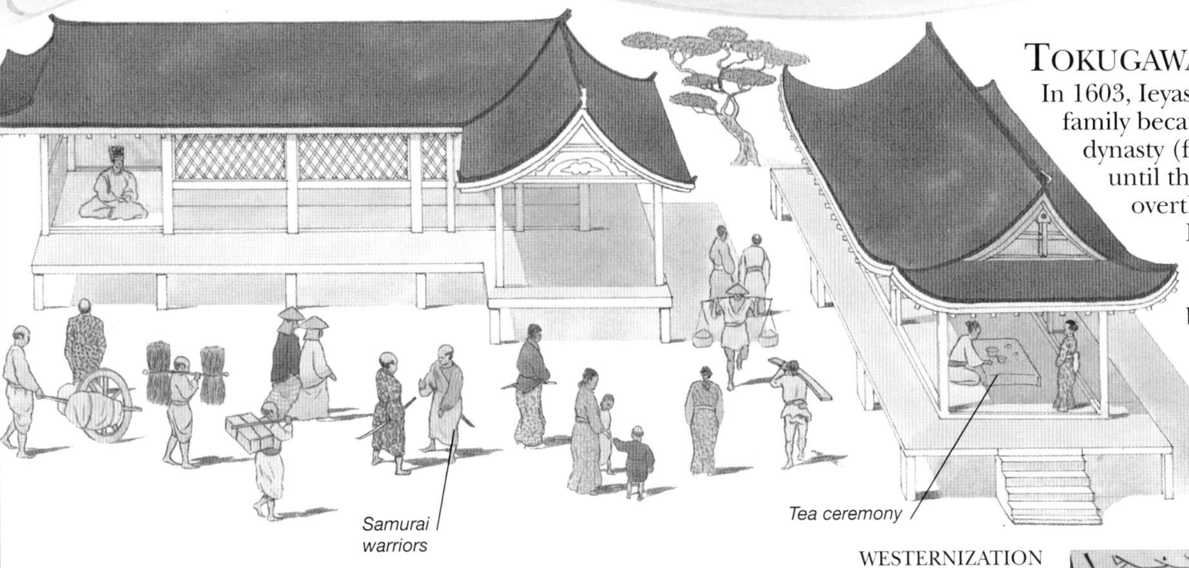

TOKUGAWA DYNASTY

In 1603, Ieyasu of the Tokugawa family became shogun. His dynasty (family) ruled Japan until the shogunate was overthrown in 1868. Ieyasu put down the Christian movement which had been brought in by Saint Francis Xavier. Foreigners were expelled, and contact with the outside world was forbidden.

WESTERNIZATION

In 1853, Commodore Matthew Perry of the U.S. Navy sailed into Tokyo Bay and demanded that Japan end its isolation and begin trading with the outside world. Dramatic changes followed. The shogunate ended, and the young emperor Meiji took power. Within 50 years, Japan became one of the world's leading industrial and economic powers. Factories and railways were built, a national education system was set up, and students were sent abroad to learn about Western life.

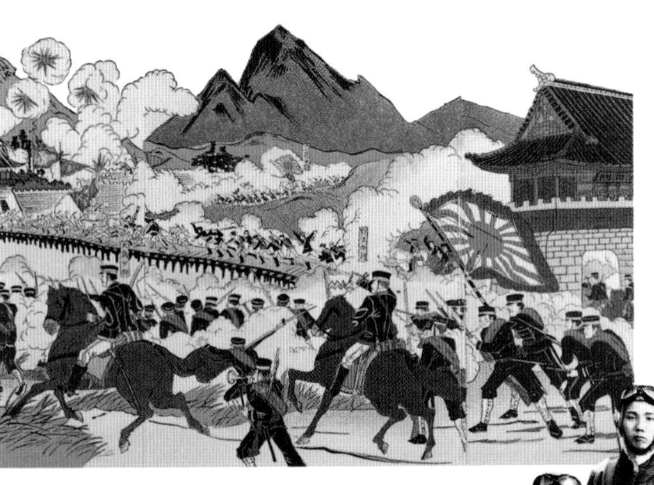

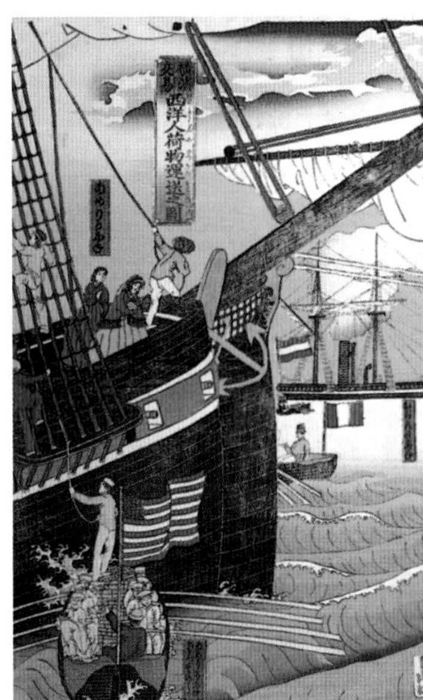

SINO-JAPANESE WAR

Japan went to war with China in 1894-95 over the control of Korea, and then with Russia in 1904-5 in order to gain colonies in Taiwan, Korea, and China. Both wars revealed the new Westernized Japan to be a powerful force in world affairs.

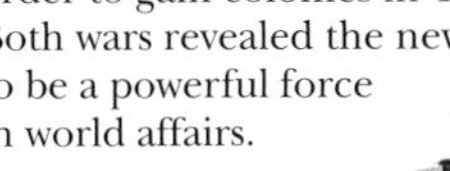

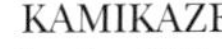

KAMIKAZE

In the 13th century, a storm destroyed the Mongol fleet and saved Japan from invasion. Japanese called the storm kamikaze, meaning "divine wind". During World War II, the Japanese used kamikaze pilots, who crashed their bomb-laden planes on to American warships. These "suicide pilots" believed that they, like the storm, were saving Japan, and were blessed by the emperor, whom they believed to be divine.

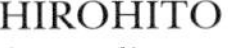

HIROHITO

According to tradition, the first emperor of Japan was descended from the sun goddess and took power around 660 B.C. An unbroken line of descent then stretched to Hirohito, who in 1926 became the 124th emperor. In 1946, after the Japanese defeat in World War II, Hirohito publicly rejected the divinity of the emperor. He died in 1989. His son Akihito became emperor in 1990.

Find out more

China, history of
Japan
Nuclear age
World war I
World war II

JESUS CHRIST

ONE OF THE WORLD'S MAJOR RELIGIONS – Christianity – was inspired by a man named Jesus Christ. We know about Jesus from the New Testament gospels, which were written by Matthew, Mark, Luke, and John, men who knew him. The gospels declare that Jesus was a Jew born in Bethlehem, in the Roman province of Judea, and was believed to be the Son of God. At the age of 30 he began to travel around Palestine (then under Roman rule) preaching a new message. He told stories called parables to explain his ideas. The gospels also describe miracles – amazing things he did such as raising the dead. However, some people thought his ideas might cause rebellion against Roman rule. He was arrested, tried, and sentenced to death. When Jesus appeared to his disciples (closest followers) after his death, they were convinced that God had raised him from the dead. The Christian church was founded on the belief, and soon his ideas swept across the Roman Empire.

NATIVITY
The birth of Jesus, which took place in a stable in Bethlehem, is called the Nativity. Every year, on 25 December, Christians celebrate Jesus' birthday.

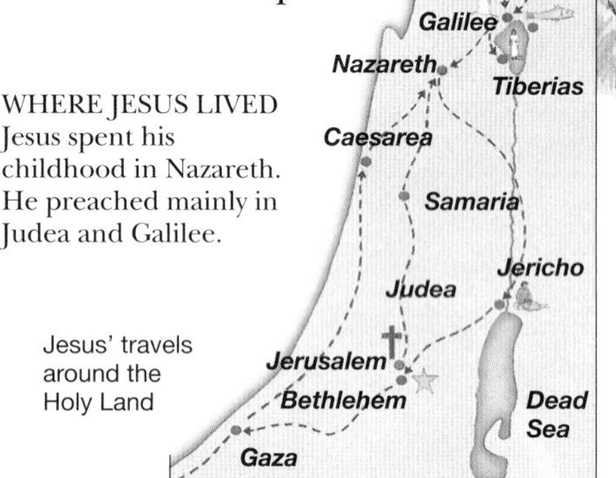

WHERE JESUS LIVED
Jesus spent his childhood in Nazareth. He preached mainly in Judea and Galilee.

SERMON ON THE MOUNT
Jesus taught that God was a kind, loving father, and that people should not fight back when attacked but should "turn the other cheek". He stressed the importance of love. His Sermon on the Mount contained new ideas describing how ordinary people who were humble, gentle, and poor would go to heaven. He also taught his followers a special prayer – the Lord's Prayer.

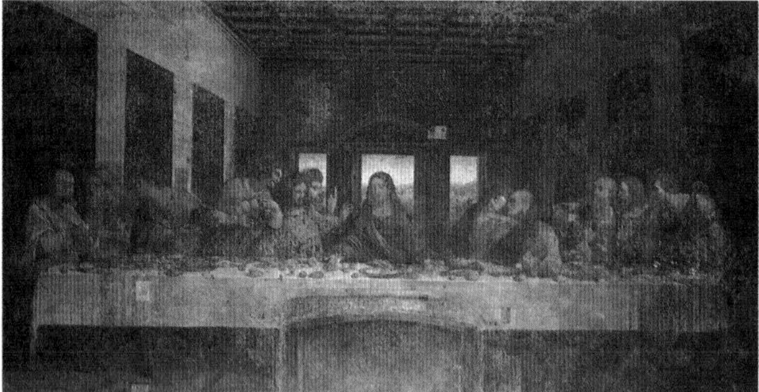

LAST SUPPER
Near the end of his life Jesus shared a last supper with his 12 disciples. Using bread and wine as symbols of his body and blood, Jesus told them to remember him by this feast. To this day, the last supper is re-enacted during communion, when Christians take wine and wafers of bread as part of church services.

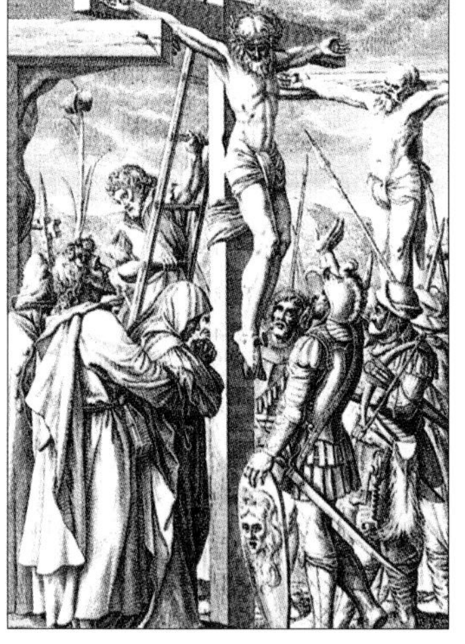

CRUCIFIXION
Jesus was accused of treason against Rome and tried by the Roman governor, Pontius Pilate. He was sentenced to be crucified – nailed to a cross on a hill called Calvary, outside Jerusalem. After his death his body was sealed in a tomb.

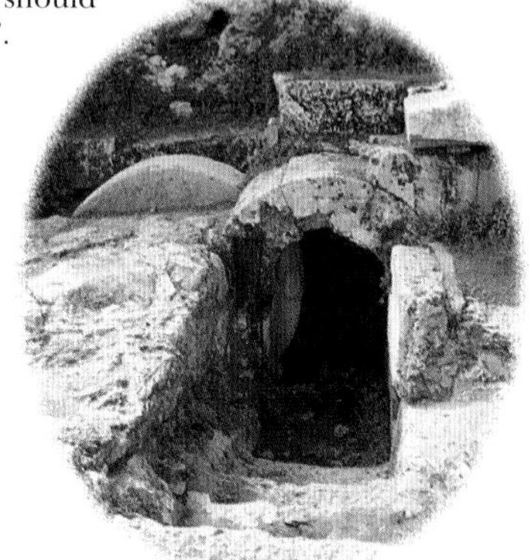

RESURRECTION
On Sunday morning, three days after Jesus' death, the tomb in which his body had been placed was found empty. The gospels of Matthew, Mark, Luke, and John tell how he appeared to his disciples and, after 40 days of teaching them, rose to heaven.

Find out more
CHRISTIANITY
RELIGIONS

Joan of Arc

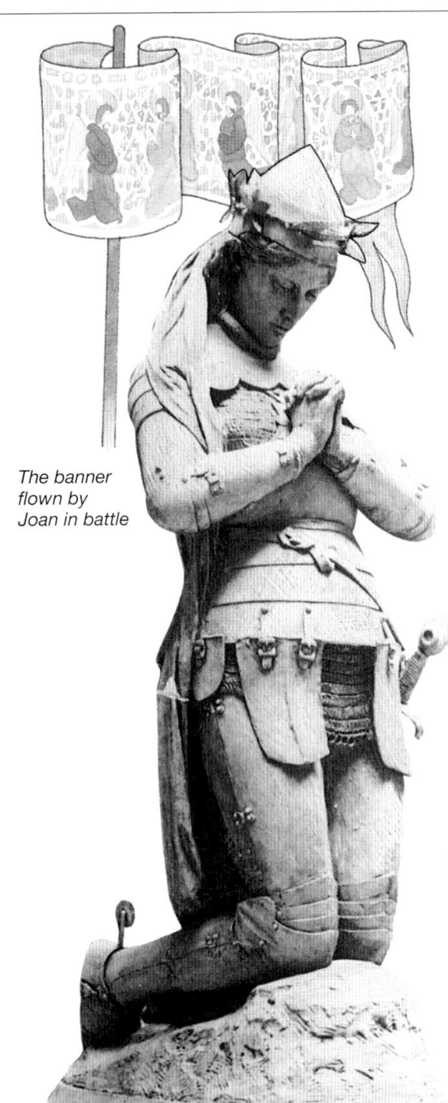

The banner flown by Joan in battle

IN THE EARLY 15TH CENTURY the French finally defeated the English, who had ruled much of their country. The warrior who led them into battle was a woman who has since become one of the best-loved heroines of French history. Joan of Arc was born into a farming family in 1412. She could not read or write, but she was inspired and stubborn, and could debate with educated people. As a young girl, Joan heard "voices" of saints and angels. The voices told her that she must restore the rightful king to the throne of France. Joan convinced the heir to the throne (the Dauphin) – who later became King Charles VII – to support her. In 1429, when only 17, she led the French army to victory at Orléans. Joan led her country's troops in other successful battles, but in 1430 she was caught by a powerful group of French people from Burgundy. They sold her to the English, who imprisoned her and put her on trial as a heretic – a person who does not believe in the official teachings of the Church. Joan was found guilty, and on 30 May, 1431, she was executed in Rouen by being burned at the stake. After her death the English were driven out of France, and Joan's reputation as a heroine flourished. Legends about Joan became widespread, and in 1920 she was made a saint.

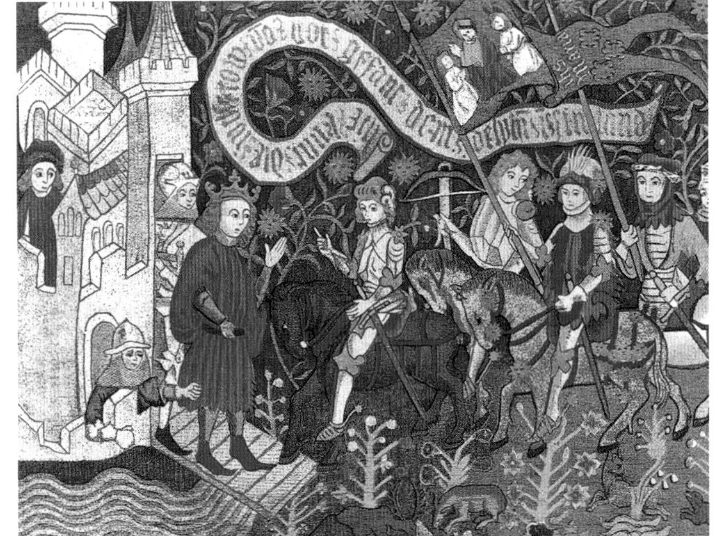

MEETING THE DAUPHIN
This contemporary tapestry shows Joan's arrival at the Château of Chinon in February 1429, in the company of six armed men. She is greeted by the Dauphin Charles, who wears a golden crown – a token of his claim to the disputed French throne.

The Maid of Orleans

Joan of Arc was a brave fighter who wore a suit of armour like a man. She was deeply religious, and prayed for guidance before going into battle. She was known as the "Maid of Orléans" because she led the French army to victory at Orléans.

JOAN'S HELMET
Joan may have worn this helmet in battle against the English. There is a hole in the side made by an arrow or a crossbow bolt.

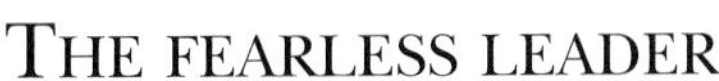

The Fearless Leader

Joan demonstrated that previous French defeat had resulted from military error and that, with better tactics, victories were possible. At first the troops were reluctant to follow Joan, but they soon realized that they won when obeying her commands. Joan's first victory was the lifting of the English siege of Orléans in 1429, which swelled the troops' confidence in their young leader. The Orléans victory was followed by similar success at Jargeau, Meung, Beaugency, and Patay. Her thrilling run came to an end when she was captured at Compiègne on 24 May, 1430.

Joan leads the French troops into battle at Orléans.

CROSS OF LORRAINE
During World War II (1939-45), France was occupied by Germany, partly under German military control and partly under a pro-German French government. The fighters of the French Resistance movement adopted the cross of Lorraine, originally Joan of Arc's symbol, because they shared her aim – to rid their country of foreign domination.

Find out more

FRANCE, HISTORY OF
HUNDRED YEARS WAR

JUDAISM

JEWISH FESTIVALS

Yom Kippur (Day of Atonement) Tenth day of New Year; holiest of festivals, with 24 hours of fasting.

Purim (Feast of Lots) Early spring festival.

Passover (Pesach) Eight-day spring festival.

Shavuot (Feast of Weeks) Harvest festival in early summer.

Rosh Hashanah (New Year) Early autumn.

Sukkoth (Feast of Tabernacles) Nine-day autumn festival.

Hanukkah (Festival of Lights) Eight-day winter festival.

THE HISTORY OF THE JEWISH PEOPLE and of their religion, Judaism, are closely linked. All Jews believe in one God who, more than 4,000 years ago, made a special agreement with their ancestor, Abraham. They were to become God's chosen people. In return they promised to obey his laws and to spread his message to others. Jews believe that a Messiah, God's messenger, will one day come to transform the world into a better place and to restore the ancient Jewish kingdom that was destroyed in the 6th century B.C. Judaism aims for a just and peaceful life for all people on earth. Jewish scriptures explain that to achieve this aim, correct behaviour is very important. Orthodox Jews – those who interpret the scriptures very strictly – obey many rules about their day-to-day activities, including how to dress and what to eat. For example, they do not eat pork or shellfish. Many Jews, however, are not orthodox and apply the rules less strictly. For all Jews, Hebrew is the language of worship. It is also the national language of Israel, the Jewish homeland. However, Jews live and work all over the world, speaking many different languages. Their strong family life and the laws which guide them unite them wherever they live.

Jews light candles in a menorah, or branched candlestick, during Hanukkah.

Jewish men wear a skull cap called a yarmulke or kipa.

During prayers Jewish men wear a tallith, or prayer shawl, over their shoulders.

The Talmud contains instructions for following the Jewish way of life.

TALMUD

Jewish religious leaders are called rabbis. They are responsible for teaching and explaining the laws of Judaism. They study two holy books: the Talmud (right), and the Torah which is kept as a scroll. The Talmud contains instructions for following a Jewish way of life and understanding Jewish laws.

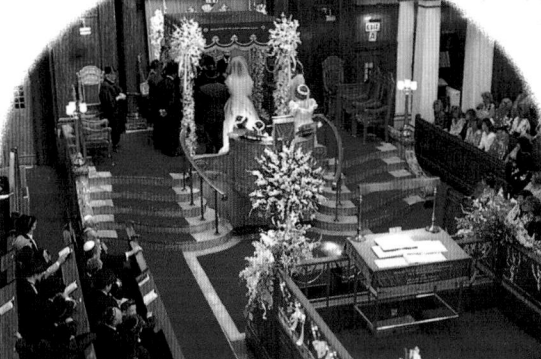

SYNAGOGUE
Jews worship in the synagogue. Prayer, study, and special family occasions such as weddings and bar and bat mitzvahs (the celebrations of children becoming adult Jews) take place here. A *minyan* (quorum of 10 males) is required to formally recite Kaddish (memorial prayers) and read from the Torah.

TORAH

The first five books of the Hebrew Bible – the Torah (left) – contain the laws of Judaism and the early history of the Jewish people. Other sections of the Hebrew Bible contain the psalms, the words of the prophets, and other holy writings. For Jews, the Torah is the most important of books.

Find out more

FESTIVALS
ISRAEL
RELIGIONS

JOHN F. KENNEDY

AN ASSASSIN'S BULLET abruptly ended the promise that John Fitzgerald Kennedy brought to the US presidency. His family name meant politics in their hometown of Boston. Kennedy graduated from Harvard University, then served in the US Navy. After the war, Kennedy launched his political career, serving first in the House of Representatives, then in the Senate. In 1956, he began a long campaign for the presidency, which ended with his winning by a small margin in 1960. He brought youth and vigour to the White House, and his wife Jackie became a fashion icon.

1917 Born in Brookline, Massachusetts, USA.

1940 Graduates from Harvard University.

1941-45 Serves in US Navy during World War II.

1945 Wins election to US House of Representatives.

1952 Elected to US Senate.

1953 Marries Jacqueline Bouvier.

1960 Elected 35th President of the US.

1961 Berlin Wall divides East and West Berlin.

1962 Presides over the Cuban missile crisis.

1963 Assassinated in Dallas, Texas.

THE KENNEDY DYNASTY

Kennedy was born into America's most glamorous and famous political dynasty. His grandfather was a state senator in Massachusetts, and his father served as ambassador to Great Britain. His mother's father was mayor of Boston and a US congressman. Three of the nine Kennedy children developed political careers: John; Robert, who became attorney general during his brother's presidency, then served as a US senator for New York until his own assassination in 1968; and Edward (known as Ted), who has represented Massachusetts in the Senate since 1962.

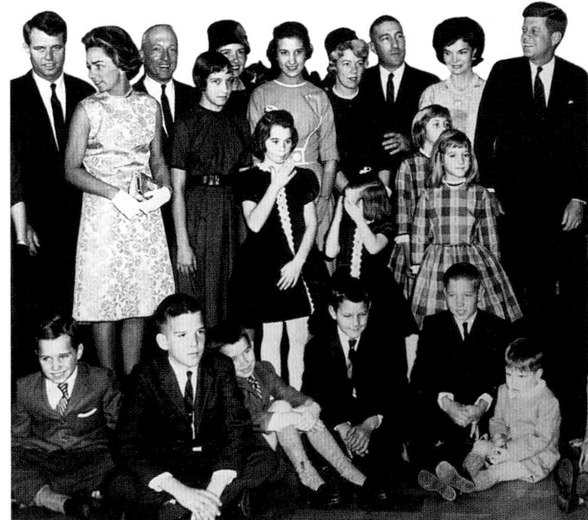

In his time, President Kennedy was the youngest president of the United States, and the first Roman Catholic to hold the office.

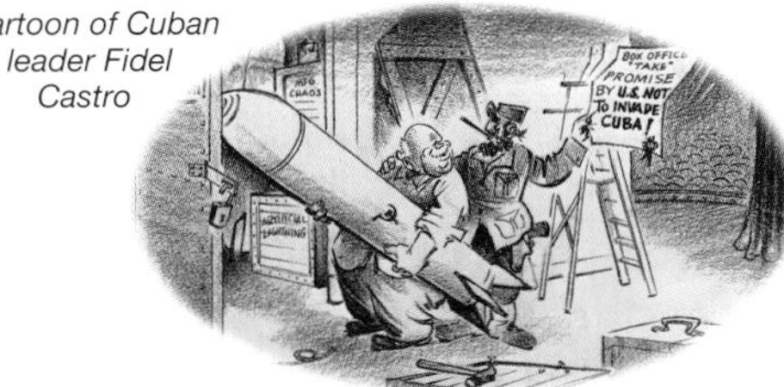

Cartoon of Cuban leader Fidel Castro

CUBAN MISSILE CRISIS

When satellites revealed Soviet missiles in Cuba within striking distance of several US cities, Kennedy ordered a naval blockade. For 13 days, the world was on the brink of war, until the missiles were withdrawn.

WARTIME HERO

Kennedy served in the US Navy during World War II. After saving his crew in an encounter with a Japanese destroyer near the Solomon Islands, he was awarded a medal for bravery.

John Kennedy was also awarded the Purple Heart, a medal given to those wounded in action.

KENNEDY'S ASSASSINATION

In 1963, Kennedy and his wife, campaigning in Texas, rode an open-top car through Dallas. Shots rang out and Kennedy slumped down. He died half an hour later. Police arrested Lee Harvey Oswald, who denied the shooting. Two days later, as Oswald was taken to jail, he was killed by a lone gunman in front of a nationwide television audience.

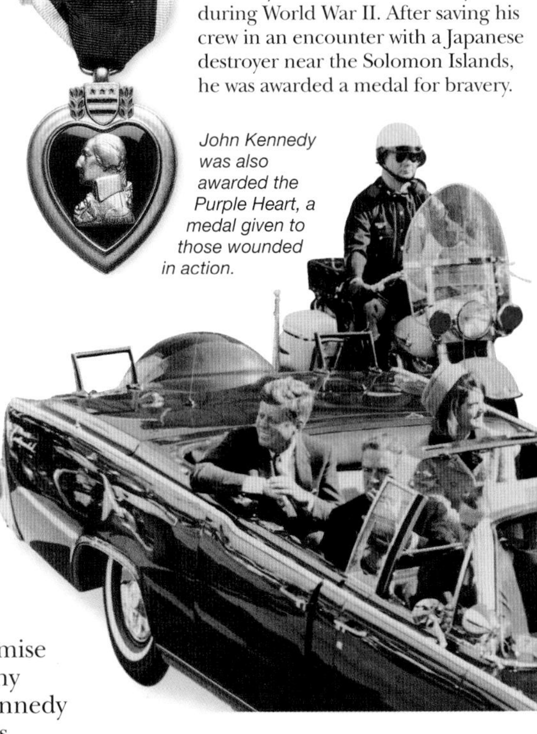

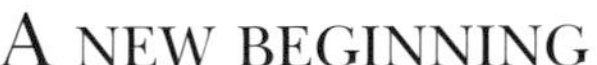

A NEW BEGINNING

Kennedy campaigned for president with the promise of a new frontier for Americans. Although many voters worried about his lack of experience, Kennedy defeated Richard Nixon. In his inaugural address, Kennedy urged Americans to, "Ask not what your country can do for you – ask what you can do for your country." During Kennedy's short time in office, the US had its first manned space flights, the civil rights movement brought equality closer for African Americans, and the testing of atomic bombs was outlawed.

Find out more

COLD WAR
GOVERNMENT AND POLITICS
WORLD WAR II

MARTIN LUTHER KING

IN 1963 A BAPTIST MINISTER from Alabama, United States, led 250,000 people in a march on Washington, D.C., and delivered a moving and powerful speech. He was Martin Luther King, Jr., and his mission in life was to achieve equality and freedom for black Americans through peaceful means. Under his leadership the civil rights movement won many victories against segregation laws; laws that prevented blacks from voting, separated blacks from whites in schools and other places, and gave white people better opportunities and more freedom. Martin Luther King encouraged people to practise non-violent protest: demonstrations, "sit-ins", and peaceful disobedience of the segregation laws. King went to jail several times and faced constant threats of violence and death, but he continued to work for civil rights. Some white people hated him because he was black, and some black people disliked him because he refused to use more extreme and violent methods. King was assassinated in 1968, but his dream of a country without racial discrimination lives on today. In 1986, the United States began to observe a national holiday in his name.

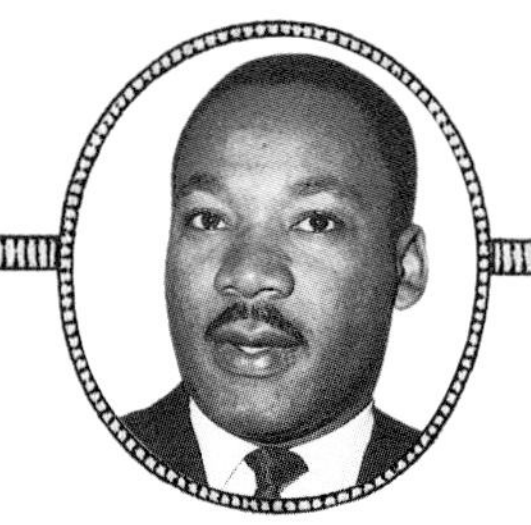

1929 Born, Atlanta, USA.

1954 Baptist minister.

1955 Philosophy Doctorate.

1955-56 Leads Montgomery bus boycott.

1957 Southern Christian Leadership Conference.

1961 Freedom Rides to support desegregation.

1963 March on Washington, D.C.

1964 Nobel Peace Prize.

1965 Selma-Montgomery march.

1968 Assassinated.

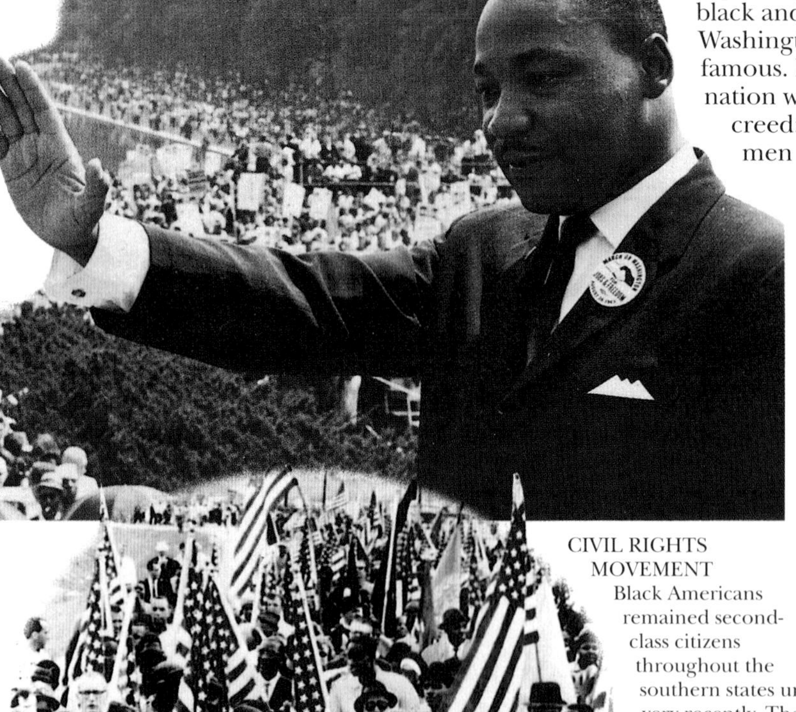

PUBLIC SPEAKER
Martin Luther King's words inspired millions of Americans, black and white. At the August 1963 march on Washington, King made a speech that has since become famous. He said: "I have a dream that one day this nation will rise up and live out the true meaning of its creed: We hold these truths to be self-evident; that all men are created equal."

CIVIL RIGHTS MOVEMENT
Black Americans remained second-class citizens throughout the southern states until very recently. They were not allowed to vote, and restrictions were placed on where they could sit in buses and restaurants. During the late 1950s, a movement arose which demanded equal rights for all Americans. Martin Luther King and others organized non-violent protests designed to force changes in the law. In 1964-65, racial discrimination was finally outlawed throughout the United States.

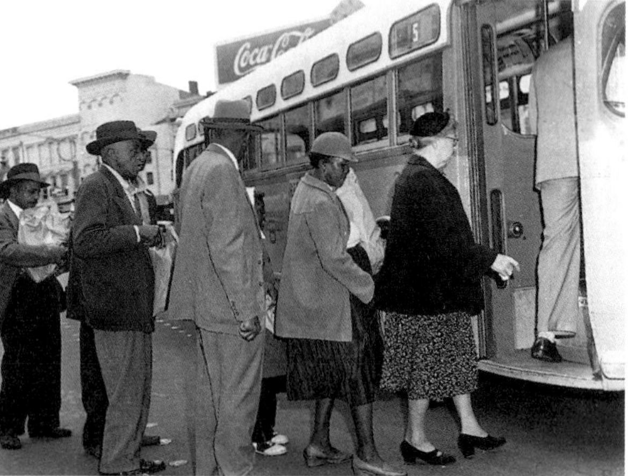

BUS BOYCOTT
In December 1955, Rosa Parks, a black seamstress who worked in an Alabama department store, was arrested for refusing to give up a bus seat reserved for white people. For one year, Martin Luther King and his friends persuaded people to boycott (refuse to use) every bus in Montgomery, Alabama, until the segregation of the bus seats was declared illegal.

Find out more

AMERICAN CIVIL WAR
HUMAN RIGHTS
SLAVERY
UNITED STATES OF AMERICA, history of

KITES AND GLIDERS

CHINESE KITES
Flowing, painted tails in the shape of dragons, birds, and butterflies are typical of traditional Chinese kites. This centipede-like kite is made from 15 round paper and bamboo kites strung together.

NO FLYING machine is as old as the kite. People in China were flying silk kites more than 3,000 years ago, and legends tell how in 202 B.C. General Huan Theng terrified his enemies with kites whose taut strings wailed eerily in the breeze. Fifteen hundred years later, Marco Polo, the great Italian traveller, came back from China with tales of vast kites that hoisted prisoners into the air to test the wind. In Europe, children have played with toy kites for more than 1,000 years. Gliders owe their origins to kites, and they too are old. In about 1800, the English inventor George Cayley found that a kite with arched wings and a tail could glide through the air without a breeze to lift it or a string to guide it. Later, Cayley built a glider large enough to carry a person. This rough prototype (test model) was the forerunner not only of the streamlined gliders of today but of all winged aircraft.

Without a line to hold it at the correct angle to the wind, a kite would not be able to fly.

FLAT KITES
The oldest and simplest kites are diamond-shaped and have flat frames. They can also be strung together to make spectacular writhing serpents.

DELTA KITES
Triangular "delta" kites are simple to build and fly well in light winds. Hang gliders are based on the delta kite.

HANG GLIDERS
The hang glider is the cheapest and simplest form of aircraft, and hang gliding is becoming an increasingly popular sport. When a hang glider takes to the air, the fabric of the wings arches up to give an aerofoil shape, like an ordinary aircraft wing. Without this, the craft would plummet, not glide, through the air.

BOX KITE
Elaborate box kites have a frame that may be a combination of squares, triangles, and rectangles. Box kites are the most stable fliers of all.

The wing is made from lightweight dacron fabric stretched over a long aluminium tube. On some hang gliders, curved spars help give the wing its aerofoil shape.

The pilot hangs under the wing and steers by shifting body weight to one side or the other.

Straps hold the pilot safely in position.

Gliders have long, thin wings which give a lot of lift (upward force) but keep air resistance to a minimum.

Eventually the glider loses height and lands.

The pilot looks for isolated clouds, which often indicate a thermal.

GLIDERS

Because a glider has no engine, it ultimately can fly only downwards. Modern gliders are streamlined and made of light fibreglass so that they lose height very slowly. However, a glider needs help to fly far. To take off, an aeroplane or a truck tows the glider into the air. Then the pilot looks for pockets of rising warm air, called thermals, to keep the glider flying high in the sky.

Once the glider is high enough, the pilot releases the winch line, and the glider flies free.

Warm air rising over a city or a sun-warmed field carries the glider upward in a spiral.

As the truck moves off, the glider rises into the air.

Find out more
AIRCRAFT
CHINA, HISTORY OF
PLASTICS

KNIGHTS AND HERALDRY

A THOUSAND YEARS AGO men who fought in battle on horseback were called knights. At first they were just powerful warriors who terrified the enemy's foot soldiers. But by the 13th century the knights of western Europe had an important role in society. They fought in the armies of the king or queen in return for land. Knights also protected the peasants who lived and worked on the land, and in exchange the peasants gave the knights their service and produce. Heraldry developed as a way of identifying knights in battle. Armour completely covered the knights' faces and bodies, and they all looked alike. Thus, each knight chose "arms" – a unique coloured pattern or picture which everyone could recognize. He displayed his arms on a linen tunic worn over his armour. This was his "coat of arms". The chosen pattern remained in the knight's family and was passed on from father to son.

Argent a mullet azure

Vert a lily or

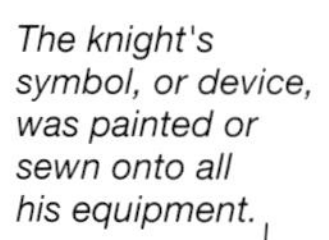

Ermine a cross crosslet gules

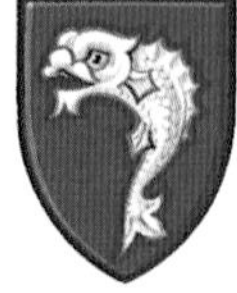

Azure a dolphin argent

Sable a bee or

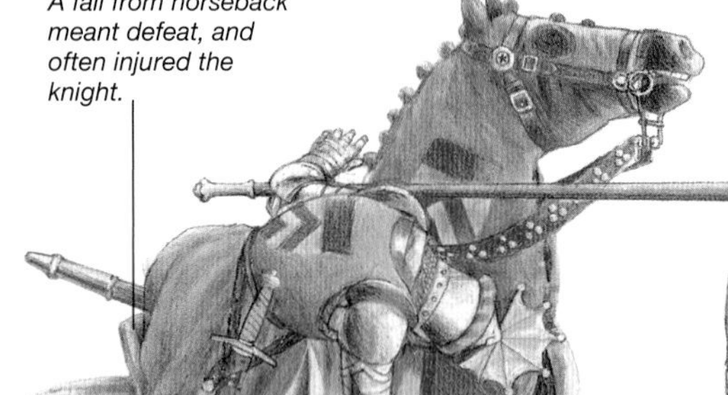

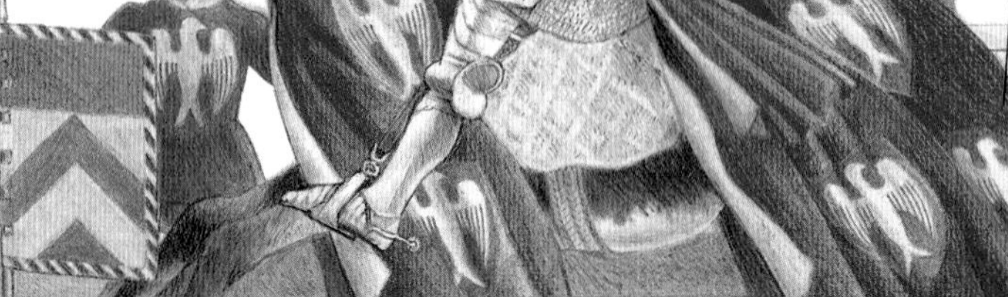

A fall from horseback meant defeat, and often injured the knight.

The knight's symbol, or device, was painted or sewn onto all his equipment.

TOURNAMENTS AND JOUSTING

Tournaments began in France in the middle of the 11th century as peacetime training exercises for knights. They soon developed into major events with elaborate rules. Teams of knights fought fierce mock battles over great areas of land, and the losing side paid a ransom or handed over valuable possessions. During the 13th century, tournaments became better organized and took place in a single field. Only two knights jousted at a time, or fought with blunt weapons. Later, tilting replaced jousting and the knights used lances to knock their rivals to the ground.

CHIVALRY

The period between the 11th and 14th centuries is often known as the "age of chivalry". Knights of the time were supposed to follow a special code of chivalry – a system of rules about honour, obedience to God and the king, and protecting the weak. In reality, many knights forgot the code. They honoured only people of noble birth and stole from the poor and weak.

Gules a lion rampant or

Or a chief indented purpure

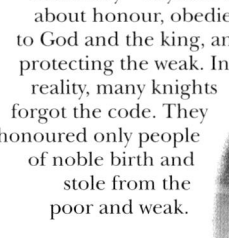

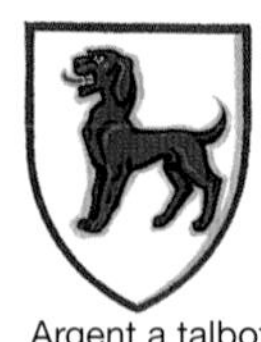

Argent a talbot statant sable

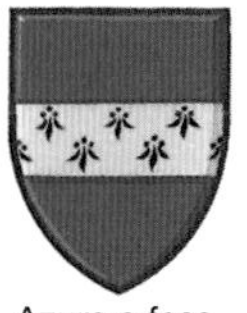

Azure a fess erminois

Gules a lymphad argent

Azure an owl argent

Vair a chevron sable

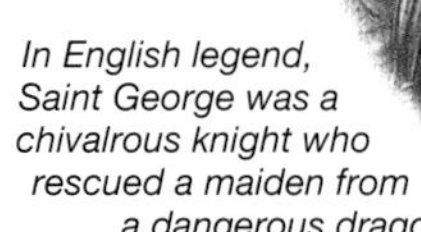

In English legend, Saint George was a chivalrous knight who rescued a maiden from a dangerous dragon.

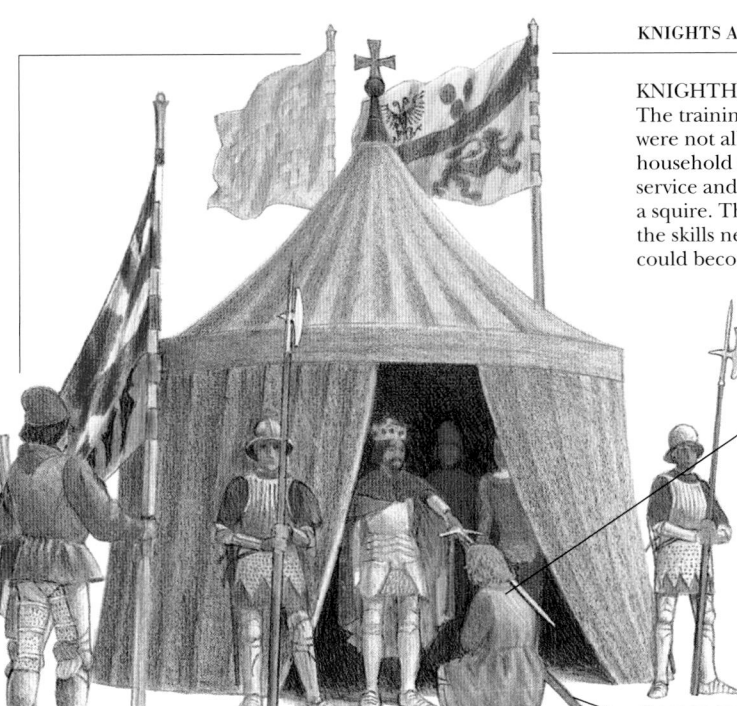

KNIGHTHOOD

The training to become a knight started at seven years of age. Girls were not allowed to become knights, but boys began as pages in the household of their father's lord. Pages learned the rules of knightly service and how to use weapons. At the age of 15 or 16, a page became a squire. The squire was the personal servant to his master and learned the skills needed for fighting on horseback. After five years the squire could become a knight. At first this was an honour that any knight could bestow on a squire. Today, only English kings and queens can grant knighthoods, but the title is a formal one given to people who deserve national recognition and has lost most of its original meaning.

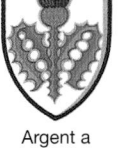

Dubbing a squire, or tapping him on the shoulders with a sword, made him into a knight.

Once he became a knight, the squire had to supply his own equipment.

Argent a thistle proper

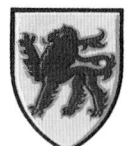

Or a lion passant gules

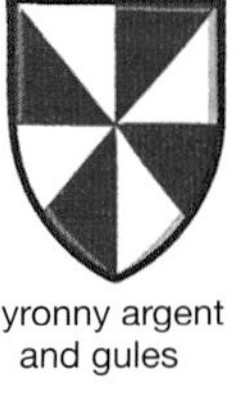

Gyronny argent and gules

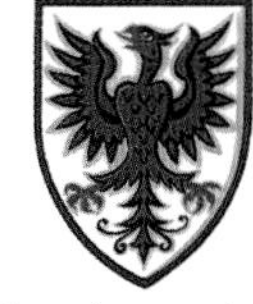

Argent an eagle displayed sable

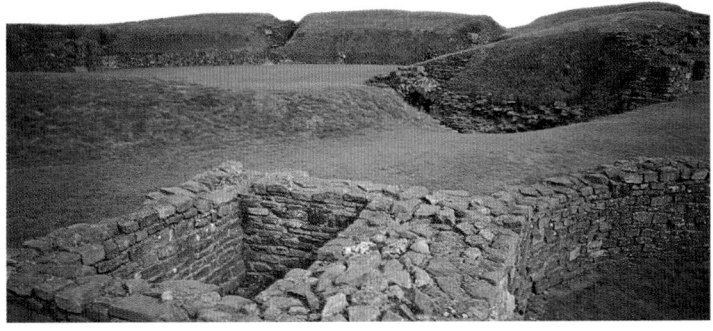

Sable a cross engrailed or

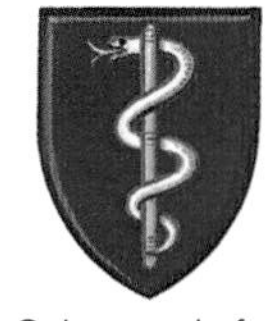

Gules a rod of Aesculapius or

Azure a harpy or

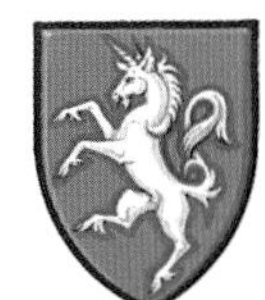

Vert a unicorn rampant argent

THE KNIGHTS OF THE ROUND TABLE

King Arthur and his knights are said to have held their court at a round table in the ancient capital of Camelot. If it really did exist, Camelot was probably built in the west of Britain some fifteen centuries ago. According to legend, Arthur led his band of Celtic knights in battle against Saxon invaders. The knights of Camelot became heroes and had many adventures.

Caerleon Castle, Wales, possible site of Camelot

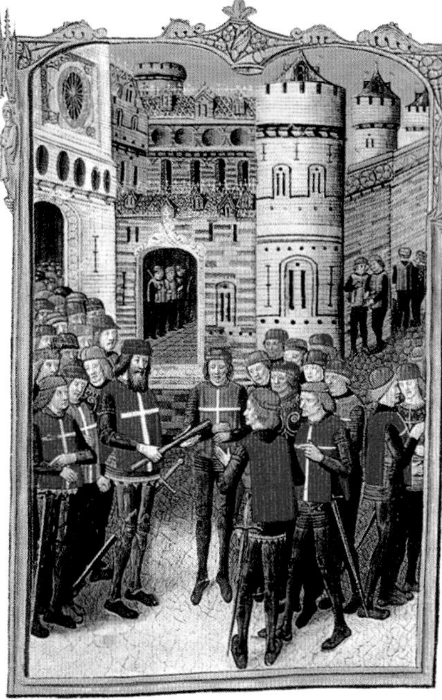

KNIGHTS HOSPITALLERS

Knights from northwest Europe fought in the Crusades – a series of religious wars between Christians and Muslims that took place in the Middle East during the 12th and 13th centuries. The warriors formed powerful alliances, one of which was the Knights Hospitallers. This group set up hospitals along the Crusaders' routes to war.

NAMING SHIELDS

The blazon, or description, below each shield names the field and charge and gives their colours and other details in a language based on medieval French.

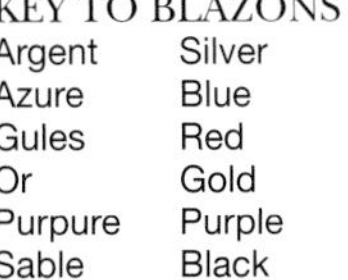

KEY TO BLAZONS

Argent	Silver
Azure	Blue
Gules	Red
Or	Gold
Purpure	Purple
Sable	Black
Vert	Green

The charge is a dragon vert (green). He is sitting "sejant" – with forepaws on the ground.

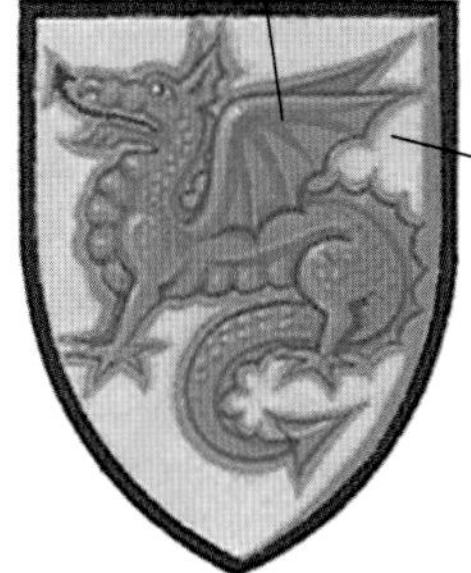

The field on this shield is or (gold).

Or a dragon sejant vert

Shields

Each knight displayed his arms on a shield. The shield had two parts: the field, or surface, painted in a plain colour or a pattern; and the charge, which displayed a symbol, such as an animal or bird. The arms appeared everywhere on the knight's equipment. Sometimes the area above the shield design might show an image of a helmet with a crest, silk wreath, and mantling (a cloth for protection from the sun). The knight's motto, or slogan, could also be added below the shield. The full combination of designs was called a heraldic achievement (a herald was an expert in arms).

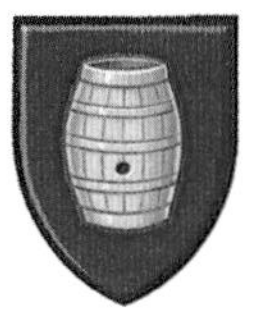

Gules a barrel palewise or

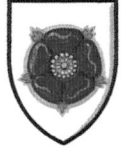

Argent a rose gules

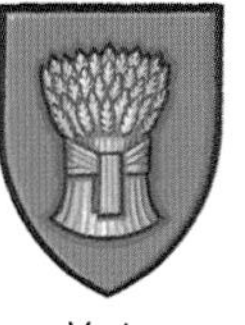

Vert a garb or

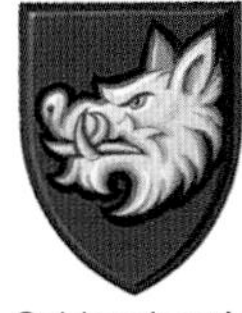

Sable a boar's head erased or

Find out more

Armour
Castles
Crusades
Medieval Europe
Weapons

KOREA

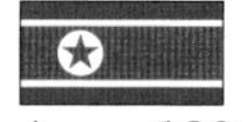

The Korean peninsula is bordered by China and, in the far northeast, Russia. On the west it is bordered by the Yellow Sea and, in the east, by the Sea of Japan. The peninsula is divided, along the 38th parallel, into North and South Korea.

THE KOREAN PENINSULA has a long history of invasion and occupation by its two powerful neighbours, China and Japan. In 1948, it was divided into Communist North and pro-American South, and the invasion of the South by the North led to the Korean War (1950-53). The war devastated both countries, but their subsequent histories have been very different. South Korea, once a rural society, became a major industrial power, and one of the world's leading ship-builders and car manufacturers. It also became a centre of high technology and electronics. The economy of the North, an isolated and repressive Communist regime, is a marked contrast. Heavy industry has created severe pollution and nationwide electricity blackouts are common. In 1995 and 1996, floods wrecked harvests, and many people suffered terrible hardship.

NORTH KOREA

Area: 120,540 sq km (46,540 sq miles)
Population: 22,700,000
Capital: Pyongyang
Languages: Korean, Chinese
Religions: Non-religious, traditional beliefs, Ch'ondogyo, Buddhist
Currency: North Korean Won

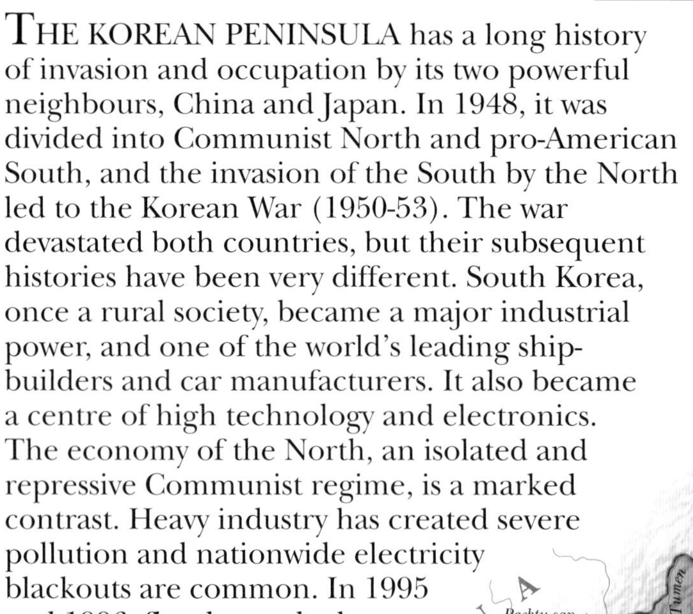

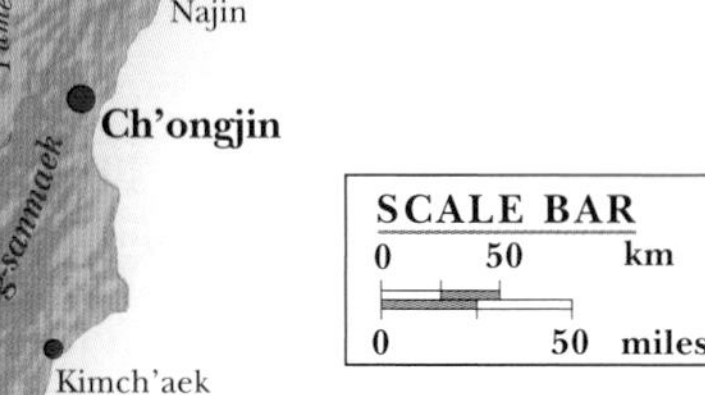

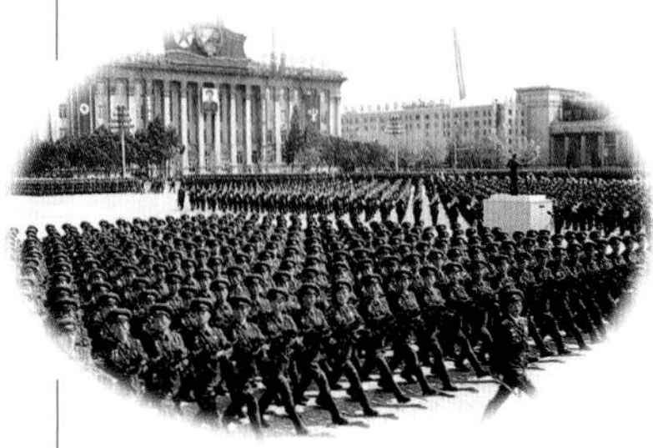

NORTH KOREA

The independent Communist republic of North Korea invaded the South in 1950, leading to the Korean War (1950-53). The border that now divides the two countries is the most militarized in the world. North Korea now has one of the world's largest military organizations, a huge army and an advanced arms industry. Its military might is regularly displayed at regimented parades.

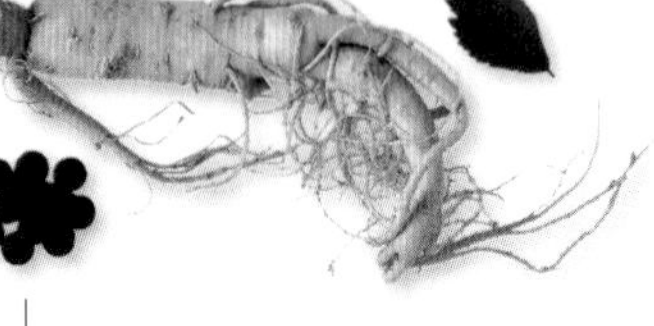

GINSENG
Korea is a major exporter of the valuable ginseng root, believed to improve health, and promote long life and vigour.

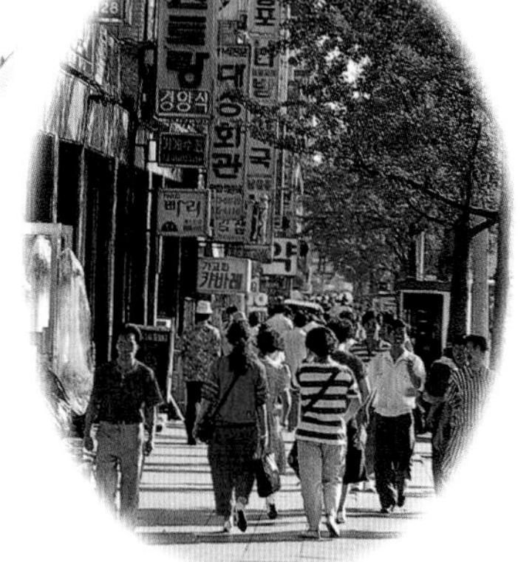

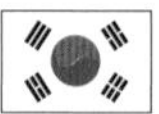

SOUTH KOREA

Area: 99,020 sq km (38,232 sq miles)
Population: 47,700,000
Capital: Seoul
Languages: Korean, Chinese
Religions: Mahayana Buddhist, Protestant, Roman Catholic, Confucianism
Currency: Won

SEOUL

Seoul was the capital of Korea from 1394 to 1948, when it became capital of South Korea. It is a fast-expanding city of over 10 million people. The orderly, rectangular street patterns of the centre give way to sprawling suburbs on the low surrounding hills. Seoul is a major commercial and manufacturing centre, with many small-scale textile factories. It is congested with traffic, and pollution is becoming a major problem.

Find out more

ARMIES
ASIA
ASIA, HISTORY OF
COMMUNISM
JAPAN, HISTORY OF

LAKE AND RIVER WILDLIFE

THE WATER IN LAKES and rivers is teeming with all kinds of life. Grasses, reeds, and other plants grow along the water's edge, providing food and shelter for insects, nesting birds, and mammals such as water voles and muskrats. In rivers, the fast-flowing water sweeps away plants, but in lakes, tiny floating plants are food for small creatures such as water fleas and shrimps, which are in turn eaten by bigger fish. Larger floating waterweeds provide shade for basking fish. Fallen leaves, animal droppings, and rotting plant matter form a rich mud at the bottom of rivers and lakes, where worms, snails, and other small organisms live. Today, many lakes and rivers are suffering from serious pollution. Industrial chemicals, farm fertilizers, untreated sewage, and a host of other damaging substances discharged into lakes and rivers have upset or destroyed the natural wildlife balance.

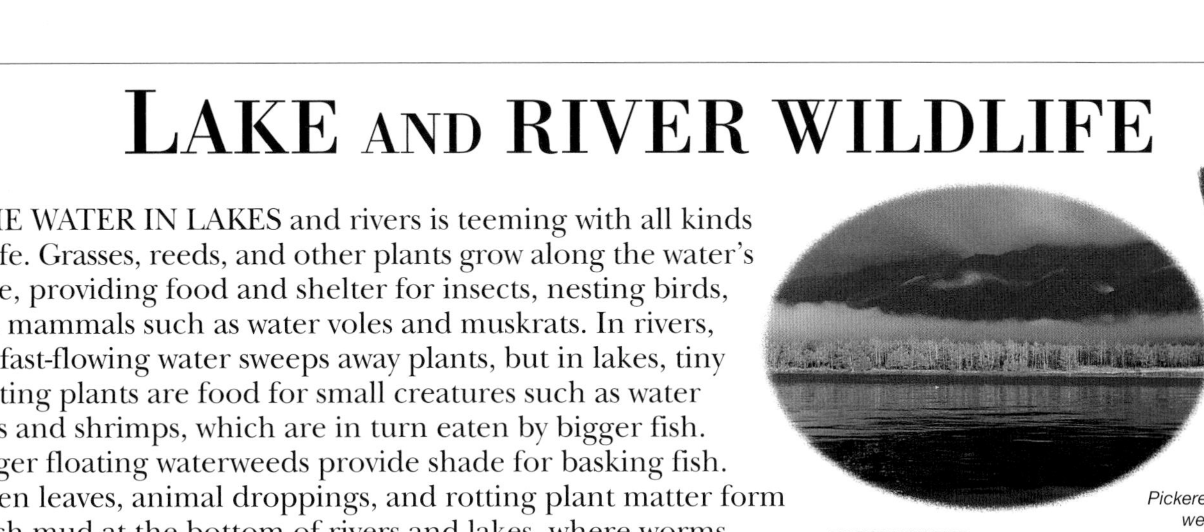

FRESH WATER
The water in lakes and rivers is called fresh water. Although it makes up only about 0.03 per cent (that is, 1 part in 3000) of all the water on Earth, fresh water is home to thousands of different plants and animals.

Pickerell weed grows at the water's edge of lakes and rivers.

MUSKRAT
The muskrat is a rodent that usually eats water plants but also feeds on small animals such as fish, frogs, and freshwater shellfish.

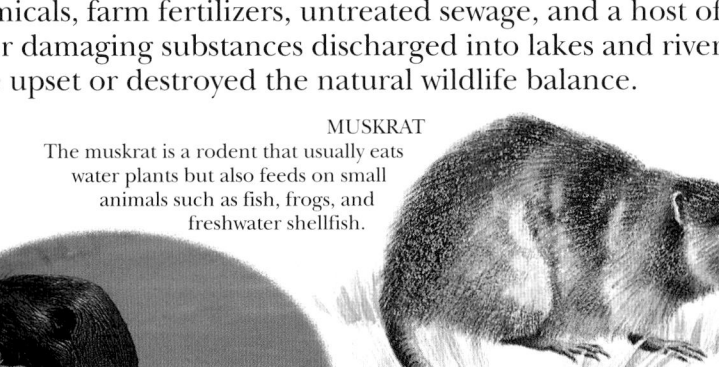

Muskrat swims powerfully with its webbed back feet and uses its long, hairless tail as a rudder for steering.

RUDDY DUCK
The ruddy duck is found in open waters in many parts of Europe. It has a stiff, upward-pointing tail and dives in search of plants, small water insects, larvae, and worms.

GIANT OTTER
The largest member of the otter family lives in South America. The giant otter grows to more than 1.5 m (5 ft) long including its tail. It hunts catfish, piranha, and other fish. Unlike other otters, the giant otter prefers to stay in streams and pools and is not often seen on land. Today, this otter is very rare and is on the official list of endangered species.

PIKE
The northern pike is a large, fearsome predator with a huge mouth and sharp teeth for seizing many kinds of fish, as well as frogs, water birds, and small mammals. Pike live in lakes and slow-moving rivers; the biggest pike grow to more than 1 m (3 ft) long.

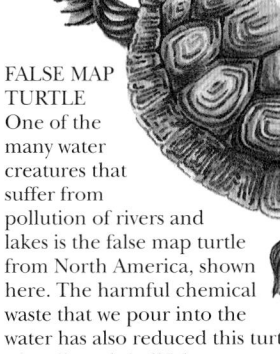

FALSE MAP TURTLE
One of the many water creatures that suffer from pollution of rivers and lakes is the false map turtle from North America, shown here. The harmful chemical waste that we pour into the water has also reduced this turtle's food of snails and shellfish.

RIVER PLANTS

The speed of the water in a river has a great effect on the wildlife. In a fast river the water sweeps the river bed clean of sand and mud, leaving only pebbles. Nothing can grow in the middle of a river, and the river bank consists mainly of plants such as willows that hang over the water. In a slow river, sand and mud can settle, and plants such as irises take root more easily.

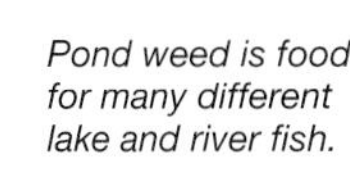

Pond weed is food for many different lake and river fish.

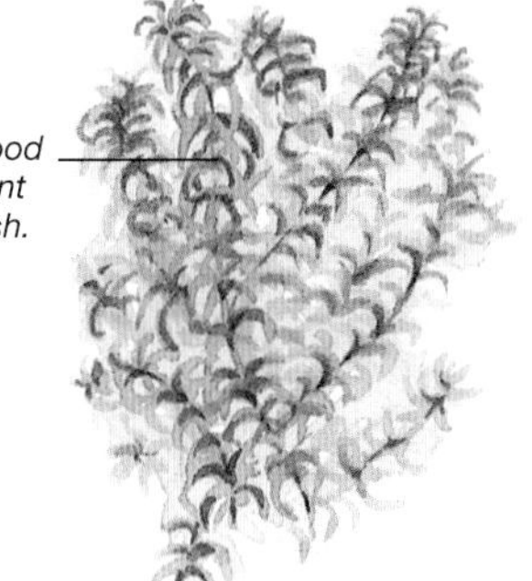

CRAYFISH
The crayfish, found in rivers, is a freshwater relative of sea-living lobsters. It is active mainly at night and walks along the river bed on its four pairs of legs, eating a wide range of food, from plant matter to worms, shellfish, and small fish.

Lake wildlife

Trees such as willows and alders line the edge of many lakes; rushes, tussock sedges, reeds, and other marshy plants grow closer to the water. Plants such as water lilies and water horsetails grow in the shallow water and stick up above the surface. Each type of plant is food for a different assortment of animals.

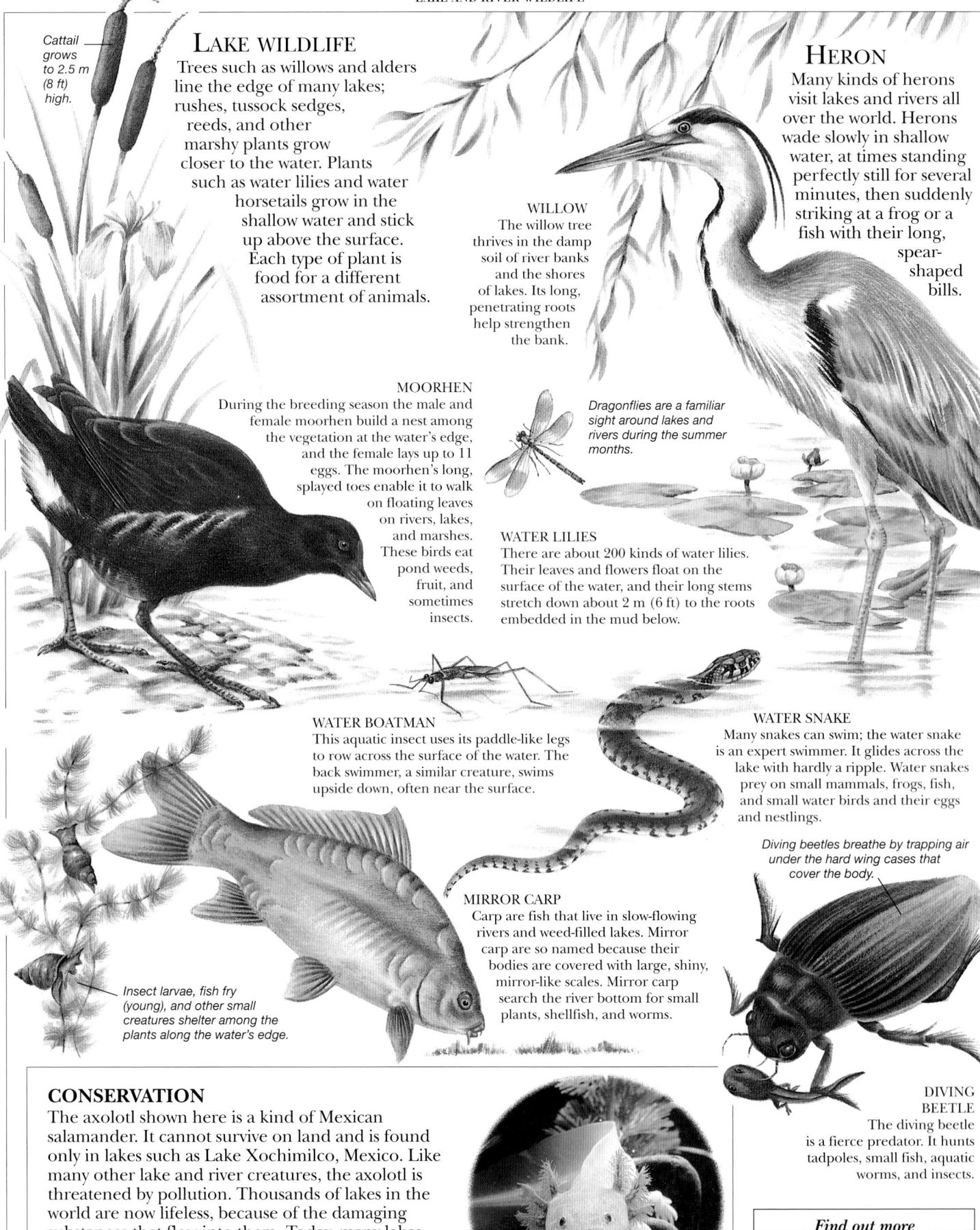

Cattail grows to 2.5 m (8 ft) high.
Dragonflies are a familiar sight around lakes and rivers during the summer months.

Diving beetles breathe by trapping air under the hard wing cases that cover the body.

Heron

Many kinds of herons visit lakes and rivers all over the world. Herons wade slowly in shallow water, at times standing perfectly still for several minutes, then suddenly striking at a frog or a fish with their long, spear-shaped bills.

WILLOW

The willow tree thrives in the damp soil of river banks and the shores of lakes. Its long, penetrating roots help strengthen the bank.

MOORHEN

During the breeding season the male and female moorhen build a nest among the vegetation at the water's edge, and the female lays up to 11 eggs. The moorhen's long, splayed toes enable it to walk on floating leaves on rivers, lakes, and marshes. These birds eat pond weeds, fruit, and sometimes insects.

WATER LILIES

There are about 200 kinds of water lilies. Their leaves and flowers float on the surface of the water, and their long stems stretch down about 2 m (6 ft) to the roots embedded in the mud below.

WATER BOATMAN

This aquatic insect uses its paddle-like legs to row across the surface of the water. The back swimmer, a similar creature, swims upside down, often near the surface.

WATER SNAKE

Many snakes can swim; the water snake is an expert swimmer. It glides across the lake with hardly a ripple. Water snakes prey on small mammals, frogs, fish, and small water birds and their eggs and nestlings.

MIRROR CARP

Carp are fish that live in slow-flowing rivers and weed-filled lakes. Mirror carp are so named because their bodies are covered with large, shiny, mirror-like scales. Mirror carp search the river bottom for small plants, shellfish, and worms.

DIVING BEETLE

The diving beetle is a fierce predator. It hunts tadpoles, small fish, aquatic worms, and insects.

CONSERVATION

The axolotl shown here is a kind of Mexican salamander. It cannot survive on land and is found only in lakes such as Lake Xochimilco, Mexico. Like many other lake and river creatures, the axolotl is threatened by pollution. Thousands of lakes in the world are now lifeless, because of the damaging substances that flow into them. Today, many lakes and rivers are being turned into nature reserves in order to protect the birds, fish, mammals, and other wildlife they contain.

Axolotl means "water beast".

Find out more

Animal senses
Ducks, geese, and swans
Fish
Frogs and other amphibians
Snakes

LAKES

WATER FROM RIVERS, MOUNTAIN SPRINGS, and rain fills hollows in the ground and forms lakes, which are areas of water surrounded by land. Lakes also form in depressions dug out of the ground by glaciers, or in holes in limestone rocks. Some lakes are artificial: reservoirs are lakes made by building dams across rivers. Several landlocked seas such as the Caspian Sea and the Dead Sea are really lakes. The Caspian Sea, which lies between Europe and Asia, is the world's biggest lake. Its surface covers an area almost as large as Japan.

Lakes sustain a wealth of plant and animal life and are often surrounded by fertile land. Freshwater lakes provide water for towns and cities, and recreation areas for swimming, sailing, and water-skiing. Large lakes, such as the Great Lakes in North America, are used to transport goods in ships. However, lakes do not last forever. Silt and plants can fill up a lake over a period of years and turn it into a swamp.

SALTY LAKES
Salt collects in lakes that have no outlet, such as the Dead Sea between Israel and Jordan. The water is so salty that people can float in it without swimming.

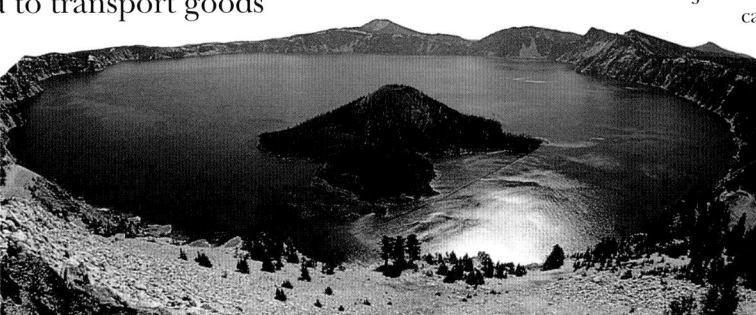

VOLCANIC LAKES
Rainwater fills the volcanic crater at the summit of Mount Mazama, Oregon, United States, to form Crater Lake. It is 589 m (1,932 ft) deep, making it the deepest lake in the United States.

KINDS OF LAKES

Lakes form in hollows dug by glaciers during the Ice Age, and in places where glaciers have left barriers of rock across valleys. Water dissolves huge holes in limestone regions, which often fill with rainwater to create lakes. Lakes can also form in volcanic craters.

FRESHWATER LAKES
The water in freshwater lakes is not salty like the sea, because the lakes are constantly fed and drained by rivers. The largest group of freshwater lakes are the Great Lakes in the United States and Canada. Lake Superior (left) is the largest of the Great Lakes.

SWAMPS AND MARSHES

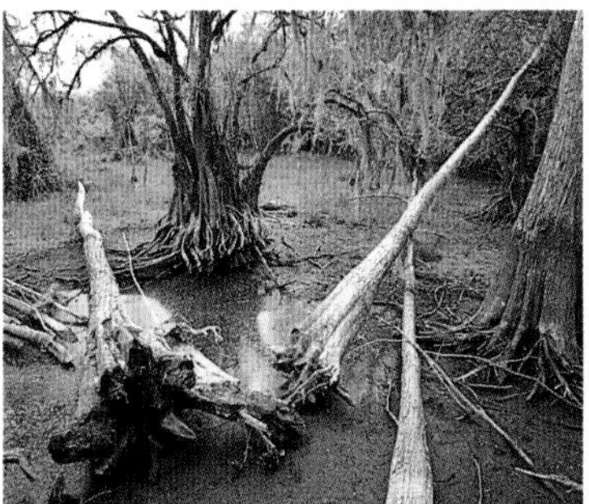

The Everglades is a large region of swamps in the United States. Swamps, or marshes, can form at the edge of a lake where the ground is soaked with water or covered with shallow water. They also form on land where water cannot drain away.

THE LIFE OF A LAKE

Lakes are not permanent features of the landscape. They may come and go as their water supply rises and falls. Lakes can slowly fill with soil and stones washed down from the land above the lake. The outlet river may deepen and drain the lake.

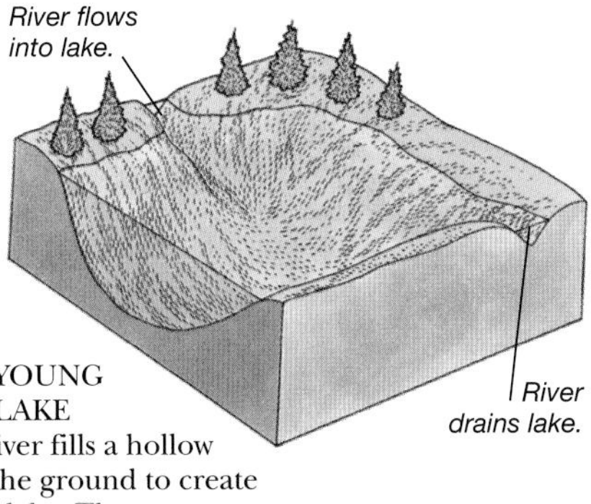

River flows into lake.
River drains lake.

1 YOUNG LAKE
A river fills a hollow in the ground to create the lake. The water flows through the lake, running out into another river.

2 SHRINKING LAKE
The river carries soil, which falls to the bottom as it enters the lake. A layer of soil builds up along the edge of the lake.

Soil and mud build up at sides and bottom of lake.

Plants grow on the damp, fertile soil.

3 DYING LAKE
The soil layers extend into the lake. Plants grow and the layers become land. This continues until the lake vanishes.

Find out more
DAMS
GLACIERS AND ICECAPS
LAKE AND RIVER WILDLIFE
MARSH AND SWAMP WILDLIFE
RIVERS
WATER

LANGUAGES

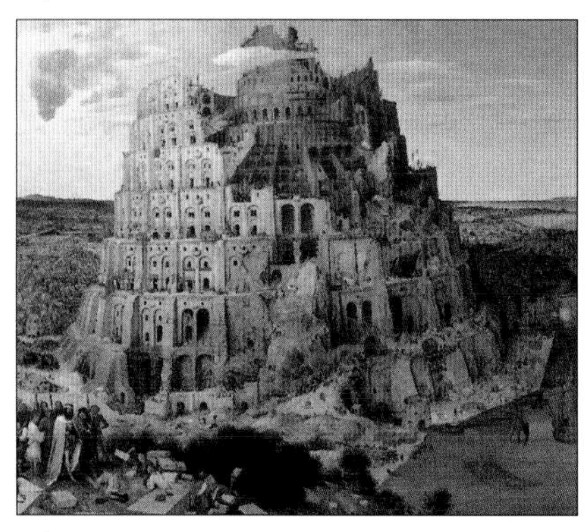

TOWER OF BABEL
At the beginning of this Bible story, everyone spoke the same language. But when people tried to build a tower to reach heaven, God became angry. He made many languages so people could not understand and help one another.

OUR ABILITY TO TALK is one of the skills that makes humans different from the rest of the animal world. Some mammals and birds have simple "languages" of just a few noises, but human speech is much more highly developed. In English, for example, most people use a vocabulary (a list of words) of about 5,000 words in talking, and 10,000 in writing. A language is a way of organizing spoken sounds to express ideas. Human language developed over thousands of years, and people in different countries use different languages. Some languages share words with the languages of nearby countries. For instance, book is *libro* in both Italian and Spanish, and *livre* in French; in English we get the word library from the same source. There are now some 5,000 different languages and many dialects – local versions of major languages.

English is spoken by 330 million people as a first language, and by about 600 million as a second or third language.

About two thirds of China's population, 850 million people, speak Mandarin Chinese.

France once ruled many countries in West Africa, and people there still speak French as well as their local languages.

There are at least 845 languages in India. Hindi and English are the official languages.

Some people have no difficulty in learning foreign languages and can speak several fluently; the record is about 28.

There are about 700 languages in Papua New Guinea.

Mandarin Chinese
English
Russian
Spanish
French
Portuguese
Arabic
Other

LATIN
For many centuries, educated people of many nationalities spoke Latin as well as their native, or first, language. Throughout Europe, scholars, governments, and the Christian Church used Latin.

COMMON LANGUAGES

A map of national languages shows how European nations have explored the world: for example, English settlers took their language to the United States, Canada, Australia, and New Zealand. Spain conquered much of South America, and Spanish is still spoken there. But many people using these languages also have their own local language, which is part of their native culture.

SIGN LANGUAGE

Human speech and hearing make language possible. People who have difficulty speaking or hearing cannot use a spoken language. Instead, they communicate using hand signals. There are signs and gestures for all the common words, and signs for individual letters.

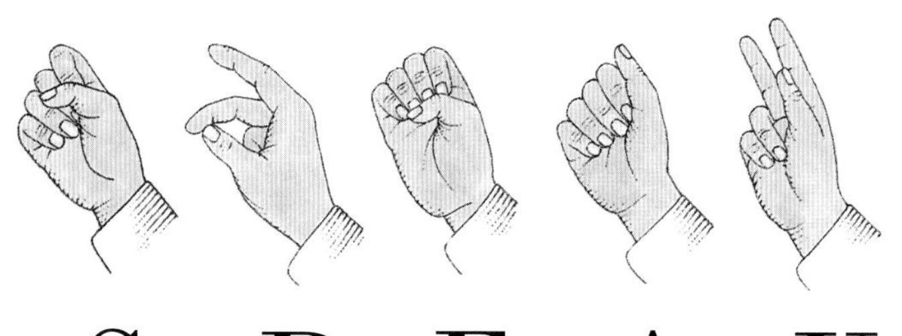

S P E A K

Find out more
ALPHABETS
EDUCATION
SIGNS AND SYMBOLS

LASERS

IF SOMEONE ASKED YOU what is the brightest, most intense light of all, you might say sunlight. You would be wrong. The light from lasers is even brighter; in fact, it is the brightest light known. A laser produces a pencil-thin beam of coloured light that can be so intense that it will burn a hole through steel, or so straight and narrow that it can be aimed precisely at a tiny mirror on the moon, more than 384,000 km (238,000 miles) away.

A scientist named Theodore Maiman built the first laser in 1960. Maiman created the beam by flashing ordinary light into a special rod of synthetic ruby. Today's lasers work with many other materials, as well as ruby. Gas lasers, for instance, use gases such as argon, which gives a low-power beam ideal for delicate surgery. By contrast, powerful solid-state lasers produce a beam with solid rods of crystals such as emerald.

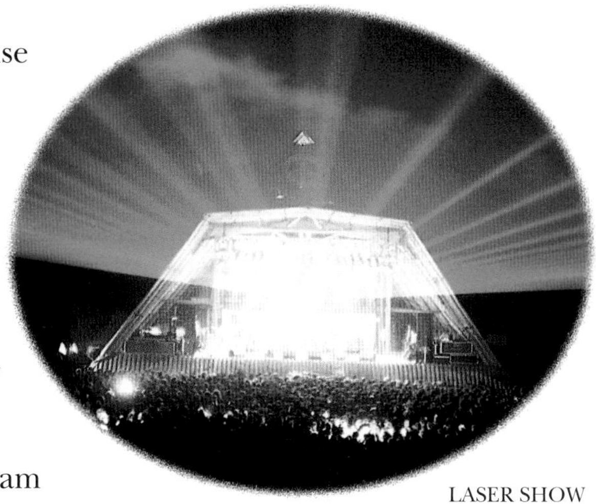

LASER SHOW
Multicoloured lasers produce spectacular light shows for rock concerts and public celebrations.

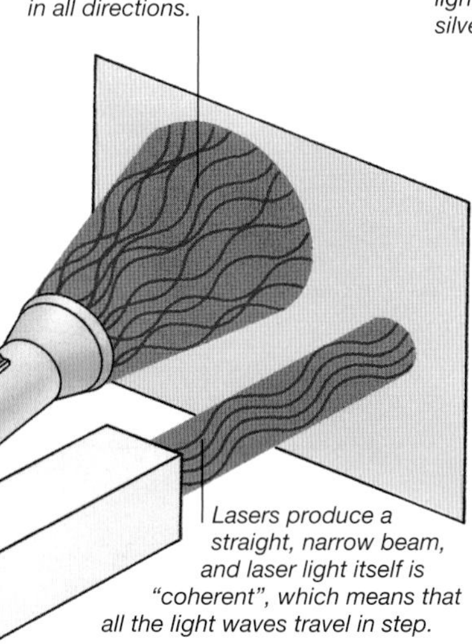

In ordinary light, such as that from a flashlight, light waves are jumbled up together and spill out in all directions.

Lasers produce a straight, narrow beam, and laser light itself is "coherent", which means that all the light waves travel in step.

Laser light bounces back and forth between the mirrors at either end of the tube. Some light gets through the half-silvered mirror at the front.

Gas atoms in laser tube produce laser light.

Tube contains mixture of gases, such as helium and neon.

Electric discharge excites the gas atoms into firing off photons.

Gas laser

This laser sends out a continuous beam of light. "Pulsed" lasers emit the beam in regular rapid bursts.

LASER

An electric spark gives energy to atoms in the laser tube. This extra energy makes some atoms fire off photons – tiny bursts of light. These photons hit other atoms, making them fire off photons too. Mirrors reflect the photons back and forth along the tube, making them bump into more atoms as they go. Some of the photons surge through a "partial" mirror at the front of the laser to form the beam.

An atom has electrons moving around its nucleus.

Electrical energy from power supply boosts an electron into a different energy state.

When the electron returns to its original state, it gives out a photon of laser light.

Laser light hits other atoms, which in turn produce laser light.

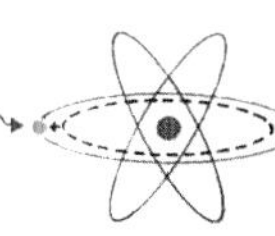

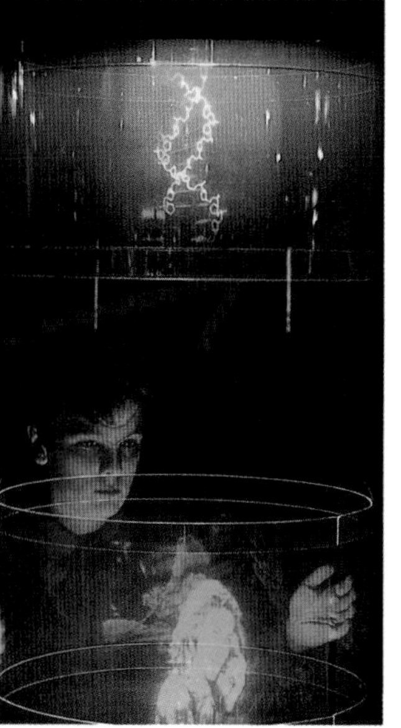

HOLOGRAMS

A hologram is a photograph made with laser light. When you look at a hologram, you see a three-dimensional view of the object, just as with the real thing. Holograms are made by splitting a laser beam into two. One beam, the reference beam, goes straight to the photographic film; the other hits the object of the hologram first, breaking up its neat pattern of light waves. The film records the way the disturbed "object" beam upsets the undisturbed reference beam, producing a three-dimensional image.

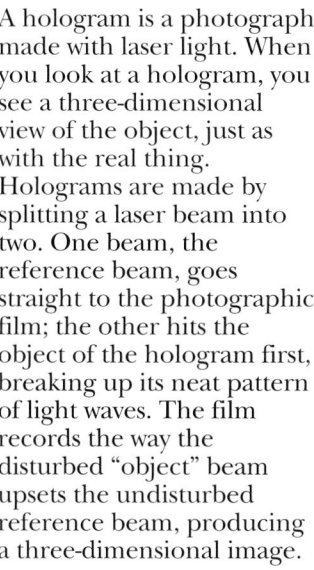

USES OF LASERS
Lasers are used in industry to drill steel and engrave microchips with speed and precision; by engineers to line up bridges and skyscrapers with pinpoint accuracy; in phone networks to carry calls swiftly and clearly through optical fibres; and by doctors to treat cancer and perform delicate eye operations.

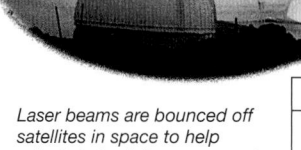

Laser beams are bounced off satellites in space to help scientists track the movement of the Earth's continents.

Find out more

GAS
GEMS AND JEWELLERY
LIGHT
SHOPS AND SHOPPING
SOUND RECORDING

LAW

EVERY SOCIETY HAS its own set of laws to safeguard the rights of its citizens and to balance individual freedom against the needs of the people in general. On the simplest level, there are laws to protect citizens from attack or robbery as they walk along the street. These and other similar rules are called criminal laws. However, the law does much more than provide simple protection. It also settles arguments between individuals. For example, if you believe that you have bought damaged goods, and the person who sold them disagrees, the law must decide who is right. The branch of law that deals with arguments such as these is called civil law. The law is very complex because it must meet the different needs and expectations of society's millions of members. It includes not only civil and criminal branches, but also other smaller divisions, such as family law, which settles arguments when people divorce. Understanding the law takes a long time; lawyers, who apply and interpret the law, study for many years. Most lawyers specialize in just one area of the law.

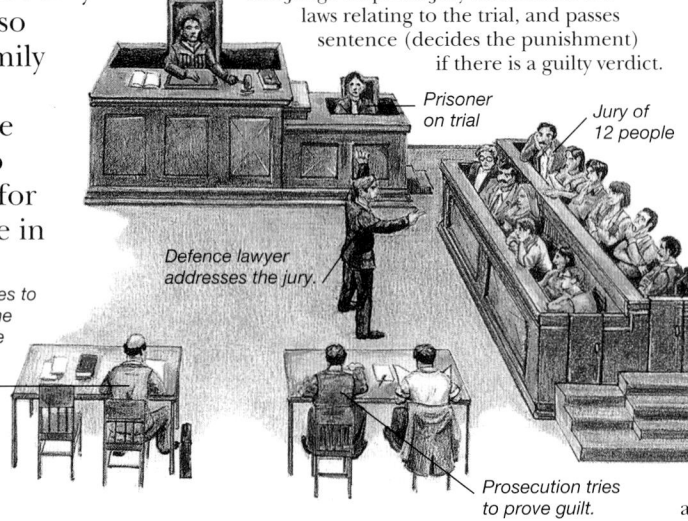

FAIR AND JUST LAW
A statue representing justice wears a blindfold to show that the law does not favour any one person. However, not all law is good law, for governments can make laws that remove freedoms as well as ones that safeguard them. The scales show that justice weighs opposing evidence in the same way that a balance weighs goods. The sword represents punishment.

JUDGES
The judge helps the jury understand the laws relating to the trial, and passes sentence (decides the punishment) if there is a guilty verdict.

Prisoner on trial

Jury of 12 people

Defence lawyer addresses the jury.

Defence tries to convince the jury that the prisoner is not guilty.

Prosecution tries to prove guilt.

DEATH PENALTY
In past centuries a serious crime was punishable by death and, until the mid-19th century, hangings were public. Some countries still apply the death penalty, and in Europe people were executed for murder up to the mid-20th century.

JURY TRIAL

A person accused of a serious crime has the right to a trial by jury, a group of men and women (usually 12) chosen at random from the community. A prosecuting lawyer tries to convince the jury that the defendant – the accused person – is guilty. A defence lawyer sets out to prove the defendant's innocence. Witnesses tell the court what they know about the crime. The jury listens to the facts, or evidence, and decides whether the prosecution has proved guilt.

WORLD LAW

International problems call for worldwide co-operation. Air disasters, for example, may involve companies and individuals from many countries. Lawyers must agree on ways of establishing liability (blame) and compensating people for loss. Many countries share extradition treaties, so that criminals such as terrorists can be sent home for trial if they are caught elsewhere.

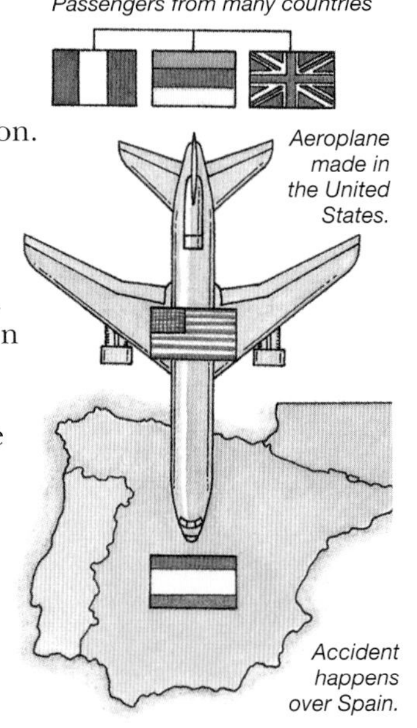

Accident happens over Spain.

ALTERNATIVES TO PRISON
Electronic tags locked to the ankles of criminals keep them at home and out of trouble. A box placed next to the offender's telephone monitors the range of the tag. If the wearer of the tag moves too far away, the box dials up a police central computer and sounds the alarm.

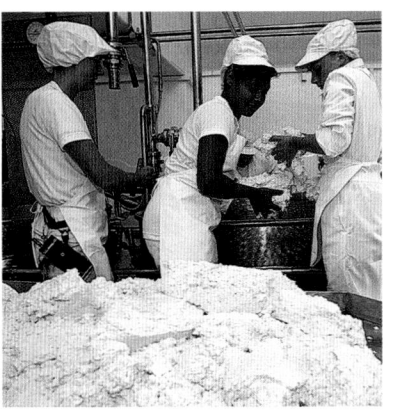

Offenders learn useful skills by following a schedule of duties such as working in the kitchen.

PRISON AND PUNISHMENT
People found guilty of serious crimes usually go to prison. This is to deter them from criminal activity in future and to protect others from danger for the term of their sentence. Prisons also aim to reform offenders – for example by teaching skills to improve their employment prospects on release.

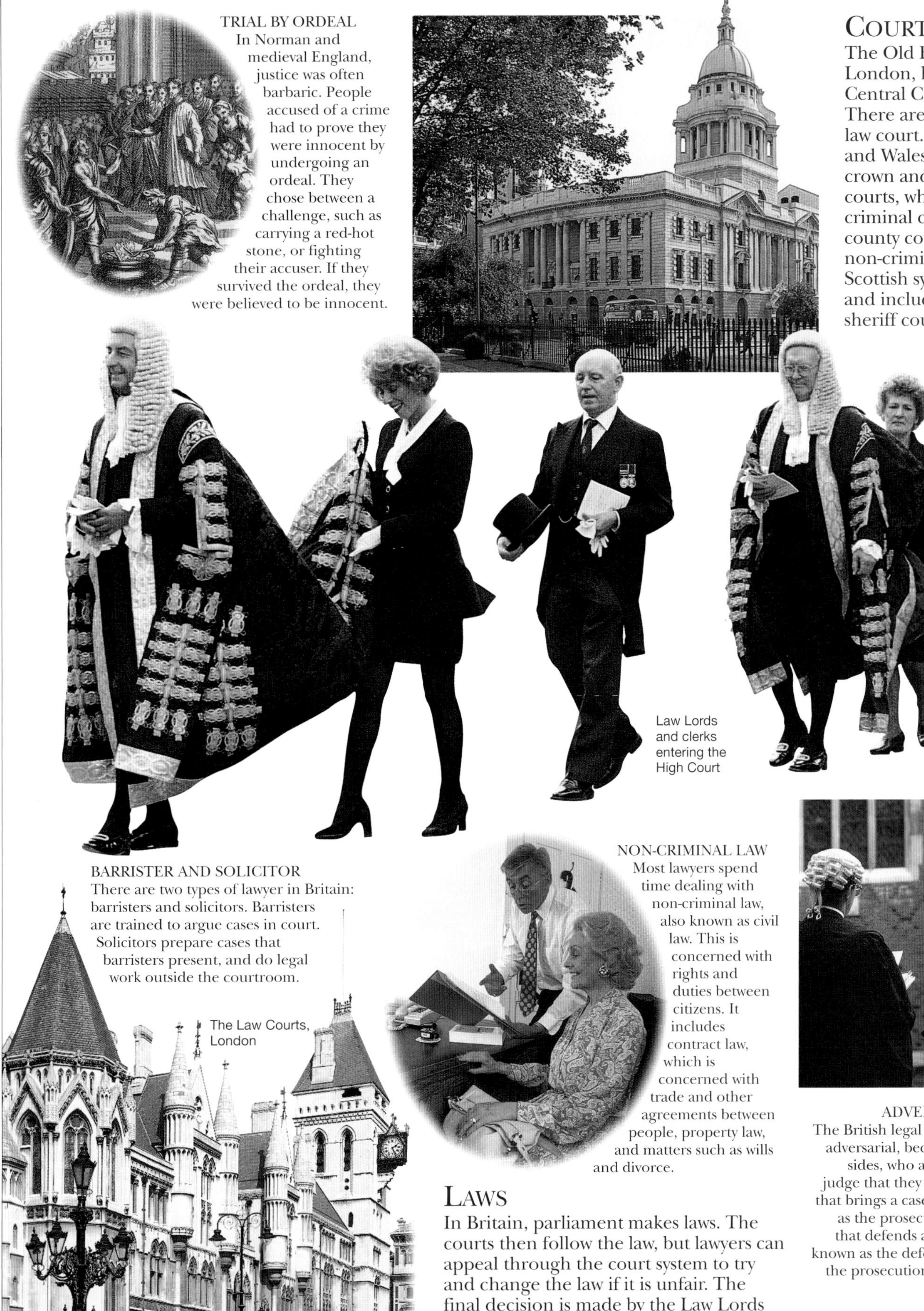

TRIAL BY ORDEAL
In Norman and medieval England, justice was often barbaric. People accused of a crime had to prove they were innocent by undergoing an ordeal. They chose between a challenge, such as carrying a red-hot stone, or fighting their accuser. If they survived the ordeal, they were believed to be innocent.

COURTS

The Old Bailey, in London, houses the Central Criminal Court. There are many types of law court. In England and Wales these include crown and magistrate's courts, which handle criminal cases, and county courts for civil or non-criminal cases. The Scottish system differs, and includes district and sheriff courts.

Law Lords and clerks entering the High Court

BARRISTER AND SOLICITOR
There are two types of lawyer in Britain: barristers and solicitors. Barristers are trained to argue cases in court. Solicitors prepare cases that barristers present, and do legal work outside the courtroom.

The Law Courts, London

NON-CRIMINAL LAW
Most lawyers spend time dealing with non-criminal law, also known as civil law. This is concerned with rights and duties between citizens. It includes contract law, which is concerned with trade and other agreements between people, property law, and matters such as wills and divorce.

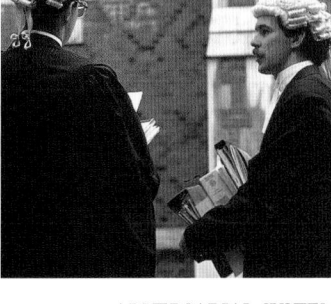

LAWS

In Britain, parliament makes laws. The courts then follow the law, but lawyers can appeal through the court system to try and change the law if it is unfair. The final decision is made by the Law Lords who sit in the House of Lords. British law is based on common law, which dates back to the Anglo-Saxons. Court decisions are based on precedent – previous decisions made on similar court cases.

ADVERSARIAL SYSTEM
The British legal system is known as adversarial, because there are two sides, who argue to convince a judge that they are right. The side that brings a case to court is known as the prosecution, and the side that defends a charge in court is known as the defence. In civil cases, the prosecution is often known as "the plaintiff".

Find out more
ANGLO-SAXONS
GOVERNMENT AND POLITICS
POLICE

Leonardo da Vinci

A HIGHLY TALENTED ARTIST and scientist, Leonardo da Vinci was years ahead of his time. He was one of the greatest figures in the movement called the Renaissance, the revival of art and learning that began in Italy in the 15th century. Today, many people remember Leonardo for painting some of the most famous pictures of his time, but he achieved a great deal more than this. He designed castles and weaponry, invented machines, studied physics and mathematics, and made accurate scientific drawings of plants, animals, and the human body. He was probably one of the world's greatest all-round geniuses.

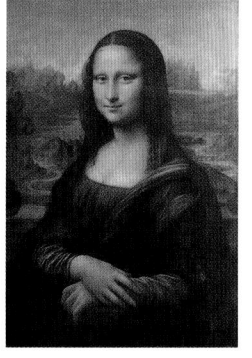

MONA LISA
Leonardo's best-known portrait is of Mona Lisa, the wife of a rich Florentine. The painting is famous for Mona Lisa's haunting smile, and for the softly blended colours, an effect known as *sfumato*. The painting is in the Louvre gallery in Paris.

1452 Born near the village of Vinci, in Italy.

1466 Moves to Florence; works in studio of the artist Verrochio.

1482 Works as architect, engineer, and painter in Milan, in northern Italy.

1503 Begins *Mona Lisa*.

1503 Designs famous flying machine.

1513 Makes pioneering study of lenses and optics.

1515 Studies anatomy.

1516 Dies in France.

Machinery

Leonardo's notebooks are crammed with designs for ingenious machines. Some of these devices, such as a pump, an armoured car, and a machine for grinding lenses, could actually have been built and used. Others, like his famous "ornithopter" flying machine with its flapping wings, would never have worked, but they were still ahead of their time.

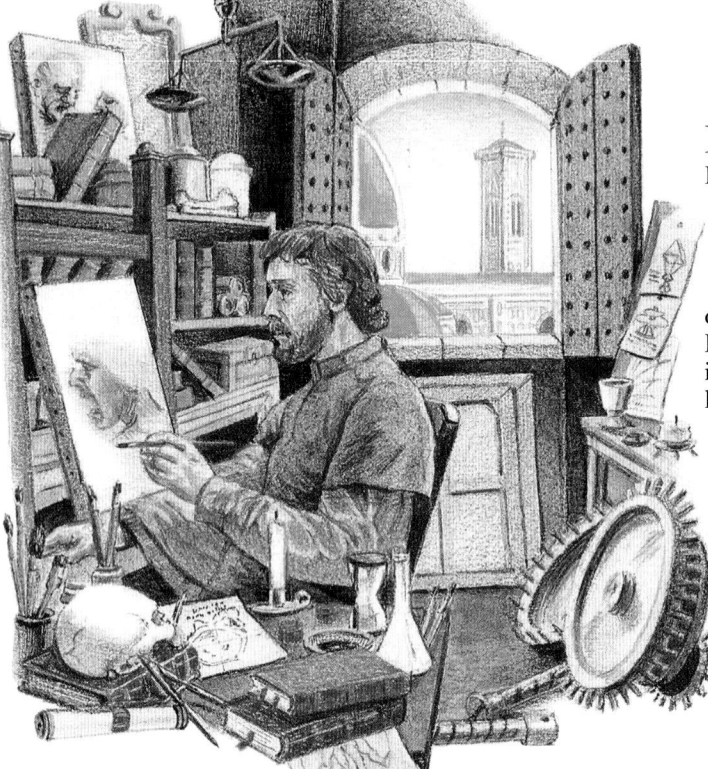

Renaissance man

In Leonardo's time, people believed it was possible for a person to become highly skilled in all branches of learning – such a person was called a "Renaissance man". Leonardo produced new ideas in practically every area he studied. He wrote down many of these ideas in a series of beautifully illustrated notebooks.

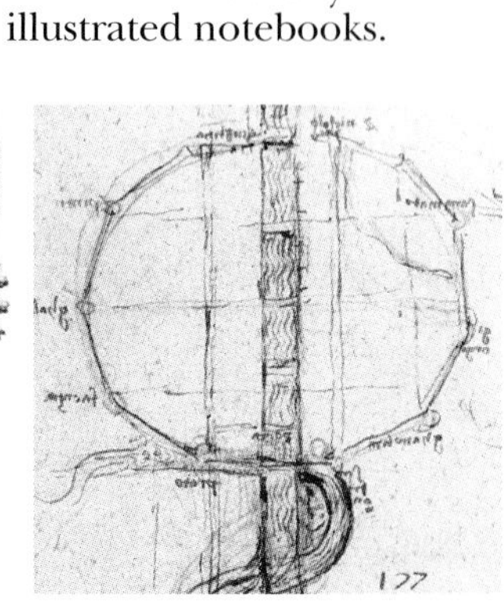

ARCHITECTURE
Buildings and town planning fascinated Leonardo. He designed an "ideal city" which was never built. The streets of the city were arranged in a grid pattern, like a modern American town. He also designed bathhouses, together with drainage networks and systems for rubbish collecting, which were unknown at the time.

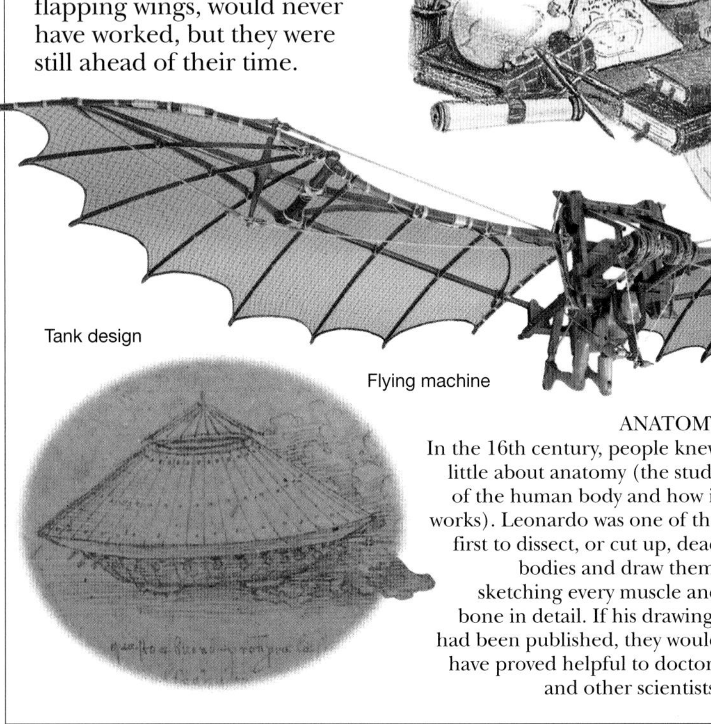

ANATOMY
In the 16th century, people knew little about anatomy (the study of the human body and how it works). Leonardo was one of the first to dissect, or cut up, dead bodies and draw them, sketching every muscle and bone in detail. If his drawings had been published, they would have proved helpful to doctors and other scientists.

Find out more
DRAWING
HELICOPTERS
RENAISSANCE

LEWIS AND CLARK

IN 1804, U.S. PRESIDENT Thomas Jefferson sent Meriwether Lewis and William Clark to lead an expedition to explore the wild and largely unknown lands west of Missouri to the Pacific Ocean. Their instructions were to explore and chart the region, to make contact with Native Americans, and to find out if there was a water link between the Atlantic and Pacific oceans. Lewis and Clark were not experienced explorers, but they successfully led a band of about 40 men, travelling by boat, horse, and foot, some hazardous 13,000 km (8,000 miles) to the Pacific and back. They returned home as heroes with important exciting new information about the region, which later encouraged U.S. expansion westward.

MERIWETHER LEWIS
Lewis (1774-1809) was private secretary to President Jefferson. Co-leader of the expedition, he served as the party's naturalist, collecting animal and plant specimens.

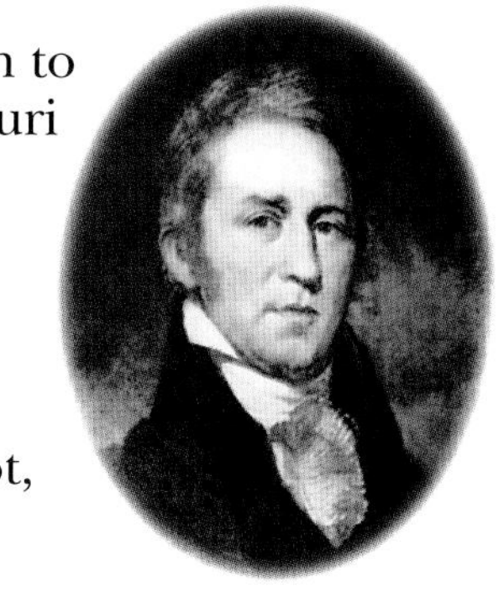

WILLIAM CLARK
Clark (1770-1838) was a lieutenant in the army. He resigned in 1796 but rejoined the army in 1804 to go westward with Lewis. Although untrained, he mapped accurate routes for the expedition and assembled records of the journey for publication.

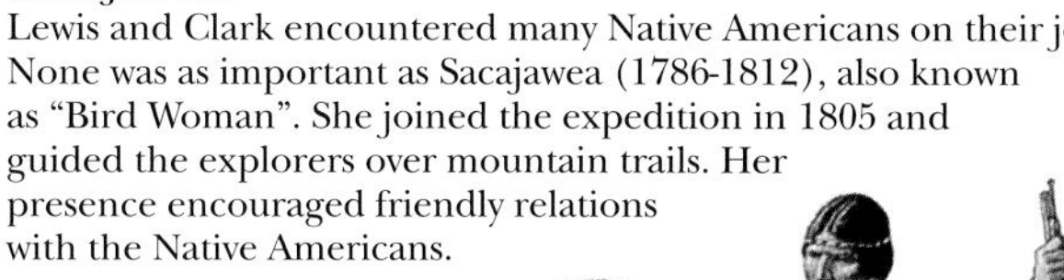

SACAJAWEA
Lewis and Clark encountered many Native Americans on their journey. None was as important as Sacajawea (1786-1812), also known as "Bird Woman". She joined the expedition in 1805 and guided the explorers over mountain trails. Her presence encouraged friendly relations with the Native Americans.

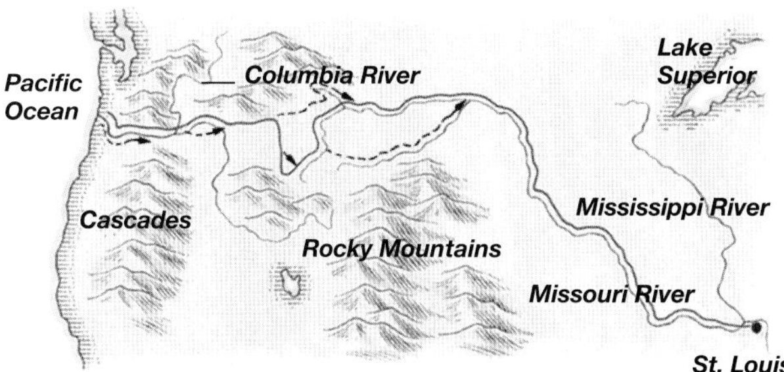

ROUTE OF THE EXPEDITION

The expedition left St. Louis on 14 May 1804, travelling along the Missouri River by boat. In November the explorers reached what is now North Dakota, where they spent the winter with native Mandans. In April 1805, they continued up the Missouri. Leaving the river they struggled on a perilous journey over the Rocky Mountains, then paddled up the Columbia River, finally reaching the Pacific in November. They spent the winter on the Pacific coast, before retracing their steps, arriving back in St. Louis on 23 September 1806.

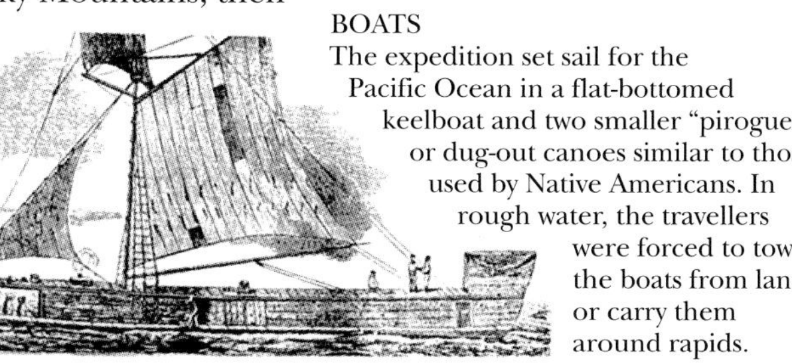

BOATS
The expedition set sail for the Pacific Ocean in a flat-bottomed keelboat and two smaller "pirogues", or dug-out canoes similar to those used by Native Americans. In rough water, the travellers were forced to tow the boats from land or carry them around rapids.

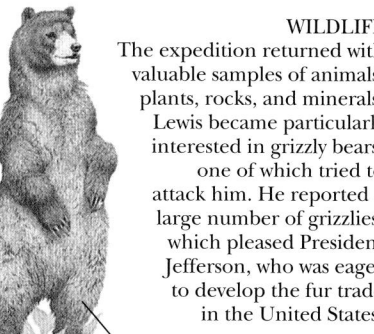

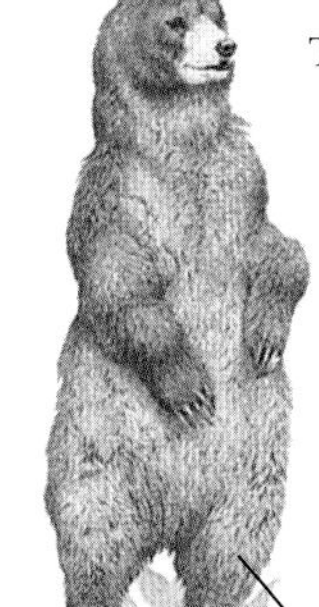

WILDLIFE
The expedition returned with valuable samples of animals, plants, rocks, and minerals. Lewis became particularly interested in grizzly bears, one of which tried to attack him. He reported a large number of grizzlies, which pleased President Jefferson, who was eager to develop the fur trade in the United States.

Grizzly bear

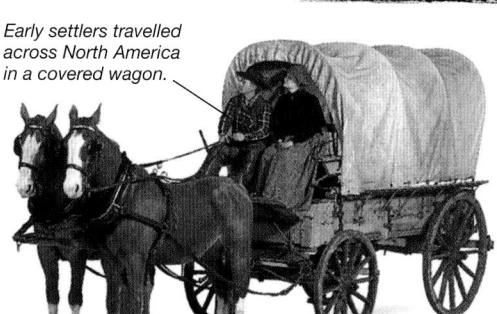

Early settlers travelled across North America in a covered wagon.

WESTWARD EXPANSION

Lewis and Clark's expedition proved there was no direct water link between the Atlantic and Pacific oceans. However, Lewis and Clark's information about the diversity and richness of the lands attracted hundreds of traders and settlers to the West. From the 1840s, increasing numbers made their way on the long journey westward in covered wagons, or prairie schooners.

Find out more

BEARS AND PANDAS
NATIVE AMERICANS
NORTH AMERICAN WILDLIFE
UNITED STATES OF AMERICA
UNITED STATES, HISTORY OF

LIGHT

WITHOUT LIGHT, life on Earth would be impossible. Sunlight provides the energy to make plants grow and keep all living things alive. Light itself is a form of energy which travels as tiny packets of electromagnetic energy called photons. When photons enter our eyes they stimulate special light-sensitive cells so that we can see. Other forms of energy which travel as electromagnetic waves include radio waves, x-rays, and microwaves in microwave ovens. Just as there is a spectrum of colours in light, there is also an electromagnetic spectrum. In fact, light waves are also a type of electromagnetic wave, and the colours in light form a small part of the electromagnetic spectrum. Light waves and all other electromagnetic waves travel at 300,000 km (186,000 miles) per second, which is so fast that they could circle the world almost eight times in a second. Nothing in the universe can travel faster than light.

LIGHT BULB
In the middle of every electric light bulb is a tiny spiral of tungsten wire called the filament. When an electric current is sent through the filament, it warms up so much that it glows white hot. It is the brightly glowing filament that produces light.

Filament made of tungsten metal

Bulb is filled with an inert gas such as argon to keep the filament from catching fire and burning out, as it would do in air.

Filament and electric terminals are sealed into an airtight glass bulb.

Electrical contact is made when the bulb terminal is screwed into the socket.

The explosion of gunpowder inside a firework produces a burst of coloured light.

Nuclear reactions inside the centre of the Sun produce intense heat and light. All stars produce light from nuclear reactions.

BRIGHTNESS OF LIGHT

The further you are from a light, the less bright it will seem. This is because light spreads out in all directions from its source. So when you are far away, the light is spread over a wide area. Many stars, for instance, are much brighter than our Sun, but their light is spread out over so vast an area that by the time it reaches us, the stars do not even seem as bright as a candle.

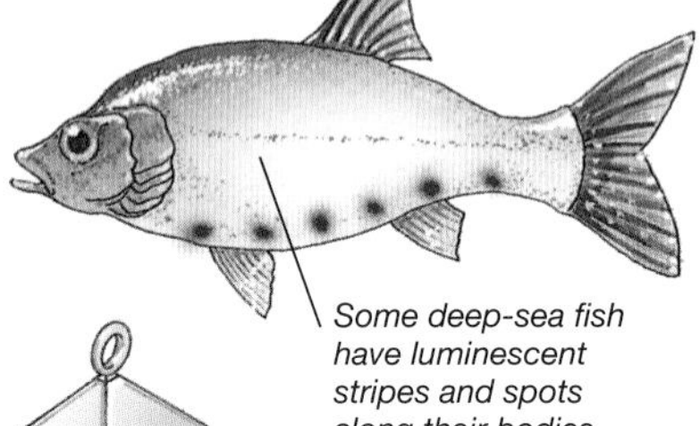

Some deep-sea fish have luminescent stripes and spots along their bodies that give out light.

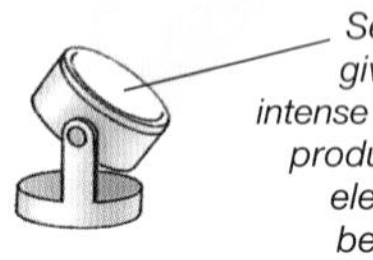

Searchlights give out very intense light, often produced by an electric spark between two pieces of carbon.

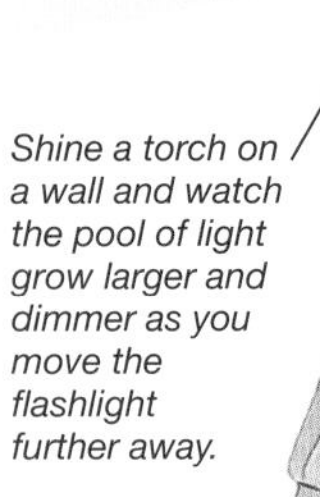

Shine a torch on a wall and watch the pool of light grow larger and dimmer as you move the flashlight further away.

A candle is a wide source of light, so it produces a fuzzy shadow.

Candles and lanterns give out light.

When things burn they give out light as well as heat.

SOURCES OF LIGHT

Many different objects give off light. The Sun, electric light bulbs, and fireworks are incandescent, which means they glow because they are hot. But not all lights are hot. Chemicals, not heat, produce the glowing spots on the bodies of some deep-sea fish. All cool lights, including fluorescent lights, are called luminescent.

LIGHT AND SHADOW
Light travels in straight lines, so, in most cases, it cannot go around obstacles in its path. When light rays hit a solid object, some bounce back and some are absorbed by the object, warming it up a little. The area behind receives no light rays and is left in shadow.

FLUORESCENT LIGHT
A lot of energy in an electric light bulb is wasted as heat. Fluorescent tubes are cooler and more economical. When an electric current is passed through the gas in the tube, gas atoms emit invisible, ultraviolet light. The ultraviolet light strikes phosphors – chemicals in the tube's lining – and makes them glow with a brilliant white light.

MIRRORS

Light passes easily through transparent substances such as glass and water, but not through opaque objects such as paper. Most opaque objects have a rough surface which scatters light in all directions. However, a mirror has a smooth surface, so it reflects light in a regular way. When you look at your face in a mirror, the light bounces straight back, producing a sharp image. Most mirrors are made of glass; your face is reflected from a shiny metal coating at the back of the mirror, not from the glass.

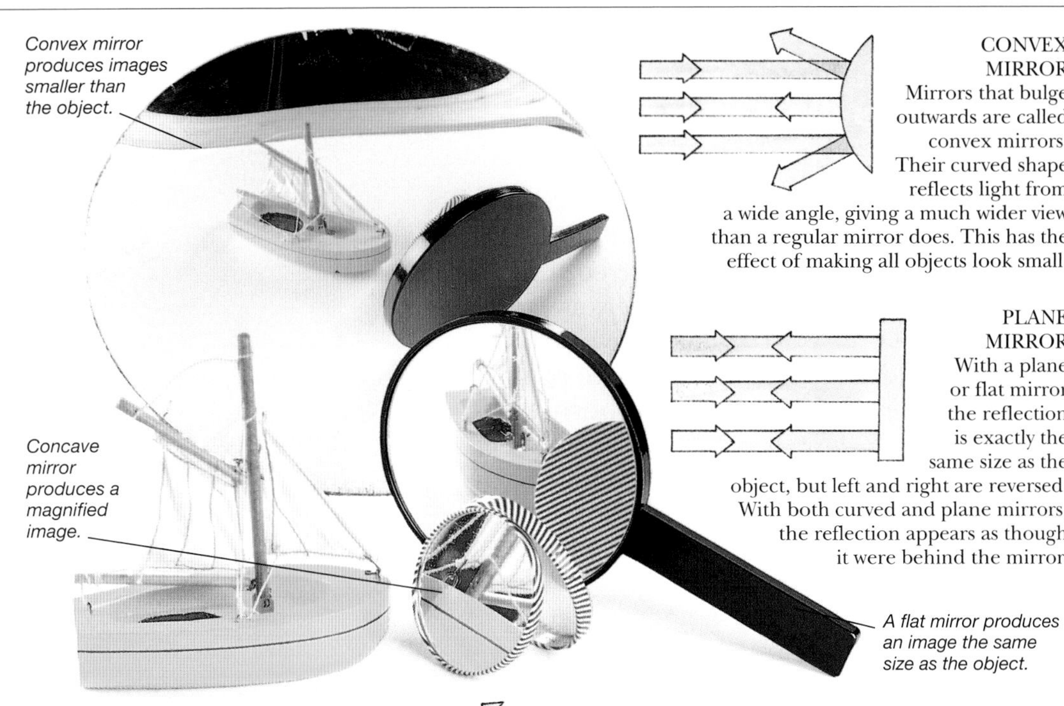

Convex mirror produces images smaller than the object.
Concave mirror produces a magnified image.
A flat mirror produces an image the same size as the object.

CONVEX MIRROR
Mirrors that bulge outwards are called convex mirrors. Their curved shape reflects light from a wide angle, giving a much wider view than a regular mirror does. This has the effect of making all objects look small.

PLANE MIRROR
With a plane or flat mirror the reflection is exactly the same size as the object, but left and right are reversed. With both curved and plane mirrors, the reflection appears as though it were behind the mirror.

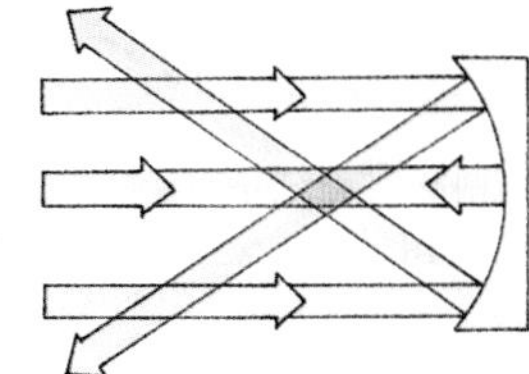

CONCAVE MIRROR
A concave mirror, which is curved inwards, forms two kinds of image. If the object is close to the mirror, the reflection is larger than the real thing. If the object is far away, the image formed is small and upside down.

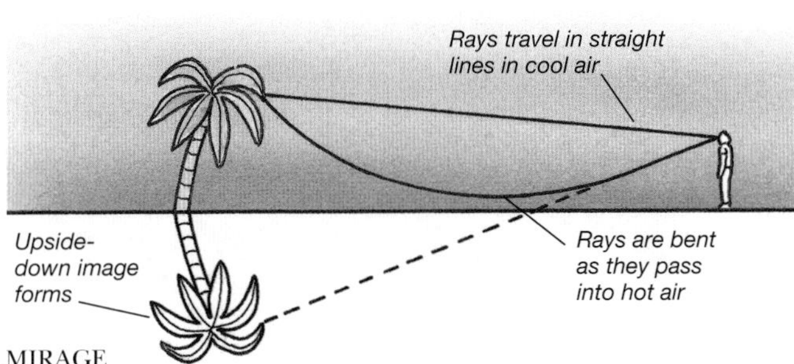

Rays are bent as they pass into hot air

MIRAGE
In the hot desert, weary travellers are often fooled by the sight of an oasis. The oasis appears on the horizon, only to vanish as the travellers hurry towards it. What they have seen is an illusion called a mirage. In the example above, light rays travelling from the palm tree are bent upwards by the warm air. The observer's eyes interpret the light as having travelled in a straight line so he sees a watery reflection of the tree on the ground.

LENSES AND REFRACTION

Glasses, cameras, telescopes, and microscopes use lenses to create particular kinds of images. The lenses in a telescope, for example, produce a magnified view of a distant object. All lenses work on the principle that although light always travels in straight lines, it travels slower through glass than through air. If a light ray strikes glass at an angle, one side of the ray will hit the glass just before the other and will slow down earlier. The effect is to bend the light ray slightly, just as a car pulls to one side if it has a puncture. This bending of light is called refraction.

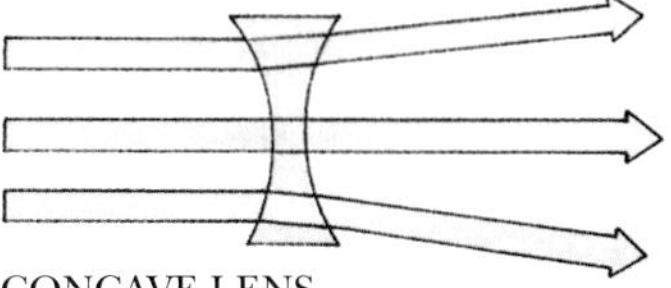

CONCAVE LENS
A concave lens is thicker at the edges than in the centre, so it spreads light rays out. If you look through a concave lens, everything appears smaller.

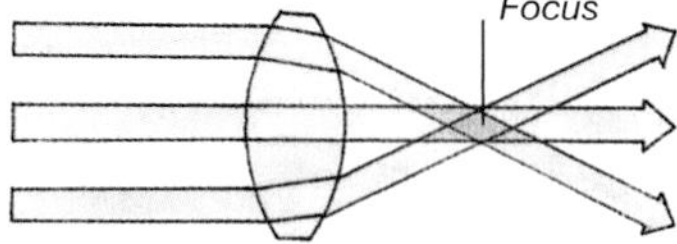

CONVEX LENS
Convex lenses bring light rays together. At the focus, where light rays from a distant object meet, they form an image of the object which can be seen on a screen.

Magnifying glasses are convex lenses.

Light refracts when it passes through water, because the water slows it down. This makes objects look as though they are bent.

FIBRE OPTICS

Fibre optic cables are channels that carry light. They are flexible so they can carry light around corners. The fibres are long, thin filaments of glass; the light bounces back and forth along the inner surface of the glass. Fibre optics are valuable for seeing into awkward places. Doctors can use fibre optic endoscopes to see inside a patient's body without opening the body up.

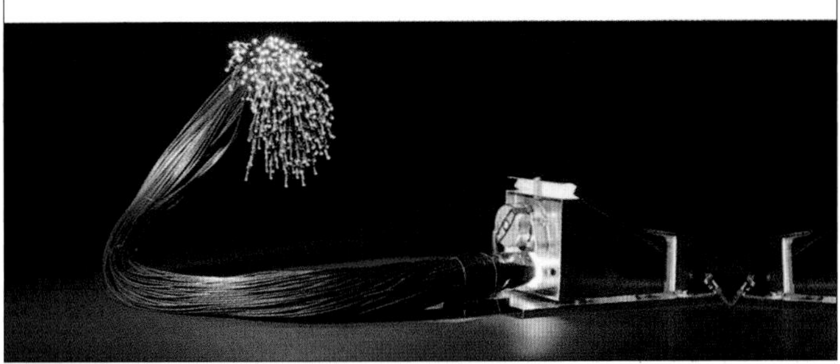

Find out more

CAMERAS
COLOUR
EYES
LASERS
PHOTOGRAPHY
PLANTS
SUN

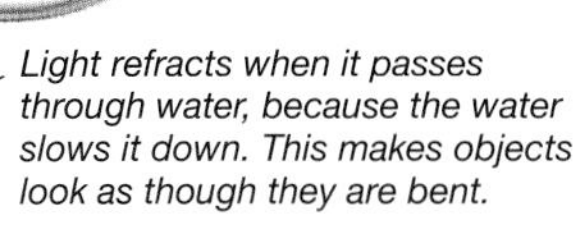

ABRAHAM

LINCOLN

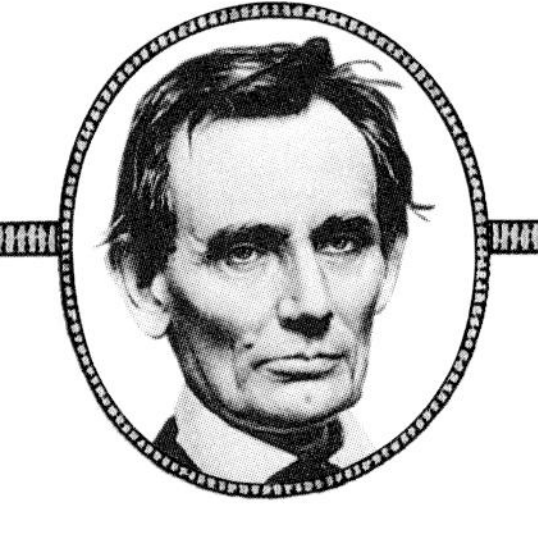

1809 Born in Kentucky.

1831 Moves to New Salem, Illinois, where he worked as a storekeeper, surveyor, and postmaster while studying law.

1834 Elected to state legislature.

1836 Qualifies as a lawyer.

1842 Marries Mary Todd.

1846 Elected to Congress.

1855, 1859 Runs unsuccessfully for Senate.

1860 Elected president.

1861 Mobilizes 75,000 volunteers to put down the southern rebellion.

1863 Issues Emancipation Proclamation.

1864 Re-elected president.

1865 Assassinated.

ONE OF THE MOST FAMOUS PRESIDENTS in history is Abraham Lincoln. But when he was elected in 1860, less than half the country supported him, and he remained very unpopular with many people for the entire five years of his presidency. Lincoln did not approve of slavery, and many landowners in the southern United States still kept slaves. As a result of his election, 11 southern states left the Union and declared themselves an independent Confederacy, or alliance. Civil war then broke out between the Union and the Confederacy. Lincoln was a capable war leader. He struggled to keep the remaining states united behind his leadership. Many people in his own government opposed him. But in 1865 he led the Union states to victory. Afterwards, Lincoln tried to repair the damage done by the war and bring together the two opposing sides.

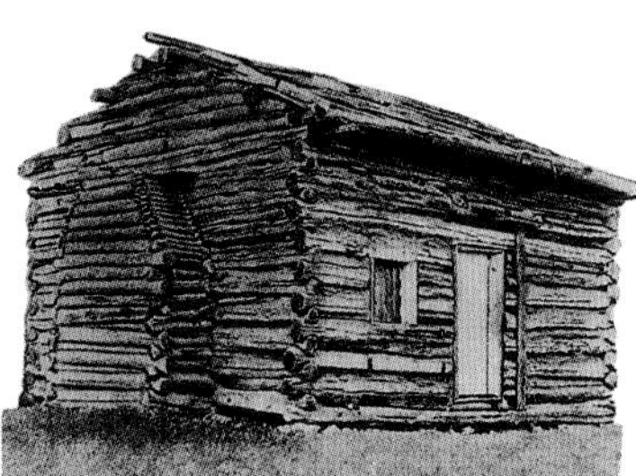

LINCOLN'S BIRTHPLACE
This log cabin in Kentucky, United States, is a replica of the birthplace of Abraham Lincoln. The poverty of Lincoln's childhood influenced his political ideas.

GETTYSBURG ADDRESS

Abraham Lincoln was famous for his speeches. In 1863, he attended the dedication of a national cemetery on the site of the Civil War battlefield in Gettysburg, Pennsylvania. He made a speech known as the Gettysburg Address. He hoped that "these dead shall not have died in vain".

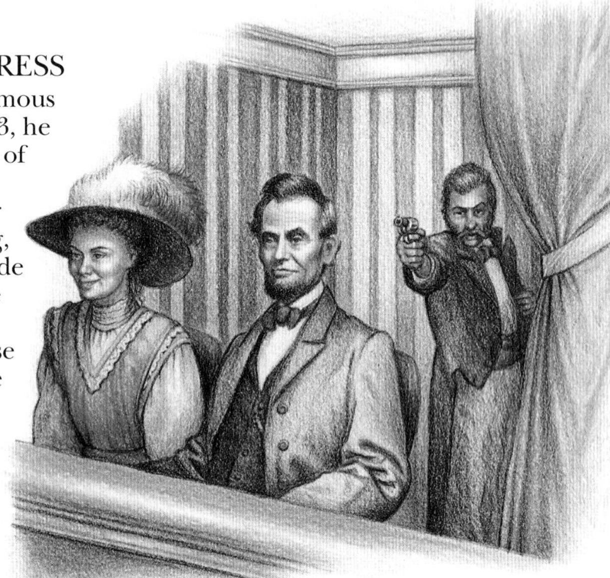

THE DEATH OF LINCOLN
On 14 April 1865, Abraham Lincoln was watching a play at Ford's Theatre in Washington, D.C. John Wilkes Booth, an actor who supported the southern states in the Civil War, crept quietly into the president's box and shot him. The president died of his wounds the next day.

ABOLITION

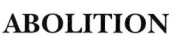

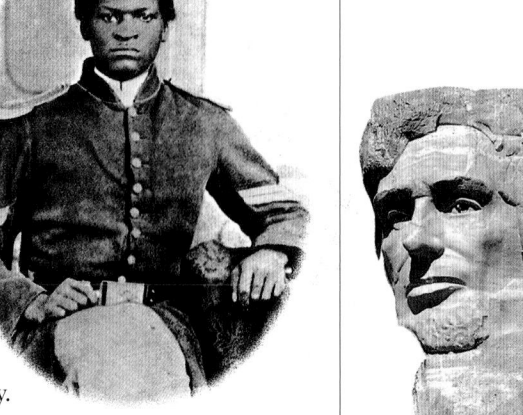

The move to abolish slavery in the United States grew under Lincoln. Led by white middle-class Northerners, many freed slaves joined the abolition movement. Some, such as Andrew Scott (right), fought in the Union army during the Civil War. Slaves fled from South to North (and freedom) via the Underground Railroad – a secret escape route. Harriet Tubman, a famous pioneer of the railroad, helped 300 slaves to escape in this way.

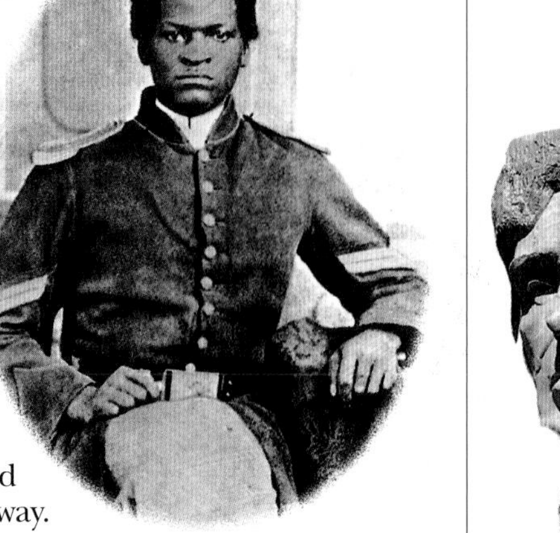

MOUNT RUSHMORE
The faces of four American presidents – George Washington, Thomas Jefferson, Theodore Roosevelt, and Abraham Lincoln – are carved out of rock on the side of Mount Rushmore in the Black Hills of South Dakota, United States.

Find out more

AMERICAN CIVIL WAR
SLAVERY
TUBMAN, HARRIET
UNITED STATES OF AMERICA, history of

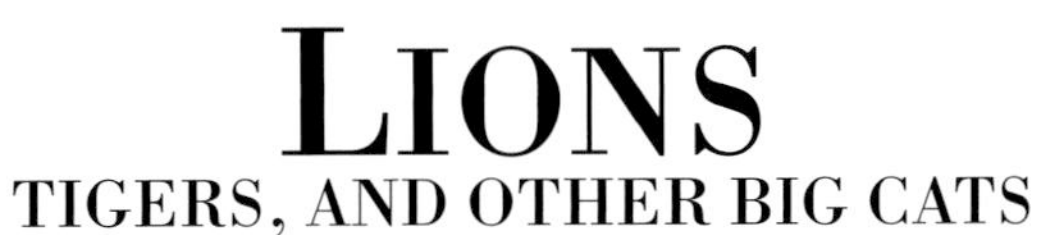

LIONS
TIGERS, AND OTHER BIG CATS

CUBS
Like all young big cats, tiger cubs have pale markings when they are born. After a few months, the pale stripes change to black and orange.

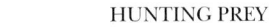

FEW CREATURES ARE HELD in such awe as lions, tigers, cheetahs, and leopards, which we often call the big cats. These agile predators have strong, razor-sharp teeth and claws, muscular bodies, and excellent senses. Their beautiful striped and spotted fur breaks up their outline and camouflages them, allowing them to ambush unwary zebras, giraffes, and other prey. There are seven kinds of big cats. The tiger is the largest. A fully grown tiger may measure more than 3 m (10 ft) from nose to tail; a fully grown lion is almost as big.

The first large cats lived 45 million years ago. Many, including the lion, cheetah, and leopard, still inhabit parts of Africa. Snow leopards and lions dwell in the mountains and forests of Asia. Jaguars are the largest of the big cats in North and South America. They are equally at home swimming in lakes or climbing trees.

HUNTING PREY
Lions live mainly on savannas (grassy plains) and scrubland, and the females do most of the hunting. This picture shows two adult lionesses charging at a young gazelle, separating it from the rest of the herd.

LION PRIDE

Lions are the only big cats that live in groups, called prides, which may be up to 30 strong. The pride roams over an area of 100 sq km (40 sq miles) or more, depending on the abundance of prey in the area. The large male lions protect the pride's territory against other prides. The lions also defend the females against other males.

Lion has a thick, shaggy mane.

Large, strong canine teeth for tearing prey

Large feet and sharp claws

The dominant male is the strongest member of the pride. It can measure 2.5 m (8 ft) in length, and 1 m (3 ft) high at the shoulder.

SKULL AND TEETH
Lions and other big cats have short, strong skulls with powerful jaws. Their spear-like canine teeth are used to grab hold of the victim's flesh. The large molar teeth tear flesh and gristle as the jaw opens and closes.

CARNIVORES
Lions, tigers, and other big cats are true carnivores (flesh eaters). Lions usually eat large prey such as antelopes and zebras. One giraffe is often enough to feed a whole pride of lions.

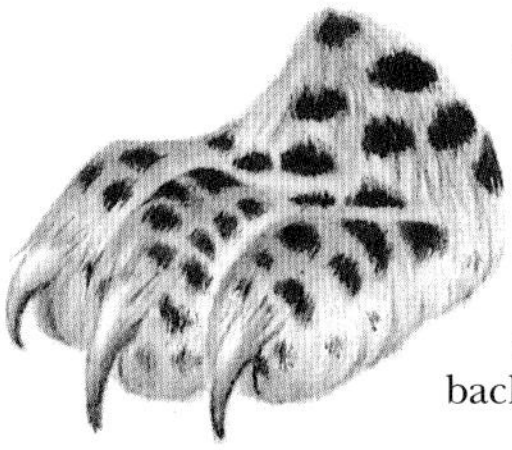

CLAWS OUT
When a cat pounces on a victim or climbs up into a tree, it unsheathes its sharp claws. Muscles in the feet pull the claws out and draw back the sheaths.

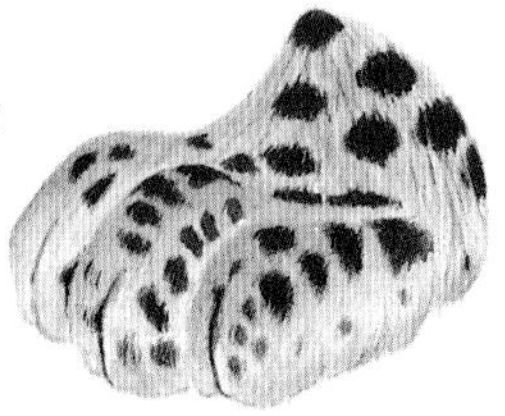

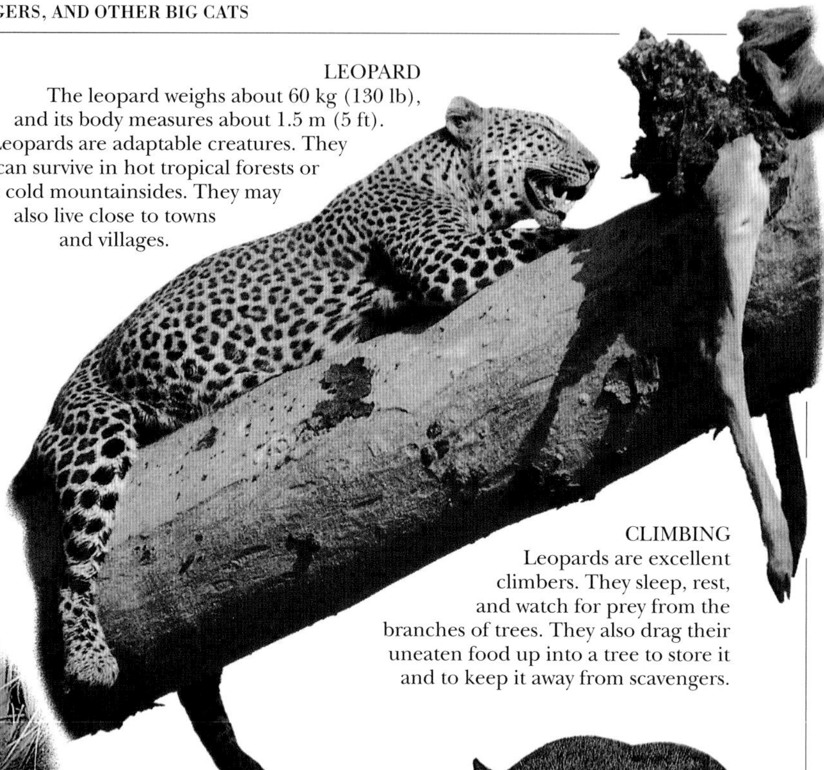

LEOPARD
The leopard weighs about 60 kg (130 lb), and its body measures about 1.5 m (5 ft). Leopards are adaptable creatures. They can survive in hot tropical forests or on cold mountainsides. They may also live close to towns and villages.

CLAWS IN
Most of the time, a cat's claws are protected in muscular sheaths. This keeps the claws sharp and less likely to break. The claws are extended when the cat cleans its feet.

CLIMBING
Leopards are excellent climbers. They sleep, rest, and watch for prey from the branches of trees. They also drag their uneaten food up into a tree to store it and to keep it away from scavengers.

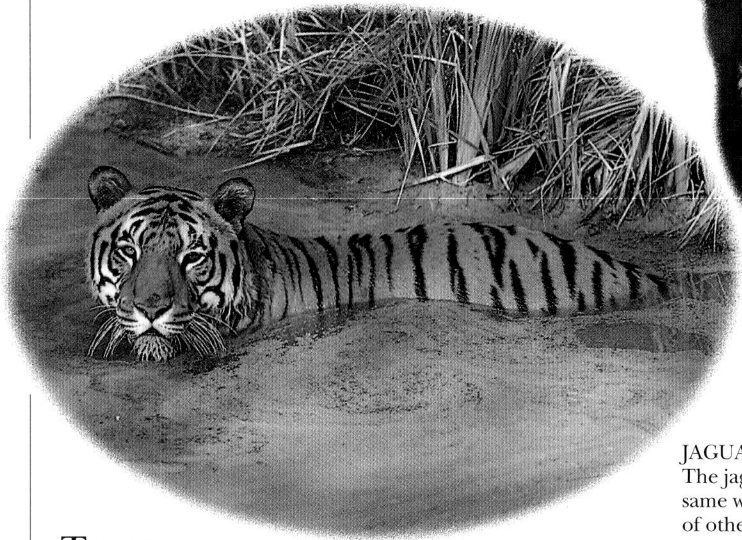

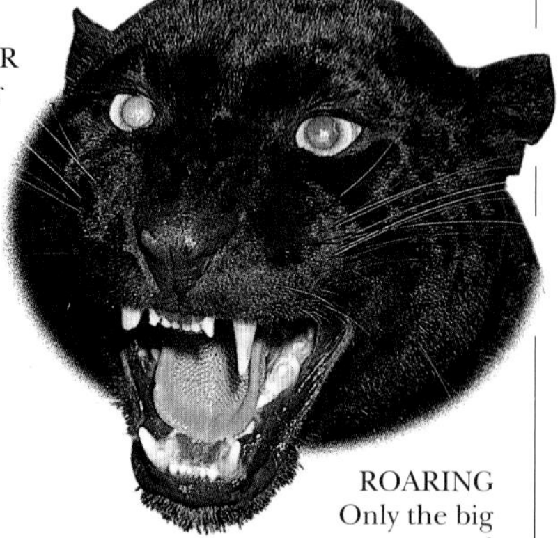

PANTHER
The black panther (right) is a leopard with dark colouring. In daylight, its spots show black in its dark grey-brown fur.

JAGUAR
The jaguar (below) stalks its prey in the same way as the tiger. Jaguars eat a variety of other creatures, including tapirs, fish, frogs, rodents, sloths, and small caimans (South American crocodiles).

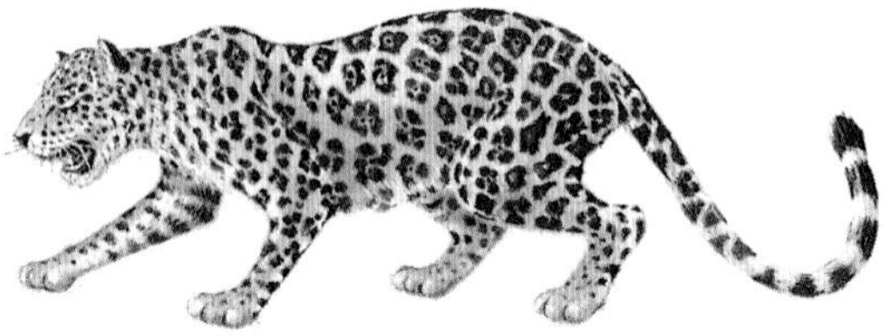

Tiger

Unlike most cats, the tiger does not mind water. A tiger sometimes pulls its dead prey near the water's edge, because it needs to take frequent drinks during a meal. Tigers stalk their prey through dense undergrowth, then bound over the last 15 m (50 ft) or so, taking their victim by surprise. On average, a tiger consumes about 18 kg (40 lb) of meat a day.

ROARING
Only the big cats can roar, and they do so loudly, although the jaguar and snow leopard roar only rarely. The roar is a way of expressing anger, and warns other creatures to keep away.

Cheetah

No animal can outrun a cheetah over a short distance. Cheetahs can speed along at about 100 km/h (60 mph) – as fast as a car. Unlike other cats, the cheetah's claws are always extended, because it has no sheaths to withdraw them into. This gives the cheetah extra grip as it starts its run. If a stalking cheetah is detected before it gets within about 180 m (600 ft) of its prey, it does not make the final dash.

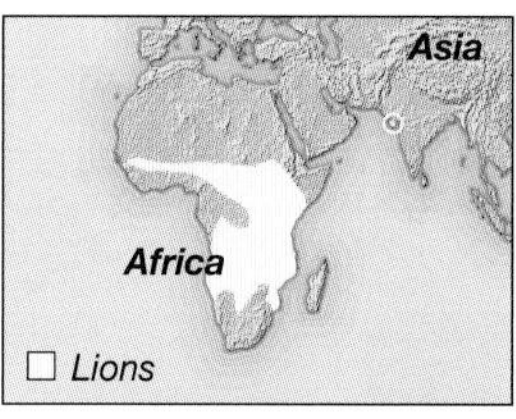

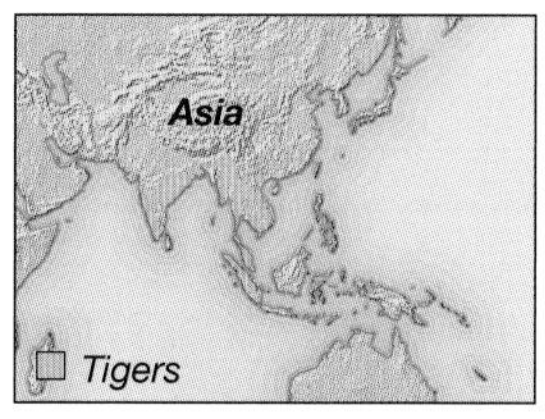

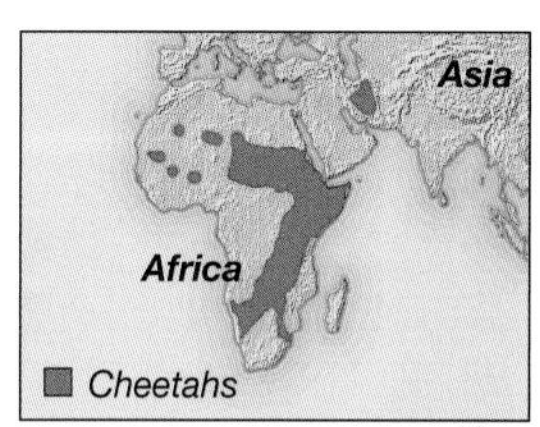

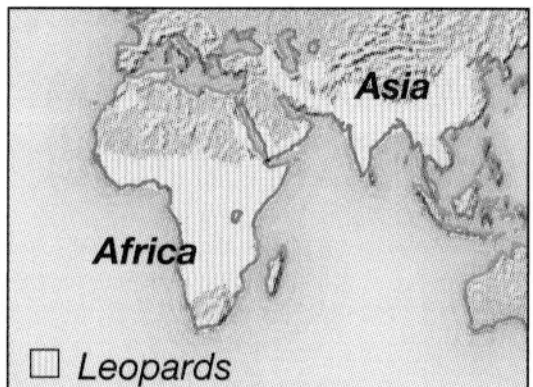

Conservation

Leopards and other big cats have been overhunted for their fur and because they attack livestock and, very rarely, people. The trade in big cats and fur products is now banned by an international agreement. The maps show the main areas of the world where these big cats still live.

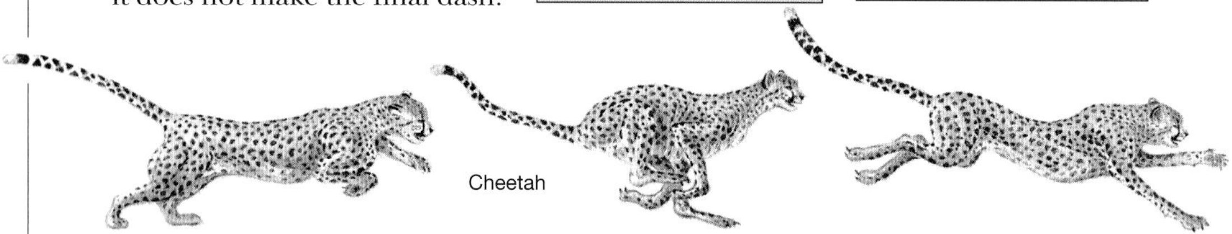

Cheetah

Find out more

African wildlife
Animals
Camouflage, animal
Cats
Conservation and endangered species
Mammals
Zoos

LITERATURE

LITERATURE INCLUDES PLAYS, poems, novels, and short stories. It is writing that carries strong and lasting value through offering the reader important insights into the nature of human emotions. For example, the English playwright William Shakespeare (1564-1616) often based his plays on old or well-known stories, and because Shakespeare was a very skilled writer and had a great understanding of human nature, his plays still excite audiences of all nationalities hundreds of years after they were written. Literature can be powerful, as it can express the writer's thoughts, ideals, and beliefs. Authors, or writers, have often used literature to protest injustice in the world, make a social criticism, and influence the opinions of peoples or governments. For instance, in *The Grapes of Wrath*, American novelist John Steinbeck (1902-68) drew public attention to the suffering of homeless farmers fleeing from Oklahoma to California during the Great Depression of the 1930s.

GULLIVER'S TRAVELS

English author Jonathan Swift (1667-1745) wrote *Gulliver's Travels* in 1726. Although he did not write the book for children, the first two parts have long been popular with young people.

When the people of Lilliput find Gulliver sleeping in their land, they tie him down on the ground so that he cannot move.

The arrogant and petty-minded Lilliputians represent the ruling class of 18th-century England.

PLOT

The collection of events that occur in a work of literature is called the plot. *Gulliver's Travels* tells the story of Lemuel Gulliver, a ship's surgeon. In the first part, Gulliver is shipwrecked in an imaginary land called Lilliput, where the people are only a few centimetres tall. In the second tale, he meets the giants of Brobdingnag. In the third story, Gulliver visits various strange lands. Finally he is marooned among the Houyhnhnms – a race of horses that are wiser and more intelligent than their repulsive human servants, the Yahoos. Rejected by the Houyhnhnms, Gulliver returns to England, where he is no longer able to tolerate the company of other humans.

The Lilliputian politicians discuss new wars against their enemies.

THEME

Writers use their plots and characters to explore key themes such as love, death, morality, and social or political issues. *Gulliver's Travels* seems just an adventure story, but the underlying theme is 18th-century England, where the Lilliputians and other nationalities represent different types of people with their good and bad qualities.

CHARACTERS

An essential part of most literature is the writer's description of the characters – the people who take part in the plot. A writer portrays a character's personality by describing how they react to events in the story. For example, Swift shows that Gulliver was a kindhearted man by describing how he entertained the tiny Lilliputian people: "I would sometimes lie down, and let five or six of them dance on my Hand. And at last the Boys and Girls would venture to come and play at Hide and Seek in my Hair."

ORAL LITERATURE

Long before writing was invented, storytelling, or oral literature, was used to pass on myths and history. The heroine of a traditional Arabic story called *The Thousand and One Nights* is a storyteller named Scheherazade (right). Her cruel husband vows to kill her in the morning, but she charms him with a tale and so delays her death. Each night she tells another story and lives for one more day. After many stories her husband changes his mind and spares Scheherazade's life.

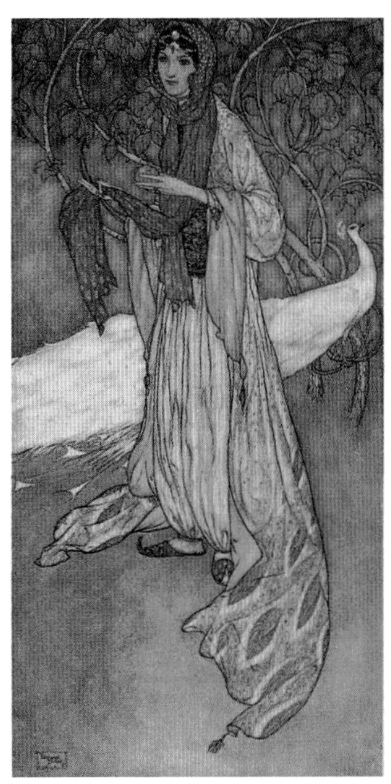

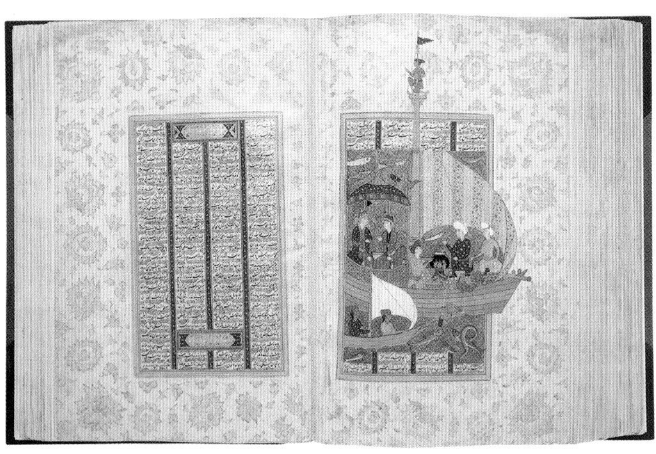

This copy of the *Book of Kings* is written in Arabic script.

EPICS AND SAGAS

Epics and sagas tell of legendary heroes and their deeds. An epic tells the story as a long poem, while a saga is written in prose. The national Persian epic, the *Book of Kings (Shah-nameh)* by Firdausi (c.935-1020), is 1,000 years old, and tells the story of Persian kings and their battles against monsters in mythical times. Other great epics include Homer's *Iliad* and *Odyssey*; Virgil's *Aeneid*; *Beowulf*, a 10th-century epic written in Old English; and John Milton's *Paradise Lost* and *Paradise Regained*.

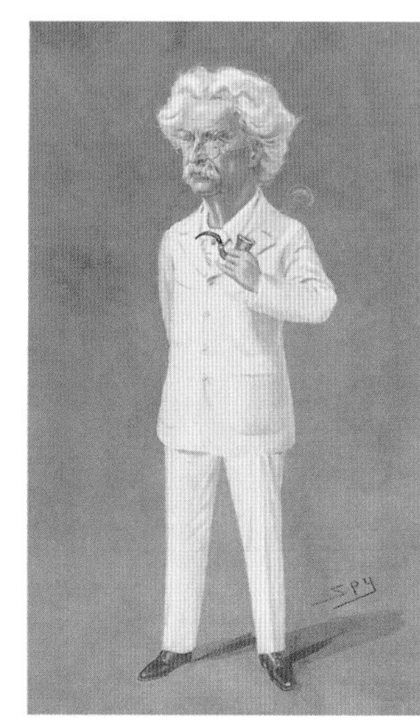

BIOGRAPHY

A biography is a book that describes a person's life. In an autobiography the author writes of his or her own life. US writer Mark Twain (right) was portrayed in J. Kaplan's biography *Mr. Clemens and Mark Twain* (the title refers to Twain's real name, Samuel Langhorne Clemens).

Poetry

Poetry is different from other forms of literature because it usually has rhythm and rhyme. In a rhythmic poem, such as a song, the accents or beats in each line follow a pattern that is repeated in each verse. In poems that rhyme, lines end with words that sound similar. One of the world's greatest poets was the American Walt Whitman (1810-92), whose poems express a great love of his country and its people. His collection of poems *Leaves of Grass* (1855) is considered one of his best works.

Novels

A novel is a long story about fictional (unreal) characters, which is written in prose. This form of writing only began in the early 17th century, and has had a dramatic rise in popularity because there are novels to suit all tastes. Some offer insights into everyday life, and some tell of fantastic adventures that keep you turning the pages. American author Louisa May Alcott wrote *Little Women* (1868-69), which tells the story of four sisters and their lives. This remains one of the best-loved children's books ever written. Many successful modern authors are now rewarded with high incomes from sales of their books, as well as from cinema films based on their novels.

Louisa May Alcott

Drama

Literature that is written to be performed by actors is called drama. Different countries have their own forms of drama. There is little scenery in Japanese Noh drama (below), which was first performed in the 14th century. The all-male actors use dance, mime, and masks for each performance, which can last for several hours. Noh drama is influenced by the religious beliefs of Buddhism and Shintoism.

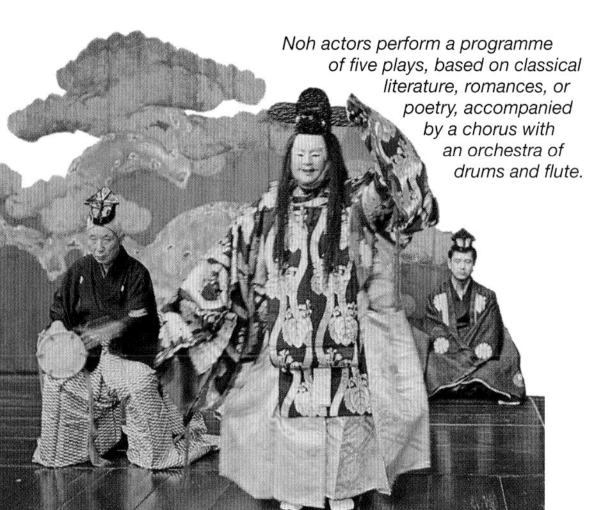

Noh actors perform a programme of five plays, based on classical literature, romances, or poetry, accompanied by a chorus with an orchestra of drums and flute.

STORIES

Most stories describe a single incident or events that take place over a short period of time. There are children's stories about every subject ranging from adventures to ghosts. One of the best-known story writers was the Danish author Hans Christian Andersen (1805-75), who wrote tales such as *The Emperor's New Clothes* and *The Ugly Duckling*.

A Hans Christian Andersen story, The Princess and the Pea, *tells how a single pea beneath a heap of mattresses keeps a princess awake all night.*

Find out more

Books
Printing
Theatre
Writers and poets

LITERATURE

LITERATURE WRITTEN IN ENGLISH FIRST APPEARED during the eighth century. The earliest literature was written in Old English, but after the Norman invasion of 1066 the language altered until it became a form called Middle English. Eventually, the language evolved into the modern English we speak and write today. As British society changed, so did its literature. Popular styles ranged from the riddles of the 17th-century Metaphysical poets to the amusing satires of the 18th-century political and social observers. Writers inspired by Shakespeare's works wrote for the theatre. Perhaps the greatest success of all is the novel, whose content caters for every reader – from humour to tragedy, from historical romance to science fiction.

Geoffrey Chaucer

THE BEGINNINGS

The earliest major work is the poem *Beowulf*, written in the 8th century A.D. The most famous writer of the Middle Ages is Geoffrey Chaucer (1340-1400). His *Canterbury Tales* is a series of stories in verse told by pilgrims journeying to Canterbury. Each story matches the character of its teller.

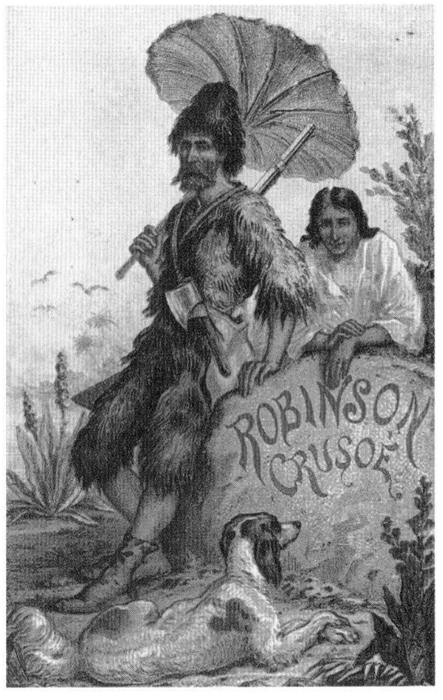

EARLY PROSE

Prose stories developed from the medieval romances and fables. An early prose writer was Daniel Defoe (1660-1731), whose story *Robinson Crusoe* (1719) tells of a castaway's adventures.

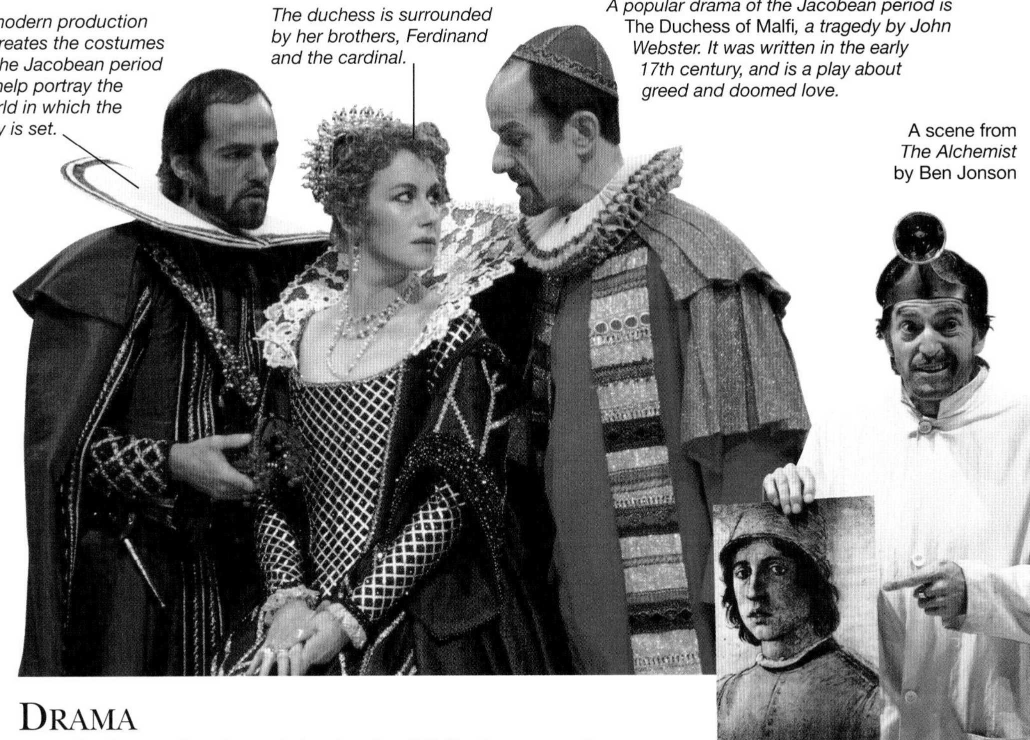

A modern production recreates the costumes of the Jacobean period to help portray the world in which the play is set.

The duchess is surrounded by her brothers, Ferdinand and the cardinal.

A popular drama of the Jacobean period is The Duchess of Malfi, *a tragedy by John Webster. It was written in the early 17th century, and is a play about greed and doomed love.*

A scene from *The Alchemist* by Ben Jonson

DRAMA

British drama has its origins in the Biblical scenes that monks acted out in church. The Elizabethan Age was the highpoint of British drama. The first playhouses were built in London and people flocked to see popular works by dramatists such as William Shakespeare and Christopher Marlowe. Jacobean theatre was characterized by its dark tragedies, while the Restoration period was known for its comedies. After a period of decline, British drama was resurrected in the late Victorian period. In the 20th century, a boom in commercial theatre led to a diversity of theatrical styles.

JACOBEAN DRAMA

Drama written during the reign of James I (ruled 1603-25) is famous for its spectacle and violent action. Revenge was a common theme. Well-known dramatists include Ben Jonson, John Webster, and Francis Beaumont.

SCOTTISH AND WELSH LITERATURE

Early stories were written in the native languages of Scotland and Wales. From the 16th century onwards, many authors wrote in English. Scottish writers include Sir Walter Scott, Robert Burns, and Robert Louis Stevenson. The poet Dylan Thomas is the most popular Welsh literary figure.

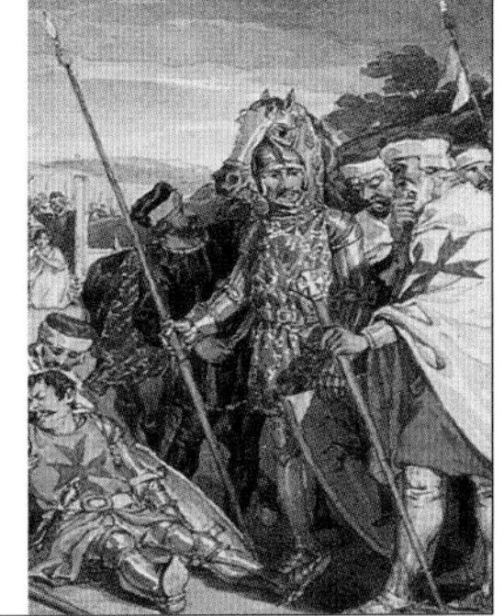

Illustration from *Ivanhoe* by Sir Walter Scott

THE ROMANTICS

In the early 19th century, poets such as John Keats, Percy Bysshe Shelley, and Lord Byron began to write with greater passion and emotion. They stressed the value of their personal experience, wrote about the natural world, and tried to imitate the speech of ordinary people in their poetry. A famous Romantic poet was William Wordsworth (1770-1850), who lived in the Lake District and was inspired by the region's wild beauty.

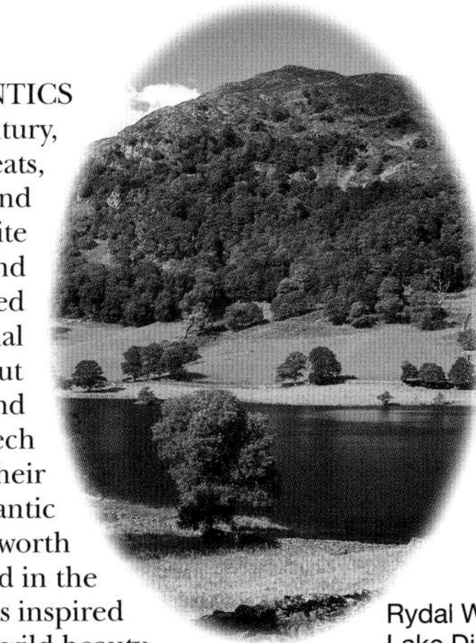

Rydal Water, Lake District

MODERN POETRY

English poetry is now more varied than ever before. Many of today's poets do not follow old-fashioned rules of rhyme and metre. They use a variety of kinds of language – from street slang to the forms of English used in different regions and by diverse ethnic groups. Some poets write their work to be performed in front of an audience, often to the accompaniment of music.

Dub poets such as Benjamin Zephaniah (left) and Linton Kwesi Johnson write poetry that follows the rhythms of reggae music.

LYRIC POETRY

The words of songs are known as lyrics because lyric poetry was originally written to be sung. A lyric poem is a short poem that expresses the thoughts and feelings of its poet. It can deal with any subject, from something the poet has seen to a momentous event. A dramatic battle in the Crimean War inspired Alfred, Lord Tennyson to write "The Charge of the Light Brigade" in 1854.

NOVEL

Since its initial appearance in the 18th century, the novel has become the most popular type of British literature. Victorian novelists, such as Jane Austen, Elizabeth Gaskell, Thomas Hardy, and Charles Dickens, wove long, gripping stories around memorable characters. In the 20th century, novelists from D.H. Lawrence to George Orwell kept the form popular, and used it to tackle important issues of the day.

BRONTE SISTERS

Some of the finest novels of the 19th century were written by the three Brontë sisters – Charlotte (1816-55), Emily (1818-48), and Anne (1820-49). Their novels depict women's lives and relationships with a frankness that was considered radical at the time of their original publication.

Anne wrote Agnes Grey *(1847) and* The Tenant of Wildfell Hall *(1848).*

Charlotte wrote Jane Eyre *(1847).*

Emily wrote Wuthering Heights *(1847).*

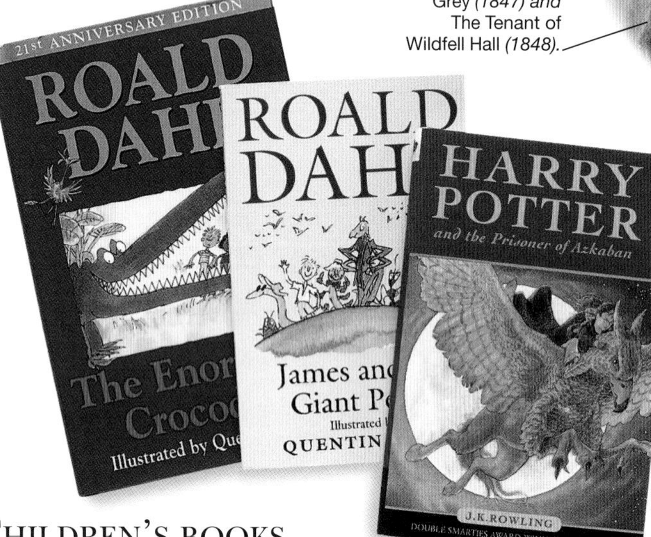

DETECTIVE STORIES

For more than a hundred years, millions of readers have enjoyed trying to solve the mysteries in detective stories. A detective story features a central character – usually an amateur detective – who has to solve one or more crimes. As a result, these books are also called "whodunnits". The first popular detective was Sherlock Holmes, who appeared in several books by Sir Arthur Conan Doyle (1859-1930). Other popular authors include Wilkie Collins, Agatha Christie, Ruth Rendell, and Ian Rankin.

CHILDREN'S BOOKS

Many authors write books especially for children. Successful children's books often share key ingredients – stories that engage you, a good mix of characters, and plenty of surprises. The most popular children's writers, such as Roald Dahl (1916-90), combine all these features and add something special of their own – in Dahl's case, a nasty character or two who get what they deserve.

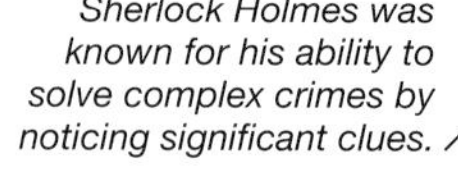

Sherlock Holmes was known for his ability to solve complex crimes by noticing significant clues.

UK LITERATURE

c. 700-1500 Authors write in Old and Middle English.

1533-1603 Poetry and drama develop during the Elizabethan period.

1603-25 Jacobean dramatists write dark tragedies. Poets develop the Metaphysical style.

1728 Alexander Pope writes a satirical poem *The Dunciad.*

1749 Henry Fielding writes *Tom Jones*, an early novel.

1798 *Lyrical Ballads* by S.T. Coleridge and William Wordsworth launches the Romantic movement.

1840s The novel develops rapidly into a major form.

1913 D.H. Lawrence publishes *Sons and Lovers.*

1922 T.S. Eliot's poem "The Waste Land" sets a fresh standard for modern poetry. James Joyce's *Ulysses* offers new scope to the novel.

1960s Feminism brings a new prominence to literature written by women.

Find out more

LITERATURE
POETRY
THEATRE
UNITED KINGDOM, HISTORY OF
WRITERS AND POETS

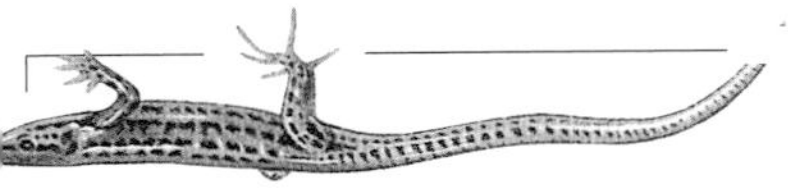

LIZARDS

THE LARGEST GROUP of reptiles is the lizard family, with about 4,300 kinds. Lizards live in almost every habitat except the open sea and the far north. The huge Komodo dragon is the largest, and tiny geckos are the smallest – some are less than 2 cm (1 in) long. A typical lizard such as the iguana has a slim body, a long tail, legs that splay out sideways, and five-toed feet. There are many variations, however; skinks are often extremely long, with short legs. They seem to move effortlessly through loose soil with a wriggling motion. Snake-lizards are even more snake-like, with no front legs and small, paddle-shaped back legs. Several kinds of lizards, including the slow-worm, have lost their limbs during the course of evolution. Like other reptiles, most female lizards lay eggs, which they bury in the soil or hide under rocks until the young hatch.

Long tail for balance

Typical scaly skin like other reptiles, such as snakes and crocodiles

Outstretched claws give extra balance.

Lizards can hear through their ear openings.

Green iguana

CRESTED WATER DRAGON

This lizard is found in Asia and lives mainly in trees that grow close to water. Like most lizards, the water dragon is able to swim. Unlike most other lizards, however, which move on all four legs, the crested water dragon runs on two legs if it is threatened, which gives it more speed on land.

LIZARD TAILS

In the same way that a starfish regrows its arms, a lizard can regrow its tail. When a predator such as a bird or cat grabs a lizard by its tail, the lizard sheds the tail in order to escape. The vertebrae (backbones) along the tail have cracks in them, so the tail breaks off easily. The broken-off part of the tail often twitches for a few minutes, confusing the enemy while the lizard runs away. The tail grows back to its original length in about eight months.

Tree skink has lost the end of its tail.

Tail has regrown fully within a few months.

Loose skin around neck looks like a huge collar.

The more the frilled lizard opens its mouth, the more the frill expands.

Tail waves around to frighten enemy.

FRILLED LIZARD

The Australian frilled lizard has a flap of loose skin around its neck which folds flat along the body. The lizard raises the frill to make itself look bigger in order to scare away a predator. It also waves its tail and head around to alarm its enemy, then scuttles away.

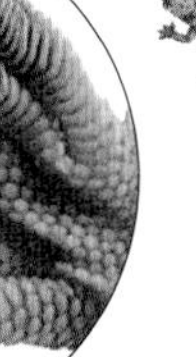

Tokay gecko

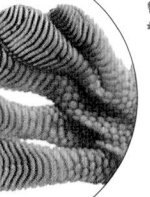

TOKAY GECKO

The pads on the feet of the tokay gecko are covered with about one million microscopic hair-like structures which help the gecko grip on to surfaces. The rubber soles of plimsolls and walking boots look like the soles of the gecko's feet.

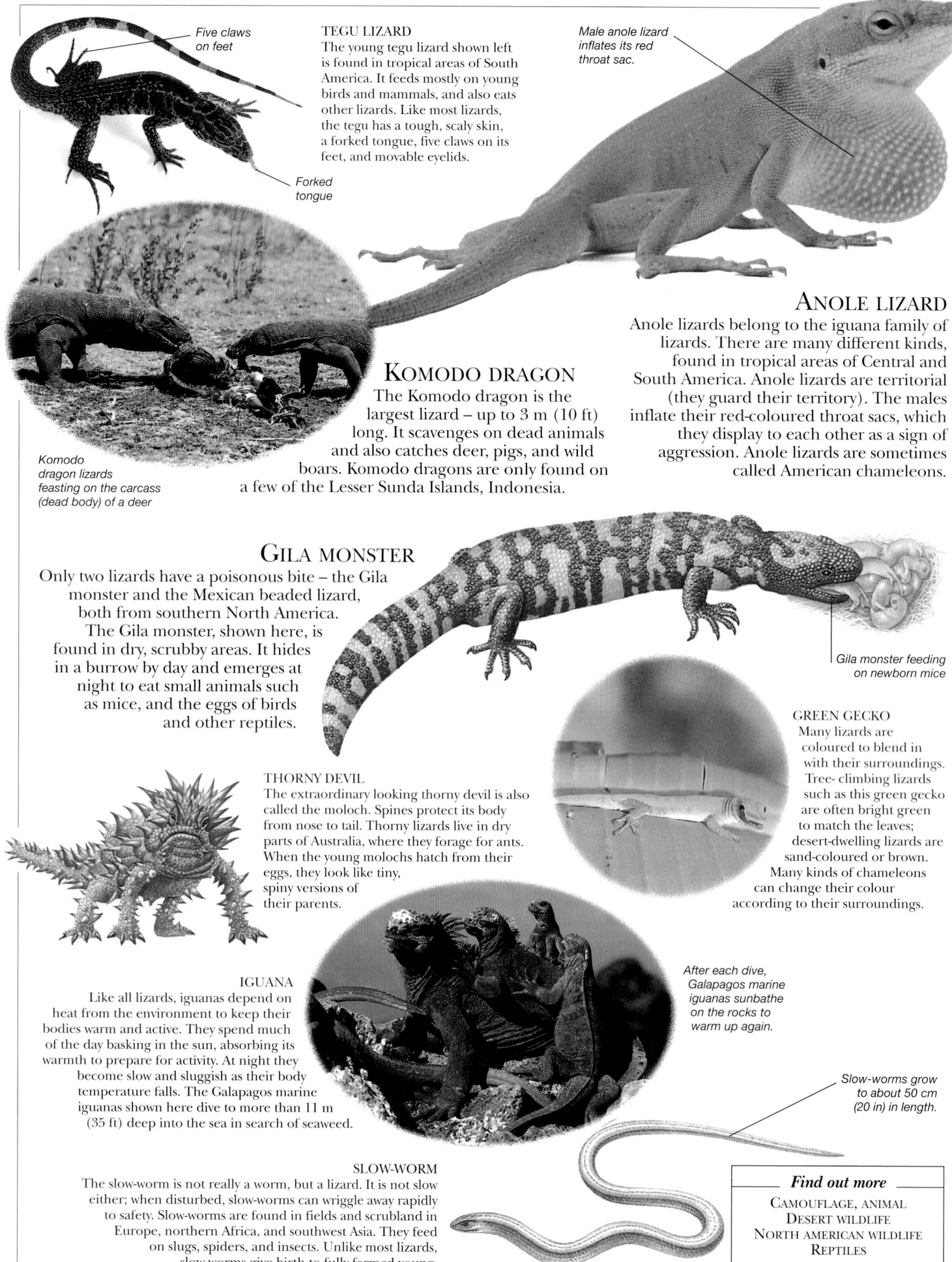

Slow-worms grow to about 50 cm (20 in) in length.

TEGU LIZARD

The young tegu lizard shown left is found in tropical areas of South America. It feeds mostly on young birds and mammals, and also eats other lizards. Like most lizards, the tegu has a tough, scaly skin, a forked tongue, five claws on its feet, and movable eyelids.

Anole lizard

Anole lizards belong to the iguana family of lizards. There are many different kinds, found in tropical areas of Central and South America. Anole lizards are territorial (they guard their territory). The males inflate their red-coloured throat sacs, which they display to each other as a sign of aggression. Anole lizards are sometimes called American chameleons.

Komodo dragon

The Komodo dragon is the largest lizard – up to 3 m (10 ft) long. It scavenges on dead animals and also catches deer, pigs, and wild boars. Komodo dragons are only found on a few of the Lesser Sunda Islands, Indonesia.

Komodo dragon lizards feasting on the carcass (dead body) of a deer

Gila monster

Only two lizards have a poisonous bite – the Gila monster and the Mexican beaded lizard, both from southern North America. The Gila monster, shown here, is found in dry, scrubby areas. It hides in a burrow by day and emerges at night to eat small animals such as mice, and the eggs of birds and other reptiles.

Gila monster feeding on newborn mice

GREEN GECKO

Many lizards are coloured to blend in with their surroundings. Tree- climbing lizards such as this green gecko are often bright green to match the leaves; desert-dwelling lizards are sand-coloured or brown. Many kinds of chameleons can change their colour according to their surroundings.

THORNY DEVIL

The extraordinary looking thorny devil is also called the moloch. Spines protect its body from nose to tail. Thorny lizards live in dry parts of Australia, where they forage for ants. When the young molochs hatch from their eggs, they look like tiny, spiny versions of their parents.

IGUANA

Like all lizards, iguanas depend on heat from the environment to keep their bodies warm and active. They spend much of the day basking in the sun, absorbing its warmth to prepare for activity. At night they become slow and sluggish as their body temperature falls. The Galapagos marine iguanas shown here dive to more than 11 m (35 ft) deep into the sea in search of seaweed.

After each dive, Galapagos marine iguanas sunbathe on the rocks to warm up again.

SLOW-WORM

The slow-worm is not really a worm, but a lizard. It is not slow either; when disturbed, slow-worms can wriggle away rapidly to safety. Slow-worms are found in fields and scrubland in Europe, northern Africa, and southwest Asia. They feed on slugs, spiders, and insects. Unlike most lizards, slow-worms give birth to fully formed young.

Find out more

Camouflage, animal
Desert wildlife
North American wildlife
Reptiles

LOUIS XIV

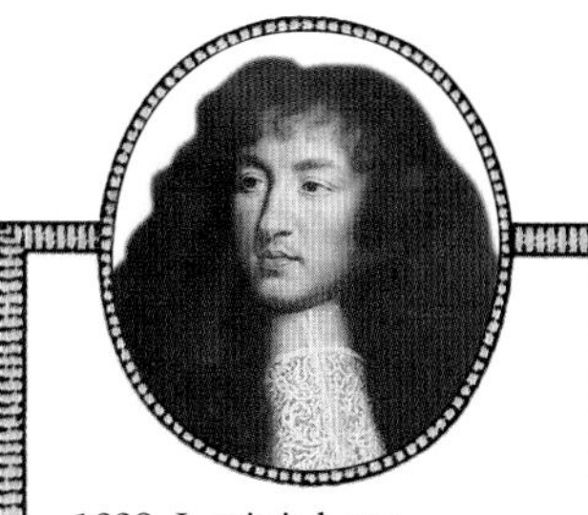

1638 Louis is born.

1643 Louis becomes king.

1662 Louis moves court to Versailles.

1667-68 War of Devolution. France fights Dutch for control of Netherlands. Gains part of Flanders.

1701 War of Spanish Succession. France fights for control of Spanish empire.

1713 Peace of Utrecht ends War of Spanish Succession and marks decline of France's power.

1715 Louis dies.

IN 1643 LOUIS XIV became king of France. He ruled for 72 years and made his country the most powerful in Europe at that time. While Louis was still young, his mother and his chief minister, Cardinal Mazarin, ruled on his behalf. During this time the nobility rose up against the throne and tax policies in a rebellion called the Fronde. However, when Louis was 23, he took complete charge of France and ruled as an absolute monarch, making all decisions himself. He moved his court to Versailles, just outside Paris, and appointed Jean Colbert, a French statesman, as his finance minister. Under Colbert's control, trade and industry flourished. Louis XIV fought a series of wars and increased the territory of France. But the many wars cost France a lot of money, and the country became nearly bankrupt. Taxes were raised to pay off debts, causing much hardship among the poor.

VERSAILLES PALACE

The palace at Versailles was magnificent. Its many rooms included a hall of mirrors that was 73 m (240 ft) in length and lavishly decorated. Formal gardens with fountains and sculpted hedges surrounded the palace. Louis spent one tenth of all France's wealth on its upkeep. Even so, many parts of the palace were overcrowded, dark, and cold. Today, Versailles palace is open to the public.

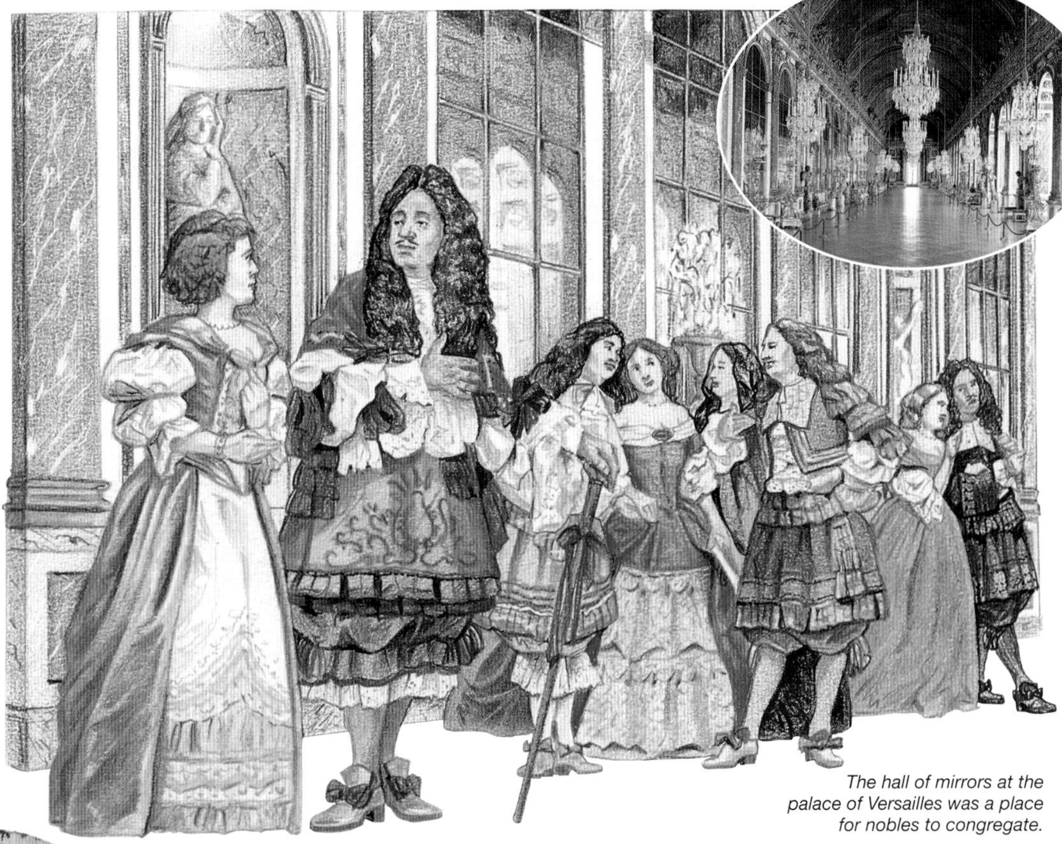

The hall of mirrors at the palace of Versailles was a place for nobles to congregate.

SUN KING

Louis XIV surrounded himself with splendour. His court was a centre for the great writers, artists, and musicians of the time. He said of himself *"L'état c'est moi"* or "I am the state". Louis was given the nickname "the Sun King" after the Greek god Apollo, who was also a patron of the arts.

Detailed embroidery on chair typical of Louis XIV style of furniture

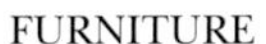

FURNITURE

Louis XIV employed groups of expert craftsworkers to make furniture for his palace at Versailles. The style of the furniture, such as this walnut chair, was elaborate and ornate. It became known as the Louis XIV style.

Find out more

FRANCE, HISTORY OF
FRENCH REVOLUTION

LOW COUNTRIES

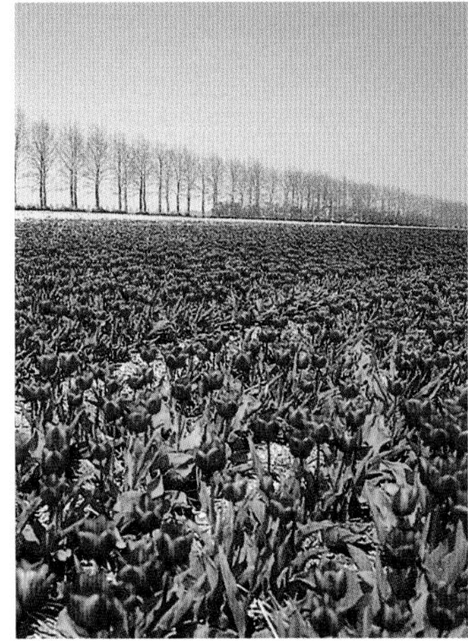

BULB FIELDS
The Dutch have been famous for their flower bulbs since the 16th century, when tulips first arrived in Europe from the Middle East. In spring, fields of spring flowers are a spectacular sight. Fresh cut flowers are flown all over the world.

SMALL AND DENSELY populated, the Low Countries are highly developed industrial nations with thriving economies. Nearly one-third of the Netherlands lies below sea level. Over the last four centuries, Dutch engineers have reclaimed land by pushing back the North Sea with a network of barriers, or dykes. In northern Belgium, the land is also flat and low-lying, although to the south it rises towards the forested uplands of the Ardennes. Belgium only became independent in the 19th century. It is divided by language; Dutch (Flemish) is spoken in the north, while French is spoken in the south. Farming is important throughout the region. The fertile land and cool, rainy climate is ideally suited to dairy and arable farming. Major industries produce iron and steel, natural gas, clothing, textiles and electrical goods. The tiny country of Luxembourg has the highest living standards in Europe, and is known as a major banking centre.

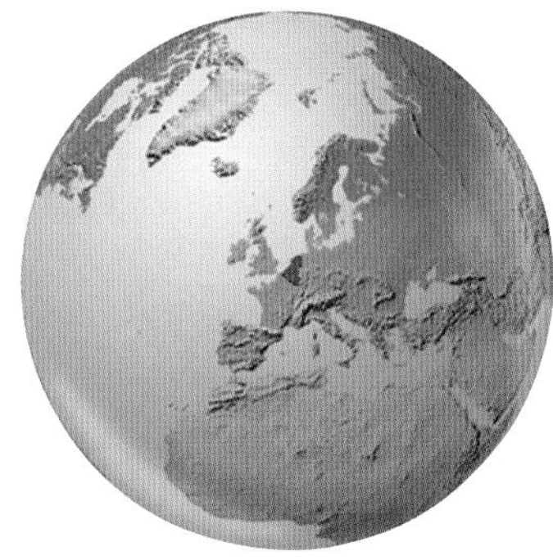

The Low Countries lie in northwest Europe, with Germany to the east and France to the south. To the west, lies the North Sea.

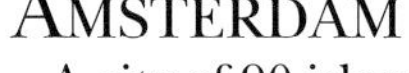

AMSTERDAM

A city of 90 islands, connected by 1,000 bridges, Amsterdam is linked by canal to the North Sea. The city became important in the Middle Ages, and many of the churches, towers, and gabled merchants' houses of the old city still stand. In the 17th century, Amsterdam was the financial capital of the world. Since 1945, new suburbs have been built on polders (reclaimed land), tripling the size of the city.

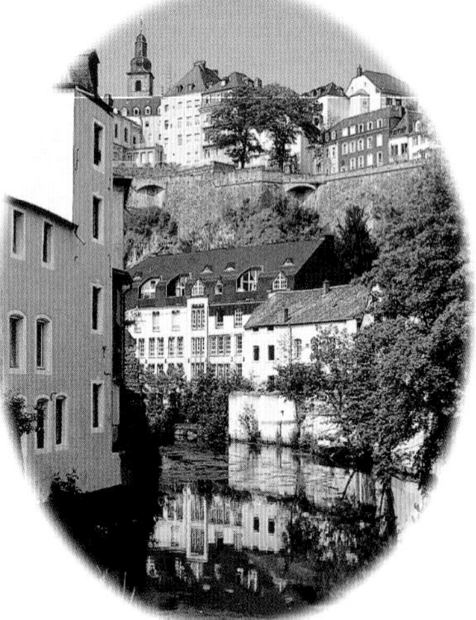

LUXEMBOURG
The capital of Luxembourg stands on a sandstone plateau, cut into deep ravines by the Alzette river. The Old Town centres on the Grand Ducal Palace (1572), the cathedral and the Town Hall. Luxembourg is a thriving industrial and banking centre.

LAND RECLAMATION
Over the centuries, low-lying land has been reclaimed from the sea. Engineers built dykes to enclose areas of shallow water, which were then drained. From the 14th century, windmills were used to drain water and pump it into canals. On the windswept lowlands, windpower was very effective, although it has now been replaced by steam and electric pumps. However, storms and high tides are still a major threat to the people of the Netherlands.

Porters carry trays of cheese at the famous market in Alkmaar.

CHEESE

Much of the cheese produced in the Netherlands is made from the milk of cows, which graze on areas of reclaimed land. The country's most famous cheeses are Gouda and Edam, with its rind of red wax.

Windmills tap the energy of the wind by means of sails mounted on a rotating shaft.

Find out more
EUROPE
EUROPEAN UNION
FLOWERS AND HERBS
PORTS AND WATERWAYS
WORLD WAR I

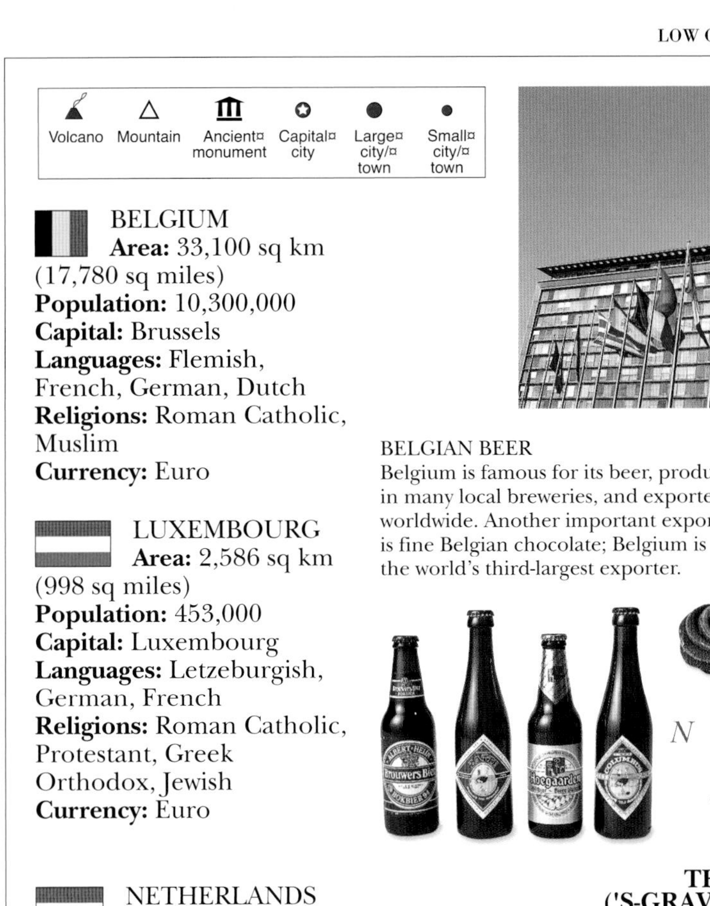

BELGIUM
Area: 33,100 sq km (17,780 sq miles)
Population: 10,300,000
Capital: Brussels
Languages: Flemish, French, German, Dutch
Religions: Roman Catholic, Muslim
Currency: Euro

LUXEMBOURG
Area: 2,586 sq km (998 sq miles)
Population: 453,000
Capital: Luxembourg
Languages: Letzeburgish, German, French
Religions: Roman Catholic, Protestant, Greek Orthodox, Jewish
Currency: Euro

NETHERLANDS
Area: 37,330 sq km (14,410 sq miles)
Population: 16,100,000
Capital: Amsterdam, The Hague ('s-Gravenhage)
Languages: Dutch, Frisian
Religions: Roman Catholic, Protestant, Muslim
Currency: Euro

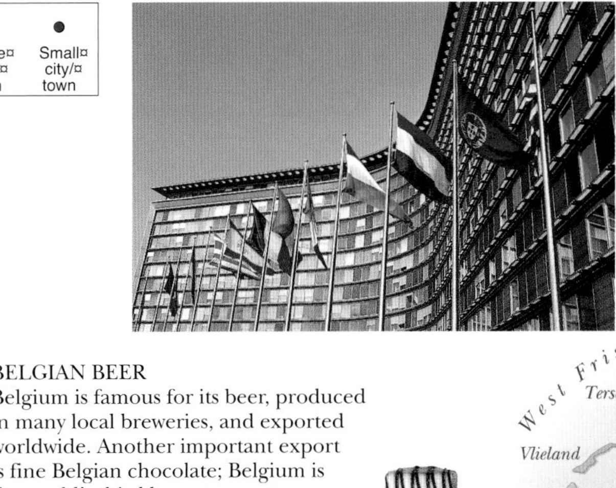

EU HEADQUARTERS
In 1957, all three countries were founding members of the European Economic Community (EEC). Brussels is now the administrative headquarters of the European Union (EU), while Luxembourg is the headquarters of the European Investment Bank and the Court of Justice.

BELGIAN BEER
Belgium is famous for its beer, produced in many local breweries, and exported worldwide. Another important export is fine Belgian chocolate; Belgium is the world's third-largest exporter.

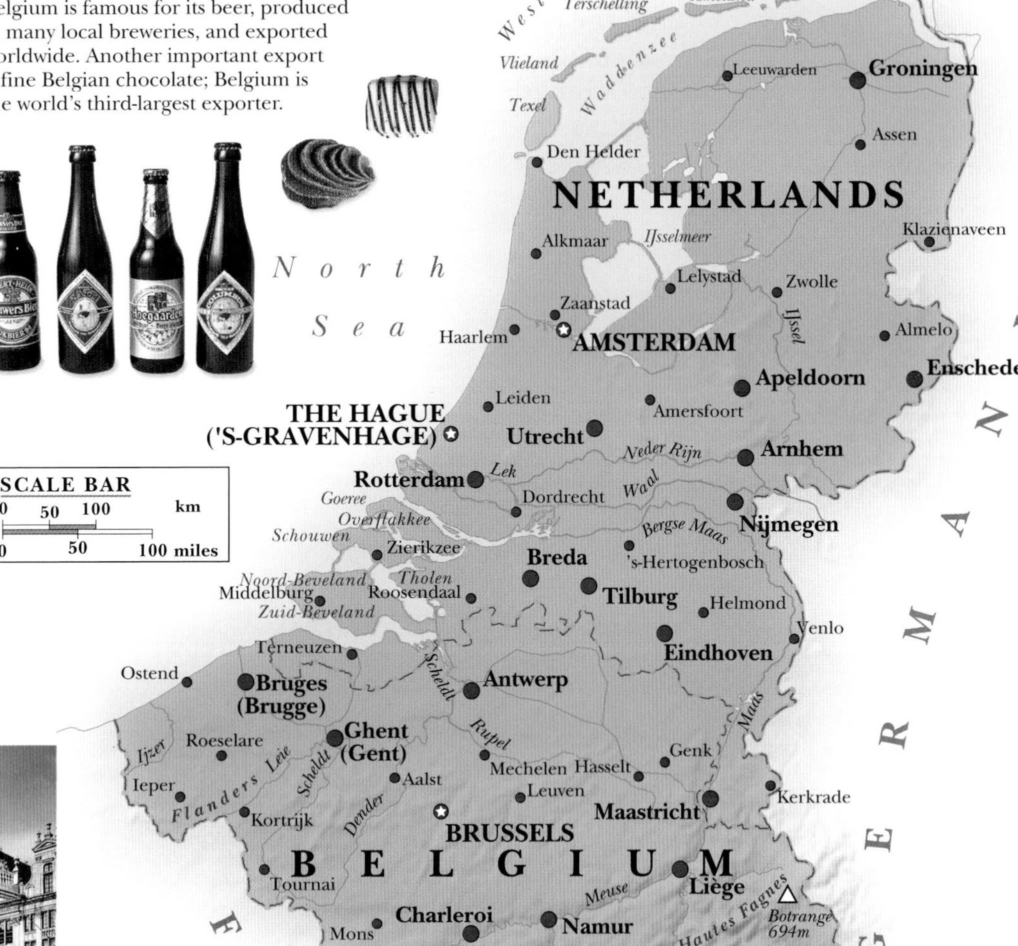

BRUSSELS

Brussels, the capital of Belgium, is an international economic and financial centre. The city expanded rapidly in the 19th century, and became the centre of Belgium's growing steel, chemical, and textile industries. The Grand Place (above) is the heart of the Old Town. Brussels is now a major financial centre, with its own Stock Exchange.

WAR CEMETERY
The Flanders region of southwest Belgium is imprinted with memories of World War I. One of the costliest battles of the four-year war was Passchendaele in 1917, where an estimated 800,000 Allied and German troops were killed. Vast war cemeteries, such as Tyne Cot near Ieper (left), attract many visitors.

HISTORY OF THE LOW COUNTRIES

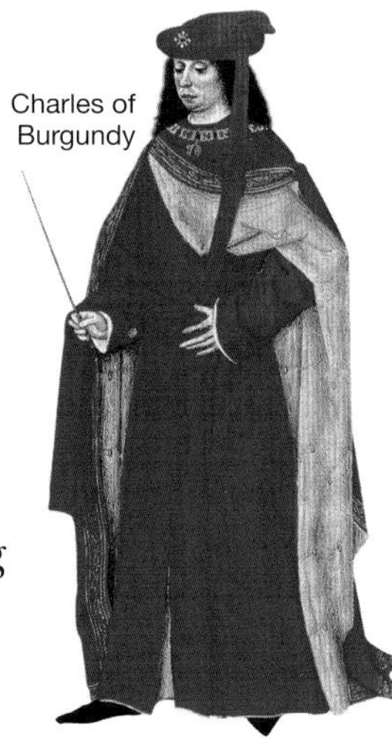

BURGUNDY AND SPAIN
In 1400s, Burgundy ruled the Low Countries. In 1516, Charles, Duke of Burgundy became king of Spain, bringing the Low Countries under Spanish rule.

THE NETHERLANDS, BELGIUM, AND LUXEMBOURG were once thought of as a single region, called the Low Countries. From the 1100s to the 17th century, the area was ruled by Europe's major powers, Germany, France, and Spain. In 1568, the northern region (what is now the Netherlands) turned to Protestantism and rebelled against Catholic Spain. Spain finally recognized the Netherlands' independence in 1648, and the country flourished throughout the 1600s. France regained its power over the region in the 18th century, ruling until the fall of Napoleon in 1815, when the Netherlands, Belgium, and the Duchy of Luxembourg united as the Kingdom of the Netherlands. Belgium declared its independence in 1830, and Luxembourg in 1890. Today, all three countries thrive as founder members of the European Community.

Dutch East Indiaman, or ocean-going cargo ship

Merchants checking cargoes of spices, gold, and china

THE GOLDEN CENTURY

In the 1600s, the Netherlands grew rich on international trade and exploration, so the period was known as "the Golden Century". Amsterdam was the trading centre and money market of the western world, taking over from Antwerp, Belgium, which was captured by the Spanish in 1576. Rich merchants built large houses along Amsterdam's canals.

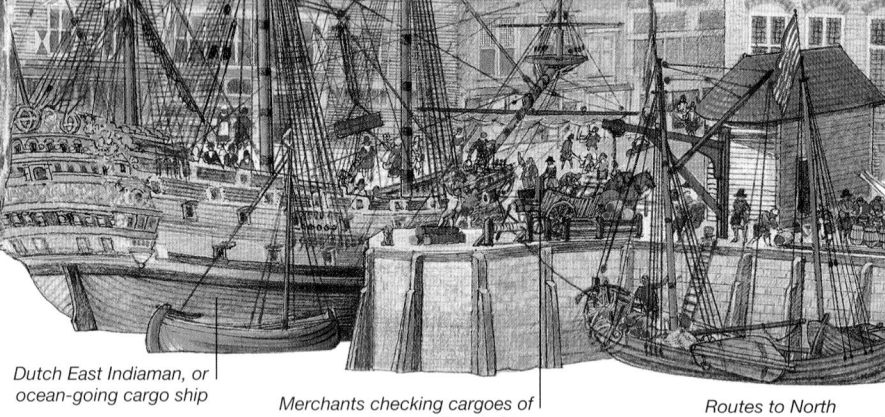

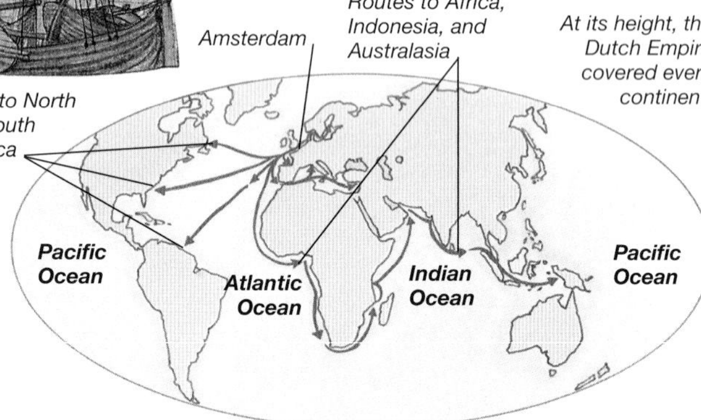

At its height, the Dutch Empire covered every continent.

TULIPMANIA
The tulip was brought to Europe from Turkey in the 16th century and soon became fashionable. A craze called "tulipmania" swept through the Netherlands between 1634 and 1637. People invested money in tulips, and the price for rare bulbs went up until they were worth more than gold. When prices fell, many people were ruined.

LOW COUNTRY COLONIES
The Dutch East Indies (now Indonesia), set up in the early 17th century, was the largest of the Low Country colonies. In 1634, the Dutch captured the Antilles (Curaçao, Aruba, Bonaire, Saba, St. Eustatius, and St. Martin Island) from Spain. By 1674, they had taken Surinam from Britain.

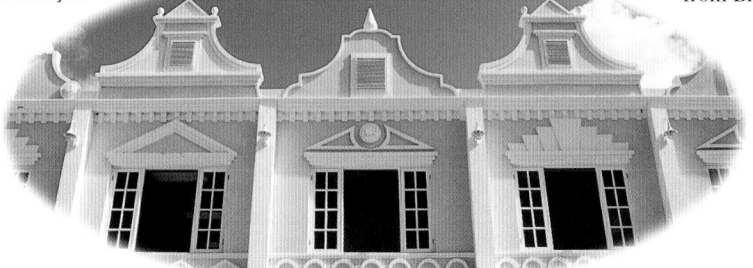

Dutch architecture in Caribbean colours on the island of Curaçao.

THE GREAT TRADERS
The Netherlands became a leading sea power in the 17th century, finding new trade routes. The Dutch East India Company was founded in 1602 to trade with Indonesia and southern Africa. The Dutch West India Company, founded in 1621, opened routes to America, Australasia, and West Africa.

HOLDING BACK THE SEA
Much of the Low Countries, especially the Netherlands, is below sea level. For centuries, the Dutch have fought to hold back the North Sea, building large earth walls called dykes to prevent flooding. They also set up thousands of windmills across the country to pump water away from the land along canals. Today, electric pumps are used.

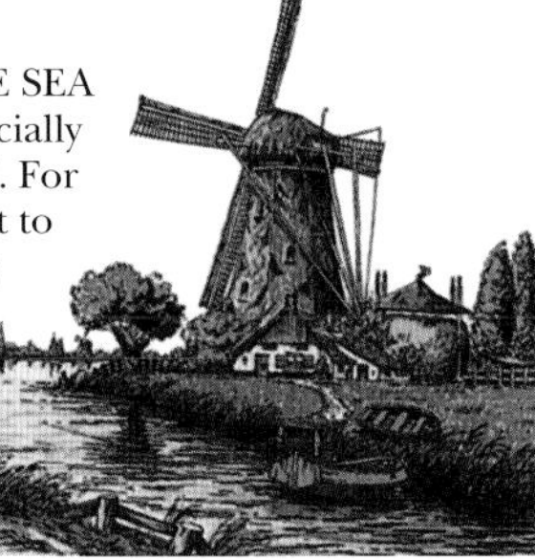

NEW AMSTERDAM
In 1624, the Dutch West India Company set up the colony of New Netherland in northern America. They built its capital, New Amsterdam, on the island of Manhattan, which they bought from Native Americans for goods worth 60 Dutch guilders. In 1664, the English took over the colony by force, and renamed it New York.

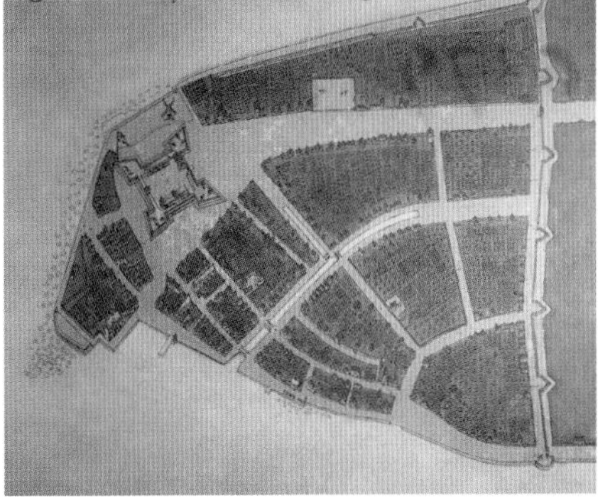

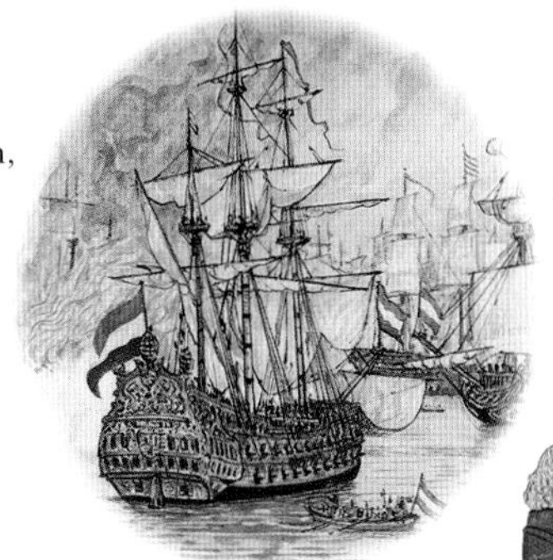

ANGLO-DUTCH WARS
Between 1652 and 1674, the Dutch and the English fought three wars for the control of sea trade routes. The Dutch won, even after France joined in to help England in 1670. England signed a truce with the Dutch in 1674.

CONGRESS OF VIENNA
After Napoleon's defeat at Waterloo in 1815, the other European powers were determined to prevent the French from becoming so powerful again. They met at the Congress of Vienna in 1815, and decided to make the Low Countries stronger to stop France expanding in that direction. The Netherlands and Belgium were joined together as the Kingdom of the Netherlands, ruled by Prince William VI of the Netherlands as King William I and Grand Duke of Luxembourg.

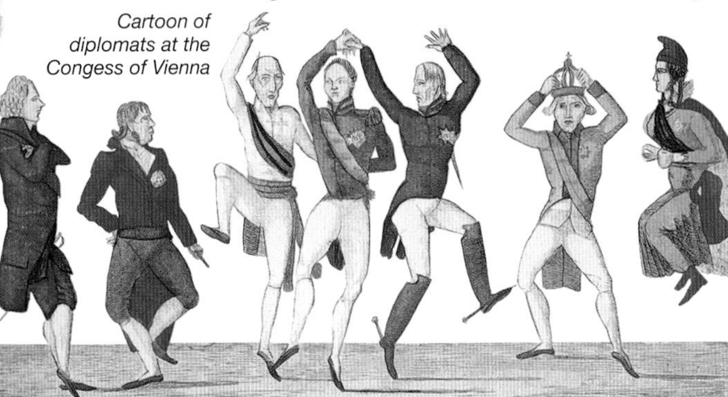

Cartoon of diplomats at the Congess of Vienna

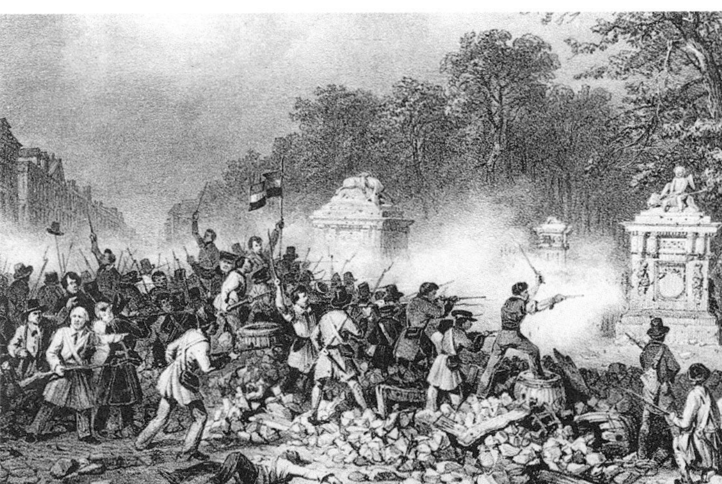

Belgian independence

Belgium remained under Spanish rule when the Netherlands declared its independence in 1568, so it followed Catholic beliefs and traditions. In 1830, Belgium revolted against the Protestant Netherlands, and seized its independence under Charles Rogier. Fighting lasted only a month, then the people elected Prince Leopold of Saxe Coburg as their first king, Leopold I.

Tank warfare in World War II

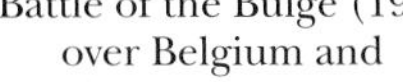

THE BATTLEFIELD OF EUROPE
The Low Countries have been the site of many of Europe's battles. Napoleon saw defeat at Waterloo, in Belgium. In World War I, the battles of Ypres, Mons, and Namur were fought in Belgium; in World War II, the Battle of the Bulge (1944) was fought all over Belgium and Luxembourg.

Modern Luxembourg is a very prosperous country.

Luxembourg

The name Luxembourg comes from a word meaning "little castle". Luxembourg began life as a castle (built in 963) but later it became a duchy (ruled by a duke) until the Netherlands took it over in 1443. In 1815, it was made a Grand Duchy, ruled by the Netherlands. In 1890, Queen Wilhelmina came to the Netherlands' throne, and as Luxembourg's laws did not allow women to rule, the Grand Duchy ended the alliance. Today Luxembourg is a separate, independent country.

LOWLAND HISTORY

1300s-1400s Burgundy rules the region.

1516 Charles of Burgundy becomes king of Spain.

1648 Spain recognizes Dutch independence.

1652-74 Anglo-Dutch Wars.

1652 Dutch settlers arrive in South Africa.

1776 Dutch side with America in US War of Independence.

1795-1814 France controls the Netherlands.

1815 Belgium and the Netherlands unite.

1830 Belgium declares independence.

1890 Luxembourg declares independence.

1914-18 Belgium fights with Allies in World War I; the Dutch remain neutral.

1948 Benelux – an economic trading association between Belgium, Netherlands and Luxembourg – formed.

1957 Benelux countries sign Treaty of Rome to set up European Economic Community (EEC).

1967 Benelux countries are founder members of EU.

Find out more
EUROPEAN UNION
EUROPE, HISTORY OF
NAPOLEONIC WARS

LUNGS AND BREATHING

WE NEED OXYGEN TO LIVE, and we get oxygen by breathing air. When we breathe in, air is sucked through the nose or mouth, down the windpipe, and into the lungs, two powerful organs in the chest. The lungs absorb as much oxygen from the air as possible. The oxygen travels in the blood from the lungs to every part of the body. Our bodies use oxygen to burn up the food we eat and convert it into energy. Then the harmful carbon dioxide is breathed out of the body by the lungs. The whole process is called respiration. The lungs, together with the airways, throat, and nasal passages, form the respiratory system. Each lung is surrounded by a thin covering or membrane called the pleura. The lungs themselves contain air tubes, blood vessels, and millions of tiny air sacs called alveoli. If you spread these air sacs out flat, they would cover the area of a tennis court.

HOW WE MAKE SOUNDS
We use the air flowing in and out of our lungs to make sounds. We speak, shout, laugh, and cry by making air flow over two small leathery flaps called the vocal cords. These are in the larynx (voice box), in the lower part of the throat. Muscles in the throat stretch the flaps tighter to change from low notes to high notes.

Air flows in through the nose and mouth, down the throat, along the trachea (windpipe), and into the lungs.

Pharynx (throat)

Larynx (voice box) at top of trachea

Trachea (windpipe)

The rib cage is flexible, so the lungs can expand and shrink when we breathe.

Trachea divides into two main bronchi.

Lung

Bronchiole

Bronchi continue to branch and divide.

Diaphragm is a dome-shaped sheet of muscle

Alveolus

Capillary blood vessels

BREATHING

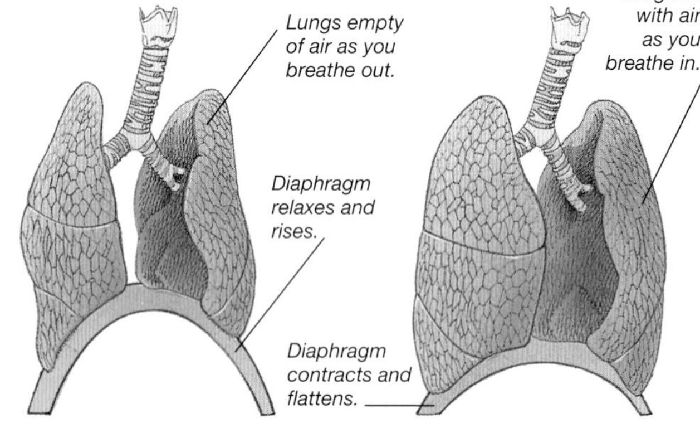

Lungs empty of air as you breathe out.
Lungs fill with air as you breathe in.
Diaphragm relaxes and rises.
Diaphragm contracts and flattens.

BREATHING OUT
When you breathe out, the diaphragm and chest muscles relax. The lungs are spongy and elastic, so they spring back to their smaller size after they have been stretched. This blows air back out of the lungs.

BREATHING IN
When you breathe in, the diaphragm contracts (becomes flatter) and pulls down the base of the lungs. Muscles between the ribs contract to swing the ribs up and out. These actions stretch and enlarge the lungs, so that air is sucked in.

Air space inside alveolus

The alveoli are grouped together like bunches of grapes. Tiny tubes called bronchioles bring fresh oxygen-containing air to the alveoli.

LUNGFISH
Most animals that live on land have lungs. Many water animals, however, including most fish, breathe using feathery flaps called gills. Oxygen in the water passes through the thin gill coverings to the blood inside the fish's body. The lungfish shown here is an unusual animal because it has lungs and gills, so it can breathe in both ways and can survive out of water for a long time.

ALVEOLUS
Each alveolus is surrounded by a network of very fine blood vessels called capillaries. Oxygen passes from the air space inside the alveolus, through the lining, and into the blood. Carbon dioxide passes in the opposite way.

Find out more
BRAIN AND NERVES
HEART AND BLOOD
HUMAN BODY
MUSCLES AND MOVEMENT
OXYGEN
SKELETONS

MACHINES

INCLINED PLANE
Simple machines reduce the effort needed to move or lift an object, but the object has to travel a greater distance. The simplest machine is the ramp, or inclined plane. You need less force to push an object with a downwards load up an inclined plane than you need to lift it straight up. This is because the object moves a greater distance along the plane. The gentler the slope, the further you have to push, but the easier it is.

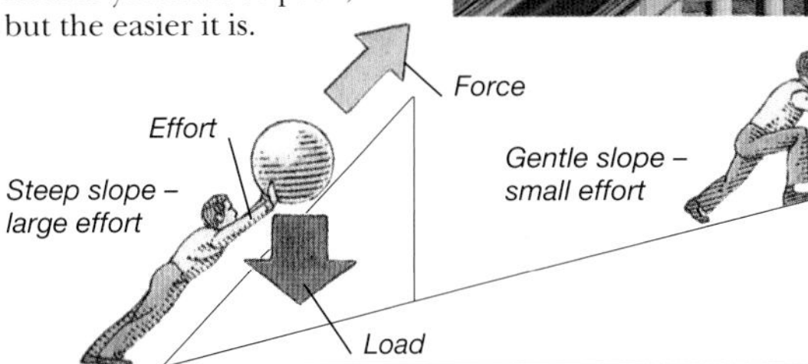

WHAT DO A SAW and a computer have in common? Both are machines. One is simple and the other is very complex, but both are tools that do work for us. Machines perform tasks that we would find difficult or even impossible to do. You cannot cut through wood with your bare hands, for example, but it is easy with a saw. Likewise, a computer can do calculations rapidly that would take you an enormous amount of time. All machines need a source of energy. Mechanical machines, such as a corkscrew, use the energy of movement. A motor or a person's muscles drive the machine with a certain amount of force called the effort. The machine then applies this movement but produces a larger force to move a load. For example, your fingers operate a can opener, but the blade of the can opener moves with much more force than that produced by your fingers. Many hand-powered machines help us perform tasks for which we do not have enough strength. They use devices known as simple machines. These include levers, gears, pulleys, and screws.

SCREW

A screw moves forward a shorter distance than it turns. It therefore moves forward with a much greater force than the effort needed to turn it. The screw bites into the wood with great force and is held strongly.

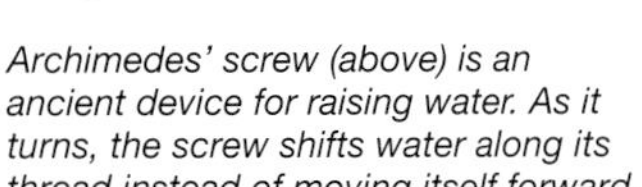

Archimedes' screw (above) is an ancient device for raising water. As it turns, the screw shifts water along its thread instead of moving itself forward.

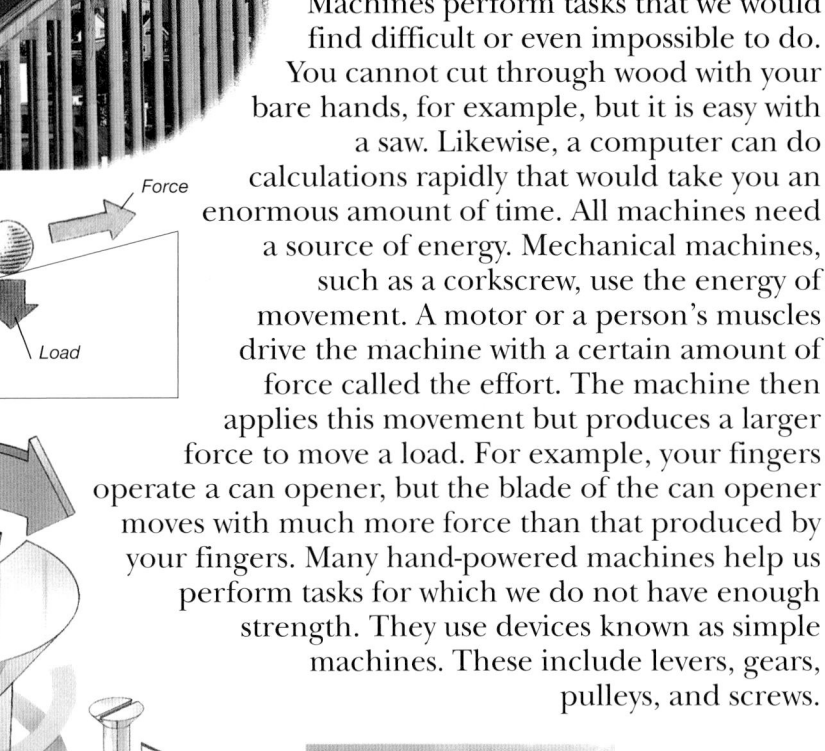

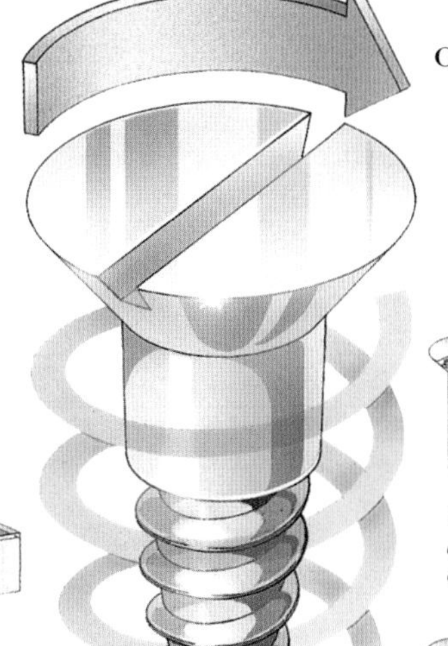

The screw makes use of the principle of the inclined plane.

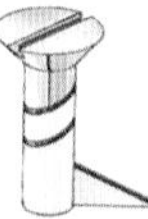

The thread of the screw is like a slope wrapped around a cylinder.

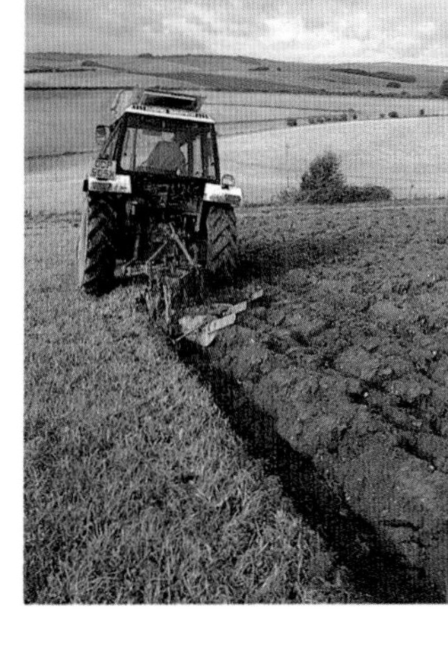

PLOUGH
The plough has a cutting blade that bites into the soil and a V-shaped blade that turns the soil over.

PERPETUAL MOTION

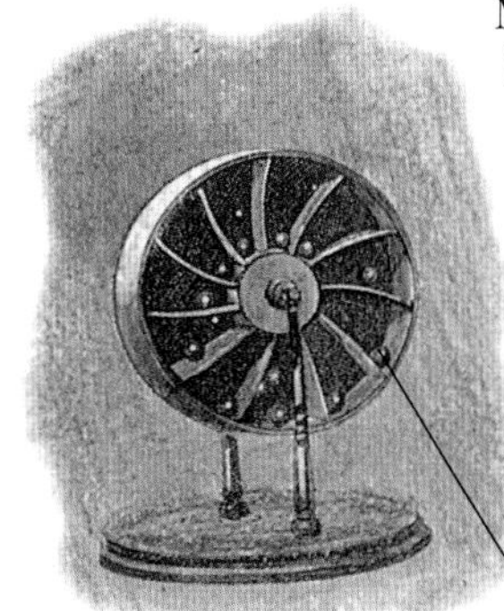

Many inventors have tried to build a machine that,once started, would never stop. It would run on its own without any source of energy. However, such a perpetual motion machine is impossible. This is because all machines lose some energy as they work. Without a constant source of energy, a machine always slows down and stops.

In this machine, the motion of the balls was supposed to keep the wheel turning.

WEDGE
The wedge is a form of inclined plane. Instead of moving a load along a slope, the wedge is a slope that pushes a load aside or upward as it moves forward. The wedge pushes with greater force than the effort needed to move the wedge. Sharp blades are thin wedges that make cutting an easy task.

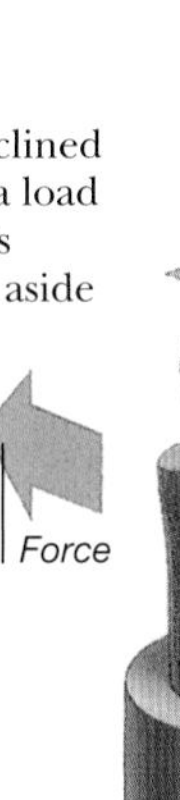

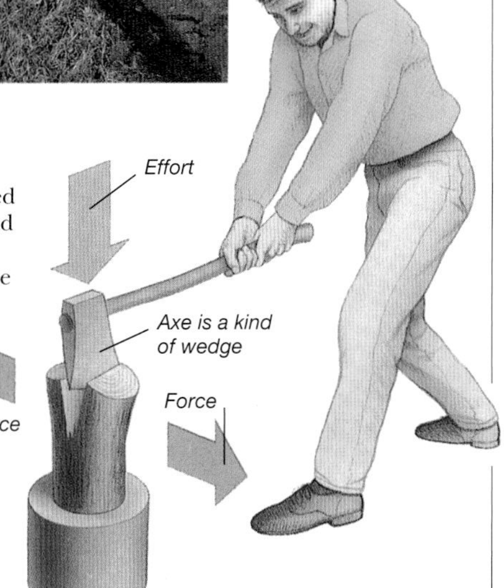

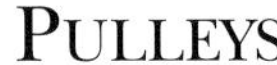

PULLEYS

Lifting a heavy load is easy with a pulley system. It contains a set of wheels fixed to a support. A rope goes around grooves in the wheels. Pulling the rope raises the lower wheel and the load. A pulley system allows you to lift a heavy load with little effort, but you must pull the rope a large distance to raise the load by a small amount.

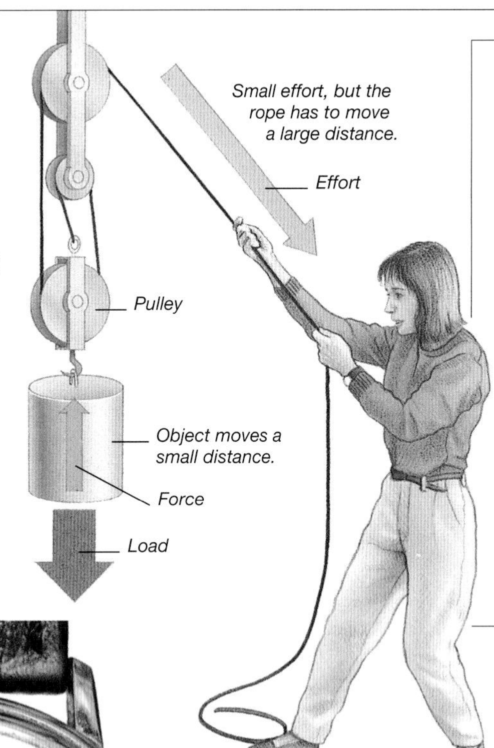

AUTOMATIC MACHINES

Many machines do not need to be operated by people. These are automatic machines. They contain mechanisms or computers to control themselves. These machines may simply perform a set task whenever it is required; automatic doors, for example, open as people arrive. Other machines are able to check their own work and change the way they operate to follow instructions. One example is an aircraft autopilot, which guides the plane through the skies.

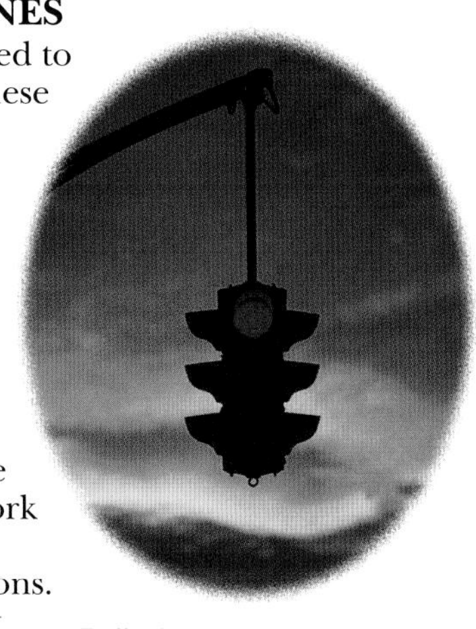

Traffic lights are machines that control traffic automatically.

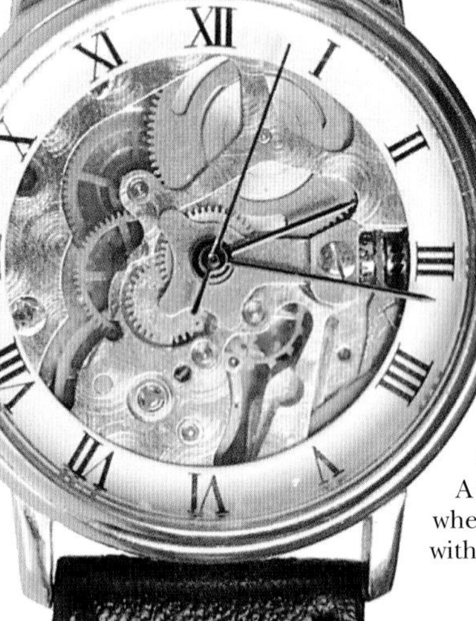

Mechanical clocks and watches contain gears that turn the hands at different speeds.

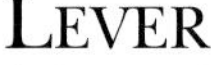

GEARS
Gears are intermeshing toothed wheels. They can increase force or speed depending on the relative size of the wheels and their number of teeth. A gearwheel driven by a smaller wheel turns less quickly than the smaller wheel but with greater force. A wheel driven by a larger wheel turns faster but with less force.

LEVER

A long stick propped up on a small object (a fulcrum) helps you move a heavy load. The stick is a simple machine called a lever. Pushing down on the end furthest from the fulcrum raises the other end with greater force, helping you move the load. Other kinds of levers can increase either the force applied to, or the distance moved by, a load.

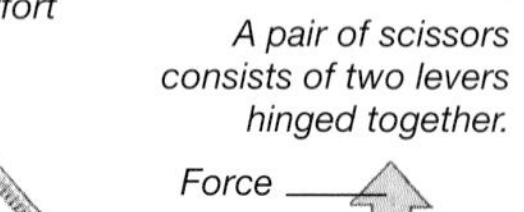

A pair of scissors consists of two levers hinged together.

There are three types of lever. A crowbar is called a first-class lever. The fulcrum is between the load and the effort, which is the force that you apply.

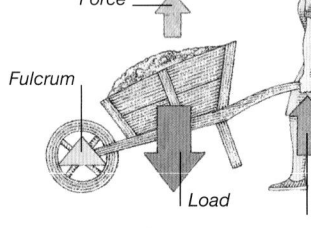

A wheelbarrow is a second-class lever. The load lies between the fulcrum and the effort.

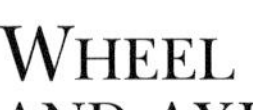

WHEEL AND AXLE

Several machines use the principle of the wheel and axle. One example is the winch, in which a handle (the wheel) turns a shaft (the axle) that raises a load. The handle moves a greater distance than the load rises. The winch therefore lifts the load with a greater force than the effort needed to turn the handle.

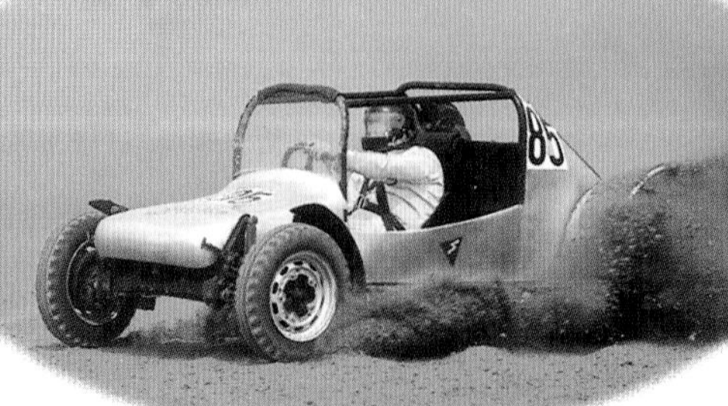

STEERING WHEEL
The steering wheel on a car is an example of the wheel and axle. The shaft turns with greater force than the effort needed to turn the steering wheel.

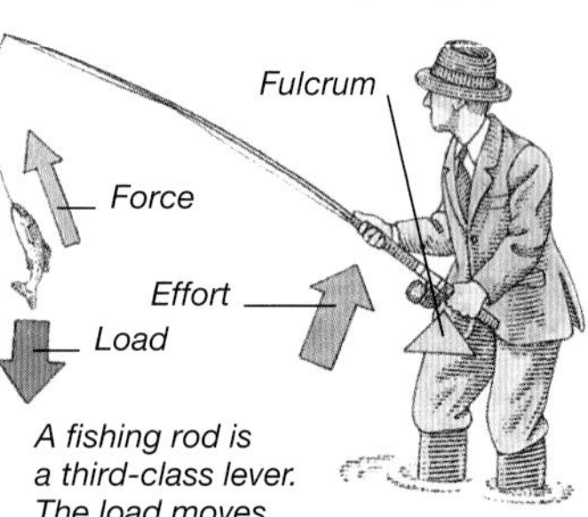

A fishing rod is a third-class lever. The load moves a greater distance than the effort, but with less force. The effort pushes between the load and the fulcrum.

Find out more
ENGINES
FACTORIES
INDUSTRIAL REVOLUTION
ROBOTS
TECHNOLOGY

MAGAZINES

WHATEVER YOUR INTEREST, you'll find a magazine that tells you more about it. Like newspapers, new issues of a magazine go on sale regularly – usually weekly or monthly. But magazines last longer than newspapers. Often, two or three people read the magazine before discarding it. And some magazines, such as scientific journals, are more like reference books. Their buyers keep them to refer to months or even years later. The simplest magazines, such as neighbourhood newsletters, are sheets that have been roughly photocopied and stapled together. Other magazines cover topics with a wide appeal. They are printed in colour on glossy paper and have many pictures. The editor-in-chief decides what goes into the magazine. Other editors and journalists write the features and articles. The art director is responsible for the style and look of the magazine. Designers choose pictures and lay out the pages.

LIFE MAGAZINE
The first magazines began in Europe in the 17th century. But modern magazines started only when it was possible to print photographs on their pages. One of the greatest picture magazines is *Life*, which first appeared in 1936. *Life* tells stories with a series of pictures and few words.

COMICS
Children and adults read comics. The word comic is short for comic strip, because the first comics were collections of comic strips from newspapers. They were originally called funnies. A new type of comic, containing adventure stories, first appeared in the 1930s and led to the many different comics of today.

Superman, one of the world's best-known comic-strip heroes, first appeared in Action Comics in 1938.

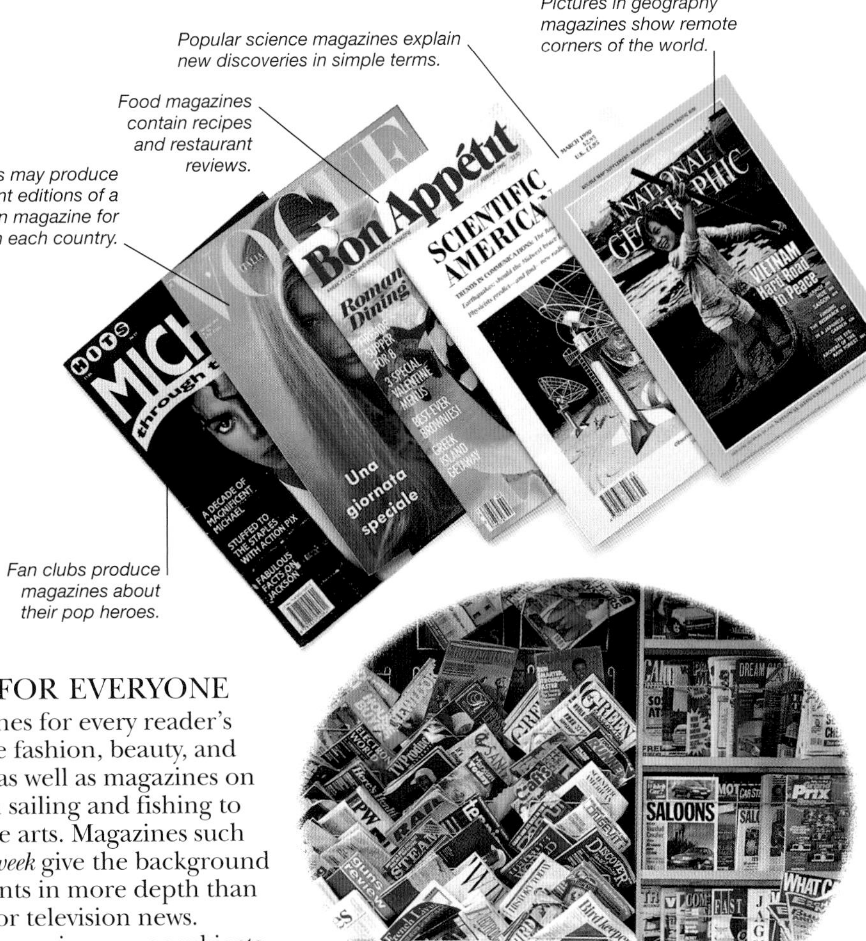

Pictures in geography magazines show remote corners of the world.

Popular science magazines explain new discoveries in simple terms.

Food magazines contain recipes and restaurant reviews.

Publishers may produce different editions of a fashion magazine for readers in each country.

Fan clubs produce magazines about their pop heroes.

MAGAZINES FOR EVERYONE

There are magazines for every reader's interest. There are fashion, beauty, and family magazines as well as magazines on every activity from sailing and fishing to computers and the arts. Magazines such as *Time* and *Newsweek* give the background to current events in more depth than newspapers or television news. Specialist magazines cover subjects such as science or hobbies. Fanzines are magazines about pop stars. Trade magazines are for businesses such as publishing, banking, or engineering.

NEWS STANDS
At a news stand you can choose from a huge range of national and foreign magazines on subjects such as politics, fashion, and lifestyle.

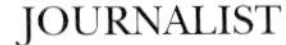

JOURNALIST
Magazines are sometimes called journals, so the editors and writers who create them are called journalists. An editor decides what will appear in the magazine and chooses the writer. The writer carries out research or interviews and writes the article. Then the editor corrects errors and makes sure the article fits into the space on the page.

Find out more
ADVERTISING
CARTOONS
NEWSPAPERS

MAGNA CARTA

IN 1215, KING JOHN OF ENGLAND signed a document known as Magna Carta, or Great Charter. The document, which was complicated, set out rules and conditions for ruling the country, and was a major event in the history of English government. Magna Carta resulted from disagreements between King John and his barons. The barons wanted to be more involved in the government of England, while John wanted to keep power for himself, and angered them by imposing heavy taxes. Some barons rebelled, and drew up a list of demands that John was forced to accept, and which became Magna Carta. The charter mainly concerned the rights of barons, but it did promise justice to all. It is seen as a step towards making the monarchy answerable to the law.

KING JOHN
The youngest son of Henry II, King John (r. 1199-1216) was weakened by wars with France and quarrels with the pope and the English Church.

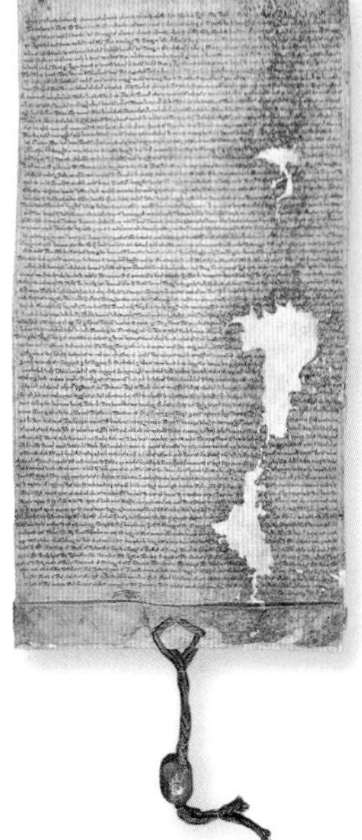

THE CHARTER
The original charter was on parchment and carried King John's seal. There were 63 clauses, setting out the duties of the king and subjects. The king's right to tax the barons was limited, and the rights of the Church were guaranteed. Four copies of Magna Carta survive today.

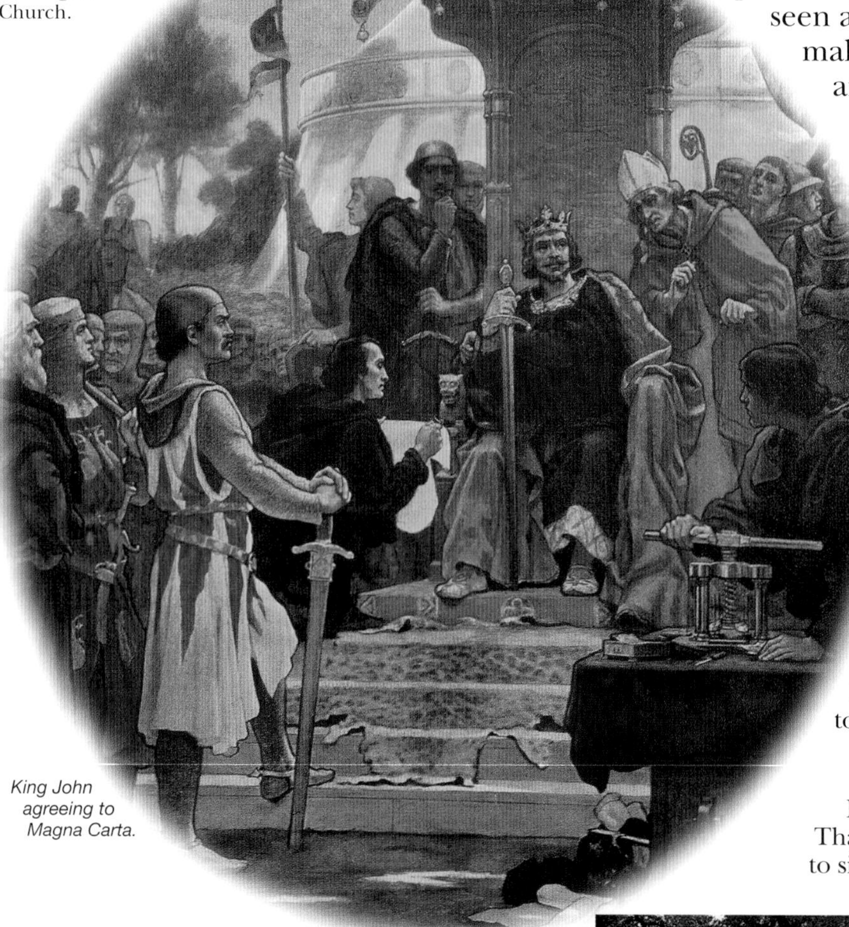

King John agreeing to Magna Carta.

SEALING THE CHARTER

King John had agreed to grant the barons all their demands. In the last month of negotiations, Archbishop Langton persuaded the barons to include some clauses that benefited the king's subjects. On 15 June 1215, John set his Great Seal on a draft version of the charter, called the Articles of the Barons. A final version was ready by 19 June. Twenty-five barons were appointed to see that it was carried out. Magna Carta was reissued several times. In the 1640s, during the English Civil War, it was used to criticise King Charles I.

RUNNYMEDE

It was at Runnymede, a meadow beside the River Thames, that King John met the barons and agreed to sign Magna Carta. The site, chosen because it was midway between the king's residence, Windsor Castle, and the barons' assembly point in the town of Staines, has been preserved as an open space ever since. The memorial commemorating the charter was presented in 1957 by the American Bar Association.

STEPHEN LANGTON
Churchman Stephen Langton (1165-1228) was a close friend of Pope Innocent III. The pope made Langton a cardinal in 1206 and, two years later, helped him to be elected as Archbishop of Canterbury, an appointment which King John opposed. Langton supported the barons against the king and helped them to persuade the king to agree to the charter. Langton wrote a large part of the text of Magna Carta.

Find out more

ENGLISH CIVIL WAR
HUMAN RIGHTS
UNITED KINGDOM, HISTORY OF

MAGNETISM

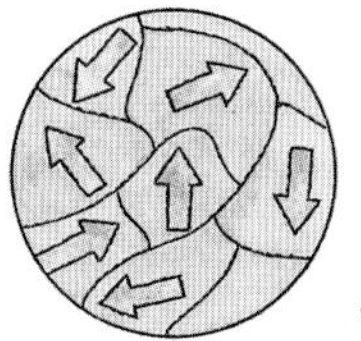

ORIGIN OF MAGNETISM
Iron contains millions of tiny magnets called magnetic dipoles. Normally, all the dipoles point in different directions so their magnetism cancels out. In a magnet, the dipoles point the same way so that their magnetism combines.

MAGNETIC FIELD
The area around a magnet in which its magnetic force works is called its magnetic field. For instance, a paper clip is pulled towards the magnet (right) when it is placed within the magnetic field of the magnet.

All magnets attract iron and steel objects but not plastic or wooden ones.

THE FORCE of magnetism is invisible, yet you can see its power when a magnet drags a piece of metal towards it. A material that attracts certain metals such as iron is called a magnet. Materials that are attracted by a magnet are called magnetic. Every magnet has two poles – places at which magnetic objects cluster. The Earth itself is a huge magnet; its magnetic poles are close to the geographical North and South Poles. One pole of a magnet is attracted to the Earth's northern magnetic pole and is called the magnet's north pole; the other is attracted to the south and is called the magnet's south pole. Materials that retain their magnetism all the time are called permanent magnets. An electric current flowing in a coil of wire produces a magnet called an electromagnet that can be switched on and off. Electromagnets are used in electric motors, loudspeakers, and many other devices.

MAGNETIC POLES

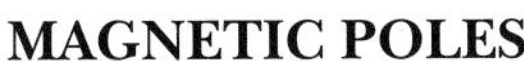

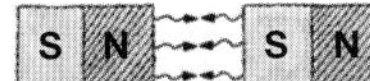

The north pole of one magnet and the south pole of another magnet attract each other.

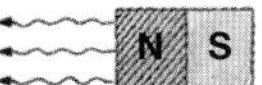

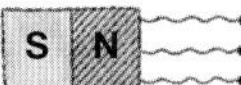

A magnetic pole, such as a south pole, repels (pushes away) another pole of the same kind.

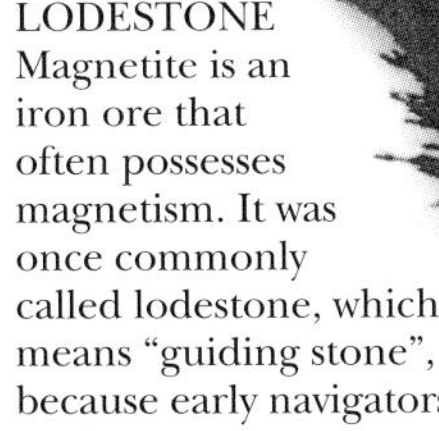

LODESTONE
Magnetite is an iron ore that often possesses magnetism. It was once commonly called lodestone, which means "guiding stone", because early navigators used it as a compass.

The geographical North and South Poles lie on the Earth's axis, which is the line around which the Earth spins.

The pattern of lines shows the Earth's magnetic field. The field is strongest where the lines are closest together.

The magnetic north and south poles lie a small distance away from geographical North and South.

GEOMAGNETISM
The Earth produces a magnetic field which makes it seem as though it has a huge "bar" magnet inside it. Electric currents flowing within the Earth's liquid iron core cause the Earth's magnetism, which is called geomagnetism.

ELECTROMAGNETS
An electromagnet is a coil of wire. An electric current within the coil creates a magnetic field. The field can be made stronger by winding the wire around a piece of iron. Turning off the current switches off the magnetic field. Some cranes use an electromagnet instead of a hook.

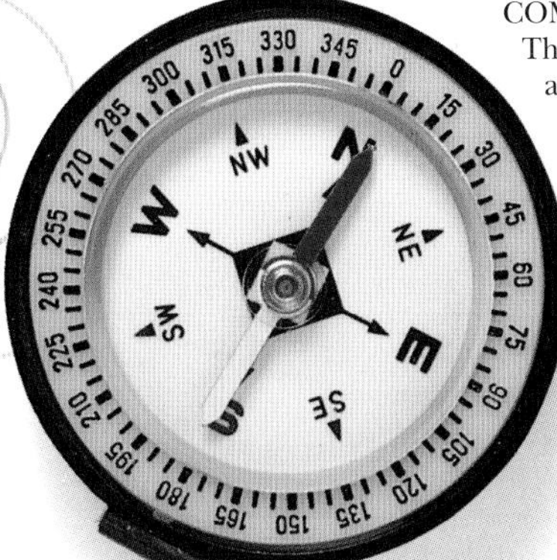

COMPASS
The needle inside a magnetic compass is a thin, light magnet, balanced so that it swings freely. The needle's north pole points towards the Earth's magnetic north pole, which is very close to the geographical North. People use magnetic compasses to navigate at sea and on land.

Find out more
EARTH
ELECTRICITY
MAPS
NAVIGATION

MAMMALS

THE ANIMAL GROUP CALLED MAMMALS includes the heaviest, tallest, and fastest animals on land – the elephant, the giraffe, and the cheetah. Mice, whales, rhinoceroses, bats, and humans are also mammals. Like birds, mammals are warm-blooded (endothermic), but three features set them apart from all other creatures. All mammals are covered in fur or hair, all feed their young on milk, and all have a unique type of jaw. The jawbone helps us to identify the fossilized bones of prehistoric mammals that lived on Earth millions of years ago. Mammals are also members of the group known as vertebrates because they all have vertebrae (backbones). Today there are more than 5,000 kinds of mammals, including carnivores (flesh eaters) such as tigers; herbivores (plant eaters) such as rabbits; and omnivores (flesh and plant eaters) such as bears. Cattle, sheep, goats, and most other farm animals are mammals, and many pets are mammals too, including cats, dogs, and guinea pigs. Mammals live nearly everywhere. They are found on land, in the sea, and in the sky, from the coldest Arctic to the most searing heat of the desert.

MARSUPIAL YOUNG
Marsupials are very tiny when they are born. At birth, a kangaroo is less than 2.5 cm (1 in) long. It crawls through its mother's fur into a pocket-like pouch on the abdomen, where it attaches itself to her teat and suckles milk.

A mammal's body is covered in fur.

A kangaroo's large tail is so strong that it can act as a prop for the kangaroo to lean on.

Young male joey

PLACENTAL MAMMALS

Most mammals, including monkeys, cats, and dogs, are called placental mammals because the young develop inside the mother's womb, or uterus, and are fed by means of the placenta. The placenta is a specialized organ embedded in the wall of the womb. It carries nutrients and other essential materials from the mother's blood to the baby's blood. These nutrients help the young to grow and develop. After the young are born, the placenta comes out of the uterus as afterbirth.

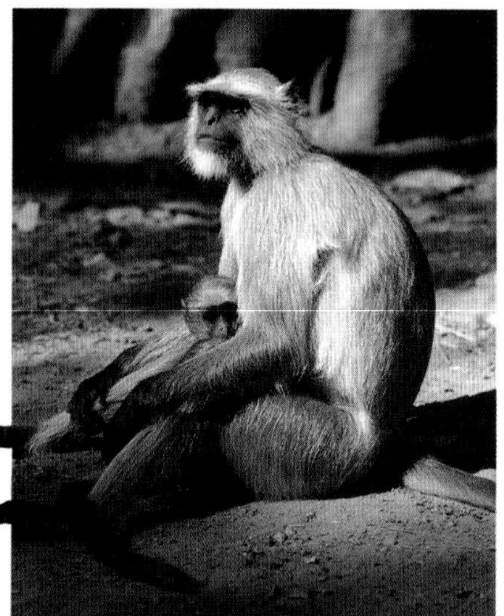

PRIMATES

Monkeys, apes, and humans belong to a group called primates. Primates are able to grasp with their hands. Most primates have thumbs and big toes, with flat fingernails rather than claws. Members of the primate group range in size from the mouse lemur, which weighs only 60 g (2 oz), to the gorilla, which weighs up to 275 kg (610 lb).

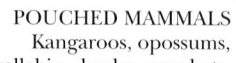

POUCHED MAMMALS
Kangaroos, opossums, wallabies, koalas, wombats, and bandicoots are all known as marsupials, or pouched mammals. These animals carry their young in their pouches until the young are able to fend for themselves. Once it has left the pouch, the joey (young kangaroo) returns to the pouch to suck milk. Marsupials are found in Australia and New Guinea, South America, and North America. A few marsupials, such as the shrew opossum of South America, do not have pouches.

MONOTREME MAMMALS
Three kinds of mammals lay eggs. They are called monotreme mammals, and include the platypus and the two types of echidna (spiny ant-eater). All are found in Australasia. After about 10 days, the young hatch out of the eggs, then feed on their mother's milk.

SPINY ANTEATER
The short-beaked spiny ant-eater, or echidna, lays a single egg in a temporary pouch on its abdomen. The young echidna hatches, then sucks milk from mammary glands on its mother's abdomen.

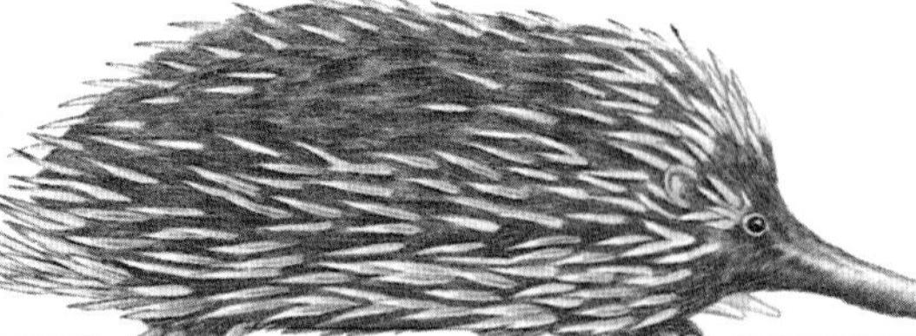

MAMMAL GROUPS

There are about 27 main groups of mammals, some of which are shown below. Rodents make up half of all mammals; bats account for a quarter. There are only three kinds of elephant, and the aardvark is in a group of its own.

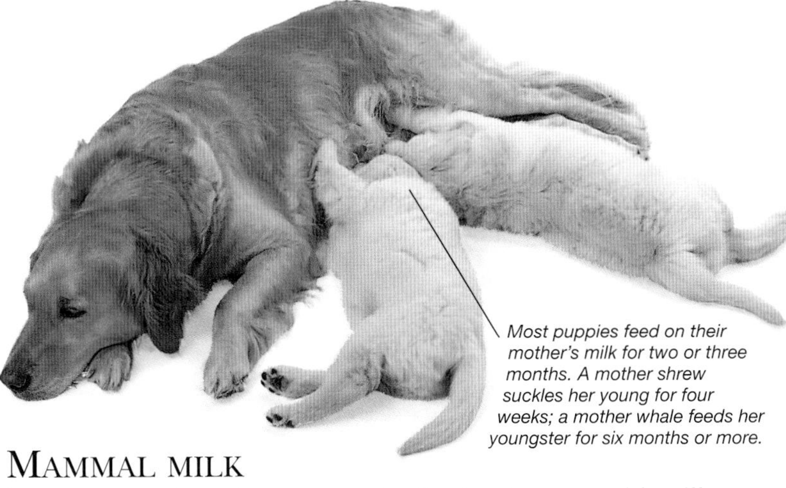

Most puppies feed on their mother's milk for two or three months. A mother shrew suckles her young for four weeks; a mother whale feeds her youngster for six months or more.

MAMMAL MILK

Mammals are the only creatures that feed their young with milk. When the female is about to give birth, she starts to produce milk in mammary glands on the chest or abdomen. When the young are born, they suck the milk from the mother's teats. Mother's milk is an ideal food for the young – warm and nourishing, and full of special substances which protect the young from disease. As the babies grow larger and stronger, they take less milk and begin to eat solid foods. This process is called weaning.

GESTATION

The time between mating and birth, when the young develop in the mother's womb, is called the gestation or pregnancy period. In general, large mammals have longer pregnancies and fewer young than small mammals.

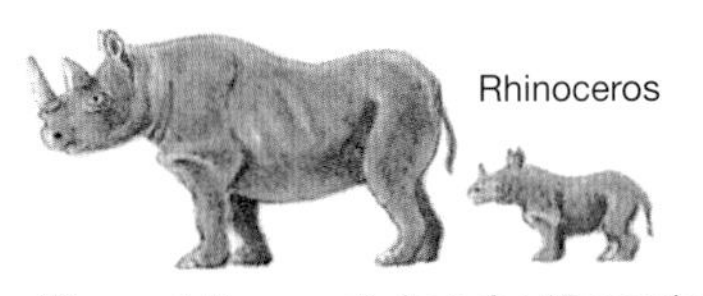

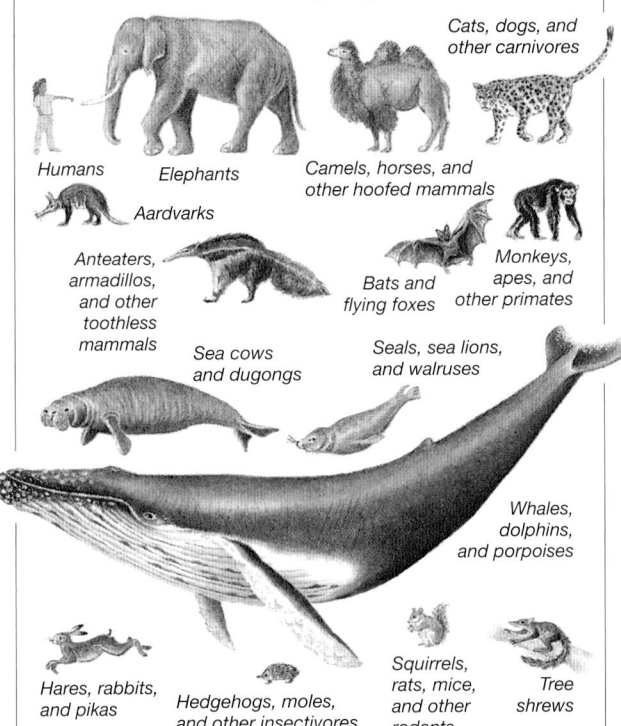

The gestation usually lasts for 15 months; one young is born.

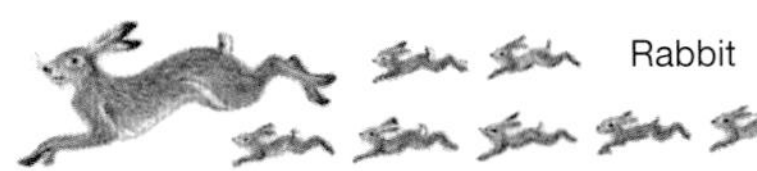

Gestation usually lasts for 30 days; as many as eight young are born in a litter.

Dirty fur harbours pests and also lets heat escape, so many mammals spend time cleaning or grooming their fur.

HAIR AND FUR

Fur or hair protects the mammal's skin from injury and the sun's rays. It also keeps heat in and moisture out. The colours and patterns of the fur provide camouflage. Water-dwelling mammals such as beavers have special oily, waterproof fur. The porcupine's spines are modified hairs and the rhinoceros's horn is made from strong hairs tightly packed together.

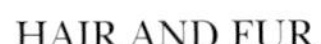

ARMADILLO

Some mammals, such as armadillos and pangolins, have reptile-like scales instead of fur. The scales, or scutes, of an armadillo are made of a type of horn and bone that grows from the skin. Hairs grow between the scutes and also cover the animal's soft-skinned underbelly.

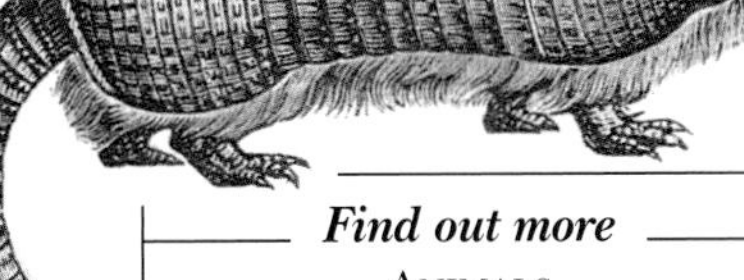

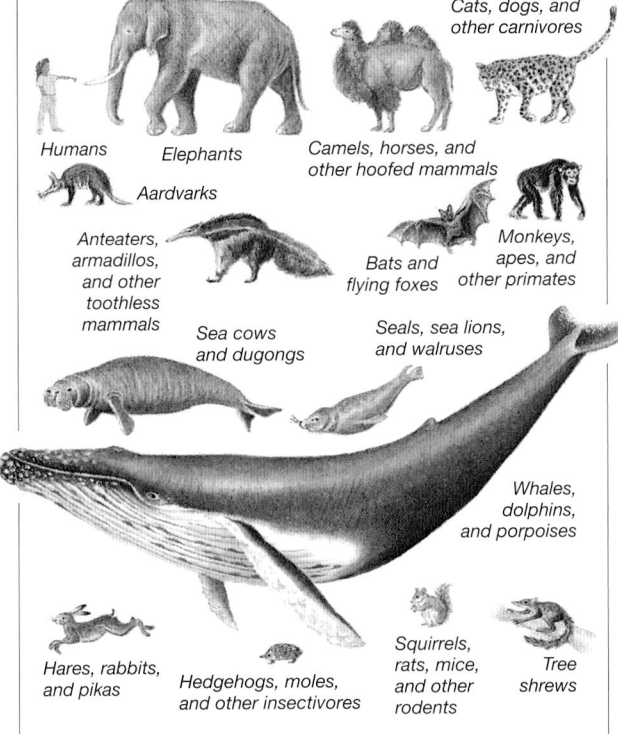

BODY TEMPERATURE

Mammals and birds are called warm-blooded animals because they can maintain a high body temperature even in cold conditions. Mammals do, however, need plenty of food to provide the energy for warmth. The heat to warm a mammal is produced by chemical reactions in the body, particularly in the muscles.

Huskies are able to stay warm in deep snow because of their thick fur.

Find out more

ANIMALS
ANIMAL SENSES
AUSTRALIAN WILDLIFE
FARM ANIMALS
FLIGHT, ANIMAL
HIBERNATION
PREHISTORIC LIFE

NELSON

MANDELA

IN FEBRUARY 1990 the 72-year-old Nelson Mandela walked into freedom after spending more than 27 years in prison. He had spent his life opposing the white-led South African government, which practised the policy of apartheid, or separate development of the races. Within four years Mandela led his party, the African National Congress (ANC), to victory in the general election and became the first-ever black president of a multiracial, democratic South Africa. By the time he retired in 1999 he was one of the most famous and deeply-loved political leaders in the world.

1918 Born in Mvezo, Transkei.

1942 Gained law degree; practises in Johannesburg.

1952 Becomes deputy national president of the ANC.

1962 Imprisoned as a leader of the ANC.

1964 Sentenced to life imprisonment and sent to Robben Island (until 1985).

1990 Released from prison.

1993 Wins Nobel Peace Prize.

1994 Elected first black president of South Africa.

1999 Steps down as president.

AFRICAN NATIONAL CONGRESS

In 1912, the African National Congress was formed to protect the interests of the black population of South Africa. It tried to achieve a multiracial, democratic country through peaceful means, but the South African government thought it was revolutionary, and banned it in 1961. From 1952, Mandela was a senior member of the organization. He became its leader in 1991.

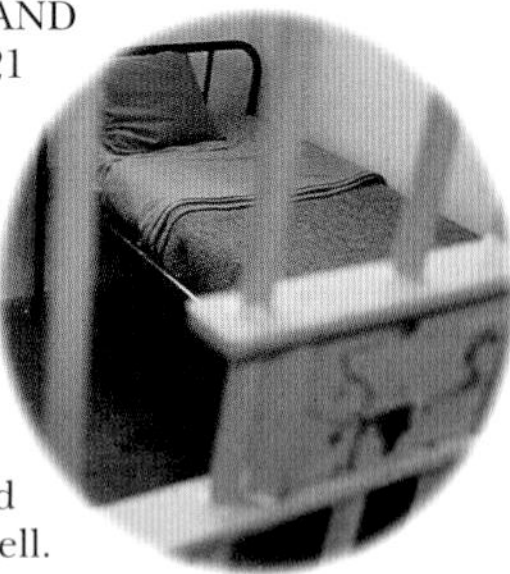

ROBBEN ISLAND
Nelson Mandela spent 21 of his 27 years in prison on Robben Island, a high-security prison off the coast of Cape Town. He broke rocks in the quarry, and studied with other ANC prisoners. Now the prison is closed, and people visit Mandela's cell.

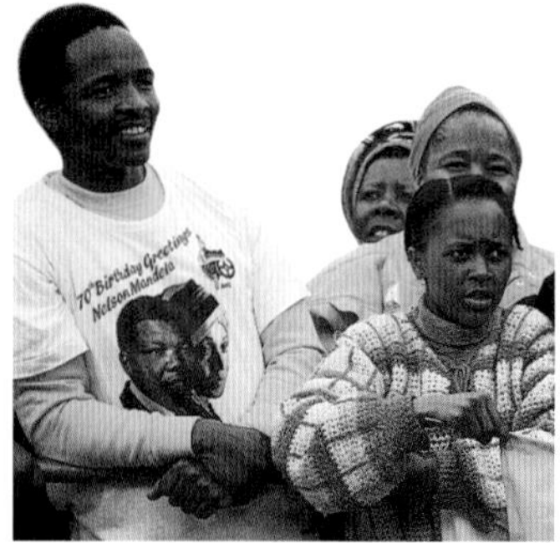

FREE NELSON MANDELA
People campaigned worldwide to free Mandela from prison. They boycotted (refused to buy) South African goods, such as fruit and wine, and demonstrated against the South African government. In 1988, a huge rock concert was held at London's Wembley Stadium to mark Mandela's 70th birthday.

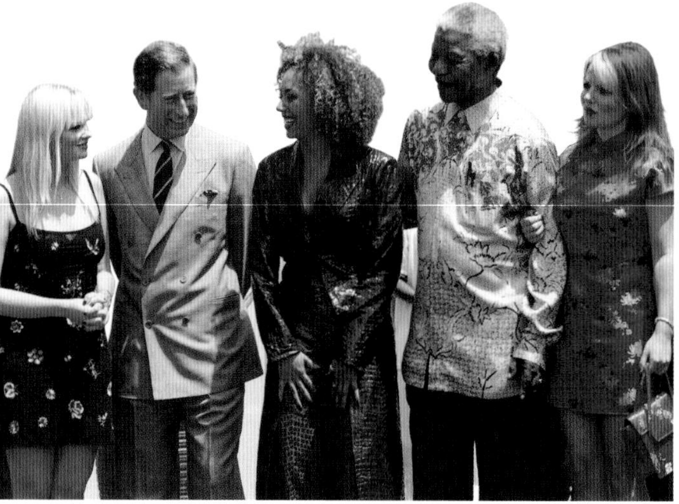

TRUTH AND RECONCILIATION
In order to heal the wounds left by apartheid, Mandela set up the Truth and Reconciliation Commission. Nobel Peace Prize winner, Archbishop Desmond Tutu, ran the Commission. It examined the events of the apartheid era, and tried to reconcile (bring together) former enemies.

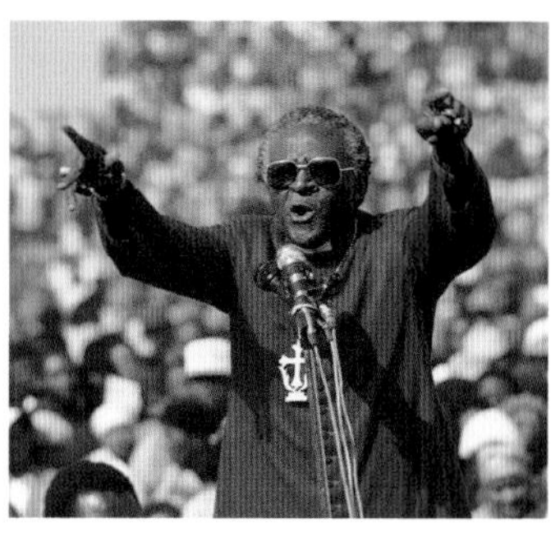

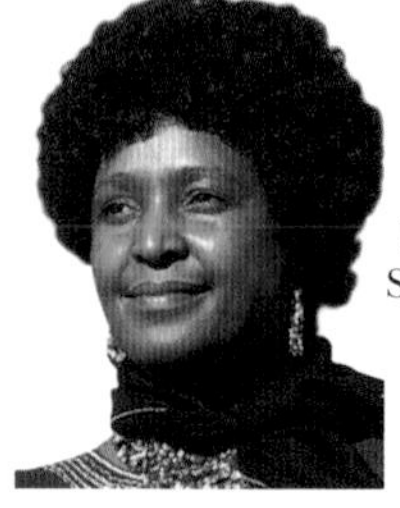

WINNIE MANDELA
In 1961, Mandela married Winnie Mdikizela (b. 1934). She campaigned for his release, but her political activities were controversial. They divorced in 1996.

PRESIDENT

The first multiracial elections in South Africa were held in 1994. Mandela led the ANC to a huge victory, and became president. He worked to obtain peace, and unite all the peoples of his troubled country. When famous people – including the Prince of Wales and the Spice Girls – came to see him, he always wore one of his distinctive shirts.

Find out more

AFRICA, HISTORY OF
HUMAN RIGHTS
SOUTH AFRICA, HISTORY OF

MAO ZEDONG

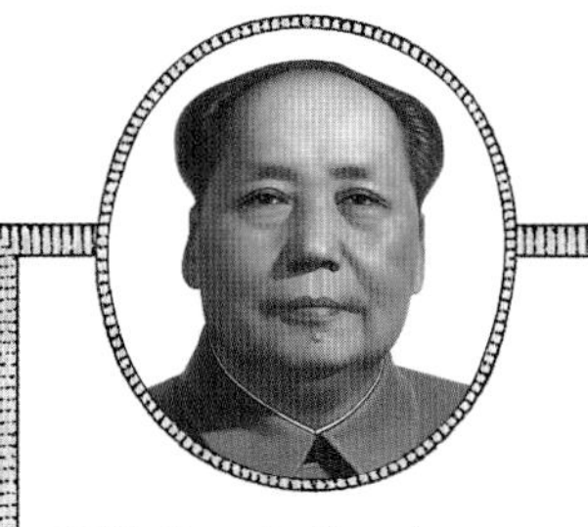

1893 Born in Shaoshan, Hunan province.

1921 Founding member of Chinese Communist Party.

1928 Establishes Chinese Soviet (Communist) Republic in Kiangsi province.

1934-35 Leads The Long March.

1945-49 Leads Communists in fight to overthrow Nationalist government.

1958 Great Leap Forward

1966-69 Cultural Revolution

1976 Dies.

ONE MAN TRANSFORMED CHINA from a backward peasant society into one of the most powerful nations in the world. That man was Mao Zedong. Mao was born to a peasant family, and as a young man he travelled widely, observing the conditions of the poor. He became interested in Communism as a way to improve people's lives and, in 1921, helped set up the Chinese Communist Party. There followed a long period of struggle between the Communists, led by Mao, and the Nationalist Party (who believed in strong national government), led by Chiang Kai-shek. The struggle ended in a civil war. In October 1949, the Communist Party was victorious and took power in China. Mao proclaimed China a People's Republic. Under his leadership, the Communists put everything under state control. Mao's face became a familiar sight. Since his death in 1976, many people have criticized Mao for causing the deaths of millions during his rule.

LONG MARCH

In October 1934, Mao led his Communist supporters from their stronghold, Juichin, in Kiangsi province to Yenan in Shensi province in northwest China. Kiangsi was under attack from Chiang Kai-shek. More than 100,000 people marched for more than a year, covering 9,700 km (6,000 miles). Only 8,000 marchers survived the ordeal.

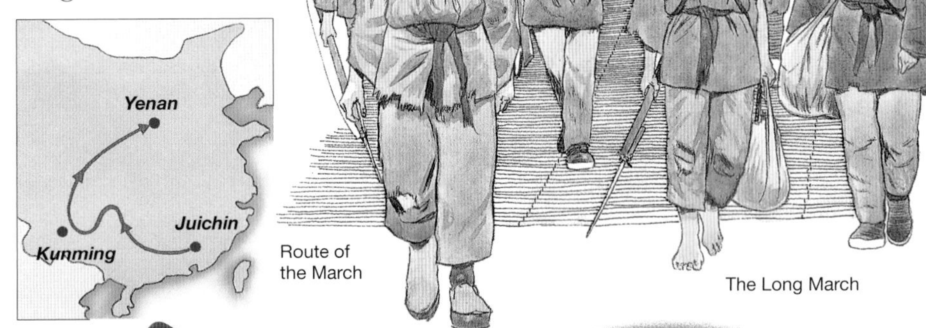

Route of the March

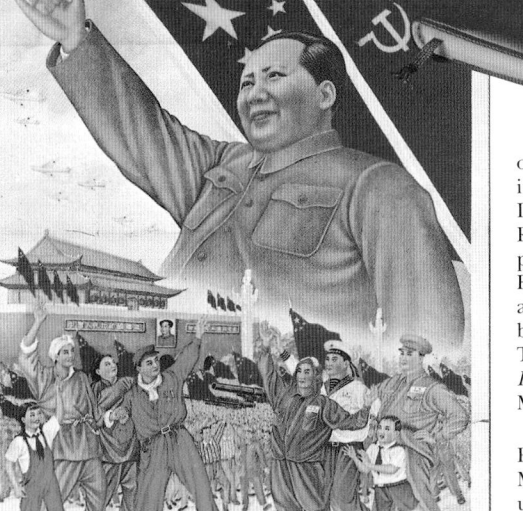

The Long March

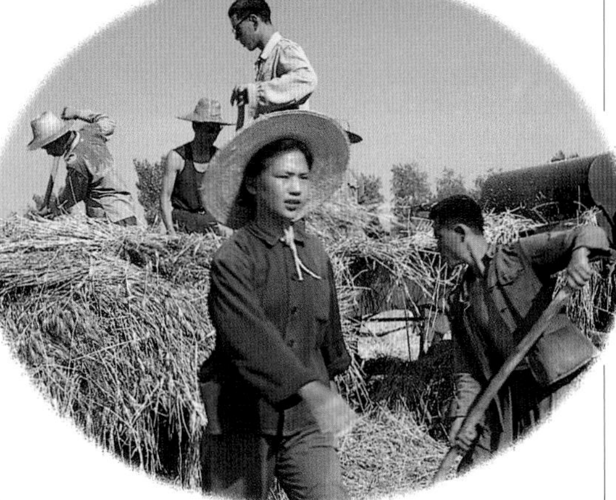

CULTURAL REVOLUTION

After the failure of the Great Leap Forward, Mao lost influence inside the Communist Party. In 1966, he launched the Cultural Revolution, a campaign to regain power and get rid of foreign influences. For three years, China was in turmoil as every aspect of society was criticized by the Red Guards, followers of Mao. They armed themselves with the *Little Red Book*, which contained Mao's thoughts.

GREAT LEAP FORWARD

In 1958 Mao launched a plan to improve the Chinese economy. The Great Leap Forward, as it was called, set up huge agricultural communes and encouraged the growth of small, labour-intensive industries. However, the policy failed and led to millions of deaths through famine.

PERSONALITY CULT

Mao Zedong encouraged a cult of his personality to unite the country. His round face with the familiar mole on the chin adorned every public building in China. He was praised as the father and leader of his nation, and huge rallies were held at which he addressed his followers.

Find out more

CHINA, HISTORY OF
COMMUNISM

MAPS

MAPPA MUNDI
An English priest created the Mappa Mundi, or map of the world, between 1280 and 1300. It shows how Christians of that time viewed their world but was of little use to travellers. For religious reasons, Jerusalem is at the centre, and east is at the top of the map.

EARLY TRAVELLERS FOUND THEIR WAY by asking directions from strangers they met. Their guides created the first maps by scratching rough drawings of the route on the ground. Maps still show the positions of different places, but travellers today need many different maps. For local journeys, they use large-scale maps which cover a small area but show lots of detail. For longer journeys, travellers may use a small-scale map that shows a larger area in less detail, or they may use an atlas (a book of maps) of whole countries. There are also special-purpose maps; political maps, for example, show legal boundaries. Utility companies need large-scale maps to show them where to dig for power lines and water pipes. Sailors use a special kind of map, called a chart, which shows coastlines and water depths.

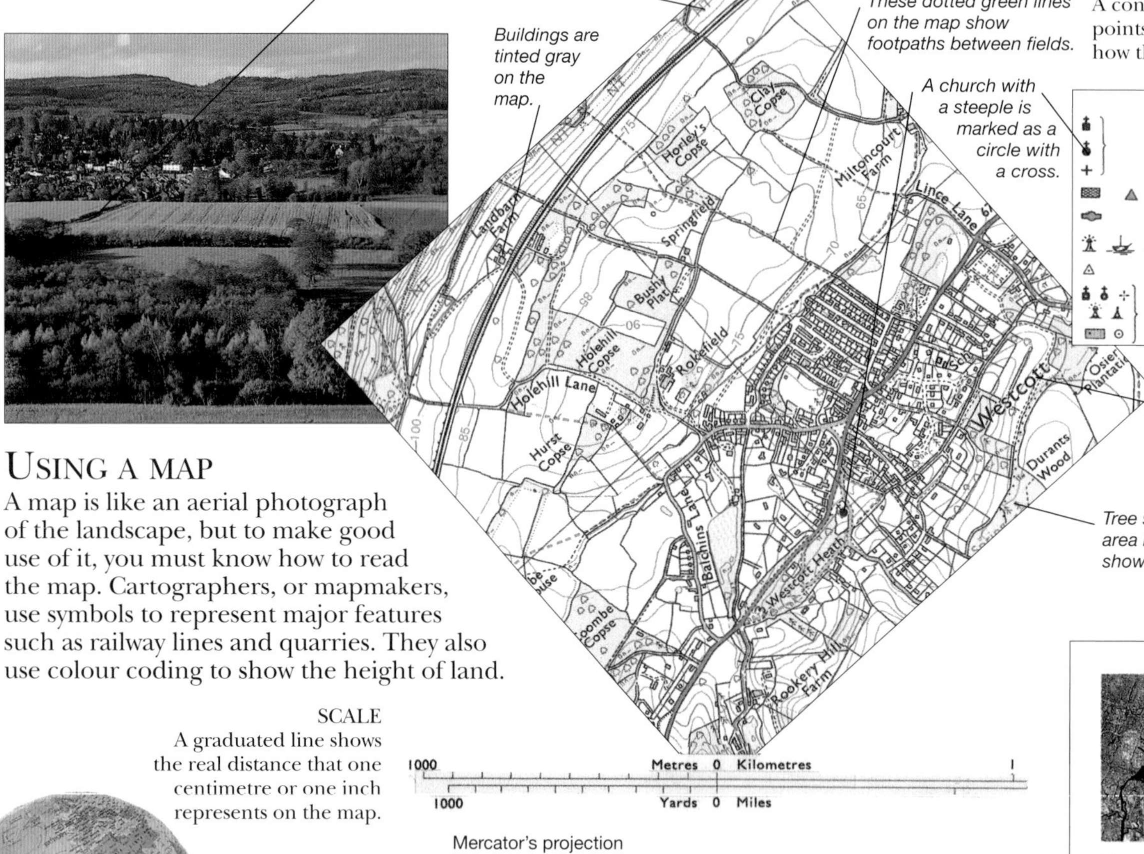

Map shows the landscape that appears in the photograph.
The steeper the hill, the closer together the contours are.
These dotted green lines on the map show footpaths between fields.
Buildings are tinted gray on the map.
A church with a steeple is marked as a circle with a cross.
The bigger a place is, the bigger its name is printed on the map.
Tree symbols show that an area is wooded; they also show different types of trees.
Clay Copse
Horley's Copse
Miltoncourt Farm
Lince Lane
Landbarn Farm
Springfield
Bushy Place
Holehill Copse
Holehill Lane
Rokefield
Westcott
Hurst Copse
Durants Wood
Balchins Lane
Westcott Heath
Rookery Hill Farm
1000 Metres 0 Kilometres 1
1000 Yards 0 Miles

CONTOURS
A contour line on the map joins points of equal height and shows how the land slopes.

LEGEND
Many maps have a panel called a legend explaining what the symbols and colours mean. These symbols save space, so that map-makers can include more information.

USING A MAP

A map is like an aerial photograph of the landscape, but to make good use of it, you must know how to read the map. Cartographers, or mapmakers, use symbols to represent major features such as railway lines and quarries. They also use colour coding to show the height of land.

SCALE
A graduated line shows the real distance that one centimetre or one inch represents on the map.

The equator is 0° latitude.

LONGITUDE AND LATITUDE
Lines of longitude, or meridians, run between the North and South Poles on a world map showing you how far east or west you are. Longitude is measured in degrees from the meridian that runs through Greenwich, England. Lines of latitude are parallel to the equator and show how many degrees north or south you are.

Mercator's projection

Peters' projection

MERCATOR'S PROJECTION
To represent the round Earth on a flat sheet of paper, mapmakers use a projection. Imagine a glass globe with a light at its centre. The light projects shadows of the continents onto a flat screen. All projections distort the world's shape, areas or distances. The most familiar world map is Gerhard Mercator's projection made in 1569. This shows the correct shapes of the continents but distorts their areas. Arno Peters' projection, published in 1973, distorts the shapes of countries but shows their true areas. It counteracts the focus on Europe encouraged by Mercator, whose map makes Europe look bigger than it really is.

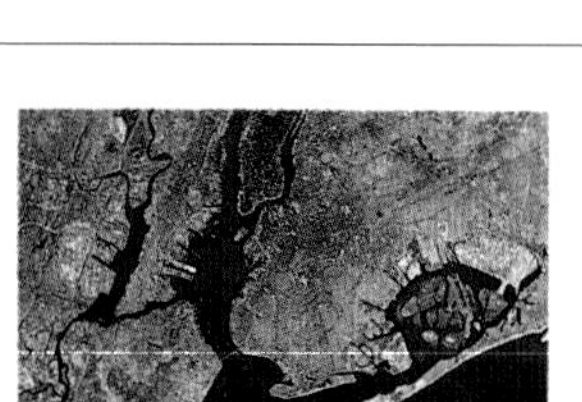
New York area from a satellite

SATELLITE MAP

Satellites can now map every part of the world. Their sensors send video photographs of the Earth's surface to ground stations, which turn them into maps.

Find out more

EXPLORERS
MAGNETISM
NAVIGATION
SATELLITES

MARSH AND SWAMP WILDLIFE

THE SALT AND FRESHWATER habitats of swamps and marshland are called wetlands. Marsh and swamp wildlife includes crocodiles, frogs, birds, fish, and countless plants. At different times of the year the water level of marshes and swamps rises and falls. In summer the land dries up, and in winter it floods. Wetlands are usually unsuitable for large mammals – except the African swamps where hippopotamuses live. Smaller mammals such as muskrats live in North American swamps, and the European marshes are home to many birds. The main plant life consists of reeds, rushes, saw grass, and cattail. Large trees are found only in the tropical mangroves, where the trees form dense thickets. Willows and other waterside trees grow in the higher, drier ground around the marsh.

CONSERVATION
Farming and industry threaten many swamplands, but some animals, such as the marsh harriers shown here, are protected. They live in the Coto Doñana National Park in Spain – one of Europe's most important wetlands.

PROBOSCIS MONKEY
This large-nosed monkey lives among the mangrove trees of river and coastal swamps. The proboscis monkey is a good swimmer. Proboscis monkeys eat leaves, flowers, and fruit.

PELICAN
These fish-eating birds build their nests in remote marshland areas. Some species breed on the ground, some in trees. Others, such as spot-billed and Dalmatian pelicans, are very rare, because of destruction of their nesting sites.

Front fins help the mudskipper walk on mud and grip roots.

COTTONMOUTH
Most snakes are good swimmers and climbers, and they can travel through swamps with ease in search of prey. The cottonmouth, also called the water moccasin, is a North American swamp dweller with a very poisonous bite.

SWAMP RABBIT
This large rabbit from North America can swim well and dives to escape from predators. Swamp rabbits eat water plants, grasses, and other vegetation.

Swamp mud is usually so dense and waterlogged that, unlike normal soil, it contains almost no oxygen. The roots of mangrove trees stick up above the mud, to absorb the oxygen they need to grow.

MARSHLAND

Marshes are nursery areas for many insects whose larvae live in water, such as dragonflies and mosquitoes. Insect larvae and worms form the main diet of many fish and water birds. Frogs, toads, and tadpoles are also eaten by larger creatures.

MUDSKIPPER
This unusual fish has a store of water in its large gill chambers which allows it to live out of water for long periods. From time to time it skitters over the mud to a pool to take in a new supply of water.

MANGROVE SWAMPS
Mangroves are trees that grow in muddy tropical swamps. Some kinds of mangrove trees grow in fresh water; others tolerate salty water and grow on the coast or in river estuaries. Their roots and trunks trap mud, and their seeds begin to grow while they are still attached to the parent tree. When the seeds drop into the mud, they quickly establish roots so they are not washed away.

Archer fish adjusts its aim if it misses, and fires again.

ARCHER FISH
The archer fish spits drops of water at insects on over-hanging twigs. The insects fall off the twigs, into the water, where the fish gulps them down.

The drops of water hit the insect like tiny bullets.

Find out more

BIRDS
FISH
MONKEYS AND APES
RABBITS AND HARES
SEASHORE WILDLIFE
SNAKES

Materials

Ever since early humans started using tools, about 2.5 million years ago, materials have played an important part in our lives. This is because everything we use is made from some sort of material. A material is anything that is used to make something; it is not just a woven fabric like the material in your clothes. Buildings, cars, and furniture are all made from materials of one kind or another. Some materials are natural, such as the stone and timber of a house. Others are artificial, like the plastic used to make the keyboard of a computer. Natural materials can also be further divided into categories such as minerals, metals, and organics. Every material has its own properties, making it better suited for some jobs than others, and scientists are always inventing more materials.

METAL
Because they are tough and hard-wearing, metals have been used for centuries. Pure metals such as iron are natural elements. Metals can also be mixed to make alloys, which are usually stronger than pure metals.

Racket frame made of plastic containing graphite.

Sports clothes made from synthetic nylon and polyester, and natural cotton.

Sunglasses made from plastic.

Cap made from natural cotton fabric.

Socks made from natural fibres.

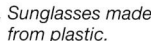

Drink can made from aluminium metal.

RUBBER
Some materials, such as rubber, exist in natural and synthetic forms. Natural rubber is the gummy sap of rubber trees. It is expensive to produce, so scientists have found ways to copy its chemical make-up and produce it more cheaply.

Chair made from wood, a tough natural material.

Tennis balls made from rubber with a woollen felt coating.

Paper made from wood pulp.

Shoes made from canvas, with rubber soles for flexibility.

Glass

Some containers are made from glass, a tough material that lets light through and resists heat. Glass is made from sand, which is crushed quartz, a natural mineral that forms glassy crystals. Glassmakers melt sand, then cool it quickly so it solidifies without forming crystals.

Organics

Any materials that come from plants or animals are known as organic. They include bone, leather, wool, cotton, and wood. Throughout history, people have used organic materials to make a whole range of objects, from furniture and artefacts, to clothes and musical instruments. Each organic material has its own particular properties. Wool, for instance, is warm, strong, and absorbent.

Flax plants, used to make linen

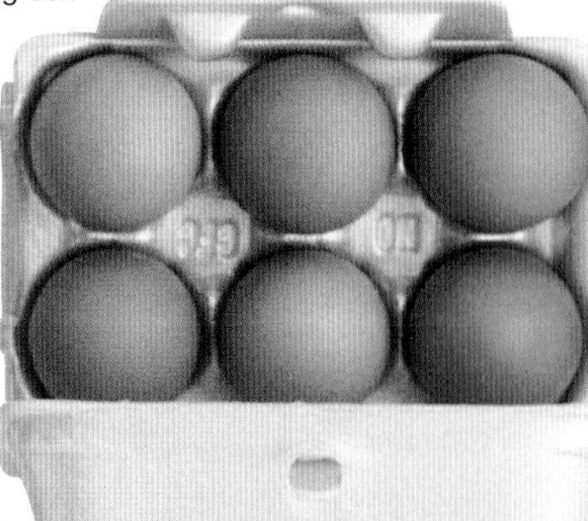

Plastic egg box

PLASTICS
There are many kinds of plastic. Some copy natural materials, but others are specially designed for new applications. The word "plastic" actually means "capable of being moulded", and it is this property that makes plastics so useful. Some plastics melt when heated and are easily formed into shapes. Others are heated to make them set, so they can be used for objects that become hot, such as kettles.

Find out more
Glass and ceramics
Metals
Plastics
Textiles

MATHEMATICS

PROBABILITY THEORY
Probability theory is the analysis of chance. For instance, if you repeatedly roll two dice, you can use probability theory to work out how often you can expect a certain number to come up.

SENDING A SPACECRAFT to a distant planet is like trying to throw a stone at an invisible moving target. Space scientists do not use trial and error; instead they use the science of mathematics to direct the spacecraft precisely to its target. Mathematics is the study of number, shape, and quantity. There are several different branches of mathematics, and they are valuable both in science and in everyday life. For instance, arithmetic consists of addition, subtraction, multiplication, and division of numbers; it helps you work out the change when you buy something. Geometry is the study of shape and angle; it is useful in carpentry, architecture, and many other fields. Algebra is a kind of mathematical language in which problems can be solved using symbols in place of varying or unknown numbers. Branches of mathematics that relate to practical problems are called applied mathematics. However, some mathematicians study pure mathematics – numerical problems which have no known practical use.

INFINITY

Pure mathematicians study the fundamental ideas of numbers and shapes. One such idea is the concept of infinity, which means "never-ending". The pattern shown above is called a fractal. It is produced by a computer according to a strict formula (rule). You can enlarge any part of the pattern again and again, but you will still get a pattern that is just as intricate. The pattern is infinitely complex.

SYMMETRY

A symmetrical object is made up of alike parts. Many symmetrical patterns and shapes occur in nature. A starfish exhibits lateral symmetry, since one of its arms looks the same when reflected in a line drawn along its length. This line is called an axis. The starfish also displays rotational symmetry, as it looks the same when rotated around its central point.

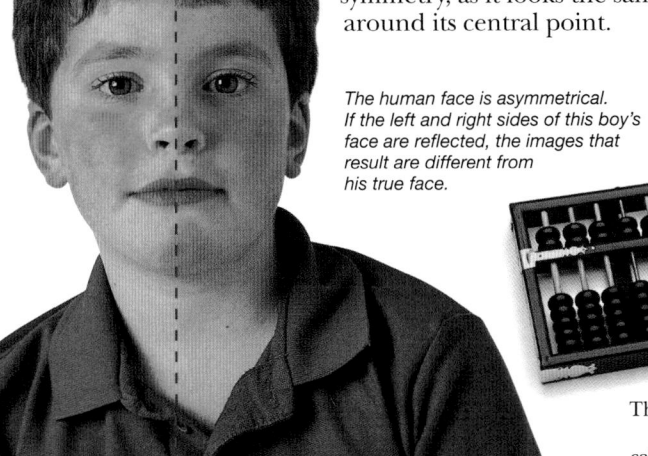

The human face is asymmetrical. If the left and right sides of this boy's face are reflected, the images that result are different from his true face.

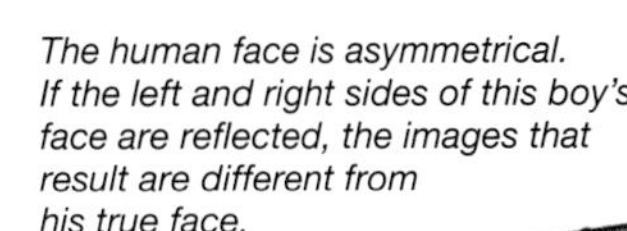

ABACUS
The abacus, or counting frame, is an ancient calculating device which comes from China. It consists of rows of beads that represent units of tens, hundreds, and thousands. The abacus is worked by moving the beads along the rows. People in Asian countries still use the abacus as a rapid tool for adding, subtracting, multiplying, and dividing.

EUCLID

The ancient Greek mathematician Euclid (c. 330-275 B.C.) was the first to formulate theories on the nature of shapes and angles. His book *Elements* outlined the principles of geometry, and its theories were accepted for centuries. Euclid found many practical uses for geometry, such as in optical science.

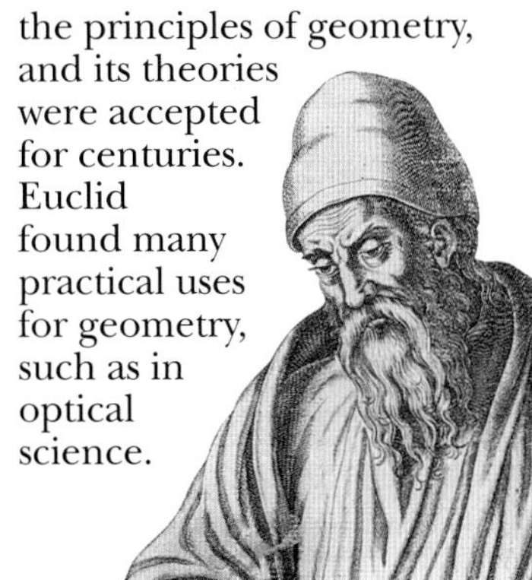

PARTS OF A CIRCLE
A circle is a shape in which every point on its circumference, or outside margin, is the same distance from the centre. The diameter is the line that exactly bisects a circle, passing through the centre. The distance from the centre to the circumference is the radius. The slice of circle between two radii is a sector, and the part of the circumference that bounds a sector is an arc.

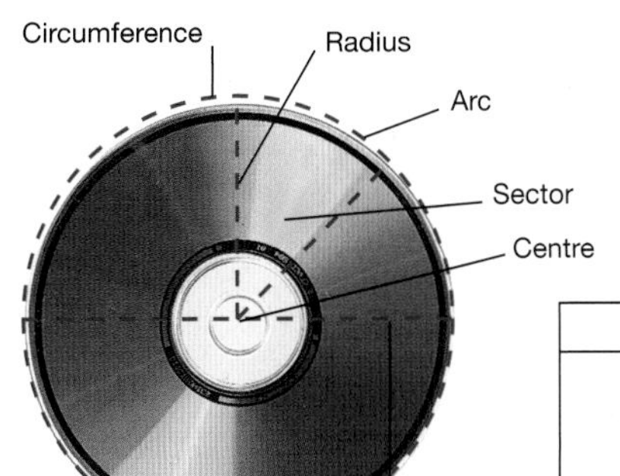

Find out more

COMPUTERS
GEOMETRY
NUMBERS
WEIGHTS AND MEASURES

MAYA

DEEP IN THE TROPICAL FORESTS of Mexico, the Mayan people created one of the most amazing ancient civilizations, which reached its height between A.D. 250 and 900. The Maya built cities with huge stone temples. Each city was the centre of a separate kingdom, with a king who was treated like a god. The Maya were great scholars who developed systems of mathematics and astronomy. They even created their own writing system and used it to carve inscriptions about their history on stone plaques that they set up in their cities. Despite their sophistication, the Maya had only the simplest technology. They used stone tools, and did not know about the wheel. By the 1500s the Spanish had conquered the region.

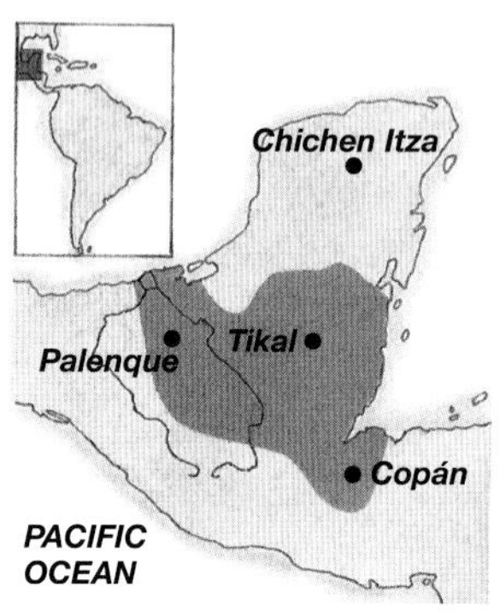

MAYAN CIVILIZATION
The Maya came from the Yucatan Peninsula and the highlands to the south, in what is now eastern Mexico. They also built cities in parts of modern Guatemala and Honduras.

FLINT CARVING
Craftworkers made their tools out of stones such as flint or obsidian (a black, naturally occurring glass). They could work these materials to make a sharp edge. The Maya became highly skilled at this type of stoneworking, and made intricate carvings in strange shapes to show off their skill. Many were made to place in graves or as offerings to the gods.

Outer shell of stone concealed earth base and royal tomb.

Temple contains historic inscriptions.

Priests used the main staircase.

People taking part in ceremonies could stand on the main stepped levels.

PALENQUE

The Temple of the Inscriptions at Palenque was a famous Mayan pyramid. Deep inside the base was a secret chamber containing the tomb of a local king, Pacal, who died in about A.D. 684. In the temple on top of the pyramid were stone tablets carved with glyphs that recorded the history of the local kings up to Pacal's reign. Its ruins still exist today.

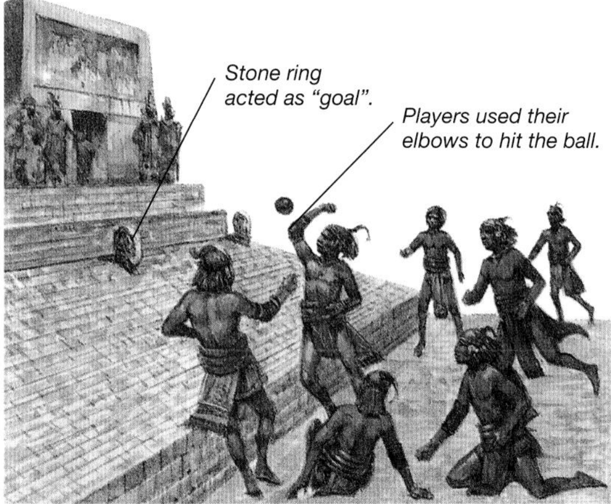

Stone ring acted as "goal".

Players used their elbows to hit the ball.

GLYPHS
Mayan writing was made up of a series of signs, which archaeologists call glyphs. Many of the glyphs were simplified pictures of the objects they stood for. Some represented sounds, which were used to build up words. Others were symbols that stood for different numbers. The Maya used glyphs to record their calendar, and to write inscriptions about their history.

Glyph describing a Mayan noble woman called Lady Xoc

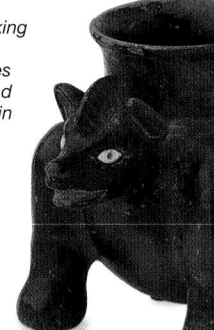

BALL GAME
Many cities had a ball court where people played a game with a rubber ball. Players wore padded clothing, and were only allowed to touch the ball with their hips, arms, or elbows. The aim was to get the ball through a small stone ring at the side of the court. Players who lost were sometimes put to death.

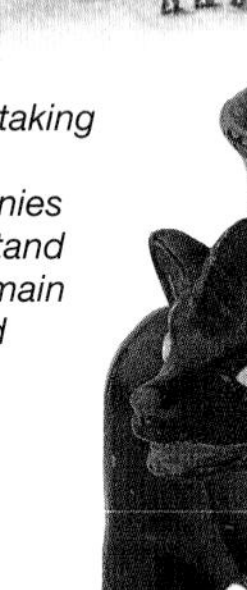

Pot shaped like a jaguar

BLOOD SACRIFICE
Some Mayan communities believed that their gods would be pleased if people were killed in their honour. They also saw sacrificial blood as food for the gods. In some places a pot shaped like a jaguar, a beast sacred to the Maya, was used to collect the blood.

Find out more
BRONZE AGE
CENTRAL AMERICA
WHEELS

MEDICINE

TWO HUNDRED AND FIFTY YEARS AGO, most people lived no longer than 35 years. Today, in the industrialized parts of the world, the average lifespan has increased to more than 70 years. Better food and hygiene have helped, but one of the main reasons for this change is the advances made in medicine. Medicine is the branch of science concerned with the prevention, diagnosis (identification), and treatment of disease and damage to the human body. Medical scientists are constantly searching for new ways of treating diseases. Treatments include drugs, radiation therapy, and surgery. Preventive measures, such as vaccinations against infections, are becoming an increasingly important part of modern medicine.

DIAGNOSIS
A doctor's first step with a sick patient is to diagnose the illness. This can be done in various ways – by asking the patient about his or her symptoms (physical feelings), by making a physical examination of the ill person, and by carrying out medical tests if necessary.

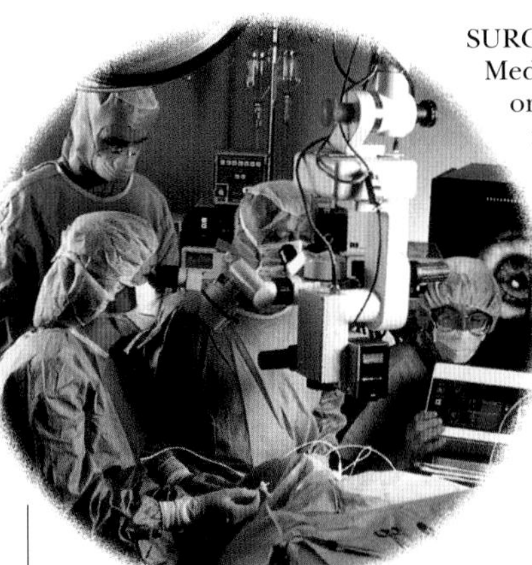

SURGERY
Medical treatments may include drugs or surgery. Surgery is the branch of medicine that involves operating, or cutting into the body, to treat the cause of an illness. Today surgery is so advanced that surgeons can sometimes repair or replace organs such as the kidneys and the heart.

BRANCHES OF MEDICINE

Medicine is a huge subject and nobody can hope to know it all. Thus doctors, nurses, and other medical workers often become expert in a single area of medicine, a process which can take years and years of study.

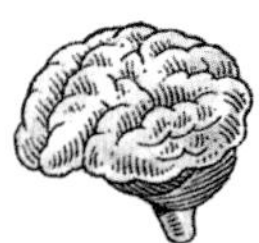

Neurology is concerned with disorders of the brain and nerves.

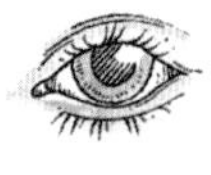

Ophthalmology is the treatment of disorders of the eyes.

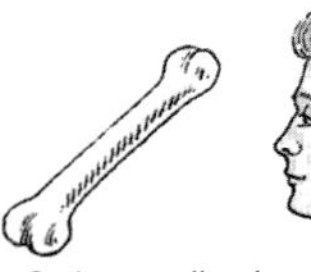

Orthopaedics is the care of the spine, bones, joints, and muscles.

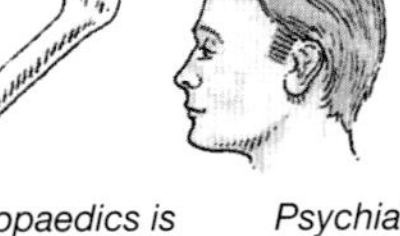

Psychiatry is the study of mental health problems.

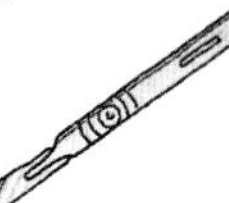

Cutting into the body to cure illness is called surgery.

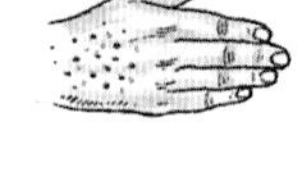

Dermatology is concerned with the skin and skin diseases.

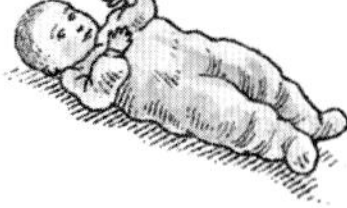

Paediatrics is the medical care of children.

RECOVERY
Recovery from an illness or an operation may take only a few hours or as long as several weeks. Much depends on the severity of the illness and the impact the treatment has on the body.

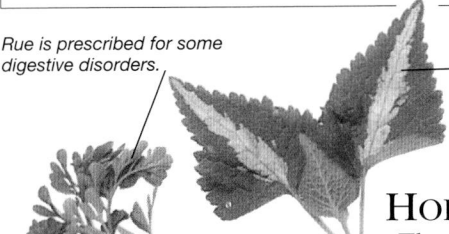

Rue is prescribed for some digestive disorders.

Catmint is a cold cure that was first used by prehistoric people.

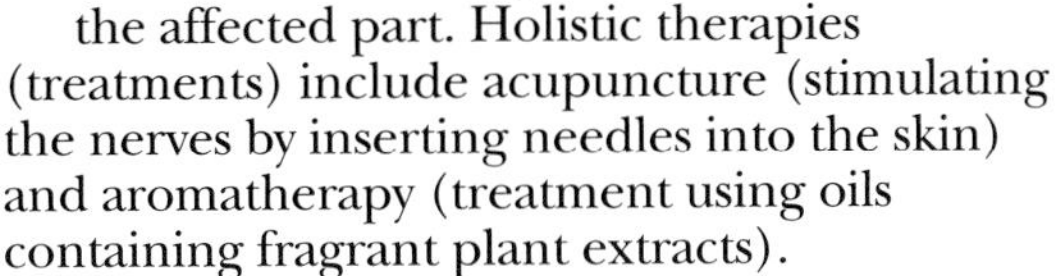

Mint is used for settling a stomach upset.

HOLISTIC MEDICINE

The word *holistic* means "of the whole". The principle of holistic medicine is to treat the whole person – body and mind – rather than just the affected part. Holistic therapies (treatments) include acupuncture (stimulating the nerves by inserting needles into the skin) and aromatherapy (treatment using oils containing fragrant plant extracts).

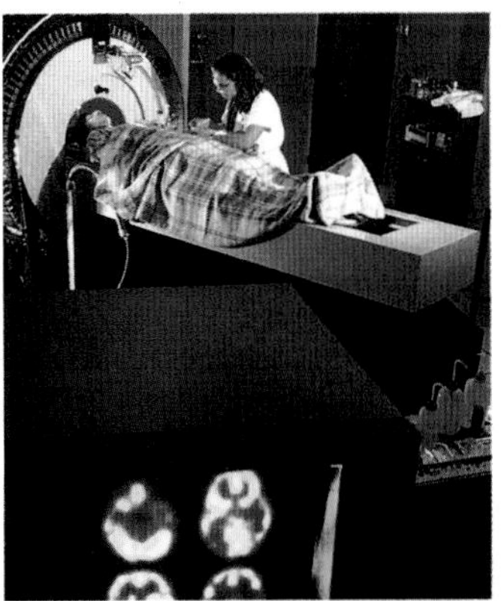

Doctors use brain scanners to check patients for tumours or damage to the brain.

MEDICAL TECHNOLOGY

Modern medicine makes use of a wide range of technology. Latest developments include body scanners which use a strong magnetic field or ultrasound (very high-frequency sound waves) to produce an image of the interior of the human body. Such equipment has revolutionized medicine.

Find out more

DISEASE
DOCTORS
DRUGS
FIRST AID
HEALTH AND FITNESS
HOSPITALS
MEDICINE, HISTORY OF

HISTORY OF MEDICINE

SINCE THE EARLIEST TIMES, people have looked for ways of curing their illnesses. Early people believed that disease was a punishment from the gods. They also believed that priests and magicians could heal them. In Ancient Greece, people visited temples when they were ill and sacrificed animals to Asclepius, the Greek god of healing. They also drank and bathed in medicinal waters and followed strict diets in the hope of being cured. During the fifth century B.C. the Greek doctor Hippocrates declared that it was nature, not magic, that caused and cured disease. Hippocrates was famed as "the father of medicine", and he and his followers wrote many medical books. The spirit of enquiry, which was part of the Renaissance (a cultural movement in 14th-century Europe), encouraged experiments that put European medicine on a firm scientific basis. Many people began to question the traditional ideas about medicine. Scientists such as Vesalius (1514-1564) began to study the bodies of dead people to learn more about disease and how to treat it. Since then, there have been many more discoveries in medicine, and the battle against disease continues.

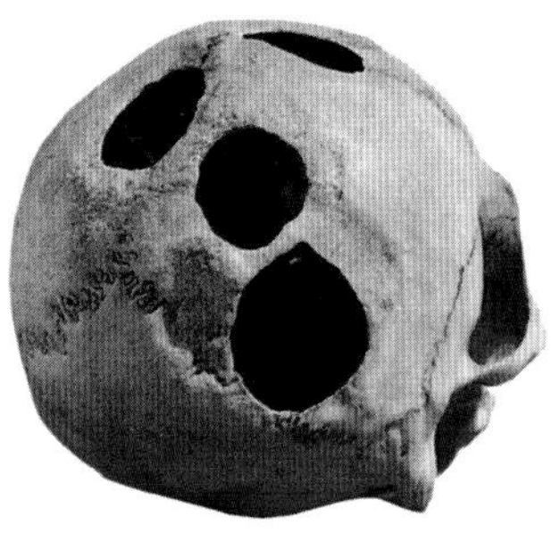

TREPANNING
Ten thousand years ago, the first doctors, tried to cure an ill person by cutting a hole in his or her skull. Healers believed that the hole in the head released evil spirits that caused pain. This was known as trepanning.

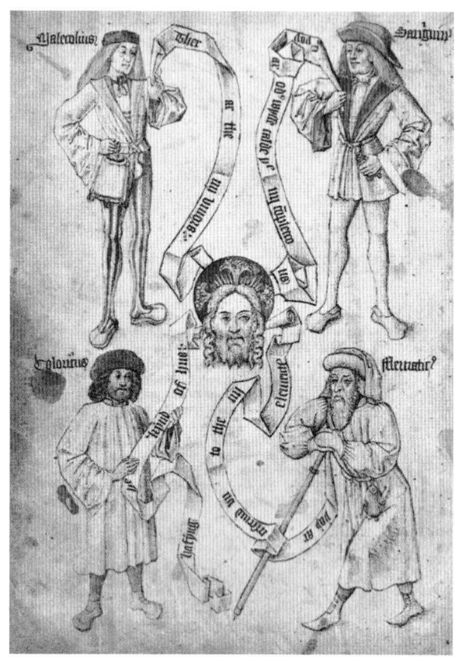

HUMOURS
The Greek physician Galen (c. A.D. 130-200) introduced the idea that the body contained four fluids called humours – blood, phlegm, yellow bile, and black bile. He believed that a person's mood depended on which of these four fluids ruled the body, and that if the fluids were not balanced, illness would result.

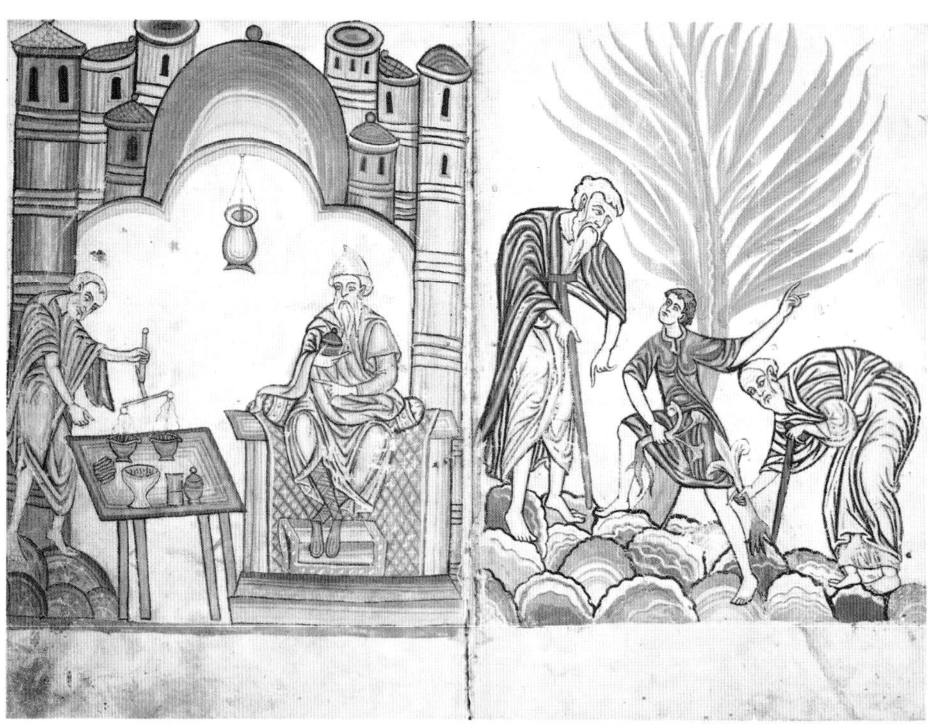

HERBALISM

For thousands of years, people have used herbs and plants in healing. Herbalists wrote lists of herbs and their uses. Monks were also famed for their knowledge of herbs. The first pharmacists, called apothecaries, used herbs to make potions, or medicines. But in Europe during the Renaissance many herbalists were accused of being witches. Many people are now turning to herbs as a natural way of treating illnesses.

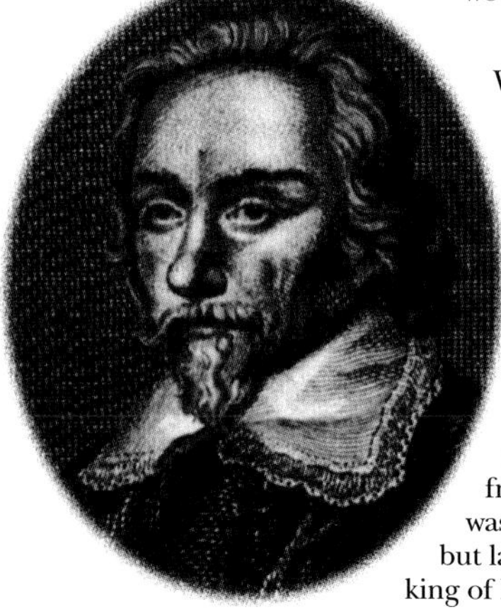

WILLIAM HARVEY
In 1628, an English doctor named William Harvey (1578-1657) discovered that blood constantly circulates around the body. He described how blood is pumped by the heart into the arteries and returns to the heart in the veins. He showed that valves in the veins stop the blood from flowing backwards. At first, Harvey was scorned for contradicting old ideas, but later he became physician to Charles I, king of England.

Harvey drew detailed diagrams to explain his theory of circulation.

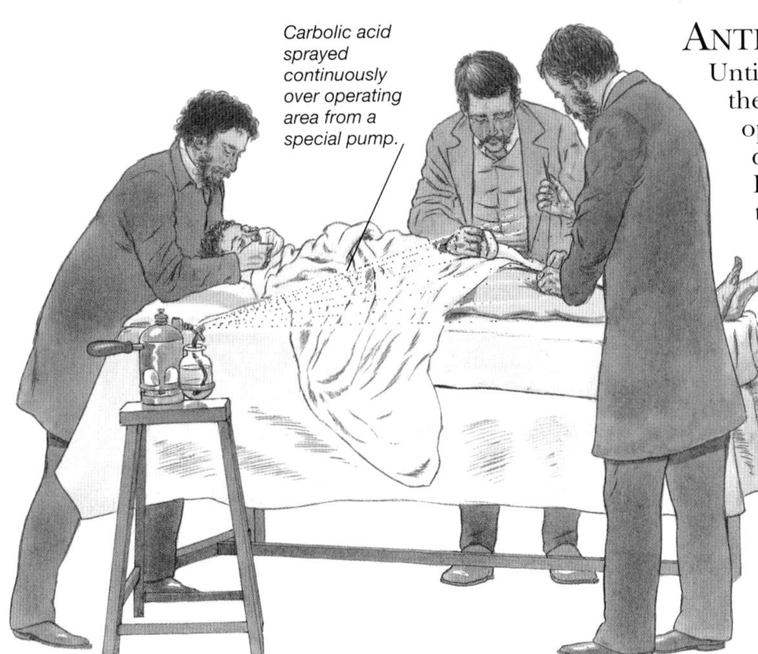

Carbolic acid sprayed continuously over operating area from a special pump.

ANTISEPTICS

Until the late 19th century, surgeons did not wash their hands or their medical instruments before operating on a patient. Many patients died from deadly infections following an operation. Joseph Lister (1827-1912), an English surgeon, guessed that infection with bacteria might be the cause of these deaths. In 1865, Lister developed an antiseptic spray called carbolic acid. This spray could destroy bacteria in the operating room, so there was a dramatic drop in the number of deaths following operations.

Leeches are parasites that attach themselves to a host. They secrete a substance that stops blood clotting while they feed on it.

BLOOD-LETTING

Doctors once believed that too much blood in the body was the cause of disease. They removed the excess blood by blood-letting. Doctors either cut open a vein to let the blood out, or they applied bloodsucking creatures called leeches to the body. The leech attached itself to the patient with its sucker, made a wound, then sucked out blood. The exact spot for blood-letting depended on what was wrong with the patient.

ALEXANDER FLEMING

Bacteria cause many of the illnesses that affect humans, so for years scientists tried to find a substance that would kill bacteria but would not harm human tissue. The Scottish bacteriologist Alexander Fleming (1881-1955) was the first person to identify an antibacterial substance. Fleming carried out his research in a laboratory at St. Mary's Hospital, London. In 1928, Fleming noticed that a mould that had accidentally developed on a dish of bacteria culture caused the bacteria to die. In 1941, the researchers Howard Florey and Ernst Chain purified the mould, *Penicillium*, to produce penicillin, the world's first antibiotic. Penicillin is widely used in the treatment of many diseases, including meningitis and pneumonia. Fleming shared the 1945 Nobel Prize for medicine with Florey and Chain.

HISTORY OF MEDICINE

c. 8000 B.C. Early healers practise trepanning.

400s B.C. Hippocrates, a Greek, begins scientific medicine.

1543 Vesalius publishes first scientific study of human body.

1615 Santorio, an Italian doctor, designs mouth thermometer.

1683 Anton van Leeuwenhoek, a Dutch scientist, discovers bacteria.

1796 Edward Jenner gives first smallpox vaccination.

1816 Rene Laennec, a French doctor, invents stethoscope.

1842 American surgeon, Horace Long, operates using general anaesthetic.

1895 Wilhelm Roentgen, a German physicist, discovers x-rays, which enable doctors to see inside the human body.

1898 Polish-born Marie Curie and her husband, Pierre Curie of France, discover the chemical element radium to treat cancer.

1928 Scottish bacteriologist, Alexander Fleming, discovers penicillin.

MEDICAL PIONEERS

Through the centuries many people have shaped modern medicine. The Flemish doctor Vesalius produced accurate drawings of the human body; Dutchman Anton van Leeuwenhoek (1632-1723) first discovered microbes, now called bacteria; and the English doctor Edward Jenner (1749-1823) discovered vaccinations – a way of preventing certain diseases by injection.

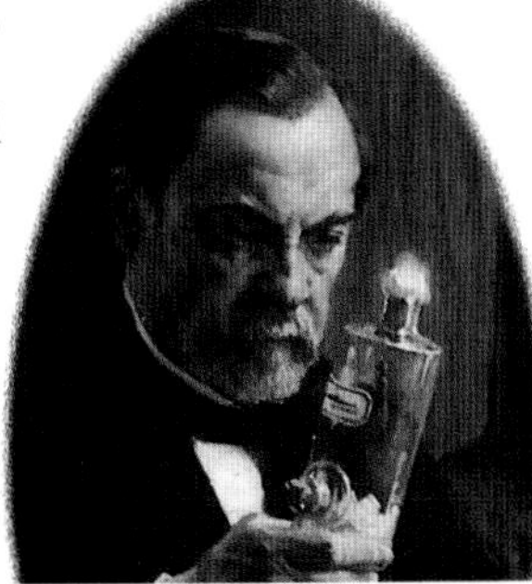

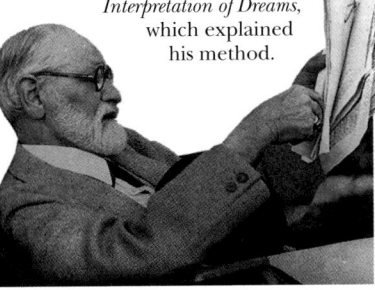

LOUIS PASTEUR
Frenchman Louis Pasteur (1822-1895) showed that bacteria caused disease. He invented pasteurization – the heating of milk and beer to destroy harmful bacteria.

SIGMUND FREUD
The Austrian doctor Sigmund Freud (1856-1939; below) was interested in finding out how the mind works. He treated patients with mental disorders by listening to them talk about their dreams and thoughts. This treatment was called psychoanalysis. In 1900, Freud published *The Interpretation of Dreams*, which explained his method.

Find out more
DRUGS
EGYPT, ANCIENT
GREECE, ANCIENT
MEDICINE

MEDIEVAL EUROPE

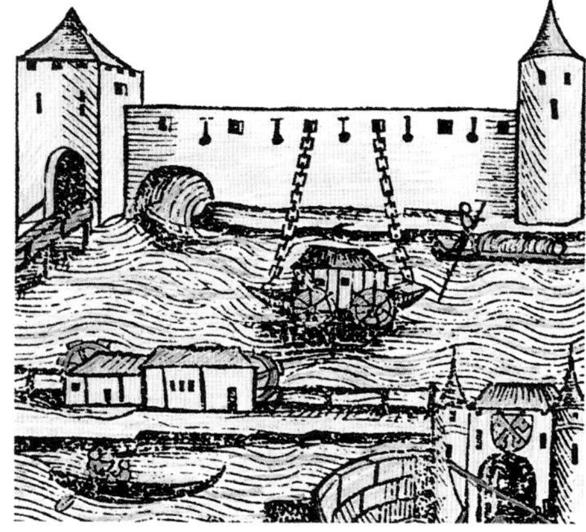

FAIRS
Great fairs were held every year in towns, such as Winchester, England, which were on important trade routes. Merchants travelled from all over Europe to sell their goods at these fairs.

LORDS AND LADIES feasting in castle banquet halls, peasants working on the land, knights in armour – all these are associated with a time in European history known as the medieval period or the Middle Ages. This was a time of great change in western Europe between the 5th and 15th centuries. During the 5th century the Roman Empire fell, to be replaced by invading German tribes. Western Europe then broke up into many kingdoms. Trade collapsed, and people had to make their living from the land. Gradually, powerful landowners or lords emerged and the feudal system developed. The early medieval period of Europe is sometimes called the Dark Age because the learning of Ancient Greece and Rome almost disappeared. But the Christian Church gave leadership to the people. Trade gradually improved. By about the 13th century the Middle Ages had reached their height. Feudalism governed society, and monasteries (where monks lived) were the centres of learning. The medieval times came to an end in the 15th century when the Renaissance swept through Europe.

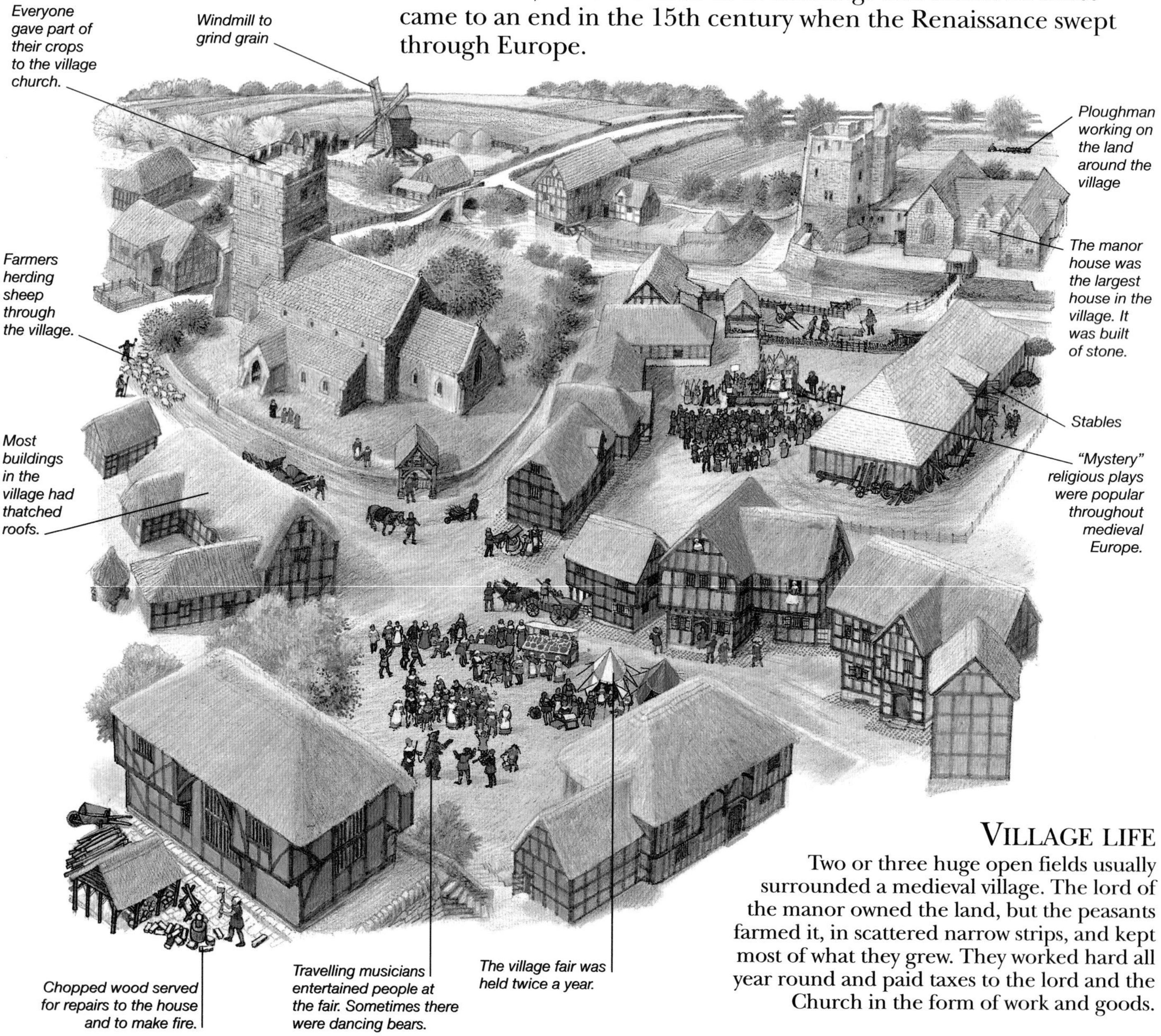

Everyone gave part of their crops to the village church.

Windmill to grind grain

Ploughman working on the land around the village

Farmers herding sheep through the village.

The manor house was the largest house in the village. It was built of stone.

Stables

Most buildings in the village had thatched roofs.

"Mystery" religious plays were popular throughout medieval Europe.

Chopped wood served for repairs to the house and to make fire.

Travelling musicians entertained people at the fair. Sometimes there were dancing bears.

The village fair was held twice a year.

VILLAGE LIFE

Two or three huge open fields usually surrounded a medieval village. The lord of the manor owned the land, but the peasants farmed it, in scattered narrow strips, and kept most of what they grew. They worked hard all year round and paid taxes to the lord and the Church in the form of work and goods.

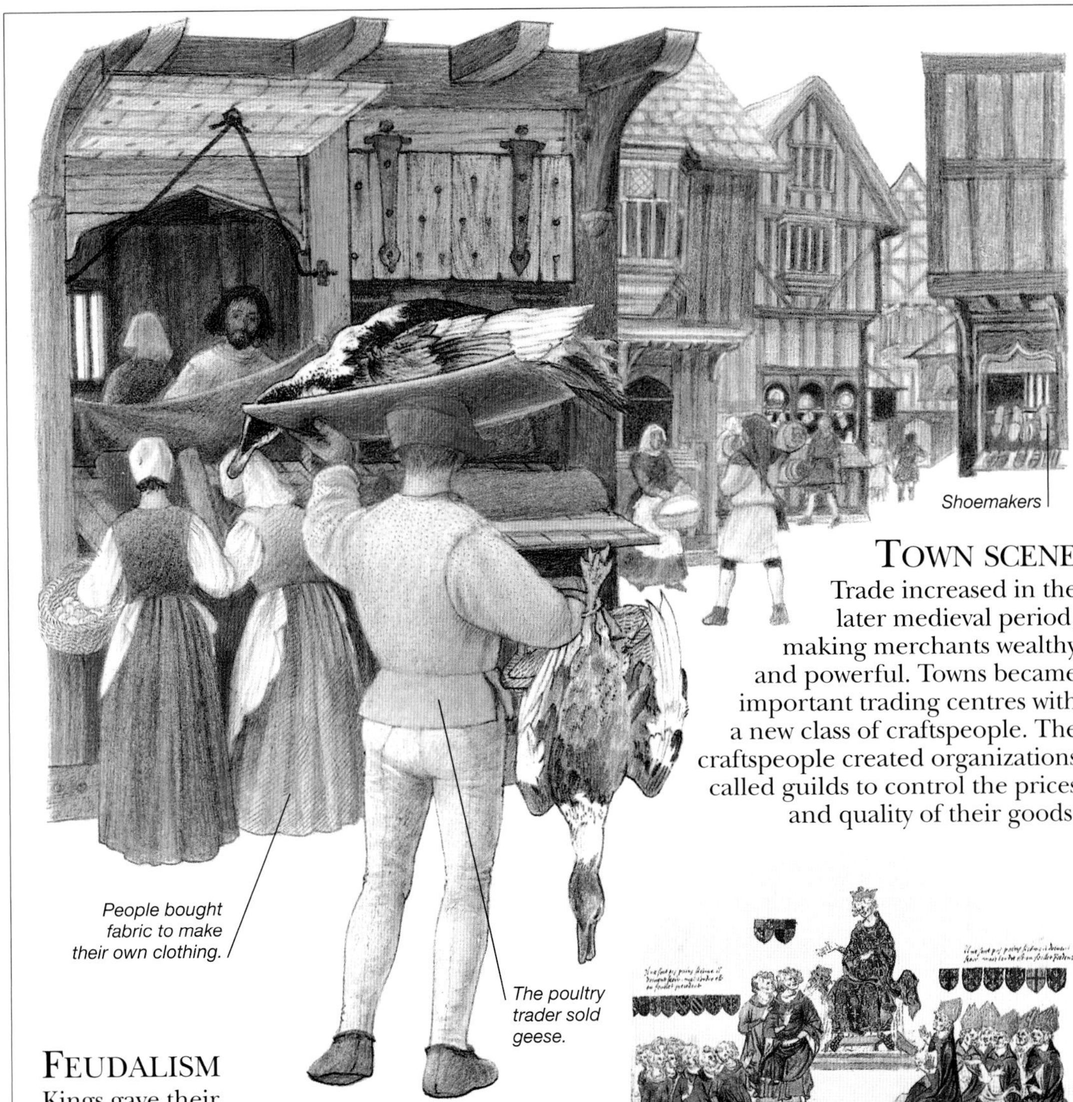

Shoemakers

TOWN SCENE

Trade increased in the later medieval period, making merchants wealthy and powerful. Towns became important trading centres with a new class of craftspeople. The craftspeople created organizations called guilds to control the prices and quality of their goods.

People bought fabric to make their own clothing.

The poultry trader sold geese.

FEUDALISM

Kings gave their vassals – powerful nobles – tracts of land called fiefs. In return for this land the vassals fought for the king when required. The vassals divided their land into manors (estates), which they gave to lesser nobles and knights. In return, the knights and lesser nobles worked for the lord of the manor, and had to fight for him when called on.

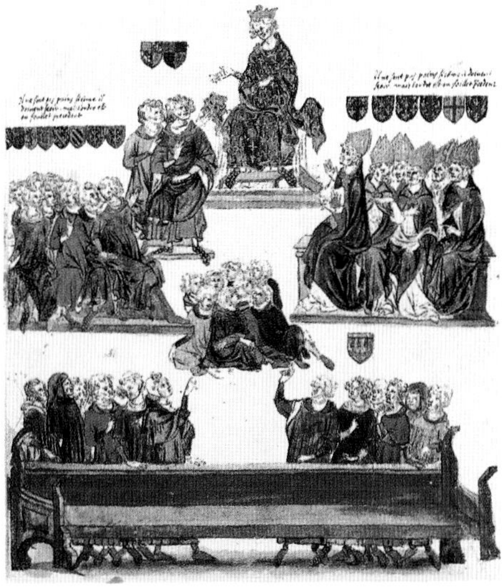

14th-century manuscript (right) shows feudal structure, with the king at the top.

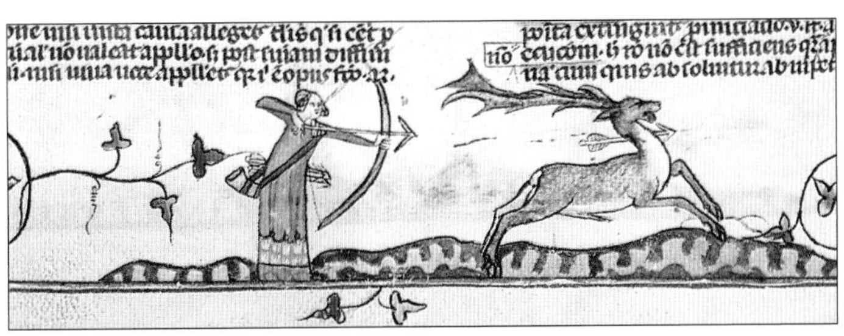

Hunting (above) was a popular sport for upper-class medieval women.

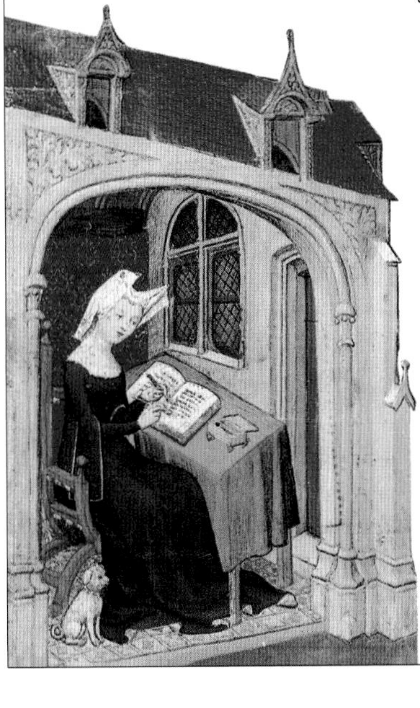

A French medieval woman, Christine de Pisan (left), earned her living as a writer.

WOMEN

Peasant women worked very hard all their lives. They brought up their children, spun wool and wove clothing, and helped with all the farmwork. Upper-class women also led busy lives. They often ran the family estates while their husbands were away travelling around their lands, fighting against neighbouring lords, or on a Crusade to the Holy Land. Women also nursed the sick and provided education for children in their charge.

MEDIEVAL EUROPE

A.D. 400 Roman empire begins to decline.

450 German tribes – Angles, Jutes, and Saxons – settle in Britain.

480s Franks set up kingdom in Gaul (now France).

800 Charlemagne, king of the Franks, unites western Europe.

900-1000s Europe is divided into feudal estates; there is widespread poverty and disease in the region.

1066 Normans conquer England.

1000s-1200s High Middle Ages: trade improves, population grows, towns develop, and learning flourishes.

c. 1100 First universities are founded.

1215 Magna Carta: English barons win power and rights from King John.

1300-1500 Late Middle Ages.

c. 1320 Renaissance, a rebirth of arts and learning, begins in Italy.

1337 Hundred Years' War begins between England and France.

1348 Black Death, a killing plague, reaches Europe. Eventually, it wipes out one third of the population of Europe.

1378-1417 Great Schism: Catholic Europe is divided in support of two different popes, Urban VI and Clement VII.

1454 Johannes Gutenberg, a German, develops movable type. Printing begins in Europe.

Find out more

BLACK DEATH
CHURCHES AND CATHEDRALS
KNIGHTS AND HERALDRY
MONASTERIES
RENAISSANCE
ROMAN EMPIRE

METALS

IMAGINE A WORLD WITHOUT METALS. There would be no cars or aeroplanes, and skyscrapers would fall down without the metal frames that support them. Metals have countless uses because they possess a unique combination of qualities. They are very strong and easy to shape, so they can be used to make all kinds of objects from ships to bottle tops. All metals conduct electricity. Some are ideal for wires and electrical equipment. Metals also carry heat, so they make good cooking pots. These qualities can be improved by mixing two or more metals to make alloys. Most metallic objects are made of alloys rather than pure metals. There are more than 80 kinds of pure metals, though some are very rare. Aluminium and iron are the most common metals. A few metals, such as gold, occur in the ground as pure metals; the rest are found as ores in rock. Metals can also be obtained by recycling old cars and tins. This reduces waste and costs less than processing metal ores.

Gold watch

Mercury thermometer

Copper wire

Silver-plated frame

PURE METALS

The rarity and lustre of gold and silver have been prized for centuries. Other pure metals have special uses. Electrical wires are made of copper, which conducts electricity well. Mercury, a liquid metal, is used in thermometers.

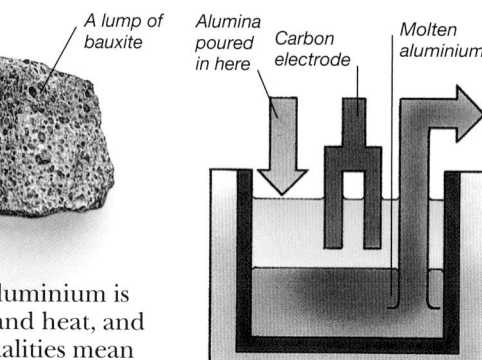

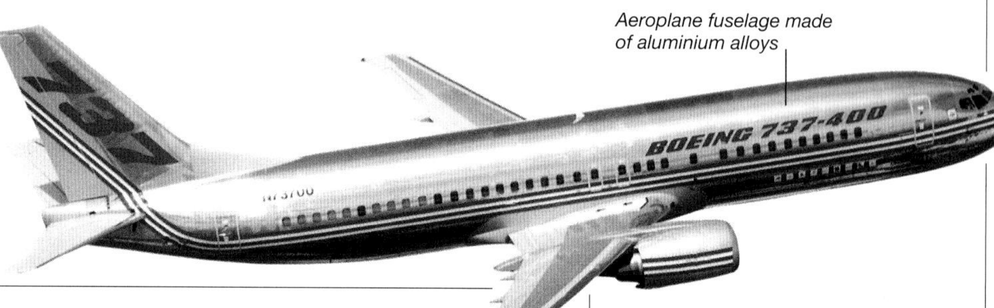

Aeroplane fuselage made of aluminium alloys

ALUMINIUM

The most common metal in the Earth's crust is aluminium. The metal comes from an ore called bauxite, which contains alumina, a compound of aluminium and oxygen. Aluminium is light, conducts electricity and heat, and resists corrosion. These qualities mean the metal and its alloys can be used in many things, including aircraft and bicycles, window frames, paints, saucepans, and electricity supply cables.

A lump of bauxite

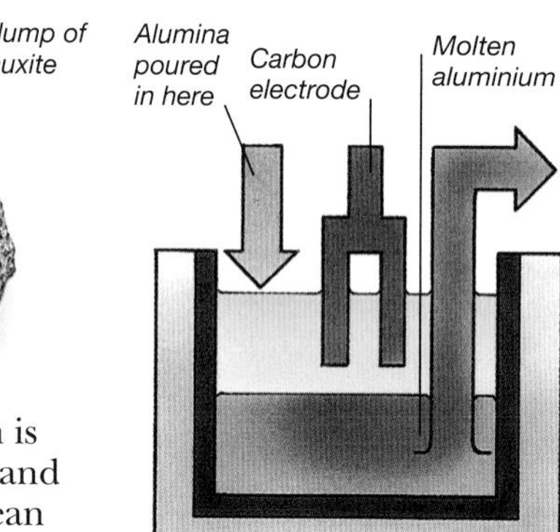

ELECTROLYSIS
Passing an electric current through alumina separates it into aluminium and oxygen. This process is called electrolysis.

Thin, flexible aluminium foil is useful for cooking and storing food because it is nonreactive and can stand high temperatures.

ALLOYS

Most metal objects are made of steel or other alloys. This is because alloys are often stronger or easier to process than pure metals. Copper and tin are weak and pliable, but when mixed together they make a strong alloy called bronze. Brass is a tough alloy of copper and zinc that resists corrosion. Alloys of aluminium are light and strong and are used to make aircraft.

METAL FATIGUE
Metals sometimes fail even though they may be very tough and strong. Corrosion weakens some metals, as in the case of rusty steel. Repeated bending can cause metal parts to break, an effect called metal fatigue.

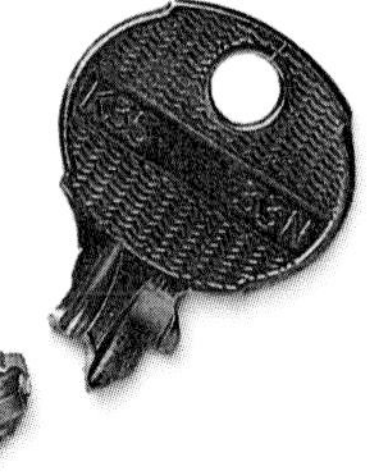

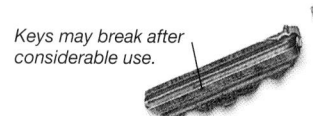

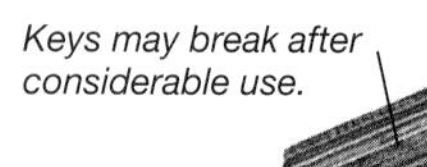
Keys may break after considerable use.

METALWORKING

There are many ways of shaping metal. Casting is one method of making objects such as metal statues. Hot, molten metal is poured into a mould where it sets and hardens into the required shape. Metal can also be pressed, hammered, or cut into shape.

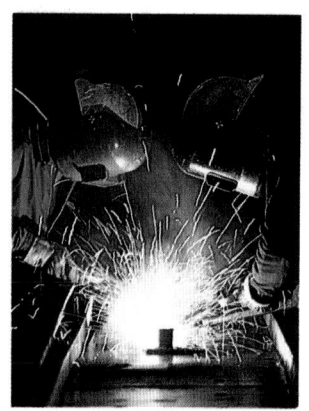

WELDING
Metal parts can be joined by welding. Welders apply heat, from a gas flame or an electric spark, to the edges of two pieces of metal. The heat causes the edges to melt so that they can be joined together.

Find out more

BRONZE AGE
IRON AGE
IRON AND STEEL
ROCKS AND MINERALS
SCULPTURE

MEXICO

THE WEALTH OF MEXICO has traditionally come from the land. Precious metals lie buried in the mountains and rich crops grow in the valleys. Oil flows from wells on the coast. The Mexican people began to exploit these advantages centuries ago. Farming supported most of the people, and from the country's mines came silver to make beautiful jewellery. The mineral wealth of the country attracted invading European soldiers in the 16th century, and Spain ruled Mexico for three centuries. A revolt against Spanish rule gave the Mexican people independence in 1821. The discovery of oil early in the 20th century brought new wealth to Mexico. The government invested this in new factories, and in social services to relieve hunger and improve health and education. In 1994, the North American Free Trade Agreement (NAFTA) reduced trade barriers between Mexico, Canada, and the United States, promising long-term economic benefits. However, the border between Mexico and the US has been strengthened as a result of US concern over the estimated 850,000 illegal crossings each year.

Mexico is part of the continent of North America and lies between the United States to its north and Central America to its south.

José Guadalupe Posada (1852–1913) drew humorous illustrations, many of which supported the Mexican revolution.

POLITICS AND REVOLUTION
Mexico was a Spanish colony from 1521 to 1821, when it became an independent republic. After a long period of political unrest, there was a revolution in 1910, in which half a million people died. From 1929, the Institutional Revolutionary party governed Mexico, but in 2000 it lost the presidential election for the first time. Mexico is now a fully functioning democracy.

MEXICO CITY

More than 18 million people live in and around Mexico City, the capital of Mexico, making it one of the most populated cities in the world. The city lies 1.6 km (1 mile) above sea level in a natural basin surrounded by mountains. These mountains trap the pollution from the city's industries. As a result, Mexico City is one of the world's most unhealthy cities, with an inadequate water supply, a lack of housing, and the constant threat of earthquakes adding to its many problems.

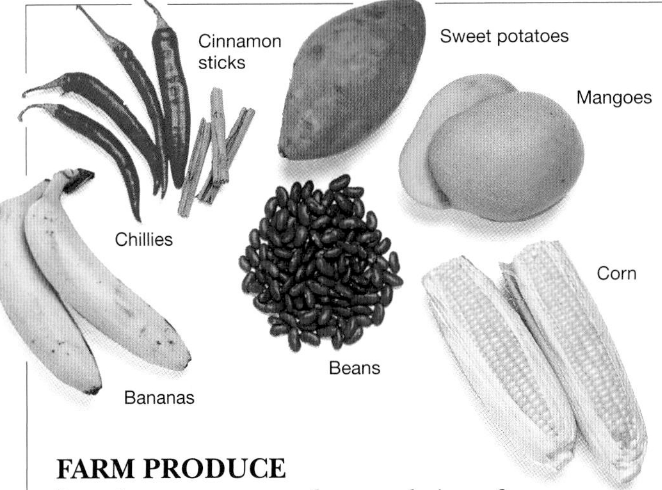

FARM PRODUCE

Less than one-quarter the population of Mexico lives and works on the land, growing staple or food crops. Increasingly, however, farmers are growing coffee, cotton, sugar, and tomatoes for export. These cash crops take vital land away from the crops that the Mexican people themselves need for food. Most of the farmers are members of co-operatives, pooling their limited resources to help one another.

Mexican artisans are skilled at making fine jewellery from the precious metals found in their country.

MINERAL WEALTH
Copper, silver, zinc, mercury, and other valuable metals are among the many minerals found in Mexico. Oil is the country's most important resource. In 1974, vast new reserves were discovered in the south of the country.

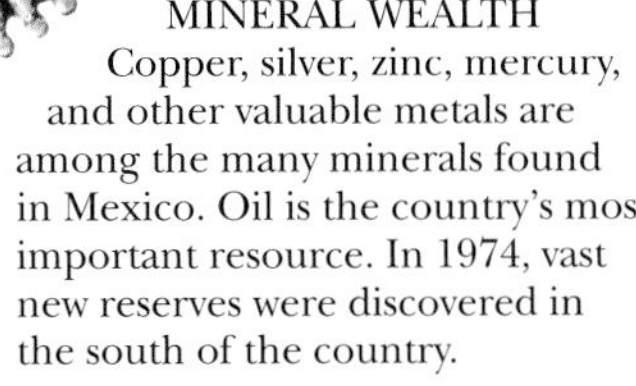

Find out more

CONQUISTADORS
NORTH AMERICA
VOLCANOES

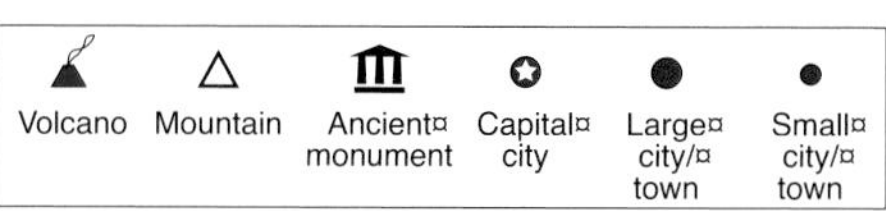

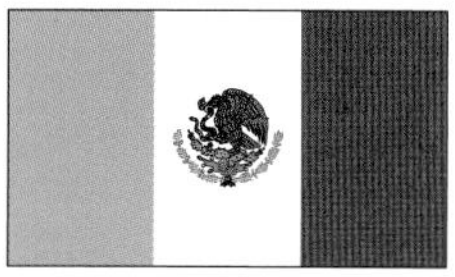

STATISTICS

Area: 1,958,200 sq km (756,061 sq miles)
Population: 104,000,000
Capital: Mexico City
Languages: Spanish, Nahuatl, Maya, Zapotec, Mixtec, Otomi, Totonac, Tzotzil, Tzeltal
Religions: Roman Catholic, Protestant
Currency: Mexican peso
Main occupations: Subsistence farming, manufacturing, oil production
Main exports: Oil, cotton, machinery, coffee
Main imports: Machinery, vehicles, chemicals

SIERRA MADRE

The main mountain system of Mexico, the Sierra Madre, runs 2,400 km (1,500 miles) southeast from the border with the United States. There are three ranges, in the east, south, and west, and they enclose Mexico's central plateau. Mexico's third highest mountain, Volcán Iztaccihuatl (right), is in the Sierra Madre del Sur, the southern range. The mountain has three separate summits, and its name means "White Woman" in the Aztec language, because the peaks resemble a woman wearing a hood.

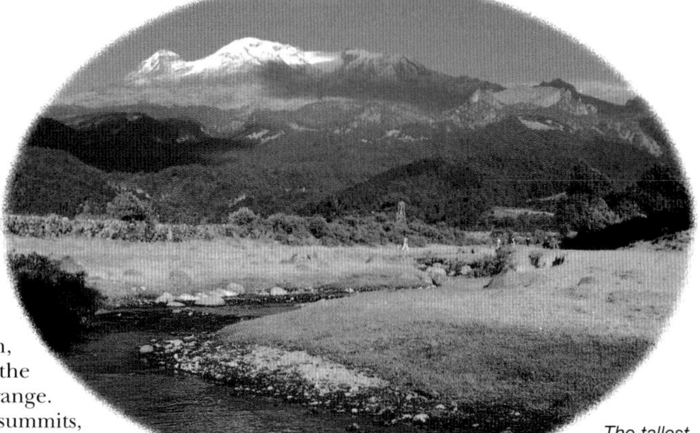

The tallest peak of Volcán Iztaccihuatl rises to 5,268 m (17,274 ft).

POPULATION

Most of northern Mexico is sparsely populated due to the hot, dry climate and lack of cultivable farmland. As people have migrated from the countryside in search of work, the cities have grown dramatically; almost 75 per cent of Mexicans now live in urban areas. Mexico city is home to almost a quarter of the population and is one of the world's largest cities. Rapid, unplanned growth has led to poor sanitation and water supplies.

GUANAJUATO

Spanish prospectors searching for gold founded Guanajuato (below) in 1554. The town is the capital of Guanajuato state in the mountains of central Mexico and rises more than 2,050 m (6,726 ft) above sea level. It is built in a ravine and has steep, winding streets.

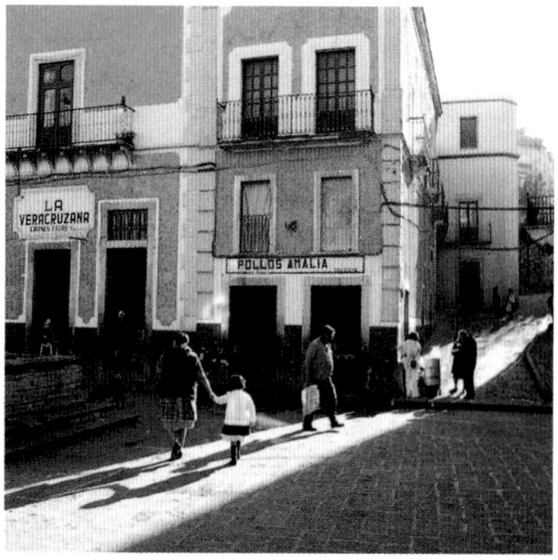

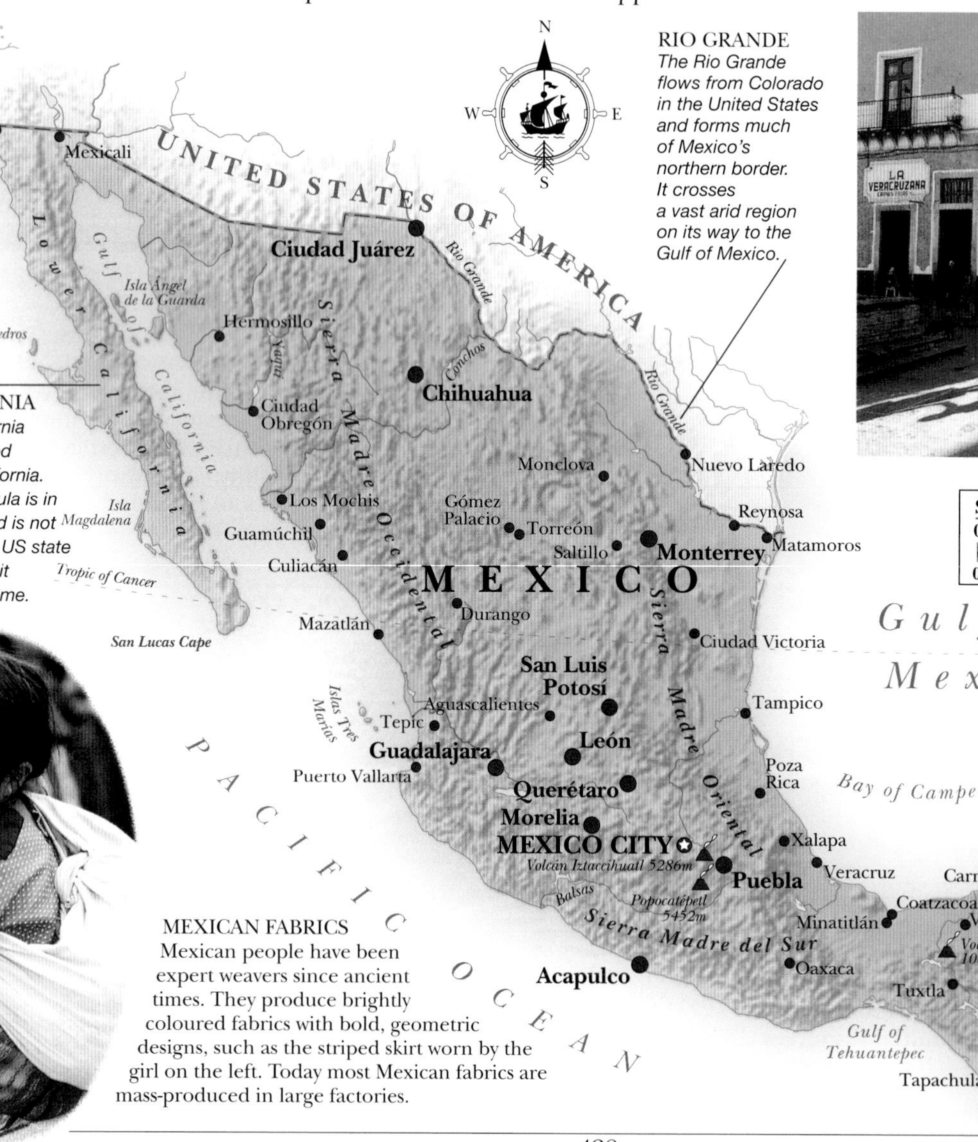

RIO GRANDE

The Rio Grande flows from Colorado in the United States and forms much of Mexico's northern border. It crosses a vast arid region on its way to the Gulf of Mexico.

BAJA CALIFORNIA

Baja California is also called Lower California. The peninsula is in Mexico, and is not part of the US state with which it shares a name.

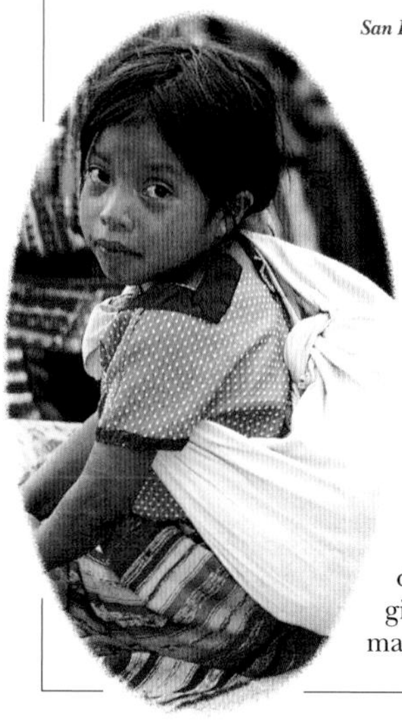

SCALE BAR

0 200 400 km

0 200 400 miles

MEXICAN FABRICS

Mexican people have been expert weavers since ancient times. They produce brightly coloured fabrics with bold, geometric designs, such as the striped skirt worn by the girl on the left. Today most Mexican fabrics are mass-produced in large factories.

MICE
RATS, AND SQUIRRELS

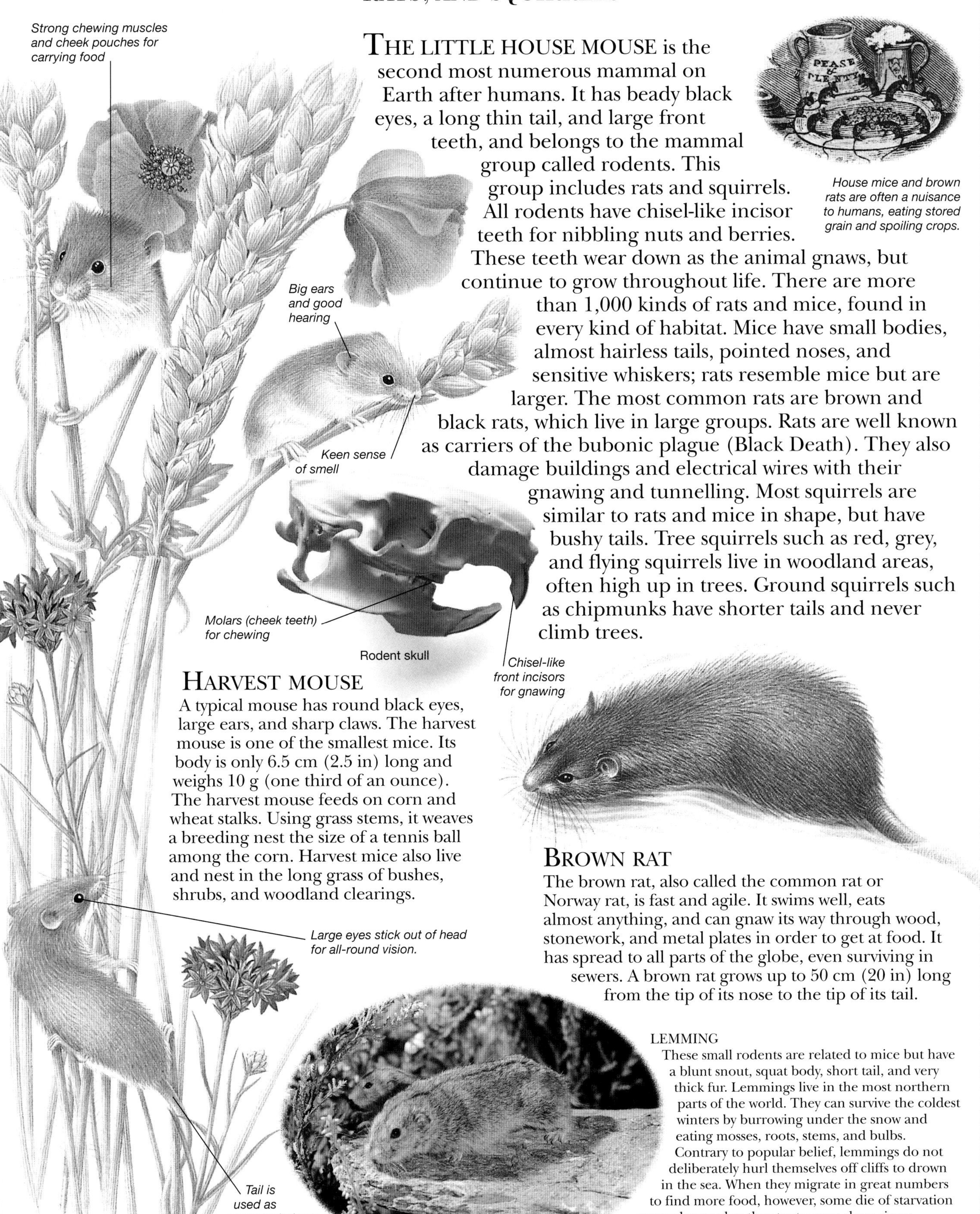

Strong chewing muscles and cheek pouches for carrying food
Big ears and good hearing
Keen sense of smell
Molars (cheek teeth) for chewing
Rodent skull
Chisel-like front incisors for gnawing
Large eyes stick out of head for all-round vision.
Tail is used as a counterbalance.

House mice and brown rats are often a nuisance to humans, eating stored grain and spoiling crops.

THE LITTLE HOUSE MOUSE is the second most numerous mammal on Earth after humans. It has beady black eyes, a long thin tail, and large front teeth, and belongs to the mammal group called rodents. This group includes rats and squirrels. All rodents have chisel-like incisor teeth for nibbling nuts and berries. These teeth wear down as the animal gnaws, but continue to grow throughout life. There are more than 1,000 kinds of rats and mice, found in every kind of habitat. Mice have small bodies, almost hairless tails, pointed noses, and sensitive whiskers; rats resemble mice but are larger. The most common rats are brown and black rats, which live in large groups. Rats are well known as carriers of the bubonic plague (Black Death). They also damage buildings and electrical wires with their gnawing and tunnelling. Most squirrels are similar to rats and mice in shape, but have bushy tails. Tree squirrels such as red, grey, and flying squirrels live in woodland areas, often high up in trees. Ground squirrels such as chipmunks have shorter tails and never climb trees.

HARVEST MOUSE

A typical mouse has round black eyes, large ears, and sharp claws. The harvest mouse is one of the smallest mice. Its body is only 6.5 cm (2.5 in) long and weighs 10 g (one third of an ounce). The harvest mouse feeds on corn and wheat stalks. Using grass stems, it weaves a breeding nest the size of a tennis ball among the corn. Harvest mice also live and nest in the long grass of bushes, shrubs, and woodland clearings.

BROWN RAT

The brown rat, also called the common rat or Norway rat, is fast and agile. It swims well, eats almost anything, and can gnaw its way through wood, stonework, and metal plates in order to get at food. It has spread to all parts of the globe, even surviving in sewers. A brown rat grows up to 50 cm (20 in) long from the tip of its nose to the tip of its tail.

LEMMING

These small rodents are related to mice but have a blunt snout, squat body, short tail, and very thick fur. Lemmings live in the most northern parts of the world. They can survive the coldest winters by burrowing under the snow and eating mosses, roots, stems, and bulbs. Contrary to popular belief, lemmings do not deliberately hurl themselves off cliffs to drown in the sea. When they migrate in great numbers to find more food, however, some die of starvation or are drowned as they try to cross deep rivers.

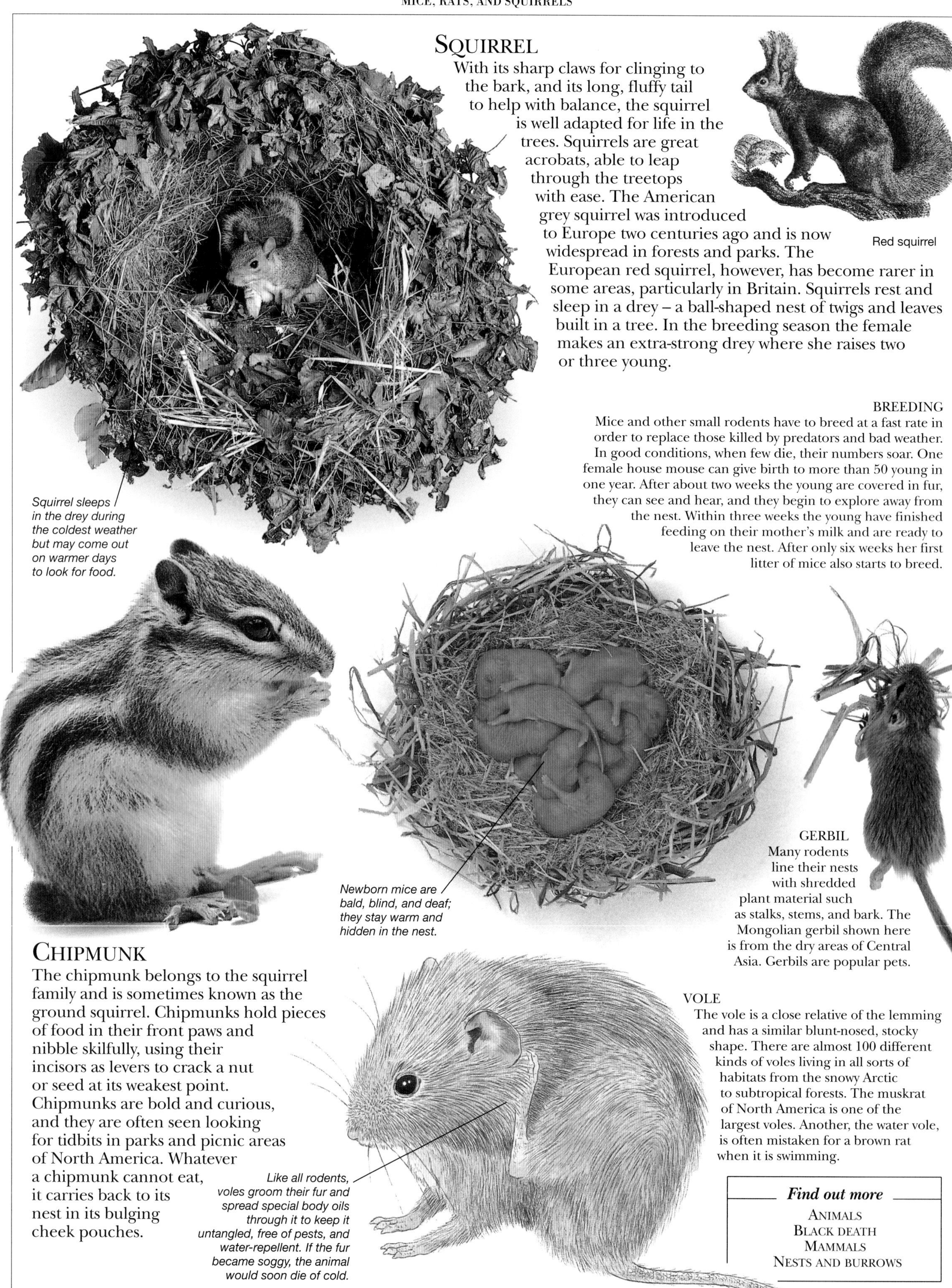

Squirrel

With its sharp claws for clinging to the bark, and its long, fluffy tail to help with balance, the squirrel is well adapted for life in the trees. Squirrels are great acrobats, able to leap through the treetops with ease. The American grey squirrel was introduced to Europe two centuries ago and is now widespread in forests and parks. The European red squirrel, however, has become rarer in some areas, particularly in Britain. Squirrels rest and sleep in a drey – a ball-shaped nest of twigs and leaves built in a tree. In the breeding season the female makes an extra-strong drey where she raises two or three young.

Squirrel sleeps in the drey during the coldest weather but may come out on warmer days to look for food.

BREEDING

Mice and other small rodents have to breed at a fast rate in order to replace those killed by predators and bad weather. In good conditions, when few die, their numbers soar. One female house mouse can give birth to more than 50 young in one year. After about two weeks the young are covered in fur, they can see and hear, and they begin to explore away from the nest. Within three weeks the young have finished feeding on their mother's milk and are ready to leave the nest. After only six weeks her first litter of mice also starts to breed.

Newborn mice are bald, blind, and deaf; they stay warm and hidden in the nest.

GERBIL

Many rodents line their nests with shredded plant material such as stalks, stems, and bark. The Mongolian gerbil shown here is from the dry areas of Central Asia. Gerbils are popular pets.

Chipmunk

The chipmunk belongs to the squirrel family and is sometimes known as the ground squirrel. Chipmunks hold pieces of food in their front paws and nibble skilfully, using their incisors as levers to crack a nut or seed at its weakest point. Chipmunks are bold and curious, and they are often seen looking for tidbits in parks and picnic areas of North America. Whatever a chipmunk cannot eat, it carries back to its nest in its bulging cheek pouches.

VOLE

The vole is a close relative of the lemming and has a similar blunt-nosed, stocky shape. There are almost 100 different kinds of voles living in all sorts of habitats from the snowy Arctic to subtropical forests. The muskrat of North America is one of the largest voles. Another, the water vole, is often mistaken for a brown rat when it is swimming.

Like all rodents, voles groom their fur and spread special body oils through it to keep it untangled, free of pests, and water-repellent. If the fur became soggy, the animal would soon die of cold.

Find out more
Animals
Black death
Mammals
Nests and burrows

MICROSCOPES

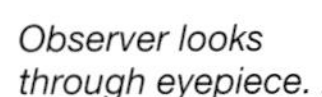

Observer looks through eyepiece.

Objective lenses of different power can be swung into position when needed.

The objective lens produces an image which the eyepiece magnifies (makes larger).

The object being studied rests on a glass slide.

Condenser lenses concentrate a beam of light onto the object.

A strong beam of light strikes a mirror under the microscope. The beam shines onto the object from below.

WITHIN ALL OBJECTS there is a hidden world, much too tiny for us to see. With the invention of the microscope in the 16th century, scientists were able to peer into this world and unravel some of the great mysteries of science. They discovered that animals and plants are made of millions of tiny cells, and later were able to identify the minute organisms called bacteria that cause disease. Early microscopes consisted of a single magnifying lens; today's microscopes have several lenses and can be used to see very tiny objects. Electron microscopes are even more powerful. Instead of light they use a beam of electrons – tiny particles which are normally part of atoms – to magnify objects many millions of times. Scientists use electron microscopes to study the smallest of living cells and to delve into the structure of materials such as plastics and metals.

Optical microscopes can reveal living cells such as these cells which come from a human cheek. They are magnified more than 200 times.

OPTICAL MICROSCOPE

The optical, or light, microscope has two main lenses: the objective and the eyepiece. High-quality microscopes contain several additional lenses which help to give a clear, bright image. Different objectives can be fitted which give a range of magnification from about 10 times to 1,500 times normal size.

INVENTING THE MICROSCOPE

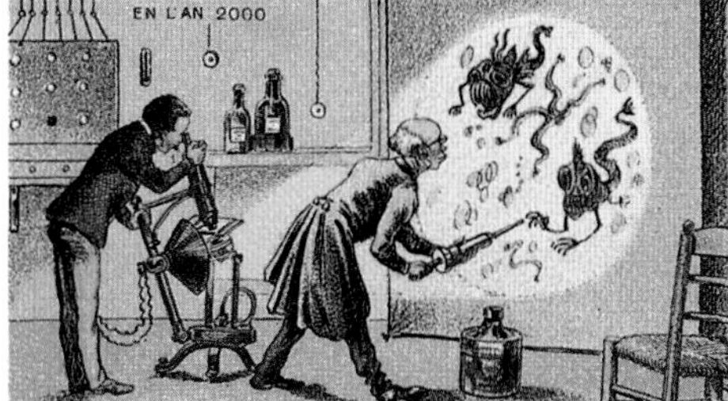

Although the Romans used magnifying lenses about 2,000 years ago, the first true microscope appeared around 1590, built by Dutch spectacles makers Hans and Zacharias Janssen. In 1663, English scientist Robert Hooke studied insects and plants with a microscope. He found that cork was made up of tiny cells, a discovery of great scientific importance. Microscopes aroused great interest in microscopic life, as this old etching shows.

ELECTRON MICROSCOPES
Objects must be cut into thin slices in order to see them with a microscope. However, a scanning electron microscope can magnify a whole object such as this ant (right), which is about 15 times normal size.

With a scanning electron microscope the image appears on a monitor screen.

IMAGING ATOMS
Special electron microscopes can show individual atoms, which are so small that a line of 0.5 million atoms would only span the width of a human hair. This piece of silicon (above) is magnified 45 million times, revealing its atoms.

Find out more

ATOMS AND MOLECULES
BIOLOGY
MICROSCOPIC LIFE

MICROSCOPIC LIFE

Dust mite

ALL AROUND US there are living things that we cannot see because they are too small. They float in the air, they swim in puddles and oceans, and they coat rocks, soil, plants, and animals. Microscopic life includes bacteria and viruses; single-celled animals, called protoctists; and single-celled plants, called algae. It also includes the microscopic stages in the lives of larger plants and animals, such as the tiny pollen grains of flowers and the spores of mushrooms. From bacteria to algae, all are so small that we can see them only through a microscope. Viruses, which are the smallest and simplest of all living things, must be magnified one million times before we can see them. Microscopic life has a crucial role to play. Plankton consists of millions of algae and protozoa, and is an important food for water creatures. Bacteria in soil help to recycle nutrients. Some microscopic life, such as viruses, can cause disease.

DUST MITE

This microscopic animal can be found in everyone's home. It lives among dust, fluff, cat fur, and bits of dirt. Dust mites eat the dead skin you shed every day.

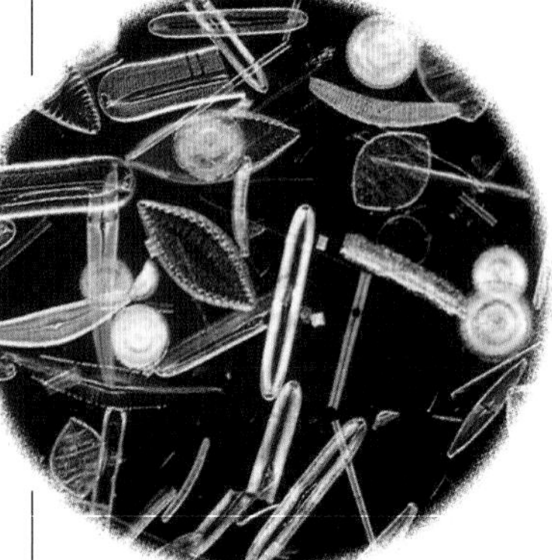

DIATOM
Microscopic plants called diatoms live in lakes, rivers, and oceans. There are thousands of different kinds of diatoms, providing food for many insects and water creatures. Diatoms live and grow by using sunlight and the nutrients in the water. Around their bodies are strong shell-like walls made of silica – the same material found in sand grains.

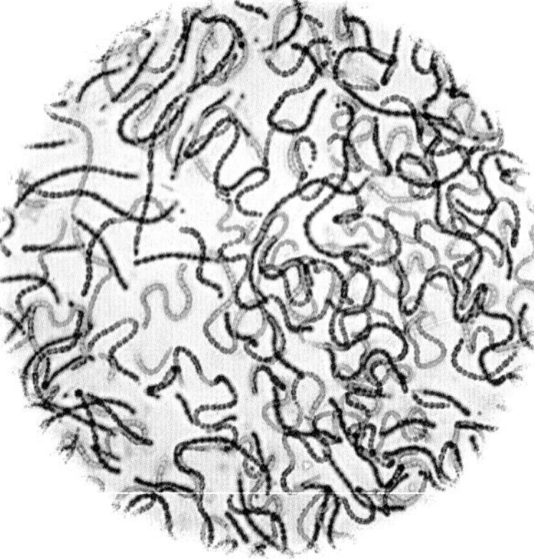

ALGAE
The slimy scum that you see on the surface of a stagnant pond is blue-green algae. These algae are not true plants. They are more closely related to bacteria. Blue-green algae were among the first forms of life to appear on Earth more than 2,000 million years ago.

AMOEBA

The amoeba is a single-celled organism. It lives in ponds and puddles. We need to magnify an amoeba at least one thousand times before we can see it. The amoeba moves by stretching out a part of its body known as a pseudopod, or "false foot". The rest of the body then flows into the pseudopod. Amoebas feed by engulfing prey such as bacteria with their pseudopods; then the whole body flows over the prey.

Amoeba divides in half, forming two daughter cells.

Nucleus – control centre of amoeba

Food is stored in a small bag called the food vacuole.

Pseudopod (false foot)

Cell membrane, the skin around the cell

HOW AN AMOEBA REPRODUCES
To reproduce, the amoeba divides into two. This is called fission. First the nucleus splits in two, then the rest of the body divides in half to form two separate amoebas. These are called daughter cells.

POLLEN
Microscopic grains of pollen grow on the male part of a plant, called the stamen. Each kind of plant has a different type of pollen grain with its own pattern and shape.

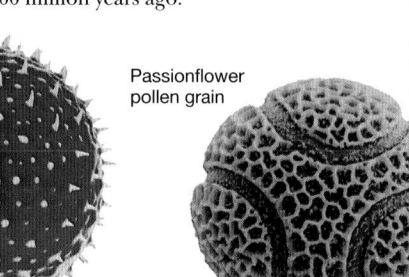

Hollyhock pollen grain

Passionflower pollen grain

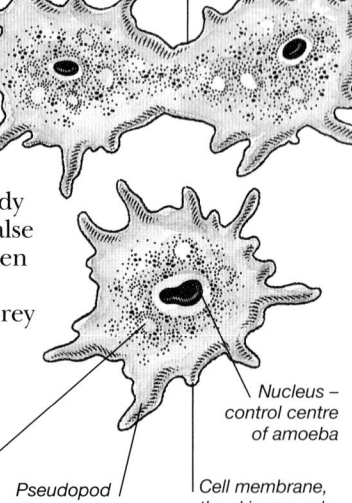

Find out more

DISEASE
HUMAN BODY
MICROSCOPES
OCEAN WILDLIFE

MIDDLE EAST

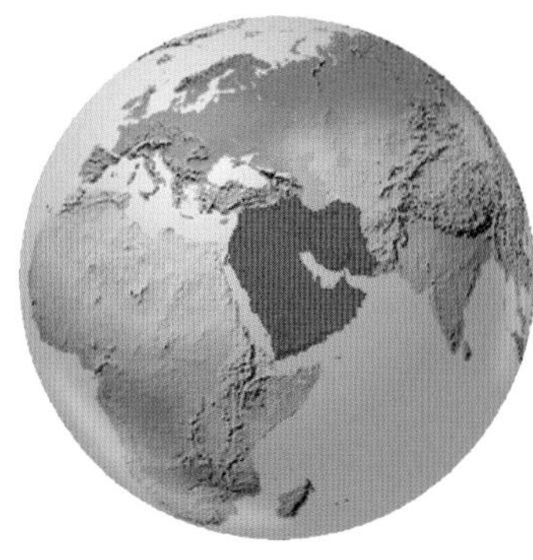

The Middle East consists of 15 independent countries. They sit at the crossroads of three great continents – to the northwest lies Europe, to the southwest is Africa, to the north and east are the Caucasus and Central Asian republics, all part of Asia.

LESS THAN 100 YEARS AGO, many of the inhabitants of the Middle East were Bedouins – desert-dwelling nomads who lived in tents and led their animals in search of food. The rest of the population lived in small towns and villages and made a living as farmers or craftsworkers. Almost everyone was poor and uneducated. Today, the lives of their children and grandchildren have been transformed by the discovery of oil. Many people have grown rich from the new industries and services related to oil production and refining. In some countries, notably Kuwait and Bahrain, there is free education and medical care for everyone. Oil transformed the international importance of the Middle East as well. The region had little influence in world affairs. Now it controls one quarter of the world's oil production, and decisions made in the Middle East affect the economies of Europe, America, and Asia. But despite this massive change, traditional customs have not been completely abandoned, and the religion of Islam continues to dominate daily life throughout the Middle East, as it has done for more than 1,300 years.

WATERWAYS

Rising in the mountains of Turkey, the Tigris and Euphrates rivers irrigate the almost rainless land of the Middle East as they flow in parallel to the Persian Gulf. The fertility of the Euphates-Tigris Delta, known as Mesopotamia in ancient times, gave rise to the world's first cities.

MODERNIZATION

The discovery of oil brought great wealth and rapid industrial and social change to the Middle East. But governments in the region recognize that the oil will eventually run out. So they have spent some of the money they earned from selling oil in encouraging and modernizing local industry and business. Many Middle East countries have also invested in property and businesses in other nations throughout the world.

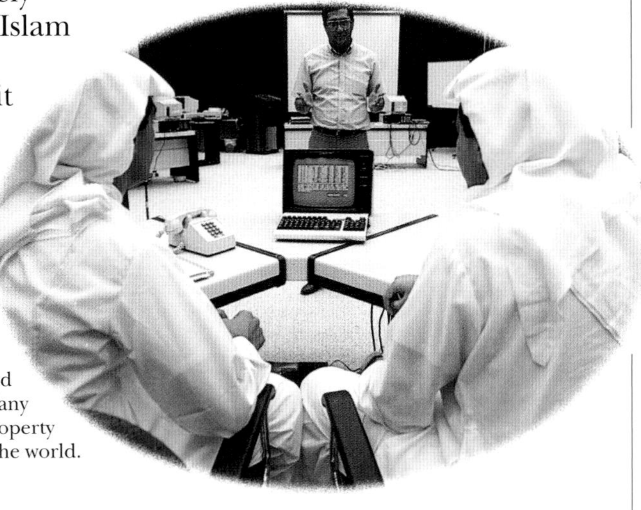

At a banking school in the Middle East, students learn the skills that will help them modernize business in their country.

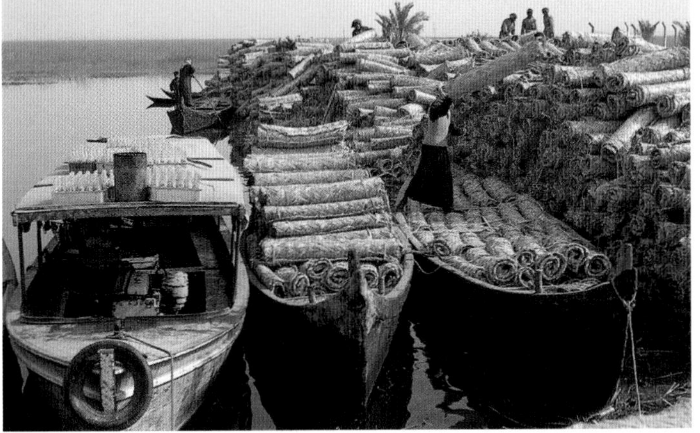

The areas of desert bordering the Euphrates and Tigris rivers are swamps and marshlands. Here, small boats replace the camel as the most common means of transport.

LANDSCAPE AND CLIMATE

Most of the Middle East consists of hot, dry, rocky deserts. A crescent of fertile land stretches west from the Tigris and Euphrates rivers through northern Iraq and Syria and then south into Lebanon and Israel. Turkey and Iran are mountainous, as are the southern parts of the Arabian peninsula. In the southeast of Saudi Arabia lies the Rub' al Khali, a vast, uninhabited sandy desert known as the Empty Quarter.

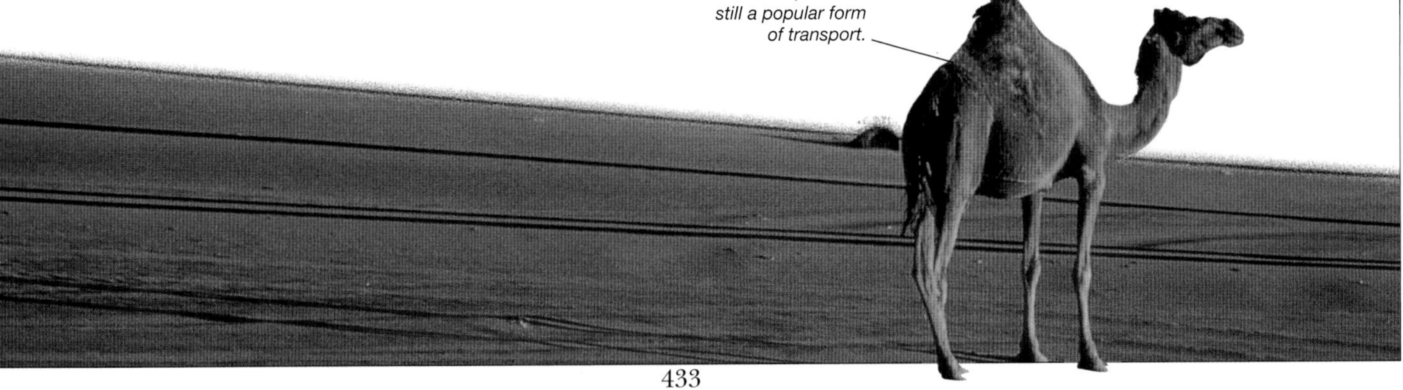

Camels are well adapted to the harsh conditions of the Middle East, and are still a popular form of transport.

SUEZ CANAL

More than 160 km (100 miles) in length, the Suez Canal links the Mediterranean Sea and the Red Sea. The canal took ten years to build, and when completed in 1869, it cut more than 11,000 km (7,000 miles) from the distance that sailing ships travelled to reach the Far East. Today, nearly 50 ships pass through the canal each day. The Suez Canal is an important trade route and has often been at the centre of conflict in the Middle East. The waterway has been closed by war and political disagreements several times, most recently by the Arab-Israeli Six Day War of 1967.

The Suez Canal is not wide enough for ships travelling in opposite directions to pass each other. Vessels must travel in convoy (above), passing only at by-passes, where stretches of the canal has been doubled.

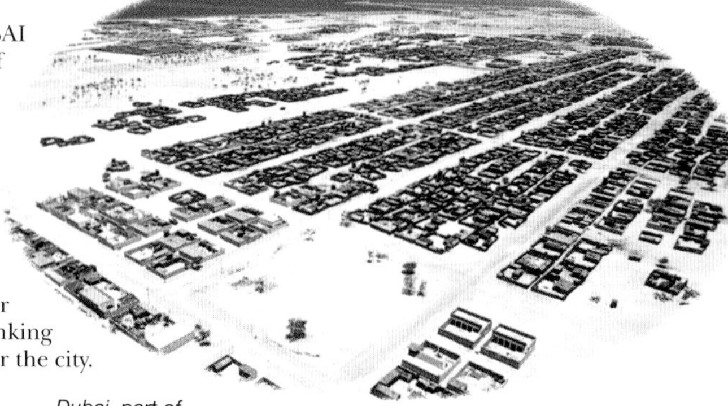

DUBAI

The city-state of Dubai on the Gulf has a modern centre, but on the outskirts it merges into the surrounding desert. Rainfall on the Arabian Peninsula where Dubai stands averages less than 100 mm (4 in) a year, and in most places the only natural water comes from underground springs. Desalination plants turn salt water from the Gulf into a supply of drinking water for the city.

Dubai, part of the federation of United Arab Emirates, is generally flat with large areas covered by dunes and barren rock.

Splendid architecture, financed by revenue from oil, can be found in Abu Dhabi (below).

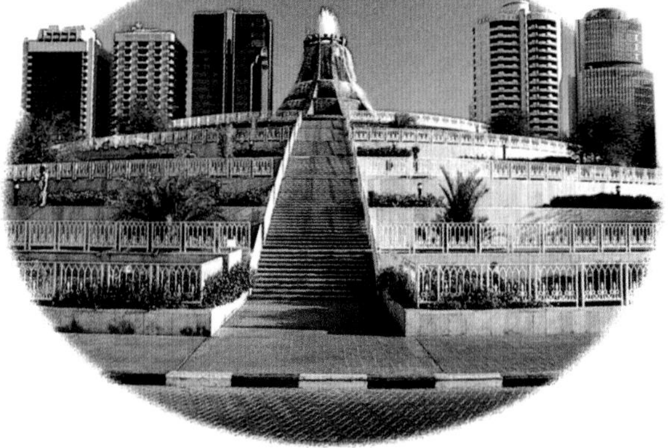

ABU DHABI

The rulers of many Middle East states invested income from sales of oil to improve the living conditions of their people and develop the economies of their nations. In the 1960s the city of Abu Dhabi was just a fishing village on the Gulf. Today it is the capital city of the Abu Dhabi sheikdom in the United Arab Emirates, complete with an international airport and high-rise downtown area. Abu Dhabi's revenues from oil royalties give it one of the world's highest per capita incomes.

UNITED ARAB EMIRATES

Like many Middle East nations, the United Arab Emirates has no democratic government. Instead, the country is ruled by a group of wealthy emirs (kings) who have absolute power over their people. Each emir controls his individual emirate, or kingdom, but they meet in the Federal Supreme Council of Rulers to make decisions that affect the whole country. Today, oil provides most of the country's wealth, but shipping has traditionally been important, and there are major ports at Abu Dhabi, Dubai, and Sharjah.

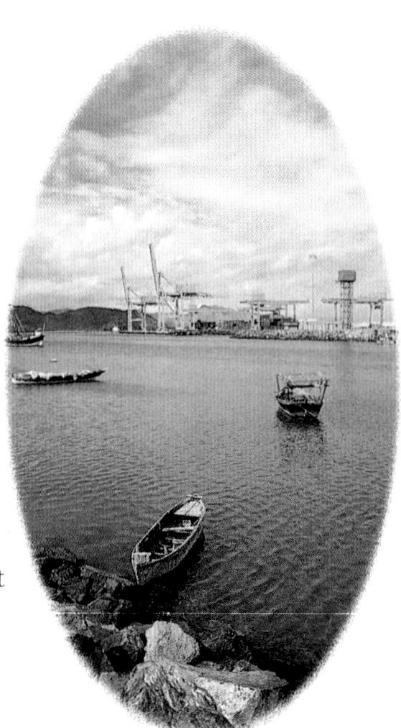

The port at Sharjah is built to accommodate the most modern container ships.

Muslim guerrillas fight in the streets of Lebanon.

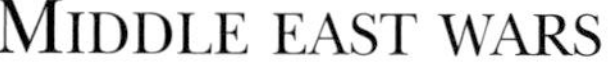

MIDDLE EAST WARS

Bitter wars have caused much suffering and death in the Middle East. Israel and its Arab neighbours have fought four wars over the last 60 years. Iran and Iraq were constantly at war throughout the 1980s, and Lebanon was devastated by a civil war. In 1991 UN forces defeated Iraq after the Iraqis invaded Kuwait. In 2003 American and British forces invaded Iraq and overthrew the dictator Saddam Hussein.

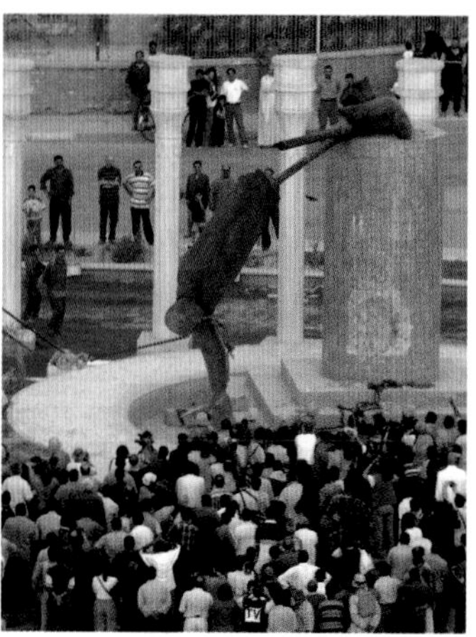

A statue of the former Iraqi dictator Saddam Hussein is toppled in a square in central Baghdad after the 2003 invasion.

Find out more

DESERTS
IRAN
ISLAM
ISRAEL
OIL

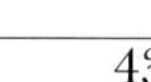

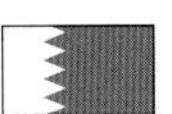

BAHRAIN
Area: 680 sq km (263 sq miles)
Population: 724,000
Capital: Manama

CYPRUS
Area: 9,251 sq km (3,572 sq miles)
Population: 802,000
Capital: Nicosia

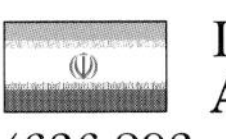

IRAN
Area: 1,648,000 sq km (636,293 sq miles)
Population: 68,900,000
Capital: Tehran

IRAQ
Area: 438,320 sq km (169,235 sq miles)
Population: 25,200,000
Capital: Baghdad

ISRAEL
Area: 20,700 sq km (7,992 sq miles)
Population: 6,400,000
Capital: Jerusalem

JORDAN
Area: 89,210 sq km (34,440 sq miles)
Population: 5,500,000
Capital: Amman

KUWAIT
Area: 17,820 sq km (6,880 sq miles)
Population: 2,500,000
Capital: Kuwait

LEBANON
Area: 10,400 sq km (4,015 sq miles)
Population: 3,700,000
Capital: Beirut

OMAN
Area: 212,460 sq km (82,030 sq miles)
Population: 2,900,000
Capital: Muscat

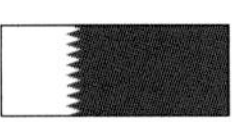

QATAR
Area: 11,000 sq km (4,247 sq miles)
Population: 610,000
Capital: Doha

SAUDI ARABIA
Area: 2,149,690 sq km (829,995 sq miles)
Population: 24,200,000
Capital: Riyadh

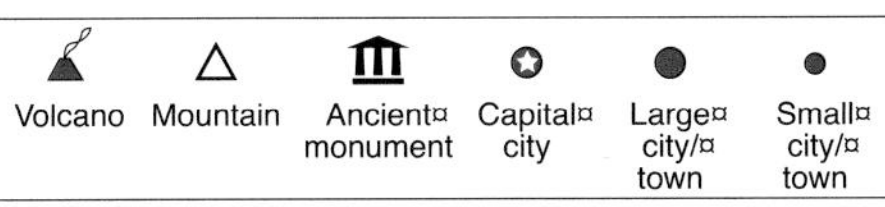

SYRIA
Area: 185,180 sq km (71,500 sq miles)
Population: 17,800,000
Capital: Damascus

TURKEY
Area: 769,630 sq km (297,154 sq miles)
Population: 71,300,000
Capital: Ankara

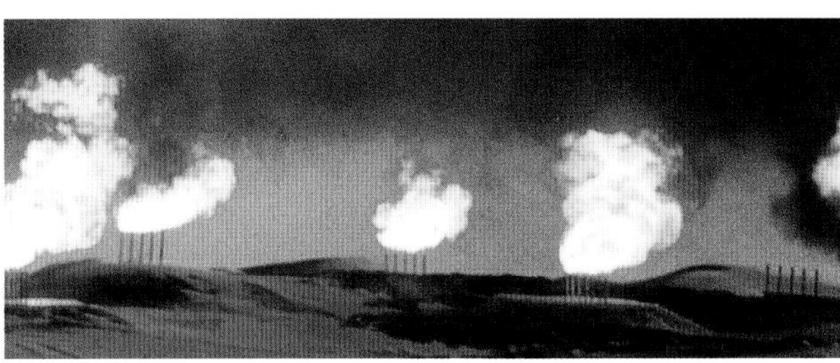

Oil industry

Deposits of oil and natural gas were first discovered in the Gulf in the early 1900s. Today, more than half the world's oil reserves are located in the Gulf. The oil industry has made several of the countries very rich, particularly Saudi Arabia, the United Arab Emirates, Bahrain, and Kuwait.

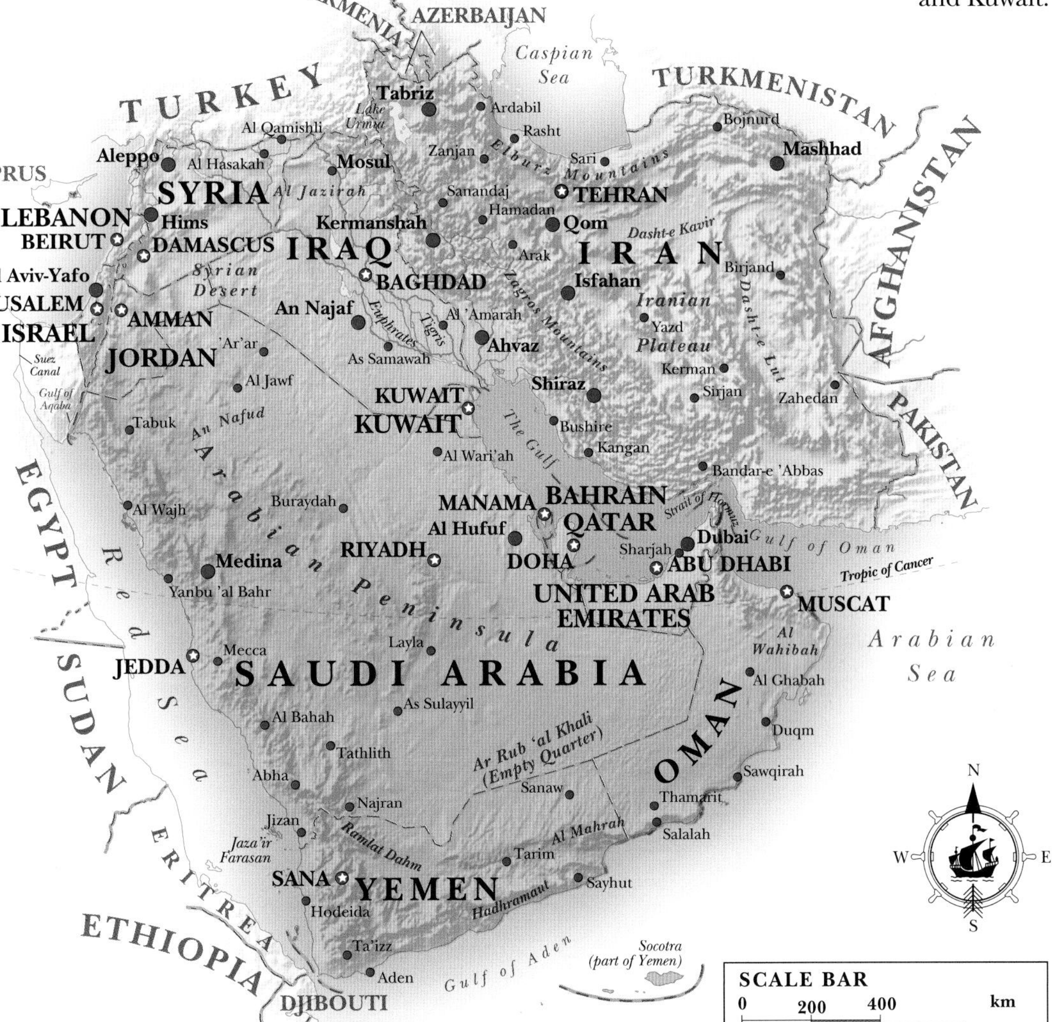

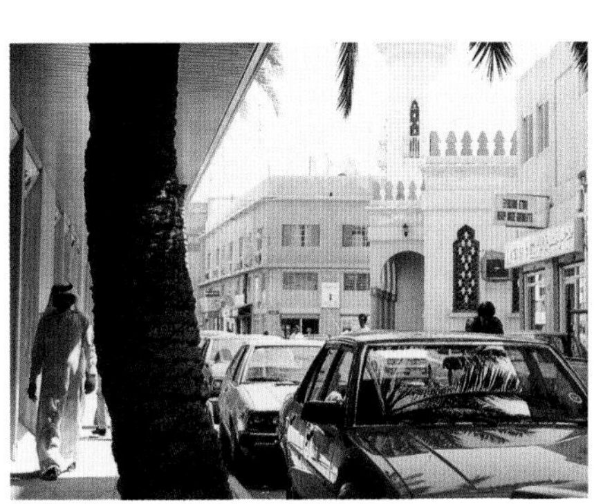

The roofs of buildings in Bahrain extend across pavements, providing shade from the scorching sun.

BAHRAIN
The island of Bahrain is little more than 50 km (30 miles) long. Oil wells and refineries provide employment for many people, but tourism is important, too; in 1986 a causeway was opened, linking Bahrain to Saudi Arabia. Since then, many visitors from neighbouring Gulf States with strict Islamic laws, have visited Bahrain to enjoy its liberal lifestyle.

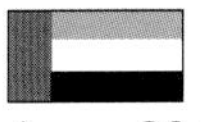

UNITED ARAB EMIRATES
Area: 83,600 sq km (32,278 sq miles)
Population: 3,000,000
Capital: Abu Dhabi

YEMEN
Area: 527,970 sq km (203,849 sq miles)
Population: 20,000,000
Capital: Sana

ANIMAL

MIGRATION

MANY ANIMALS LIVE in the same areas all their lives, rarely going far. But others undertake migrations – long journeys in search of food, warmth, or a suitable place to breed and raise young. Some animals migrate seasonally. During the dry season, for example, buffaloes may set off in search of water holes or fresh pasture. Some creatures migrate to avoid the harsh winter cold; others to avoid the scorching summer Sun. Migration can cover thousands of kilometres and often involves a return journey. Birds such as cuckoos and swallows, for instance, spend the summer in Europe and winter in Africa. Some animals, such as locusts, migrate only when they become so numerous that the area can no longer support them.

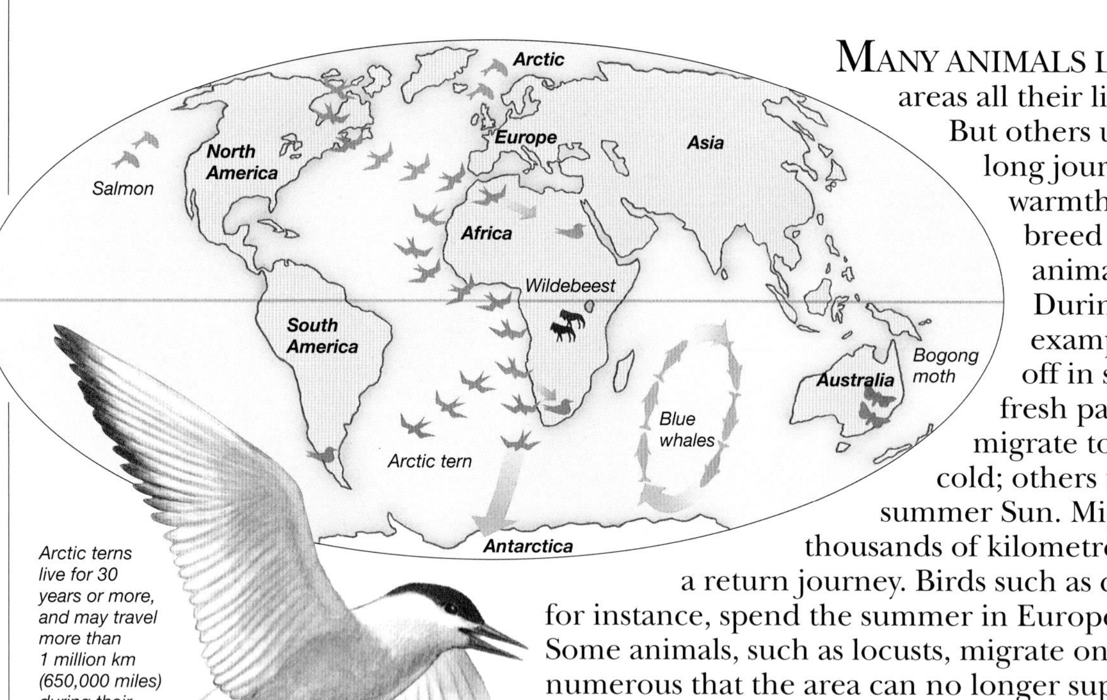

Arctic terns live for 30 years or more, and may travel more than 1 million km (650,000 miles) during their lifetime.

ARCTIC TERN
The longest migration in the world is made by the Arctic tern. This champion migrator travels from the top of the globe to the bottom each year and back again. Arctic terns spend the summer in the Arctic, where they rear their young and feed on insects, fish, and shellfish. After the short summer they fly south, and some reach the Antarctic. The direct journey is 15,000 km (9,000 miles), yet many terns go even farther, flying east across the North Atlantic, then west across the South Atlantic. After another summer near the South Pole, they migrate north again.

NAVIGATION

Some animals seem to navigate, or find their way, by following the position of the Sun, Moon, or stars. Others may have a built-in compass that senses the Earth's magnetic field or the electric field of ocean currents. Scientists are not sure how animals know where to migrate, especially young animals that have never made the journey before.

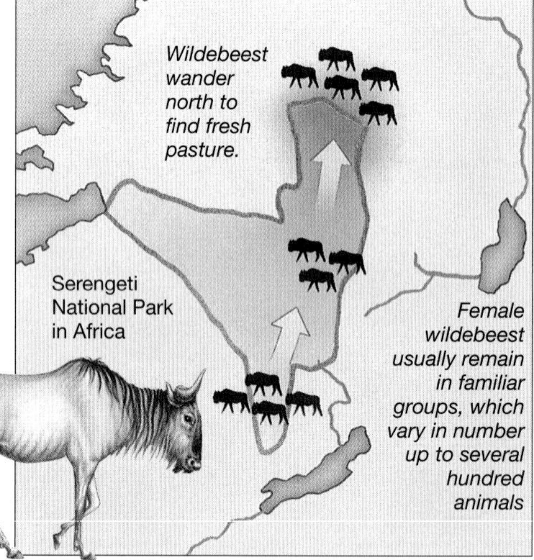

Wildebeest wander north to find fresh pasture.
Serengeti National Park in Africa
Female wildebeest usually remain in familiar groups, which vary in number up to several hundred animals

WILDEBEEST
During the dry season in Africa, huge herds of gnus (also called wildebeest) set out in search of fresh grassland and water. Sometimes they travel more than 1,500 km (1,000 miles) before they reach a suitable place.

SALMON
Salmon hatch from eggs in rivers and streams, then swim to the ocean, where they spend most of their lives. As adults they migrate thousands of kilometres back to the river where they were born, to breed. They are so sensitive to the chemicals in the stream where they hatch that they can find their way back to the same spot even after a few years. Salmon are powerful swimmers, and leap out of the water as they fight their way upstream.

Spring: Adult bogong moths migrate to mountain regions above 1,200 m (4,000 ft).

Summer: Adults gather in mountain caves and among rocks to rest during the hot, dry season.

Autumn: Adult moths wake and fly down to the lowlands to lay eggs.

BOGONG MOTH
Some animals migrate in summer rather than winter. During the hot, dry summer in southeast Australia, bogong moths sleep in cool caves and rock crevices high in the mountains. This type of hibernation is called aestivation. In autumn the moths fly down over the lowlands. Some keep flying when they reach the coast, and perish at sea.

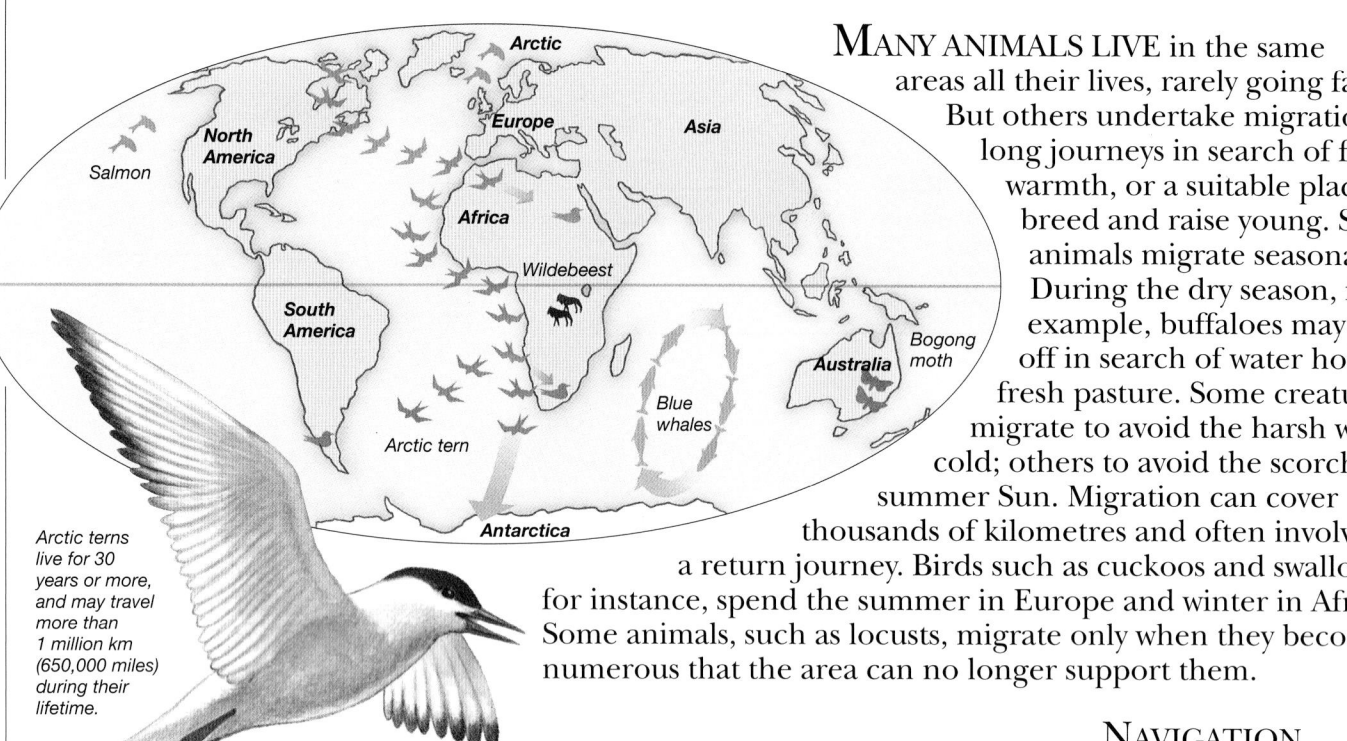

Find out more
ANIMALS
BIRDS
BUTTERFLIES AND MOTHS
FISH
HIBERNATION

MILITARY AIRCRAFT

JUST A FEW YEARS after the Wright brothers' historic first powered flight of 1903, aeroplanes took to the air as weapons of war. These early aircraft were fragile machines made only of wood and fabric held together with steel wire, and were armed with one or two machine guns. By the end of World War I in 1918, military aircraft had developed into large, long-range bombers for attacking distant cities or military installations, and small, manoeuvrable fighters for destroying enemy aircraft. However, these machines seem primitive by comparison with military aircraft of today. The latest aeroplanes are built of the lightest, strongest materials, powered by jet engines which drive them through the air as fast as a rifle bullet, and armed with a fearsome array of weaponry. They are also very adaptable; with only minor modifications a single aircraft may be used as a fighter, as a bomber, or for aerial reconnaissance (scouting) operations.

FIGHTER AIRCRAFT

Generally considered to be one of the world's most advanced fighter aircraft, the F-15E *Eagle* is equipped with sophisticated electronic instruments for detecting and attacking other aircraft and ground targets. The aeroplane has a top speed of more than 3,000 km/h (1,850 mph) and can fly to a height of 18,000 m (60,000 ft), which is twice that of Mount Everest.

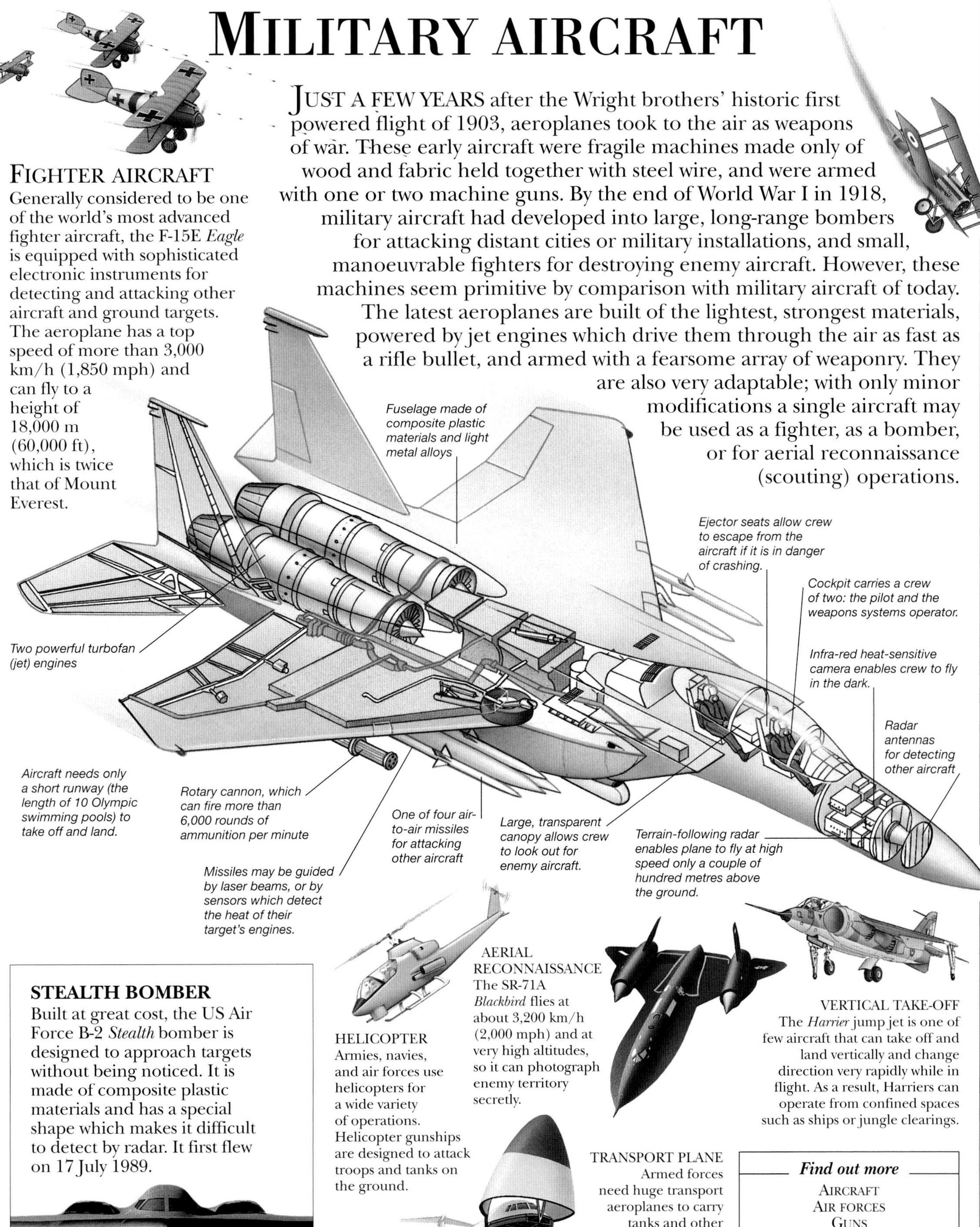

Fuselage made of composite plastic materials and light metal alloys
Ejector seats allow crew to escape from the aircraft if it is in danger of crashing.
Cockpit carries a crew of two: the pilot and the weapons systems operator.
Infra-red heat-sensitive camera enables crew to fly in the dark.
Radar antennas for detecting other aircraft
Two powerful turbofan (jet) engines
Aircraft needs only a short runway (the length of 10 Olympic swimming pools) to take off and land.
Rotary cannon, which can fire more than 6,000 rounds of ammunition per minute
One of four air-to-air missiles for attacking other aircraft
Large, transparent canopy allows crew to look out for enemy aircraft.
Terrain-following radar enables plane to fly at high speed only a couple of hundred metres above the ground.
Missiles may be guided by laser beams, or by sensors which detect the heat of their target's engines.

STEALTH BOMBER

Built at great cost, the US Air Force B-2 *Stealth* bomber is designed to approach targets without being noticed. It is made of composite plastic materials and has a special shape which makes it difficult to detect by radar. It first flew on 17 July 1989.

HELICOPTER

Armies, navies, and air forces use helicopters for a wide variety of operations. Helicopter gunships are designed to attack troops and tanks on the ground.

AERIAL RECONNAISSANCE

The SR-71A *Blackbird* flies at about 3,200 km/h (2,000 mph) and at very high altitudes, so it can photograph enemy territory secretly.

VERTICAL TAKE-OFF

The *Harrier* jump jet is one of few aircraft that can take off and land vertically and change direction very rapidly while in flight. As a result, Harriers can operate from confined spaces such as ships or jungle clearings.

TRANSPORT PLANE

Armed forces need huge transport aeroplanes to carry tanks and other equipment into battle. Aircraft of this type can carry loads weighing over 150 tonnes (about 150 tons).

Find out more

AIRCRAFT
AIR FORCES
GUNS
HELICOPTERS
ROCKETS AND MISSILES
WORLD WAR I
WORLD WAR II

MINOANS

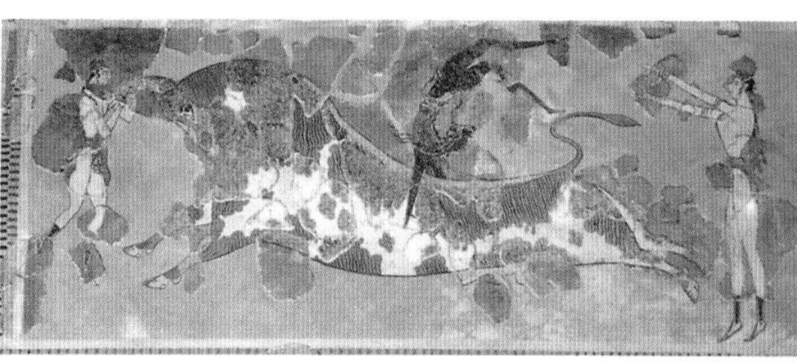

BULL DANCE
Young Minoan men and women performed life-threatening acrobatic feats, probably for religious reasons. They took turns leaping through the horns of a charging bull. After the dance they sacrificed the bull and spread its blood on the land. Few would have survived this type of sport.

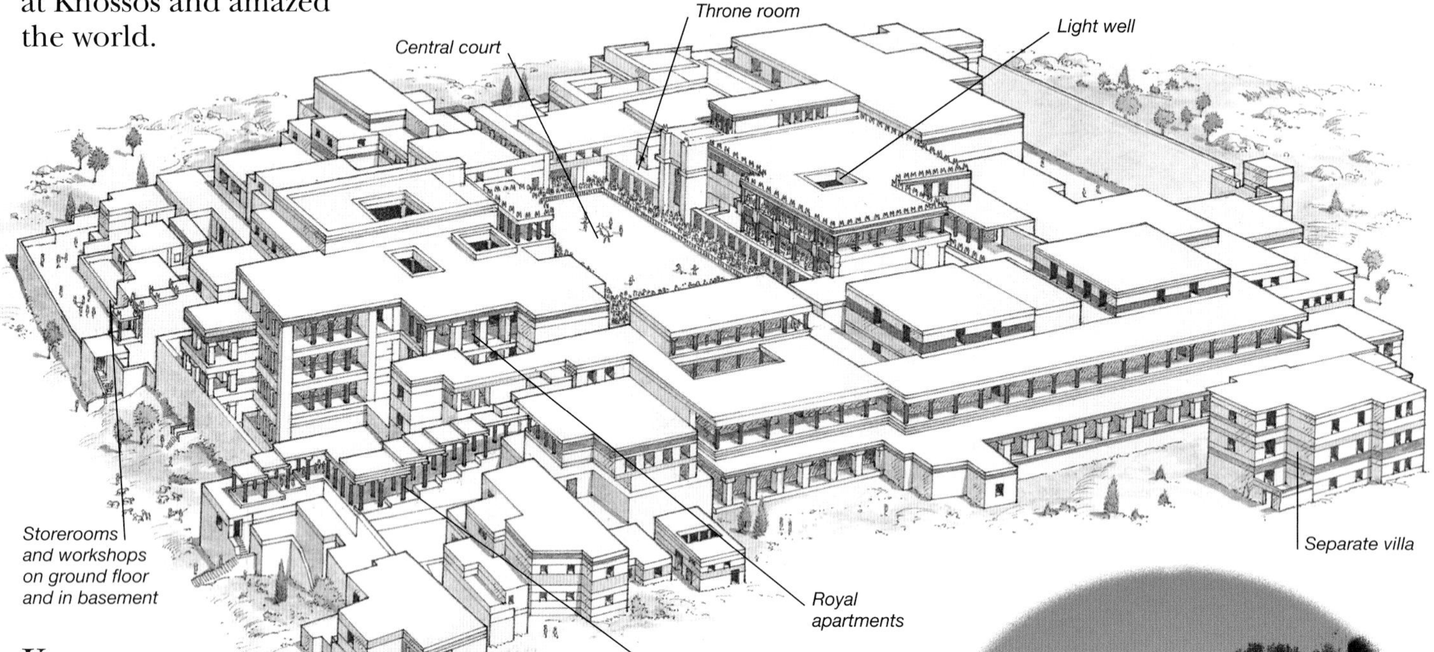

FOR NEARLY A THOUSAND YEARS a glittering civilization dominated the Mediterranean. Its people were known as the Minoans, after their legendary king Minos. In about 6000 B.C. settlers had travelled from mainland Greece to the island of Crete. Blessed with rich soil and a fruitful sea, these people became prosperous and developed a rich culture that reached its height between 2200 B.C. and 1500 B.C. They built huge palaces, such as the palace at Knossos, their main city. The Minoans were great seafarers. They traded throughout the Mediterranean region and with Egypt, carrying passengers, wine, oil, cloth, and bronze in their ships. They grew wheat, vines, and olives, and herded sheep on the mountain slopes. Quite suddenly, a huge volcanic eruption devastated the Minoan civilization. It was not until early 20th century that an archaeologist uncovered the palace at Knossos and amazed the world.

Throne room

Light well

Central court

Storerooms and workshops on ground floor and in basement

Separate villa

Royal apartments

Red-painted pillars supported flat roof.

KNOSSOS

The main Minoan palace at Knossos was five storeys high in places and contained more than 1,300 rooms. The walls bore colourful paintings showing scenes from Minoan life. The palace itself contained rooms with religious shrines, workrooms for craftsworkers, store-rooms, and living quarters.

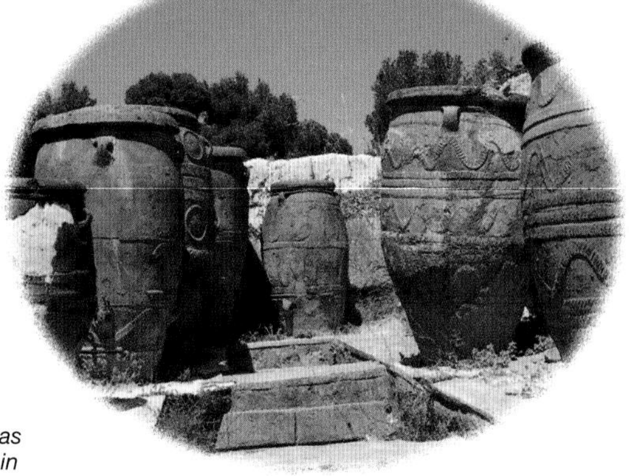

Cyclonia

Crete

Knossos

Phaestos

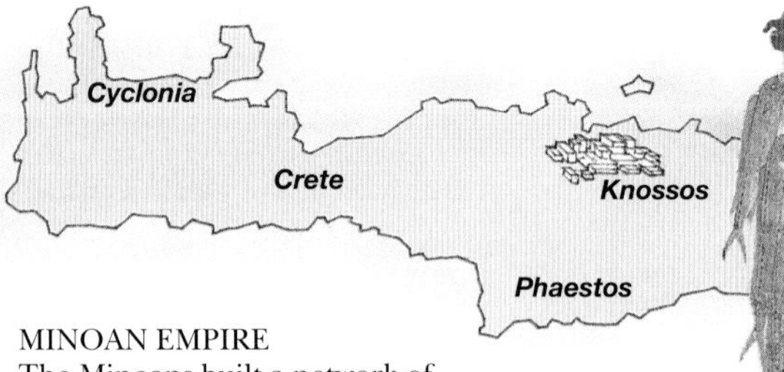

MINOAN EMPIRE
The Minoans built a network of towns on the island of Crete and set up many trading posts around the shores of the eastern Mediterranean. After the volcanic eruption on the nearby island of Thera in about 1550 B.C., peoples from mainland Greece overran Crete. They were called Mycenaeans. The Minoan civilization then went into decline.

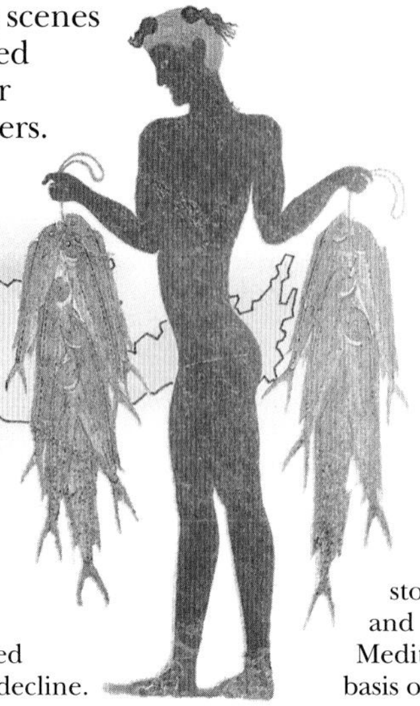

Fresco of fisherboy was discovered in a house on the island of Thera. (Fresco is the ancient art of painting on plaster.)

FISHING
Minoan sailors fished the stormy waters around Crete and traded all over the eastern Mediterranean. Fishing was the basis of the Minoan economy.

MINOAN POTTERY
The Minoans produced outstanding pottery. They used potter's wheels to make eggshell-thin, finely decorated pots and huge storage jars called pithoi (above). Oil, wine, and grain were kept in the pithoi.

Find out more
EGYPT, ANCIENT
GREECE, ANCIENT

MONASTERIES

DURING THE MIDDLE AGES men who wanted to devote their lives to the Christian religion often became monks and entered a monastery. They promised to give up all their possessions and never to marry. They followed a hard routine of worship and work. Monks attended up to eight services each day in the abbey church. Regular hours were set aside for working, praying, studying, and recreation. Most monks never left their monastery. They grew their own food, raised their own animals, and made most of the things they needed. Monasteries helped the sick and gave food to the poor. They were also important centres of learning.

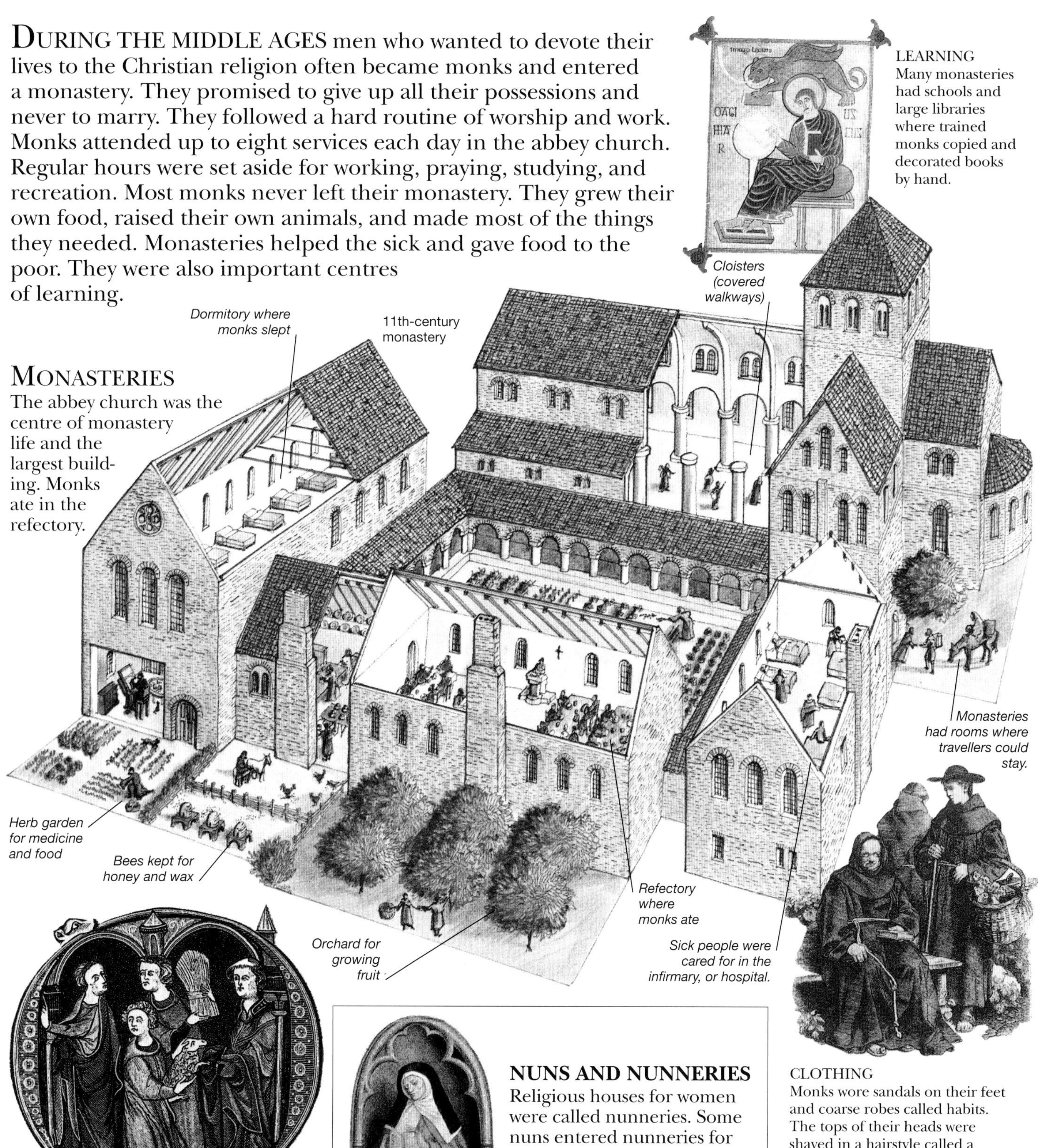

Dormitory where monks slept
11th-century monastery
Cloisters (covered walkways)
Monasteries had rooms where travellers could stay.
Herb garden for medicine and food
Bees kept for honey and wax
Orchard for growing fruit
Refectory where monks ate
Sick people were cared for in the infirmary, or hospital.

LEARNING
Many monasteries had schools and large libraries where trained monks copied and decorated books by hand.

MONASTERIES

The abbey church was the centre of monastery life and the largest building. Monks ate in the refectory.

ORDERS OF MONKS
Different types, or orders, of monks organized their lives in different ways. Some orders devoted most of their time to prayer and meditation; others spent more time at physical work.

NUNS AND NUNNERIES

Religious houses for women were called nunneries. Some nuns entered nunneries for religious reasons; others went to escape from brutal husbands. Nuns taught, prayed, and studied, and followed the same hard routine as monks. Some orders were very strict; others were more relaxed.

CLOTHING
Monks wore sandals on their feet and coarse robes called habits. The tops of their heads were shaved in a hairstyle called a tonsure; this represented Christ's crown of thorns.

Find out more

CHRISTIANITY
CHURCHES AND CATHEDRALS
MEDIEVAL EUROPE
RELIGIONS

Money

The next time you are about to buy something, look at your money. Coins and notes are just discs of metal and sheets of paper, yet the shop accepts them as payment for useful, valuable goods. Money is a token which people trade for goods of an agreed value, and strange objects have been used for money throughout the world. Tibetans once used blocks of dried tea! It does not really matter what you use as money, provided everyone can reach an agreement about what it is worth. Many early coins were made from precious metals, such as gold and silver, but in 11th-century China, paper bank notes, or bills, first appeared. Unlike gold, bank notes had no real value. However, the bank that issued them promised to exchange them for gold. English bank notes still have the same promise printed on them. The United States government stopped exchanging bills for gold in 1971.

MINT
A government-controlled factory called a mint produces coins and paper money. Each coin is stamped with a special design, including its value, and often the year of manufacture. This stamping process is known as "minting".

Some Native Americans used wampum belts made of clamshell beads for money.

The first Chinese coins were made of bronze in the shape of tools, such as the head of a hoe.

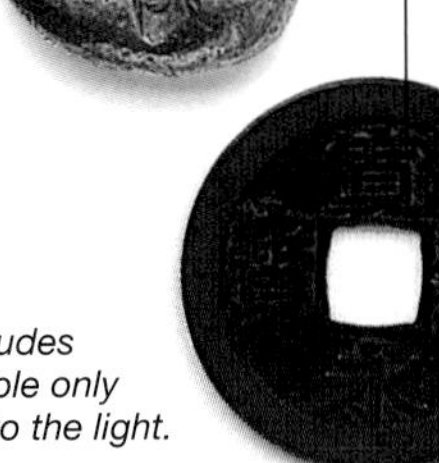

The weight of a coin made of precious metal indicates its value.

A strip of plastic or metal thread is embedded in the paper.

Specially made paper includes a watermark, which is visible only when the note is held up to the light.

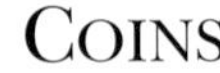

The loops and whirls are machine-engraved and extremely difficult to copy.

The metal of a modern coin is almost worthless, so the value of the coin is stamped on it.

Coins

People from ancient Lydia (now Turkey) were the first to make coins, about 2,700 years ago. Their coins were made from electrum, a mixture of gold and silver. Today, coins are used only for small denominations (sums of money). Paper money is used for larger sums, because notes are more difficult to forge than coins.

Bank notes

Governments issue bank notes and guarantee their value. It is a crime for anyone else to copy and print bank notes. The crime is called forgery, or counterfeiting, and bank notes have complicated designs to make copying difficult. Thomas De La Rue & Company is one of the world's most successful bank note printers. Their specimen note includes various security features which make their notes very difficult to copy.

BANKS
Most people deposit, or store, their money in a bank. Banks keep this money safe in a vault or lend it to their other customers. The bank has an account, or record, of how much each of its customers has deposited. Banks pay out notes and coins when their customers need money to make purchases. People with bank accounts can also buy things by writing cheques – notes which the bank promises to exchange for cash.

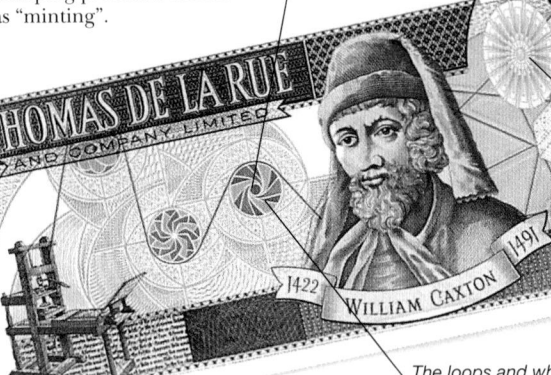

All credit cards have to be signed by the user and can be used only by that person.

Many credit cards incorporate holograms which are difficult to copy.

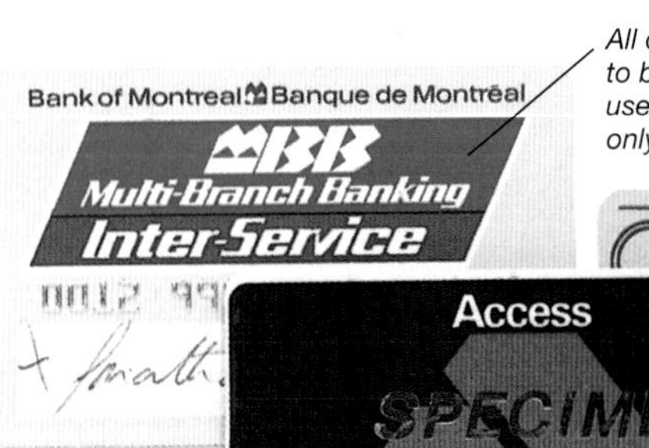

The raised letters imprint your name and card number on the receipt.

CREDIT CARDS
A credit card is a piece of plastic that can be used in place of money. When you use it to buy something, you sign a receipt. The credit card company pays for the goods, and you pay the credit card company a month or so later. Credit cards are carefully made to reduce the risk of forgery or misuse.

Find out more

Rocks and minerals
Shops and shopping
Stock exchange
Trade and industry

Mongol empire

In the late 1100s a masterful chieftain united a group of wandering tribes into a powerful army. He was called Genghis Khan; the tribes were the Mongols. All were toughened by a harsh life spent herding on the treeless plains of northeastern Asia. Determined to train the best army of his time, Genghis built up a formidable cavalry force. Using new weapons such as smoke bombs and gunpowder, they were invincible. In 1211, the Mongols invaded China, then swept through Asia. They moved at incredible speed, concentrating their forces at critical moments. All their military operations were planned to the smallest detail. Looting and burning as they came, they struck terror into the hearts of their enemies. In 1227, Genghis Khan died, leaving a huge empire to his four sons, who extended it through Asia Minor into Europe. However, the empire broke apart as rival khans (Mongol kings) battled for control.

GENGHIS KHAN
Temüjin (1162-1227) was the son of a tribal chief. His father was murdered when Temüjin was still a child, and when he grew up he defeated his enemies, united all other tribes under his control, and took the title Genghis Khan, "prince of all that lies between the oceans". He aimed to conquer the world.

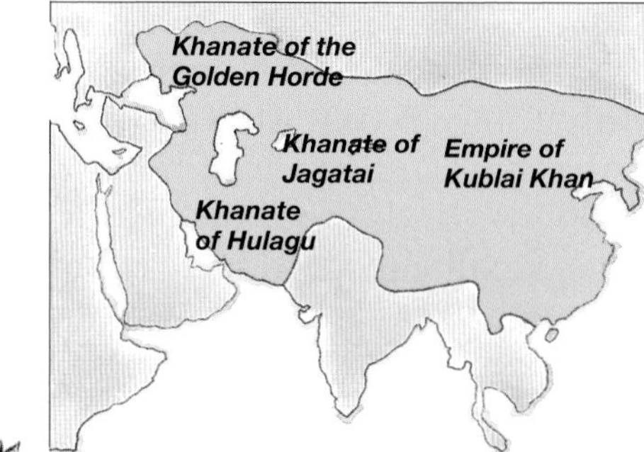

Mongol khanates

After Genghis's death, the Mongol Empire divided into four khanates, or states, with different rulers. Kublai, grandson of Genghis, ruled the eastern khanate. The smaller western empires, although briefly united in the 1300s by Tamerlane the Great, gradually disintegrated.

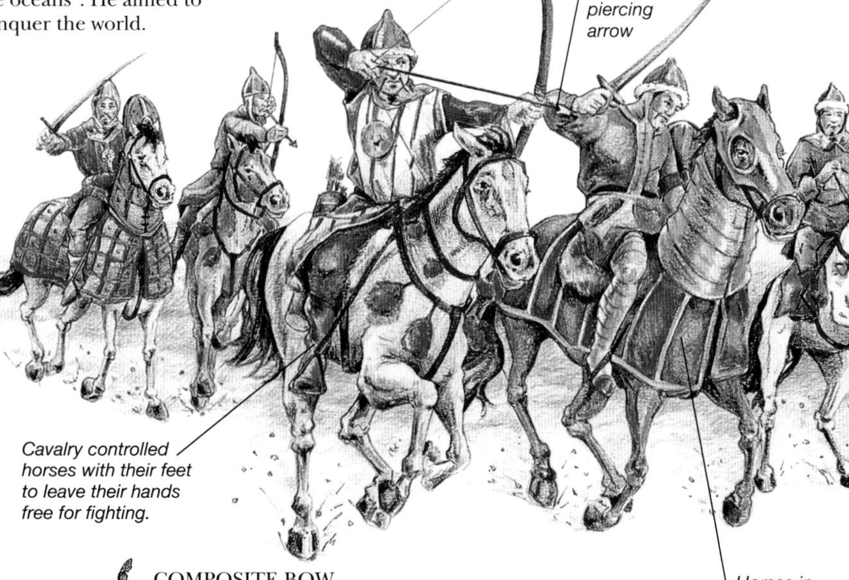

Armour-piercing arrow

Cavalry controlled horses with their feet to leave their hands free for fighting.

Horses in battle gear

COMPOSITE BOW
Mongols made their deadly bows out of wood, horn, and sinew, which gave the bows incredible power. The Mongols were superb archers, able to string, aim, and fire at full gallop. They developed armour-piercing arrows, whistling arrows for signalling, and even arrows tipped with grenades.

Strung bow

Unstrung bow

YURTS
Tribes wandered the Mongolian steppes following their herds of sheep, goats, cattle, and horses. They lived in circular tents called yurts, which they took with them when they moved. The women drove wagons which held the yurts; the men hunted, looked after the herds, and traded for grain and metal. Mongols of today still live in yurts.

MONGOL EMPIRE

1206 Temüjin unites all the tribes of Mongolia.

1219 Mongols invade Persia.

1223 Mongols invade Russia.

1237 Batu, grandson of Genghis Khan, invades north Russia.

1240 Batu invades Poland and Hungary.

1260 Mamelukes, Egyptian warriors, defeat Mongols.

1279 Kublai Khan defeats China.

1370 Tamerlane the Great conquers the western khanates.

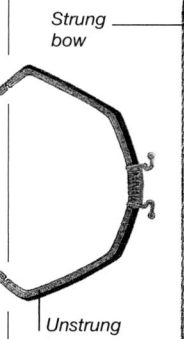

Find out more

China, history of
Explorers
Russia, history of

MONKEYS AND APES

AMONG THE MOST INTELLIGENT creatures on Earth are the apes – chimpanzees, gorillas, gibbons, and orang-utans. They have large brains, long arms, fingers, and toes, and their bodies are covered in hair. In body shape and intelligence these creatures resemble humans. Apes and humans both belong to the larger group known as Primates. Closely related to apes are monkeys, a larger group of animals that includes baboons, macaques, colubuses, and marmosets. Monkeys and apes have a similar body plan, although monkeys tend to be smaller. A pygmy marmoset weighs only 150 g (5 oz), whereas a huge male "silverback" gorilla weighs as much as 180 kg (400 lb). Both monkeys and apes have a rounded face, small ears, and large eyes which face forward. They use their front limbs like arms, and their hands can grasp strongly and manipulate delicately. Most monkeys have tails, which they use as a counterbalance as they swing through trees. In some monkeys the tail is strong and prehensile (grasping); apes, however, have no tails. Apes and monkeys feed on a variety of foods, including fruit, leaves, insects, and birds' eggs.

ORANG-UTAN

The richly coloured orang-utan is found in the forests of Borneo and Sumatra in southeast Asia. Orang-utans spend most of their time high up in the trees searching for fruit, shoots, leaves, and insects. They live alone, except where there is plenty of food.

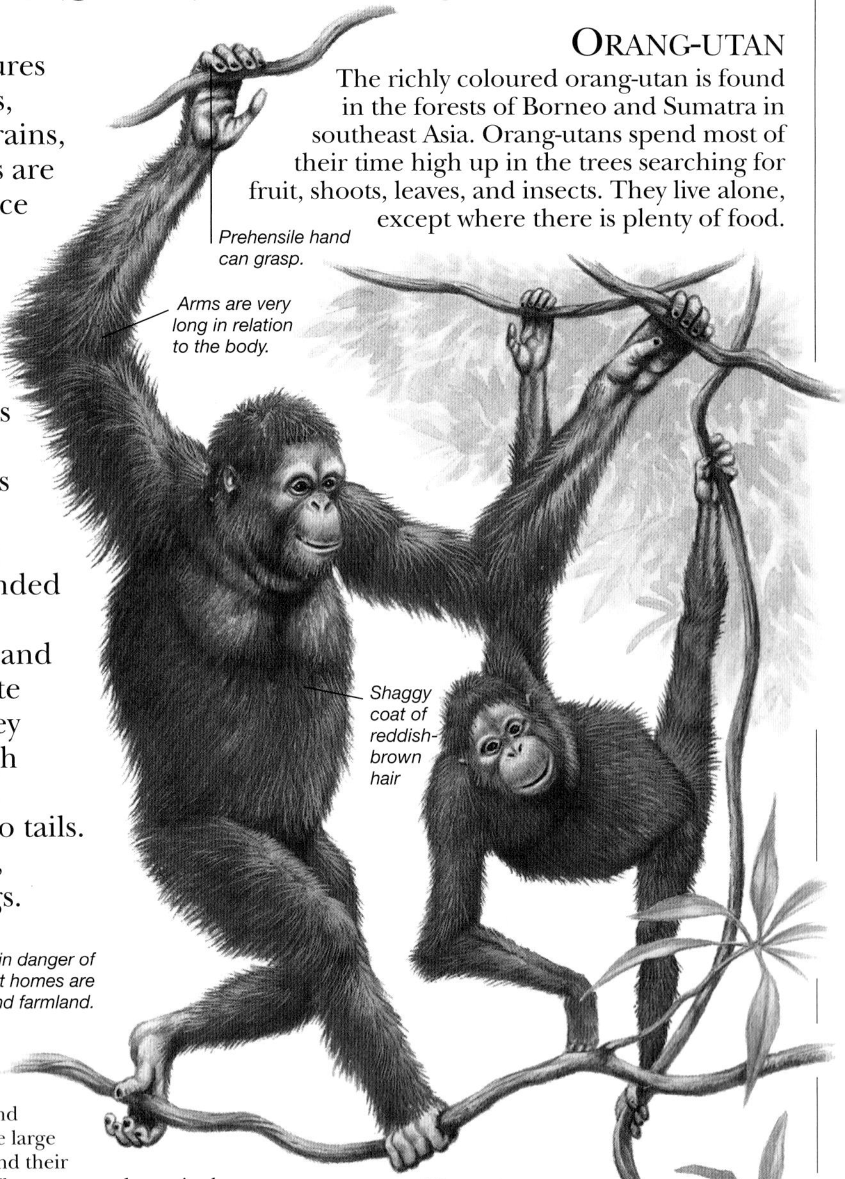

Prehensile hand can grasp.

Arms are very long in relation to the body.

Shaggy coat of reddish-brown hair

Today, orang-utans are in danger of extinction because their forest homes are being cleared for timber and farmland.

GORILLA

Measuring up to 2 m (6 ft) in height, gorillas are the largest apes. Gorillas are slow, gentle creatures – unless disturbed – and they spend their time resting and eating leaves, stems, and shoots. Gorillas live in small family groups that travel slowly through the forest, eating some but not all of the food in one place before moving on to another area.

BREEDING

A gorilla group contains between five and 10 animals. There is one large male, several females, and their young of various ages. The young are born singly; a female gives birth about every four years.

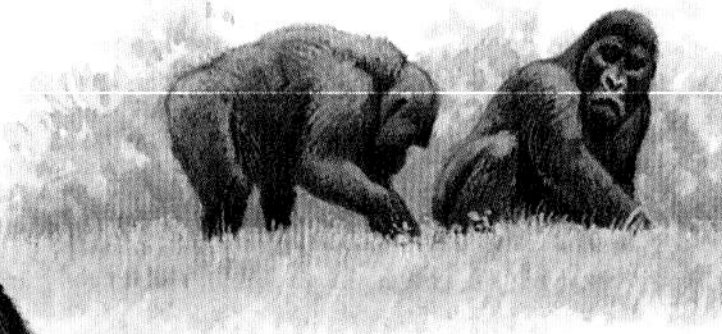

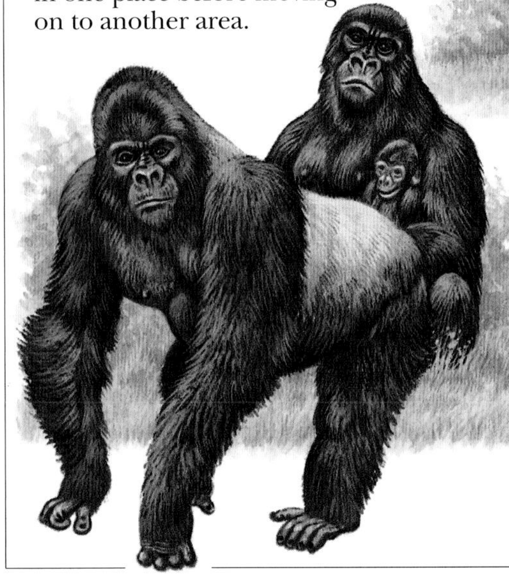

PRIMATES

All monkeys and apes belong to the mammal group called primates. Other primates include bush babies, pottos, tarsiers, and humans. Today, many primates, including gibbons and the other apes, are on the official list of endangered species.

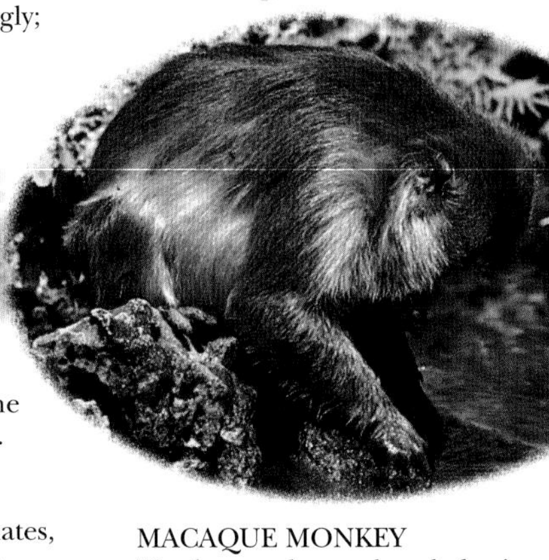

MACAQUE MONKEY

Monkeys and apes show behaviour that we describe as "intelligent". These creatures communicate well, have good memories, and are able to solve problems. A famous example is the Japanese macaque monkey, which discovered that by washing its food in water it could get rid of the dirt and sand on it. Other members of the troop saw what the monkey was doing and copied it.

GIBBON

A gibbon's muscular arms and hands are so long that the knuckles touch the ground even when the gibbon stands upright. Gibbons live in family groups of a male, a female, and two to four young. There are 14 kinds of gibbon; the largest is the siamang, which weighs about 10 kg (22 lb). The siamang is so heavy that it cannot swing out to the tips of thin branches as other gibbons can.

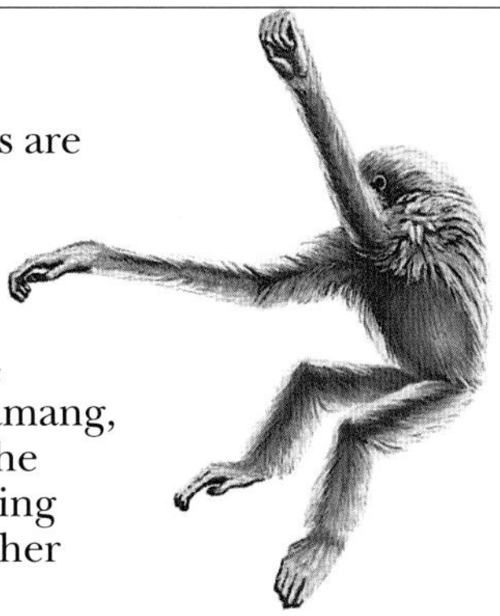

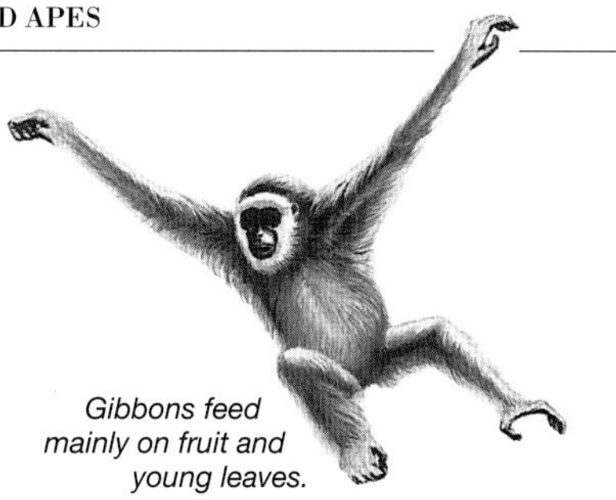

Gibbons feed mainly on fruit and young leaves.

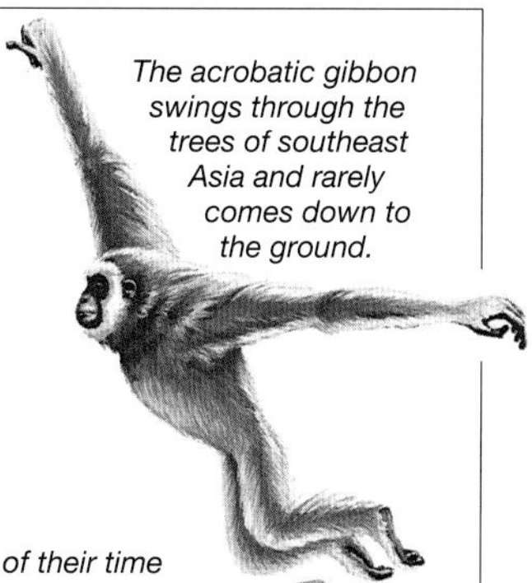

The acrobatic gibbon swings through the trees of southeast Asia and rarely comes down to the ground.

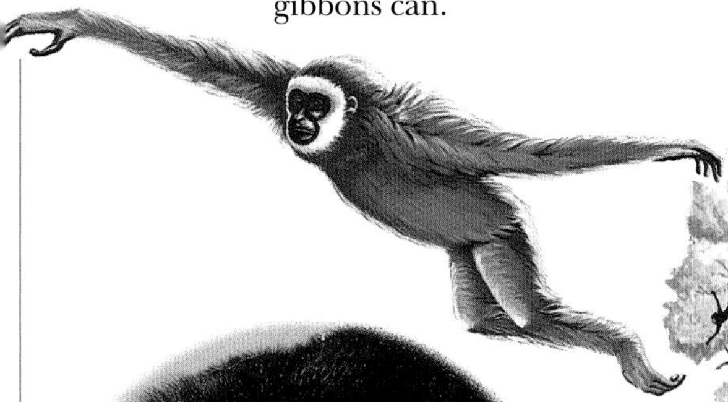

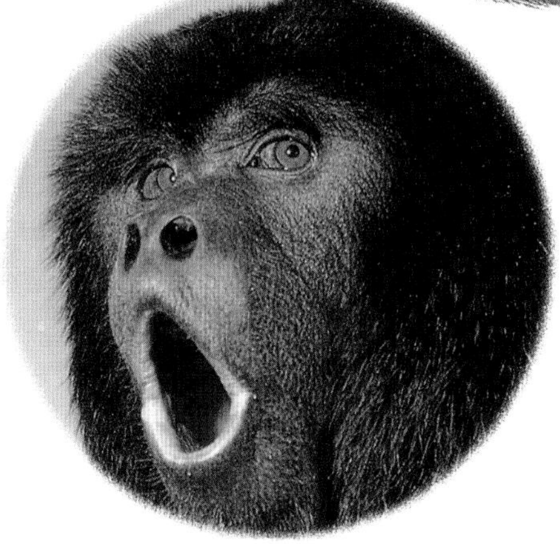

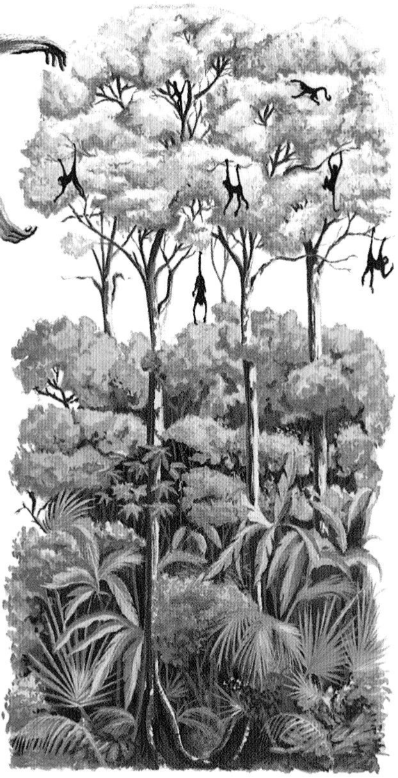

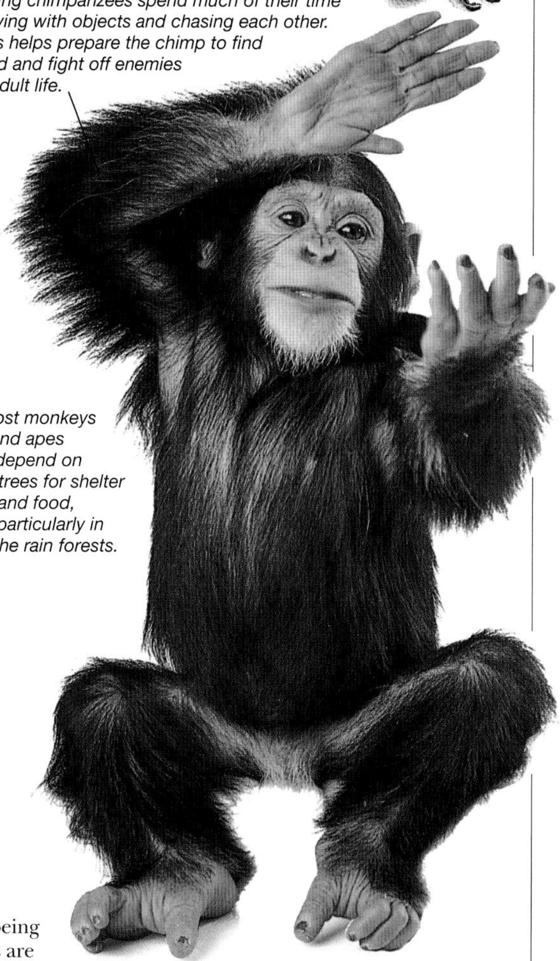

Young chimpanzees spend much of their time playing with objects and chasing each other. This helps prepare the chimp to find food and fight off enemies in adult life.

Most monkeys and apes depend on trees for shelter and food, particularly in the rain forests.

COMMUNICATION

Many monkeys communicate by sounds. The howler monkey of South America produces extremely loud howling noises using its specialized larynx (voice box). These sounds warn other howler troops to stay out of the group's territory. The leading male howler is usually the main shouter and can be heard nearly 3 km (2 miles) away.

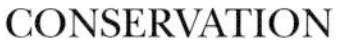

CONSERVATION

The forests where monkeys and apes live are being cut down at a great speed. Newly planted trees are soon removed for timber, so they do not provide homes for the local wildlife. Dozens of different kinds of monkeys are at risk. Among them is the woolly spider monkey of Brazil. Some non-profit organizations have taken up their cause. Their three-point programme works through rescue and rehabilitation, conservation education, and research.

CHIMPANZEE

Chimpanzees are the animals which remind us most of ourselves – because of their facial expressions and the way they play games, make tools, and solve puzzles. Chimpanzees live in groups which sometimes fight with neighbouring groups. Their main foods are fruit, leaves, seeds, flowers, insects, and sometimes larger creatures such as monkeys and deer. Chimpanzees live deep in the forests and open grassland of Africa. Pygmy chimps or bonobos are found only in the thick forests of the Democratic Republic of Congo (Zaire).

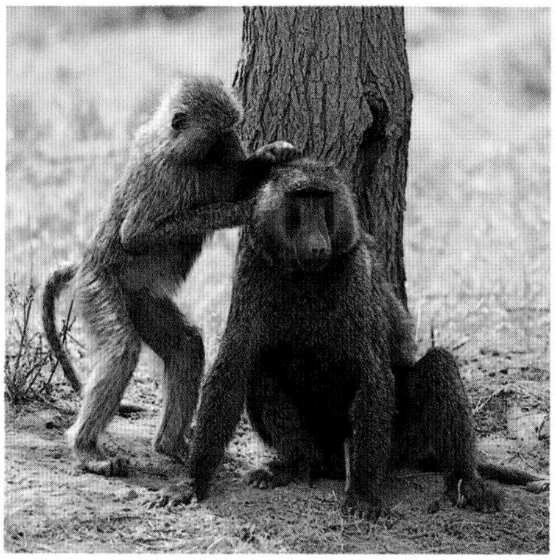

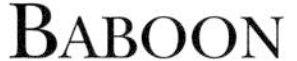

BABOON

The African baboon can climb but usually walks or gallops on all fours. Baboons are easy to study because they live in open country, and scientists have learned much about their social life. Baboons live in troops. Each troop is based around senior females and their offspring. Growing males tend to live alone while they are maturing. When a male becomes an adult he joins a troop, but has to battle with other males to establish his rank. The troop protects itself against predators such as lions and against other baboon troops that stray into its territory.

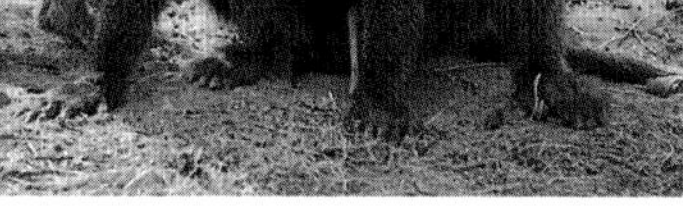

Find out more

AFRICAN WILDLIFE
ANIMALS
CONSERVATION and endangered species
FOREST WILDLIFE
MAMMALS

Moon

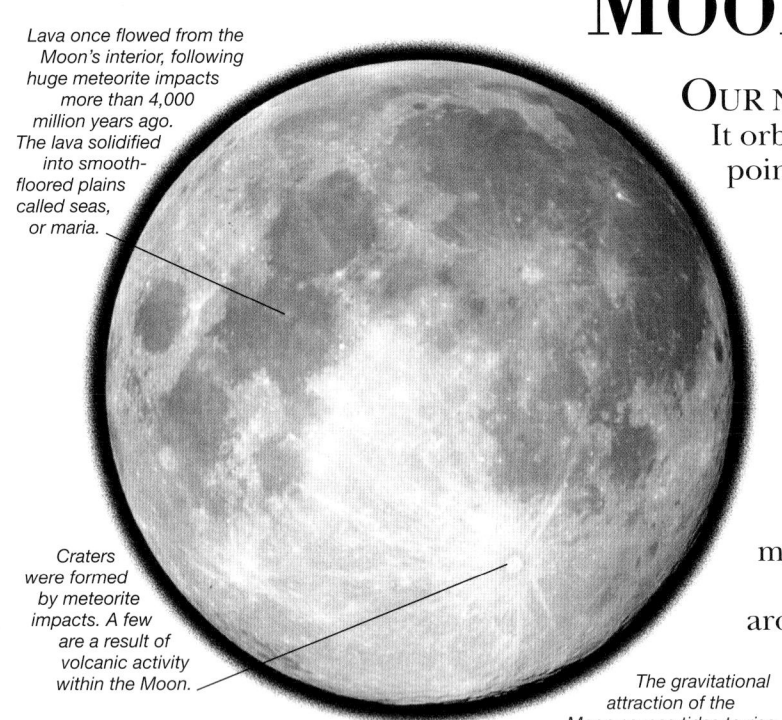

Lava once flowed from the Moon's interior, following huge meteorite impacts more than 4,000 million years ago. The lava solidified into smooth-floored plains called seas, or maria.

Craters were formed by meteorite impacts. A few are a result of volcanic activity within the Moon.

OUR NEAREST NEIGHBOUR in space is the Moon. It orbits, or circles, the Earth keeping the same face pointed towards us. The Moon is a hostile place. It has no atmosphere to keep the temperature constant, as Earth does. Instead, temperatures range from a scorching 115°C (240°F) during the Moon's day to an icy -160°C (-260°F) at night. There is no water, so no plants or animals can live there. Great plains stretch over the Moon's surface, dotted with huge mountains and scarred by numerous craters. The Moon does not produce light of its own. We see the Moon because it acts like a huge mirror, reflecting light from the Sun. The Moon is a natural satellite – something that orbits around a planet or a star. There are many moons circling the other planets in the solar system.

BIRTH OF THE MOON
There have been many theories to explain the formation of the Moon. Scientists have suggested that the Moon may be a piece of the Earth that broke away millions of years ago. Today, however, most astronomers believe that the Moon was formed when an asteroid the size of Mars struck the Earth about 4.5 billion years ago.

The gravitational attraction of the Moon causes tides to rise and fall in the Earth's oceans.

1 New moon (moon invisible)
2 Crescent moon
3 Half moon (first quarter)
4 Gibbous moon (waxing)
5 Full moon
6 Gibbous moon (waning)
7 Half moon (last quarter)
8 Old moon

Moon seen from here

PHASES OF THE MOON
As the Moon orbits the Earth, different shapes, or phases, appear, depending on the amount of the sunlit side of the Moon that is visible from Earth.

LUNA 3
Until 1959, the far side of the Moon had never been seen. In October of that year, the Russian space probe *Luna 3* (right) sent back the first photographs of this part of the Moon.

OTHER MOONS

Our solar system contains more than 150 known moons. Nearly all circle the giant outer planets and are made of ice mixed with rock. The largest planet, Jupiter, has at least 63 moons, three of them larger than our own moon. One, Io (seen alongside Jupiter, left), is alive with active volcanoes. Another, Ganymede, is the largest satellite in the solar system. Some of Saturn's moons are very small and orbit in the outer sections of the planet's rings.

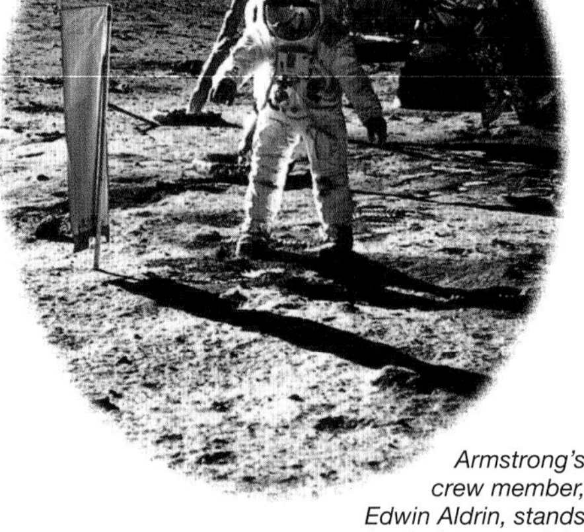

Armstrong's crew member, Edwin Aldrin, stands by the lunar module.

LUNAR LANDINGS
In 1966, the Russian *Luna 9* spacecraft made the first controlled landing on the Moon. It was only three years later, in July 1969, that American astronaut Neil Armstrong climbed down from the *Apollo 11* lunar module to become the first person on the Moon.

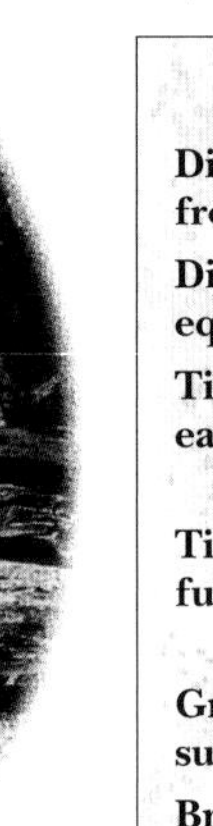

MOON FACTS

Distance from Earth	384,401 km (238,855 miles)
Diameter at equator	3,477.8 km (2,160.5 miles)
Time for each orbit	27 days, 7 hours, 43 minutes
Time between full moons	29 days, 12 hours, 43 minutes
Gravity at surface	1/6 of Earth's surface gravity
Brightness	1/425,000 brightness of Sun

Find out more
ASTRONOMY
EARTH
OCEANS AND SEAS
PLANETS
SPACE FLIGHT

WILLIAM
MORRIS

1834 — **1834** Born in Walthamstow, England.

1853-56 Joins Pre-Raphaelite Brotherhood.

1861 Founds a company of fine-art workmen.

1869-70 Writes *The Earthly Paradise*.

1877 Founds the Society for the Protection of Ancient Buildings.

1891 Sets up the Kelmscott Press.

1896 Dies at Kelmscott in Oxfordshire.

THE 19TH-CENTURY CRAFTSMAN and thinker William Morris first trained as an architect, but became a painter, furniture maker, wallpaper and fabric designer, writer, lecturer, printer, poet and political activist. Morris believed that everyday objects should be beautiful as well as useful, and that they should be made by craftspeople, not on a factory production line. He was also a socialist who believed that everybody had the right to art, education, and freedom in their lives. His interest in medieval art led him to join the Pre-Raphaelite Brotherhood, a group of young artists who wanted to return to the way people had painted before the Renaissance. Many people still find Morris's political ideas inspiring. A number of his designs for fabrics are still popular.

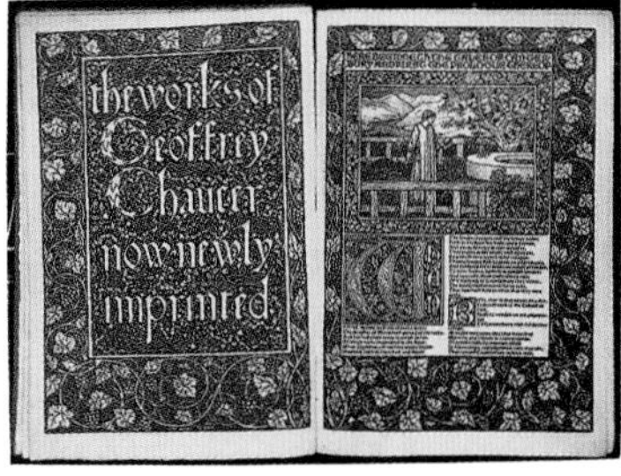

KELMSCOTT PRESS
Morris set up the Kelmscott Press in 1891, at Hammersmith, London to print his own books. He designed three styles of type for them.

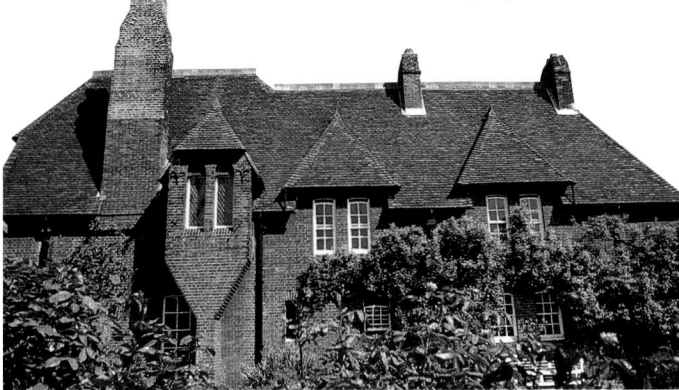

THE RED HOUSE
In 1859 architect Philip Webb (1831-1915) designed a house at Bexley Heath, Kent, for Morris and his new wife. It was built in red brick in an informal style, and furnished and decorated by Morris and his friends.

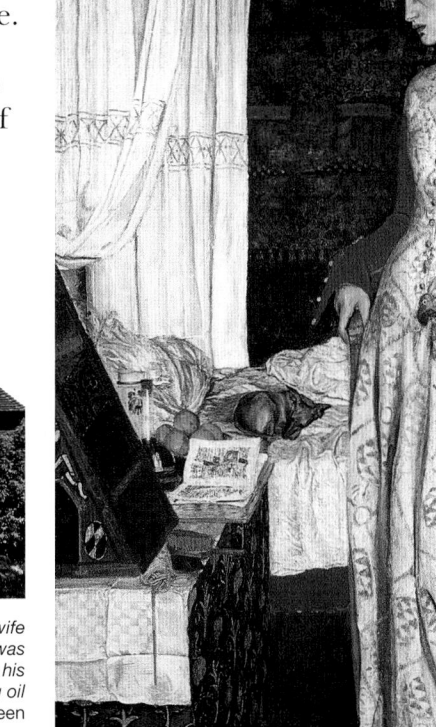

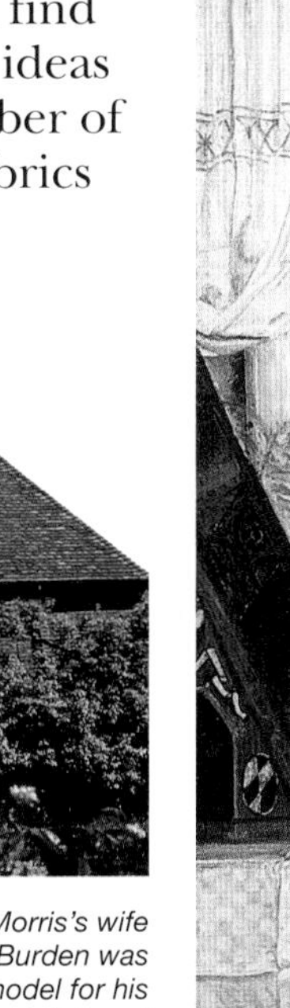

Morris's wife Jane Burden was the model for his only surviving oil painting, Queen Guenevere.

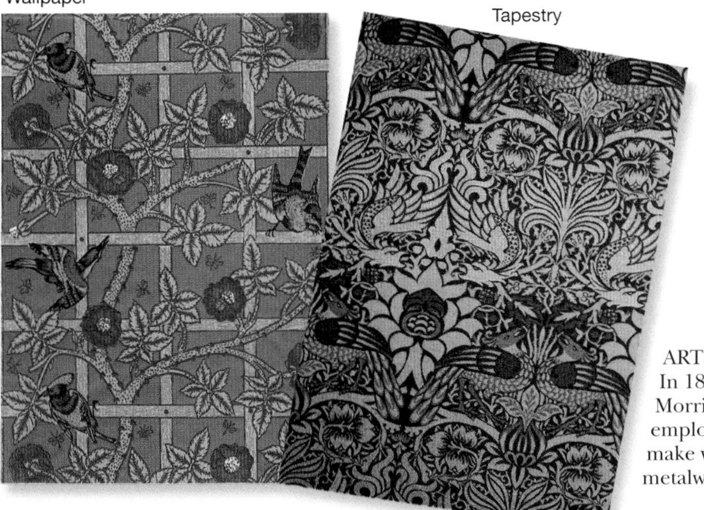

Wallpaper

Tapestry

CRAFTSMAN AND SOCIALIST

Morris believed that the industrial revolution was taking away the dignity of people's labour. He formed a national group, the Socialist League, and lectured widely on the need for change. His views on art and handicraft went together with his thoughts about the nature of a good and just society.

ARTS AND CRAFTS
In 1861 Morris founded a company, Morris, Marshall, Faulkner & Co., that employed artist-craftsmen to design and make wallpaper, furniture, stained glass, metalwork, tapestries, and carpets.

Find out more
DESIGN
PAINTERS, UK
RENAISSANCE

MOSSES, LIVERWORTS AND FERNS

HORSETAILS
Horsetails are fern-like plants with no flowers. About 300 million years ago, forests of giant horsetails grew up to 46 m (150 ft) high. Their remains have turned into coal.

MISTY TROPICAL RAIN FORESTS and moist, shady woodlands shelter some of the simplest land plants. These are mosses and liverworts, also seen on logs, stone walls, and garden lawns. They are quite different to other plants. They have no true root systems, flowers, or seeds. Instead, mosses and liverworts have tiny rootlets that absorb only a small amount of water from the soil, and short-stemmed leaves that take in moisture from the air. There are 11 different types of non-flowering plants.

Ferns are also flowerless. They are an ancient group of plants that have grown on Earth for more than 300 million years. Unlike mosses and liverworts, ferns do have true roots, with tubes inside their stems that carry water to the leaves. The giant tree ferns are the largest of all ferns. They grow up to 20 m (65 ft) high and look like palm trees. The smallest ferns in tropical rain forests are tiny, with leaflike fronds less than 1 cm (0.5 in) long. Ferns grow in most kinds of soil, but not in hot desert sand.

Carpet of moss covers wet bark on log.

HOW MOSS REPRODUCES
The leafy moss plant has male and female organs. The fertilized spores grow in the brown spore-containing capsules, which are held above the leaves on long stalks.

FERN

A new fern frond gradually unfurls. When it is mature, brown dots called sori appear on the frond. These sori contain spores. The spores grow into tiny heart-shaped plants, which bear male and female organs.

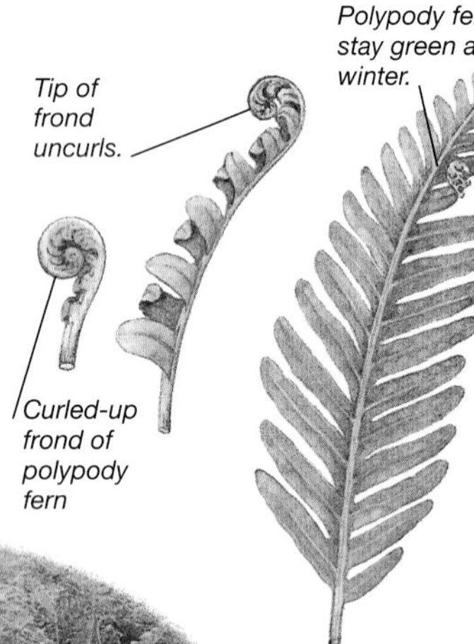
Tip of frond uncurls.
Curled-up frond of polypody fern
Polypody fern fronds stay green all winter.

Sori are on the underside of fern frond.

Fern

MOISTURE-LOVING PLANTS

Mosses and liverworts grow beside streams and rivers because they need the moisture from the water. They do not have roots to absorb water from the soil and pass it to their leaves. Instead, their leaves take in moisture from the air.

Liverwort

BRACKEN
Bracken is found on every continent except Antarctica. It has far-reaching roots and underground stems, and spreads quickly across grassland and woodland. Bracken is a nuisance to many farmers and gardeners because it is very difficult to remove once it has become established.

Bracken spreads into a pasture, reducing the grazing area.

LIVERWORT

The liverwort grows close to the ground, from which it soaks up moisture. Some liverworts, mosses, and ferns grow on trees and other plants, which they cling to for support.

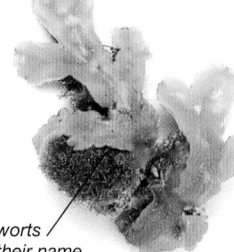

Liverworts take their name from their shape, which looks like the human liver.

BOG MOSS

Sphagnum moss is one of the few plants found in wet, marshy areas. It grows very well in swamps, forming wet, spongy hummocks. As the sphagnum dies, it rots slowly, and over many centuries turns into mossy peat below the surface.

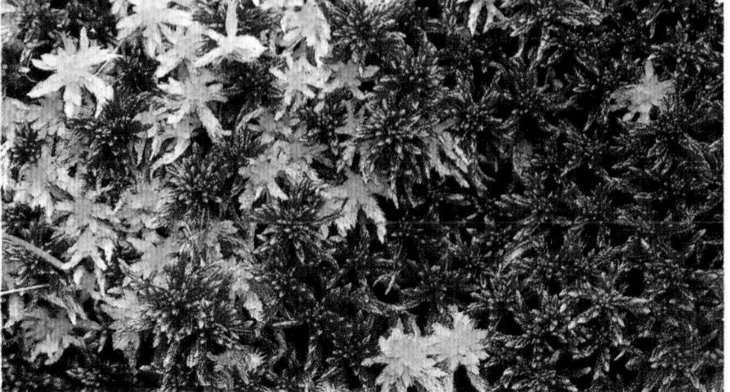

Find out more
FOREST WILDLIFE
MARSH and swamp wildlife
PLANTS
SOIL

Mountains

Continents collide and grind against one another, while hot, molten rock bubbles beneath the Earth's surface. These powerful forces thrust up mountains reaching as high as 8 km (5 miles). Many mountains are still growing, and those that formed long ago are slowly wearing away. Some mountains are volcanoes, made of layers of solidified lava which build up as the volcano erupts. There are mountains under the oceans and on other planets. The highest known mountain is on Mars; it is three times as high as Mount Everest.

The Earth has two vast mountain ranges. The Rocky Mountains and Andes run through North and South America; the mighty Himalayas, Alps, and Atlas Mountains stretch across Asia, Europe, and North Africa. These mountains are "young": they formed during the last 50 million years. Other ranges, such as the Urals in Russia, are much older and lower. The forces of erosion have worn them down since they were first formed more than 200 million years ago.

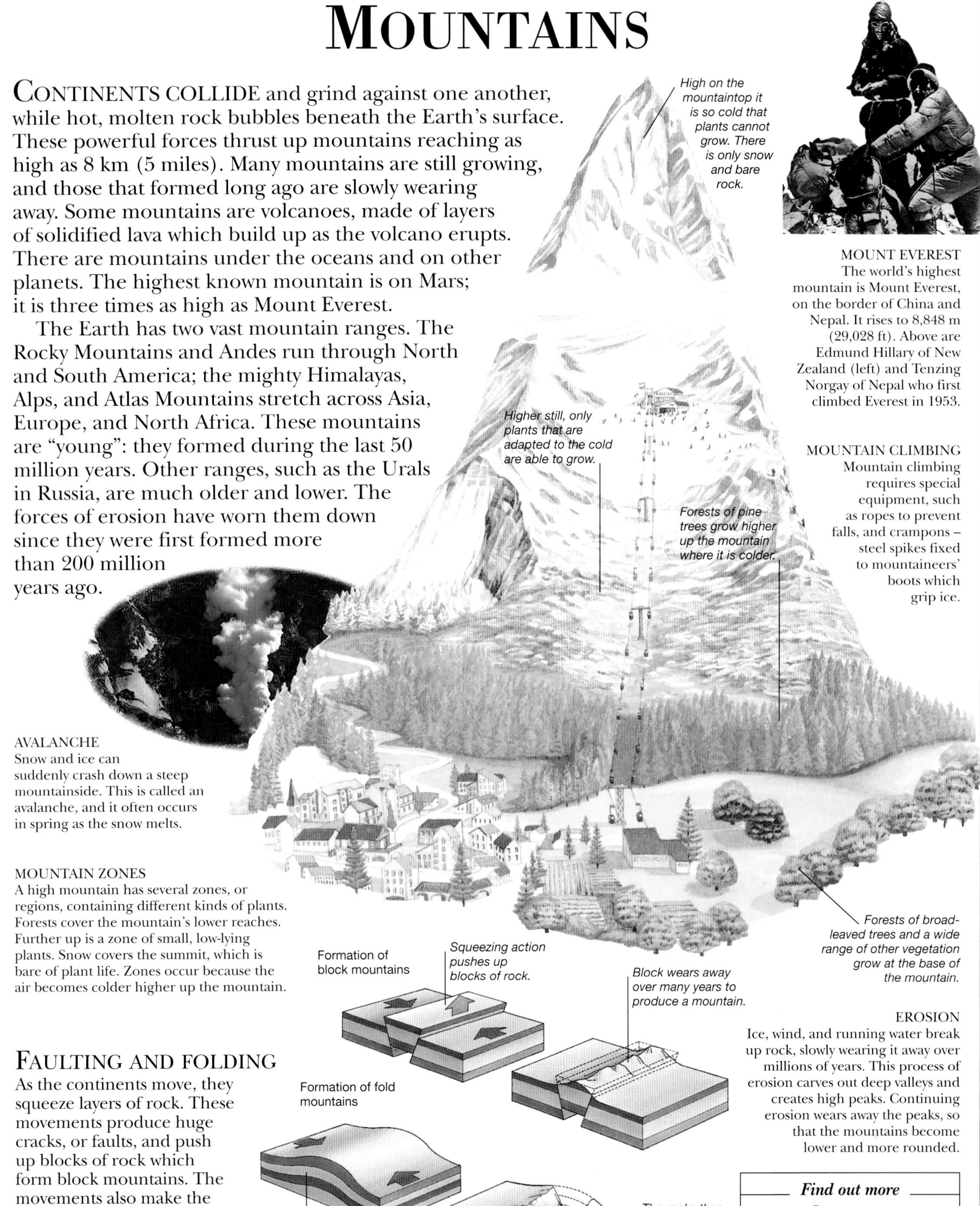

High on the mountaintop it is so cold that plants cannot grow. There is only snow and bare rock.
Higher still, only plants that are adapted to the cold are able to grow.
Forests of pine trees grow higher up the mountain where it is colder.
Forests of broad-leaved trees and a wide range of other vegetation grow at the base of the mountain.
Formation of block mountains
Squeezing action pushes up blocks of rock.
Block wears away over many years to produce a mountain.
Formation of fold mountains
As layers of rock are squeezed, they form zigzag folds.
The rocks then crack and wear away at the top of the curve, forming jagged mountains.

MOUNT EVEREST
The world's highest mountain is Mount Everest, on the border of China and Nepal. It rises to 8,848 m (29,028 ft). Above are Edmund Hillary of New Zealand (left) and Tenzing Norgay of Nepal who first climbed Everest in 1953.

MOUNTAIN CLIMBING
Mountain climbing requires special equipment, such as ropes to prevent falls, and crampons – steel spikes fixed to mountaineers' boots which grip ice.

AVALANCHE
Snow and ice can suddenly crash down a steep mountainside. This is called an avalanche, and it often occurs in spring as the snow melts.

MOUNTAIN ZONES
A high mountain has several zones, or regions, containing different kinds of plants. Forests cover the mountain's lower reaches. Further up is a zone of small, low-lying plants. Snow covers the summit, which is bare of plant life. Zones occur because the air becomes colder higher up the mountain.

EROSION
Ice, wind, and running water break up rock, slowly wearing it away over millions of years. This process of erosion carves out deep valleys and creates high peaks. Continuing erosion wears away the peaks, so that the mountains become lower and more rounded.

Faulting and folding

As the continents move, they squeeze layers of rock. These movements produce huge cracks, or faults, and push up blocks of rock which form block mountains. The movements also make the Earth's surface buckle, forming fold mountains. Dome mountains appear when molten granite pushes the rock above it into a huge hump.

Find out more

Continents
Glaciers and icecaps
Mountain wildlife
Oceans and seas
Volcanoes

MOUNTAIN WILDLIFE

LAMMERGEIER
The lammergeier is one of the biggest vultures. It has a wingspan of about 3 m (10 ft) and soars over the high mountain peaks of Africa, Asia, and Europe. This bird of prey feeds mostly on carrion (bodies of dead animals).

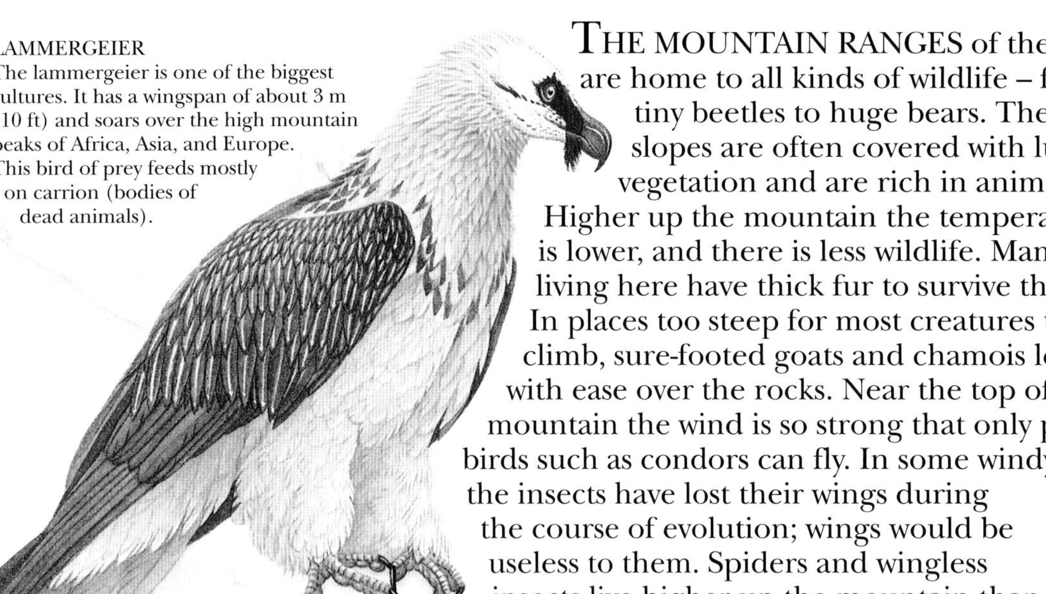

THE MOUNTAIN RANGES of the world are home to all kinds of wildlife – from tiny beetles to huge bears. The lower slopes are often covered with lush vegetation and are rich in animal life. Higher up the mountain the temperature is lower, and there is less wildlife. Mammals living here have thick fur to survive the cold. In places too steep for most creatures to climb, sure-footed goats and chamois leap with ease over the rocks. Near the top of the mountain the wind is so strong that only powerful birds such as condors can fly. In some windy areas the insects have lost their wings during the course of evolution; wings would be useless to them. Spiders and wingless insects live higher up the mountain than any other creature. As you climb higher the temperature drops by 3.6°C (6.5°F) for every 300 m (1,000 ft) of height. Above about 2,400 m (8,000 ft) small shrubs grow, bent and twisted by the icy winds. Higher up still, only mosses and lichens grow, and at the very top there is permanent snow and ice.

CONSERVATION
Wildlife parks protect mountain animals such as the bobcat shown here. In the past people hunted the bobcat for its fur; today this cat is an endangered species.

This map shows the main mountain ranges of the world.

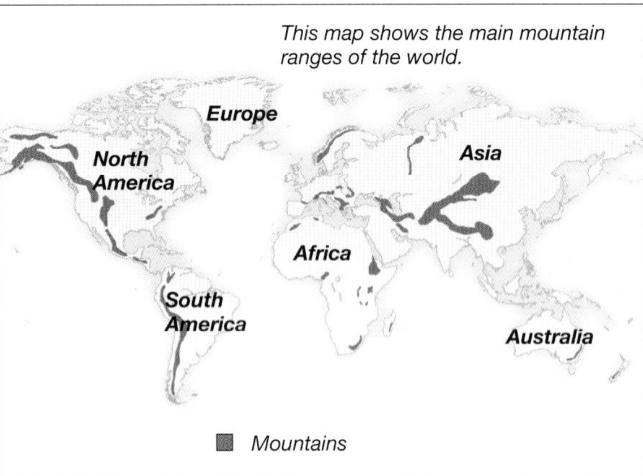

CHAMOIS

A rubbery hoof pad allows the chamois to grip stony surfaces with ease as it leaps nimbly among rocks in search of grasses, herbs, and flowers. Chamois live in groups of up to 30 females and young. The males live alone except in the breeding season.

The mountain goat is a North American relative of the European chamois. Its body is more thickset and sturdy, and it is three times the weight of a chamois. The mountain goat moves slowly and deliberately through deep snow.

MOUNTAIN PLANTS
High up where trees do not grow, alpine flowers bloom in the short summer. The word *alpine* means above the tree line. The leaves of most alpine flowers grow low and flat so they are protected from the bitter winds. These flowers are pollinated mainly by flies, butterflies, and other insects that have survived the winter as eggs or as adults under the snow.

The trumpet gentian is named for its deep trumpet of petals. It grows in stony places and in damp, short turf at heights of 3,000 m (10,000 ft), in the Alps, Pyrenees, and Apennines of Europe.

Today the edelweiss is a protected plant in many areas.

SPECTACLED BEAR
The only bear in South America is the spectacled bear, so-named because of the markings around its eyes. It lives in the Andes Mountains and is found in warm, moist forests and mountains at heights of 3,500 m (11,500 ft). Spectacled bears eat a wide range of foods, including leaves, fruits, insects, eggs, small deer, and other mammals.

The alpine longhorn beetle shown here suns itself on mountain flowers and feeds on their pollen.

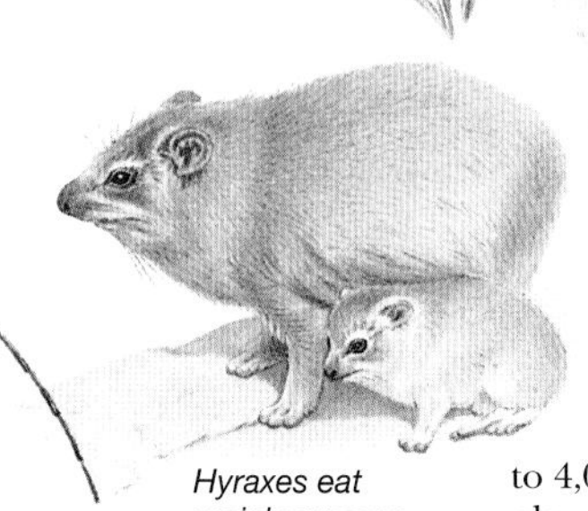

Hyraxes eat mainly grasses.

ROCK HYRAX
The small, furry, stoutly built hyrax of Africa is the closest living relative of the elephant – the largest animal on land. Rock hyraxes live at heights of up to 4,000 m (13,300 ft) in rocky places such as Mount Kenya.

Find out more
BEARS AND PANDAS
CONSERVATION and endangered species
EAGLES and other birds of prey
LIONS, TIGERS, and other big cats
MOUNTAINS

MUHAMMAD

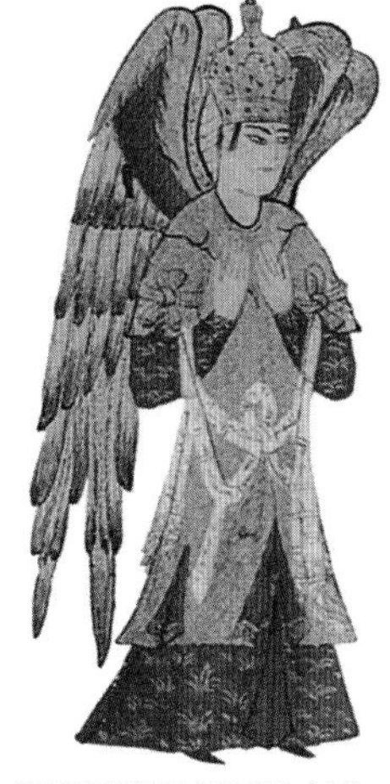

PROPHET OF ISLAM
The Angel Gabriel told Muhammad that he had been chosen by God to be a prophet, in the same way as Moses and Abraham before him.

DURING THE 600s, one man founded what was to become one of the world's great religions. His name was Muhammad, and the religion was Islam. Muhammad came from Mecca in southwestern Arabia (now Saudi Arabia), and was born into one of the city's Arab clans around A.D. 570. Orphaned at an early age, he became a merchant and married Khadija, a wealthy widow, with whom he had three daughters. At the time, the Arab people worshipped many gods and prayed to idols and spirits. Muhammad came to believe that there was only one God, named Allah, and that he had been chosen to be Allah's prophet. Muhammad's family and friends were the first to share his beliefs, but his views angered the people of Mecca and he was forced to flee to Medina, a city north of Mecca. There he proclaimed the principles of Islam and won many converts. After a series of holy wars, Muhammad and his followers conquered Mecca in 630. Missionaries spread the message of Islam far and wide, and by the time of Muhammad's death in 632, Arabia was an Islamic state.

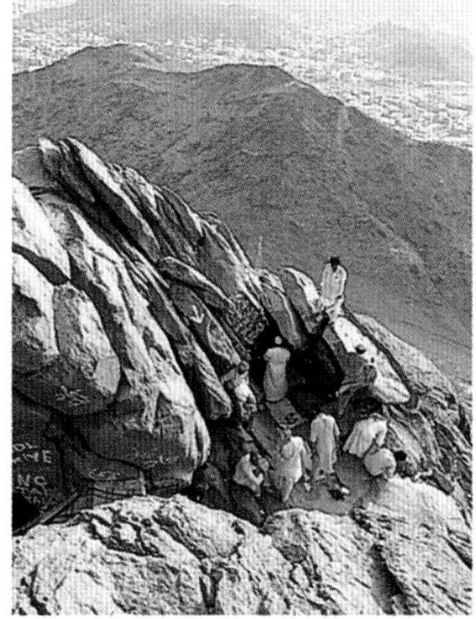

MOUNT HIRA
At age 40, Muhammad began to meditate in a cave on Mount Hira, north of Mecca. Here he had a vision in which the Angel Gabriel spoke the words of God to him and told him that he was to preach that people should believe in only one God – Allah. The teachings of Allah were revealed to Muhammad in a series of visions throughout his life.

HEGIRA

People came to Mecca to worship and trade at the Kaaba, a huge shrine that contained hundreds of idols. Muhammad was persecuted when he spoke out against the worship of idols. In 622, he fled with a few of his followers to Medina. Their journey is called the Hegira (meaning "flight" or "migration"). Today, the Kaaba is a holy shrine for Muslims (followers of Islam). It is surrounded by a great mosque (Muslim temple) and visited by thousands of pilgrims each year.

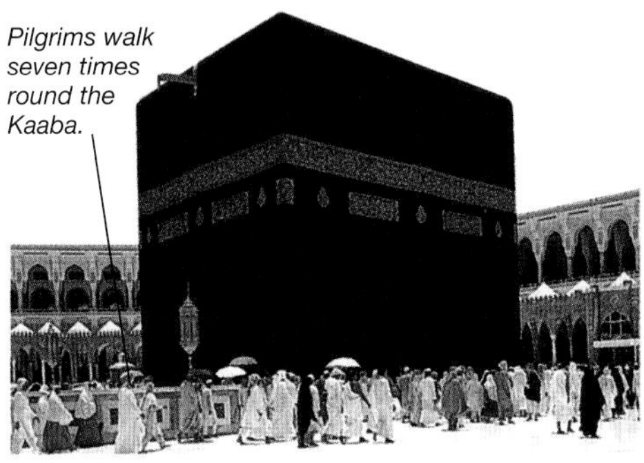

Pilgrims walk seven times round the Kaaba.

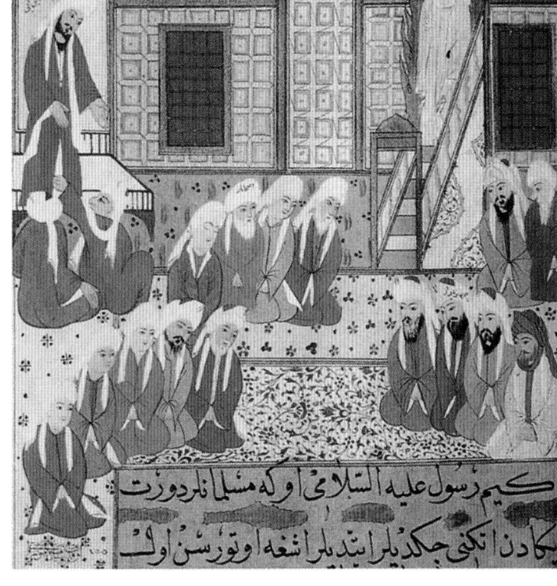

MUHAMMAD'S TEACHINGS
Muhammad did not claim to be divine. He believed that he was the last of the prophets and that he had received messages from God, which he had to pass onto others. He taught that there is only one God, that people should be obedient to God's will, and that all people were equal. He also preached against the selfishness of the rich, the unjust treatment of women, slaves, and poor people, and cruelty to animals. In 632, knowing that his life was coming to an end, he led a farewell pilgrimage to Mecca. There he delivered a famous sermon on the most important principles of Islam.

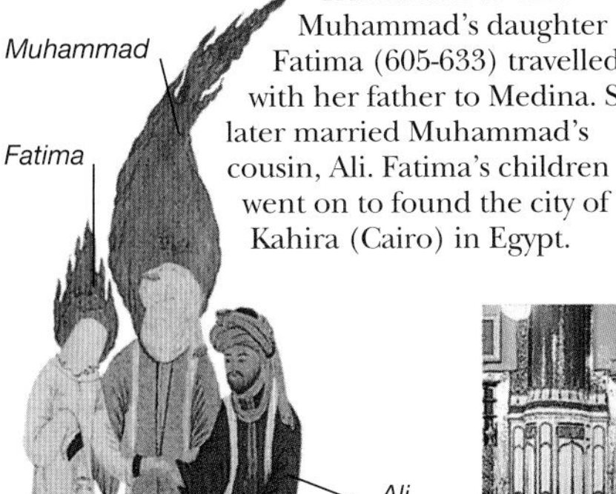

Muhammad
Fatima
Ali

FATIMA AND ALI
Muhammad's daughter Fatima (605-633) travelled with her father to Medina. She later married Muhammad's cousin, Ali. Fatima's children went on to found the city of Kahira (Cairo) in Egypt.

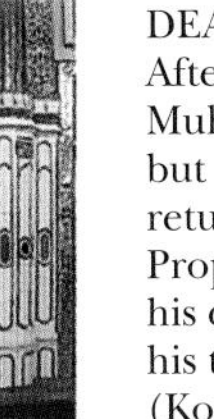

DEATH OF MUHAMMAD
After the farewell pilgrimage, Muhammad went back to Medina, but died within a few days of his return. His tomb lies in the Prophet's Mosque at Medina. After his death, his followers wrote down his teachings in the Qur'an (Koran), the holy book of Islam.

MUHAMMAD

c. A.D. 570 Born in Mecca.

595 Marries Khadija, a wealthy widow.

610 Has a vision of the Angel Gabriel telling him to proclaim a new faith, Islam.

613 Begins preaching to the people of Mecca.

622 Leaves Mecca and travels to Medina.

624 Meccan army defeated at Battle of Badr by much smaller Muslim force.

630 Conquers Mecca.

632 Dies in Medina.

Find out more
ISLAM
RELIGIONS

MUSCLES AND MOVEMENT

EVERY MOVEMENT YOU MAKE is powered by muscles. Muscles are controlled by nerve signals from the brain. There are three main types of muscle – skeletal, smooth, and cardiac. Skeletal muscle is also called striated muscle, and it covers the bones of the skeleton. It is attached to the bones by long cords called tendons. When the muscle contracts, or shortens, it moves the bone. Skeletal muscles are also called voluntary muscles because they can be controlled at will. Smooth muscle is found in the digestive system, bladder, and blood vessels. It is called involuntary muscle because it works automatically, even when you are asleep. Cardiac muscle is found only in the heart. All muscles need energy in order to work properly. Blood carries oxygen and glucose (sugar) to muscles to provide them with fuel. As a muscle works harder, it needs more fuel, so the heart pumps faster to supply it with more blood.

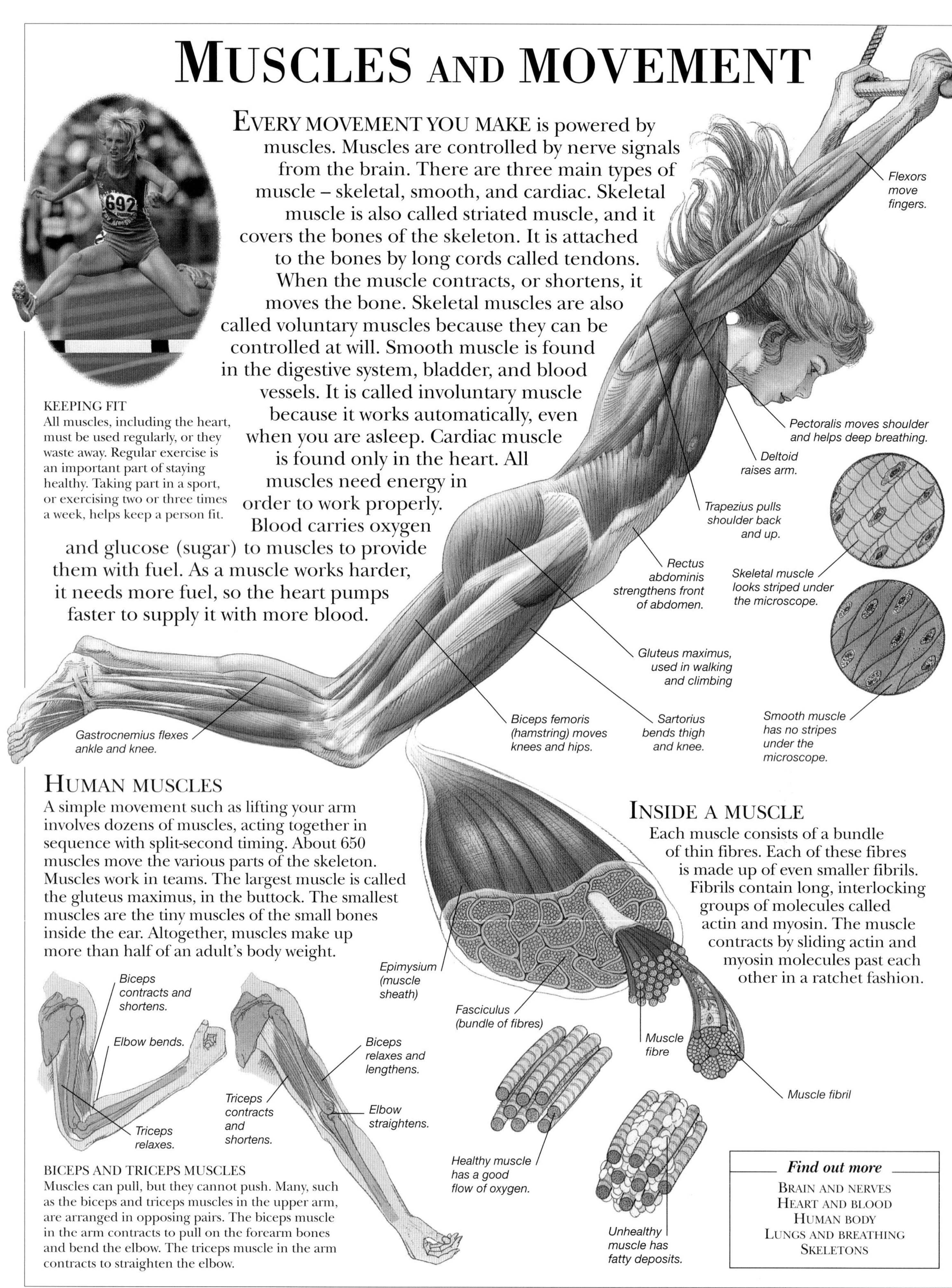

692
Flexors move fingers.
Pectoralis moves shoulder and helps deep breathing.
Deltoid raises arm.
Trapezius pulls shoulder back and up.
Rectus abdominis strengthens front of abdomen.
Skeletal muscle looks striped under the microscope.
Gluteus maximus, used in walking and climbing
Smooth muscle has no stripes under the microscope.
Biceps femoris (hamstring) moves knees and hips.
Sartorius bends thigh and knee.
Gastrocnemius flexes ankle and knee.
Epimysium (muscle sheath)
Fasciculus (bundle of fibres)
Muscle fibre
Muscle fibril
Healthy muscle has a good flow of oxygen.
Unhealthy muscle has fatty deposits.
Biceps contracts and shortens.
Elbow bends.
Triceps relaxes.
Biceps relaxes and lengthens.
Triceps contracts and shortens.
Elbow straightens.

KEEPING FIT
All muscles, including the heart, must be used regularly, or they waste away. Regular exercise is an important part of staying healthy. Taking part in a sport, or exercising two or three times a week, helps keep a person fit.

HUMAN MUSCLES

A simple movement such as lifting your arm involves dozens of muscles, acting together in sequence with split-second timing. About 650 muscles move the various parts of the skeleton. Muscles work in teams. The largest muscle is called the gluteus maximus, in the buttock. The smallest muscles are the tiny muscles of the small bones inside the ear. Altogether, muscles make up more than half of an adult's body weight.

BICEPS AND TRICEPS MUSCLES
Muscles can pull, but they cannot push. Many, such as the biceps and triceps muscles in the upper arm, are arranged in opposing pairs. The biceps muscle in the arm contracts to pull on the forearm bones and bend the elbow. The triceps muscle in the arm contracts to straighten the elbow.

INSIDE A MUSCLE

Each muscle consists of a bundle of thin fibres. Each of these fibres is made up of even smaller fibrils. Fibrils contain long, interlocking groups of molecules called actin and myosin. The muscle contracts by sliding actin and myosin molecules past each other in a ratchet fashion.

Find out more
BRAIN AND NERVES
HEART AND BLOOD
HUMAN BODY
LUNGS AND BREATHING
SKELETONS

MUSEUMS AND LIBRARIES

This is how the ISBN appears.

ISBN BOOK CODE
Every book has an ISBN (International Standard Book Number). This number, in the form of a barcode, carries all the information that a library needs to catalogue a book correctly.

BUILDINGS THAT ARE USED FOR COLLECTING and displaying works of art or interesting objects are known as museums. Some museums contain general collections; others are more specialist. Museum staff, called curators, acquire and care for exhibits. They also study and keep records of the collection, preserve and restore exhibits, and make sure they are displayed to the public in an informative way. Libraries are collections of books and documents. The librarian's job includes classifying the books by subject, and ensuring that books can be found easily on the shelves. The first museums and libraries date back to ancient times. Today, people can visit museums and libraries in most towns for information on a huge range of topics.

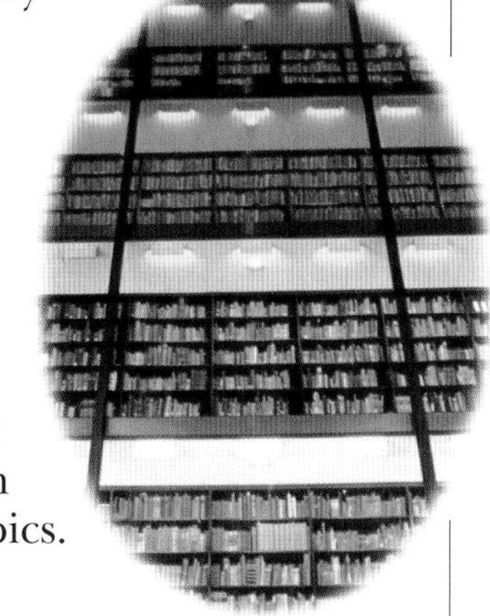

This working model of a grain pit is hand-driven, enabling visitors to interact with the process.

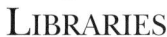

Children are allowed to touch and move the museum exhibit.

School party investigating an interactive exhibit at the Science Museum, London.

INTERACTIVE MUSEUM

The first publically funded museums were set up in the 19th century. Exhibits were displayed in glass cases, and could not be touched. Today, especially in science museums, interactive displays using working models and computer technology encourage a more "hands-on" approach. Audio-visual guides also make a museum visit exciting.

LIBRARIES

The first public library opened in Athens, Greece, in 330 B.C. Until the 18th century, most libraries were reference libraries, where people could read books, but not take them away. Today, lending libraries let people borrow books to read at home.

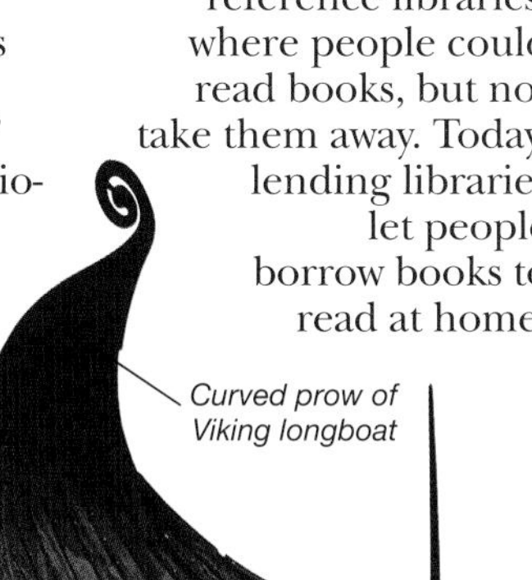

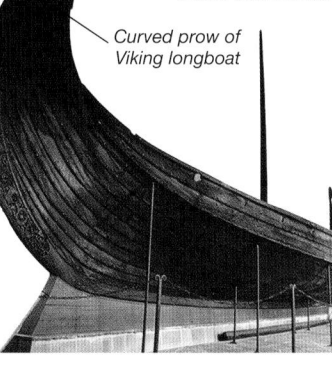

Curved prow of Viking longboat

SPECIALIST MUSEUMS
Many museums specialize in one particular area. These include science museums, natural history museums, and those that concentrate on one particular period of history, such as the time of the Vikings. Many smaller museums started life as private collections, specializing in the interests of the original collector.

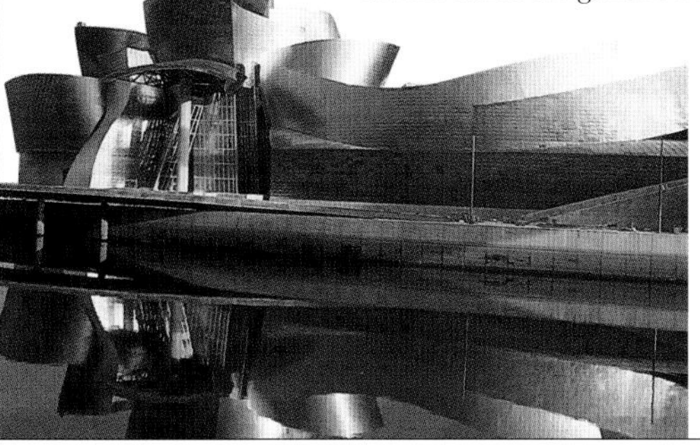

The Guggenheim Museum building is a work of art in itself.

ART GALLERIES
Museums that specialize in works of art are called art galleries. Major art galleries usually contain a range of different artworks, but some concentrate on one artist, or the art of a particular period. The new Guggenheim Museum in Bilbao, northern Spain, displays 20th-century American and European art.

LOCAL COLLECTIONS
The major national collections and specialist museums are usually found in the capital or big cities of the world, from the National Museum in Phnom Penh, Cambodia, through to the Natural History Museum, in England. However, small towns and villages often contain a museum that houses a purely local collection.

Find out more
BOOKS
EDUCATION
PAINTERS
REFERENCE BOOKS

MUSHROOMS
TOADSTOOLS, AND OTHER FUNGI

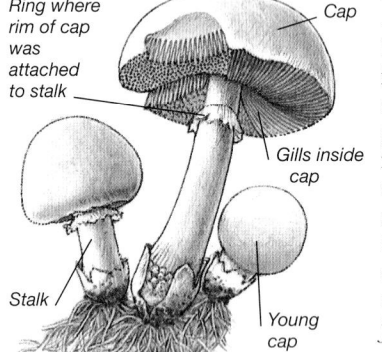

Champignon mushrooms grow in a ring in meadows and in gardens. Many people used to believe these were magic fairy rings.

BRIGHTLY COLOURED TOADSTOOLS, delicate mushrooms, and the furry green mould on a rotting piece of bread all belong to a unique group of organisms called fungi. Fungi are neither plants nor animals. They are the great decomposers of the natural world. Fungi feed by releasing chemicals called enzymes which rot away whatever they are feeding on. The dissolved nutrients and minerals are absorbed and recycled by the fungi. Many kinds of fungi grow in damp woodlands and lush, grassy meadows, especially during autumn. There is no scientific difference between mushrooms and toadstools, but toadstools are often more colourful, and some are extremely poisonous. The part of a mushroom that we eat is called the cap. It contains spores – minute cells which grow into new mushrooms when they are released from the cap. Some harmful fungi cause diseases on plants and ringworm in humans. Yeast is a fungus used to make bread dough rise. Another fungus is used to make the antibiotic drug penicillin.

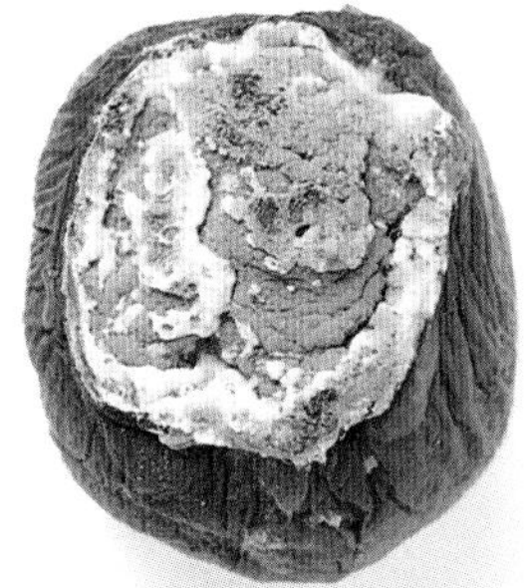

MOULD
The decaying parts of plants and animals are rotted away by pinmould, which grows on damp bread, and is the blue mould growing on this peach.

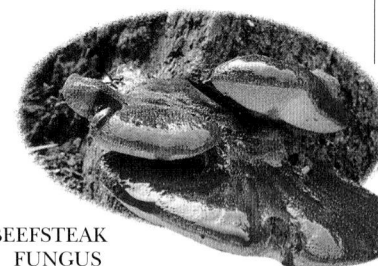

BEEFSTEAK FUNGUS
This fungus grows on trees. It is called the beefsteak bracket because it looks like a piece of undercooked steak.

Ring where rim of cap was attached to stalk

Cap

Gills inside cap

Stalk

Young cap

Spores are released from between the gills of mature caps.

EDIBLE FUNGI

Many mushrooms and other fungi are edible; some are not only delicious but also are a good source of minerals and fibre. Cultivated mushrooms are farmed in dark, damp sheds on beds of peat. Collecting wild fungi to eat can be very dangerous. Some deadly poisonous fungi look just like edible mushrooms.

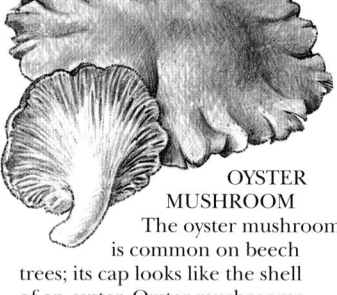

OYSTER MUSHROOM
The oyster mushroom is common on beech trees; its cap looks like the shell of an oyster. Oyster mushrooms are tasty and keep well when they are dried.

FIELD MUSHROOM
During the autumn, field mushrooms spring up overnight in damp pastures and meadows.

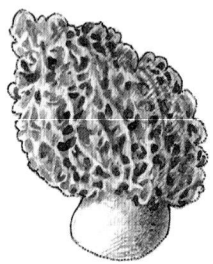

MOREL
Prized for its flavour, the morel's cap is crisscrossed with patterned ridgework.

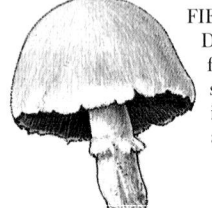

CHANTERELLE
The funnel-shaped cap of the chanterelle mushroom is yellow and smells like an apricot. It is found in oak, beech, and birch woods. It grows slowly, preserves well, and is much prized by chefs.

GIANT PUFFBALL
When the giant puffball ripens, its top breaks open, and clouds of tiny spores puff out with the slightest breeze or the smallest splattering of rain.

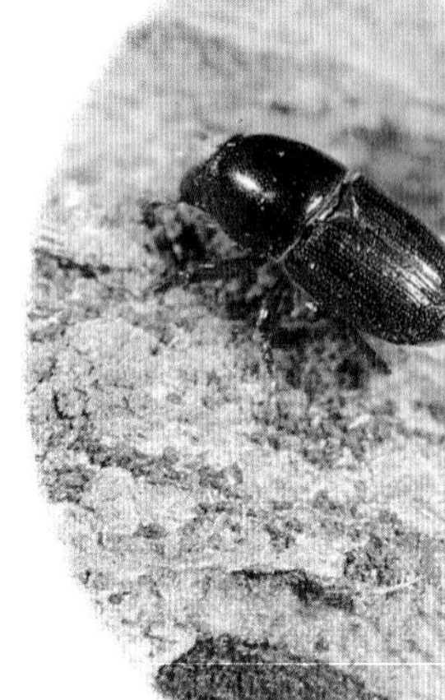

DUTCH ELM DISEASE
Dead and dying elm trees are a familiar sight in Europe and North America. A deadly fungus carried on the bodies of elm bark beetles, which live on elm trees, has killed millions of trees. The fungus grows through the bark, blocking the water-carrying tubes inside the trunk.

POISONOUS FUNGI

People die every year from eating poisonous fungi. Some of these are brightly coloured toadstools which are easily recognized. Others, such as the destroying angel, look harmless, but cause death rapidly if they are eaten.

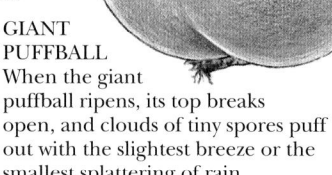

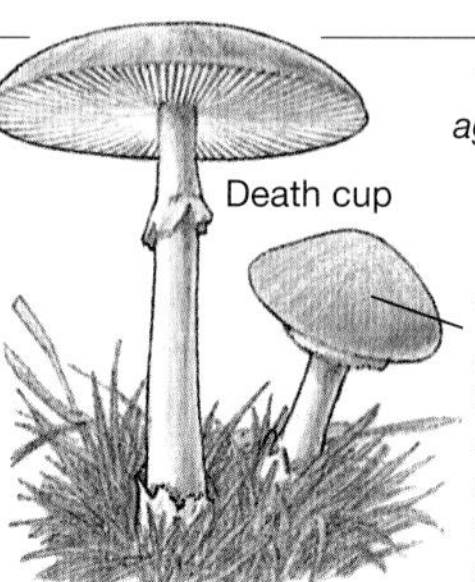

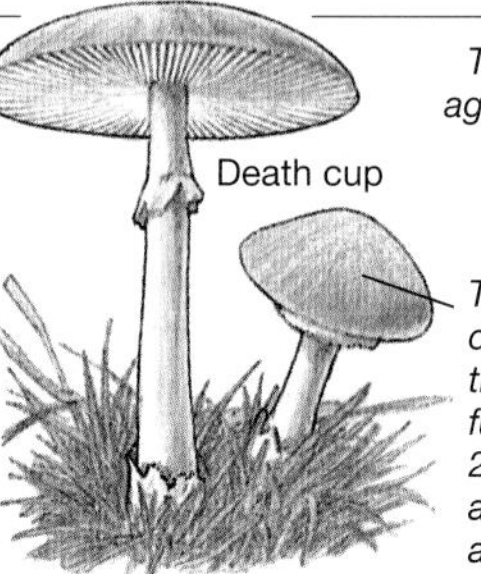

Death cup

The harmless-looking death cup is one of the most poisonous fungi. Less than 28 g (1 oz) can kill a person in only a few hours.

The bright red fly agaric toadstool is poisonous. Small amounts can cause unconsciousness.

Fly agaric

Find out more

DRUGS
FOOD
FOREST WILDLIFE
PLANTS
SOIL

MUSIC

MUSICIANS MAKE MUSIC by carefully organizing sounds into a regular, pleasing pattern that anyone can appreciate. Notes are the starting point for all music. A note is a regular vibration of the air which musicians create with musical instruments or with their voices. The more rapid the vibration, the higher the pitch of the note – the higher it sounds to a listener. Certain notes sound better together than others. Most music uses these notes, organized into a scale. A scale is a series of notes that increase gradually and regularly in pitch. Musicians usually play or sing notes at fixed time intervals. We call this regular pattern of notes the rhythm or meter of the music. A melody or tune is a combination of the rhythm, the notes the musician plays, and their order. The melody is the overall pattern that we hear and remember – and whistle or hum days or perhaps weeks later.

Ancient musicians of Ur in Sumer (now Iraq) played lutes, flutes, pipes, and percussion instruments.

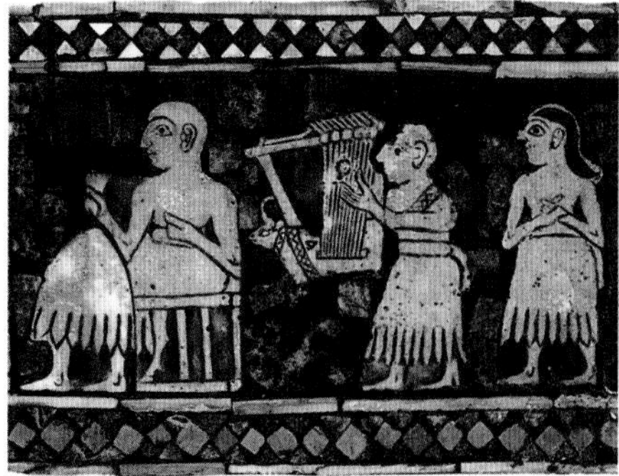

THE FIRST MUSIC

The chanting of prehistoric people was probably the earliest music. The oldest surviving musical instruments are mammoth bones from northern Eurasia; musicians may have banged them together or blown them to make notes about 35,000 years ago.

The clef shows the pitch at which to play the music. This is the treble clef.

The key signature shows which key the music is in. A key is a series of related notes.

Allegro

The speed of the music is often written in Italian. Allegro means "quickly".

A curved tie line joining two identical notes means they must be played as one unbroken note.

The shape of each note tells the musician how long to play it. This is a quarter note.

The time signature shows the musician the meter in which to play the piece. This is four-four or common time.

Rests show where the musician should pause.

When eighth notes are next to each other their hooks are usually joined together.

All music is divided into equal measures, each of which has the same number of beats, as indicated by the time signature. The bar marks the end of the measure.

mf

Dynamic markings indicate how loudly to play the music – mf *stands for mezzo forte, or moderately loud.*

A crescendo shows that the music gets gradually louder.

The position of the notes on or between the five horizontal staff lines indicates their pitch. Musicians use letters of the alphabet as names for each of the eight notes in an octave.

c d e f g a b c

NOTATION

Composers need a way of writing down the music they create. Musical notation is a code of symbols and signs that records every aspect of the music. Monks were the first to use musical notation in the 9th century, to help them remember the tunes of holy songs. The system in use today had developed fully by about A.D. 1200.

JAZZ

The essential ingredient of jazz is improvisation – the musicians make up some or all of the music as they play it. Black musicians created the very first jazz music at the beginning of the 20th century in New Orleans, U.S.A. Jazz is a mixture of blues, religious gospel, and European music.

Charlie "Bird" Parker (1920-55) popularized a new form of jazz, called "bebop", in the 1940s.

CHAMBER MUSIC

Classical – rather than pop – music for small groups of instruments is called chamber music. Chamber music was so called because it began as music for enjoyment in chambers, or rooms, in the home. Composers wrote different types of music for theatres or churches. Today, performances of chamber music often take place in concert halls.

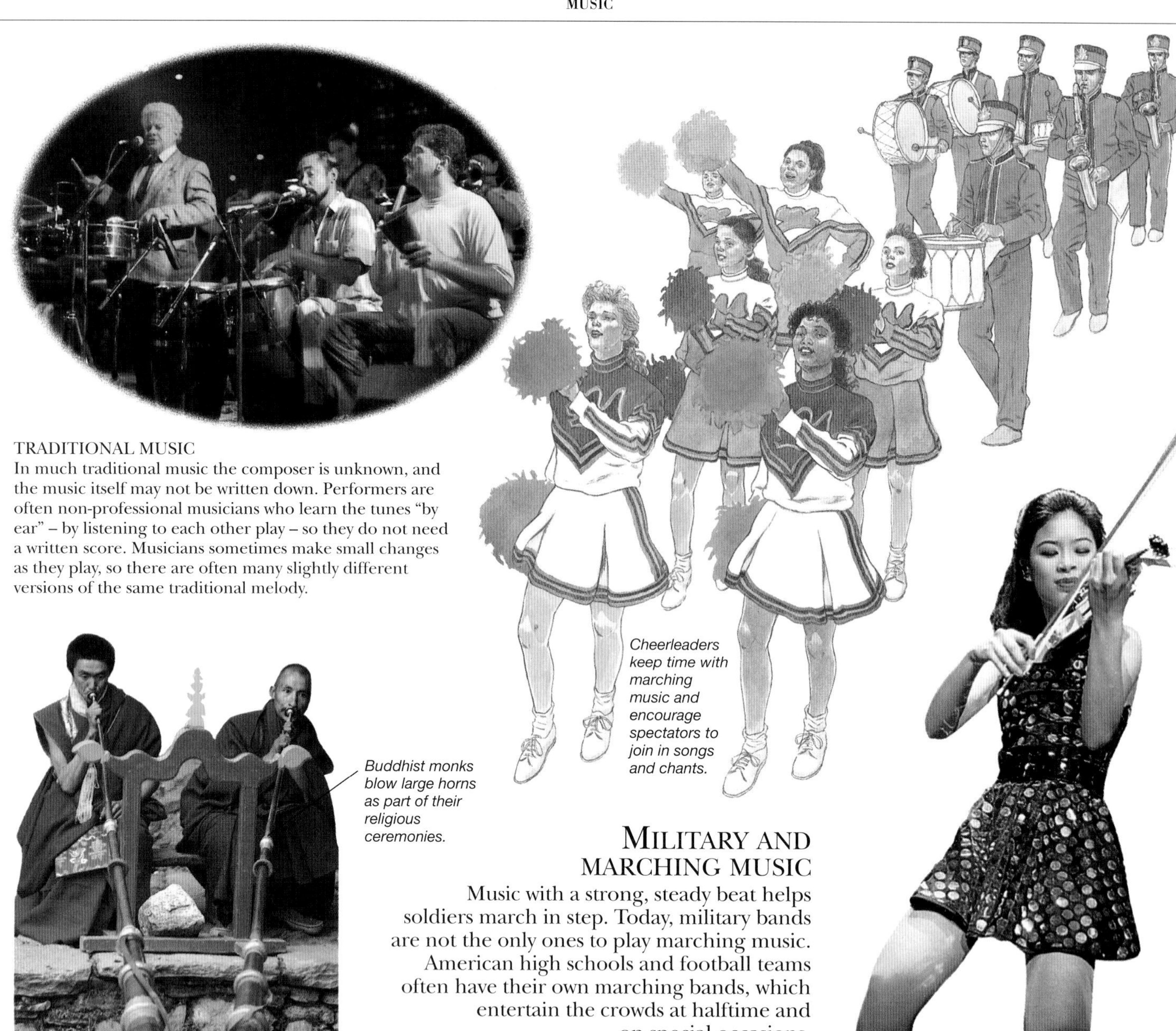

TRADITIONAL MUSIC
In much traditional music the composer is unknown, and the music itself may not be written down. Performers are often non-professional musicians who learn the tunes "by ear" – by listening to each other play – so they do not need a written score. Musicians sometimes make small changes as they play, so there are often many slightly different versions of the same traditional melody.

Cheerleaders keep time with marching music and encourage spectators to join in songs and chants.

Buddhist monks blow large horns as part of their religious ceremonies.

RELIGIOUS MUSIC
Music has always played an important part in religion. In religious ceremonies, music inspires people to think about their God or gods. It accompanies religious songs and sacred dances. Composers also choose religious themes for music that is not part of worship: *Messiah* by the German composer George Frideric Handel (1685-1759) sets part of the Bible to music.

MILITARY AND MARCHING MUSIC

Music with a strong, steady beat helps soldiers march in step. Today, military bands are not the only ones to play marching music. American high schools and football teams often have their own marching bands, which entertain the crowds at halftime and on special occasions.

ROCK MUSIC

During the 1950s a new form of popular music was heard for the first time. Rock and roll songs had a powerful beat and words that young people could relate to. This form of music began in the United States, where it grew from traditional rhythm and blues played by black musicians. Over the years it has influenced many other musical forms.

American-born singer Elvis Presley (1935-77) sold millions of rock and roll records and starred in 33 movies.

CLASSICAL MUSIC
Classical music has become increasingly popular in recent years, partly thanks to the efforts of young musicians such as violinist Vanessa Mae. Mae started writing her own music at age nine, and by age 18 had made several records and performed in classical concerts all over the world. She has also mixed classical with modern by combining the sounds of acoustic and electric violins.

Find out more
COMPOSERS
MUSICAL INSTRUMENTS
OPERA AND SINGING
ORCHESTRAS
ROCK AND POP

MUSICAL INSTRUMENTS

THE POUNDING BEAT of an electric guitar might seem far removed from the delicate trill of a classical violin, yet these two instruments make their different sounds in a similar way. Both use a stretched string to create the vibrations we hear as music. The guitar and the violin evolved in a similar manner, but they actually belong to different families of musical instruments. String instruments such as the violin make their notes when the musician plucks the strings or draws a stretched bow – a bundle of horsehair – across them. Electric instruments, such as the electric guitar, produce weak vibrations that must be amplified for the audience to hear the music. There are five other groups: woodwind, percussion, brass, keyboard, and electronic. This short list includes a huge variety: some instruments, such as the hollow wooden flute, are very simple; others, such as the synthesizer, are highly complex.

STRING INSTRUMENTS

Vibrating strings stretched across these instruments make the musical note: the finer the string and the shorter its length, the higher the note. The size of the instrument also affects its sound. The small violin, for example, produces higher sounds than the large double bass. Musicians pluck the strings of guitars, harps, and lutes, and usually use a bow to play the violin, viola, cello, and double bass.

WOODWIND INSTRUMENTS

Blowing into a woodwind instrument makes the air inside vibrate; this produces the musical notes. Covering the holes in the tube with fingers or keys changes the length of the vibrating air, producing different notes. The instruments with the shortest tubes, such as the piccolo, make the highest notes. Other woodwind instruments are the bassoon, English horn, saxophone, clarinet, oboe, and flute.

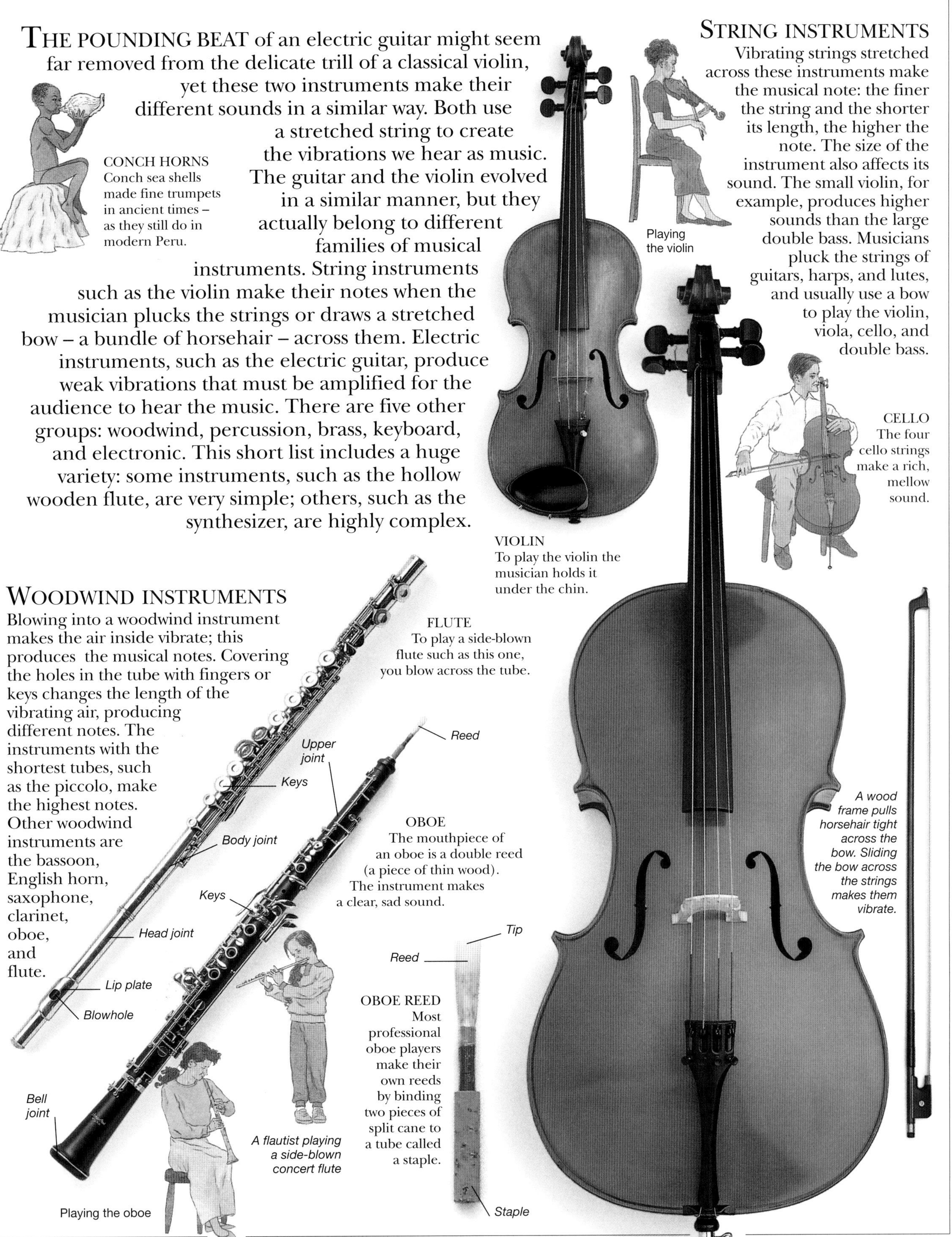

CONCH HORNS Conch sea shells made fine trumpets in ancient times – as they still do in modern Peru.

Playing the violin

CELLO The four cello strings make a rich, mellow sound.

VIOLIN To play the violin the musician holds it under the chin.

FLUTE To play a side-blown flute such as this one, you blow across the tube.

OBOE The mouthpiece of an oboe is a double reed (a piece of thin wood). The instrument makes a clear, sad sound.

OBOE REED Most professional oboe players make their own reeds by binding two pieces of split cane to a tube called a staple.

A wood frame pulls horsehair tight across the bow. Sliding the bow across the strings makes them vibrate.

A flautist playing a side-blown concert flute

Playing the oboe

Brass

Some of the most exciting sounds in music come from brass instruments. This group includes the French horn, trumpet, bugle, cornet, trombone, and tuba. The instruments are long tubes of brass or other metal curved around for easier handling. Sounds produced by the musician's lips on the mouthpiece vibrate down the tube. Pressing the valves opens more of the tube, making the pitch of the note lower. The trumpet has a long history. When the Egyptians buried King Tutankhamun more than 3,000 years ago, they placed a trumpet in his tomb.

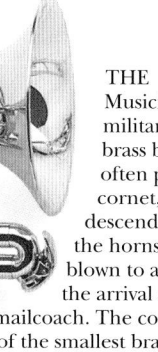

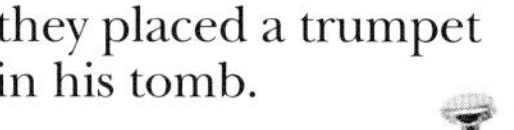

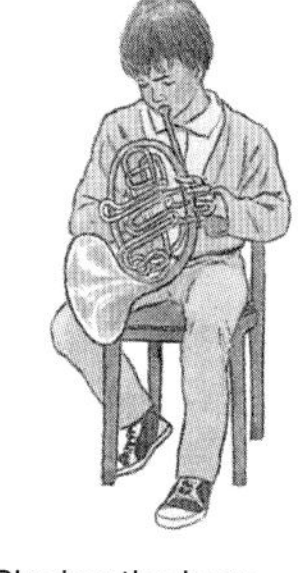

Playing the horn

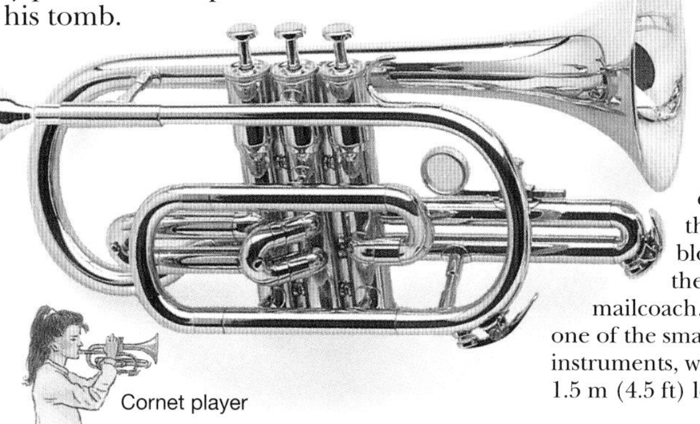

THE CORNET Musicians in military and brass bands often play the cornet, which is descended from the horns that were blown to announce the arrival of a mailcoach. The cornet is one of the smallest brass instruments, with a tube about 1.5 m (4.5 ft) long.

Cornet player

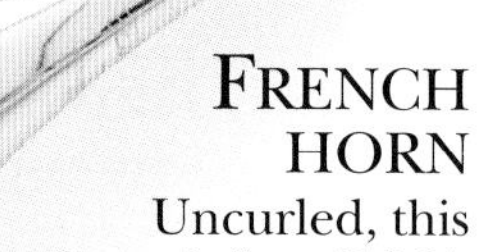

French horn

Uncurled, this horn is 5 m (16 ft) long. It developed from an 18th-century hunting horn and makes a rich, warm sound. The Austrian composer Wolfgang Amadeus Mozart created four pieces of music for the French horn.

Percussion

Bells, gongs, and drums are percussion instruments and there are many more, because all over the world people find different objects, such as beads and seeds, that make a noise when beaten or shaken. Some percussion instruments, such as the xylophone and timpani, are tuned to play definite notes.

SNARE DRUM The wire spring on the bottom skin of the snare drum vibrates when the player strikes the top skin.

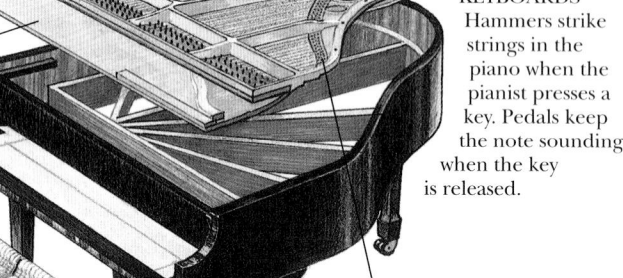

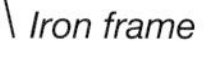

KEYBOARDS Hammers strike strings in the piano when the pianist presses a key. Pedals keep the note sounding when the key is released.

TRADITIONAL INSTRUMENTS

Musicians in symphony orchestras play only a few of the world's vast range of musical instruments. Many more are used in the traditional or folk music of individual countries. Some of these instruments developed unique shapes in different parts of the world, as musicians explored the music-making potential of local materials. However, some are remarkably similar: the bagpipes are played in Europe, Asia, and Africa.

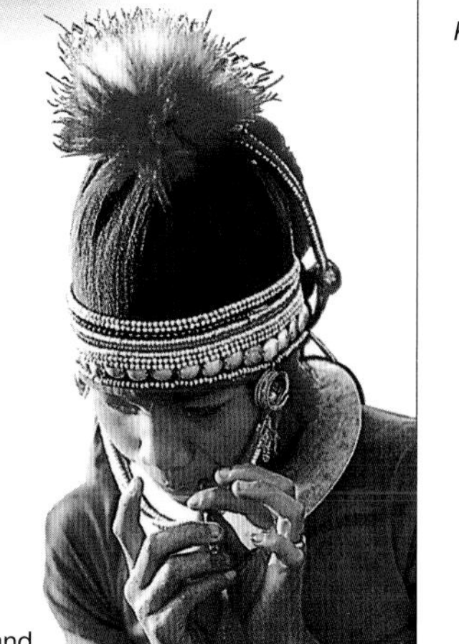

A flute player from Thailand

Electronic instruments

These instruments can produce an exciting array of sounds, by either simulating existing instruments or synthesizing completely new sounds. The musician can feed sounds into the memory of the instrument and then play them back together to simulate a whole orchestra.

Find out more

Composers
Music
Orchestras
Rock and pop

MYTHS AND LEGENDS

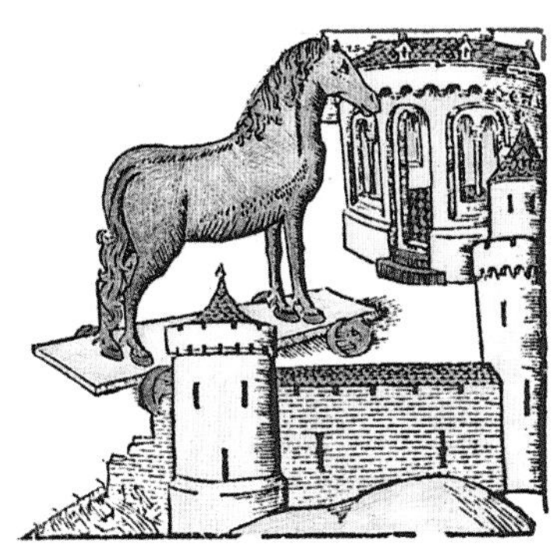

THE TROJAN HORSE LEGEND
Greek soldiers conquered the besieged city of Troy by hiding in a huge wooden horse. When the Trojans took the horse inside the city walls, the Greeks emerged and conquered Troy.

BEFORE THERE WERE ANY BOOKS, storytelling was an important way of passing on knowledge and beliefs from one generation to the next. Often, the stories took the form of myths which explained mysteries of nature, such as the origins of thunder. Ancient peoples told stories about gods and goddesses, and about human heroes with special powers. These myths became part of art and literature. Legends, though, were often based on real people and real-life events. To make a better tale, parents exaggerated the details as they repeated the legends to their children. Every country has its own legends. Paul Bunyan, the hero of stories told by North American lumberjacks, supposedly carved out the Grand Canyon by dragging his pick behind him. Sometimes, legendary monsters were created, such as the werewolf which appears in stories from many cultures.

SUN GODS

The same myths can be found in widely different cultures thousands of kilometres apart. This is because natural things such as the rain, the sea, and the moon are common to everyone. Many peoples worshipped sun gods: Surya in India and Apollo in Ancient Greece were both believed to ride across the sky in chariots of flame.

The Indian sun god, Surya – as painted on a doorway in Jaipur, India

The Egyptian sun god, Ra

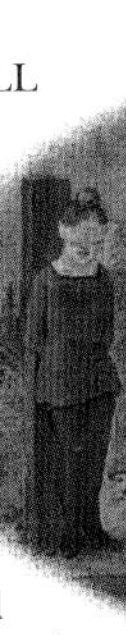

WILLIAM TELL
A famous Swiss legend describes how William Tell insulted his country's hated Austrian rulers. His punishment was to shoot an apple balanced on his son's head. He succeeded, and later led a revolt against Austrian rule.

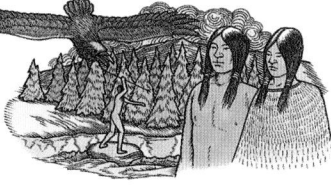

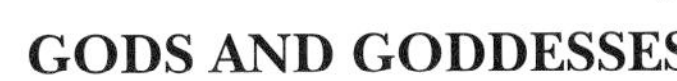

CREATION MYTHS

Most peoples used myths to explain how the world may have begun. This Native American myth was told by members of the Kwakiutl tribe.

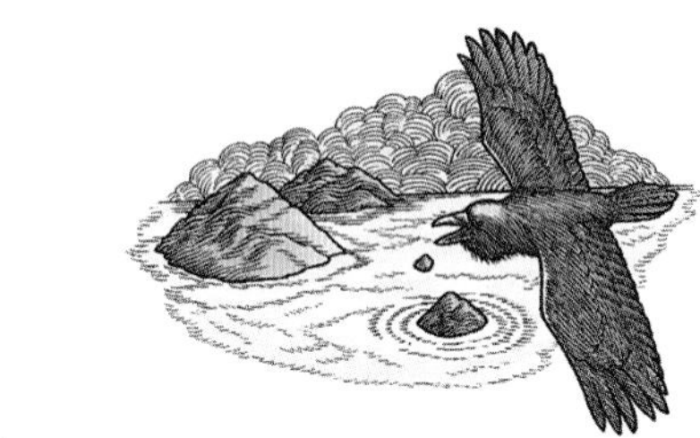

A raven, flying over water, could find nowhere to land. He decided to create the world by dropping small pebbles to make islands.

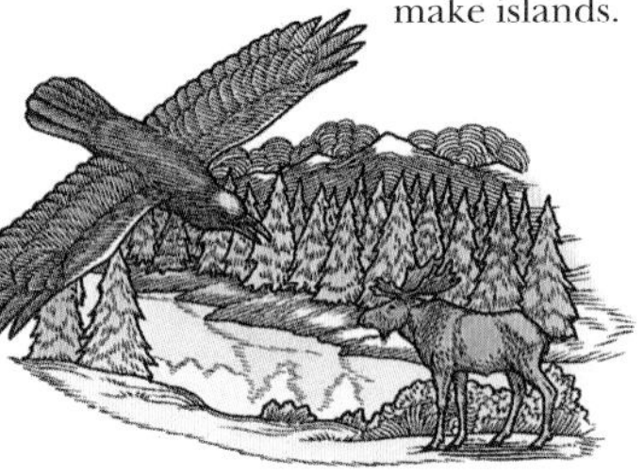

Then he created trees and grass. Beasts lived in the forest, birds flew in the air above, and the sea was filled with fish.

After many failed attempts, the raven succeeded in making the first man and woman out of clay and wood. At last, his world was complete.

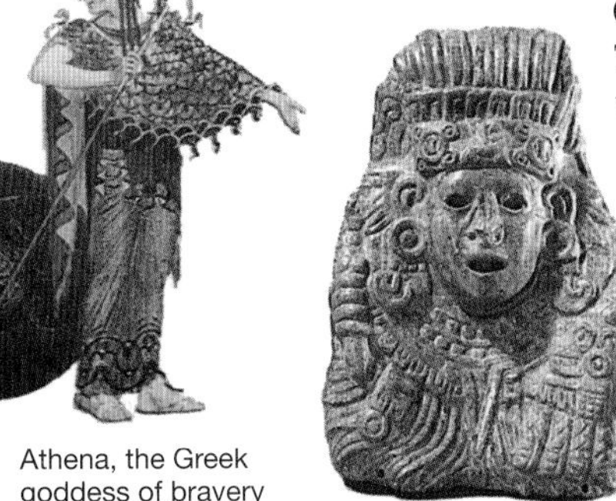

GODS AND GODDESSES

The ancient Greeks worshipped many gods and goddesses. The goddess Athena took part in battles and loved bravery. Athens, the capital of Greece, is named after her. Quetzalcoatl appears in Mexican mythology as one of the greatest Aztec gods. As god of air, Quetzalcoatl created the winds that blew away the rain.

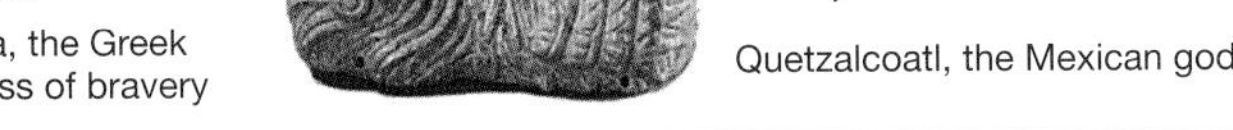

Athena, the Greek goddess of bravery

Quetzalcoatl, the Mexican god of air

Find out more
GREECE, ANCIENT
LITERATURE
RELIGIONS

NAPOLEON BONAPARTE

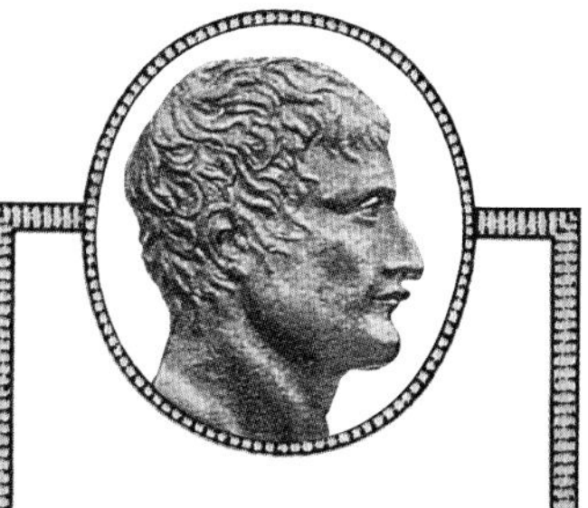

15 August 1769 Born on the island of Corsica.

1779-84 Military school

1799 Becomes ruler of France.

1804 Crowned Emperor.

1812 Defeated in Russia.

1814 Exiled to island of Elba in the Mediterranean.

1815 Returns to France; defeated at Waterloo.

5 May 1821 Dies in exile on the island of St. Helena.

IN A LAVISH CEREMONY IN 1804, Napoleon Bonaparte crowned himself Emperor of the French. He was an unlikely figure to lead his country, and spoke French with a thick Corsican accent. Yet he was one of the most brilliant military leaders in history. Napoleon first caught the public eye in 1793, when he commanded an attack against the British fleet occupying the French port of Toulon. In 1795 he crushed a revolt in Paris and soon led the French armies to victory in Italy. By 1799, Napoleon was strong enough to take power with the help of the army. He made himself First Consul and restored the power of the French government after the chaos left by the French Revolution. He introduced many social reforms, laying the foundations of the French legal, educational, and financial systems. Napoleon was a military genius who went on to control Europe from the English Channel to the Russian border. But he suffered a humiliating defeat in Russia, and when the British and Prussians beat him at the Battle of Waterloo in 1815, Napoleon was sent out of France into exile on a British island in the South Atlantic. He died six years later.

NAPOLEONIC EMPIRE

At the height of his power in 1812, Napoleon ruled Europe from the Baltic to the south of Rome, and his relations ruled Spain, Italy, and parts of Germany. The rest of Germany, Switzerland, and Poland were also under French control, and Denmark, Austria, and Prussia were allies. Only Portugal, Britain, Sweden, and Russia were independent.

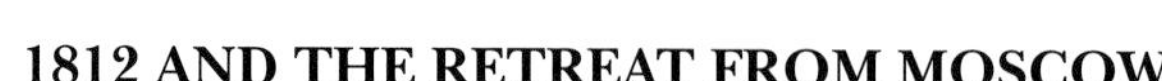

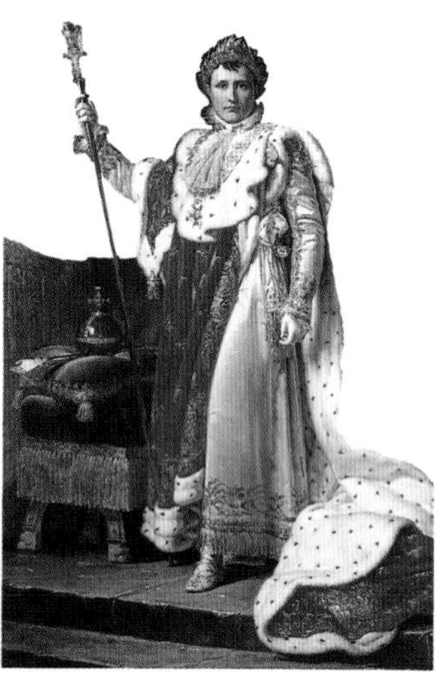

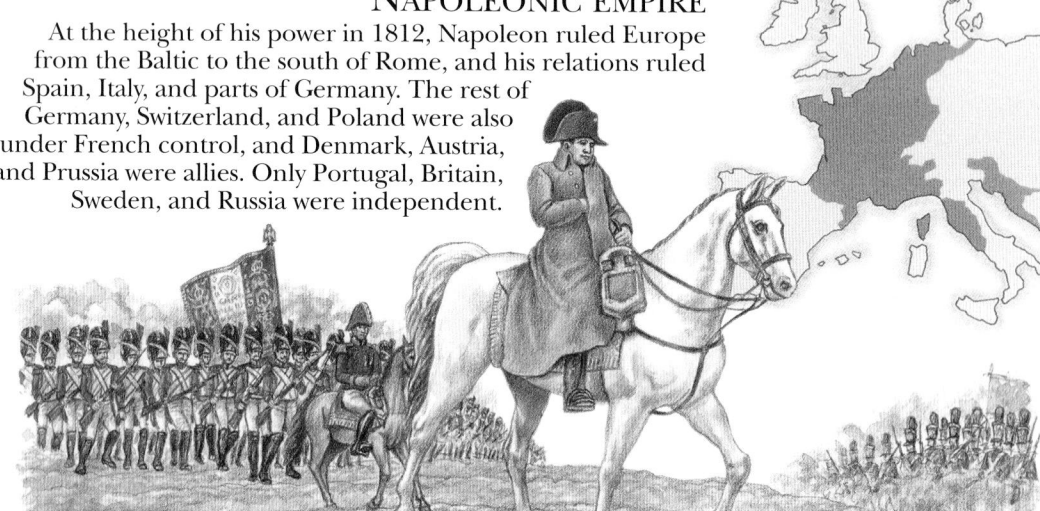

EMPEROR
On 2 December 1804, Napoleon crowned himself Emperor of the French in a ceremony at Notre Dame Cathedral in Paris. He had already changed his Italian-sounding name, Buonaparte, to the French name of Bonaparte. Now he was to be known as Napoleon I.

1812 AND THE RETREAT FROM MOSCOW

Napoleon invaded Russia in June 1812 with a force of more than 500,000 men. The Russians retreated, drawing the French army deeper into the country. Napoleon captured the capital, Moscow, but was forced to retreat because he could not supply his army. The harsh Russian winter killed many troops as they returned to France.

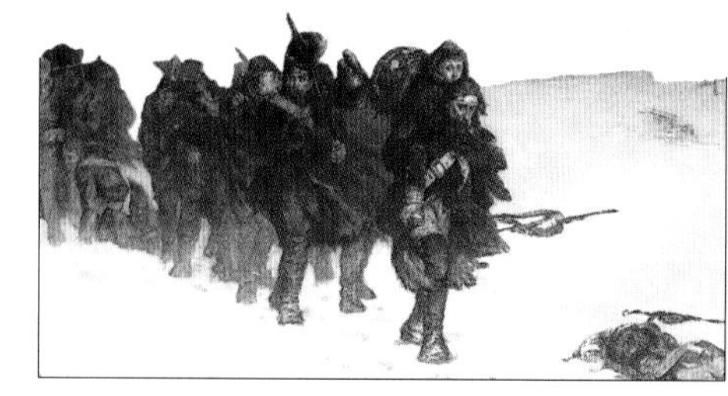

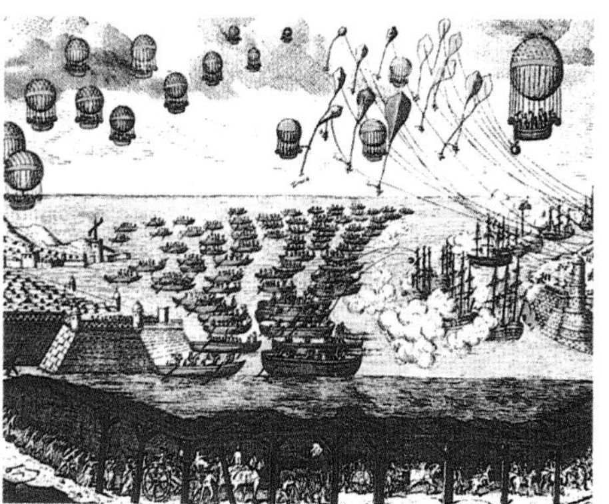

INVASION OF ENGLAND
In 1805 Napoleon assembled an army of 140,000 soldiers by the English Channel and drew up plans to invade England which he called "a nation of shopkeepers". These plans included crossing the Channel by ship and balloon, and digging a tunnel under the sea. The invasion was cancelled when the British admiral Nelson defeated the French fleet at the Battle of Trafalgar.

Find out more

FRANCE, HISTORY OF
FRENCH REVOLUTION
NAPOLEONIC WARS

Napoleonic Wars

Two centuries ago a series of bloody wars engulfed Europe, causing hardship to millions of people and disrupting trade. Sparked off by the French Revolution, the Napoleonic Wars began in 1792 and continued for nearly a quarter of a century. On one side was revolutionary France, and on the other the old kingdoms of Britain, Austria, Russia, and Prussia. At first the countries encircling France fought the new republic because they wanted to put down the Revolution. But after Napoleon became ruler in 1799, the French conquered most of Europe, until only Britain remained free. The French army was the most powerful in Europe, but paying the troops required high taxes. Too few people volunteered to join the army, so the government had to force people to fight. These measures were unpopular in the countries that France occupied, and led to revolts in Spain and elsewhere.

SPANISH CAMPAIGN
Napoleon invaded Spain in 1808 and put his brother on the Spanish throne. The Spanish fought back with what they called a guerrilla or "little war". Many were executed or died in the fighting.

NAPOLEONIC WARS

1792 France declares war on Austria.

1793 France declares war on Britain, Holland, and Spain.

1799 Napoleon takes power.

1803 Britain declares war on France.

1805 Napoleon defeats Russians and Austrians.

1806 Defeats Prussians.

1807 Defeats Russians at Friedland.

1808 France occupies Spain and Portugal.

1812 Napoleon's invasion of Russia ends in disaster.

1813 Austrians, Prussians, and Russians defeat Napoleon at Leipzig.

1814 Napoleon exiled to island of Elba, off Italy.

1815 Napoleon escapes, marches on Paris. Final defeat at Waterloo.

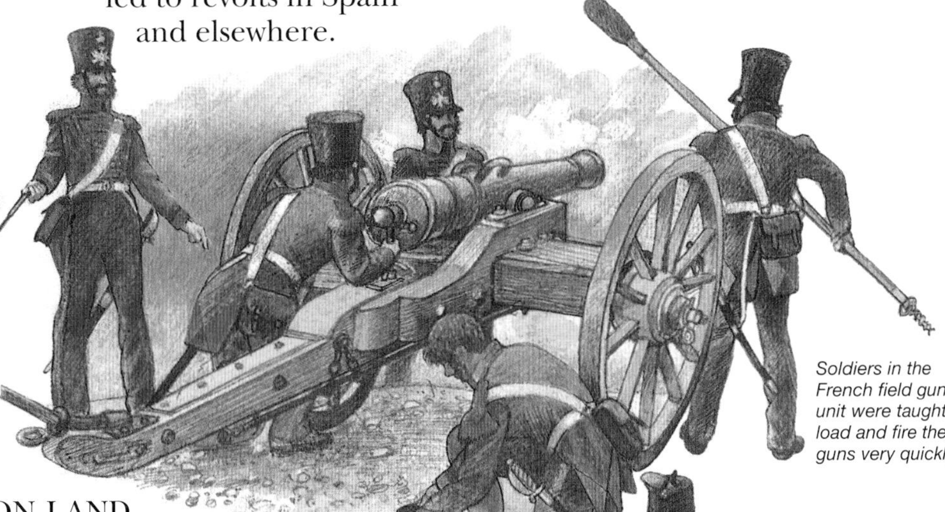

Soldiers in the French field gun unit were taught to load and fire their guns very quickly.

War on land

Napoleon organized his army brilliantly. His genius lay in making the right decisions at the right time and in using his forces in the most effective way. With superior tactics he often beat far larger forces.

Battle of Trafalgar

Horatio Nelson was an admiral in the British navy. At the battle of Trafalgar in 1805, Nelson destroyed the French fleet by attacking in a fan formation, rather than by sailing side by side, as the French had expected. He died in the battle.

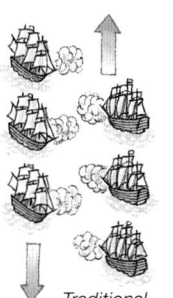

Traditional sea battle

How Nelson attacked the French fleet

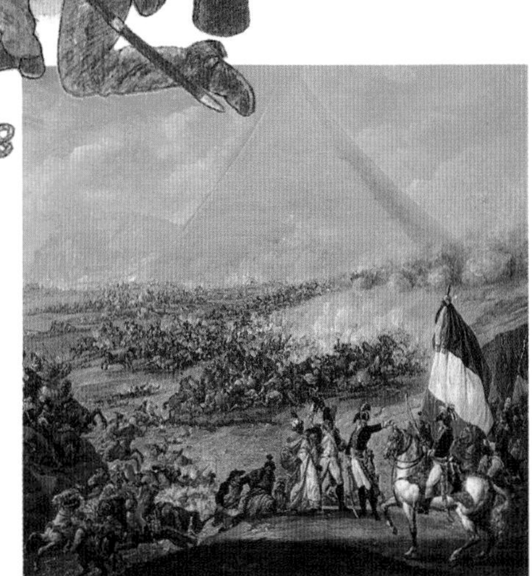

BATTLE OF THE PYRAMIDS
In July 1798, Napoleon conquered Egypt, which was then part of the Ottoman Empire. At the Battle of the Pyramids he defeated the Mamelukes who ruled the country.

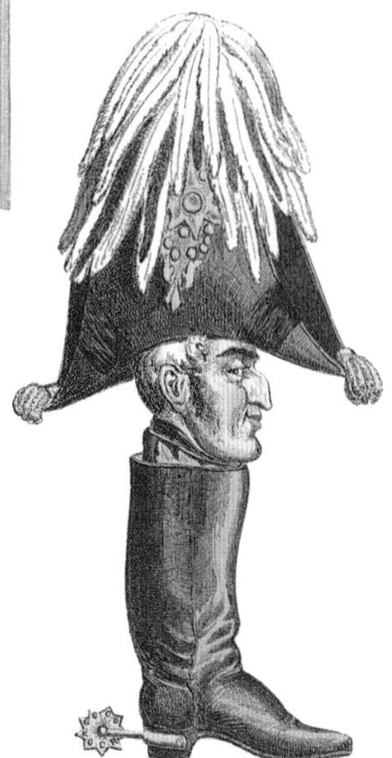

DUKE OF WELLINGTON
"A Wellington Boot, or the Head of the Army." Cartoons made fun of everyone who took part in the wars, including the Duke of Wellington, the British army commander who defeated Napoleon at Waterloo.

Find out more

France, history of
Napoleon Bonaparte
Spain, history of

NATIONAL PARKS

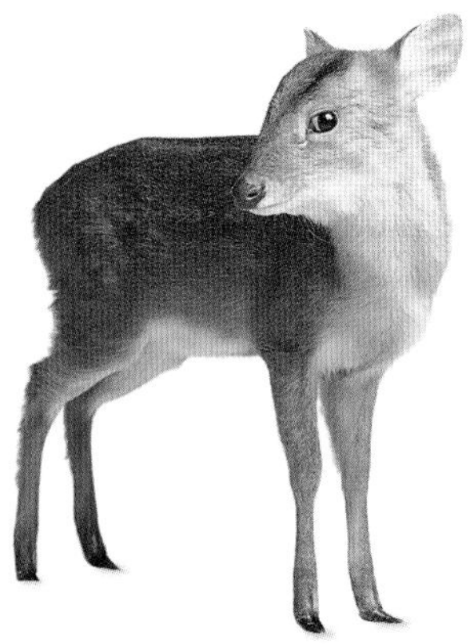

WILDLIFE
Animals, birds, and flowers, sometimes rare varieties, flourish in the national parks because the parks and their wildlife are strictly protected.

THE NATIONAL PARKS contain some of the most stunning landscapes in England, Scotland, and Wales. National parks are protected zones, specially set up by an Act of Parliament of 1949, to conserve and protect areas of natural beauty. Much of the land in national parks is privately owned, but the act says that the public must be able to visit and enjoy them. Each park has a staff of wardens, who work with farmers and residents to preserve the area. Northern Ireland does not have national parks, but it has scenic conservation areas. There are eight national parks in England, three in Wales, and two in Scotland.

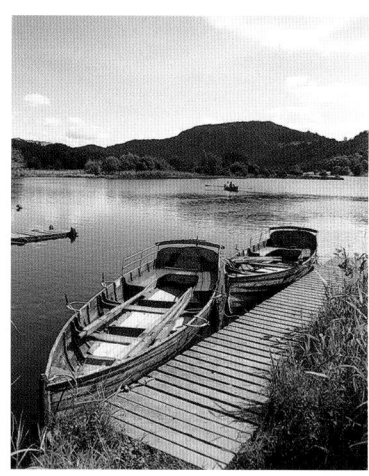

LEISURE IN THE PARKS
The national parks are like a massive playground for the people of Britain. Walkers and climbers, birdwatchers and sightseers make around 100 million visits to the national parks each year. Most come for just a day, and picnic sites are popular. Park rangers and volunteers maintain the national parks, and provide information for the millions of visitors.

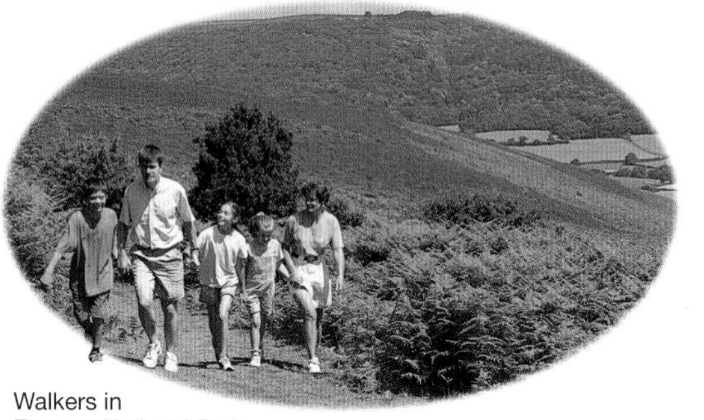

Walkers in Exmoor National Park

OUTSTANDING NATURAL BEAUTY

Some of the most beautiful countryside in Britain is inside the national parks. The wilderness of Dartmoor, the peaks of Snowdonia, and the slopes of the Lake District are all within national parks. To protect the appearance of the parks, strict rules control what can be built within their boundaries. Development is limited, and must not spoil views or be out of place.

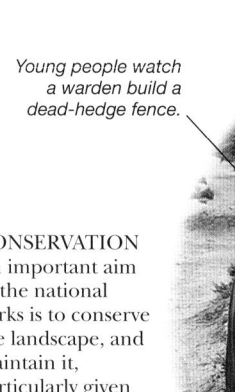

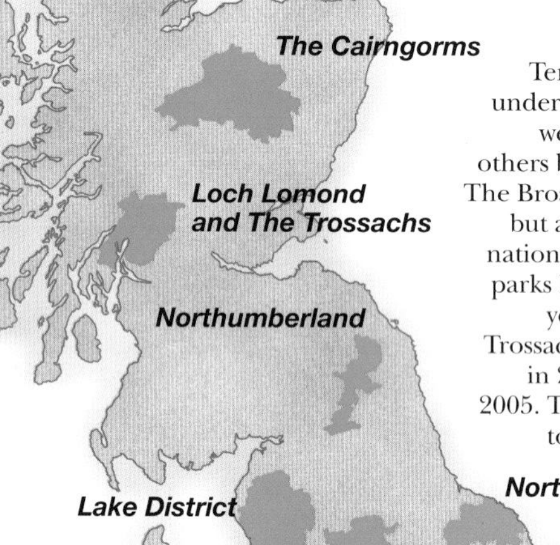

LOCATION OF PARKS
Ten national parks were set up under the 1949 Act. The first four were created in 1951, and the others before the end of the 1950s. The Broads were not included then, but are today considered to be a national park. Three new national parks have been created in recent years: Loch Lomond and the Trossachs in 2002, the Cairngorms in 2003, and the New Forest in 2005. The South Downs is planned to become a national park in the future.

Young people watch a warden build a dead-hedge fence.

CONSERVATION
An important aim of the national parks is to conserve the landscape, and maintain it, particularly given the numbers of visitors. Staff use environmentally friendly materials and, sometimes, traditional craft-based techniques to carry out repairs, such as mending fencing and building dry-stone walls.

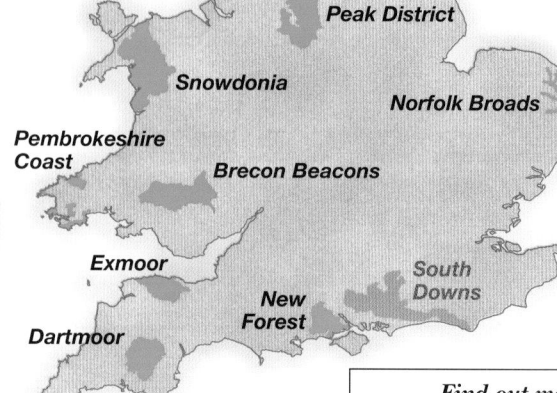

Find out more
ENGLAND
TOURISM AND TRAVEL
WALES

NATIVE AMERICANS

THE FIRST PEOPLE to live in North America arrived from Asia more than 20,000 years ago. They wandered over the Bering Strait, which was a land bridge at the time and now separates Asia and North America, following animals they were hunting. Gradually these early people settled into different tribes. Over the centuries the tribes developed organized societies. During the 1500s, Europeans arrived in North America for the first time. They thought they were in the "Indies", or Asia, so they called the native Americans "Indians", a misleading name. The Europeans wanted land and threatened the existence of native North Americans. The natives fought many wars with the new settlers. During the 1800s, the tribes resisted when the United States government tried to make them leave their homelands. After a bitter struggle the native Americans were moved onto reservations – areas of land set aside for them – where many still live today.

Smoke flap open for ventilation

Straight poles are bound together at the top to form a cone shape.

Bison hide was used to make the tepee cover.

Lodge pins made from bone held the hides together.

Paintings that told a story decorated the hides.

Door flap

WOMEN
Women played an important part in the life of a tribe. They provided the food, made the clothes, and raised the children. The women of the Hopi Indians of the Southwest also owned the houses and organized the village.

TEPEES

The Sioux and other tribes on the Great Plains lived in tepees. Tepees were made of bison hides stretched over a wooden frame and were easy to put up. Flaps at the top of the tepee could be opened to allow smoke from the fire to escape.

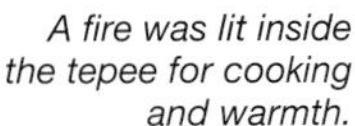

A fire was lit inside the tepee for cooking and warmth.

GERONIMO
One of the most successful native chiefs in leading resistance to the "white man" was Geronimo (1829-1909), of the Chiricahua Apache Indians. Geronimo led raids across the southwestern states and into Mexico. In 1886, he was captured and exiled to Florida. Later he was released and became a national celebrity.

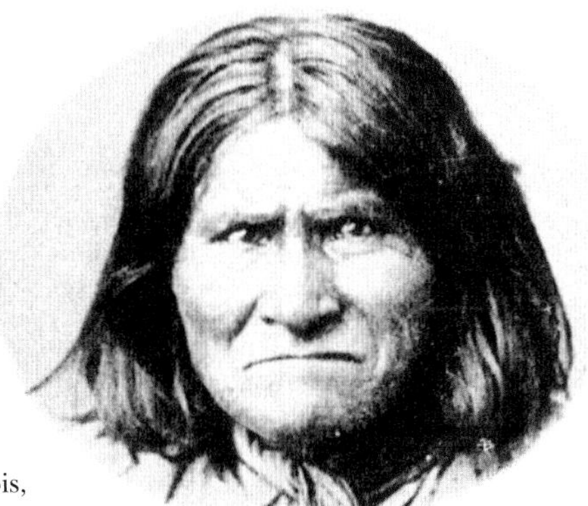

TRIBES
The native peoples of North America belonged to numerous tribes. Most of them hunted, fished, and farmed. Among the best known tribes are the Cheyenne, Comanche, and Sioux, who lived on the Great Plains; the Apache, Navajo, and Pueblo, who lived in the Southwest; and the Iroquois, Huron, and Cherokee, who lived in the East.

SIGN LANGUAGE

Each tribe of the natives spoke its own language. But people from different tribes were able to communicate with each other using a special sign language they all understood.

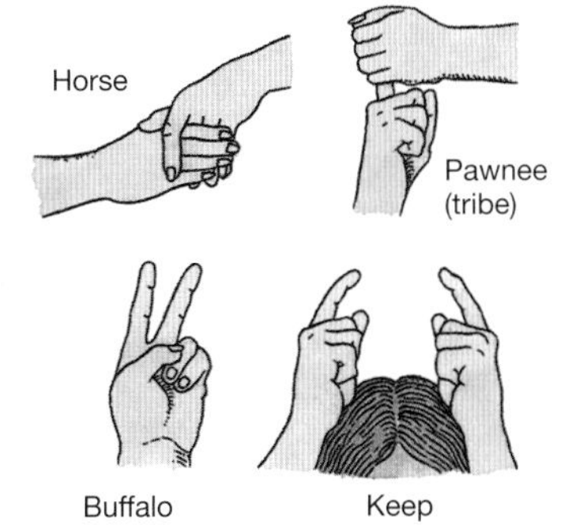

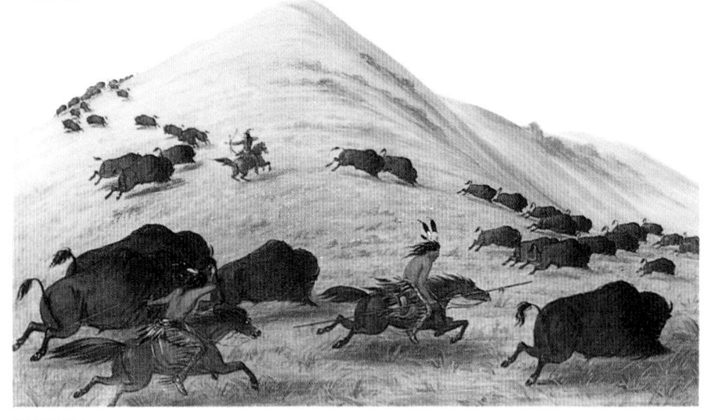

SIOUX
The Sioux lived on the Great Plains. They hunted bison on horseback, using the skins for clothing and tepees, the meat for food, and the bones and horns for tools. The Sioux were noted for their bravery and fighting skills, and fought a long series of battles with European settlers and gold miners who took over their territory in the 1880s. In 1876, the Sioux defeated the US cavalry at the now famous Battle of the Little Bighorn in Montana. Eventually the Sioux were driven onto reservations.

CANOES

Northern tribes who lived by rivers and lakes, such as the Penobscot and Malecite, built canoes from the bark of birch trees. These strong, fast canoes were light enough to be carried overland when they could not be paddled.

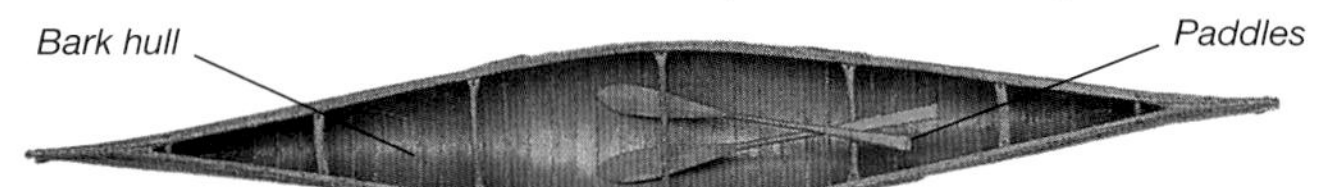

WEAPONS

Natives used bows and arrows, knives, and clubs as weapons. Many also carried tomahawks. During the 16th century, they got rifles from European traders.

Bow made of wood

Quiver used for holding arrows

Bow case holds the bow when not in use.

Tomahawks were axes with stone or iron heads. It was the Europeans who first made a combined axe blade and tobacco pipe.

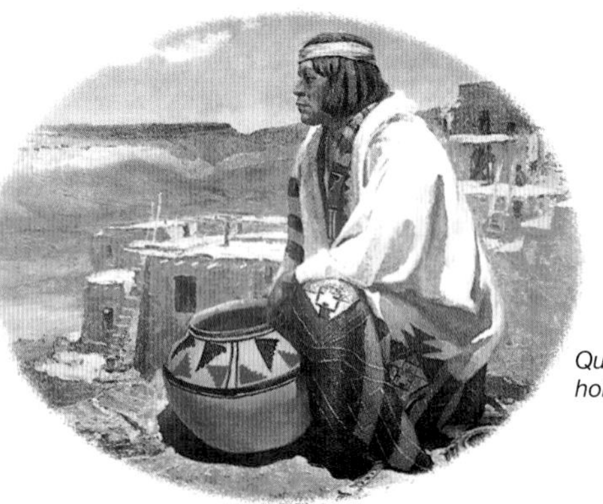

PUEBLOS
The Pueblos were a peaceful tribe that lived in the southwest. They farmed vegetables for food and were skilled craftsworkers, weaving brightly-coloured cloth from home-spun cotton and making pots. Their multi-storeyed houses were built of stone or adobe (sun-dried clay bricks) and were occupied by several families. Today, many Pueblos live on reservations in Arizona and New Mexico.

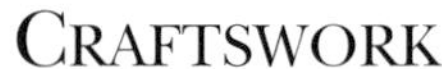

CRAFTSWORK

Many natives were skilled craftsworkers. They produced beautifully decorated clothes and head-dresses. This pair of men's moccasins, from the Blackfeet tribe of western Canada, are made of stitched leather decorated with leather thongs and embroidered with coloured beads.

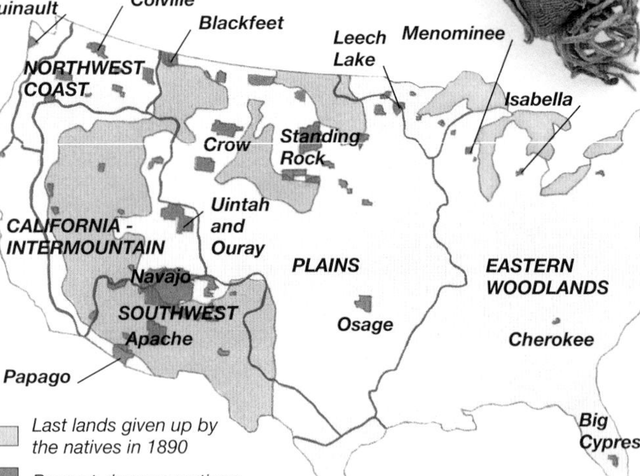

TRIBAL LANDS
Before the Europeans arrived, the natives occupied most of what later became the United States. The tribes were roughly grouped into six geographical regions. European settlement gradually forced the natives to the west and southwest, so that by 1890 they were living on a few scattered reservations.

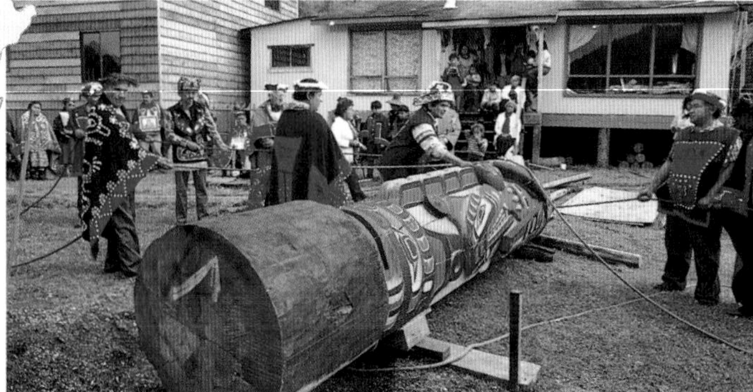

MODERN RESERVATIONS
The 1.5 million natives in the United States live on reservations that they govern themselves. The Navajo reservation, for example, covers over 6 million hectares in Arizona, New Mexico, and Utah. Recently, several tribes, such as the Pacific Northwest Coast Indians, have protested successfully and regained lost land.

Find out more
AZTECS
CANADA, HISTORY OF
INCAS
SIGNS AND SYMBOLS
UNITED STATES OF AMERICA, history of

NAVIES

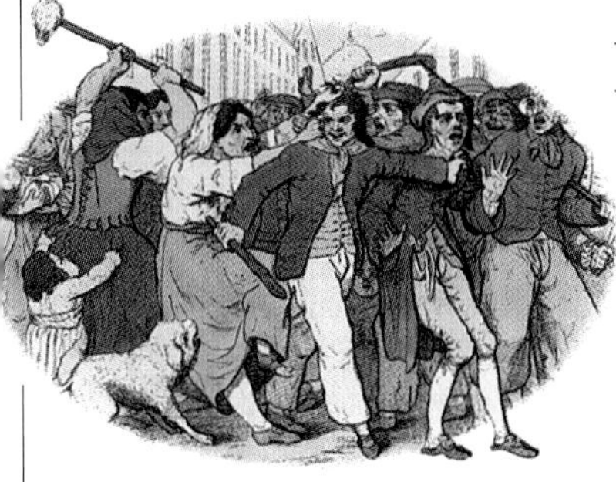

PRESSGANG
An 18th-century sailor's life was harsh, and few volunteered. The pressgang forced or "impressed" men to join the navy. The sailors in the pressgang kidnapped those who refused to join.

IN THE DAYS BEFORE cars and aircraft, sea travel was the fastest way to get around the world. However, it was also dangerous: pirates robbed cargo ships, and in wartime, opposing countries raided each other's vessels. The Ancient Greeks, Persians, and Romans were among the first to build ships for war at sea. In the 16th century, European nations organized navies as a way of protecting civilian shipping from attack. They used the ships to defend cargo and passenger vessels visiting their new colonies overseas. In wartime, modern navies do their traditional job. They guard merchant ships and sail out in groups, or fleets, to attack the enemy until the sea is secure for trade again. Naval ships also transport soldiers to the war zone and supply invasion forces with food and ammunition. In peacetime the oceans are safe for shipping, so navies train for war and are useful in other ways. Sailors help with rescue work after an earthquake or hurricane. Navies also pay goodwill visits to promote friendship between countries.

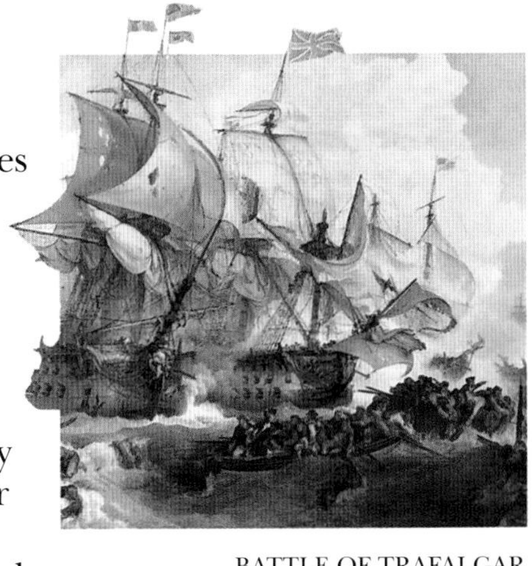

BATTLE OF TRAFALGAR
The first navies relied on wind power, and sea battles were tests of both fighting and sailing skills. At the Battle of Trafalgar in 1805, the British navy defeated a combined French and Spanish fleet, sinking or capturing more than half the enemy ships.

AIRCRAFT CARRIERS

Fighter planes based on aircraft carriers defend the fleet from enemy air attack. The runway deck is short, so a catapult gives aeroplanes added power for take-off. Carriers are huge and have few guns, and other warships must protect them in battles.

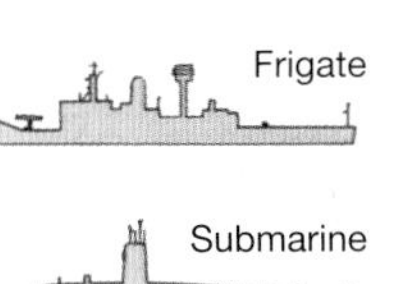

Aircraft carrier
Destroyer
Frigate
Submarine
Patrol craft

NAVAL SHIPS
A navy needs many different ships. Aircraft carriers act as floating airfields. Fast-moving destroyers and frigates attack enemy ships. Nuclear submarines defend the fleet and carry missiles to hit targets on land. Patrol craft are very fast and are used to defend ports and other land sites.

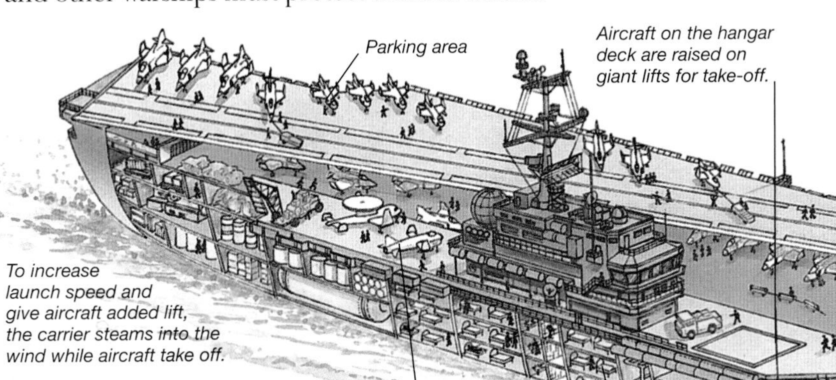

Parking area
Aircraft on the hangar deck are raised on giant lifts for take-off.
Take-off area is short, so steam catapults give aircraft extra speed.
To increase launch speed and give aircraft added lift, the carrier steams into the wind while aircraft take off.
Aircraft wings fold to save storage space.
Crew's living quarters

USS *FORRESTAL*
A typical aircraft carrier, such as the USS *Forrestal* of the United States navy, carries about 90 aircraft. Most are fighters, but one fifth are used as supply planes or for scouting. Most of the interior of the ship is taken up by hangars, repair areas, and ammunition stores.

UNIFORMS

Each nation has its own naval uniform, carrying information about the person wearing it. There are many different tasks on board a ship; jobs also vary from ship to ship. These uniforms therefore vary too. For example, a gunner on a destroyer wears a helmet, and a deck hand on an aircraft carrier wears goggles and earphones.

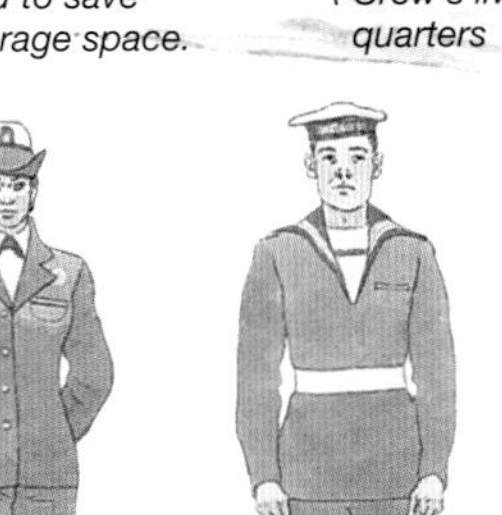

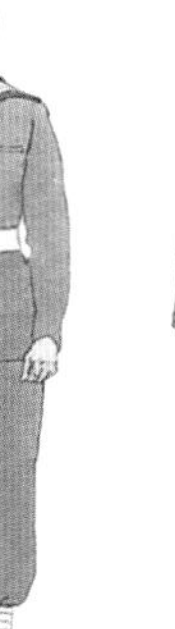

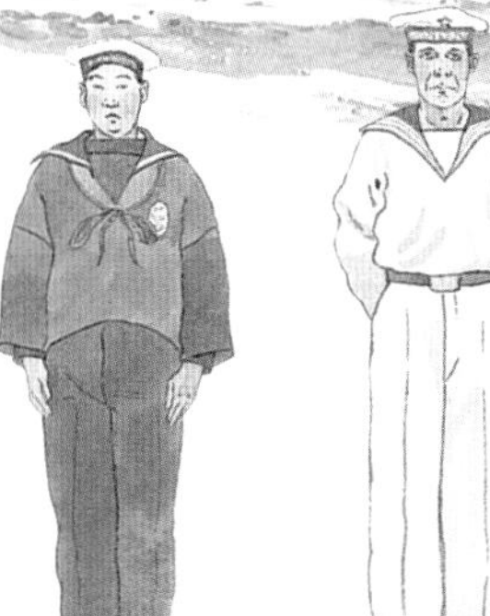

United States
United Kingdom
China
Russia

Find out more

NAVIGATION
SHIPS AND BOATS
WARSHIPS
WORLD WAR I
WORLD WAR II

NAVIGATION

EVEN IN A CITY with signs and street names to help you, it is easy to get lost. But imagine you were out in the open country or sailing in a boat without a map. How would you find your way? The earliest sailors faced this problem as they made their voyages of discovery. The answer was to watch the Sun by day and the stars by night. Because the Sun always rises in the east and sets in the west, sailors could work out which direction they were travelling in. The position of stars in the sky also gave them their direction: Polaris, the North Star, for instance, is almost in line with the Earth's North Pole. Navigation is the process of working out where you are and in what direction you are travelling. This can be on land, at sea, or in the air. Today, navigators have many aids to help them find their way. There are detailed maps of almost every part of the world, and electronic systems which use radar and satellites can fix the position of an aircraft or ship to within a few hundred metres. Such advances in navigation make even the longest journey easy and safe.

MAP AND COMPASS
Marks on a map show paths, hills, and other features. A magnetic compass shows which way to point a map so that it represents the landscape. The Chinese first used magnetic compasses about 1,000 years ago; about 2300 B.C. the first map was drawn in Babylon.

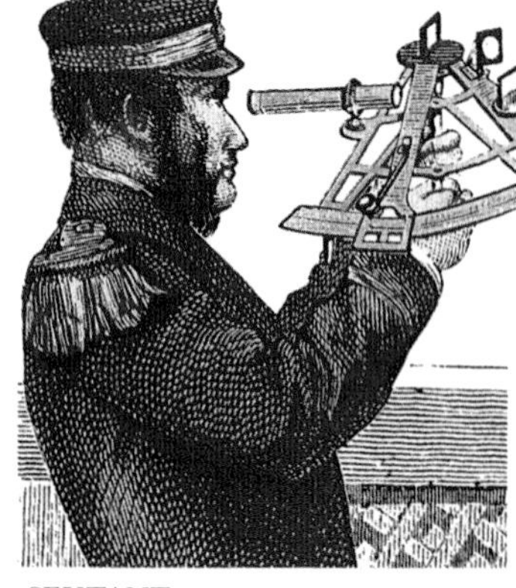

SEXTANT
For more than 250 years, navigators have used a device called a sextant. A sextant gives a measurement of the angle between two objects in the sky, such as two stars. From this angle, it is possible to calculate the position of a ship or an aircraft.

NAVIGATION SYSTEMS

Today, ships and aircraft routinely travel around the world without danger of becoming lost. Navigators use a gyrocompass, which gives the direction in which they are travelling even more precisely than a magnetic compass. In addition, ships and aeroplanes are packed with electronic navigation systems which guide them automatically.

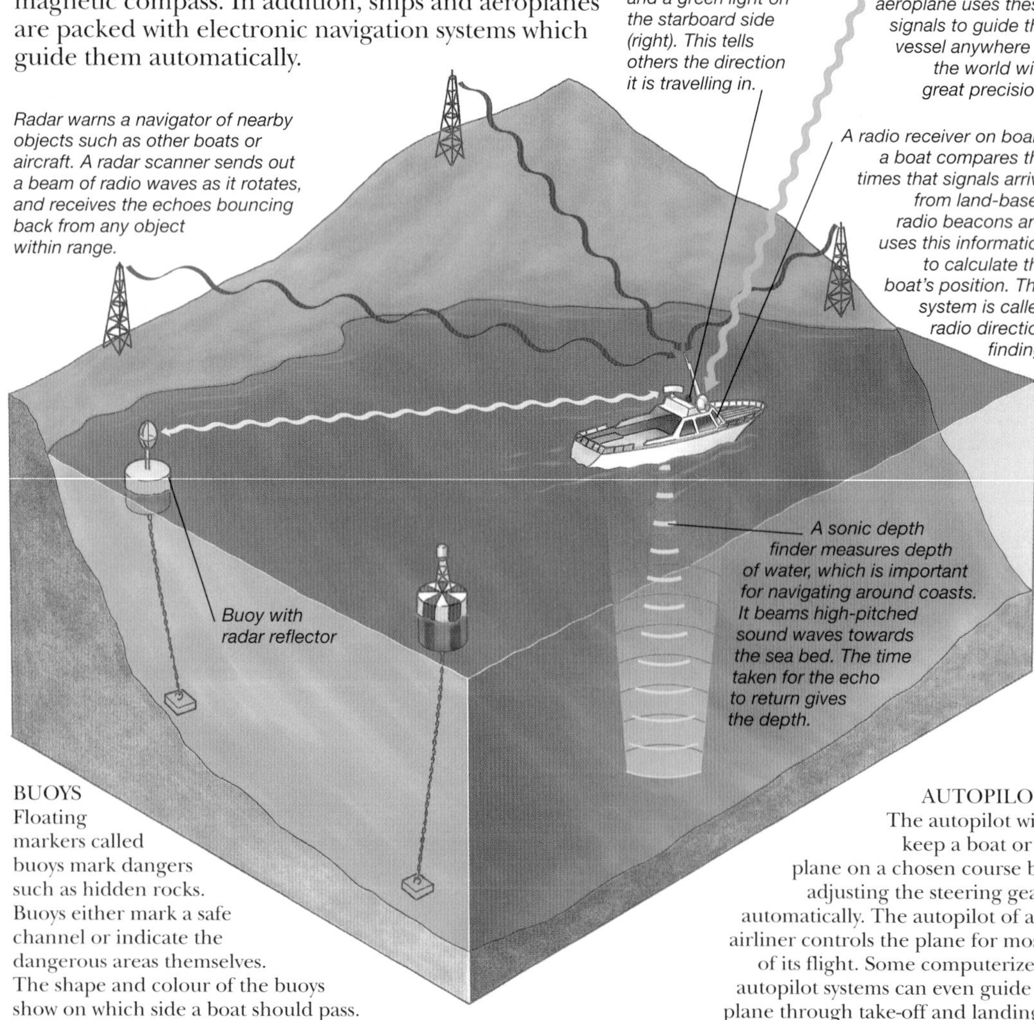

For safety, a boat or aircraft travelling at night carries a red light on the port side (left) and a green light on the starboard side (right). This tells others the direction it is travelling in.
Navigation satellites beam radio signals to Earth. A computer on board a boat or aeroplane uses these signals to guide the vessel anywhere in the world with great precision.
Radar warns a navigator of nearby objects such as other boats or aircraft. A radar scanner sends out a beam of radio waves as it rotates, and receives the echoes bouncing back from any object within range.
A radio receiver on board a boat compares the times that signals arrive from land-based radio beacons and uses this information to calculate the boat's position. This system is called radio direction finding.
A sonic depth finder measures depth of water, which is important for navigating around coasts. It beams high-pitched sound waves towards the sea bed. The time taken for the echo to return gives the depth.
Buoy with radar reflector

BUOYS
Floating markers called buoys mark dangers such as hidden rocks. Buoys either mark a safe channel or indicate the dangerous areas themselves. The shape and colour of the buoys show on which side a boat should pass.

AUTOPILOT
The autopilot will keep a boat or a plane on a chosen course by adjusting the steering gear automatically. The autopilot of an airliner controls the plane for most of its flight. Some computerized autopilot systems can even guide a plane through take-off and landing.

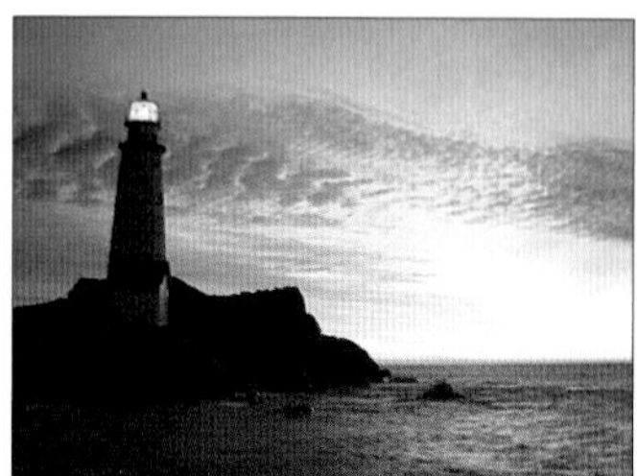

LIGHTHOUSE
Coastal waters can be dangerous because of rocks or tides. Lighthouses send out a bright beam of light to warn ships. The interval at which the light flashes identifies the lighthouse and so helps navigators find their position.

Find out more

AIRCRAFT
MAGNETISM
MAPS
RADAR
SATELLITES
SHIPS AND BOATS

NESTS AND BURROWS

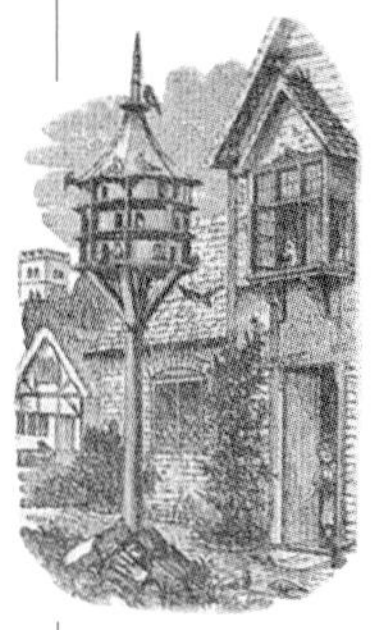

Nesting boxes and dovecotes encourage many birds to breed in the same place each year.

MOST ANIMALS need shelter and a place to bring up their young. A nest in a tree or a burrow underground protects an animal against predators and extremes of temperature. Many creatures, including birds and squirrels, build nests. Some creatures weave complicated nests. The harvest mouse makes a ball-shaped nest among corn stalks, where it rests and sleeps. Other animals, including birds, build a nest only during the breeding season, in which they lay eggs or give birth to live young. They line the nest with moss, grass, fur, or feathers to keep it warm and dry. Rabbits and foxes dig burrows, or tunnels, in the ground; a desert tortoise digs a burrow in which to hide from the midday sun. Some burrows are shallow; others, such as rabbit warrens, are deep, with escape routes, dead ends, and a separate burrow for the breeding nest.

Natural building materials from the surrounding area, such as lichens, help camouflage the nest.

Nest has a soft, thick lining of moss, hair, and feathers to keep eggs warm.

Wagtail weaves twigs and stems together to strengthen the nest.

NESTS

Many birds spend weeks making a nest in a sheltered place. Each kind of bird has its favourite materials, such as twigs, grass, or fur. Each also chooses a particular place to make the nest, such as a tree or a spot on the ground. A pied wagtail, for example, often builds its nest around farm buildings and uses twigs, straw, leaves, and moss, with a lining of hair and feathers. A grey wagtail builds its nest beside fast-flowing water and uses grasses and moss, with a lining of hair.

Flamingo nests are cone-shaped and made of mud.

FLAMINGO

Many animals, such as these African flamingos, nest in large groups called colonies. When a predator approaches, flamingos make such a noise that few predators dare to enter the colony. In a flamingo colony there is safety in numbers.

TRAP-DOOR SPIDER

The trap-door spider digs a small burrow in loose soil and hides in it. Using silk that it produces from its body, the spider glues particles of soil together to make a neatly fitting, well-disguised door. As an insect or other prey passes by, the spider flips open the door and grabs the victim.

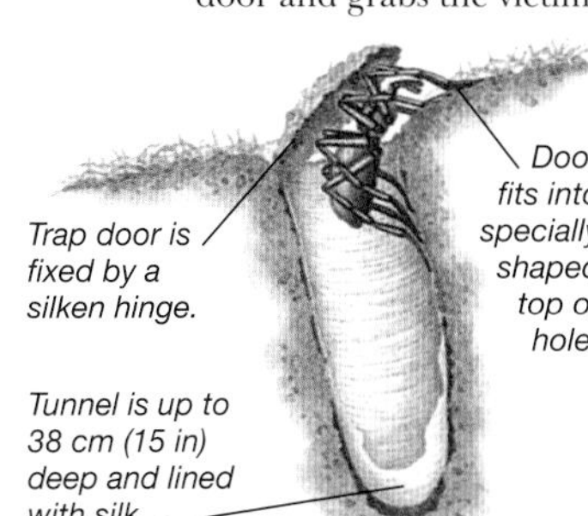

Trap door is fixed by a silken hinge.
Door fits into specially shaped top of hole.
Tunnel is up to 38 cm (15 in) deep and lined with silk.

Young platypuses stay in the breeding nest in a burrow underground and suckle milk from their mother for up to four months.

PLATYPUS BURROW

The Australian platypus digs a complex breeding burrow up to 20 m (66 ft) long in the riverbank. Here, the female lays eggs and raises the young when they hatch. Each time the platypus enters or leaves the burrow to feed, it digs its way out and rebuilds the series of doors made of mud along the tunnel to protect its young from intruders.

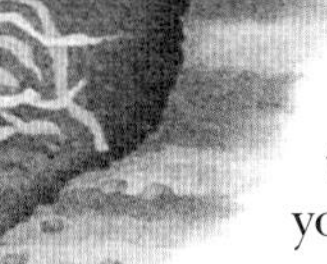

Find out more

ANTS AND TERMITES
BEES AND WASPS
BIRDS
MICE, RATS, AND SQUIRRELS
RABBITS AND HARES

NEWSPAPERS

THE PAGES OF A NEWSPAPER keep everyone in touch with local, national, and world events. Newspapers provide more details about events than television news programmes have time for, and stories in the paper cover a wide range of topics. In addition to news, there is information about politics, the arts, sports, fashion, business, technology, and the environment. Newspapers also contain opinions or points of view; some newspapers support a political party, and others try to remain independent. Local newspapers concentrate on events in one city or neighbourhood; national newspapers sell countrywide and cover events at home and abroad. A big newspaper has a large staff of editors, reporters, feature writers, cartoonists, photographers, typesetters, printers, and many others who work through the night to deliver the latest news each morning. Many newspapers are now also published on the Internet.

THE BROADSIDE
Before the first newspaper was published in 17th-century Germany, people read the news in "broadsides". These were single sheets of printed paper.

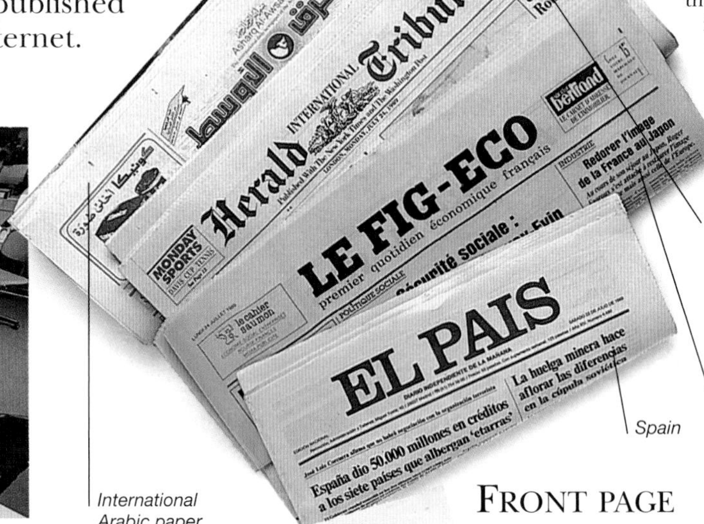

ON THE NEWS STAND
Every country has its own newspapers. Some are published daily, others weekly. Some sell millions of copies a day, others just a few thousand a week. Each newspaper has a unique format – a special type style and general layout that sets it apart from others on the news stand.

NEWS ROOM
The heart of a newspaper is the news or editorial room. Here, national news and reports from all over the world come pouring in via the telephone, fax machine, and Internet. Here, too, reporters write their stories, assistant editors check them, and editors make decisions about how important each story is and what to include in the newspaper.

FRONT PAGE
Big headlines and photographs of important, newsworthy events feature on the front page. In an eventful day the editor may need to change the leading story several times before the last copies of the paper are printed. Front pages carry the news that makes history – the outbreak of war, for example, or a major disaster, such as the sinking of the *Titanic*.

Short pieces of text called captions explain what is happening in the pictures.

PRINTING PRESS
The thunder of the press as it prints newspapers each night shakes the floor. Huge reels of paper up to 8 km (5 miles) long roar through the press. Some machines can print, fold, cut, and stack more than 1,000 newspapers a minute. Lorries and trains rush them to news stands so people can buy them first thing in the morning.

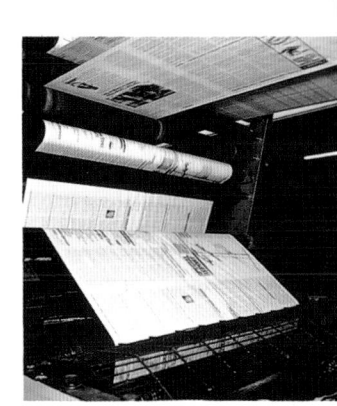

Find out more
ADVERTISING
CARTOONS
INFORMATION TECHNOLOGY
MAGAZINES
PRINTING

NEW ZEALAND

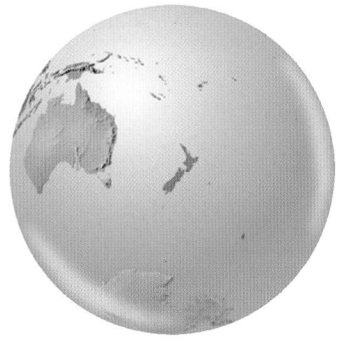

New Zealand lies in the Pacific Ocean, east of Australia. There are two large islands – the North Island and the South Island – and many smaller ones, making a total area of 268,670 sq km (103,733 sq miles).

THE ISLAND NATION of New Zealand is a fascinating mixture of cultures and peoples. Maori people were the original inhabitants of the country, which they call Aotearoa, and they still live there, together with the descendants of the early British settlers and immigrants from other European and Asian countries. Only 3.9 million people live in New Zealand, and there are few large towns. The people are young – more than half of them are less than 35 years old – and the number of births per 1,000 of population is among the highest of all developed nations. A former British colony, New Zealand became fully independent in 1947. It is a leading Pacific nation and has strong links with many of the small islands in the region, such as Niue. The landscape of New Zealand is varied. There are towering mountains, glaciers, volcanoes, lakes, hot springs, sandy beaches, rolling hills, and plains.

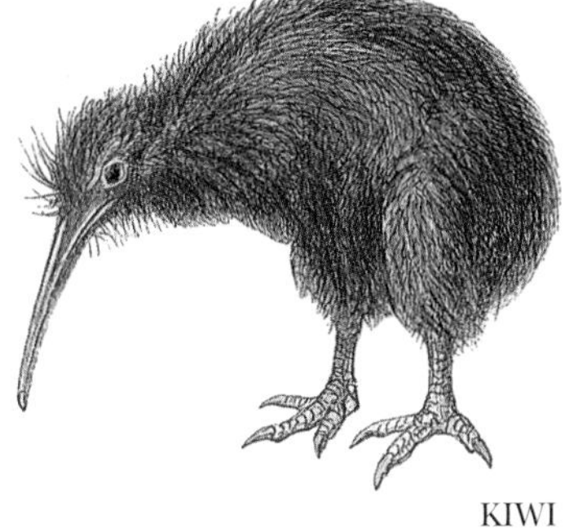

KIWI
New Zealand lies far from other land masses, and as a result its wildlife has developed in an unusual way. The kiwi, which cannot fly, is the most famous of all New Zealand creatures. There are several other species of flightless birds.

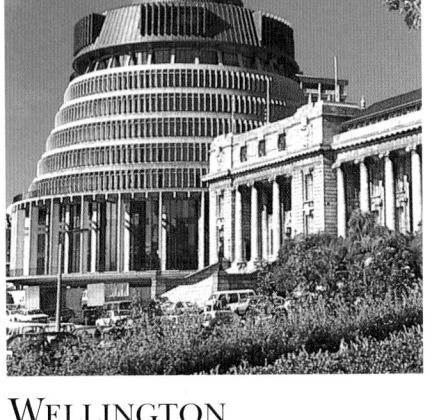

WELLINGTON

The capital of New Zealand is Wellington, which stands at the southern tip of the North Island. The city lies around a large natural harbour and is a busy port. Older wooden buildings stand close to recent structures built in a more modern style.

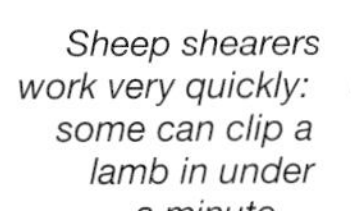

Sheep shearers work very quickly: some can clip a lamb in under a minute.

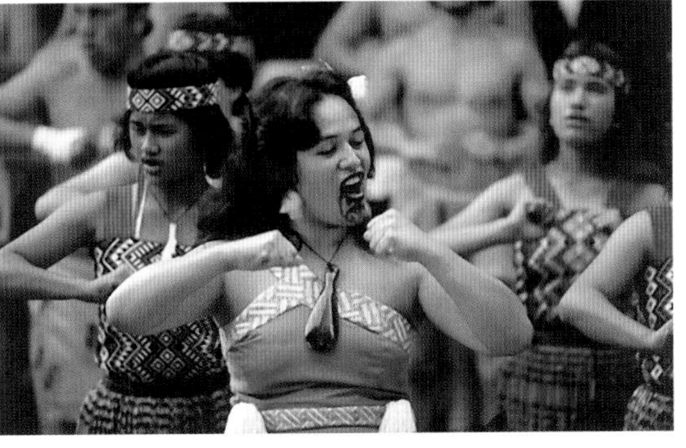

MAORI CULTURE
The Maoris, a Polynesian people, arrived in New Zealand around 950 A.D. from islands in the Pacific. Today their descendants keep alive the rich culture of wood carving, weaving, and music and dance, which they brought with them.

FARMING

New Zealand has a warm, moist climate which is ideal for many types of farming. Sheep and cattle ranching are the biggest businesses. There are two cattle and 13 sheep for every human in New Zealand. The country exports more dairy produce and lamb than any other nation and is the second largest exporter of wool. Over the past 15 years production of other crops, such as kiwi fruit, oranges, and lemons, has increased. Newly built fishing boats have helped New Zealand's fleet increase its catch, and today the country is a major seafood exporter.

SOUTH ISLAND

Although the South Island is the largest New Zealand island, it has fewer inhabitants than the North Island. The western side of the island is covered by the Southern Alps, a region of mountains and glaciers, parts of which have not been explored. The rest of the island consists of farmland, grazing land for sheep and cattle, and a few ports and coastal cities.

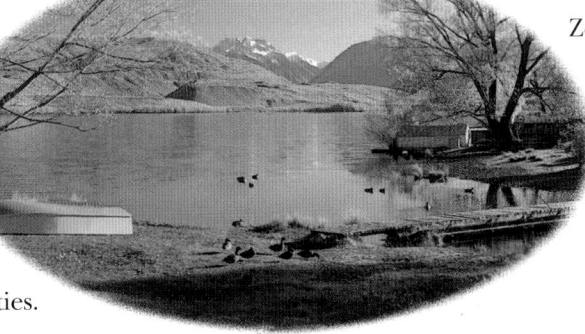

Find out more

FOOTBALL AND RUGBY
MOUNTAINS
NEW ZEALAND, HISTORY OF
OSTRICHES AND EMUS
PACIFIC OCEAN

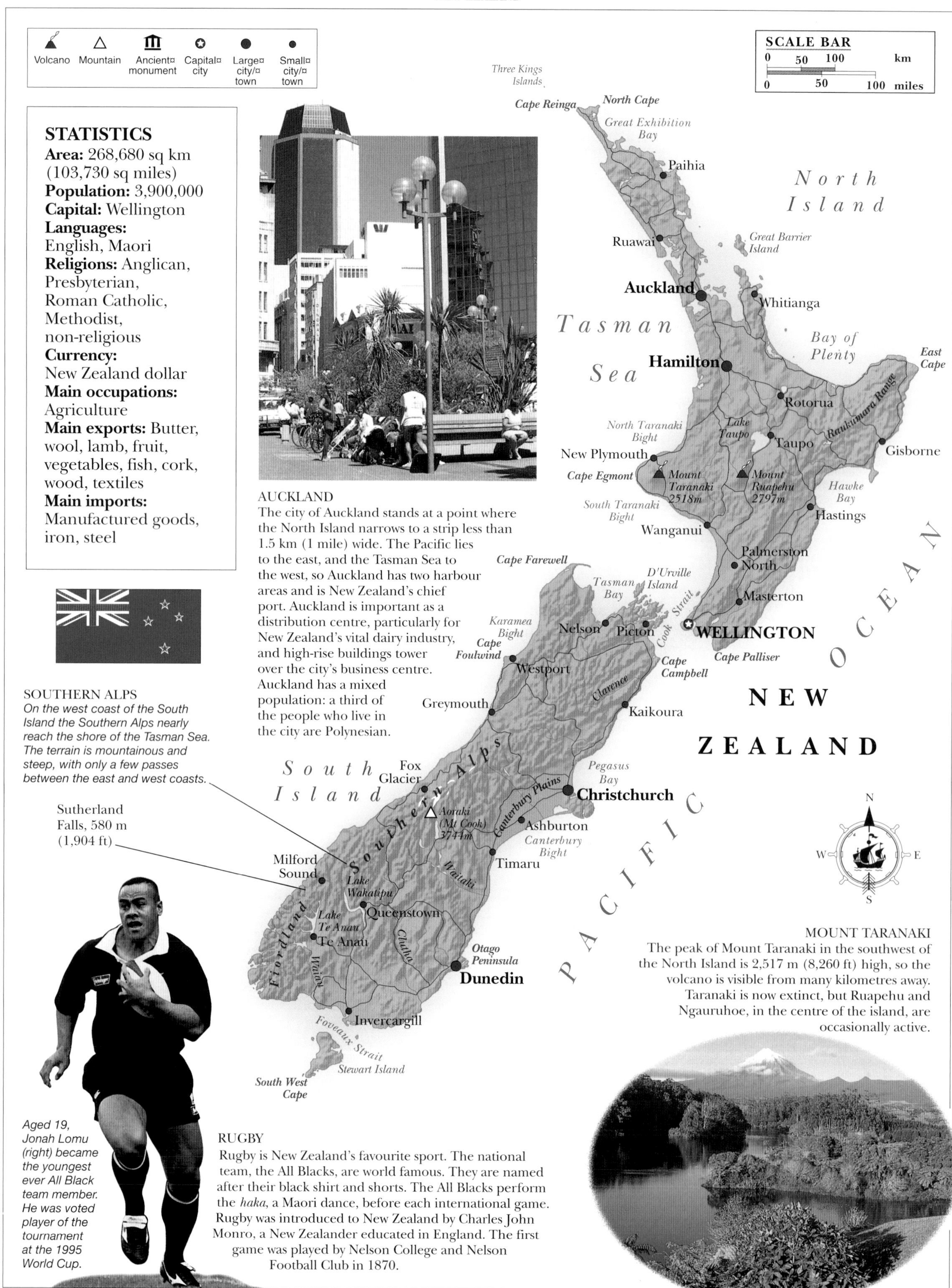

STATISTICS

Area: 268,680 sq km (103,730 sq miles)
Population: 3,900,000
Capital: Wellington
Languages: English, Maori
Religions: Anglican, Presbyterian, Roman Catholic, Methodist, non-religious
Currency: New Zealand dollar
Main occupations: Agriculture
Main exports: Butter, wool, lamb, fruit, vegetables, fish, cork, wood, textiles
Main imports: Manufactured goods, iron, steel

AUCKLAND
The city of Auckland stands at a point where the North Island narrows to a strip less than 1.5 km (1 mile) wide. The Pacific lies to the east, and the Tasman Sea to the west, so Auckland has two harbour areas and is New Zealand's chief port. Auckland is important as a distribution centre, particularly for New Zealand's vital dairy industry, and high-rise buildings tower over the city's business centre. Auckland has a mixed population: a third of the people who live in the city are Polynesian.

SOUTHERN ALPS
On the west coast of the South Island the Southern Alps nearly reach the shore of the Tasman Sea. The terrain is mountainous and steep, with only a few passes between the east and west coasts.

Sutherland Falls, 580 m (1,904 ft)

MOUNT TARANAKI
The peak of Mount Taranaki in the southwest of the North Island is 2,517 m (8,260 ft) high, so the volcano is visible from many kilometres away. Taranaki is now extinct, but Ruapehu and Ngauruhoe, in the centre of the island, are occasionally active.

Aged 19, Jonah Lomu (right) became the youngest ever All Black team member. He was voted player of the tournament at the 1995 World Cup.

RUGBY
Rugby is New Zealand's favourite sport. The national team, the All Blacks, are world famous. They are named after their black shirt and shorts. The All Blacks perform the *haka*, a Maori dance, before each international game. Rugby was introduced to New Zealand by Charles John Monro, a New Zealander educated in England. The first game was played by Nelson College and Nelson Football Club in 1870.

HISTORY OF NEW ZEALAND

NEW ZEALAND

c. A.D. 950 First Maoris arrive.

1642 Dutch navigator Abel Tasman visits islands.

1769-77 British explorer Captain James Cook visits islands four times.

1814 British missionaries arrive.

1840 British settlement established in Wellington. Treaty of Waitangi.

1844-70 Land wars between Maoris and British settlers.

1852 Britain grants New Zealand self-government.

1863 Gold Rush draws many immigrants from Europe.

1893 Women get to vote.

1898 State pensions given.

1907 New Zealand becomes an independent dominion in the British Empire.

1914-18, 1939-45 Troops fight with Britain in two world wars.

1960s Troops fight with Americans in the Vietnam War.

1985 New Zealand joins its Pacific neighbours in declaring the region a nuclear-free zone.

ABOUT 1,000 YEARS AGO, a group of people ventured ashore on a string of islands in the South Pacific. These people were the Maoris, and they had travelled in canoes across the Pacific Ocean from the distant islands of Polynesia to a land they called Aotearoa. For about 700 years, the Maoris lived on the islands undisturbed. In 1642, the Dutch Explorer Abel Tasman visited the islands, and named them New Zealand, after a province in the Netherlands. Soon, American, Australian, and European sealers and whalers were exploiting the rich coastal waters, and in 1840, the British founded the first European settlement. The Maoris fought protest wars until 1870, when they lost control of their lands. As a British colony, New Zealand grew wealthy by exporting its agricultural produce. In 1907, New Zealand became independent. More recently, New Zealand has formed several alliances with its neighbours in the South Pacific to keep the region free from nuclear weapons.

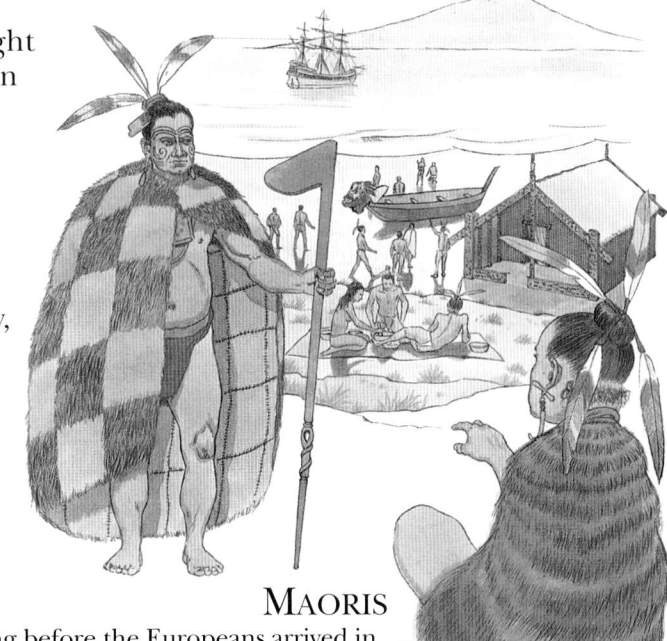

MAORIS

Long before the Europeans arrived in New Zealand, the Maoris had established a thriving agricultural community. They grew sweet potatoes and caught fish and fowl. They wore colourful clothes woven from flax. They lived in houses made of rushes and wood. Today, more than 500,000 Maoris still exist, most of whom live in the North Island.

Traditional Maori cloak made out of feathers

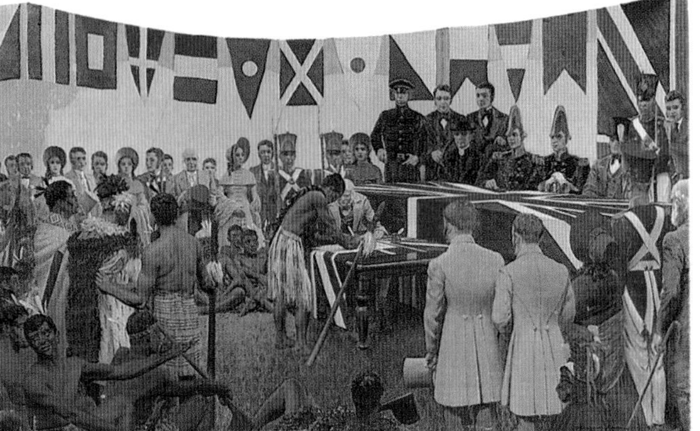

TREATY OF WAITANGI
In 1840, the Maoris granted sovereignty, or ownership, of their country to Britain. In return, Britain promised protection of their rights and property. New Zealand then became a colony of the British Empire.

Protestors try to interrupt the path of a nuclear submarine.

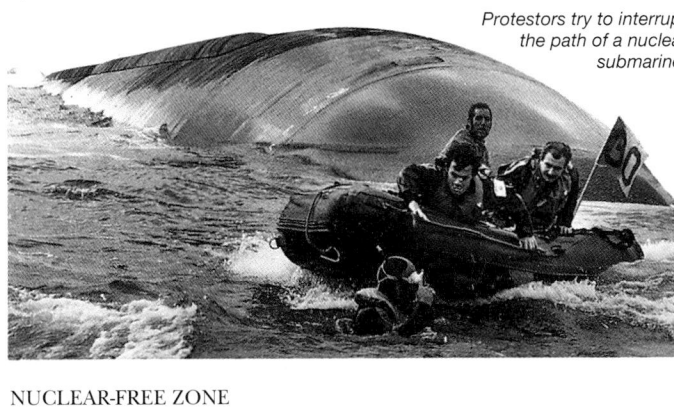

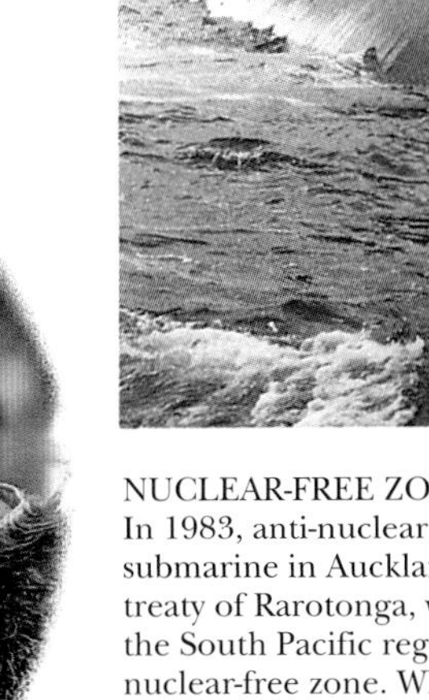

INDEPENDENCE
In 1852, Britain granted new Zealand self-government. The country gave pensions to workers and was the first in the world to give women the right to vote. In 1907, New Zealand gained full independence, but ties with Britain remained strong. The British monarch, Queen Elizabeth II, seen here with Prince Philip in a traditional Maori cloak, is the nation's head of state.

NUCLEAR-FREE ZONE
In 1983, anti-nuclear protesters blockaded the USS *Phoenix* nuclear submarine in Auckland Harbour. In 1985, New Zealand signed the treaty of Rarotonga, which declared the South Pacific region to be a nuclear-free zone. When France continued to carry out nuclear tests in Mururoa Atoll, in the South Pacific Ocean, these were fiercely opposed by other Pacific countries.

Find out more

BRITISH EMPIRE
COOK, JAMES
NEW ZEALAND

FLORENCE
NIGHTINGALE

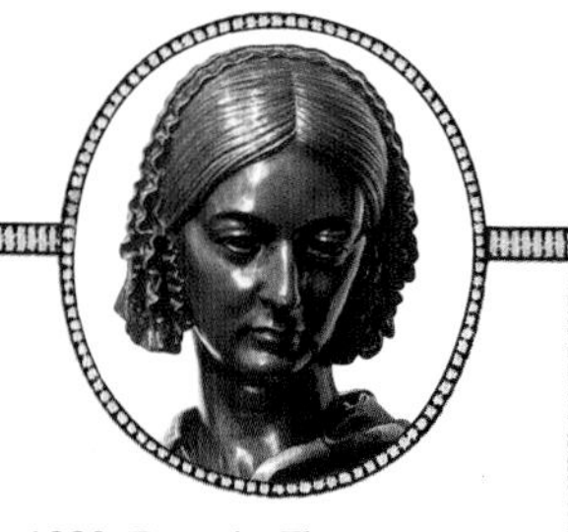

1820 Born in Florence, Italy.

1853 Supervises women's hospital, London.

1854 Goes to Crimea to nurse soldiers.

1856 Returns to England.

1859 Publishes *Notes on Nursing*.

1860 Sets up world's first training school for nurses, in London.

1907 Becomes first woman to receive Order of Merit.

1910 Dies, aged 90.

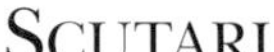

THE FOUNDER OF MODERN nursing, Florence Nightingale was a remarkable woman. She reformed nursing practice, and revolutionized healthcare. Florence Nightingale came from a wealthy family, and received a good education. Her parents were horrified when she said she wanted to be a nurse. Nursing in the 19th century was dirty and dangerous, and nurses tended to be poor, uneducated women. However, she was a determined woman, and, in 1853, began work supervising a women's hospital in London. The following year, she went to the Crimean War, where she completely reorganized the military hospital at Scutari, Turkey, reducing death rates dramatically. She returned to England as a heroine, and worked for nursing reforms until her death.

THE LAMP
Florence Nightingale was nicknamed "The Lady with the Lamp" because she carried a lamp through the wards.

Florence Nightingale walked through the wards, checking that soldiers were comfortable and free of pain.

SCUTARI

When Florence Nightingale arrived at the military hospital in Scutari, she found appalling conditions. Rats and lice infested the hospital, medical supplies were almost non-existent, and wounded soldiers were effectively left to die of neglect. With her team of workers and money raised by the British public, Nightingale washed and painted wards, cleared drains, set up laundries, bought in supplies, and introduced strict nursing discipline. Male army doctors resented her, but death rates dropped from 40 to 2 per cent.

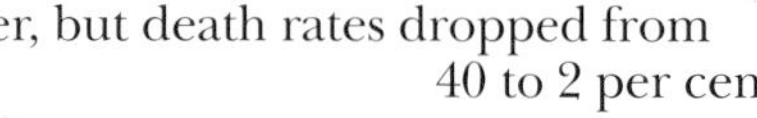

Florence Nightingale in the Military Hospital at Scutari, Turkey

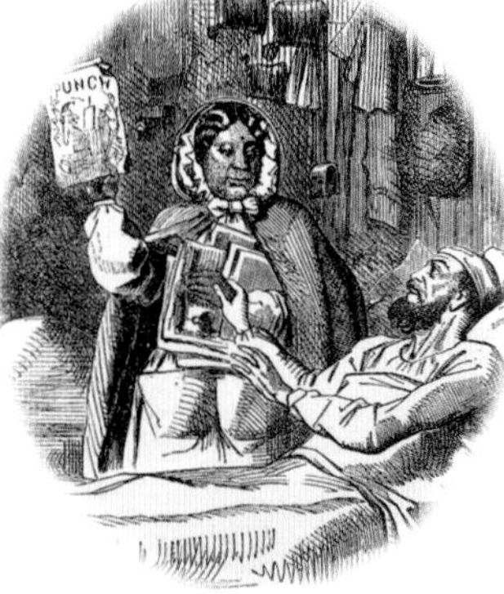

MARY SEACOLE
Born in Jamaica, Mary Seacole (1805-81) gained nursing experience during fever epidemics. In 1854, she volunteered to nurse in the British army, but was refused, probably because she was black. Undaunted, she went to the Crimea, where she nursed the wounded on the battlefield.

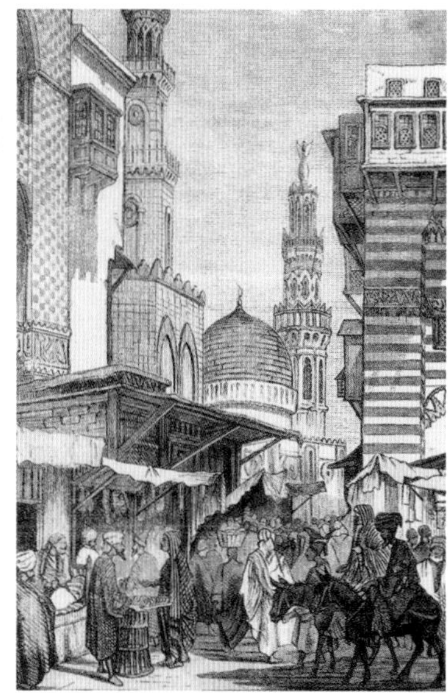

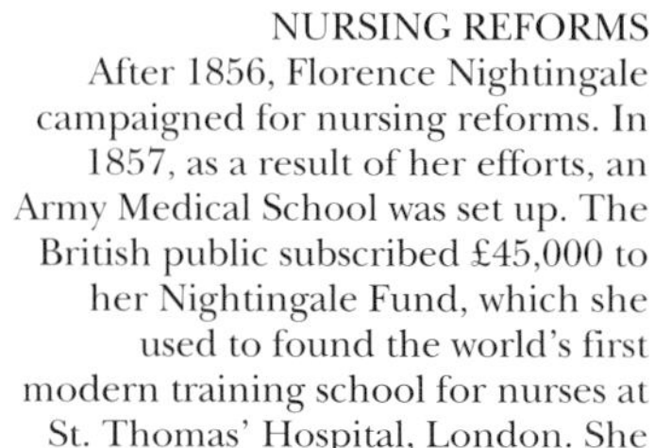

NURSING REFORMS
After 1856, Florence Nightingale campaigned for nursing reforms. In 1857, as a result of her efforts, an Army Medical School was set up. The British public subscribed £45,000 to her Nightingale Fund, which she used to found the world's first modern training school for nurses at St. Thomas' Hospital, London. She personally drew up the curriculum.

YOUNG FLORENCE
From an early age, Florence Nightingale wanted activity and challenge. But, as a young middle-class woman, she was supposed to play the piano and entertain, rather than work. In her diary, she wrote of her boredom. Finally, when she was 30, she began her career, spending time with the nursing Sisters of St. Vincent in Alexandria, Egypt.

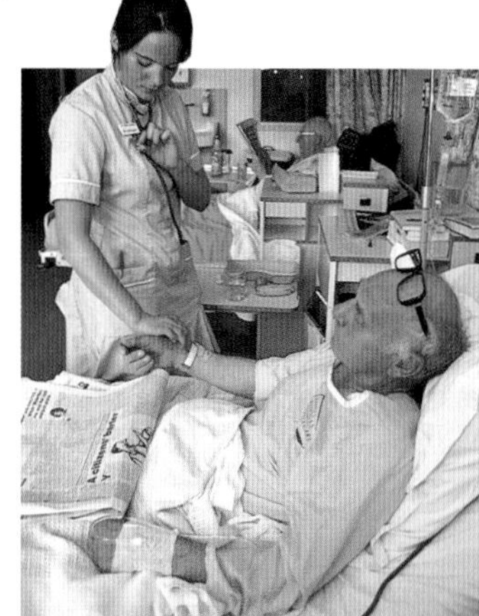

Find out more

MEDICINE, HISTORY OF
VICTORIANS
WOMEN'S RIGHTS

NORMANS

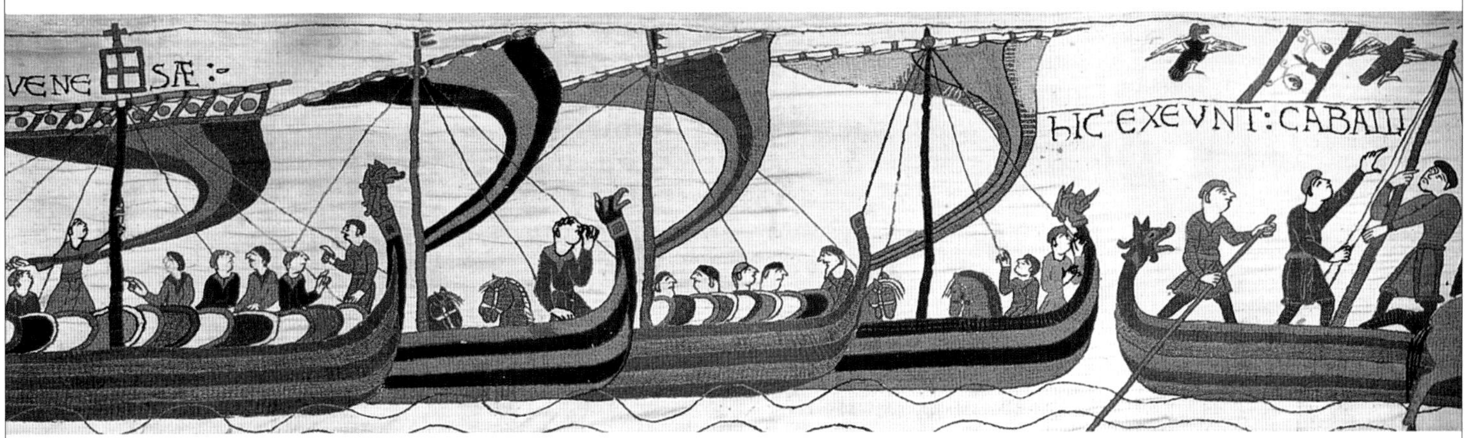

BAYEUX TAPESTRY
Dating to the 11th century, the Bayeux tapestry was produced to record the Norman Conquest of England. It shows scenes of battle, and can be seen today at Bayeux, in France.

TODAY, SOLID STONE CASTLES in England, Sicily, and France stand as reminders of the Normans, warriors from northern France, who transformed Europe during the 11th and 12th centuries. The Normans were descendants of the Norsemen, or Vikings, and were formidable fighters. They settled in northern France during the early 900s in an area now known as Normandy. The Normans were not only warriors but also skilled administrators. Their dukes created a complex and efficient society, dividing their kingdom into areas called fiefs. A knight controlled each fief. The Normans reached their height of power under William, Duke of Normandy, who led the conquest of England in 1066. They quickly transformed England into a Norman kingdom, building castles to defend their conquests, as well as churches, monasteries, and cathedrals. The Normans continued to rule England until 1154. After this, the Saxons and Normans began to merge into one nation. In 1204 the king of France conquered Normandy and took it over.

WILLIAM THE CONQUEROR

William, Duke of Normandy (c. 1028-87), was a brilliant, but ruthless general and administrator. He led the Norman invasion of England and, after defeating the Saxon king, Harold II, was crowned king of England.

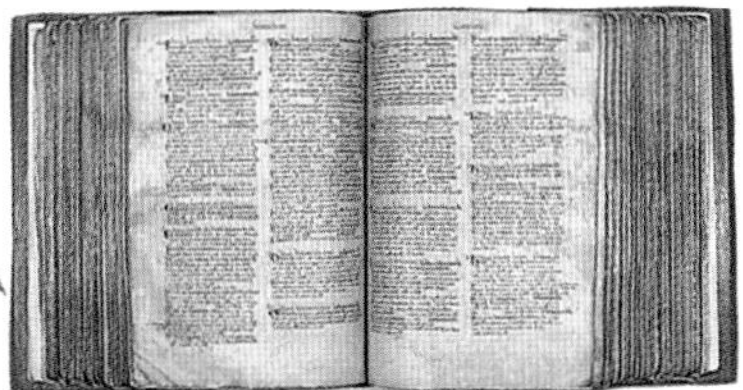

DOMESDAY BOOK
In 1085, King William I ordered a complete survey of England. Known as the Domesday Book, it contained thorough details of people, goods, animals, and lands for every single village in the country.

Sovereign states
SCOTLAND
Unconquered territory
Conquered territory
IRELAND
WALES
ENGLAND
Paris
BRITTANY
AQUITAINE

EMPIRE
At their height of power under Henry II (reigned 1154-89), the Normans had conquered northern France, England, southern Italy, and Sicily. They did not survive as a separate group, but merged with the peoples they had conquered.

ARCHITECTURE

The Normans were skilled architects. They built strong castles to guard their conquests, such as the Tower of London, which stands to this day. They also built churches, cathedrals, and monasteries. Norman churches have intricately carved arches over the doors and windows, and massive walls and pillars.

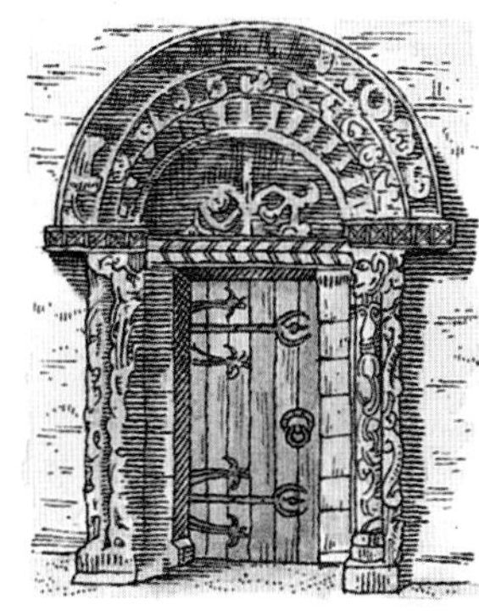

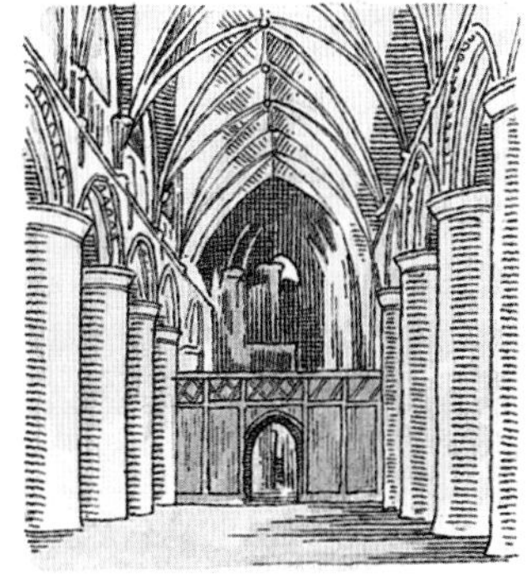

Find out more
BRITAIN, ANCIENT
CASTLES
FRANCE, HISTORY OF
UNITED KINGDOM, HISTORY OF
VIKINGS

NORTH AFRICA

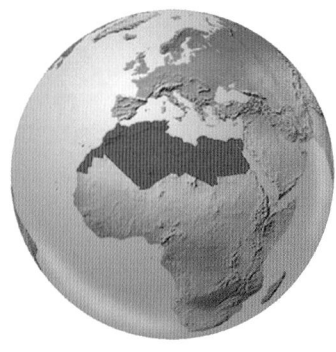

The North African coast occupies the southern shores of the Mediterranean, where the climate is mild and the land fertile. The Atlas Mountains and the rolling hills of Algeria and Tunisia lie between the coast and the sand seas and barren rocks of the Sahara.

THE COUNTRIES OF NORTH AFRICA have suffered many invasions, from the Romans to the French and British. But the conquest by the armies of Islam in the 7th century was to have a major impact on the region, giving it a shared religion, language, and sense of identity. Much of North Africa is dominated by the largest desert on Earth, the Sahara. It is sparsely populated by dwindling numbers of nomads. Most people live along the fertile coastal strip on the banks of the Nile. Cities increasingly attract migrants from the country – Cairo is the fastest-growing city in the Islamic world with a population of over 15 million. In Algeria and Libya, the desert has revealed hidden riches – vast reserves of oil are fuelling modernization programmes. Many tourists visit Morocco, Tunisia, and Egypt, attracted by ancient ruins, medieval cities, and baking hot beaches.

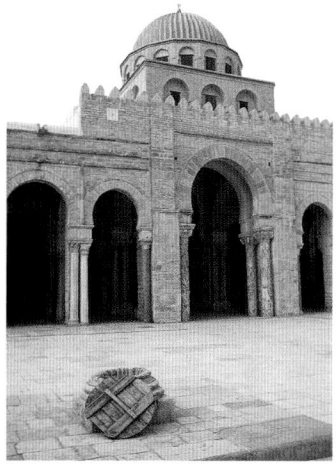

KAIROUAN
When Islamic Arabs conquered North Africa in the 7th century, they founded many cities that are still important today. The walled city of Kairouan, in Tunisia, is a sacred shrine for Muslims in Africa. The Great Mosque was built in the 9th century. Its imposing marble courtyard, where the people pray, is surrounded by columns.

NILE AGRICULTURE

The River Nile floods every summer, carrying rich mud from the highlands of Ethiopia and Sudan to the arid deserts of Egypt. It was this annual miracle that provided the foundations of Ancient Egyptian civilization. Today, nearly 99 per cent of the Egyptian population live along the green and fertile land on the banks of the Nile. Egypt is a leading producer of dates, melons, and cotton. Most Egyptian farmers use centuries-old methods; donkeys and asses are still used to pull heavy loads and carry water.

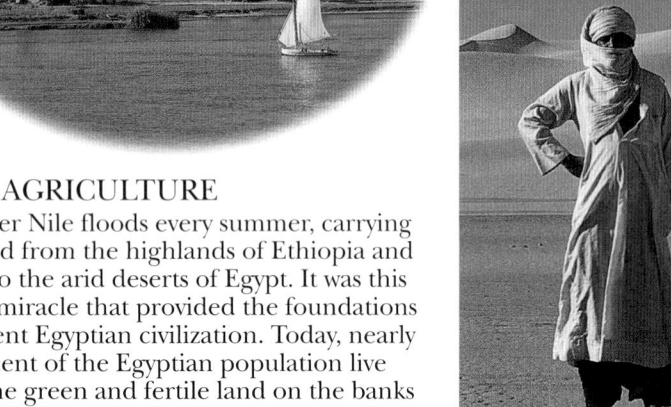

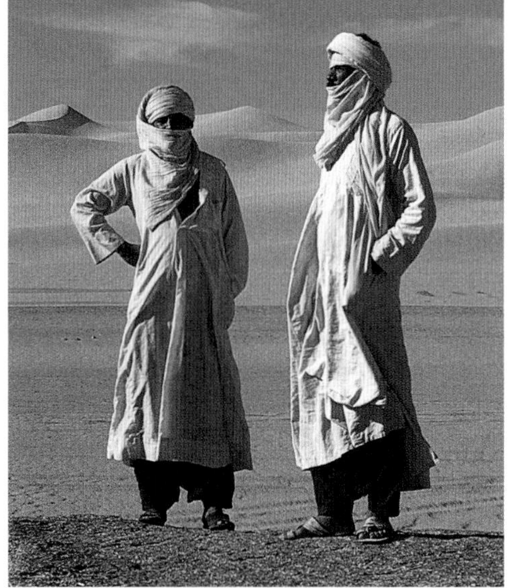

People who live in the desert regions of Africa, such as these Berber men (left), wear loose clothes to keep cool, and veils to protect themselves from the wind-blown sands of the desert.

BERBERS

The Berbers are the original people of Northwest Africa. They were converted to Islam in the 8th century. Arab invaders drove them into the Atlas Mountains where many still live in remote villages. In the Sahara, Berber live a nomadic life herding camels, sheep, and goats.

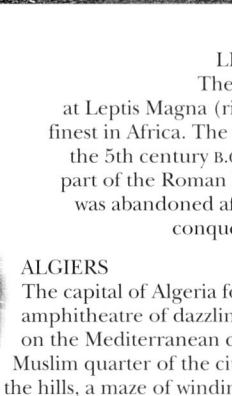

LEPTIS MAGNA
The Roman ruins at Leptis Magna (right) are the finest in Africa. The city dates to the 5th century B.C. It became part of the Roman Empire and was abandoned after the Arab conquest in 643 A.D.

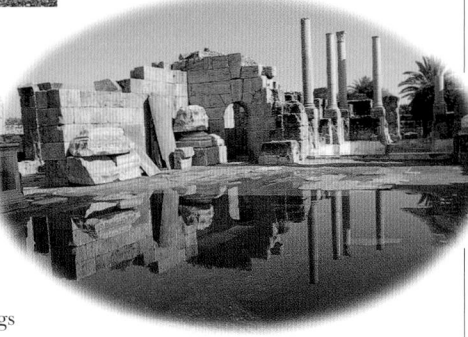

ALGIERS
The capital of Algeria forms a vast amphitheatre of dazzling white buildings on the Mediterranean coast. The old Muslim quarter of the city sprawls across the hills, a maze of winding streets and high-walled houses. The French colonial quarter, with its public squares and tree-lined avenues, is found near the harbour. The French captured the city, an unruly centre of Mediterranean piracy, in 1830. They left in 1962.

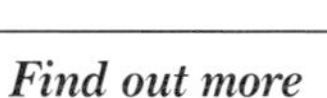

Find out more

AFRICA
AFRICA, HISTORY OF
DESERTS
ISLAM

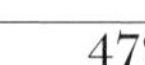

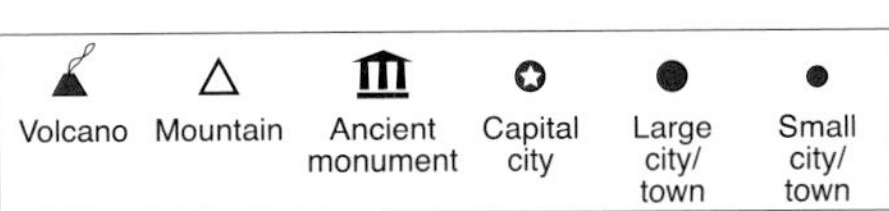

ALGERIA
Area: 2,381,740 sq km (919,590 sq miles)
Population: 31,800,000
Capital: Algiers

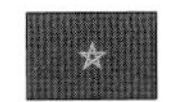

MOROCCO
Area: 698,670 sq km (269,757 sq miles)
Population: 30,600,000
Capital: Rabat

EGYPT
Area: 1,001,450 sq km (386,660 sq miles)
Population: 71,900,000
Capital: Cairo

TUNISIA
Area: 163,610 sq km (63,170 sq miles)
Population: 9,800,000
Capital: Tunis

LIBYA
Area: 1,759,540 sq km (679,358 sq miles)
Population: 5,600,000
Capital: Tripoli

WESTERN SAHARA
Area: 266,000 sq km (102,703 sq miles)
Population: 273,000
Capital: Laayoune
Status: disputed territory occupied by Morocco

SCALE BAR
0 200 400 km
0 200 400 miles

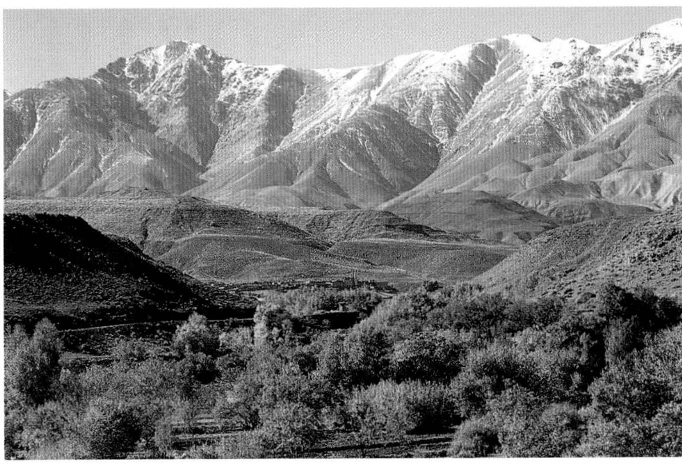

ATLAS MOUNTAINS

The Atlas Mountains are a group of ranges, running roughly parallel to the Mediterranean coast. They stretch 2,410 km (1,500 miles) from southeast Morocco to northeast Tunisia. The High Atlas Mountains rise to 4,165 m (13,655 ft) at the summit of Jbel Toubkal. Mountain reservoirs provide water for lowland farmers and many tourists visit the Middle Atlas range for winter sports.

RIVER NILE
The Nile is the world's longest river. It flows 6,695 km (4,158 miles) to the Mediterranean Sea.

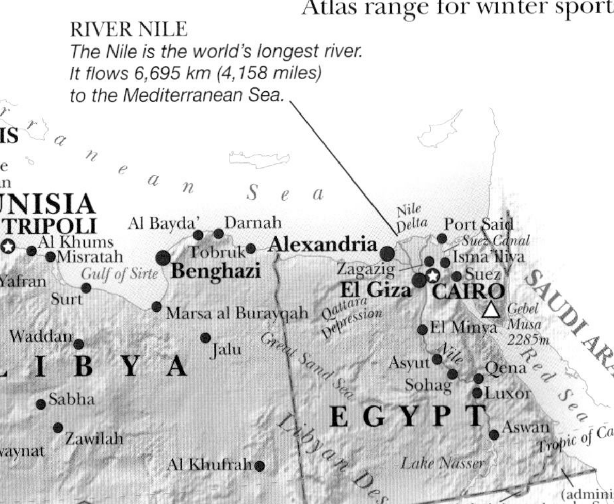

OILFIELDS
The oil reserves of Libya were discovered in the 1950s. Profits from oil were invested in industry and agriculture. New roads, railways, schools, and hospitals were also built. In the 1980s, oil accounted for 99 per cent of Libyan exports. The government has been trying to improve industrial and agricultural outputs in order to reduce this over-dependence on oil.

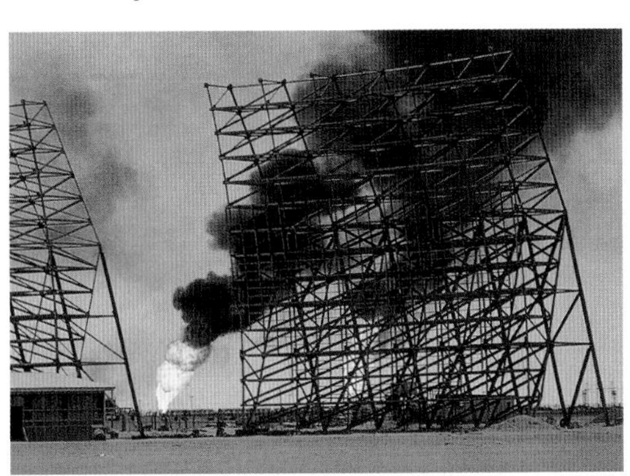

WEAVING
Morocco is famous for its colourful, hand-knotted carpets. Berbers weave carpets, tent hangings, and even produce embroidered boots (left).

SOUK

The souk (market) is the commercial heart of North African towns. Each trade is located in a particular street. Smelly trades, such as tanning leather, are always located as far away from the mosque as possible.

NORTH AMERICA

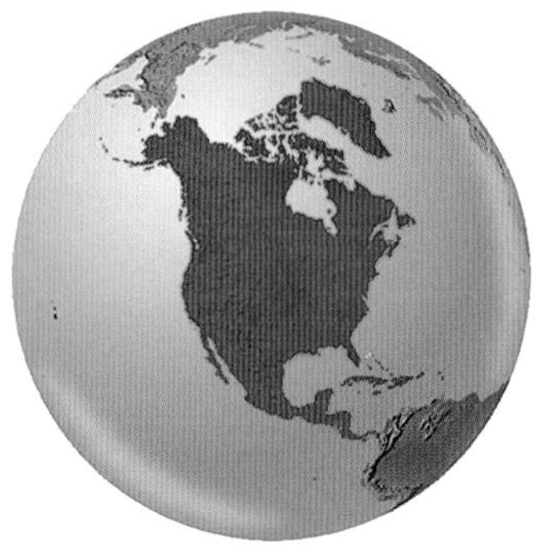

The North American continent stretches from the Arctic Circle to the Tropics and is flanked by the Atlantic, Pacific, and Arctic Oceans. The five Great Lakes of North America form the largest area of fresh water in the world.

THE NORTH AMERICAN continent is a region of great contrasts. Impressive mountain chains – the Appalachians and Rockies – run down its east and west coasts, enclosing a vast, and mostly flat, landscape, criss-crossed by mighty rivers such as the Mississippi and Missouri. The north is blanketed with coniferous forests. The central Great Plains are grasslands, once grazed by huge herds of buffalo. In the north the Arctic region is permanently frozen, while in the south arid deserts and rocky canyons bake in year-round sunshine. Tropical forests cover southern Mexico, and in the southeastern USA, semi-tropical wetlands harbour many endangered species. Native Americans are descendants of the peoples who first settled the continent over 25,000 years ago. They were displaced by European colonists who explored and settled on the continent from the 16th century. Successive waves of immigrants, first from Europe, and then from the rest of the world, continued to settle in North America, drawn by its wealth of natural resources, its fertile prairies, and its vibrant cities – home to most of its population.

THE BIG FREEZE

Severe winter weather is common in the centre of the continent, especially around the Great Lakes, which often freeze over in winter. Chicago, on Lake Michigan, is prone to severe snowstorms, which can cut off the city. In 1998, a freak icestorm in the Canadian Great Lakes region froze power lines, blacking out the area for several days.

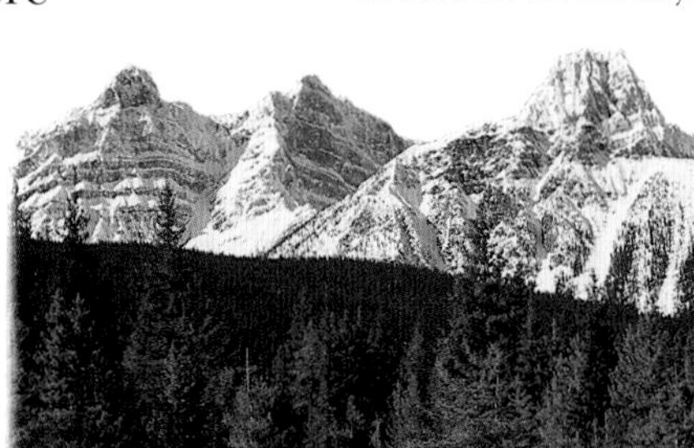

ROCKIES

The Rocky Mountains form the backbone of the American continent, separating the great plains of the east from the high plateaux and basins of the west. Stretching from the Canadian Arctic to New Mexico, they are highest in Colorado, where some 254 mountains are over 4,000 m (13,000 ft). The highest point, Mt Elbert, is 4,312 m (14,149 ft).

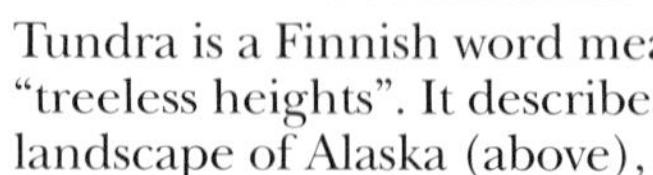

TUNDRA IN ALASKA

Tundra is a Finnish word meaning "treeless heights". It describes the landscape of Alaska (above), where the only vegetation is lichens, mosses, turf and low-lying shrubs. The average temperature is below freezing and in winter it can plummet to -32°C (-89.6°F). These low temperatures leave a layer of permanently frozen soil which can reach depths of 1,525 m (5,000 ft).

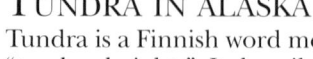

AUTUMN IN NEW ENGLAND

The climate of North America ranges from the hot rainforests of Yucatán to the frozen Arctic. The eastern coast of the USA has four distinct seasons. The colours of autumnal leaves, especially the bright red of the maple, is a famous sight which attracts many tourists.

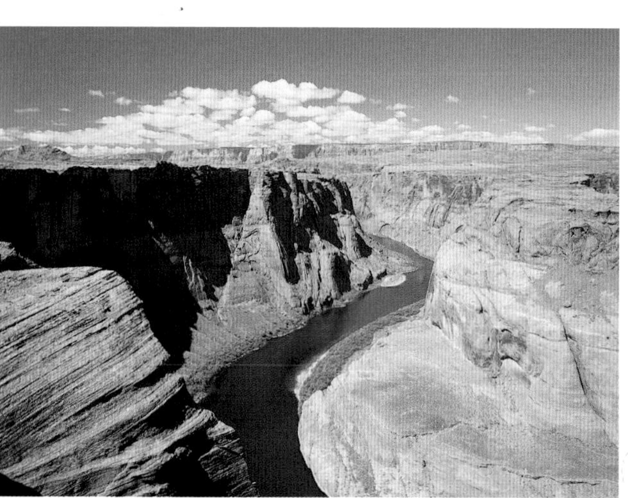

GRAND CANYON

Canyons are dramatic, deep rock formations created by the eroding flow of a river. The most famous is the Grand Canyon in Arizona, formed by the Colorado River. It is 350 km (220 miles) long, and plunges to depths of 1,820 m (5,970 ft). The processes of erosion started about 5-6 million years ago. Some of the rocks at the base are 2 billion years old – the oldest rocks known in the USA.

Limestone, sandstone, shale and granite are eroded at different speeds, giving the Grand Canyon its distinctive layered colours.

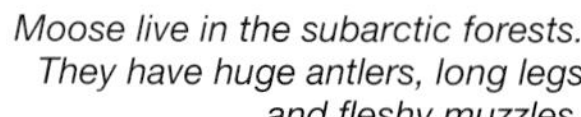

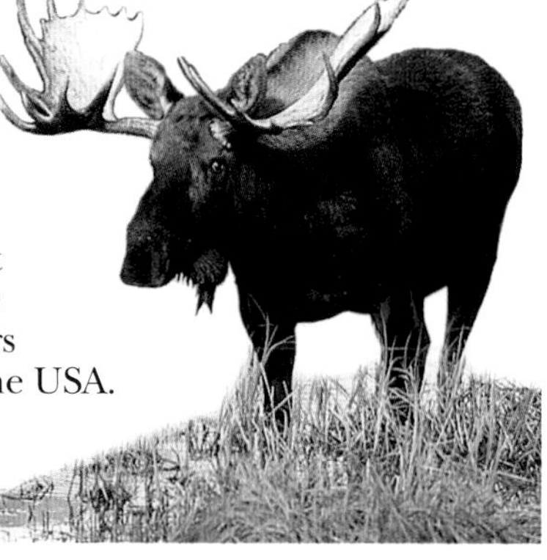

Moose live in the subarctic forests. They have huge antlers, long legs and fleshy muzzles.

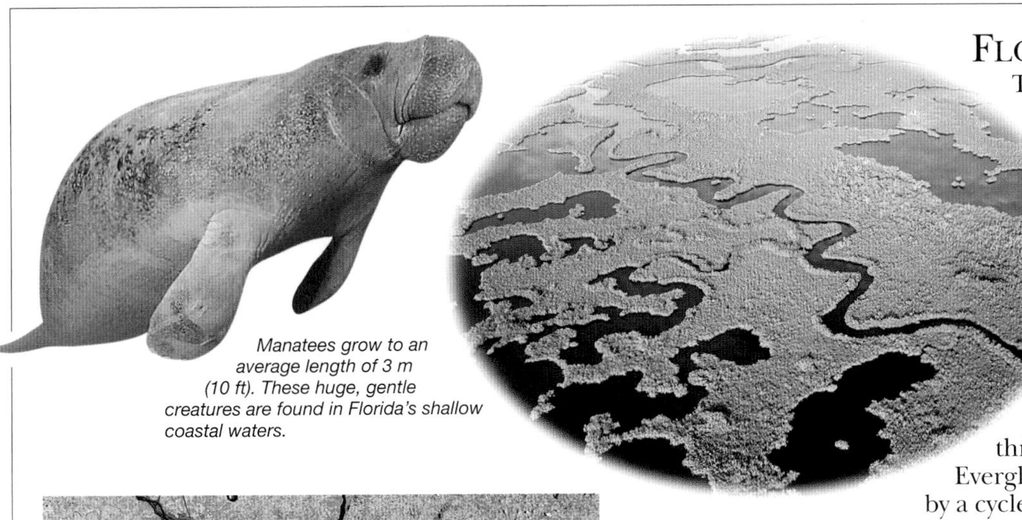

Manatees grow to an average length of 3 m (10 ft). These huge, gentle creatures are found in Florida's shallow coastal waters.

FLORIDA EVERGLADE

The Everglades (left) is a vast area of semi-tropical marshland which stretches across the southwestern part of Florida. A series of low islands, called "hammocks", are home to a great variety of trees, ranging from tropical hardwoods, such as mahogany, to bay trees, eucalyptus and mangroves. Over 400 species of bird are found in the Everglades, and other animals such as alligators, tree frogs, and otters thrive in the swampy conditions. The Everglades' unique ecosystem is supported by a cycle of dry winters and wet summers.

MISSISSIPPI

At 6,020 km (3,740 miles) long, the Mississippi is the main river artery of the USA and one of the busiest commercial waterways in the world. It rises in northern Minnesota, flowing south and receives the waters of the Missouri and Ohio rivers in its middle reaches. It drains into the Gulf of Mexico, where it forms a delta which is moving the shoreline out to sea at a rate of nearly 10 km (6 miles) every 100 years.

This satellite image (above) shows the Mississippi and Missouri rivers converging at St Louis during flooding in 1993.

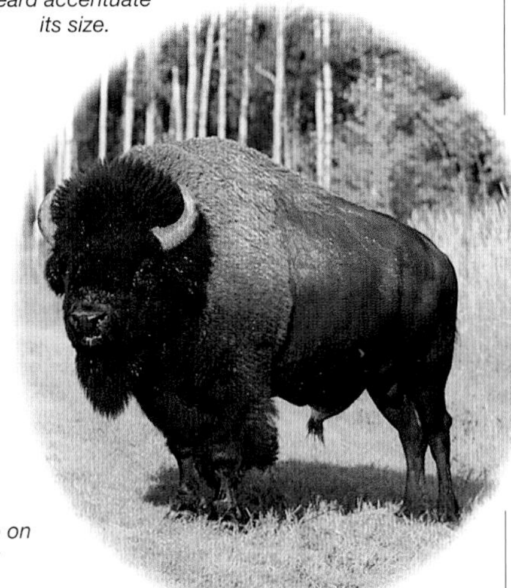

This bison's thick hair and beard accentuate its size.

GREAT PLAINS

The Great Plains, which stretch across the centre of North America, were once areas of grassland (prairie) grazed by huge herds of buffalo (bison). Over-hunting wiped out the buffaloes and, as the frontier of pioneer settlement moved further west throughout the 19th century, the Plains were settled by farmers. Today, this is one of the most intensively farmed regions in the world, a vast producer of both maize and wheat.

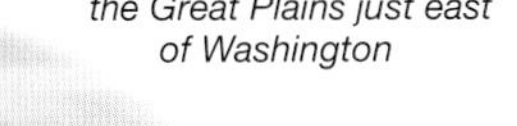

A barn and yellow canola crop on the Great Plains just east of Washington

BISON

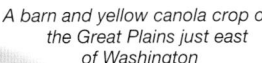

The so-called American buffalo that used to roam the Great Plains of North America is actually a bison. A fully grown bison stands 2 m (6.6 ft) high and weighs more than 900 kgs (1,985 lbs). Traditionally the bison provided food and clothing for the Native Americans living on the Plains. Up until the 18th century, the bison population flourished as the Native American method of hunting had little effect on numbers. It was not until the "white man" arrived with rifles that the herds were dramatically reduced. During construction of the railways in the 19th century, whole herds were shot to feed the rail workers. Today, only 40,000-50,000 bison remain. Most live in reserves, protected by American law.

URBAN LIFE

Much of the North American continent, such as the drier south and west, is sparsley populated, but there are great concentrations of population and industry in urban areas – especially in the temperate regions along the coasts and the shores of the Great Lakes. New York (right) lies at the centre of a vast conurbation of cities, which stretches from Boston to Washington D.C. Accessible to both the Atlantic Ocean and the Hudson River, New York developed as a major port. Today, it is the USA's main financial, commercial, and cultural centre. Toronto is the largest urban area in Canada. It is an important commercial, financial, and industrial centre. The city and its surrounding area produce more than half of Canada's manufactured goods.

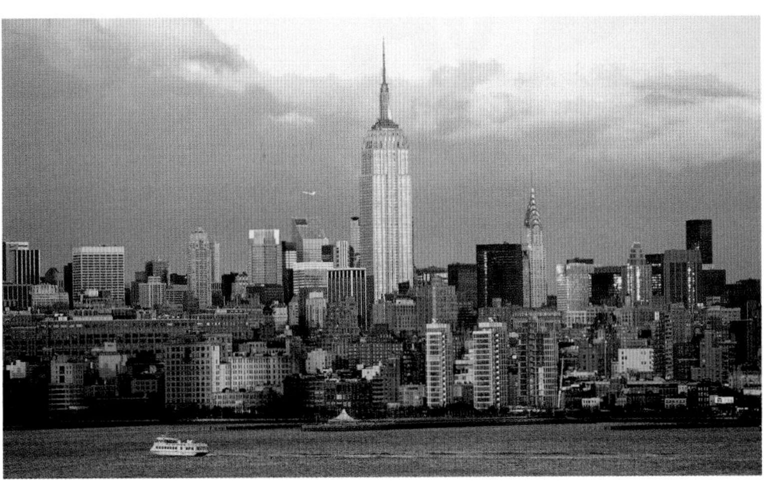

BALD EAGLE
The bald eagle, the only eagle native to North America, has been the US national bird since 1782. It has a wingspan of 2 m (7 ft), and is found mainly along the coasts. It is a protected species in the USA.

OIL RIG

The USA has an abundance of natural resources, including oil, coal, and minerals. Oil was found along the coast of East Texas in 1901. After Alaska, Texas is the USA's main oil-producing state. Oil is transported to refineries on the Gulf Coast by pipeline, tanker, and train. Houston is the capital of the oil business, although it is also the centre of high-tech industries and home to the space shuttle programme.

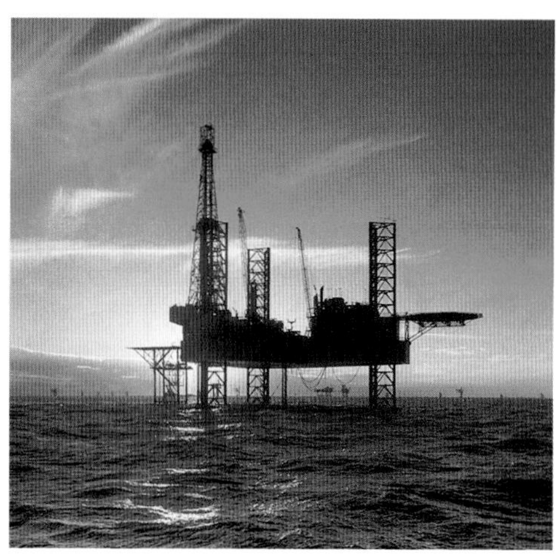

NATIVE AMERICANS

The first people to settle North America crossed into the continent from Asia more than 25,000 years ago. As they settled, they adapted to many different climatic conditions, resources, and terrain. Today, after centuries of conflict with European settlers, many Native Americans now live on Government reservations. The Navajo are the largest tribe in the USA. Most of them live in a large reservation in the Southwest. The tribe is famous for weaving and silverwork and many of their hand-made artefacts are sold to tourists.

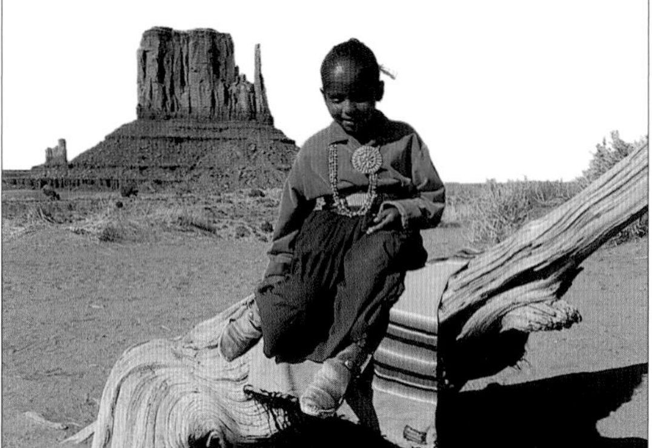

NATURAL HAZARDS

A chain of volcanoes stretches from the US-Mexican border to the southern end of South America. Popocatapetl, one of Mexico's many dormant volcanoes, is 5,452 m (17,888 ft) high, with a crater 152 m (500 ft) deep. Central Mexico is also vulnerable to earthquakes, which often hit the country's most heavily populated regions. In 1985, an earthquake in Mexico City killed some 9,500 people.

El Castillo, the temple-pyramid at Chichén-Itzá is 22m (73ft) high. It stands in the main plaza of the city.

DESERT

The barren deserts of the Southwest are harsh and arid places, swept by fierce wind eddies and baked by searing heat. Only the hardiest animals, such as snakes, lizards, and reptiles, can survive these conditions. Spiny-leaved Joshua trees thrive in the desert, and can live for up to 1,000 years.

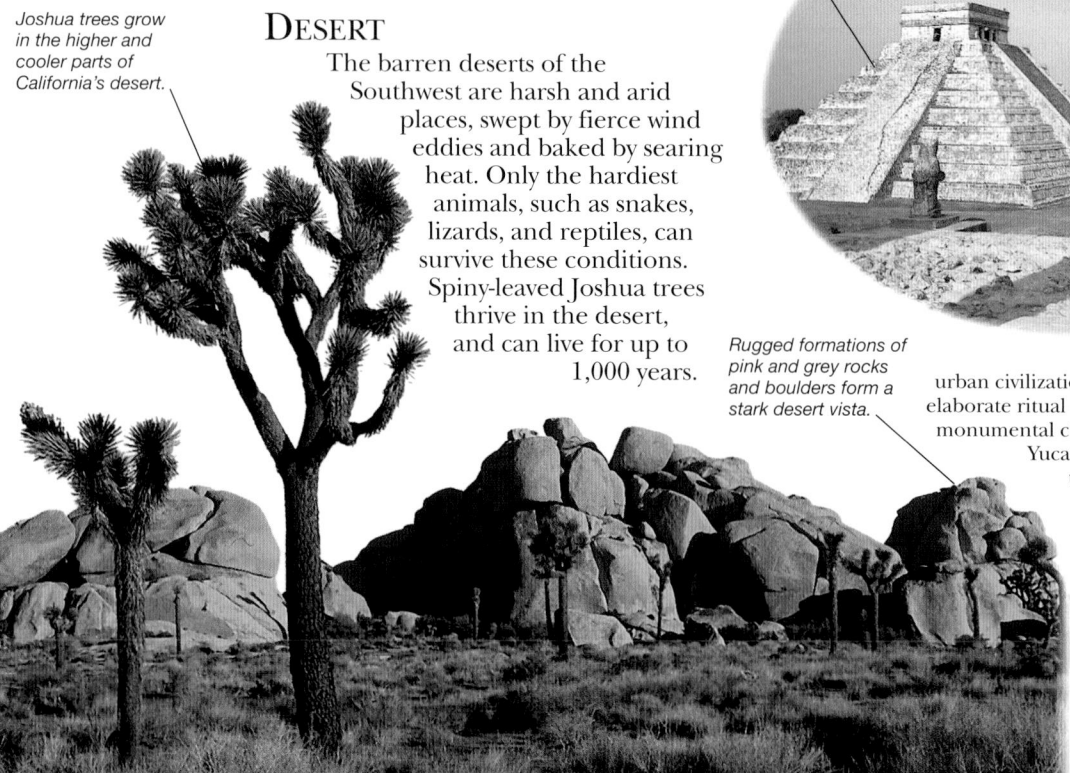

Joshua trees grow in the higher and cooler parts of California's desert.

Rugged formations of pink and grey rocks and boulders form a stark desert vista.

CHICHEN-ITZA
The history of Mexico's urban civilizations dates back to c. 1150 B.C., and the elaborate ritual centres of the Olmec. The Maya built monumental cities and temples in the jungles of the Yucatán from c. 200 A.D. They are thought to be the first American civilization to develop a writing system. The Mayan pyramid-temple at Chichén Itzá dates to the 12th century A.D.

Find out more

CANADA
MEXICO
NORTH AMERICAN WILDLIFE
UNITED STATES OF AMERICA

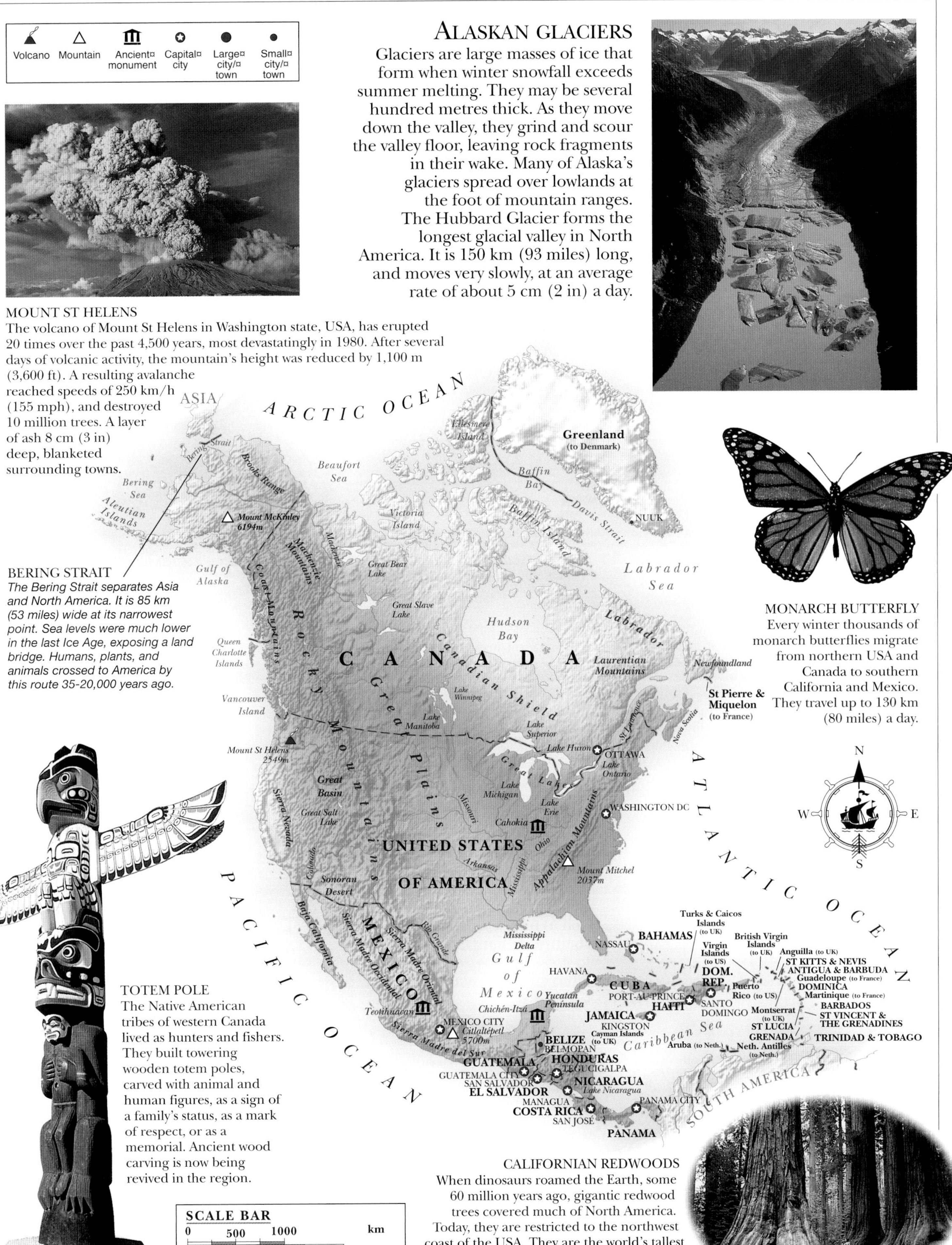

ALASKAN GLACIERS

Glaciers are large masses of ice that form when winter snowfall exceeds summer melting. They may be several hundred metres thick. As they move down the valley, they grind and scour the valley floor, leaving rock fragments in their wake. Many of Alaska's glaciers spread over lowlands at the foot of mountain ranges. The Hubbard Glacier forms the longest glacial valley in North America. It is 150 km (93 miles) long, and moves very slowly, at an average rate of about 5 cm (2 in) a day.

MOUNT ST HELENS
The volcano of Mount St Helens in Washington state, USA, has erupted 20 times over the past 4,500 years, most devastatingly in 1980. After several days of volcanic activity, the mountain's height was reduced by 1,100 m (3,600 ft). A resulting avalanche reached speeds of 250 km/h (155 mph), and destroyed 10 million trees. A layer of ash 8 cm (3 in) deep, blanketed surrounding towns.

BERING STRAIT
The Bering Strait separates Asia and North America. It is 85 km (53 miles) wide at its narrowest point. Sea levels were much lower in the last Ice Age, exposing a land bridge. Humans, plants, and animals crossed to America by this route 35-20,000 years ago.

MONARCH BUTTERFLY
Every winter thousands of monarch butterflies migrate from northern USA and Canada to southern California and Mexico. They travel up to 130 km (80 miles) a day.

TOTEM POLE
The Native American tribes of western Canada lived as hunters and fishers. They built towering wooden totem poles, carved with animal and human figures, as a sign of a family's status, as a mark of respect, or as a memorial. Ancient wood carving is now being revived in the region.

CALIFORNIAN REDWOODS
When dinosaurs roamed the Earth, some 60 million years ago, gigantic redwood trees covered much of North America. Today, they are restricted to the northwest coast of the USA. They are the world's tallest trees, reaching heights of 112 m (368 ft).

NORTH AMERICAN WILDLIFE

This map shows the main kinds of habitat in North America.

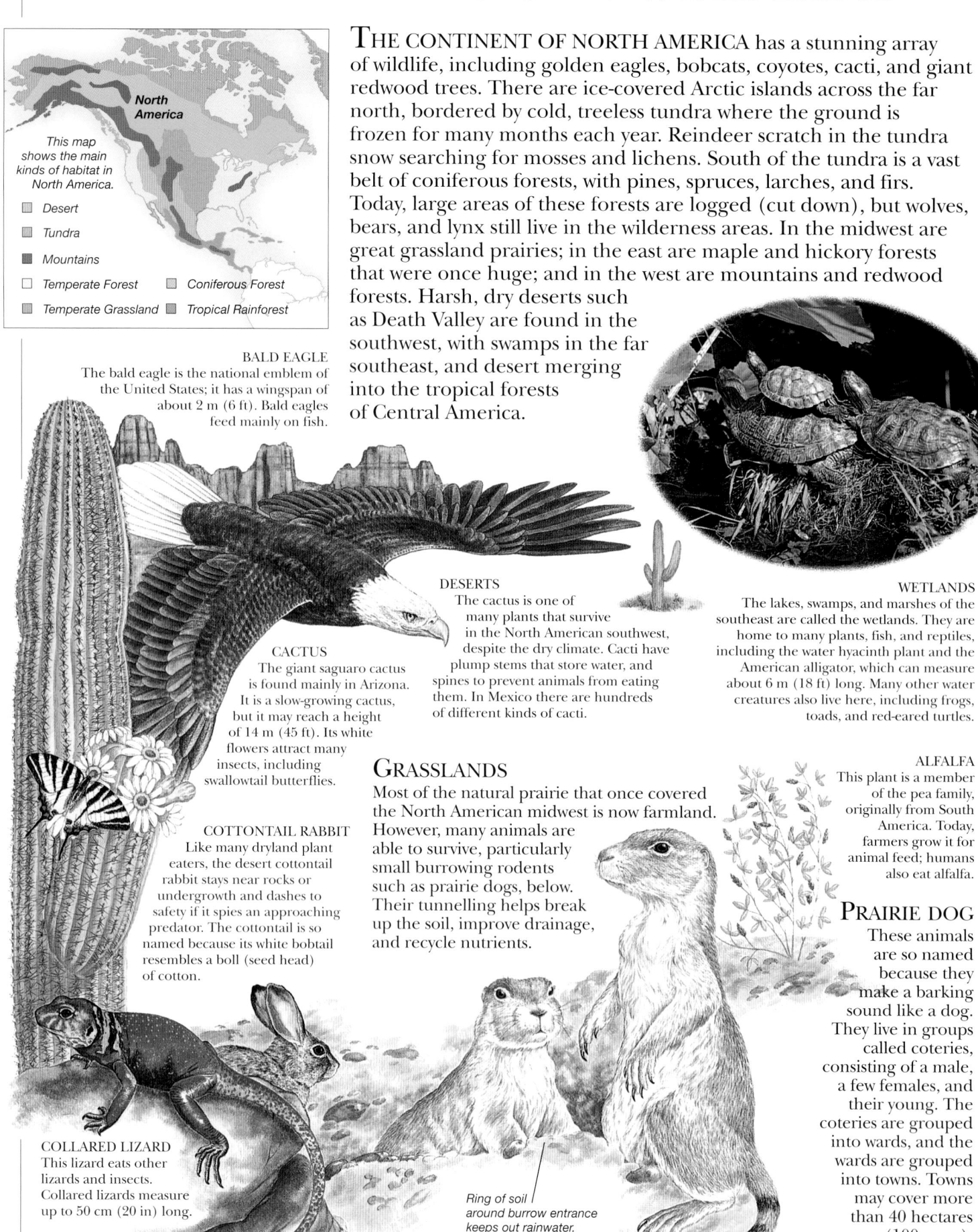

Temperate Grassland
Tropical Rainforest
Ring of soil around burrow entrance keeps out rainwater.

THE CONTINENT OF NORTH AMERICA has a stunning array of wildlife, including golden eagles, bobcats, coyotes, cacti, and giant redwood trees. There are ice-covered Arctic islands across the far north, bordered by cold, treeless tundra where the ground is frozen for many months each year. Reindeer scratch in the tundra snow searching for mosses and lichens. South of the tundra is a vast belt of coniferous forests, with pines, spruces, larches, and firs. Today, large areas of these forests are logged (cut down), but wolves, bears, and lynx still live in the wilderness areas. In the midwest are great grassland prairies; in the east are maple and hickory forests that were once huge; and in the west are mountains and redwood forests. Harsh, dry deserts such as Death Valley are found in the southwest, with swamps in the far southeast, and desert merging into the tropical forests of Central America.

BALD EAGLE
The bald eagle is the national emblem of the United States; it has a wingspan of about 2 m (6 ft). Bald eagles feed mainly on fish.

DESERTS
The cactus is one of many plants that survive in the North American southwest, despite the dry climate. Cacti have plump stems that store water, and spines to prevent animals from eating them. In Mexico there are hundreds of different kinds of cacti.

WETLANDS
The lakes, swamps, and marshes of the southeast are called the wetlands. They are home to many plants, fish, and reptiles, including the water hyacinth plant and the American alligator, which can measure about 6 m (18 ft) long. Many other water creatures also live here, including frogs, toads, and red-eared turtles.

CACTUS
The giant saguaro cactus is found mainly in Arizona. It is a slow-growing cactus, but it may reach a height of 14 m (45 ft). Its white flowers attract many insects, including swallowtail butterflies.

GRASSLANDS

Most of the natural prairie that once covered the North American midwest is now farmland. However, many animals are able to survive, particularly small burrowing rodents such as prairie dogs, below. Their tunnelling helps break up the soil, improve drainage, and recycle nutrients.

ALFALFA
This plant is a member of the pea family, originally from South America. Today, farmers grow it for animal feed; humans also eat alfalfa.

COTTONTAIL RABBIT
Like many dryland plant eaters, the desert cottontail rabbit stays near rocks or undergrowth and dashes to safety if it spies an approaching predator. The cottontail is so named because its white bobtail resembles a boll (seed head) of cotton.

PRAIRIE DOG

These animals are so named because they make a barking sound like a dog. They live in groups called coteries, consisting of a male, a few females, and their young. The coteries are grouped into wards, and the wards are grouped into towns. Towns may cover more than 40 hectares (100 acres).

Temperate Forest

COLLARED LIZARD
This lizard eats other lizards and insects. Collared lizards measure up to 50 cm (20 in) long.

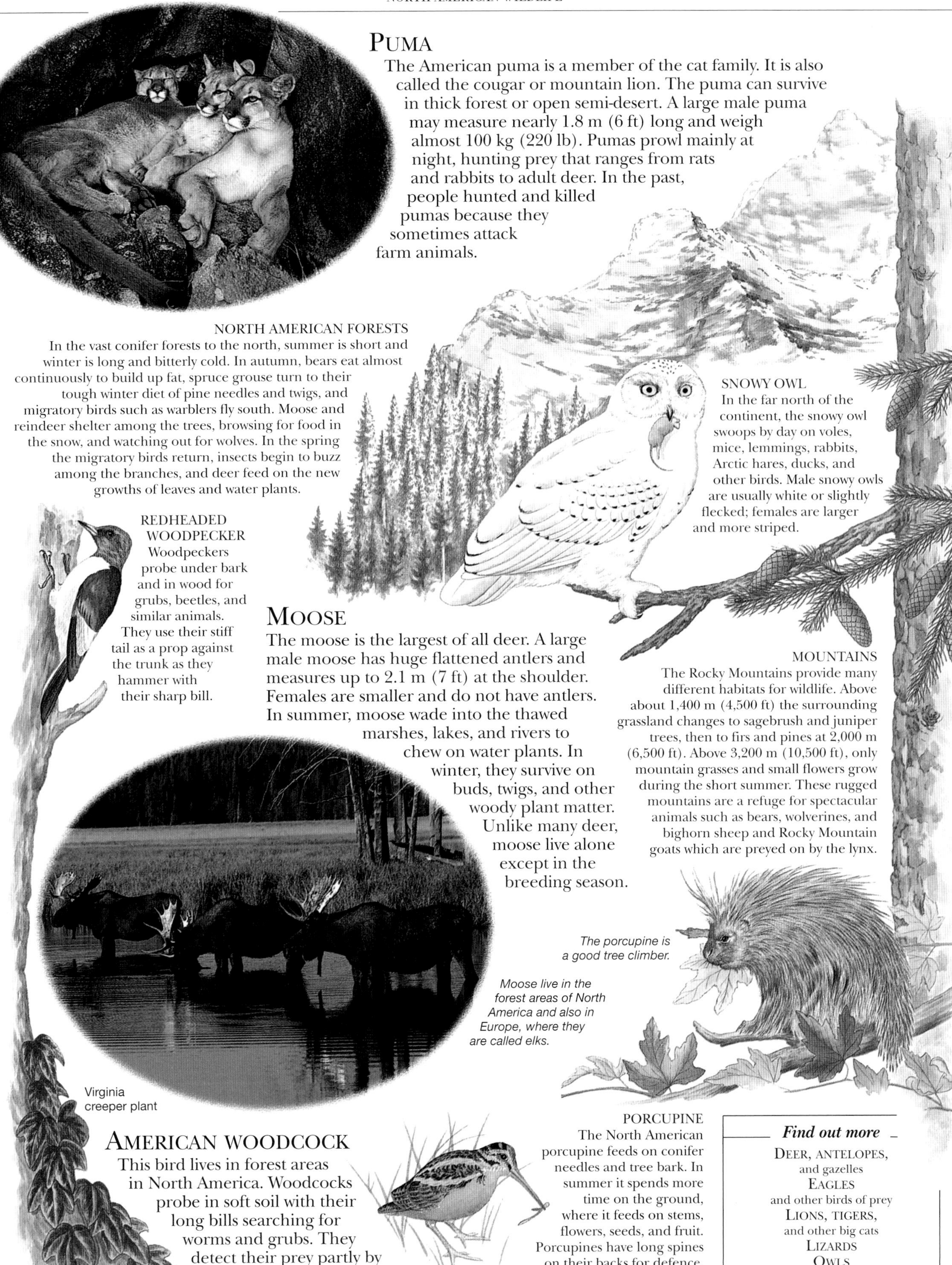

Puma

The American puma is a member of the cat family. It is also called the cougar or mountain lion. The puma can survive in thick forest or open semi-desert. A large male puma may measure nearly 1.8 m (6 ft) long and weigh almost 100 kg (220 lb). Pumas prowl mainly at night, hunting prey that ranges from rats and rabbits to adult deer. In the past, people hunted and killed pumas because they sometimes attack farm animals.

NORTH AMERICAN FORESTS
In the vast conifer forests to the north, summer is short and winter is long and bitterly cold. In autumn, bears eat almost continuously to build up fat, spruce grouse turn to their tough winter diet of pine needles and twigs, and migratory birds such as warblers fly south. Moose and reindeer shelter among the trees, browsing for food in the snow, and watching out for wolves. In the spring the migratory birds return, insects begin to buzz among the branches, and deer feed on the new growths of leaves and water plants.

SNOWY OWL
In the far north of the continent, the snowy owl swoops by day on voles, mice, lemmings, rabbits, Arctic hares, ducks, and other birds. Male snowy owls are usually white or slightly flecked; females are larger and more striped.

REDHEADED WOODPECKER
Woodpeckers probe under bark and in wood for grubs, beetles, and similar animals. They use their stiff tail as a prop against the trunk as they hammer with their sharp bill.

Moose

The moose is the largest of all deer. A large male moose has huge flattened antlers and measures up to 2.1 m (7 ft) at the shoulder. Females are smaller and do not have antlers. In summer, moose wade into the thawed marshes, lakes, and rivers to chew on water plants. In winter, they survive on buds, twigs, and other woody plant matter. Unlike many deer, moose live alone except in the breeding season.

MOUNTAINS
The Rocky Mountains provide many different habitats for wildlife. Above about 1,400 m (4,500 ft) the surrounding grassland changes to sagebrush and juniper trees, then to firs and pines at 2,000 m (6,500 ft). Above 3,200 m (10,500 ft), only mountain grasses and small flowers grow during the short summer. These rugged mountains are a refuge for spectacular animals such as bears, wolverines, and bighorn sheep and Rocky Mountain goats which are preyed on by the lynx.

The porcupine is a good tree climber.

Moose live in the forest areas of North America and also in Europe, where they are called elks.

Virginia creeper plant

American woodcock

This bird lives in forest areas in North America. Woodcocks probe in soft soil with their long bills searching for worms and grubs. They detect their prey partly by smell, and by using the sensitive tip of the bill.

PORCUPINE
The North American porcupine feeds on conifer needles and tree bark. In summer it spends more time on the ground, where it feeds on stems, flowers, seeds, and fruit. Porcupines have long spines on their backs for defence. Although they look like hedgehogs, the two animals are not related.

Find out more
DEER, ANTELOPES, and gazelles
EAGLES and other birds of prey
LIONS, TIGERS, and other big cats
LIZARDS
OWLS
RABBITS AND HARES

NORTHERN IRELAND

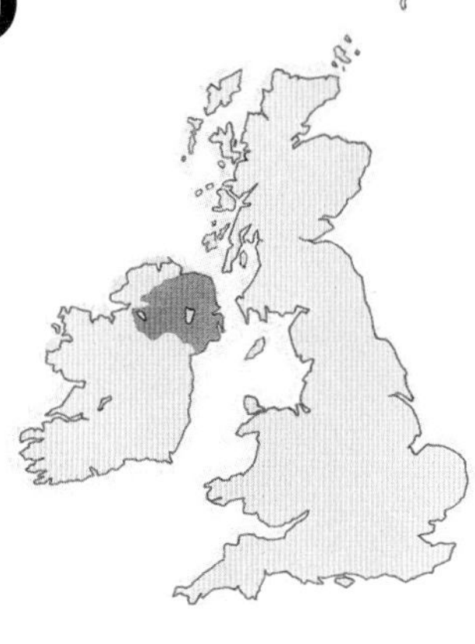

Northern Ireland occupies the northeastern part of Ireland. It is bordered by the Republic of Ireland to the south and west, with the Irish Sea to the east.

LYING JUST ACROSS THE IRISH SEA from Scotland, Northern Ireland is part of the United Kingdom. It covers an area of 14,121 sq km (5,452 sq miles), and has a population of just over 1.7 million people, split between a Protestant majority and a slightly smaller number of Roman Catholics. Also known as Ulster, Northern Ireland consists of the six counties of Antrim, Londonderry, Tyrone, Fermanagh, Armagh and Down. Remaining part of the United Kingdom when southern Ireland split away in 1920, Northern Ireland has had a troubled history, dominated by religious and political conflict. Since the late 1990s, peace initiatives have been taking place. In 1998, Catholics and Protestants agreed to share power in a self-governing assembly, but it has proved difficult to make this arrangement work.

BELFAST

Belfast is the biggest city in Northern Ireland, and capital of the province. Sitting on the northeast coast, Belfast is a major UK port and manufacturing centre, which was once world famous for its engineering works and shipyards. The *Titanic,* for instance, was built in Belfast. Political troubles have divided the city in recent years.

GIANT'S CAUSEWAY

A major landmark, the Giant's Causeway lies off the coast of County Antrim on the north coast. The thousands of rocks that make up the Causeway are shaped like hexagons, or eight-sided columns. They were created when lava from underground volcanoes cooled in the sea some 60 million years ago. Its name comes from a legend that giants built a causeway to Scotland so they could cross the Irish Sea.

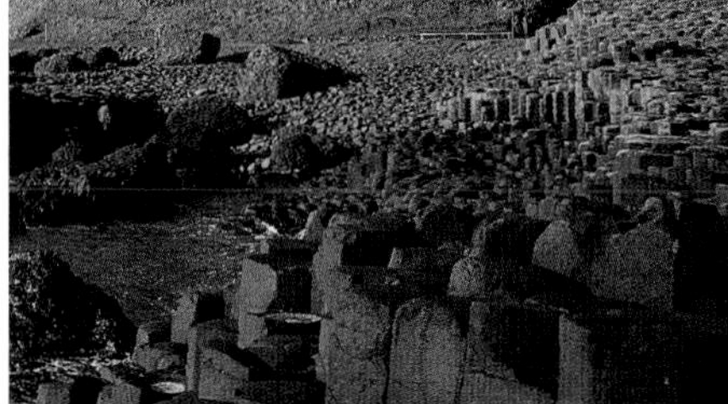

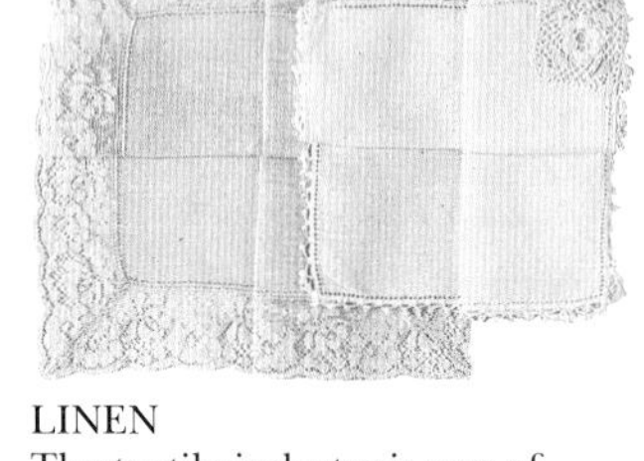

LINEN

The textile industry is one of Northern Ireland's chief industries. Linen-making is traditional. Woven from flax, linen from Northern Ireland is among the finest in the world. Farming and engineering are also important to the economy.

MUSIC

There is a long tradition of music-making in Northern Ireland, and many famous musicians have been born there. Music varies from the pipe and drum bands of the Orange Order, through to traditional Gaelic music and more modern pop music.

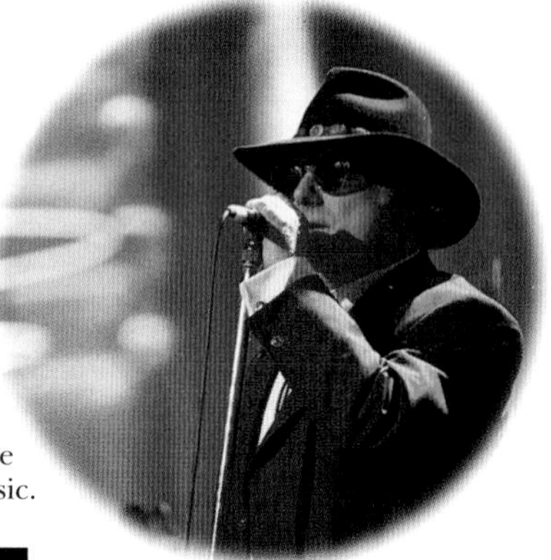

The famous singer Van Morrison grew up in Northern Ireland.

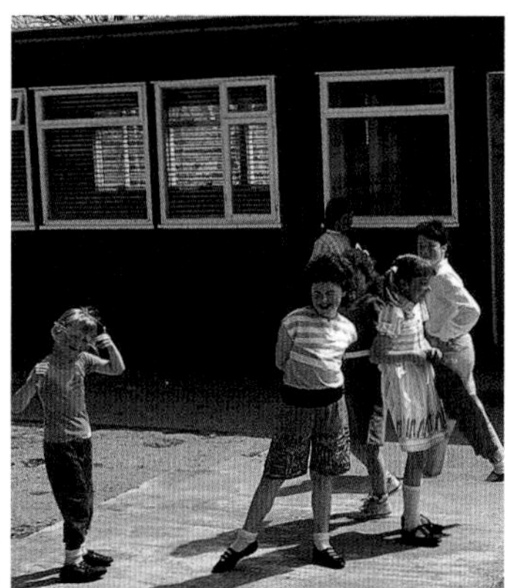

PEOPLE

Many of Belfast's children have grown up surrounded by violence, caused by the long-running conflict between Protestants and Roman Catholics. Most Protestants wish to remain part of the United Kingdom, although some favour self-government. Many Catholics would like to unite with the Republic of Ireland in the south.

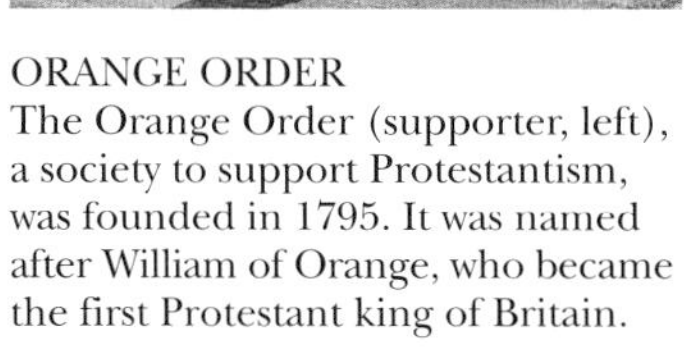

ORANGE ORDER

The Orange Order (supporter, left), a society to support Protestantism, was founded in 1795. It was named after William of Orange, who became the first Protestant king of Britain.

Find out more

IRELAND, HISTORY OF
UNITED KINGDOM
UNITED KINGDOM, HISTORY OF

NUCLEAR AGE

IN 1945, THE FIRST atomic bombs were dropped on the Japanese cities of Hiroshima and Nagasaki. The years since 1945 have sometimes been called the nuclear age because the knowledge that nuclear bombs can destroy civilization has affected political decisions and attitudes towards war. The term nuclear age also describes the growth of nuclear energy. In 1953, U.S. President Eisenhower launched the Atoms for Peace campaign to develop nuclear power for peaceful uses, such as generating electricity. At first nuclear energy was welcomed; today many people believe that it is dangerous. The nuclear arms "race" between the United States and the Soviet Union, which began in 1945, caused political tension for years. By the 1980s, the United States and the Soviet Union owned enough nuclear weapons to destroy every living thing on the Earth. Many people wanted to rid the world of nuclear weapons, and in the late 1980s both superpowers began to disarm.

NUCLEAR FISSION
In 1939, the German scientists Fritz Strassman (above left) and Otto Hahn discovered that energy could be created by splitting uranium atoms into two. This process, called nuclear fission, was later developed to produce the energy to create electricity and the explosion to make a nuclear bomb.

HIROSHIMA
On 6 August 1945, an American warplane dropped an atomic bomb on the city of Hiroshima to force Japan to surrender in World War II. The city was destroyed, and about 130,000 people were killed. The people of Hiroshima commemorate the event every year in "Peace City", a place where the ruins have been left untouched in memory of those killed.

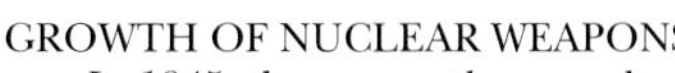

GROWTH OF NUCLEAR WEAPONS
In 1945, there were three nuclear weapons in existence. By 1962, the number had risen to about 2,000. By 1990, the total number had grown to about 25,000. Together, these weapons had one million times more power than the bomb dropped on Hiroshima. The United States and the Soviet Union owned the most nuclear weapons, but six other countries also developed nuclear arms: Britain, France, China, India, Pakistan, and Israel.

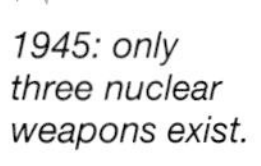

1945: only three nuclear weapons exist.

1962: the number of nuclear weapons is in the thousands.

1990: the number of nuclear weapons is over 25,000.

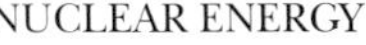

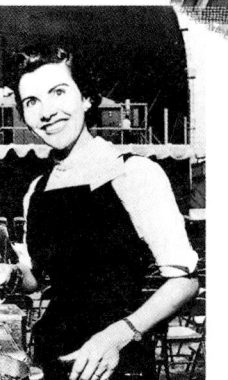

NUCLEAR ENERGY
In 1954, the world's first nuclear power station opened in the Soviet Union. Today there are about 440 nuclear power stations producing 15 per cent of the world's energy. Above is a 1950s cooking demonstration: a woman cooks hamburgers using electricity produced by atomic power.

ANTI-NUCLEAR MOVEMENTS
Opposition to nuclear weapons began in the 1950s as people realized that nobody would survive a nuclear war. Throughout the world people adopted the peace symbol (left) as they demonstrated against nuclear weapons.

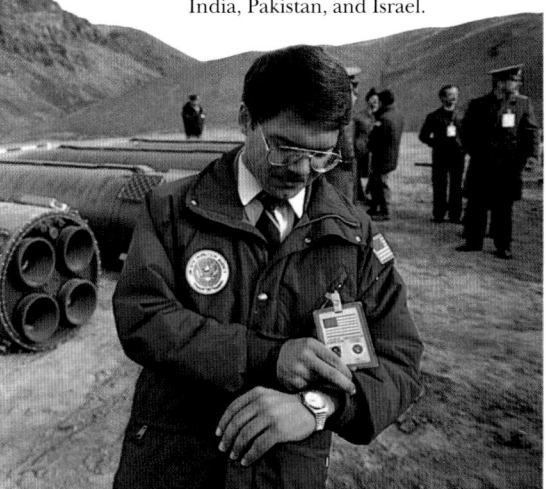

NUCLEAR DISARMAMENT
During the late 1980s, the United States and the former Soviet Union discussed nuclear disarmament. In 1987, U.S. President Reagan and Soviet Premier Gorbachev agreed to dismantle some intermediate-range nuclear weapons (left). In 1993, U.S. President Bush and Russian President Yeltsin signed a treaty agreeing to reduce their nuclear arsenals by two-thirds within ten years.

Find out more

NUCLEAR ENERGY
SOVIET UNION, HISTORY OF
UNITED STATES OF AMERICA, history of
WORLD WAR II

NUCLEAR ENERGY

THE ATOMS THAT MAKE UP everything in the universe are the source of a huge amount of energy called nuclear energy. Nuclear energy produces the searing heat and light of the Sun, the deadly explosions of nuclear weapons, and vast amounts of electricity in nuclear power stations. Nuclear energy is based on the fact that matter and energy are different forms of the same thing, and one can be converted into the other. In a nuclear reaction, a tiny amount of matter changes into an enormous amount of energy. The nuclear reaction occurs in the nuclei (centres) of atoms. This can happen in two ways: when the nucleus of a heavy atom splits, in a process called fission, and when two lightweight nuclei join together, in a process called fusion. In nuclear weapons, fission or fusion occurs in a split second. By contrast, nuclear power stations produce electricity from fission reactions that work at a controlled rate.

Experimental nuclear fusion reactor near Oxford, England

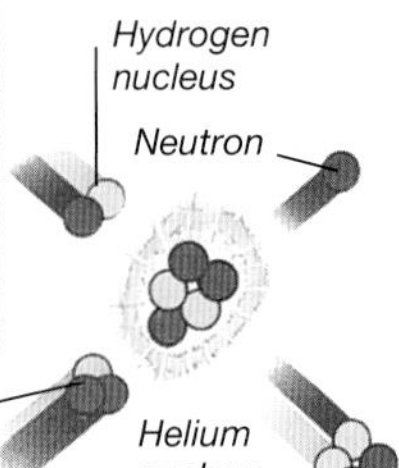

NUCLEAR FUSION
Scientists are trying to build reactors that use nuclear fusion, a process which produces less dangerous waste than nuclear fission (below). Nuclear fusion occurs when hydrogen atoms smash together and join to form heavier atoms of helium. However, nuclear fusion is extremely difficult to achieve. Hydrogen atoms must be held by a magnetic field and heated to a temperature higher than that in the Sun's centre for fusion to occur.

Neutron hits nucleus of uranium atom.

Fission occurs, releasing energy and neutrons.

NUCLEAR FISSION
Nuclear power stations produce energy from the fission of atoms of uranium dioxide. The impact of a particle called a neutron makes an atom of uranium split. This releases heat energy and two or three neutrons. The neutrons strike other uranium atoms and make them divide. Soon, many atoms begin to split, producing a huge amount of energy.

Reactor core contains pellets of uranium dioxide fuel held in fuel rods. Two thimble-sized pellets would produce enough electricity for a person for one year.

Pump for high-pressure water system

If neutrons travel too rapidly, they bounce off uranium atoms without producing fission. The fuel is surrounded by water, which slows the neutrons down so they produce fission. A material that slows neutrons in a reactor is called a moderator.

Control rods absorb neutrons and slow down the nuclear reaction. In an emergency, the control rods drop into the reactor core and shut off the nuclear reaction.

The high-pressure water flows through pipes in a steam generator which transfers its heat to a separate water system. The water in this second system boils to form steam.

Water is pumped around the reactor core at high pressure in a sealed circuit. The nuclear reactions heat the water to more than 300°C (570°F), but the high pressure keeps it from turning into steam.

Steam spins turbines that drive generators, producing electricity.

A third water circuit acts as a coolant, changing the steam back into water which returns to the steam generator once again.

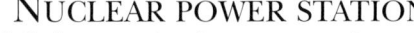

Pressurized water reactor (PWR)

Protective clothing worn when handling nuclear waste

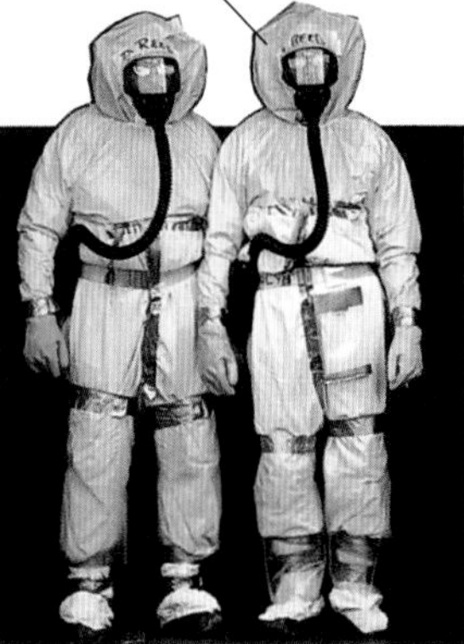

NUCLEAR RADIATION

Some waste from nuclear power stations is radioactive – it produces deadly nuclear radiation consisting of tiny particles or invisible waves that can damage living cells. Some radioactive waste may last for thousands of years, so it is buried underground in sealed containers. Many people are concerned about the dangers of nuclear waste and are demanding an end to nuclear energy production.

NUCLEAR POWER STATION

A fission reaction becomes continuous only if there is a certain amount of fuel present, called the critical mass. In a nuclear reactor, rods contain uranium fuel. The fuel rods are placed close together to provide the critical mass that starts the reaction.

Find out more

ATOMS AND MOLECULES
ENERGY
NUCLEAR AGE
PHYSICS
RADIOACTIVITY
SOVIET UNION, HISTORY OF
WEAPONS

NUMBERS

WHEN WE WANT TO KNOW how many things we have, or measure how large something is, we use numbers. Numbers are symbols that describe an amount. There are only ten number symbols: 0, 1, 2, 3, 4, 5, 6, 7, 8, and 9, but they can be put together in many different ways to make other numbers of any size. As well as counting and measuring, numbers can also be used to work out time and distances, or to put things in order. The skill of working with numbers is called arithmetic. Early humans probably used their fingers and thumbs to count. Because we have ten digits – eight fingers and two thumbs – we developed a system of counting that was based on tens. This is called the decimal system, after the Latin word for ten. Numbers are just as important as words for passing on information. They can be written down, so that other people can read and use them.

FRACTIONS
Sometimes the number 1 has to be divided into portions. Parts of a whole number are called fractions.

COUNTING

When people needed to count higher than ten, they used objects such as pebbles to represent multiples of ten. So, five pebbles and three fingers stood for the number 53. Making calculations with pebbles led to the invention of the abacus, and later the slide rule, and calculator.

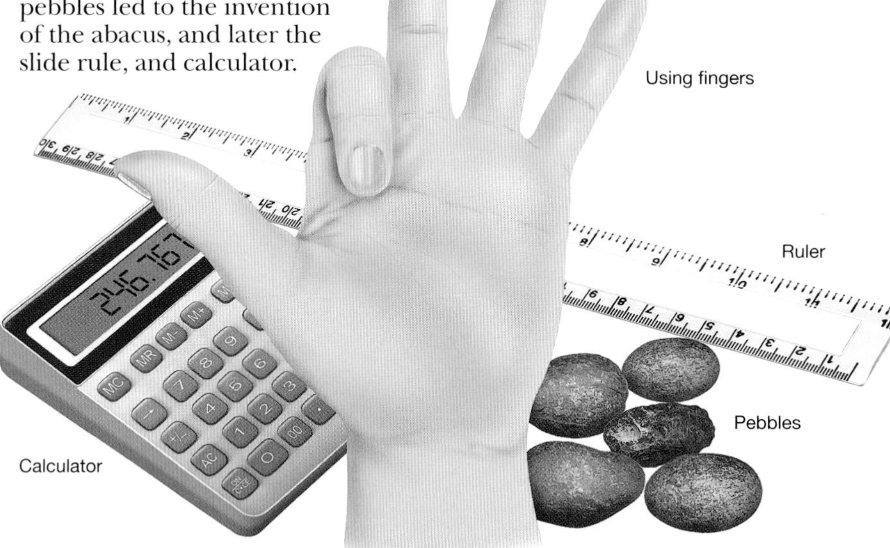

Using fingers

Ruler

Pebbles

Calculator

Cardinal numbers

A fraction, two-thirds

A decimal fraction, ten and sixty-five hundredths

NUMBERS IN HISTORY
People have invented many different ways of representing numbers with symbols. The modern decimal system has now been taken up all over the world, but older systems are still used in a few places. Even the Ancient Roman system is used sometimes, especially on clock faces.

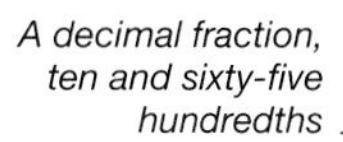

The Babylonians invented a number system based on ten about 3,500 years ago, but the symbols took a long time to write down.

I II III IV V VI VII VIII IX X

The Ancient Roman number system goes back to about 500 B.C. It is an awkward system, but it is still sometimes used today.

In about 200 B.C. the Hindus used a number system based on ten. About 1,400 years ago they modified it to include zero.

By the 15th century, Hindu-Arabic numbers had replaced Roman numerals as the most popular number system.

0 1 2 3 4 5 6 7 8 9 10

Today, most countries use a modern version of the Hindu-Arabic number system, because it makes calculations easy.

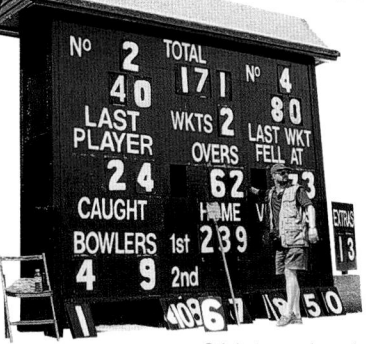

Cricket scoreboard

TYPES OF NUMBER

Whole numbers that stand for quantities, such as 1, 2, or 3, are called cardinal numbers. Numbers that put things in order, such as 1st, 2nd, or 3rd, are known as ordinal numbers. In a fraction, the number below the line shows how many parts the whole is divided into; the number above shows how many of those parts are being described.

USING NUMBERS
If you look around, you will see how numbers are used in everyday life. For example, scoreboards, speed limits, distances, prices, TV channels, and the time of day are all shown using numbers. Page numbers in the index of this book show where to find the topics that interest you. Money is also divided into units to make it simple to understand.

Find out more
COMPUTERS
GEOMETRY
MATHEMATICS
STATISTICS

OCEANS AND SEAS

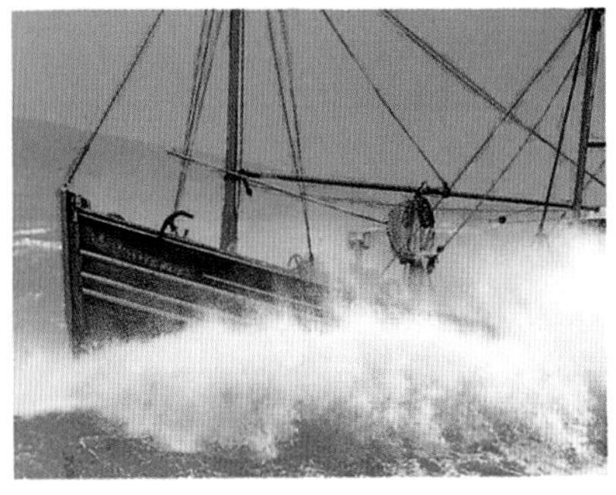

OCEAN HUNTERS
Fishing boats sail the oceans and seas to bring us the fish and other sea creatures that we eat. The best fishing grounds are in shallow seas, where the water teems with fish. But catches must be controlled; otherwise the numbers of fish will fall as the fish fail to breed.

YOUR FEET MAY BE RESTING firmly on the ground, but more than two thirds of our planet is covered with water. Oceans and seas make up 71 per cent of the Earth's surface. They influence the climate, supply us with food, power, and valuable minerals, and provide a home for a fascinating range of plant and animal life.

The oceans and seas began millions of years ago when the Earth cooled from its original molten state. Water vapour escaped from inside the Earth in volcanic eruptions, cooled, and fell as rain. It filled vast hollows and basins surrounding rocky land masses. These gradually moved around to form the continents and oceans as they exist today. As rivers formed on the land and flowed into the seas, they dissolved minerals from the rocks, making the oceans and seas salty.

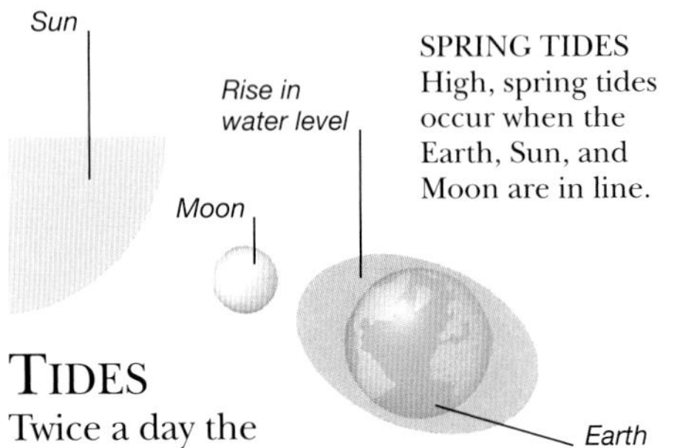

SPRING TIDES
High, spring tides occur when the Earth, Sun, and Moon are in line.

TIDES

Twice a day the level of the seas rises and falls. These changes in level are called tides. They are caused mainly by the pull of the Moon's gravity on the Earth. When the Moon lies directly over the ocean, its gravity pulls the water towards it. Water also rises on the opposite side of the Earth, because the Earth itself is pulled towards the Moon.

THE WORLD'S OCEANS AND SEAS
Oceans are vast bodies of water, usually separating the continents. The Pacific Ocean, which is the largest and deepest, lies between America and Asia and covers more than a third of the globe. The others, in order of size, are the Atlantic, Indian, and Arctic oceans. The Arctic Ocean lies between the land masses around the North Pole and is largely covered by ice. Seas, bays, and gulfs are smaller bodies of water that lie between arms of land, or between islands and land masses. Some, such as the Caspian and Dead seas, are entirely surrounded by land and are really not seas but large lakes.

Pacific Ocean
Indian Ocean
North Pacific Ocean
South Atlantic Ocean
Atlantic Ocean
Indian Ocean

The Pacific, Atlantic, and Indian oceans surround Antarctica. This area is sometimes called the Antarctic Ocean.

The Arctic Ocean is an ice-covered ocean at the North Pole.

OCEAN CURRENTS

The water in the oceans is constantly moving in great circular streams, or currents, which can flow about as fast as you walk. Winds blow the surface layer of the oceans to form these currents, which carry warm or cold water along the shores of continents, greatly affecting the weather there. Sometimes, currents flow deep below the surface, moving in the opposite direction to surface currents. For example, surface currents carry warm water away from the equator, while currents deep beneath the sea bring cold water back to the equator. Most seas have strong currents. But the waters of the Sargasso Sea, which lies in the North Atlantic Ocean, are almost still, causing the sea to become choked with seaweed.

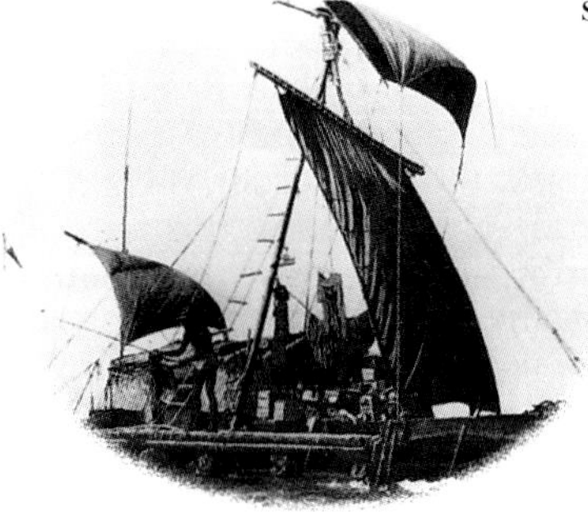

THE *KON TIKI* EXPEDITION
Early peoples may have used the currents to travel across oceans. In 1947 the *Kon Tiki* expedition, led by Norwegian explorer Thor Heyerdahl, tested this theory by sailing a light wooden raft from Peru to the Polynesian Islands.

GULF STREAM
Water heated by the Sun flows out from the Gulf of Mexico. This warm current crosses the Atlantic Ocean and flows around the shores of western Europe. There the winter weather is mild, while places on the other side of the ocean away from the current are freezing cold.

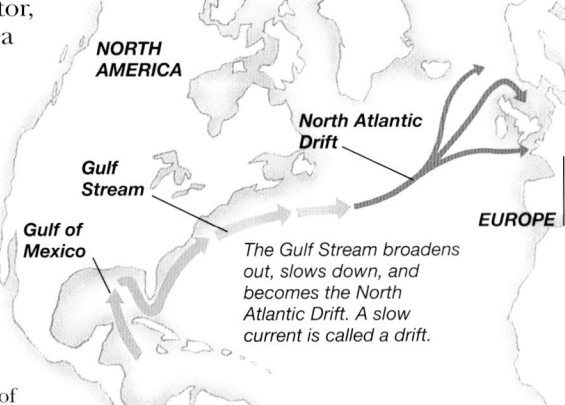

NORTH AMERICA
North Atlantic Drift
Gulf Stream
Gulf of Mexico
EUROPE

The Gulf Stream broadens out, slows down, and becomes the North Atlantic Drift. A slow current is called a drift.

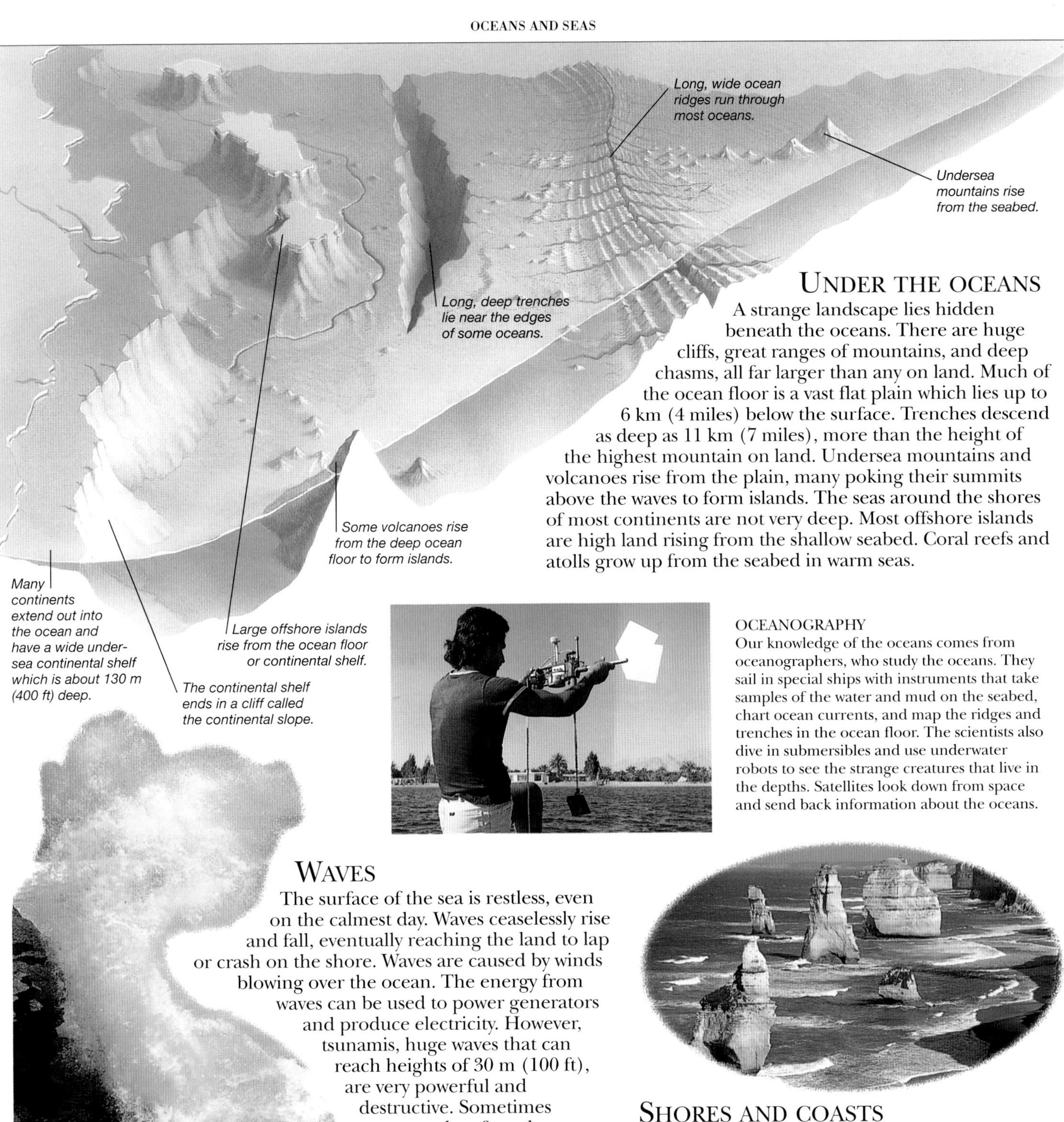
Long, wide ocean ridges run through most oceans.
Undersea mountains rise from the seabed.
Long, deep trenches lie near the edges of some oceans.
Some volcanoes rise from the deep ocean floor to form islands.
Many continents extend out into the ocean and have a wide undersea continental shelf which is about 130 m (400 ft) deep.
Large offshore islands rise from the ocean floor or continental shelf.
The continental shelf ends in a cliff called the continental slope.

Under the oceans

A strange landscape lies hidden beneath the oceans. There are huge cliffs, great ranges of mountains, and deep chasms, all far larger than any on land. Much of the ocean floor is a vast flat plain which lies up to 6 km (4 miles) below the surface. Trenches descend as deep as 11 km (7 miles), more than the height of the highest mountain on land. Undersea mountains and volcanoes rise from the plain, many poking their summits above the waves to form islands. The seas around the shores of most continents are not very deep. Most offshore islands are high land rising from the shallow seabed. Coral reefs and atolls grow up from the seabed in warm seas.

Oceanography

Our knowledge of the oceans comes from oceanographers, who study the oceans. They sail in special ships with instruments that take samples of the water and mud on the seabed, chart ocean currents, and map the ridges and trenches in the ocean floor. The scientists also dive in submersibles and use underwater robots to see the strange creatures that live in the depths. Satellites look down from space and send back information about the oceans.

Waves

The surface of the sea is restless, even on the calmest day. Waves ceaselessly rise and fall, eventually reaching the land to lap or crash on the shore. Waves are caused by winds blowing over the ocean. The energy from waves can be used to power generators and produce electricity. However, tsunamis, huge waves that can reach heights of 30 m (100 ft), are very powerful and destructive. Sometimes wrongly referred to as tidal waves, tsunamis are in fact caused by earthquakes and volcanic eruptions.

Shores and coasts

High land at the shore ends in cliffs, and low land slopes gently to form beaches. The waves hurl stones at the base of cliffs, causing rocks to fall and form coasts with bays and headlands. Strange rock formations and caves may result. The waves batter the rocks and break them up into pebbles and then into sand. Beaches form at the base of cliffs, and the sea also sweeps pebbles and sand along the shore to form beaches elsewhere.

Water reaches base of circle in trough of wave.

Water reaches top of circle in crest of wave.

Crest topples over to break on shore.

How waves move

The water in a wave does not move forwards. It moves in a circle, so the water only goes up and down as a wave passes. The approaching shore holds back the base of the wave, making the top of the wave move faster to break on the shore.

Find out more

Continents
Deep-sea wildlife
Earthquakes
Fishing industry
Indian ocean
Ocean wildlife
Seashore wildlife

OCEAN WILDLIFE

LIFE BEGAN IN THE OCEANS millions of years ago. Today, oceans cover 71 per cent of the planet's surface and provide homes for countless fish, octopuses, seals, sharks, and jellyfish. Ocean wildlife is at its richest in the warm shallow waters of coral reefs, where dazzlingly colourful angelfish and butterfly fish live. In deeper waters, whales, dolphins, and porpoises are found. Most plants and animals live close to the water's surface. Sunlight filters through the surface, allowing microscopic organisms such as diatoms to flourish. An intricate web of small animals feeds on these tiny organisms; larger sea creatures eat the smaller ones, and so on, up the food chain to the large predators such as sharks. Today, many marine plants and animals are threatened; we dump chemical wastes in the oceans, fertilizers flow into the oceans from rivers, and we catch so many fish that fish-eating sea mammals such as seals and dolphins have to compete with us for their food.

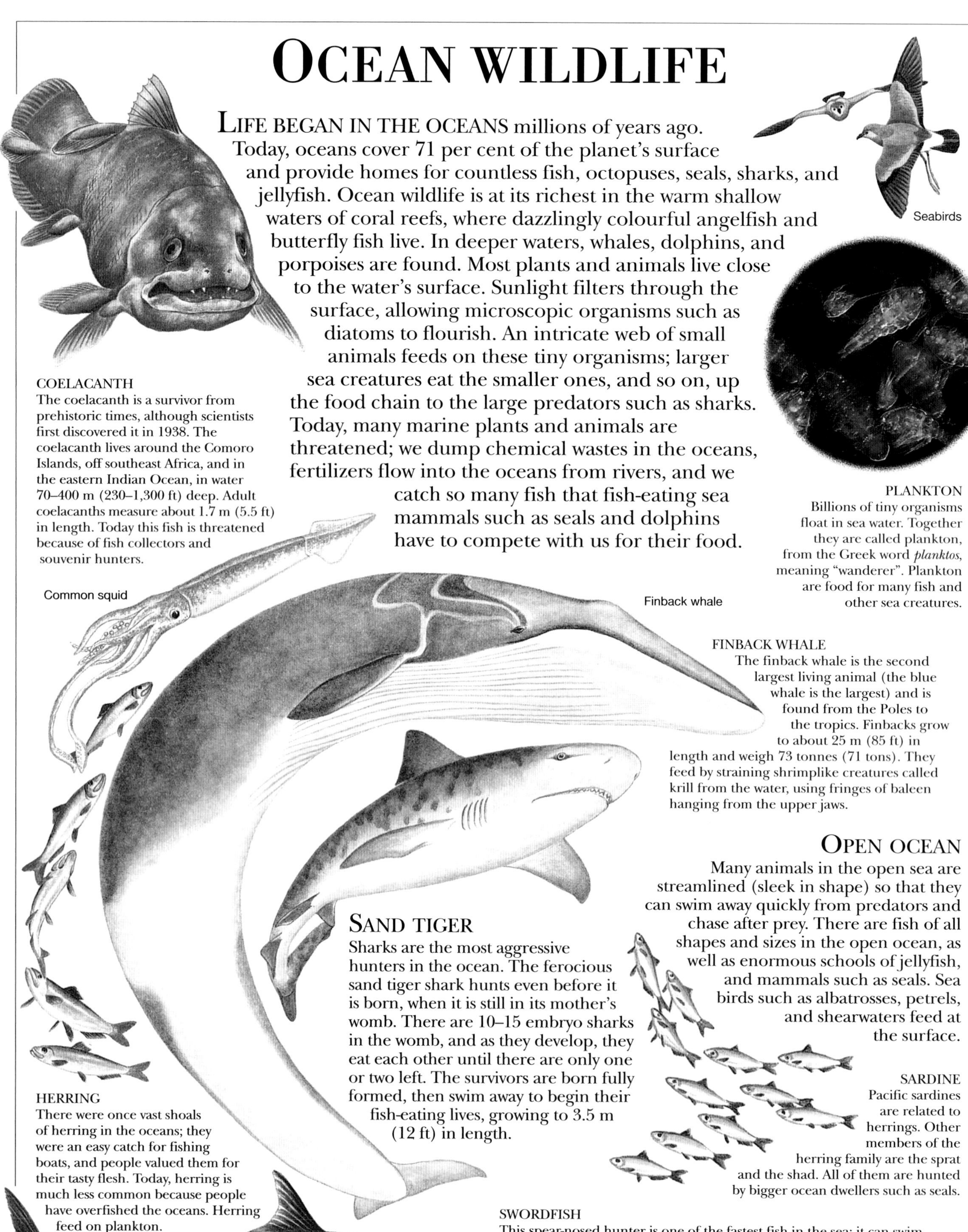

COELACANTH
The coelacanth is a survivor from prehistoric times, although scientists first discovered it in 1938. The coelacanth lives around the Comoro Islands, off southeast Africa, and in the eastern Indian Ocean, in water 70–400 m (230–1,300 ft) deep. Adult coelacanths measure about 1.7 m (5.5 ft) in length. Today this fish is threatened because of fish collectors and souvenir hunters.

PLANKTON
Billions of tiny organisms float in sea water. Together they are called plankton, from the Greek word *planktos*, meaning "wanderer". Plankton are food for many fish and other sea creatures.

FINBACK WHALE
The finback whale is the second largest living animal (the blue whale is the largest) and is found from the Poles to the tropics. Finbacks grow to about 25 m (85 ft) in length and weigh 73 tonnes (71 tons). They feed by straining shrimplike creatures called krill from the water, using fringes of baleen hanging from the upper jaws.

OPEN OCEAN

Many animals in the open sea are streamlined (sleek in shape) so that they can swim away quickly from predators and chase after prey. There are fish of all shapes and sizes in the open ocean, as well as enormous schools of jellyfish, and mammals such as seals. Sea birds such as albatrosses, petrels, and shearwaters feed at the surface.

SAND TIGER

Sharks are the most aggressive hunters in the ocean. The ferocious sand tiger shark hunts even before it is born, when it is still in its mother's womb. There are 10–15 embryo sharks in the womb, and as they develop, they eat each other until there are only one or two left. The survivors are born fully formed, then swim away to begin their fish-eating lives, growing to 3.5 m (12 ft) in length.

HERRING
There were once vast shoals of herring in the oceans; they were an easy catch for fishing boats, and people valued them for their tasty flesh. Today, herring is much less common because people have overfished the oceans. Herring feed on plankton.

SARDINE
Pacific sardines are related to herrings. Other members of the herring family are the sprat and the shad. All of them are hunted by bigger ocean dwellers such as seals.

SWORDFISH
This spear-nosed hunter is one of the fastest fish in the sea; it can swim in bursts at speeds of 95 km/h (60 mph). The swordfish resembles the marlin and sailfish, and weighs up to 675 kg (1,500 lb). Swordfish injure their prey with sideways slashes of the sword, and then devour them.

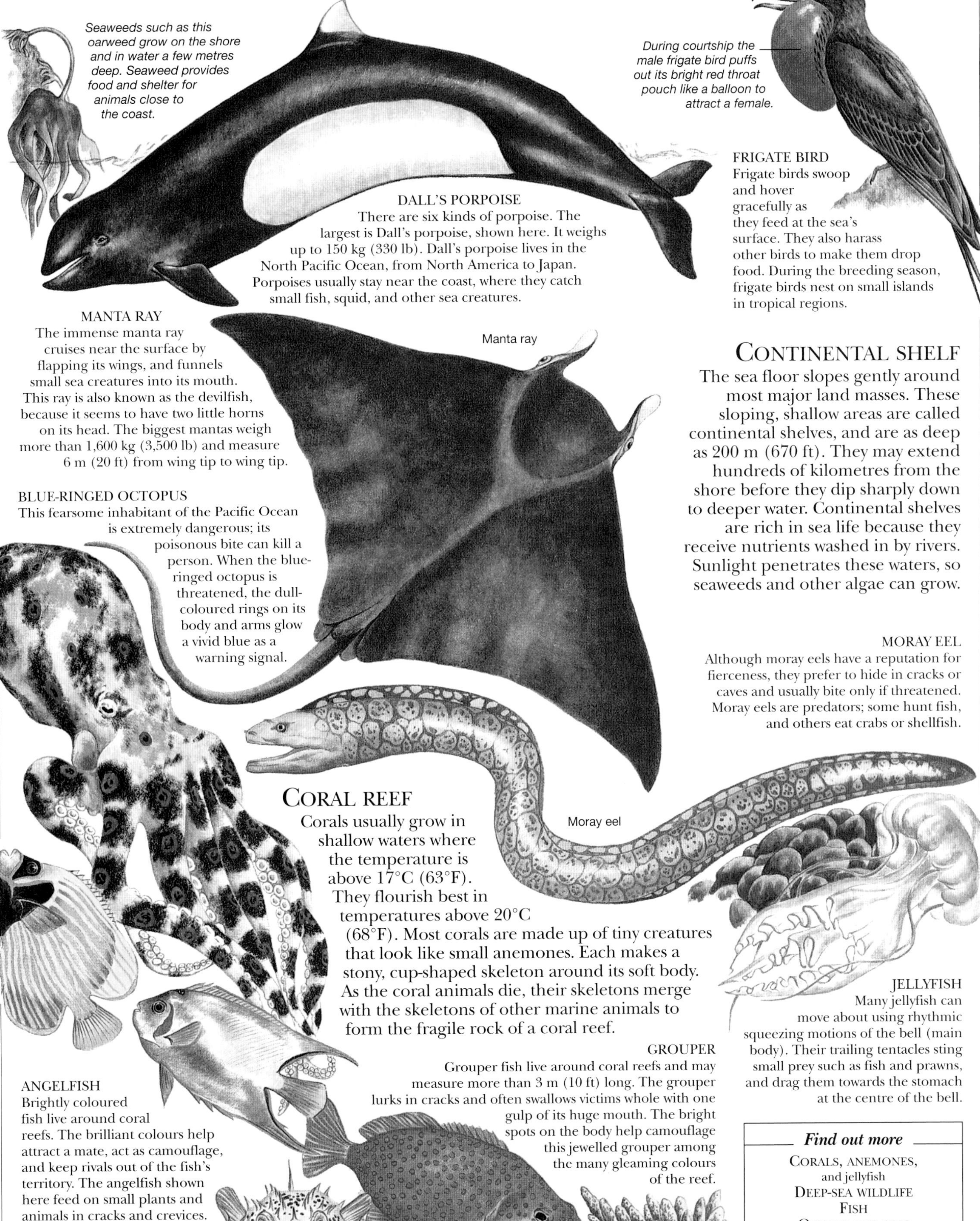

Seaweeds such as this oarweed grow on the shore and in water a few metres deep. Seaweed provides food and shelter for animals close to the coast.

During courtship the male frigate bird puffs out its bright red throat pouch like a balloon to attract a female.

DALL'S PORPOISE
There are six kinds of porpoise. The largest is Dall's porpoise, shown here. It weighs up to 150 kg (330 lb). Dall's porpoise lives in the North Pacific Ocean, from North America to Japan. Porpoises usually stay near the coast, where they catch small fish, squid, and other sea creatures.

FRIGATE BIRD
Frigate birds swoop and hover gracefully as they feed at the sea's surface. They also harass other birds to make them drop food. During the breeding season, frigate birds nest on small islands in tropical regions.

MANTA RAY
The immense manta ray cruises near the surface by flapping its wings, and funnels small sea creatures into its mouth. This ray is also known as the devilfish, because it seems to have two little horns on its head. The biggest mantas weigh more than 1,600 kg (3,500 lb) and measure 6 m (20 ft) from wing tip to wing tip.

Continental shelf

The sea floor slopes gently around most major land masses. These sloping, shallow areas are called continental shelves, and are as deep as 200 m (670 ft). They may extend hundreds of kilometres from the shore before they dip sharply down to deeper water. Continental shelves are rich in sea life because they receive nutrients washed in by rivers. Sunlight penetrates these waters, so seaweeds and other algae can grow.

BLUE-RINGED OCTOPUS
This fearsome inhabitant of the Pacific Ocean is extremely dangerous; its poisonous bite can kill a person. When the blue-ringed octopus is threatened, the dull-coloured rings on its body and arms glow a vivid blue as a warning signal.

MORAY EEL
Although moray eels have a reputation for fierceness, they prefer to hide in cracks or caves and usually bite only if threatened. Moray eels are predators; some hunt fish, and others eat crabs or shellfish.

Coral reef

Corals usually grow in shallow waters where the temperature is above 17°C (63°F). They flourish best in temperatures above 20°C (68°F). Most corals are made up of tiny creatures that look like small anemones. Each makes a stony, cup-shaped skeleton around its soft body. As the coral animals die, their skeletons merge with the skeletons of other marine animals to form the fragile rock of a coral reef.

JELLYFISH
Many jellyfish can move about using rhythmic squeezing motions of the bell (main body). Their trailing tentacles sting small prey such as fish and prawns, and drag them towards the stomach at the centre of the bell.

GROUPER
Grouper fish live around coral reefs and may measure more than 3 m (10 ft) long. The grouper lurks in cracks and often swallows victims whole with one gulp of its huge mouth. The bright spots on the body help camouflage this jewelled grouper among the many gleaming colours of the reef.

ANGELFISH
Brightly coloured fish live around coral reefs. The brilliant colours help attract a mate, act as camouflage, and keep rivals out of the fish's territory. The angelfish shown here feed on small plants and animals in cracks and crevices.

In self-defence, the porcupine fish swallows water and swells into a ball shape with its spines poking outwards.

Find out more
CORALS, ANEMONES, and jellyfish
DEEP-SEA WILDLIFE
FISH
OCEANS AND SEAS
SEALS AND SEA LIONS
SHARKS AND RAYS
WHALES AND DOLPHINS

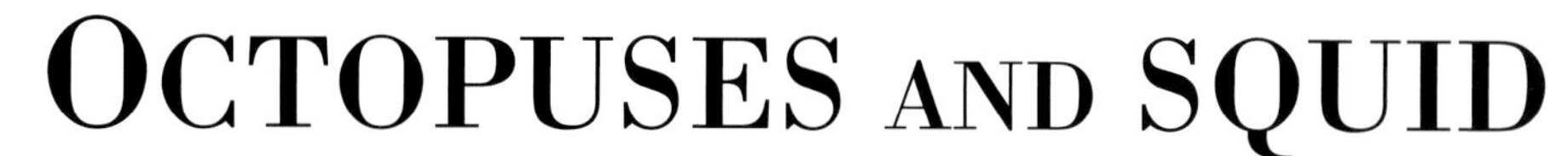

OCTOPUSES AND SQUID

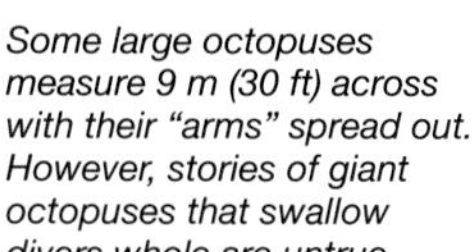

Some large octopuses measure 9 m (30 ft) across with their "arms" spread out. However, stories of giant octopuses that swallow divers whole are untrue.

SEA CREATURES SUCH AS THE OCTOPUS and squid have always held a strange fascination for humans. With their powerful tentacles and strange shape, they were once thought of as sea monsters. Octopuses and squid are clever, active creatures, the biggest and most intelligent of all the invertebrates (animals without backbones). They have sharp eyesight, a large brain, fast reactions, and the ability to remember. Octopuses, squid, and their relatives the cuttlefish, are molluscs, related to shelled animals with soft bodies such as snails and clams. Unlike snails and clams, octopuses, squid, and cuttlefish have no outer shells, though squid have a very thin shell called a pen inside the body. The white oval cuttlebones of cuttlefish are often seen washed up on beaches. An octopus has eight "arms" covered with suckers, which it uses for moving around. Squid and cuttlefish have eight short "arms" and two long tentacles, which curl and uncurl. They use their arms as rudders for swimming and their tentacles for catching prey.

Water can be squirted out through siphon for jet-propelled movement.

Mouth is on underside; it has a horny "beak" for cutting food, and saliva that contains poison.

Each "arm" has two rows of powerful suckers for moving, feeling, and grabbing prey.

COMMON OCTOPUS

The common octopus lurks in caves or crevices during the day. It emerges at night to hunt for crabs, shellfish, and small fish. It has a hard, beaklike mouth and a rough tongue.

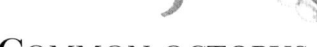

CUTTLEFISH

Octopuses, squid, and cuttlefish can change colour in less than a second. This can provide camouflage so that the creature blends in with its surroundings. The dappled red colouring of the cuttlefish shown here is a good disguise among the coral. Change of colour may also indicate a change of mood – a male cuttlefish turns black with rage when it is angry.

INK CLOUD

Octopuses and squid have an ink gland attached to their digestive system. To confuse an enemy, they squirt ink out of the siphon and cannot be seen behind the dark, watery screen. This ink was once used by artists and is called sepia, which is also the scientific name for cuttlefish.

Common squid

GIANT SQUID

Measuring 20 m (60 ft) in length including its tentacles, the giant squid is the world's largest invertebrate. It is an important source of food for sperm whales.

SQUID

With its torpedo shape, the common squid is an especially fast swimmer. Powerful muscles inside the body squirt water rapidly through the siphon, pushing the creature along through the water.

Find out more

ANIMALS
DEEP-SEA WILDLIFE
OCEAN WILDLIFE

OIL

WITHOUT OIL, modern life would grind to a halt. Oil is needed to make the fuels that drive cars, lorries, diesel trains, ships, and aircraft. Power stations burn oil to produce much of the world's electricity, and many homes use oil-burning boilers for heating. Oil is also very important because it is needed to make plastics, textiles, and other useful products. Oil is a dark, thick liquid which lies deep underground and beneath the sea bed. Oil wells are bored to obtain oil, which is also called crude oil or petroleum. Crude oil contains a mixture of chemicals and many different types of oil. Lubricating oil is made from crude oil. It helps machine parts slide easily so that the machine works well.

OFFSHORE OIL
Rigs drill wells down to oil deposits, and production platforms bring the oil to the surface. The platforms either float on the sea or stand on the sea bed.

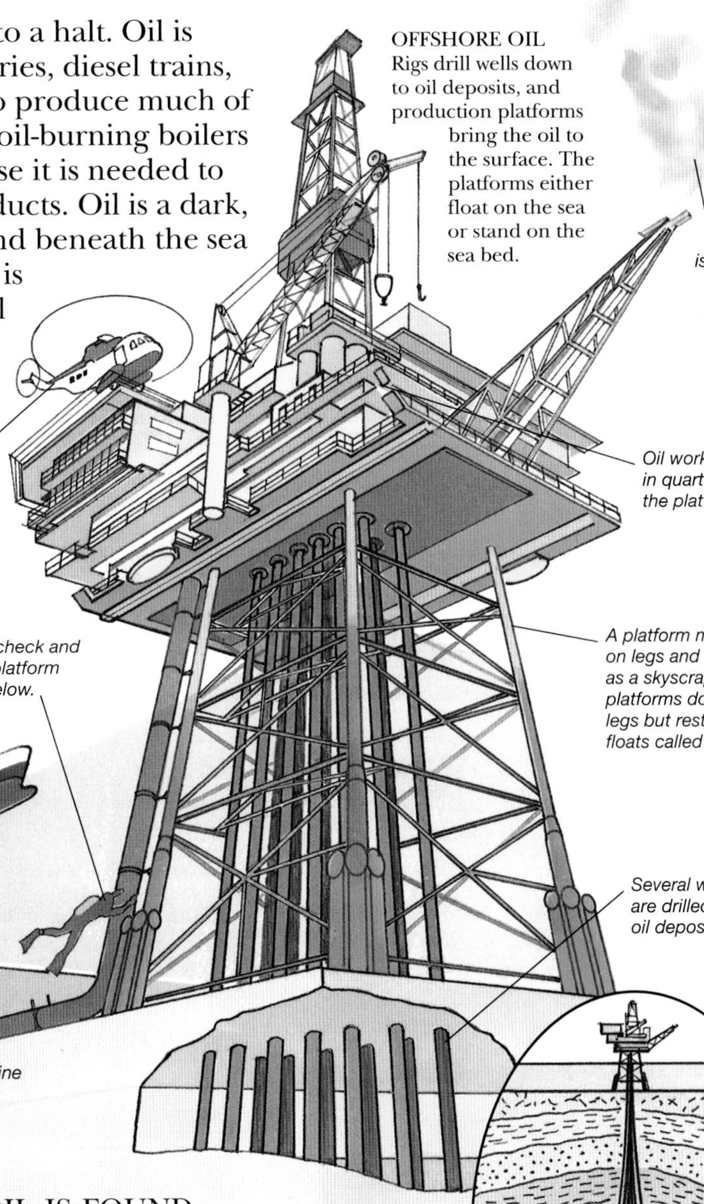

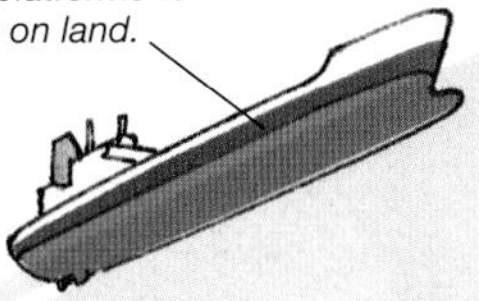

Some gas from the oil is burned off as a safety precaution.

Oil workers are ferried to production platform by helicopter.

Oil workers live in quarters on the platform.

OIL REFINERY
The crude oil that comes from a deposit is a mixture of chemicals and many kinds of oil. Crude oil is taken to an oil refinery, where it is heated. This makes the oil break down, or separate, into petrol and other fuels, lubricating oils, chemicals, and bitumen for making roads.

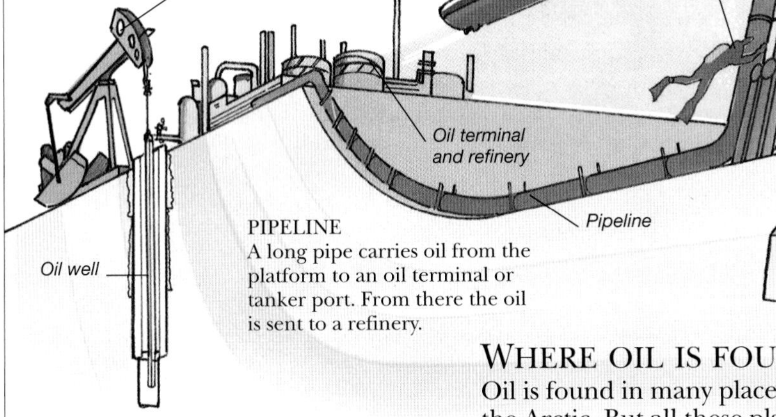

Huge oil tankers carry oil from offshore platforms to refineries on land.

Divers check and repair platform from below.

A platform may stand on legs and be as tall as a skyscraper. Some platforms do not have legs but rest on huge floats called pontoons.

Nodding donkey

Several wells are drilled to an oil deposit.

Oil terminal and refinery

Pipeline

Oil well

PIPELINE
A long pipe carries oil from the platform to an oil terminal or tanker port. From there the oil is sent to a refinery.

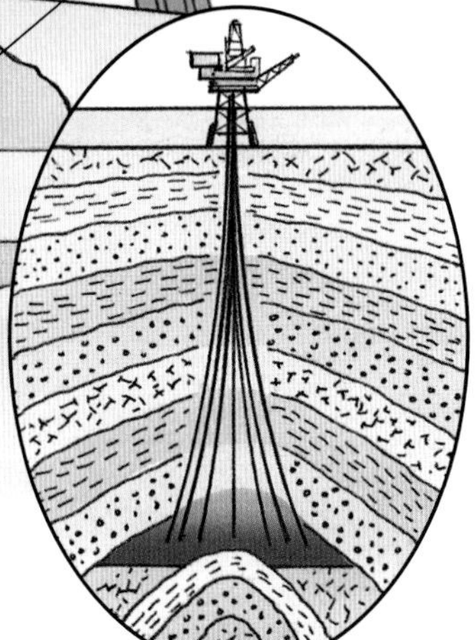

WHERE OIL IS FOUND

Oil is found in many places, from the Middle East to the Arctic. But all these places were once covered by the sea. Tiny sea plants sank to the sea bed and were buried in mud. The mud turned into layers of rock. Heat from the rocks warmed the plants over millions of years and changed them into oil and natural gas.

OIL WELL
An oil well is a shaft that is drilled to obtain oil. The oil flows up the shaft from the deposit far below. On land, a machine called a nodding donkey pumps up the oil.

VEGETABLE OILS
Plants and vegetables, such as olives, peanuts, sunflowers, and corn, provide valuable oils. Olive oil is made by crushing ripe olives; sunflower oil comes from sunflower seeds. These oils are used in cooking, and sunflower oil is used to make margarine. Factories treat plant and vegetable oils to make other products, such as soap and paints.

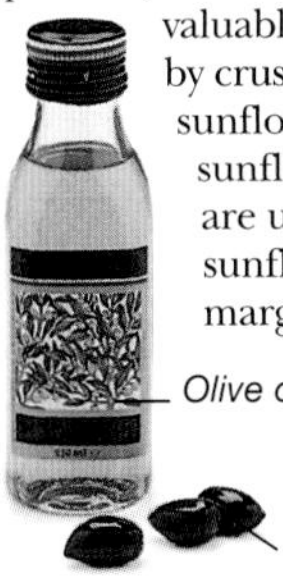

Olive oil

Olives

CHEMICALS FROM OIL

An oil refinery produces many chemicals from crude oil, which are called petro-chemicals. Factories use these chemicals to make plastics, textiles, and other products. Polythene, for example, is made from a gas that comes from oil. Chemicals from oil are also used to make drugs, fertilizers, detergents, and dyes and paints in all colours.

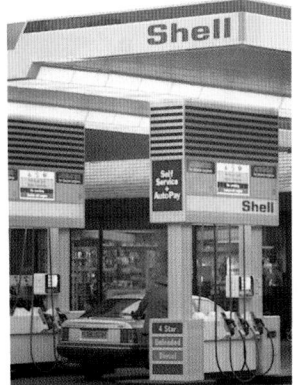

PETROL
Petrol is one of the most important of all oil products. Diesel fuel is another kind of motor fuel made from oil.

Find out more

GAS
GEOLOGY
PLASTICS
ROCKS AND MINERALS
TEXTILES

OLYMPIC GAMES

Five interlocking rings make up the Olympic symbol.

EVERY TWO YEARS, the world's best athletes compete in the Summer or Winter Olympics. About 10,000 athletes from nearly 200 nations take part in the Summer Olympics, in more than 25 sports. The Winter Games are smaller, with 1,800 athletes from nearly 80 countries competing in seven sports.

The inspiration for today's Olympics came from Ancient Greek games of more than 2,000 years ago. The modern Olympics began in Athens, Greece, in 1896. Individual excellence and team achievement are the theme of the Olympic Games, and not competition between nations. The International Olympic Committee (IOC) chooses a city, not a country, to host the games. No one country "wins" the games, and there is no prize money. Instead, individuals and teams compete for gold (first place), silver (second), and bronze (third) medals – as well as for the glory of taking part.

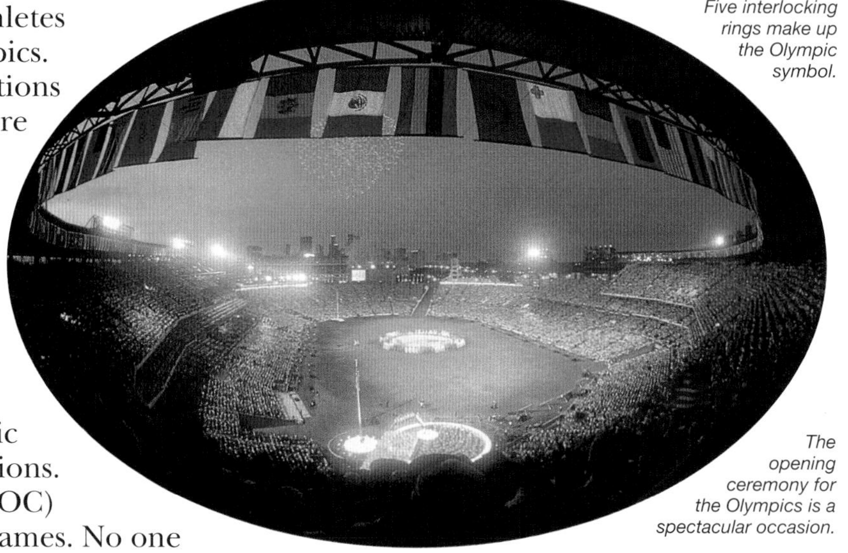

The opening ceremony for the Olympics is a spectacular occasion.

OLYMPIC FLAME

The Olympic Games open with a spectacular ceremony. The most important part is the lighting of the Olympic Flame with a burning torch. Teams of runners carry the torch from Olympia, in Greece, site of the ancient games, to the stadium where the games are to be held. This ceremony dates back to 1928, when Baron Pierre de Coubertin, founder of the modern Olympics, urged the athletes to "keep alive the flame of the revived Olympic spirit".

Ski jumping, shown here, is one of the most exciting events in the Winter Olympics.

ANCIENT GAMES

The ancient Olympics began as a religious festival. At first they consisted of just one race, but at their height the games lasted five days and included sports such as wrestling and chariot racing. Only men could compete in, or watch the ancient Olympics. Women held their own games in honour of the goddess Hera.

POLITICS AND THE GAMES

The huge international audience for the Olympics ensures that any political protests, or terrorist acts that may occur, gain maximum publicity. In 1968, winning athletes raised clenched fists to show that they supported a campaign to give black people more power. Four years later, an act of terrorism caused the deaths of 11 Israeli athletes at Munich, Germany.

The black power salute

WINTER OLYMPICS

A separate Winter Games takes place every four years, midway between two Summer Olympics. It includes ice and snow sports such as skating and skiing.

The Games include a variety of team and individual sports. New ones are added, and old ones are sometimes dropped.

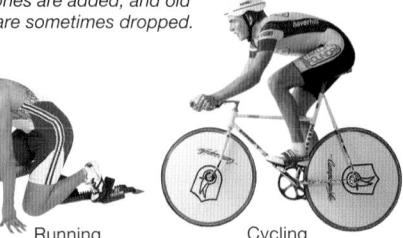

Running

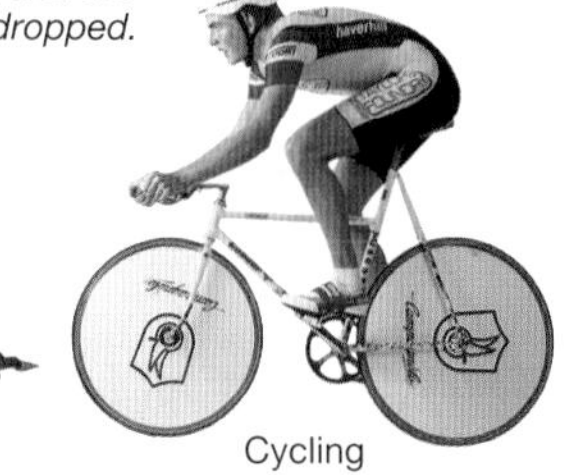

Cycling

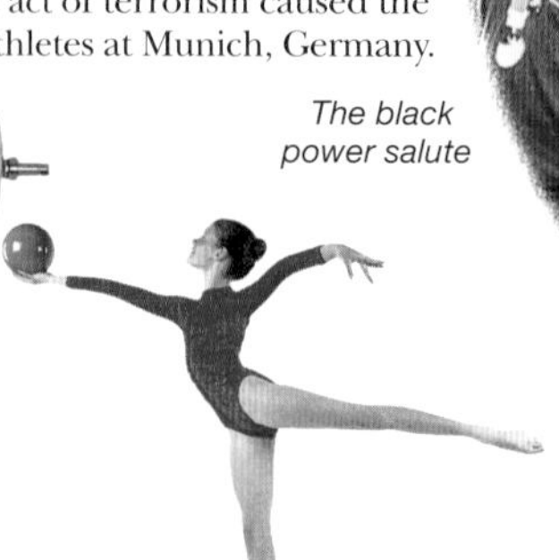

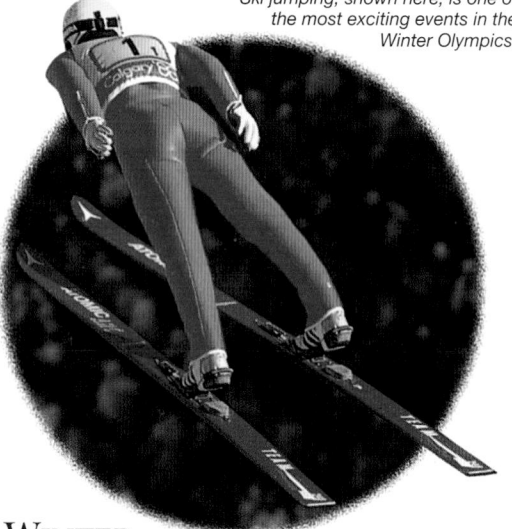

Weightlifting

Gymnastics

Find out more

ATHLETICS
BALL GAMES
GREECE, ANCIENT
GYMNASTICS
SPORTS

OPERA AND SINGING

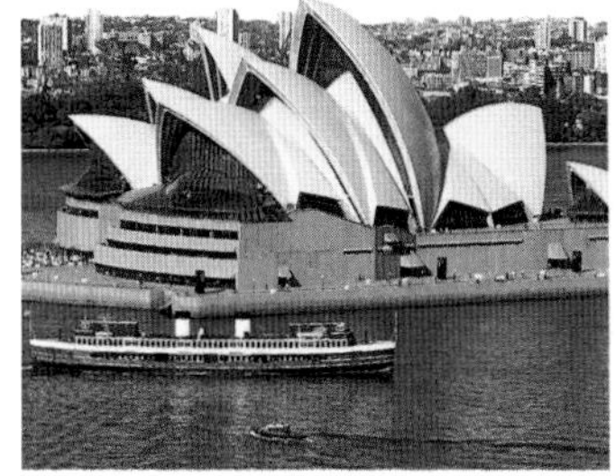

SYDNEY OPERA HOUSE
This striking opera house overlooking Sydney Harbour in Australia caused much debate when it opened in 1973. It was designed to match the shape of ships in the harbour. Hanging ceilings beneath the roofs create the right acoustics.

THE HUMAN VOICE is a versatile musical instrument that has inspired many composers to write beautiful solo songs and works for groups of singers, or choirs, as well. Every voice is unique. Some women have a high soprano voice; others a deep, rich contralto. The male voice can range from a very high countertenor to a low bass. There are also variations in between. In the Middle Ages monks sang as part of their religious life, and wandering troubadours sang poetic songs of bravery and love. In the 17th century a new form of sung drama called opera began in Italy. New musical forms required trained voices, and by the 18th century great professional singers were delighting audiences everywhere. Today, singers perform all kinds of historical music, but constantly explore new ways of using their voices.

GRAND OPERA

In grand opera every word is sung. Most of the main characters have an opportunity to show off their voices by singing arias, or solos. Some arias, such as "One fine day" from Puccini's *Madame Butterfly*, are very well known. Operas composed by Puccini, Verdi, Wagner, and Mozart also include fine music for the chorus, a group of opera singers who are not featured in solos.

FAMOUS SINGERS

The greatest opera singers are those who can touch the emotions of their audience. Some, like Nellie Melba, moved people with the beauty of their voices. Maria Callas brought characters such as Aida and Tosca to life through superb acting as well as singing. Singers such as Kiri Te Kanawa and Placido Domingo sing popular songs as well as opera.

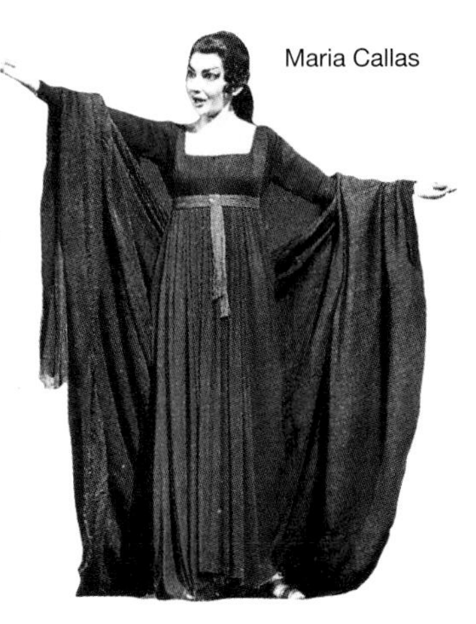

Maria Callas

MUSICALS

Musical comedies first became popular in the United States at the beginning of this century. Like opera, they have solos and a chorus, but the stories are mostly spoken. Spectacular dance routines are an important ingredient in musicals such as composer and conductor Leonard Bernstein's *West Side Story*. Many successful musicals are later made into films.

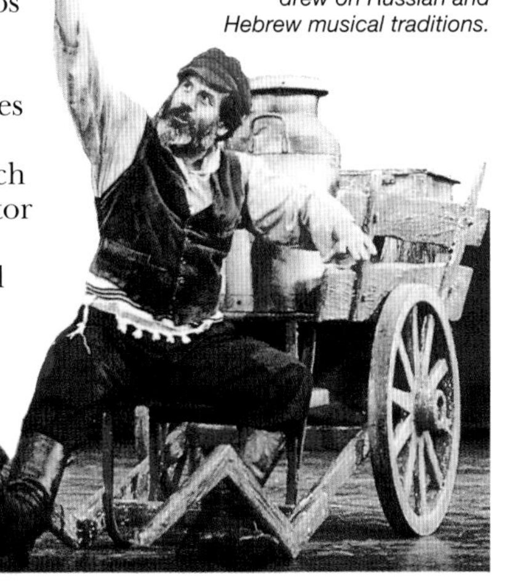

The film Fiddler on the Roof *drew on Russian and Hebrew musical traditions.*

FIDDLER ON THE ROOF
Popular musicals can turn performers into stars. Topol (above) found fame in *Fiddler on the Roof*, directed by choreographer Jerome Robbins.

WORK SONGS

In the days before steam was used to power ships, special songs called sea chanties or shanties were a popular accompaniment to heavy work. Singing them helped the sailors keep a steady, repetitive rhythm as they hauled on ropes to lift a sail or raise the anchor.

Find out more
COMPOSERS
MUSIC
ORCHESTRAS
THEATRE

ORCHESTRAS

THE THRILLING SOUND made by an orchestra is no accident. An orchestra is not just a random collection of instruments brought along by the musicians; it is a carefully planned group of different families or types of instruments. Each family has its own part to play in the performance of a piece of music. The symphony orchestra is the largest group of musicians who perform together. They play four main sections of instruments: strings, woodwinds, brass, and percussion. Orchestras in the past were not so well organized, and for a long time musicians simply played whatever instruments they owned. But in the 18th century, composers wanted to make sure that their music would sound the same whenever it was played. So they wrote on the piece of music which instruments of the orchestra should play each part of the tune. By the early 20th century the form of the symphony orchestra was established, and many large cities in Russia, the United States, and Europe had their own symphony orchestras.

GAMELAN
Indonesian orchestras are called gamelans. Most of the instruments belong to the percussion family: gongs, metallophones, xylophones, and gong-chimes. Flutes, two-string fiddles, and zithers complete the gamelan, which has about 30 players.

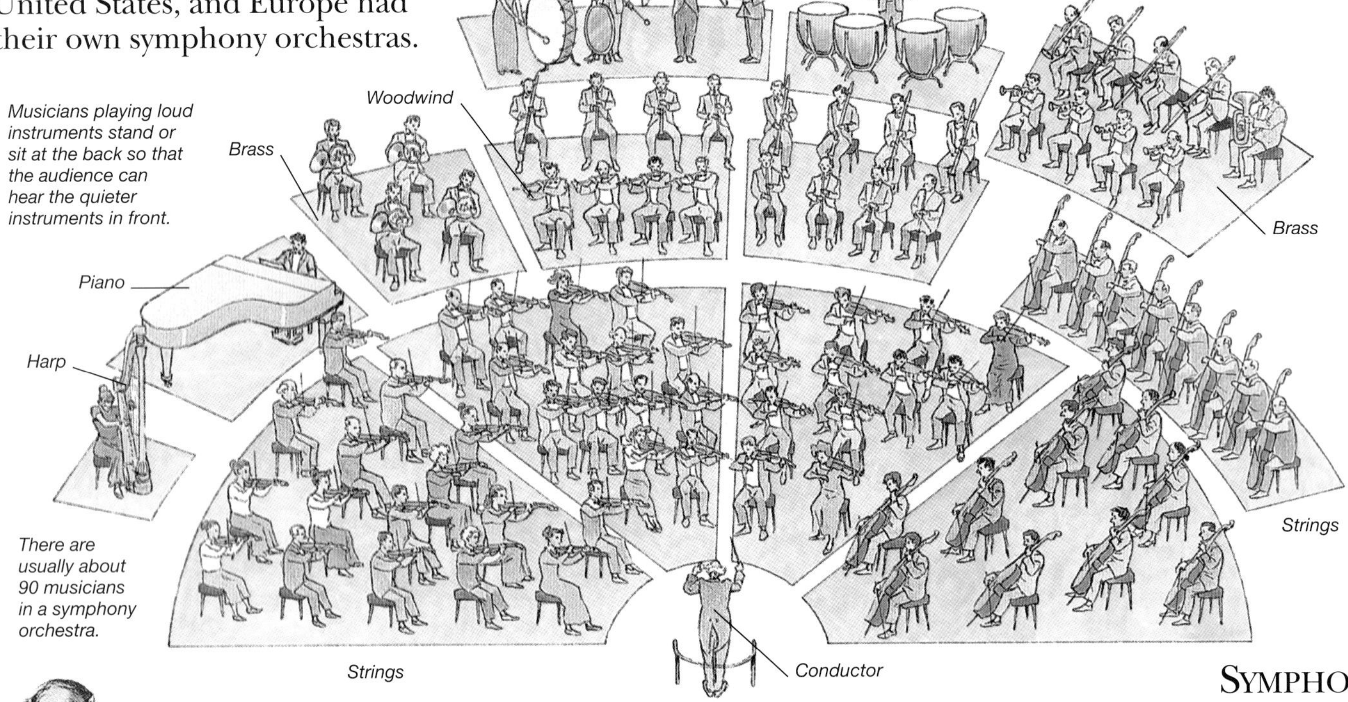

Musicians playing loud instruments stand or sit at the back so that the audience can hear the quieter instruments in front.

There are usually about 90 musicians in a symphony orchestra.

SYMPHONY ORCHESTRA

Great composers such as Wolfgang Amadeus Mozart (Austria) and Ludwig van Beethoven (Germany) wrote major pieces of orchestral music called symphonies. Symphony orchestras take their name from this sort of music, but they also play other kinds of classical music, film and television scores, and pop songs.

THE CONDUCTOR

The conductor uses hand motions or a baton – a small stick – to give the orchestra the tempo, or speed, of the music. Conductors don't just direct the orchestra like a police officer directing traffic; they interpret the composer's music, so that each performance is special. Arturo Toscanini (1867-1957), shown here, was an exciting conductor.

The pattern of movement of the conductor's baton indicates the rhythm of the music to the orchestra.

2 beats in a bar

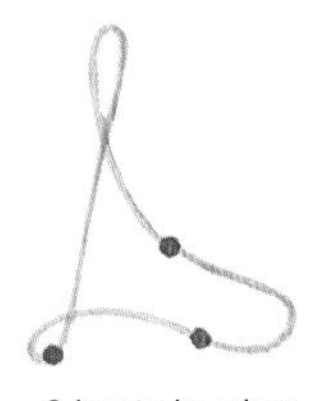

3 beats in a bar

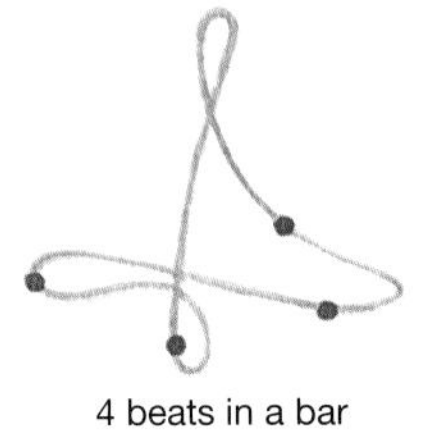

4 beats in a bar

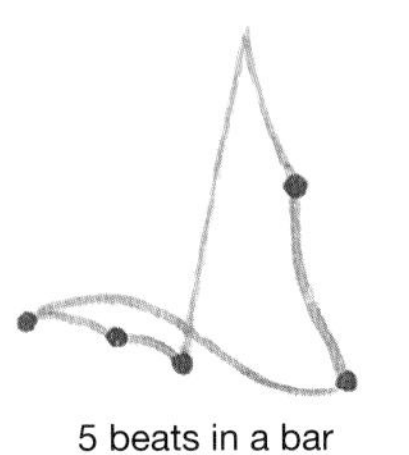

5 beats in a bar

Find out more
COMPOSERS
MUSIC
MUSICAL INSTRUMENTS
OPERA AND SINGING

OSTRICHES AND EMUS

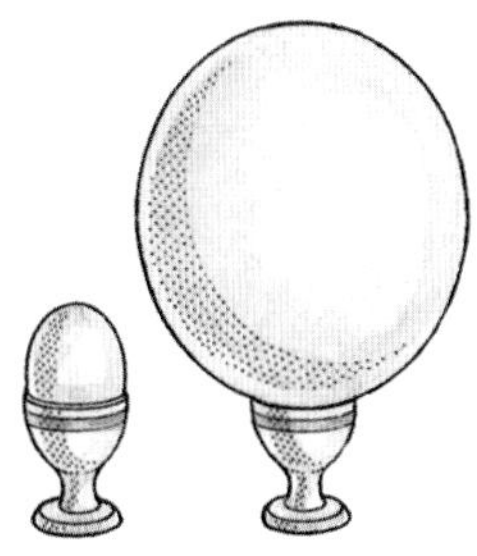

BIGGEST EGG
An ostrich egg is 20 cm (8 in) long and 30 times heavier than a hen's egg. This makes ostrich eggs the largest bird's eggs in the world.

THERE ARE MANY KINDS of birds that cannot fly, including ostriches and emus, and most of these birds are large. Ostriches are the biggest of all living birds, at more than 2.5 m (8 ft) high. They live in the dry grassland areas of Africa, and their feathers are soft and fluffy because they are not needed for flying. Ostrich eggs are the biggest of any living bird. The egg shells are only 3 mm (⅛ in) thick but very hard. Ostriches and emus are speedy runners on land, and emus also swim well. The emu is a well-known pest to farmers in Australia, where it tramples on wheat fields. Other flightless birds include the secretive cassowary, which lives in the dense forests of Australasia, and the kiwi, which is found only in New Zealand. Kiwis are about 30 cm (1 ft) high, with tiny, useless wings. The rhea, a fast-running flightless bird, lives in the grassland areas of Brazil and Argentina in South America. Rheas gather in large flocks in winter.

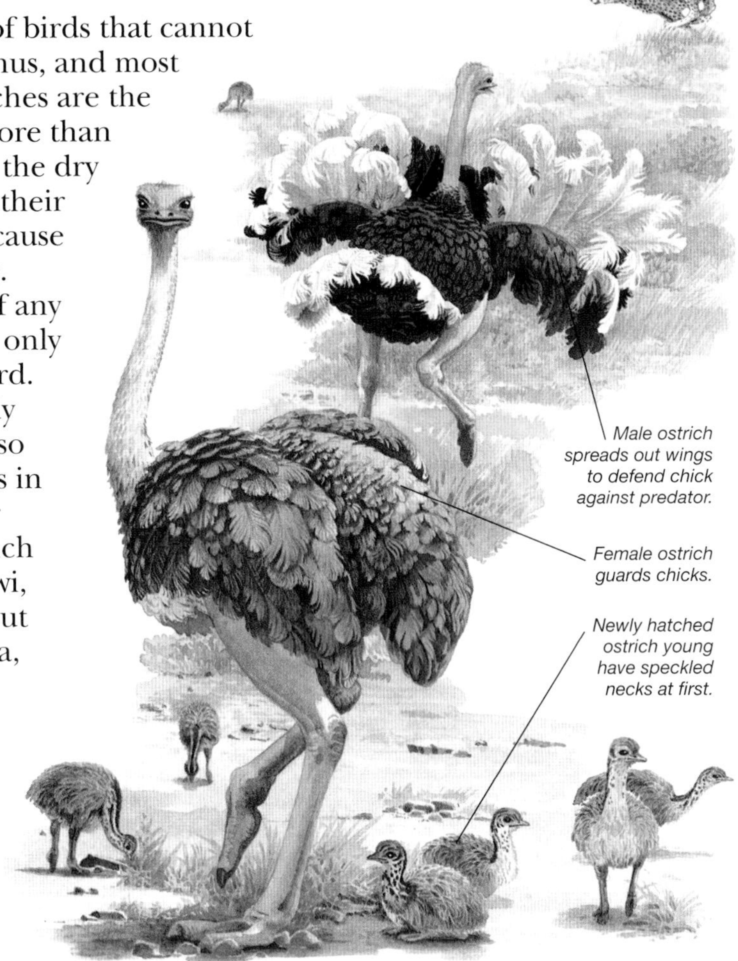
Male ostrich spreads out wings to defend chick against predator.
Female ostrich guards chicks.
Newly hatched ostrich young have speckled necks at first.

OSTRICH CHICKS

Both ostriches guard the chicks, but the male usually looks after the eggs until they hatch. Within a month of hatching, the young ostrich chicks can run fast and feed themselves. Adult ostriches have strong, powerful legs and large, flexible feet for running quickly.

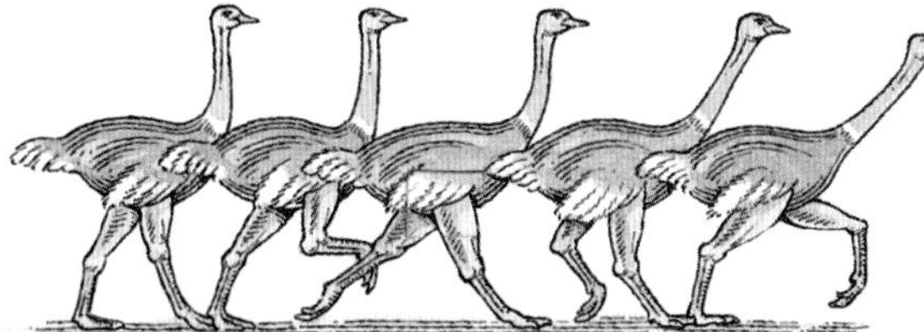

FASTEST BIRD ON LAND
The ostrich runs faster than any other bird and faster than most animals. It can run at 50 km/h (30 mph) for several minutes and may reach 70 km/h (45 mph) in short bursts.

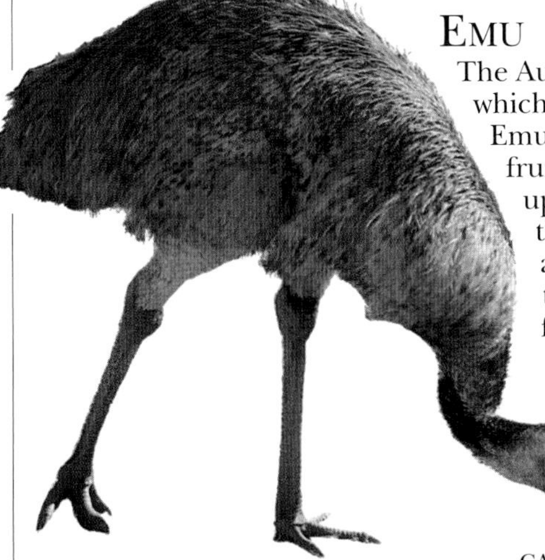

EMU

The Australian emu grows to 2 m (6 ft) tall, which makes it the second-largest living bird. Emus eat a varied diet of seeds, leaves, fruit, shoots, and insects. The female lays up to 15 green eggs in a shallow nest on the ground. The newly hatched young are striped and stay with their parents for the first 18 months.

CASSOWARY
Three different kinds of cassowary live in Australasia, wandering the dense, dark forests in search of fruit and seeds. The female common cassowary usually lays about five bright green eggs in a shallow nest lined with leaves. The male cassowary sits on the eggs to keep them warm and stays with the chicks after they hatch for up to one year.

RHEA
The male rhea makes a shallow nest called a scrape which can contain up to 60 eggs. This Darwin's rhea is about 1 m (3 ft) tall.

Find out more
AUSTRALIAN WILDLIFE
BIRDS
GRASSLAND WILDLIFE

OTTOMAN EMPIRE

DURING THE LATE 13TH CENTURY, a group of nomadic Turkish tribes settled in Anatolia, in modern Turkey. They were led by Osman, their first sultan, or ruler. He gave his name to the Ottoman Empire – one of the greatest empires in the world. The empire expanded through war and alliance with neighbours, and by purchasing land. By 1566, it had spread along the Mediterranean Sea across the Middle East to the Persian Gulf. The Ottomans owed their success to their military skill. Their armies included many Christian recruits organised into groups of highly trained foot soldiers called Janissaries. The empire grew wealthy on the trade it controlled throughout the Middle East. Art and architecture flourished within its borders. Discontent with Ottoman rule, and widespread famine eventually weakened the empire, and it declined during the 19th century before it finally collapsed in 1918. The country of Turkey emerged out of its ruins.

SULEIMAN THE MAGNIFICENT
The greatest of all Ottoman sultans was Suleiman I (1495-1566), known as Suleiman the Magnificent. During his reign the Ottoman Empire reached the height of its power. A patron of the arts, Suleiman reformed the educational and legal systems.

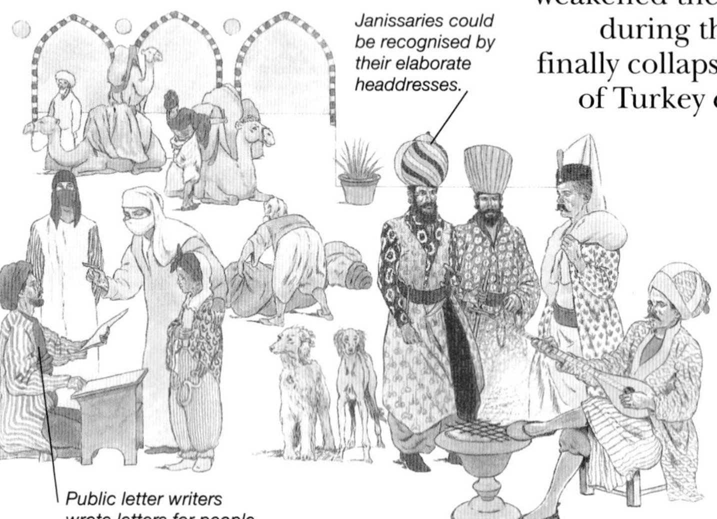
Janissaries could be recognised by their elaborate headdresses.
Public letter writers wrote letters for people.

THE OTTOMANS

Although the Ottomans were Muslims, they allowed Christians and Jews to practise their own religions and tolerated the many different peoples who lived within their empire. The sultans lived in great luxury and wealth and encouraged the arts and learning. Ottoman women had to live in a separate section of the household called a harem.

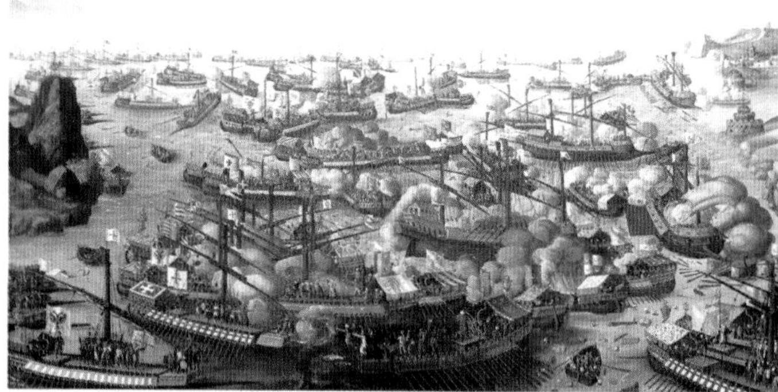

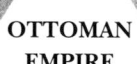

BATTLE OF LEPANTO
To stop the growth of Ottoman power, Pope Pius V formed a Christian league that included Spain, Venice, Genoa, and Naples. In 1571 the Christian forces defeated the Turks at the Battle of Lepanto, off the coast of Greece. The defeat was the first major setback to the Ottoman Empire and ended Turkish naval power in the Mediterranean Sea.

SICK MAN OF EUROPE
During the 19th century, the Ottoman Empire lost its grip on its European possessions and was in danger of falling apart. The empire became known as the "Sick Man of Europe".

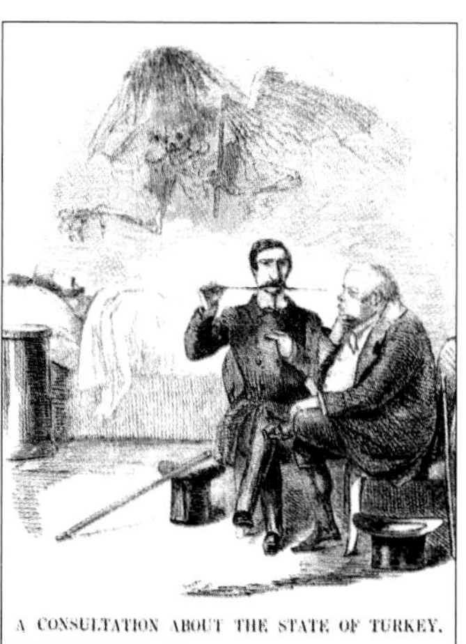
A CONSULTATION ABOUT THE STATE OF TURKEY.

A 19th-century cartoon mocks at the declining state of the Ottoman Empire.

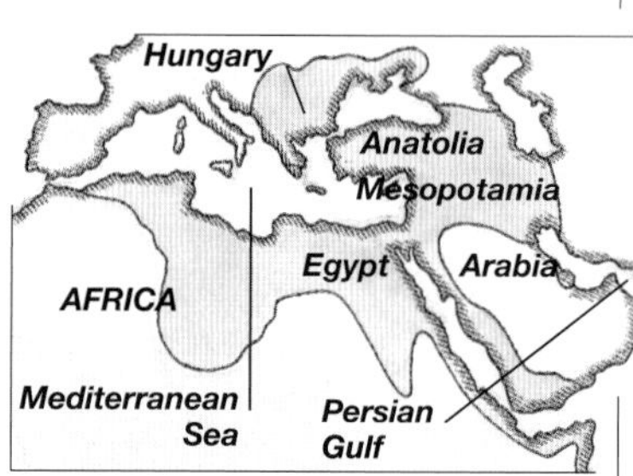

Ottoman Empire at its greatest extent

OTTOMAN EMPIRE

1281-1324 Osman founds Ottoman Empire.

1333 Ottomans capture Gallipoli, Turkey, giving them a foothold in Europe.

1453 Ottomans capture city of Constantinople (now Istanbul), the capital of the Byzantine Empire; the city becomes the capital of the new empire.

1566 Ottoman Empire reaches its greatest extent.

1571 Christian navy destroys Turkish fleet at Lepanto.

1697-1878 Russia slowly expels the Turks from the lands around the Black Sea.

1878-1913 Turks expelled from most of their European possessions.

1914-18 Ottoman Empire fights with Germany and Austria in World War I.

1918 Troops of several allied nations including Britain and Greece occupy the Ottoman Empire.

1922 Last sultan is overthrown. Turkey is declared a republic.

Find out more

BYZANTINE EMPIRE
ISLAM

Outlaws and Bandits

People who live outside the law are called outlaws or bandits. They do not just break one or two laws: their whole way of life is illegal, or against the law. Some outlaws and bandits are criminals who hope to get rich by stealing. Many of the famous bandits of the Wild West lived like this. It was easy for them to avoid getting caught, because there were so few people to enforce the law. But other outlaws are "social bandits". They are outlaws because they try to change and improve society. Many countries have laws that benefit rich and powerful people and punish the poor and weak. These are the laws that social bandits break. Social bandits often escape capture for many years because many ordinary people support them. From their supporters the bandits can get food and shelter. There have been social bandits in most countries of the world at one time in their history. Some have become legendary figures, and people still tell stories of their daring deeds.

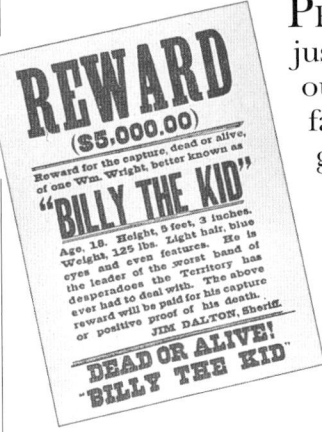

REWARD
($5,000.00)
Reward for the capture, dead or alive, of one Wm. Wright, better known as
"BILLY THE KID"
Age, 18. Height, 5 feet, 3 inches. Weight, 125 lbs. Light hair, blue eyes and even features. He is the leader of the worst band of desperadoes the Territory has ever had to deal with. The above reward will be paid for his capture or positive proof of his death.
JIM DALTON, Sheriff.
DEAD OR ALIVE!
"BILLY THE KID"

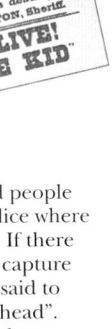

REWARDS
Rewards encouraged people to tell lawmen or police where outlaws were hiding. If there was a reward for the capture of an outlaw, he was said to have "a price on his head". Rewards were printed on posters such as the one above.

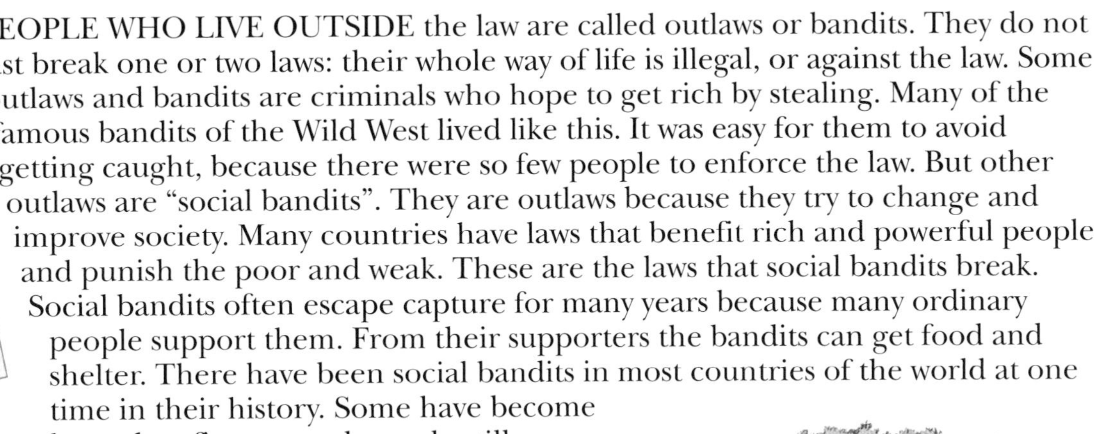

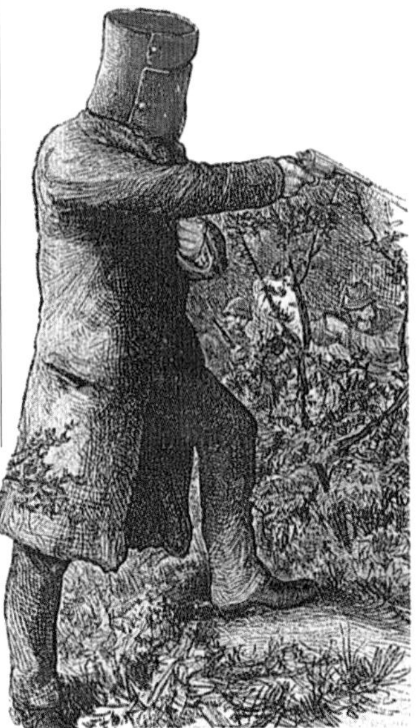

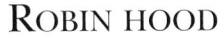

NED KELLY
Australian outlaw Ned Kelly (1855-80) was the son of a convict who had been sent to Tasmania as punishment for crimes in Ireland. He took up crime, and soon the British-led police were on his trail. Kelly and his gang became outlaws after they shot three policemen in 1878. Local people hid them, but the police trapped the gang in a hotel in 1880. Protected by homemade armour, Ned (left) tried to shoot his way out. The police caught him, and he was executed.

Robin Hood

One of the most famous outlaws was Robin Hood. People believe he lived in England around 1300. He and his band of followers, or "merry men", hid in Sherwood Forest, close to Nottingham. They defended the peasants from the unjust rule of the landowners. Robin Hood robbed rich people so that he could give their money and possessions to the poor.

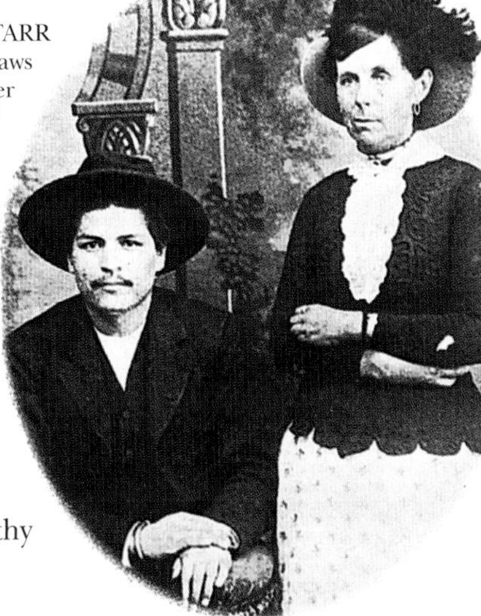

BELLE STARR
One of the handful of female outlaws was Belle Starr. She was the partner of several male outlaws and shared their lives of crime. In 1880, she and a Cherokee Native American named Sam Starr had a ranch in Oklahoma. It became a hideout for outlaws. An unknown killer shot Belle Starr in 1889.

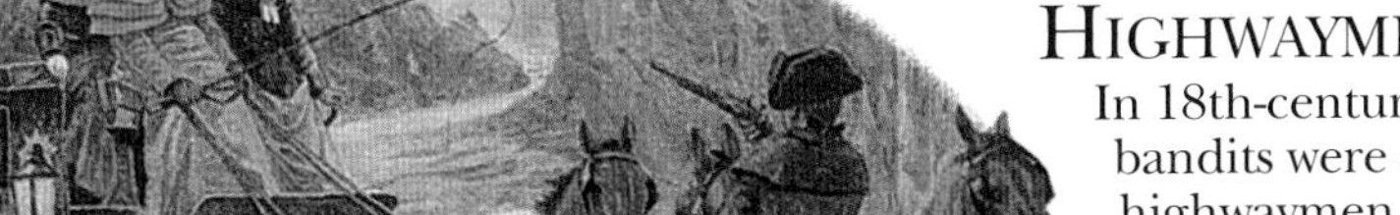

Highwaymen

In 18th-century England, bandits were called highwaymen. They stopped stagecoaches on lonely roads and robbed the wealthy travellers inside. The most famous of the highwaymen was Dick Turpin (1705-39). He robbed coaches on the busy roads to the northeast of London. He had a reputation for generosity and for giving away the valuables that he stole.

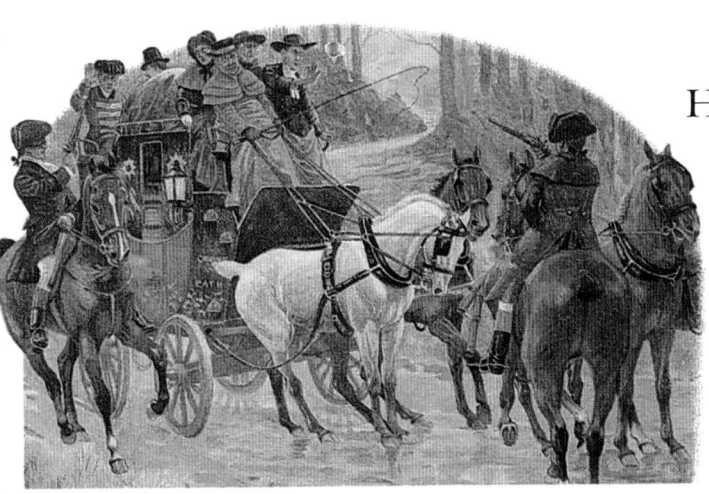

Find out more
Australia, history of
Myths and legends
Pirates

OWLS

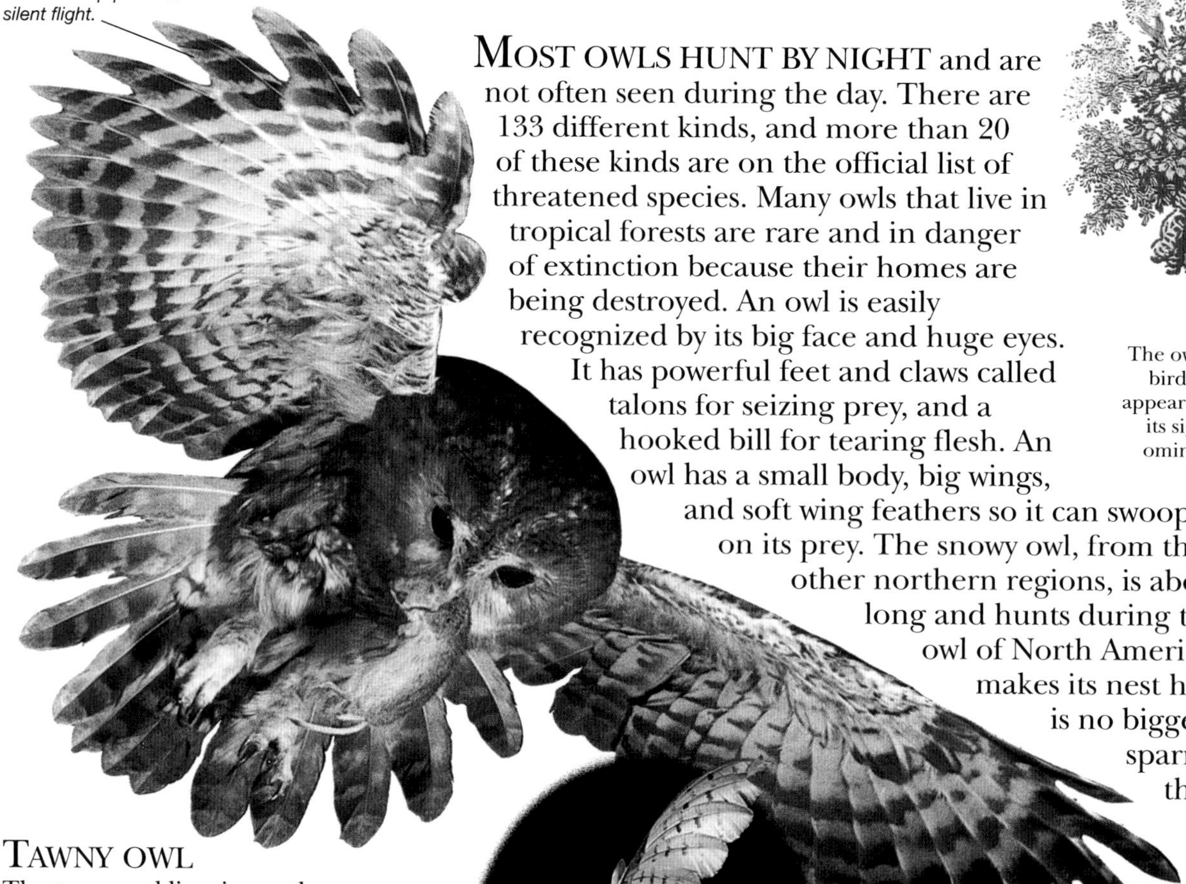

Fringed edges on wing feathers help produce silent flight.

MOST OWLS HUNT BY NIGHT and are not often seen during the day. There are 133 different kinds, and more than 20 of these kinds are on the official list of threatened species. Many owls that live in tropical forests are rare and in danger of extinction because their homes are being destroyed. An owl is easily recognized by its big face and huge eyes. It has powerful feet and claws called talons for seizing prey, and a hooked bill for tearing flesh. An owl has a small body, big wings, and soft wing feathers so it can swoop down silently on its prey. The snowy owl, from the Arctic and other northern regions, is about 60 cm (2 ft) long and hunts during the day. The elf owl of North America, which makes its nest hole in a cactus, is no bigger than a sparrow. Eagle owls, the largest owls, weigh about 4 kg (9 lb).

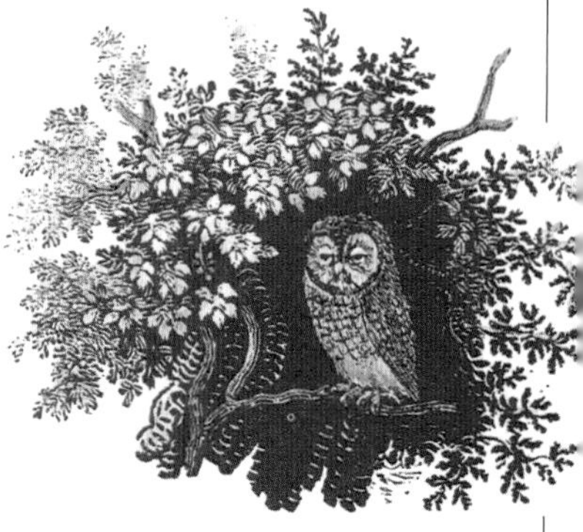

WISE BUT OMINOUS
The owl is known to be a wise bird, as it has an intelligent appearance. In some cultures, its sighting is believed to be ominous (sign of bad luck).

TAWNY OWL

The tawny owl lives in northern Asia and Europe and hunts all sorts of small mammals and birds. Its prey also includes worms, snails, and even fish.

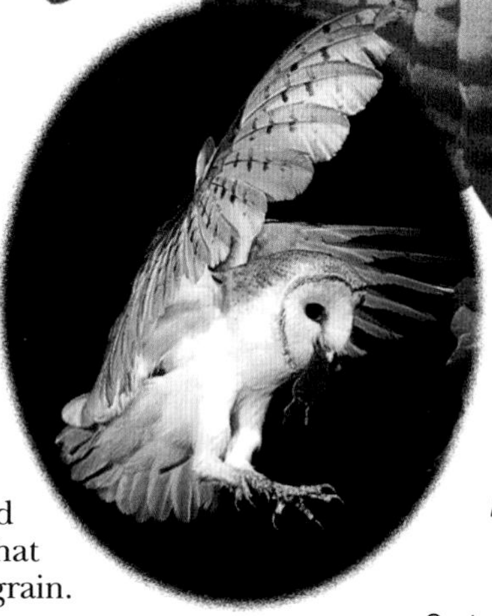

BARN OWL

Throughout the world the barn owl is known as the farmer's friend because it catches rats and mice that live in barns and eat grain.

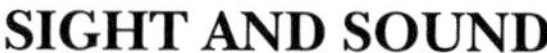

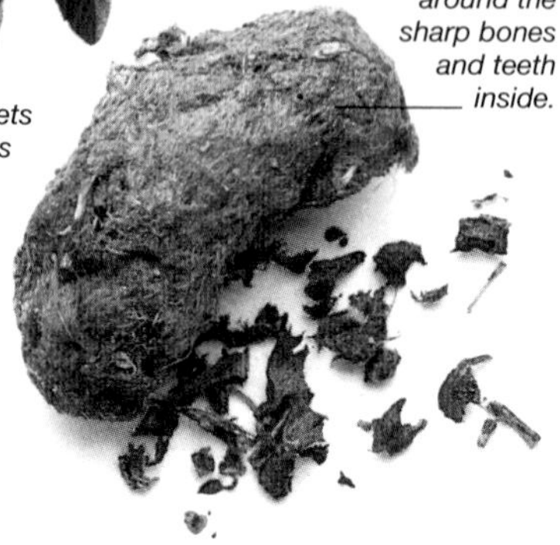

This pellet has soft fur, hair, and feathers wrapped around the sharp bones and teeth inside.

Tawny owl pellets also contain the remains of other birds, such as the starling skull and lower bill shown here.

Contents of owl pellet

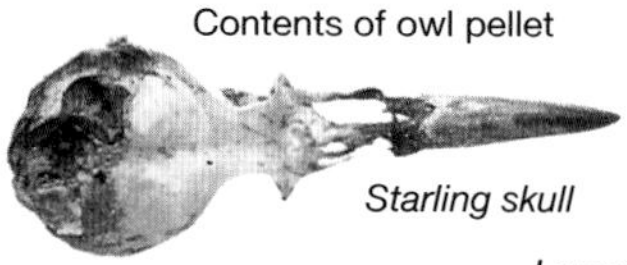

Starling skull

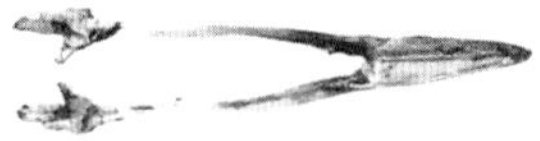

Lower bill

Remains of three field mice

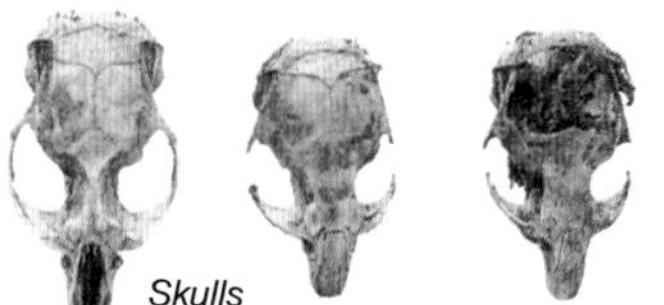

Skulls

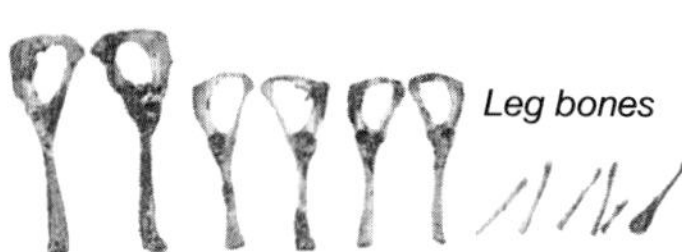

Leg bones

Hip bones

OWL PELLETS
Owls swallow their prey whole, but do not digest the bones, fur, feet, or beaks. Instead, the owl regurgitates, or coughs up, these remains in the form of pellets which fall to the ground under the owl's roost, where it perches. Take a pellet apart, and you can tell what the owl has eaten recently.

SIGHT AND SOUND

Owls have good eyesight and hearing. Their eyes are at the front of the head, so they can see ahead with both eyes, unlike most birds, whose eyes are on each side of the head. Owl eyes cannot swivel in their sockets, but the bird has a very flexible neck, and can turn its head right around to see behind – as shown by this eagle owl.

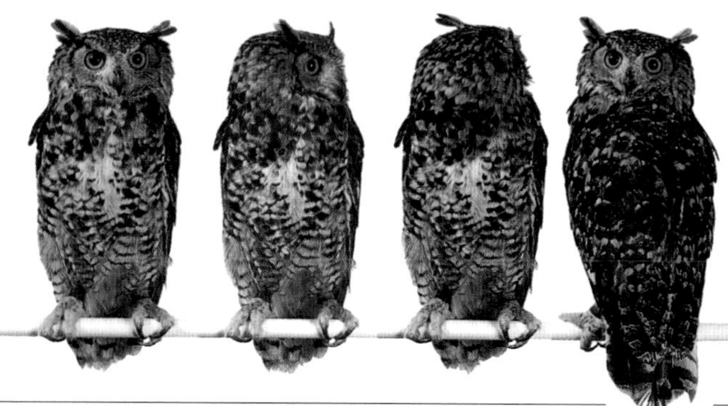

Find out more

BIRDS
EAGLES
and other birds of prey
FLIGHT, ANIMAL
NORTH AMERICAN WILDLIFE

OXYGEN

WE CANNOT SEE, SMELL, or taste oxygen, yet without oxygen, none of us could survive longer than a few minutes. It is fortunate, then, that oxygen is the most common substance on Earth. Oxygen is a gas. Mixed with other gases, it makes up about one fifth of the air we breathe. Most of the oxygen in the world, though, does not float free as a gas. Instead, the oxygen is bound up in combination with other substances – in a solid or liquid form. This is because oxygen is chemically reactive: it readily combines with other substances, often giving off energy in the process. Burning is an example of oxygen at work. When a piece of timber burns, oxygen is combining with the wood and giving off heat. Oxygen is also found in water, combined with atoms of another gas, hydrogen. Oxygen can be extracted from water by passing an electric current through it. The electricity breaks the water into its parts (the gases oxygen and hydrogen), and oxygen bubbles off.

RESPIRATION
Our bodies need oxygen to release the energy consumed when we use our muscles. The oxygen we breathe in is used to "burn" the food we eat, producing energy. This process is called respiration. Blood carries the oxygen from the lungs, which extract it from the air, to the muscles where it is needed.

BURNING

Nothing can burn without oxygen. In outer space there is no air or oxygen, so it would be impossible to light a fire. The rocket motors used to launch spacecraft need oxygen to burn the rocket fuel and propel the craft upwards. Spacecraft therefore carry their own supply of pure oxygen which mixes with the fuel in the rocket motor. When anything burns in pure oxygen, it produces a very hot flame. In welding machines a fuel gas is burned with pure oxygen, producing a flame hot enough to melt metals.

OXYGEN CYCLE
Breathing air or burning fuel removes oxygen from the atmosphere and gives off carbon dioxide. Plants do the reverse. During the day, they produce energy for growth by the process of photosynthesis. The green parts of the plant take in sunlight, water, and carbon dioxide to make new cells, and give off oxygen. So oxygen continually passes into and out of the air. This is called the oxygen cycle.

People and animals breathe in oxygen.

Green plants absorb carbon dioxide breathed out by living creatures.

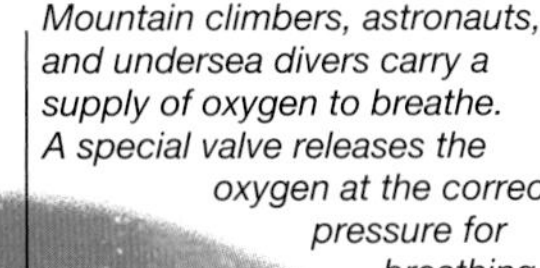

Mountain climbers, astronauts, and undersea divers carry a supply of oxygen to breathe. A special valve releases the oxygen at the correct pressure for breathing.

OXYGEN IN WATER
Sea water contains dissolved oxygen. Fish use this oxygen to breathe. Water flows over their gills, which extract the oxygen. Unlike other fish, some sharks can breathe only when moving in the water. To avoid suffocating, they must swim constantly, even when asleep.

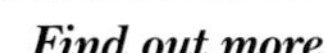

Find out more

AIR
CHEMISTRY
FIRE
HUMAN BODY
PLANTS

PACIFIC OCEAN

ON A MAP OF THE PACIFIC OCEAN, the sunny, tropical Pacific islands look like tiny grains of sand scattered on the sea. The first adventurous settlers of these islands sailed from Southeast Asia. They spread gradually across the region, travelling over the vast expanses of ocean in their light wooden sailing boats. Today the islands are divided into three main groups: Micronesia to the north, Melanesia to the south, and Polynesia to the east. There are twelve independent countries in the Pacific, including Fiji, Tonga, and Nauru, one of the world's smallest nations. Europeans first arrived in the Pacific in the 16th century, and a number of islands maintain strong links with Europe. New Caledonia, for instance, is French. Many Pacific islanders lead lives that have barely changed for centuries, but there are a number of important modern industries, including large-scale fishing and mining, as well as tourism.

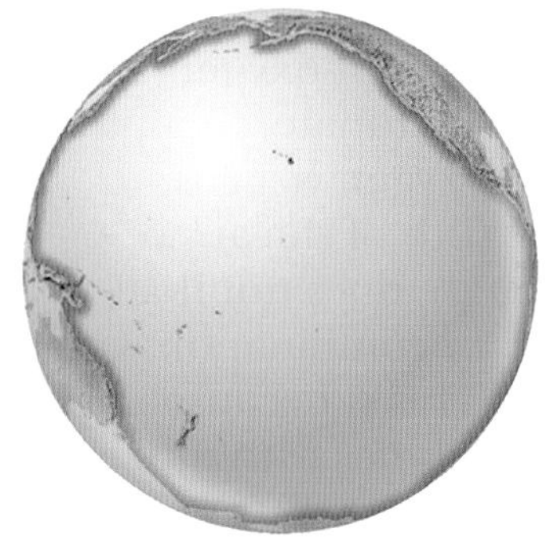

There are some 25,000 Pacific islands, but only a few thousand are inhabited. They stretch across the central part of the Pacific Ocean, straddling the equator and occupying an area larger than the whole of Asia. To the west and southwest lie Southeast Asia, Australia, and New Zealand; North and South America are to the east.

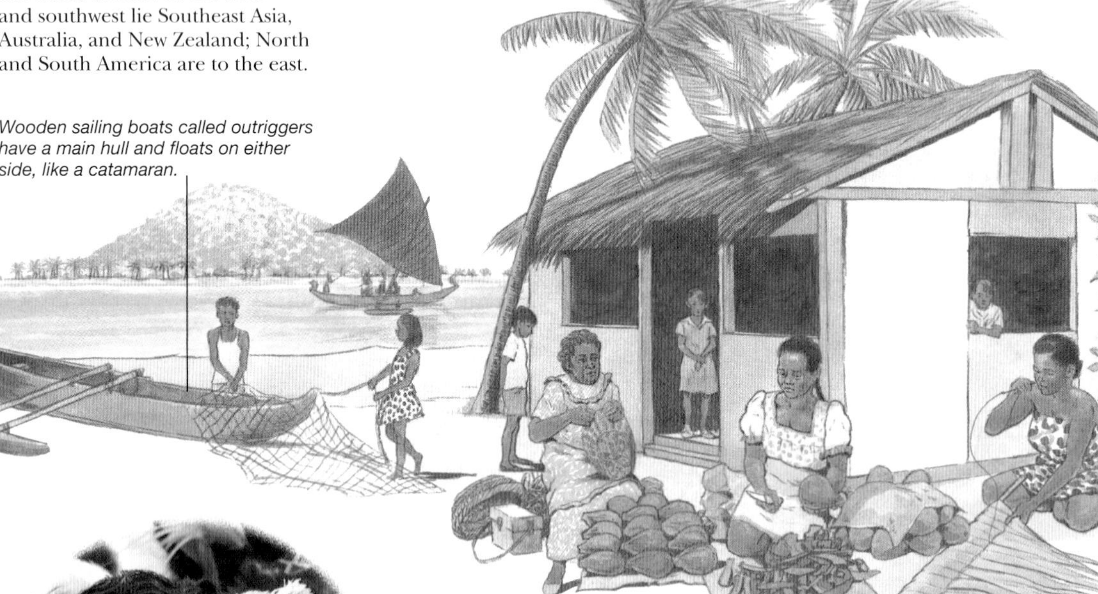

Wooden sailing boats called outriggers have a main hull and floats on either side, like a catamaran.

ISLAND LIFE

Many Pacific islands are very small. They are the tops of submerged mountains. Coral reefs protect them from the Pacific waves. On the remoter islands, people live much as their ancestors did. Their simple houses have thatched roofs made of palm fronds. Families keep pigs and chickens and grow fruit and vegetables. They use traditional boats for fishing and for trade between the islands.

Those taking part in the spectacular traditional dances of Papua New Guinea wear costumes decorated with feathers and beads.

PAPUA NEW GUINEA

New Guinea, one of the world's largest islands, is part of Melanesia. Half of it belongs to Indonesia and is called Irian Jaya. The other half is a mountainous independent country called Papua New Guinea. Its thick tropical forests are the home of many remote tribes who have little contact with the outside world.

United States military bases cover virtually all of some Pacific Islands, mainly in Micronesia.

EASTER ISLAND

Tiny, remote Easter Island is one of the furthest east of the Pacific islands. A Dutch admiral gave the island its name when he landed there on Easter Day in 1722. More than 1,000 years ago the islanders' Polynesian ancestors carved mysterious stone statues, which still dot the dry, barren landscape.

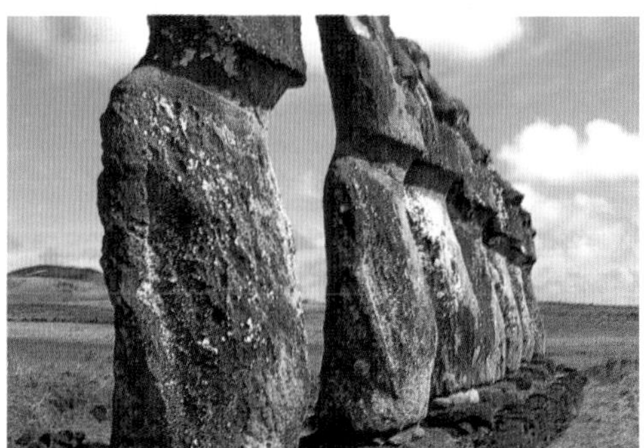

There are more than 600 of these huge heads on Easter Island, some over 20 m (65 ft) tall.

WAKE ISLAND

The United States controls a number of Pacific islands, including Wake Island (above) and Midway, which was the scene of a major battle in World War II. The islands of Hawaii form one of the 50 states of the United States.

Find out more

OCEANS AND SEAS

WORLD WAR II

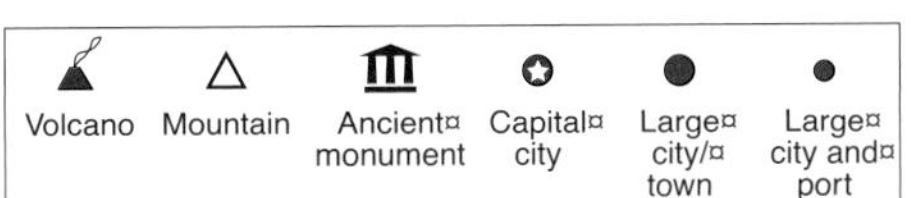

STATISTICS
Area: 790,225 sq km (305,106 sq miles)
Population: 7,820,900
Number of independent countries: 12
Languages: English, local languages and dialects
Religions: Protestant, Roman Catholic, Hindu
Highest point: Mount Wilhelm (Papua New Guinea) 4,509 m (14,793 ft)
Main occupations: Agriculture, fishing

FIJI
Area: 18,270 sq km (7,054 sq miles)
Population: 839,000
Capital: Suva
Currency: Fiji dollar

KIRIBATI
Area: 710 sq km (274 sq miles)
Population: 98,500
Capital: Bairiki
Currency: Australian dollar

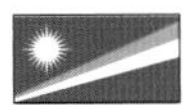

MARSHALL ISLANDS
Area: 181 sq km (70 sq miles)
Population: 56,400
Capital: Delap District
Currency: U.S. dollar

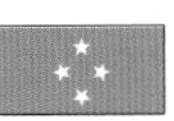

MICRONESIA
Area: 2,900 sq km (1,120 sq miles)
Population: 108,100
Capital: Palikir
Currency: U.S. dollar

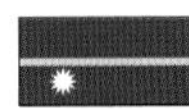

NAURU
Area: 21.2 sq km (8.2 sq miles)
Population: 12,600
Government Centre: Yaren
Currency: Australian dollar

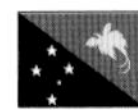

PAPUA NEW GUINEA
Area: 462,840 sq km (178,700 sq miles)
Population: 5,700,000
Capital: Port Moresby
Currency: Kina

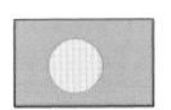

PALAU
Area: 497 sq km (192 sq miles)
Population: 19,700
Capital: Koror
Currency: U.S. dollar

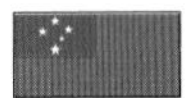

SAMOA
Area: 2,840 sq km (1,027 sq miles)
Population: 178,000
Capital: Apia
Currency: Tala

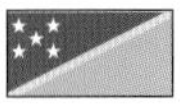

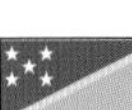

SOLOMON ISLANDS
Area: 289,000 sq km (111,583 sq miles)
Population: 477,000
Capital: Honiara
Currency: Solomon Islands dollar

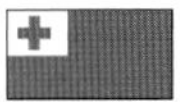

TONGA
Area: 750 sq km (290 sq miles)
Population: 108,100
Capital: Nuku'alofa
Currency: Tongan pa'anga

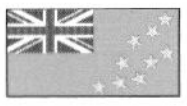

TUVALU
Area: 26 sq km (10 sq miles)
Population: 11,300
Capital: Fongafale
Currency: Australian dollar

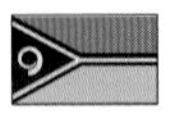

VANUATU
Area: 12,190 sq km (4,706 sq miles)
Population: 212,000
Capital: Port-Villa
Currency: Vatu

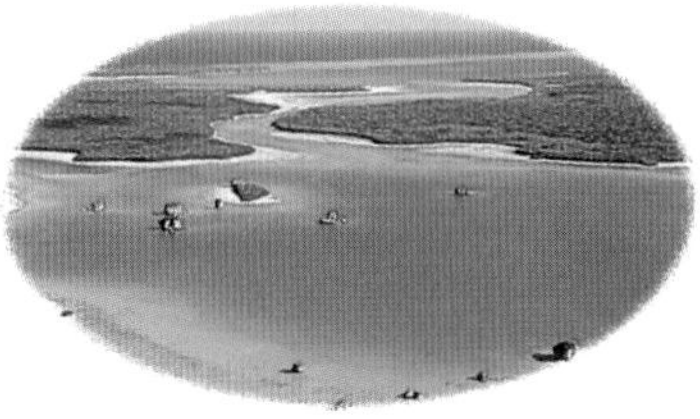

NEW CALEDONIA
The Isle of Pines (above) is one of the smallest inhabited islands in the New Caledonia group. Like many of the Pacific Islands, New Caledonia is governed by a larger, more powerful country. France rules New Caledonia, and French aid provides one-third of the country's income. Most of the rest comes from the export of nickel – the islands have 40 per cent of the world's reserves of the metal.

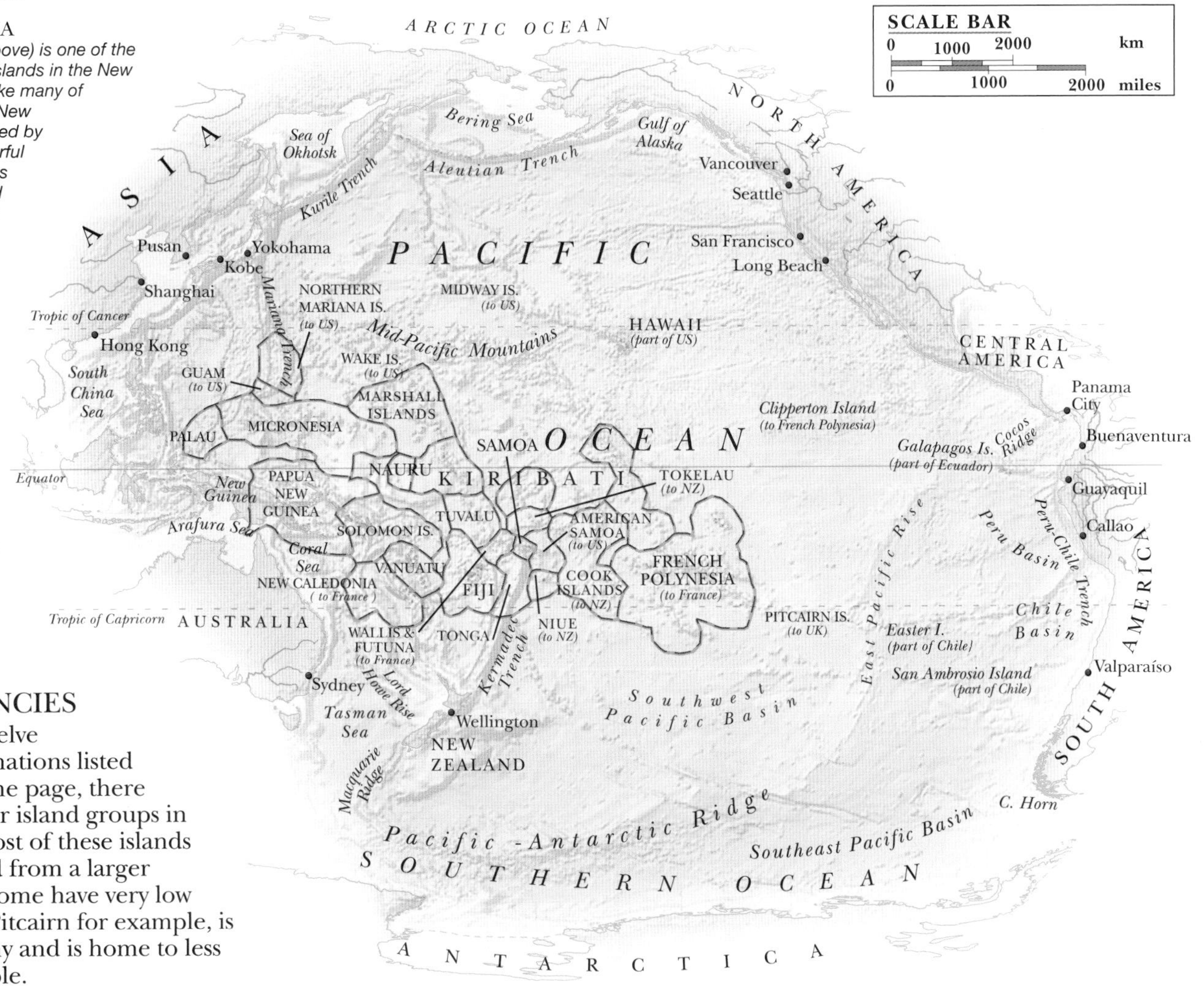

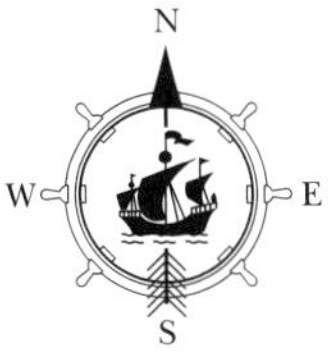

SCALE BAR
0 1000 2000 km
0 1000 2000 miles

ARCTIC OCEAN
ASIA
NORTH AMERICA
PACIFIC OCEAN
Sea of Okhotsk
Bering Sea
Gulf of Alaska
Aleutian Trench
Kurile Trench
Vancouver
Seattle
San Francisco
Long Beach
Pusan
Yokohama
Kobe
Shanghai
Mariana Trench
NORTHERN MARIANA IS. (to US)
MIDWAY IS. (to US)
Mid-Pacific Mountains
HAWAII (part of US)
Tropic of Cancer
Hong Kong
South China Sea
GUAM (to US)
WAKE IS. (to US)
MARSHALL ISLANDS
CENTRAL AMERICA
Panama City
PALAU
MICRONESIA
Clipperton Island (to French Polynesia)
Cocos Ridge
Buenaventura
SAMOA
Galapagos Is. (part of Ecuador)
Equator
NAURU
KIRIBATI
TOKELAU (to NZ)
Guayaquil
New Guinea
PAPUA NEW GUINEA
TUVALU
AMERICAN SAMOA (to US)
Callao
Arafura Sea
SOLOMON IS.
East Pacific Rise
Peru Basin
Peru-Chile Trench
Coral Sea
VANUATU
FRENCH POLYNESIA (to France)
NEW CALEDONIA (to France)
FIJI
COOK ISLANDS (to NZ)
Tropic of Capricorn
AUSTRALIA
WALLIS & FUTUNA (to France)
TONGA
NIUE (to NZ)
PITCAIRN IS. (to UK)
Easter I. (part of Chile)
Chile Basin
SOUTH AMERICA
Kermadec Trench
San Ambrosio Island (part of Chile)
Valparaíso
Sydney
Lord Howe Rise
Southwest Pacific Basin
Tasman Sea
Wellington
NEW ZEALAND
Macquarie Ridge
Pacific-Antarctic Ridge
C. Horn
Southeast Pacific Basin
SOUTHERN OCEAN
ANTARCTICA
N
W
E
S

DEPENDENCIES

Besides the twelve independent nations listed at the top of the page, there are many other island groups in the Pacific. Most of these islands depend on aid from a larger country, and some have very low populations. Pitcairn for example, is a British colony and is home to less than 100 people.

PAINTERS

ARTISTS USE PAINT in the same way that writers use words to convey ideas on paper. Painters capture the likeness of a face or a flower, but they can do much more than just paint a realistic image. Painters work skilfully with colour, texture, and shape to create all kinds of eye-catching images of the world as they see it. Every culture throughout history has produced its own great painters, from Giotto in the 14th century to Picasso in the 20th century. There have been many different groups, or movements, in painting, such as classicism, cubism, and pop art. Painters change the way we see the world. Rembrandt's portrait paintings, for example, are powerful studies from real life, whereas Salvador Dali's strange surrealist (dreamlike) landscapes are drawn from his imagination. Painters use all kinds of paint to create a picture – thick blobs of oil colour daubed onto a canvas with a palette knife; delicate brushstrokes of water-colour on a sheet of paper. Some painters dab paint on with sponges, rags, even their fingers; others flick paint onto a surface. Whatever the medium (materials) used, each great painter has his or her own distinctive style.

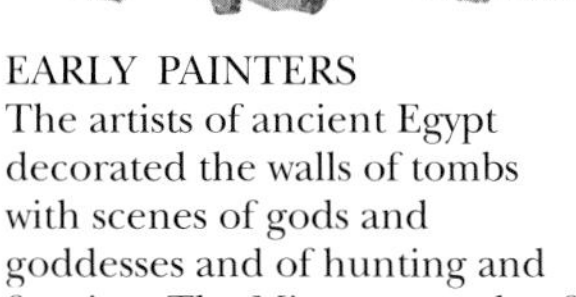

EARLY PAINTERS
The artists of ancient Egypt decorated the walls of tombs with scenes of gods and goddesses and of hunting and feasting. The Minoan people of early Greece painted their houses and palaces with pictures of dancers, birds, and flowers. Roman artists painted gods and goddesses and scenes from classical mythology.

People in medieval paintings sometimes look stiff and expressionless, like the figures in this 11th-century picture (left) of an emperor, a saint, and an angel.

MEDIEVAL PAINTERS
Up until the 14th century, Western artists painted mostly Christian subjects – the life of Christ and the saints. Painters used rich colours and thin layers of gold to make these religious paintings. These early artists used different methods of painting people from later Western painters, but although the paintings may look flat to us, they are no less powerful. Artists worked on wood panels for altarpieces and painted directly on church walls.

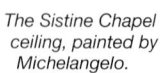

The Sistine Chapel ceiling, painted by Michelangelo.

RENAISSANCE

One of the greatest periods in European painting was the Renaissance, which reached its height in Italy in the early part of the 16th century. During the Renaissance, painters developed more realistic styles of painting. They studied perspective and the human body, painted more realistic landscapes, and developed portrait painting.

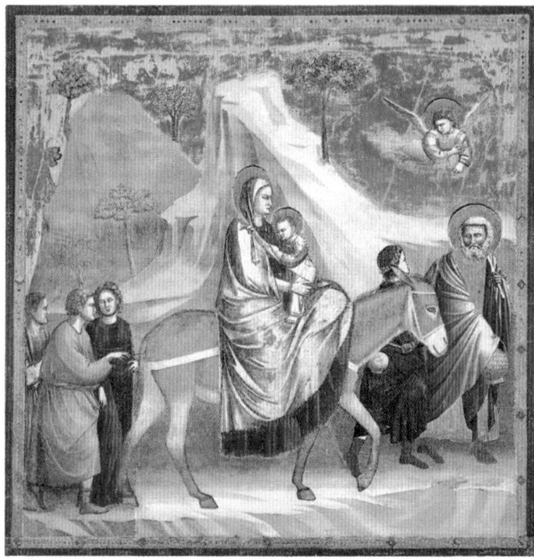

MICHELANGELO

Michelangelo Buonarroti (1475-1564) is one of the best-known Italian Renaissance painters. Much of his work was for Pope Julius II, who commissioned him to paint the ceiling of the Sistine Chapel in the Vatican, in Rome, between 1508 and 1512.

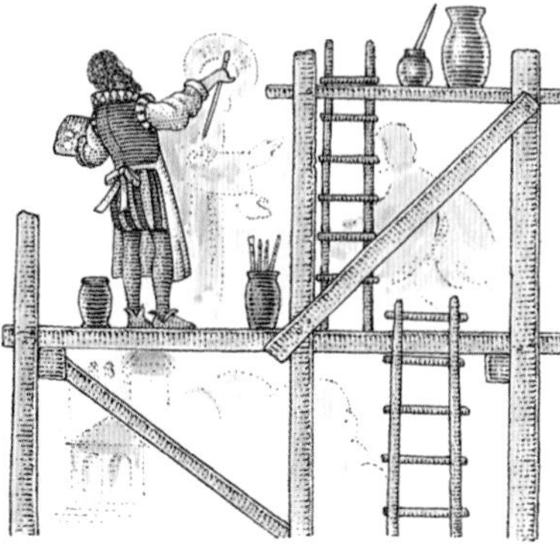

Michelangelo had difficulty in reaching certain parts of the ceiling in the Sistine Chapel, so he built a scaffold and sometimes lay on his back to paint.

GIOTTO

The Italian artist Giotto (c.1266-1337) painted at the beginning of the Renaissance. He brought a new sense of naturalness to paintings. The painting shown above is called *The Flight into Egypt.* It shows Mary and Jesus on a donkey being led by Joseph.

REMBRANDT

Most people know the Dutch artist Rembrandt H. van Rijn (1606-69) only by his first name. He is well known for his portraits which are full of expression. The painting shown here is one of many self-portraits.

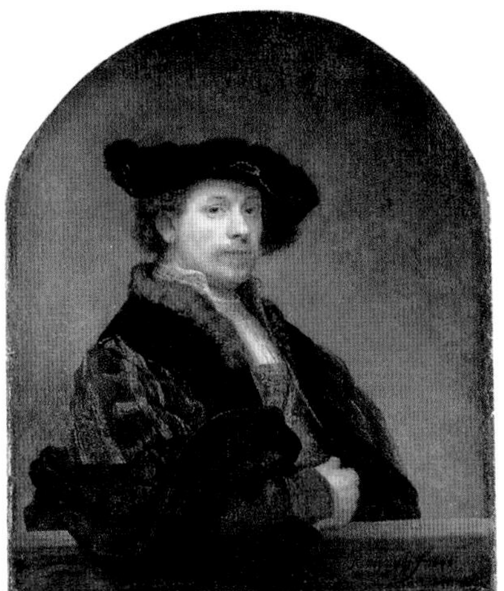

ROMANTIC MOVEMENT

During the late 18th and early 19th centuries, painters such as the French artist Eugène Delacroix (1798-1863) began a new style of painting, which became known as the Romantic Movement. The romantics used bright colour and a free handling of paint to create their dramatic pictures. The English painter J.M.W. Turner (1775-1851) painted landscapes and seascapes flooded with light and colour.

EASTERN PAINTERS

While European art was developing, Eastern artists were evolving their own styles of painting. The Chinese observed nature accurately and painted exquisite pictures with simple brushstrokes in ink on silk and paper. Some Japanese artists, such as Hokusai (1760-1849), made beautiful prints.

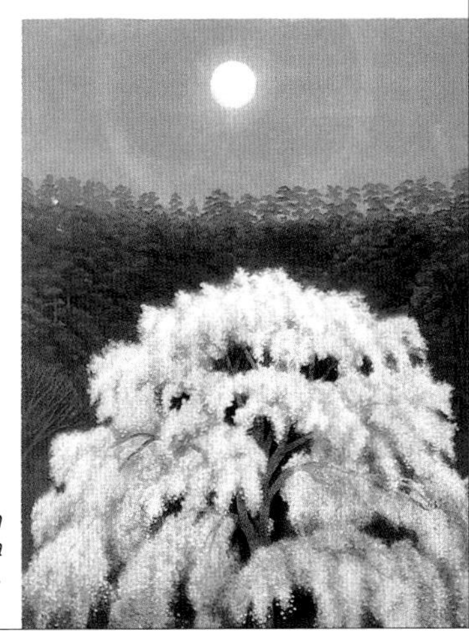

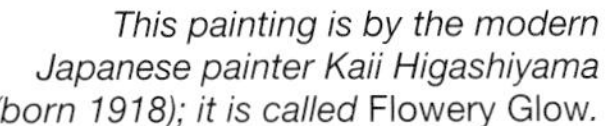

This painting is by the modern Japanese painter Kaii Higashiyama (born 1918); it is called Flowery Glow.

PICASSO

Many people believe that the Spanish painter Pablo Picasso (1881-1973) was the most creative and influential artist of the 20th century. From a very young age, Picasso was extremely skilful at drawing and painting. His restless personality led him to paint in many different styles. One style was his "blue period" of painting, when he concentrated on blue as the main colour for his pictures. In 1907, Picasso painted a picture called *Les Demoiselles D'Avignon*, which shocked many people – it was a painting of human figures represented by angular and distorted shapes. This led to a style of painting called cubism.

This is a detail from the painting by the French artist Fragonard (1732-1806) called The Swing.

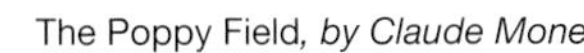

The Poppy Field, *by Claude Monet*

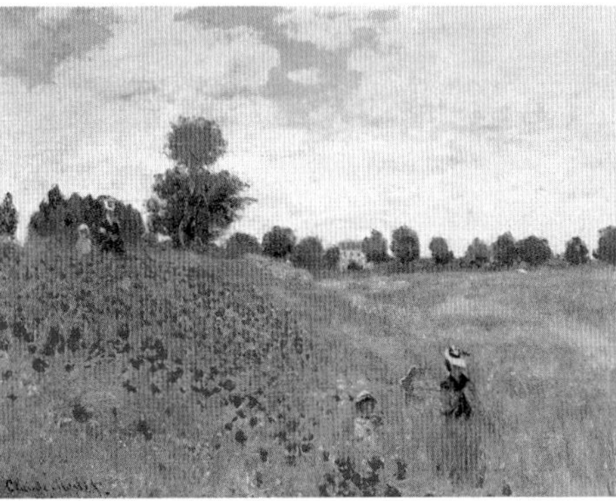

This photograph shows Picasso with a painting of his children, Claude and Paloma. He is on his way to show this painting at an exhibition of his work.

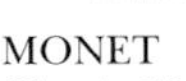

MONET

Claude Monet (1840-1926) was the leader of the impressionists. He painted many pictures of the flowers in his garden at Giverny and in the French countryside, including the picture above right, called *The Poppy Field*. Seen close up, the picture consists of many brushstrokes of different colours, but from a distance the dabs of colour come together to form a field of red flowers.

IMPRESSIONISM

At an exhibition in Paris in 1874 a painting by the French artist Claude Monet caused an uproar. Art critics and the public were used to seeing realistic objects in pictures, but Monet and his fellow artists, known as impressionists, painted in dabs of colour to create the effect of light and shade. Other great artists of the impressionist movement were Camille Pissarro, Pierre Auguste Renoir, Edgar Degas, Mary Cassatt, and Alfred Sisley.

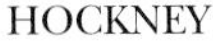

HOCKNEY

David Hockney (born 1937) is a well-known British painter. He is famous for his pictures of California, especially paintings of swimming pools such as this one, called *A Bigger Splash*. Hockney works with many different materials, including photographs and colour photocopies.

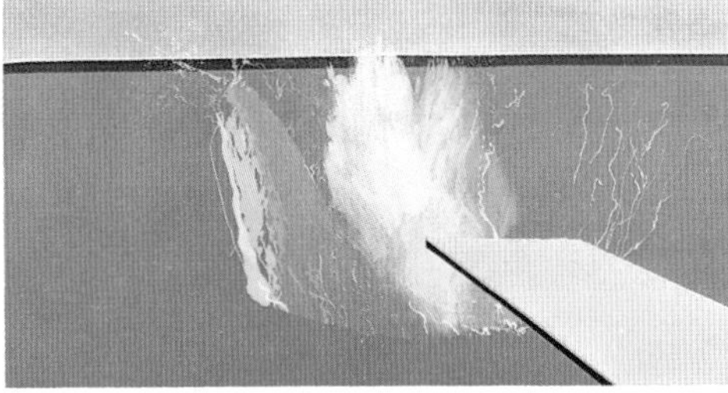

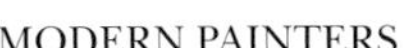

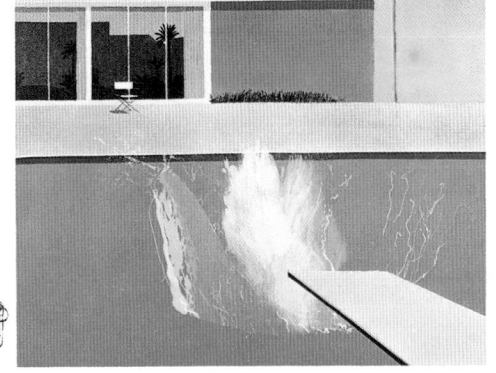

MODERN PAINTERS

Since the beginning of the 20th century, painters have experimented with different ways of creating pictures. Picasso and Georges Braque stuck fabric, sand, and newsprint on to canvases to make collages. Piet Mondrian painted in straight lines and right angles. Action painting was developed by the American artist Jackson Pollock, who splashed paint onto huge canvases on his studio floor.

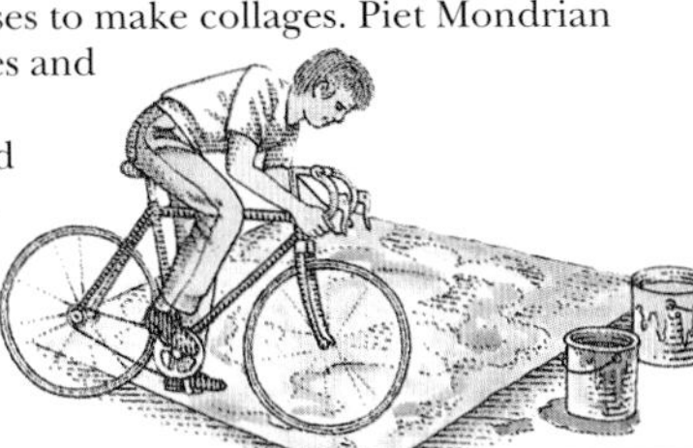

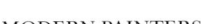

Find out more

DRAWING
LEONARDO DA VINCI
MORRIS, WILLIAM
PAINTING
RENAISSANCE
SCULPTURE

Painters

Today, British painters are known all over the world for shocking the public with new ways of looking at the things around them. In fact, British artists have been surprising their public for hundreds of years. They may not seem shocking today, but the tiny miniature portraits of Tudor times, the freely painted landscapes of Constable, and the brightly coloured paintings of the Pre-Raphaelites amazed everybody when they were first shown. This is because artists in Britain, while valuing past achievements, have often turned their backs on the art of earlier years, to try new styles and develop fresh techniques. Their paintings and sculptures live on in galleries and museums, to tell us about the past, to show how styles have changed, and to entertain us.

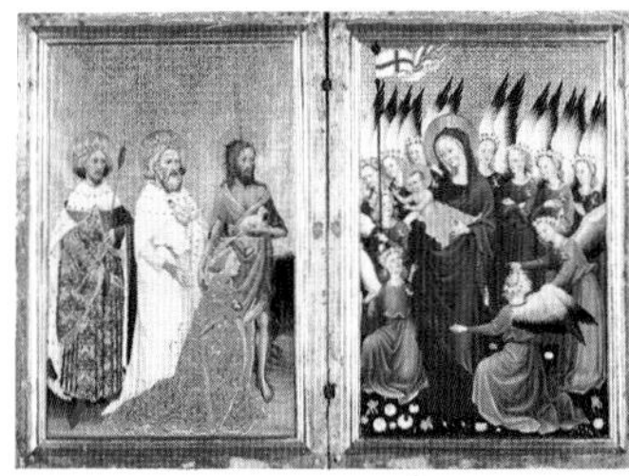

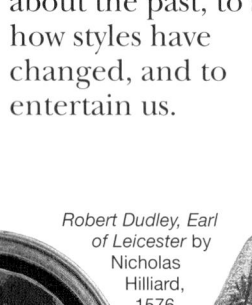

MEDIEVAL PAINTING
The Wilton Diptych, a two-panel altarpiece that belonged to English King Richard II (1377-99), is one of the masterpieces of British medieval art. It shows the king, his features portrayed in beautiful detail, kneeling before the Virgin Mary.

NICHOLAS HILLIARD
Many 16th- and 17th-century artists painted miniatures – tiny, highly detailed portraits a few centimetres across. Nicholas Hilliard (1547-1619), who painted lords and ladies of the royal court, was the greatest miniaturist.

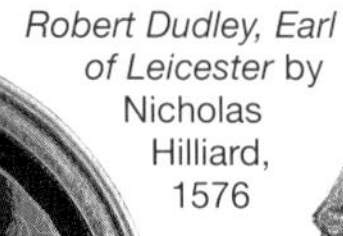

Robert Dudley, Earl of Leicester by Nicholas Hilliard, 1576

Detail from *The Painter's Daughters Chasing a Butterfly* by Thomas Gainsborough, late 1750s

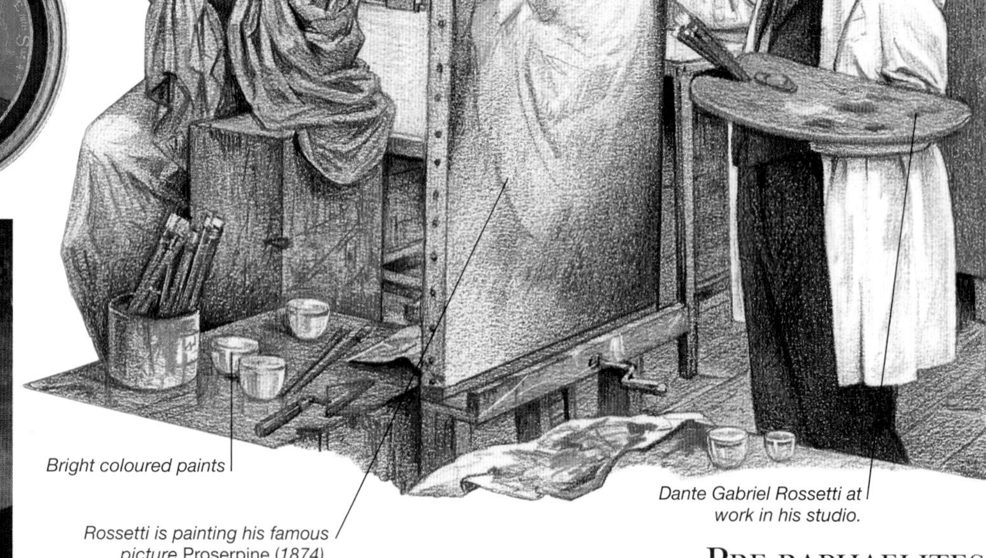

Bright coloured paints

Dante Gabriel Rossetti at work in his studio.

Rossetti is painting his famous picture Proserpine *(1874).*

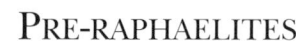

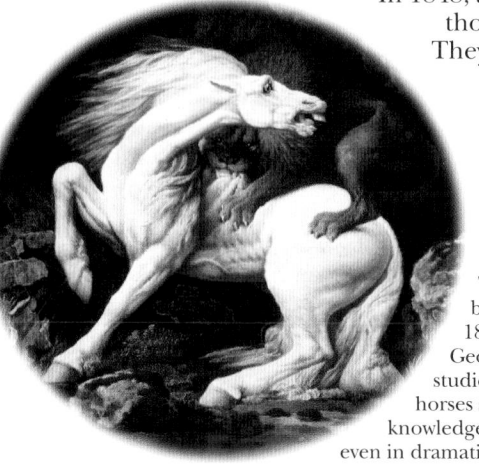

Pre-Raphaelites

In 1848, a group of artists rebelled against what they thought to be the dullness of 19th-century art. They wanted to work more realistically, to paint scenes from everyday life, and use bright colours, like the Italian artists who lived before Raphael (1483-1520). They were called the Pre-Raphaelites, and included artists such as John Millais (1829-96) and Dante Gabriel Rossetti (1828-82).

Portraiture

Painting people is called portraiture. The greatest British portrait painters were Sir Joshua Reynolds (1723-92) and Thomas Gainsborough (1727-88). Reynolds produced grand portraits of rich people, Gainsborough specialized in elegant figures posed in a landscape background. He was famed for his delicate brushwork.

ANIMAL ART
The British have always been fascinated by animals, but did not produce great animal paintings until the 18th century. The breakthrough came when artist George Stubbs (1724-1806) started to make detailed studies of animal muscles and bones. He even dissected horses so that he could draw their anatomy. Stubbs's knowledge helped him to paint the creatures with realism, even in dramatic works such as his Lion Devouring a Horse.

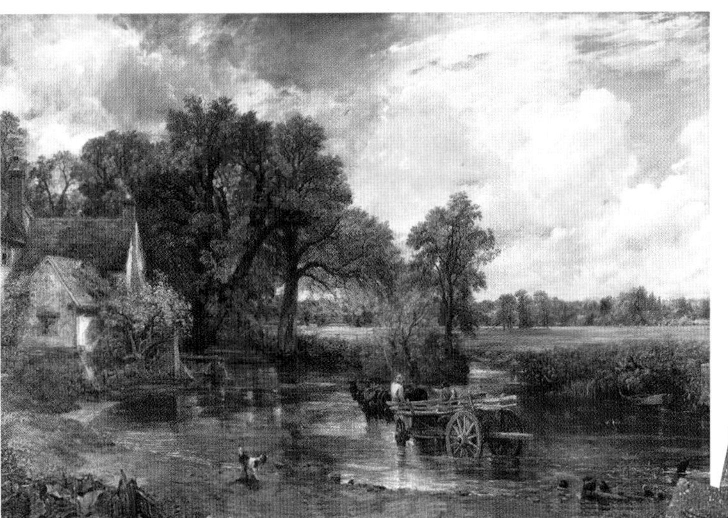

ILLUSTRATION

Some artists specialize in illustrating books, using their skills to bring characters and scenes to life. Before photography, book illustrators were in great demand. Two of the best known were John Tenniel (1820-1914), illustrator of Lewis Carroll's Alice books, and "Phiz" (Hablot Browne, 1815-82), who illustrated novels by Charles Dickens.

John Tenniel illustration from *Alice in Wonderland*

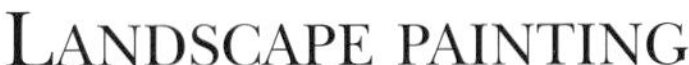

LANDSCAPE PAINTING

The British landscape, with its fields, woods, and streams, fascinated the painters of the 19th century. John Constable (1776-1837) painted the fields and ever-changing skies of his native East Anglia. Large-scale landscapes, such as *The Hay Wain*, made him famous, but today people also admire his sketches, with their rapid, free brushstrokes.

TURNER

J.M.W. Turner (1775-1851) may have been the greatest landscape painter of all. His use of colour is dazzling, and in his oil paintings and watercolours, the individual details of the landscape often seem to dissolve in shimmering, brilliant light.

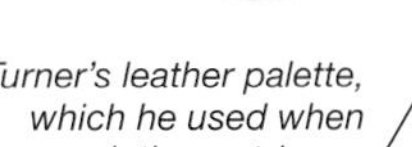

Turner's leather palette, which he used when painting outdoors.

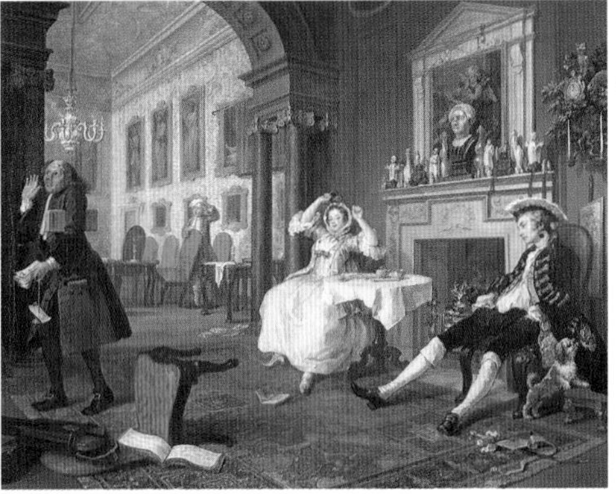

HOGARTH

William Hogarth (1697-1764) was one of Britain's most versatile painters. He was known both for his portraits and for paintings and engravings that satirized the manners of the times. His famous series of paintings, *Marriage à la Mode* shows what happens when a fashionable marriage goes wrong.

BRIDGET RILEY

"Op", or optical, art was the name given to the dazzling black-and-white paintings produced in the 1960s by artists such as Bridget Riley (b. 1931). It was called optical because it tricked the eye. Riley's pictures, which she later also painted in colour, consist of flat patterns which look as if they are moving across the surface of the canvas, or as if the canvas is curved.

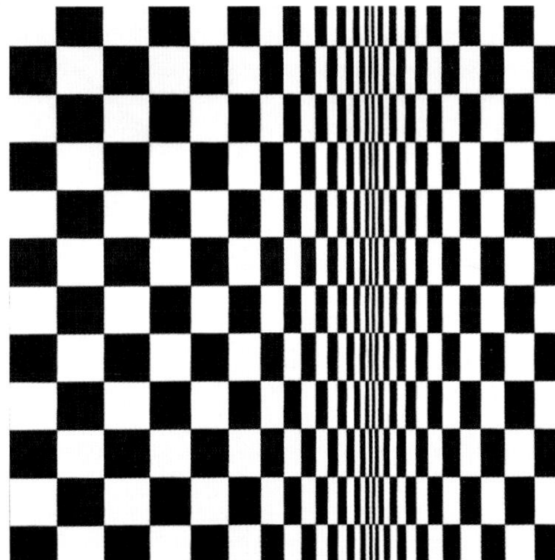

Movement in Squares (1961)

BRIT ART

During the 1980s and 1990s, a group of young British artists became famous all over the world. A leading member of this "Brit art" group was Damien Hirst, best known for his sculpture consisting of a sheep in a tank of preserving fluid. His later work included dot paintings.

Argininosuccinic Acid by Damien Hirst (1995)

Find out more

LITERATURE
PAINTERS
PAINTING

PAINTING

SINCE PREHISTORIC PEOPLE first applied natural pigments to cave walls, artists have painted to express themselves. Paintings can be important historical documents, providing clues as to how people dressed at the time of the painting and what their customs and interests were. Training is not necessary in order to paint, but it can help in learning basic techniques. A painting can be done with oil paints, watercolours, or as a fresco – that is, painting onto wet plaster. The type of paint depends on what the powdered pigment or colour is mixed with to allow it to be brushed onto the painting. Oil paints use a vegetable oil such as linseed or poppy oil. Before oil paints were developed in the 15th century, artists made tempera paintings in which the pigments were mixed with an emulsion such as egg yolk. Artists may paint onto almost any surface: from rock and wood to fabric, paper, metal, plastics – even skin. They may also choose any subject, such as a still life or something abstract like random shapes.

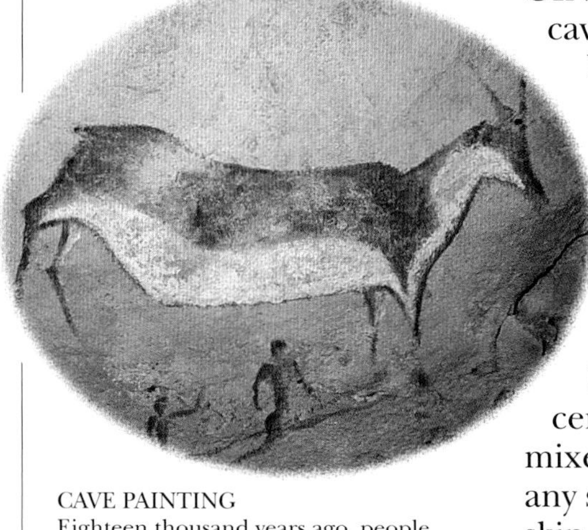

CAVE PAINTING
Eighteen thousand years ago, people used burned bones and wood, and different-coloured earth mixed with water or animal fat, to paint scenes on cave walls. South African bushmen produced this cave painting. It shows men hunting an eland, a type of deer.

OIL PAINTING

Oil paint has the advantage of drying slowly. This gives the artist time to change things on the painting while the paint is still wet, and makes it easier to blend colours and tones or even scrape off the paint where it is not working successfully. Oil paint can be applied thickly or thinly. It is flexible enough to be built up in layers to produce a particular effect. The paint is applied to a canvas (a piece of fabric stretched onto a frame) with brushes, a painting knife, or the fingers.

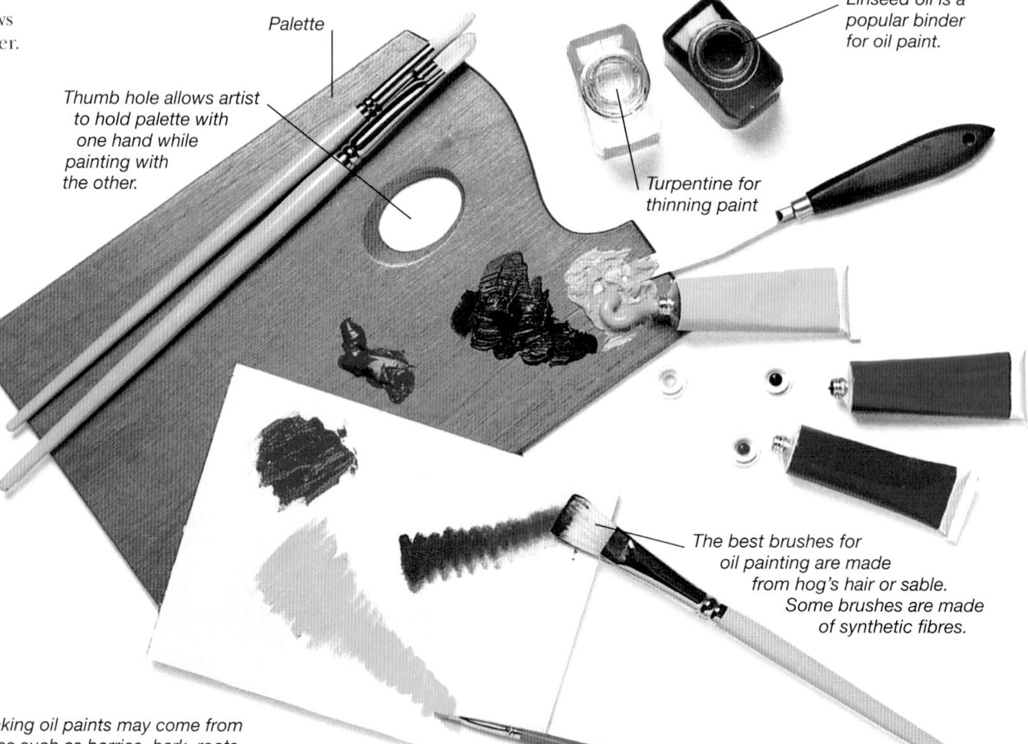

Palette

Thumb hole allows artist to hold palette with one hand while painting with the other.

Linseed oil is a popular binder for oil paint.

Turpentine for thinning paint

The best brushes for oil painting are made from hog's hair or sable. Some brushes are made of synthetic fibres.

Pigments for making oil paints may come from natural sources such as berries, bark, roots, and earth, or from petroleum and metals.

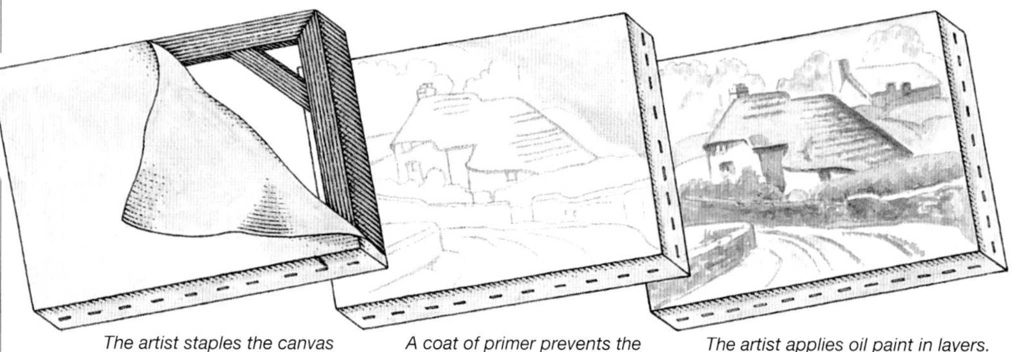

The artist staples the canvas to a wooden frame. This makes the canvas taut.

A coat of primer prevents the canvas from absorbing the paint; then an outline is done.

The artist applies oil paint in layers. When dry, the painting will be coated with varnish to protect it against dirt.

PREPARING FOR OIL PAINTING
Linen or cotton canvas is a popular surface or "support" for oil painting. Before beginning, the canvas must be specially prepared (left). Once it is ready, the painter can begin to apply layers of paint. Some artists draw outlines in charcoal or pencil on the canvas first; others put the paint straight on. Oil paint can be thinned down with turpentine to produce an effect rather like a watercolour.

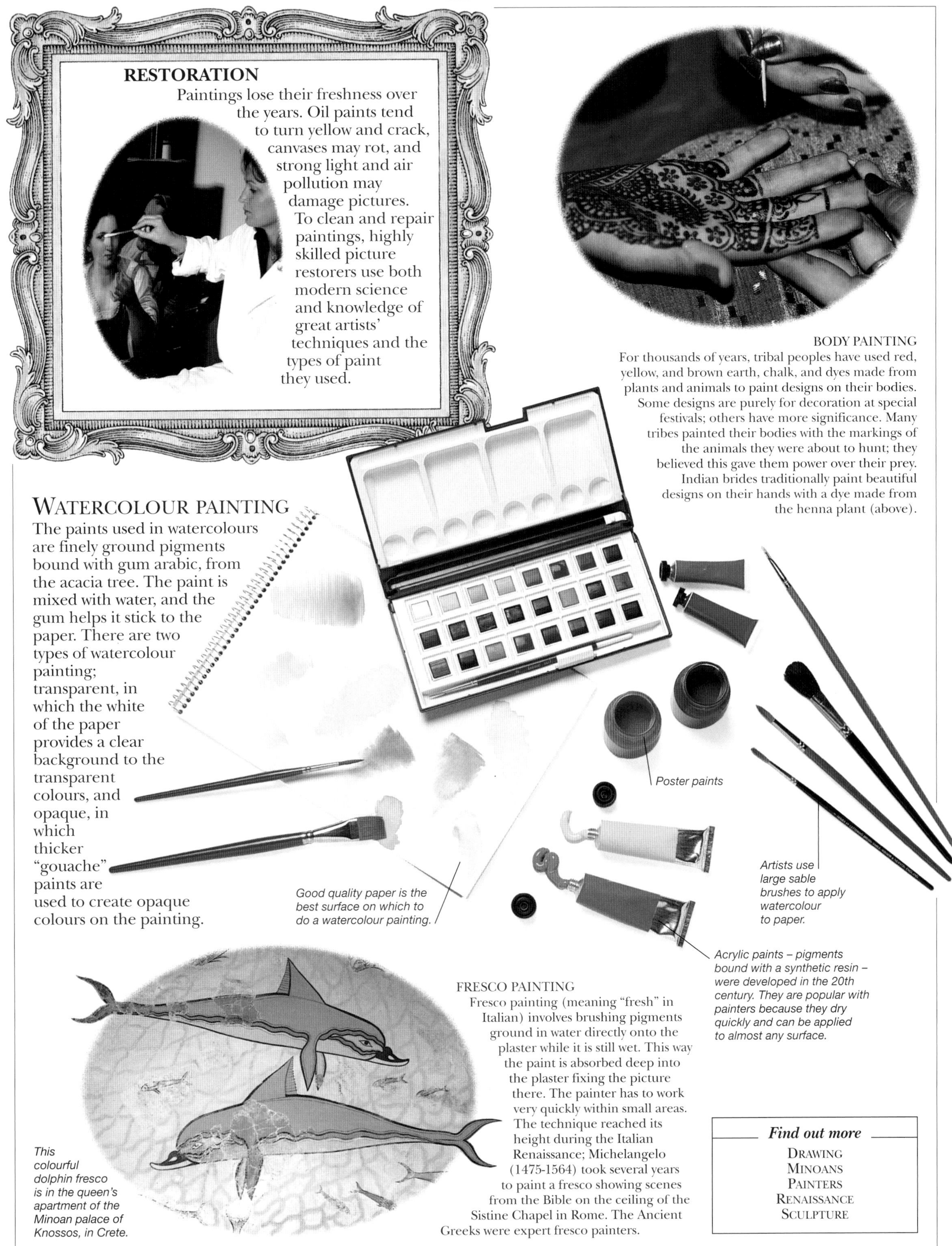

RESTORATION

Paintings lose their freshness over the years. Oil paints tend to turn yellow and crack, canvases may rot, and strong light and air pollution may damage pictures. To clean and repair paintings, highly skilled picture restorers use both modern science and knowledge of great artists' techniques and the types of paint they used.

BODY PAINTING

For thousands of years, tribal peoples have used red, yellow, and brown earth, chalk, and dyes made from plants and animals to paint designs on their bodies. Some designs are purely for decoration at special festivals; others have more significance. Many tribes painted their bodies with the markings of the animals they were about to hunt; they believed this gave them power over their prey. Indian brides traditionally paint beautiful designs on their hands with a dye made from the henna plant (above).

WATERCOLOUR PAINTING

The paints used in watercolours are finely ground pigments bound with gum arabic, from the acacia tree. The paint is mixed with water, and the gum helps it stick to the paper. There are two types of watercolour painting; transparent, in which the white of the paper provides a clear background to the transparent colours, and opaque, in which thicker "gouache" paints are used to create opaque colours on the painting.

Poster paints

Artists use large sable brushes to apply watercolour to paper.

Good quality paper is the best surface on which to do a watercolour painting.

Acrylic paints – pigments bound with a synthetic resin – were developed in the 20th century. They are popular with painters because they dry quickly and can be applied to almost any surface.

FRESCO PAINTING

Fresco painting (meaning "fresh" in Italian) involves brushing pigments ground in water directly onto the plaster while it is still wet. This way the paint is absorbed deep into the plaster fixing the picture there. The painter has to work very quickly within small areas. The technique reached its height during the Italian Renaissance; Michelangelo (1475-1564) took several years to paint a fresco showing scenes from the Bible on the ceiling of the Sistine Chapel in Rome. The Ancient Greeks were expert fresco painters.

This colourful dolphin fresco is in the queen's apartment of the Minoan palace of Knossos, in Crete.

Find out more

DRAWING
MINOANS
PAINTERS
RENAISSANCE
SCULPTURE

PANKHURST FAMILY

IN THE YEARS LEADING UP TO WORLD WAR I, the cry of "votes for women" was front-page news. Thousands of long-skirted women marched, demonstrated, and fought for their right to vote. Three fearless women inspired them: Emmeline Pankhurst and her daughters, Christabel and Sylvia. They were not the first to demand votes for women, but they used completely new methods. In 1903 they founded the Women's Social and Political Union (WSPU). At a time when women were supposed to live quiet, respectable lives, the Pankhursts declared war on Parliament for refusing the vote to women, fought with police, and even went to prison for their cause.

1858 Emmeline born.
1880 Christabel born.
1882 Sylvia born.
1903 WSPU founded, Manchester.
1905 Christabel arrested for the first time.
1911 WSPU attacks on property.
1912 Christabel flees to Paris.
1928 Emmeline dies.
1958 Christabel dies.
1960 Sylvia dies.

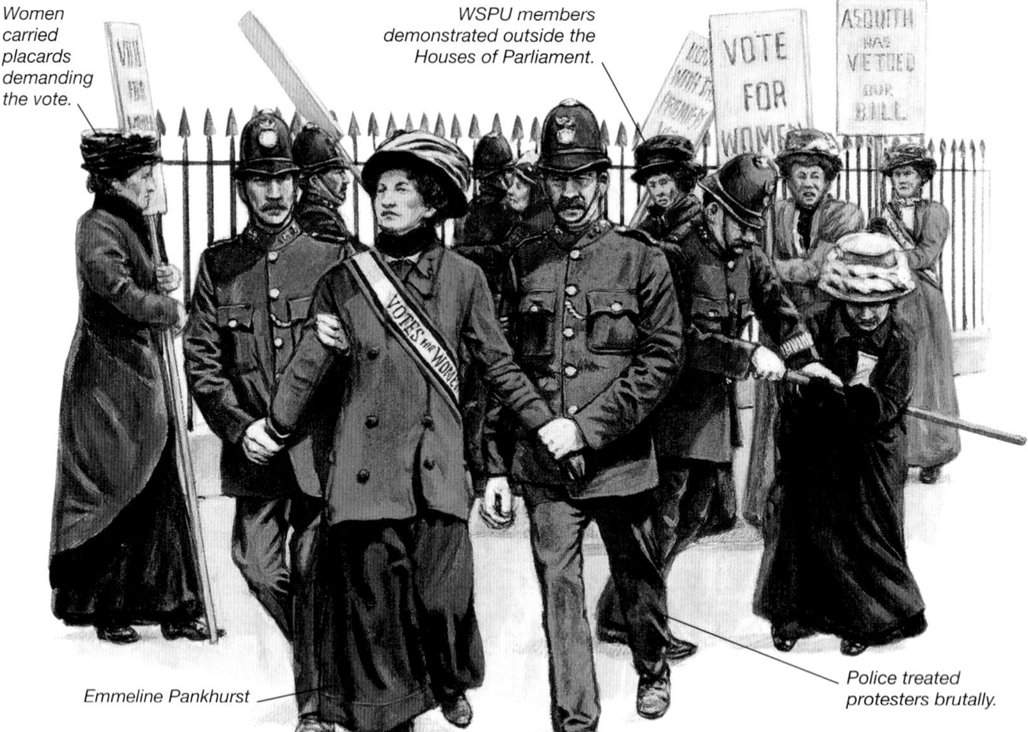
Women carried placards demanding the vote.
WSPU members demonstrated outside the Houses of Parliament.
VOTE FOR WOMEN
ASQUITH HAS VETOED OUR BILL
Emmeline Pankhurst
Police treated protesters brutally.

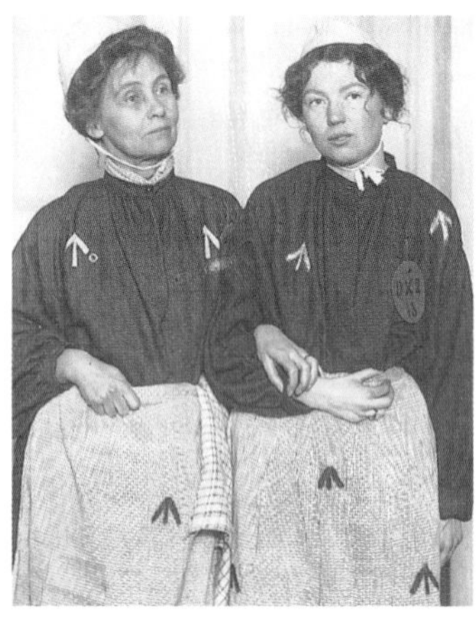

EMMELINE AND CHRISTABEL
Both women, shown here in prison clothes, were forceful personalities and brilliant organizers. Christabel (right) trained as a lawyer, but because she was a woman was not allowed to practise. Emmeline, her mother, was an inspiring speaker.

WSPU

The Pankhursts founded the Women's Social and Political Union (WSPU). Its aim was to get the vote "by any means". The WSPU used daring tactics and thousands of women joined in the fight. Emmeline inspired them; Christabel led them like an army commander. They heckled politicians, attacked property, and hundreds were arrested.

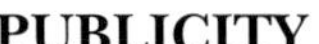

PUBLICITY

The Pankhursts publicised their cause brilliantly. They adopted three distinctive colours: green (for hope); purple (for dignity); and white (for purity). WSPU members carried these colours at all times, as sashes, badges, or banners, so people recognized them immediately. Today, these are still the colours of the women's movement.

WSPU badge designed by Sylvia Pankhurst

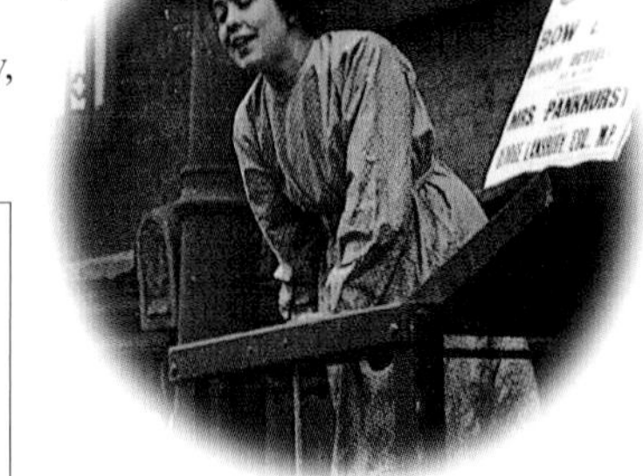

SYLVIA PANKHURST
A dedicated campaigner, Sylvia went to prison 13 times. She was a talented artist, and designed WSPU banners and badges. She worked with poor women in London's East End, and fell out with Emmeline and Christabel because she believed the WSPU was too middle class.

CASTING THE FIRST VOTE
In 1914, World War I began, and the WSPU split. Emmeline and Christabel supported the war effort; Sylvia opposed it. After the war, in 1918, women finally won their right to vote, largely thanks to the Pankhursts. Christabel stood for Parliament, but did not win a seat.

Find out more
GOVERNMENT AND POLITICS
HUMAN RIGHTS
WOMEN'S RIGHTS
WORLD WAR I

Paper

TEAR A PIECE OF PAPER, and you will see tiny fibres along the tear. These are plant fibres, and a piece of paper contains millions of them stuck together. Paper may also contain other materials, such as a filler to make it stiff, resin to keep ink from soaking into the fibres, and dye to colour the paper. Using different materials produces different kinds of paper, from stiff, heavy cardboard to light, fluffy tissues. The plant fibres in paper come mainly from trees. Millions of trees are cut down every year to provide us with paper, and new trees are planted in their place. Rags are also used to make some paper, and waste paper can be reused to make new paper. Recycled paper is paper made completely or partly from waste paper. Making paper in this way saves forests, uses much less energy, and reduces air and water pollution. Paper is named after papyrus, a reed-like plant which the Ancient Egyptians used as a writing material more than 5,000 years ago. The Chinese invented the paper that we use about 2,000 years ago. But wasps have been making paper for much longer. They chew up wood and plant fibres to make paper nests.

ORIGAMI
Folding a sheet of paper into a decorative shape is called origami. The art of origami is at least 300 years old and began in Japan.

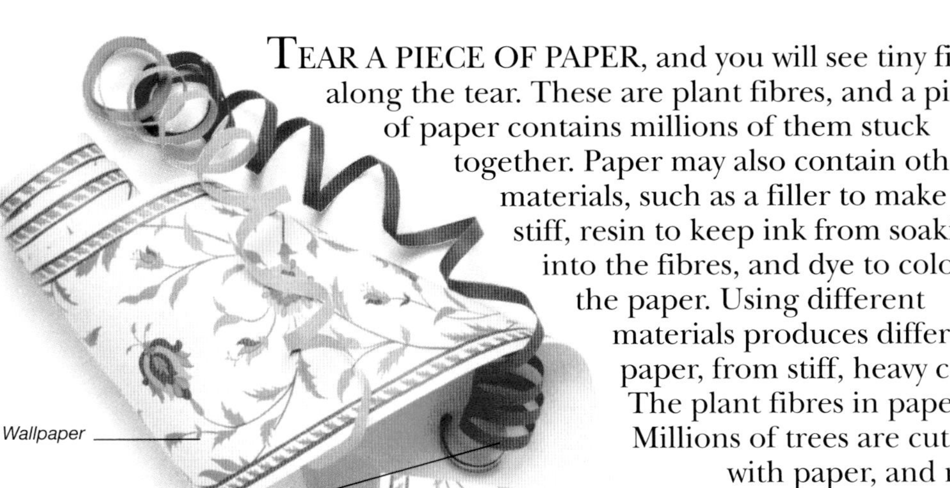

DECORATION
Wallpaper gives a special look to a room. The pattern is printed on the surface of heavy paper or pressed paper. People hang paper decorations at parties and other festive occasions.

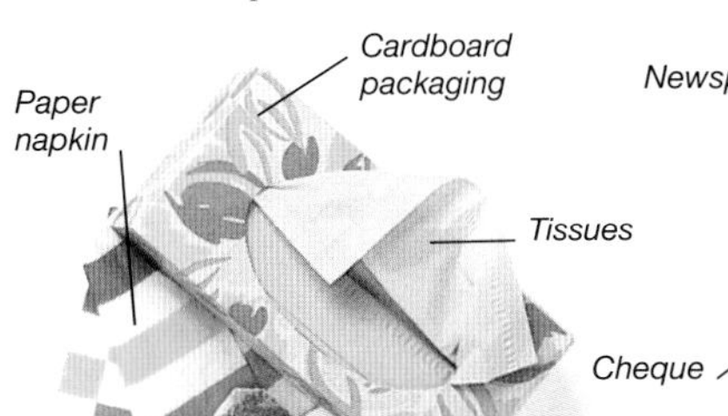

Newspaper
Cheque
Photograph

PAPER IN THE HOME
Paper is good for tasks such as cleaning because it can be thrown away after use. Light paper soaks up liquid and is used to make tissues and paper towels.

INFORMATION
A huge amount of information is recorded on paper, either as printed words and pictures or as photographs. People also use paper for money, in the form of banknotes and cheques.

Paper making

A paper mill is a large factory that turns trees into big rolls of paper. The trees are ground up and mixed with water to make wood pulp. A machine then presses and rolls a layer of pulp into paper.

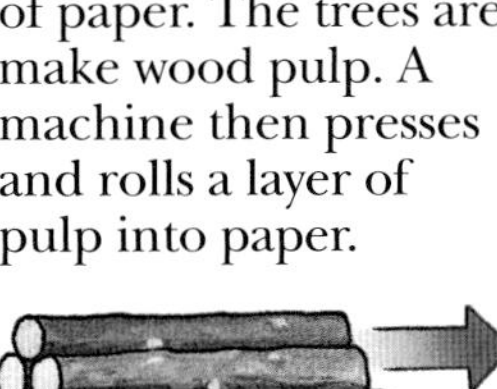

Trees are cut down and sawn into logs. The logs are then sent to paper mills.

The bark is removed and the logs are cut into tiny chips.

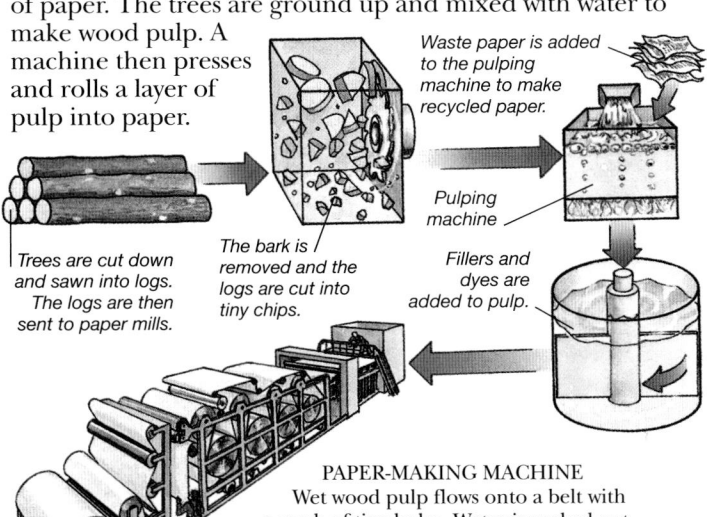

Waste paper is added to the pulping machine to make recycled paper.

Pulping machine

Fillers and dyes are added to pulp.

PAPER-MAKING MACHINE
Wet wood pulp flows onto a belt with a mesh of tiny holes. Water is sucked out, and the wet paper passes through rollers and heated cylinders that press and dry it. The finished paper is wound onto a large roll.

Writing paper
Note- paper
Wrapping paper
Handmade paper

Paper types

There are many different types of paper. They range from the most delicate handmade papers to the toughest cardboard, and they have many uses. The colour, strength, and texture of the paper can be changed by printing and dyeing, and by mixing it with materials such as wax or plastic.

TREES FOR PAPER
A big tree has to fall to provide each person with a year's supply of paper. A new tree is planted in its place, usually at a special tree farm. It takes between 15 and 50 years for a freshly planted tree to grow large enough to be used for paper making.

Find out more
BOOKS
NEWSPAPERS
POLLUTION
PRINTING
TREES

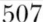

PEASANTS REVOLT

IN JUNE 1381, A MAJOR UPRISING occurred in England when angry peasants marched on London in protest against an unfair poll tax and harsh working conditions. Known as the Peasants' Revolt, it was the most important uprising by ordinary people in English history. The leaders were Wat Tyler, Jack Straw, and John Ball, a former priest. They led 100,000 men from Kent and Essex to London burning buildings and looting along the way. They also murdered the Archbishop of Canterbury, and some government ministers. Richard II, the 14-year-old king, met the peasants at Smithfield and agreed to abolish serfdom and the poll tax. Most peasants dispersed, but Tyler was killed. After the revolt, Richard failed to keep his promises, but such a heavy poll tax was not imposed again, and serfdom gradually disappeared.

WAT TYLER AND JACK STRAW
Wat Tyler led the Kentish rebels. Jack Straw, a thresher, led a group who set fire to buildings, including the palace of John of Gaunt, the king's uncle.

MORE REVOLTS

Rebellions broke out in St Albans, Hertfordshire, Bury St. Edmonds, Suffolk, Cambridgeshire, Huntingdonshire, Norfolk, and Sussex. Most of the outbreaks were fairly short-lived. The violence frightened the government and after the revolt Jack Straw and John Ball were executed.

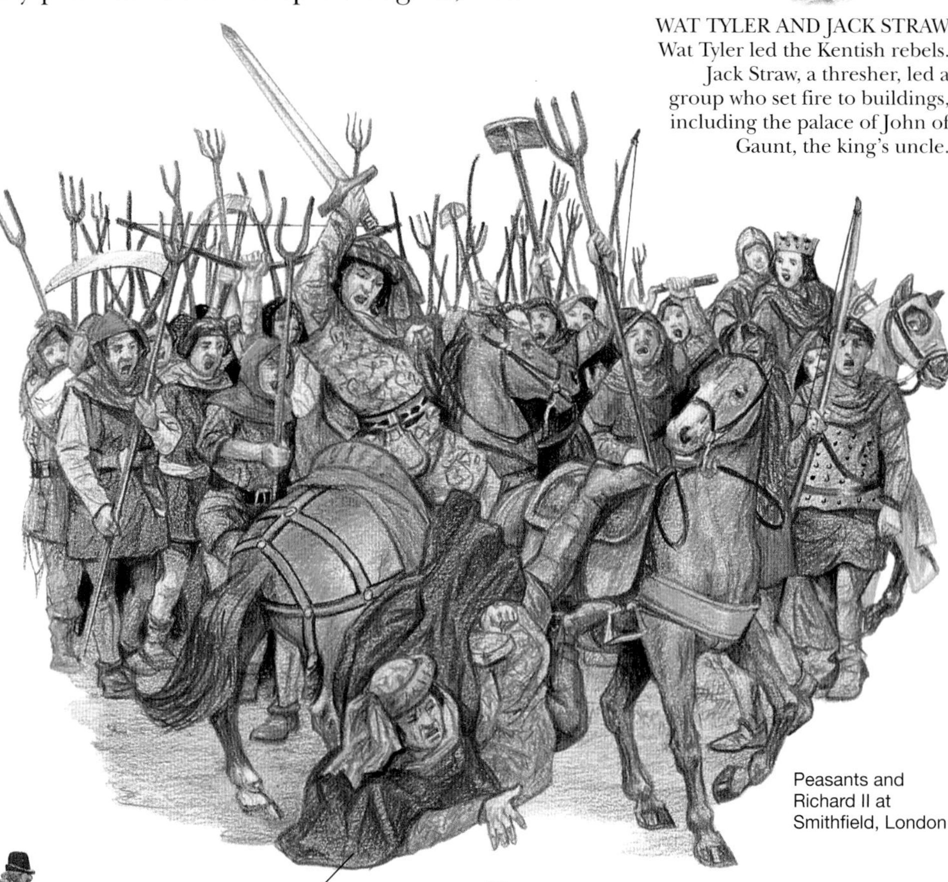

Peasants and Richard II at Smithfield, London

Wat Tyler falls from his horse and is killed.

Gold noble

Groat

POLL TAX
Poll means "head", and the poll tax was levied on every person over the age of 14. In 1377, parliament imposed a poll tax of one groat to meet the costs of the Hundred Years War. In 1380, it was raised to one shilling (5p) per head, a huge amount then. This sparked off the revolts.

RICHARD II
Grandson of Edward III, Richard II (1367–1400) became king in 1377, aged 10. He used courage and daring to suppress the Peasants' Revolt. He was deposed by Henry IV in 1400 and was either murdered or died of starvation.

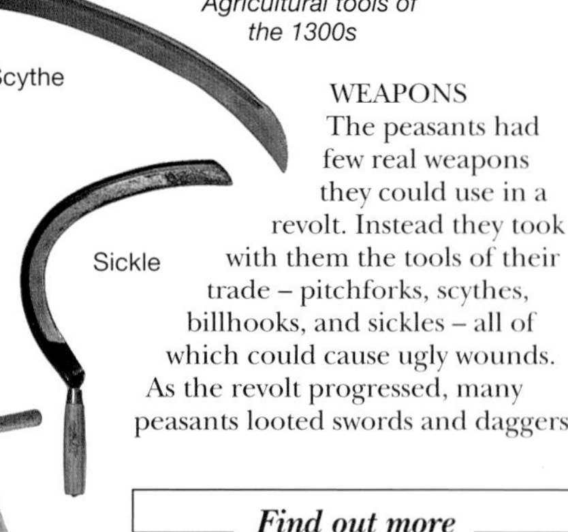

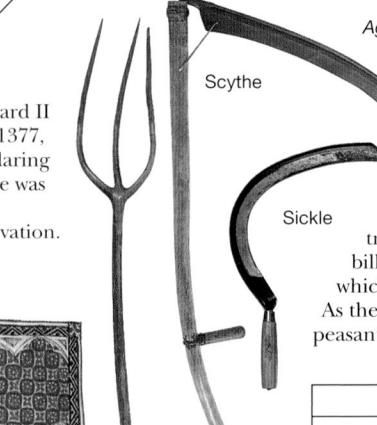

Agricultural tools of the 1300s

WEAPONS
The peasants had few real weapons they could use in a revolt. Instead they took with them the tools of their trade – pitchforks, scythes, billhooks, and sickles – all of which could cause ugly wounds. As the revolt progressed, many peasants looted swords and daggers.

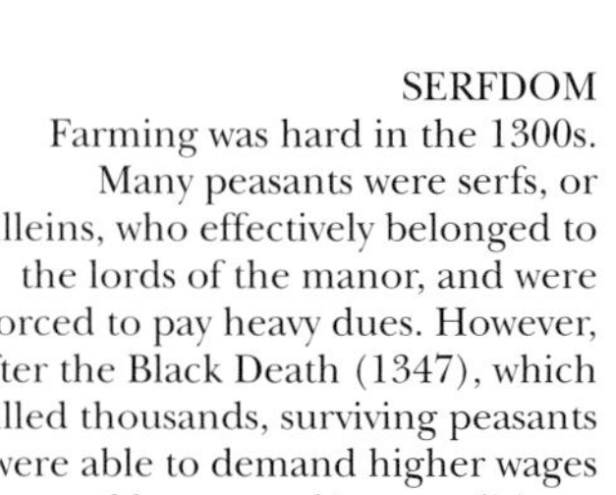

SERFDOM
Farming was hard in the 1300s. Many peasants were serfs, or villeins, who effectively belonged to the lords of the manor, and were forced to pay heavy dues. However, after the Black Death (1347), which killed thousands, surviving peasants were able to demand higher wages and better working conditions.

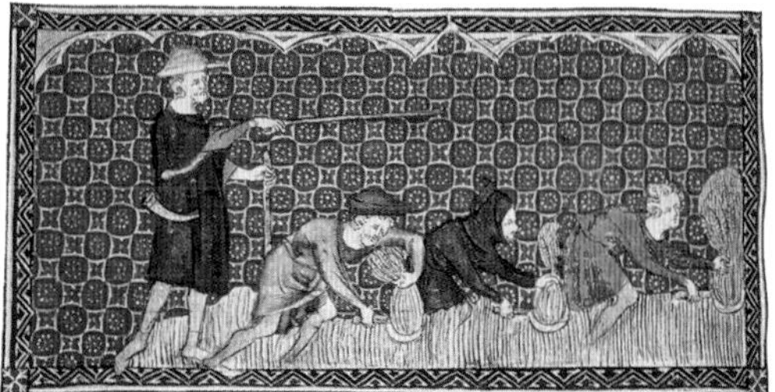

Find out more
BLACK DEATH
FARMING, HISTORY OF
HUNDRED YEARS WAR
MEDIEVAL EUROPE
WEAPONS

ANCIENT
PERSIANS

MORE THAN 3,000 YEARS AGO, the present-day country of Iran was home to various tribes, including the Medes and the Persians. For many years, the Medes ruled the area, but in 549 B.C. Cyrus, the Persian king of a small state called Ashan, conquered the Medes and set out to create a vast kingdom. Within 30 years Persia had become the most powerful nation in the world, and the Persian Empire covered all of Mesopotamia, Anatolia (Turkey), the eastern Mediterranean, and what are now Pakistan and Afghanistan. For more than 200 years the Persian Empire was the greatest the world had ever seen. The Persians were skilled warriors, horse riders, and craft workers. They were also highly organized. Under Darius I, also called Darius the Great, the empire was divided into provinces called satrapies. A network of roads linked the provinces and enabled people to trade easily. Darius introduced a postal system and a single currency to unify the empire. The empire flourished until the Greek leader Alexander the Great conquered Persia in 331 B.C.

CYRUS THE GREAT
Cyrus (ruled 549-529 B.C.) founded the Persian Empire. During his reign many different peoples, including Babylonians, Egyptians, Greeks, and Syrians, lived in the Persian Empire.

People bringing gifts to the royal palace

Reliefs show people arriving for a festival on New Year's Day

PERSEPOLIS

In about 520 B.C. Darius I began to build the city of Persepolis. Building continued in the reign of Xerxes I (486-465 B.C.). Persepolis was the site of many beautiful buildings, including the royal palace. The city was used only once a year at New Year, when the peoples of the empire brought tributes (gifts) to the king.

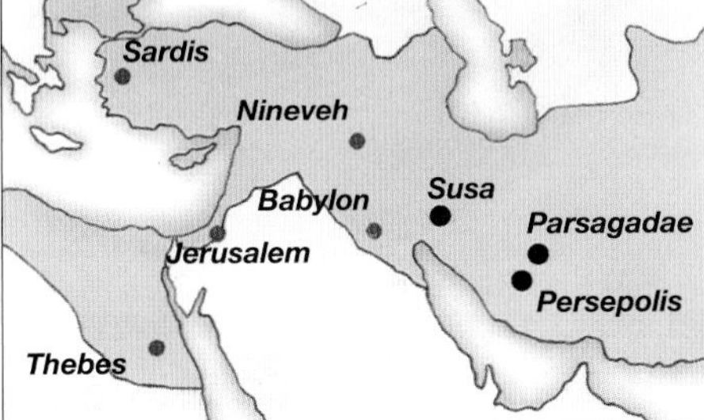

PERSIAN EMPIRE
At its height, the Persian Empire stretched from the borders of India to the River Nile in Egypt. The city of Susa was the administrative capital of the empire, Persepolis was the royal capital, and Parsagadae was the city where kings were crowned.

ZOROASTRIANISM
The Persian people followed the teachings of a prophet named Zoroaster, who lived from about 628 to 551 B.C. Zoroastrianism was the main religion in Persia until the country became Muslim in the 7th century A.D.

Zoroastrian priests carried a mace with a bull's head as a symbol of the priests' religious battle against evil.

Remains of Persepolis include statues such as the carved head of this horse in the Central Palace.

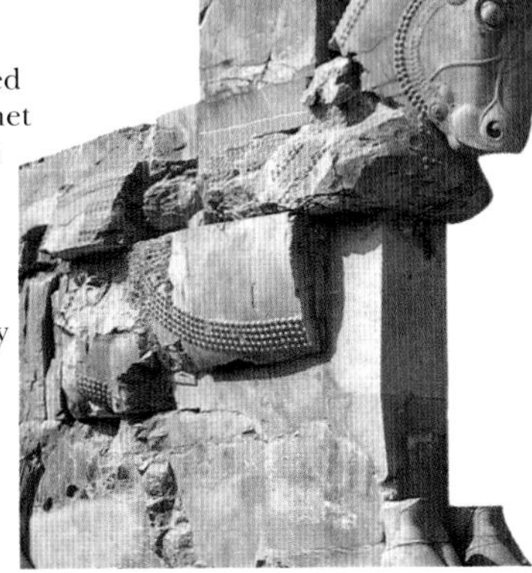

PERSEPOLIS TODAY
When Alexander the Great invaded the Persian Empire, he burned Persepolis to the ground. But the ruins of the city, including the royal palace, can still be seen today in southern Iran.

ANCIENT PERSIANS

549 B.C. Cyrus the Great defeats the Medes peoples and forms the Persian Empire.

538 B.C. Cyrus conquers the Babylonian Empire.

529 B.C. Cyrus dies.

525 B.C. Persians conquer Egypt.

521-486 B.C. Reign of Darius the Great.

510 B.C. Persians invade southeast Europe and central Asia.

500-449 B.C. Persian Wars between Persian Empire and Greek states, because Persian kings felt threatened by the democracy of Greece.

490 B.C. Greeks defeat Persians at the Battle of Marathon.

480 B.C. Greek navy defeats Persians at the Battle of Salamis.

334 B.C. Alexander the Great invades Persia.

331 B.C. Alexander defeats Persians at the Battle of Gaugamela. Persian Empire collapses.

Find out more

ALEXANDER THE GREAT
ASSYRIANS
BABYLONIANS
GREECE, ANCIENT
MIDDLE EAST

PETS

LIKE TRUSTED FRIENDS, pets give us comfort and affection. In return, pets need people to provide food and shelter and care for their health. Pets are tame animals kept for companionship or because they are attractive to look at. Humans first tamed animals for their milk or meat 11,000 years ago, but people have kept pets only since about 2000 B.C. At that time the Ancient Egyptians tamed hyenas, cats, and even lions for company. Choosing the right pet is an important decision. Some pets, such as large dogs, need space to run around, so it is cruel to keep them in a city home. Cats thrive almost anywhere, but enjoy exploring outdoors. And many pets need very little attention or space – there's room in even the smallest home for a fish tank or a birdcage.

CATS
Mammals make rewarding pets because they are affectionate and often become fond of their owners. Cats and dogs are the most common pets; there are more than 50 million pet cats in the United States alone.

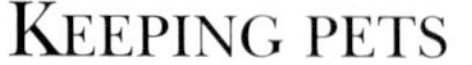

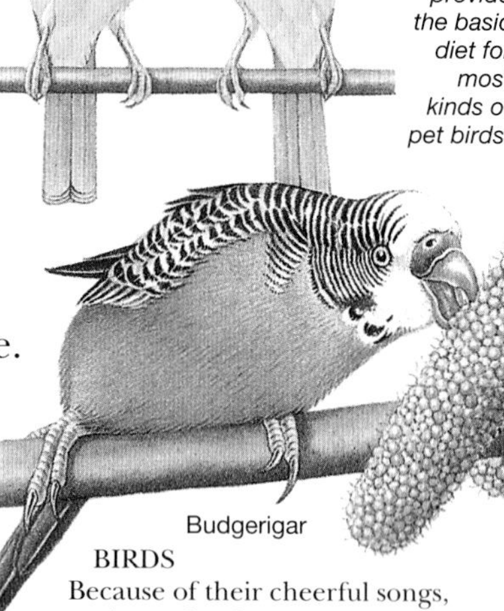

Canaries

Seeds and fruit provide the basic diet for most kinds of pet birds.

Budgerigar

BIRDS
Because of their cheerful songs, canaries make charming pets. Some cage birds, especially parrots and mynah birds, can be trained to imitate human speech. The world's most talkative bird was an African grey parrot that knew more than 800 words.

KEEPING PETS

In their natural habitat, animals look after themselves. But few pets can hunt or exercise in a natural way. It is therefore important to understand a pet's requirements and give it what it needs to stay healthy. Exercise and a suitable diet are most important, but all pets also need a clean living area and the care of a vet when they get sick.

Hamsters exercise by running inside a wheel.

The hamster drinks from a drip feeder.

Hamsters keep their teeth sharp by gnawing, so their cages have to be made with sturdy metal bars.

Hamsters eat dried food such as seeds and nuts, as well as fresh vegetables.

BREEDING PETS
All pets may produce young if adult males and females are put together. In a large aviary (above), birds will pair off and make nests, just as they do in the wild. For especially valuable pets, breeding pairs are carefully selected, since the best males and females usually produce the best young.

GUINEA PIGS
In warm weather guinea pigs can live in outdoor cages and feed on fresh grass. Some special breeds have long, glossy coats, which have to be kept well brushed. Guinea pigs are not actually pigs at all, but small rodents, which originated in South America.

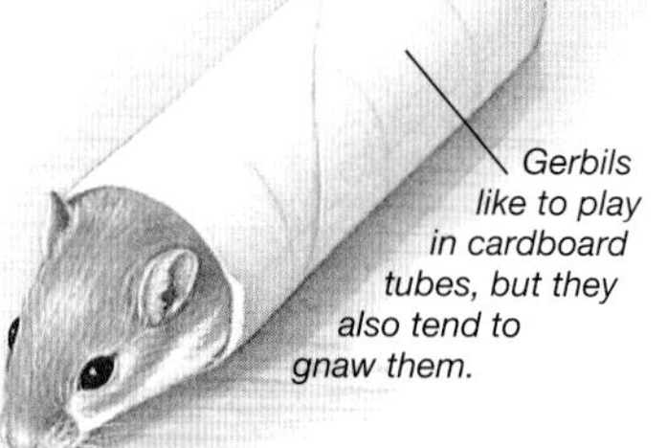

Gerbils like to play in cardboard tubes, but they also tend to gnaw them.

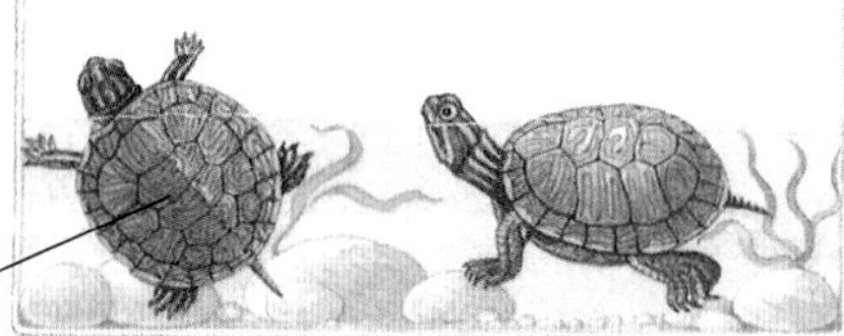

Terrapins like to swim, so they have to be kept in tanks containing pools of water.

TRAINING
Any pet that lives outside a cage has to be trained so that it does not soil the home. Without training, dogs can be especially destructive and even dangerous.

At dog shows, prizes are awarded to the most well-trained dogs.

UNUSUAL PETS
Almost any animal could be a pet, but unusual pets require special care and some knowledge about how these animals live and behave in the wild.

Pythons kill their prey by strangling them. If handled correctly, they make good pets.

Find out more
CATS
DOGS, WOLVES, AND FOXES
FARM ANIMALS
HORSES, ZEBRAS, AND ASSES
VETERINARIANS

PHOENICIANS

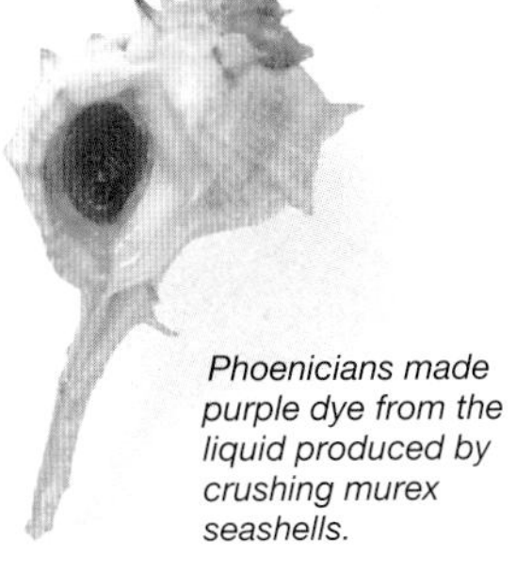
Phoenicians made purple dye from the liquid produced by crushing murex seashells.

A TINY GROUP OF CITIES perched along the coast of the Mediterranean produced the most famous sailors and traders of the ancient world. These seafaring people were called the Phoenicians. The cities of Phoenicia were linked by the sea, and they traded in many goods, including purple dyes, glass, and ivory. From 1200 to 350 B.C. the Phoenicians controlled trade throughout the Mediterranean. They spread their trading links to many points around the coast. Their most famous trading post was Carthage on the north coast of Africa. During its history, Phoenicia was conquered by several foreign empires, including the Assyrians, Babylonians, and Persians. These foreign rulers usually allowed the Phoenicians to continue trading. But in 332 B.C. Alexander the Great conquered Phoenicia, and Greek people came to live there. The Greeks brought their own culture with them, and the Phoenician culture died out.

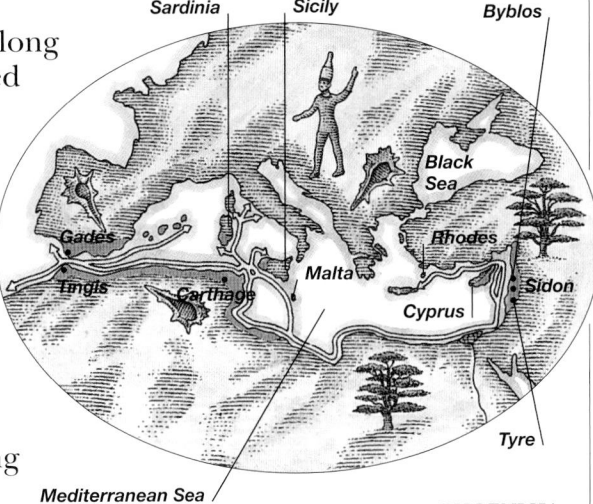

Sardinia
Sicily
Byblos
Black Sea
Gades
Rhodes
Tingis
Carthage
Malta
Sidon
Cyprus
Tyre
Mediterranean Sea

PHOENICIA
Phoenicia lay on the coast of the eastern Mediterranean roughly where Lebanon is today. The Phoenicians spread throughout the Mediterranean, to Carthage, Rhodes, Cyprus, Sicily, Malta, Sardinia, Gades (Cadiz), and Tingis (Tangier).

When arriving at a new place to trade, the Phoenicians would lay their goods out on the beach and let the local people come and look at what they had brought.

Sculptures show that Phoenician men wore distinctive conical hats.

Phoenicians traded in a vast array of goods from the Mediterranean, including metals, farm animals, wheat, cloth, jewellery, and gemstones.

Phoenician glassware, such as this glass jar, was a luxury in the ancient world.

PHOENICIAN SHIPS

The Phoenicians' ships were famous all over the Mediterranean, and were the main reason for the Phoenicians' success as traders. The ships had oarsmen, sails, and heavy keels, which enabled them to sail in any direction.

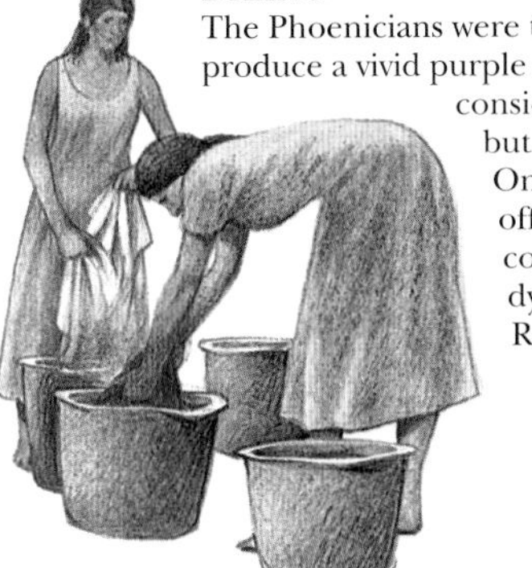

DYEING
The Phoenicians were the only people who knew how to produce a vivid purple dye from murex shells. The dye was considered to be exceptionally beautiful but it was also very expensive. Only high government officials, for example, could wear purple dyed cloth in the Roman Empire.

PHOENICIAN GLASSWARE
Ancient Egyptians made glass many years before the Phoenicians did, but Egyptian glass was cloudy, whereas Phoenician glass was clear. The Phoenicians were able to make clear glass because their sand contained large amounts of quartz.

BYBLOS

The Phoenician port of Byblos was famous for its trade in papyrus – a kind of paper made in Egypt by pressing together strands of papyrus reeds. The Greeks called papyrus *biblos* after the port of Byblos. A number of our words concerned with books, such as Bible, and bibliography (a list of books), come from *biblos*.

The papyrus reed grows in the warm, damp conditions of the River Nile in Egypt.

Find out more
ALEXANDER the great
ALPHABETS
ASSYRIANS
BABYLONIANS
GREECE, ANCIENT
PERSIANS, ANCIENT
SUMERIANS

PHOTOGRAPHY

MORE THAN TWO HUNDRED million times a day, a camera shutter clicks somewhere in the world to take a photograph. There are family snapshots capturing happy memories, dramatic news pictures, advertising and fashion shots, pictures of the planet beamed back from satellites in space, and much more. The uses of photography are numerous, and new applications are being found all the time. The first photographs were made by coating sheets of polished metal with light-sensitive chemicals, but the image appeared in dull, silvery grey and could only be seen from certain angles. During the 19th century, new processes were invented for spreading the chemicals onto a glass plate or onto a film of cellulose (a kind of plastic). Eventually, photographs could be made in either black-and-white or full colour. Film is still in use today, although it is fast being replaced by digital photography. Digital cameras use a light-sensitive chip, instead of film, and store pictures as digital image files that can be transferred to a computer. There, they can be altered before being printed or sent anywhere in the world via the Internet.

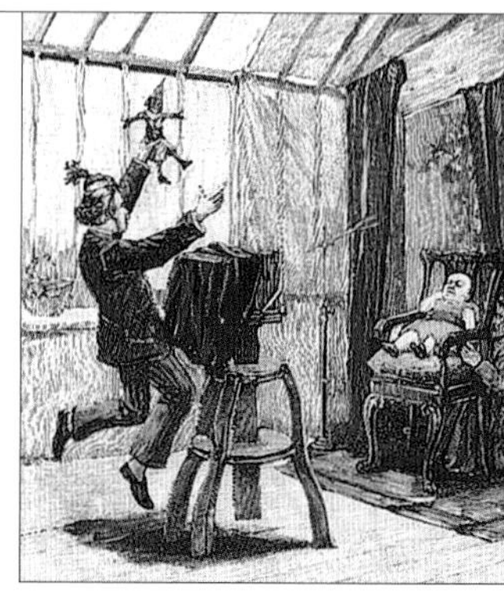

A 19th-century photographer tries to hold a baby's attention while he struggles to operate his bulky camera.

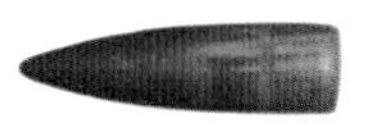

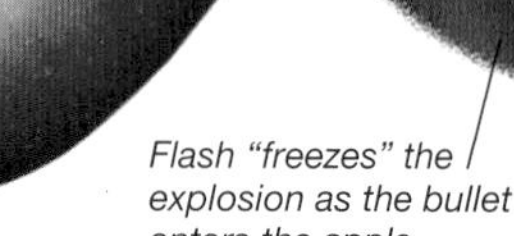

HIGH-SPEED PHOTOGRAPHY
With the use of special cameras and lights, high-speed photography can reveal movement too fast for the eye to see. A brief burst of light from an electronic flash, lasting less than one millionth of a second, freezes objects moving at hundreds of kilometres per hour.

Flash "freezes" the explosion as the bullet enters the apple.

HISTORY OF PHOTOGRAPHY

A Frenchman named Joseph Niépce took the first photograph in 1826. The exposure took eight hours to make, and the picture was fuzzy and dark. In 1837, another Frenchman, Louis Daguerre, discovered how to make sharp photographs in a few minutes. Just two years later an English scientist, William Fox Talbot, invented the process that is still used for developing films today. In the early days, cameras were bulky, and for each picture photographers had to carry a separate glass plate. Then, in 1888, American George Eastman invented the Kodak camera. It was small and light and came loaded with a roll of film rather than plates. Taking a picture became so easy that anyone could try it.

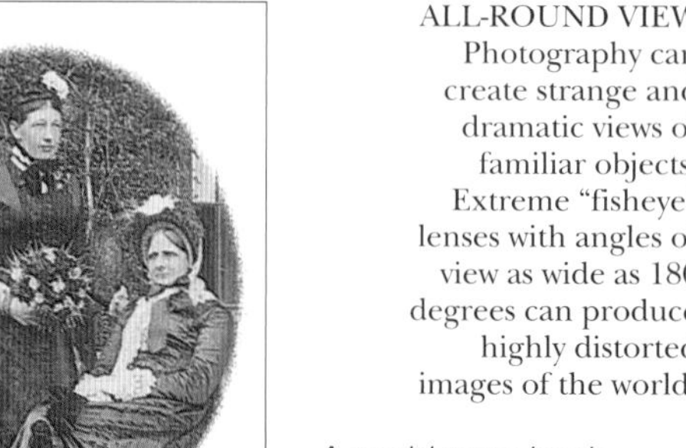

People in early portraits often look uncomfortable and stiff because they had to keep still for several minutes.

The Kodak Box Brownie was so simple that Eastman claimed even a child could use it.

ALL-ROUND VIEW
Photography can create strange and dramatic views of familiar objects. Extreme "fisheye" lenses with angles of view as wide as 180 degrees can produce highly distorted images of the world.

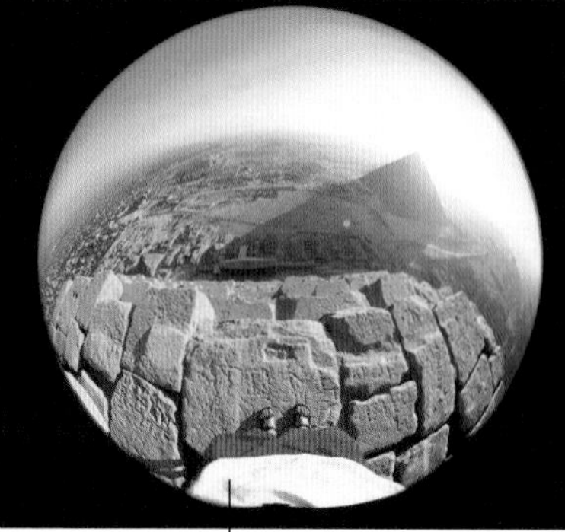

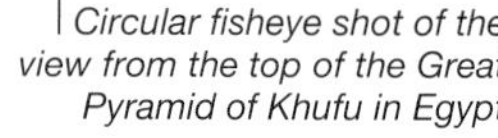

Circular fisheye shot of the view from the top of the Great Pyramid of Khufu in Egypt

A special macro lens is needed to focus at distances as close as this.

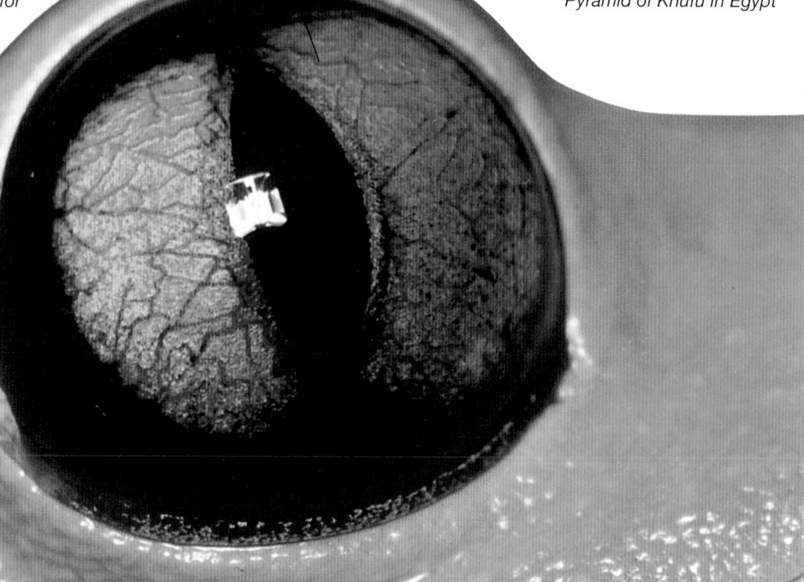

CLOSE-UP PHOTOGRAPHY
Macro, or close-up, photography magnifies tiny details barely visible to the naked eye, such as the beautiful gold-coloured eye of a leaf frog (right).

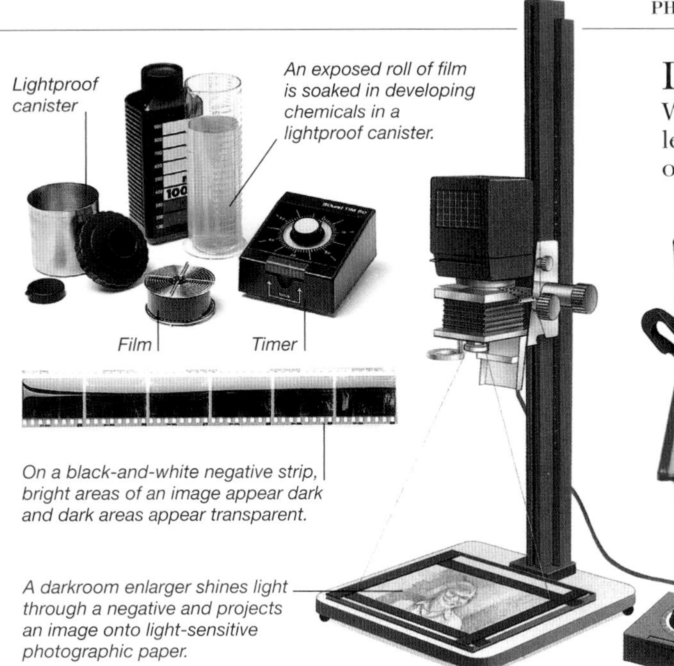

Lightproof canister

An exposed roll of film is soaked in developing chemicals in a lightproof canister.

Film

Timer

On a black-and-white negative strip, bright areas of an image appear dark and dark areas appear transparent.

A darkroom enlarger shines light through a negative and projects an image onto light-sensitive photographic paper.

Developing and printing

When a picture is taken with a traditional camera, light enters the lens briefly and strikes the film. Each grain of light-sensitive silver on the film is subtly changed by the light that falls on it, and an invisible image is recorded. The film must be processed before the picture can be seen. It is immersed in a bath of chemicals called developer. This turns the exposed silver salts into silver metals. The developed film is then washed and "fixed" to create a negative or transparency that is no longer affected by light. In a darkroom the image is enlarged by projecting it onto light-sensitive paper, which in turn must be developed to make a print.

The exposed print is developed and fixed in the same way as film.

Digital photgraphy

A digital camera does not use film at all. Instead, it contains a light-sensitive image sensor – a chip made up of millions of tiny silicon photo diodes, each of which records the brightness and colour of the light falling on it when the picture is taken. The picture information is translated into digital data and stored on the camera's memory card from where it can be printed or downloaded to a computer.

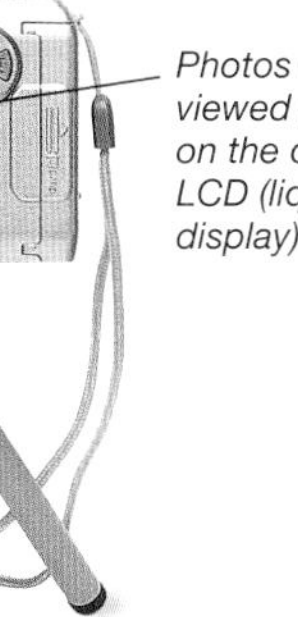

Photos can be viewed immediately on the camera's LCD (liquid crystal display) screen.

Mini tripod

Connection cable

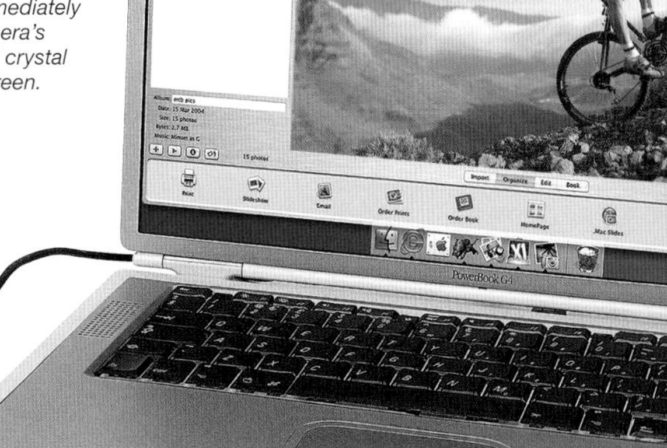

Photo-management software

Laptop computer

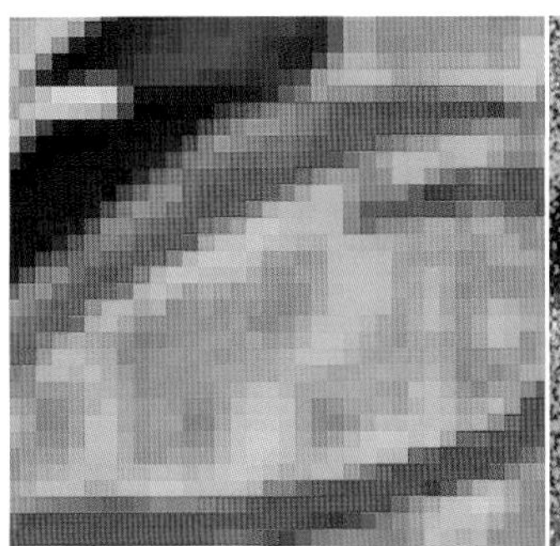

A digital image enlarged until it becomes "pixellated"

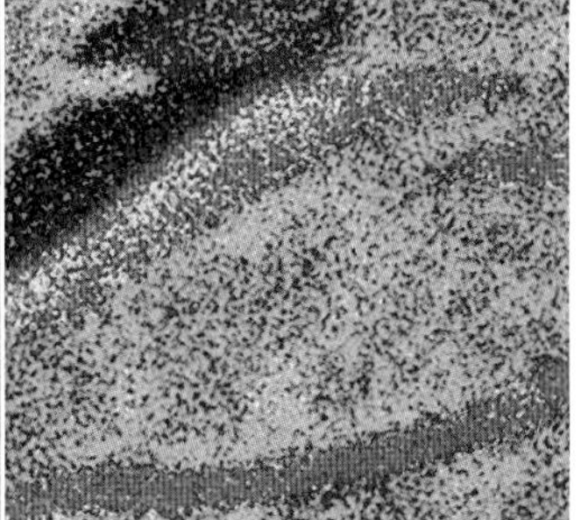

Film grain magnified until it becomes visible

DIGITAL AND FILM IN CLOSE-UP

Both digital and film images are made up of minute blocks of colour, so small that they are normally invisible to the naked eye. However, it is possible to see individual pixels when a digital photograph is enlarged on screen and to see separate grains when film or a photographic print is viewed under a microscope or magnifying glass.

Camera phones

Most new mobile phones have built-in digital cameras, capable of taking photographs and recording short video clips. Both pictures and movies can be sent immediately to other mobile phones or transferred wirelessly to TVs, computers, printers, and other digital devices. As image quality improves, many people may choose to use a single device to combine the functions of phone, email, palmtop, camera, video camcorder, and music player.

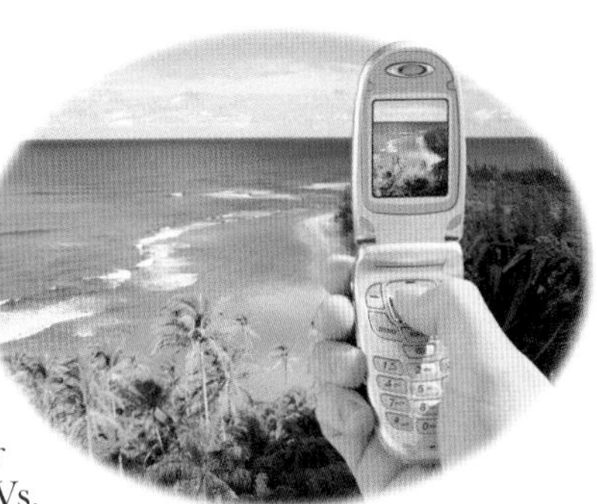

Find out more

CAMERAS
COLOUR
FILMS
LIGHT
TELEVISION AND VIDEO

PHYSICS

THE SCIENCE OF PHYSICS used to be called natural philosophy, which means thinking about and investigating the natural world. Physicists seek to understand and explain the universe from the largest, most distant galaxy to the tiniest invisible particle. Great physicists have wrestled with fundamental questions such as what is it that holds us to the Earth, what is time, and what is inside an atom. Physicists work with theory and experiment. They conduct experiments and then think of a theory, or idea, that explains the results. Then they try new experiments to test their theory. Some theories have become so good at explaining nature that many people refer to them as the laws of physics. For example, one such law states that nothing can travel faster than the speed of light. The German-born physicist Albert Einstein (1879-1955) proposed this in 1905 as part of his revolutionary theory of relativity.

BRANCHES OF PHYSICS

Physics is the science of energy and matter (the materials of which everything is made). There are several branches of physics. They cover a range of subjects from atoms to space.

ASTROPHYSICS
Astronomers use physics to find out about the origins and interiors of the Sun and stars. This branch of physics is called astrophysics.

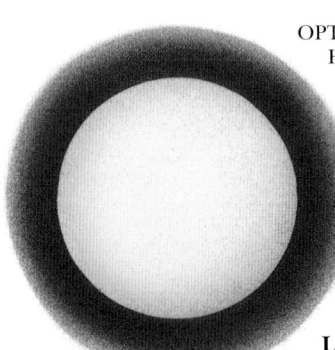

OPTICS AND THERMAL PHYSICS
Heat and light are important forms of energy: the Sun sends out light and heat that make life possible on Earth. The physics of light is called optics; the branch of physics concerned with heat is called thermal physics.

STATICS
Statics is the branch of physics concerned with calculating and understanding forces that support buildings and bridges.

Satellites transmit radio waves for long-distance communication.

Laws of mechanics are put to use to design and run a car.

Coal is burned to produce electricity.

MECHANICS
The study of force and movement is a branch of physics known as mechanics.

ELECTRICITY
One of the most useful forms of energy is electricity. Physicists study the nature of electricity and find ways of using it in electrical appliances, microchips, and computers.

ELECTROMAGNETISM
Physicists have discovered a group of mostly invisible rays called electromagnetic waves. Electromagnetism is the physics of the relationship between magnetism and electric currents.

KINETIC THEORY
Physicists use the idea of molecules to explain the way solids, liquids, and gases behave. This branch of physics is called kinetic theory.

Accelerator speeds up atomic particles and forces them to collide.

MAGNETISM
Physicists study magnets and the forces that magnets produce. This includes the Earth's magnetism, which comes from the movements of the molten metal core at the centre of the Earth.

Sound waves reflected from the ocean floor bring back information about deep-sea structures.

QUANTUM MECHANICS
Energy can only exist in tiny packets called quanta. This idea is very important in the study of atoms, and it has given rise to a branch of physics called quantum mechanics.

ACOUSTICS
The science of sound is called acoustics. Physicists can use sound to study the interior of the Earth and the oceans.

NUCLEAR PHYSICS
Physicists are constantly searching for a greater understanding of the particles that make up the nucleus (centre) of an atom. This branch of physics is called nuclear physics.

Atomic particles crash into each other to release vast amounts of energy.

GEOPHYSICS
The interior of the Earth is hidden from us, but physicists have discovered that there is great heat and pressure beneath the Earth's crust, which sometimes erupts in volcanoes. Geophysics is the branch of physics concerned with the Earth.

LANDMARKS IN PHYSICS

200s B.C. Greek scientist Archimedes explains floating and the way levers work.

1687 English physicist Isaac Newton puts forward the laws of motion and gravity.

1900 German physicist Max Planck introduces quantum theory.

1905 German physicist Albert Einstein publishes his theory of relativity.

1938 German physicists Fritz Strassmann and Otto Hahn split the atom.

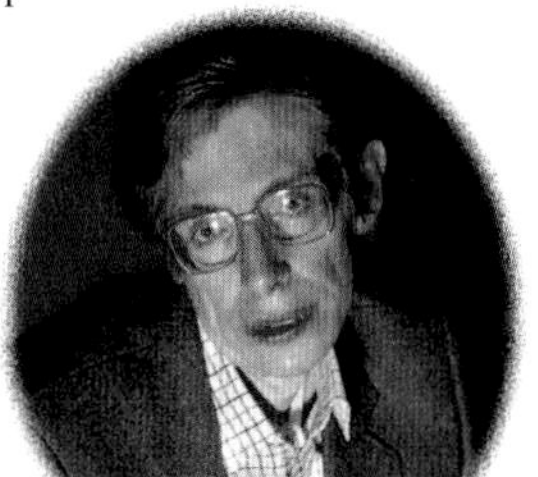

English physicist Stephen Hawking (born 1942) developed new theories about the nature of matter, black holes in space, and the origin of the universe that have opened doors to new possibilities in physics.

Find out more

EINSTEIN, ALBERT
ELECTRICITY
FORCE AND MOTION
GRAVITY
HEAT
LIGHT
MAGNETISM
SCIENCE
SOUND

PILGRIMS

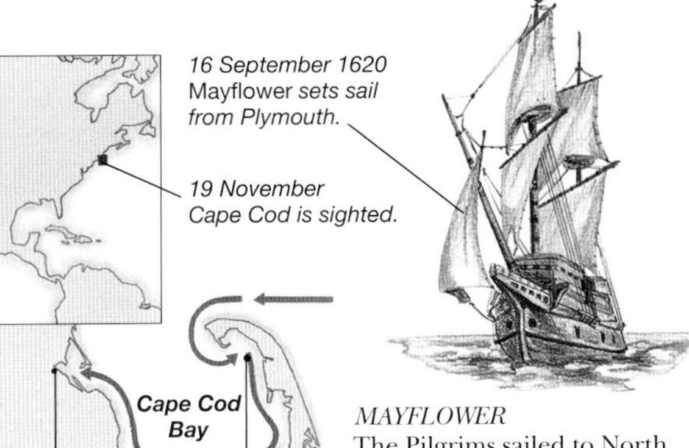

21 November *Mayflower anchors in Provincetown harbour.*

26 December Plymouth colony founded, Massachusetts.

MAYFLOWER
The Pilgrims sailed to North America in a two-masted ship, the *Mayflower*. The ship was about 30 m (90 ft) long and was built to carry wine and other cargo.

ON A BLUSTERY SEPTEMBER DAY in 1620, a small ship set sail from the port of Plymouth, England, bound for North America. The 102 settlers on board hoped that in the New World they could worship freely in their own way, which they had not been able to do in England. Because of their Puritan faith, and because they started one of the colonies that would later grow into the United States, the group became known as the Pilgrims. The Pilgrims landed in what is now Massachusetts and established a settlement called Plymouth. The first winter was hard. The settlers had little food, and it was difficult to farm and fish. But with help from the local Native Americans, the settlement eventually prospered. The Pilgrims replaced their wooden homes with more secure dwellings and started trading furs with the Native Americans. More groups of Puritans came to join the original settlers; together they created one of the first successful European settlements in North America.

EARLY SETTLEMENT

The first settlements in Plymouth were built of wood from the local forests. The chimneys were made of sticks held together with clay, and the roofs were waterproofed with bark.

Splitting logs to make planks

Food had to be cooked in the open.

Every member of the family had to work hard to build a house and plant crops for food.

The Pilgrims held prayer meetings outside until they built churches.

GOVERNMENT
The early Plymouth settlers elected their own government which met annually to make laws and levy taxes.

PURITANISM
The Puritan religion stressed hard work and obedience and disapproved of frivolity and idleness.

PURITANS
The people known as the Puritans wished to purify the Church of England of its pomp and ritual. They dressed in simple clothes and tried to live in accordance with the Bible.

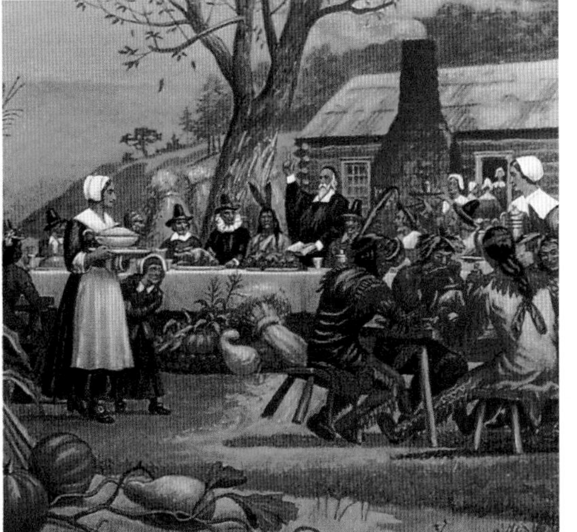

THANKSGIVING
In the autumn of 1621, the Pilgrims celebrated their first successful harvest. They invited the local Native Americans to join them in a feast of thanksgiving. Thanksgiving, which became a national holiday in 1863, is celebrated in the United States on the fourth Thursday in November.

Find out more
EXPLORERS
FESTIVALS
UNITED STATES OF AMERICA, history of

PIRATES

IN TALES ABOUT PIRATES, shady figures row through the moonlight to bury treasure on tropical islands. The reality of a pirate's life, though, was very different from the storybook version. Most pirates were simply criminals who robbed ships at sea and often murdered the crews. Pirates first appeared when trading ships began to cross the Mediterranean about 4,000 years ago. They have flourished ever since in every ocean of the world, but were particularly active from 1500 to 1800. Some pirates, such as Blackbeard, cruised the Caribbean Sea, which was also called the Spanish Main. Others, such as Captain Kidd, attacked ships in the Indian Ocean. Sometimes countries at war encouraged piracy, but only against enemy shipping. They called the pirate ships privateers and gave them letters of marque – official licences to plunder enemy ships. Till recently, pirates existed in the South China Sea. They robbed families fleeing by boat from Vietnam.

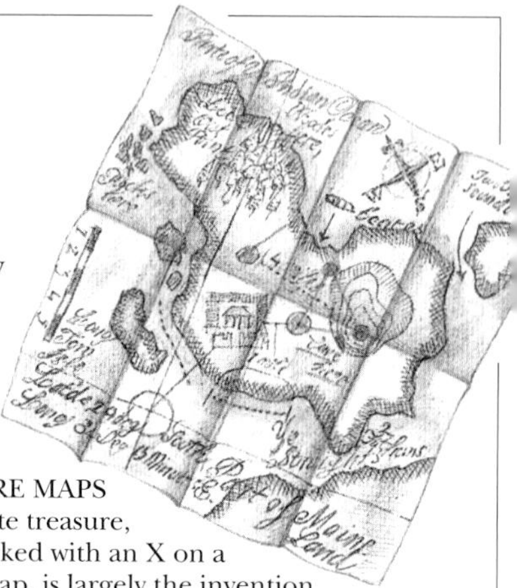

TREASURE MAPS
Buried pirate treasure, marked with an X on a map, is largely the invention of adventure writers. Most of the time pirates attacked lightly armed merchant ships, stealing food and weapons.

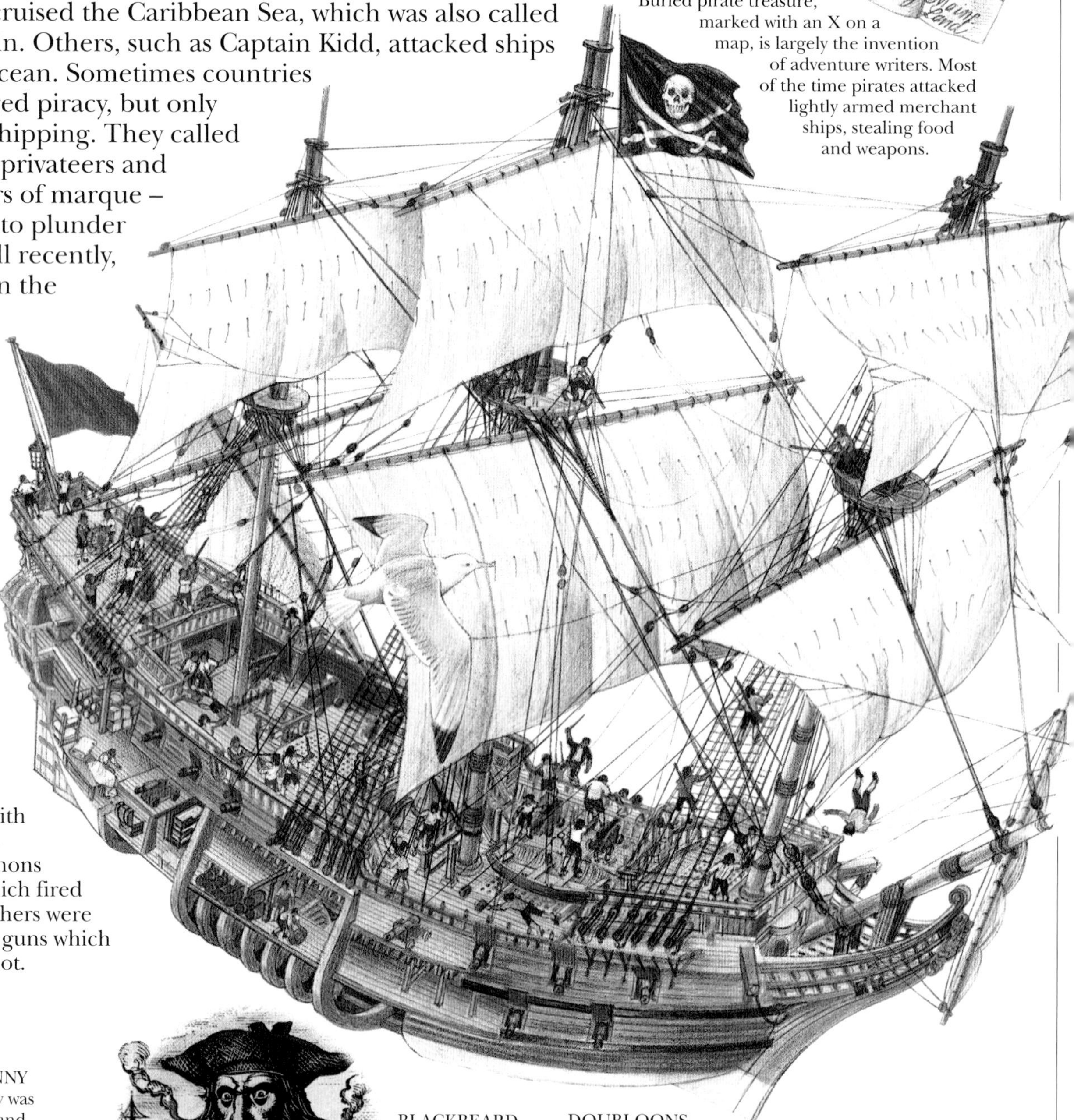

PIRATE SHIPS

Traditional pirate vessels were generally small, fast, and manoeuvrable. They floated high in the water so they could escape into shallow creeks and inlets if pursued. They were armed with as many cannons as possible. Some cannons were heavy guns which fired large metal balls; others were lighter swivel guns which fired lead shot.

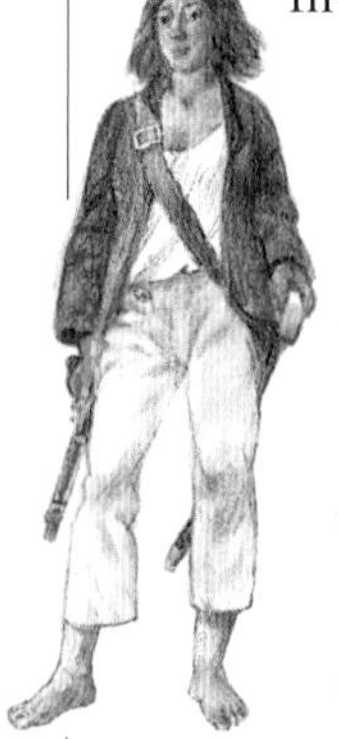

ANNE BONNY
Anne Bonny was born in Ireland. She fell in love with the pirate "Calico Jack" Rackham and sailed with him. On a captured ship she met another woman pirate, Mary Read. The women pirates were arrested in 1720 but escaped the gallows, as they were both expecting babies.

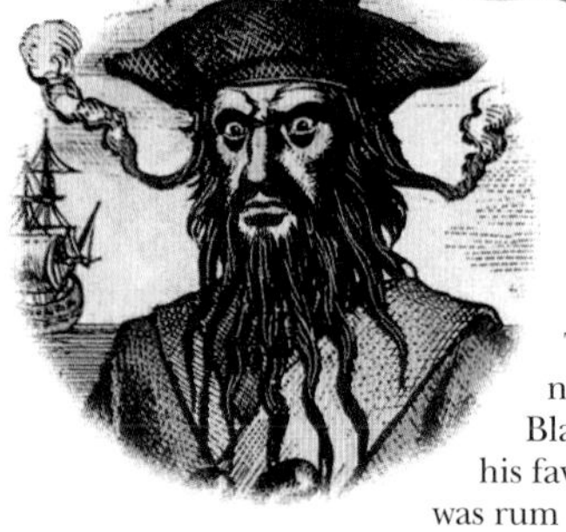

BLACKBEARD
One of the most terrible pirates was Edward Teach. His nickname was Blackbeard, and his favourite drink was rum and gunpowder. In battle he carried six pistols and wore burning matches twisted into his hair. He died on a British warship in 1718.

DOUBLOONS
The pirate's currency was a Spanish gold dollar called the doubloon. Doubloons were also called *doblón de a ocho,* meaning pieces of eight, because each was worth eight Spanish gold escudos.

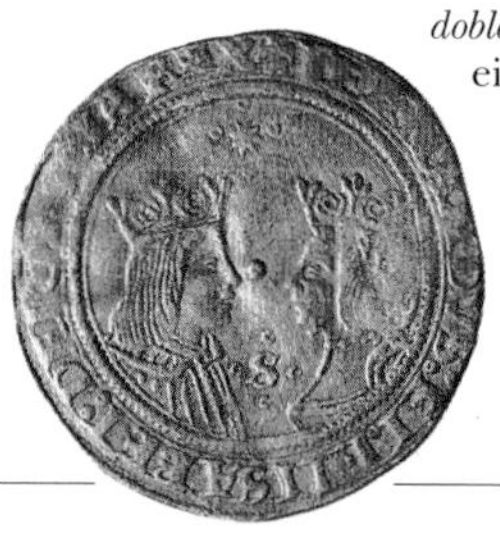

Find out more
OUTLAWS AND BANDITS

PLANETS

THE EARTH IS one of nine roughly spherical objects that move around our Sun. These objects are planets – vast balls of rock, metal, and gases that orbit a star. All planets travel in the same direction around the Sun, each revolving in an elliptical (oval) orbit. Through a telescope, the planets appear as discs of light moving across the night sky. They do not, however, produce light themselves, but reflect light from the Sun. Some planets, such as Earth and Venus, are surrounded by a layer of gas called an atmosphere. The largest planets, such as Jupiter and Saturn, are also surrounded by rings. The planets vary greatly in temperature: Mercury, closest to the Sun, is hotter than an oven by day; Pluto, at the edge of the solar system, is at night five times colder than a deep-freeze. As far as we know, Earth is the only planet in our solar system that supports life. However, there are millions of stars similar to our Sun in the universe, many believed to have their own planets. It is possible that some of these also support life forms.

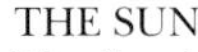

JUPITER
Jupiter is the largest planet in the solar system. It has no solid surface as it is made up of a mixture of liquids and gases, with belts of swirling gas forming an atmosphere around it. It is a cold planet, surrounded by a ring of dust, and orbited by more than 60 moons.

THE SUN
The Sun is a star – a vast ball of hot gas, far larger than any of the planets.

MARS
Mars is a small, dry planet with a red, rocky surface. It is cold – about -23°C (-9°F) – and has two polar caps of ice and frozen gas. Mars has two tiny moons named Phobos and Deimos.

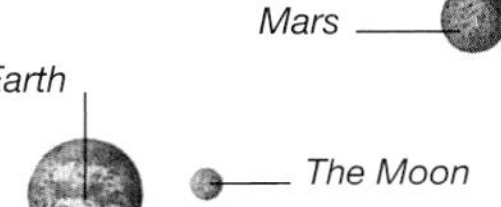

MERCURY
Mercury is so close to the Sun that it has no atmosphere or oceans. It has a rocky surface that rises to a temperature of about 350°C (662°F).

VENUS
Thick clouds cover the whole surface of Venus. They trap the Sun's heat, making Venus the hottest planet in the solar system. The surface temperature of Venus is about 480°C (896°F).

EARTH
The Earth has an atmosphere of air and oceans filled with water. The Earth's average temperature is 22°C (72°F). A source of energy and liquid water are essential for life on the planet. If the Earth were hotter, the water would evaporate; if it were colder, the water would freeze.

ASTEROIDS

Thousands of tiny bodies called asteroids orbit the Sun, mainly travelling in a belt between Mars and Jupiter. Dating from the earliest days of the solar system, most asteroids are lumps of rock and metal just a few kilometres in diameter. Jupiter's gravitational pull can send asteroids into erratic orbits, causing them to collide with planets and other asteroids. Many objects made of ice and rock are also known to exist in the Kuiper Belt, an area in the solar system beyond the orbit of Neptune.

PLANET PICTURES

Space technology has shown us what the other planets in the solar system look like and what they are made of; it has also established that these other planets are unlikely to support life. The images shown right and at the foot of the next page were taken from a variety of spacecraft.

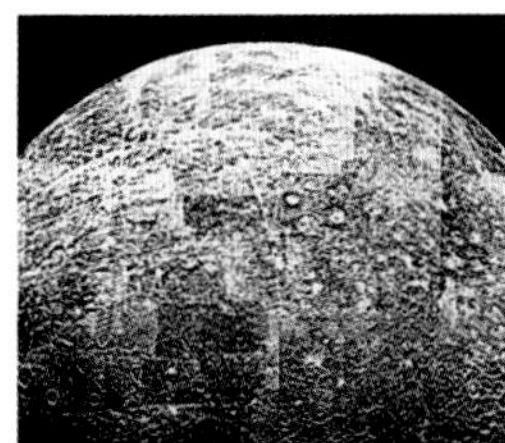

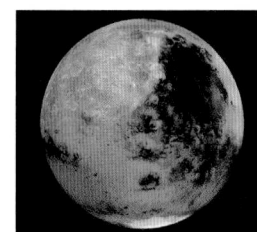

The heavily cratered surface of Mercury is revealed in this composite photograph taken by the space probe Mariner 10.

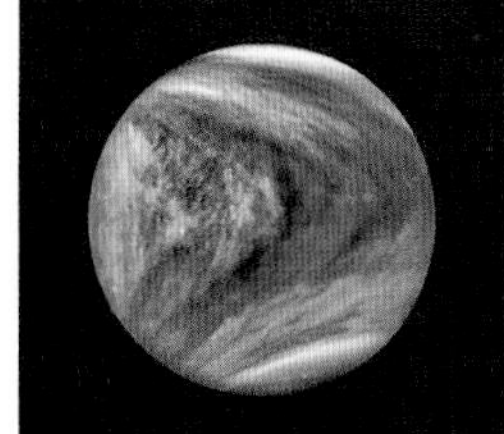

Photograph taken by the Pioneer-Venus *probe shows thick yellowish clouds covering the surface of Venus.*

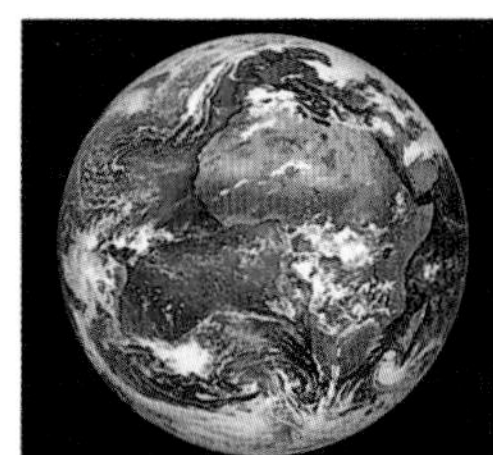

Picture of the Earth taken by the Meteosat *weather satellite. Colours have been enhanced using a computer.*

Picture of Mars constructed from 100 images taken by the Viking 1 *space probe.*

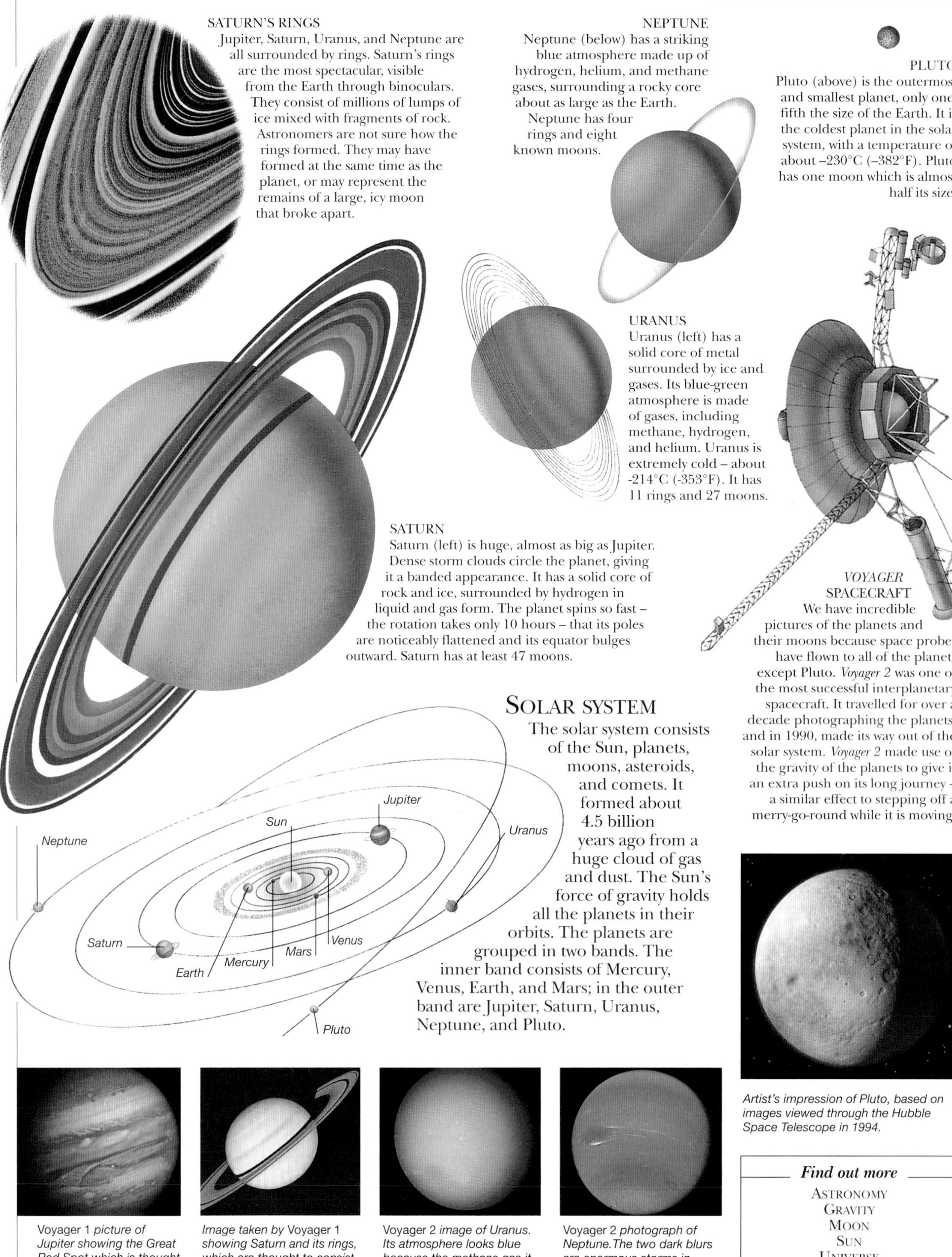

SATURN'S RINGS
Jupiter, Saturn, Uranus, and Neptune are all surrounded by rings. Saturn's rings are the most spectacular, visible from the Earth through binoculars. They consist of millions of lumps of ice mixed with fragments of rock. Astronomers are not sure how the rings formed. They may have formed at the same time as the planet, or may represent the remains of a large, icy moon that broke apart.

NEPTUNE
Neptune (below) has a striking blue atmosphere made up of hydrogen, helium, and methane gases, surrounding a rocky core about as large as the Earth. Neptune has four rings and eight known moons.

PLUTO
Pluto (above) is the outermost and smallest planet, only one-fifth the size of the Earth. It is the coldest planet in the solar system, with a temperature of about –230°C (–382°F). Pluto has one moon which is almost half its size.

URANUS
Uranus (left) has a solid core of metal surrounded by ice and gases. Its blue-green atmosphere is made of gases, including methane, hydrogen, and helium. Uranus is extremely cold – about -214°C (-353°F). It has 11 rings and 27 moons.

SATURN
Saturn (left) is huge, almost as big as Jupiter. Dense storm clouds circle the planet, giving it a banded appearance. It has a solid core of rock and ice, surrounded by hydrogen in liquid and gas form. The planet spins so fast – the rotation takes only 10 hours – that its poles are noticeably flattened and its equator bulges outward. Saturn has at least 47 moons.

VOYAGER SPACECRAFT
We have incredible pictures of the planets and their moons because space probes have flown to all of the planets except Pluto. *Voyager 2* was one of the most successful interplanetary spacecraft. It travelled for over a decade photographing the planets, and in 1990, made its way out of the solar system. *Voyager 2* made use of the gravity of the planets to give it an extra push on its long journey – a similar effect to stepping off a merry-go-round while it is moving.

SOLAR SYSTEM

The solar system consists of the Sun, planets, moons, asteroids, and comets. It formed about 4.5 billion years ago from a huge cloud of gas and dust. The Sun's force of gravity holds all the planets in their orbits. The planets are grouped in two bands. The inner band consists of Mercury, Venus, Earth, and Mars; in the outer band are Jupiter, Saturn, Uranus, Neptune, and Pluto.

Artist's impression of Pluto, based on images viewed through the Hubble Space Telescope in 1994.

Voyager 1 *picture of Jupiter showing the Great Red Spot which is thought to be a huge storm.*

Image taken by Voyager 1 *showing Saturn and its rings, which are thought to consist of a mixture of ice and rock.*

Voyager 2 *image of Uranus. Its atmosphere looks blue because the methane gas it contains cuts out red light.*

Voyager 2 *photograph of Neptune.The two dark blurs are enormous storms in Neptune's atmosphere.*

Find out more

ASTRONOMY
GRAVITY
MOON
SUN
UNIVERSE

PLANTS

LIFE ON EARTH could not exist without plants. Humans and animals need plants for food and oxygen. The cereal you eat for breakfast, the orange juice you drink, even the jeans you wear, are all derived from plants. Trees provide us with wood for fuel, furniture, and tools. In almost every country, flowers and vegetables are grown by the millions for food and pleasure. Scientists use plants to make drugs such as digitalis (from foxglove) and morphine (from poppies). Plants range from tiny mosses to gigantic coniferous trees so tall you cannot see their tops. What they all have in common is their unique ability to capture and use the Sun's light as an energy source. This process is called photosynthesis, and it powers all plant life and growth. About 400,000 plants are already known to us, from rare exotic flowers to common garden vegetables. Even more plants await discovery, especially in tropical regions. Today, however, more than 25,000 different trees, flowers, and other plants are in danger of extinction due to the destruction of their natural habitats.

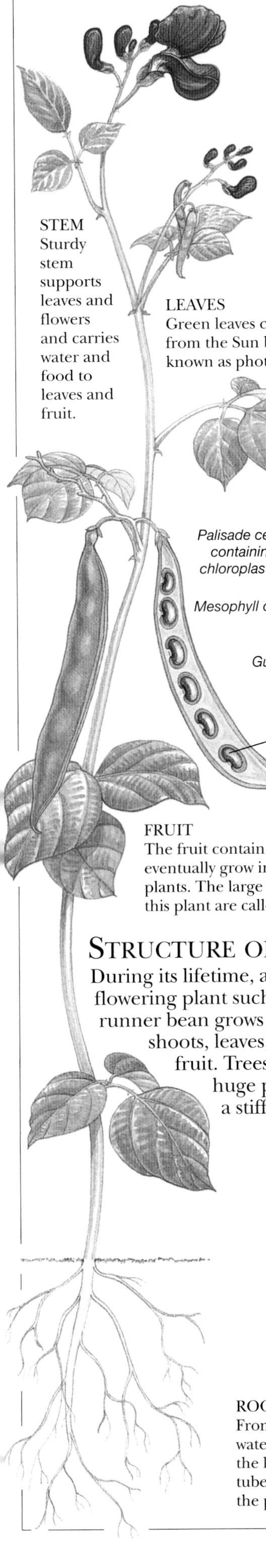

FLOWERS
The flowers of a plant contain both male and female reproductive parts, the pollen and ovule cells. If pollinated the ovule develops into a seed.

STEM
Sturdy stem supports leaves and flowers and carries water and food to leaves and fruit.

LEAVES
Green leaves capture light energy from the Sun by the process known as photosynthesis.

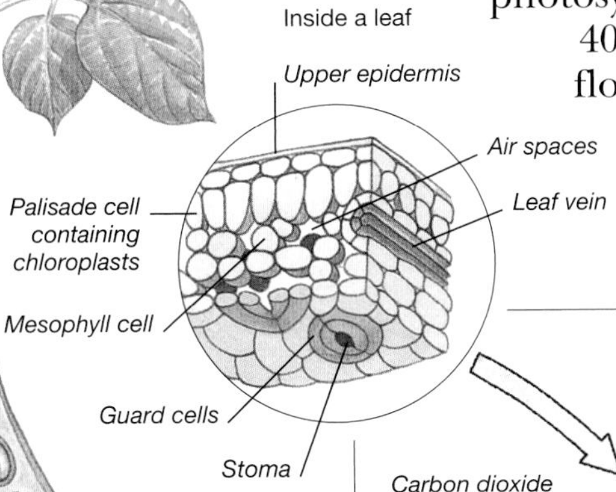

FRUIT
The fruit contain seeds which eventually grow into new plants. The large fruit on this plant are called beans.

STRUCTURE OF A PLANT

During its lifetime, a typical flowering plant such as this runner bean grows a stem, roots, shoots, leaves, flowers, and fruit. Trees, which are huge plants, have a trunk – a stiff, woody stem full of fibres.

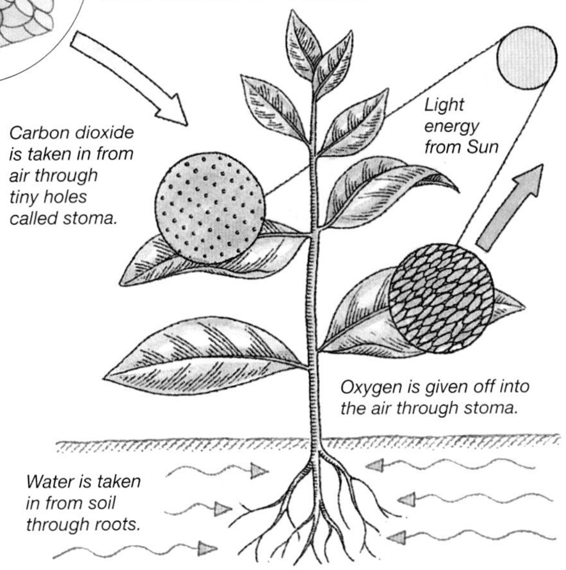

PHOTOSYNTHESIS

In order to grow, plants use energy from sunlight. This process is called photosynthesis. A green substance called chlorophyll is contained in the cells of a plant's leaves. Chlorophyll captures energy in the light waves from the Sun, then carries out chemical reactions in which carbon dioxide gas from the air is combined with water from the soil. This process creates sugars and other substances which the plant uses for energy and growth.

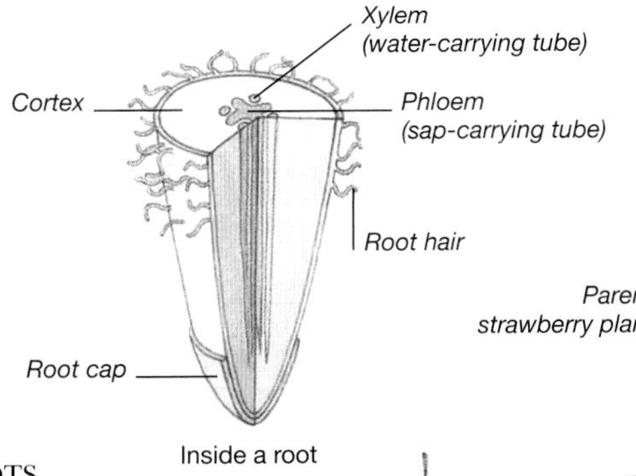

ROOTS
From the soil, the roots take in water and minerals which pass to the leaves and fruit through tiny tubes in the stem. Roots also anchor the plant firmly in the ground.

REPRODUCTION

Most plants reproduce sexually. Pollen fertilizes the ovules in the ovaries, which ripen into fruit that contains seeds. Other plants, such as the potato, reproduce asexually. They grow by tubers which develop into new plants that look like the parent plant.

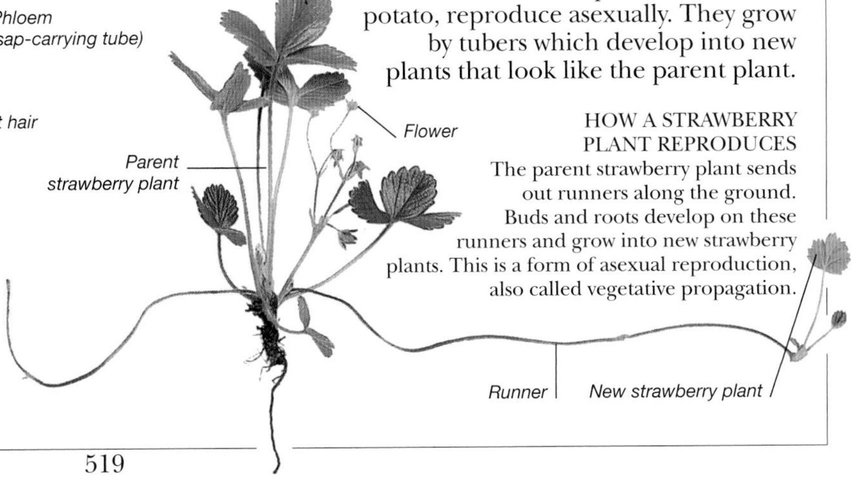

HOW A STRAWBERRY PLANT REPRODUCES
The parent strawberry plant sends out runners along the ground. Buds and roots develop on these runners and grow into new strawberry plants. This is a form of asexual reproduction, also called vegetative propagation.

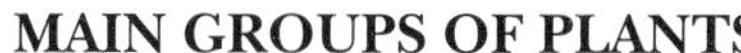

MAIN GROUPS OF PLANTS

The plant kingdom is made up of many different groups. These groups are divided into flowering and non-flowering plants, as shown here.

Seaweed is an alga that grows in sea water and attaches itself to rocks.

Moss grows on logs and walls and in moist, shady woodland areas.

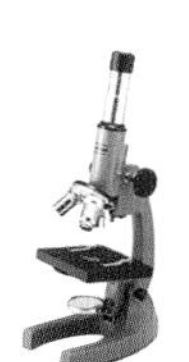

Microscopic plants are so small that we can see them only through a microscope.

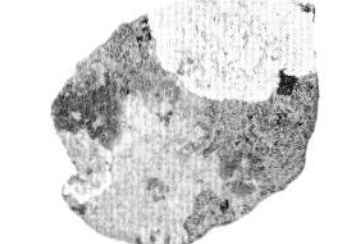

Lichen is now classified as a fungi. It has no true leaves, stems, or roots.

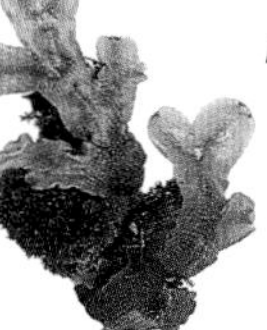

Liverworts are small non-flowering plants related to mosses.

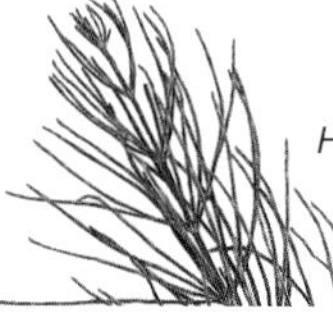

Horsetails were among the earliest plants on Earth.

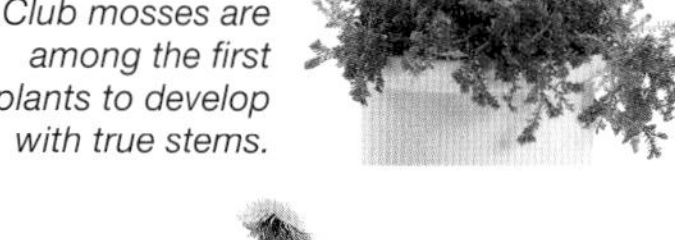

Club mosses are among the first plants to develop with true stems.

Coniferous trees include fir trees and pine trees. They are also called evergreen trees.

Ferns grow in all parts of the world. Some are as large as trees; others are tiny and look like moss.

Weeds are unwanted flowering plants that include dandelions, nettles, and buttercups.

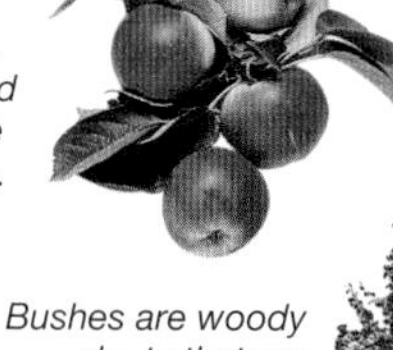

Fruit trees provide many kinds of fruit, including apples, lemons, and bananas. All are rich in vitamins.

Vegetables are edible flowering plants that are rich in vitamins and minerals. They include carrots, potatoes, spinach, tomatoes, and beans.

True flowering plants include roses, tulips, and other garden plants.

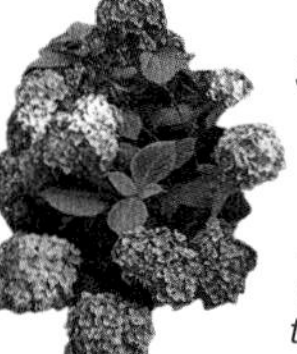

Bushes are woody plants that are smaller than trees. They usually have one main stem.

Herbs have scented leaves. They include basil and oregano.

Grasses include lawn grass and cereals such as wheat, rice, barley, and corn.

Deciduous trees are also called broadleaved trees. They lose their leaves each autumn.

Shrubs are woody plants with more than one main branch growing from the ground.

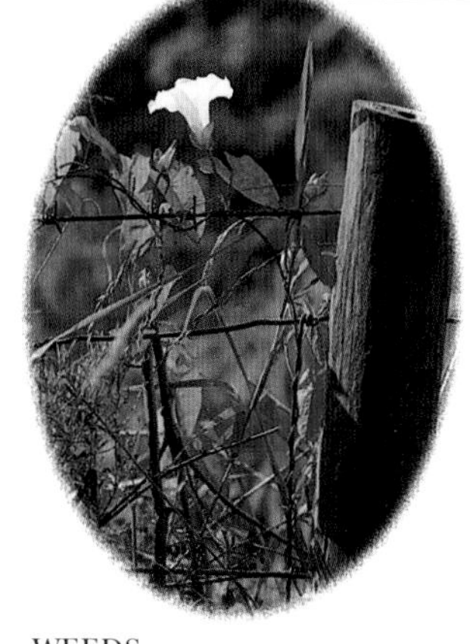

WEEDS

A weed is simply a plant growing where it is troublesome to humans. Most weeds grow fast, come into flower quickly, then spread their seeds. Some weeds, such as the convolvulus shown above, have pale, delicate flowers; others are colourful, such as the dandelions and buttercups that grow on lawns.

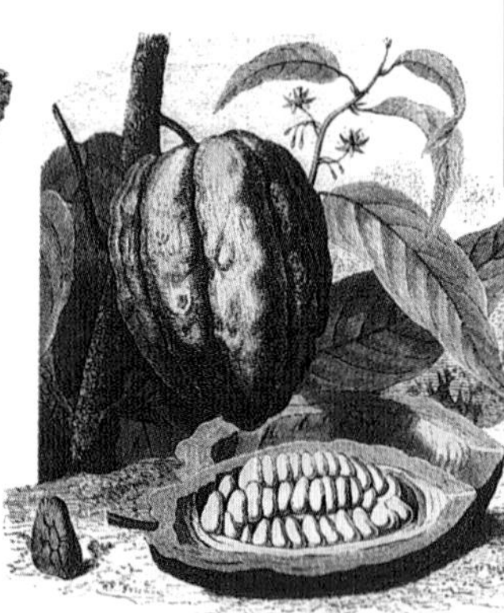

Food from plants

We grow plants for food on farms and in gardens, too. Food plants include cereals such as rice, fruit such as oranges, and vegetables such as carrots. Spices such as cinnamon are parts of plants and are used for flavouring. Some plant parts cannot be eaten because they are bitter, sour, or poisonous. Potatoes are an important food crop, but we eat only the tuber that grows underground. The fruit and leaves of the potato plant, which grow above ground, are poisonous.

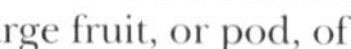

CHOCOLATE

Inside every large fruit, or pod, of the tropical cacao tree are about 40 cacao beans. These beans are roasted, shelled, then ground into a paste. The cacao paste is mixed with sugar at a high temperature to make chocolate.

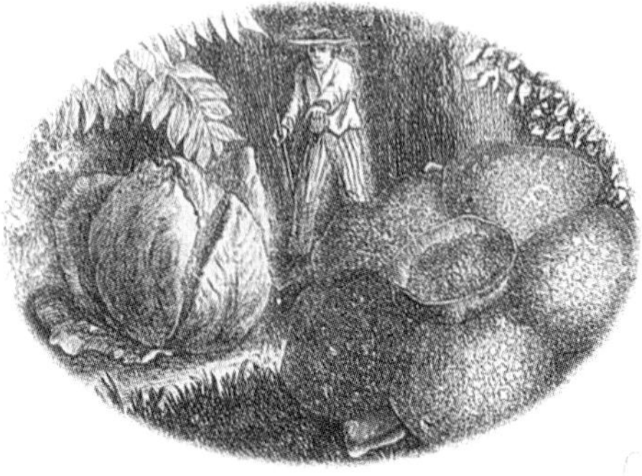

THE BIGGEST FLOWER

The giant rafflesia is a parasitic plant. It has no leaves and draws its food from the liana creepers it lives on. It has the world's largest flower, at 1 m (3 ft) across. Because of its smell, it is also called the stinking giant.

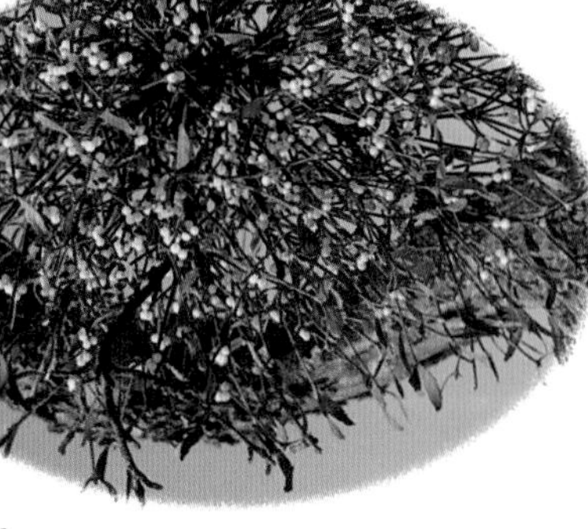

MISTLETOE

This plant "steals" its food and energy by growing and feeding on trees. It grows high up in the branches, and its roots grow into the bark and absorb the tree's nutrients.

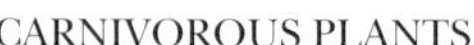

CARNIVOROUS PLANTS

Some plants obtain extra food from animals. One plant, commonly called the Venus's-flytrap, usually grows in swamps, where the soil is poor. Flesh-eating or carnivorous plants trap and digest insects and other small creatures.

Venus's-flytrap flower

The flytrap shuts in one fiftieth of a second, when trigger hairs at the base of each leaf are moved.

When a small creature touches sensitive hairs on the leaves of the Venus's-flytrap, the leaves snap shut with one of the fastest movements in the plant world.

Find out more

FLOWERS AND HERBS
FRUITS AND SEEDS
GRASSES AND CEREALS
MOSSES, liverworts, and ferns
SOIL
TREES

PLASTICS

MANY MATERIALS that we use are natural materials, such as cotton, wool, leather, wood, and metal. They come from plants or animals, or they are dug from the ground. Plastics can be used in place of natural materials, and they are used to make clothes, parts for cars, and many other products. Plastics are synthetic materials, which means that they are made from chemicals in factories. The chemicals come mainly from oil, but also from natural gas and coal. An important quality of plastics is that they are easy to shape. They can be used to make objects of all kinds as well as fibres for textiles. Extra-strong glues, long-lasting paints, and lightweight materials that are stronger than metal – all of these products are made of plastics with special qualities. None can be made with natural materials.

BAKELITE
Bakelite was invented in 1909 by the American chemist Leo Baekeland. It was the first plastic to be made from synthetic chemicals.

PVC
Electrical wires have a coating of flexible PVC (polyvinyl chloride), which is also used to make inflatable toys.

KINDS OF PLASTICS

There are thousands of different plastics. Some of the most common types are shown here.

POLYTHENE
Plastic bags are often made of polythene, a plastic that can be made into a tough, flexible film. When produced in thicker layers, polythene is also used to make bottles, bowls, and other household containers.

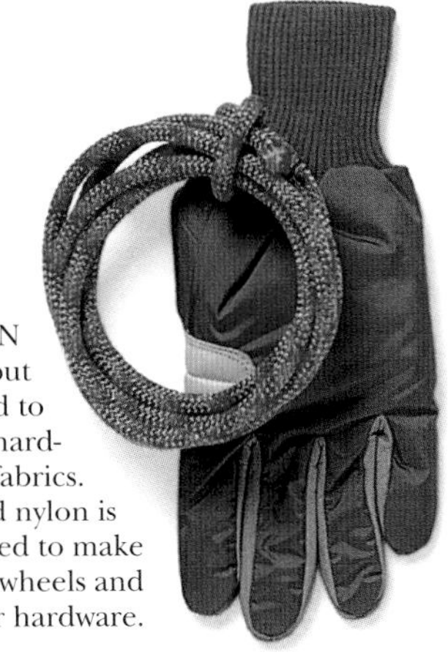

NYLON
Fibres of nylon, a strong but flexible plastic, are used to make ropes and hard-wearing fabrics. Solid nylon is used to make gearwheels and other hardware.

Molecule of polythene

POLYMERS

Plastics are polymers, which are substances with molecules composed of long chains of atoms. This is why the names of plastics often begin with poly, which means "many". Long molecules give plastics their special qualities, such as flexibility and strength.

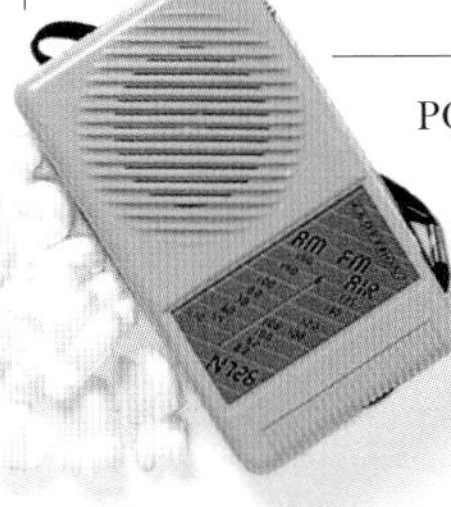

POLYSTYRENE
Packaging made from polystyrene is light and rigid. Tough plastics often contain polystyrene.

BEECH STARSHIP 1
In aircraft, composites can be used to replace many metal parts. This aircraft is made almost entirely of composites which are highly resistant to corrosion and cracking.

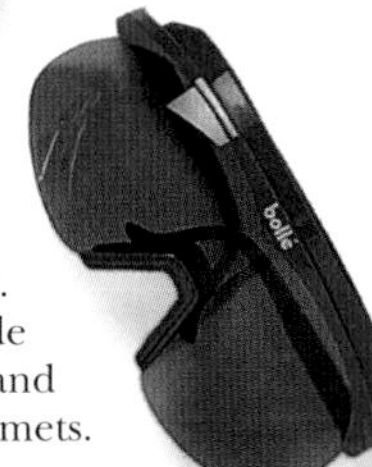

POLYCARBONATE
Goggles need to be clear and strong, two qualities of polycarbonate plastic. Other uses include car lights and crash helmets.

COMPOSITES

Strong fibres are put into tough plastics to create materials called composites, (right) which are very strong yet light and easily shaped. Thin fibres of glass, carbon, or Kevlar (a strong plastic) are used.

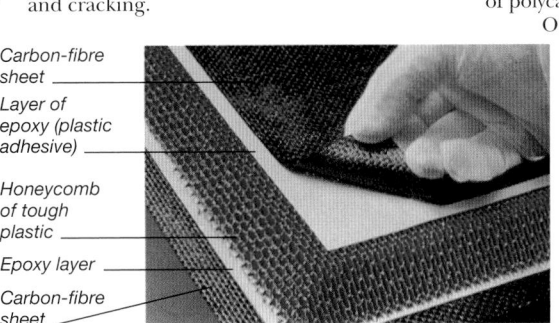

Carbon-fibre sheet
Layer of epoxy (plastic adhesive)
Honeycomb of tough plastic
Epoxy layer
Carbon-fibre sheet

Find out more
ATOMS AND MOLECULES
CHEMISTRY
COAL
MATERIALS
OIL
TEXTILES

POETRY

THE VERY FIRST LITERATURE produced by any culture is usually poetry. Poetry is written in language that is strong and vivid enough to be memorable and to provoke a lasting, and often emotional, response from the reader. All poems are written in lines. Many poems rhyme, have a regular rhythm, and use figures of speech such as metaphor to make the language different to that used in everyday speech, but this is not always the case. These varying patterns and the way they are used allow poets to create different moods, from fast-moving and witty to sad and slow. The most important thing about a poem is that it should make a strong impression on the reader. Although we read poems today, much ancient poetry was passed on by oral (spoken) traditions.

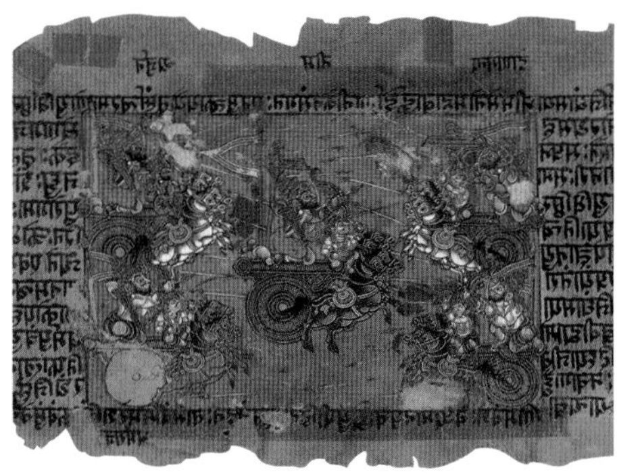

MAHABHARATA
The longest poem ever written is the Indian epic called the *Mahabharata*. It has more than 90,000 couplets (pairs of rhyming lines) and was written in ancient Sanskrit by various writers, before the 4th century A.D. It tells many stories about the ancient Indian kingdom of Kurukshetra.

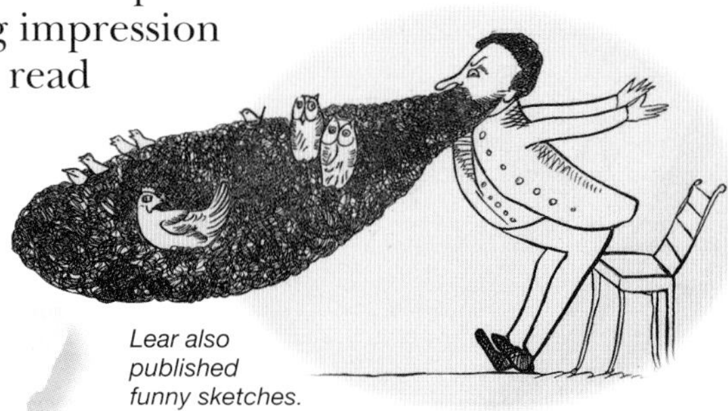

Lear also published funny sketches.

LIMERICKS
The limerick is a type of funny five-line poem made popular in the 19th century by British writer Edward Lear (1812-88). Limericks can be written on any subject, but always begin with a line like "There once was a person from..."

Stanza from *The Tiger* by William Blake

Stressed syllable — *Unstressed syllable*

Ti|ger! Ti|ger! burn|ing bright (A)
In the fo|rests of the night, (A)
What im|mor|tal hand or eye (B)
Could frame thy fear|ful sym|metry? (B)

Pairs of lines rhyme with each other, creating a pattern AABB

— U *Trochee*
— U U *Dactyl*
U — *Iamb*
AABB *Rhyme scheme*
Foot
| *Scansion break*

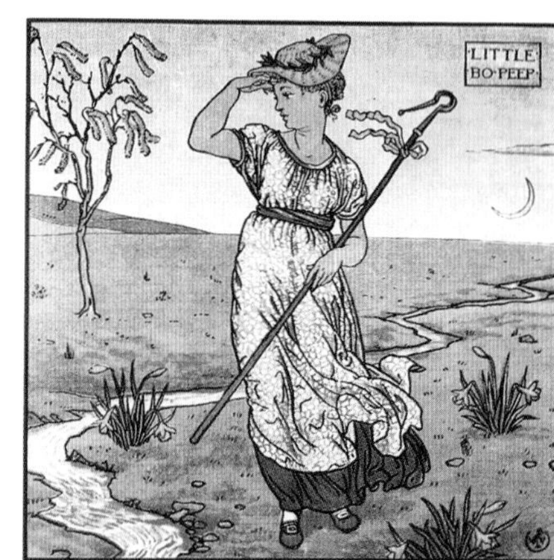

NURSERY RHYME
Children have been singing and reciting nursery rhymes such as "Little Bo Peep" for hundreds of years. Most of the verses have changed little, although there are variations in different regions and countries. No one knows who wrote these poems. Some of them seem to describe real events, but others may be political ideas or jokes about important people, disguised as harmless children's rhymes.

POETIC FORMS

Traditional poetry is written in verse lines. They contain repeating patterns of stressed (emphasized) and unstressed syllables (units of sound in a word), put together in different ways. These patterns of syllables are called "feet". There are different names for each kind of foot. The way the lines rhyme makes another set of patterns, called a rhyme scheme. Groups of rhyming lines are called stanzas and there may be several of them in a poem. Breaking down a poem into its separate parts is called scanning or scansion.

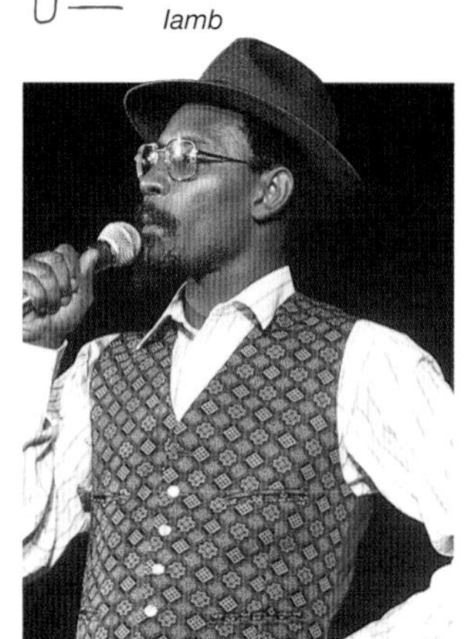

Performance poet Linton Kwesi Johnson often uses music in his work.

PERFORMANCE POETRY
Poetry is written to be read aloud. Like medieval bards (singing poets), who sang their own lyrics, many modern poets prefer to perform their work in public in theatres, cafés, clubs, or wherever people gather to be entertained. Poets such as British writer Linton Kwesi Johnson (b. 1952), for example, act out the scenes and characters in their work, making poetry entertaining for people who may not have enjoyed reading verse before.

Find out more
LITERATURE
LITERATURE, UK
WRITERS AND POETS

POLAR EXPLORATION

THE COLDEST PLACES on Earth were also the very last to be explored. At the North and South Poles fierce, icy winds lash the surrounding masses of snow. The first European explorers to reach the Poles risked their lives in the attempt, and some of them never returned. They used primitive equipment and simple transport. Explorers travelled part of the way by ship, then used skis for the remaining distance, carrying their equipment on sledges pulled by husky dogs or ponies. They faced terrible hazards. The low temperatures made frostbite common, and they had to carry with them everything they needed, including enough food for the long journey to the Pole and back. These early explorers used the position of the sun to tell them when they had reached their goal, because there were no landmarks in the polar landscapes. Later explorers had the advantage of more modern vehicles, but it was not until the middle of the 20th century that both polar regions had been fully explored.

ROBERT PEARY
Robert Peary (1856-1920) was the first person to reach the North Pole on 6 April 1909, together with one other American and four Inuits.

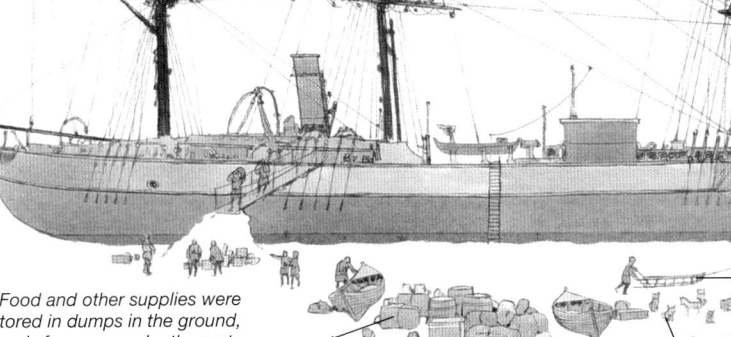

Scott's ship *Discovery*

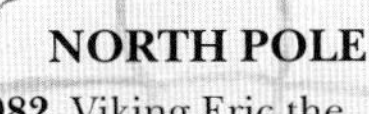

Sledges travelled easily over the ice.

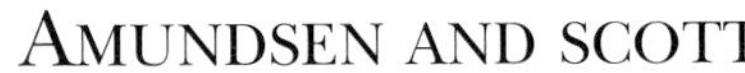

Food and other supplies were stored in dumps in the ground, ready for recovery by the party returning from the Pole.

Scott's expedition took only a few dogs, and instead used ponies to haul sledges.

NORTH POLE

982 Viking Eric the Red discovers Greenland.

1607 Hudson tries to sail around northern Canada.

1827 Sir William Parry tries to reach the Pole using dog sledges.

1893-96 Norwegian ship freezes in pack ice and drifts close to the Pole.

1909 Peary reaches Pole.

1926 First flight to Pole.

1959 US submarine *Skate* surfaces at Pole.

SOUTH POLE

1820 First sighting of Antarctic continent.

1821 A Russian sails around Antarctica, and an American sets foot on it.

1911 Five expeditions race to the Pole; Roald Amundsen wins.

1928 First aeroplanes used in Antarctica.

AMUNDSEN AND SCOTT

In 1912 the specially built wooden ship *Discovery* took an expedition led by British Captain Robert Scott (1868-1912) to within 1,450 km (900 miles) of the South Pole. When Scott's party reached the Pole, they discovered that they were not the first. A Norwegian team led by Roald Amundsen (1872-1928) had arrived at the South Pole on 14 December 1911, well ahead of their British rivals. Scott's group died before they could complete their return journey.

Early explorers' clothing

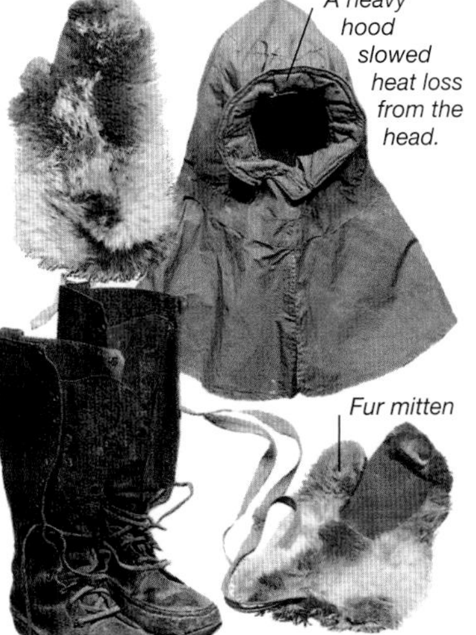

A heavy hood slowed heat loss from the head.

Fur mitten

Goggles prevented sunlight from dazzling the explorers.

MODERN RESEARCH
Today explorers have been replaced by scientists who carry out research at the Poles using more advanced equipment, but in the same harsh and unfriendly environment.

Find out more
ANTARCTICA
ARCTIC
EXPLORERS
GLACIERS AND ICECAPS

POLAR WILDLIFE

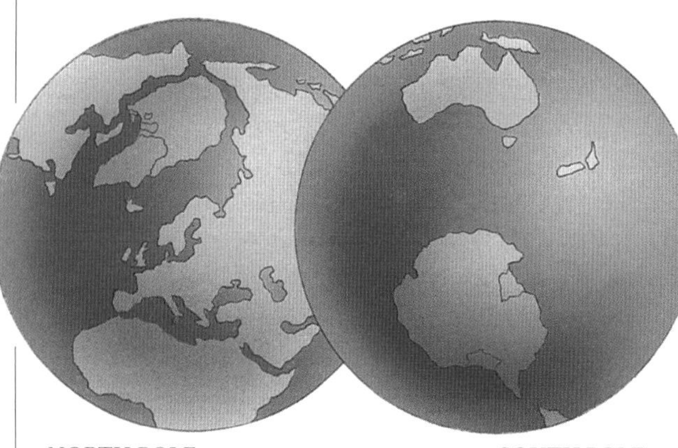

NORTH POLE
In the central Arctic Ocean at the top of the globe, there are vast areas of drifting ice several metres thick.

SOUTH POLE
At the bottom of the globe, the continent of Antarctica is almost completely covered by a massive sheet of ice.

THE NORTH AND SOUTH POLES are the coldest places on Earth. But despite freezing temperatures, icy water, and biting winds, many different plants and animals live near the Poles and are found nowhere else in the world. All survive because they have adapted to the harsh conditions. Plants in these regions are low-growing, to protect them from the cold wind, and they complete their life cycle during the few short weeks of summer. Polar animals, too, have adapted to the cold conditions; some have thick fur or feathers; others have a layer of fatty blubber to conserve body warmth. The biggest animals, the great whales, roam the waters of Antarctica, near the South Pole, and the largest bear, the polar bear, lives in the Arctic, near the North Pole. Many other warm-blooded animals, including wolves, foxes, reindeer, hares, and lemmings, also live here. Polar animals are often white in colour for camouflage on the ice. The cold seas are also teeming with life, particularly in summer. Around Antarctica, ocean currents bring up nutrients from the deep sea to feed the plankton, which in turn feeds animals such as krill.

ARCTIC SKUA
The skua snatches food from other birds such as gulls and puffins. It pesters them in midair until they drop their catch of fish.

NARWHAL
The narwhal belongs to the whale family. It hunts in small groups among pack ice searching for cod, flatfish, shrimps, and squid. Narwhals have only two teeth. In the male, the left tooth usually develops into a tusk, which can measure up to 2.5 m (8 ft) long.

POLAR BEAR CUBS
Young polar bears are born in winter in a den made by their mother under the snow. The cubs stay in the den for four months, feeding on their mother's milk, then begin to learn how to hunt. The cubs leave their mother at about two years old.

BEARDED SEAL
Bearded seals live all around the Arctic region, mainly in shallow water. They eat shellfish on the seabed, as well as crabs and sea cucumbers. In the breeding season, male bearded seals make eerie noises under water. The female seals give birth to pups on ice floes in the spring.

HOODED SEAL
In summer, hooded seals migrate north to the waters around Greenland. They hunt deep-water fishes such as halibut and redfish, as well as squid. They spend the winter further south, off northeastern North America, resting on ice floes and rarely coming onto land.

The male hooded seal inflates the hood – a sac of loose skin on its nose – to scare off other males.

POLAR BEAR

The huge polar bear is covered in thick, water-repelling fur, except for its footpads and the tip of its nose. Polar bears have an excellent sense of smell for locating prey, and they can bound across the ice at great speed. An adult polar bear weighs about half a tonne. It is so strong that a single blow of its paw can kill a person.

Polar bears eat seals, fish, birds, and small mammals. They also scavenge on the carcasses (dead bodies) of whales.

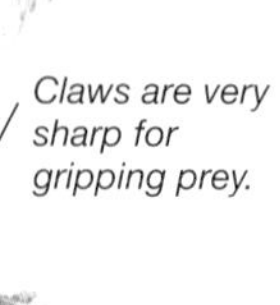

Claws are very sharp for gripping prey.

Conservation

Today, polar bears and whales are protected from hunting by law. But many polar animals are still threatened by oil spills from ships and by over-fishing. Fishing boats catch huge quantities of fish, which affects the numbers of animals that depend on fish for food.

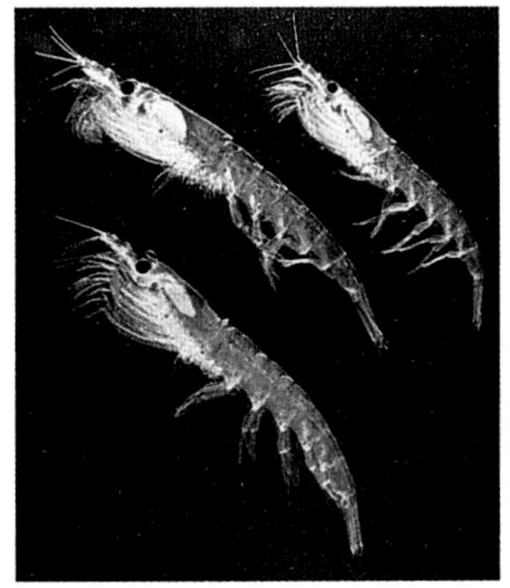

KRILL
The shrimp-like creatures shown left are called krill. They are the main food for baleen (whalebone) whales, such as the blue whale, which scoop up thousands of krill from the ocean every day.

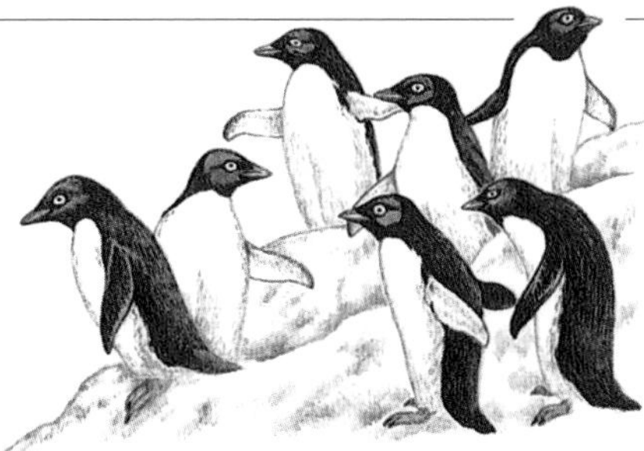

Penguins

There are 17 different kinds of penguins; all live in the southern hemisphere. Penguins cannot fly, but they are expert swimmers and divers. They can speed along in the water after fish and squid using their flipper-shaped wings.

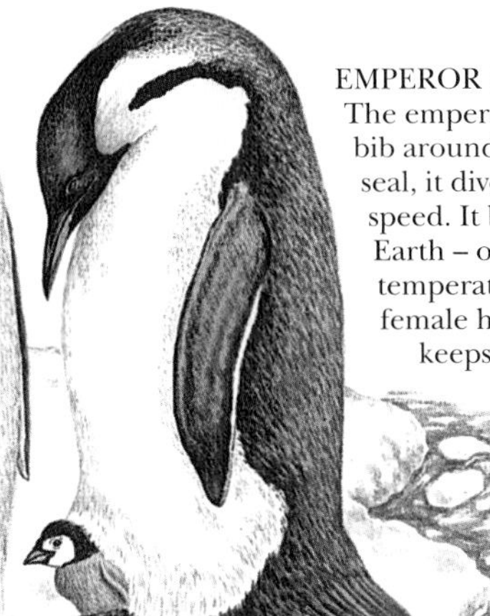

EMPEROR PENGUIN
The emperor penguin has a bright orange bib around its neck. To escape the leopard seal, it dives out of the water with great speed. It breeds in the coldest place on Earth – on Antarctic ice where the average temperature is -20°C (-4°F). After the female has laid an egg, the male penguin keeps it warm between his feet and belly for about 60 days. The newborn chicks stay warm by standing on their parents' feet.

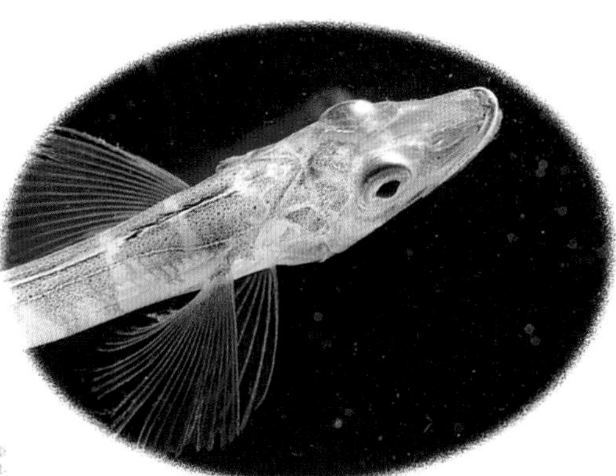

ICE FISH
The blood of most fish freezes solid at about –35°C (-32°F), and the waters in the polar regions sometimes drop even lower. The ice fish, also called the crocodile fish, has special chemicals in its blood to stop it from freezing.

LEOPARD SEAL
The four main kinds of seals around Antarctica are the leopard, crabeater, Ross, and Weddell seals. The leopard seal measures up to 3 m (10 ft) in length. It patrols the pack ice and island coasts hunting for penguins and other seals, especially crabeater seals.

Tundra

The lands on the edge of the Arctic Ocean are bleak and treeless. This region is called the tundra. The brief summer in the Arctic allows small plants such as sedges, cushion-shaped saxifrages, heathers, mosses, and lichens to grow. These plants provide food for many insects and the grazing caribou. Birds such as snow geese breed along the shores and migrate south in autumn.

There is little life on the continent of Antarctica itself, apart from a few mosses, lichens, and tiny creatures such as mites.

MUSK OX
The musk ox is a type of goat. It is the only large mammal that can survive winter on the tundra. The musk ox's thickset body has dense underfur and a thick, shaggy outer coat of tough hairs. Musk oxen stand together in a herd for warmth and as protection against predators such as wolves.

SNOW GOOSE
About 100 kinds of birds migrate to the tundra to breed in spring. Snow geese arrive two weeks before there are any plants to eat, but they have a store of body fat which allows them to make a nest and lay eggs before they eat. Later they feed the chicks on the newly growing grasses.

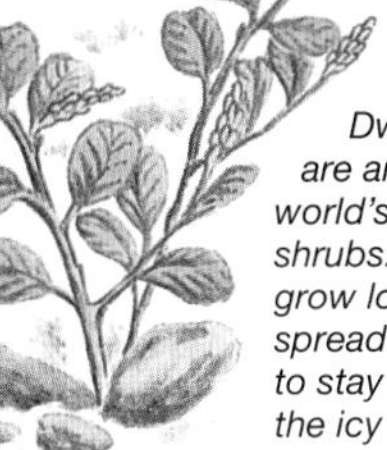

Dwarf willows are among the world's smallest shrubs. They grow low and spread sideways to stay out of the icy winds.

ARCTIC SAXIFRAGE
The cushion shapes of tundra flowers such as saxifrage and crowberry help prevent the plants from freezing. These plants also provide shelter for the tiny creatures living inside them.

Find out more
Antarctica
Arctic
Bears and pandas
Fish
Seabirds
Seals and sea lions
Whales and dolphins

Police

ALL SOCIETIES HAVE RULES OR LAWS to protect the rights of their citizens. In a few communities the people themselves enforce the laws and identify and catch anyone who breaks them. But in most societies law enforcement is the job of the police. Police officers have many different duties, including chasing dangerous criminals, stopping motorists who drive too fast, and patrolling neighbourhood streets. Some work in offices, carefully studying information for clues in order to solve a crime. The police arrest people suspected of committing a crime, then charge the suspects (accuse them of the crime) and hand them over to the courts for trial. The police must be careful to enforce only existing laws and not to arrest people for imagined crimes. In some countries, such as the United States, the police are civilians who are employed by the government. In other countries the police are similar to soldiers. In many nations the government uses the police to hold on to power and to stop political opposition.

PEELERS
British police officers first appeared in the early 19th century. Politician Sir Robert Peel (1788-1850), shown above, argued for their introduction to try to make London a more law-abiding city. People nicknamed these first policemen "peelers" or "bobbies" after the founder of the force.

Detectives

Police officers with special training in investigating crime are called detectives. When a crime has been committed, one detective takes charge of the investigation. Detectives interview witnesses – people who saw the crime happen – and search for evidence. First they look for evidence that will help track down the person who committed the crime. When they have arrested a suspect, detectives look for evidence that will support their suspicions.

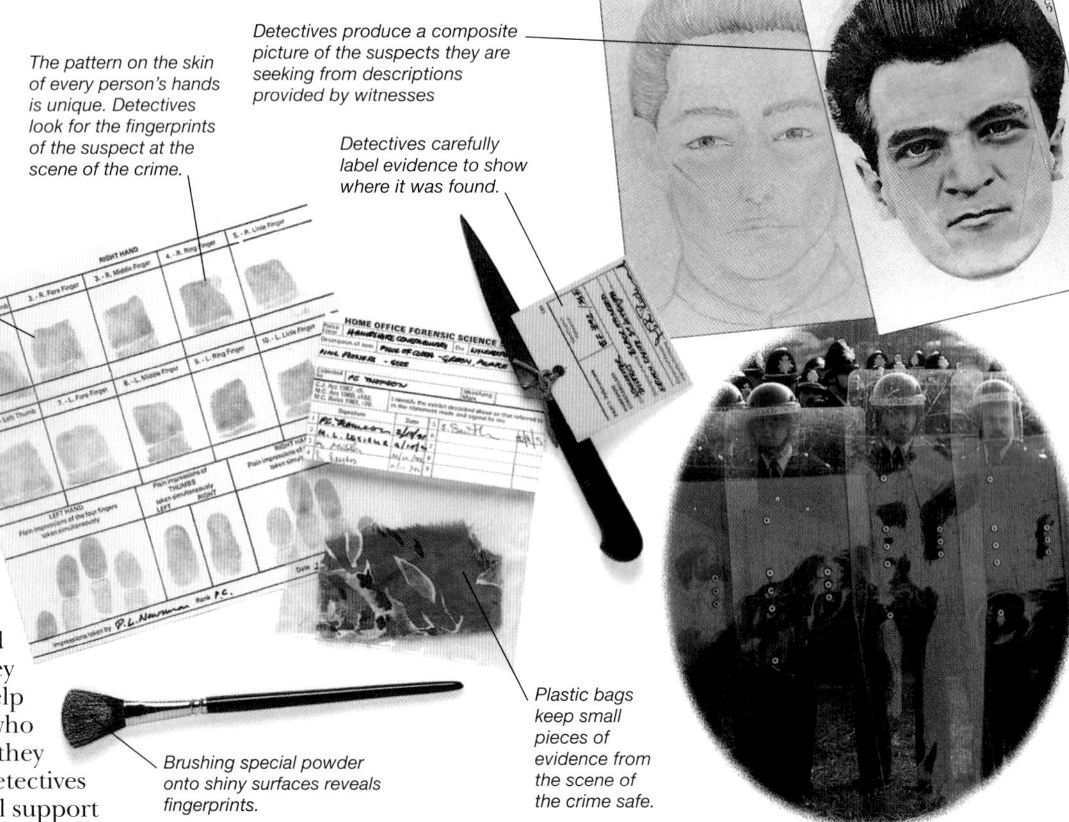

Detectives produce a composite picture of the suspects they are seeking from descriptions provided by witnesses

The pattern on the skin of every person's hands is unique. Detectives look for the fingerprints of the suspect at the scene of the crime.

Detectives carefully label evidence to show where it was found.

Police keep fingerprint records of every known criminal.

Brushing special powder onto shiny surfaces reveals fingerprints.

Plastic bags keep small pieces of evidence from the scene of the crime safe.

UNIFORMED POLICE
Detectives often wear ordinary clothes, but most police officers wear a uniform. The uniform enables members of the public to recognize the police officers. In some countries traffic police wear a completely different uniform from the criminal investigation police. A uniform must be practical, with pockets for a two-way radio, notebooks, handcuffs, a truncheon, and other equipment. In some countries, such as the United States, the police are armed. In other countries, such as Britain, police do not usually carry guns.

Japan | Zimbabwe | United Kingdom | Thailand

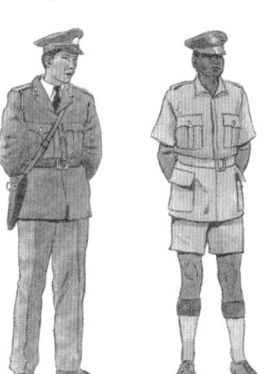

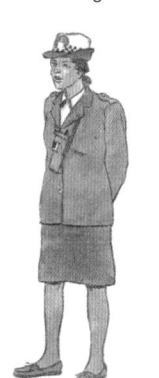

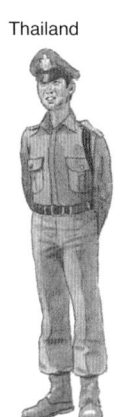

RIOT POLICE
Sometimes large demonstrations or marches become violent. The demonstrators may loot shops or attack members of the public. Riot police move in to control such disturbances. They try to stop the violence by arresting the worst troublemakers and dispersing the crowd so that peace returns. Some riot police are specially trained personnel; others are regular officers equipped with special riot equipment including helmets, full-length shields to protect the body, and heavy truncheons.

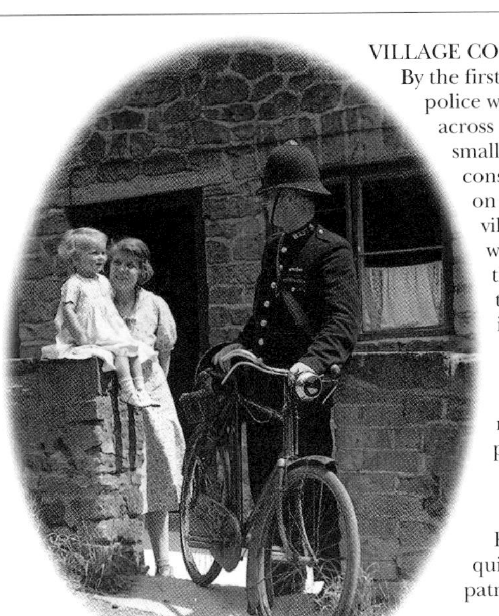

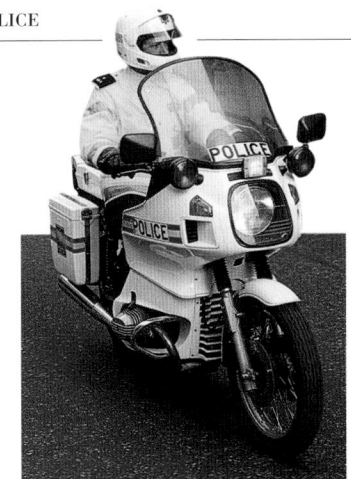

VILLAGE CONSTABLE
By the first half of the 1900s the police were well established across Britain and many small villages had a local constable who patrolled on foot or by bicycle. The village "bobby", as he was called, often lived in the village and knew the names of all the inhabitants. Policing has changed in recent years and very few small communities now have their own police officer.

TRAFFIC POLICE
The main responsibility of the traffic police is to enforce the rules of the road. They use special electronic radar equipment to track the speed of moving cars, and breathalysers to measure the amount of alcohol consumed by suspected drunk drivers. Traffic police also direct the traffic, help pedestrians cross the road, and provide assistance at road accidents.

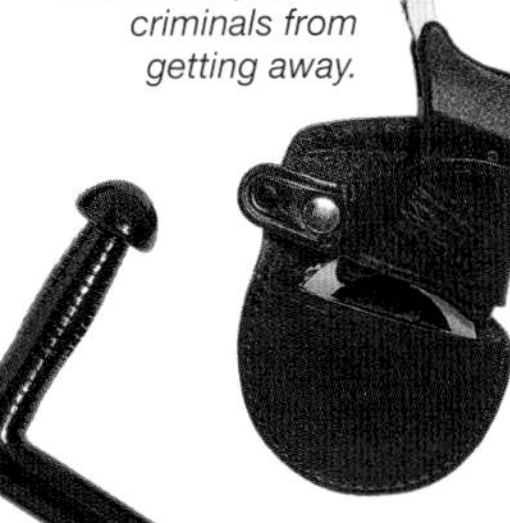

Handcuffs prevent criminals from getting away.

MODERN POLICE EQUIPMENT
Police officers use motorbikes and cars to get around quickly. Many forces also use helicopters. Officers on patrol carry long batons, which offer better protection than the older, shorter truncheons. Two-way radios enable them to respond quickly and to summon help. In big cities, riot police wear plastic visors and carry shields. Only special weapons officers carry guns and wear body armour.

Baton with side handle

SECURITY CAMERAS
The police use technology to try to prevent crime. More and more cities and towns are installing security cameras to watch over streets. The cameras are operated from control rooms and new computers can identify criminals automatically. The film can be used as evidence in court.

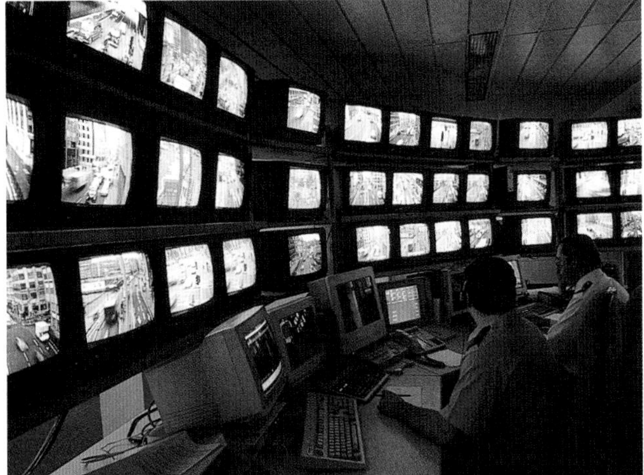

Police camera

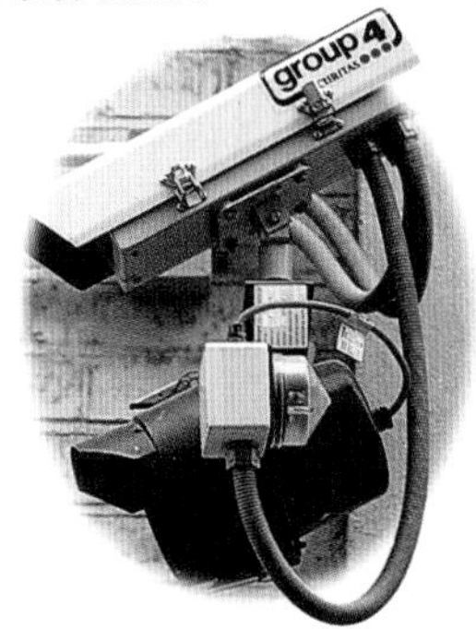

Modern police

Today all police information, including details of crimes and criminals, is stored on a central computer system. This makes it easy to access the information when trying to solve a crime or trace a criminal. Police forces are trying to recruit more women and people from black and Asian communities in an effort to reflect British society.

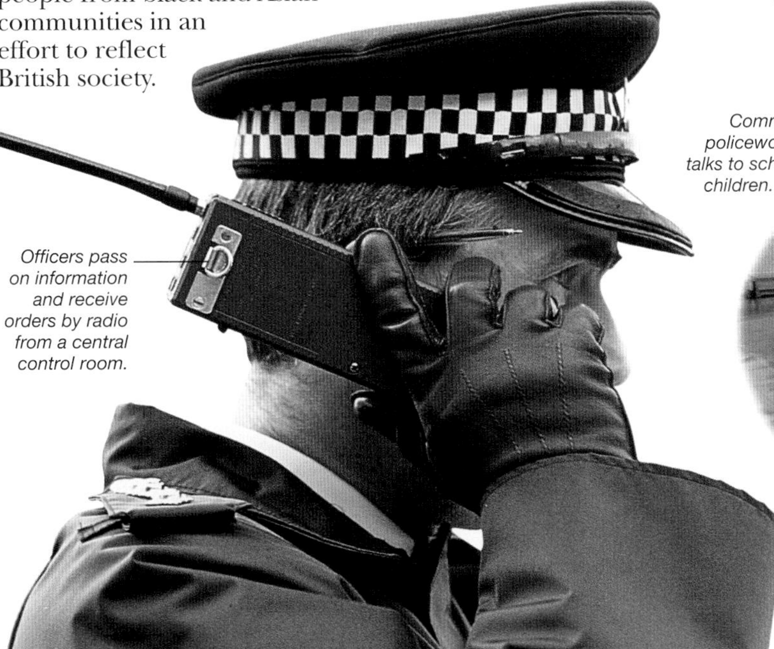

Officers pass on information and receive orders by radio from a central control room.

Police officers on the beat wear uniforms that show their rank. Police detectives wear ordinary clothes.

COMMUNITY POLICING
The job of a community officer involves working in a certain area of a town or city, called a beat, with the purpose of getting to know the residents and finding out what problems they may be experiencing. Duties include visiting old people and making sure their homes are safe, helping children cross the road, and going into schools.

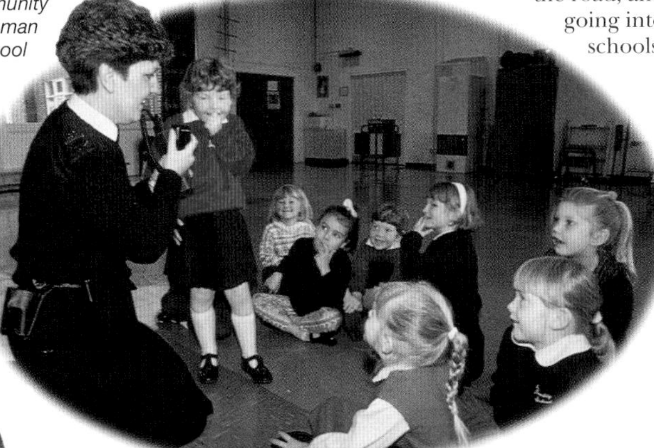

Community policewoman talks to school children.

Find out more
Computers
Information technology
Law

Pollution

Oil on beaches, vehicle exhaust fumes, litter, and other waste products are called pollutants, because they pollute (dirty) our environment. Pollutants can affect our health and harm animals and plants. We pollute our surroundings with all kinds of chemical waste from factories and power stations. These substances are the unwanted results of modern living. Pollution itself is not new – a hundred years ago factories sent out great clouds of poisonous smoke. Today, there are many more factories and many more pollutants. Pollution has spread to the land, air, and water of every corner on Earth, even to Antarctica and Mount Everest. Scientists are worried that the gases released by factories and vehicles are even changing the atmosphere and causing the surface temperature of the planet to heat up. We can reduce pollution by recycling waste and using biodegradable materials that eventually break down in the soil.

ACCIDENTAL POLLUTION
As well as everyday pollution, there is also accidental pollution – for example, when a ship leaks oil and creates a huge oil slick in the ocean. This kind of pollution causes damage to the environment and kills millions of fish and sea birds, like the oil-covered birds shown above.

ATMOSPHERIC POLLUTION
Ozone is a kind of oxygen present in the atmosphere. It forms a protective layer that blocks out the Sun's ultraviolet radiation, which can cause skin cancer in humans. Chemicals called CFCs (chlorofluorocarbons) destroy the ozone.

GLOBAL WARMING
Burning fossil fuels releases carbon gases into the atmosphere. They act like the panes of glass in a greenhouse, trapping the heat. Many scientists now believe that the Earth is becoming too warm. If the Earth becomes just a few degrees warmer, sea levels will rise, drowning low-lying coastal cities.

ACID RAIN
Vehicle exhausts produce fumes that contain nitrogen oxides. The coal we burn in power stations produces sulphur dioxide. When these two substances mix with water in the air, they turn into acids, then fall as acid rain. Acid rain damages trees, eats into buildings, and kills wildlife in rivers. Today, it is possible to reduce the amount of sulphur dioxide given off by power stations, but the process is expensive.

Farmers spray crops with fertilizers to help them grow, and pesticides to control pests and weeds, but these chemicals harm the other kinds of wildlife that live and feed on the crops.

Many factories release pollutants as a by-product.

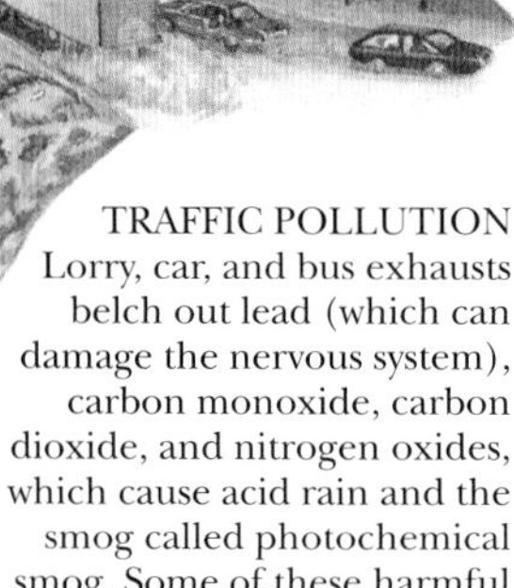

Ships leak oil into the sea, which is harmful to sea creatures.

TRAFFIC POLLUTION
Lorry, car, and bus exhausts belch out lead (which can damage the nervous system), carbon monoxide, carbon dioxide, and nitrogen oxides, which cause acid rain and the smog called photochemical smog. Some of these harmful substances are reduced by special catalytic converters attached to vehicle exhausts.

Every day we drop litter on the ground – sweet wrappers, paper bags, empty tin cans, bottles, and cigarette packets. Litter is ugly, unhygienic, and a fire risk, and it can kill animals that eat it.

RECYCLING

If we save the glass, metal, plastics, and paper that we use every day, they can be recycled and used again. This helps preserve the Earth's natural resources. Recycling cuts down litter, reduces air and water pollution, and can save energy. Many towns have "bottle banks" to collect glass for recycling.

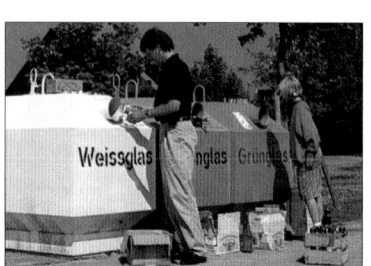

Waste dumping

In many parts of the world people bury toxic (poisonous) chemicals and other dangerous waste products. These substances leak into the soil and water, killing wildlife. We treat the seas as waste dumps, and the North Sea is now seriously polluted. For the wildlife in the seas to survive, we must produce less harmful waste products.

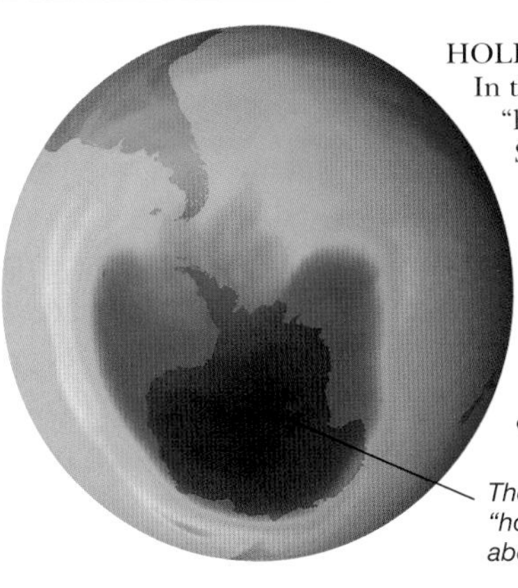

The dark patch is the "hole" in the ozone layer above the Antarctic.

HOLES IN THE OZONE LAYER

In the late 1970s, scientists detected "holes" in the ozone layer above the South and North Poles. Probably caused by air pollutants, such as CFCs and methane, the "holes" seemed to be growing larger. In 1987, more than 30 countries signed an agreement called the Montreal Protocol, which has sharply reduced the production of CFCs worldwide.

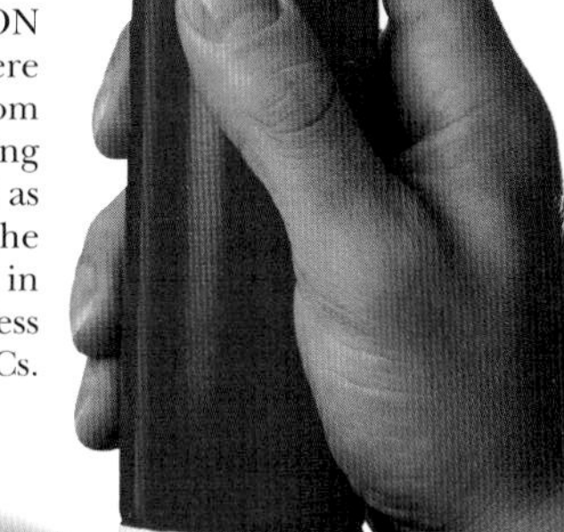

An aerosol is a mixture of product and propellant.

The can is pressurized by the propellant gas.

HOUSEHOLD POLLUTION

Some of the polluting gases that were destroying the ozone layer came from household devices. The most damaging were chlorofluorocarbons (CFCs), used as propellants in aerosol cans and inside the cooling systems of refrigerators. Today, in the move to reduce pollution, less harmful gases have replaced CFCs.

Cleaning up

Neutralizing chemicals can be used to clean up pollution. Spilt oil, for example, can be countered with detergents. But unfortunately these chemicals can do just as much damage as the original spill. Sometimes the only way to clean up is to physically remove the pollutant. Sadly the damage is often already done, although it may not be very obvious.

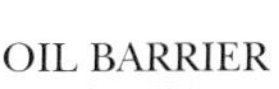

Where possible, mechanical scoops remove spilt oil sludge.

Special V-shaped paddles are used to push the oil sludge into heaps.

OIL BARRIER

Crude oil is a particularly harmful chemical pollutant. However, because oil floats on water, an oil slick created by a spillage from a wrecked tanker can be contained by barriers. The oil must then be dispersed or collected quickly because, if it is left, it will eventually thicken and sink. Also, oil barriers cannot withstand storms.

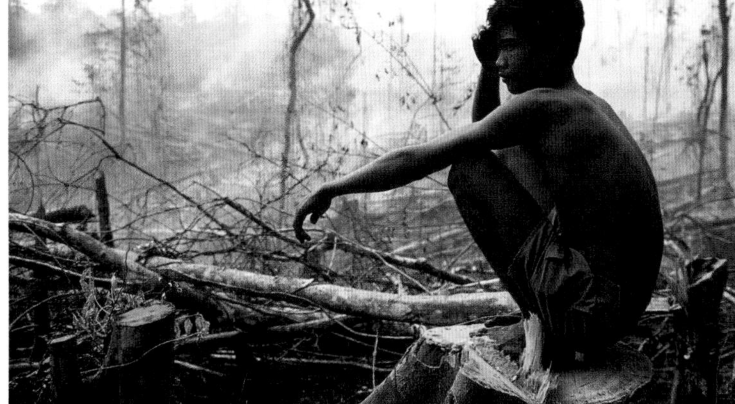

ENERGY SAVING

Much of the pollution that we produce is the result of burning fossil fuels in power plants and motor vehicles. Generators and engines can be made more efficient so that they use less fuel. Individuals too can save energy and reduce pollution by making use of energy-efficient light bulbs and other appliances in the home, and by using cars less.

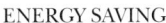

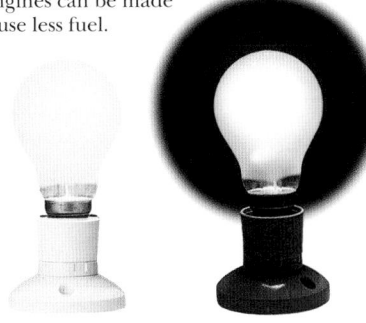

Energy-saving lamps reduce pollution, but just switching off lights helps even more.

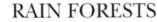

RAIN FORESTS

Since 1945, more than half of the world's rain forests have been destroyed. They are cut down for timber or burnt to clear space for farmland. Burning produces carbon dioxide, contributing to global warming. Scientists are increasingly concerned about the impact of this on the environment.

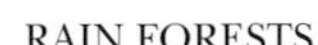

Find out more

ATMOSPHERE
CLIMATES
CONSERVATION and endangered species
ENERGY

PORTS AND WATERWAYS

SHIPS LOAD AND UNLOAD their cargoes at ports, or harbours – sheltered places on coasts or rivers with cranes and warehouses to handle ships, passengers, and goods. Road and rail connections link the ports with inland areas. The earliest ports were simply landing places at river mouths. Here ships were safe from storms, and workers on board could unload cargo into smaller boats for transport upriver. Building walls against the riverbanks created wharfs to make loading easier. In the 18th and 19th centuries, port authorities added docks – deep, artificial pools – leading off the rivers. Ships and boats use waterways to sail to inland towns or as shortcuts from one sea to another. Waterways can be natural rivers, or artificial rivers called canals. One of the world's largest waterway systems, based on the Mississippi River links the Great Lakes with the Gulf of Mexico. It includes 24,000 km (15,000 miles) of waterways.

Navigation lights guide ships safely into the port.

Because oil burns easily, oil tankers use special terminals to unload their cargo.

Huge tanks at the terminal store the oil until it is needed.

Ships and boats unload at wharfs.

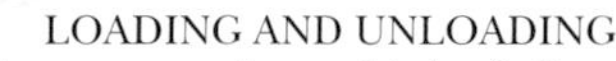

LOADING AND UNLOADING
Ships carry nearly two thirds of all goods in containers, but many items do not fit neatly inside them. Cranes lift these individual large pieces of cargo on and off the ships. Loose cargo such as grain is sucked up by huge pumps and carried ashore through pipes. Vehicles drive onto special ships known as "ro-ros": roll-on, roll-off ferries.

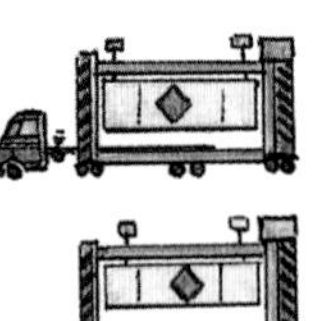

CONTAINERS
A special wheeled crane handles containers. It lifts them off the ship and can either stack them nearby or lower them onto the back of a truck. Cranes, ships, and trucks around the world have the same size fittings so that they can move containers easily between different countries.

DOCKS

Huge gates at the entrance to the docks maintain the water level inside. The warehouses and cranes of the old-style docks are disappearing today as more ships carry goods in containers – large steel boxes of standard size that are easy to stack and move.

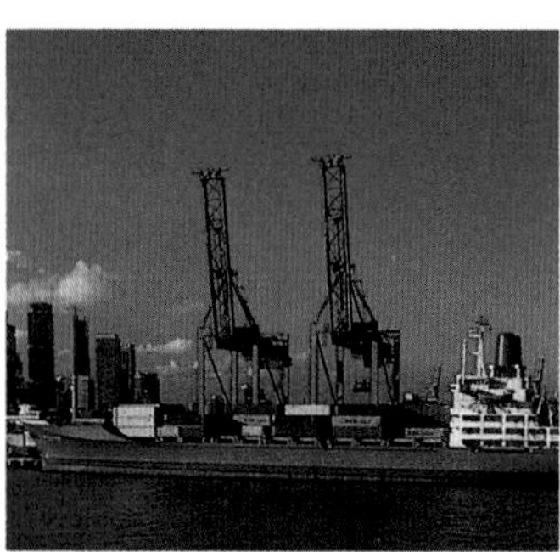

SINGAPORE
At the centre of the sea routes of southern Asia lies Singapore, one of the busiest ports in the world. Its large, modern docks handle goods from all over the world. Many large ships from Europe and the Americas unload their cargoes here into smaller vessels for distribution to nearby countries.

LOCKS

To raise or lower ships from one water level to another, canals and harbours have locks. If a ship is going to a lower water level, the lock fills with water and the ship sails in. Closing the upper gates and letting out the water gradually lowers the ship to the level of the water outside the lower gates.

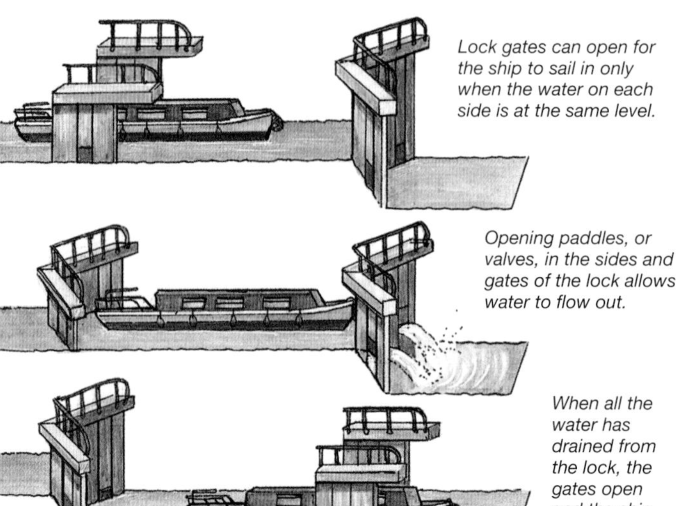

Lock gates can open for the ship to sail in only when the water on each side is at the same level.

Opening paddles, or valves, in the sides and gates of the lock allows water to flow out.

When all the water has drained from the lock, the gates open and the ship can continue on its way.

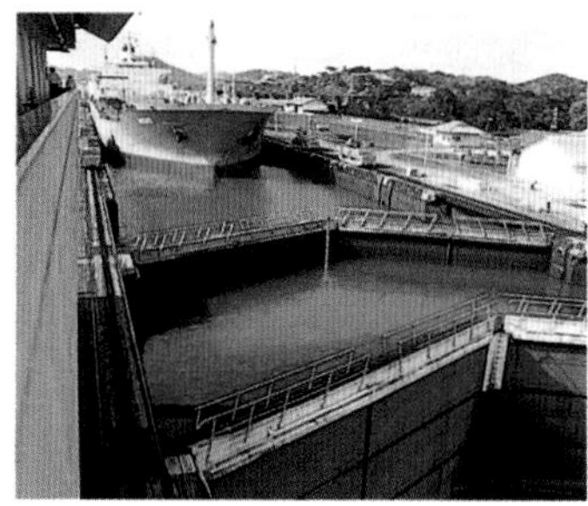

PANAMA CANAL
Ships travelling around the South American coast from the Caribbean Sea to the Pacific Ocean must sail nearly 10,000 km (6,000 miles). So the United States built a huge canal through Panama in Central America where the Pacific and the Caribbean are just 82 km (51 miles) apart. The canal opened in 1914.

Find out more
NAVIGATION
SHIPS AND BOATS
TRADE AND INDUSTRY

PORTUGAL

PORTUGAL'S LONG ATLANTIC coast has shaped its destiny as a seafaring nation. It is a land with few natural resources, and its economy has traditionally been based on fishing and farming. The grapes that grow on the moist, fertile slopes of the Douro river produce fine wines and port, while olives, cork trees, and tinned fish are also major exports. Today, Portugal is becoming more industrialized, and its textile industry is expanding. Although it has a good internal road network, its transport links to its eastern neighbour, Spain, are poor, and most heavy goods are still moved by ship. Tourism, especially to the mild south coast, is increasingly important.

On the southwestern side of the Iberian peninsula, which it shares with Spain, Portugal is the westernmost country in mainland Europe. It also includes the Azores and Madeira, two self-governing island groups in the Atlantic Ocean.

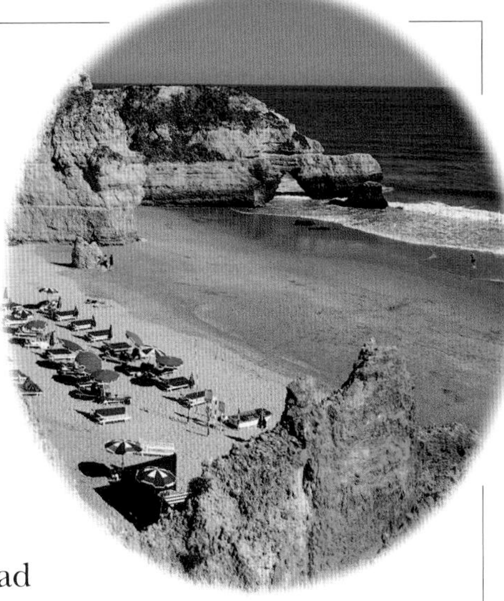

ALGARVE

The fertile coastal lowlands in the south of Portugal are densely inhabited. Inland, the mainly agricultural economy is based on corn, figs, olives, almonds, and grapes. Many fishing villages line the coast. In recent years, these quiet backwaters have been transformed by tourism (above). Some traditional villages have been completely swallowed up by tourist development. Tourists come for mild winters, fine scenery and some of the best golf courses in Europe.

Port is a sweet dessert wine, made by adding brandy to the fermenting grapes.

VINEYARDS

Vineyards blanket the terraced hills that line the valley of the Douro river (left). The grapes harvested here are used to make Portugal's distinctive wines and famous fortified wine, which is named "port" after Porto, a major town on the Douro estuary. Grapes are transported down the river by barge to the towns of Porto and Villa Nova da Gaia, where the wine is blended and matured in casks and bottles and shipped all over the world. The island of Madeira is also famous for its wine, which is heated over a period of six months by a combination of hot water pipes and the rays of the sun. It is then fortified with brandy, which helps to give Madeira wine a richer flavour.

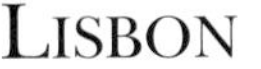

LISBON

Portugal's capital and main port lies on the banks of the Tagus river, 13 km (8 miles) from the coast. Baixa, the historic city centre (below), lies on the north bank. In 1755, most of the city was destroyed by an earthquake and completely rebuilt. Today, it is the bustling commercial heart of the city. Lisbon's manufacturing centre, dominated by large cement and steel works, lies on the south bank.

CORK CULTIVATION

Portugal is the world's leading producer of cork, made from the bark of the cork oak tree. Trees are first stripped of cork at 15 to 20 years old, and then every 10 years thereafter. Cork is used to make stoppers for bottles and jars.

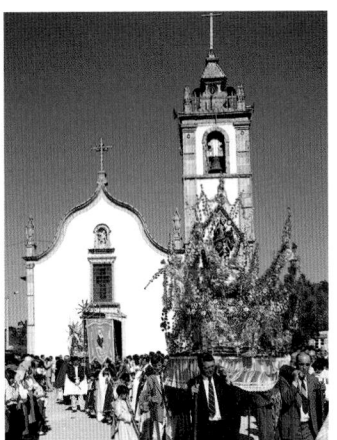

FESTIVALS

Portugal is a Roman Catholic country; many villages hold an annual festival to mark a particular saint's day or religious holiday. Colourful parades march through the streets, accompanied by the Portuguese guitar (a type of mandolin), and the entire village comes together for a lavish meal, with music and dancing. Plaintive folk songs (*fados*) are famous throughout Portugal.

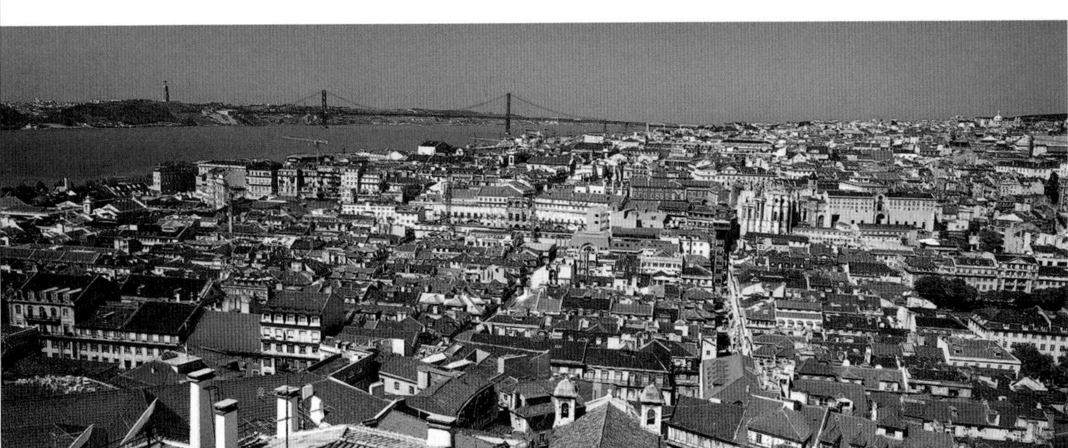

Find out more

EUROPE, HISTORY OF
PORTUGAL, HISTORY OF

STATISTICS

Area: 92,390 sq km (35,670 sq miles)
Population: 10,100,000
Capital: Lisbon
Languages: Portuguese
Religions: Roman Catholic, Protestant
Currency: Euro
Main occupations: Finance, tourism, manufacturing, agriculture
Main exports: Clothes, shoes, wine, tomatoes, citrus fruit, cork, sardines, tungsten, copper, tin
Main imports: Oil

FISHING
Fishing has always been important in Portugal, and many fishing villages are located along its long Atlantic coast. Small fishing boats net large catches of tuna, anchovies, sardines, oysters and mackerel, which are then processed in coastal factories. Portugal has become a major exporter of tinned pilchards and sardines. The national Portuguese dish is *bacalháo*, dried, salted cod, which is caught by offshore Portuguese fleets in the Atlantic.

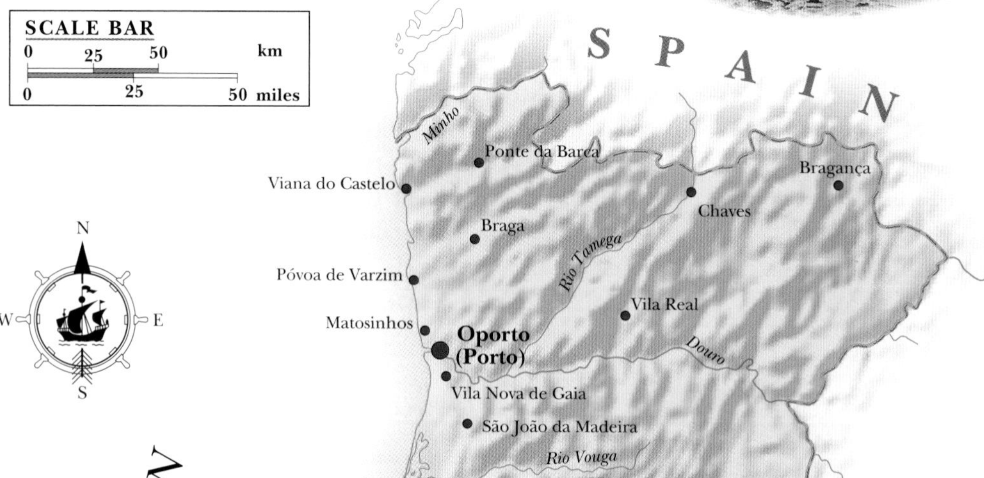

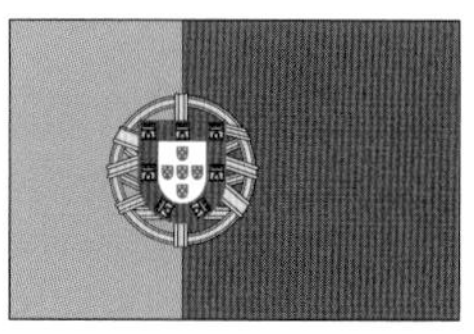

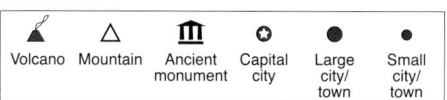

FARMING

On the whole, the land in Portugal is fertile and well-watered, although in the far south it is very arid. A wide range of crops are grown: wheat, rye, oats, barley, olives, figs, grapes and tomatoes. Goats and sheep are found throughout Portugal, and are well adapted to the arid south. Most farms are small, family-owned and use very traditional farming methods. In the Alentejo region in the south (below), some of the land is being successfully farmed by village cooperatives.

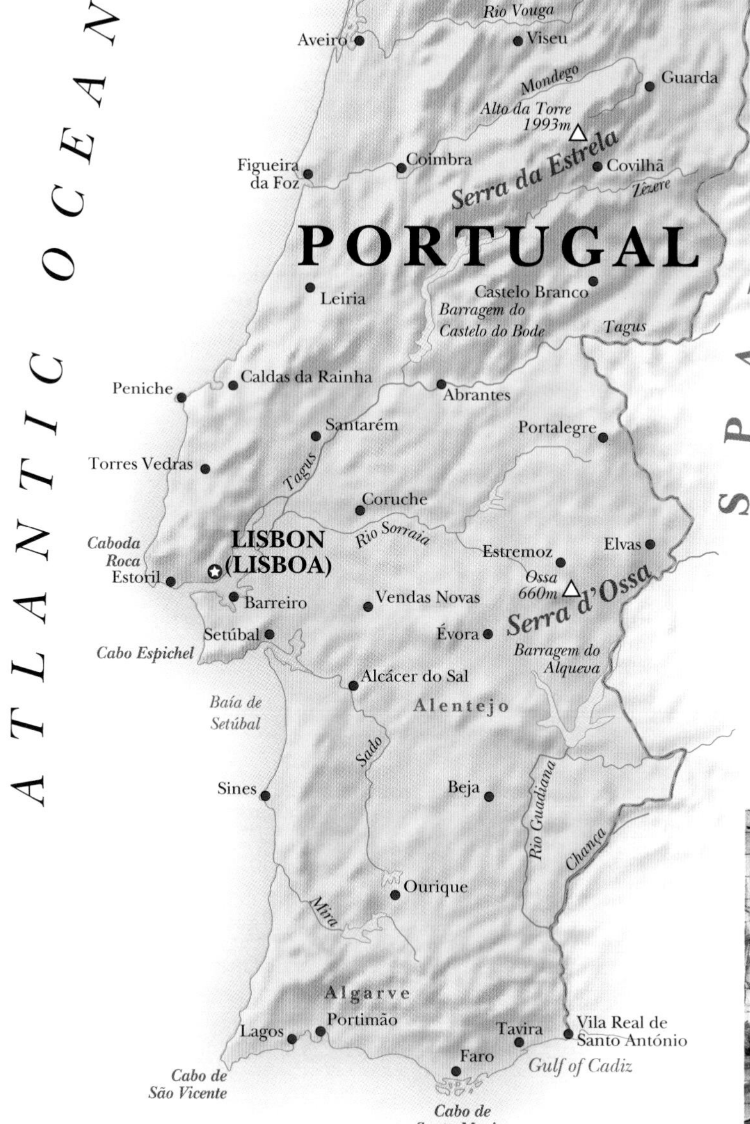

CERAMICS
This glazed, ceramic *azulejos* tile comes from the Minho in the north. These tiles, painted with pictorial scenes, have been used for centuries to decorate walls.

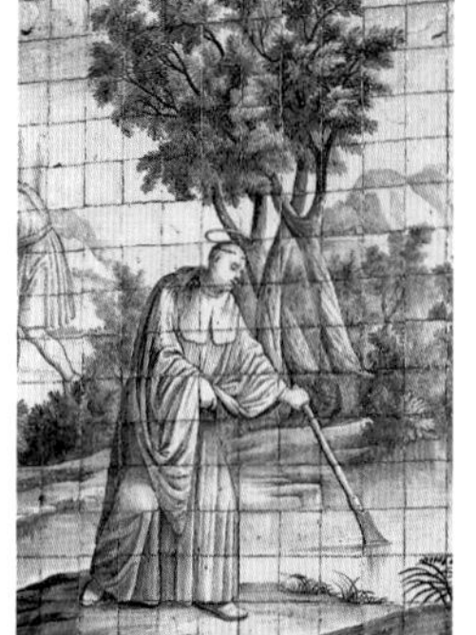

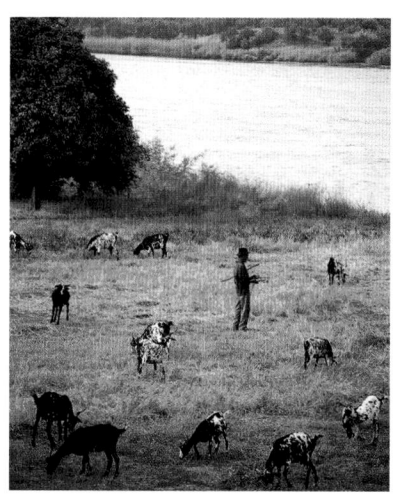

HISTORY OF PORTUGAL

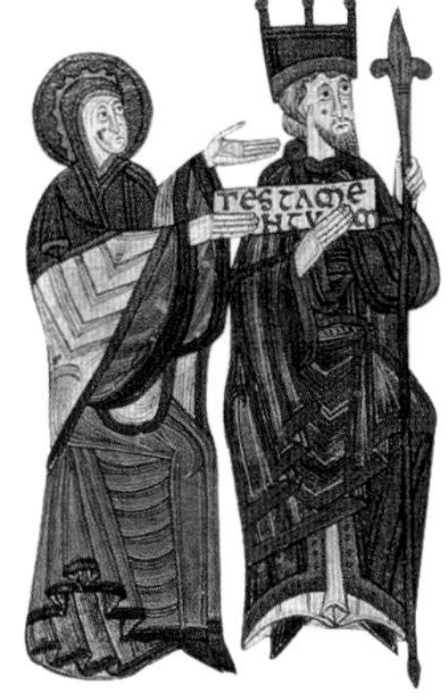

PART OF THE IBERIAN peninsula, Portugal only became a separate country in the 1100s. When the Romans colonized the area, they called it Lusitania. The Moors took over the region in the 700s, and Portugal thrived under their rule. In the 1400s, Portuguese explorers set up a great empire in competition with Spain, which occupied Portugal in the 16th century. In 1910, Portugal became a republic. Ruled by a dictatorship for some years, Portugal has been a democracy since 1974.

AFONSO III
Portugal emerged as an independent country in the 11th century, but the Moors still occupied the southern region. In 1248, Afonso III became king, and finally drove the Moors out of Portugal.

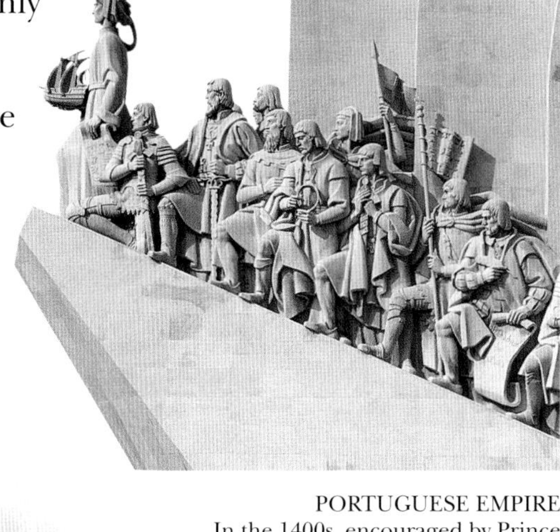

PORTUGUESE EMPIRE
In the 1400s, encouraged by Prince Henry the Navigator (son of John I, the King of Portugal), Portuguese navigators made long voyages of exploration around the world. In 1498, Vasco da Gama led four ships to Calicut in India, and two years later Pedro Álvares Cabral reached Brazil. Soon Portugal ruled a vast empire with lands in southern Asia, Africa, and Brazil.

REVOLT

In 1580, Philip II of Spain conquered Portugal. The Portuguese resented this, but were unable to rebel successfully until 1640, by which time Spain was greatly weakened by a war with France. John, Duke of Braganza, Portugal's greatest landowner, led the revolt against Spain. The Spaniards were driven out, and John was crowned John IV, first king of the House of Braganza, which ruled Portugal until the monarchy ended in 1910.

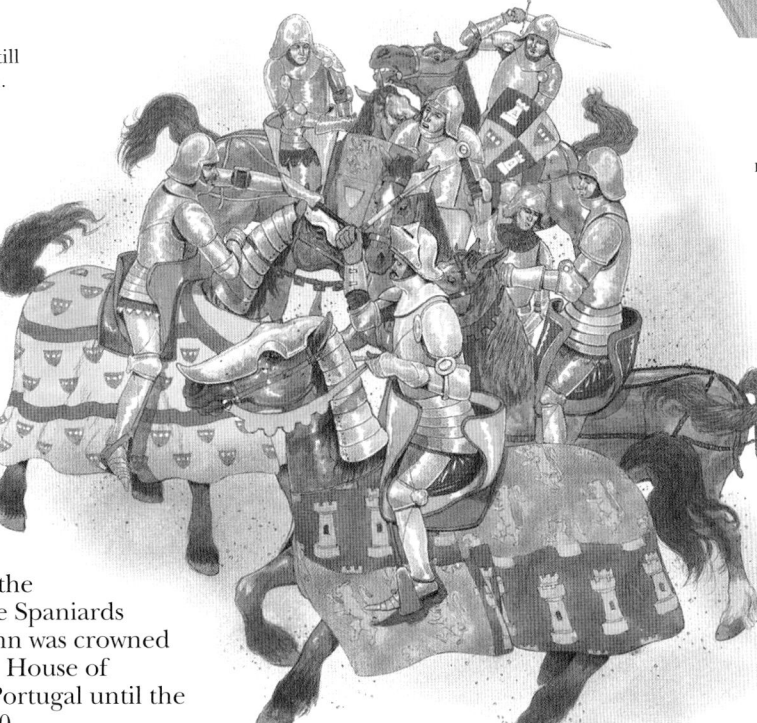

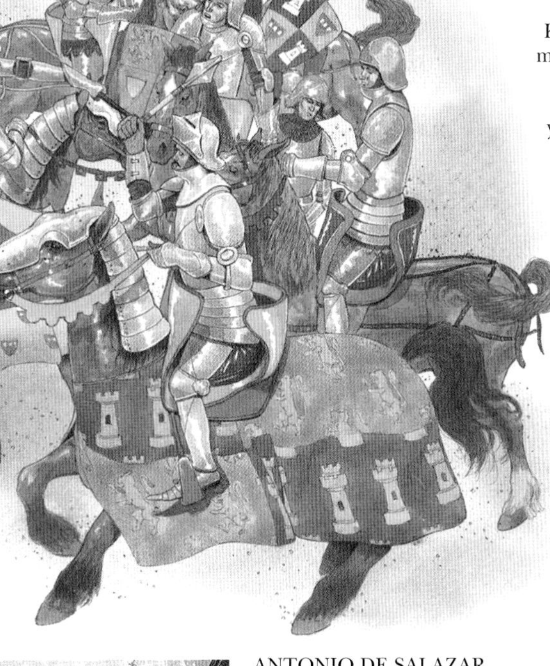

Battle scene during the Portuguese revolt

PORTUGAL

201 B.C. Romans colonize Iberian peninsula.

700s Moors (Muslims from North Africa) occupy Portugal.

1100s Christians drive out Moors; Portugal becomes a separate country from Spain.

1419 Portuguese begin exploring overseas.

1494 Treaty of Tordesillas: Spain and Portugal divide the world.

1500 Portugal claims Brazil

1580-1640 Spain rules Portugal.

1822 Portugal loses Brazil.

1910 Portugal becomes a republic.

1974 Military coup overthrows dictatorship.

1986 Portugal joins European Union.

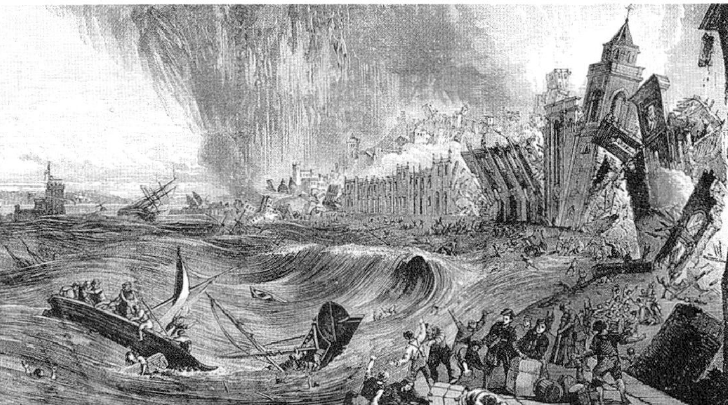

LISBON EARTHQUAKE

In 1755, a massive earthquake destroyed the low-lying part of Lisbon, Portugal's capital, killing more than 60,000 people. São Jorge Castle, once the home of Portuguese kings, survived because it was on a hill. The Marquis of Pombal, Portugal's prime minister (1756-77), had the city rebuilt.

ANTONIO DE SALAZAR
Portugal's prime minister from 1932, António de Oliviera Salazar ruled as a dictator until 1968, when he retired after a stroke. He was succeeded by Marcello Caetano. In 1974, a military coup overthrew the regime.

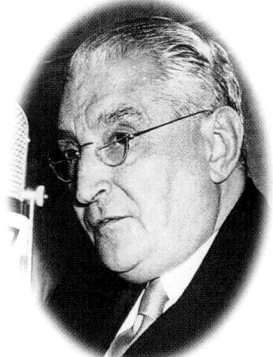

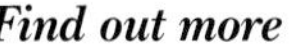

Find out more
DEMOCRACY
EARTHQUAKES
EXPLORERS
SPAIN, HISTORY OF

POTTERY

HEATING CLAY DUG FROM THE GROUND transforms it from oozing wet mud to the strong, hard, waterproof material that we call pottery. Pottery has many uses because its properties are so different from those of clay. The potter (pot maker) can easily mould the soft clay into a wide variety of shapes, from flat plates for eating, to deep jars for storage. Firing, or baking the pot, sets its shape forever. The potter's art is very old. The first potters worked in the Middle East 9,000 years ago. They made simple pressed pots and coiled pots as shown below left. And 3,500 years ago potters started to use small turntables, now called potter's wheels, to make their pots perfectly round. We know this because pottery does not decay in the ground as wood does. Archaeologists use pottery fragments to learn about the people who made the pots centuries ago.

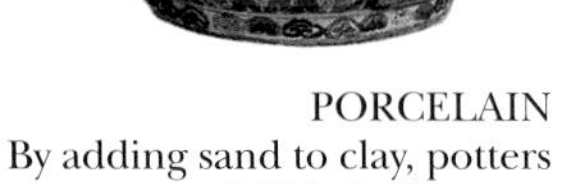

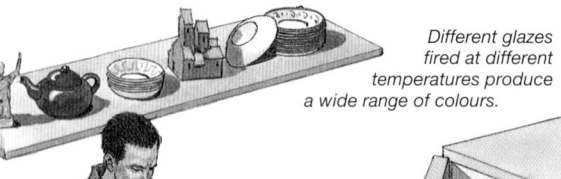

PORCELAIN
By adding sand to clay, potters create a special kind of pottery called porcelain. The sand turns to glass in firing, making the porcelain almost translucent. The Chinese invented porcelain more than 1,200 years ago, but their art remained a secret until the 18th century.

PRESSED POTS
A potter can make many identical pots by pressing clay into a plaster mould.

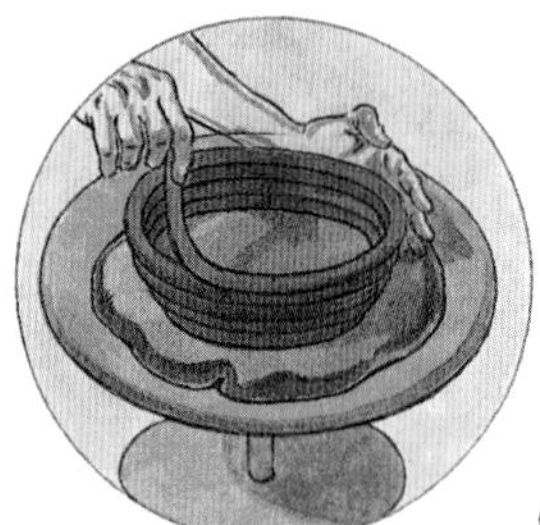

COILED POTS
Pots can be made without a wheel by coiling long, thin rolls of clay.

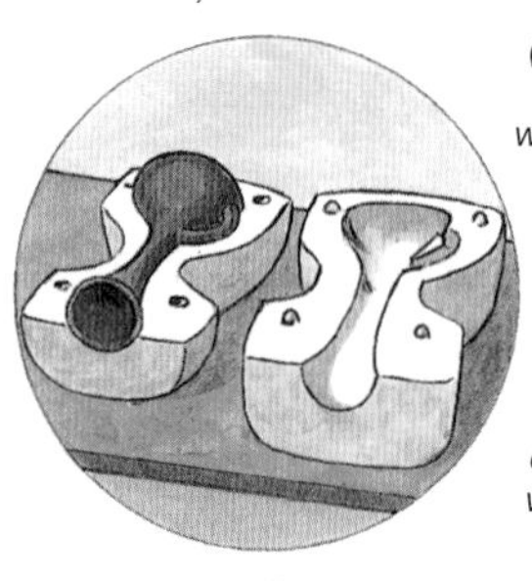

SLIP CASTING
Pouring liquid clay (slip) into the plaster mould of a pot coats the inside. When dry, the clay forms a perfect replica of the mould.

MAKING POTS

There are three main stages in making pots: shaping the clay, firing, and glazing. Potters use many different methods of shaping clay. To make perfectly circular objects, they "throw" the pot from a lump of clay on a revolving wheel. As the wheel spins, the potter uses both hands to draw the lump of clay upward and form the sides of the vessel.

FIRING
Pots must dry out after shaping. Then the potter stacks them carefully in the kiln – a big oven. Gas or electricity heats the kiln to more than 600°C (1,100°F) to turn the dry, brittle clay into rigid pottery. To make pots, the potter must control the temperature of the firing and how long it lasts.

Different glazes fired at different temperatures produce a wide range of colours.

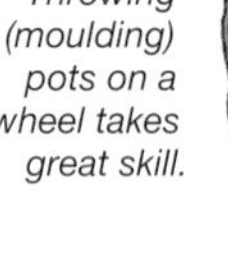

Throwing (moulding) pots on a wheel takes great skill.

Potters must keep their hands wet while they mould the clay.

The lump of clay must be centred on the wheel, or it will wobble out of control.

Dry pottery waiting to be fired.

Clay is stored in large bins, covered with plastic or wet cloth. This keeps the clay moist and easy to work.

The potter measures the firing temperature with a special thermometer or by placing small ceramic cones in the kiln. The cone melts when the temperature is high enough to fire the pots.

GLAZING
After the first firing, pottery is porous – water can still seep through it. Glazing the pottery completely seals its surface with a very hard, glasslike coating. Glaze is a mixture of metal oxides and minerals in water. The potter dips the pot into the glaze or pours the glaze on. The glaze dries, then the pot goes back into the kiln for a second firing. This melts the glaze and makes it stick to the pot.

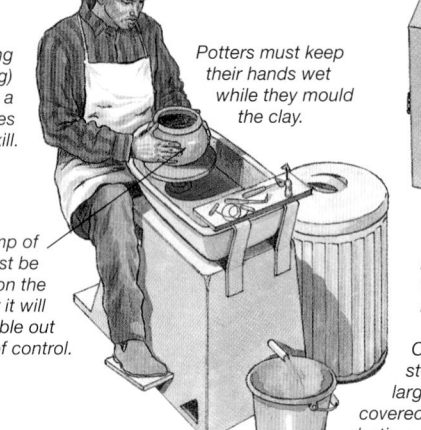

Glazing makes the pot more attractive and seals its surface.

Before glazing their pots, potters decorate them with slip, underglaze colours, or enamel.

TRADITIONAL POTTERY

Potters in every culture have shaped and decorated their pots in unique ways. Many made useful pots such as bowls and cooking vessels. But craft potters as far apart as South America and Korea also made objects for decoration and enjoyment, including beads and musical instruments.

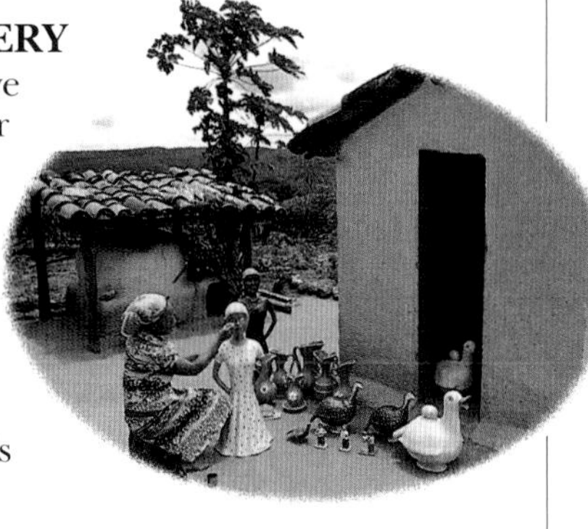

Find out more

CHINA, HISTORY OF
GLASS AND CERAMICS
ROCKS AND MINERALS

PREHISTORIC LIFE

WHEN PLANET EARTH FORMED more than 4,600 million years ago, there was no life. Torrential storms raged, lightning bolts flashed, volcanoes poured out poisonous gases, and there was no atmosphere to protect the Earth from the sun's radiation. Slowly, warm shallow seas formed. In these seas the first forms of life appeared, protected by the water. We call these early beginnings "prehistory" because they happened before written history. Fossils – the preserved remains of plants and animals – provide the only records of prehistoric life. We know from fossils more than 2,000 million years old that some of the earliest forms of life were bacteria. Gradually, plants called blue-green algae evolved, or developed. These produced oxygen – the gas that plants and animals need for life. Oxygen was released into the air from the sea and formed a protective blanket of ozone in the atmosphere. The ozone screened out the sun's radiation, and living things began to invade the land and take to the air. Millions of kinds of animals and plants have existed since the first signs of life – some, such as insects, have thrived; others, such as the dinosaurs, have died out as the Earth's environment has changed.

2,000 MILLION YEARS AGO
The earliest forms of life were bacteria and blue-green algae. The algae grew in rings or short columns called stromatolites, which are fossilized in rocks. Today, stromatolites still form in shallow tropical seas.

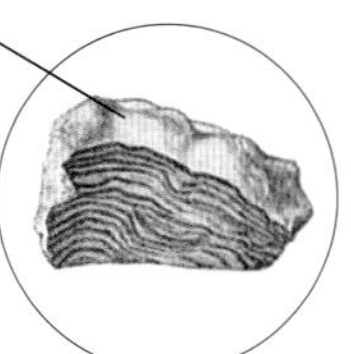

Some of the earliest remains of the life on Earth are fossils called stromatolites.

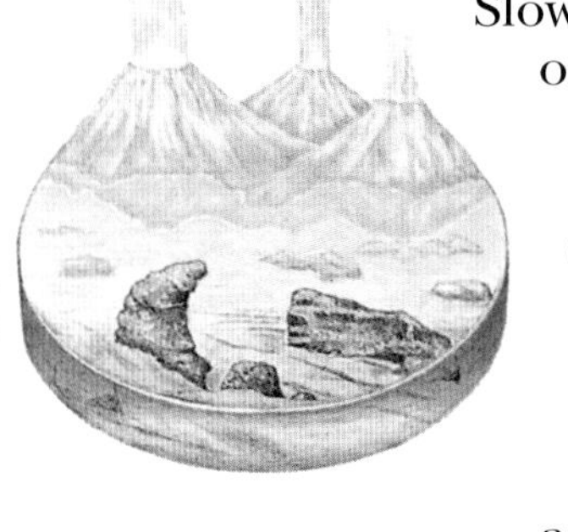

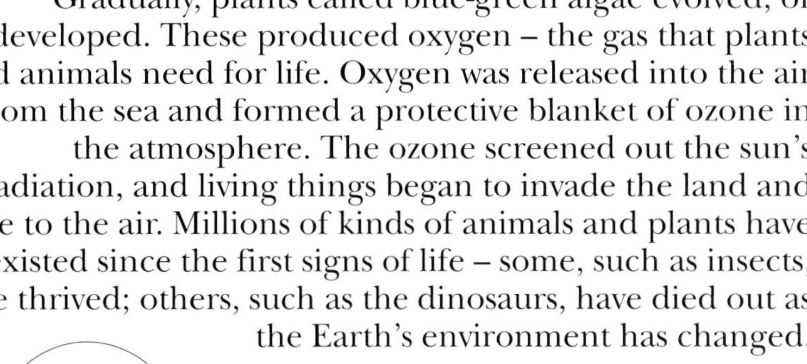

600 MILLION YEARS AGO
Rare fossils of soft-bodied creatures show us that many different animals had evolved by this time. They included the first kinds of jellyfish, corals, sea pens, and worms.

Sea pens existed 600 million years ago.

450 MILLION YEARS AGO
Fossils from this time are much more common, because animals had developed hard shells that preserved well. They include trilobites, nautiloids, sea urchins, and giant eurypterids, or sea scorpions, more than 2.5 m (8 ft) long.

Trilobites were common 450 million years ago. They are ancient relatives of crabs.

One of the first fishes, about 390 million years old

390 MILLION YEARS AGO
Fish were the first creatures with backbones. They evolved quickly into many different kinds. Gradually, they developed jaws and fins. The first small land plants, such as mosses, appeared on the swampy shores.

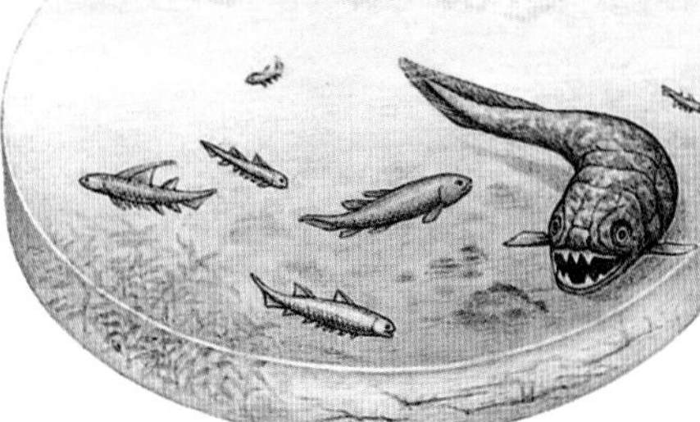

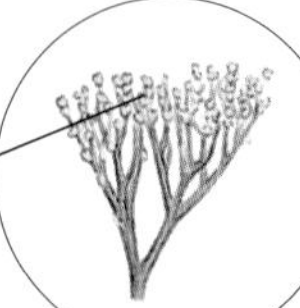

Cooksonia was one of the first land plants to appear on Earth.

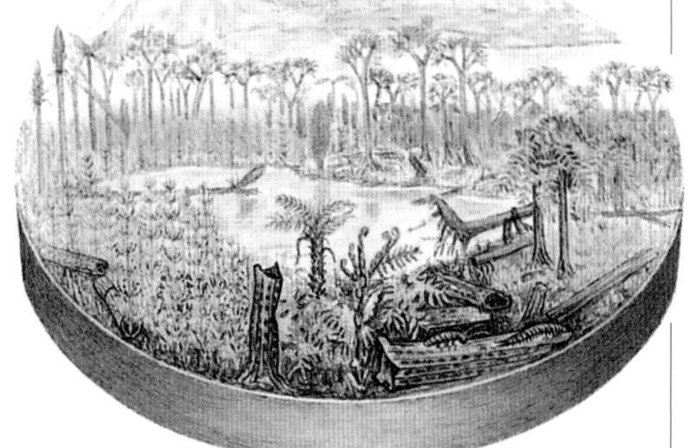

350 MILLION YEARS AGO
As plants became established on land, they were soon followed by the first land animals, such as millipedes and insects. Woody trees that looked like conifers stood more than 30 m (100 ft) high. Sharks and many other fish swam in the seas.

HOW WE KNOW THE AGE OF FOSSILS

Stages	*Million years ago (mya)*
Quaternary period	2 mya–today
Tertiary period	65–2 mya
Jurassic and Cretaceous periods	195–65
Triassic period	230–195
Carboniferous and Permian periods	345–230
Devonian period	395–345
Ordovician and Silurian periods	500–395
Cambrian period	570–500
Pre-cambrian period	4,000–570

Scientists called palaeontologists find out how old a fossil is from the age of the rocks around it. This is called relative dating. They also measure the amounts of radioactive chemicals in the rocks and fossils to find out when they formed. This is called absolute dating.

Prehistoric time is divided into different stages, called eras, which are further divided into periods. Each of these stages lasted for many millions of years. If you dig deep down into the Earth's surface, you can find fossils of animals and plants that lived during the different periods.

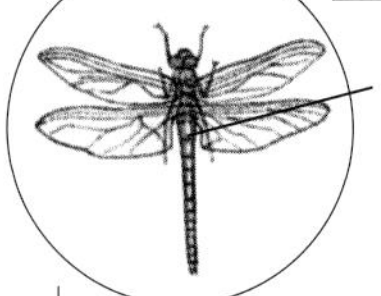

Insects such as the dragonfly evolved about 350 million years ago.

300 MILLION YEARS AGO
The first amphibians had crawled out from the water about 50 million years earlier. Gradually, they developed stronger limbs and thicker skins, so they could live on land. They still had to return to the water to lay their eggs. Giant ferns and horsetails grew in the warm swamps.

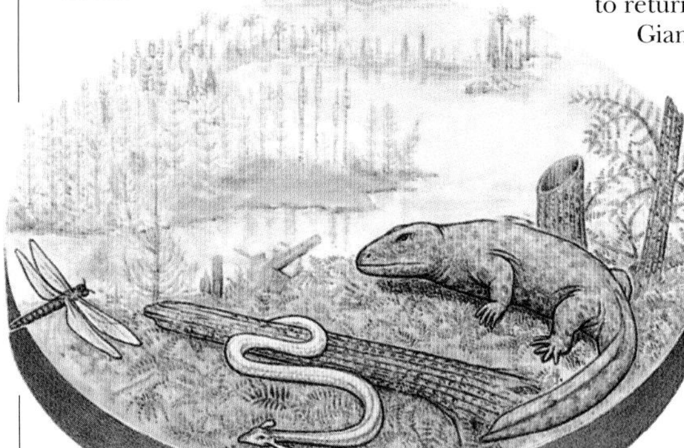

150 MILLION YEARS AGO
Dinosaurs ruled the land. Reptiles such as plesiosaurs ruled the seas, and other reptiles, the pterosaurs, flew in the air. There were also birds and mammals at this time. Ammonites were common in the seas.

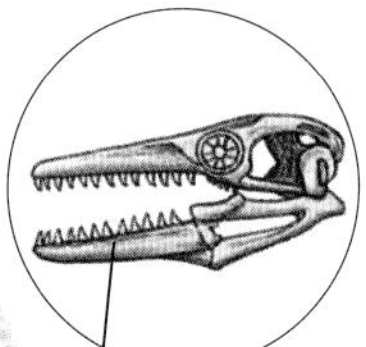

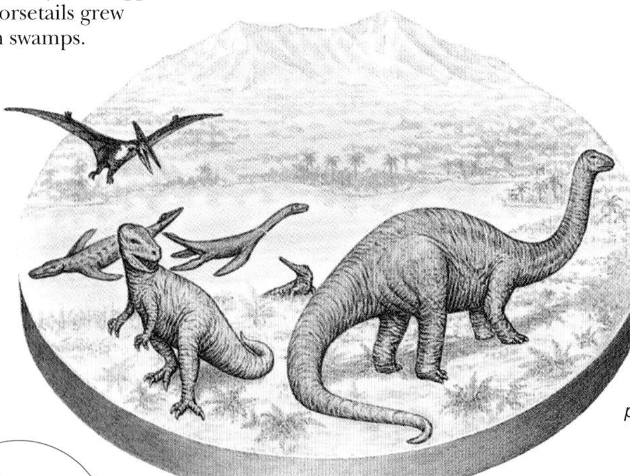

Mosasaur was one of the first sea reptiles. Its sharp teeth show that it was a meat eater, and it probably hunted fish.

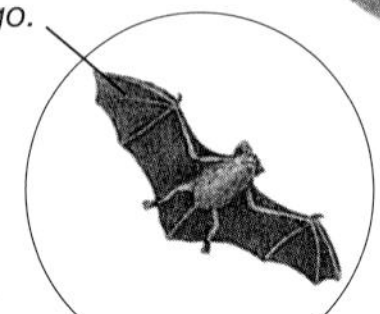

The first bats existed about 50 million years ago.

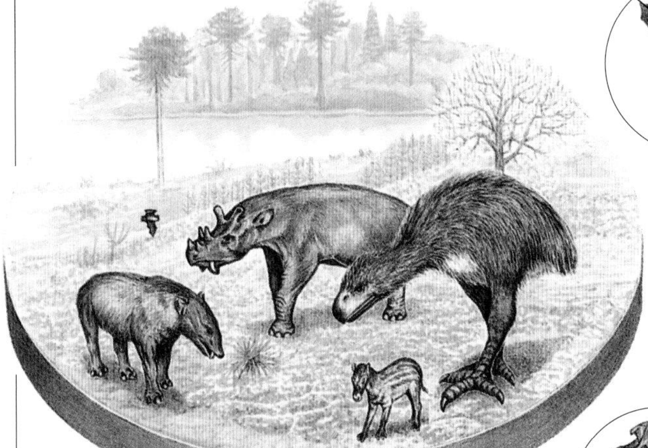

65 MILLION YEARS AGO
Trees with blossoms, such as the magnolia, began to appear on Earth more than 100 million years ago. Later, about 65 million years ago, dinosaurs and many other living things became extinct (died out). During the next few million years different kinds of mammals and birds became more common.

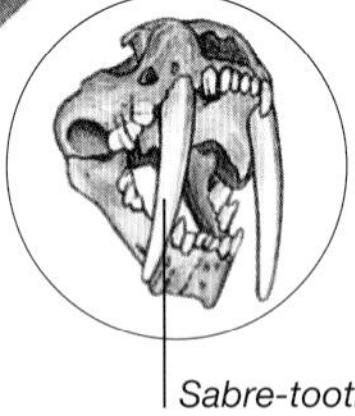

Sabre-toothed cats existed 19 to 2 million years ago. Their huge teeth enabled them to attack and kill large prey.

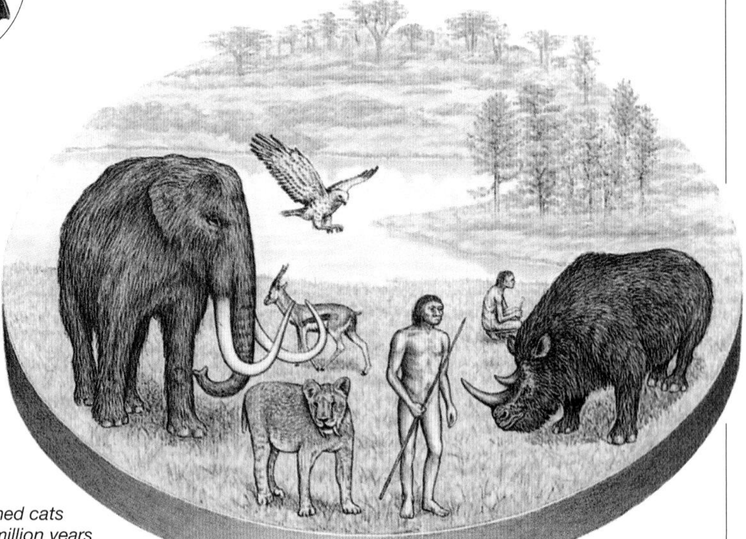

EXTINCTION

There is concern over the fact that many animals and plants are in danger of dying out, or becoming extinct. But ever since life began, animals and plants have died out, to be replaced by others. This process is part of nature. As the conditions on Earth change, some living things cannot adapt; they eventually become extinct. Scientists believe that 99 per cent of all the different plants and animals that ever lived have died out naturally. In prehistoric times there were mass extinctions when hundreds of different things died out together. These extinctions were often due to dramatic changes in climate. About 225 million years ago, 90 per cent of all the living things in the sea died out. Today, animals and plants are dying out more quickly because humans damage and destroy the areas where they live.

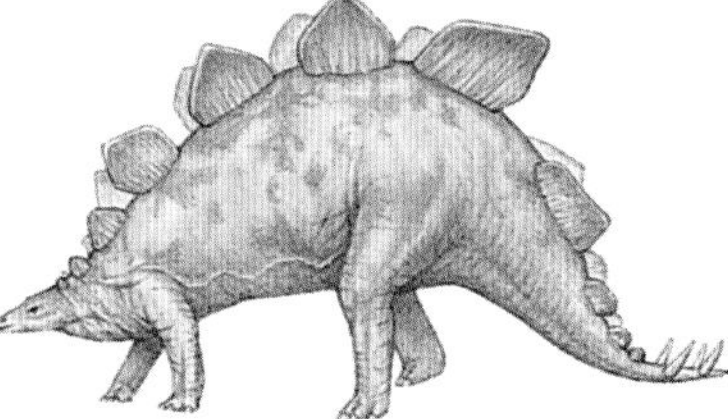

STEGOSAURUS
This dinosaur lived about 150 million years ago in North America. It became extinct about 140 million years ago.

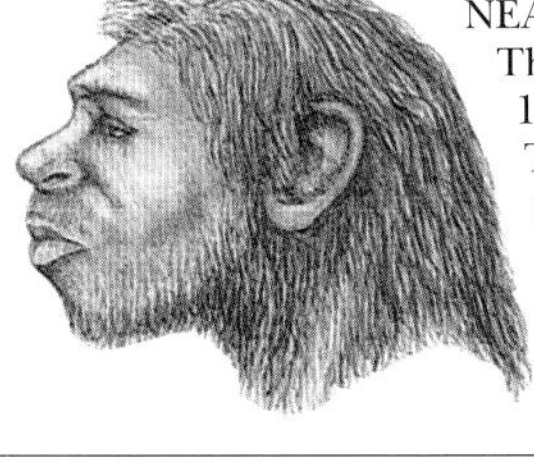

NEANDERTHAL PEOPLE
These people lived from about 120,000–35,000 years ago. They were the immediate, and smaller, predecessors of *Homo sapiens* (modern humans). As humans evolved (developed), these people died out.

GREAT ICE AGE

About 2 million years ago, several ice ages gripped the Earth, with warmer stretches between. Humans evolved – probably in Africa – and spread around the world. In the north, they hunted woolly mammoths, woolly rhinos, and sabre-toothed cats. About 18,000 years ago, ice sheets covered much of northern Europe, northern Britain, and North America.

Find out more
COAL
DINOSAURS
EVOLUTION
FOSSILS
PREHISTORIC PEOPLES

PREHISTORIC PEOPLES

PREHISTORIC PEOPLES

c. 7,000,000 B.C. Apes and hominids begin to evolve in different ways.

c. 2,500,000 B.C. First stone tools made. Palaeolithic (Old Stone) Age begins.

c. 1,500,000 B.C. *Homo erectus* appears.

c. 125,000 B.C. First Neanderthals (an early form of *Homo sapiens* – "wise man") develop.

c. 50,000 B.C. First modern people, *Homo sapiens*, develop.

c. 8,000 B.C. Neolithic (New Stone) Age begins.

c. 7,000 B.C. Farming villages and pottery.

c. 3,500 B.C. Sumerians in Mesopotamia develop writing. Sumerians begin to live in cities.

c. 3,000 B.C. Metal tools and weapons begin to replace stone.

COMPARED WITH the rest of life on Earth, human beings arrived quite recently, after the dinosaur age and the age of mammals. The whole story of human evolution is incomplete, because many parts of the fossil record have never been found. Human-like mammals first emerged from the ape family about five million years ago in central Africa. They came down from the trees and began to walk on two legs. Hominids, or early humans, were more apelike than human and lived in the open. Over millions of years they learned to walk upright and developed bigger brains. These large brains helped them to develop language and the ability to work together. Hominids lived in groups and shared work and food, wandering through the countryside gathering fruits, roots, nuts, berries, and seeds, and hunting animals. Standing upright left their hands free to make tools and weapons, shelters and fire. They lived in caves and in shelters made from branches and stones. These early humans spread slowly over the rest of the world and soon rose to dominate life on Earth.

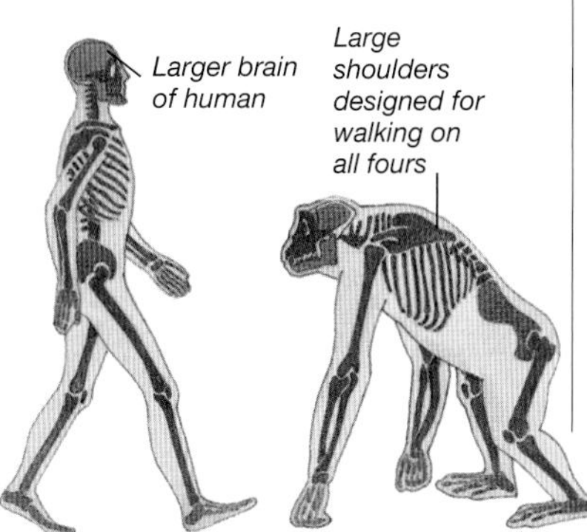

HUMAN OR APE?
Humans have smaller jaws and larger brains than apes. The human hand has a longer thumb; apes have longer fingers. The human pelvis and thigh allow upright motion, giving the spine an S-shaped curve. Human legs are longer than arms; apes have the reverse. Unlike apes, humans cannot use their big toes as extra thumbs; the foot has adapted to walking and can no longer grasp.

WISDOM TOOTH
Early people needed wisdom teeth in order to eat roots and berries. Today, we no longer need wisdom teeth, and many people do not even develop them.

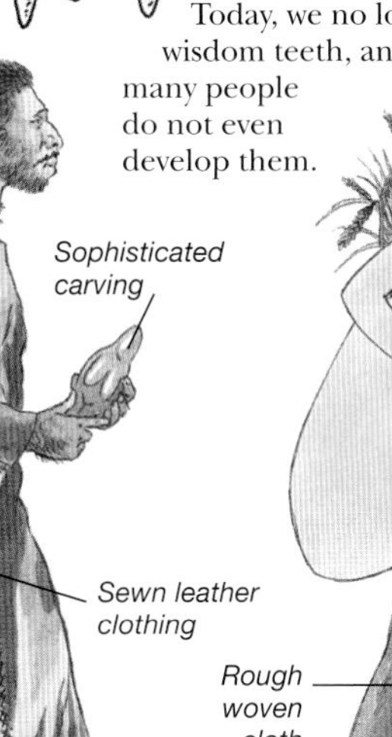

Lucy's remains were found at Hadar.

Lucy gathered fruit to eat.

Fossil remains of the earliest hominids have all been found in East Africa.

Simple stone tool

Homo habilis

Homo erectus made more advanced tools, such as this spear.

Simple clothing

Homo erectus

Sophisticated carving

Sewn leather clothing

Neanderthal man

Rough woven cloth

Modern people wear shoes.

LUCY
In 1974, archaeologists discovered a complete fossil hominid skeleton in Ethiopia, northeastern Africa. She was nicknamed Lucy, after the Beatles' song *Lucy in the Sky with Diamonds.* Lucy was 3 million years old. Although nearly human, she was probably not one of our direct ancestors.

When alive, Lucy was about the same height as a 10-year-old girl, and weighed 30 kg (66 lb).

FROM HOMINIDS TO HUMANS

About 2.5 million years ago hominids called *Homo habilis* (meaning "handy man") shaped crude stone tools and built rough shelters. Other, more advanced hominids, called *Homo erectus*, moved out of Africa into Europe and Asia. They lived in camps, made use of fire, and probably had a language. After the Ice Age, Neanderthals lived in Europe. Neanderthals looked much like people today, wore clothes, made flint tools and fire, and buried their dead. They vanished about 30,000 years ago and were replaced by "modern people", who invented farming about 9,000 years ago and began to settle down in communities. Shortly after, the first civilizations began.

MODERN PEOPLE
When humans learned to domesticate animals and grow crops, they stopped wandering and settled down on farms. Thus towns began to develop.

Find out more
ARCHAEOLOGY
BRONZE AGE
EVOLUTION
PREHISTORIC LIFE
STONE AGE

PRINTING

HAVE YOU EVER THOUGHT about how many times you look at print each day? Printed words and pictures have found their way into almost every part of our lives: on advertisements, road signs, food labels, records, clothes, newspapers, and, of course, in books such as this. Today, we take this information for granted, but before the invention of printing, all information had to be laboriously written by hand, and only a few people had access to education. The introduction of printing caused a revolution. Printing means that numerous identical copies of words and pictures can be made quickly and cheaply. Printing presses use a mirror image of the original to apply ink to paper, cardboard, and other materials. In the old days, printers used to set type (form words) in "hot" metal. They put pages together from metal blocks, each one of which printed either a single letter or a single line of text. Nowadays, entire complex pages like this one can be printed from sheets of transparent film or from digital text-and-image files created on a computer.

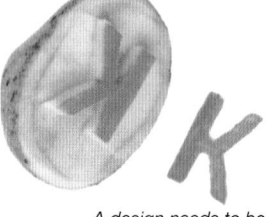

A design needs to be engraved in reverse (as a mirror image) to print the right way.

1 TYPESETTING
To set the type for a book, the words are typed into a computer. The computer sends signals to a machine containing a laser that prints the words onto a plastic, light-sensitive film, called the type film.

2 COLOUR SEPARATION
All the colours and illustrations in a book are reproduced with just four coloured inks; each is printed with a plate made from a separate film. To make the separate films (called colour separations), all the pictures are laid on a spinning drum. A laser scans over the pictures four times – once for each separation.

Original picture containing all colours

Yellow colour separation

Cyan colour separation

Magenta colour separation

Black colour separation

3 PRINTING PRESS
The printing plates are made photographically, by shining light through the type and colour films so that the details are recorded by the plate's light-sensitive coating. Each of the plates is treated with chemicals to bring out the print image, then fitted onto rollers in the printing press. There are four plates altogether, one for each of the coloured inks. As the paper runs through the press, it passes over each of the four inked plates in turn. These plates add the four colours one by one. Separate rollers run over the plates and keep them wet with fresh ink. The paper emerges at the far end as printed pages in full colour.

Adding yellow ink

Adding cyan ink

Adding magenta ink

Adding black ink

Page printed with yellow ink only.

Final printed page built up from yellow, cyan, magenta, and black inks.

After the paper is printed on one side, it is fed back through the press for printing on the other side.

FOUR-COLOUR PRINTING
All the colours you see on this page are made up of dots printed with just four different coloured inks: yellow, cyan (green-blue), magenta (blue-red), and black. More colours are sometimes used for high-quality prints, but this costs more, since most printing presses are set up to print in four colours only.

THE HISTORY OF PRINTING

In A.D. 868, the Chinese were printing books using carved wooden blocks. In about 1440, Johannes Gutenberg of Germany developed movable type, in which separate pieces of type print each letter on a handpress (right). This process remained in use for 350 years until the invention of power-driven presses which allowed books to be printed more easily.

Gutenberg and his press

Find out more
BOOKS
COLOUR
NEWSPAPERS
PAPER

PUPPETS

THE PUPPET SHOW is one of the oldest forms of theatre, and each age has produced new traditions. In Africa, China, and India puppets were used in early times to dramatize legends and religious stories. In the 18th century the Bunraku puppets of Japan acted out dramatic stories to the words of a narrator with the puppeteers in full view. Punch and Judy in England and Petrushka in Russia are puppets that grew out of the characters of Italian comedy of the 16th to 18th centuries. There are many different ways to work a puppet. It takes just one hand to work simple finger puppets, but some complicated Japanese puppets require three operators. Puppets sometimes comment on what is going on in the real world and can be quite mischievous. Modern puppeteers such as the late Jim Henson, the creator of the Muppets, have replaced the strings and rods of traditional puppets with electronic mechanisms.

MARIONETTES
String puppets, or marionettes, require two hands and great skill. The operator controls the puppet by moving a wooden bar to which the strings are attached. Some strings are linked to synchronize movements; for example, raising one leg lowers the other.

FINGER PUPPETS

Making a finger puppet is simple – and operating one is just as easy. With a little practice, you can stage a whole puppet play using just the fingers of both hands.

Several operators are needed to control the body puppet.

A television set shows the operator what the viewer sees.

The puppet's eyes can open and close.

So that the mouth can move, it is attached to the frame by hinges.

The person inside the puppet can hear directions from the operator.

The puppet is moved by a cable link to the operator.

BODY PUPPETS

Life-size puppets are a real team effort. The person inside the suit manoeuvres the limbs while other operators control the face. The puppet is made from foam rubber over a rigid frame, so it is very light and easy to move.

SHADOW PUPPETS
In this ancient form of puppetry the operator holds the puppet close to a screen. The light behind casts a shadow which the audience can see from the other side of the screen. Javanese puppets such as this one can be more than 1 m (3 ft) tall. The arms are moved by rods held from below. These puppets are traditionally made from buffalo hide and are brightly coloured in golds, reds, and blues.

The television camera films only the puppet; Jim Henson (centre) and the other operators below remain hidden.

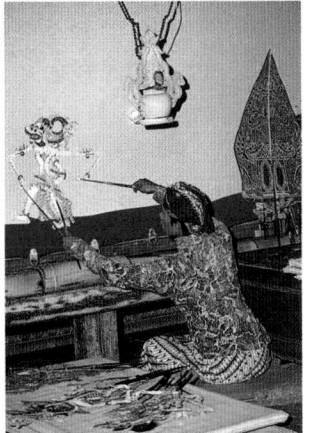

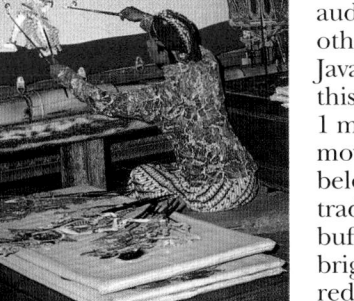

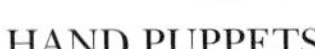

HAND PUPPETS
Glove puppets are very simple to operate. A hand inside makes the puppet move, with the index finger supporting and turning the head. The arms of these Muppets are moved by a combination of glove and rod techniques.

Find out more
THEATRE

PUZZLES

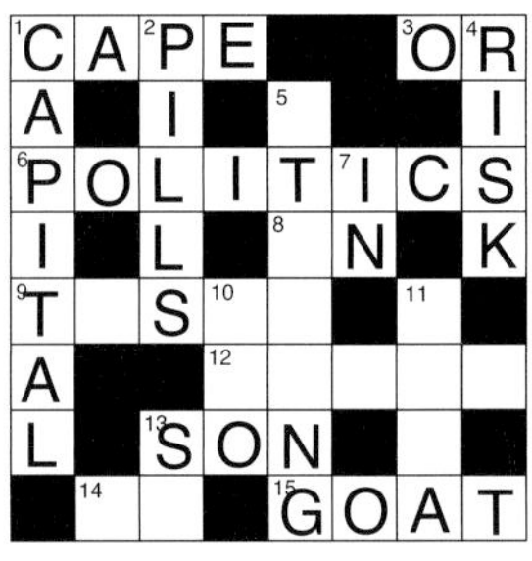

CROSSWORD PUZZLES
Crosswords are word puzzles. You must solve two sets of numbered clues correctly to fill in the blanks that fit across and down the grid.

ANYTHING THAT CONFUSES THE BRAIN until a solution can be found may be called a puzzle. The human brain is good at solving puzzles. Some scientists believe that the human race developed so successfully because of people's curiosity and ability to understand and solve problems. Nowadays, survival does not depend so much on problem-solving, and most puzzles are made for amusement. They can take many forms, from verbal and visual puzzles, such as crosswords and jigsaw puzzles, to three-dimensional puzzles, such as mazes, Rubik's cubes, and virtual reality games. Some puzzles, such as riddles or brain teasers, require a lot of thought to solve. When we read a crime novel or watch a suspense film, we are also solving puzzles, following clues to find out who did it. Mysteries in the real world are also called puzzles. Most are eventually solved by science, but some, such as the puzzle of the Bermuda Triangle, have still to be explained.

JIGSAW PUZZLES

These puzzles are named after the jigsaw, the tool once used to make the puzzles by cutting out the pieces from sheets of wood. Most "jigsaw puzzles" today are punched out of cardboard, using tools called cutting dies. Jigsaws may be simple or very difficult, have as few as four or as many as 10,000 pieces, and can be made to suit any age. Jigsaws are visual puzzles. Putting them together teaches patience and concentration.

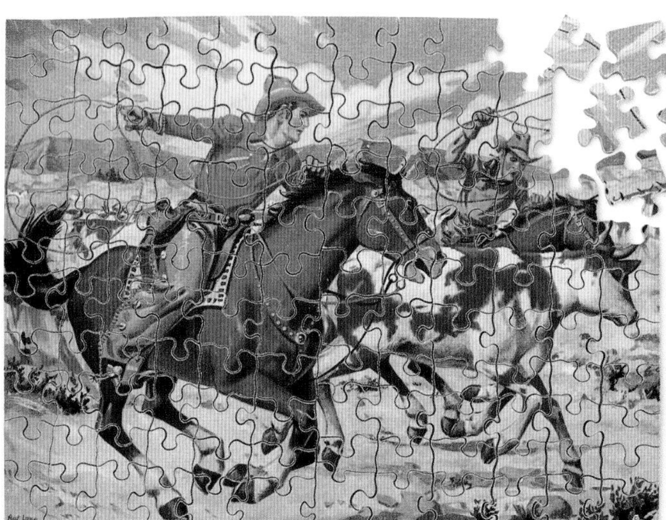

A viewing device allows the game player to see a three-dimensional picture.

A world of virtual reality as seen by the game player.

MAZES

The misleading pathways of maze puzzles test your sense of direction and ability to think logically, while in a confusing situation. The aim is to reach the centre of the maze, and then to try to make your way out again. In Ancient Egypt and Greece, mazes were built as prisons, but modern mazes are for fun.

COMPUTER GAMES
In many computer games, players follow puzzling quests or solve clues to move on to the next stage. Virtual reality games challenge players to solve puzzles outside the real world.

BRAIN ACTIVITY

Most of us enjoy the challenge of a puzzle because of the way our brains work. Human intelligence makes us curious, so we become determined to find the solution to the puzzle. The stimulation of tackling and solving a puzzle makes our brains release chemicals called endorphins, which make us feel pleased or happy.

The midbrain is used to process language.

The cerebrum controls reasoning and judgement.

The medulla oblongata controls our metabolism.

The cerebellum controls our muscular reflexes.

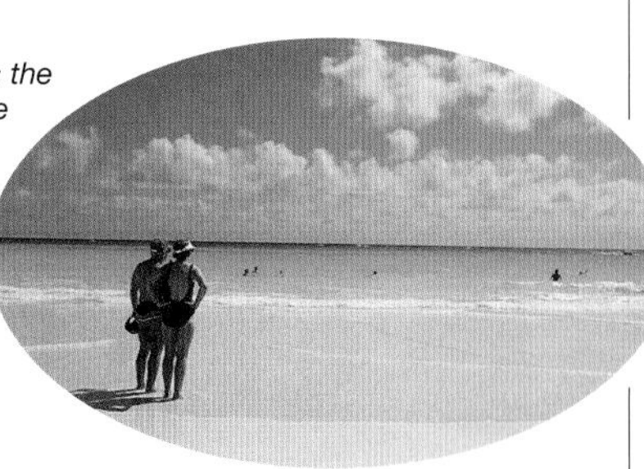

Looking out towards the Bermuda Triangle

BERMUDA TRIANGLE
An unusually high number of aircraft and ships are mysteriously lost in a triangular area between Bermuda, Florida, and Puerto Rico in the Atlantic Ocean. The "Bermuda Triangle" was first described in 1964. The area is particularly busy and prone to dramatic weather changes, so ships and planes that disappeared could have crashed or been sunk. So far no-one has come up with a satisfactory explanation.

Find out more
ATLANTIC OCEAN
BRAIN AND NERVES
COMPUTERS
GAMES

RABBITS AND HARES

ONE FEMALE wild rabbit produces more than 20 young each year, making the common rabbit one of the most numerous mammals. Originally from Europe, rabbits are now found in every region except Antarctica. In many places they are serious pests to farmers because they eat crops, but in recent years a disease called myxomatosis has reduced their numbers. The common rabbit belongs to a large group of animals called lagomorphs. They include hares, cottontails, and a small, furry creature called the pika. Rabbits and hares are fast, agile runners. They can walk but usually hop at great speeds. Rabbits and hares have sensitive whiskers and sharp senses. They also have long rodent-like front teeth to gnaw grass, roots, and leaves. Rabbits and hares have an unusual method of double digestion. They eat food, digest some of it, expel soft droppings, and then eat these to obtain more nutrients. Finally they leave small, hard pellets on the ground. Rabbits build burrows; hares live in open country. Young hares are born covered in fur with their eyes open; newborn rabbits are bald at first, and their eyes are closed.

Small white tail is used as a danger signal to other rabbits.

Large ears swivel to find direction of a sound.

Whiskers help rabbit find its way in tunnels and at night.

Body is about 40 cm (16 in) long.

Eyes stick out for all-round vision.

COMMON RABBIT

Most common rabbits usually stay within 140 m (450 ft) of their warren. Although rabbits usually feed at twilight and at night, they sometimes come above ground by day. Rabbits nibble grasses and other plants, cropping them close to the ground. Each rabbit spends much time grooming its coat with its claws, tongue, and teeth to remove dirt and the fleas that may carry the disease called myxomatosis.

PIKA

The pika, found in Asia and North America, is much smaller than its relative, the rabbit. In summer it breaks off stems of grass, leaves them to dry in the sun, then piles the dried grass into tiny haystacks. The pika uses the dried grass as a food store during the winter months.

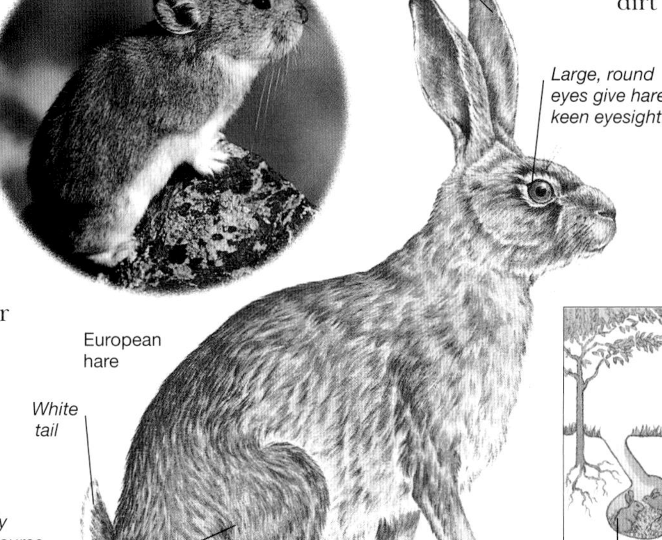
Long ears and excellent hearing
Large, round eyes give hare keen eyesight.
European hare
White tail
Body measures more than 50 cm (20 in) in length.
Hare has long, slim front legs.
Long, powerful back legs

WARREN

The warren is a system of tunnels dug among tree roots or in a bank or sand dune. It is home to about 10 adult rabbits and their young. Other smaller burrows in the rabbits' territory are used in emergencies. A doe (female rabbit) often raises her kits (young) in a separate tunnel called a stop.

Rabbit warren has many entrances and escape routes.

Female and young live in a stop.

Some tunnels are dead ends.

HARE

Hares are larger and longer than rabbits, with longer hind legs and ears. Male hares are called jacks, and females are called jills. The jill gives birth to two or three young, called leverets. While the mother is away feeding, the young crouch in a shallow scoop in the grass called a form. The young are well camouflaged – as long as they keep perfectly still.

JACK RABBIT

Despite its name, the North American jack rabbit is actually a hare. Jack rabbits are speedy animals; some can run at more than 80 km/h (50 mph), outpacing many other creatures. In hot deserts jack rabbits lose excess heat through their huge ears. The black-tailed jack rabbit causes much damage by eating crops in the western part of North America.

Find out more

ANIMALS
CAMOUFLAGE, ANIMAL
MAMMALS
NESTS AND BURROWS
WEASELS, STOATS, and martens

RADAR

FROM HUNDREDS OF KILOMETRES AWAY, a radar operator can track the movements of ships and aircraft even in dark or cloudy conditions. Radar finds objects by bouncing high-frequency radio waves off them and detecting the reflected waves. Radar is an extremely valuable tool. It helps aircraft find their way safely through crowded skies, warns weather forecasters of approaching storms, and reduces the risk of collisions at sea. Astronomers use radar to study the planets, while armies, air forces, and navies use radar for aiming missiles and locating opposing forces.

In the 1930s, a group of British scientists headed by Sir Robert Watson-Watt (1892-1973) developed an early radar system. During World War II (1939-45), this system gave early warning of bombing attacks, which allowed defending aircraft time to take to the air.

Radar in aircraft's nose detects bad weather.

When transponder detects radar pulses, it beams out its return pulse.

Plane reflects radar pulses back to antenna.

Secondary radar system picks up pulses from the aircraft's transponder.

Pulses from secondary radar scanner

Pulses from primary radar scanner

Radar antenna spins slowly to scan for aircraft in all directions.

RADAR
The word radar stands for "radio detecting and ranging".

RADAR SYSTEMS
There are two main types of radar systems: primary radar, which detects a radar "echo", and secondary radar, which detects a pulse transmitted by the target. Secondary radar is important for air traffic control. Airliners carry a transponder, a device which sends out a signal whenever a pulse from an air traffic control radar system strikes the plane. The transponder signal carries information such as the aircraft's identity, height, and speed.

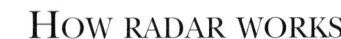

HOW RADAR WORKS

A radar antenna sends out short bursts, or pulses, of radio waves. Between pulses the antenna listens for a return signal which has bounced off the target plane or ship. The direction in which the antenna is pointing gives the direction of the target. The delay between the transmitted pulse and the return pulse shows the distance of the target.

Ship's radar

Radar image of coastline

Yellow line indicates direction of ship's travel.

RADAR SCREEN
A radar screen inside a ship or aircraft displays a computer-generated map of the nearby land and sea. A central dot indicates the position of the ship or plane; other craft are represented by symbols on the screen.

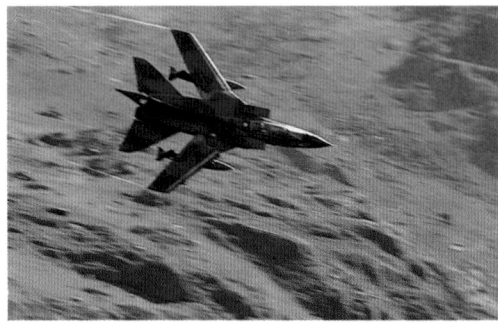

MILITARY RADAR
Long-range ground-based radar scans the skies for intercontinental missiles; radar on high-altitude planes searches for low-flying aircraft approaching beneath the long-range beams. High-speed fighter aircraft have some of the most advanced radar systems. The radar scans the ground ahead so that the plane can fly rapidly just above the treetops and attack an enemy without warning.

Radio waves from speed trap

Radio waves bounce back off speeding car.

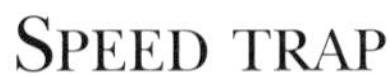

SPEED TRAP

Police officers use radar to measure the speed of passing cars. A radar scanner sends out a beam of radio waves which bounce off an approaching car. The car's forward movement squeezes up the waves, so the reflected signal has a fractionally shorter wavelength than the original signal. The radar set measures the change in wavelength and calculates the car's speed.

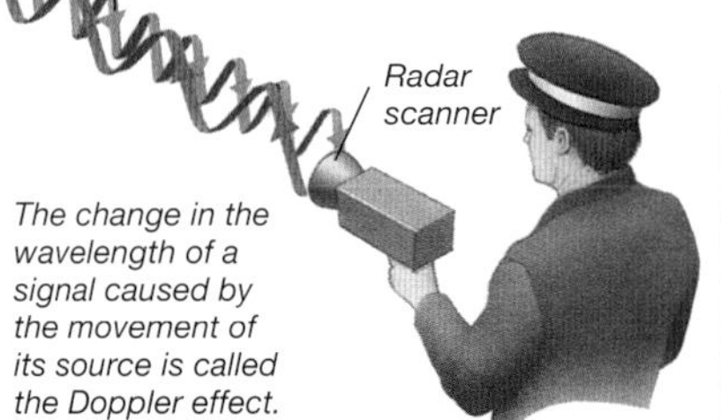

Radar scanner

The change in the wavelength of a signal caused by the movement of its source is called the Doppler effect.

Find out more

AIRCRAFT
AIRPORTS
MILITARY AIRCRAFT
NAVIGATION
RADIO

RADIO

EARLY RADIO WAS often called "the wireless" because radio uses invisible waves instead of wires to carry messages from one place to another. Today, radio waves are an important means of communicating sounds and pictures all over the world. Within the circuits of a radio transmitter, rapidly varying electric currents generate radio waves of different lengths that travel to a radio receiver. Radio waves are a type of electromagnetic (EM) wave, similar to light and x-rays. Like these waves, radio waves travel at the speed of light, 300,000 km (186,000 miles) per second, nearly one million times the speed of sound waves. Radio waves can travel through the air, solid materials, or even empty space, but are sent most efficiently by putting the transmitting antenna on high ground like a hill.

MORSE CODE
Early radio signals consisted of beeps, made by tapping a key. Operators tapped out a message using a series of short and long beeps called Morse code, invented by Samuel Morse (1791-1872) in 1837.

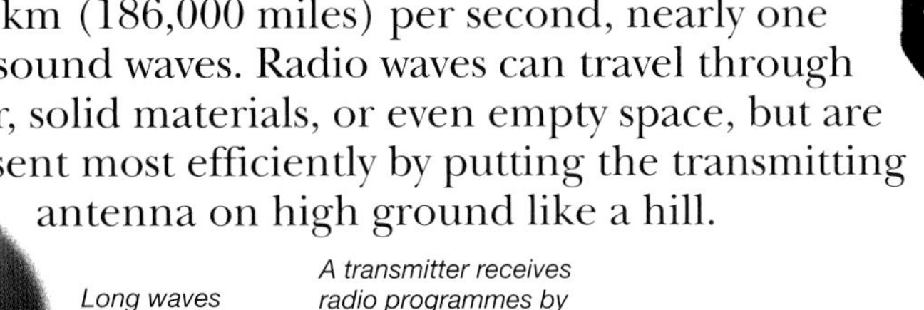

RADIO STUDIO
A microphone converts sound waves from the announcer's voice into electrical signals, which are then transmitted as radio waves.

Long waves (30-300 kHz) can travel 1,000 km (about 600 miles). They are used for national broadcasts and to send information to ships.

A transmitter receives radio programmes by cable from the studio. The transmitter antenna beams radio waves that spread out like ripples in water.

Communications satellites pick up and rebroadcast radio programmes using super-high-frequency waves with frequencies of more than 3 million kHz.

Television programmes are carried on UHF (ultra-high-frequency) radio waves (300,000-3,000,000 kHz).

Dish sends and receives radio waves

VHF (very-high-frequency) radio waves (30,000-300,000 kHz) move in straight lines so they cannot travel over the horizon. Police, fire brigade, and citizens' band radios use VHF waves for short-range communications.

Many radio stations transmit programmes on the medium-wave band. These medium-frequency (300-3,000 kHz) channels are restricted to within a few hundred kilometres.

International radio stations and amateur radio enthusiasts use short-wave radio signals. Short waves (3,000-30,000 kHz) can travel great distances. They bounce around the world, reflected off the Earth's surface and a layer of the atmosphere called the ionosphere.

RADIO FREQUENCIES
Radio waves consist of rapidly oscillating (varying) electric and magnetic fields. The rate of oscillation is called the frequency of the wave, measured in hertz (Hz). One Hz equals one oscillation per second; one kilohertz (kHz) equals 1,000 hertz. Bands of certain frequencies are used to transmit different kinds of information.

RADIO RECEIVER
When radio waves reach the antenna of a radio set, they produce tiny varying electric currents in the antenna. As the tuner knob is turned, an electronic circuit selects a single frequency from these currents corresponding to a particular radio channel. This signal is amplified (boosted) to drive the loudspeaker, which then converts the signal into sound waves.

PIONEERS OF RADIO

In 1864, Scottish physicist James Clerk Maxwell developed the theory of electromagnetic waves, which are the basis of radio. In 1888, Heinrich Hertz, a German physicist, discovered radio waves. Italian Guglielmo Marconi (1874-1937, right) created the first radio system in 1895, and in 1901 he transmitted radio signals across the Atlantic.

Find out more

ASTRONOMY
NAVIGATION
RADAR
TELEPHONES
TELEVISION AND VIDEO

RADIOACTIVITY

SOME ELEMENTS GLOW in the dark. We cannot always see the glow because our eyes are not sensitive to it, but it is still present. The glow is radiation, a form of energy, like the light and heat that we generate from electricity. Unlike heat and light, radiation is generated inside the substance itself, which is radioactive. Radioactive means producing radioactivity. A radioactive substance, such as uranium, is made up of big, unstable atoms. Some of the particles that form the atoms break away in a process called radioactivity. They are radiated as rays of alpha or beta particles, or as gamma waves. Eventually atoms reach a stable state, stop decaying, and the substance is no longer radioactive. This process can take millions of years.

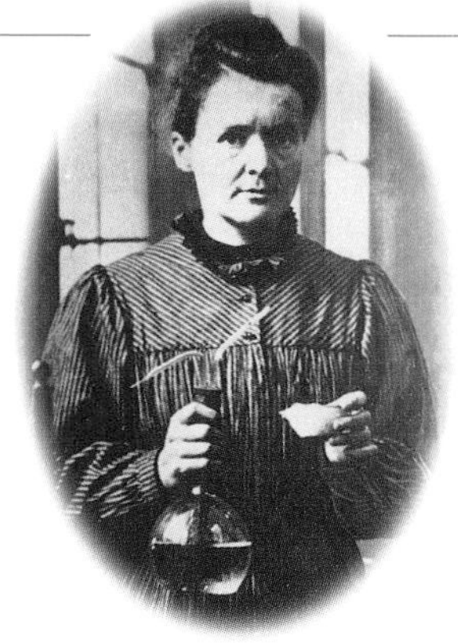

MARIE CURIE
Polish-born Marie Curie (1867-1934), and husband, Pierre, won the 1903 Nobel physics prize for discovering radioactivity. She did not know it was harmful, and died from radiation poisoning.

Large alpha particle

Small beta particle

High-frequency gamma radiation wave

Alpha radiation

Beta radiation

Gamma radiation

GEIGER COUNTER
A geiger counter consists of a gas-filled tube, and a meter. It can detect radioactivity.

TYPES OF RADIOACTIVITY

Radioactive substances give off three types of radiation: alpha, beta, and gamma. Alpha particles are larger than those of beta radiation, so cannot penetrate as far. Gamma radiation is a very high frequency wave and can pass through most materials. Only direct collisions with atoms can stop it. Shields to protect people from gamma radiation are made from dense material such as lead.

SOURCES OF RADIATION

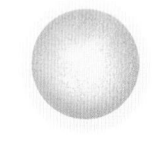

The Sun emits a type of radiation that includes radiant heat, and all the colours of visible light. This radiation is called electromagnetic radiation.

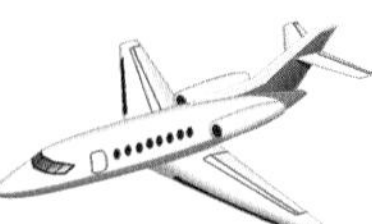

Objects such as this aircraft reflect the Sun's electromagnetic radiation as light waves.

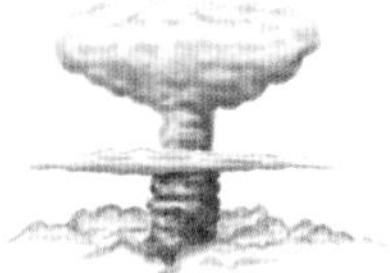

The explosion of a nuclear weapon produces both electromagnetic and radioactive radiation, with devastating effect.

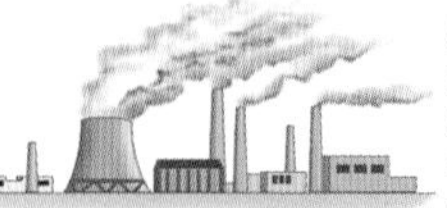

In a nuclear power station, the heat produced by radioactivity is used to make steam and drive an electricity generator.

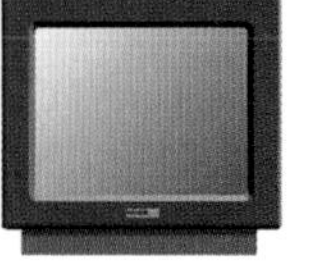

Television sets and computer monitors work by converting electrical energy into the visible electromagnetic radiation that we call light.

RADIOGRAPHY

Radioactive substances also produce x-rays. These are like gamma rays, but with a longer wavelength. In 1895, German scientist Wilhelm Roentgen (1845-1923) discovered x-rays could pass through the body, but dense tissue such as bone stopped them. This meant that broken bones and hard objects could be detected inside people, and photographed in the process known as radiography.

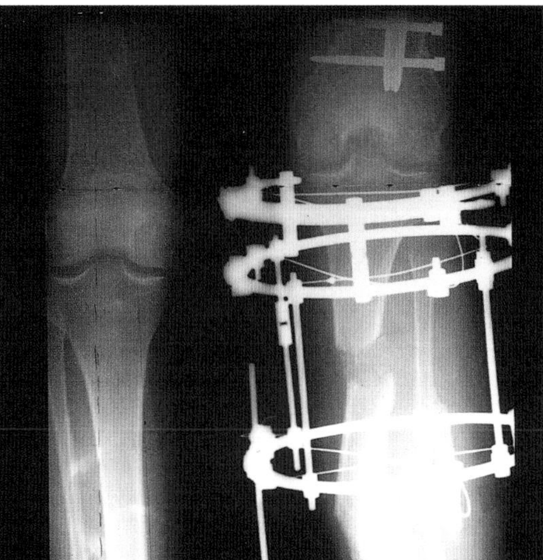

Radiation damage has caused this rare mutation of yellow eyes.

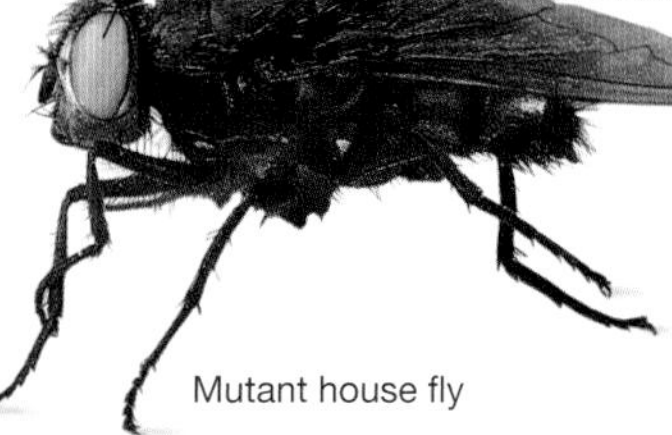

Mutant house fly

GENE MUTATION
Alpha and beta particles, x-rays, and gamma rays produced by radioactivity can damage living things, because they alter the DNA of genes. This can result in life-threatening diseases such as cancer. It can also lead to mutations, or changes, in the next generation.

Find out more

ATOMS AND MOLECULES
GENETICS
NUCLEAR ENERGY
X-RAYS

RAIN AND SNOW

THE WATER THAT FALLS from the sky as rain or snow is taking part in a continuous cycle. It begins when the water on the Earth's surface evaporates, or dries out, and enters the air as invisible water vapour. Rising air carries the vapour into the sky. The air cools as it rises, and the water vapour turns into tiny water droplets. These droplets are so small that they float in the air, and a cloud forms. A rain cloud contains millions of water droplets which merge together to form larger drops. When these drops become too large and heavy to float, they fall to the ground as rain and the cycle starts all over again. If the air is very cold, the water in the cloud freezes and forms snowflakes or hailstones. However, rainfall and snowfall are not equal all over the world. Deserts have hardly any rain at all; tropical regions can have so much rain that there are severe floods, while in the polar regions snow falls instead of rain.

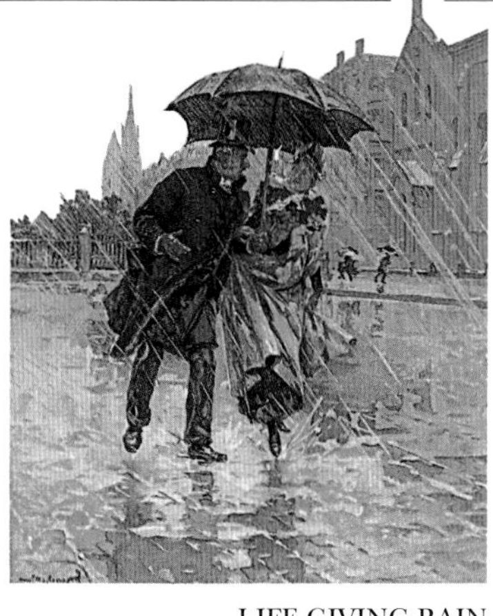

LIFE-GIVING RAIN
Rain is vital to life on Earth. Plants need water to grow, providing food for us and other animals. Rain also fills the rivers and lakes which provide our water supply.

WATER CYCLE

Water enters the air from lakes, rivers, seas, and oceans through the process of evaporation. In addition, plants, animals, and people give out water vapour into the atmosphere. The vapour stays in the air for an average time of 10 days and then falls as rain or snow. It joins the sea, rivers, and underground water-courses, and the cycle begins once more.

Trees and other plants release water vapour into the air from their leaves.

Cloud begins to form from water vapour in the atmosphere.

Water joins rivers and streams and flows down to the sea.

Water droplets fall from a cloud especially over high ground where the air is cooler. The general name for rain, snow, sleet, hail, mist, and dew is precipitation.

Water seeps underground through a layer of porous rock and flows down to the sea.

Wind and the sun's heat cause water to evaporate from the oceans and other large areas of water.

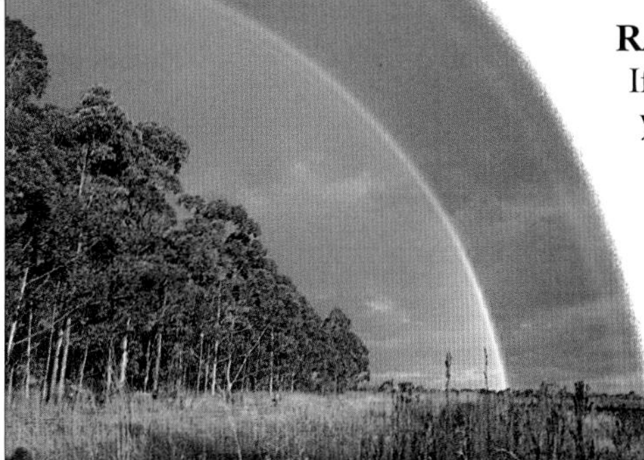

RAINBOW

If the sun shines on a shower of rain, you may see a rainbow if you are looking towards the rain and the sun is behind you. The raindrops in the shower reflect the sun's light back to you. As the sunlight passes through the raindrops, it splits up into a circular band of colours. You see the top part of this circle as a rainbow.

SNOW AND HAIL

In cold weather, the water in a cloud freezes and forms ice crystals. These crystals stick together and fall as snowflakes. The snow may melt slightly as it falls, producing sleet. In some clouds, strong air currents can toss frozen raindrops up and down. Each time they rise and fall, the frozen drops collect more ice crystals and water, and frozen layers build up like the skin around an onion. Eventually they become so heavy that they fall to the ground as hailstones.

ICE CRYSTAL
A microscope reveals that snowflakes are made of tiny six-sided ice crystals. No two crystals are exactly the same.

Find out more

COLOUR
RIVERS
STORMS
WATER
WEATHER
WIND

REFERENCE BOOKS

WHEN PEOPLE NEED INFORMATION about a subject, they quite often use a reference book. Reference books, unlike novels, provide factual information on all sorts of subjects, from the meanings of individual words, to facts about history, science, and the world around us. Reference books may include information on one subject only, or a variety of subjects. They may be general reference books, or specialist books such as dictionaries, atlases, and encyclopedias. Most reference books contain not only words, but also maps, illustrations, photographs, and diagrams, which make subjects easier to understand. Many also include cross-references that direct readers to pages in the book covering related topics, and an index, at the back of the book, so readers can look up specific topics. Reference books need regular updating and revising.

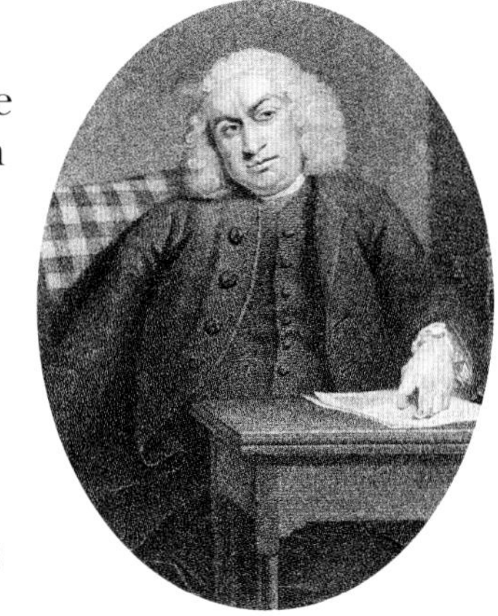

EARLY DICTIONARIES
In Ancient Greece, dictionaries were used to provide explanations of difficult or obscure words. In 1755, the writer Samuel Johnson, published *A Dictionary of the English Language*. It was the standard dictionary of the English language for more than a century.

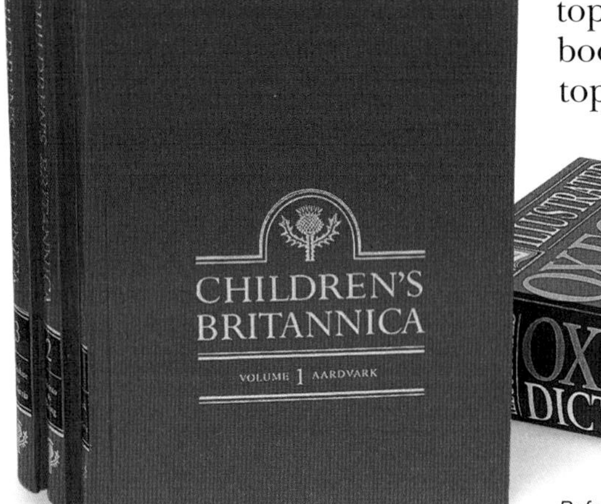

Reference books usually have hard covers to make them more resistant to wear and tear.

ENCYCLOPEDIA

An encyclopedia is a book containing information on people, places, things, and events, and may consist of one or more volumes. General encyclopedias, such as this book, cover a wide range of topics. Specialist encyclopedias focus on a particular area of study. A music encyclopedia, for example, covers only musical topics. The Ancient Greek philosopher Aristotle produced an encyclopedia c. 300 B.C.

HOW A DICTIONARY WORKS

A dictionary is an alphabetical list of words that gives the spelling, pronunciation, and meaning of each word. Every dictionary is designed to match the needs of its users. Dictionaries for young people, for instance, may include pictures. Specialist dictionaries contain only those words relevant to a particular subject, such as scientific or technical words.

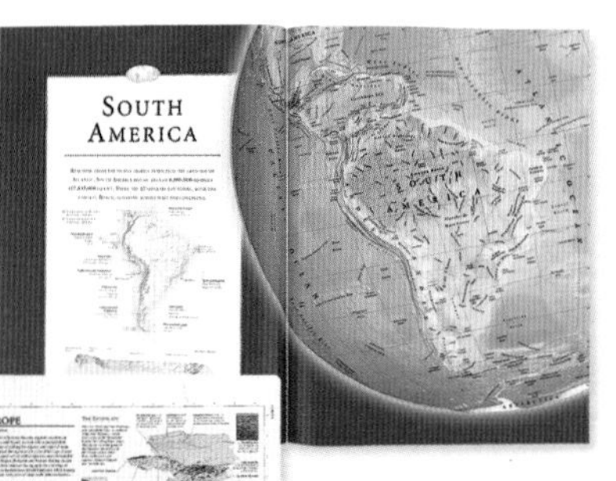

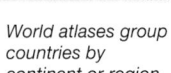

World atlases group countries by continent or region.

ATLASES
An atlas is a collection of maps. Traditional atlases include maps that show physical features, such as rivers, mountains, and deserts, as well as towns, cities, and roads. Maps can also show population, and the distribution of resources and crops. Some atlases specialize in subjects such as astronomy.

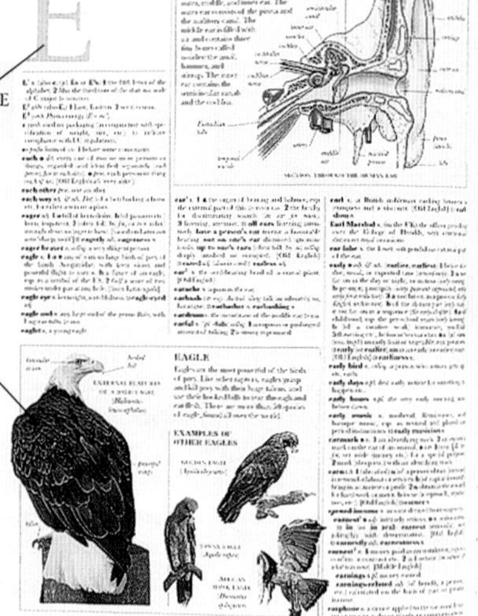

Large initial indicates that the section contains only words that begin with this letter.

Illustration provides a visual guide to the word.

ELECTRONIC FORMAT
Many reference books are now published as CD-ROMs, or on the Internet. Electronic formats allow enormous amounts of information to be put on a single disc. Users of the Internet can access up-to-date facts with ease and convenience.

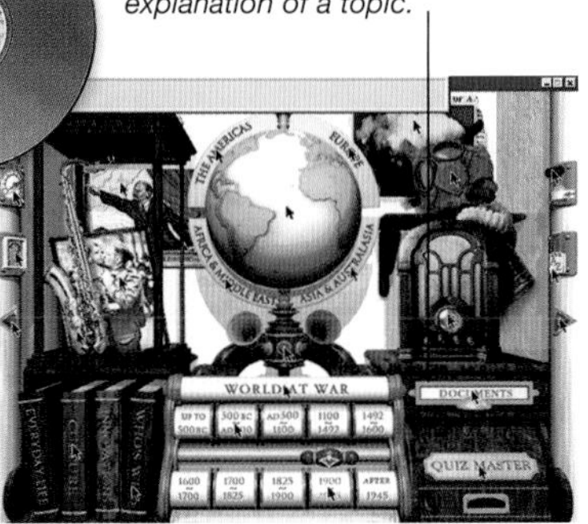

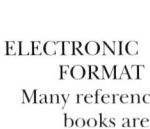

Sound and moving images can be included with the text to achieve a more effective explanation of a topic.

Find out more
BOOKS
EDUCATION
INFORMATION TECHNOLOGY
LITERATURE
MAPS

REFORMATION

ON 31 OCTOBER 1517, German monk Martin Luther pinned a list of 95 theses, or complaints, on a church door in Wittenberg, Saxony. This sparked off a movement known as the Reformation because its followers demanded the reform of the Catholic Church, then the most powerful force in Europe. Many, like Luther, believed it was corrupt, and attacked its wealth and the sale of indulgences (pardons for sins). In 1521, Luther was expelled from the Church. He set up his own church which became known as Protestant because its followers "protested" against what they felt were the errors of the Catholic Church. Protestantism spread through Europe. Then, in a movement called the Counter-Reformation, the Catholic Church began to reform itself. The Counter-Reformation led to religious persecution and bitter civil wars.

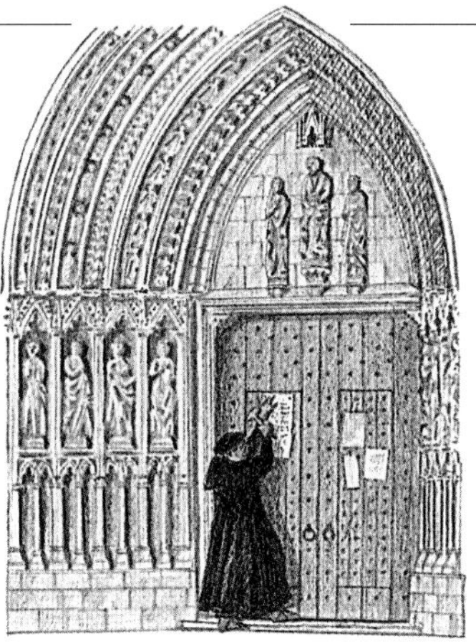

MARTIN LUTHER
Martin Luther (1483-1546) inspired the Reformation. He attacked the sale of indulgences and said that no amount of money paid to the clergy could pardon an individual for his sins. Only through faith could people be saved.

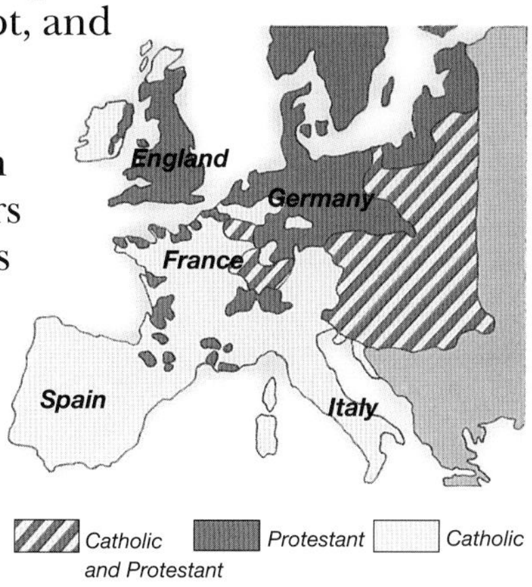

PROTESTANTISM
By 1560, Europe had two main religions – Roman Catholic and Protestant. Protestantism began in Germany. Many German rulers adopted the new religion so that they could break away from the control of the Pope and the Holy Roman Emperor (the "political" Catholic ruler).

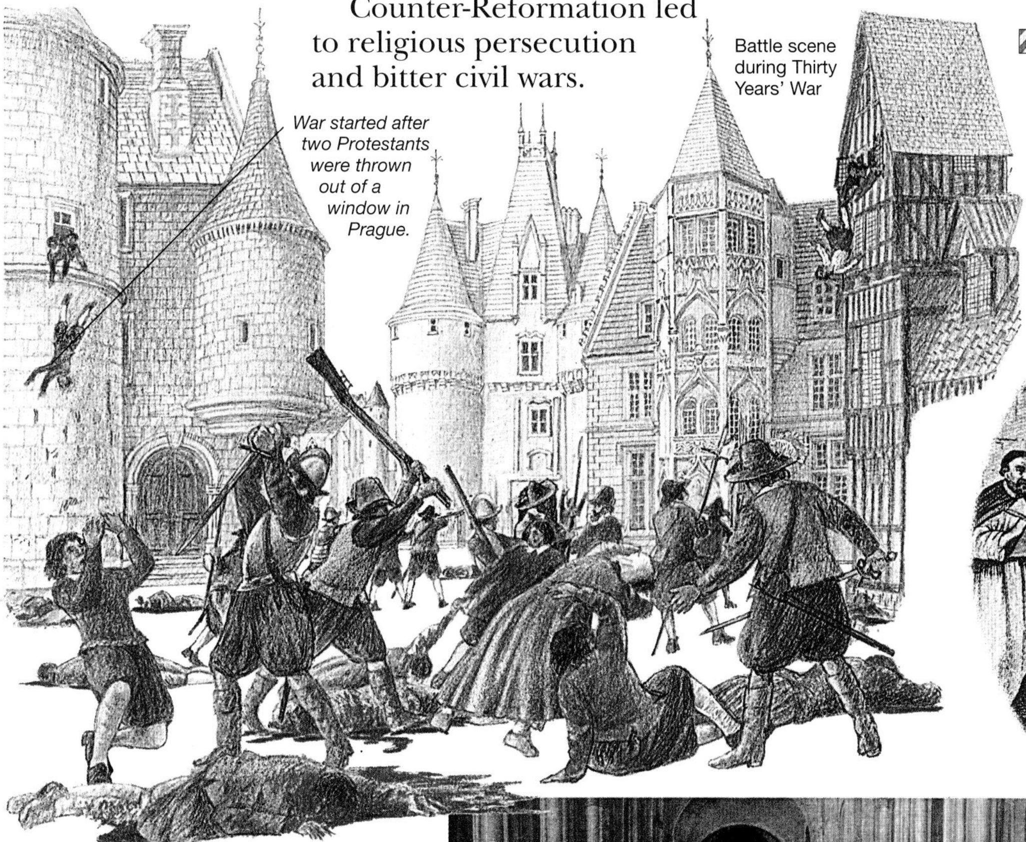

THIRTY YEARS' WAR
The Thirty Years' War lasted from 1618 to 1648. It began as a religious struggle between Catholics and Protestants in Germany. Then it grew into a war between the Hapsburg rulers of the Holy Roman Empire and the kings of France for possession of land. In 1648, by the Peace of Westphalia, the Protestants won the struggle.

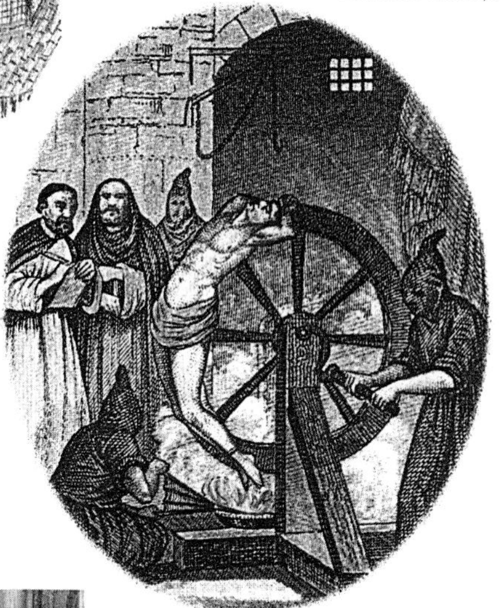

INQUISITION
In 1231, the Pope set up the Inquisition – a special organization that searched out and punished heretics (those who did not conform to the Catholic faith). Inquisitors arrested, tortured, and executed alleged heretics and witches (above). During the Reformation, 300 years later, the Inquisition tried to crush the new Protestant churches, but failed.

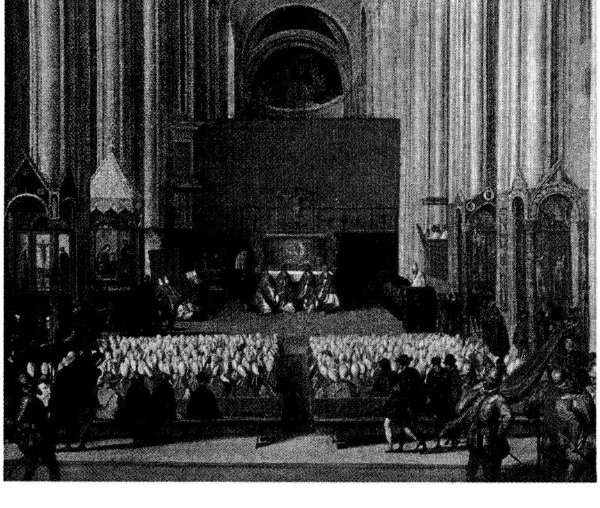

COUNCIL OF TRENT
The Counter-Reformation began when Catholic leaders met at the Council of Trent in 1545. The council established the main principles of Catholicism and set up places for training priests and missionaries. During this time the Jesuits, an important teaching order founded in 1534, became popular.

Find out more
EUROPE
FRANCE, HISTORY OF
GERMANY, HISTORY OF
HAPSBURGS
UNITED KINGDOM, HISTORY OF

RELIGIONS

PEOPLE HAVE ALWAYS SEARCHED for answers to life's mysteries and unexpected events. This questioning may have led to the growth of religions, to give meaning to life and death. Most religious people believe in a god or several gods. Gods are thought of as supreme beings who created the world or who control what happens in it. Religions may be highly organized, and teach people how to live, with a set of beliefs and rituals to follow. There may be special places in which to worship, and a spiritual leader for guidance. Some religions believe there is a spirit or a god in every object, from animals to rocks. Many believe in a life after death. Other religions have less formal rules, and people follow beliefs in their own way. The world's six major organized religions are Christianity, Judaism, Islam, Hinduism, Buddhism, and Sikhism.

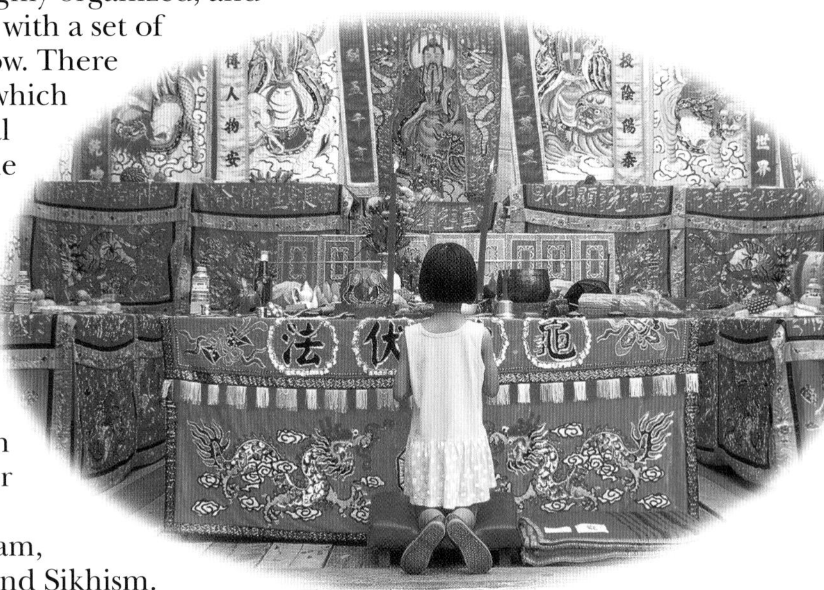

MOTHER GODDESSES
Pregnant female figures found at ancient holy sites were probably worshipped as a symbol of the making of new life.

RELIGION AND ART
Many people use art, architecture, and sculpture to convey their religious ideas, and to show the important icons of their religion. This Christian sculpture of the Virgin Mary holding Jesus shows her crowned as the Queen of Heaven.

GODS
Many religions worship either a single God, or several gods. There may be myths or stories associated with the god, which demonstrate an important lesson. Ganesha (right) is the Hindu god of wisdom. According to legend, his father accidentally cut off his head and in desperation replaced it with that of an elephant.

WORSHIP AND PRAYER

Each religion has its own system of worship and prayer. Worship shows reverence towards a god or deity, in a public ceremony or service. It often takes place in a special building, such as a mosque or church. Prayers can be spoken or thought during worship or in private, and are a thanksgiving or request to a god or holy object. The girl above prays during the Buddhist Festival of Hungry Ghosts in Singapore.

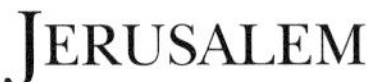

JERUSALEM

Jerusalem is sacred to three religions. Jews pray at the Wailing Wall, the ruins of a temple destroyed in A.D. 70. The Dome of the Rock mosque is holy to Muslims as the place where Prophet Muhammad rose to heaven. The Church of the Holy Sepulchre is built on the site of the crucifixion and burial of Jesus Christ.

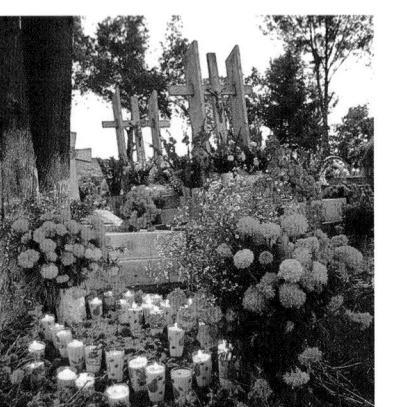

DEATH AND HEAVEN
Many faiths believe that the human body is a temporary container for the soul. After death the soul may be reborn in another body or go to heaven as a reward for good deeds on earth. Most religions have special rituals or funerals to honour and remember the dead, such as the Day of the Dead in Mexico (above). Candles are lit to help dead relatives find their way to the land of the living.

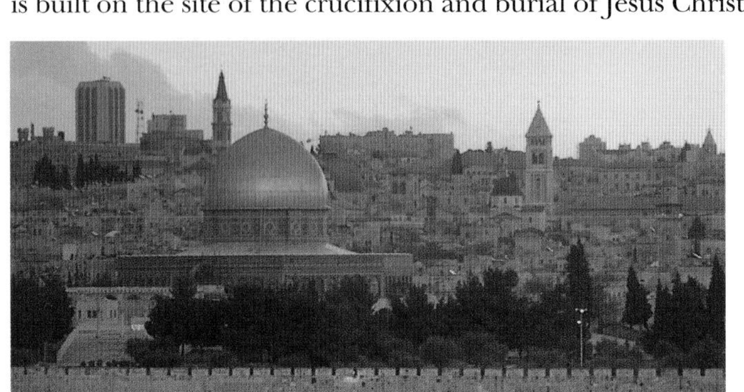

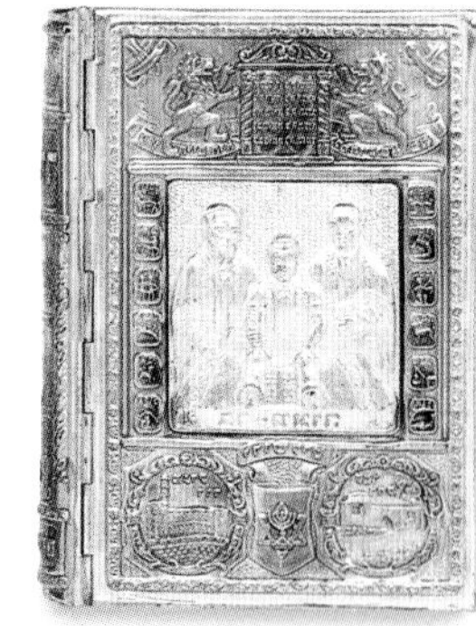

SACRED TEXTS
Many religions have texts which teach and guide. Muslims read the Qur'an, Christianity is based on the Bible, Buddhists follow the Dharma, and the Talmud (above) is central to Judaism.

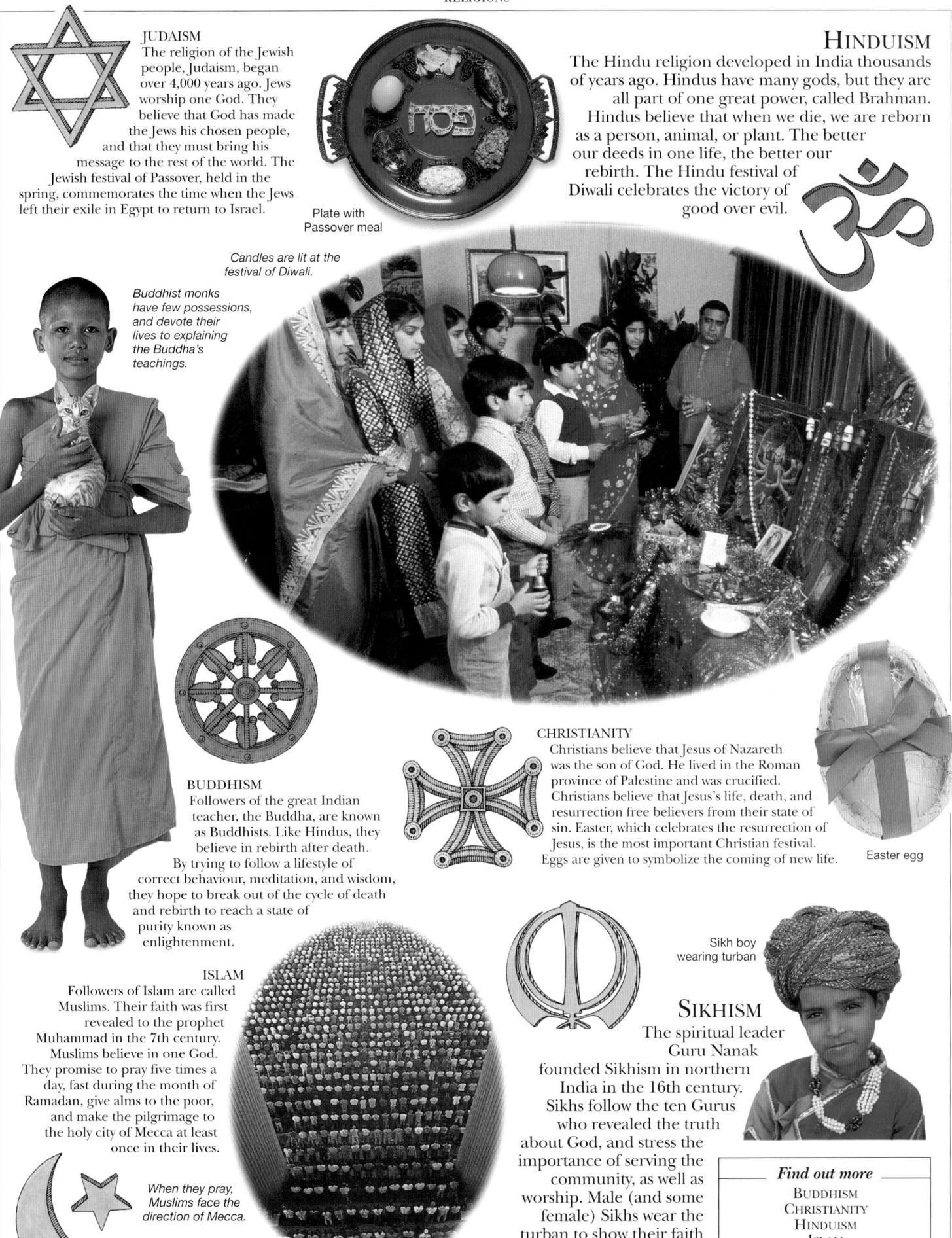

JUDAISM
The religion of the Jewish people, Judaism, began over 4,000 years ago. Jews worship one God. They believe that God has made the Jews his chosen people, and that they must bring his message to the rest of the world. The Jewish festival of Passover, held in the spring, commemorates the time when the Jews left their exile in Egypt to return to Israel.

Plate with Passover meal

HINDUISM

The Hindu religion developed in India thousands of years ago. Hindus have many gods, but they are all part of one great power, called Brahman. Hindus believe that when we die, we are reborn as a person, animal, or plant. The better our deeds in one life, the better our rebirth. The Hindu festival of Diwali celebrates the victory of good over evil.

Candles are lit at the festival of Diwali.

Buddhist monks have few possessions, and devote their lives to explaining the Buddha's teachings.

BUDDHISM
Followers of the great Indian teacher, the Buddha, are known as Buddhists. Like Hindus, they believe in rebirth after death. By trying to follow a lifestyle of correct behaviour, meditation, and wisdom, they hope to break out of the cycle of death and rebirth to reach a state of purity known as enlightenment.

CHRISTIANITY
Christians believe that Jesus of Nazareth was the son of God. He lived in the Roman province of Palestine and was crucified. Christians believe that Jesus's life, death, and resurrection free believers from their state of sin. Easter, which celebrates the resurrection of Jesus, is the most important Christian festival. Eggs are given to symbolize the coming of new life.

Easter egg

ISLAM
Followers of Islam are called Muslims. Their faith was first revealed to the prophet Muhammad in the 7th century. Muslims believe in one God. They promise to pray five times a day, fast during the month of Ramadan, give alms to the poor, and make the pilgrimage to the holy city of Mecca at least once in their lives.

When they pray, Muslims face the direction of Mecca.

Sikh boy wearing turban

SIKHISM

The spiritual leader Guru Nanak founded Sikhism in northern India in the 16th century. Sikhs follow the ten Gurus who revealed the truth about God, and stress the importance of serving the community, as well as worship. Male (and some female) Sikhs wear the turban to show their faith and their membership of the Sikh community.

Find out more

BUDDHISM
CHRISTIANITY
HINDUISM
ISLAM
JUDAISM

RENAISSANCE

ITALY IN THE 15TH CENTURY was an exciting place. It was here that educated people began to develop new ideas about the world around them and rediscovered the arts and learning of Ancient Greece and Rome. For a period of about 200 years that became known as the Renaissance (rebirth) people made great advances in education, technology, and the arts. Helped by the invention of printing, the Renaissance gradually spread from Italy to the rest of Europe. Although the Renaissance mainly affected the wealthy, it had a huge impact on the way that everybody lived and perceived the world around them. The Renaissance produced great artists such as Michelangelo and Raphael. It also produced a new way of thinking called humanism, as scholars and thinkers such as Erasmus began to challenge the authority of the Roman Catholic Church. Humanism gave human beings more importance. It meant that artists such as Leonardo da Vinci began to produce realistic images instead of symbolic scenes. Scientists challenged old ideas about the nature of the universe, and conducted pioneering experiments.

COPERNICUS
By observing the movement of planets and stars, astronomers such as Nicolaus Copernicus (1473-1543) began to challenge ideas about the solar system which had been accepted since the time of the Ancient Greeks. Copernicus was first to suggest that the Earth revolves every 24 hours and that it travels around the Sun once a year. Many people did not accept his findings until many years later.

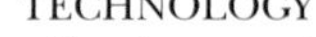

TECHNOLOGY
Renaissance scientists invented or developed new scientific instruments to help them in their work. The armillary sphere, a skeleton sphere with the Earth in the centre, was used to measure the position of the stars. Galileo invented the useful proportional compass, which could be set at any angle.

Armillary sphere

Proportional compass

Galileo at work

GALILEO
Galileo Galilei (1564-1642) was an Italian astronomer and physicist. He disproved many of the Ancient Greek thinker Aristotle's theories, including the theory that heavy objects fall faster than light ones. He perfected a refracting telescope and observed that the Earth and all the planets of the solar system revolve around the Sun.

RENAISSANCE MUSIC

When the first music was printed in Italy in the late 15th century, new musical styles began to spread throughout Europe. Non-religious music became more common, showing the influence of the humanist approach to life which characterized the Renaissance period. Music became more harmonious and melodic than before. William Byrd (1543-1623), left, was the first Englishman to have his music printed in England. He was a well known organist, first at Lincoln Cathedral, and then later at the Queen Elizabeth I Chapel Royal in London. He was also a composer, and developed the first madrigals (music for singing without any accompanying instruments).

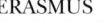

ERASMUS
Desiderius Erasmus (1466-1536), a Dutch priest, wanted to reform the Roman Catholic Church. He criticized the superstitions of the clergy, and published studies of the Old and New Testaments, giving a better understanding of the Bible. A leading humanist, he questioned the authority of the Church – a shocking idea at the time.

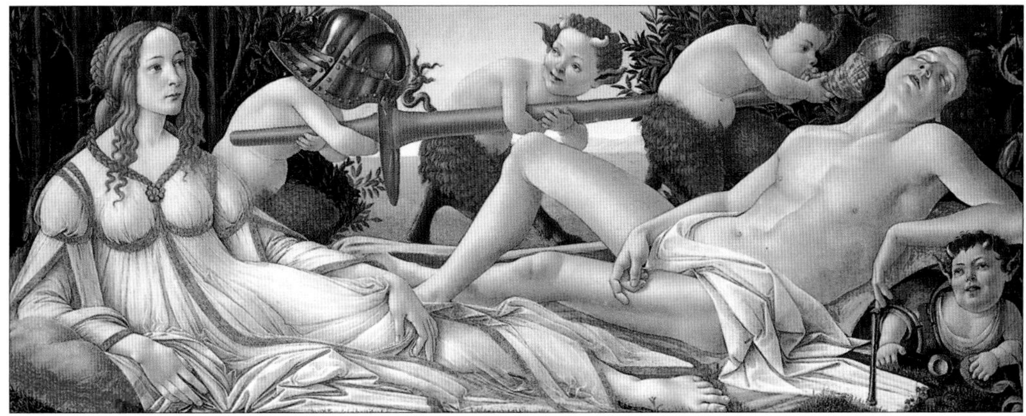

BOTTICELLI
The paintings of Sandro Botticelli (1444-1510) show many of the features typical of Renaissance art: clear lines, even composition, and an emphasis on human activity. Renaissance artists painted realistic, mythological, and Biblical subjects. Most tried to make their paintings as realistic as possible by using perspective to give scenes an appearance of depth. Above is the Botticelli painting *Venus and Mars.*

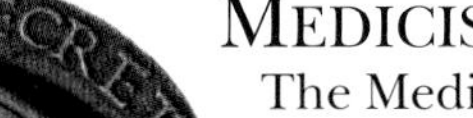

MEDICIS

The Medicis were a great banking family who ruled Florence for more than 300 years. They became very powerful. Many of them, particularly Lorenzo "the Magnificent" (1449-92), encouraged artists such as Michelangelo, and helped them financially.

MICHELANGELO
Michelangelo (1475-1564) was a very skilled Italian artist and sculptor. His marble statue of David (left) is one of the finest examples of Renaissance sculpture. People admired the statue's youthful strength and beauty, which demonstrated the new realistic style of art.

Dome rises more than 120 m (400 ft) from the floor of the church.

Begun in 1505, the building took 150 years to complete.

ST. PETER'S

Situated in Vatican City, Rome, Italy, St. Peter's Church has a rich history. Ten different architects worked on its construction. Michelangelo designed the dome. The Italian architect Bernini (1598-1680) designed the inside of the church and the majestic piazza outside the church. St. Peter's houses many fabulous works of art, and marble and detailed mosaics decorate the walls.

SCULPTURE
Renaissance sculptors made great use of marble, copying the style of Ancient Roman statues. A new understanding of anatomy inspired sculptors to carve nude figures, with accurate depictions of muscles and joints. Some sculptors even dissected corpses to discover how the human body works.

ARCHITECTURE
Renaissance architecture was modelled on classical Roman building styles. Architects featured high domed roofs, vaulted ceilings, decorative columns, and rounded arches in their buildings. One of the most influential architects was Andrea Palladio (1508-80). The classical designs used by Palladio for his many villas and palaces were widely copied by later architects.

RENAISSANCE

1420-36 Architect Filippo Brunelleschi develops the system of perspective.

1430-35 Donatello's sculpture of David is the first large nude statue since the Roman Empire.

1480-85 Sandro Botticelli paints *The Birth of Venus.*

1497 Leonardo da Vinci paints *The Last Supper.*

1501 Petrucci publishes first printed music in Venice.

1501-04 Michelangelo sculpts *David.*

1502 Leonardo paints the *Mona Lisa.*

1505 Architect Donato Bramante begins the new St. Peter's in Rome. Completed in 1655.

1508 Artist Raphael begins to decorate the Pope's apartments in the Vatican.

1508-12 Michelangelo decorates the Sistine chapel.

1509 Erasmus writes *In Praise of Folly*, criticizing the Church.

c.1510 Renaissance art in Venice reaches its peak with artists such as Titian, Veronese, and Tintoretto.

1513 Death of Pope Julius II.

1532 Niccolo Machiavelli's book *The Prince* is published, suggesting how a ruler should govern a state.

1543 Astronomer Copernicus claims that the Earth and the other planets move around the sun.

1552 Architect Palladio begins to build the Villa Rotunda in Venice.

1564 Death of Michelangelo.

1593 Galileo develops the thermometer.

1608 Galileo develops the telescope.

Find out more
ARCHITECTURE
ITALY, HISTORY OF
LEONARDO DA VINCI
PAINTERS
SCULPTURE

Reproduction

For life to continue on Earth, humans and other animals must produce young. The process of creating new life is called reproduction. Human beings reproduce in much the same way as other mammals. From birth, a woman has many tiny pinhead-sized ova (egg cells) in two glands inside the abdomen called ovaries. From puberty onwards, one of these egg cells is released each month as part of the menstrual cycle. Throughout life, a man produces small tadpole-shaped cells called sperm in sex organs called the testes. During sexual intercourse, sperm cells leave the man's body and enter the woman's body, swimming towards her ovaries. If a sperm meets a ripe egg cell, the two join together. This is called fertilization. The egg cell can only be fertilized for about three days after ovulation. Fertilization makes the egg cell begin to develop in the woman's uterus. During the following nine months the tiny egg develops into a fully formed baby, ready to be born.

FOETUS
A developing baby, or foetus, lives inside the uterus, cushioned from bumps, bright lights, and noise by a surrounding fluid called the amniotic fluid. However, the baby can hear the regular thump of the mother's heartbeat and the gurgling of food in her intestines.

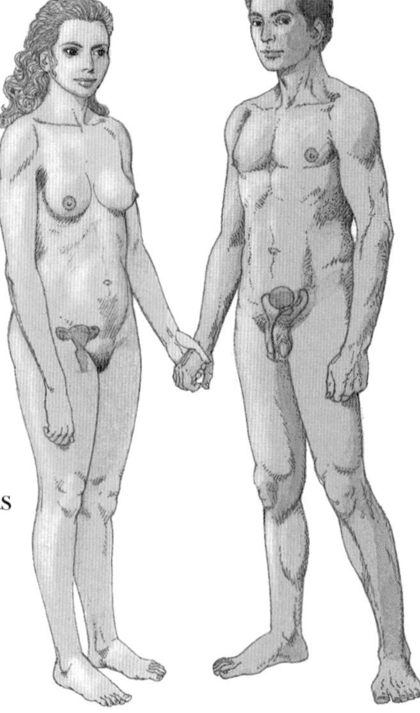

SEX ORGANS
The main female sex organs, the ovaries, are inside the abdomen. The main male organs, the testes and penis, hang outside the abdomen. Other differences between males and females, such as the woman's breasts, are called secondary sexual characteristics.

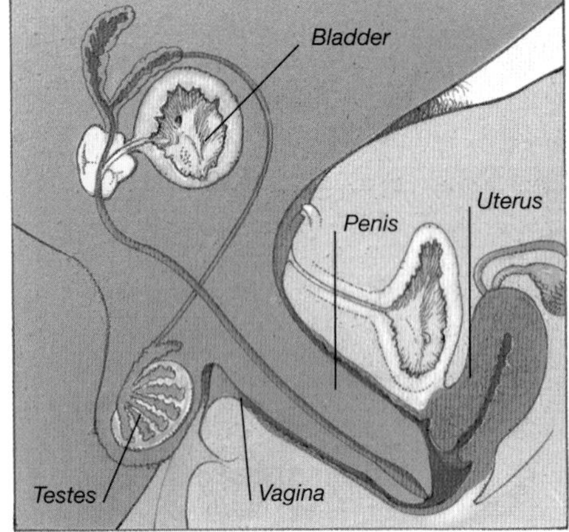

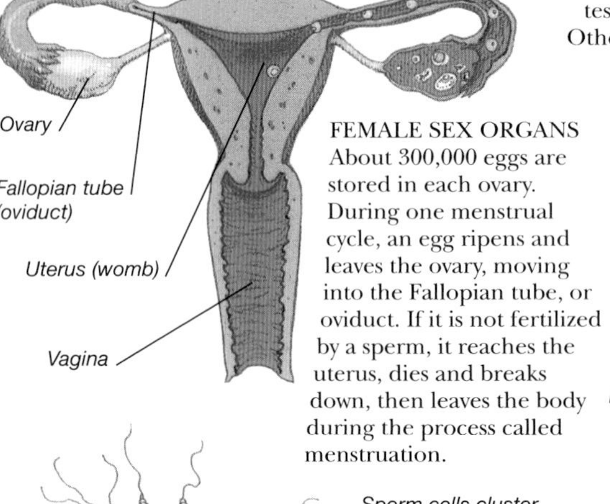

FEMALE SEX ORGANS
About 300,000 eggs are stored in each ovary. During one menstrual cycle, an egg ripens and leaves the ovary, moving into the Fallopian tube, or oviduct. If it is not fertilized by a sperm, it reaches the uterus, dies and breaks down, then leaves the body during the process called menstruation.

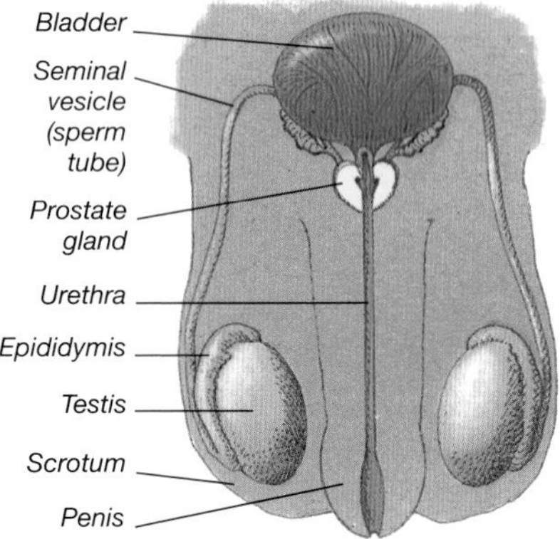

MALE SEX ORGANS
Each testis makes more than 250 million sperm cells every day. The cells are stored in the testis itself and in a long, winding tube called the epididymis. If they are not released, they break down and are reabsorbed into the bloodstream.

Sexual intercourse

During sexual intercourse, the man's penis becomes stiff enough to insert into the woman's vagina, which also enlarges. After a while muscular contractions squeeze sperm cells from the man's testes out of the penis and into the vagina, in a fluid called semen. This process is called ejaculation. The sperm cells swim through the uterus, propelled by their tails, and travel along the Fallopian tube. Sometimes, one of these sperm cells reaches the egg cell and fertilizes it, resulting in pregnancy.

Sperm cells cluster around egg cell in Fallopian tube.

Only one sperm penetrates egg to fertilize it.

Fertilized egg divides into two cells within 36 hours, four within 48 hours, then eight, and so on. Barrier around dividing cells keeps out other sperm cells.

FERTILIZATION
An egg cell begins to divide and develop into a baby only when it is joined by a sperm cell. After intercourse, hundreds of sperm cells may reach the egg, but only one breaks through the outer layer. Once this occurs, genetic material in the sperm – the instructions needed to make a new human – joins the genetic material inside the egg. The coming together of sperm and egg and their genes is called fertilization, or conception.

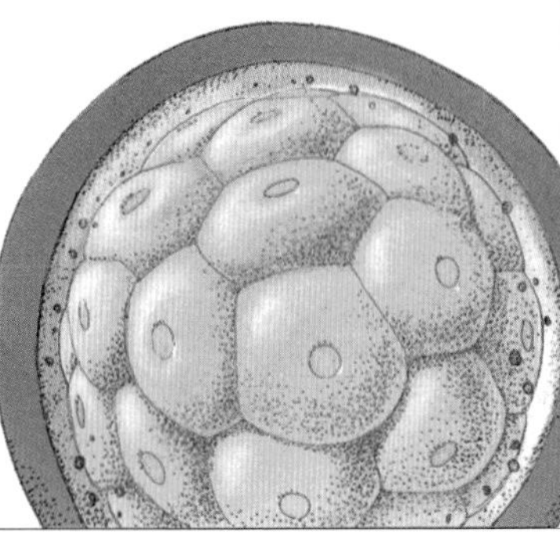

Embryo enters uterus about three days after fertilization as a solid ball of 16-32 cells.

PREGNANCY

About one week after fertilization, the ball of cells embeds itself in the blood-rich lining of the uterus where it absorbs nutrients. The cells continue to divide and change, forming the first body tissues such as blood vessels and nerves. Gradually the ball of cells folds and twists into the basic body shape of the baby. Meanwhile, other cells form the placenta, a saucer-shaped organ, in the lining of the uterus. The placenta is fed with blood from the mother, and oxygen and nutrients pass to the baby through the umbilical cord. This lifeline consists of three blood vessels; the largest vein carries nutrients and oxygen-rich blood to the baby, and the smaller ones carry waste and blood low in oxygen back to the placenta.

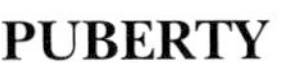

5 WEEKS
The developing baby is now about 10 mm ($1/2$ in) long. It has a recognizable head, back, and heart, and the beginnings of a mouth and eyes. The limbs are forming as small buds. At this stage, the developing baby is called an embryo.

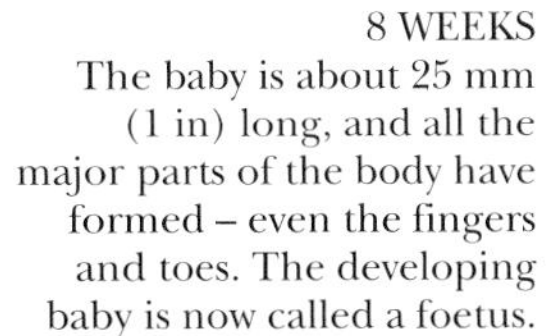

8 WEEKS
The baby is about 25 mm (1 in) long, and all the major parts of the body have formed – even the fingers and toes. The developing baby is now called a foetus.

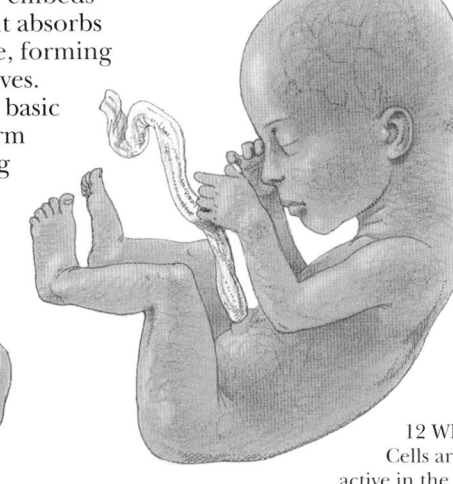

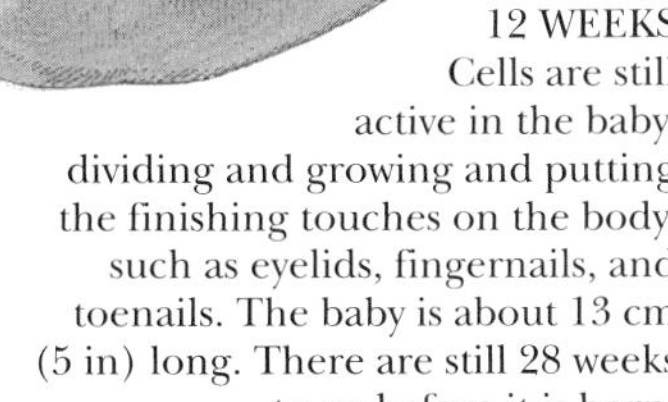

12 WEEKS
Cells are still active in the baby, dividing and growing and putting the finishing touches on the body, such as eyelids, fingernails, and toenails. The baby is about 13 cm (5 in) long. There are still 28 weeks to go before it is born.

BIRTH

Birth is the process that ends pregnancy and carries a baby out of the uterus, usually after 38-42 weeks of pregnancy. When the baby has reached full term (left), it is about 50 cm (20 in) long. Labour is triggered by the hormone oxytocin and by changes in the level of other hormones in the mother's blood. During labour the cervix widens to allow birth to take place, and powerful contractions in the uterus push the baby out through the vagina, usually head first. If a baby is born feet first it is called a breach birth. The baby then takes its first breaths and the umbilical cord is cut. The placenta is expelled from the uterus a few minutes later as afterbirth.

PUBERTY

Babies and children have sex organs, but they are not able to release egg or sperm cells. At puberty, which generally starts when people are between 10 and 15 years old, chemicals called sex hormones are released into the bloodstream from hormonal glands. These sex hormones cause the sex organs to mature (become fully developed). Other changes occur at this time too, particularly a spurt in growth.

In a boy, the testes produce a sex hormone called testosterone. This makes hair grow on the face and body. It also makes the voice deeper, encourages muscle development, and sets off production of sperm.

In a girl, the ovaries produce progesterone and oestrogen, which cause the breasts to develop and fatty tissue to form, giving the body a more rounded shape. From puberty onwards, a woman's body also undergoes a monthly process called the menstrual cycle or period, as shown below. Changing levels of hormones thicken the uterus lining and enrich it with blood, which will nourish a fertilized egg if it implants.

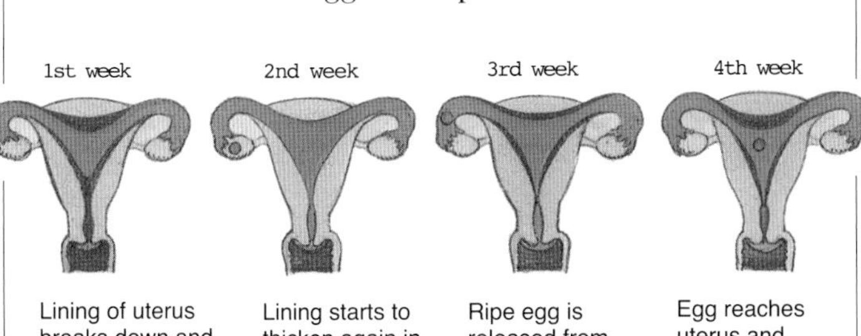

Lining of uterus breaks down and passes out of the vagina as menstrual blood flow, called menstruation.

Lining starts to thicken again in preparation for next egg. Next egg begins to ripen in ovary.

Ripe egg is released from ovary. Egg can be fertilized for up to 36 hours in Fallopian tube.

Egg reaches uterus and implants if fertilized, or breaks down if not fertilized.

PREMATURE BABIES
If a baby is born before the 37th week of pregnancy it is called premature and may have difficulty breathing. The baby is placed in an incubator and monitored very carefully until it is strong enough to breathe for itself.

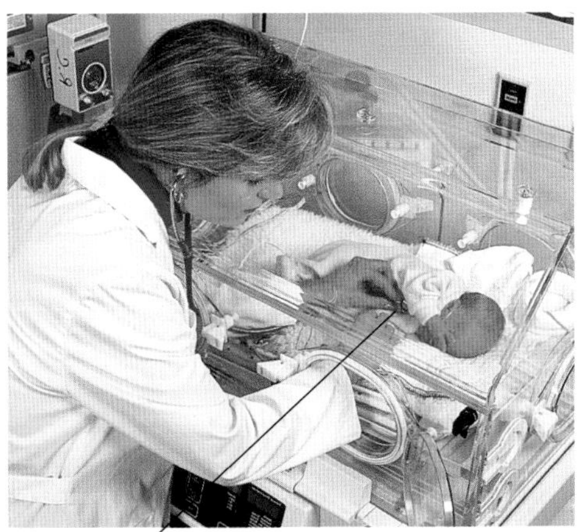

A doctor checks the heartbeat of a premature baby in its incubator.

Find out more
ANIMALS
HUMAN BODY

REPTILES

SCALY-SKINNED ANIMALS such as alligators, turtles, and snakes are called reptiles. Some reptiles live in water and some on land; most are found in the warmer parts of the world. There are six main groups; lizards, snakes, worm lizards, turtles and tortoises, crocodiles and alligators, and the tuatara. Tortoises and turtles are the only reptiles with shells. Lizards make up the largest group, with about 4,300 different kinds, yet there is only one kind of tuatara. Reptiles are among the most ancient of all animals. The ancestors of today's reptiles were the dinosaurs. Dinosaurs roamed the Earth for about 150 million years, then suddenly died out 65 million years ago. Today, there are more than 8,000 kinds of reptiles, from the long reticulated python, measuring 10 m (33 ft), to the tiny dwarf gecko, only 33 mm (1.3 in) in length. Unlike warm-blooded (endothermic) mammals, reptiles are cold-blooded (ectothermic) – they need the warmth of the Sun to give them the energy to move.

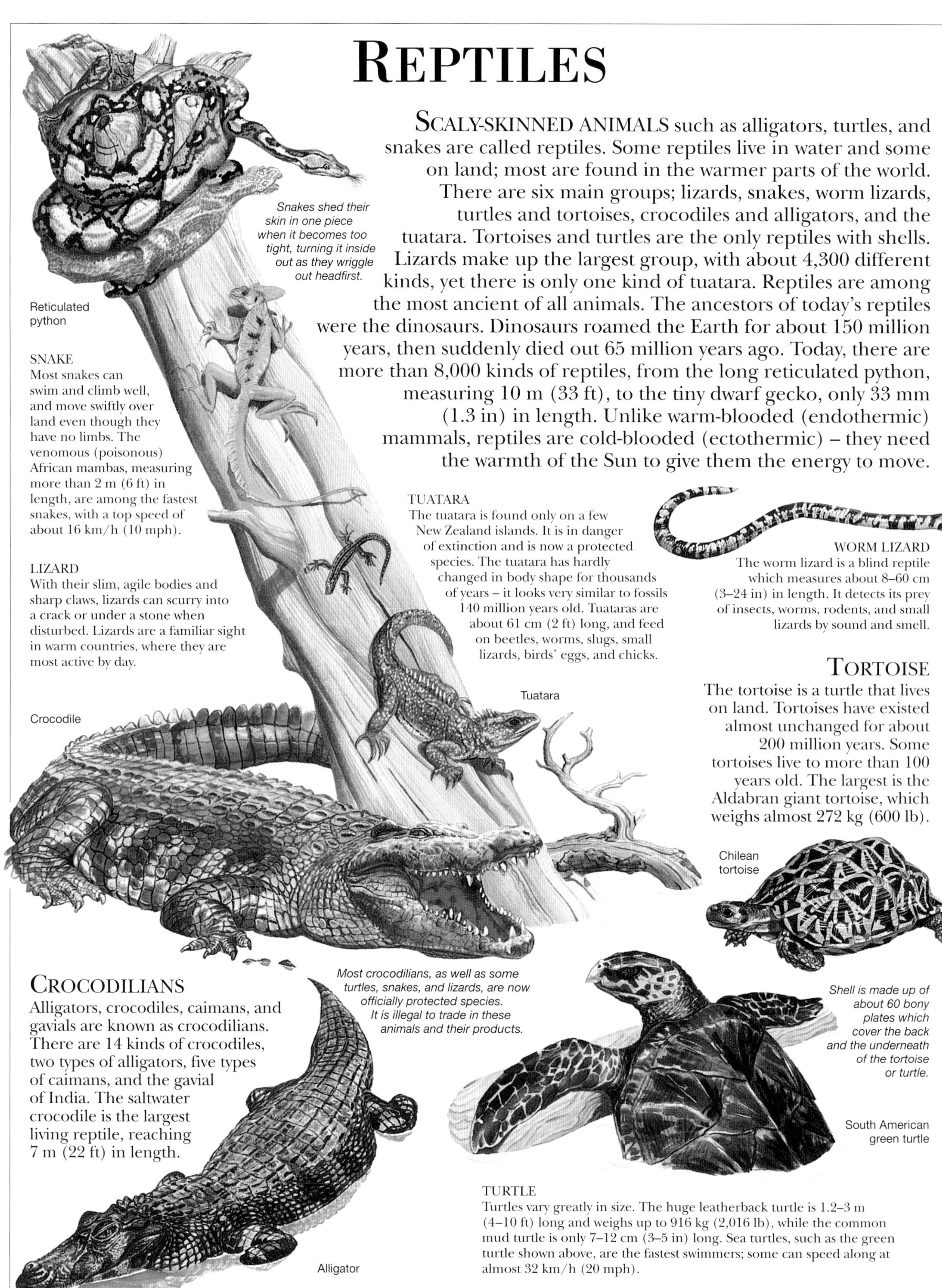

Snakes shed their skin in one piece when it becomes too tight, turning it inside out as they wriggle out headfirst.

SNAKE
Most snakes can swim and climb well, and move swiftly over land even though they have no limbs. The venomous (poisonous) African mambas, measuring more than 2 m (6 ft) in length, are among the fastest snakes, with a top speed of about 16 km/h (10 mph).

LIZARD
With their slim, agile bodies and sharp claws, lizards can scurry into a crack or under a stone when disturbed. Lizards are a familiar sight in warm countries, where they are most active by day.

TUATARA
The tuatara is found only on a few New Zealand islands. It is in danger of extinction and is now a protected species. The tuatara has hardly changed in body shape for thousands of years – it looks very similar to fossils 140 million years old. Tuataras are about 61 cm (2 ft) long, and feed on beetles, worms, slugs, small lizards, birds' eggs, and chicks.

WORM LIZARD
The worm lizard is a blind reptile which measures about 8–60 cm (3–24 in) in length. It detects its prey of insects, worms, rodents, and small lizards by sound and smell.

TORTOISE

The tortoise is a turtle that lives on land. Tortoises have existed almost unchanged for about 200 million years. Some tortoises live to more than 100 years old. The largest is the Aldabran giant tortoise, which weighs almost 272 kg (600 lb).

CROCODILIANS

Alligators, crocodiles, caimans, and gavials are known as crocodilians. There are 14 kinds of crocodiles, two types of alligators, five types of caimans, and the gavial of India. The saltwater crocodile is the largest living reptile, reaching 7 m (22 ft) in length.

Most crocodilians, as well as some turtles, snakes, and lizards, are now officially protected species. It is illegal to trade in these animals and their products.

Shell is made up of about 60 bony plates which cover the back and the underneath of the tortoise or turtle.

TURTLE
Turtles vary greatly in size. The huge leatherback turtle is 1.2–3 m (4–10 ft) long and weighs up to 916 kg (2,016 lb), while the common mud turtle is only 7–12 cm (3–5 in) long. Sea turtles, such as the green turtle shown above, are the fastest swimmers; some can speed along at almost 32 km/h (20 mph).

Breeding

Most reptiles lay eggs, from which the young hatch. Snake and lizard eggs usually have a leathery, flexible shell.The eggs of crocodiles and tortoises are hard and rigid, and the temperature at which the eggs are incubated determines the sex of the hatchling. The loggerhead turtle, shown here, digs a deep hole in the beach sand and lays its eggs under the cover of darkness. The eggs take several weeks to hatch and are at risk from foxes and monitor lizards, which dig them up and eat them. After hatching, the young turtles have to avoid sea birds and crabs as they scuttle down to the sea.

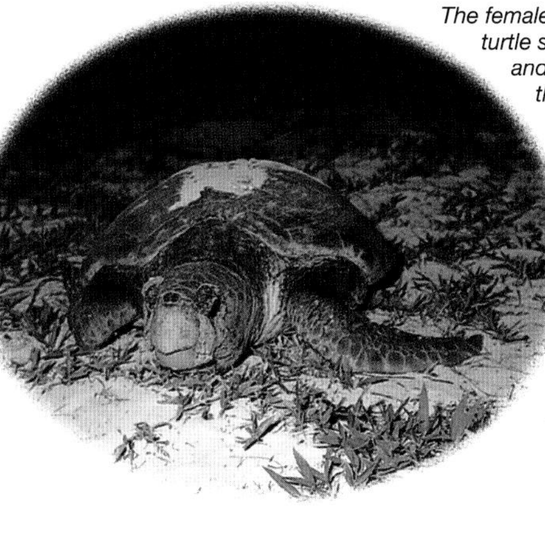

The female loggerhead turtle swims ashore and crawls up the beach at night to lay eggs.

The female turtle lays about 100 eggs in the sand.

BLUE-TONGUED SKINK
The reptiles tongue has several uses. Lizards and snakes use it to detect their surroundings. The tongue flicks out to pick up chemicals in the air and carries them back to Jacobson's organs, special sensory organs in the roof of the mouth. When in danger, the Australian blue-tongued skink opens its mouth wide, thrusts out its bright blue tongue, hisses, and puffs up its body to frighten away a predator.

SCALES
A reptile's scaly skin provides good protection against predators and stops the animal from drying out. The arrangement of the scales helps scientists identify species. Some reptiles, such as chameleons, have special cells in the skin. These cells make the coloured pigments inside the skin expand or contract. This is how the chameleon changes its colour, for camouflage.

WALL GECKO
Wall geckos have tiny, sticky pads on their toes, which enable them to run up smooth glass windows and upside-down across the ceiling.

Some geckos are smaller than the human palm.

Temperature regulation

We often describe reptiles as cold-blooded, but this is not strictly true. Reptiles cannot generate body heat internally, in the way that mammals do, but they can control their body temperature by their behaviour. Reptiles bask in the Sun to absorb warmth, then hide in the shade when they become too hot.

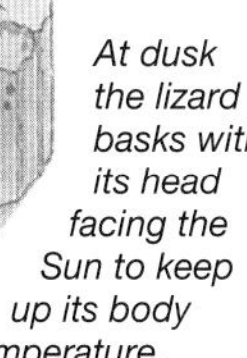

During the hot midday Sun the lizard stays in the shade to avoid overheating.

At dawn the lizard sunbathes with the length of its body facing the Sun to absorb maximum heat.

At dusk the lizard basks with its head facing the Sun to keep up its body temperature.

Largest and smallest reptiles

The saltwater crocodile is the largest reptile, although some snakes, such as the reticulated python, are longer, growing to 10 m (33 ft) in length. The largest lizard is the Komodo dragon, a type of monitor lizard. The smallest of all reptiles are some kinds of geckos, only about a centimetre long when fully grown.

Coelophysis

The first reptiles appeared on Earth more than 300 million years ago and gradually took over from amphibians as the largest animals on land. Dinosaurs, such as the *Coelophysis* shown here, were early reptiles that evolved about 200–220 million years ago. *Coelophysis* was about the size of an adult human.

Coelophysis *probably hunted lizard-like reptiles and other small animals of the time.*

Find out more

ANIMALS
CROCODILES AND ALLIGATORS
DINOSAURS
LIZARDS
SNAKES

RHINOCEROSES
AND TAPIRS

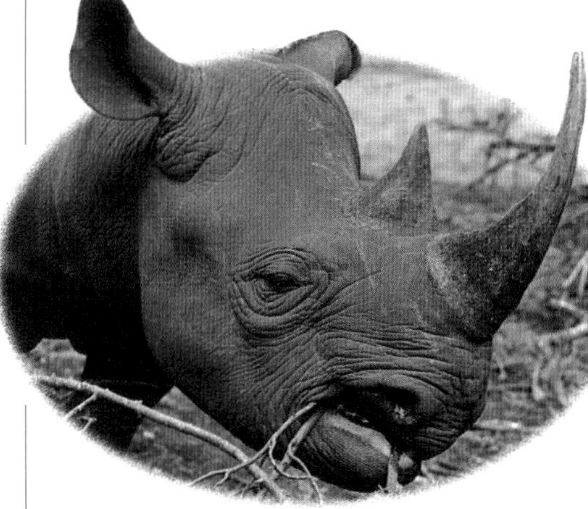

BLACK RHINOCEROS

The black rhinoceros shown here is slightly smaller than the white rhinoceros. Black rhinos are found in central and southern Africa. They cannot focus clearly on things further than about 30 m (100 ft) away and sometimes charge at suspicious objects. Black rhinoceroses feed mainly at night on trees and bushes. They grasp the leaves and shoots with their long, hooked lips.

THE FIRST RHINOCEROSES existed about 30 million years ago and some evolved into the largest land mammals that ever lived. Today, few creatures are in such a desperate plight as the rhinoceros. Thousands have been killed for their horns, and all are on the official list of endangered species. Rhinoceroses are herbivores, or plant eaters. There are five different kinds – the white and black rhinoceroses of Africa, and the Indian, Javan, and Sumatran rhinoceroses of Asia. Rhinos usually live on their own, unless they are mothers with young calves. They are short-sighted animals, but have good hearing and an excellent sense of smell. Tapirs are closely related to rhinoceroses. They are stout, pig-like mammals that live mainly in forests. Tapirs are most active at night, when they feed on plants. They are good swimmers and spend much of their time in water. Tapirs are rare in many areas today, because of overhunting by humans.

WHITE RHINOCEROS
With a weight of more than two tonnes, this is the second-largest animal on land (the elephant is largest). It is very shortsighted and sometimes charges at objects it does not recognize. It snips off grasses and other ground plants with its broad, blunt lips. White rhinoceroses are poached for their horns, which some people believe have medicinal properties.

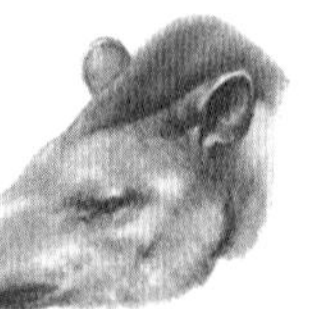

American tapir

Black rhinoceros

White square-lipped rhinoceros

FACES
Black rhinoceroses have long, hooked upper lips. The white rhinoceros has a square-shaped mouth. Tapirs have an elongated snout, used as a snorkel when the animal is in water.

RHINOCEROS HORN
Horn is made of hairlike fibres pressed together into a hard mass; there is no bone inside. The Indian rhinoceros (right) and the Java rhinoceros have only one horn; the other kinds of rhinoceros have two horns.

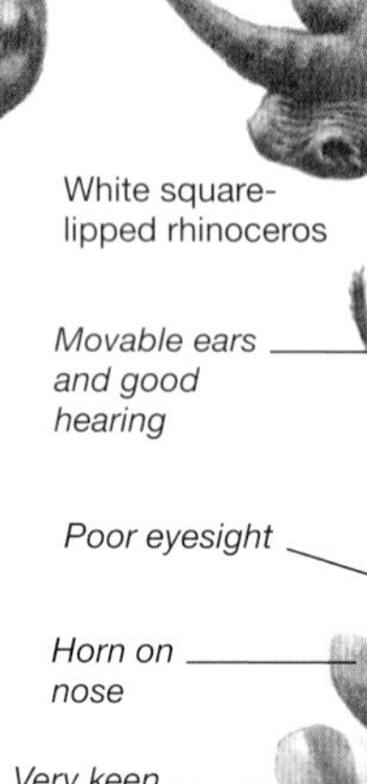

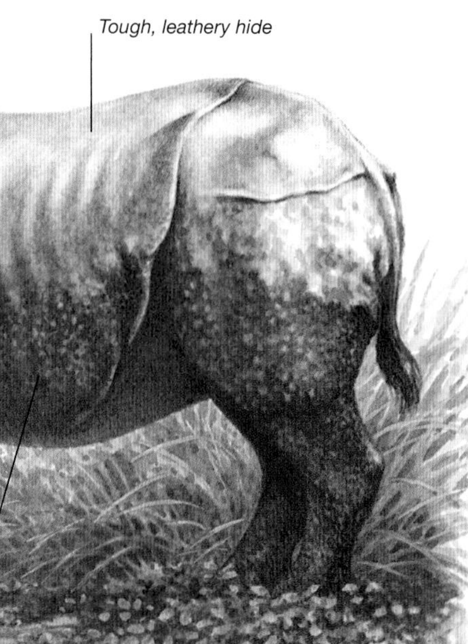

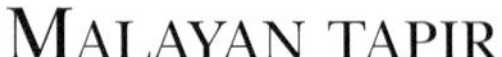

Mud baths keep rhinoceroses cool, and coat their skin for protection against biting insects.

RHINOCEROS HIDE
Rhinoceros skin, or hide, is extremely thick and tough. It hangs in flat sheets, with folds and creases around the legs and neck. It looks like a suit of armour on the Indian rhinoceros shown here. Only the Sumatran rhinoceros has hair on its body; all other rhinoceroses are bald.

MALAYAN TAPIR

Tapirs give birth to one young after a gestation (pregnancy) of 400 days. A newborn Malayan tapir has a spotted coat which gives good camouflage in the dappled forest undergrowth. At about six months, the spots and stripes fade and the tapir begins to look like its parents. An adult tapir has a large white patch on its black body, which helps to break up the animal's shape in dim light.

Find out more
AFRICAN WILDLIFE
ANIMALS
CONSERVATION AND endangered species
MAMMALS

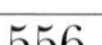

RIVERS

Rain feeds the river system.

WATER RUNS DOWN from high ground, cutting out a channel in the rock as it moves. This flowing water forms a river, which can be fed by a melting glacier, an overflowing lake, or a mountain spring. Rivers shape the landscape as they flow: the water sweeps away soil and eventually creates deep valleys in the land. One of the world's deepest valleys, cut by the River Kali Gandak through the Himalayas, is 5.5 km (3.4 miles) deep. Rivers also flow deep underground, slowly wearing away limestone rocks to form caves.

Rivers are important for transport and as a source of water, which is why most big cities lie on rivers. The longest rivers are the River Nile in Africa, which is 6,670 km (4,145 miles) long, and the River Amazon in South America, which is 6,448 km (4,007 miles) long.

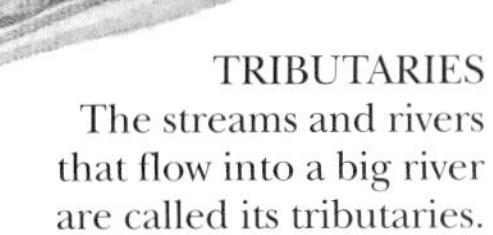

TRIBUTARIES
The streams and rivers that flow into a big river are called its tributaries.

WATERFALL
The river plunges over a shelf of hard rock to form a waterfall.

RIVER SYSTEM

Small rivers and streams feed a large river with water. A river system consists of the whole group of rivers and streams. A watershed, or high ridge, separates one river system from another. Streams flow in opposite directions on either side of a watershed.

GORGE
The waterfall slowly wears away the rock, cutting a deep gorge.

RAPIDS
Fast, swirling currents form where water flows down a steep slope. These parts of the river are called rapids.

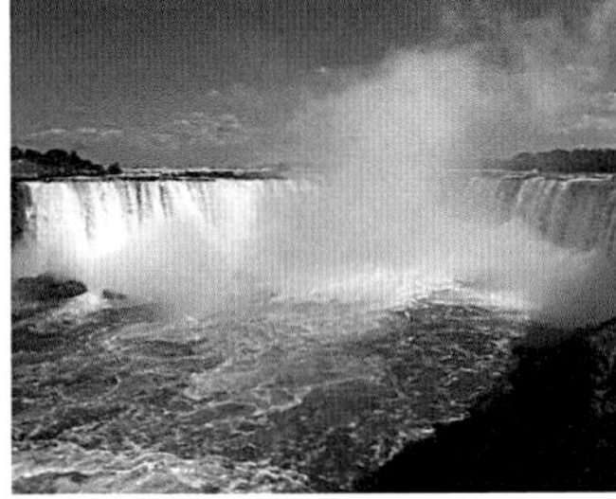

NIAGARA FALLS
The Niagara River plunges almost 55 m (180 ft) at Niagara Falls, which is situated on the border of the United States and Canada.

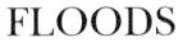

RIVER VALLEY
The river carries along stones and mud, which grind against the river-bed and sides, deepening and widening the V-shaped valley.

Weathering on the valley sides breaks up soft rock and soil. This material falls into the river and is carried away by the current.

OXBOW LAKE
The river cuts through the neck of a loop by wearing away the bank. Material is deposited at the ends of the loop, eventually forming a lake.

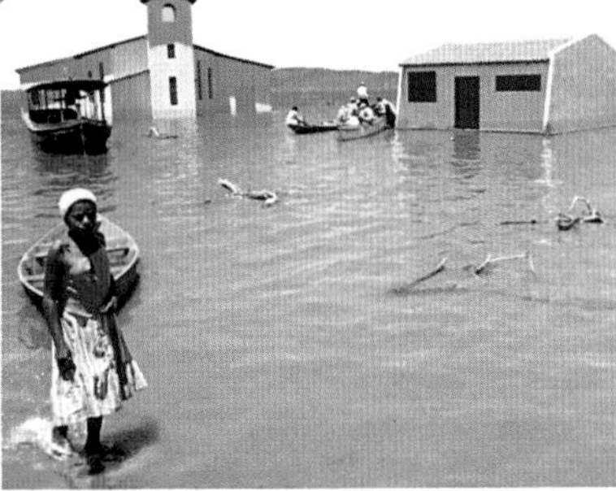

FLOODS
Rivers can overflow with heavy rain, or when water surges up from the sea. Flooding is severe in low-lying places, such as parts of Brazil in South America, which are often hit by tropical storms. Destruction of surrounding forests may be increasing the flow of water, making floods worse.

FLOOD PLAIN
Further down the river, the valley flattens out. This area, called the flood plain, is sometimes submerged during floods. The river runs through the plain in loops called meanders.

USES OF RIVERS

Great rivers that flow across whole countries carry boats that take goods from place to place. Some rivers have dams which build up huge stores of water in reservoirs. This water is used to supply towns and cities, irrigate crops, and generate electricity in hydroelectric power stations. Rivers are also a source of fish, but many rivers are now polluted by farms and factories.

DELTA
The river sometimes fans out into separate streams as it reaches the sea. The streams dump mud which forms an area of flat land called a delta.

Some rivers do not form deltas, but flow into the sea through a single wide channel called an estuary.

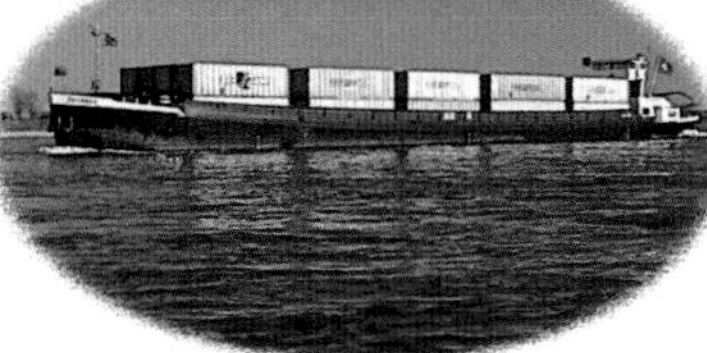

RIVER RHINE
The River Rhine is an important trade route. Barges carry goods between towns in northern Europe.

Find out more

DAMS
GLACIERS AND ICECAPS
LAKE AND RIVER WILDLIFE
LAKES
RAIN AND SNOW
WATER

ROADS AND MOTORWAYS

THE UNITED STATES has more roads than any other country. They stretch more than 6 million km (almost 4 million miles). You would have to drive non-stop at 80 km/h (50 mph) for almost nine years to travel all of them. Great networks of roads and motorways cover most countries. Major motorways link cities, and minor roads crisscross cities and towns to reach neighbourhoods and homes. Cars, coaches, and buses speed along roads and motorways carrying people from place to place. Trucks and lorries bring the goods that we buy in shops. In most countries, motorists drive on the right-hand side of the road. In some countries, including Britain, India, Japan, and Australia, motorists drive on the left. Most large cities contain systems of one-way streets which help traffic to flow smoothly.

ANCIENT ROADS

The Ancient Romans were great road builders. They constructed a system of roads throughout their European empire about 2,000 years ago. These and many other old roads still exist, now surfaced for motor vehicles. Ancient roads were also trade routes. From as early as the 3rd century B.C., the Silk Road was used to bring silk from China across Asia to Europe.

Narrow roads twist through the countryside and over hills, often following old tracks and paths.

Flyovers allow vehicles to change roads without crossing other lines of traffic.

MOTORWAYS

Motorways carry traffic non–stop between cities and around city centres. They are very wide, usually with three lanes in each direction, so they can carry large amounts of traffic. A central barrier separates the two sides of the road.

Bypass carries traffic around the edge of the city, avoiding the city centre.

ROAD BUILDING

To build a major road that carries heavy traffic, bulldozers first clear and level the ground and build embankments or dig trenches if necessary. Drains are laid to carry rainwater away, and the road is then built in several layers. One or more layers of crushed stone are placed on the soil. The top layer can be made of concrete, or a "blacktop" of tar and stone chips. Steamrollers squash down each layer to make it firm.

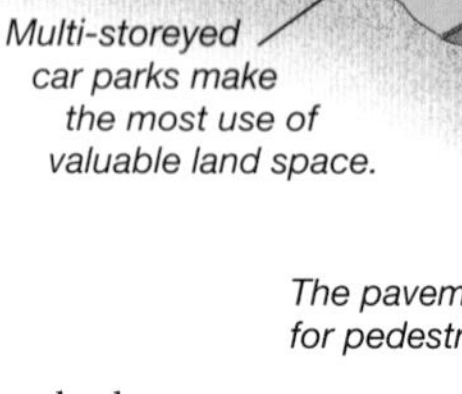

Multi-storeyed car parks make the most use of valuable land space.

The pavement is for pedestrians.

Tarmac or concrete

Layers of crushed stone

Compressed soil

Traffic meets at crossroads, and the vehicles on one road yield to those on the other road.

Pedestrianized street in which vehicles are forbidden

Pedestrian crossing

Bicycle lane

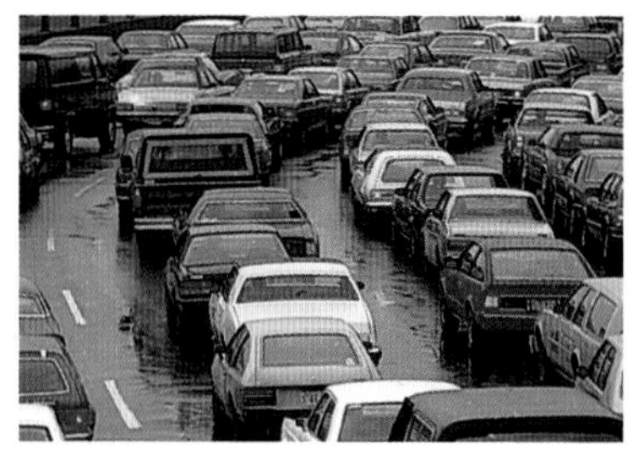

TRAFFIC JAM

By the year 2025, there will be an estimated one billion cars on the world's roads. This will mean an increase in traffic congestion.

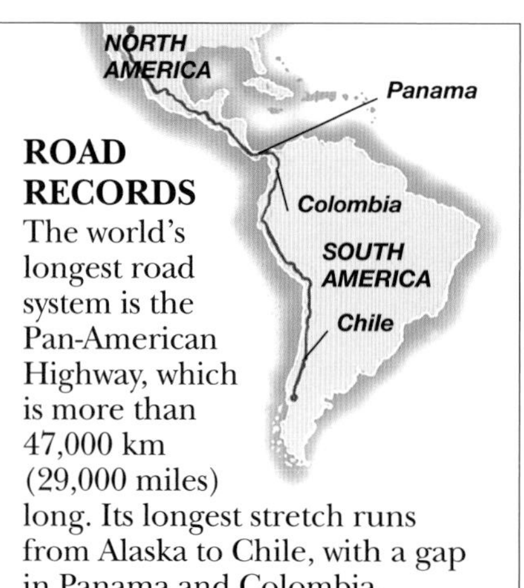

ROAD RECORDS

The world's longest road system is the Pan-American Highway, which is more than 47,000 km (29,000 miles) long. Its longest stretch runs from Alaska to Chile, with a gap in Panama and Colombia.

TRAFFIC CONTROL

Road signs, such as speed limits and warnings of hazards ahead, help make the traffic move more safely. Road markings keep traffic in lanes, and traffic signals keep vehicles from colliding at crossroads. Police officers monitor busy roads using video cameras, and computers control city traffic, operating groups of signals to speed traffic flow and prevent jams.

Find out more

BRIDGES
BUILDING
CITIES
ROMAN EMPIRE
TUNNELS

Robots

WHEN PEOPLE THINK OF ROBOTS, they often imagine the metal monsters of science fiction movies. However, most robots at work today look nothing like this. A robot is a computer-controlled machine that carries out mechanical tasks. The Czech playwright Karel Capek invented the word *robot*, which comes from a Czech word meaning "forced labour". Indeed, robots do jobs that would be dangerous or boring for people to do. Many factories have robots that consist of a single arm that is fixed in one spot. The robot simply repeats a task that it has been instructed to perform, such as spray-painting car parts. Today, engineers are developing much more sophisticated robots. These robots can move around, and their electronic detectors enable them to sense their surroundings. They also have "intelligence", which means that they can respond to what they see and hear and make decisions for themselves. Intelligent robots are designed to act as guards and firemen, and may travel into space to study distant worlds.

SCIENCE FICTION ROBOTS
The robots of science fiction, such as C3-P0 from the film *Star Wars*, are often anthropoid (human-like). In reality, anthropoid robots are rare. However, Japanese engineers have built experimental robots with two legs.

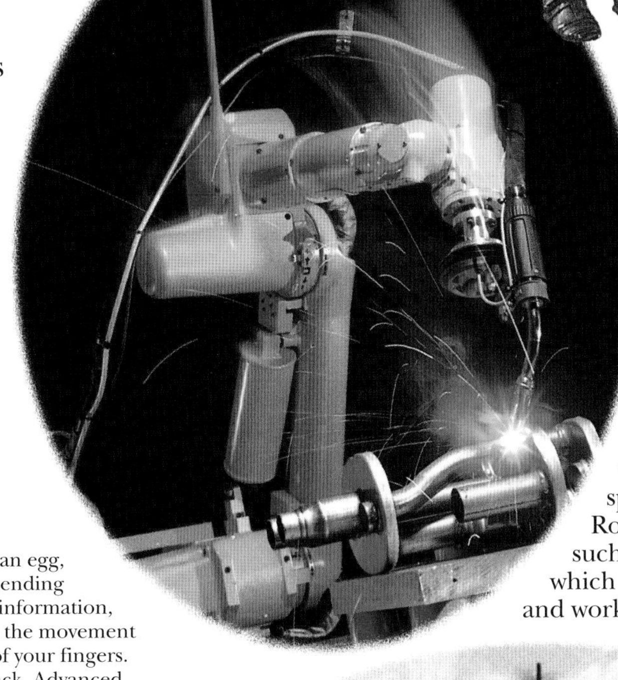

Robot arm

Sophisticated robots work in factories, assembling, spraying, and welding components (parts). A skilled welder or painter will have programmed the robot by leading it (or a similar robot) through the task. Some robots can understand simple spoken instructions too. Robots often have sensors such as laser vision systems which help the robots to find and work on complex parts.

Held too tightly – loosen grip.

Brain sends nerve signals to muscles in the hand, adjusting the strength of the grip so the egg is neither dropped nor squashed.

Held too loosely – tighten grip.

Touch sensors in your hand detect how hard you are pressing on the egg.

FEEDBACK
When you pick up an egg, your senses begin sending signals to your brain. From this information, your brain automatically adjusts the movement of your hand and the pressure of your fingers. This adjustment is called feedback. Advanced robots control their actions by feedback from electronic detectors such as lasers, television cameras, and touch sensors.

SPACE ROBOT
In January 2004, two unmanned exploration rovers, *Spirit* (right) and *Opportunity*, touched down on Mars. They photographed the planet and analysed samples of rock. Robot space probes such as these are designed to obey instructions from controllers on Earth, but decide for themselves how to carry out the orders.

Space probes need to be able to work independently because radio instructions could take minutes or even hours to travel from Earth.

This bomb disposal robot runs on tracks so that it can climb into awkward places. It carries cameras to send back pictures to the operator, and a gun for detonating the bomb.

REMOTE CONTROL
Mobile robots do dangerous jobs such as repairing and dismantling nuclear reactors and detonating concealed bombs. These robots are remotely controlled – a human operator controls the general actions of the robot from a safe distance, and onboard computers control detailed movements.

Find out more

COMPUTERS
FACTORIES
TECHNOLOGY

ROCK AND POP

Bono and The Edge, members of Irish rock band U2.

A NEW TYPE OF MUSIC EMERGED IN THE USA in the 1950s. First known as rock and roll, it is now called rock music. It drew on many different musical styles including folk, gospel, blues, country and western, classical, and world music. The main thing that distinguished rock music from any previous music was that it was played, and often written by, young people rebelling against the music and lifestyles of their parents. Pop music is a softer style of rock. Image is very important in the world of rock and pop, with fans identifying with particular groups or singers by copying their clothes and hairstyles, and rock and pop is listened to all over the world. Millions of people of all ages buy and play rock and pop music. It is a mass-market industry.

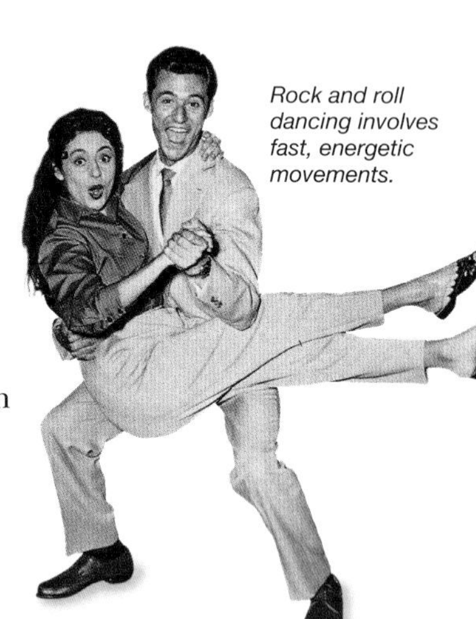

Rock and roll dancing involves fast, energetic movements.

ROCK AND' ROLL

Teenagers in the 1950s rebelled against the slow, romantic music that their parents liked. They wanted their own kind of music to listen to: loud, fast, rhythmic songs which they could, literally, rock and roll to on a Saturday night.

INSTRUMENTS

The first rock and roll bands were formed in the 1950s, with Bill Haley and the Comets' hit Rock Around the Clock launching the new music style. The new bands featured electric guitars and drum kits, giving their music great volume and rhythm. Since then, the classic band line-up has consisted of a singer, lead guitarist, rhythm guitarist, bass guitarist, and drummer.

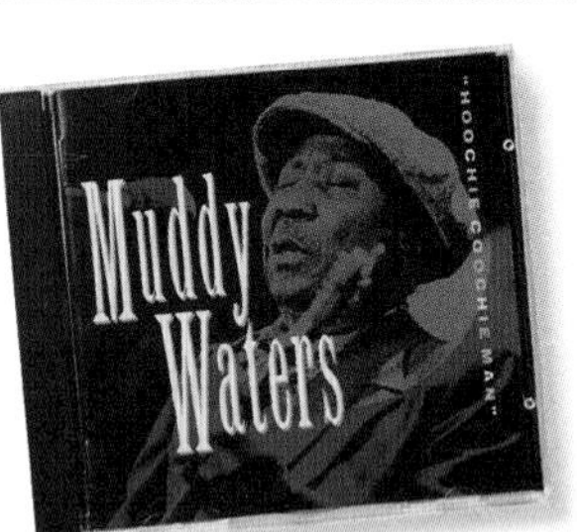

RHYTHM AND BLUES

In the 1940s, US blues musician Muddy Waters (1915-83), and others, took the haunting blues music of rural black America and played it fast and loud on electric guitars. This new music – rhythm and blues – influenced rock music.

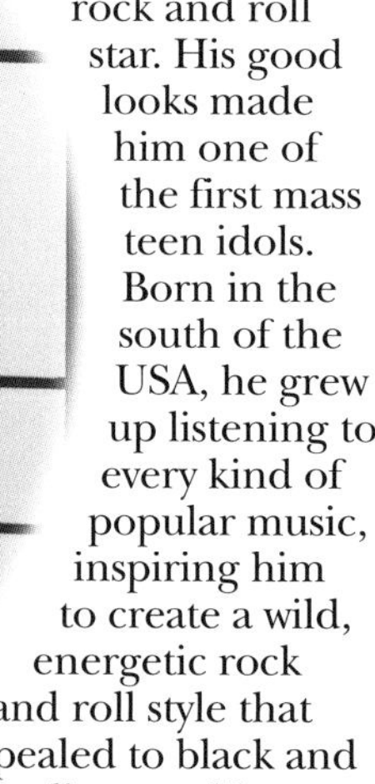

ELVIS PRESLEY

Singer Elvis Presley (1935-77) was the first international rock and roll star. His good looks made him one of the first mass teen idols. Born in the south of the USA, he grew up listening to every kind of popular music, inspiring him to create a wild, energetic rock and roll style that appealed to black and white audiences alike.

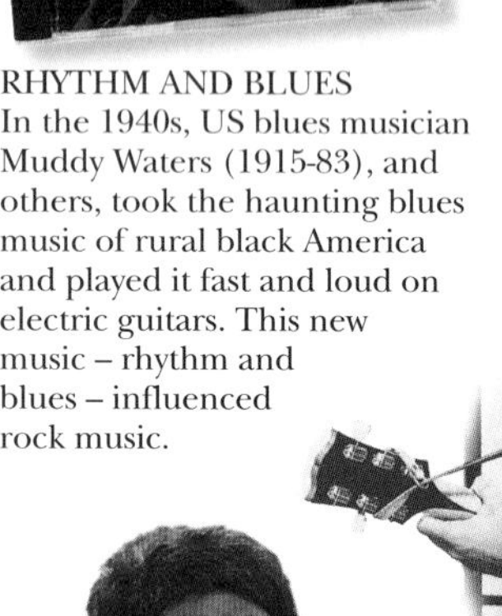

Aretha Franklin

SOUL MUSIC

Written and performed by black US musicians such as Marvin Gaye (1939-84) and Otis Redding (1941-67), soul music was a fusion of blues and gospel music. Many soul musicians, notably Aretha Franklin (b. 1942), began by singing gospel music in church. Franklin sings soul music with similar power and emotion.

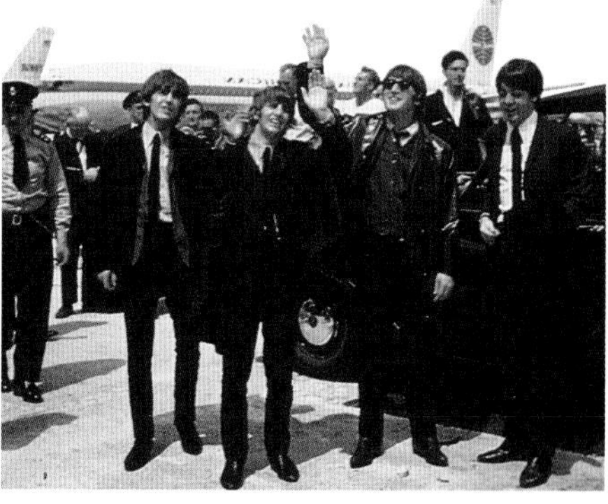

THE BEATLES

Four young musicians from Liverpool, England – John Lennon, Paul McCartney, George Harrison, and Ringo Starr – first recorded together in 1962. By 1964 their group, the Beatles, was the biggest rock band in the world. They broke up in 1970, but their songs are still hugely popular today.

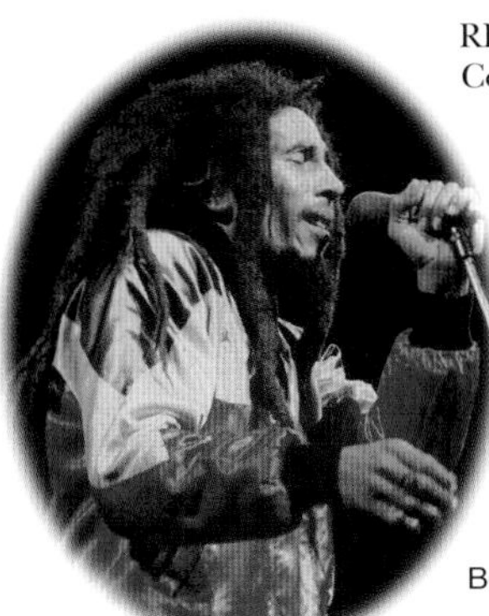

REGGAE
Coming from the Caribbean island of Jamaica, reggae music is influenced by jazz, gospel, rhythm and blues, and soul. It is an infectious music combining catchy melodies with words of strength and hope. The most important reggae star, Bob Marley (1945-81), turned reggae into an international music.

Bob Marley

Woodstock attracted over 400,000 people.

The festival was held on a farm site.

Woodstock music festival

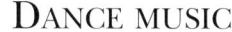

Rock festivals

Rock festivals began in the 1960s on the west coast of the USA, when thousands of people turned up to hear free, all-day concerts. The most famous festival ever took place at Woodstock, New York State, in 1969, with performers such as Jimi Hendrix, Janis Joplin, and The Who. Today, most festivals are large, commercially organized events, where you can hear a wide range of rock and pop bands.

ROCK AND POP

1951 First rock and roll records.

1954 Elvis Presley records *That's All Right*, his first single.

1955-58 Elvis has a run of 14 million-selling records, including *Heartbreak Hotel*.

1962 Beatles record *Love Me Do*, their first single.

1964 Beatles have top five singles in US charts.

1965 Bob Dylan introduces electric guitar to folk music.

1967 Aretha Franklin makes her first soul records.

1969 Woodstock festival.

1975 Bob Marley becomes major international star with *No Woman No Cry*.

1976 Punk music erupts.

1983 Madonna's first album.

1995 "Britpop" dominates the UK charts.

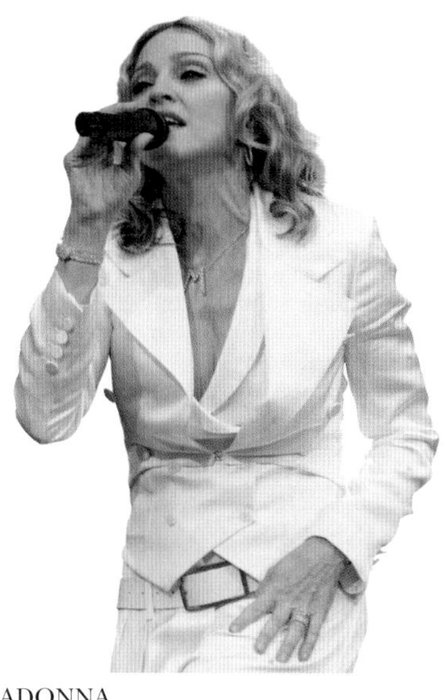

MADONNA
US singer Madonna (b. 1958) started out in the early 1980s, singing simple pop songs. She soon became one of the most successful recording artists of recent years, with huge-selling albums. Her fame is partly due to her ever-changing image.

Dance music

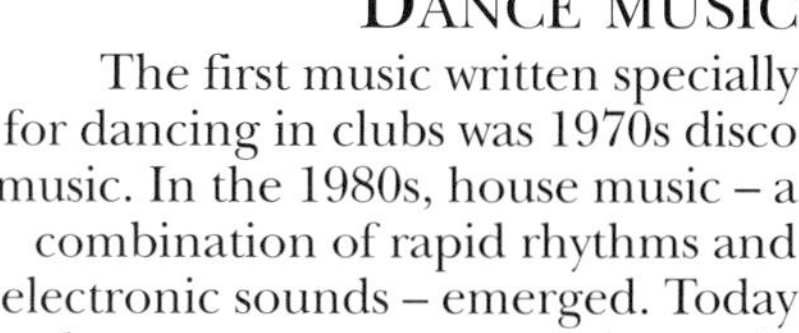

The first music written specially for dancing in clubs was 1970s disco music. In the 1980s, house music – a combination of rapid rhythms and electronic sounds – emerged. Today there are many types of electronic music, including house, breakbeat, and drum and bass.

Norman "Fatboy Slim" Cook.

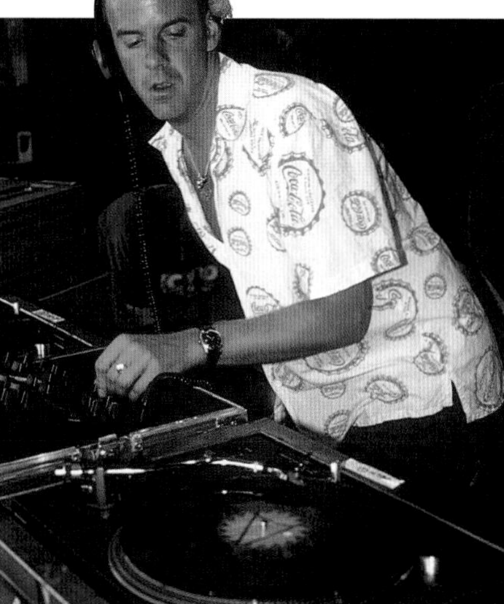

OutKast is one of the most popular mainstream hip hop acts.

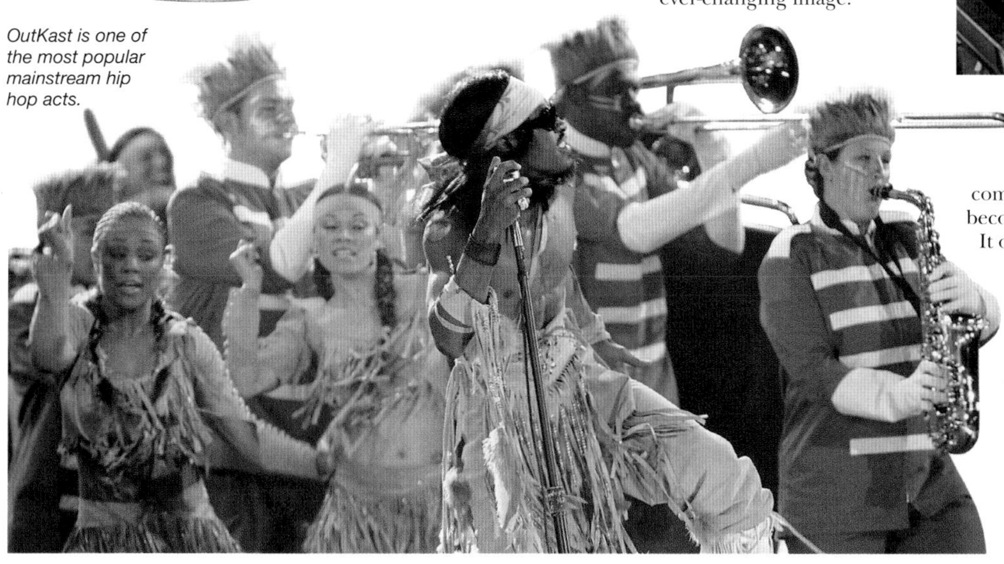

HIP HOP
Hip hop is a type of popular music, which began in the African American communities of New York in the 1970s and has become hugely successful around the world. It often features effects produced using turntables, samples from other records, and rhythmic vocals known as rap. OutKast, a duo from Atlanta, Georgia, USA, are one of the most successful hip hop acts ever, having sold more than 20 million albums worldwide.

Find out more
Dance
Music
Musical instruments

ROCKETS AND MISSILES

THE INVENTION OF THE ROCKET ENGINE was a landmark in history. Not only did it give humans a tool with which to explore space, but it also produced the missile, a weapon of terrible destructive power. A rocket engine is the most powerful of all engines. It has the power to push a spacecraft along at more than 40,000 km/h (25,000 mph), the speed necessary for it to break free from Earth's gravity. In a rocket engine, fuel burns to produce gases that rush out of the nozzle at the back, thrusting the rocket forward. However, unlike other engines, rockets do not need to use oxygen from the air to burn their fuel. Instead they carry their own supply of oxygen, usually in the form of a liquid, so that they can operate in space where there is no air. There is one major difference between a missile and a space rocket: missiles carry an explosive warhead instead of a satellite or human cargo.

Third stage fires for about 12 minutes, carrying its satellite payload into orbit about 320 km (200 miles) above the Earth's surface.

Once first stage has run out of fuel, it falls away and second stage takes over, burning for about two minutes.

First stage propels rocket for about three minutes, by which time rocket is more than 50 km (30 miles) above the Earth.

A few seconds after takeoff, booster fuel is expended.

SPACE ROCKET

Most space rockets are made up of several stages, or segments, each with its own rocket engines and propellant, or fuel. By detaching the stages as they are used, the rocket can reach higher speeds because its weight is kept to a minimum. There are two main types of rocket propellant: solid and liquid. Solid fuel burns rapidly and cannot be controlled once ignited. But rockets powered by liquid propellant can be controlled by opening and closing valves that adjust the flow of fuel into the engine.

NUCLEAR MISSILES

Deadly nuclear warheads and precise navigational systems make nuclear missiles the most dangerous weapons in the history of warfare. A single warhead has the power to destroy a large city and cause millions of deaths. Nuclear missiles can be launched from submarines, aircraft, trucks, and hidden underground launch sites.

ARIANE ROCKET

Vehicle equipment bay contains satellite that is being carried into orbit.

Guidance systems keep rocket on the correct course.

Third stage with one liquid-propellant rocket

Tank containing oxidizer, a liquid that contains oxygen

Tank containing highly inflammable liquid fuel

Pumps push fuel and oxidizer to the nozzle, where they burn and produce a violent rush of hot gases that push the rocket upwards.

Second stage with one liquid-propellant rocket

Two solid-propellant and two liquid-propellant strap-on booster rockets give space rocket an extra push in the first part of its flight.

First stage with four liquid-propellant rocket engines

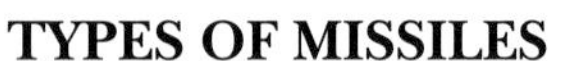

TYPES OF MISSILES

Huge intercontinental ballistic missiles (ICBMs) blast up into space and come down on their targets thousands of kilometres away. However, not all rocket-powered missiles travel into space; many have replaced guns for short-range attacks on tanks, ships, and aircraft. Many of these missiles home in on their targets automatically.

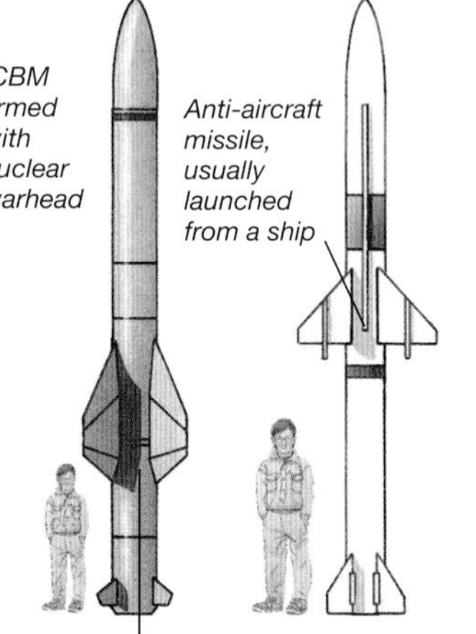

ICBM armed with nuclear warhead

Anti-aircraft missile, usually launched from a ship

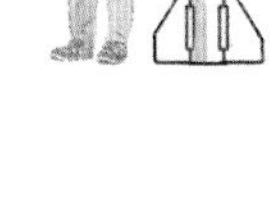

Radar-guided anti-ship missile. It can be launched from the air, from land, or from a warship.

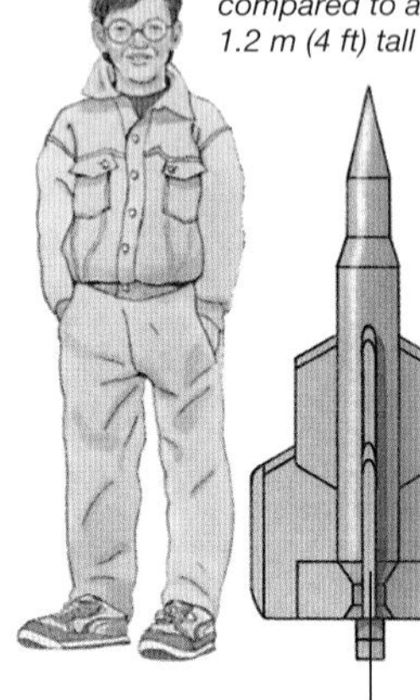

Size of rockets compared to a child 1.2 m (4 ft) tall

Anti-tank missile, guided to target by remote control

DEVELOPMENT OF ROCKETS

In the 13th century, the Chinese used a simple type of rocket powered by gunpowder to scare enemy horses. Six hundred years later, Englishman Sir William Congreve developed a gunpowder rocket that the English forces used during the Napoleonic Wars. During World War II (1939-45), German scientist Wernher von Braun invented the first successful long-range rocket, the V-2, the forerunner of the ICBM.

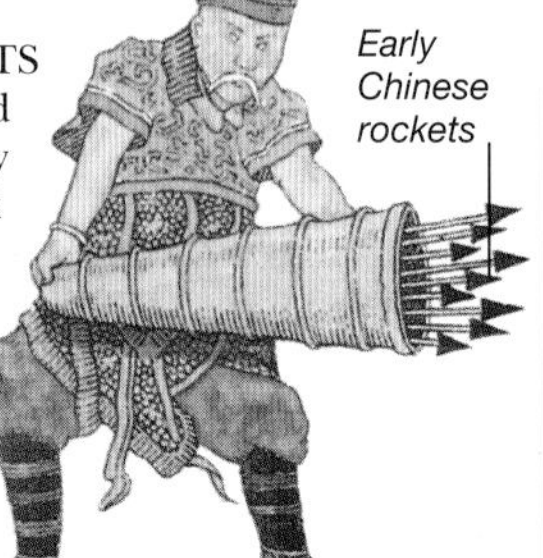

Early Chinese rockets

Find out more

MILITARY AIRCRAFT
NAPOLEONIC WARS
NUCLEAR AGE
NUCLEAR ENERGY
SPACE FLIGHT
SUBMARINES
WEAPONS
WORLD WAR II

ROCKS AND MINERALS

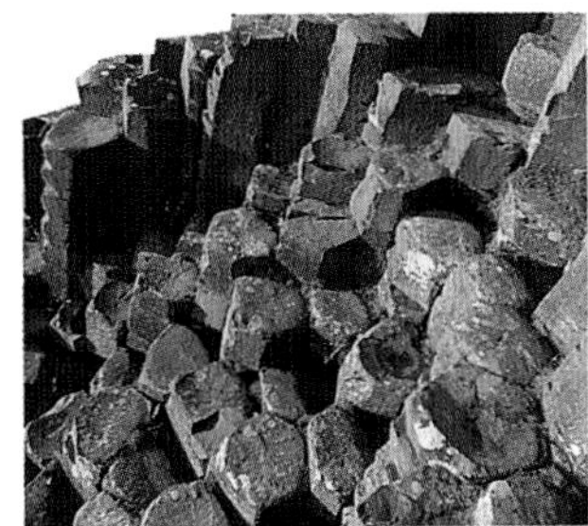

GIANT'S CAUSEWAY
The steps of this unusual rock formation in Northern Ireland are made of columns of basalt, rock which developed when lava from a volcano cooled and set. The rock cracked into columns as it cooled.

WE LIVE ON THE SURFACE of a huge ball of rock, the Earth. The landscape everywhere is made up of rocks. Most are covered by soil, trees, or grass. Others, such as Uluru (Ayers Rock) in Australia, a massive lump of sandstone 348 m (1,142 ft) high, rise from the ground and are visible. The oldest rocks on Earth are about 3,800 million years old. Other rocks are much more recent, and new rocks are forming all the time. All rocks contain substances called minerals. Marble consists mainly of calcite, for example, and granite contains the minerals mica, quartz, and feldspar.

Rocks form in different ways: from molten rock within the Earth, from the fossils of animals and plants, and by the action of heat and pressure on ancient rocks inside the Earth. But no rocks, however hard, last forever on the Earth's surface. They are slowly eroded, or worn away, by the action of wind, rain, and other weather conditions.

HOW ROCKS FORM

All rocks started out as clouds of dust in space. The dust particles came together and formed the rocks that make up the planets, moons, and meteorites. There are now three main kinds of rocks on the Earth's surface: igneous, sedimentary, and metamorphic rocks. Each kind of rock forms in a different way.

Mud and pebbles are buried and squashed together, producing a hard sedimentary rock called conglomerate.

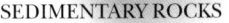

Bubbles of gas trapped in the lava created holes in this piece of rock.

When lava from a volcano cools on the Earth's surface, it forms basalt.

IGNEOUS ROCKS
Deep underground the heat is so intense that some rock is molten (melted). When it cools, this molten rock, or magma, sets hard to produce an igneous rock. This may happen underground, or the magma may rise to the surface as lava and solidify.

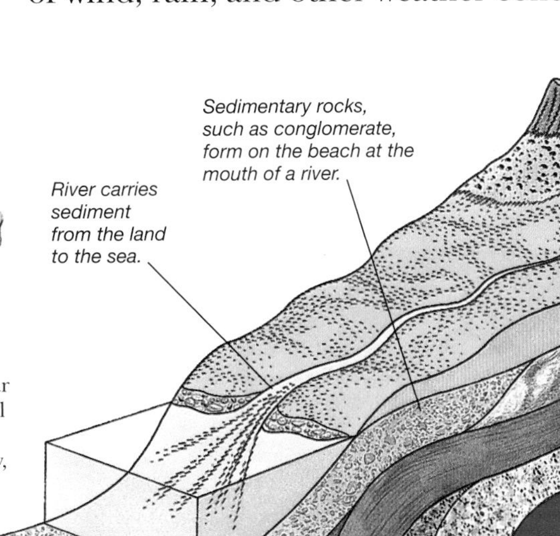

Lava flows from a volcano and solidifies, forming basalt, an igneous rock.
Sedimentary rocks, such as conglomerate, form on the beach at the mouth of a river.
River carries sediment from the land to the sea.
Red-hot magma heats surrounding limestone, turning it into marble.
Hot magma solidifies, forming granite, an igneous rock.
Shale forms from clay at the river bed.

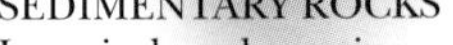

SEDIMENTARY ROCKS
Ice, wind, and running water wear away rocks into pebbles and small particles called sediment. Layers of sediment containing sand, clay, and animal skeletons are buried and squeezed so that they slowly change into hard rocks called sedimentary rocks.

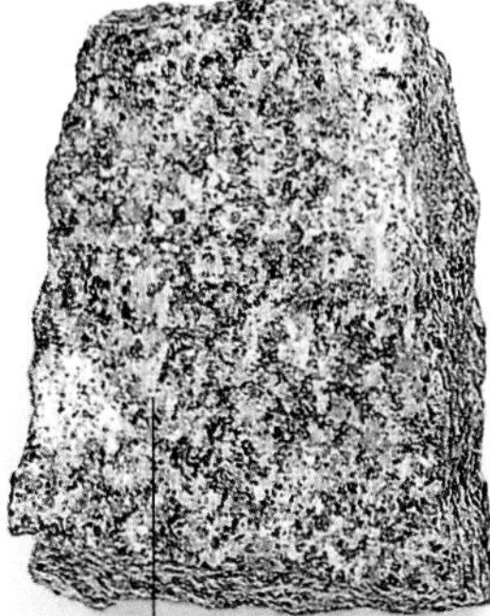

When magma slowly cools deep underground, it often forms granite, a hard rock which is used as a building material.

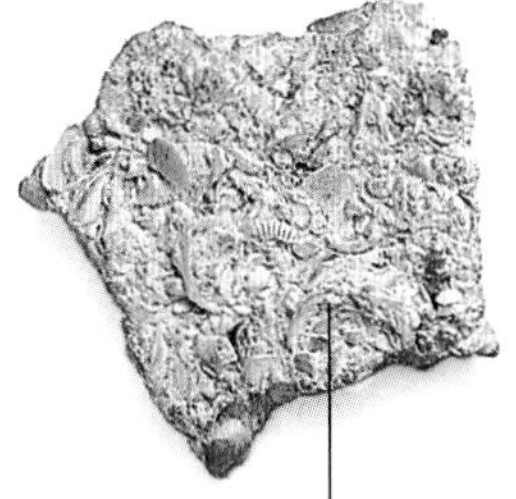

Limestone contains the remains of shellfish. Chalk, another kind of limestone, is made of the skeletons of sea animals.

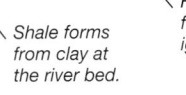

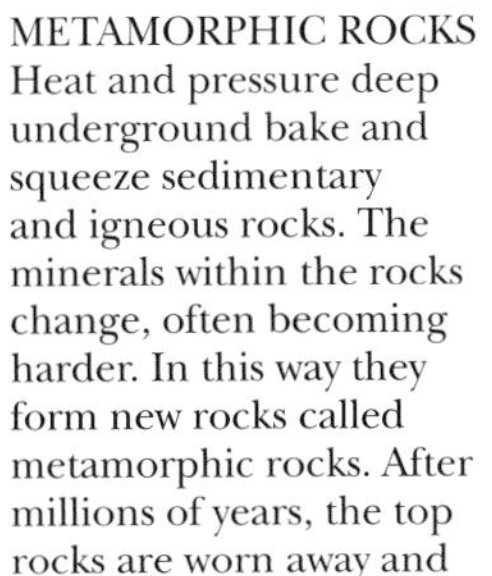

Clay forms shale, a sedimentary rock that crumbles easily. This rock is slate, the metamorphic rock which forms from shale.

METAMORPHIC ROCKS
Heat and pressure deep underground bake and squeeze sedimentary and igneous rocks. The minerals within the rocks change, often becoming harder. In this way they form new rocks called metamorphic rocks. After millions of years, the top rocks are worn away and metamorphic rocks appear on the surface.

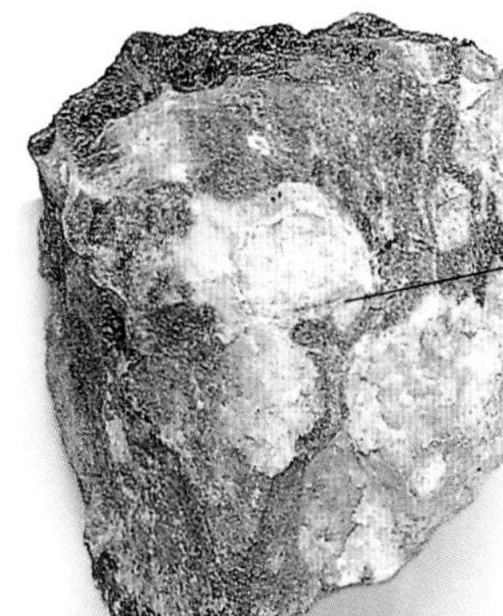

Heating and compressing limestone turns it into marble, a hard metamorphic rock.

MINERALS

An impressive rock collection will feature rocks that contain beautiful mineral crystals. Minerals are the different substances of which rocks are made. For example, limestone and marble contain the white mineral calcite. Minerals include precious stones such as diamonds, and ores – minerals that contain metals such as iron and aluminium. Almost all metals are produced by mining and quarrying ores, and then treating the ores to extract their metals.

DESERT ROSE
The mineral gypsum forms petal-shaped crystals in deserts and dry regions. This happens as water dries up, leaving mineral deposits behind. The crystals often look like flowers, so they are called desert roses or gypsum flowers.

TURQUOISE
Jewellers cut beautiful gemstones and ornaments from turquoise, a blue-green mineral that often runs in a thin vein through other rocks.

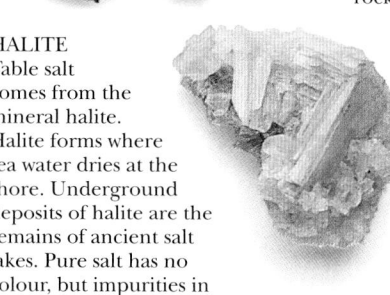

HALITE
Table salt comes from the mineral halite. Halite forms where sea water dries at the shore. Underground deposits of halite are the remains of ancient salt lakes. Pure salt has no colour, but impurities in halite give it a pink colour.

SULPHUR
Yellow crystals form when molten sulphur cools. Large underground deposits in places such as the United States provide sulphur for making rubber and chemicals.

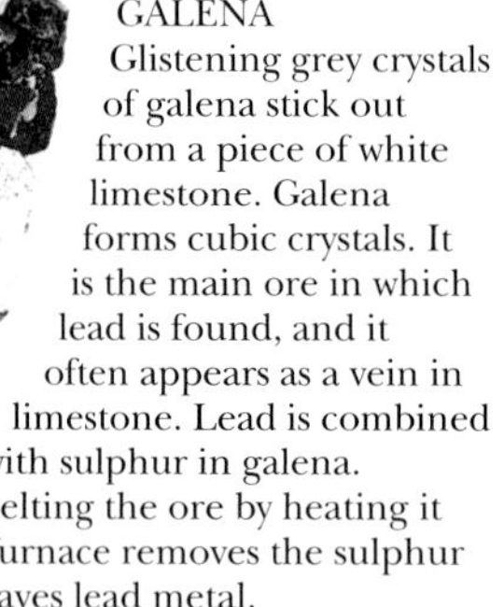

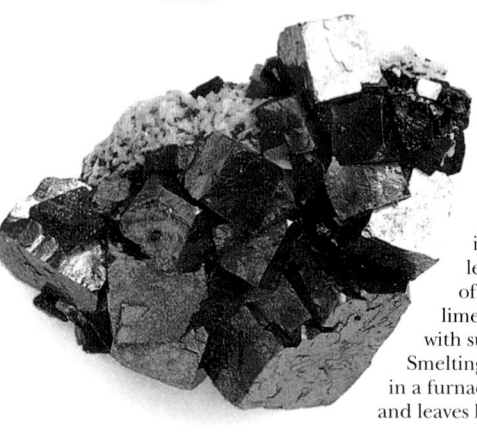

GALENA
Glistening grey crystals of galena stick out from a piece of white limestone. Galena forms cubic crystals. It is the main ore in which lead is found, and it often appears as a vein in limestone. Lead is combined with sulphur in galena. Smelting the ore by heating it in a furnace removes the sulphur and leaves lead metal.

CRYSTALS

Minerals often form crystals – solids which grow in regular shapes with flat sides. Light sparkles from crystals because they are often transparent and have smooth, shiny surfaces. Each mineral forms crystals with particular shapes, such as columns and cubes. Crystals grow from molten minerals or minerals that are dissolved in liquids, such as water.

Hexagonal crystals form in six-sided columns.

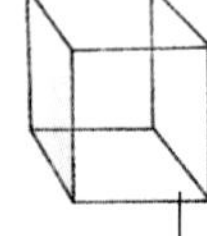

Cubic crystals form in four-sided columns.

Some minerals, such as solecite, form needle-shaped crystals.

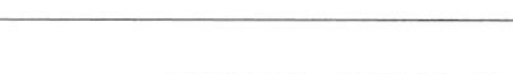

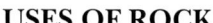

Crystals form in columns, such as in this piece of the mineral beryl.

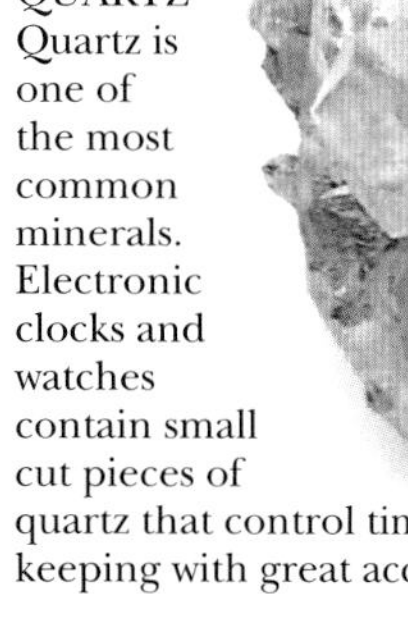

QUARTZ
Quartz is one of the most common minerals. Electronic clocks and watches contain small cut pieces of quartz that control time-keeping with great accuracy.

USES OF ROCK

Rocks in one form or another surround us in towns, cities, and the countryside. Hard rocks such as granite, sandstone, and limestone provide good building materials for houses and walls, and roads contain fragments of crushed rock. Soft rocks have uses too. Heating clay or shale with crushed limestone produces cement for making concrete and laying bricks. Bricks themselves are made by baking clay in moulds.

The first tools were made of stone. Early people broke pieces of rocks and stone to make sharp cutting implements such as axes.

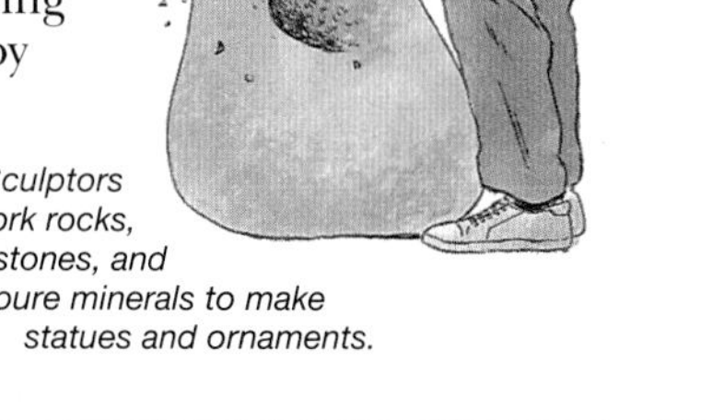

Sculptors work rocks, stones, and pure minerals to make statues and ornaments.

Find out more

ATOMS AND MOLECULES
CLOCKS AND WATCHES
COMETS AND METEORS
FOSSILS
GEMS AND JEWELLERY
GEOLOGY
VOLCANOES

ROMAN EMPIRE

TWO THOUSAND YEARS AGO a single government and way of life united most of western Europe, the Middle East, and the north coast of Africa. The Roman Empire was based on good organization and centralized control. Towns in different countries were planned in exactly the same way. A network of stone-paved roads (parts of which remain today) connected every area to Rome. The reign of the first emperor, Augustus, began a long period of stability known as the Pax Romana, or Roman Peace, which lasted for about 200 years. Strong border defences manned by the Roman army protected the empire, while a skilled civil service governed it. Trade flourished and the people were united. The empire reached the height of its power in about A.D. 200 and then began to decline slowly. It was divided into two parts in 284. In 476, barbarian tribes conquered the Western Empire (based in Rome). The Eastern Empire (based in Constantinople, now called Istanbul, Turkey) continued until 1453.

GRAFFITI
The Romans were fond of making fun of each other. This caricature was found on a wall in Pompeii. It is a mockery of a leading local citizen – probably a noble, judging from his laurel wreath.

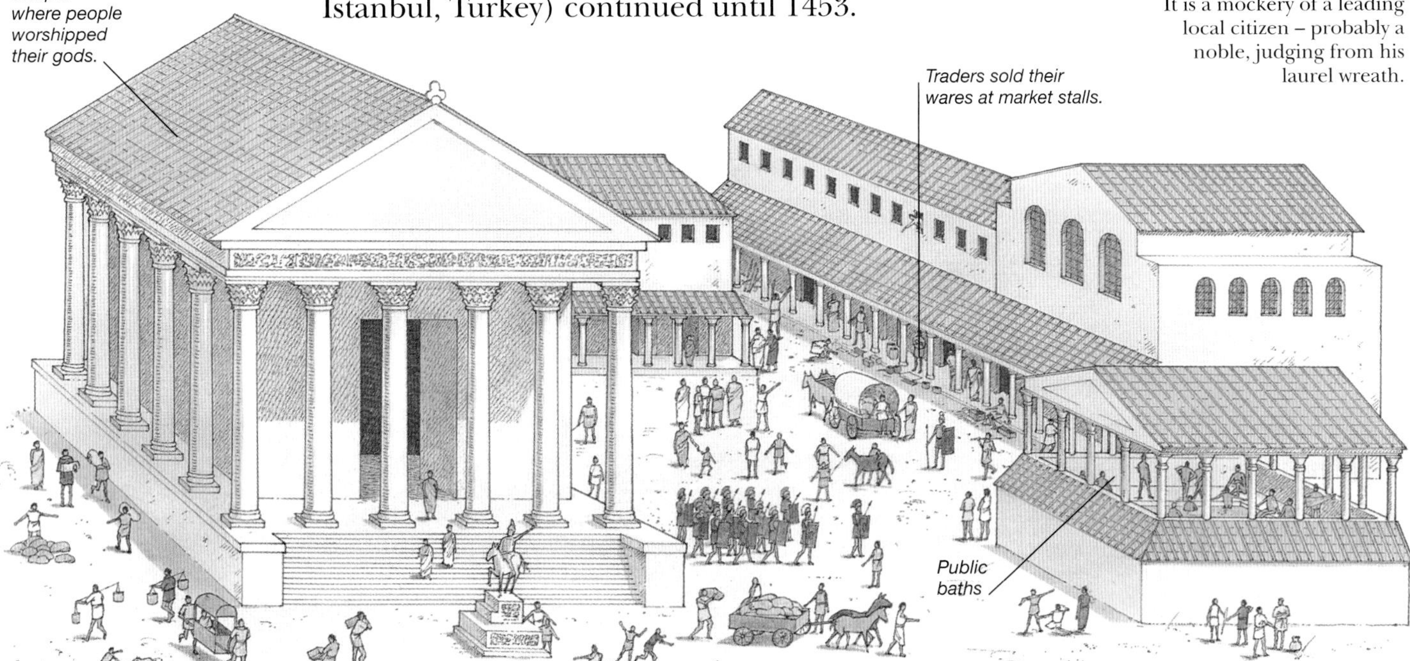
Temple where people worshipped their gods.
Traders sold their wares at market stalls.
Public baths

CITY LIFE

Roman cities were carefully planned with straight streets, running water, and sewers. The forum, or central market-place, was surrounded by shops, law courts, and the town hall. The rich, always Roman citizens, lived in fine villas; the poor lived in apartment-style buildings. There were many temples. Most of the hard work was done by slaves, who had none of the rights granted to citizens, such as access to the baths.

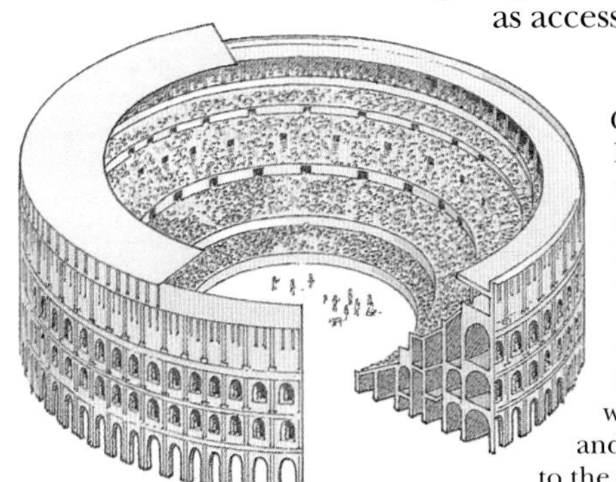

COLOSSEUM
Emperors paid for expensive public games, such as chariot racing, in order to be popular with the crowds. In Rome a massive theatre called the Colosseum held 45,000 people, who watched gladiators and wild animals fight to the death.

ROMAN BATHS

The Romans loved bathing. They scraped off the dirt, rubbed oil into their skin, relaxed in steam rooms, swam in warm pools, and plunged into icy water.

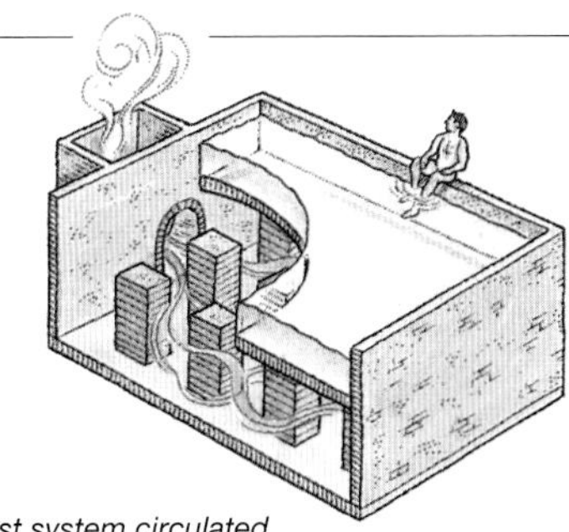

The hypocaust system circulated hot air under the floors and through the walls to heat houses and baths.

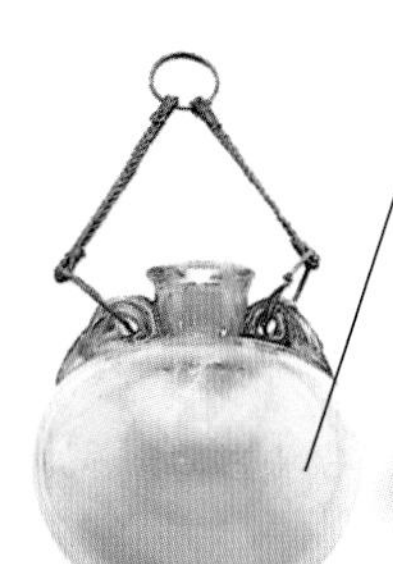

People rubbed oil, which they carried in oil flasks, on their bodies.

Bathers scraped the sweat and dirt off their bodies with strigils.

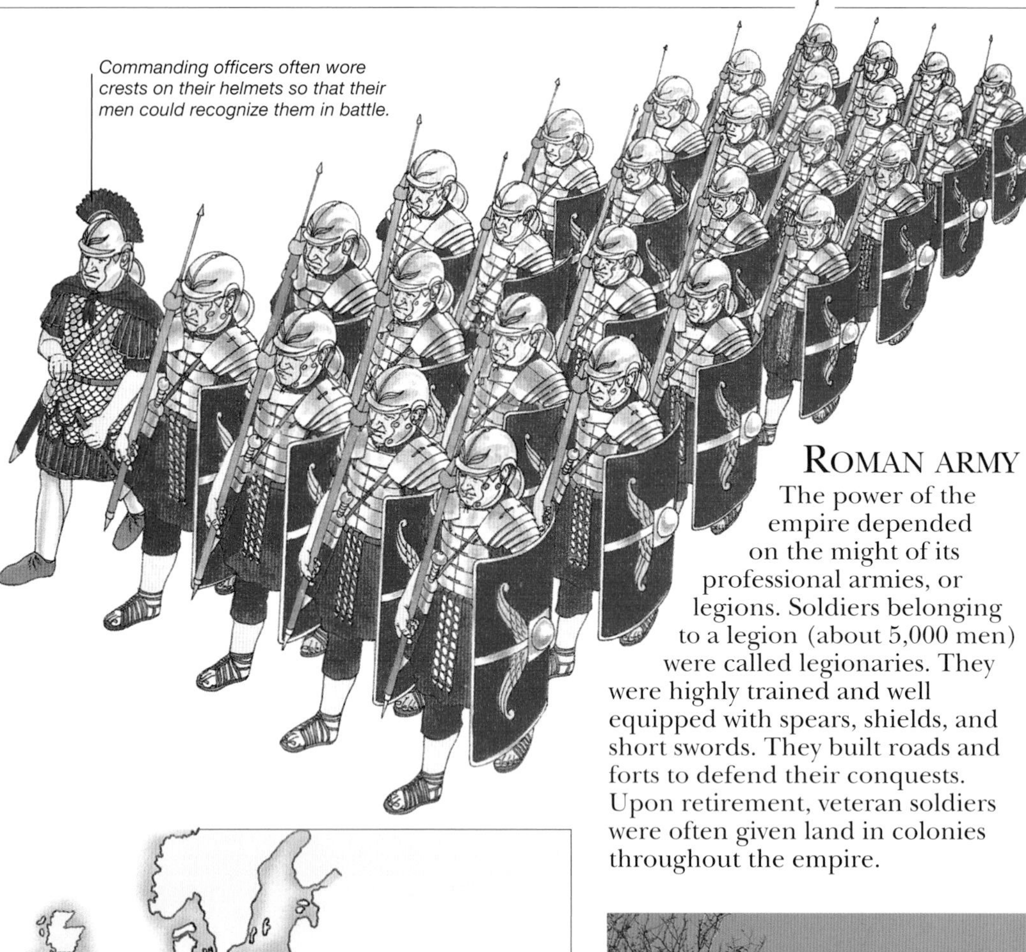

Commanding officers often wore crests on their helmets so that their men could recognize them in battle.

ROMAN ARMY

The power of the empire depended on the might of its professional armies, or legions. Soldiers belonging to a legion (about 5,000 men) were called legionaries. They were highly trained and well equipped with spears, shields, and short swords. They built roads and forts to defend their conquests. Upon retirement, veteran soldiers were often given land in colonies throughout the empire.

ROMAN EMPIRE

c.753 B.C. First settlement built.

509 B.C. Etruscans driven out of Rome. Republic established.

275 B.C. Italy conquered. Expansion overseas begins.

146 B.C. Destruction of Carthage gives Rome control of Spain and North Africa.

71 B.C. Slaves revolt, led by Spartacus.

52 B.C. Gaul (France) conquered by Julius Caesar.

44 B.C. Caesar assassinated.

27 B.C. Augustus becomes first emperor.

A.D. 43 Claudius conquers Britain.

A.D. 117 Empire reaches its greatest size.

A.D. 284 Empire splits into two halves.

A.D. 410 Visigoths sack Rome.

A.D. 476 Western part of the Empire falls.

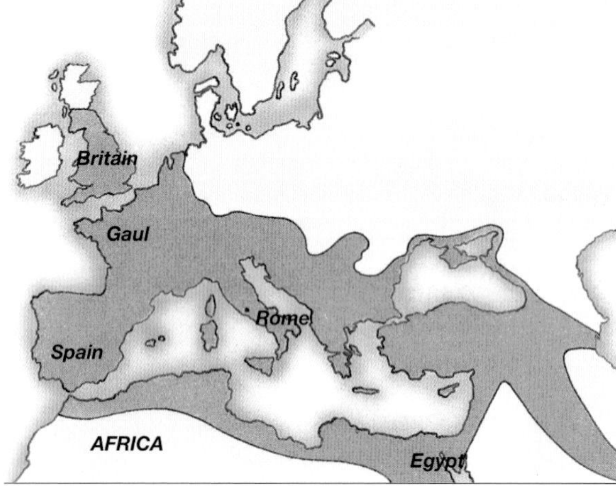

THE ROMAN EMPIRE
At its height the Roman Empire stretched from the Middle East to Britain. The inhabitants were of many different races and spoke many different languages.

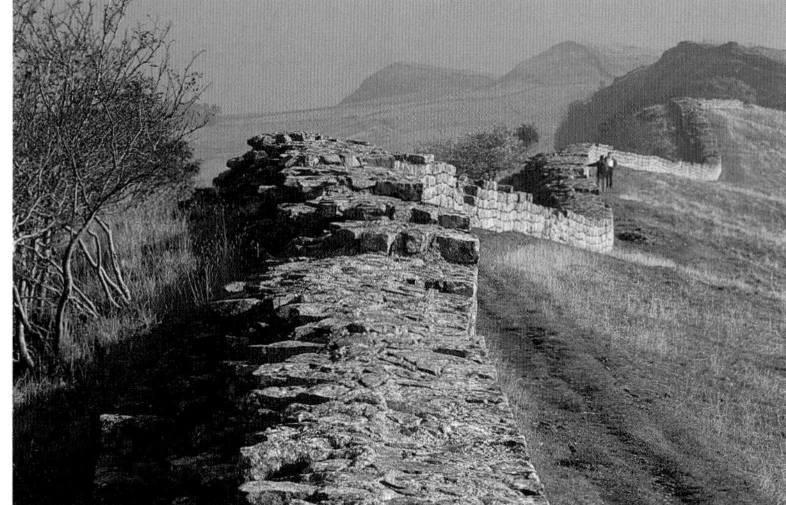

HADRIAN'S WALL
The emperor Hadrian ordered a wall to be built across northern Britain to defend Roman lands from the fierce, unconquered tribes who lived in the mountains of Scotland. The wall, parts of which can still be seen today, was 120 km (75 miles) long, and studded with forts. The army built defensive ditches, fortress bases, and signal towers along it.

TECHNOLOGY AND CRAFTS

The Romans were highly skilled engineers and craftworkers. Their towns had water supplies and drains, and rich people lived in centrally heated houses. The houses often had detailed mosaics on the floors. Artisans worked with glass, metals, bone, and clay to make beautiful objects that have lasted to this day.

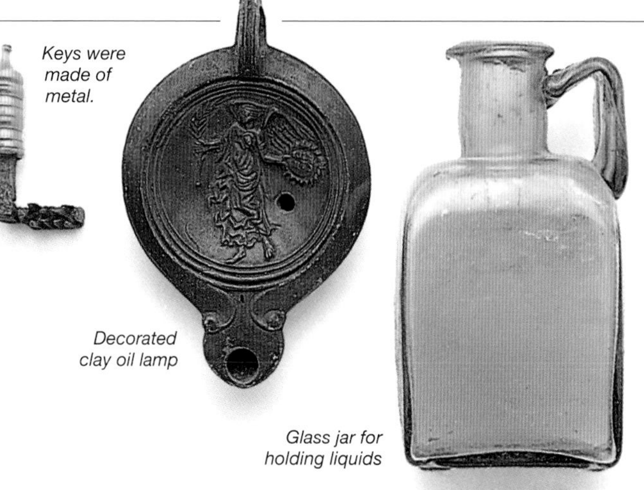

Keys were made of metal.

Decorated clay oil lamp

Glass jar for holding liquids

Find out more
ARMIES
BARBARIANS
BYZANTINE EMPIRE
CAESAR, JULIUS
ITALY, HISTORY OF

FRANKLIN DELANO
ROOSEVELT

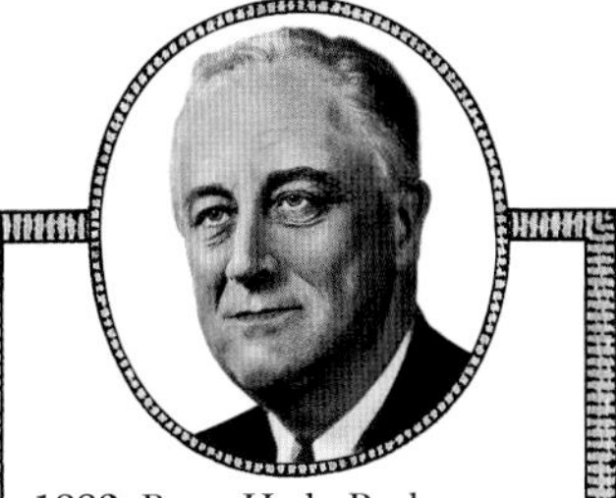

1882 Born Hyde Park, New York.

1905 Earns law degree.

1910 Elected to New York state senate.

1913-20 Assistant secretary of the navy.

1920 Runs for vice president.

1921 Afflicted by polio.

1928 Elected governor of New York.

1932 Elected president of the United States.

1933 Institutes New Deal.

1936, 1940, 1944 Re-elected president.

1941 United States enters World War II after Japanese bomb Pearl Harbor naval base, Hawaii.

1945 Roosevelt dies just before the end of the war.

IN 1932 THE UNITED STATES was at one of its lowest points in history. Thirteen million people – nearly one third of the country's work force – were unemployed. Then a new president was elected with a mission to make Americans prosperous again. When Franklin Delano Roosevelt was disabled by polio in the summer of 1921, it appeared to be the end of a promising political career. But Roosevelt was a fighter and, helped by his wife, Eleanor, he regained the partial use of his legs. In 1928 he was elected governor of New York, then ran for president in 1932. He won a landslide victory, and for 13 years – the longest time any United States president has ever served – Roosevelt worked to overcome the effects of unemployment and poverty, telling Americans that "the only thing we have to fear is fear itself". He launched the New Deal – a series of social reforms and work programmes. During World War II, Roosevelt proved to be an able war leader, and with his Soviet and British allies he did much to shape the postwar world.

FIRESIDE CHATS
President Roosevelt was an expert communicator who used the then new medium of the radio to explain his controversial policies to the nation. These informal "fireside chats" established firm links between the President and the American people.

NEW DEAL

During the Depression of the 1930s, Roosevelt promised a New Deal. The government provided jobs for the unemployed and tried to return the country to prosperity. New laws were passed that provided better conditions for workers and pensions for retired workers.

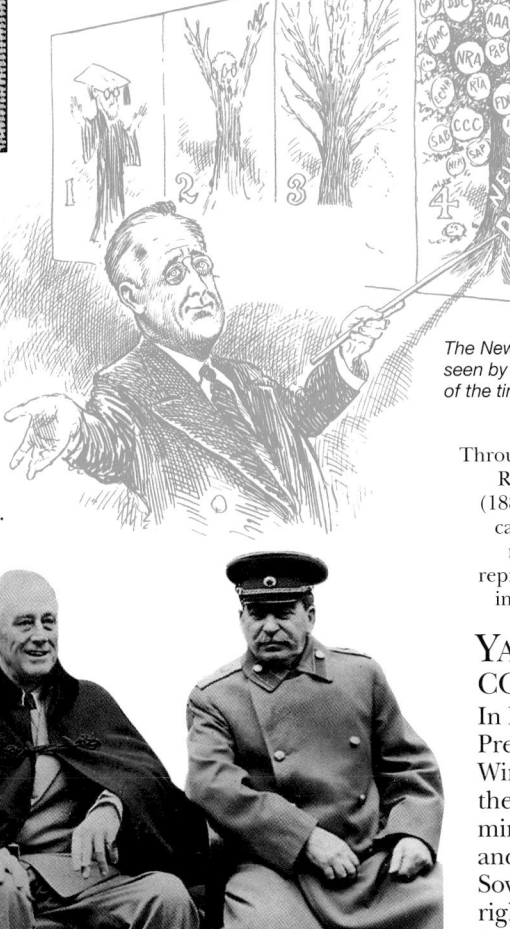

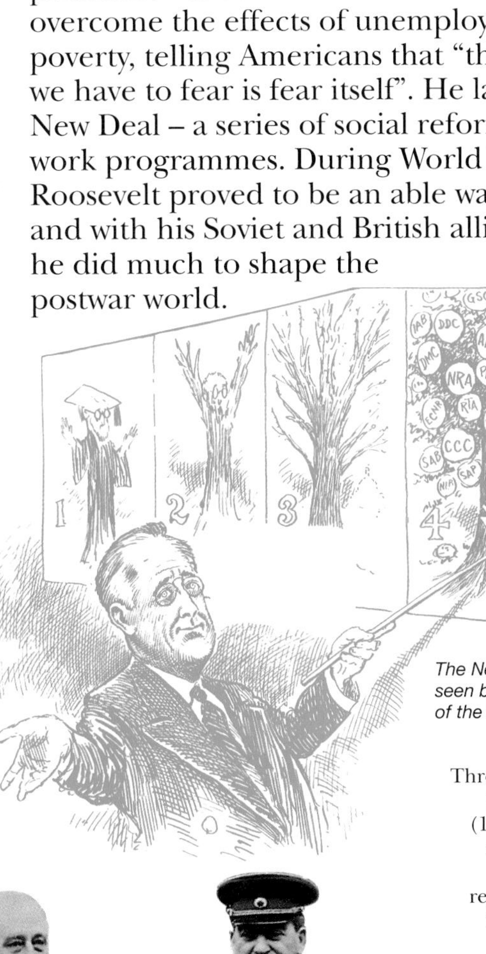

The New Deal as seen by a cartoonist of the time.

ELEANOR ROOSEVELT
Throughout her life President Roosevelt's wife, Eleanor (1884-1962), was a tireless campaigner for human rights. After 1945 she represented her country in the United Nations.

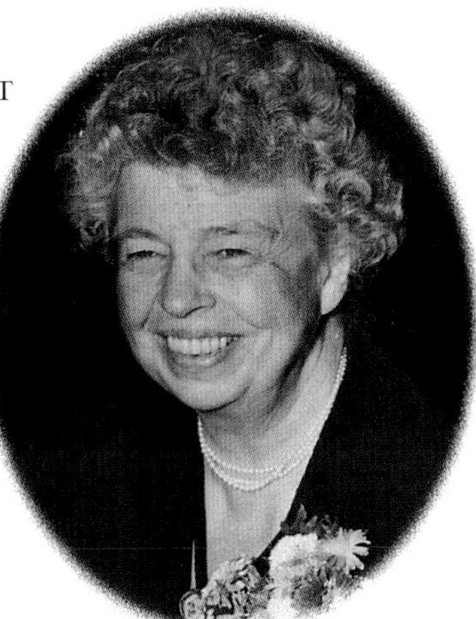

YALTA CONFERENCE

In February 1945, President Roosevelt, Winston Churchill, the British prime minister (far left), and Joseph Stalin, Soviet premier (far right), met in the Soviet resort of Yalta to discuss the postwar world. Together they decided to set up the United Nations.

Find out more
DEPRESSION of the 1930s
UNITED NATIONS
UNITED STATES OF AMERICA, history of
WORLD WAR II

RUSSIAN FEDERATION

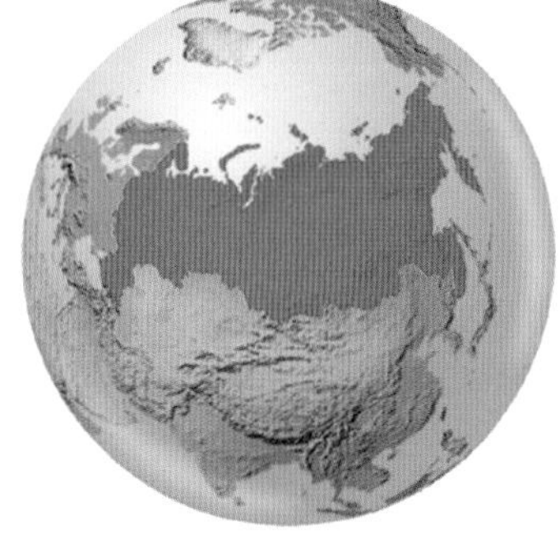

The Russian Federation stretches from eastern Europe in the west across the entire width of Asia to the Pacific Ocean in the east, and from the Arctic Circle in the north to Central Asia in the south.

THE LARGEST NATION in the world is the Russian Federation. Also called Russia, it consists of 20 autonomous (self-governing) republics, and more than 50 other regions. It covers one-tenth of the earth's land area – one-third of Asia, and two-fifths of Europe. Russia has a very varied climate and a landscape that ranges from mountains in the south and east to vast lowlands and rivers in the north and west. The population is varied too, although most of the 143 million people are of Russian origin and speak the Russian language. The Russian Federation came into being in 1991 after the break up of the Soviet Union, or U.S.S.R. After 1991, the Russian people experienced greater political freedom but also economic hardship as their country changed from a state-planned to a free-market economy. The Russian Federation has vast agricultural resources. It is also rich in minerals, and has considerable industry. Although many people in Russia are very poor, the country now has some of the world's richest billionaires.

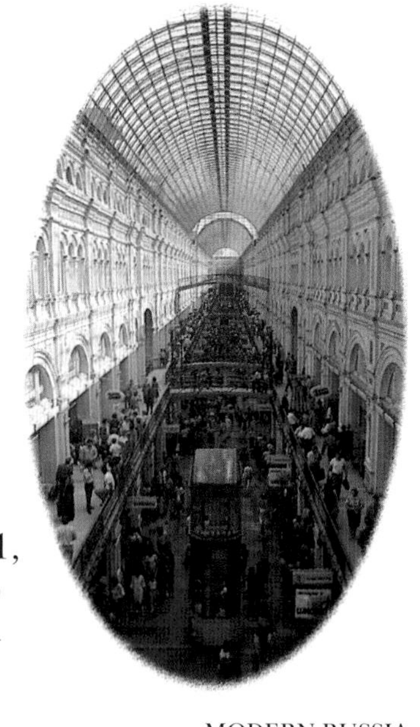

MODERN RUSSIA
Large Russian cities look similar to cities elsewhere in the world, but the bright lights hide economic problems. Both luxury and essential goods are often in short supply. Lining up for food (above) is a daily occupation, and clothes and consumer goods are scarce and often of poor quality. Most homes are rented from the government, but housing is in limited supply, which means that overcrowding is common.

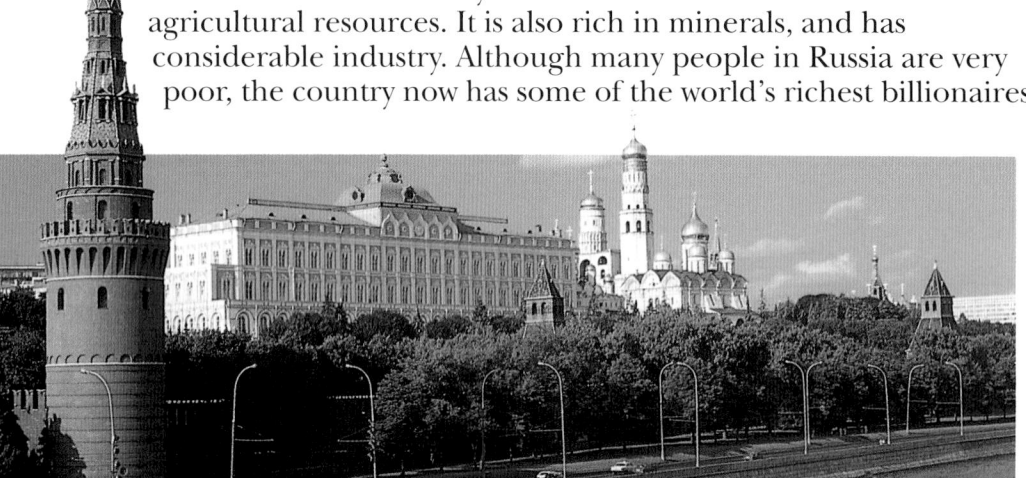

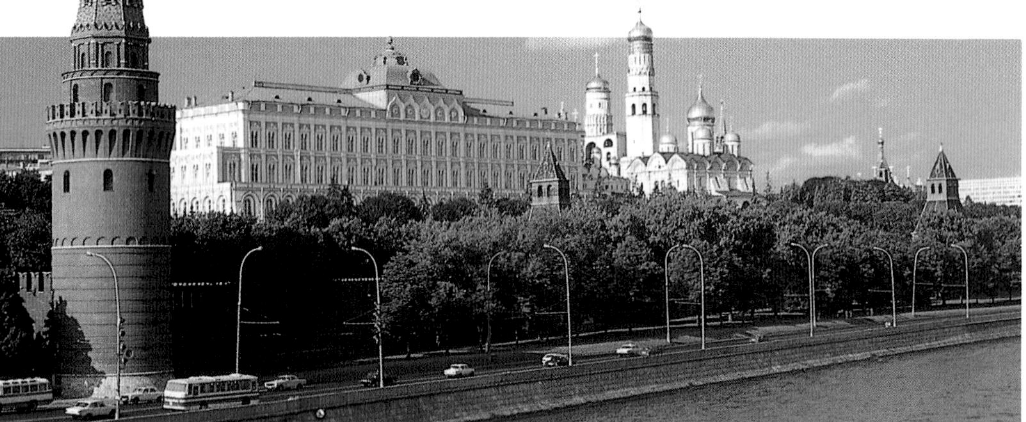

MOSCOW

The capital city of the Russian Federation is Moscow. It was founded during the 12th century. At the city's heart, on the banks of the Moscow river, lies the Kremlin. This is a walled fortress housing all the government buildings. Within these walls lies the impressive Red Square. The stunning St. Basil's Cathedral stands at the southern end of the square. It was built in the 16th century to celebrate a military victory.

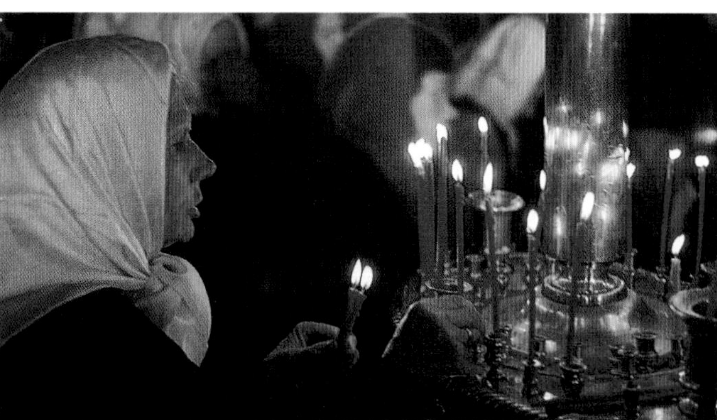

RUSSIAN ORTHODOX CHURCH
The chief religion in Russia is the Russian Orthodox Church. Under Communism, all religions were persecuted. In the late 1980s, freedom of worship returned to Russia, and today millions of people worship without fear (above). The Russian Federation also contains many Muslims, Jews, and Buddhists.

ST. PETERSBURG
The second-largest city in the Russian Federation, St. Petersburg has a population of 4.5 million. Before 1917, St. Petersburg (called Leningrad from 1924 to 1991) was the capital of Russia. It still contains many beautiful, historical buildings, such as the Hermitage Art Gallery, once the summer palace of the czars.

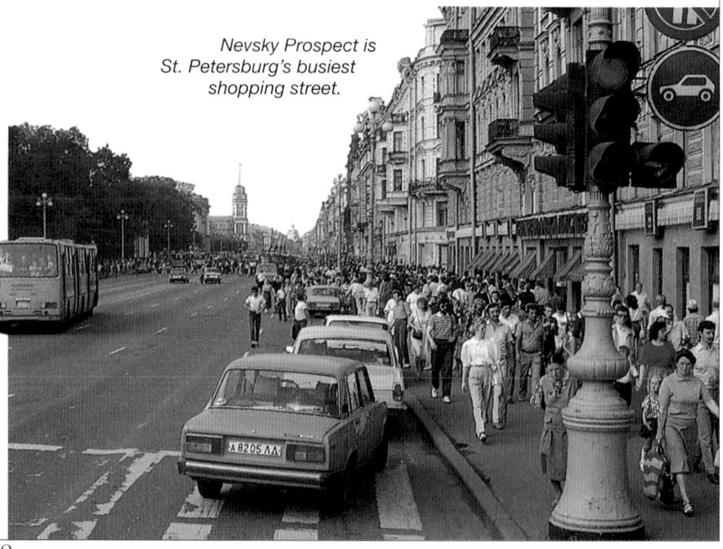

Nevsky Prospect is St. Petersburg's busiest shopping street.

AGRICULTURE

Most agriculture in the Russian Federation takes place on the fertile Russian plain that stretches from the western border into Central Asia. Here, farmers produce wheat and other cereals, meat, dairy products, wool, and cotton. The Russian Federation is one of the world's biggest cereal producers, but often fails to grow enough food to feed its own population and has to import grain.

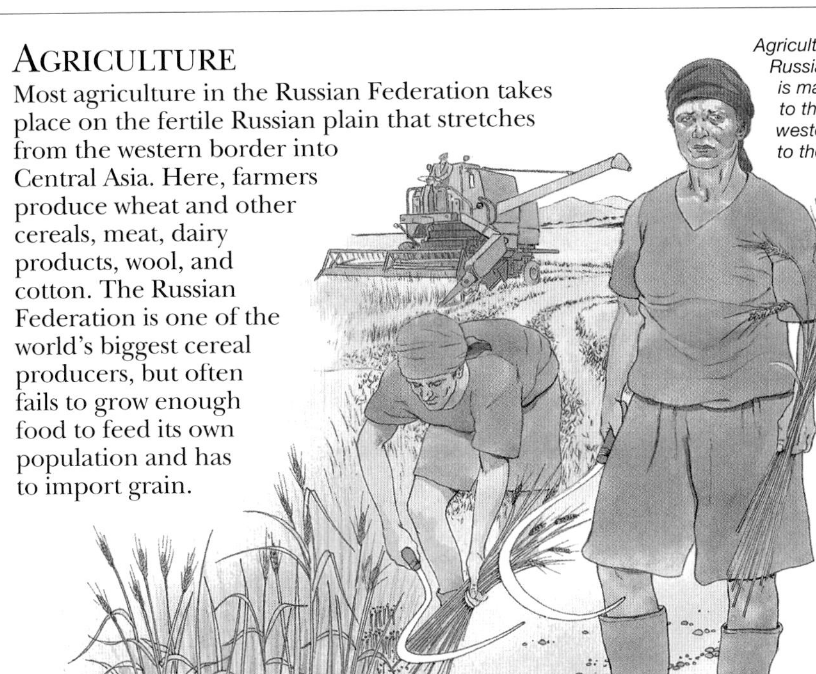

Agriculture in the Russian Federation is mainly confined to the southern and western regions due to the cold climate in the northern margins.

RUBLES AND KOPECKS

The unit of Russian money is the ruble, which is divided into 100 kopecks. Following the break up of the Soviet Union in 1991, Russia moved from a state-planned to a free-market economy. This led to economic instability and fluctuating exchange rates. In recent times the currency has begun to stabilise.

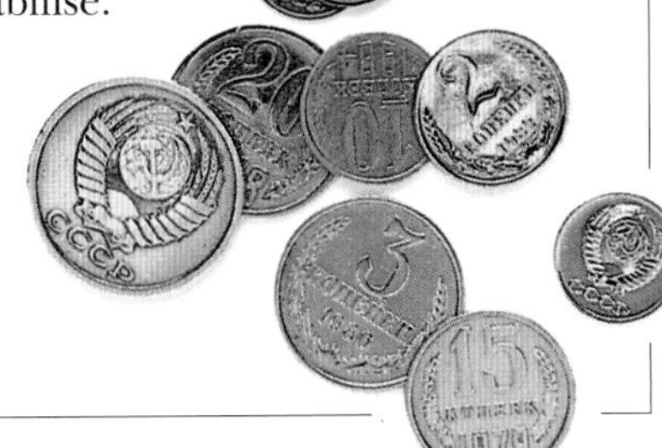

RUSSIAN PEOPLE

Most people in the Russian Federation are Russian in origin. But there are at least 100 minority groups, including Tatars, Ukrainians, Bashkirs, and Chukchis. Some, such as the Yakut hunters, shown here in traditional clothing, are Turkish in origin; other groups are Asiatic. The population is not spread evenly through this vast nation. About 75 per cent live west of the Ural Mountains; less than 25 per cent live in Siberia and the far east of the country.

The Yakut (left) are distributed across a large area centred on the Lena river. The economy of the more southerly Yakut is based on the husbandry of cattle and horses, while the Yakut further north engage in hunting, fishing, and herding.

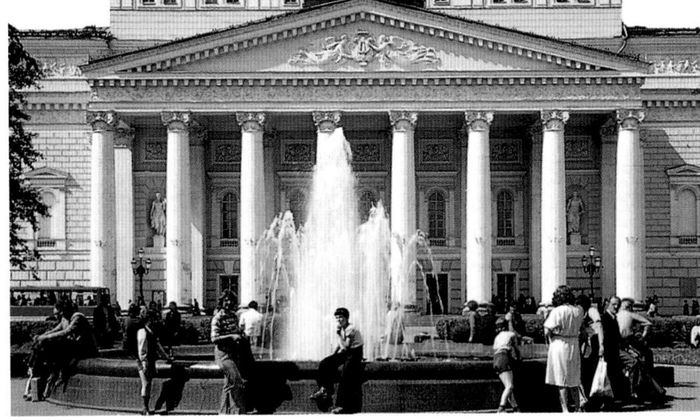

The Bolshoi Theatre, home of the Bolshoi Ballet

BOLSHOI BALLET

The world-famous Bolshoi Ballet dance company was founded in Moscow in 1773. It became famous touring the world with performances of Russian folk dances and classic ballets such as *Swan Lake*. Other Russian art forms did not enjoy the same freedom of expression under the old Soviet regime. Artists opposed to the Communist government worked in secret. For example, the novels of Aleksandr Solzhenitsyn (born 1918) were banned for many years. His most famous works, such as *The Gulag Archipelago*, were smuggled in from Europe or retyped by readers and circulated secretly.

Ленингра́д

RUSSIAN LANGUAGES

In the Russian Federation more than 112 languages including Tatar, Ukrainian, and Russian are spoken. Russian is the primary language of the majority of people in Russia, and is also used as a second language in other former republics of the Soviet Union. Russian writers use the Cyrillic alphabet, shown here.

TECHNOLOGICAL ACHIEVEMENTS

As part of the Soviet Union, Russian science developed unevenly. Today, the Russian Federation leads the world in some medical techniques, particularly eye surgery (right), but lags far behind Western Europe and the United States in areas such as computers. In the field of space research, the Soviet Union led the world, launching the first satellite in 1957, and putting the first man in space, Yuri Gagarin, in 1961. More recently, the Russians have launched the first paying passengers into space.

SIBERIA

The vast region of Siberia is in the northeast of the Russian Federation, and stretches from the Ural Mountains in the west to the tip of Alaska in the east. Although Siberia occupies nearly 80 per cent of the land area of the Russian Federation, it is thinly populated. Most Siberian people live close to the route of the Trans-Siberian Railway, which runs for 9,438 km (5,864 miles) between Moscow and Vladivostok. Much of northern Siberia lies inside the Arctic circle, and during the summer months the sun never sets, but simply dips close to the horizon at night.

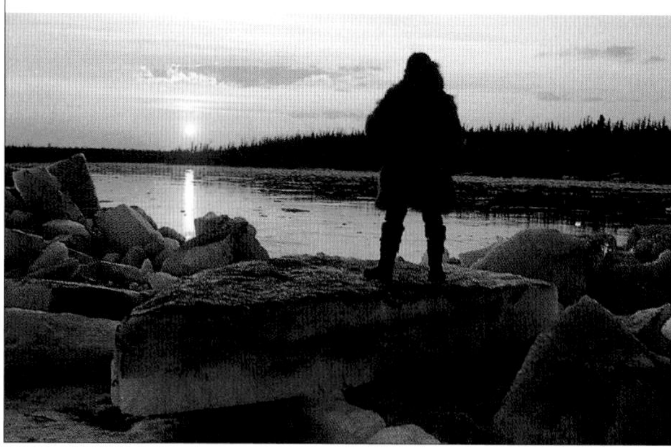

RIVER VOLGA

Russia contains Europe's longest river, the River Volga. Flowing 3,531 km (2,194 miles) from the Valdai Hills to the Caspian Sea, it is the country's leading waterway, and of great economic importance. Large boats transport oil, wheat, timber, and machinery across the country. Canals link the river to the Baltic and White Seas. The river itself is a rich source of fish, particularly sturgeon. Sturgeon's roe is pickled to make the delicacy caviar.

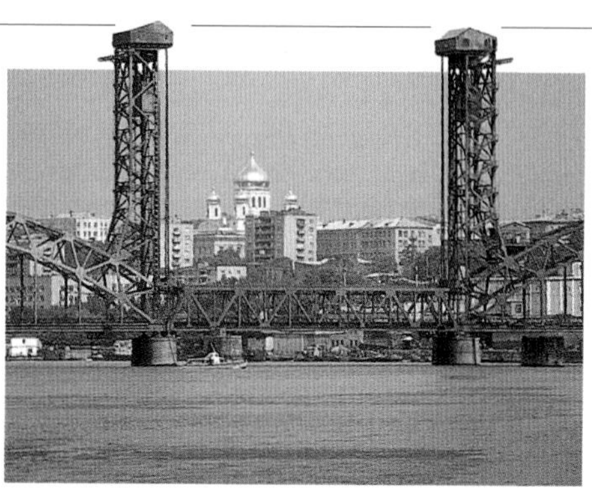

LAKE BAIKAL

With an area of 31,468 sq km (12,150 sq miles), Lake Baikal is the largest freshwater lake in the world. It is also the world's deepest lake, reaching depths of 1,940 m (6,367 ft). In recent years, logging and chemical industries have polluted the water, prompting a major campaign to protect its fragile environment.

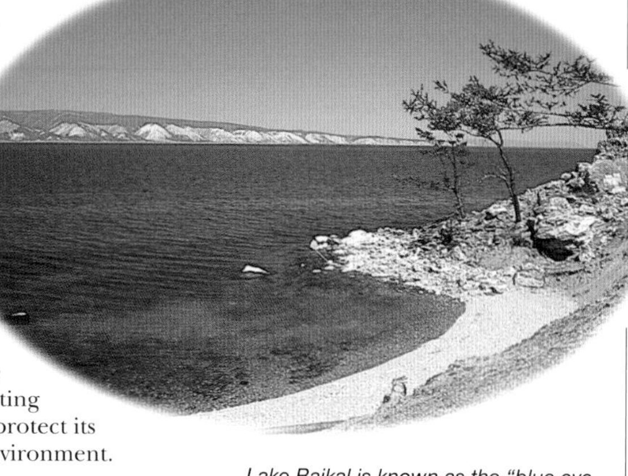

Lake Baikal is known as the "blue eye of Siberia", and contains more than 20 per cent of the world's entire supply of fresh water.

TRANS-SIBERIAN RAILWAY

The Trans-Siberian Railway links European Russia with the Pacific coast across Siberia. It is the world's longest continuous rail line, starting at Moscow and ending 9,297 km (5,777 miles) away in the Pacific port of Vladivostok. Construction of the railway enabled Siberia's mineral wealth to be exploited, and large cities have developed along its route. The journey takes eight days, and crosses eight time zones. Only one passenger train runs each way daily, but freight trains run every five minutes, day and night.

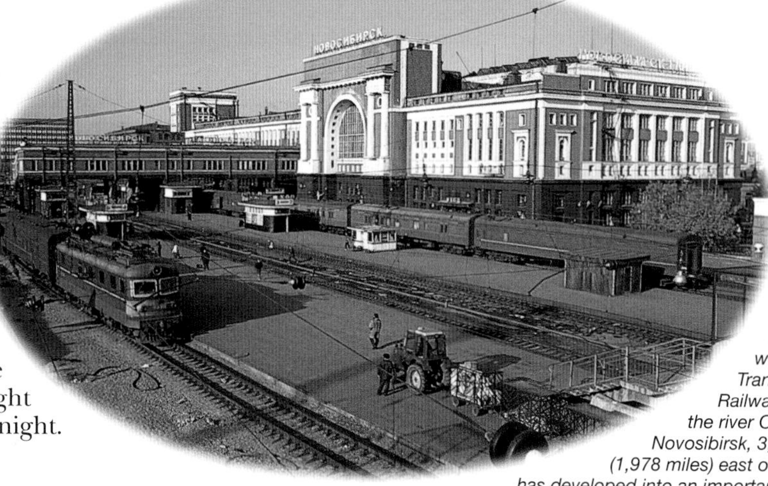

Founded in 1893, where the Trans-Siberian Railway crosses the river Ob', Novosibirsk, 3,183km (1,978 miles) east of Moscow, has developed into an important commercial centre.

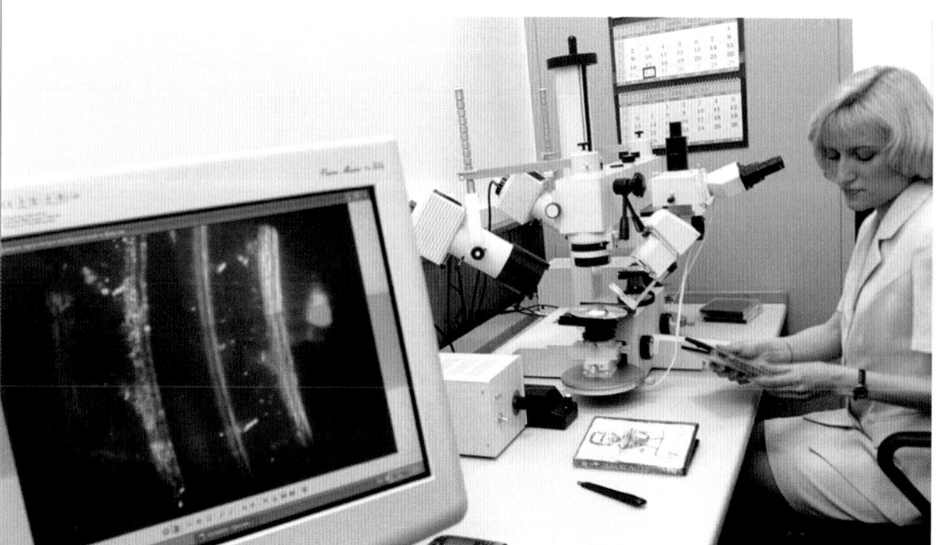

Scientist working in a laboratory to detect pirate CDs.

FEMALE WORKFORCE

Many more Russian men than women died during World War II and in the labour camps set up by the Soviet leader Stalin. As a result, women had to go out to work and many took up physical jobs traditionally done by men. In the Soviet period, good child care enabled women with children to go out to work. Today, more women in Russia hold jobs in science, technology, and engineering than in the rest of Europe, but very few reach the top jobs in these fields.

Find out more

COLD WAR
COMMUNISM
RUSSIA, HISTORY OF
RUSSIAN REVOLUTION
SOVIET UNION, HISTORY OF

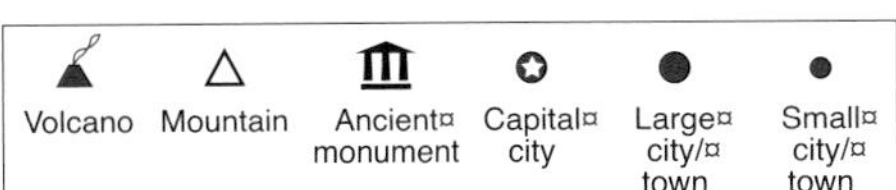

Space programme

Russia's space programme began with the launch of the Sputnik satellite in 1957. In 1965, the Russian cosmonaut Aleksei Leonov became the first person to walk in space. In 1969, the Russians lost the race with the US to land a spacecraft on the Moon. The world's most successful space station (permanent spacecraft in orbit round the Earth) was the Russian craft Mir, which orbited the earth from 1986 to 2001. It was made up of modules that were added to the station at different dates. Astronauts stayed on board for lengthy periods of time, as supplies were delivered by visiting spacecraft.

STATISTICS

Area: 17,075,400 sq km (6,592,812 sq miles)
Population: 143,000,000
Capital: Moscow
Languages: Russian
Religions: Russian Orthodox
Currency: Ruble
Main occupations: Engineering, research, agriculture
Main exports: Oil, natural gas, electricity, vodka
Main imports: Cars, machinery

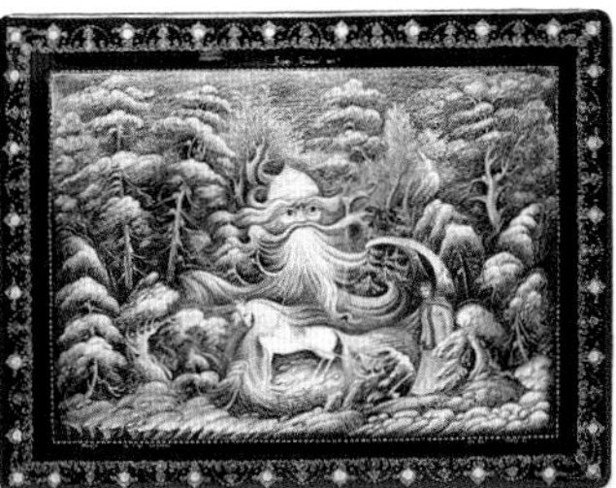

RUSSIAN LACQUERS
Lacquered boxes have been made in the Moscow region for the last four centuries. The papier mâché boxes are decorated with miniature paintings of folk stories, rural scenes, dances, forests, and fairy tales, and are then lacquered.

CAVIAR
Caviar, an expensive delicacy, is made from the tiny black eggs of the *beluga* sturgeon, a type of fish that lives in the Black and Caspian Seas. Tins of caviar are exported worldwide.

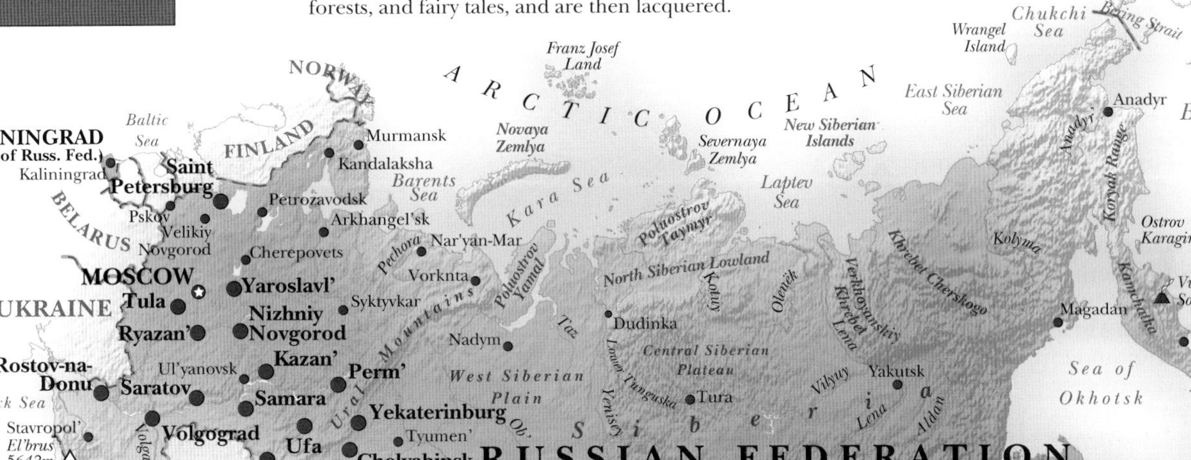

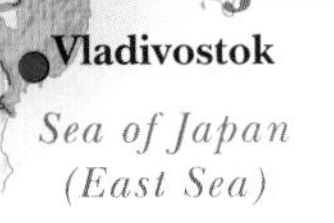

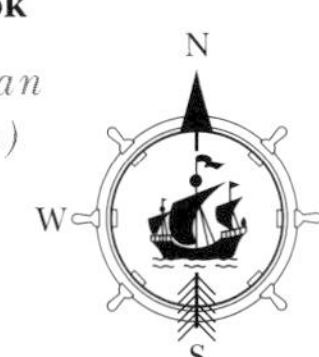

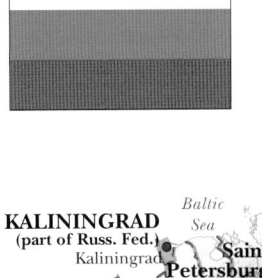

SCALE BAR
0 500 1000 km
0 500 1000 miles

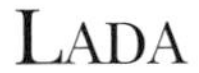

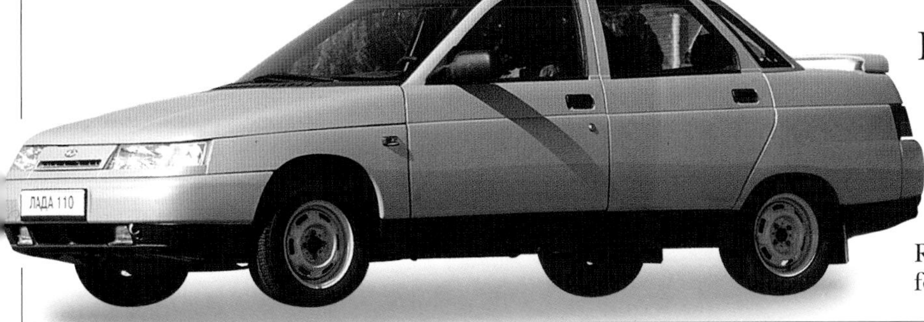

Lada

In 1965, the Russians signed a deal with the Italian car company Fiat to manufacture an economy car called the Lada in the Soviet Union. Today, Ladas, which are based on the Fiat, are exported to the West. Relatively few Russians own a car; however, the demand for luxury western cars is growing.

HISTORY OF RUSSIA

BEFORE THE NINTH CENTURY A.D., Russia consisted of scattered tribes from eastern Europe who farmed a barren landscape of marshes, forests, and steppes. In 882, the first Russian state was established at Kiev, an important trading centre. But in the 1200s, huge Mongol armies destroyed much of Russia. The Russian princes survived the attack only by brutally taxing their own people on behalf of the Mongols. Their methods began a long-lasting system of cruel government in Russia. In the 15th century, after the Mongols had withdrawn, Moscow became the capital of Russia. Over the next 300 years, the czars (emperors) conquered new lands, and Russia became the largest country in the world. However, Russia was slow to modernize, so remained backward compared with other nations. After 1900, Russia slowly began to emerge into modern life, but its newfound strength was wasted in wars. There was a huge contrast between the czar's wealth and the poverty of the people. In 1917, the Russian Revolution overthrew czarist rule. The Communists took power, and from 1917 to 1991, Russia was the largest republic in the Soviet Union. With the collapse of the Soviet Union in 1991, Russia became independent once more.

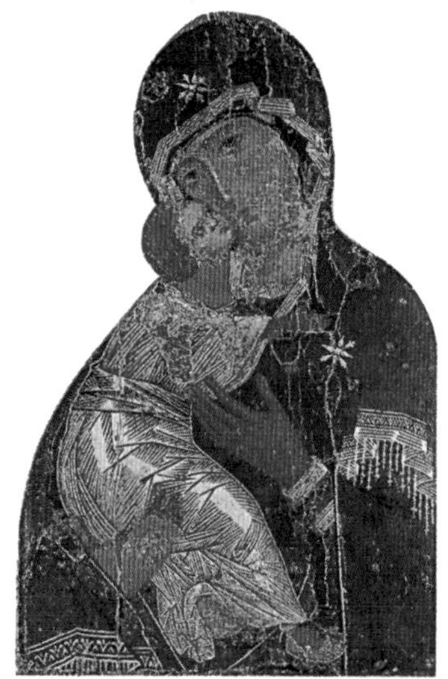

KIEV
In 882 a Viking named Oleg captured Kiev and made it the capital of Russia. After this, Russian princes, who recognized Kiev's importance as a trade route between the Baltic Sea and the Black Sea, ruled the city. In 988, Prince Vladimir I of Kiev became a Christian and made Russian Orthodoxy the state religion. In 1240, Kiev fell to the Mongols.

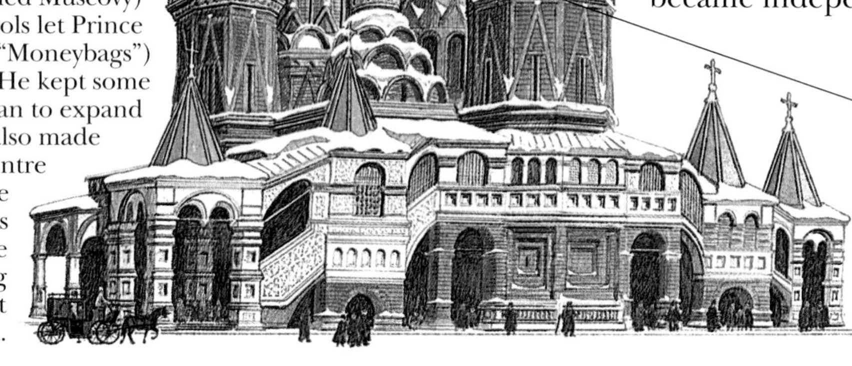

ST. BASIL'S CHURCH
In 1552, Ivan the Terrible built St. Basil's Church, Moscow. It was very ornate to show the great wealth and prosperity of Moscow. Legend has it that Ivan had the architects blinded to prevent them from designing anything as beautiful again.

The colourful decorations and onion-shaped domes on the outside of St. Basil's are typical of Russian Orthodox churches.

MOSCOW

It was under Mongol control that Moscow (then called Muscovy) rose to power. The Mongols let Prince Ivan I (nicknamed "Moneybags") collect taxes for them. He kept some of the money and began to expand Russia's territory. He also made Moscow the religious centre of Russia. Ivan III (the Great) enlarged Moscow's territory. He also drove out the Mongols, leaving Moscow the most powerful city in Russia.

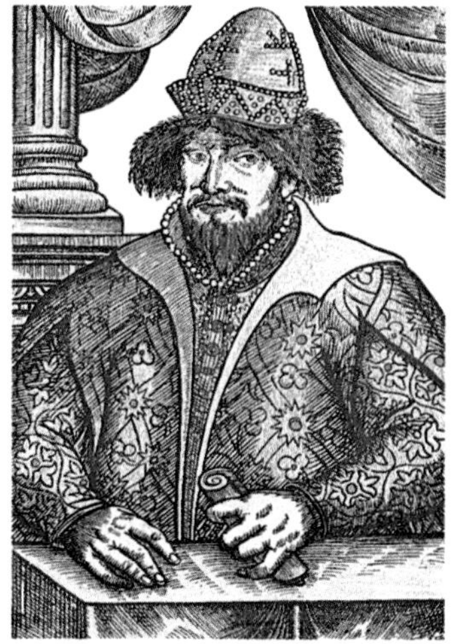

IVAN THE TERRIBLE
Under Czar Ivan IV (1530-84), Moscow gained more power. But Ivan was brutal and wicked, and earned the name Ivan the Terrible. He hated and feared the boyars (nobles) and had hundreds of them murdered. He even murdered his own son. His harsh rule brought poverty to millions and reduced the peasants to near slavery.

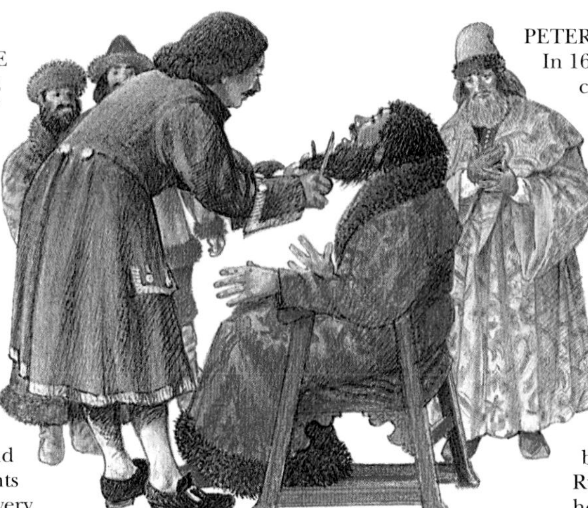

PETER THE GREAT
In 1682 Peter the Great became czar. During his reign he modernized the army, defeated Sweden, and gained control of the Baltic coast, giving Russia an outlet to the West. He built a new capital at St. Petersburg and improved industry and education. He travelled through Europe in disguise to learn about Western life and tried to modernize Russia by using Western methods. He cut off the beards of the Orthodox Russians as a symbol of all he intended to change.

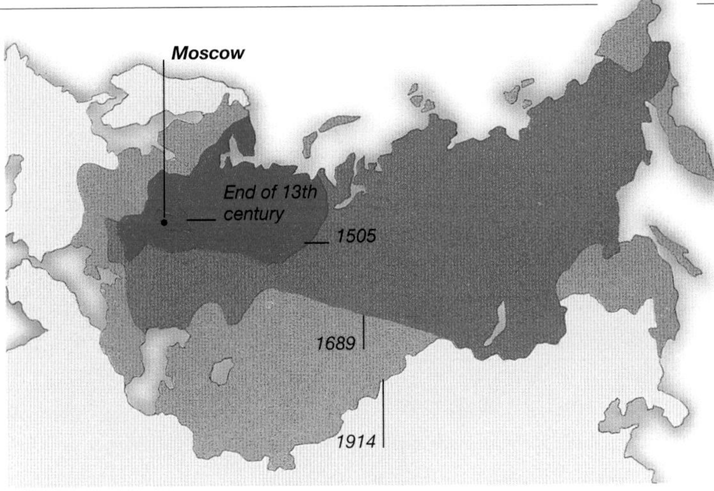

RUSSIAN EXPANSION
From the 14th century, Russia grew in size as a result of conquests. Part of the reason for this expansion was the search for a port which was ice-free all year round. The pioneers who settled in the new areas, such as Poland, lived mostly on tiny farms, scratching out a miserable existence. Power lay in the hands of the czar and a few very rich nobles. Communication across such vast distances was difficult, so the czars had no idea of the problems and poverty of their people.

RUSSIA

882 Vikings establish first Russian state at Kiev.

988 Prince Vladimir I forces all Russians to accept the Russian Orthodox faith.

1237 Mongols invade Russia.

1480 Ivan III breaks Mongol control of Russia; brings other cities under Moscow's control.

1547 Ivan IV introduces serfdom, which forces the peasants to stay in one place and work for a landowner.

1604-13 "Time of Troubles". Russia suffers civil wars as rival groups struggle for power.

1613 Michael Romanov becomes czar. Romanovs rule Russia until 1917.

1703 Czar Peter the Great begins to build his new capital at St. Petersburg. Brings in experts to modernize industry.

1774 Peasants revolt.

1812 French emperor Napoleon invades Russia. Most of his army dies in the freezing Russian winter.

1825 "Decembrist Uprising". Army officers demand an elected government.

1905 Japan defeats Russia in Russo-Japanese War. A workers' revolution forces Nicholas II to establish a parliament, called the Duma.

1914-17 Russia fights against Germany in World War I. Discontent pushes the people into revolution.

1917-91 Communists control Russia.

1991 Soviet Union collapses; Russia independent.

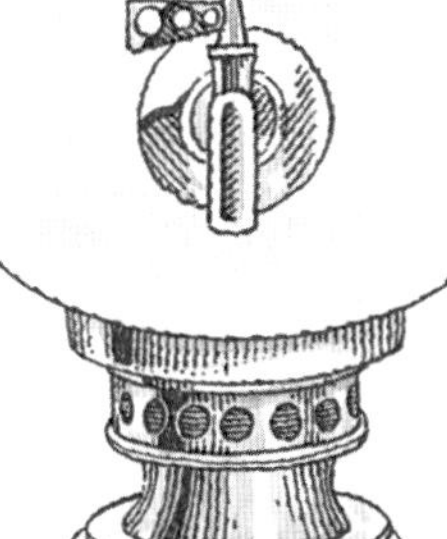

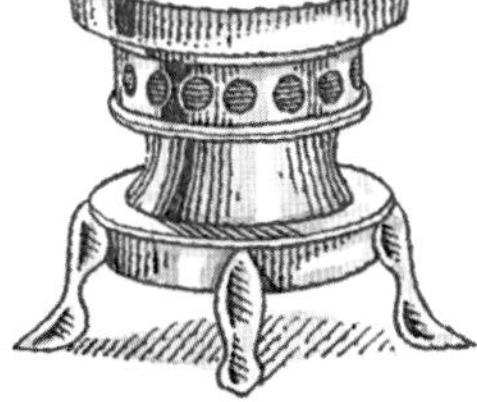

Catherine the Great

During Catherine's reign (1762-96) Russia's territory expanded. Catherine created a glittering court which was much admired outside Russia. She gave more power to the nobles but did nothing for the peasants. They were used as slave labour in distant areas and suffered untold misery.

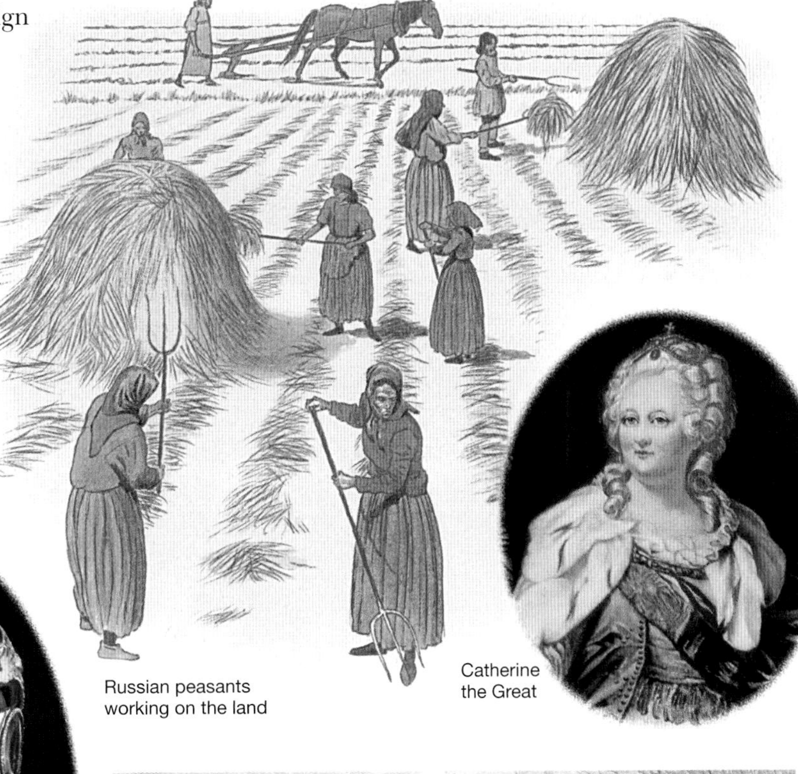

Russian peasants working on the land

Catherine the Great

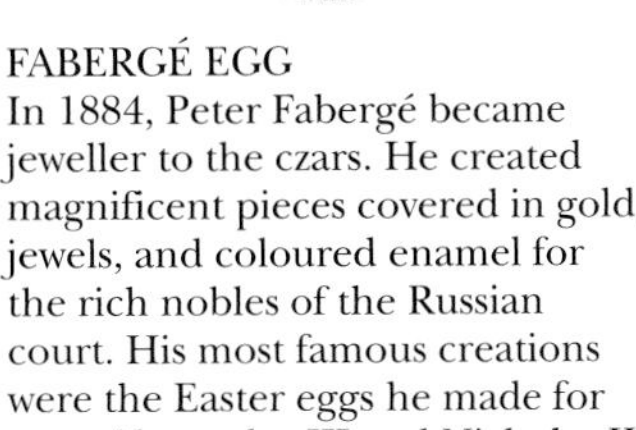

FABERGÉ EGG
In 1884, Peter Fabergé became jeweller to the czars. He created magnificent pieces covered in gold, jewels, and coloured enamel for the rich nobles of the Russian court. His most famous creations were the Easter eggs he made for czars Alexander III and Nicholas II.

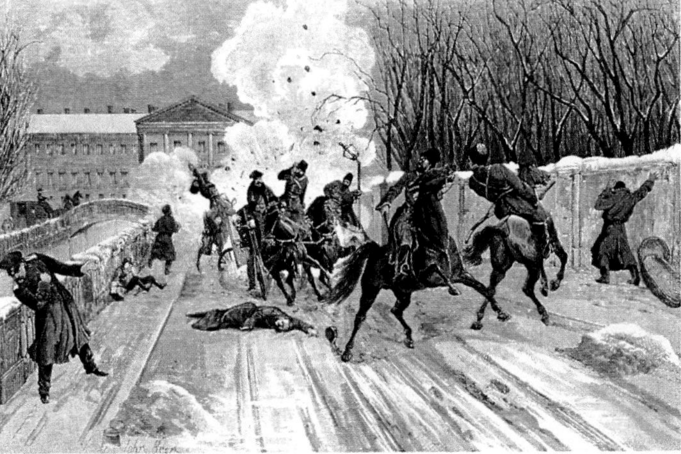

ALEXANDER II
Czar Alexander II (1818-81) realized that Russia had to keep up with the West in order to succeed. He freed the peasants and helped them buy land. But they were disappointed with the quality of their land and the high taxes they had to pay. In 1881, a revolutionary group assassinated Alexander.

Find out more

COMMUNISM
NAPOLEONIC WARS
RUSSIAN FEDERATION
RUSSIAN REVOLUTION
SOVIET UNION, HISTORY OF

RUSSIAN REVOLUTION

IN 1917, THE PEOPLE OF RUSSIA staged a revolution that was to change the course of modern history. The Russian people were desperate for change. Russia was suffering serious losses against Germany in World War I. Food and fuel were scarce. Many people were starving. Czar Nicholas II, ruler of Russia, was blamed for much of this. In March 1917 (February in the old Russian calendar) a general strike broke out in Petrograd (today St. Petersburg). The strike was in protest against the chaos caused by the war. Nicholas was forced to give up his throne, and a group of revolutionaries, called the Mensheviks, formed a provisional government. This government soon fell, because it failed to end the war. In November, the Bolsheviks, a more extreme revolutionary group, seized power. They ended the war with Germany and, led by Vladimir Lenin, set up the world's first Communist state. They declared the country a Soviet republic. This revolution was the first Communist takeover of a government. It inspired more to follow.

1905 REVOLUTION
In 1905 unarmed workers marched on Nicholas II's Winter Palace in St. Petersburg. The czar's troops fired on the crowd. Nicholas set up an elected parliament, or Duma. But the Duma had no real power, so distrust of the czar grew.

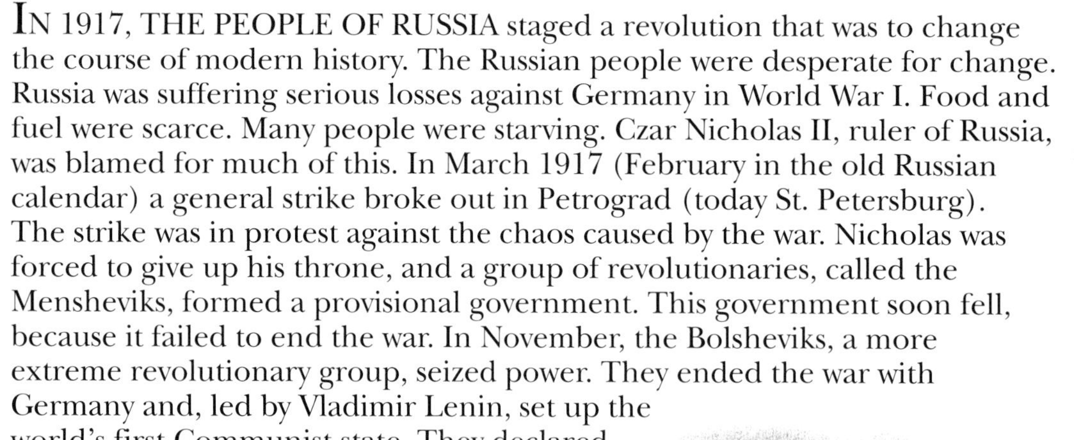

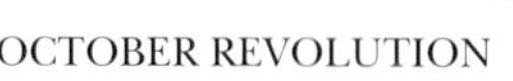

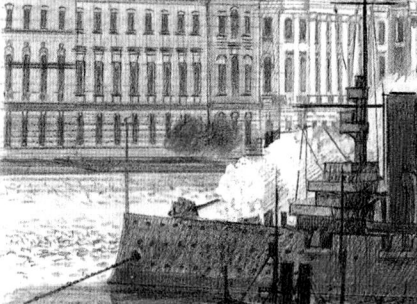

OCTOBER REVOLUTION
What is known as the October Revolution broke out on 7 November 1917 (25 October in the old Russian calendar used before the revolution). The cruiser *Aurora* fired blanks across the River Neva at the headquarters of the Menshevik government in the Winter Palace. The Bolsheviks also attacked other important buildings in Petrograd.

RUSSIAN REVOLUTION

1914 Russia joins World War I against Germany and Austria.

1916 One million Russian soldiers die after German offensive. Prices in Russia rise.

1917 March International Women's Day march in Petrograd turns into bread riot. The Mensheviks set up a provisional government. The Bolsheviks organize another government made up of committees called soviets.

July Lenin flees Russia.

October Lenin returns to Petrograd.

7 November Armed workers seize buildings in Petrograd.

15 November Bolsheviks control Petrograd.

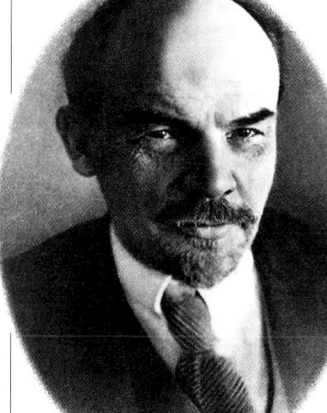

LENIN

Vladimir Lenin (1870-1924), founder of the Bolshevik party, believed in the ideas of the German writer Karl Marx. He lived mostly in exile from Russia, until the October Revolution. He was a powerful speaker whose simple slogan of "Peace, land, and bread" persuaded many Russians to support the Bolsheviks. He ruled Russia as dictator.

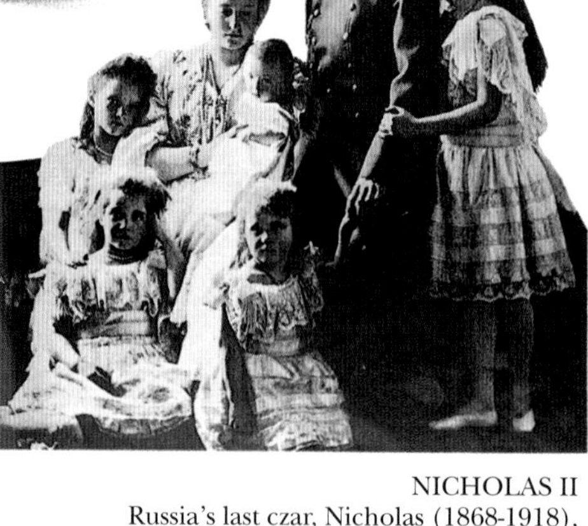

NICHOLAS II
Russia's last czar, Nicholas (1868-1918), was out of touch with his subjects. They blamed him for the Russian defeats in World War I (1914-18), where he fought at the front. His sinister adviser, a monk named Rasputin, was widely hated and feared. After Nicholas gave up the throne, he and his family were arrested. The Bolsheviks shot them all the following year.

Find out more

COMMUNISM
HUMAN RIGHTS
RUSSIA, HISTORY OF
SOVIET UNION, HISTORY OF
WORLD WAR I

Sailing and Boating

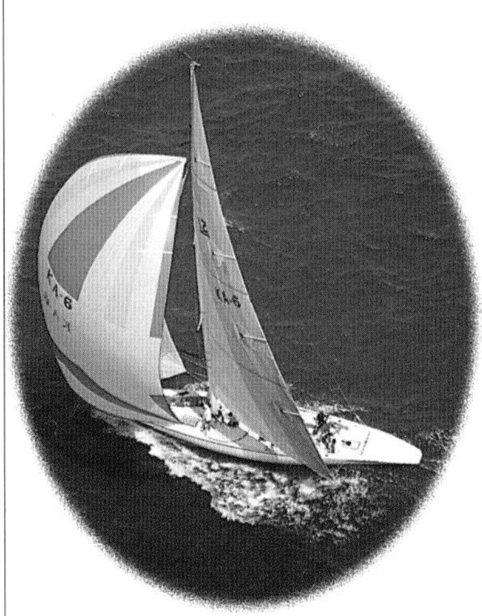

AMERICA'S CUP
One of the world's most famous ocean sailing races is the America's Cup. Two yachts, which represent two different nations, race over a triangular course, and the nation that wins receives the cup as a prize. The trophy is named for the U.S. yacht *America*, which won the cup in 1851. The New York Yacht Club kept the cup for 132 years by beating all challengers.

ONCE A VITAL MEANS of transport, sailing is now a pastime and a sport. The smallest sailing boats are one-person crafts, but ocean-going racing yachts have a crew of 20 or more. Anyone can learn to sail a simple sailing boat. There is a rudder to point it in the right direction, and a keel or centreboard to stop it from slipping sideways. The skill of sailing lies in the positioning of the sail according to the direction of the wind. Rowing and canoeing do not rely on the wind. Rowing with one oar per person is called sculling. Canoeing is a popular way of touring rivers and lakes at a leisurely pace. "White-water" canoeing is far from leisurely. Canoeists have to paddle through fast-flowing rivers while avoiding hidden rocks.

Pieces of coloured wool show the crew how the wind is blowing across the sail.

Aluminium mast is lighter and stronger than traditional timber.

Sails are made of artificial fibre such as Dacron.

The spinnaker pole supports the billowing spinnaker sail that the crew raises when the wind is behind the boat.

The centreboard drops into a slot to keep the boat on course, but lifts out so the boat can sail in shallow water.

Windows enable the crew to see through the sail.

Ropes on sailing vessels are called sheets or lines.

The mainsheet adjusts the position of the mainsail.

Tiller extension bar lets the helm turn the rudder while leaning out to balance the boat.

Rudder steers the boat through the water.

Hull is made of glass-reinforced plastic, which is lightweight but very strong.

The crew member who controls the boat's direction is called the helm.

Racing sailboat

Most races are for matched boats of the same class, or type. In this way, sailing skill and tactics determine the winner, rather than the boat's design. Even the simplest training sailboat can compete in races. Some racing sailboats require a crew of more than one.

Canoeing

The kayak, an enclosed canoe, is used for touring or racing. It is propelled with a double-bladed paddle. Canoeists use a single-bladed paddle in open canoes. In Canada canoe racers use a similar paddle and race in a high kneeling position.

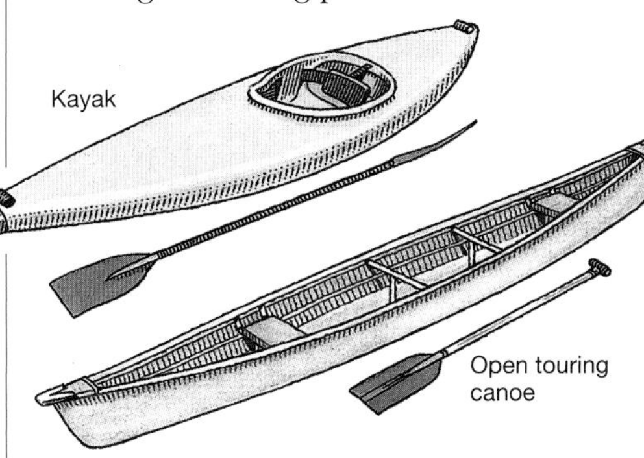

SAFETY
Sailors must always take safety precautions, such as wearing a life belt or a life jacket. A sailing boat should have a bucket for bailing out water and a paddle in case the wind drops to levels too insufficient to sail by.

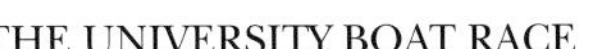

THE UNIVERSITY BOAT RACE
Every year since 1829 crews from Oxford and Cambridge universities in England have held a now-famous rowing match. The two rowing boats race over a winding 6.4-km (4-mile) course on the River Thames in London.

Find out more
NAVIGATION
PORTS AND WATERWAYS
SHIPS AND BOATS

SATELLITES

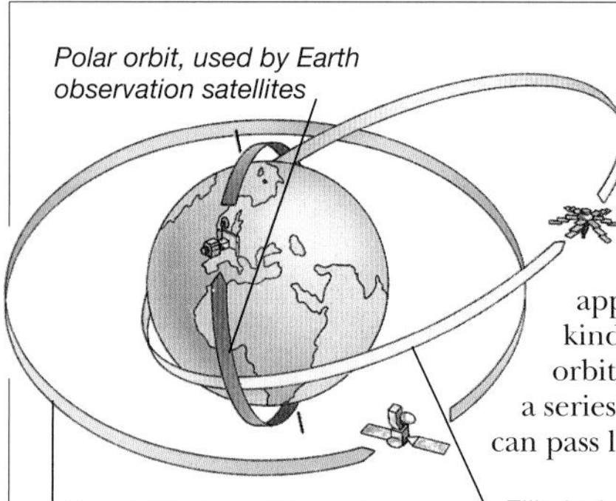

SATELLITE ORBITS
A communications satellite takes exactly 24 hours to orbit the Earth, so it appears to remain fixed over one spot. This kind of orbit is called geostationary. A polar orbit allows a satellite to see the whole Earth in a series of strips. In an elliptical orbit, a satellite can pass low over a selected part of the Earth.

Solar panels generate electricity from sunlight to power the satellite.

Radar altimeter provides data on wind speed, ocean currents, and tides.

Infra-red scanner measures water vapour in the atmosphere and the temperatures of seas and cloud tops.

Earth observation satellite *ERS-2*

Antenna for transmitting data back to Earth

WHEN AIRCRAFT and balloons first took to the skies, the people in them were amazed at their new view of the world. From hundreds of metres up they could see the layout of a large city, the shape of a coastline, or the patchwork of fields on a farm. Today, we have an even wider view. Satellites circle the Earth, not hundreds of metres, but hundreds of kilometres above the ground. From this great height, satellites provide a unique image of our planet. Some have cameras that take photographs of land and sea, giving information about the changing environment on Earth. Others plot weather patterns or peer out into space and send back data (information) about planets and stars. All of these are artificial satellites that have been launched into space from Earth. However, the word satellite actually means any object that moves around a planet while being held in orbit by the planet's gravity. There are countless natural satellites in the universe: the Earth has one, which is the Moon.

ARTIFICIAL SATELLITES

There are many types of artificial satellite. Weather satellites observe rain, storms, and clouds, and measure land and sea temperatures. Communications satellites send radio and television signals from one part of the Earth to another. Spy satellites observe military targets from low altitudes and send back detailed pictures to ground stations. Earth observation satellites monitor vegetation, air and water pollution, population changes, and geological factors such as mineral deposits.

MAPPING THE EARTH
Resources satellites take pictures of the Earth's surface. The cameras have various filters so they can pick up infra-red (heat) radiation and different colours of light. Vegetation, for instance, reflects infra-red light strongly, showing up forests and woodlands. Computer-generated colours are used to pick out areas with different kinds of vegetation and minerals.

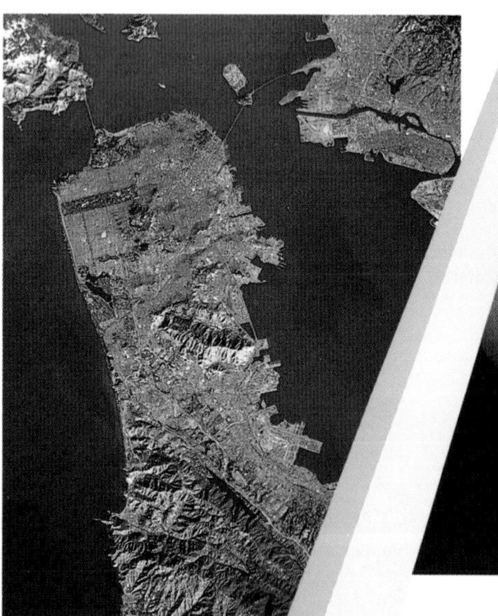

Satellite map image of San Francisco Bay, California. Clearly visible are two bridges: the Golden Gate Bridge on the left and the Bay Bridge on the right.

SPUTNIK 1
On 4 October 1957, the Soviet Union launched *Sputnik 1,* the world's first artificial satellite. *Sputnik 1* carried a radio transmitter that sent signals back to Earth until it burned up in the atmosphere 92 days later.

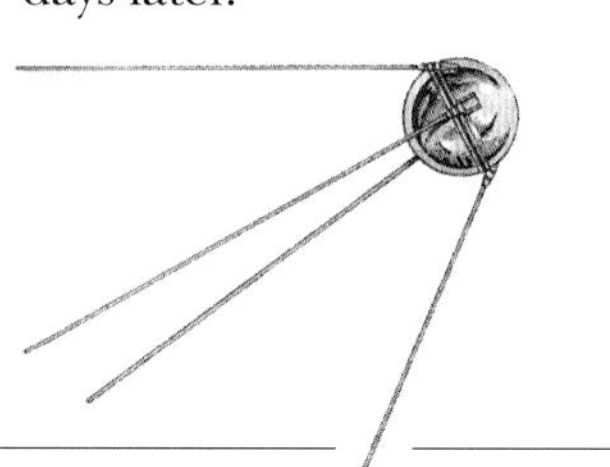

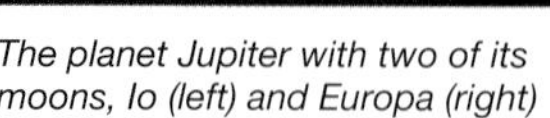

The planet Jupiter with two of its moons, Io (left) and Europa (right)

NATURAL SATELLITES
There are more than 150 known natural satellites, or moons, in the solar system. Most of these orbit (move around) the four giant outer planets: Jupiter, Saturn, Uranus, and Neptune. The largest moons are bigger than Pluto, the smallest planet; the smallest moons are only a few kilometres across and have irregular, potato-like shapes.

Find out more
ASTRONOMY
GEOLOGY
NAVIGATION
SPACE FLIGHT
TELEPHONES
TELEVISION AND VIDEO

SCANDINAVIA

AT THE FAR NORTH of Europe are the countries of Scandinavia, which have much in common yet in some ways could not be more different. Their economies are closely linked, but each uses its own currency. They are all independent nations; but in times past, several of them have been bound together in a single union. Each country has its own language, yet strong cultural ties exist between the nations. Landscapes are different, however. Denmark is flat – the biggest hill is only 173 m (567 ft) high – and most of the country is very fertile; but both Norway and Iceland are mountainous with little farmland. Sweden and Finland are dotted with lakes – more than 180,000 in Finland alone. Greenland is almost entirely covered in ice and snow. Politically, the different countries co-operate through the Nordic Council, which aims to strengthen ties between the nations. Denmark, Finland, and Sweden are members of the European Union, a trade alliance of European nations. Most Scandinavians enjoy a high standard of living and an active cultural life. Norway and Sweden award the annual Nobel Prizes for sciences, literature, and peace.

Cross country skiing is a popular sport in many parts of Scandinavia.

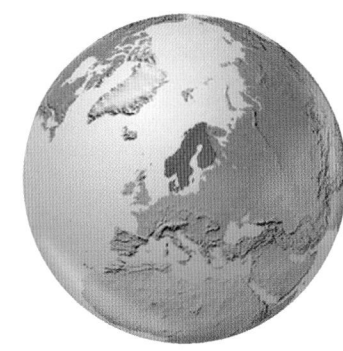

Geographically, Scandinavia consists of the Norway and Sweden peninsula. But the name is also used widely to include Denmark and Finland. The Faeroe Islands, Iceland, and Greenland are often associated with Scandinavia.

The frozen north of Scandinavia, called Lappland, is the home of 40,000 Lapplanders. Many of them live by herding reindeer for their hide and meat.

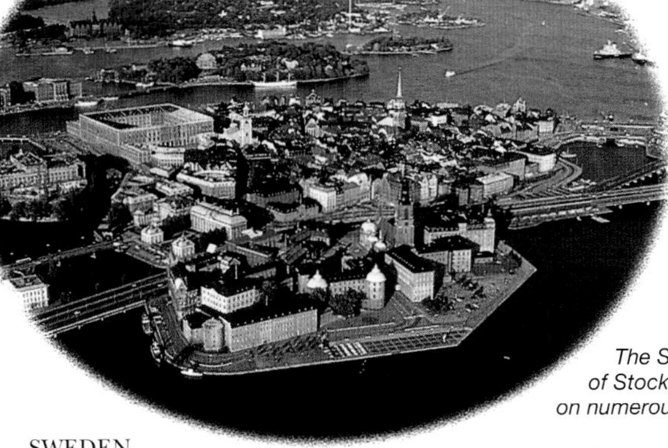

The Swedish capital of Stockholm is built on numerous islands.

FINLAND

Although Finland is part of Scandinavia, it is closely tied to the Russian Federation, and the two countries share a long frontier. Until 1917, Finland was a province of the old Russian empire. Today Finnish trade is still conducted with the Russian Federation. Forests cover two-thirds of Finland, and the paper industry dominates the economy. Shipbuilding and tourism are also important. Finland is one of the world's most northern countries, and throughout the winter months only the southern coastline is free of ice.

SWEDEN

The biggest of the Scandinavian countries, Sweden is also the wealthiest. Over the years, the Swedes have developed a taxation and social welfare system that has created a good standard of living for everybody. As a result, few people in Sweden are either very rich or very poor. The population numbers about 8.9 million, most of whom live in the south and east of the country; the mountainous north lies within the Arctic Circle and is almost uninhabited.

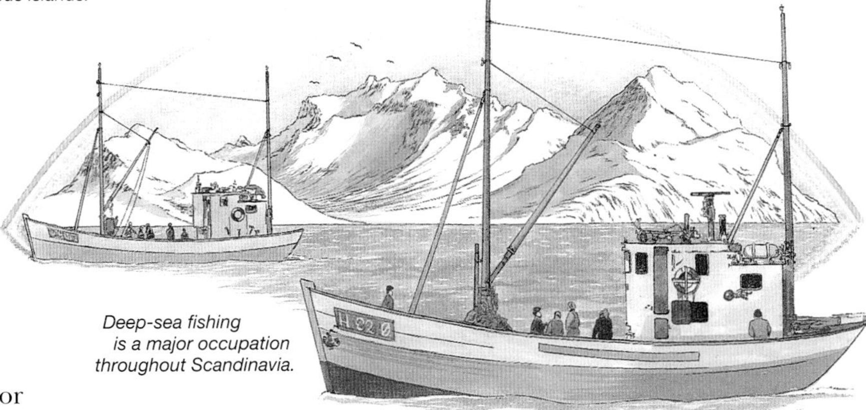

Deep-sea fishing is a major occupation throughout Scandinavia.

NORWAY

Shipping, forestry, and fishing were the traditional Norwegian industries. But in 1970, oil was discovered in the Norwegian sector of the North Sea, and the country's fortunes were transformed. Today, the 4.5 million Norwegians enjoy a high standard of living, low taxes, and almost no unemployment. But Norway has almost no natural resources apart from oil and timber. The wooded country is mountainous and indented with numerous inlets, or fjords, from the North Atlantic Ocean. These fjords make communications difficult between the cities in the south and the more sparsely populated regions in the north.

FISHING

The north Atlantic Ocean provides a rich marine harvest for Scandinavian fishermen. High-quality cod and mackerel are caught in the cold, nutrient-rich waters. Fish-farming, especially in the fjords, is on the increase in Norway, the world's largest salmon producer.

NORTH SEA OIL

Discoveries of oil and natural gas beneath the North Sea seafloor began in 1959, when a seaward extension of a major natural-gas field in the northeastern part of the Netherlands was identified. Within two decades, natural-gas production sites were located along a 100-mile band stretching from the Netherlands to eastern England. Farther north, Norway's first offshore oil field went into production in 1971. Today Norway's economy largely depends on its abundant natural resources and the country is Europe's largest oil producer. Norway is self sufficient in natural gas and oil.

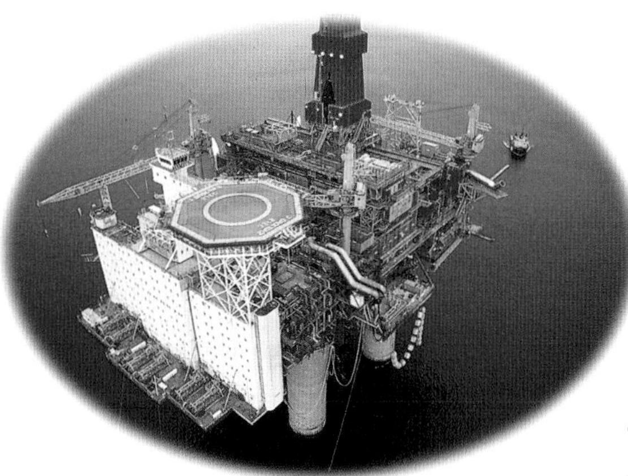

North Sea oil, produced on oil rigs such as the one pictured above, is exported globally. Norway is a world leader in the construction of drilling platforms.

SAUNAS

Finland is home to the sauna which has become a national institution. The Finns have used the steam bath for centuries as a way of cleansing and relaxing the body, and today most houses in Finland have one. A sauna is a small, very warm room which is filled with steam. The steam is produced by throwing water over hot stones periodically. As the water crackles and spits, the air fills with clouds of steam. Cooling off under a cold shower or a plunge in an icy pool (left) follows a session in the sauna, and completes the process. Saunas are traditionally fuelled by wooden logs, however they are increasingly powered by electricity, especially in Finland's cities.

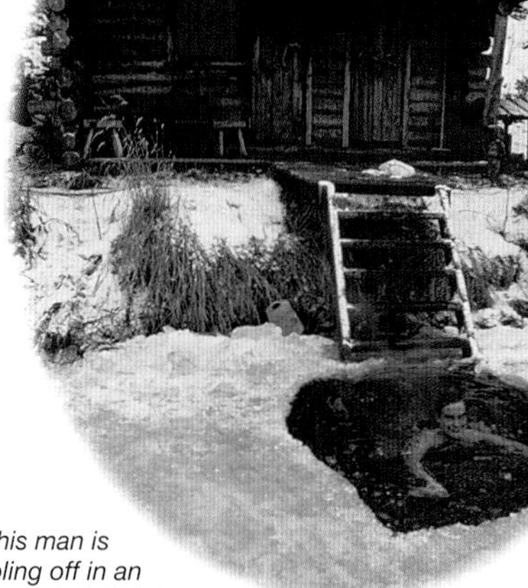

This man is cooling off in an icy pool of water after a session in a sauna.

COPENHAGEN

Copenhagen (right) is the capital of Denmark, and about one quarter of all Danish people live in and around the city. Copenhagen is on the east coast of Zealand, the largest of 482 islands that make up about 30 per cent of Denmark. The low-lying Jutland peninsula to the west makes up the rest of the land area.

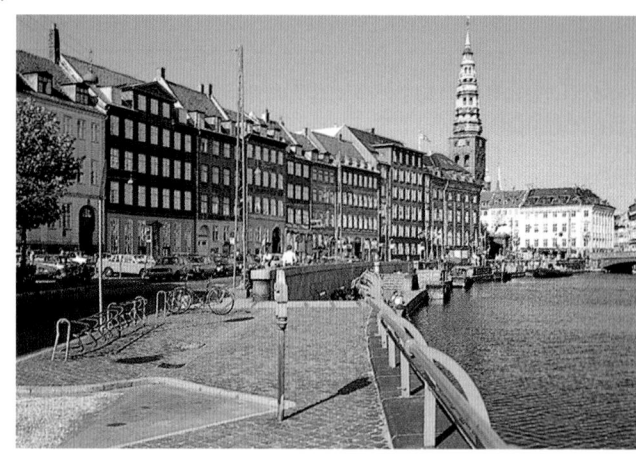

FJORDS

During the ice age, glaciers carved steep-sided valleys in the rocks along Norway's coast. As the ice melted, the North Sea flowed in, creating fjords. Glaciers have cut hundreds of fjords into Scandinavia's Atlantic coastline. Fjords are usually deeper in their middle and upper reaches than at the seaward end. The water in these inlets is calmer than in the open sea.

The tranquil waters of a Norwegian fjord. Fjords often reach great depths. The great weight of the glaciers which formed them, eroded the bottom of the valley far below sea-level. The best farming land is found in the lowland areas around fjords.

FARMING IN SWEDEN

The fertile soil in southern Sweden makes this area the most productive farming area in the country, with pig farming, dairy-farming and crops such as wheat, barley and potatoes. Many Swedish farmers belong to agricultural cooperatives which process and distribute their crops.

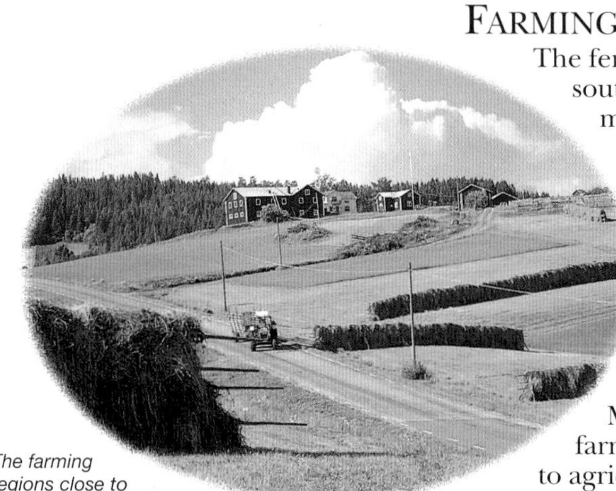

The farming regions close to the Gulf of Bothnia are best known for dairy produce.

Find out more

ANTARCTICA
ARCTIC
EUROPE
SCANDINAVIA, HISTORY OF

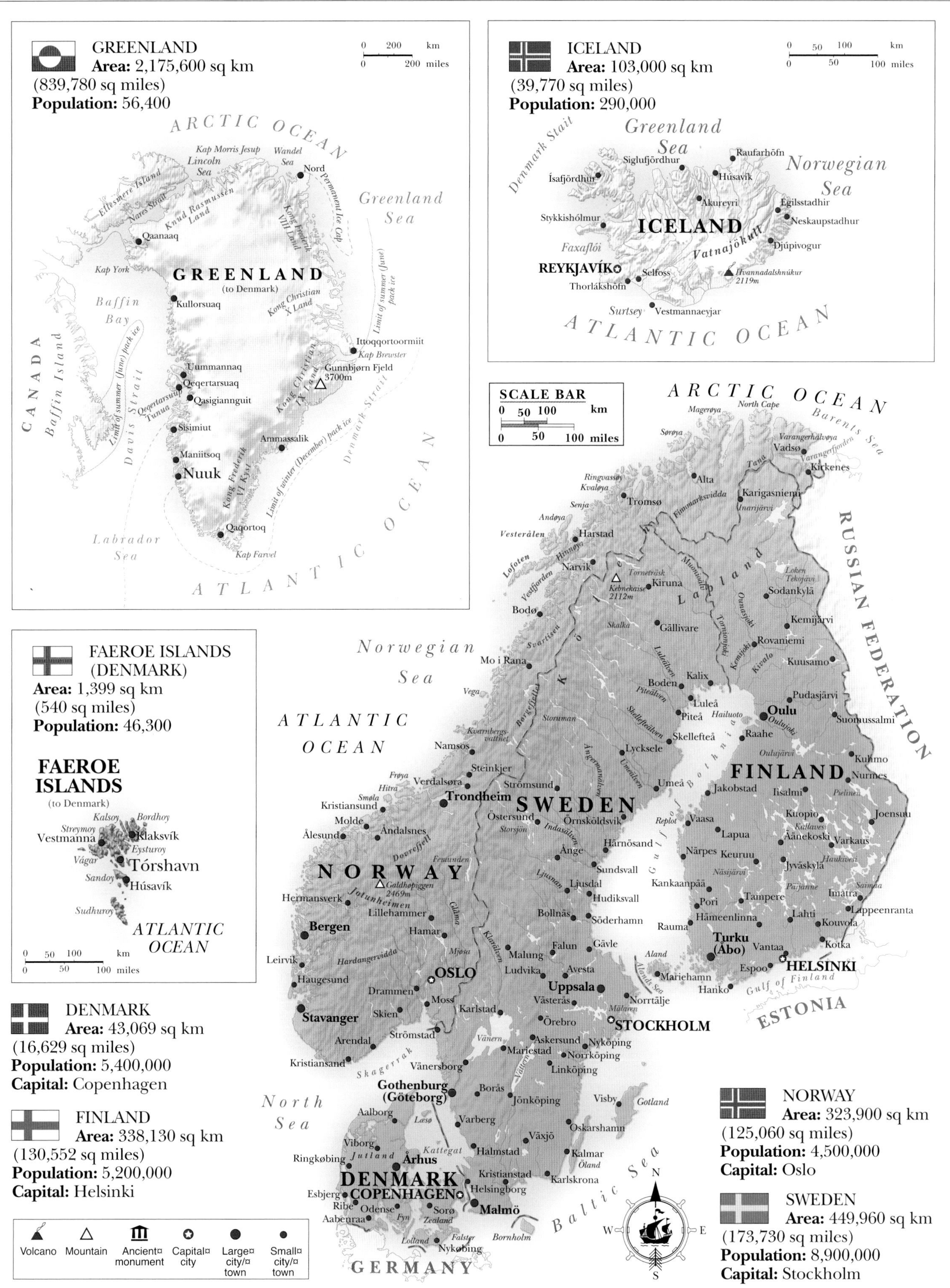
GREENLAND
Area: 2,175,600 sq km
(839,780 sq miles)
Population: 56,400
0 200 km
0 200 miles
ARCTIC OCEAN
Kap Morris Jesup
Lincoln Sea
Wandel Sea
Nord
Permanent Ice Cap
Ellesmere Island
Nares Strait
Knud Rasmussen Land
Kong Frederik VIII Land
Greenland Sea
Qaanaaq
Kap York
GREENLAND
(to Denmark)
Kong Christian X Land
Limit of summer (June) pack ice
Baffin Bay
Kullorsuaq
CANADA
Baffin Island
Limit of summer (June) pack ice
Ittoqqortoormiit
Kap Brewster
Gunnbjørn Fjeld 3700m
Uummannaq
Qeqertarsuaq
Qasigiannguit
Qeqertarsuup Tunua
Kong Christian IX Land
Davis Strait
Sisimiut
Ammassalik
Limit of winter (December) pack ice
Denmark Strait
Maniitsoq
Nuuk
Kong Frederik VI Kyst
Qaqortoq
Labrador Sea
Kap Farvel
ATLANTIC OCEAN
ICELAND
Area: 103,000 sq km
(39,770 sq miles)
Population: 290,000
0 50 100 km
0 50 100 miles
Denmark Strait
Greenland Sea
Raufarhöfn
Siglufjördhur
Norwegian Sea
Ísafjördhur
Húsavík
Akureyri
Egilsstadhir
Stykkishólmur
ICELAND
Neskaupstadhur
Faxaflói
Vatnajökull
Djúpivogur
REYKJAVÍK
Selfoss
Hvannadalshnúkur 2119m
Thorlákshöfn
Surtsey
Vestmannaeyjar
ATLANTIC OCEAN
SCALE BAR
0 50 100 km
0 50 100 miles
ARCTIC OCEAN
Magerøya
North Cape
Barents Sea
Sørøya
Varangerhalvøya
Vadsø
Varangerfjorden
Kirkenes
Tana
Alta
Ringvassøy
Kvaløya
Karigasniemi
Finnmarksvidda
Inarijärvi
Tromsø
Senja
Andøya
Vesterålen
Harstad
Hinnøya
RUSSIAN FEDERATION
Lofoten
Narvik
Torneträsk
Lokan Tekojärvi
Vestfjorden
Kebnekaise 2112m
Kiruna
Lapland
Sodankylä
Bodø
Muonioälven
Ounasjoki
Svartisen
Skalka
Gällivare
Kemijärvi
Torniojoki
Kemijoki
Rovaniemi
Norwegian Sea
Mo i Rana
Luleälven
Kitinen
Kuusamo
Kölen
Kalix
Vega
Boden
Luleå
Pudasjärvi
Piteälven
Piteå
Hailuoto
Oulu
Oulujoki
Suomussalmi
Borgefjellet
Skellefteälven
Skellefteå
Raahe
ATLANTIC OCEAN
Storuman
Kvarnbergsvattnet
Namsos
Lycksele
Oulujärvi
Kuhmo
Ångermanälven
Umeälven
Steinkjer
Frøya
Hitra
Verdalsøra
Strömsund
Umeå
FINLAND
Nurmes
Jakobstad
Smøla
Trondheim
Iisalmi
Pielinen
Kristiansund
SWEDEN
Molde
Östersund
Örnsköldsvik
Replot
Vaasa
Kuopio
Joensuu
Ålesund
Åndalsnes
Storsjön
Indalsälven
Lapua
Kallavesi
Äänekoski
Varkaus
Dovrefjell
Ånge
Härnösand
Gulf of Bothnia
Närpes
Keuruu
Femunden
Sundsvall
Näsijärvi
Jyväskylä
Haukivesi
NORWAY
Galdhøpiggen 2469m
Ljusnan
Ljusdal
Kankaanpää
Päijänne
Saimaa
Jotunheimen
Hermansverk
Hudiksvall
Pori
Tampere
Imatra
Lillehammer
Glåma
Bollnäs
Söderhamn
Hämeenlinna
Lahti
Lappeenranta
Bergen
Hamar
Klarälven
Rauma
Kouvola
Hardangervidda
Mjøsa
Falun
Gävle
Turku (Åbo)
Vantaa
Kotka
Leirvik
Malung
Aland
OSLO
Ludvika
Avesta
Espoo
HELSINKI
Haugesund
Ålands Sea
Mariehamn
Gulf of Finland
Uppsala
Hanko
Drammen
Västerås
Norrtälje
ESTONIA
Moss
Karlstad
Mälaren
Stavanger
Skien
Örebro
STOCKHOLM
Strömstad
Vänern
Askersund
Nyköping
Arendal
Mariestad
Norrköping
Kristiansand
Skagerrak
Vänersborg
Linköping
Vättern
North Sea
Gothenburg (Göteborg)
Borås
Jönköping
Visby
Gotland
Aalborg
Varberg
Læsø
Oskarshamn
Viborg
Kattegat
Växjö
Ringkøbing
Jutland
Århus
Halmstad
Kalmar
Öland
DENMARK
Kristianstad
Karlskrona
Esbjerg
COPENHAGEN
Helsingborg
Baltic Sea
Ribe
Odense
Sorø
Malmö
Aabenraa
Fyn
Zealand
Falster
Bornholm
Lolland
Nykøbing
GERMANY
N
W
E
S
FAEROE ISLANDS (DENMARK)
Area: 1,399 sq km
(540 sq miles)
Population: 46,300
FAEROE ISLANDS
(to Denmark)
Kalsoy
Bordhoy
Streymoy
Klaksvík
Vestmanna
Eysturoy
Vágar
Tórshavn
Sandoy
Húsavík
Sudhuroy
ATLANTIC OCEAN
0 50 100 km
0 50 100 miles
DENMARK
Area: 43,069 sq km
(16,629 sq miles)
Population: 5,400,000
Capital: Copenhagen
FINLAND
Area: 338,130 sq km
(130,552 sq miles)
Population: 5,200,000
Capital: Helsinki
NORWAY
Area: 323,900 sq km
(125,060 sq miles)
Population: 4,500,000
Capital: Oslo
SWEDEN
Area: 449,960 sq km
(173,730 sq miles)
Population: 8,900,000
Capital: Stockholm
Volcano
Mountain
Ancient monument
Capital city
Large city/town
Small city/town

HISTORY OF

SCANDINAVIA

HISTORICALLY, the region called Scandinavia, in northern Europe, consisted of Norway, Sweden, and Denmark. Today, Finland and Iceland are also considered part of Scandinavia. All are independent countries, but their history has been intertwined since ancient times. Seafaring Vikings were among the earliest people to live in the region of Scandinavia, more than 1,000 years ago. During the 900s the three separate nations of Denmark, Norway, and Sweden emerged for the first time. Over the next few centuries, the three countries were often united. During the 16th century, Sweden broke away to build its own empire and became a huge European power. This left Norway and Denmark closely linked. In 1814, Norway came under Swedish rule. But in 1905, Norway became an independent nation. Today, the Scandinavian nations are world leaders in environmental and health issues.

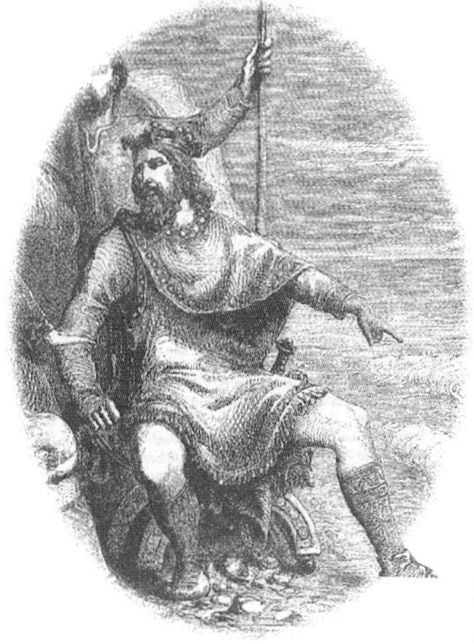

KING CANUTE
In 1014, Canute (c.995-1035) became king of Denmark. He invaded England in 1015 and conquered Norway in 1028. Canute ruled his huge empire with justice and fairness until his death.

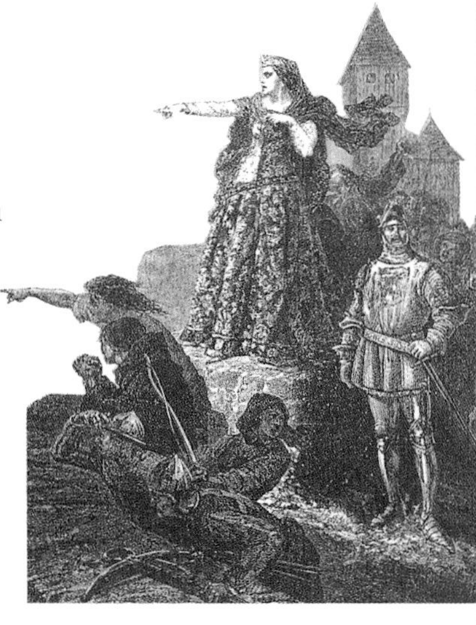

MARGARET I
Margaret I (1353-1412) became queen of Denmark (1375), Norway (1380), and Sweden (1389). In 1397 she united these countries in the Kalmar Union.

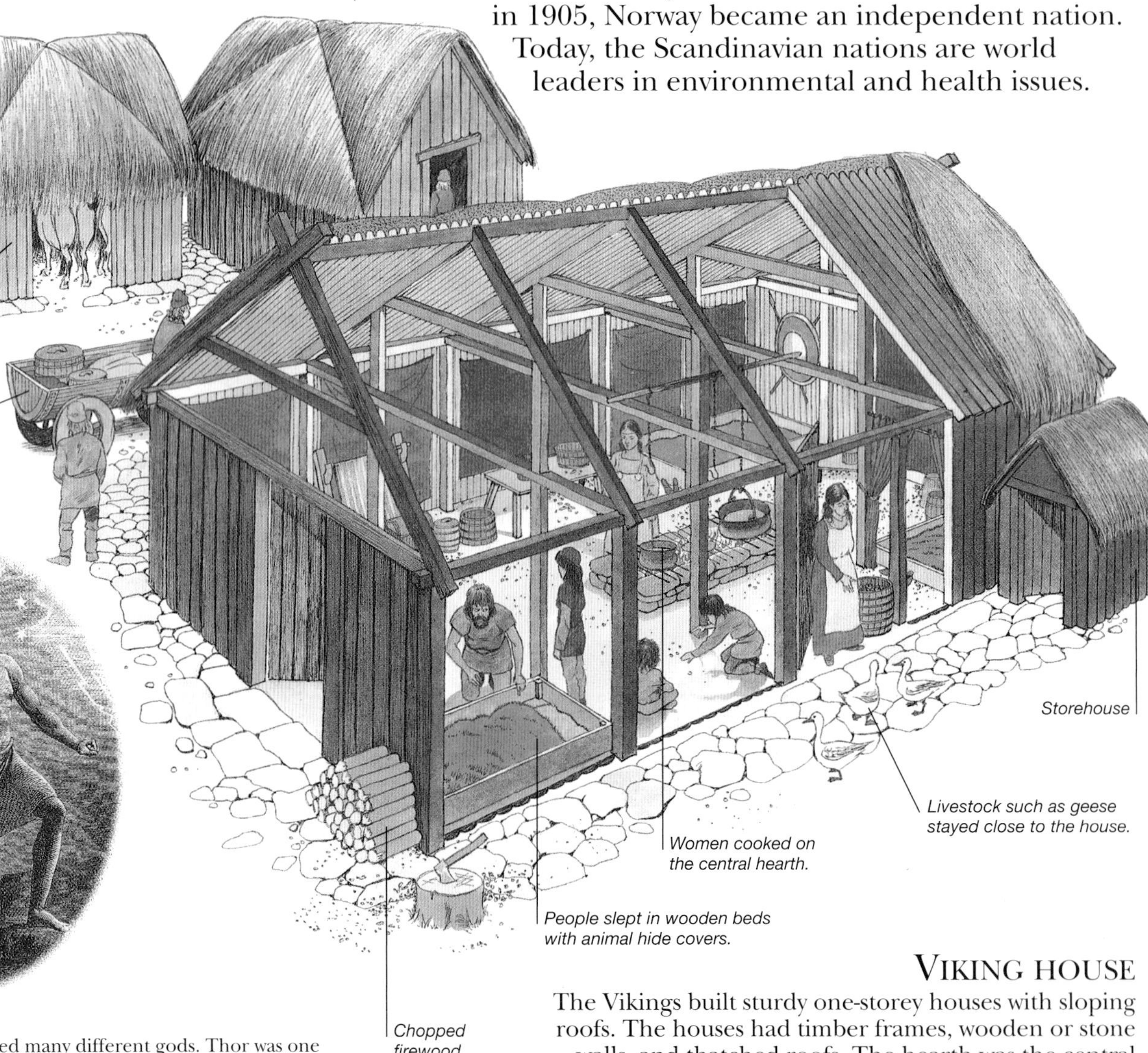

Thatched roof

Cowshed

Hollowed-out tree trunks were fixed with wheels and used as carts.

Storehouse

Livestock such as geese stayed close to the house.

Women cooked on the central hearth.

People slept in wooden beds with animal hide covers.

Chopped firewood

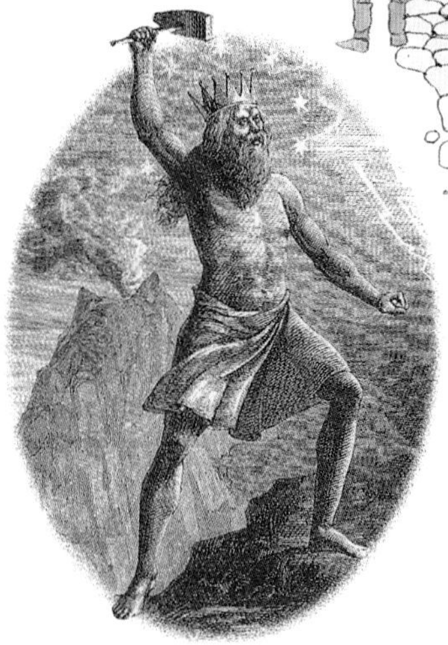

THOR
The Vikings worshipped many different gods. Thor was one of the most powerful. As ruler of the sky, he controlled the weather and was the god of thunder, lightning, rain, and storms. Vikings prayed to him for good harvests and good luck. He gave his name to Thor's day, or Thursday.

VIKING HOUSE

The Vikings built sturdy one-storey houses with sloping roofs. The houses had timber frames, wooden or stone walls, and thatched roofs. The hearth was the central feature in the house. It provided heat, light, and a place to cook. Viking houses had no windows, so the one room was usually very smoky.

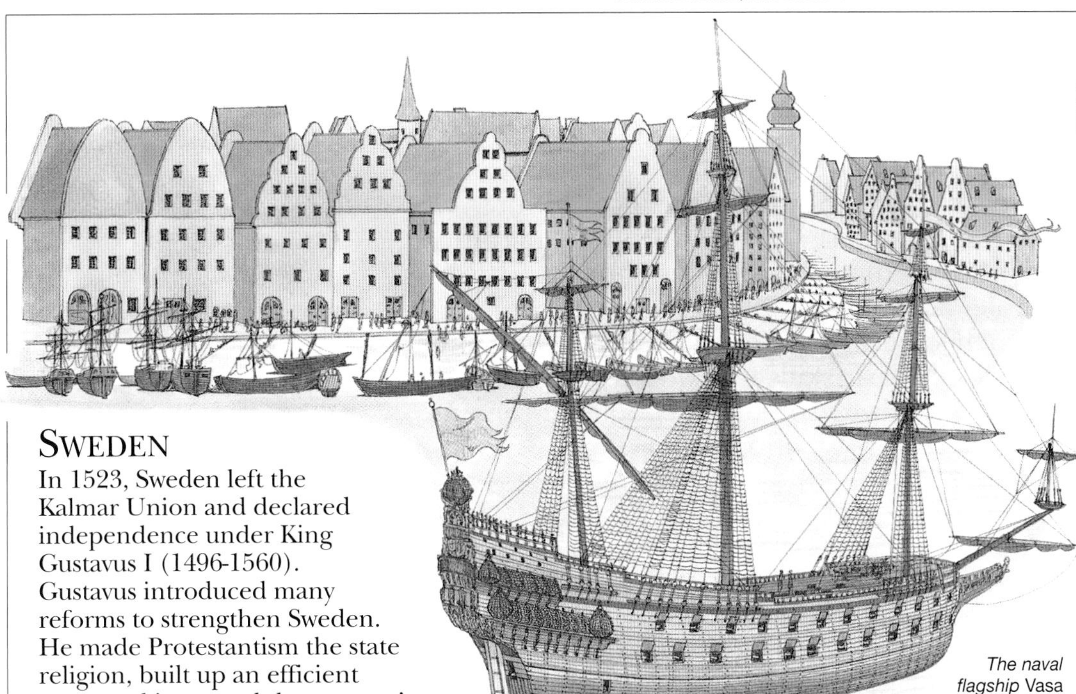

The naval flagship *Vasa* capsized in Stockholm harbour on its maiden voyage in 1628

SWEDEN

In 1523, Sweden left the Kalmar Union and declared independence under King Gustavus I (1496-1560). Gustavus introduced many reforms to strengthen Sweden. He made Protestantism the state religion, built up an efficient army, and improved the country's economy. During the reign of Gustavus II, which lasted from 1611 to 1632, Sweden became a major European power. Gustavus increased Swedish territory, gaining most of Finland from Russia. He also built a strong navy.

SCANDINAVIA

A.D. 800s-1000s Vikings raid Europe for land and trade.

1014-35 King Canute of Denmark rules vast empire.

1319 Norway and Sweden unite.

1375-1412 Margaret I rules Denmark.

1397-1523 Kalmar Union unites Denmark, Norway, and Sweden as Scandinavia.

1523 Sweden becomes independent under Gustavus I; Norway remains part of Denmark until 1814.

1500s-1700s Sweden and Russia fight for control of Finland.

1612-32 Reign of Gustavus II of Sweden; Sweden becomes major European power.

1658 Swedish power at its height.

1700-21 Great Northern War ends Swedish power in the Baltic.

1814-1905 Norway ruled by Sweden.

1901 First Nobel Prizes awarded.

1905 Norway independent.

1917 Finland declares independence from Russia following Russian Revolution.

1914-18 Scandinavian nations are neutral during World War I.

1940-45 Germany occupies Norway and Denmark during World War II.

1986 Olof Palme, Prime Minister of Sweden, assassinated.

GREAT NORTHERN WAR

Between 1563 and 1658, the Swedes fought wars with their neighbours that resulted in the Swedish domination of the Baltic Sea, an important waterway. For the next 40 years there was an uneasy peace in the region. Then, in 1700, Russia, Denmark, and Poland declared war to end Swedish power. The Great Northern War, as it was called, lasted for 21 years. The Swedes lost lands in the east to Russia.

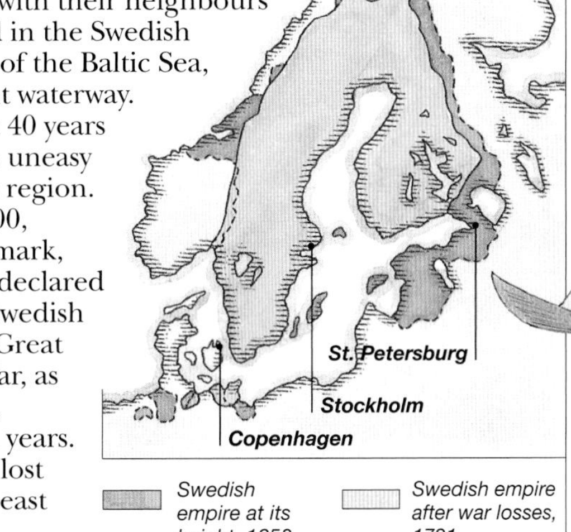

Swedish empire at its height, 1658

Swedish empire after war losses, 1721

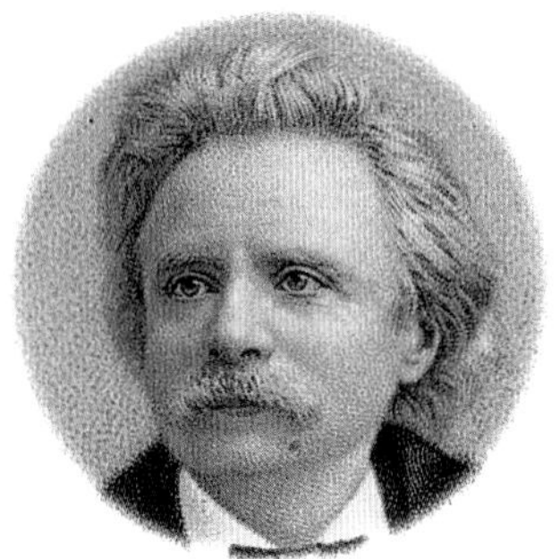

EDVARD GRIEG
During the 19th century, Sweden ruled Norway. The Norwegian composer Edvard Grieg (1843-1907) supported independence. He became known as the Voice of Norway, because he wrote patriotic music based on old Norwegian folk songs. His most famous work is music for the playwright Ibsen's *Peer Gynt*.

CHRISTIAN X
Germany invaded Norway and Denmark during World War II (1939-45). The Norwegian king, Haakon VII, went into exile in Britain, and Vidkun Quisling, a German supporter, took over. The word quisling is still used today to describe a traitor. In Denmark, King Christian X (left) led passive resistance to German rule. The Germans demanded that all Jews wear a yellow star, so Christian stated that he too would wear a star. The Danes then helped many Jews escape to neutral Sweden.

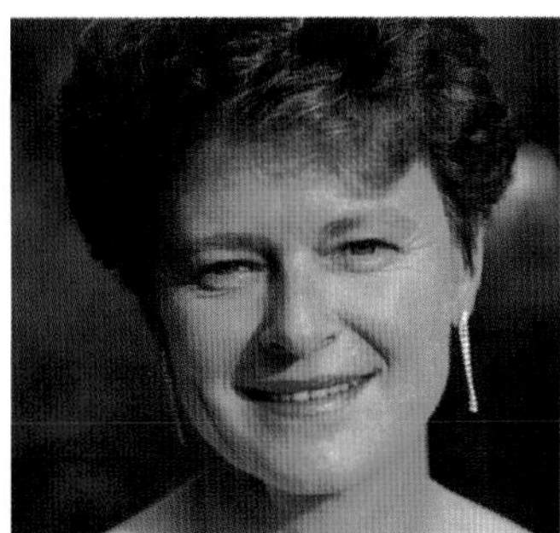

GRO BRUNDTLAND
In 1987, Norwegian Prime Minister Gro Brundtland published *Our Common Future: The Brundtland Report*, a major work that described environmental problems and their effects on the poor of the world. It also suggested solutions.

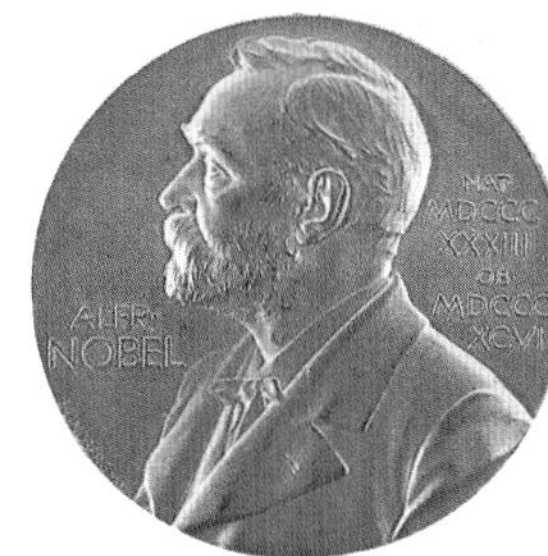

NOBEL PRIZE
Swedish chemist Alfred Nobel (1833-96) invented dynamite. He disliked its military uses, and left money in his will to fund prizes to promote peace and learning. Prizes – for physics, chemistry, medicine, literature, and peace – have been awarded since 1901.

Find out more
SCANDINAVIA
VIKINGS

Schools

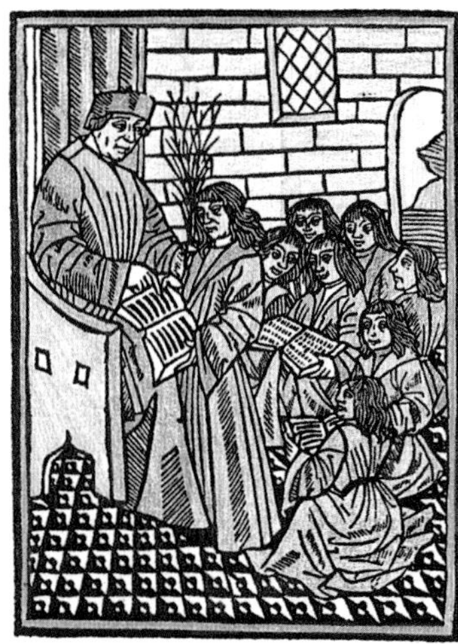

MEDIEVAL TEACHING
Discipline was strict and the school day was long for the 13th-century student. There was little reading and writing, and students learned mainly by listening to the teacher and asking questions. However, by the end of the 15th century, books of Latin grammar were a popular teaching aid.

MOST PEOPLE REMEMBER starting school. Schools vary depending on the local culture of a country, but most of us felt the same mixture of confusion and excitement on our first day at school. Many of us share other early school experiences, too. Schools all over the world aim to teach the basic skills that we need to live in society. For this reason most schoolchildren take classes in reading, writing, and arithmetic. In most Western countries, these early school years are known as primary or elementary school, because they are a preparation for later years of education. Reading skills, for example, are essential for everyone throughout their lives. In some other countries, though, school ends for many children at the age of 10, or even earlier. Schooling is expensive, and only the wealthier countries can afford to operate free schools for all children beyond the first four or five years. Even in those countries where primary education is free, many families need the extra money that younger children can earn; so millions of children work as well as – or instead of – attending school.

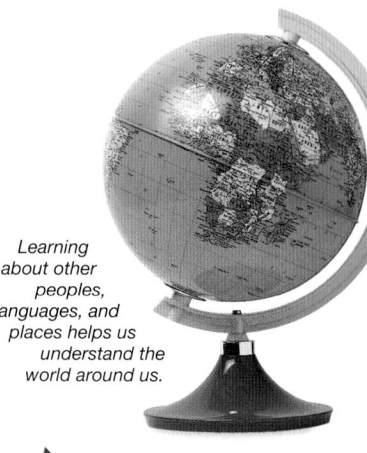

Learning about other peoples, languages, and places helps us understand the world around us.

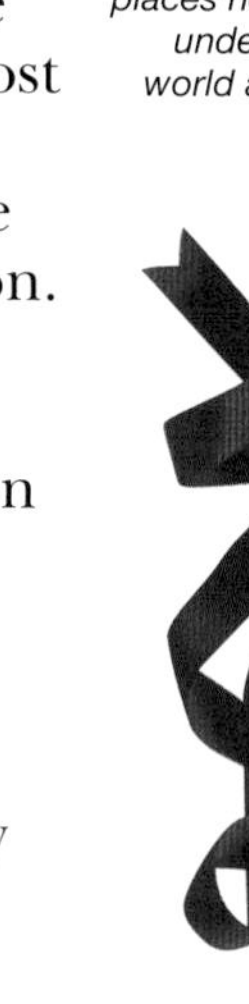

Most schoolchildren enjoy painting and sculpture; experience at school can lead to an appreciation of the great artists.

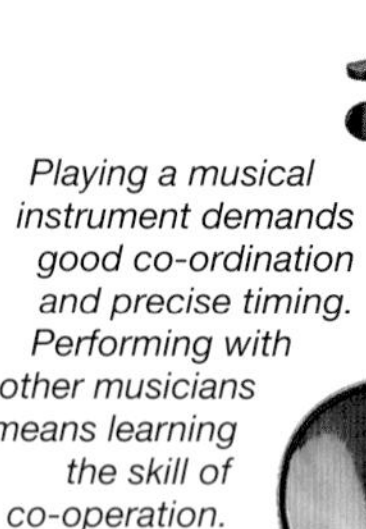

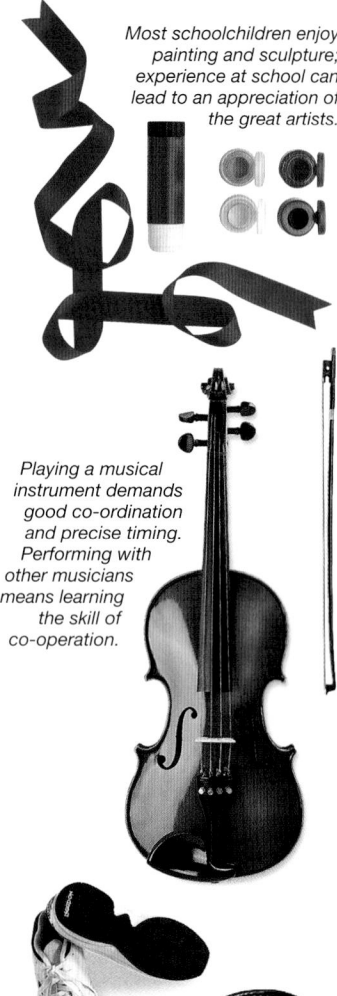

Playing a musical instrument demands good co-ordination and precise timing. Performing with other musicians means learning the skill of co-operation.

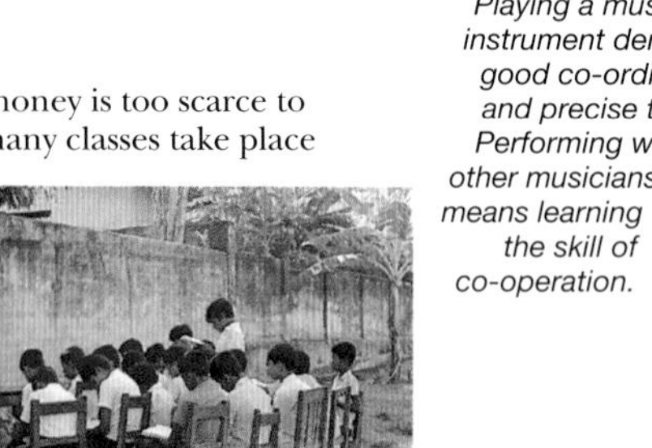

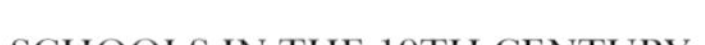

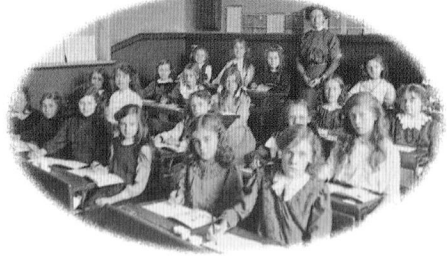

SCHOOLS IN THE 19TH CENTURY
In the last century free schooling for all became common in many European countries and in the United States. The school schedule was similar to that of today, but learning was not as exciting as it is now. For example, 19th-century teachers expected children to remember long lists of facts which they recited out loud in the classroom.

OPEN-AIR CLASSROOMS
In parts of Africa and India where money is too scarce to provide enough school buildings, many classes take place out of doors. In countries where the population is scattered, schools are far apart and children may walk several kilometres to learn. When the nearest school is very distant, as in Australia, a two-way radio brings the school to the pupil.

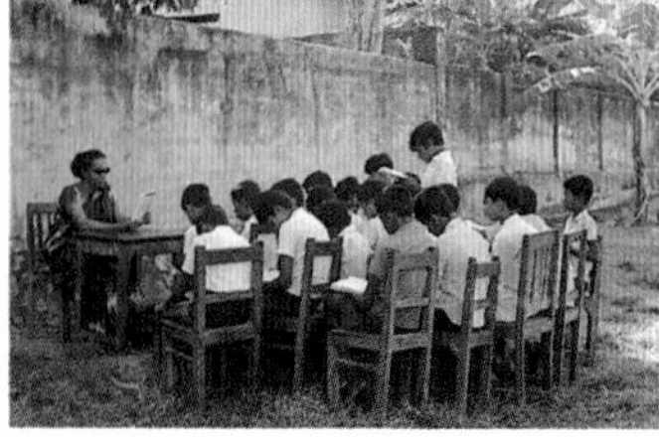

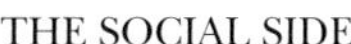

THE SOCIAL SIDE
School life includes learning to share, communicate, and get along with others. Members of a class must learn to work together and listen to other people's opinions and ideas. The school is also a place where young people learn how to make friends and cope with differences.

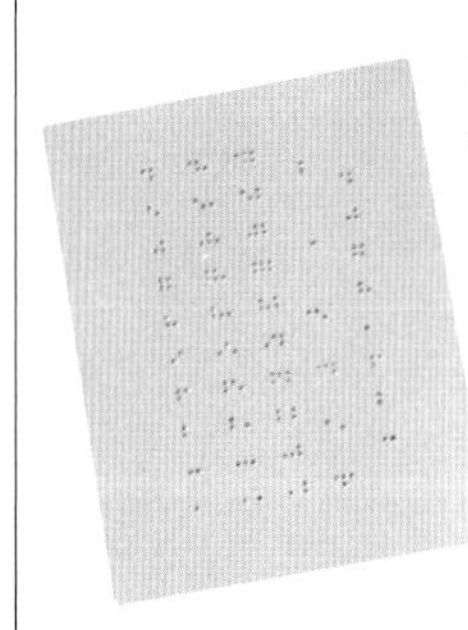

BRAILLE
Children with a physical disability may need special equipment, such as braille books, to help them study. Braille is a system of raised dots that represent words. Sight-impaired children read braille by passing their fingertips over the patterns of dots.

Regular exercise not only improves physical health, but is also vital for mental wellbeing. Physical education teaches children about discipline and endurance, and encourages both teamwork and the ability to perform as an individual.

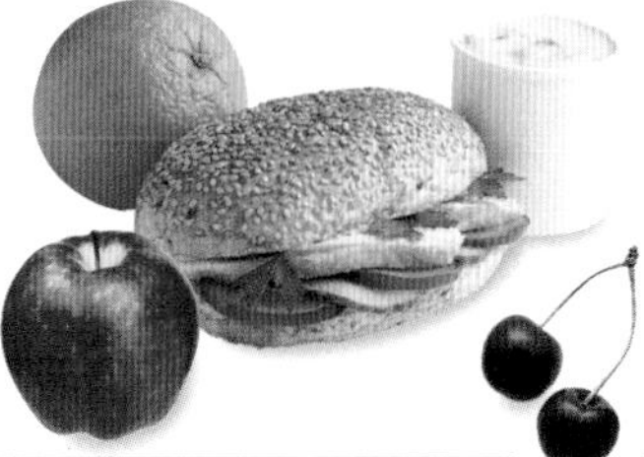

Both boys and girls study food technology – planning a meal, shopping to a budget, preparation, and presentation – as well as the essentials of a healthy and nutritious diet to prepare them for an independent adult life.

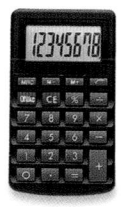

The ability to calculate and measure is essential in everyday life, as well as in many careers. Mathematical skills also improve logic and aid problem-solving in other scientific subjects.

Levels of schools

Education is compulsory in Britain between the ages of five and 16. Before five, some children attend nursery or play schools. At four or five, children go to primary schools, some of which are split into infants and juniors. Secondary education lasts until 16, with some students staying on until 18. After leaving school, many students go on to further education at college or higher education at university.

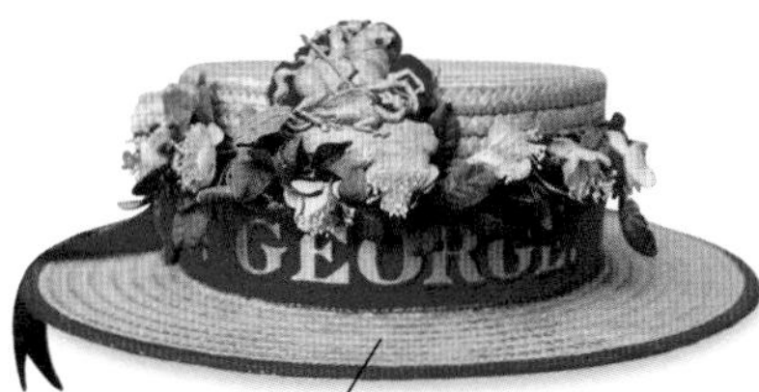

Traditional boater hat from Eton

STATE OR PRIVATE?

Most British children go to schools run by their local council or the churches. These schools are known as state schools and are free. Some children attend independent, or private schools, for which fees have to be paid. Confusingly, some of these schools, such as Eton or Winchester, are called public schools.

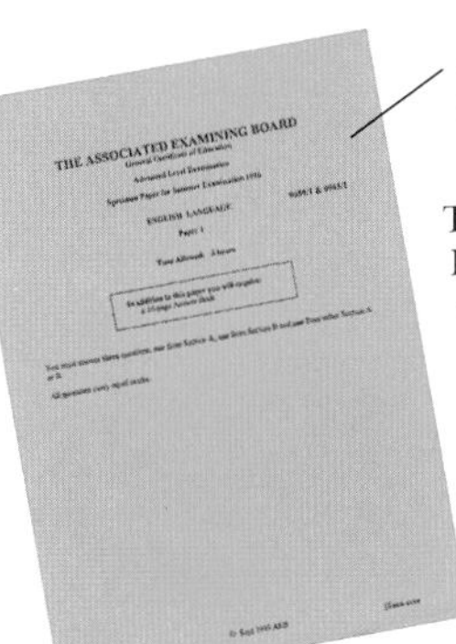

THE ASSOCIATED EXAMINING BOARD

Sample Advanced Level exam paper

THE EXAM SYSTEM

Every child has to sit exams throughout his or her school life. The most important of them are GCSEs (General Certificate of Secondary Education) and A (Advanced) levels. GCSEs are taken at the age of 16 in Year 11 at secondary school. A levels are made up of AS and A2 exams, which are taken at the end of years one and two in a school sixth form or college, usually at the ages of 17 and 18. Exams are in the form of written essays or multiple choice questions and many take into account work produced throughout the year.

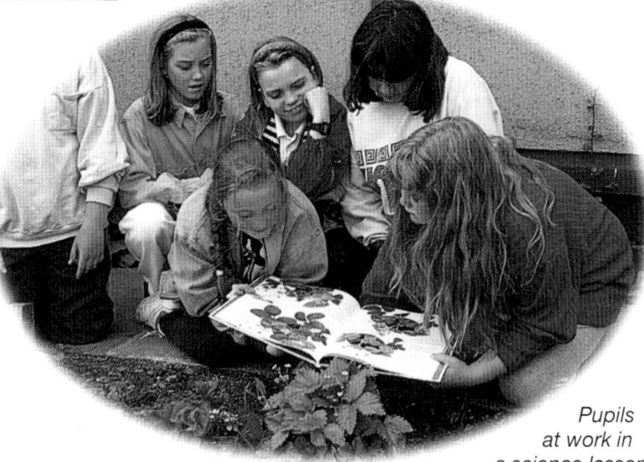

Pupils at work in a science lesson.

THE NATIONAL CURRICULUM

The National Curriculum was introduced in 1989 to ensure that every child receives a broad education across arts and sciences. The curriculum is delivered in four stages and consists of three core subjects – English (and Welsh in Wales), maths, and science – which are compulsory up to GCSE level. A range of other subjects, such as information technology and geography, are compulsory at different stages, while literacy and numeracy must be taught in all primary schools.

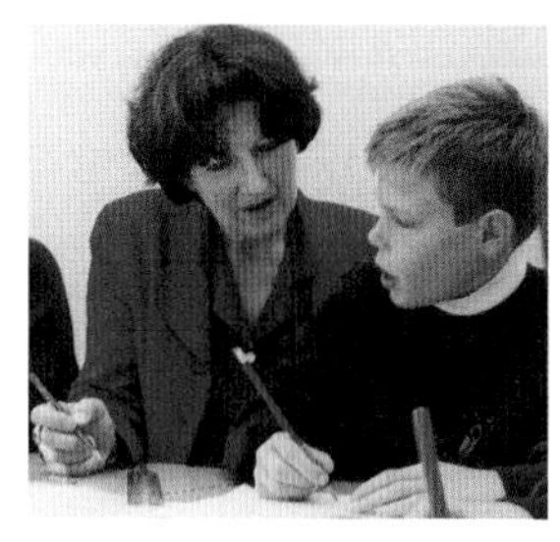

SPECIAL NEEDS

Some children need extra help to read or write. These needs are met with additional teaching support in the classroom. Children with severe difficulties, such as physical or mental disability, may be educated in special schools designed to help them learn.

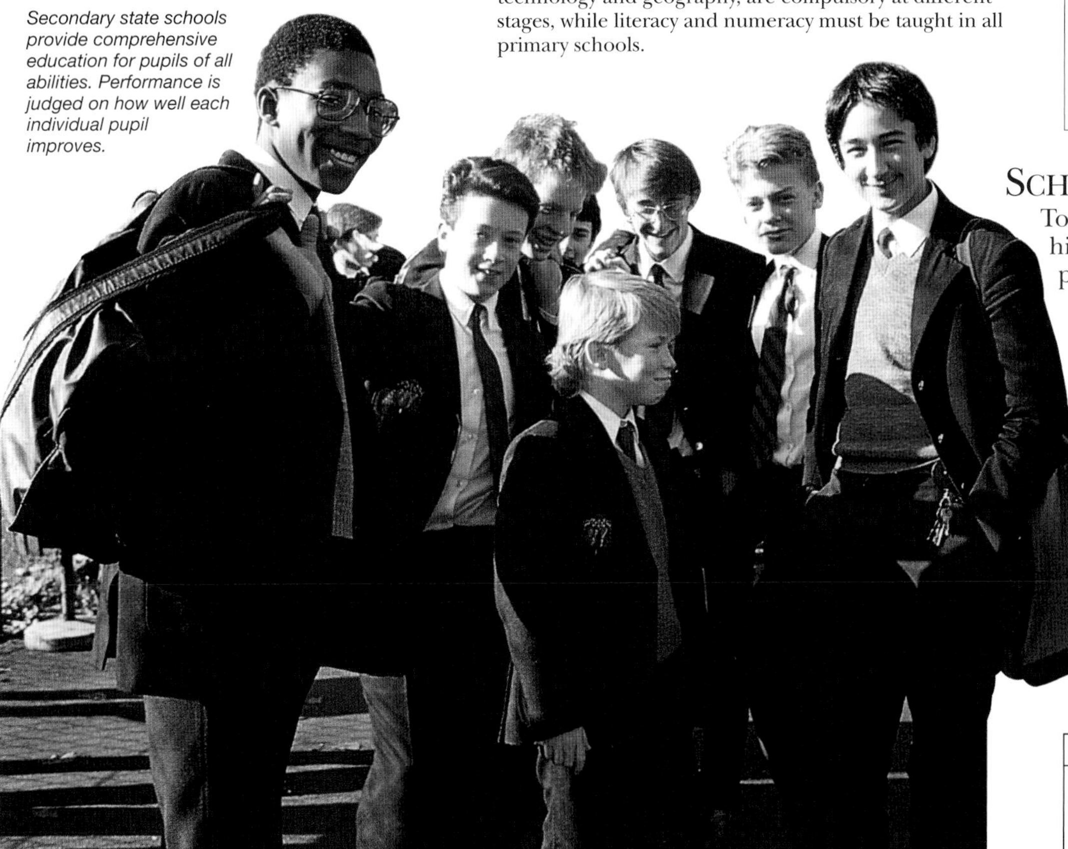

Secondary state schools provide comprehensive education for pupils of all abilities. Performance is judged on how well each individual pupil improves.

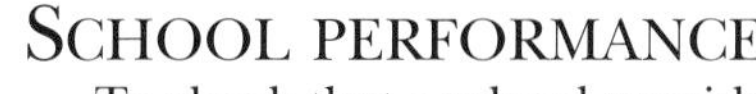

School performance

To check that a school provides high-quality education, all pupils are examined on their skills when they enter primary school. They are then assessed in English and maths at the age of 7, and science as well at the ages of 11 and 14, after finishing stages 1-3 of the national curriculum. Newspapers publish some results, so that everyone can see how well a school is performing.

Find out more

Computers
Education
Information technology

SCIENCE

A glass rod in a beaker of water looks bent because light waves travel slower through water than through air.

THERE ARE MANY FORMS OF SCIENCE, and together they study the nature and behaviour of the universe and everything in it. Science comes from the Latin word for "to know". Scientists find out what they want to know by practical methods. They observe, take measurements, make experiments, and write down the results. There are four main categories (types)of science: natural sciences, physical sciences, technological sciences, and social sciences. Natural sciences include the life sciences, such as biology and botany, and earth sciences, such as geology. Physical sciences include physics and chemistry. Technological science includes engineering, and uses information discovered by scientists to make or build things in the real world. Social sciences study people, and include anthropology and psychology. All the sciences depend on mathematics.

PHYSICS

Physics is the study of matter and energy, and how they work together. Because there are many different kinds of matter and forms of energy, there are many different branches of physics. Optics, for example, looks at the different way light waves can behave. For instance, they travel at different speeds through space, air, glass, or water.

SCIENTIFIC METHOD

Scientific method involves using observation and hypotheses (theories) to explain things, and then testing these hypotheses with experiments. To be sure that their results are accurate, scientists always follow strict rules when making an experiment. A sample of the materials used in the experiment is set aside as a "control". If the result is unusual, the control materials can be tested to make sure that they have not been changed and so affected the result of the experiment.

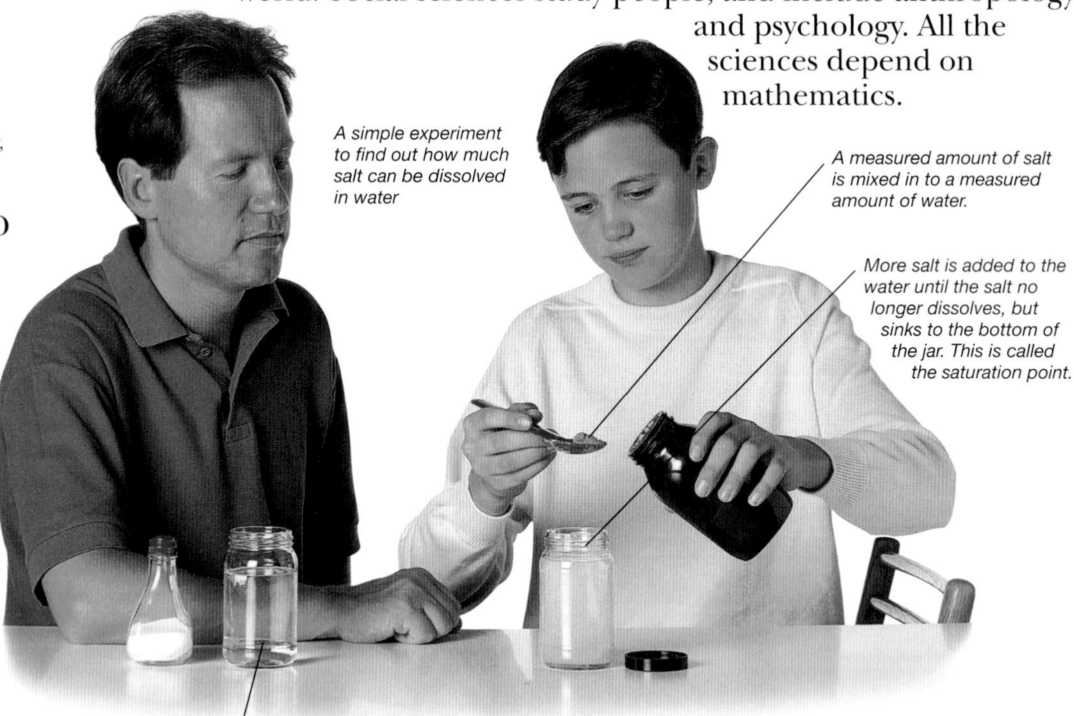

A simple experiment to find out how much salt can be dissolved in water

A measured amount of salt is mixed in to a measured amount of water.

More salt is added to the water until the salt no longer dissolves, but sinks to the bottom of the jar. This is called the saturation point.

Water and salt act as a control for the study.

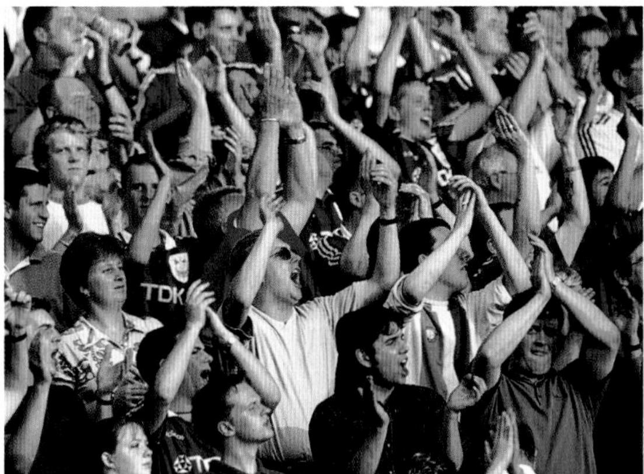

SOCIAL SCIENCES

The sciences that study people are called social sciences. There are various kinds. Anthropology is the study of life and culture of the whole of humanity. Sociology studies the way humans behave together in groups; it looks at how families work, how society is made up, what makes it change, and how the changes affect people. Psychology is also a social science, but it looks at how people behave as individuals.

Bean shoot

Shoot grows up towards the sun.

LIFE SCIENCES

Any of the sciences that study living things is called a life science. Biology is the study of life of all kinds, botany is the study of plants, and zoology is the study of animals. Because animal and plant life depend on each other, scientists also study them together. Ecology is the study of the relationships between living things of all kinds and how they fit in with and affect their environments.

Roots absorb water and nutrients.

EARTH SCIENCES

Geography and geology are earth sciences. Earth scientists study the structure of our planet and the way it changes. The study of rocks and fossils can tell us a lot about the way the planet and its life have evolved. Since Earth is a living planet, the earth sciences are linked to the life sciences.

Geologists study rocks and crystals.

Chrysocolla

Cyanotrichite

Find out more

BIOLOGY
CHEMISTRY
EARTH
PHYSICS
ROCKS AND MINERALS

HISTORY OF

SCIENCE

SPACE TRAVEL, computers, and reliable medical care are just a few of the things that owe their existence to scientists and inventors. Scientists study the natural world, from distant galaxies to tiny atoms, and try to explain what they see. The work of a scientist is based on a cycle of experiment, observation, and theorization (making theories). For instance, in the 17th century, English scientist Isaac Newton experimented with sunlight passing through a prism. From the spectrum (bands of colours) that he observed, he suggested the theory that white light is a mixture of colours. Inventors are people who think of a new idea that can be put into practice. An invention may be the result of a scientific discovery, such as the laser, which Theodore Maiman (born 1927) built because of his knowledge of light and atoms. However, this is not always the case. Early people invented the lever before they knew how it worked. Whatever their chosen fields, scientists and inventors have one thing in common: they are people of rare insight who make discoveries new to the world.

ANCIENT TIMES

Early people first invented tools about 2 million years ago. About 10,000 years ago, people began to settle in communities and started farming and building. The first civilizations grew up in the Middle East, Africa, India, and China. There, people studied the sun and stars, built simple clocks, developed mathematics, and discovered how to make metals and pottery.

This stone blade was used about 200,000 years ago in Egypt.

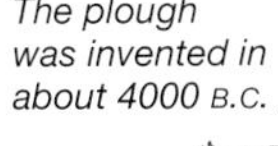

The wheel was invented in about 3500 B.C.

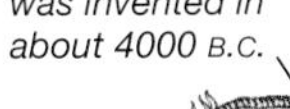

The plough was invented in about 4000 B.C.

GREEKS AND ROMANS

From about 600 B.C., the Greeks began to study their world. Great philosophers (thinkers) such as Pythagoras developed the "scientific method" – the principle of observation and experiment that is still the basis of science today. The Greeks studied mathematics and astronomy and invented simple machines. At around the same time, the Romans used Greek scientific ideas to help them build great structures.

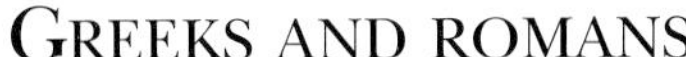

The pump was invented in the 2nd century B.C.

Hero of Greece built the first simple steam engine in the 1st century A.D.

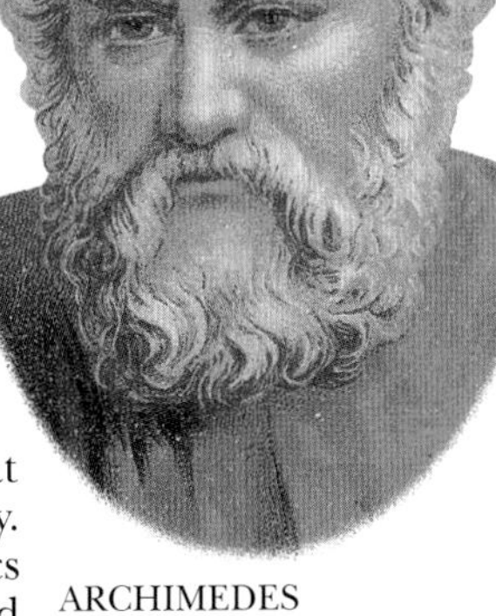

ARCHIMEDES

Greek scientist Archimedes (287-212 B.C.) explained how levers and pulleys work and discovered how things float. This idea is said to have come to him while he was in his bath.

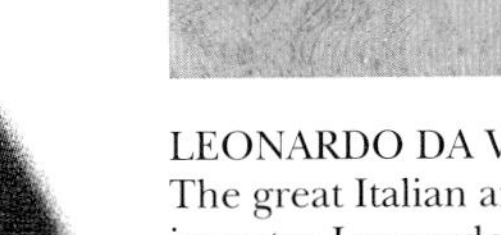

LEONARDO DA VINCI

The great Italian artist and inventor Leonardo da Vinci (1452-1519) designed many machines, including a parachute and a helicopter. However, these machines were never built.

A.D. 1000-1600

During this period, Arabic civilizations made several discoveries, particularly about the nature of light. After about A.D. 1000, people in Europe began to use the scientific method of the Ancient Greeks. Polish astronomer Nicolaus Copernicus (1473-1543) suggested that the Earth orbits the sun, and Andreas Vesalius (1514-64), a Flemish doctor, made discoveries about human anatomy.

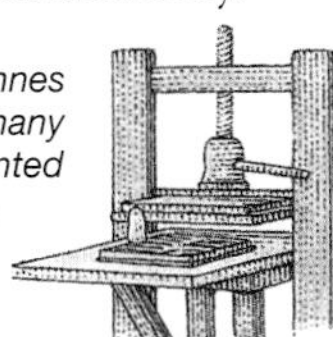

In 1438, Johannes Gutenberg of Germany (c.1398-1468) invented the modern printing process.

Archimedes's screw was a device for raising water.

A balloon first carried people in 1783.

In 1608, Dutch optician Hans Lippershey invented the telescope.

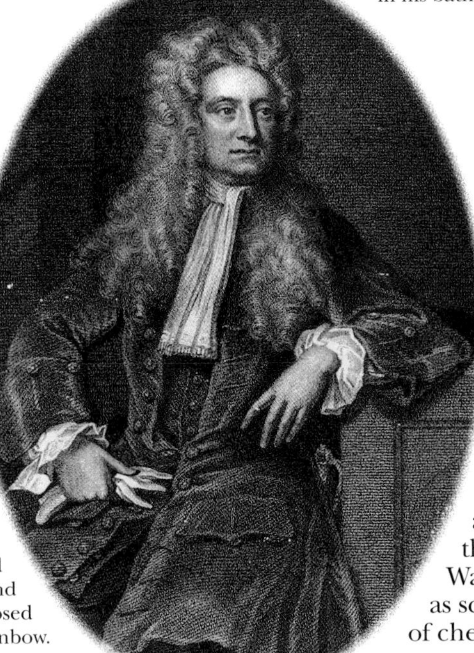

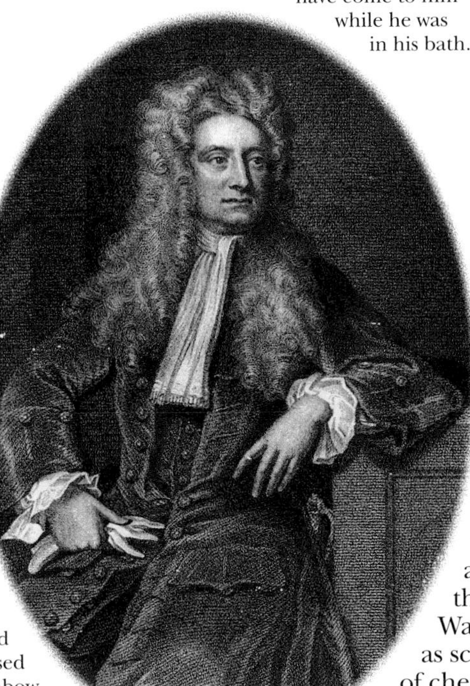

ISAAC NEWTON

In 1666, Isaac Newton (1642-1727) proposed the daring idea that gravity is a universal force, keeping planets and moons in their orbits as well as causing things to fall to the ground. Newton also put forward the famous laws of motion, and found that white light is composed of the colours in the rainbow.

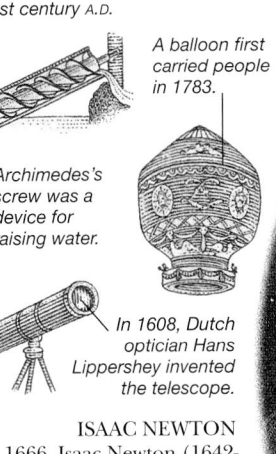

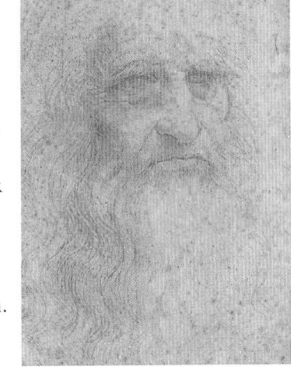

1600-1800

Italian scientist Galileo Galilei (1564-1642) made discoveries about force, gravity, and motion. Modern astronomy began in 1609 when German astronomer Johannes Kepler (1571-1630) discovered the laws of planetary motion and Galileo built a telescope to observe the heavens. During the 1700s, the first engines were built by inventors such as James Watt (1736-1819) of Scotland. Chemistry advanced as scientists discovered how everything is composed of chemical elements such as oxygen and hydrogen.

1800-1900

The invention of the battery by Italian Alessandro Volta (1745-1827) led to discoveries about electricity and magnetism by scientists such as Englishman Michael Faraday (1791-1867) and many electrical inventions such as electric light. Englishman John Dalton (1766-1844) and other scientists found out that everything is made of tiny atoms. Frenchman Louis Pasteur (1822-1895) showed that bacteria cause disease, which led to better health care. Transport advanced with the invention of locomotives, powered ships, and cars.

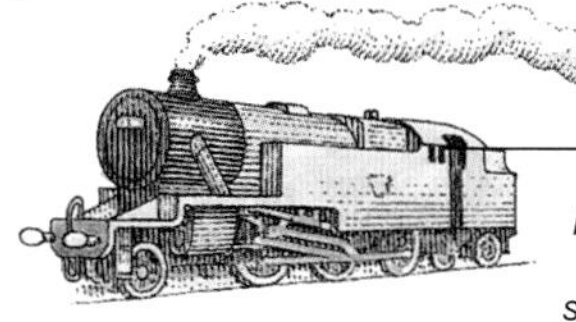

In 1804 Englishman Richard Trevithick invented the steam locomotive.

The telephone was invented by a Scottish-American, Alexander Graham Bell, in 1876.

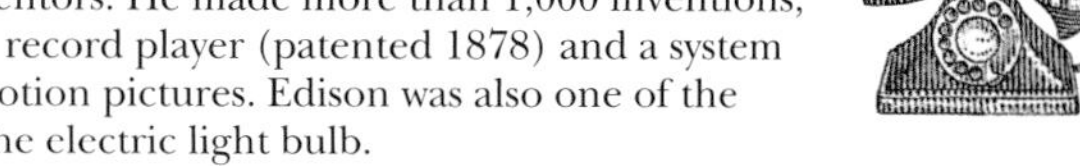

In 1895 Italian scientist Guglielmo Marconi invented radio transmission.

THOMAS EDISON
Thomas Edison (1847-1931) was one of the world's most successful inventors. He made more than 1,000 inventions, including the record player (patented 1878) and a system for making motion pictures. Edison was also one of the inventors of the electric light bulb.

1900 TO THE PRESENT

Scientists delved into the atom, finding electrons and the nucleus, and then studied the nucleus itself. This led to the invention of nuclear power and to the science of electronics, which brought us television and the computer. Scientists also explored living cells and found new ways of fighting disease. Astronomers studied stars, planets, and distant galaxies. The invention of aircraft and space flight allowed people to travel into the air and out into space.

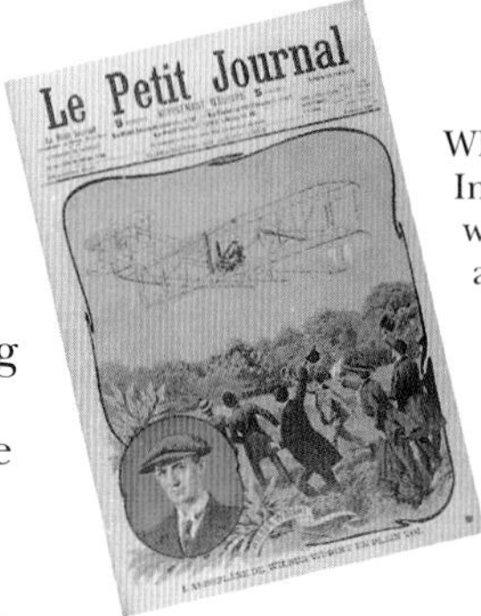

Le Petit Journal

WRIGHT BROTHERS
In 1903, the world watched in wonder as Orville Wright (1871-1948) and his brother Wilbur (1867-1912) made the first powered aeroplane flight.

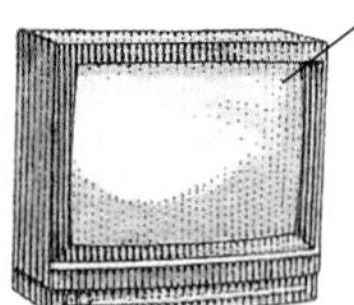

Several scientists developed television during the 1920s. The first public television service started in the 1930s.

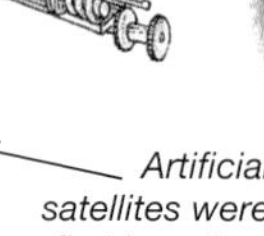

Theodore Maiman and Charles Townes invented the first working laser in 1960.

Artificial satellites were first launched in 1957.

WILLIAM SHOCKLEY
Computers, televisions, and other electronic devices depend on the transistor, invented in 1948 by a team of scientists headed by William Shockley (born 1910). Now millions of transistors can be packed into a tiny microchip.

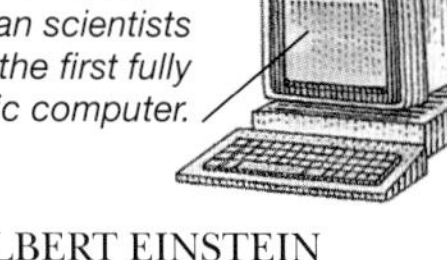

In 1946 a team of American scientists built the first fully electronic computer.

ALBERT EINSTEIN
In 1905 and 1915, the German scientist Albert Einstein (1879-1955) proposed his theories of relativity. They showed that light is the fastest thing in the universe, and that time would slow down, length would shorten, and mass would increase if you could travel at almost the speed of light. The sun's source of energy and nuclear power, and how black holes can exist in space are explained by his discoveries.

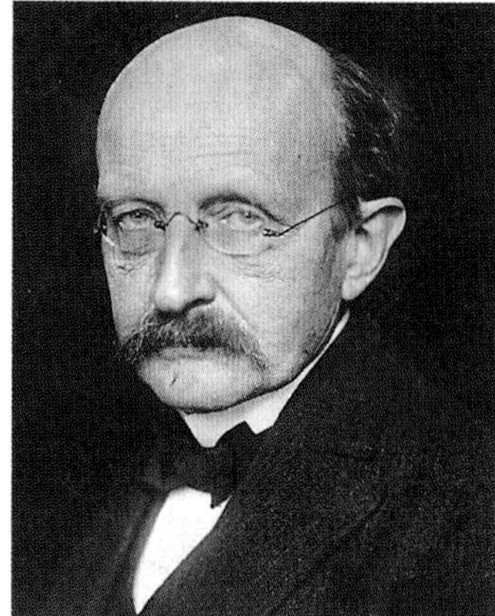

MAX PLANCK
In about 1900, German scientist Max Planck (1858-1947) published his quantum theory, which explained the nature of energy and led to many new ideas. For example, although we usually think of light as waves, quantum theory explains how light sometimes seems to behave as tiny particles called photons.

HISTORY OF SCIENCE

5000 B.C. Metal objects first made in Middle East.

400 B.C. Greek scientist Democritus suggests that all things are made of atoms.

A.D. 105 Chinese inventor Ts'ai Lun makes paper.

A.D. 650 Persians invent the windmill.

A.D. 1000 Chinese use gunpowder in warfare.

1657 Dutchman Christiaan Huygens constructs pendulum clock.

1712 English engineer Thomas Newcomen builds first practical steam engine.

1775 Englishman Joseph Priestley discovers oxygen.

1789 French scientist Antoine Lavoisier explains chemical reactions.

1803 English scientist John Dalton explains existence of atoms.

1826 Frenchman Joseph Niépce takes first photograph.

1869 Russian Dmitri Mendeleev shows relationships of elements in his periodic table.

1879 Thomas Edison (US) and Englishman Joseph Swan invent electric light bulb.

1885 German engineer Karl Benz builds first car.

1888 German scientist Heinrich Hertz discovers radio waves.

1898 French-Polish scientist Marie Curie discovers radium.

1911 English scientist Ernest Rutherford discovers nucleus of the atom.

1924 US astronomer Edwin Hubble discovers galaxies and, in 1929, the expansion of the universe.

1942 Italian scientist Enrico Fermi builds first nuclear reactor.

1959 Soviet Union launches first space probe.

1990s Global communications network established.

Find out more

BIOLOGY
CHEMISTRY
MEDICINE, HISTORY OF
PHYSICS
RENAISSANCE
SCIENCE
TECHNOLOGY

SCOTLAND

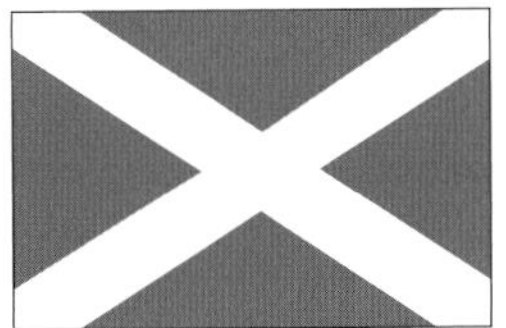

ST. ANDREW'S CROSS
The cross of St. Andrew, patron saint of Scotland, is called the saltire.

FROM EDINBURGH TO THE HIGHLANDS, the Scottish people are proud of their unique culture. Scotland is part of the United Kingdom, but has kept some of its independence. Scottish banks print their own pound notes, the legal system is different to that of England and Wales, Scottish university courses last four years, not three as in England, and Scottish students sit Higher Still examinations, not A-levels. Since 1999, Scotland has also regained its parliament. Because it is so far north, Scotland has short days in winter, but long hours of daylight in summer. The old industries have declined, but new jobs have been created in service industries and through North Sea oil.

Scotland and its islands are the most northerly parts of the United Kingdom.

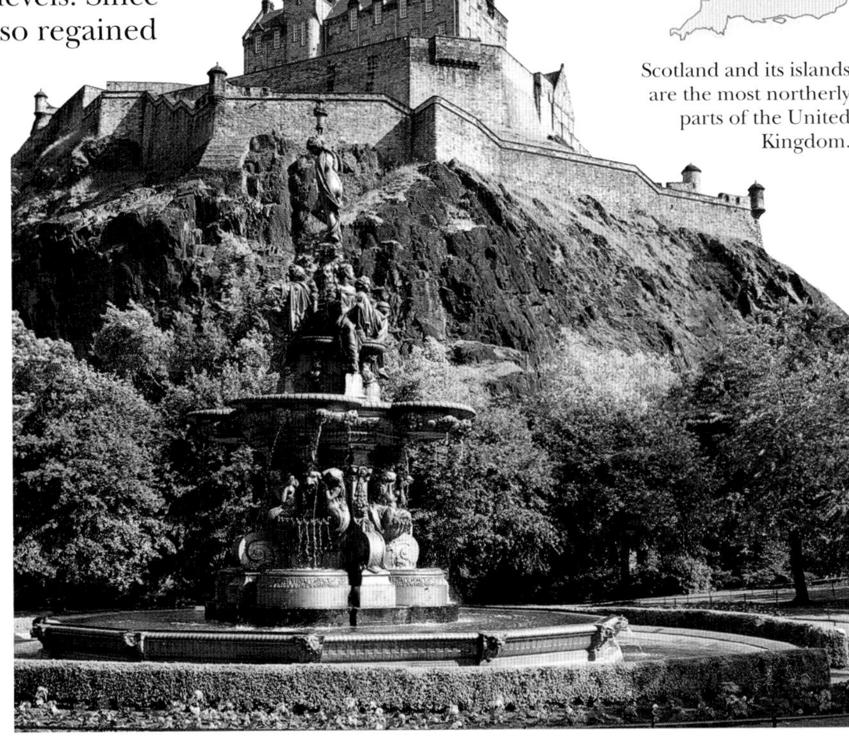

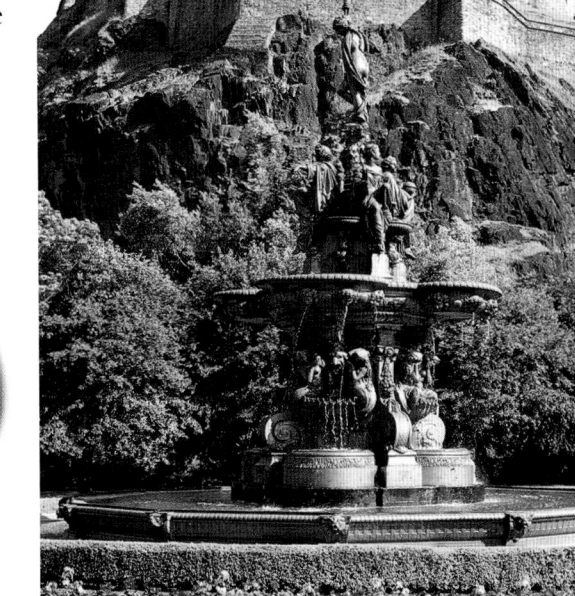

HIGHLANDS
The north of Scotland contains the Highlands, a rugged but beautiful mountainous region that includes Ben Nevis, the highest mountain in Britain, and spectacular lochs (lakes). Scotland covers an area of 78,742 sq km (30,394) sq miles). Of its population of about 5.1 million people, most live further south in the so-called Lowlands, near the cities of Glasgow and Edinburgh.

EDINBURGH

The capital of Scotland is the city of Edinburgh. The kings of Scotland used to rule the country from Edinburgh, and the newly created Scottish parliament has its home there. The volcanic crag at the centre is topped by Edinburgh Castle, and dominates the city's skyline. Every year, Edinburgh hosts an internationally renowned arts festival.

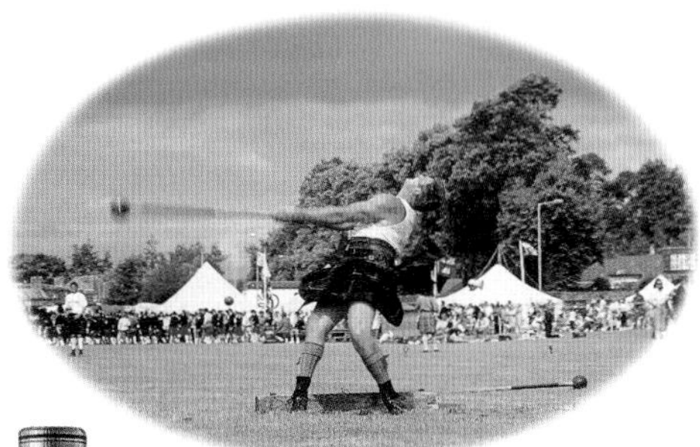

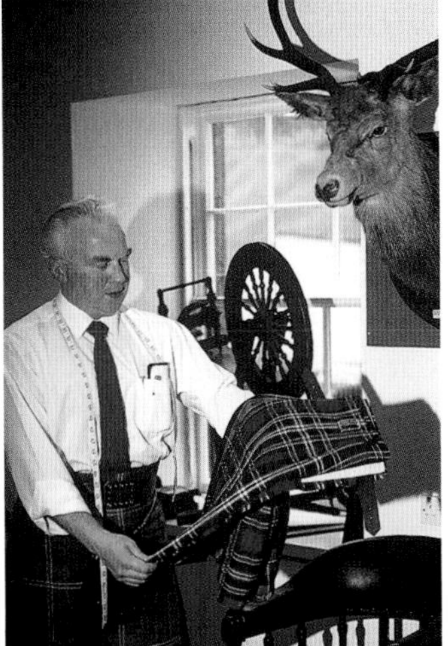

Sporran

KILTS AND SPORRANS
Tartan and kilts are unique to Scottish culture. A kilt is like a skirt and is made from tartan, a checked woollen material. Traditionally, the kilt is worn with the sporran, special shoes, and sometimes a dagger tucked into a sock. There are many different tartans. Each belongs to a special clan, or tribe.

WHISKY
Scotland is famous for its whisky. Many different distilleries across the country produce hundreds of malt whiskies varying in taste and colour. Traditional Scottish dishes include porridge, and haggis, made from spiced sheep's innards mixed with oats.

HIGHLAND GAMES
The champions of Scotland's traditional sports compete at the annual Highland Games. The Games have a long history, and include events such as putting the shot and throwing the hammer. It also includes a unique event – tossing the caber. For this, athletes compete with each other to pick up and toss (throw) the caber – a large tree trunk – as far as possible.

Find out more
STUARTS
UNITED KINGDOM
UNITED KINGDOM, HISTORY OF

SCULPTURE

BY CARVING SOLID MARBLE or pouring liquid metal, a sculptor can create art in three dimensions. Like paintings and drawings, the resulting sculpture is a vivid image from the artist's imagination. But unlike paintings, which are flat, sculpture is solid, so that you can often walk around it. Sometimes you can touch the sculpture and feel its texture. But it is the depth of sculpture that makes it so interesting. Looking at a sculpture from a different angle changes its appearance completely. For this reason, city planners often use sculpture to brighten up public parks and other outdoor places. Sculptures of people and animals are called statues. But modern sculptors also create abstract sculptures – works which do not represent any real thing but make the space they occupy more interesting, exciting, or restful.

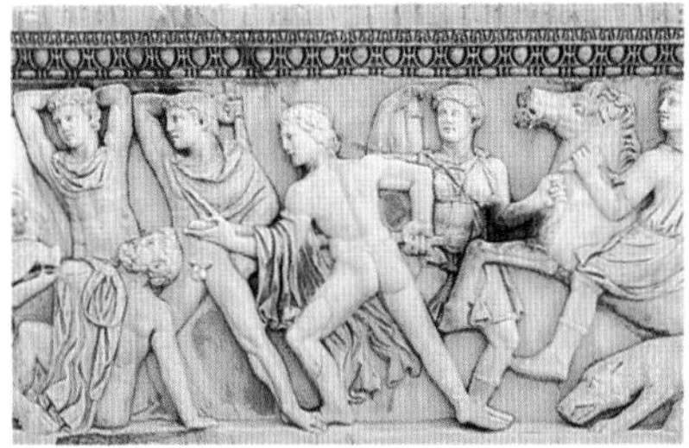

BAS-RELIEF
Not all sculptures are freestanding. Some, called bas-reliefs, are like raised pictures made of wood, metal, or stone. The sculpted figures project a bit from the background, giving a more lifelike quality. Ancient civilizations often recorded great events in their history in bas-relief panels.

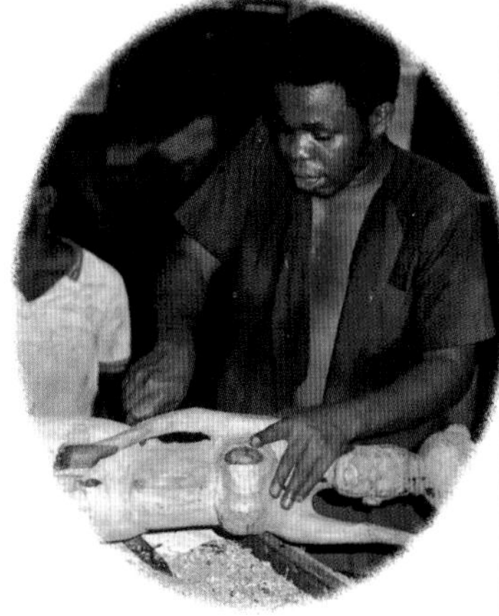

WOOD SCULPTURE
African carvers are expert in wood sculpture. They cut, shave, and polish the wood to make gleaming statues of people and forest or grassland animals. In Europe, woodcarvers decorated the insides of many churches and cathedrals. English sculptor Grinling Gibbons (1648-1720) carved fruits and flowers from wood and decorated St. Paul's Cathedral, London.

Woodcarvers hit their sharp chisels with a wooden mallet to remove large pieces of wood.

For finer work, they shave wood away by pushing the chisel with their hands.

Modelling clay is so soft that even lightweight tools can shape it.

Metal scrapers are useful for shaving the surface of set plaster.

Heavy hammer helps chip stone into shape.

SCULPTOR'S TOOLS
Because sculptors create their art from many different materials, they use a great variety of tools. Hard materials such as stone require powerful cuts from heavy chisels. But to make a sculpture that will be cast in bronze, scrapers and other small tools are all that is needed.

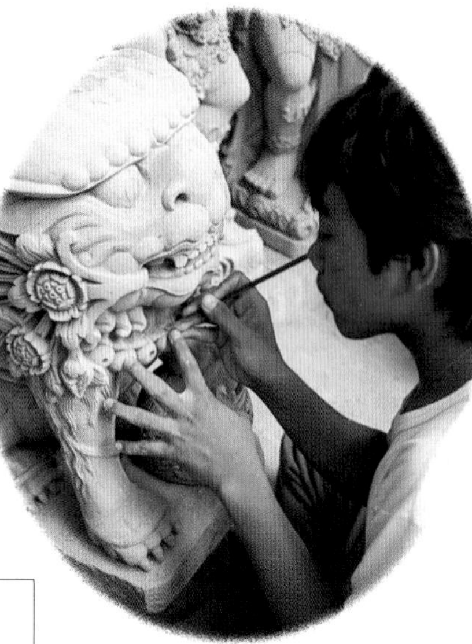

STONE SCULPTURE
Sculptors work with many kinds of stone, but marble is popular because it does not fracture unpredictably when the sculptor strikes it. Before starting work, the sculptor generally makes a plaster maquette, or small model, of the sculpture. Chipping away with chisels and hammer, the sculptor shapes the stone roughly before making the final cuts. A final polish gives the stone a beautiful finish.

BRONZE CASTING

Most cast sculptures are made of bronze – an alloy, or mixture, of copper and tin. The sculptor creates the original work in a soft material such as clay or plaster. From this master, the sculptor can make an identical copy in wax. Covering the model in plaster and heating it melts away the wax and leaves a perfect mould. Filling the mould with the molten (liquid) metal creates the sculpture. Finally, the sculptor cuts off unwanted metal and sometimes polishes the finished work.

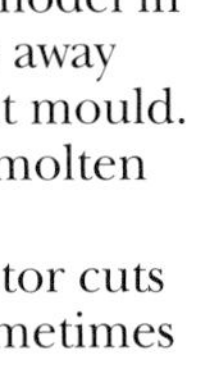

MODERN SCULPTURE

Artists sometimes use sculpture to express ideas about society. American artist Javacheff Christo (born 1935) wraps landscapes and buildings to make people think about the packaging that covers everything they buy.

By wrapping the Pont Neuf, Paris, Christo transformed this French landmark into a work of art.

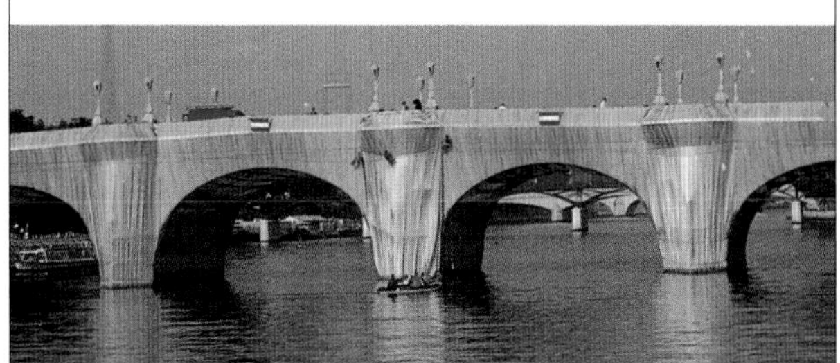

Find out more

METALS
PAINTERS
PAINTING
RENAISSANCE

SEA BIRDS

ALL KINDS OF BIRDS live near the sea, gliding over the waves and feeding along the shore or diving for fish. Sea birds belong to a number of different bird groups, all of which live near the sea. Most have webbed feet for swimming, waterproof feathers, and sharp bills for gripping slippery fish. Sea birds include razorbills and guillemots, whose small wings act like flippers for swimming. Other sea birds, such as albatrosses and petrels, have long, slim wings for soaring high in the sky. Gulls and skuas are scavengers and take almost any food, from dead flesh to other sea birds' eggs and chicks. The great skua attacks birds in midflight, making them drop their food, which it then catches. Gannets and boobies dive for fish from 30 m (100 ft). Penguins cannot fly, but they swim expertly with their wings, chasing fish in the oceans south of the equator.

Storm petrel has tube-shaped nostrils on its bill.

WANDERING ALBATROSS

There are 21 kinds of albatross, and most live south of the equator. Their wings are the longest of any bird, more than 3 m (10 ft) from tip to tip. They glide over the oceans for hours without flapping, picking fish from the water.

Long, narrow albatross wings are a perfect shape for gliding on the wind.

HERRING GULL

Noisy and aggressive, herring gulls live in Europe, North America, North Africa, and Asia. They trail after fishing boats for leftovers, visit rubbish dumps, and follow the farmer's plough to feed on worms, insects, and small mammals.

GANNET
A gannet collects grasses for its nest, then returns to the gannetry, its cliff-top breeding colony. Sometimes more than 50,000 gannets nest in the same place.

Spear-shaped bill for piercing fish

Atlantic puffin

BREEDING COLONIES

Most sea birds raise their young on cliffs and small islands. Their food is nearby, and the chicks are safe from predators on the steep ledges. The noise of a sea bird colony is deafening. Kittiwakes, cormorants, and guillemots are nesting together here, but each nest is well out of the way of all the other birds' stabbing bills.

Cormorants, kittiwakes, and guillemots share the same cliff-top nesting place.

A kittiwake's nest is made of pieces of seaweed and plant stuck together with droppings.

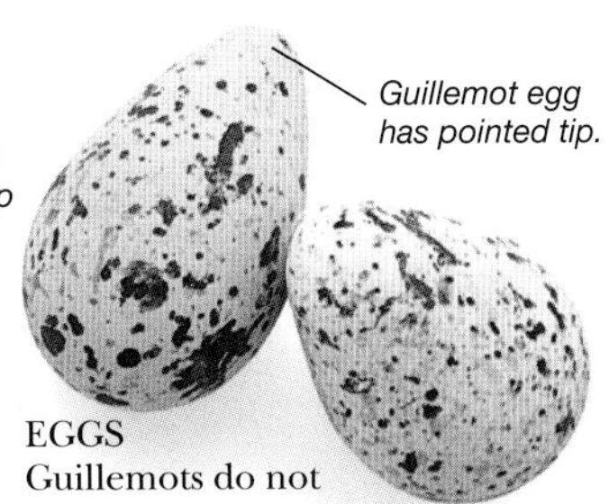

Guillemot egg has pointed tip.

EGGS
Guillemots do not make nests. Their eggs are pointed at one end, so they spin in a circle if they roll, and do not fall off the cliff edge.

PUFFIN
The Atlantic puffin can hold a dozen sand eels or small fish in its big, bright bill. When its bill is full, the puffin carries the food to its chick in the burrow.

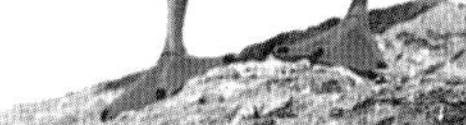

Find out more

BIRDS
FLIGHT, ANIMAL
MIGRATION, ANIMAL
SEASHORE WILDLIFE

SEALS AND SEA LIONS

WITH THEIR STREAMLINED BODIES, seals and sea lions are well equipped for life in the ocean. Despite their large size, they are speedy, energetic swimmers. A thick layer of blubber under the skin keeps them warm in cold waters, helped by their oily, glossy fur. Seals swim gracefully with alternate strokes of their back flippers. On land, however, they are clumsy without water to support their bodies, so they clamber over the shore by wriggling along on their bellies. Unlike seals, sea lions waddle along quickly on land. Sea lions also sit up on rocks, supported by their front flippers, and tuck their back flippers under their bodies. They use their front flippers like oars as they speed after fish in the sea. There are more than 30 kinds of seals and sea lions.

HARP SEAL
Newborn harp seals have white fur to camouflage them on the ice. After a few weeks their coats change to grey.

CALIFORNIA SEA LION

The best-known performing seals are California sea lions. Thousands of them live off the coast of California, in the United States. They feed on squid, fish, and other small sea creatures.

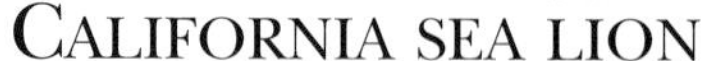

COMMON SEAL

This seal is also known as the harbour seal, as it is often seen around harbours, ports, and even a short way up rivers. Fish is its main food, and it lives around the northern shores of the Atlantic and Pacific oceans.

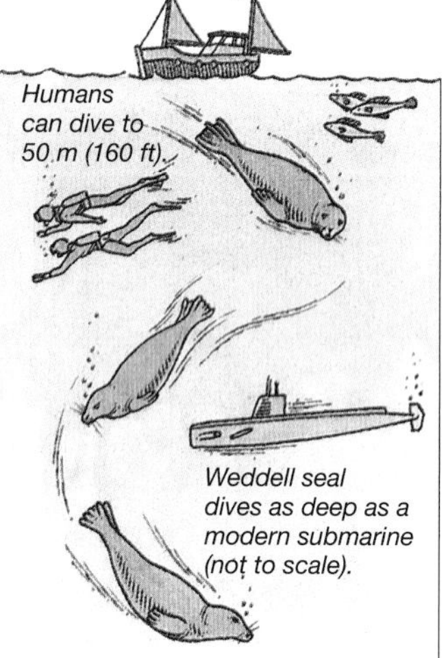
Humans can dive to 50 m (160 ft).
Weddell seal dives as deep as a modern submarine (not to scale).

WEDDELL SEAL

This seal can dive to nearly 600 m (2,000 ft), holding its breath for almost an hour. Only a submarine can dive to the same depth.

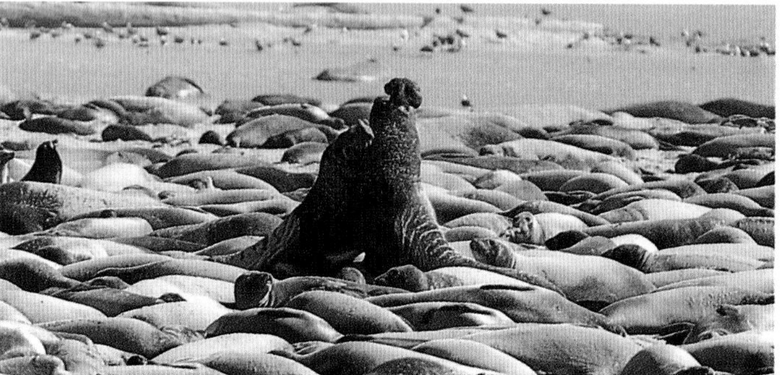

BREEDING COLONIES
Seal colonies are very crowded places during the breeding season – in spring and early summer. All kinds of seals and sea lions come ashore to breed, and live together in their hundreds. The males, or bulls, battle for a territory, as these two huge elephant seal bulls (left) are doing. Once the bulls have established their territory, the pregnant females arrive. Each female gives birth to one pup and feeds it with her milk for several weeks. At 3 tonnes (3 tons) in weight, the adult elephant seal is the heaviest member of the seal family.

WALRUS

The icy Arctic Ocean is the home of the walrus, a close relative of the seal. Males can grow to more than 3 m (10 ft) in length; females are slightly smaller. These sea mammals paddle with their back flippers and steer with the front ones. Their tough skin is 2.5 cm (1 in) thick, covered with short, coarse hairs. Females give birth to one walrus calf every other year, and it may stay with its mother for the first two years. Walruses can live for up to 40 years.

WALRUS TEETH
Walruses have huge upper canine teeth, or tusks, that grow more than 50 cm (20 in) long. Tusks are a status symbol, and the male with the largest tusks usually becomes the leader of the herd. Walruses use their strong tusks for chopping holes in the ice and for hauling themselves out of the water and on to ice floes to rest.

Find out more
ANIMALS
MAMMALS
OCEAN WILDLIFE
POLAR WILDLIFE

SEASHORE WILDLIFE

A SEASHORE is formed wherever the land meets the sea, and can be a polar ice cliff or a tropical beach. The endless motion of the waves, and the tide going in and out, means the shore changes constantly with time. Each seashore has its own selection of plant and animal life that is specially adapted to an environment governed by the rhythm of the tides. Inhabitants of the seashore must survive pounding waves, salty sea water, fresh rainwater, drying winds, and hot sunshine. Plants thrive along rocky coasts and in some muddy areas, providing food and shelter for creatures, but they cannot grow on shifting sand or pebbles. Here the inhabitants depend on the tide to bring new supplies of food, in the form of particles floating in the water. Successful seashore animal groups include molluscs and crustaceans, both of which are protected by hard casings.

SEASIDE DANGERS
Most of these baby turtles, hatching from eggs buried by their mother in the sand, will die. They are food for gulls, crabs, lizards and other hunters. Humans also steal the eggs. Conservation efforts are now being made to protect turtles.

Gulls hover over the sea looking for fish, while waders hunt around the shore.

Seagull

Many sea birds patrol the coast, searching for food or scavenging on the dead bodies of cast-up sea creatures.

Lace coral can survive harsh rubbing by the wave-washed sand grains. It provides a refuge for animals in its lacy folds.

Common starfish

SANDY BEACHES
Waves roll and tumble the tiny grains of sand on the beach. Plants cannot get a firm hold on this type of shore, so they usually grow higher up. Although the sandy beach often looks deserted, dozens of creatures are just below the surface. Sand makes an ideal hiding place for burrowing creatures. Many filter food from the sea water when the tide is in or digest tiny edible particles in the sand.

WADING BIRDS
Waders probe into sand or mud with their long, narrow bills to find shellfish and worms. Large species with the longest bills, such as the curlew (above), reach down several centimetres for deeply buried items. Smaller waders, such as the black-bellied dunlin, take food from just below the surface.

GHOST CRAB
There are hundreds of kinds of shore crabs along the world's coastlines. They are the seashore's "cleaners"; they can consume almost anything edible – living or dead. The ghost crab (above right) takes its name from its ghostly pale colour.

EGG CASES
Sharks and rays lay their eggs near the shore, anchored to seaweeds or rocks by clinging tendrils. When the young fishes hatch, the egg cases, known as "mermaid's purses", come free and are often washed up on the shore.

SAND HOPPER
Sand hoppers are crustaceans which feed on rotting vegetation. They swarm over seaweed which has washed up on shore and, when in danger, leap away on their strong back legs, hence their name.

RAZOR CLAM
So called because it looks like an old-fashioned cut-throat razor, the razor clam has a hinged shell. The mollusc inside digs quickly by pushing its strong, fleshy foot into the sand and then pulling the shell down.

The burrowing sea anemone's arms spread out to sting and catch small prey. Its stalk, up to 30 cm (12 in) long, is used to hold on to the sand.

WEEVER FISH
The weever lies half buried in the sand, waiting to gobble up small fishes, crabs, and shrimps. It has poisonous spines on its fins, which give a nasty sting if the fish is stepped on.

SAND EEL
Many animals, from puffins to herrings, feed on the sand eel shown here. In turn, the sand eel eats even smaller fishes, as well as worms and plankton. It is not a true eel, but an eel-shaped member of the perch group. It lives in shallow water.

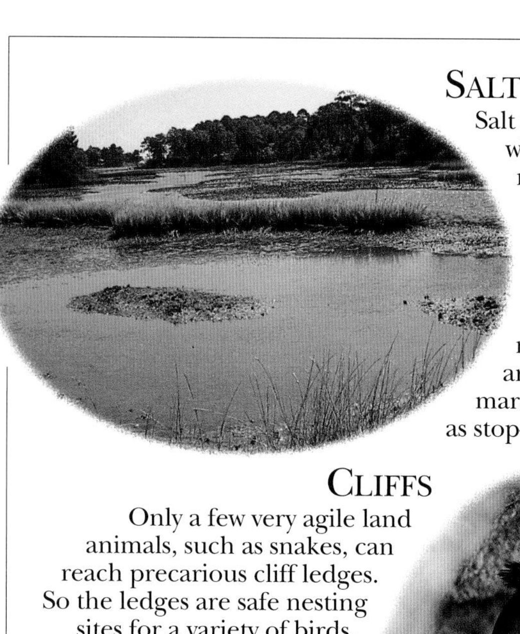

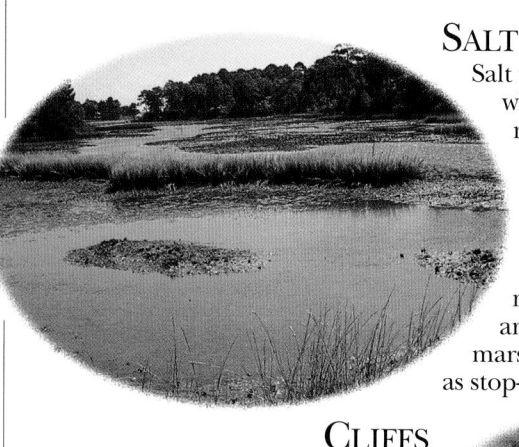

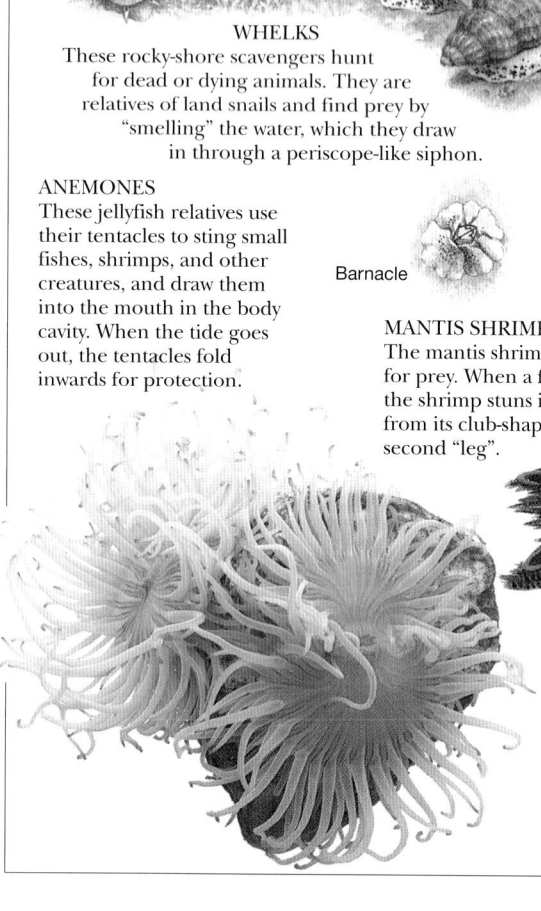

Salt marshes

Salt marshes form at the back of the shore, where the tide floods flat areas of land near a river's mouth. Plants such as cordgrass, glasswort, eelgrass, sea club rush, and sea starwort are able to survive in the salt that builds up in the soil. Birds such as geese, gulls, and terns can feed on salt marshes all year round, especially in winter, when inland areas are frozen hard. Some birds use salt marshes as summer breeding grounds, some as stop-overs while migrating.

Some large seaweeds are called kelps, such as sugar kelp and oarweed.

Cliffs

Only a few very agile land animals, such as snakes, can reach precarious cliff ledges. So the ledges are safe nesting sites for a variety of birds, from gannets to gulls, razorbills, and cormorants. A few plants, like thrift ("sea pink"), also gain a foothold, provided they can withstand strong winds and salty spray.

Seaweed

There are three main kinds of rocky-shore seaweeds, also known as algae: brown, red, and green. They do not have roots, stems, or leaves. Instead, most anchor themselves to the rocks by structures called holdfasts. The larger brown and red weeds have stem-like stipes, ending in leaflike blades known as laminae or fronds.

Periwinkles seal themselves to the rock with mucus as the tide retreats, to keep them from losing water and drying out.

ROCKY SHORES
Rocks provide a firm surface for seaweeds, and many creatures shelter among the fronds. But the weeds still face problems. Waves smash them against the hard stony surface, and they are regularly submerged by salt water, then left high and dry at low tide. Shellfish cling to the rocks, and a variety of fishes and crabs adapt themselves to the ever-changing conditions, hiding from predators in holes and crevices.

WHELKS
These rocky-shore scavengers hunt for dead or dying animals. They are relatives of land snails and find prey by "smelling" the water, which they draw in through a periscope-like siphon.

CHITON
Chitons are also called "coat of mail shells" because they look like chainmail armour. Each chiton has an eight-part shell set into its broad, fleshy body. It can grip a rock very firmly. These molluscs feed on small algae from the rock surface.

ANEMONES
These jellyfish relatives use their tentacles to sting small fishes, shrimps, and other creatures, and draw them into the mouth in the body cavity. When the tide goes out, the tentacles fold inwards for protection.

Barnacle

MANTIS SHRIMP
The mantis shrimp, a crustacean, hides in a hole waiting for prey. When a fish or other victim approaches, the shrimp stuns it by a lightning blow from its club-shaped second "leg".

Branching holdfast provides shelter for small animals

Red seaweed

SEA STAR
The biscuit sea star feeds on shellfish, sea squirts, corals, sponges, and other animals. It glides along on dozens of tiny, sucker-tipped hydraulic tube feet located on its underside.

Find out more
Corals, anemones, and jellyfish
Crabs and other crustaceans
Fish
Ocean wildlife
Sea birds
Shells and shellfish
Starfish and sea urchins

WILLIAM
SHAKESPEARE

1564 Born, Stratford-upon-Avon, England.

1582 Marries Anne Hathaway.

1592 Writes his first plays in London.

1594-99 Produces early comedies, and many history plays.

1599 Globe Theatre constructed.

1600-08 Writes many of his greatest tragedies.

1616 Dies in Stratford-upon-Avon.

THE GREATEST PLAYWRIGHT of all time was probably the Englishman William Shakespeare. He was born in Stratford-upon-Avon, where he went to school, and later married. When he was in his 20s, he went to London to work as an actor, and a playwright. His plays were very successful, and 37 of them survive. Some, such as *Hamlet*, are tragedies, serious plays that often end with the death of the hero. Others, such as *Twelfth Night*, are comedies, full of amusing characters who get into terrible difficulties that are eventually sorted out. Shakespeare also wrote histories that are based on real-life situations, such as *Henry IV*. Most of Shakespeare's plays are written in an unrhymed verse form called blank verse. They are famous worldwide for their use of language, fascinating characters, and wide appeal.

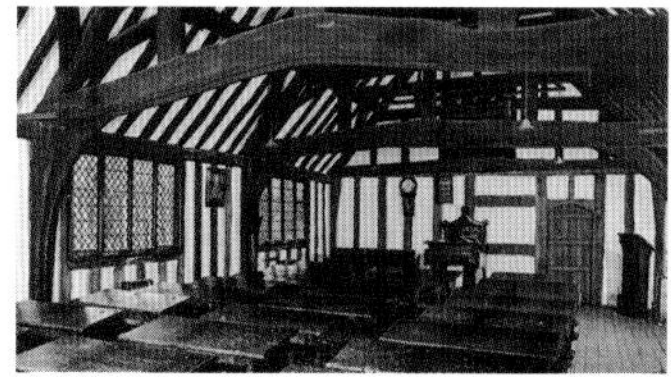

THE GRAMMAR SCHOOL
With its rows of wooden desks, the old grammar school still stands in Stratford. Shakespeare was probably educated here.

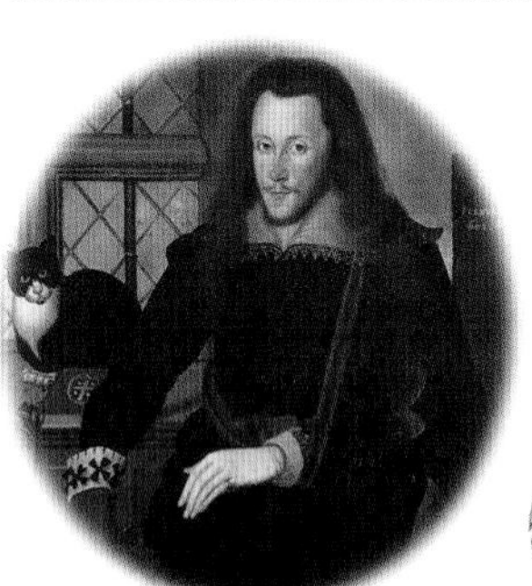

Henry Wriothesley

POETRY

Shakespeare was a fine poet, and wrote a series of 14-line love poems called sonnets. They are addressed to two different people, "a dark lady" and Mr. W.H. Scholars believe that Mr. W.H. may have been Henry Wriothesley, the Third Earl of Southampton, who was Shakespeare's patron.

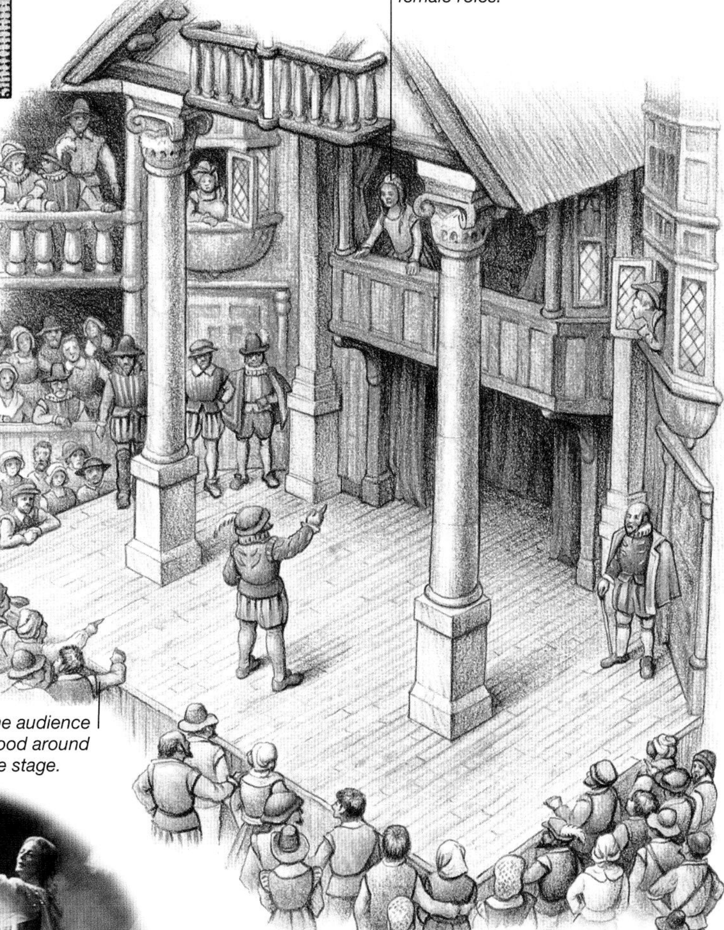
Male actors played female roles.
The audience stood around the stage.

KING'S MEN

In the 1590s, Shakespeare joined a troupe of actors called the Lord Chamberlain's Men, and became their resident writer. When James I came to the throne in 1603, they gained his support and became known as the King's Men. They had their own theatre, the Globe, near the River Thames in London.

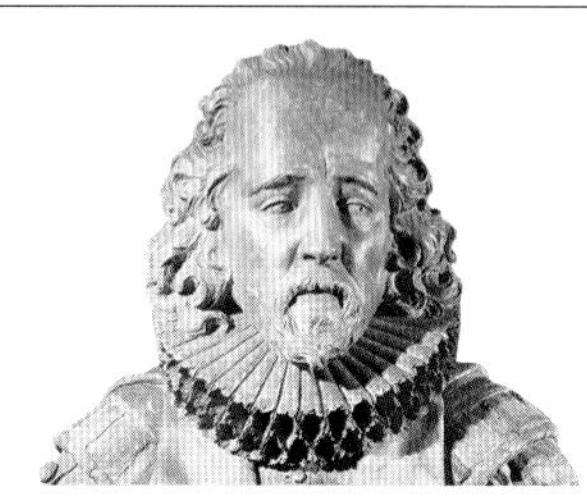

WAS IT BACON?

In the 19th century, some people thought that the learned writer Francis Bacon (1561-1626) had written Shakespeare's plays, because Shakespeare had not gone to university. But there is no real evidence that proves this.

English actress, Maggie Smith, in a performance of A Midsummer Night's Dream.

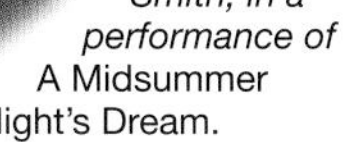

A MIDSUMMER NIGHT'S DREAM

One of Shakespeare's most popular plays, *A Midsummer Night's Dream,* is a comedy. The play has a huge cast of characters, including two young couples who fall in and out of love, a group of workmen, and the king and queen of the fairies, who create hilarious confusion with their magic.

Find out more

ELIZABETH I
LITERATURE
THEATRE
TUDORS

SHARKS AND RAYS

A PERFECT SHAPE FOR SPEED, an incredible sense of smell, and a mouth brimming with razor-sharp teeth make sharks the most fearsome fish in the sea. Sharks have existed for 350 million years, and their basic shape has hardly changed at all during this time. As adults, they have no predators and fear nothing in the ocean. The great white shark is the largest predatory fish, at more than 9 m (27 ft) in length and 2.7 tonnes (2.7 tons) in weight. Dozens of huge teeth line its jaws. The great white shark prowls the ocean, eating any kind of meat, alive or dead, and often swallows its prey in one gulp. Sharks have to keep moving in order to take in enough oxygen, and the great white travels more than 500 km (300 miles) in a day. Most fish have bony skeletons, but sharks and their relatives, the rays, have skeletons made of a substance called cartilage. Rays are flat-bodied, with a wide mouth on the underside and blunt teeth for crushing clams and other shellfish. Rays live close to the seabed and move gracefully by flapping their huge wings.

Good sense of smell for hunting

Long tail used for rounding up fish in the water

The thresher shark lashes the water with its tail to sweep fish into a group. Then, with its mouth open, the shark charges through, gobbling them up.

Excellent eyesight for spying prey

THRESHER SHARK

This shark measures 6 m (20 ft) in length. It lives mainly in the warm coastal waters of the Atlantic and Pacific oceans but sometimes strays north in summer.

FIN
A shark's dorsal (back) fin cuts the sea's surface as the shark circles before attacking. The dolphin's fin is more crescent-shaped.

Stingrays have a poison spine on the tail.

STINGRAY

There are about 100 kinds of stingrays – the biggest measures 4 m (12 ft) across.

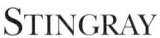

Huge wings

Shark tooth

Sharks' teeth have a serrated edge so they can saw through flesh.

TEETH
Sharks have many rows of teeth. As they grow, the teeth move from inside the mouth to the outside edge, where they are used for tearing flesh. Eventually the teeth wear away or break off, only to be replaced by the teeth behind.

SKIN
Shark skin is covered with toothlike scales, and has a texture like sandpaper.

WHALE SHARK

The harmless whale shark cruises slowly through the tropical oceans, feeding by filtering tiny floating animals (plankton) from the water. It is a peaceful creature and is the biggest fish of any kind, at 15 m (50 ft) long.

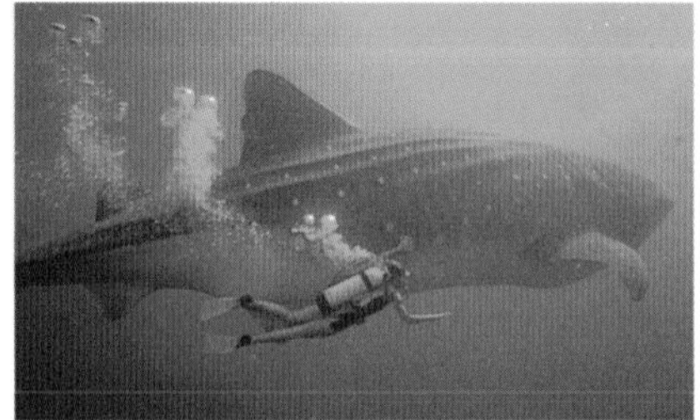

A human can swim safely with the gentle whale shark, the biggest fish in the sea.

Dorsal fin

Dorsal fin

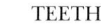

Upper lobe of caudal fin (tail)

Pectoral fin

Nostrils are excellent at detecting the smell of blood in the water.

SWIMMING MACHINE
The shark's swimming power comes from its tail. The larger upper lobe drives it down with each stroke and helps keep the body level; otherwise the creature's weight would tilt its head down. A shark cannot swivel its fins to stop quickly. It must veer to one side instead.

HAMMERHEAD
The eyes and nostrils of the hammerhead shark are on the two "lobes" of its head. Hammerheads prey on stingrays, unharmed by the poison in their spines.

Find out more

ANIMAL SENSES
ANIMALS
FISH
OCEAN WILDLIFE

SHELLS AND SHELLFISH

ALL THE WONDERFUL SHELLS you find on the seashore were once the homes of soft-bodied sea creatures. These creatures are commonly known as shellfish, although they are not fish at all, but molluscs, like slugs and snails. There are thousands of different kinds of shellfish living in the sea, including mussels, oysters, and clams. Many, such as the winkle, have small, delicate shells; others, such as the queen conch, have big, heavy shells. The shell itself is like a house, built by the shellfish. As it feeds, the shellfish extracts calcium carbonate from the water. This mineral is used by the shellfish to build up layers of shell, little by little. As the creature grows bigger, its shell grows bigger too. Some shellfish live in a single, coiled shell; others, known as bivalves, have a hinged shell with two sides that open and close for feeding.

ARGONAUT
The paper nautilus is a type of octopus which makes a thin shell to keep its eggs in. It is also known as the argonaut, after the sailors of Greek legend, because people believed they used its papery shell as a boat.

Tentacles

Head

INSIDE A SHELL
The pearly nautilus has a shell with many chambers. As it grows, the animal shuts off more chambers by building a "wall", and lives only in the last chamber.

NAUTILUS

This predator and scavenger hunts at night. It lives in the Indian and Pacific oceans, and has more than 30 tentacles for catching prey.

HOW SHELLS GROW
Shellfish hatch as larvae from eggs, then develop shells. Creatures with single coiled shells, such as this triton, grow by adding layers of shell-building material (calcium carbonate) to the open end. Hinged-shell creatures, such as cockles, add calcium carbonate to the rounded edges, in the form of coils called growth rings.

Growth rings on adult triton shell

Larva has a smooth shell.

Eggs

Young shells are tiny and have few coils.

Growth rings are slowly added to the open end.

HINGED SHELLS
The two sides of a hinged shell (bivalve) are held together by a tough ligament. Powerful muscles keep the valves closed for protection. The valves open slightly to allow the creature to breathe and feed.

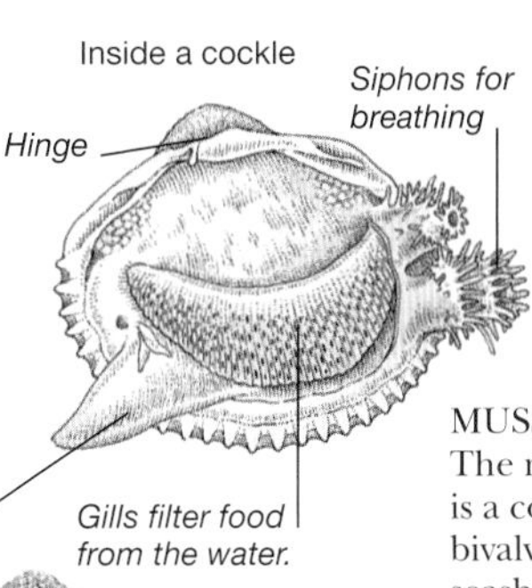

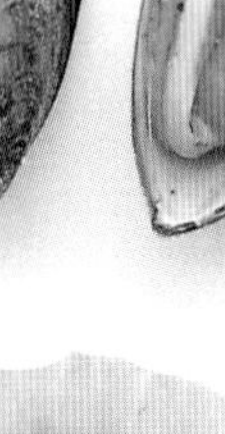

MUSSEL
The mussel is a common bivalve on many seashores.

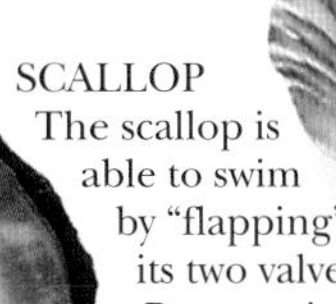

COCKLE SHELL
The ridged cockle buries itself in sand and feeds when the tide comes in.

SCALLOP
The scallop is able to swim by "flapping" its two valves. By snapping the two sides shut, it can shoot through the water to escape from a predator.

Inside a scallop

HOW A PEARL IS MADE

If a piece of grit gets lodged in an oyster's shell, the oyster covers it with mother-of-pearl (nacre), a substance lining its shell.

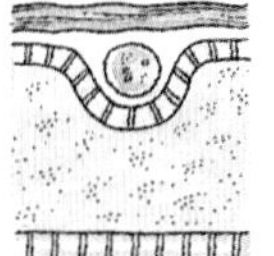

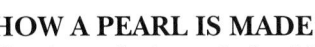

Tiny piece of grit irritates oyster.

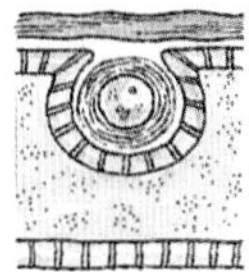

Mother-of-pearl (nacre) forms over grit.

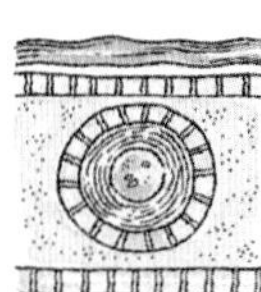

Pearl comes free, removing the irritation.

PEARL
We value oyster pearls highly because of their white, shiny appearance, but other kinds of shellfish make pearls too. The Caribbean conch makes pink pearls, and some shellfish make orange ones. The pearl shown here is a "blister pearl" on a black-lipped oyster shell.

Find out more
ANIMALS
ANIMAL SENSES
FOOD
OCEAN WILDLIFE
SEASHORE WILDLIFE

SHIPS AND BOATS

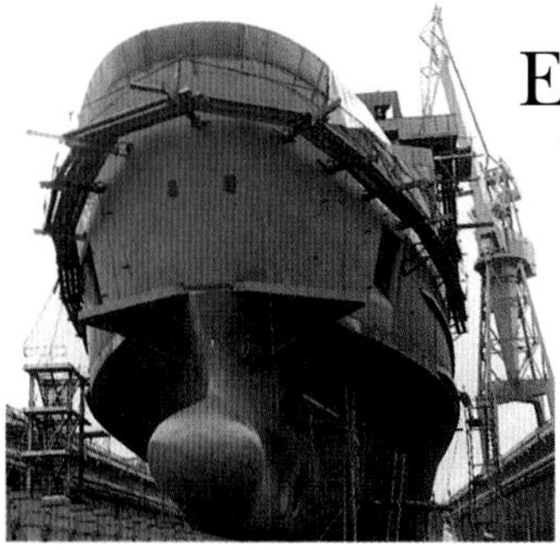

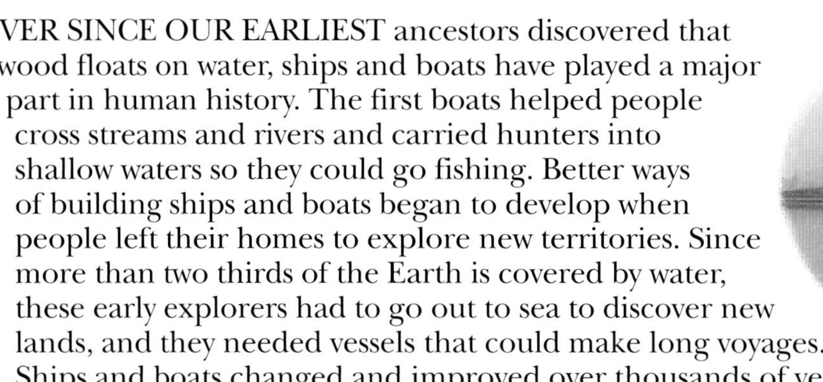

EVER SINCE OUR EARLIEST ancestors discovered that wood floats on water, ships and boats have played a major part in human history. The first boats helped people cross streams and rivers and carried hunters into shallow waters so they could go fishing. Better ways of building ships and boats began to develop when people left their homes to explore new territories. Since more than two thirds of the Earth is covered by water, these early explorers had to go out to sea to discover new lands, and they needed vessels that could make long voyages. Ships and boats changed and improved over thousands of years as distant nations began to trade and opposing navies fought battles at sea.

Today, there are thousands of different types of ships and boats. Ships are seagoing vessels; boats are generally smaller and travel on coastal or inland waters.

Traditional craft such as this Chinese junk are still used in some parts of the world.

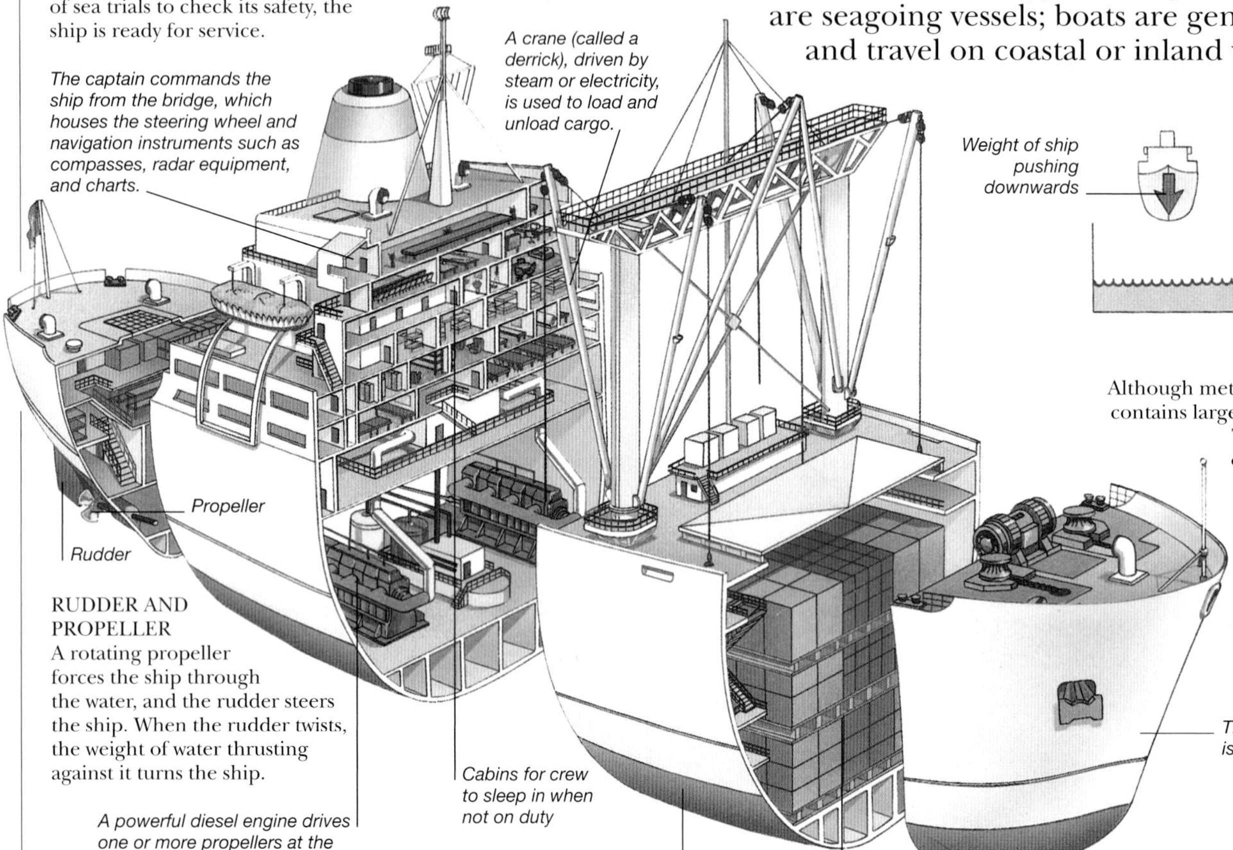

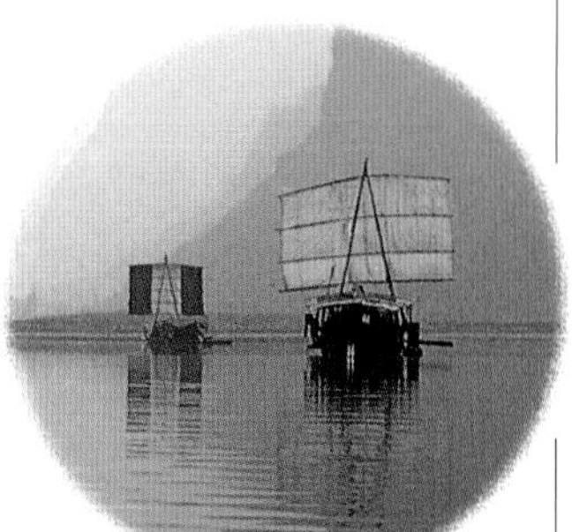

SHIPBUILDING
Modern ships are built of steel plates welded together. Ship builders make all the parts separately and finally assemble the ship in the shipyard. After months of sea trials to check its safety, the ship is ready for service.

The captain commands the ship from the bridge, which houses the steering wheel and navigation instruments such as compasses, radar equipment, and charts.

A crane (called a derrick), driven by steam or electricity, is used to load and unload cargo.

Weight of ship pushing downwards

Upthrust from water pushing upwards

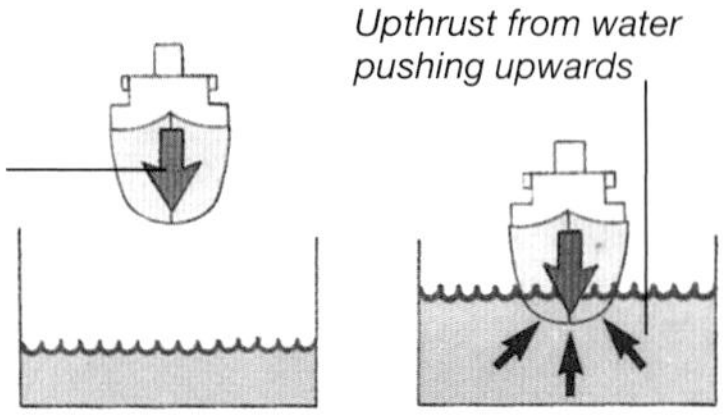

HOW SHIPS FLOAT
Although metal is very heavy, a ship contains large spaces filled with air. The hull (main body) of a ship pushes water out of the way, and the water pushes back on the ship with a force called upthrust. The upthrust balances the weight of the ship and keeps it afloat.

Propeller

Rudder

RUDDER AND PROPELLER
A rotating propeller forces the ship through the water, and the rudder steers the ship. When the rudder twists, the weight of water thrusting against it turns the ship.

A powerful diesel engine drives one or more propellers at the stern (back) of the ship.

Cabins for crew to sleep in when not on duty

Main body of the ship is called the hull.

The front end of a ship is called the bow.

Cargo is stored in a large compartment below the deck, called a hold. Large modern cargo vessels may have 12 or more holds. Ships that carry fresh food have refrigerated holds.

CARGO SHIP

Every year, cargo ships carry millions of tonnes of goods across the world's oceans. Some cargo ships, called container ships, carry huge loads piled up in large, steel boxes that stack together like building blocks. The largest ships of this kind carry more than 4,000 such containers.

KINDS OF SHIPS

There are many kinds of ships. They range from passenger vessels to cargo ships that carry goods of all types to and from the world's ports.

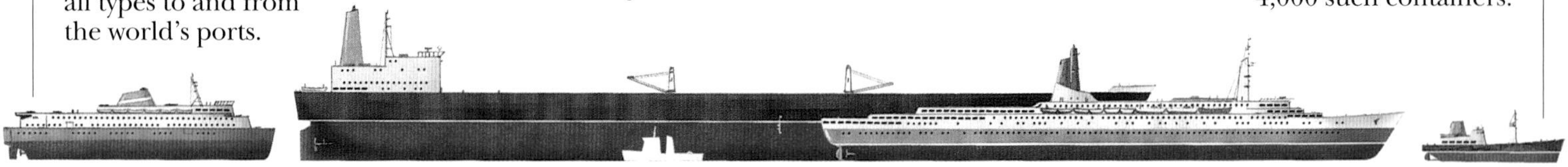

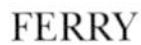

FERRY
Ferries take people and goods across a stretch of water. Large ferries carry cars, trucks, and trains as well as people.

OIL TANKER
Oil is transported at sea in huge tankers. The engines and bridge are at the stern to give more storage space.

CRUISE LINER
Liners are large ships that carry passengers on scheduled routes. Most liners are like floating hotels and take tourists on lengthy cruises.

TRAWLER
Trawlers are engine-powered fishing boats that drag a net (the trawl) along the sea bed in order to catch fish that swim near the bottom of the sea.

History of ships and boats

The development of ships began more than 6,000 years ago with rafts and reed boats, and continues today with the introduction of nuclear-powered ships and boats made of light, strong plastics.

HIDE BOAT

About 6,000 years ago the Ancient Egyptians used boats made of a wicker framework covered with animal skins. In about 3200 B.C. the Egyptians invented sails.

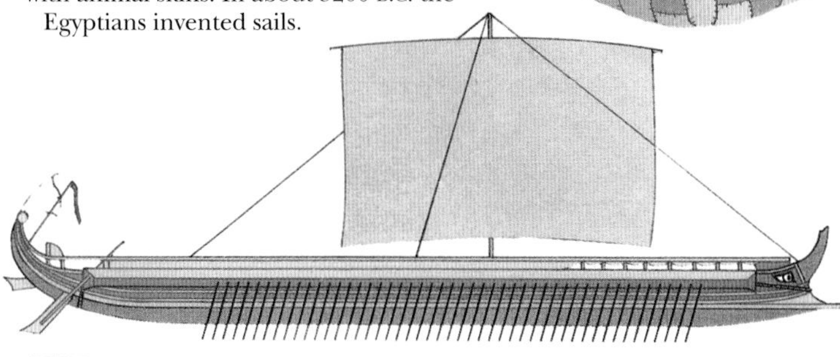

TRIREME

The Greeks invented the trireme (above) in about 650 B.C. It had sails and lines of rowers to carry it along at speed. The Romans built similar ships for trade and war.

Groups of rowers were positioned on two levels.

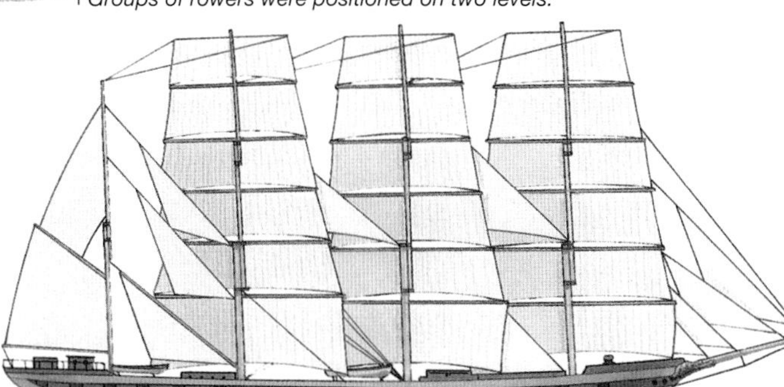

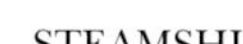

CLIPPER

Fast sailing ships called clippers (above) appeared during the 19th century, the height of the age of sailing. They carried many sails and had sleek lines to increase speed. Clippers were used mainly for trade.

STEAMSHIPS

Oceangoing steamships (below) took to the seas early in the 19th century. The earliest vessels had paddles connected to the engine and sails to gain extra speed in high winds. Ships with propellers entered service during the 1840s.

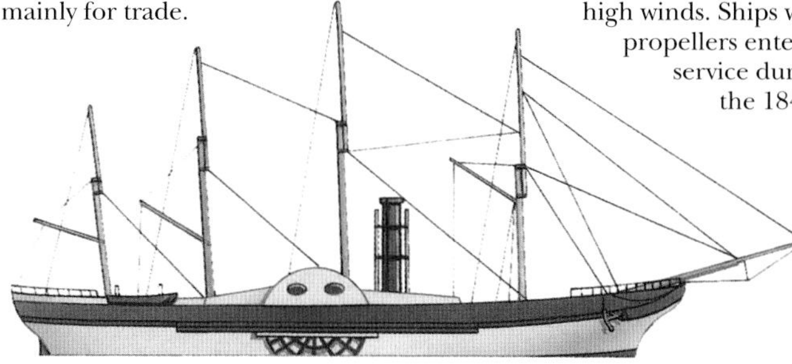

HYDROFOIL

A boat's engine has to work hard to overcome the resistance of the water. Light, fast boats called hydrofoils avoid this problem because they rise up on skis at high speeds. With the hydrofoil travelling so rapidly, water behaves as if it were a solid, so the hydrofoil skims over the water surface just like an aeroplane wing in air.

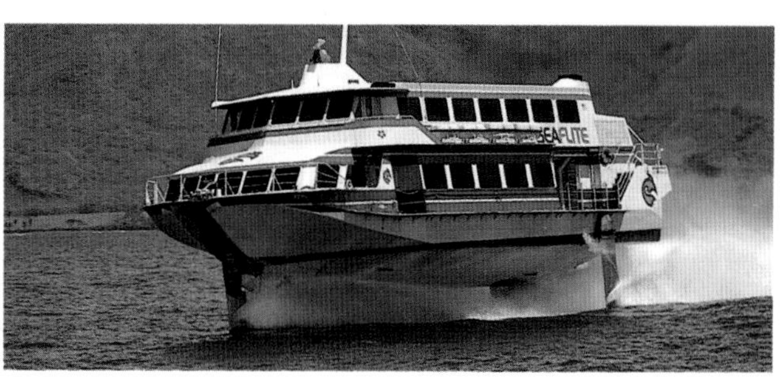

Any force can be divided into two parts at right angles to each other. The part along the length of the boat drives the boat forwards.

Air rushing past the sail produces a force that tends to move the boat at right angles to the wind.

Wind rushing past sail

Wind pushing on sail

Centreboard prevents boat from drifting with the wind and stops the boat from capsizing.

HOW A BOAT SAILS

Modern sailing boats do not need the wind behind them to move – they can travel in almost any direction. In the same way that air rushing over the wings of an aeroplane produces an upward force called lift, wind moving past a sail produces a force at right angles to the sail. Adjusting the sail makes the boat move in different directions.

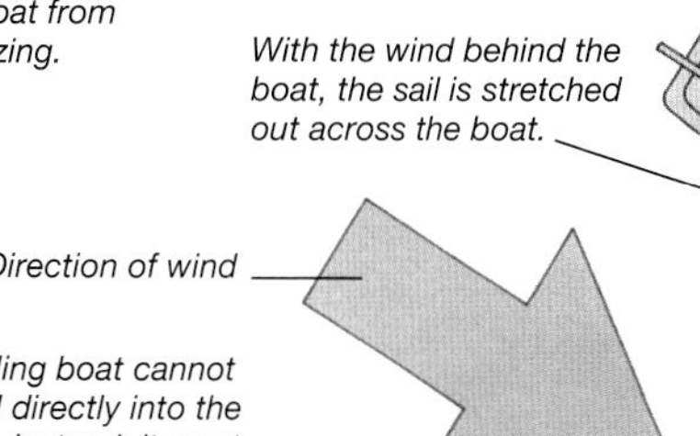

With the wind behind the boat, the sail is stretched out across the boat.

Direction of wind

Direction of movement

A sailing boat cannot travel directly into the wind. Instead, it must follow a zigzag path. This is called tacking.

The boat heads into the wind with the sail drawn in as tightly as possible.

Direction of movement

With the wind to the side of the boat, the sail is drawn in more tightly. The boat travels fastest with the wind in this position.

Kinds of boats

Different boats have different uses. Many boats, such as yachts, are pleasure craft; tugs and fishing boats, however, are the workhorses of coastal waters.

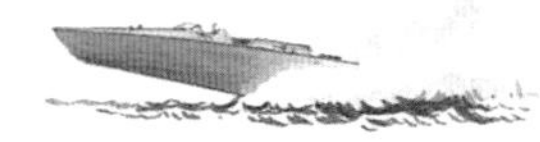

POWERBOAT

Powerboats are small, fast boats driven by powerful petrol or diesel engines. They are used either for pleasure or for racing.

TUGBOAT

Tugs tow larger vessels, guiding them through difficult or shallow waters at sea or on inland waterways such as canals.

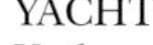

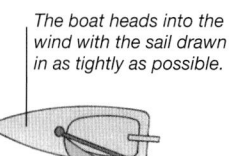

YACHT

Yachts are pleasure boats. They have engines or sails. Racing yachts are built purely for speed and are made of strong, light materials.

Find out more

NAVIES
NAVIGATION
PORTS AND WATERWAYS
SAILING AND BOATING
SUBMARINES
WARSHIPS

SHOPS AND SHOPPING

COWRIE SHELLS
People in the Pacific Islands, India, and parts of Africa once used cowrie shells as money.

IF YOU NEED TO BUY FOOD, or perhaps a book for school, there is probably a shop or a department store close to your home that sells just what you want. But shopping has not always been so easy. Shops started only with the introduction of money in Ancient China. In earlier times people used barter: in exchange for the goods they needed, they traded crops or objects they had made. The first shops sold just a few specialized products; the butcher sold meat, and the baker sold bread. In 1850 the first department store, a shop which sells many different items under one roof, opened in Paris. Self-service stores developed in the United States in the 1930s. They replaced the old methods of serving customers individually by selling prepackaged goods straight from the shelves. Modern supermarkets have car parks and provide customers with trolleys so they can shop weekly instead of daily. Nowadays you do not even have to leave home to go shopping. You can shop by post, by telephone, or through the Internet.

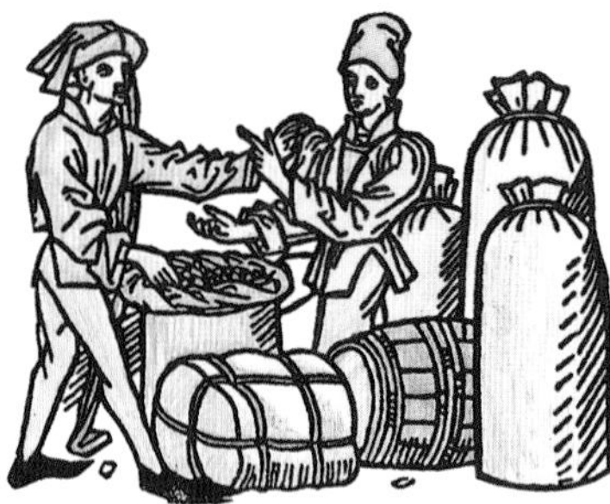

MEDIEVAL SHOPPING
In the Middle Ages shoppers liked to test the goods and argue over the price. Travelling pedlars carried their goods from place to place, selling and trading.

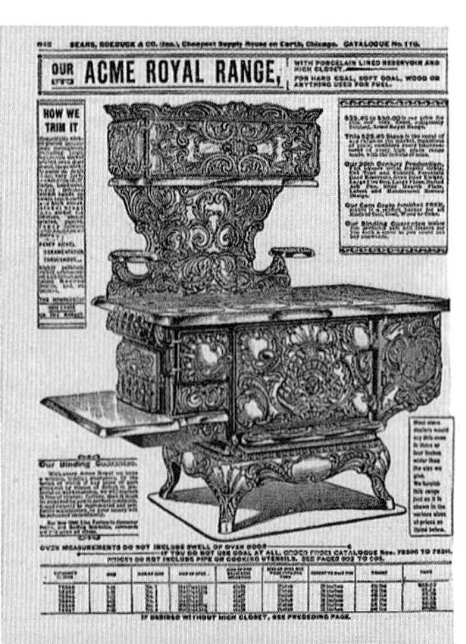

MAIL ORDER
Shopping by post has been possible for a hundred years. It was introduced for people who lived in remote areas a long way from any shops.

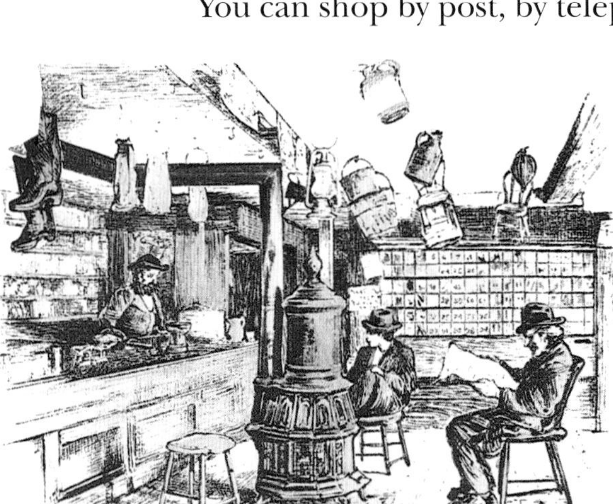

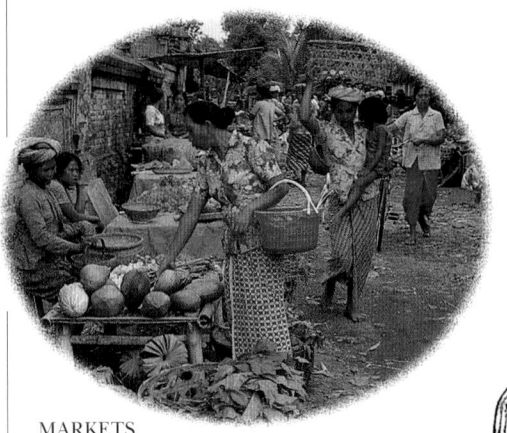

FRONTIER STORE
The frontier store supplied early American settlers with everything from food to tools. There was no packaging and little choice of goods. Supplies often ran out, and sometimes customers could not pay until they had sold their crops.

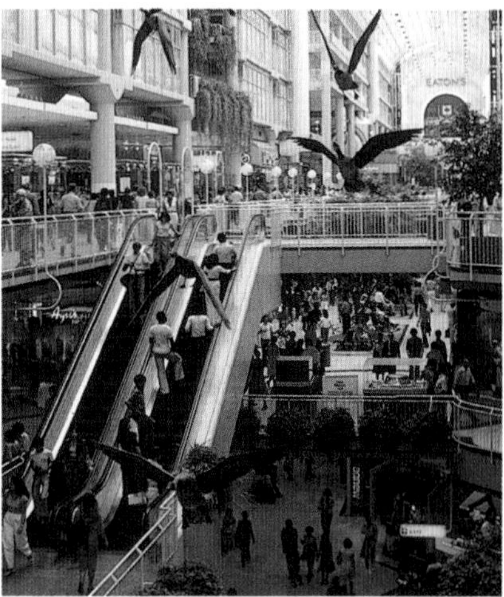

SHOPPING MALL

The modern shopping mall is a large, enclosed collection of shops. It is usually multi-storeyed and air-conditioned and has benches and restaurants to make shopping a pleasant social experience.

MARKETS
Markets are found in all parts of the world. They were the earliest kind of shops where people could bring their surplus goods to exchange or sell. They developed at important trading places where roads crossed.

BAR CODES

The packages of most modern products identify the contents both in words and with a code of black-and-white stripes. A laser scanner at the till reads the price and other information from this bar code. The till records the price, adds up the bill, and tells a central computer when to reorder the item.

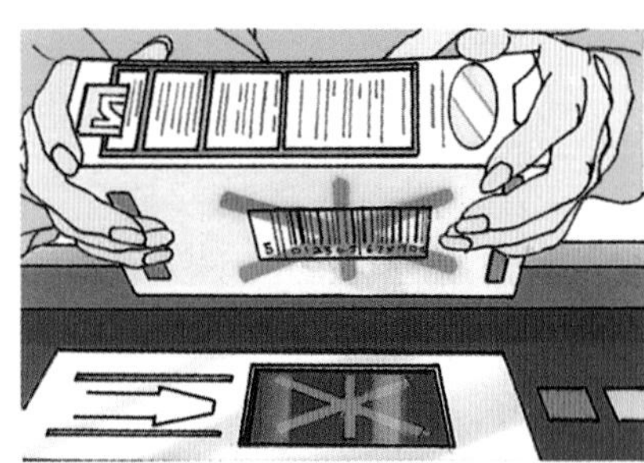

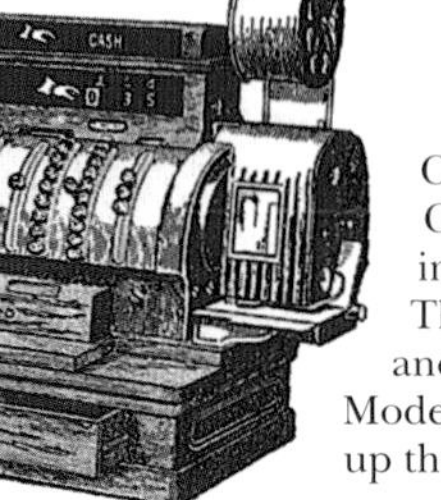

CASH REGISTERS
Cash registers, or tills, were invented in Ohio, in 1879. They recorded each sale and kept the money safe. Modern electronic tills add up the bill and print a receipt.

Find out more
ADVERTISING
MONEY
TRADE AND INDUSTRY

SIGNS AND SYMBOLS

The sun and the moon are symbols of male and female creative energy.

THERE ARE SIGNS AND SYMBOLS all around us. A sign is an object that stands for something else or points to another object. Road signs are some of the most familiar examples. Signs are usually quite easy to understand and often use simplified pictures without any words. Symbols work in a similar way, but can be more complex, and we often have to know something about how they are used to understand them fully. A good example of a symbol is the sun, which is used in different ways in different parts of the world. The sun often stands for light and warmth, but, because it helps the crops to ripen, it can also be a symbol of growth and fertility.

NATURAL SYMBOLS
Every culture uses symbols drawn from the world of nature. Plants and trees symbolize the cycle of life, from birth to death. Flowers can stand for beauty and love; herbs for the magical power of plants to heal the sick. Sun, moon, planets, and stars are often used as symbols of gods who can influence life on earth.

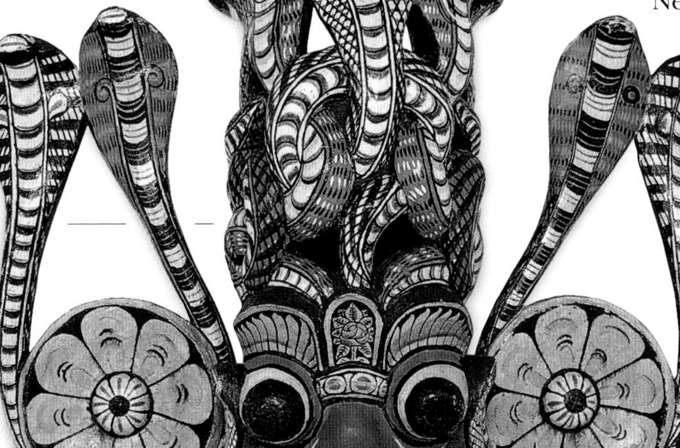

Sri Lankan mask of a snake demon, a symbol of both creation and destruction

UNIVERSAL SYMBOLS

Some symbols are so powerful that many different peoples use and understand them. Nearly everywhere, for example, the sun is a symbol of life. But some of these popular symbols change their meaning from place to place. Most peoples use the snake as a symbol, but the creature can stand for many things – life, power, lightning, cunning, or temptation.

COLOUR SYMBOLS

The same colours can mean different things to different people. For example, in the Western world, white means purity and holiness, whereas in Asia it is often the colour of mourning. Some colour symbols, such as green for "go" and red for "danger", are the same almost everywhere.

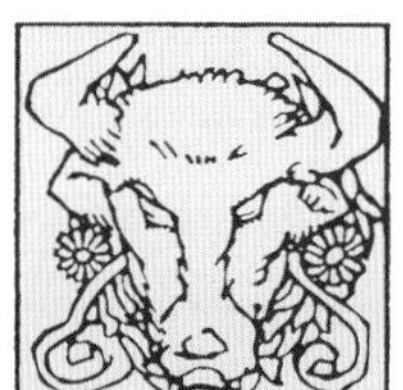

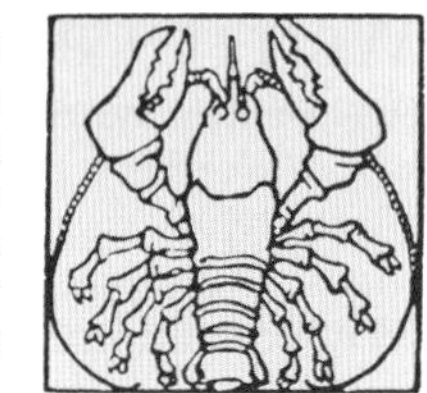

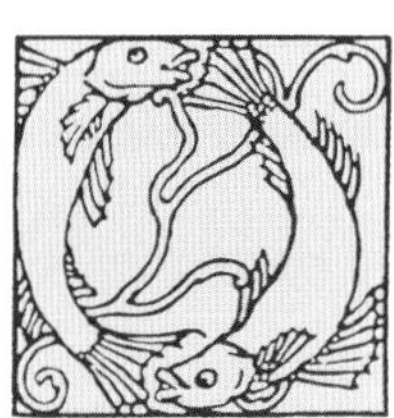

Taurus the bull, Cancer the crab, and Pisces the fish are three of the sun signs used in western astrology.

SYSTEMS OF SYMBOLS
Specialist subjects, from music to the sciences, have their own sets of symbols which work together in a system. Once you learn the symbols, you can use them like a language, to play a piece of music or work out a scientific formula. Astrology uses one of the most interesting of these systems, in which each sun sign has its own symbol.

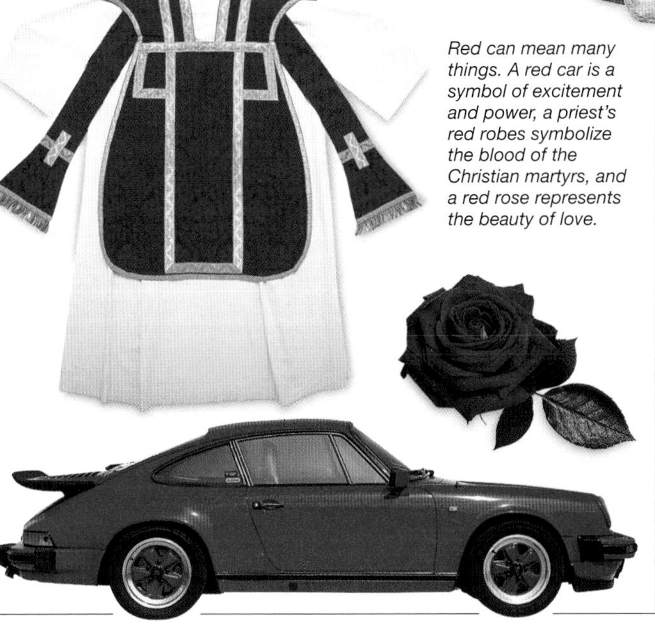

Red can mean many things. A red car is a symbol of excitement and power, a priest's red robes symbolize the blood of the Christian martyrs, and a red rose represents the beauty of love.

ANIMAL SYMBOLS

The creatures we have hunted, our farm animals, and pets – animals have always played a key role in human life. Nearly every animal, from the strong lion and noble eagle to the mischievous monkey and peaceful dove, can therefore be used as a symbol. Birds, with their ability to fly, are often seen as messengers of the gods. Amphibians and fish are common symbols of life, because of the life-giving water in which they live.

Black cats are linked with night, witches, and both good and bad luck.

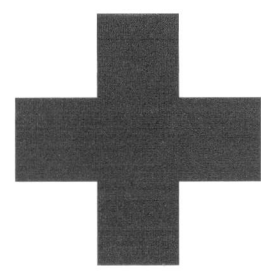

UNIVERSAL SIGNS

Many signs – for example, arrows that point the way – are so easy to understand that we forget they are signs at all. People everywhere can tell what they mean at a glance. Some signs, such as the Olympic emblem, the United Nations flag, and the Red Cross (Islamic countries use a red crescent instead), are so common that nearly everyone recognizes them.

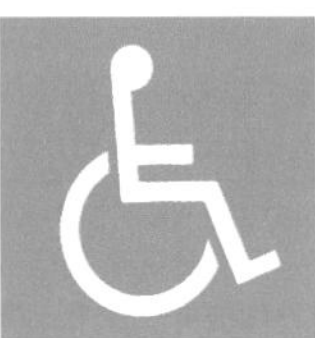

PUBLIC INFORMATION
All sorts of standard signs are used to give information in public places. These signs are designed to be easy to understand without using words, to help travellers from abroad. Most are simplified pictures, like the symbol for wheelchair access or the male and female figures used to label public toilets, but sometimes letters are used, such as the "i", which indicates a tourist information point.

MYTHOLOGY
The world's mythologies are rich stores of symbols, some of which are still used. In most mythologies, there are many gods and goddesses, each standing for one aspect of life or nature. For example, Athena was the Ancient Greek goddess of warfare and learning; her symbol was an owl. Thor was the Norse god of thunder, and his symbol was a hammer.

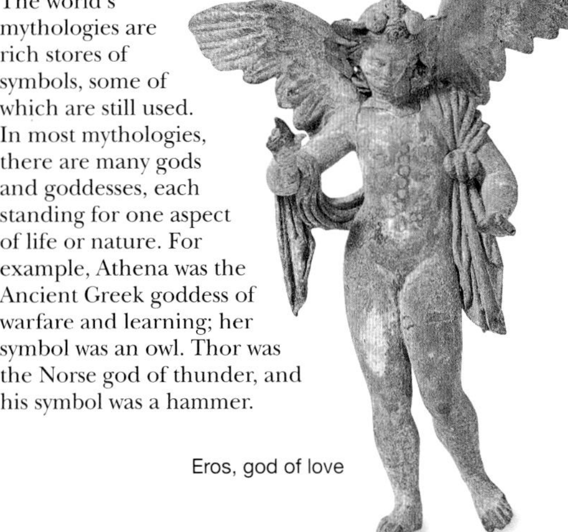

Eros, god of love

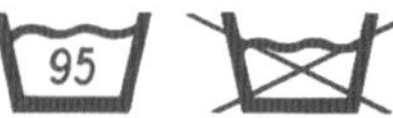

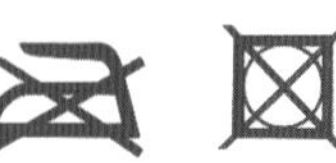

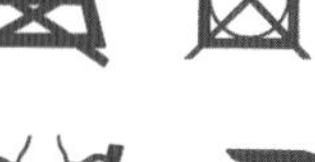

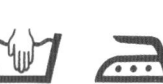

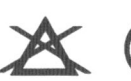

INSTRUCTION SIGNS
At work, on the road, and in the home, signs and symbols are useful ways of giving instructions. One international system of signs gives basic instructions about how to wash and care for different types of clothes and fabrics. The symbols indicate different washing temperatures and instructions for drying and ironing. A cross through a symbol means, "Do not do this".

BRAILLE

This system of printing and writing for the blind uses patterns of raised dots to stand for the different letters and numbers. Blind people read Braille by moving their fingertips along the lines of dots. The system takes its name from the blind Frenchman Louis Braille (1809-52), who invented the system during the 19th century.

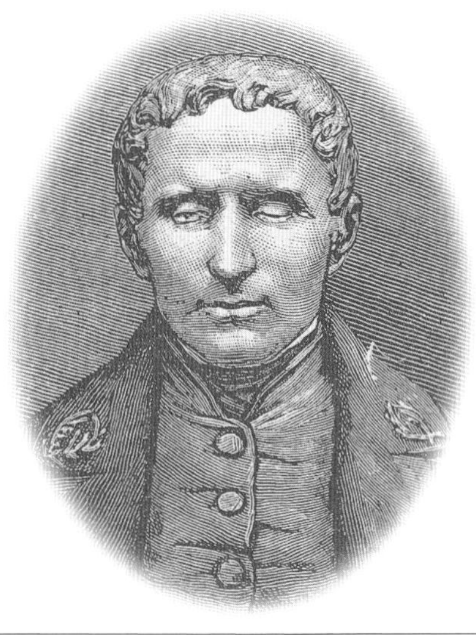

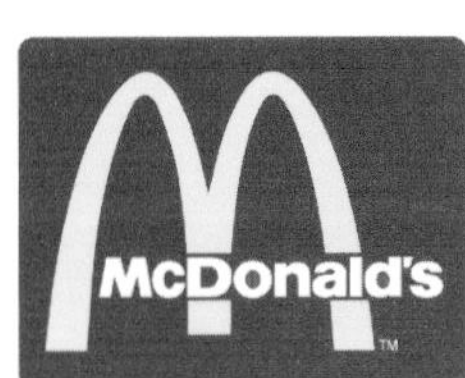

TRADEMARK
A symbol or name that identifies a company and its products can be registered as a trademark. Registering protects the trademark to prevent others from using it. One of the world's most famous trademarks, the "golden arches", belongs to McDonald's Restaurants. In 1955, one of the first McDonald's restaurants was designed with an arch either side of the building. Although they were not designed as an initial, when looked at from a certain angle the arches formed an "M" and so the golden arches became the symbol for McDonald's.

WRITTEN LANGUAGES

Any writing system is made up of a group of symbols, which can stand for whole words or parts of words. Early writing systems, such as Ancient Egyptian hieroglyphs, usually started as picture symbols standing for whole words or ideas. Some picture writing is quite recent, like the symbols shown here, which were created in Bamum, Cameroon, Africa, in the early 20th century.

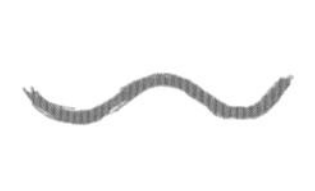
Thread

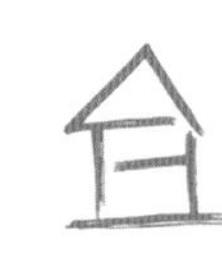
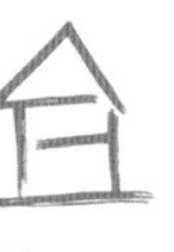
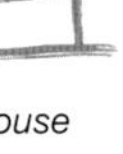
Child

House

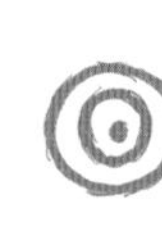

Plate

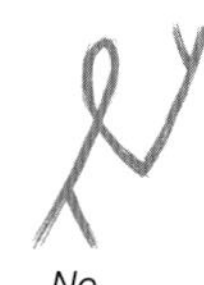
No

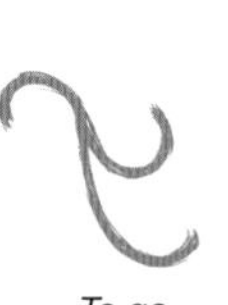
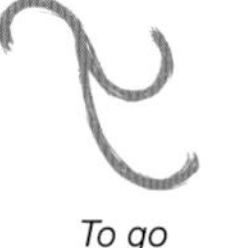
To go

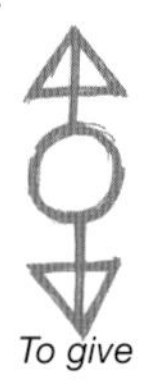
To give

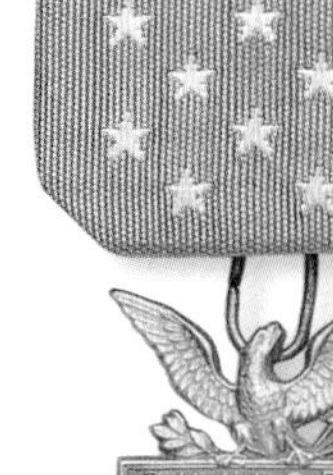

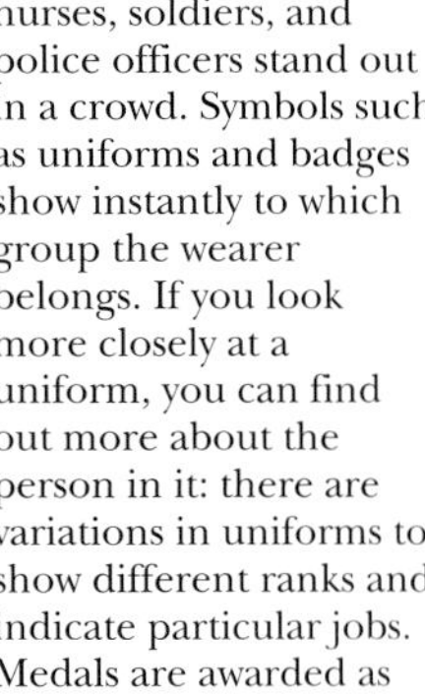

US congressional medal of honour

IDENTIFIERS
It is vital that people like nurses, soldiers, and police officers stand out in a crowd. Symbols such as uniforms and badges show instantly to which group the wearer belongs. If you look more closely at a uniform, you can find out more about the person in it: there are variations in uniforms to show different ranks and indicate particular jobs. Medals are awarded as signs of special acts of bravery or service.

TRAFFIC SIGNS
Road signs are agreed internationally, so most of them are the same the world over. Different shapes indicate different types of message. Triangular signs are used for warnings, such as signs warning of slippery roads or other hazards. Round signs are mostly for prohibitions, such as no entry or no cycling. Rectangular signs usually give directions and other information.

WARNING SIGNS
Triangular warning signs can be used for all sorts of hazards. Road users in western Europe are familiar with signs warning of cattle or deer on the road; in the Middle East, camel warnings are treated in the same way. A triangular sign with a yellow background is often used for warnings about environmental hazards such as dangerous chemicals, poisons, or radioactive material.

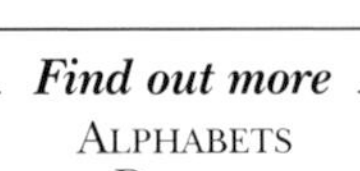

Find out more
ALPHABETS
DESIGN
MYTHS AND LEGENDS

SKELETONS

INSIDE THE HUMAN BODY, hundreds of bones link together like scaffolding to form the skeleton. Without a skeleton, the body would collapse. The skeleton holds the body rigid and gives shape to all the softer parts. It also protects the organs – the skull surrounds the brain, and the ribs act as a protective cage around the lungs and heart. The skeleton is also an anchor for the muscles, which move the different parts of the body. Bone is made of living cells surrounded by a framework of minerals, particularly calcium and phosphate, and a stringy, elastic substance called collagen. In a newborn baby, many of the bones are made of a soft, rubbery substance called cartilage. As a baby grows, the cartilage gradually turns into hard bone. Our wrists and ankles are among the last to become bone. In later life, bones gradually become more fragile and brittle, and break more easily.

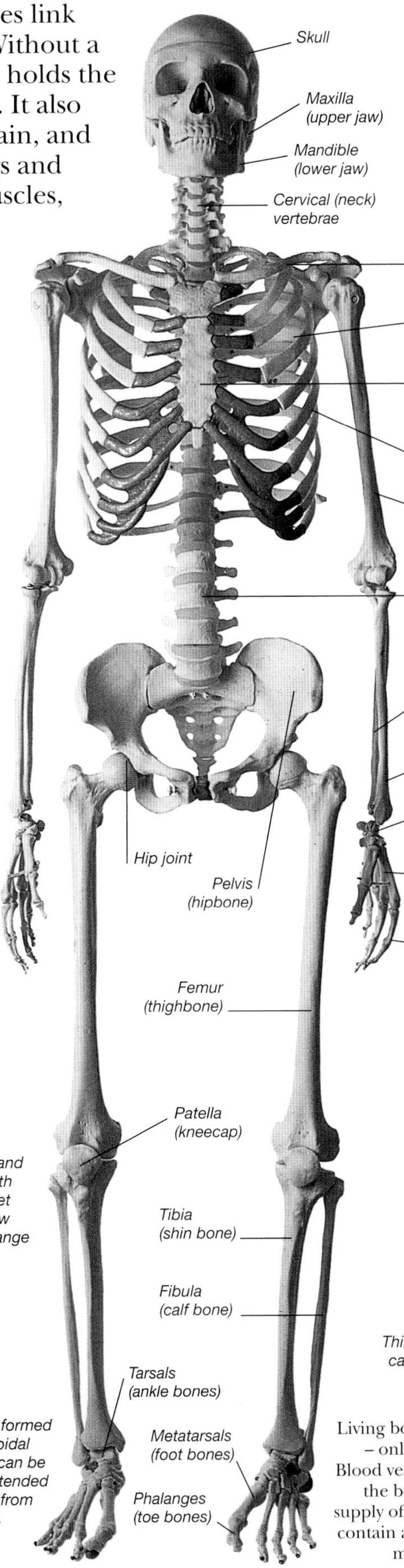

INTERNAL SKELETONS

Humans and other mammals, fish, birds, and reptiles all have an inner skeleton, or endoskeleton, made up of many separate bones. The central part of the skeleton is the spine (vertebral column or backbone). The spinal joints can move only a little, but the spine as a whole is very flexible. Some creatures, such as worms, have no bones. Instead the pressure of fluid inside their bodies helps them keep their shape. They are said to have a hydrostatic skeleton.

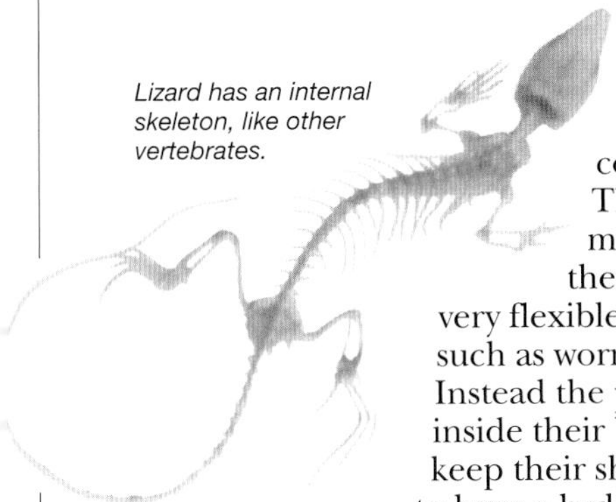

Lizard has an internal skeleton, like other vertebrates.

JOINTS

Bones are linked together at joints. There are several types of joints, including fixed, hinge, and ball-and-socket joints. Fixed joints, such as those between the separate bones in the skull, cannot move. Hinge joints, such as those in the elbow, allow movement in one direction only. Ball-and-socket joints, such as the hip, allow the bones to swing in two directions and also to twist.

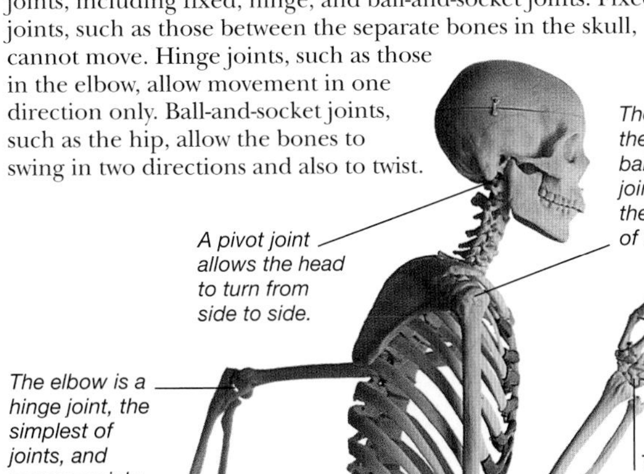

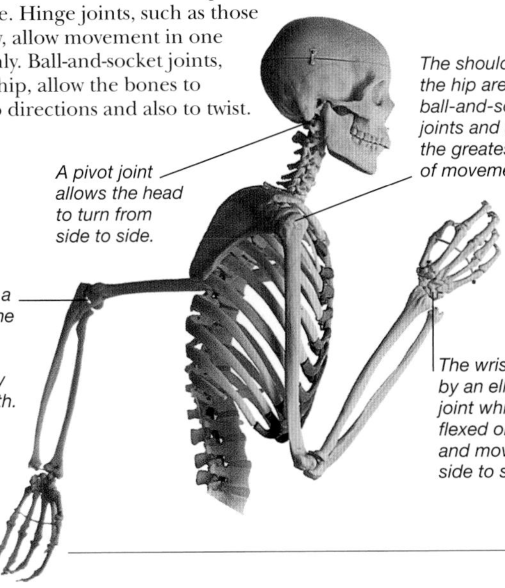

A pivot joint allows the head to turn from side to side.

The shoulder and the hip are both ball-and-socket joints and allow the greatest range of movement.

The elbow is a hinge joint, the simplest of joints, and moves mainly back and forth.

The wrist is formed by an ellipsoidal joint which can be flexed or extended and moved from side to side.

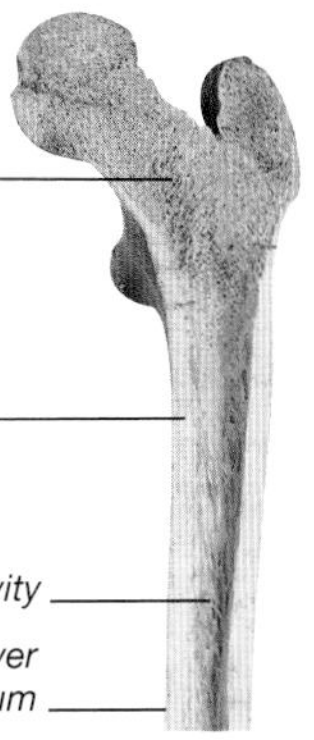

HUMAN SKELETON

There are 206 bones in the human skeleton, including 29 in the skull, 26 in the spine, 32 in each arm, 31 in each leg, and 25 in the chest. The largest bone is in the thigh, and the smallest ones are the ossicles, which are three tiny bones inside each ear.

Skull
Maxilla (upper jaw)
Mandible (lower jaw)
Cervical (neck) vertebrae
Clavicle (collarbone)
Scapula (shoulder blade)
Sternum (breastbone)
12 pairs of ribs
Humerus (upper-arm bone)
Lumbar (lower back) vertebrae
Ulna (forearm bone)
Radius (forearm bone)
Carpals (wrist bones)
Metacarpals (palm bones)
Phalanges (finger bones)
Hip joint
Pelvis (hipbone)
Femur (thighbone)
Patella (kneecap)
Tibia (shin bone)
Fibula (calf bone)
Tarsals (ankle bones)
Metatarsals (foot bones)
Phalanges (toe bones)

Soft, spongy bone inside
Hard, compact bone outside
Medullary cavity
Thin, tough outer layer called the periosteum

BONE

Living bone is tough and slightly flexible – only dead bone is white and brittle. Blood vessels pass through small holes in the bone's surface, and carry a steady supply of blood to the bone. Some bones contain a jelly-like substance called bone marrow, which makes blood cells.

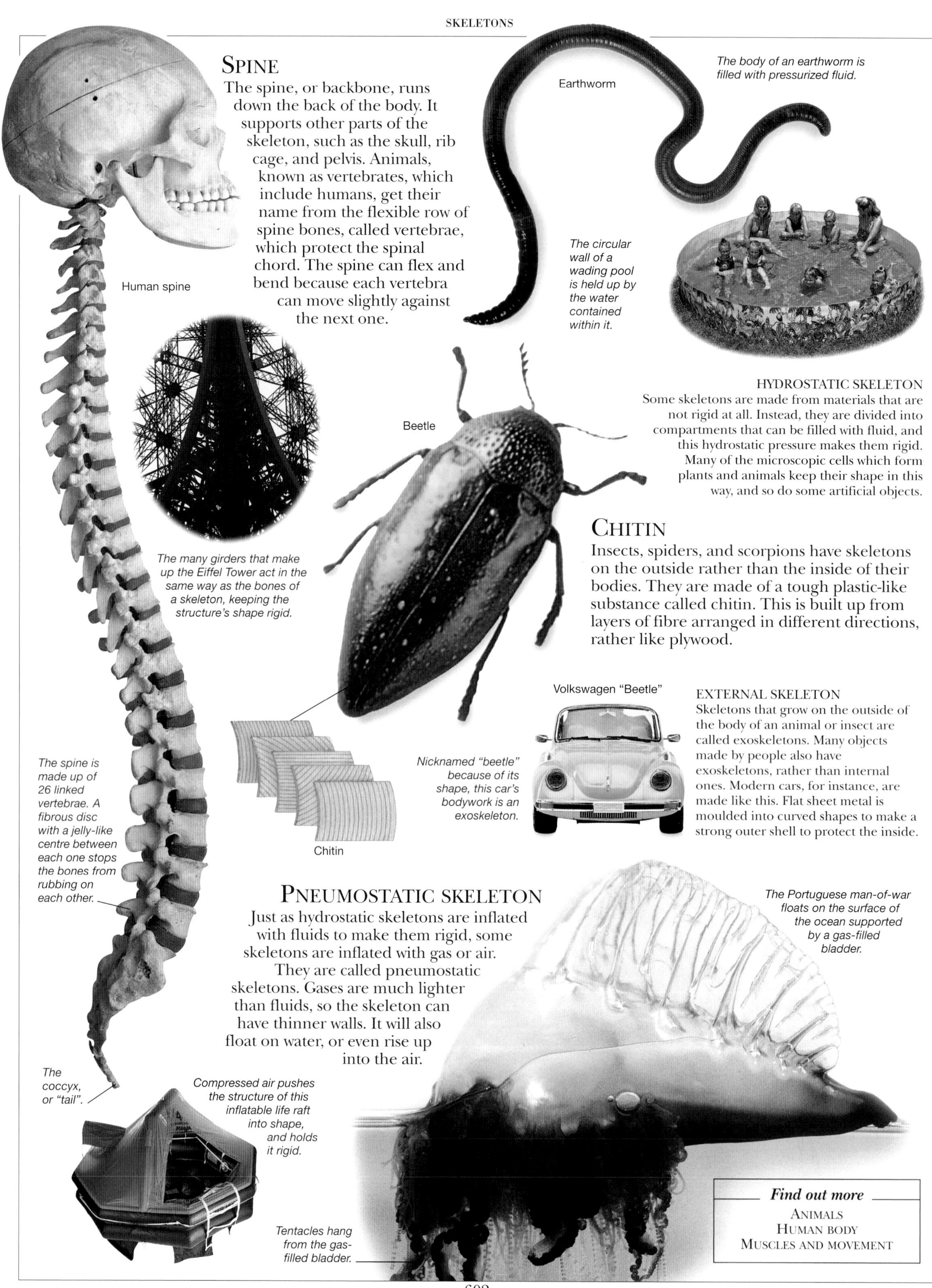

Spine

The spine, or backbone, runs down the back of the body. It supports other parts of the skeleton, such as the skull, rib cage, and pelvis. Animals, known as vertebrates, which include humans, get their name from the flexible row of spine bones, called vertebrae, which protect the spinal chord. The spine can flex and bend because each vertebra can move slightly against the next one.

The body of an earthworm is filled with pressurized fluid.

The circular wall of a wading pool is held up by the water contained within it.

HYDROSTATIC SKELETON

Some skeletons are made from materials that are not rigid at all. Instead, they are divided into compartments that can be filled with fluid, and this hydrostatic pressure makes them rigid. Many of the microscopic cells which form plants and animals keep their shape in this way, and so do some artificial objects.

The many girders that make up the Eiffel Tower act in the same way as the bones of a skeleton, keeping the structure's shape rigid.

Chitin

Insects, spiders, and scorpions have skeletons on the outside rather than the inside of their bodies. They are made of a tough plastic-like substance called chitin. This is built up from layers of fibre arranged in different directions, rather like plywood.

The spine is made up of 26 linked vertebrae. A fibrous disc with a jelly-like centre between each one stops the bones from rubbing on each other.

Nicknamed "beetle" because of its shape, this car's bodywork is an exoskeleton.

EXTERNAL SKELETON

Skeletons that grow on the outside of the body of an animal or insect are called exoskeletons. Many objects made by people also have exoskeletons, rather than internal ones. Modern cars, for instance, are made like this. Flat sheet metal is moulded into curved shapes to make a strong outer shell to protect the inside.

Pneumostatic skeleton

Just as hydrostatic skeletons are inflated with fluids to make them rigid, some skeletons are inflated with gas or air. They are called pneumostatic skeletons. Gases are much lighter than fluids, so the skeleton can have thinner walls. It will also float on water, or even rise up into the air.

The Portuguese man-of-war floats on the surface of the ocean supported by a gas-filled bladder.

The coccyx, or "tail".

Compressed air pushes the structure of this inflatable life raft into shape, and holds it rigid.

Tentacles hang from the gas-filled bladder.

Find out more

Animals
Human body
Muscles and movement

SLAVERY

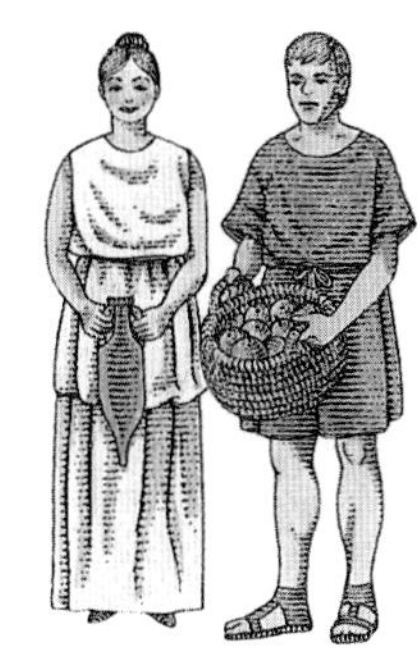

ROMAN SLAVES
Most wealthy Roman citizens owned slaves. Some slaves lived as part of the family; others were treated very badly. Some earned manumission (a formal release from slavery) through loyalty to a master.

FIVE THOUSAND YEARS AGO the Sumerians put their prisoners to work on farms as slaves. The workers had no rights and no pay, and their masters regarded them as property. In ancient Greece and Rome, slaves produced most of the goods and also worked as household servants. During the 16th century, European nations began to colonize the Americas, and imported thousands of Africans to work as slaves on their plantations and silver mines. Between 1500 and 1800, European ships took about 12 million slaves from their homes to the new colonies. By the 19th century, those against slavery set up movements in the United States, and Britain, to end it. Slavery was formally abolished in the British Empire and the United States in the mid-1800s. Sadly, it continues today in many parts of the world, most often affecting children and immigrants.

TRIANGLE OF TRADE

The British trade in slaves was known as the triangular trade. Ships sailed from British ports laden with goods such as guns and cloth. Traders exchanged these goods with African chiefs for slaves on the west coast of Africa. The slave ships then carried their cargo across the Atlantic to the Americas and the Caribbean. Here, slaves were in demand for plantation work, so the traders exchanged them for sugar, tobacco, rum, and molasses. The ships then returned to Britain carrying this cargo, which was sold at huge profits.

NORTH AMERICA
Tobacco
Ships sailed back to Europe with goods.
Britain
Ships departed from Britain carrying guns and cloth.
AFRICA
Slave coast
Ships carried slaves across the Atlantic.
SOUTH AMERICA
Rum, sugar, and molasses
Slave ship

SLAVE SHIPS
Slavers (slave traders) packed their ships with Africans to sail on what was known as the middle passage across the Atlantic. The slaves were chained and kept below deck for most of the voyage. Unclothed and underfed, thousands of Africans died on the Atlantic crossing.

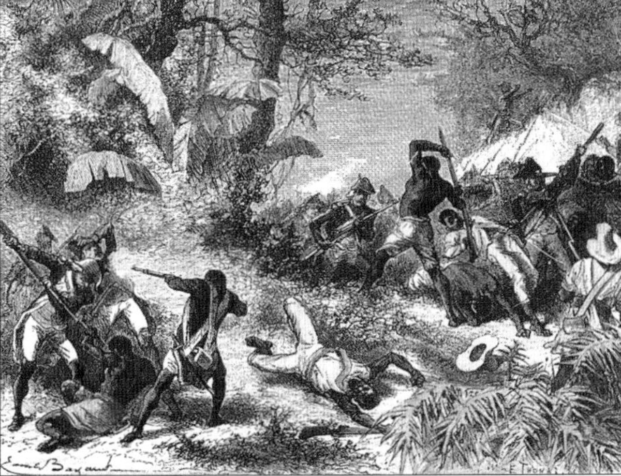

SLAVE REBELLIONS
Many Africans fought against slavery. In 1791, one of the most famous rebellions began in the French colony of Haiti. A slave named Toussaint L'Ouverture led an army of slaves against the French soldiers in a rebellion that lasted 13 years. L'Ouverture was captured and died in prison in 1803. In 1804, Haiti gained independence and became the world's first black republic.

SLAVE MARKET

Once the slaves reached the West Indies or the southern states of America, they were auctioned at a slave market. Here, they were treated like animals. Families were sometimes separated, and people were sold singly to plantation owners. Slaves were put to work on cotton, sugar, and tobacco plantations. Many received cruel treatment, and severe whipping was a common punishment for slaves who tried to escape.

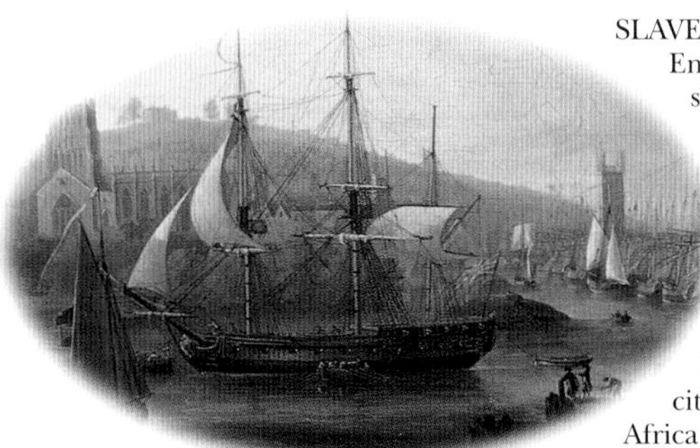

Ships in Bristol harbour

SLAVERY AND WEALTH
England dominated the slave trade, and some British cities became very rich as a result. Bristol and Liverpool, for instance, imported goods such as sugar and tobacco produced by slaves in the West Indies. Ships from both cities carried slaves from Africa to American plantations.

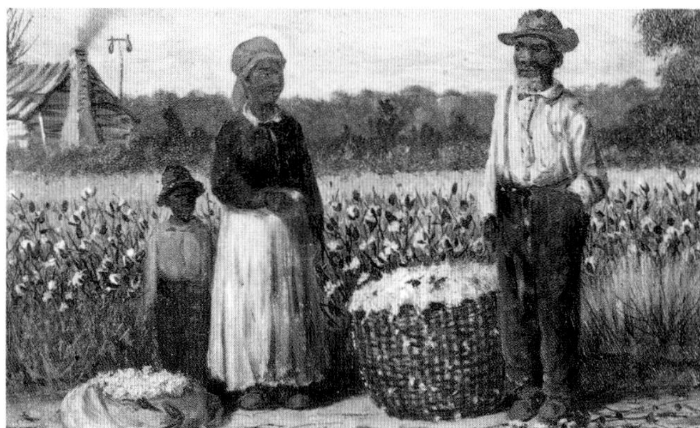

Cotton

African slave labourers were made to grow sugar in Brazil and the Caribbean. Later, tobacco was also grown. By the late 1700s there were huge cotton plantations in North America, and the British textile industry began to flourish, stimulating the Industrial Revolution. Cotton was made into cloth in Glasgow and Manchester.

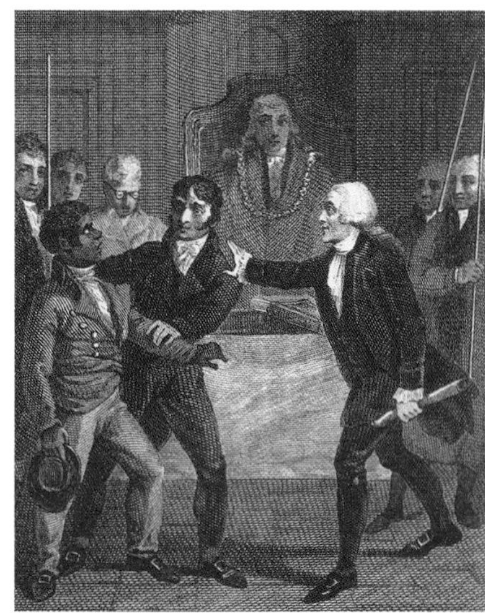

GRANVILLE SHARP
In 1772, British clerk Granville Sharp defended a black immigrant named James Somerset in a legal case known as the Somerset Case. This established that slavery was not recognized in Britain, and a slave who stepped on British soil was automatically free. The ruling was seen as officially abolishing slavery in England.

Abolitionists

On both sides of the Atlantic, Quakers, evangelical Christians, and liberal thinkers fought to abolish slavery. In Britain, Granville Sharp, and William Wilberforce (1759-1833), formed the Anti-Slavery Society in 1787-88. Members campaigned for the abolition of slavery and the freeing of all slaves. As part of the campaign, pottery owner Josiah Wedgwood produced a special medal. In 1833, the Emancipation Act freed slaves in the British Empire.

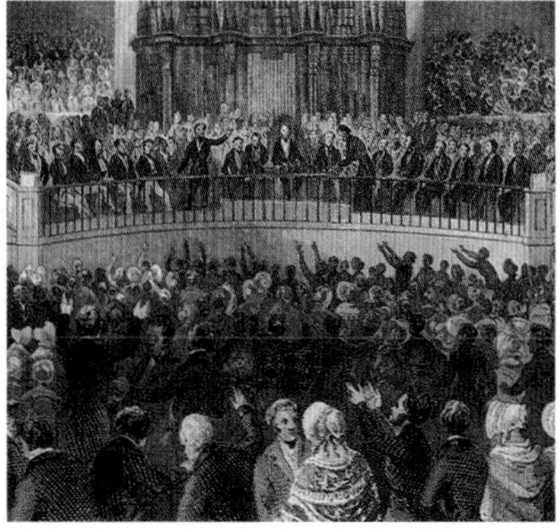

ANTI-SLAVERY MOVEMENT
In 1840, a World Anti-Slavery Convention took place in London, with delegates from the United States. Women took an active part in the abolition movement, often linking their situation with that of slaves. American feminists Lucretia Mott (1793-1880) and Susan B. Anthony (1820-1906) were leading campaigners.

OLAUDAH EQUIANO
Africans themselves played a part in the anti-slavery movement. One of the best-known African anti-slavery campaigners was Olaudah Equiano (1745-97). Born in Nigeria, he was captured with his sister when he was eleven, and taken to Britain as a servant. His autobiography was influential and is one of the earliest important works by an African written in English.

Find out more

Africa, history of
American civil war
Caribbean, history of
Industrial revolution
Tubman, Harriet

Snails and Slugs

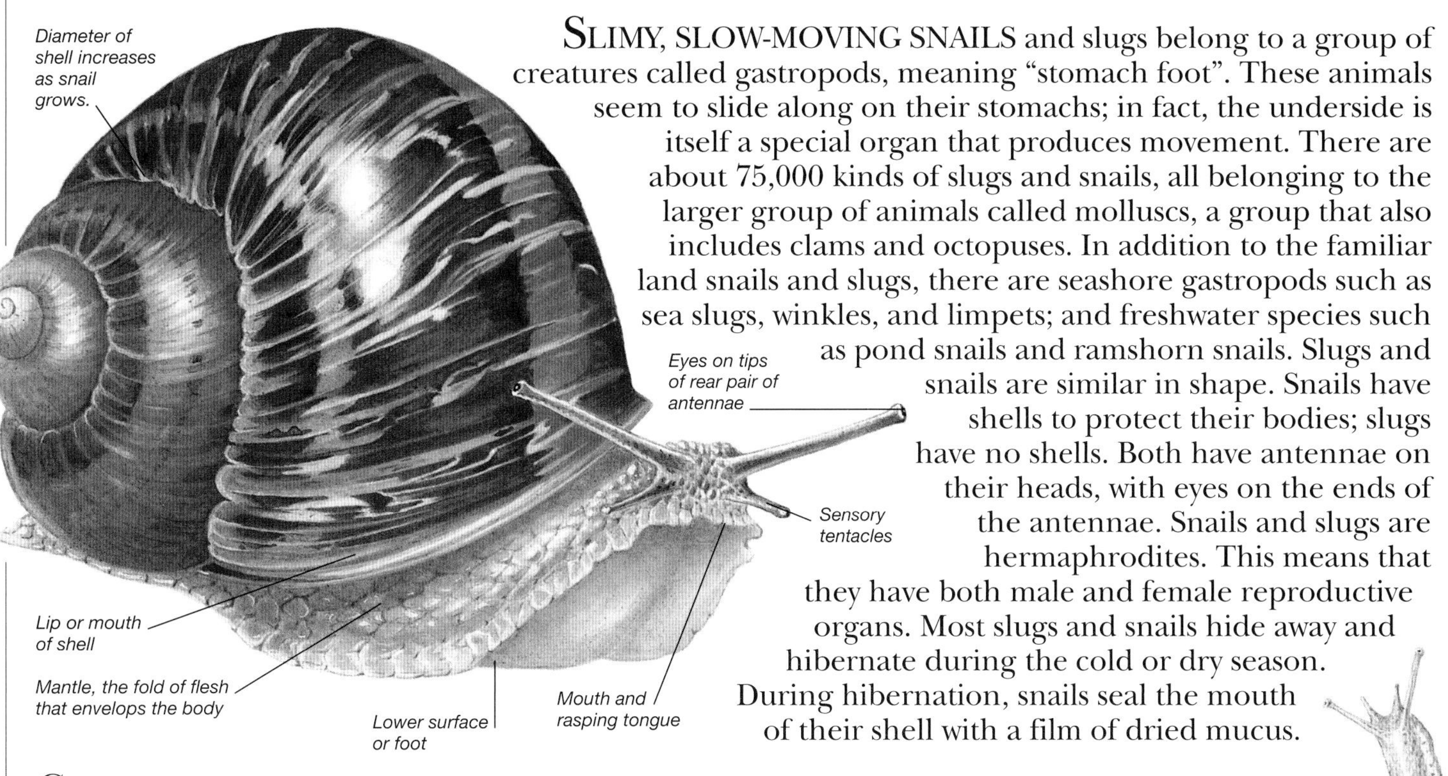

SLIMY, SLOW-MOVING SNAILS and slugs belong to a group of creatures called gastropods, meaning "stomach foot". These animals seem to slide along on their stomachs; in fact, the underside is itself a special organ that produces movement. There are about 75,000 kinds of slugs and snails, all belonging to the larger group of animals called molluscs, a group that also includes clams and octopuses. In addition to the familiar land snails and slugs, there are seashore gastropods such as sea slugs, winkles, and limpets; and freshwater species such as pond snails and ramshorn snails. Slugs and snails are similar in shape. Snails have shells to protect their bodies; slugs have no shells. Both have antennae on their heads, with eyes on the ends of the antennae. Snails and slugs are hermaphrodites. This means that they have both male and female reproductive organs. Most slugs and snails hide away and hibernate during the cold or dry season. During hibernation, snails seal the mouth of their shell with a film of dried mucus.

Garden snail

The snail's shell protects the animal from predators and prevents the soft, moist body from drying out. The shell is made of calcium carbonate and other minerals. As the snail grows, it adds more material to the mouth of the shell, making it larger. The snail's tongue is called a radula. It is small and file-like, with as many as 150,000 tooth-like denticles for rasping at plant food.

Dark-lipped banded snail has dark band around shell mouth.

YOUNG
After mating, the snail or slug lays eggs, either singly or in batches, in mucus. The young snails and slugs hatch from their eggs after about two to four weeks.

SLIME
Snails and slugs make several types of slime. As the slug crawls along, it lays down one kind of slime in patches. Another kind of slime is given off when the creature is attacked by a predator. A slug crawls by waves of muscle contractions passing along its foot.

Slug

Slugs are unpopular with gardeners because some do serious damage to plants and vegetables. Most slugs have no shells; some have a very small shell embedded in the back. Slugs avoid drying out by living in damp places and emerging only at night or after rain.

SEA SLUG
There are many beautifully coloured sea slugs in the shallow coastal waters of the world, particularly around coral reefs. Many have feathery or tufted gills for absorbing oxygen from the water. Sea slugs are predators, feeding mainly on sponges, barnacles, sea mats, and sea anemones.

TOPSHELL
The purple topshell snail lives close to the high-tide mark.

Find out more

OCEAN WILDLIFE
SEASHORE WILDLIFE
SHELLS AND SHELLFISH

Snakes

Long, legless, scaly, and slithering, snakes are a very successful group of reptiles. They are found everywhere except the coldest regions, highest mountain peaks, and a few islands. Most snakes can swim and climb well. All snakes are hunters. Some, such as pythons and boa constrictors, squeeze and suffocate their prey to death; others, such as cobras, paralyse their victims with a poisonous bite. Fast-moving snakes such as sand snakes hunt down insects, small birds, and mammals. Blind snakes are burrowers that eat ants and termites. More than 400 kinds of snakes are venomous (poisonous), but only some can give a fatal bite to humans. Deadly poisonous snakes include cobras, boomslangs, and mambas.

FANGS
The pair of hollow teeth at the front of the upper jaw are called fangs. The fangs lie flat along the jaw and swing forward when the snake strikes. Muscles pump venom from glands down the fangs into the victim.

RATTLE
Rattlesnakes are so named because they shake the tip of the tail (the rattle) to scare off predators. The rattle consists of a row of hollow tail segments which make a noise when the snake shakes them.

Rattle at tip of tail

SNAKE CHARMING
This is an ancient entertainment in Africa and Asia. Snake charmers fascinate snakes with movements that make the snakes sway to the music.

Rattlesnake

At more than 2 m (7 ft) long, the eastern diamondback is the largest rattlesnake, and the most poisonous snake in North America. The rattlesnake feeds mainly on rats, rabbits, and birds. Unlike many other snakes, which lay eggs, the rattlesnake gives birth to about 10 live young in late summer.

Snake's long belly has large scales called ventral scutes which overlap like tiles on a roof.

Emerald tree boa constricts or squeezes its prey.

MILK SNAKE
The non-venomous milk snake shown left is found all over North America, down to the north of South America. It looks similar to the poisonous coral snake, but the milk snake has yellow bands bordered by black, whereas the poisonous coral snake has black bands bordered by yellow. The milk snake hunts small mammals, birds, and other reptiles, including rattlesnakes. It coils around its prey and chokes it to death.

YOUNG SNAKES
Some snakes are described as viviparous, because they give birth to fully formed young. Others lay eggs in a burrow or under a log, leaving the young to hatch and fend for themselves. Certain kinds of pythons coil around the eggs and protect them until they hatch.

Constrictor

Boas and pythons are called constrictors because they constrict or coil around their prey and suffocate it. There are 66 kinds of boas and pythons; they include some of the largest snakes on Earth. Anacondas are boas of the Amazon region in South America. These massive snakes reach more than 8 m (25 ft) in length and weigh 225 kg (500 lbs).

The sea snake's body follows S-shaped curves, pushing sideways and backwards.

Young grass snake hatches from its egg head first and flicks its tongue to sense its surroundings.

SEA SNAKE
There are 50 kinds of sea snakes – the yellow-bellied sea snake shown left is the most common. It measures up to 80 cm (32 in) in length, preys on fish, and gives birth to about five young at sea. Sea snakes spend their lives swimming in the warm waters of the Indian Ocean, around Southeast Asia and Australia, and in the western Pacific.

Find out more
Animals
Australian wildlife
Desert wildlife
Forest wildlife
Reptiles

Soil

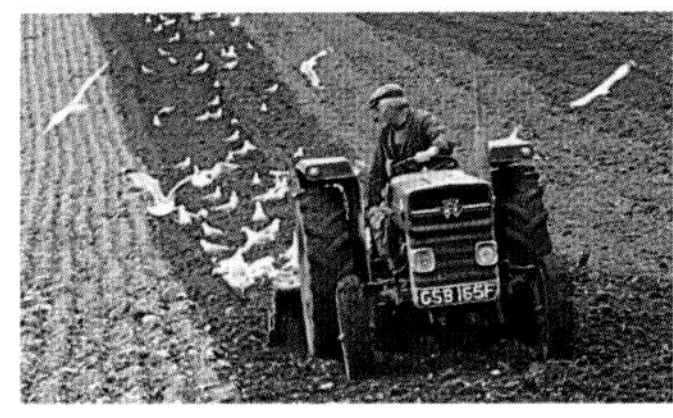

FERTILIZER
Farmers add fertilizers to poor soil. The fertilizer is rich in minerals that help the crops to grow.

If you reach down and pick up a handful of soil, you will be holding one of the Earth's most basic and valuable resources. Soil teems with life. A plot of earth the size of a small garden may contain millions of insects and micro-organisms, plus organic matter from dead or dying plants and animals. Soil provides the foundation for roots, a source of food for plants, and a home not only for burrowing animals, such as moles, but also for millions of spiders and centipedes. There are many different types of soil, from thick silt and loose sand to waterlogged mud and dry desert. Soil is formed from the wearing down of rocks and takes many years to develop. Each 6.5 sq cm (1 sq in) of soil, for instance, may take 100 to 2,000 years to form. The quality of soil varies from region to region. In hot countries such as Africa and Australia, where there is little rain, the soil is very dry. In temperate regions such as Europe and North America, much of the soil is rich and fertile. But soil can be destroyed in just a fraction of the time it takes to form. Overfarming the land, for example, has led to soil erosion in many parts of the world.

TYPES OF SOIL
Soil may be black, brown, red, yellow, orange, or cream in colour, depending on the minerals it contains. Rich, dark, peaty soil is ideal for garden plants.

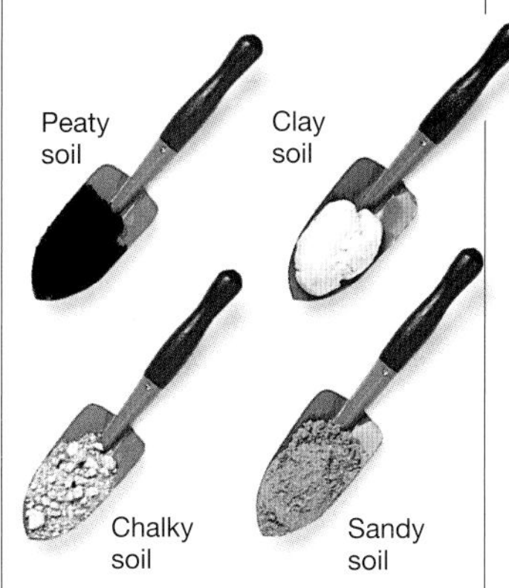

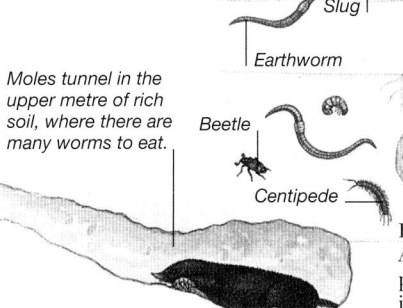

SOIL EROSION
In overfarmed areas, or where natural vegetation is removed, soil is no longer protected from rain or held in place by roots. Winds blow away the loose particles as dust, and rains wash them away as mud. The land becomes infertile and cannot support life. Today, soil erosion affects more than 513,000 sq km (198,000 sq miles) in the United States alone.

Soil layers

Soil is formed from several different layers that merge into one another. On top is a layer of humus, consisting of dead and rotting leaves. Underneath this layer is the topsoil where decayed plant and animal matter is broken down and recycled by insects, fungi, and bacteria. The subsoil layer, which contains less organic matter, lies below the topsoil and above a loose layer of partly weathered rock. A hard layer of solid bedrock lies below all the other layers.

HUMUS
Humus is the layer of decaying leaves and other plant material in the soil.

TOPSOIL
Topsoil is full of burrowing bugs, worms, and other creatures. It also gives anchorage to plants with shallow root systems.

COMPOST
Fungi, bacteria, worms, and insects thrive in a compost heap, helping the contents to decay and be recycled.

Slug
Beetle
Snail
Caterpillar
Earthworm
Beetle
Centipede
Potato tuber

Moles tunnel in the upper metre of rich soil, where there are many worms to eat.

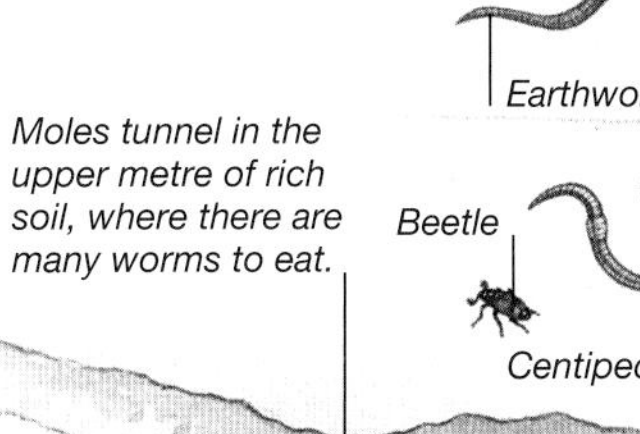

RECYCLING
All living things eventually rot away, back into the soil. The compost heap is a valuable recycler. In time, it turns domestic organic rubbish such as apple peelings, banana skins, eggshells, and grass cuttings into humus, a food supply for the soil. In this way, valuable resources are recycled.

SUBSOIL
The subsoil layer is reached only by deep-rooted plants such as trees.

POTATO
All plants, including the potato, use the energy in sunlight, mineral nutrients in the soil, water, and carbon dioxide from the air to grow. The potato plant stores its food reserves in the potatoes that we eat.

PARTLY WEATHERED ROCK ZONE
This layer of rocks has weathered and crumbled into loose chunks, and contains no organic matter.

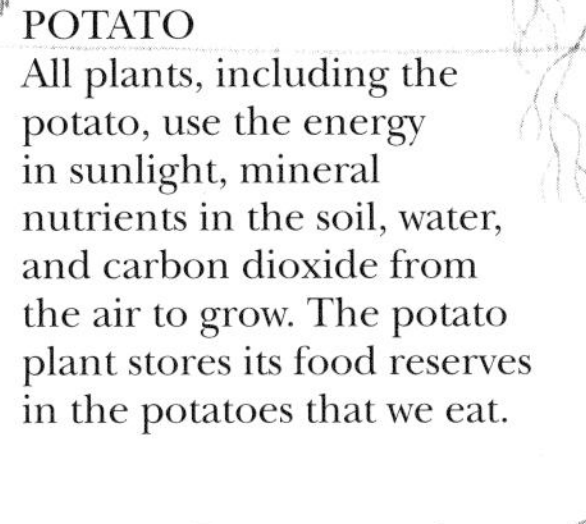

Tree roots reach into subsoil layer.

Find out more
Flowers and herbs
Mushrooms
toadstools, and other fungi
Plants
Trees

SONGBIRDS

MOST BIRDS MAKE SOME KIND OF SOUND. Some birds make loud, complicated warbles and whistles which are so pleasing to our ears that we call these birds songbirds. There are more than 5,000 kinds of songbird, also called perching birds because they perch in trees to sing. Many songbirds are small and dull-coloured, and stay hidden in trees. In dark, shady woodlands, a loud, clear singing voice is more useful for communicating with others than brightly coloured feathers. The male is usually the chief singer. He sings to show other birds where his territory is and to attract a female. Each kind of songbird has its own way of singing. Birdsongs vary from place to place, in the same way that humans pronounce words in different ways. Among the most outstanding singers are the robin chats of Africa, the warblers of Europe and Asia, and the babblers and bellbirds of Australasia.

DAWN CHORUS
As soon as the sun rises, birds finish their nightly rest and begin the day's activities. Many birds sing loudly at this time, and sing again at dusk. Each bird's song tells neighbours that it has survived the night and is still occupying its territory.

SONG THRUSH
This bird has a loud, cheerful, musical song. Its favourite singing perches include television aerials and high tree branches. Song thrushes eat snails, often breaking the shell open on a stone to extract the flesh.

ROBIN REDBREAST

During the spring, when robins have paired off to build a nest and raise young, the male robin's sweet, sad song tells intruders to stay out of his territory. The robin's warning call, a sharp *tic-tic-tic*, warns other birds of a nearby cat or hawk.

NIGHTINGALE
Many people describe the nightingale's song as the most beautiful of all. It has inspired poets and musicians through the ages. The nightingale (right) sings both day and night, but its song is noticed most at night. It makes its nest in low, tangled bushes where its eggs are well hidden in the shadows cast by leaves and branches.

BIRDSONG

There are several ways of describing a bird's song with words and symbols. Tape recordings help people learn how to identify birds by their particular songs.

SARDINIAN WARBLER
Loud, fast warbles

NIGHTINGALE
Smooth, liquid sounds

YELLOW WARBLER

In North and Central America, the yellow warbler is well known in parks and orchards. Its song often starts with three or four sweet *wheet* sounds and ends with a quick burst of high and low notes. Yellow warblers feed on caterpillars, moths, beetles, and spiders. They use their probing beaks to pick insects from leaves and bark.

Find out more
ANIMALS
BIRDS
FLIGHT, ANIMAL
MIGRATION, ANIMAL

Sound

WE LIVE IN A NOISY WORLD. The roar of city traffic, the music from a piano, the bark of a dog, all come to our ears as sound waves travelling through the air. Sound is generated when a disturbance sets air moving; for example, when someone plucks a guitar string. We hear sounds when sound waves – tiny vibrations in the air – strike our eardrums. Sound waves need a substance to travel through. This substance may be a liquid, such as water; a solid, such as brick and stone; or a gas, such as air.

Sounds such as musical notes have a certain pitch. A high-pitched sound makes the air vibrate backward and forward more times each second than a low-pitched sound. The number of vibrations per second is called the frequency of the sound and is measured in hertz (cycles per second). Humans cannot hear sounds with frequencies above about 20,000 hertz, or below about 30 hertz.

LOUDNESS AND DECIBELS
The sound of a train is louder than the sound of a whisper because the train produces larger vibrations in the air. The loudness of sound also depends on how close you are to its source. Loudness is measured in decibels (dB). A jet airliner taking off is rated at about 120 dB; the rustling of leaves is about 33 dB.

ECHOES
If you shout in a large hall or near mountains, you can hear your voice echo back to you. An echo occurs when a sound bounces off a surface such as a cliff face and reaches you shortly after the direct sound. The clarity of speech and music in a room or concert hall depends on the way sounds echo inside it.

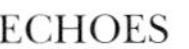

Speed of sound

Sound travels in air at a speed of about 1,224 km/h (about 760 mph). It travels more slowly when the temperature and pressure of the air are lower. In the thin, cold air 11 km (7 miles) up, the speed of sound is about 1,000 km/h (620 mph). In water, sound travels at 5,400 km/h (about 3,350 mph), much faster than in air.

The distance from one region of highest pressure to the next is called the wavelength of the sound. The higher the pitch, or frequency, of the sound, the shorter the wavelength.

Region of high-pressure air

Region of low-pressure air

The noise of the boat's engine sends sound waves through the water.

Sound waves

A sound wave consists of air molecules vibrating backward and forward. At each moment the molecules are crowded together in some places, producing regions of high pressure, and spaced out in others, producing regions of low pressure. Waves of alternately high pressure and low pressure move through the air, spreading out from the source of the sound. These sound waves carry the sound to your ears.

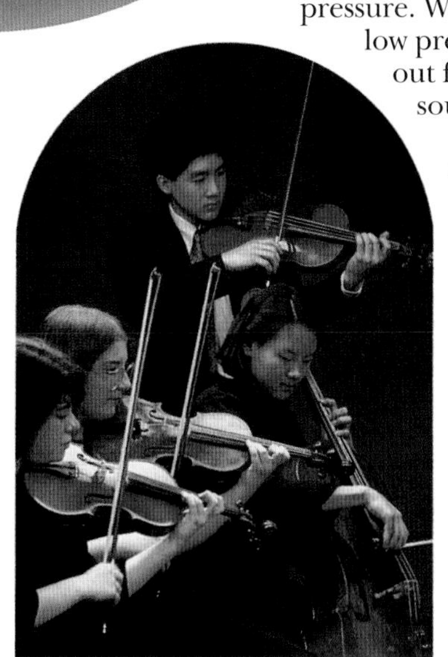

HARMONICS
In a musical note, secondary frequencies, called harmonics, are mixed with the main frequency. Harmonics are characteristic of different instruments, which is why a note played on a piano sounds different from the same note played on a violin. Harmonics bring life to the sound of musical instruments: an electronically produced sound of a single pure frequency sounds artificial and dull.

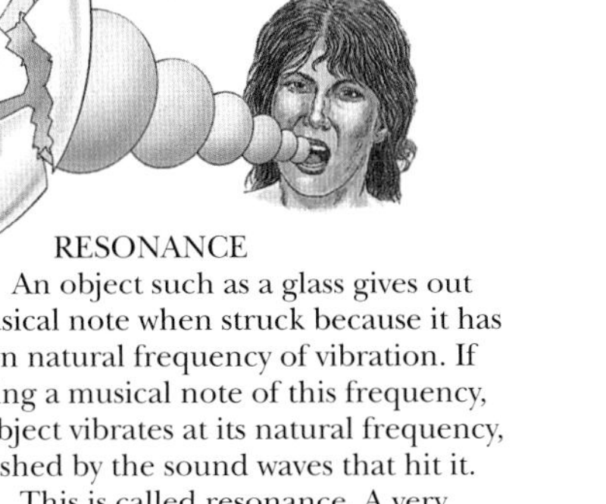

RESONANCE
An object such as a glass gives out a musical note when struck because it has its own natural frequency of vibration. If you sing a musical note of this frequency, the object vibrates at its natural frequency, pushed by the sound waves that hit it. This is called resonance. A very loud sound can make a glass resonate so strongly that it shatters.

Find out more

EARS
MUSIC
RADIO
SOUND RECORDING

SOUND RECORDING

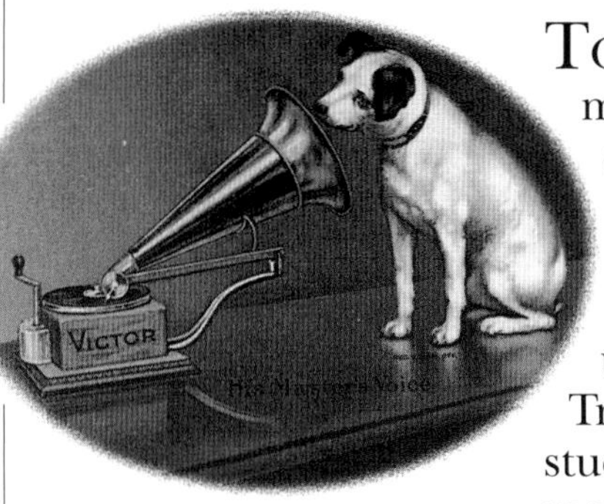

TODAY WE CAN STORE SOUND and reproduce it at will. We can hear music whenever we wish, produce "talking books" for the blind, record sounds into miniature recorders, and much more. All recording systems store sounds by making an image, or copy, of the sound waves. This image may be in the form of magnetism on a tape, the spiral groove in a record, or the pits in a compact disc. In a recording studio, sound is recorded using many microphones, each producing a recording on one track. Traditionally, these tracks were stored on magnetic tape, but most studios now store tracks on a computer. The sound engineer can modify the music on each track separately to perfect the tone and loudness of any instrument or singer. The studio recording is the master version of the music, which factories then use to make thousands of copies on compact discs, minidiscs, records, and cassette tapes.

VICTOR
His Master's Voice

RECORD PLAYER
The earliest recordings consisted of grooves cut into wax-coated cylinders. In 1887, German-American Emile Berliner first demonstrated the gramophone disc, or record. The gramophone above is the famous trademark of the record company His Master's Voice (HMV).

Whenever a coil moves within a magnetic field, a current is produced in the coil.
Protective grill prevents diaphragm from being damaged.
Permanent magnet produces magnetic field.
Fragile diaphragm made of plastic or thin metal foil
Coil of wire fixed to the diaphragm

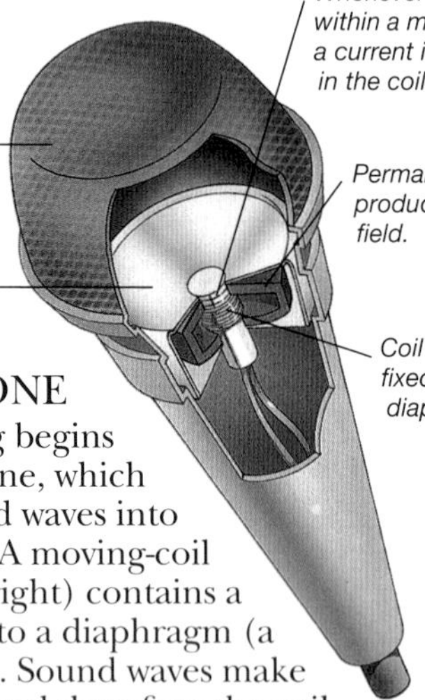

MICROPHONE

Every recording begins with a microphone, which converts sound waves into electrical signals. A moving-coil microphone (right) contains a wire coil attached to a diaphragm (a thin, flexible disc). Sound waves make the diaphragm, and therefore the coil, vibrate. The coil moves within the magnetic field of a small magnet; this movement generates an electric current in the coil. The current fluctuates in strength in the same way as the sound wave.

TAPE RECORDING
A cassette holds a spool of plastic tape coated with tiny metal grains. The grains are magnetic, and when sound is recorded onto the tape, the magnetism of the grains changes. The new magnetic pattern represents the sound.

Before a recording is made, the magnetic grains in the tape point in all directions.
Capstan and pinch roller keep the tape moving at the correct speed past the tape head.
During recording, the tape head arranges the magnetic pattern of the grains to record an image of the sound onto the tape.
Compact discs reproduce sounds of very high quality.
Metal coating on the disc reflects the laser beam into the light detector.
At a place on the CD where there is no pit, the laser beam, shown here in red, bounces back to a photocell detector that converts the light into electric current. Where there is a pit, the beam is reflected away from the detector.
Miniature laser scans underside of disc.
Photocell detector

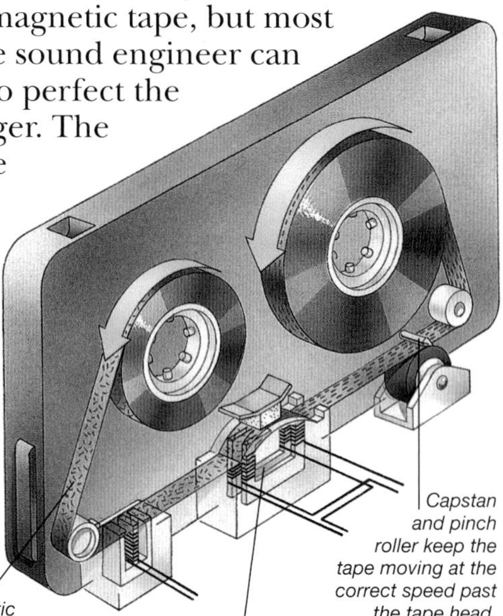

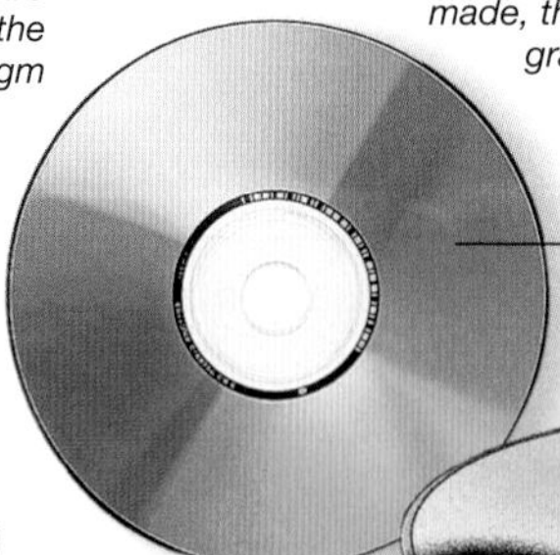

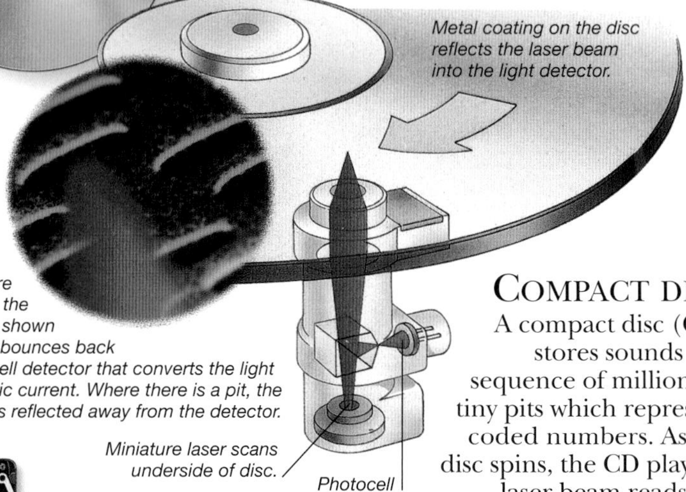

COMPACT DISC

A compact disc (CD) stores sounds as a sequence of millions of tiny pits which represent coded numbers. As the disc spins, the CD player's laser beam reads the sequence of pits and sends a signal to the loudspeaker.

An amplifier boosts the signal from the CD player before it reaches the speaker.
Loudspeakers are usually fitted in a cabinet.
Electromagnet consists of a coil of wire.
Varying field in electromagnet moves cone to and from permanent magnet.
Cone vibrates, producing sound waves.
Permanent magnet

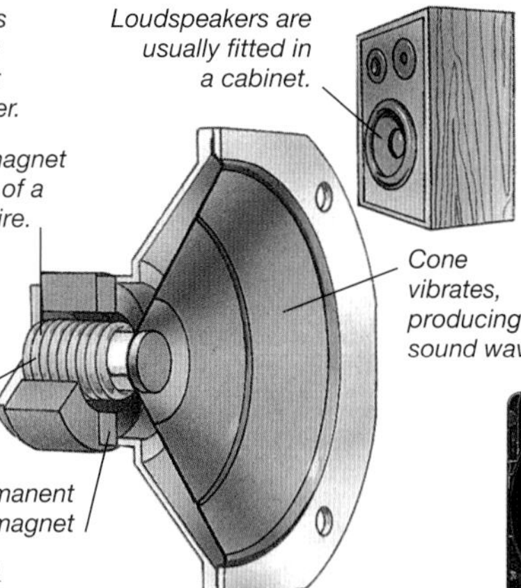

LOUDSPEAKER
A loudspeaker changes electrical signals into sound waves. Inside a loudspeaker, a varying electric current from a source such as a CD player or cassette deck powers an electromagnet, producing a varying magnetic field. This field makes a cone-shaped diaphragm vibrate, producing sound.

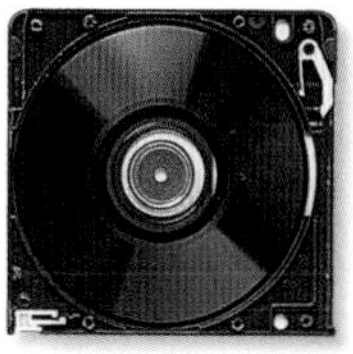

MINIDISC AND MP3
New types of data storage for sound recording are always being developed. A minidisc is a digital audio storage disc similar to a CD. However, the sound quality on a minidisc is less perfect than a CD because its small size means that data is heavily compressed. MP3 is a digital music file format that can be stored on a computer or a small portable player similar to a personal stereo. MP3 sound quality is crystal clear and near to perfect.

Find out more

BROADCASTING
LASERS
MUSIC
ROCK AND POP
SOUND

SOUTH AFRICA

AFRICA'S SOUTHERNMOST LAND, South Africa is immensely rich in natural resources, with a varied landscape and diverse animal species. In the 17th century, the Cape Town region was settled by Dutch colonists, who were soon followed by the British. From the 1830s, the Dutch (or Boers) began to penetrate the interior. Here, they clashed with the black majority, particularly the Zulus, a disciplined and effective fighting force. In the 20th century, South Africa was dominated by the white minority. The black population was deprived of the vote until 1994, when South Africa held its first multiracial, democratic elections. South Africa's diverse economy is based on mining and agriculture. It is just beginning to exploit its tourist potential. Two independent countries, Lesotho and Swaziland, marooned within South Africa, are economically dependent on their neighbour.

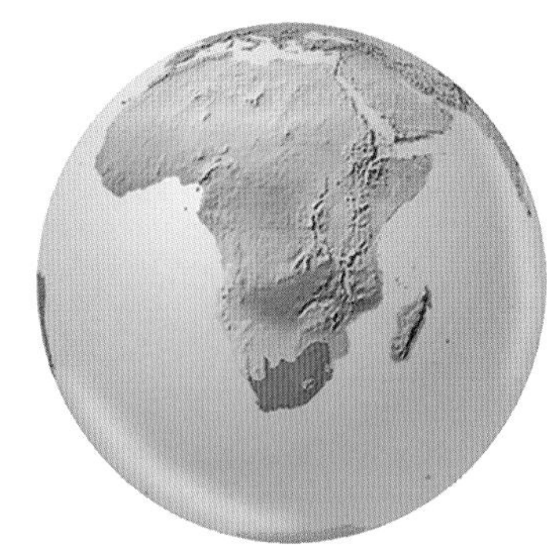

Situated at the southern tip of the African continent, South Africa is bordered by both the Atlantic and Indian Oceans. Much of the country consists of a broad plateau, bordered in the northeast by the arid Namib and Kalahari Deserts, and in the south by mountains and a sandy, coastal plain.

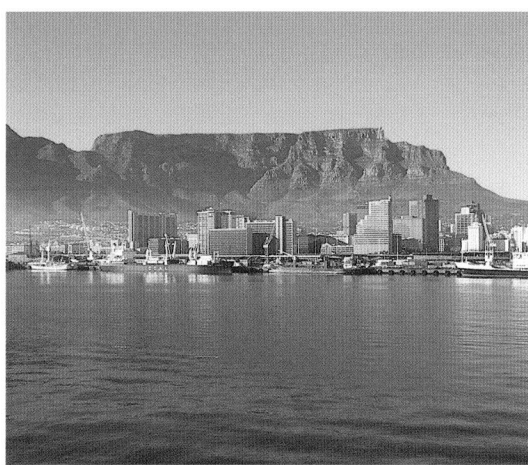

CAPE TOWN
Cape Town, home to the South African parliament, is situated along the southwestern shores of Table Bay. The town is dominated by the distinctive shape of Table Mountain, which rises to 1,005 m (3,300 ft). Cape Town was the first place to be settled by Dutch colonists in the 17th century. It was strategically placed on the main shipping routes between Europe and Asia. Today, it is still a major port and commercial centre.

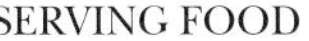

SERVING FOOD
Wooden vessels are used throughout the African continent. Bowls like this one from Lesotho are traditionally carved from a single block of wood.

THE DRAKENSBERG
The Drakensberg, or Dragon Mountains are a large range in the southeast of South Africa. They form a steep escarpment, reaching the height of 3,482 m (11,424 ft), which rises out of South Africa's central plateau. Much of South Africa's interior is dominated by tableland. This is an area of dry, rolling grassland (*veld*), with scattered trees. In places it is more than 1,200 m (3,900 ft) above sea level. It is grazed by both sheep and cattle.

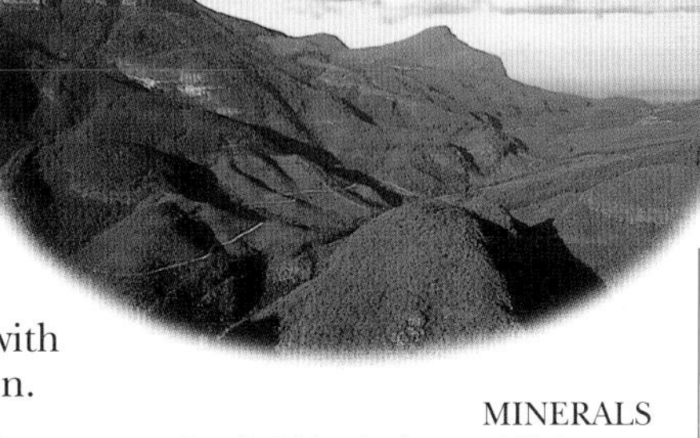

TOWNSHIPS

Until 1994, the "apartheid" system enforced the separation of the black majority from the ruling, white minority. Many black people were forced to live in purpose-built "townships", and still live there today. Soweto is a sprawling group of townships with a population of about two million. It is situated outside Johannesburg, where most of its inhabitants work, forcing them to travel long distances each day.

MINERALS
South Africa is the world's largest gold producer. It also exports large quantities of diamonds, manganese, chromium, and platinum.

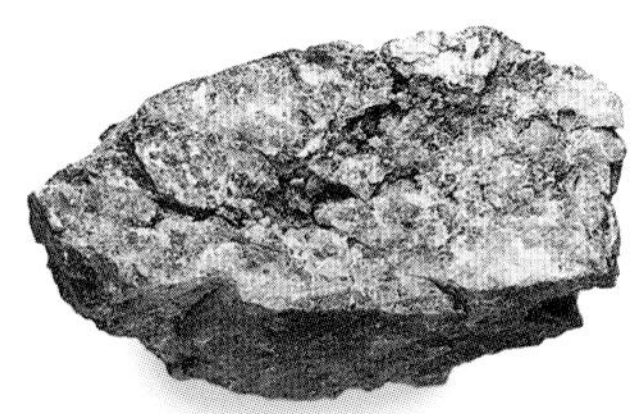

A FERTILE LAND

South Africa, with its fertile soils and warm climate, is ideally situated for agriculture. The main crops grown for export are wheat, sugar cane, potatoes, peanuts, citrus fruits, and tobacco. Sheep and cattle graze the *veld*. European settlers brought vines to South Africa in the 17th century. The Cape province is a major wine-producing area, and South African wine is exported all over the world.

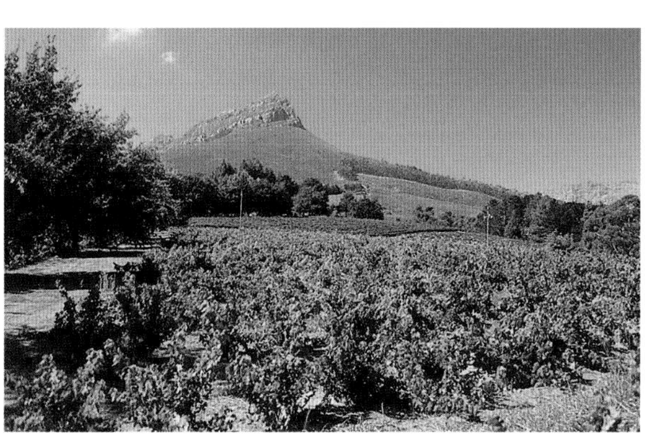

Find out more

AFRICA
AFRICA, HISTORY OF
AFRICAN WILDLIFE
ELEPHANTS
NATIONAL PARKS

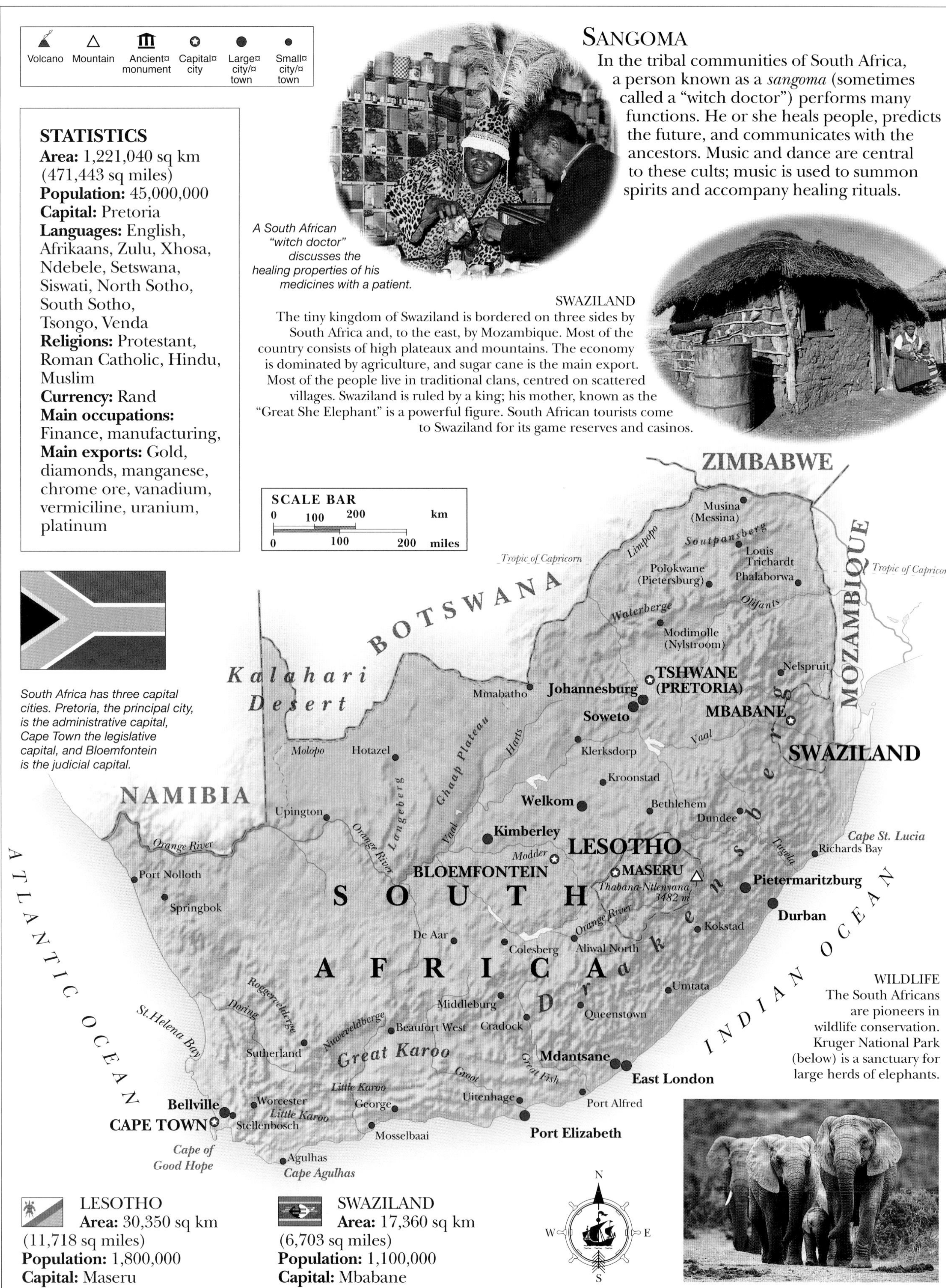

Sangoma

In the tribal communities of South Africa, a person known as a *sangoma* (sometimes called a "witch doctor") performs many functions. He or she heals people, predicts the future, and communicates with the ancestors. Music and dance are central to these cults; music is used to summon spirits and accompany healing rituals.

A South African "witch doctor" discusses the healing properties of his medicines with a patient.

STATISTICS
Area: 1,221,040 sq km (471,443 sq miles)
Population: 45,000,000
Capital: Pretoria
Languages: English, Afrikaans, Zulu, Xhosa, Ndebele, Setswana, Siswati, North Sotho, South Sotho, Tsongo, Venda
Religions: Protestant, Roman Catholic, Hindu, Muslim
Currency: Rand
Main occupations: Finance, manufacturing,
Main exports: Gold, diamonds, manganese, chrome ore, vanadium, vermiciline, uranium, platinum

SWAZILAND

The tiny kingdom of Swaziland is bordered on three sides by South Africa and, to the east, by Mozambique. Most of the country consists of high plateaux and mountains. The economy is dominated by agriculture, and sugar cane is the main export. Most of the people live in traditional clans, centred on scattered villages. Swaziland is ruled by a king; his mother, known as the "Great She Elephant" is a powerful figure. South African tourists come to Swaziland for its game reserves and casinos.

South Africa has three capital cities. Pretoria, the principal city, is the administrative capital, Cape Town the legislative capital, and Bloemfontein is the judicial capital.

WILDLIFE

The South Africans are pioneers in wildlife conservation. Kruger National Park (below) is a sanctuary for large herds of elephants.

LESOTHO
Area: 30,350 sq km (11,718 sq miles)
Population: 1,800,000
Capital: Maseru

SWAZILAND
Area: 17,360 sq km (6,703 sq miles)
Population: 1,100,000
Capital: Mbabane

HISTORY OF

SOUTH AFRICA

WHEN THE FIRST EUROPEANS settled in South Africa in the 1600s, they found a rich, fertile country long inhabited by African civilizations. The Europeans set up supply ports for ships sailing to and from India and the Far East. They moved inland, bringing them into conflict with Zulus and other African kingdoms. In 1910, South Africa became independent, but its black population was denied political power for many years. Today South Africa is a multiracial country with a black president. All races are represented in government.

ZULUS
The original inhabitants of South Africa were the Bushmen, Khoikoi, Bantus, and Zulus, who settled in the country over many thousands of years. The Zulus were fierce and warlike, living in protected homesteads made of wood with grass-thatched roofs.

Oxen pulled covered wagons through rough country.

SOUTH AFRICA

1652 Dutch establish port of Cape Town.

1814 Britain gains Cape Province from Dutch.

1836-45 Great Trek.

1852 Boers set up Transvaal, and (1854) Orange Free State.

1879 Zulu war.

1899-1902 Boer War, won by the British.

1910 South Africa becomes independent in British Empire.

1948 Nationalist Party introduces apartheid.

1960 67 Africans killed for protesting against apartheid, Sharpeville.

1994 First multiracial election.

THE GREAT TREK

The Dutch were the first Europeans to settle in South Africa, establishing Cape Town in 1652. The colony grew, but in 1814, the British took control. Relations between the Dutch farmers, known as Boers, and the British, were poor. Between 1836-45 more than 15,000 Boers trekked north, settling in Natal and the Transvaal.

Boers trekking north

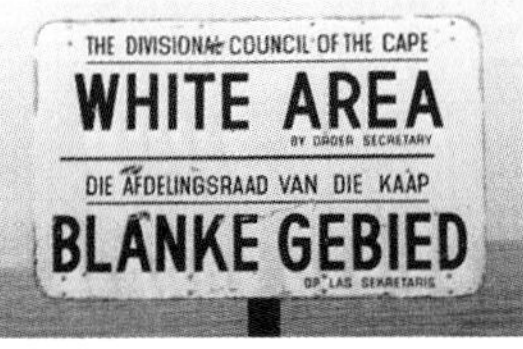
THE DIVISIONAL COUNCIL OF THE CAPE
WHITE AREA
BY ORDER SECRETARY
DIE AFDELINGSRAAD VAN DIE KAAP
BLANKE GEBIED
OP LAS SEKRETARIS

APARTHEID

In 1948, the Nationalist Party won power, and introduced a policy of apartheid, or separate development. Black and white South Africans were kept apart. Blacks were not allowed to vote in their own country, and were forced to live in poor areas called homelands.

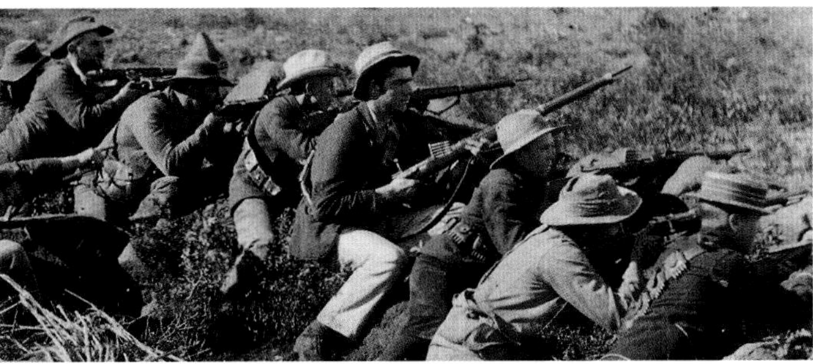

MAJORITY RULE
The African National Congress (ANC) led opposition to apartheid, with support from people worldwide. In 1990, South African president, F. W. de Klerk, began to negotiate the end of apartheid with the ANC and released Nelson Mandela from prison. Apartheid was ended. In 1994, South Africa held its first-ever multiracial elections, won by the ANC.

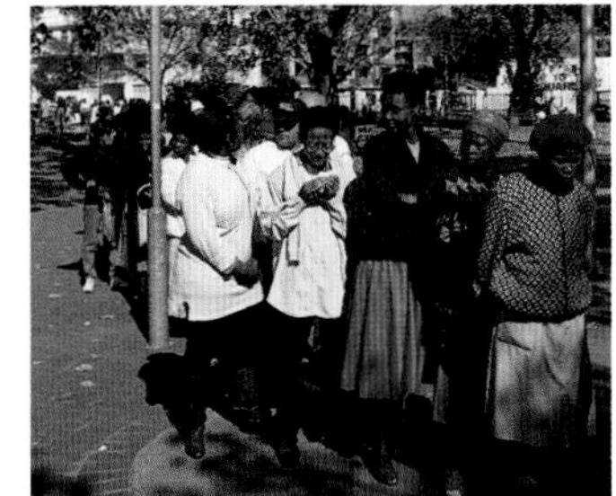

BOER WAR

In 1886, gold was discovered in the Boer-ruled Transvaal. British miners flooded into the country. The Boers felt threatened by these Uitlanders (foreigners), and, in 1899, declared war on Britain. At first they won victories, but, in 1900, the British occupied Boer lands. The Boers continued fighting, but many died in British concentration camps. In 1902, peace was declared.

Find out more

AFRICA
AFRICA, HISTORY OF
BRITISH EMPIRE
MANDELA, NELSON

South America

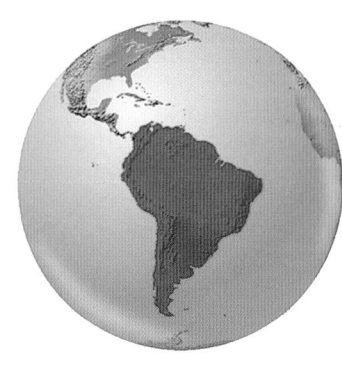

Three very different types of landscape dominate the triangular continent of South America. Along the western coast the towering Andes Mountains reach to more than 6,900 m (22,600 ft) in height. Dense rain forest covers the hot and humid northeastern area. Further south are great open plains of grass and scrub. There are huge mineral deposits and rich farming lands. Despite this, some of the 12 nations which make up the continent are among the poorest in the world.

Until about 170 years ago, Spain and Portugal ruled almost all of South America. Most people still speak Spanish or Portuguese. The population is made up of three groups: those descended from European settlers; Native Americans; and people of mixed ancestry. Many people are desperately poor and can barely afford to buy food. Large sections of the population are uneducated and cannot read or write. Many South American governments are insecure or unstable. Most have borrowed large sums of money from wealthier nations. The cost of repaying these debts makes it hard for the South American countries to develop industries which would take advantage of the natural resources.

South America lies south of the isthmus of Panama, between the Atlantic and Pacific oceans. It covers 17.8 million sq km (6.9 million sq miles).

Care of the Argentine cattle is the job of cowboys called gauchos.

Using the land

Large herds of beef cattle roam the grasslands of the Pampas, supporting the meat-packing trade in Argentina, Uruguay, and Paraguay. Corn (maize) is grown as a staple crop right across the continent. Coffee is grown as a cash crop in Brazil and Colombia, while coca plants grown in Bolivia, Peru, and Colombia, provide most of the world's cocaine, an illegal drug.

ANDES MOUNTAINS
Stretching the entire length of the continent, the Andes mountain chain is 47,250 km (4,500 miles) long. As well as mineral deposits, the Andes have rich farming land in mountain valleys and on the Altiplano, a large plateau in Peru and Bolivia.

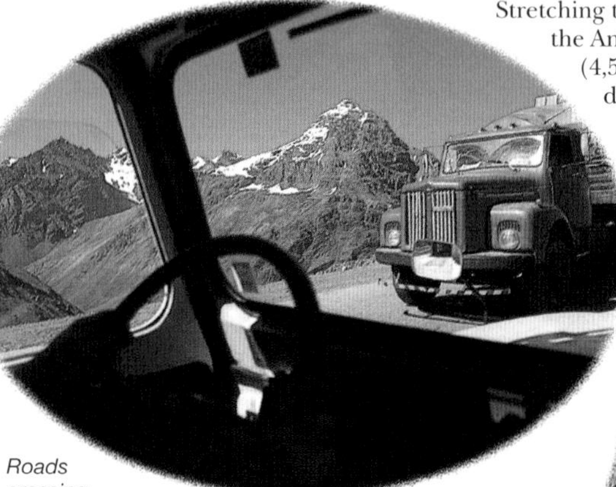

Roads crossing the Andes follow routes through the few low passes.

Peru

With a population of more than 27 million, Peru is one of the larger South American countries. It includes a long stretch of the Andes and part of the rain forest. Many people live on mountain farms and are very poor. Others work on plantations growing coffee, sugar, and cotton for export. Oil has recently been discovered and is bringing some wealth to Peru.

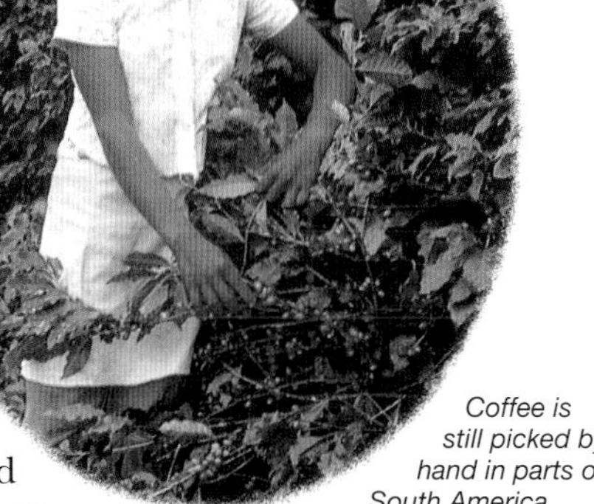

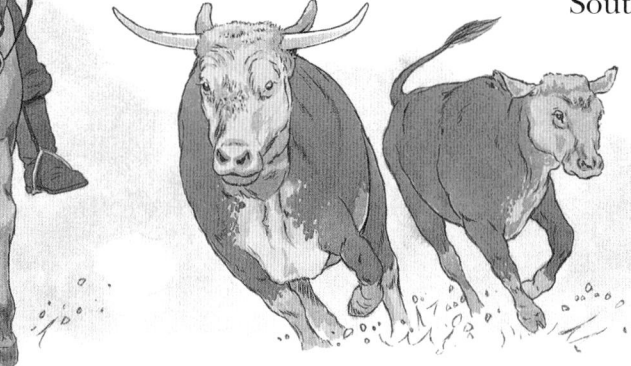

Coffee is still picked by hand in parts of South America.

Lake Titicaca

In the Andes mountains on the border between Peru and Bolivia, Lake Titicaca is the highest large lake in the world. The lake's surface is 3,812 m (12,507 ft) above sea level. Some parts are 180 m (600 ft) deep. Although large ships operate on the lake, the local people still use reed to build their traditional fishing boats.

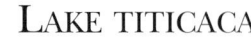

BOLIVIA

The mountain nation of Bolivia has no coastline. Its only links with the rest of the world are railways and roads running through Peru and Chile. Although there are large deposits of oil, tin, and silver in the high Andes, the nation remains very poor. About 70 per cent of the population are Aymara or Quechua Native Americans who grow just enough food in the mountains to feed themselves. Some farmers make extra money by growing the coca plant, which is processed to make the illegal drug cocaine.

A woman from Bolivia in traditional dress

SOCCER

Supported passionately, soccer is a favourite sport in most South American countries. Argentina, Brazil, and Uruguay have been very successful in international competitions. In 1930, Uruguay became the first country to host the World Cup. Uruguay also managed to win the tournament in the same year. World Cup victories in 1958, 1962, 1970, 1994, and 2002 mean that Brazil has won this fiercely contested event more times than any other country in the world.

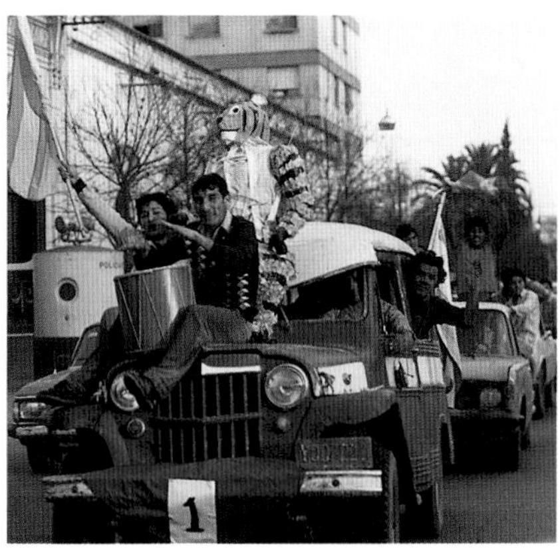

Argentinian football fans parade the streets, demonstrating support for their national soccer team. Argentina won the Fédération Internationale de Football Association (FIFA) World Cup in 1978 and 1986.

The Native Americans of South American forests live in large huts shared by many families. They sleep in hammocks hung between the posts of the huts.

Native Americans

The first peoples of South America were Native Americans. In the lowlands, Native Americans lived in small villages and gathered food from the forest, but in the Andes they built great civilizations. The arrival of European explorers destroyed these great cultures, and today only a few remote tribes still live in the forest as their ancestors did. However, the destruction of the rain forest for farming and mining threatens to eliminate these last traces of Native American society.

FALKLAND ISLANDS

Located in the Atlantic Ocean, the Falkland Islands were discovered by the English navigator John Davis, in his ship *Desire* in 1592. In 1690, the islands were named after Viscount Falkland, treasurer of the British navy. Islas Malvinas, the Argentinian name, comes from "Les Malouines", the name given to the islands by French sailors in the 1700s. The islands were occupied at various times by England, Spain, France, and Argentina.

Rockhopper, Magellanic, and Gento penguins are common on the Falkland Islands.

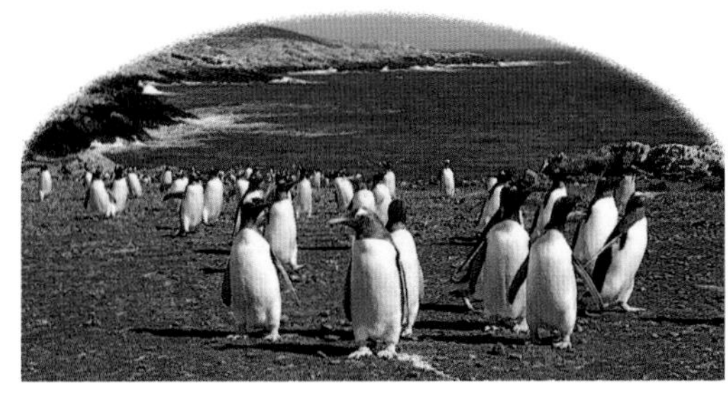

Amazon

The longest river in South America is the Amazon, which rises in the Andes and flows 6,516 km (4,050 miles) to the Atlantic. For most of its length the river flows through a rain forest which covers 6.5 million sq km (2.5 million sq miles). In recent years much of the rain forest has been cut down to provide farmland. Although the destruction continues, it is now beginning to slow down.

Find out more

Argentina
Brazil
Colombia
Football and rugby
Incas

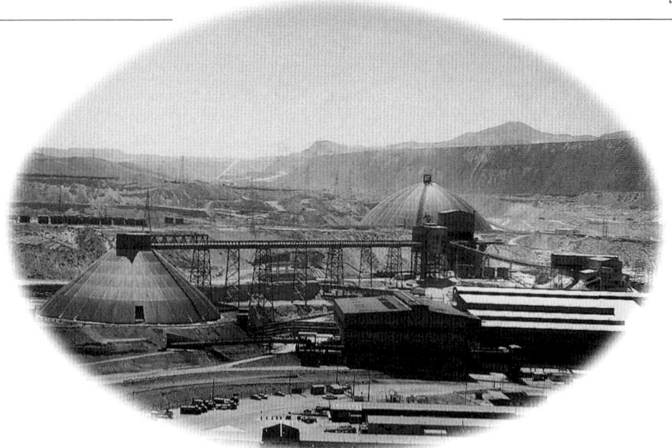

MINERALS IN CHILE
Copper is Chile's largest export. Chuquicamata (above) is the country's most productive copper mine. Metallic minerals are plentiful along the length of the Andes mountains. They are formed over thousands of years by pressure and heat during mountain-building processes. The Atacama Desert in the northern third of the country stores copper, silver, gold, and abundant deposits of sodium nitrate.

* Countries covered on other pages.

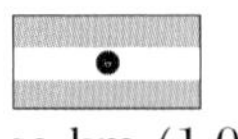

ARGENTINA *
Area: 2,766,890 sq km (1,068,296 sq miles)
Population: 38,400,000
Capital: Buenos Aires

BOLIVIA
Area: 1,098,580 sq km (424,162 sq miles)
Population: 8,800,000
Capital: Sucre, La Paz
Languages: Spanish, Quechua, Aymará
Religions: Roman Catholic
Currency: Boliviano
Main occupations: Subsistence farming, mining, trading
Main exports: Gold, silver, zinc, lead, tin, oil, natural gas

BRAZIL *
Area: 8,511,970 sq km (3,286,472 sq miles)
Population: 179,000,000
Capital: Brasília

CHILE
Area: 756,950 sq km (292,258 sq miles)
Population: 15,800,000
Capital: Santiago
Languages: Spanish, Amerindian languages
Religions: Roman Catholic, non-religious
Currency: Chilean peso
Main occupations: Mining, agriculture
Main exports: Copper, fresh fruit, fishmeal, salmon, wine, lithium, molybdenum, gold

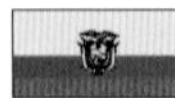

COLOMBIA *
Area: 1,138,910 sq km (439,733 sq miles)
Population: 44,200,000
Capital: Bogotá

ECUADOR
Area: 283,560 sq km (109,483 sq miles)
Population: 13,000,000
Capital: Quito
Languages: Spanish, Quechua, other Amerindian languages
Religions: Roman Catholic, Protestant, Jewish
Currency: Sucre
Main occupations: Oil production, agriculture, fishing
Main exports: Oil, bananas, fish

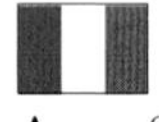

FRENCH GUIANA
Area: 83,533 sq km (32,252 sq miles)
Population: 186,900
Capital: Cayenne
Status: French department

GUYANA
Area: 214,970 sq km (83,000 sq miles)
Population: 765,000
Capital: Georgetown
Languages: English Creole, Hindi, Tamil, Amerindian languages, English
Religions: Christian, Hindu, Muslim
Currency: Guyana dollar
Main occupations: Subsistence farming, mining, forestry
Main exports: Gold, sugar, bauxite, diamond, timber, rice

PARAGUAY
Area: 406,750 sq km (157,046 sq miles)
Population: 5,900,000
Capital: Asunción
Languages: Guaraní,Spanish
Religions: Roman Catholic
Currency: Guaraní
Main occupations: Agriculture
Main exports: Energy, cotton, oilseeds, soya

PERU
Area: 1,285,220sq km (496,223 sq miles)
Population: 27,200,000
Capital: Lima
Languages: Spanish, Quechua, Aymará
Religions: Roman Catholic
Currency: Nuevo sol
Main occupations: Subsistence farming, fishing, manufacturing
Main exports: Oil, fish, cotton, coffee, textiles, copper, lead, coca leaves, sugar

SURINAM
Area: 163,270 sq km (63,039 sq miles)
Population: 436,000
Capital: Paramaribo
Languages: Pidgin English (Taki-Taki), Dutch, Hindi, Javanese, Saramacca, Carib
Religions: Christian, Hindu, Muslim
Currency: Paramaribo
Main occupations: Agriculture, forestry, mining, fishing
Main exports: Bauxite, gold, oil, rice, bananas, citrus fruits, shrimp, aluminium

URUGUAY
Area: 174,810 sq km (67,494 sq miles)
Population: 3,400,000
Capital: Montevideo
Languages: Spanish
Religions: Roman Catholic, Protestant, Jewish, non-religious
Currency: Uruguayan peso
Main occupations: Agriculture, tourism, manufacturing
Main exports: Wool, meat, rice

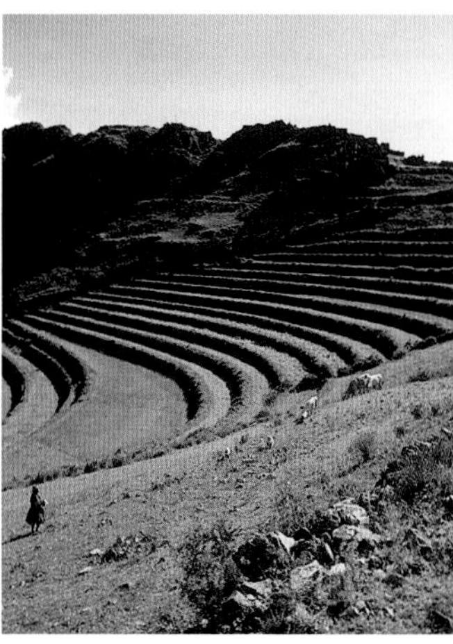

INCA TERRACES
These terraces near Cuzco, Peru, were built by the Incas to enable cultivation of the hillside. They are still farmed by descendants of the Inca people today.

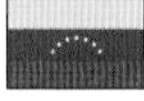

VENEZUELA
Area: 912,050 sq km (352,143 sq miles)
Population: 25,700,000
Capital: Caracas
Languages: Spanish, Amerindian languages
Religions: Roman Catholic, Protestant
Currency: Bolivar
Main occupations: Mining, agriculture, oil production
Main exports: Coal, bauxite, iron, gold, bitumen fuel, steel, aluminium, oil, coffee

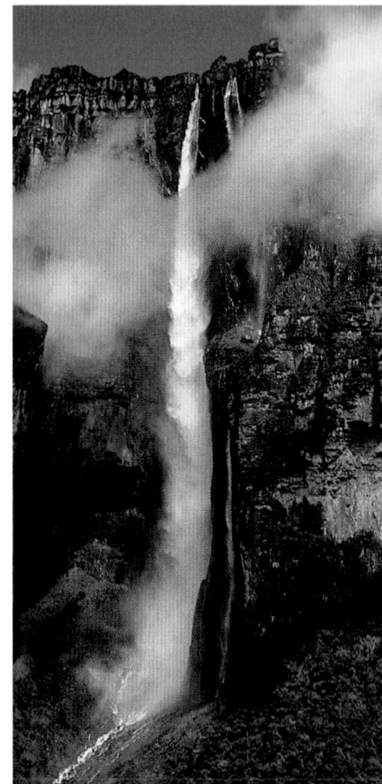

At a height of 979 m (3,212 ft), the majestic Angel Falls in Venezuela (above), is the highest uninterrupted waterfall in the world. It was named after bush pilot Jimmy Angel.

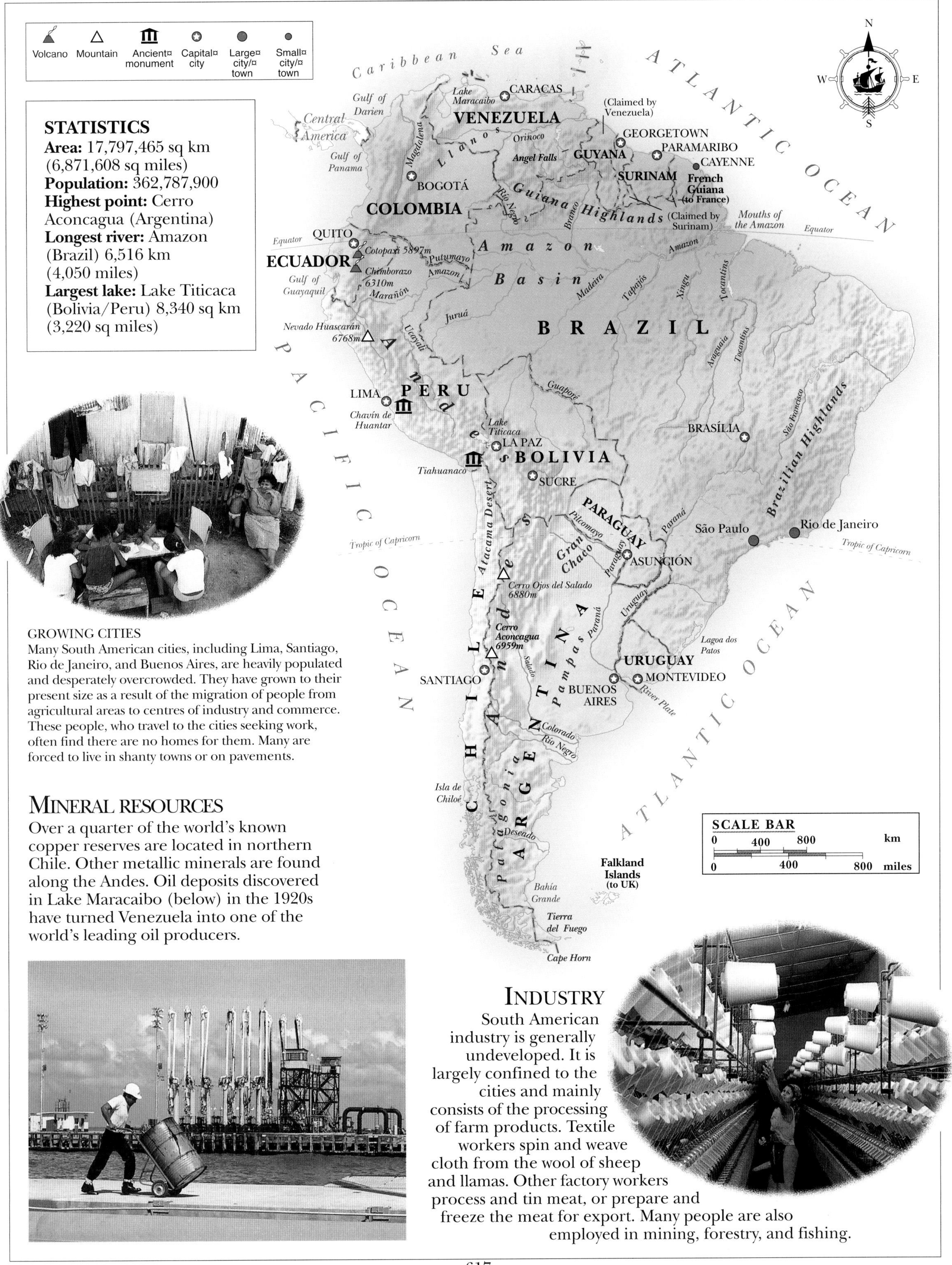

STATISTICS
Area: 17,797,465 sq km (6,871,608 sq miles)
Population: 362,787,900
Highest point: Cerro Aconcagua (Argentina)
Longest river: Amazon (Brazil) 6,516 km (4,050 miles)
Largest lake: Lake Titicaca (Bolivia/Peru) 8,340 sq km (3,220 sq miles)

GROWING CITIES
Many South American cities, including Lima, Santiago, Rio de Janeiro, and Buenos Aires, are heavily populated and desperately overcrowded. They have grown to their present size as a result of the migration of people from agricultural areas to centres of industry and commerce. These people, who travel to the cities seeking work, often find there are no homes for them. Many are forced to live in shanty towns or on pavements.

Mineral resources

Over a quarter of the world's known copper reserves are located in northern Chile. Other metallic minerals are found along the Andes. Oil deposits discovered in Lake Maracaibo (below) in the 1920s have turned Venezuela into one of the world's leading oil producers.

Industry

South American industry is generally undeveloped. It is largely confined to the cities and mainly consists of the processing of farm products. Textile workers spin and weave cloth from the wool of sheep and llamas. Other factory workers process and tin meat, or prepare and freeze the meat for export. Many people are also employed in mining, forestry, and fishing.

HISTORY OF
SOUTH AMERICA

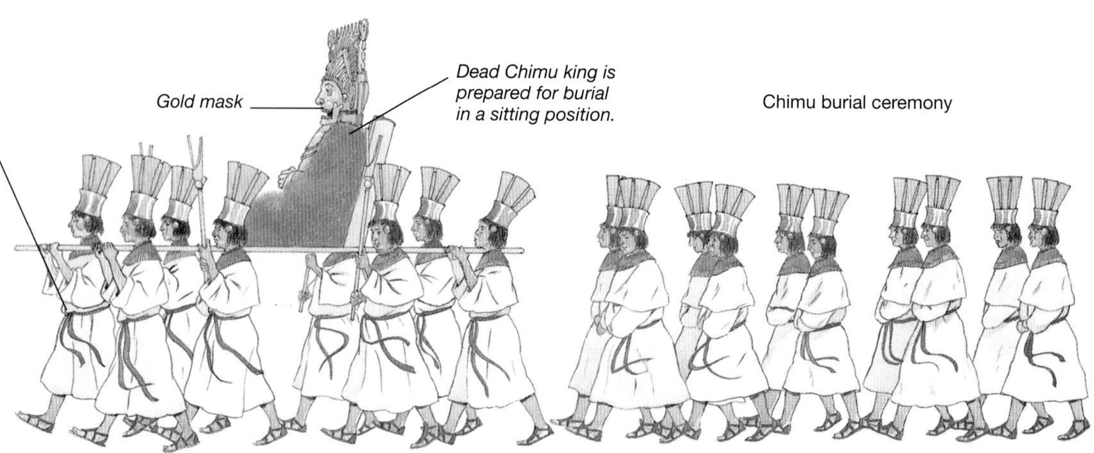

Attendants, uniformly dressed, carry the dead king on a bier.
Gold mask
Dead Chimu king is prepared for burial in a sitting position.

Chimu burial ceremony

CHIMU EMPIRE

The Chimu empire centred on the vast capital city of Chan Chan, in what is now northern Peru. The empire covered much of the Pacific coast of South America and reached the height of its power in the 15th century. In 1460, the Incas conquered the Chimu empire, and Chan Chan fell into ruin. The Chimu are remembered as a highly civilized society. The royal dead were buried with a wealth of funeral offerings.

FOR THOUSANDS OF YEARS, the continent of South America developed independently from the rest of the world. Great cultures rose and fell, among them the Nazcas, Chimus, and Incas, all of which developed highly advanced civilizations of great wealth and achievement. In 1532 the Spaniards invaded the Inca empire and within a few years ruled over most of the continent. The Portuguese established control over Brazil. Soon Spanish and Portuguese became the main languages of South America, and for the next 300 years the affairs of South America were decided in Europe. The native peoples were almost wiped out by disease and ill treatment. When Spain and Portugal became involved in the Napoleonic wars in Europe, the South Americans seized the chance to win their independence. Afterwards, the new countries were ruled by European families who had settled in South America. Many more Europeans arrived during the 19th and early 20th centuries. The nations of South America have only recently begun to control their destinities.

SOUTH AMERICA

200 B.C.-A.D. 600 Nazca empire in Peru.

600 City-states of Tiahuanaco and Huari in Peru.

1000-1470 Chimu empire in Peru.

1200 Inca empire in Bolivia, Chile, Ecuador, and Peru.

1494 Treaty of Tordesillas divides New World between Spain and Portugal.

1499-1510 Amerigo Vespucci explores coast of South America; the continent is named after him.

1530 Portuguese colonize Brazil.

1532-33 Spanish led by Francisco Pizarro conquer Inca empire.

1545 Silver discovered in Peru.

1808-25 Liberation wars: Spanish and Portuguese colonies

1822-89 Empire of Brazil

1879-84 Border wars between Peru, Chile, and Bolivia.

1932-35 War between Paraguay and Bolivia over disputed territory.

1946 Juan Perón becomes president of Argentina.

1967 Che Guevara killed in Bolivia.

Line of demarcation 1494
Portuguese territories
Spanish territories

TREATY OF TORDESILLAS

In the 1494 Treaty of Tordesillas, Spain and Portugal divided the non-European world between them. They drew a rough line down the South American continent, giving Spain the lands to the west and Portugal the lands to the east of the line.

SPANISH DOMINATION

From 1532 to 1810, Spain controlled the whole of South America apart from Portuguese-owned Brazil. The vast Spanish Empire was divided into three viceroyalties – New Granada in the north, Peru in the centre, and Rio de la Plata in the south. On the right is Santiago, the patron saint of Spanish soldiers.

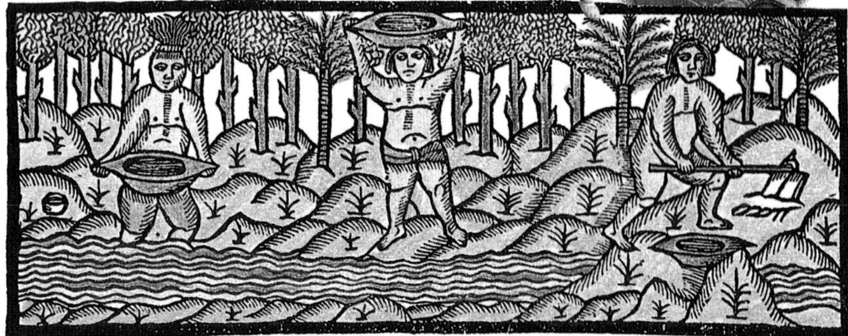

NATIVE AMERICANS

The Native Americans were put to work as slaves in the silver mines. They were also forced to labour in the big plantations of sugar and other crops that were exported to Europe. Most Native Americans died of poor conditions, overwork, and European diseases they had no immunity against.

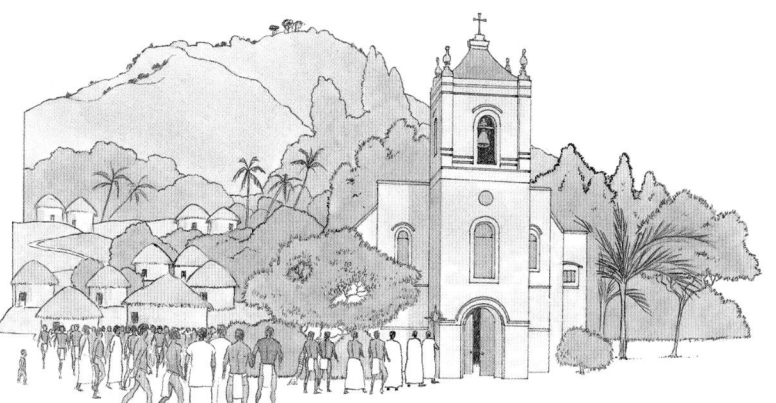

Simón bolívar

In 1808, Spain was involved in a war with French emperor Napoleon Bonaparte; the South American colonies took this opportunity to declare their independence. Led by Simón Bolívar (1783-1830) and José de San Martín (1778-1850), the colonies fought against Spanish control; all gained their freedom by 1825. Bolívar hoped to unite all of South America, but many disliked his dictatorial approach. In 1822, Brazil declared its independence from Portugal, leaving only Guiana in the north under European control.

Roman catholic church

When the Spanish arrived in South America, they brought the Roman Catholic religion with them. Catholic priests tried to stamp out local religions and convert the Native Americans to their faith. In the end the priests were forced to include parts of the old Native American religions in their services. In some places, the priests tried to protect the Native Americans against Spanish rulers who were cruel to them, but most priests upheld the Spanish colonial government. During the 20th century the Catholic Church began to take a more active role in supporting the poor against powerful landlords and corrupt governments.

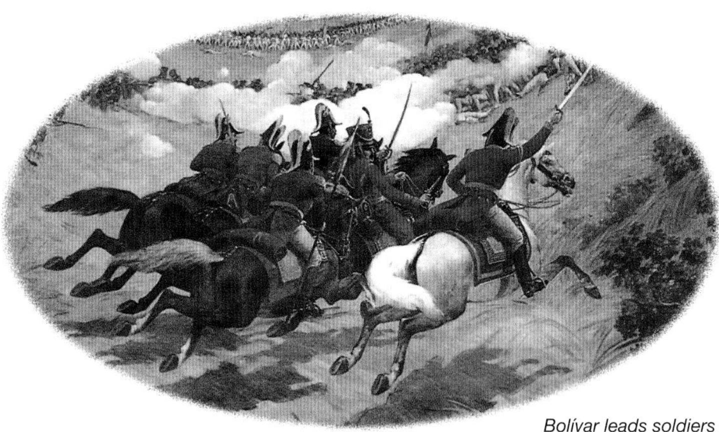

Bolívar leads soldiers into battle

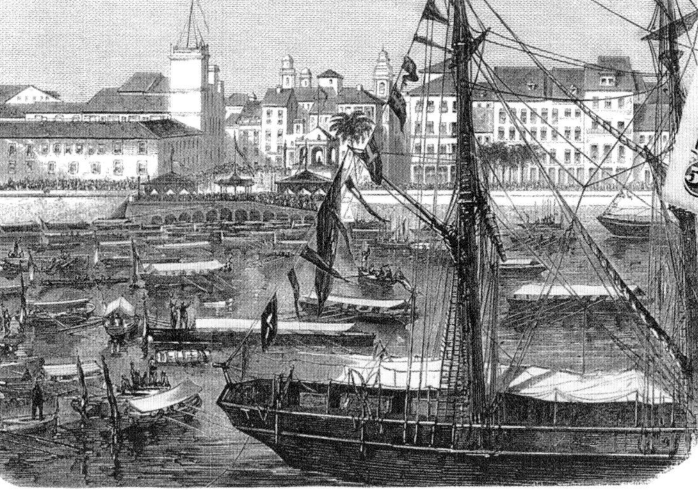

Pedro arrives in Recife (formerly Pernambuco), a prosperous town in the empire.

BRAZILIAN EMPIRE

From 1822 to 1889 Brazil was an empire. Under Emperor Pedro II (1825-1891) roads and railways were built, and the coffee and rubber industries began to prosper. Thousands of immigrants poured into the country from Italy, Portugal, and Spain. In 1888, the African slaves who had been brought over to work the plantations were freed. This angered many landowners, as they had been using the slaves as cheap labour. The landowners withdrew their support from Pedro, and in 1889 the army took over the empire and a republic was declared.

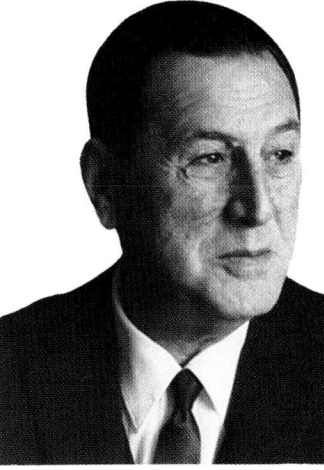

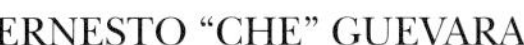

Stamp bearing a portrait of Pedro II

ERNESTO "CHE" GUEVARA

One of the most popular heroes of the 20th century, Che Guevara (1928-1967) was born into a rich Argentinian family. Guevara was a doctor before choosing to spend his life supporting revolutions against oppressive South American governments. In 1959, he helped Fidel Castro overthrow the Cuban government. Guevara served under Castro until 1965. In late 1966 he moved to Bolivia, where he based himself in the countryside among peasants. In 1967, he was killed by the Bolivian army. His death made him a hero for revolutionaries everywhere. In 1997, he was reburied in Cuba.

Juan perón

From 1946 to 1955, Argentina was ruled by President Juan Perón (1895-1974). Poor people living in the cities supported Perón and his wife, Eva. He introduced many reforms but did not allow anyone to oppose him. After the economy weakened in the early 1950s, and after Eva died (1952), Perón was much less popular. In 1955, the army overthrew him. In 1973, he again held power but died the following year. His third wife, Isabel Martínez de Perón, succeeded him as president.

Find out more

Central america
Conquistadors
Incas
South america

Southeast Asia

Southeast Asia is the part of Asia to the south of China, and east of India. The mainland portion has an area of 1.6 million sq km (640,000 sq miles). The region continues to the south as a chain of islands that separate the Pacific and Indian oceans. The island of Sumatra is 1,720 km (1,070 miles) long; other islands are tiny.

At its southeast corner, the continent of Asia extends far out into the sea, in two great peninsulas and a vast chain of islands. In this region, which is called Southeast Asia, over 543 million people live in 11 independent countries. The area has a rich and varied culture, and music and dancing are particularly important. Their performance is often governed by strict rituals and rules, some of them religious. There are several different religions in the area: most people on the mainland are Buddhist; Indonesia is chiefly Muslim; and Christianity is the religion of the Philippines. For much of this century the lives of many Southeast Asian people have been disrupted and destroyed by wars. The fighting made normal trade, agriculture, and industry impossible and turned Laos and Cambodia into the two poorest nations on Earth. In Cambodia guerrilla warfare until recently claimed the lives of soldiers and civilians. Other Southeast Asian countries, particularly the island nations, have escaped the worst fighting. These countries are now more prosperous and peaceful.

THAILAND
There are 62.8 million people in Thailand, and the country is among the wealthiest in the region. Most people in the cities work in mining and industry; in the countryside most are farmers, growing rice, sugar, and rubber trees. The country's rich heritage includes ritual temple dances and beautiful architecture.

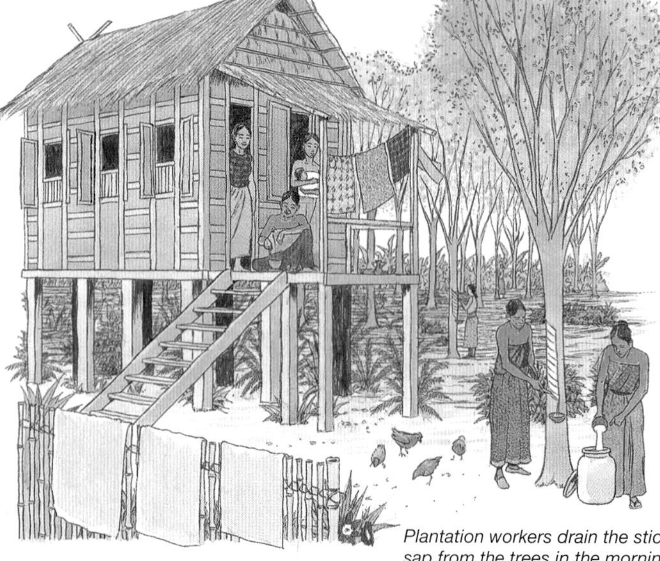

Sap is extracted by tapping – cutting or shaving the bark with a sharp knife.

Plantation workers drain the sticky sap from the trees in the morning when the flow of sap is fastest.

RUBBER
One of the most important products of Southeast Asia is rubber. The industry began about a century ago when British traders brought rubber trees to the region from Brazil. The sap of the trees is collected, then mixed with acid to form solid sheets of latex, which are hung out to dry.

Singapore City began as a small British trading station; today giant skyscrapers dominate the skyline.

Singapore

The tiny island state of Singapore occupies just 620 sq km (239 sq miles) off the coast of Malaysia. The nation is highly industrialized and very rich. Most of Singapore's 4.4 million people earn their living from industries such as textiles and electronics.

Java

The country of Indonesia is made up of 13,677 islands. Java is the most populated island, with 127 million people. Many are farmers producing large quantities of rice. The capital city, Jakarta, is a centre for the textile industry. The island has much unique wildlife, including species of tiger and rhinoceros found nowhere else.

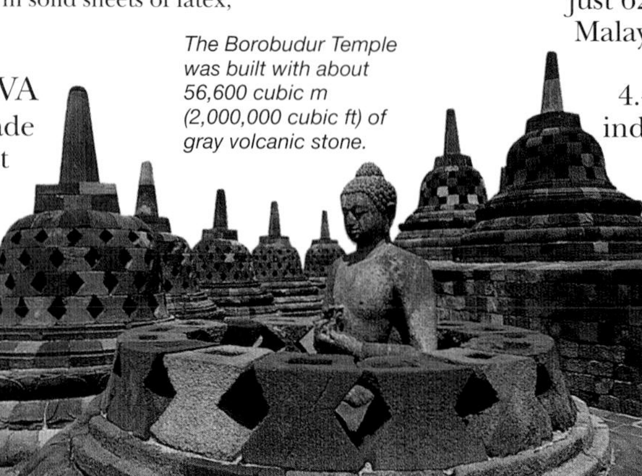

The Borobudur Temple was built with about 56,600 cubic m (2,000,000 cubic ft) of gray volcanic stone.

BOROBUDUR TEMPLE
A massive Buddhist monument in Java, the Borodubur Temple was constructed between 778 and 850 A.D. From about 1000 B.C. it was buried under volcanic ash until its discovery by the English lieutenant governor Thomas Stamford Raffles in 1814. A team of Dutch archaeologists restored the site during 1907-11, and a second restoration was completed by 1983.

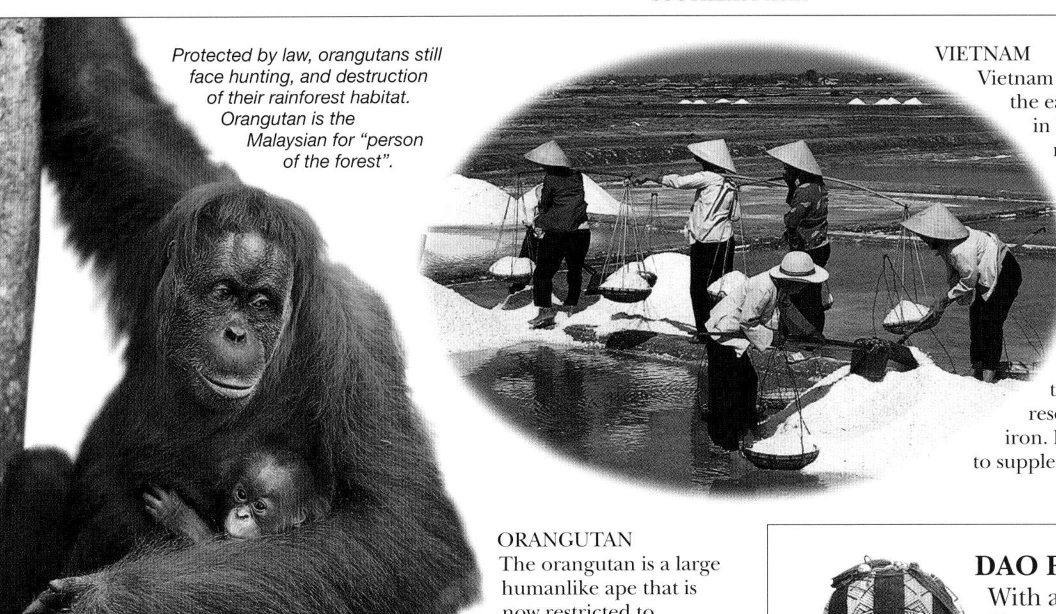

Protected by law, orangutans still face hunting, and destruction of their rainforest habitat. Orangutan is the Malaysian for "person of the forest".

VIETNAM

Vietnam is a mountainous land which occupies the eastern part of the Indo-China peninsula in Southeast Asia. Its population, which is mainly rural, mostly lives in the lowland deltas of the Red and Mekong rivers. Three-quarters of its people work in agriculture. Rice takes up more land area than all other crops produced in Vietnam put together. Other crops include rubber, maize, sugar, bananas, coconuts, pepper, tea, tobacco, and sweet potatoes. Northern Vietnam is more industrialized than the agricultural south. It has mineral resources, which include coal, salt, tin, and iron. Farmers often work in salt farms (left) to supplement their earnings from agriculture.

ORANGUTAN

The orangutan is a large humanlike ape that is now restricted to lowland swamp forests in Borneo and a small part of Sumatra. Orangutans once lived in the jungles of mainland Southeast Asia as well, but numbers have been depleted by human hunters. With its short, thickset body, long arms, and short legs, the orangutan displays many physical similarities to gorillas and chimpanzees. However, a shaggy, reddish coat, and an even greater disproportion between arm and leg lengths, sets the orangutan apart from its related primates. The male orangutan may be about 1.37 m (4.5 feet) tall and weigh about 85 kg (185 lbs) when mature, while females usually weigh about 40 kg (90 lbs).

DAO PEOPLE

With a population of 47,000, the Dao people are the eighth-largest ethnic group in Vietnam, where they inhabit all the northern bordering areas. The Dao can also be found in the neighbouring countries of China, Laos, and Thailand. The origins of the first Dao groups in Vietnam are uncertain, but it would appear that they emigrated from their native provinces of southern China in the 18th and 19th centuries.

BURMA (MYANMAR)

Burma gained independence from British colonial control in 1948 and immediately adopted a policy of political and economic isolation. Once a rich nation, the country was subsquently reduced to one of the world's poorest despite its plentiful natural resources. The Irrawaddy river basin occupies most of the country and provides rich farming land. Burma has in recent years been ruled by a military government which has excluded all foreign influences. Over 89 per cent of the population are Buddhists but in the countryside many still worship the *nats* – ancient spirits of the forest and mountains. Devotees of Buddhism pray at temples such as the Shwedagon Pagoda (below) in Yangon.

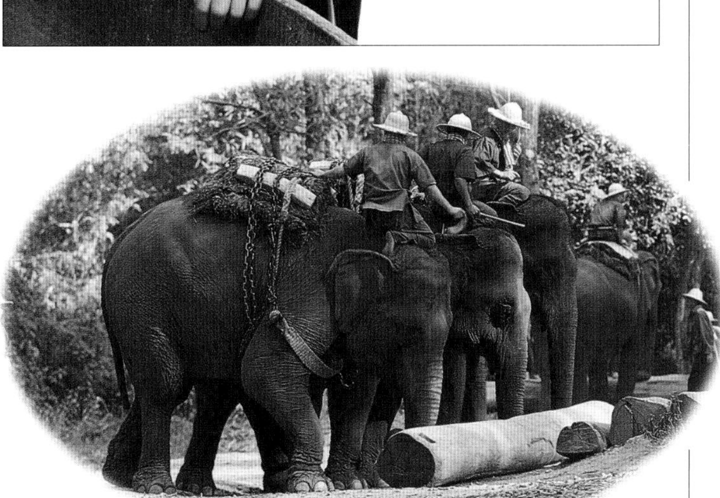

ELEPHANT SCHOOL

Elephants in Thailand are trained to work for a living. They have proved themselves to be far more cost-efficient than modern tractors. They need little fuel and do not rust or need spare parts. Tractors last for about six years, an elephant lives for 30. In addition, elephants are less harmful to the environment. They move timber and take tourists for rides in the rainforest.

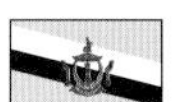

BRUNEI
Area: 5,770 sq km (2,228 sq miles)
Population: 358,000
Capital: Bandar Seri Begawan
Languages: Malay, English, Chinese
Religions: Muslim, Buddhist, Christian
Currency: Brunei dollar

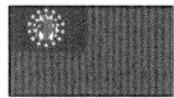

BURMA (MYANMAR)
Area: 676,550 sq km (261,200 sq miles)
Population: 49,500,000
Capital: Rangoon
Languages: Burmese, Karen, Shan, Chin, Kachin, Mon, Palaung, Wa
Religions: Buddhist, Christian, Muslim, Hindu
Currency: Kyat

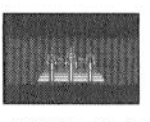

CAMBODIA
Area: 181,040 sq km (69,000 sq miles)
Population: 14,100,000
Capital: Phnom Penh
Languages: Khmer, French, Chinese, Vietnamese, Cham
Religions: Theravada Buddhist
Currency: Riel

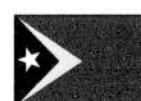

EAST TIMOR
Area: 15,007 sq km (5,794 sq miles)
Population: 778,000
Capital: Dili
Languages: Tetum, Bahasa Indonesia, Portuguese
Religions: Roman Catholic
Currency: US dollar

INDONESIA
Area: 1,904,570 sq km (735,555 sq miles)
Population: 220,000,000
Capital: Jakarta
Languages: Javanese, Madurese, Sundanese, Bahasa Indonesia, Dutch
Religions: Muslim, Protestant, Roman Catholic, Hindu, Buddhist
Currency: Rupiah

LAOS
Area: 236,800 sq km (81,428 sq miles)
Population: 5,700,000
Capital: Vientiane
Languages: Lao, Miao, Yao, Vietnamese, Chinese, French
Religions: Buddhist, Animist
Currency: New kip

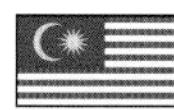

MALAYSIA
Area: 329,750 sq km (127,317 sq miles)
Population: 24,400,000
Capital: Kuala Lumpur
Languages: Malay, Chinese, Tamil
Religions: Muslim, Buddhist, Chinese faiths, Christian, traditional beliefs
Currency: Ringgit

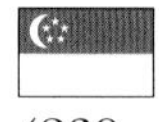

PHILIPPINES
Area: 300,000 sq km (115,831 sq miles)
Population: 80,000,000
Capital: Manila
Languages: Filipino, Cebuano, Hiligaynon, Samaran, Ilocano, Bikol, English
Religions: Roman Catholic, Protestant, Muslim, Buddhist
Currency: Philippine peso

SINGAPORE
Area: 620 sq km (239 sq miles)
Population: 4,300,000
Capital: Singapore City
Languages: Chinese, Malay, Tamil, English
Religions: Buddhist, Christian, Muslim
Currency: Singapore dollar

THAILAND
Area: 513,120 sq km (198,116 sq miles)
Population: 62,800,000
Capital: Bangkok
Languages: Thai, Chinese, Malay, Khmer, Mon, Karen, Miao
Religions: Theravada Buddhist, Muslim, Christian
Currency: Baht

VIETNAM
Area: 329,560 sq km (127,243 sq miles)
Population: 81,400,000
Capital: Hanoi
Languages: Vietnamese, Chinese, Thai, Khmer, Muong, Nung, Miao, Yao, Jarai
Religions: Buddhist, Christian, non-religious
Currency: Dông

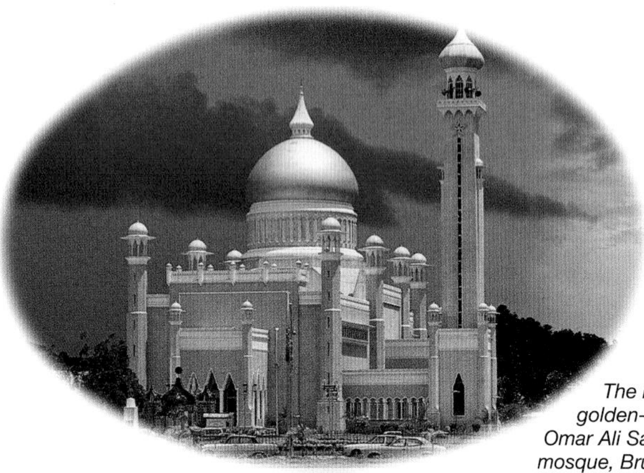

The magnificent, golden-domed Omar Ali Saifuddin mosque, Brunei

BRUNEI

Lying on the northwestern coast of the island of Borneo, Brunei is ruled by a sultan. Since gaining independence from Britain in 1984, the country has become increasingly ifluenced by Islam. Its interior is mostly rainforest and the nation's abundant oil and gas reserves have brought its citizens one of the highest standard of living in the world.

PHILIPPINES

Most of the islands in the Philippines are mountainous and forested. The Filipino people live in towns and villages on the narrow coastal plains, or on plateaus between the mountain ranges. The volcanic cone of Mount Mayon, 320 km (200 miles) southeast of Manila, is one of the most beautiful in the world. However, its beauty hides its dangerous character. The volcano is still active, and past eruptions have destroyed parts of the nearby city of Albay.

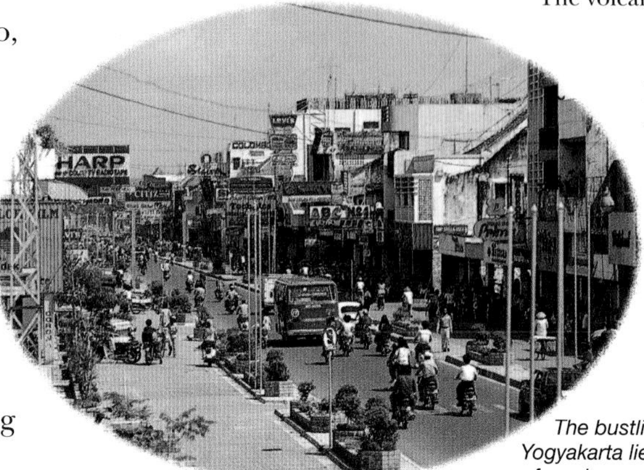

The bustling city of Yogyakarta lies at the foot of a volcano.

INDONESIA

Although more than 13,500 islands make up the Republic of Indonesia, only about 6,000 are inhabited. Most Indonesian people live in the countryside and work on farms. However, some cities are densely populated. For example, the city of Yogyakarta (left), on the southern coast of the heavily populated island of Java, has a population of about 600,000.

Find out more

ISLAM
SOUTHEAST ASIA, HISTORY OF
VIETNAM WAR

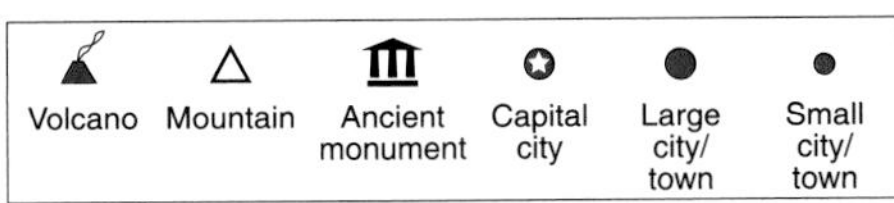

STATISTICS

Area: 4,477,761 sq km (1,728,157 sq miles)
Population: 543,336,000
No. of independent countries: 11
Religions: Buddhism, Islam, Taoism, Christianity, Hinduism
Largest city: Jakarta (Indonesia) 8,540,121
Highest point: Hkakabo Rasi (Burma) 5,885 m (19,309 ft)
Longest river: Mekong 4,184 km (2,600 miles)
Main occupation: Farming
Main exports: Sugar, fruit, timber, rice, rubber, tobacco, tin
Main imports: Machinery, iron and steel products, textiles, chemicals, fuels

POPULATION
The population on mainland Southeast Asia is concentrated in the river valleys, plateaux, or plains. The population of maritime Southeast Asia is unevenly distributed; Java is densely settled while other islands are barely occupied.

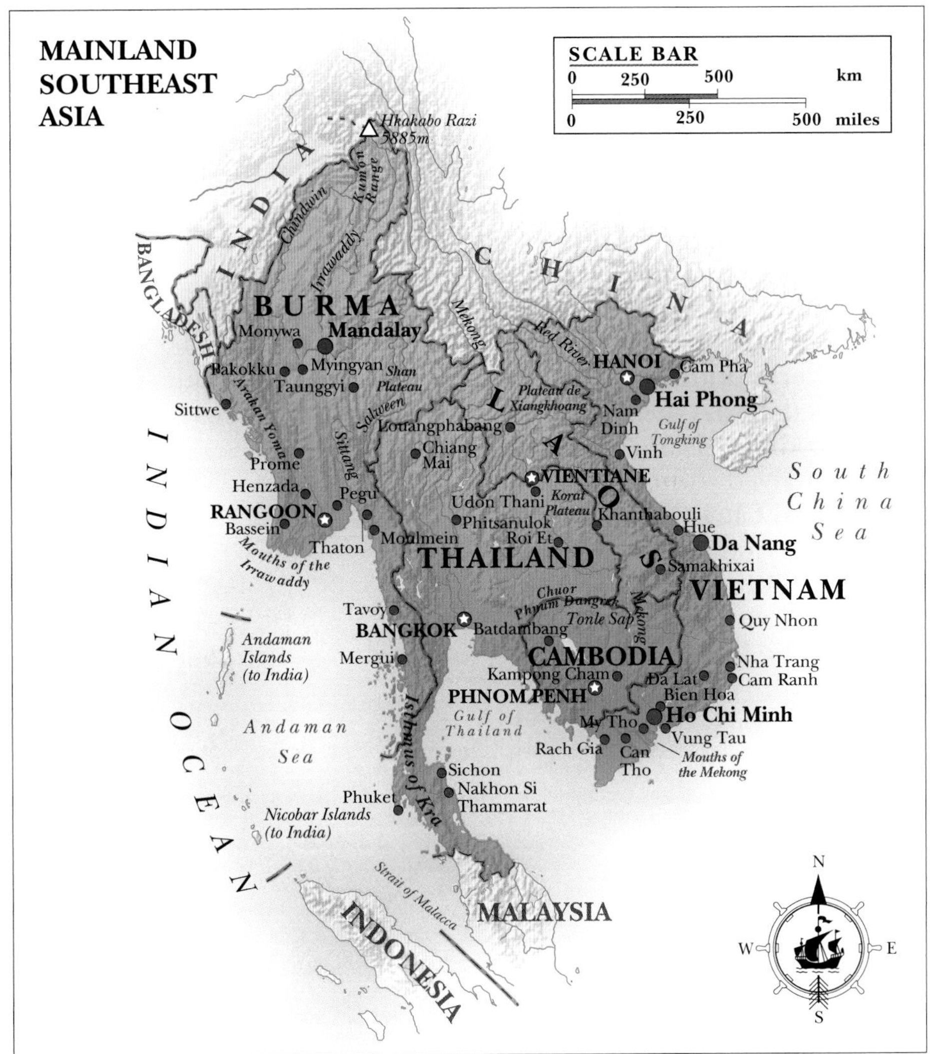

MARITIME SOUTHEAST ASIA

SCALE BAR
0 250 500 km
0 250 500 miles

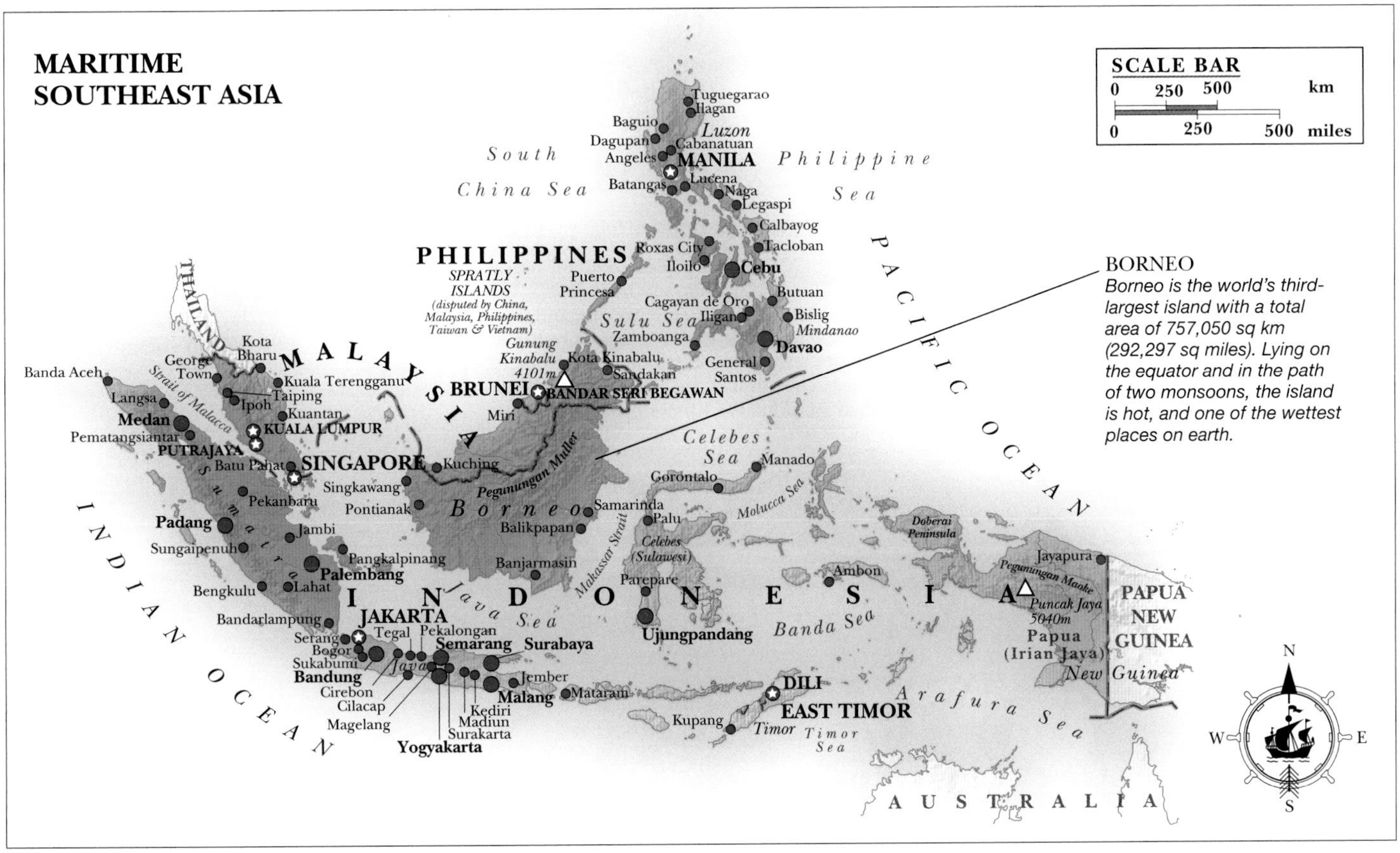

BORNEO
Borneo is the world's third-largest island with a total area of 757,050 sq km (292,297 sq miles). Lying on the equator and in the path of two monsoons, the island is hot, and one of the wettest places on earth.

HISTORY OF
SOUTHEAST ASIA

MANY COUNTRIES HAVE PLAYED A PART in the history of Southeast Asia, a region that lies between India and China, and controls the seaways from Europe and the Middle East to the Far East. In 111 B.C., the Han Empire of China overran some of Southeast Asia. Later, Chinese dynasties influenced much of Southeast Asia for the next 1,000 years. During this time, monks from India introduced Buddhism. The next arrivals were Arab traders, who sailed across the Indian Ocean in search of spices and introduced Islam. In 1511, Portuguese traders arrived from Europe, introduced Christianity, and began a period of European domination that lasted until this century. In 1940-45, the Japanese occupied the region. The Europeans regained control briefly, but soon all Southeast Asia was independent.

ANGKOR WAT

Between the 9th and 15th centuries, the Khmer empire of Cambodia dominated Southeast Asia. King Suryavarman II (reigned 1113-50) built a magnificent Hindu temple in the capital city Angkor, called Angkor Wat. All the temple buildings had reliefs showing plants, birds, animals, dancers, and battle scenes. In 1434, the Thais captured Angkor; it lay undiscovered until 1861.

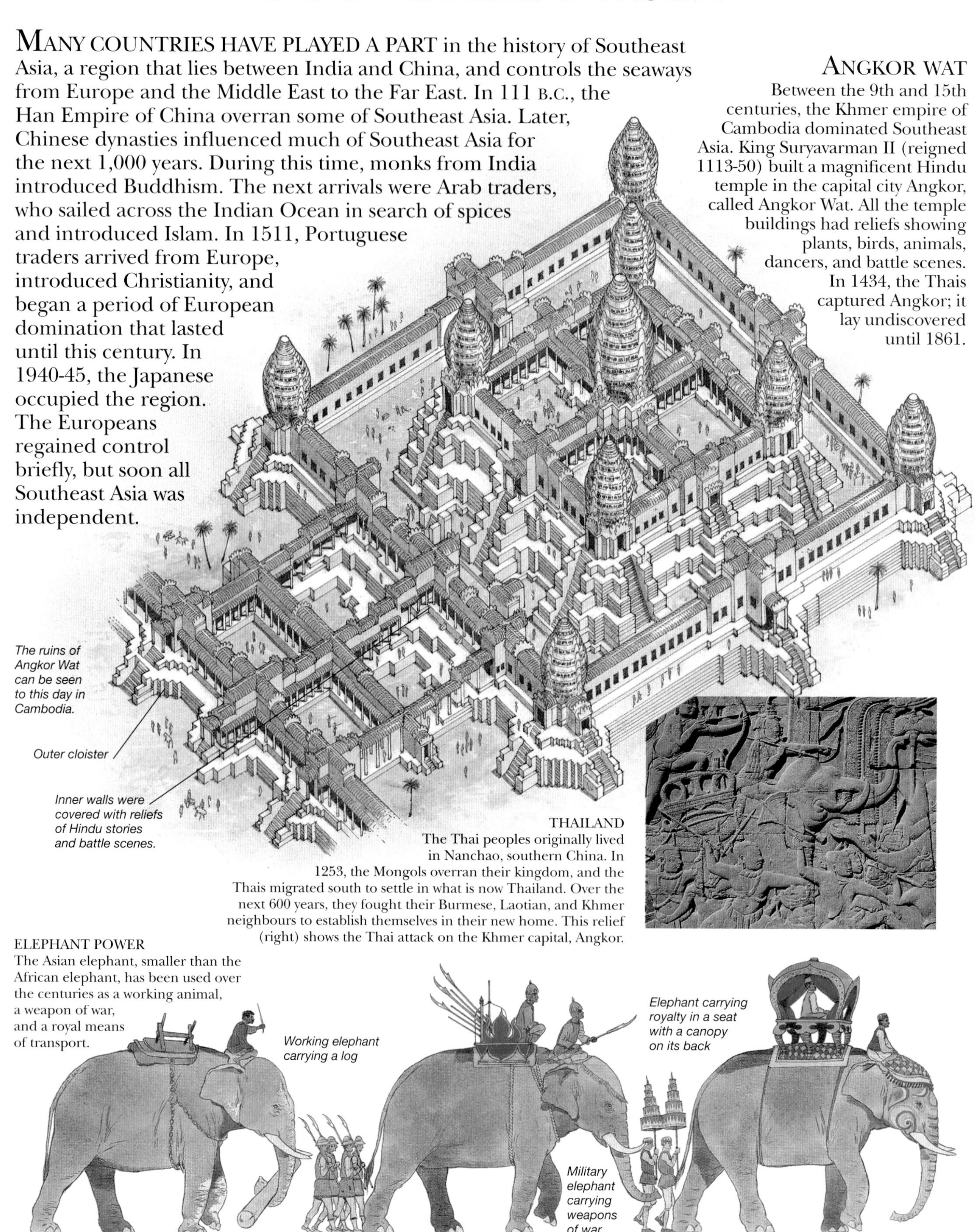

Outer cloister
Inner walls were covered with reliefs of Hindu stories and battle scenes.
Working elephant carrying a log
Military elephant carrying weapons of war
Elephant carrying royalty in a seat with a canopy on its back

The ruins of Angkor Wat can be seen to this day in Cambodia.

THAILAND

The Thai peoples originally lived in Nanchao, southern China. In 1253, the Mongols overran their kingdom, and the Thais migrated south to settle in what is now Thailand. Over the next 600 years, they fought their Burmese, Laotian, and Khmer neighbours to establish themselves in their new home. This relief (right) shows the Thai attack on the Khmer capital, Angkor.

ELEPHANT POWER

The Asian elephant, smaller than the African elephant, has been used over the centuries as a working animal, a weapon of war, and a royal means of transport.

SPICE TRADE

During the 15th century, European explorers, who arrived in the islands of Southeast Asia, were delighted to find a wide variety of spices, such as nutmeg, pepper, and cloves. Spices were in great demand for cooking in Europe, but were very expensive. As a result, first the Portuguese and the Spanish, then the Dutch and the British, fought for control of the profitable spice trade.

Rich Dutch merchants landed on Asian shores to trade with the local people.

SOUTHEAST ASIA

111 B.C. Chinese invade Vietnam; dominate northern area.

A.D. 0-500 Buddhism spreads throughout Southeast Asia.

802 Khmers establish empire in Cambodia and Laos.

1113-1150 Construction of Angkor Wat temple.

1300s Arab traders introduce Islam to Indonesia.

1434 Thais capture Angkor Wat and overrun Khmer empire.

1564 Spanish conquer Philippines.

1700 British East India Company establishes a trading base in Borneo.

1766-69 Chinese invade Burma.

1786 British East India Company establishes a base in Malaya.

1799 Dutch take over all Indonesia.

1800s Thailand is only country in region independent of Europe.

1819 Singapore founded by British merchant Sir Stamford Raffles. Becomes richest port in region.

1824-1886 British take control of Burma.

1859-1893 French take control of Vietnam, Cambodia, and Laos.

1896 Britain establishes control over Malaya.

1940-1945 Japanese occupy Southeast Asia during World War II.

1946-54 French fight to maintain control of their empire in Southeast Asia.

1948 Burma independent.

1949 Indonesia independent.

1953 Cambodia and Laos win independence from France.

1956 Civil war begins in Vietnam.

1957 Malaya independent.

1967 Formation of ASEAN (Association of Southeast Asian Nations).

1965-73 US fully involved in Vietnam War.

1975 Vietnam War ends, North Vietnamese take control.

1997 Hong Kong returned to Chinese rule.

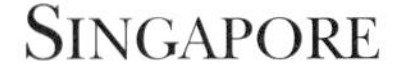

SINGAPORE

In 1824, Britain took control of the island of Singapore because it had an important harbour. But in 1942, during World War II (1939-45) Japanese troops took over the island, forcing the British to surrender (left). Several years later, Britain reoccupied the country. In 1965, Singapore became an independent nation.

INDONESIA
On 11 August 1945, Sukarno (1901-70) declared Indonesia's independence from Dutch rule and became president of the Republic of Indonesia. The Dutch transferred sovereignty four years later. By the end of the 1950s, Malaysia, Laos, Vietnam, Cambodia, and Burma had all become independent.

CORAZON AQUINO
From 1986 to 1992, Corazon Aquino was the president of the Philippines. She entered politics when her husband, Benigno, a popular political leader, was assassinated by the dictator, Ferdinand Marcos, who ruled the Philippines for 20 years. Marcos attempted to prevent Corazon from winning the country's general election. But the people rose up against him, and he was forced to flee the country.

Find out more

JAPAN, HISTORY OF
SOUTHEAST ASIA
VIETNAM WAR

CENTRAL

SOUTHEAST EUROPE

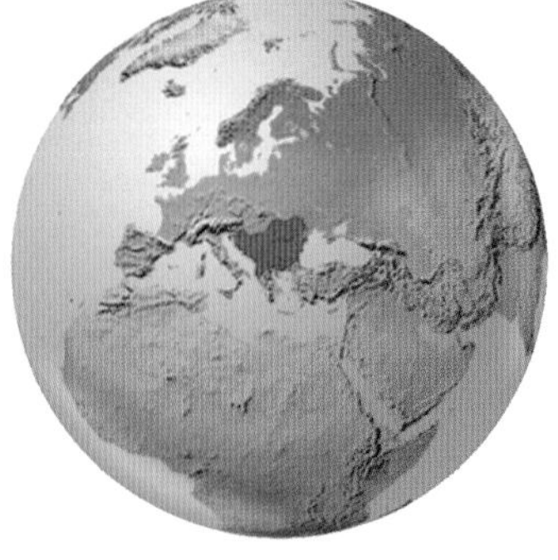

Lying to the south of the Alps, the west of the region is mountainous with deep wooded valleys. The western border is formed by the rocky coast of the Adriatic Sea. To the east lie the flat plains of the Danube, which drains into the Black Sea, and rolling steppelands.

THE NOBLE DANUBE RIVER cuts central Southeast Europe in half, providing fertile farmland along its lower course, in the heart of the region. This area of flatland, called the Danubian Plain, is surrounded by mighty mountain systems, including the Carpathians to the north, and the Balkans and Rhodope mountains in the south. Following World War II, the countries of central Southeast Europe were governed for more than 50 years by strict communist regimes, until the collapse of the Soviet Union in the early 1990s. Serbia was once part of federal Yugoslavia. The collapse of this federation led to civil war in 1991, after which five separate states emerged. Kosovo, an area in southern Serbia inhabited by Muslim Albanian Kossovans, became an autonomous region after a war in 1999.

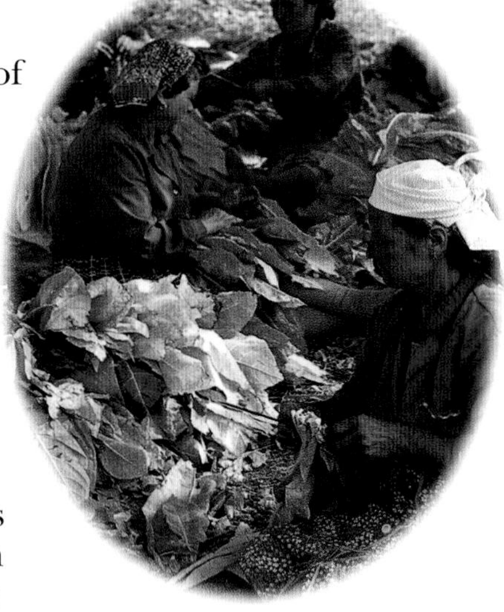

BULGARIAN TOBACCO

Bulgaria has fertile soils and a mild climate, and a wide range of crops is grown there, including cereals, sunflower seeds, grapes, and tomatoes. High-quality red wine, made from grapes grown on the Danubian plain, is exported. In the south of the country, Turkish-style tobacco is grown; it is processed in factories around the town of Plovdiv. Here, women can be seen stringing the harvested tobacco leaves together. They are then left to cure in the heat of the sun before being graded by size and colour.

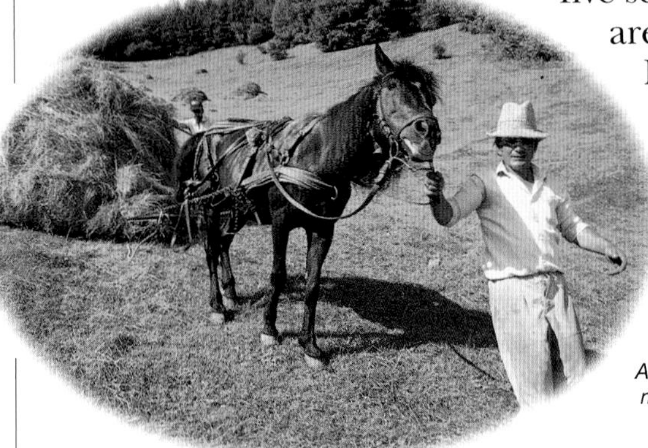

RURAL MOLDOVA

Once a part of Romania, Moldova became a Soviet state in 1940. In 1991, with the break-up of the Soviet Union, Moldova became independent. This small country is dominated by fertile rolling steppes. Most of the population works in agriculture. Warm summers and even rainfall provide ideal conditions for growing vegetables, fruits and grapes, and Moldova is internationally famous for its wines. Although the Soviets mechanized state-owned farms, there are now many small-scale farmers, who cultivate their land using traditional methods.

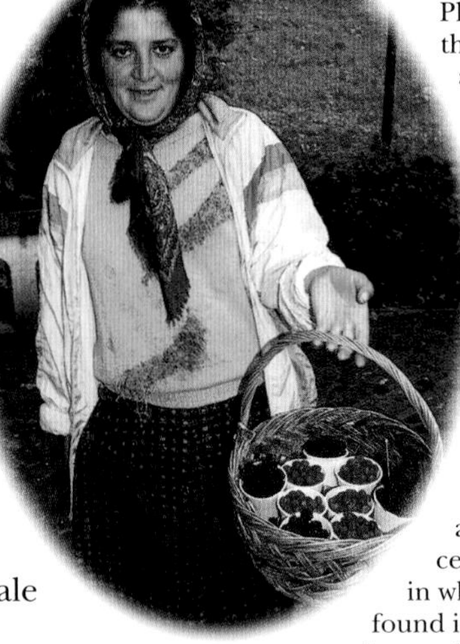

A Romanian gypsy makes a living by selling berries

GYPSIES

Romania has the largest gypsy (or Romany) population in Europe. Gypsies, who have a distinct language and culture, are thought to have originated in India, and moved to Europe via the Middle East. Traditionally, they wandered from place to place, selling goods, repairing metal utensils, and dealing in horses and livestock. They have suffered many centuries of persecution from the countries in which they settled, who found it difficult to understand their different customs and ways of life.

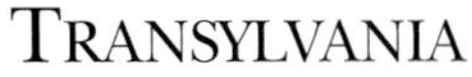

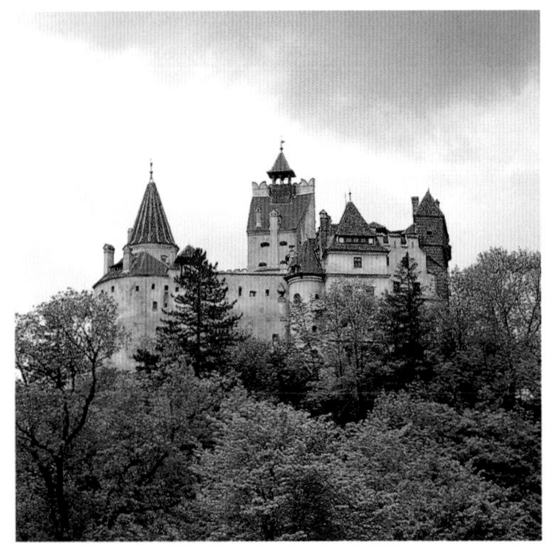

TRANSYLVANIA

The Romanian region of Transylvania is a high plateau, surrounded by the Carpathian Mountains. To the east and south the mountains form an impassable barrier. The region, with its rugged scenery and dramatic castles, has had a colourful history, passing from Hungarian to Ottoman Turkish to Hapsburg (Austrian) rule. Amongst its tyrannical rulers was the 15th-century prince, Vlad the Impaler, notorious for his cruelty. When the author Bram Stoker wrote *Dracula* in 1897, he borrowed from Slavic and Hungarian legends. His blood-sucking vampire is based on Vlad the Impaler.

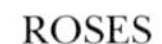

ROSES

Vast fields of roses are grown in Bulgaria. Petals are picked at dawn to produce attar, the essential oil of roses.

Find out more

COMMUNISM
DANCE
EUROPE
FLOWERS AND HERBS
TOURISM AND TRAVEL

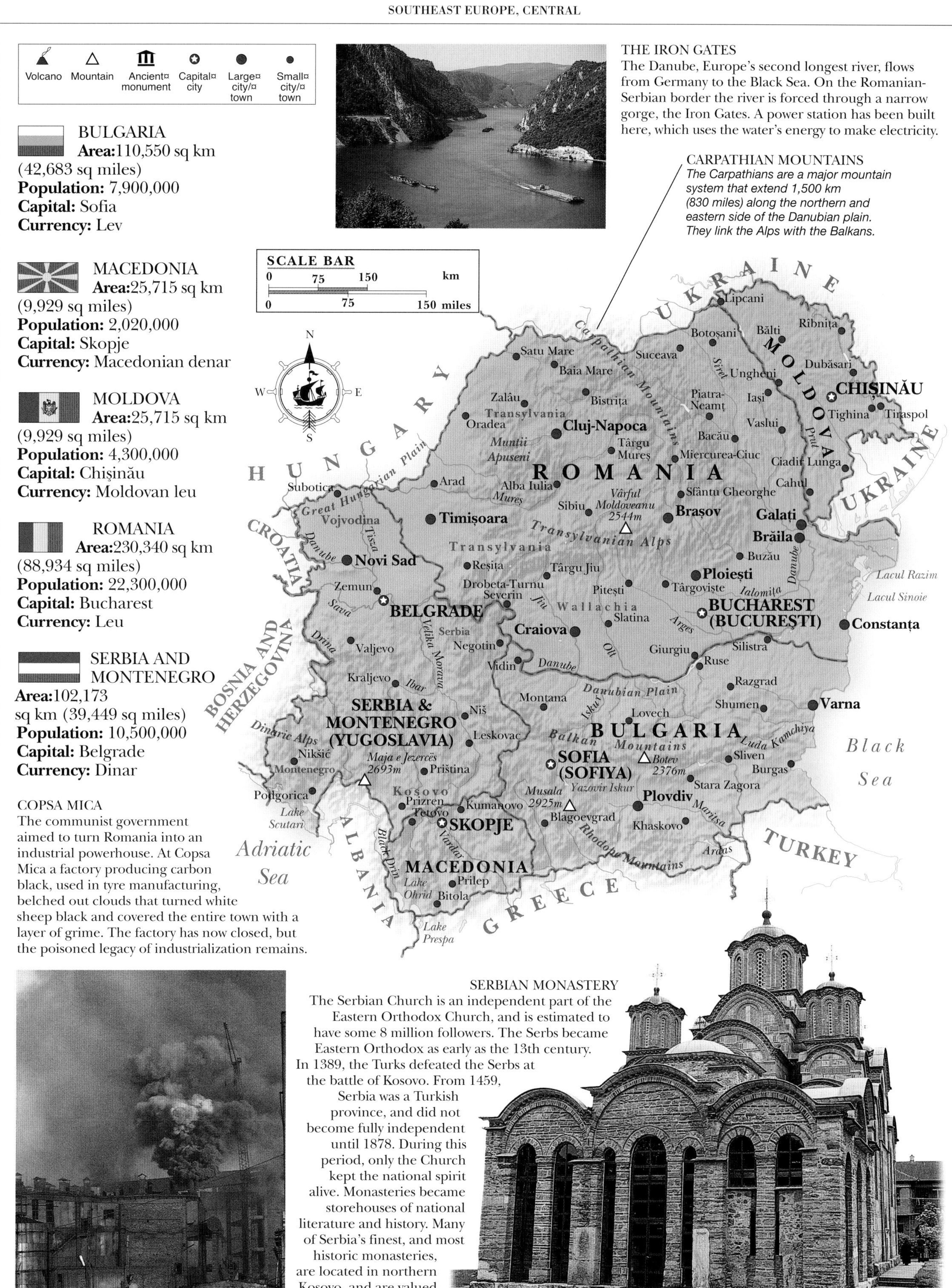

BULGARIA

Area: 110,550 sq km (42,683 sq miles)
Population: 7,900,000
Capital: Sofia
Currency: Lev

MACEDONIA

Area: 25,715 sq km (9,929 sq miles)
Population: 2,020,000
Capital: Skopje
Currency: Macedonian denar

MOLDOVA

Area: 25,715 sq km (9,929 sq miles)
Population: 4,300,000
Capital: Chișinău
Currency: Moldovan leu

ROMANIA

Area: 230,340 sq km (88,934 sq miles)
Population: 22,300,000
Capital: Bucharest
Currency: Leu

SERBIA AND MONTENEGRO

Area: 102,173 sq km (39,449 sq miles)
Population: 10,500,000
Capital: Belgrade
Currency: Dinar

THE IRON GATES
The Danube, Europe's second longest river, flows from Germany to the Black Sea. On the Romanian-Serbian border the river is forced through a narrow gorge, the Iron Gates. A power station has been built here, which uses the water's energy to make electricity.

CARPATHIAN MOUNTAINS
The Carpathians are a major mountain system that extend 1,500 km (830 miles) along the northern and eastern side of the Danubian plain. They link the Alps with the Balkans.

COPSA MICA
The communist government aimed to turn Romania into an industrial powerhouse. At Copsa Mica a factory producing carbon black, used in tyre manufacturing, belched out clouds that turned white sheep black and covered the entire town with a layer of grime. The factory has now closed, but the poisoned legacy of industrialization remains.

SERBIAN MONASTERY
The Serbian Church is an independent part of the Eastern Orthodox Church, and is estimated to have some 8 million followers. The Serbs became Eastern Orthodox as early as the 13th century. In 1389, the Turks defeated the Serbs at the battle of Kosovo. From 1459, Serbia was a Turkish province, and did not become fully independent until 1878. During this period, only the Church kept the national spirit alive. Monasteries became storehouses of national literature and history. Many of Serbia's finest, and most historic monasteries, are located in northern Kosovo, and are valued by the Serbian people.

MEDITERRANEAN

SOUTHEAST EUROPE

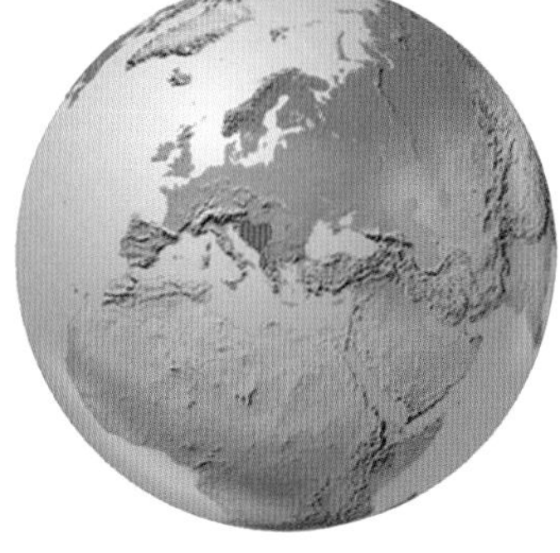

Mediterranean Southeast Europe is largely mountainous. Ranges including the Dinaric Alps run from the north to the south, parallel to the western coast. The western shores of the region are washed by the Adriatic Sea, an arm of the Mediterranean Sea.

THE LANDSCAPE of Mediterranean Southeast Europe is composed of rugged mountains, rocky coasts, and isolated valleys. The region has experienced many centuries of conflict and invasions from both Europe and Asia. Croatia, Bosnia and Herzegovenia, and Albania were once part of the Turkish Ottoman Empire. Slovenia was annexed by the Hapsburg and Austria-Hungarian Empires, and the cultural influences of these two dynasties remain. After World War II, most of Southeast Europe became part of the Communist bloc. In 1990, Slovenia elected a non-communist government which led to civil strife and the final breakup of the Yugoslavian Federation. Slovenia joined the European Union in 2004 and Croatia is a candidate for future EU membership.

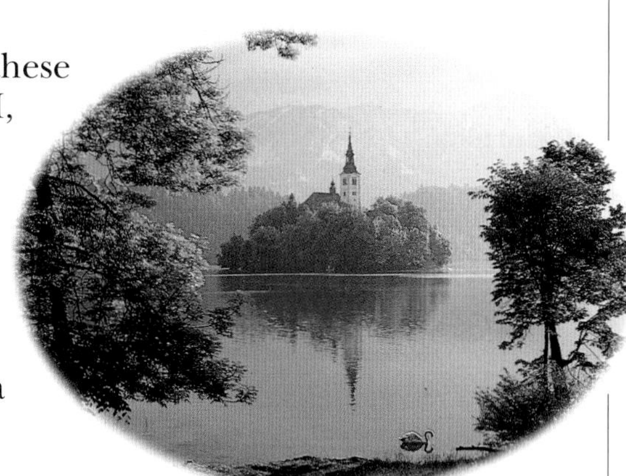

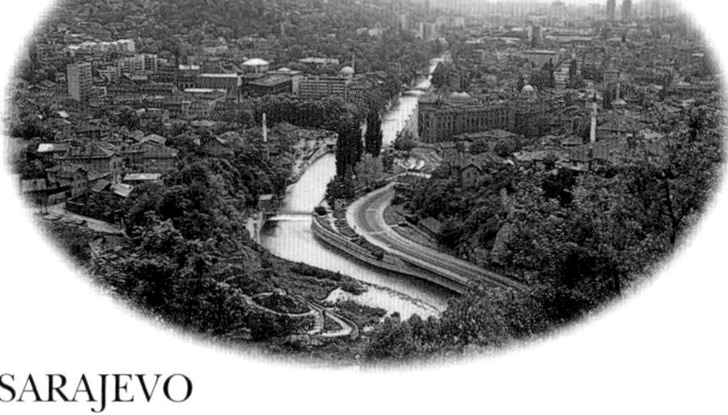

SARAJEVO

The capital of Bosnia and Herzegovina, which straddles the River Miljacka, has a strongly Muslim character, with mosques, wooden houses and an ancient Turkish market place. In 1992, when Bosnia declared independence from Yugoslavia, Sarajevo became the focus of a civil war. Thousands of Muslims were driven from the countryside by the fighting, and fled to Sarajevo. The city suffered terrible damage in 1993, when it was surrounded by Serb forces and bombarded.

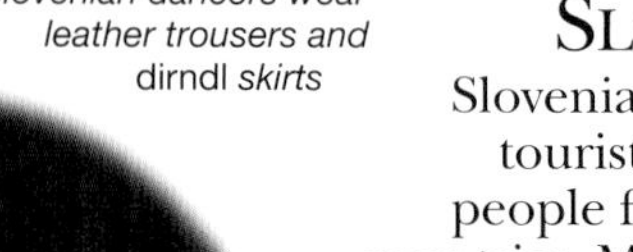

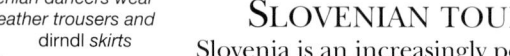

Slovenian dancers wear leather trousers and dirndl *skirts*

SLOVENIAN TOURISM

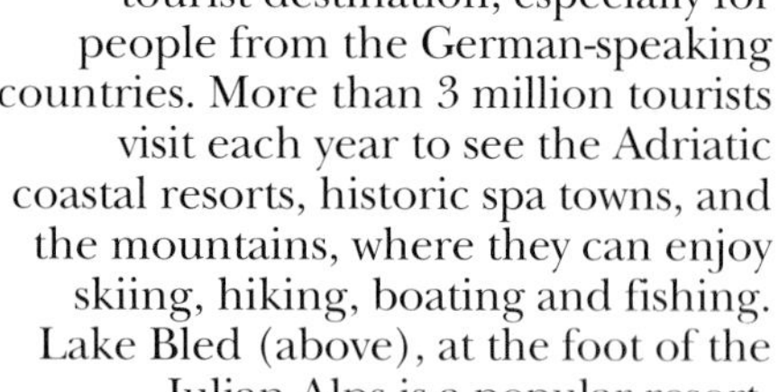

Slovenia is an increasingly popular tourist destination, especially for people from the German-speaking countries. More than 3 million tourists visit each year to see the Adriatic coastal resorts, historic spa towns, and the mountains, where they can enjoy skiing, hiking, boating and fishing. Lake Bled (above), at the foot of the Julian Alps is a popular resort, famous for bathing in summer and as a winter sports centre.

SLOVENIAN DANCERS
Slovenia shares a long history with its northern neighbour, Austria. Culturally, Slovenia has more in common with its Alpine neighbours, Switzerland and Austria, than the countries to the south. Cultural traditions are kept alive through music and dance. National costumes are distinctly Alpine.

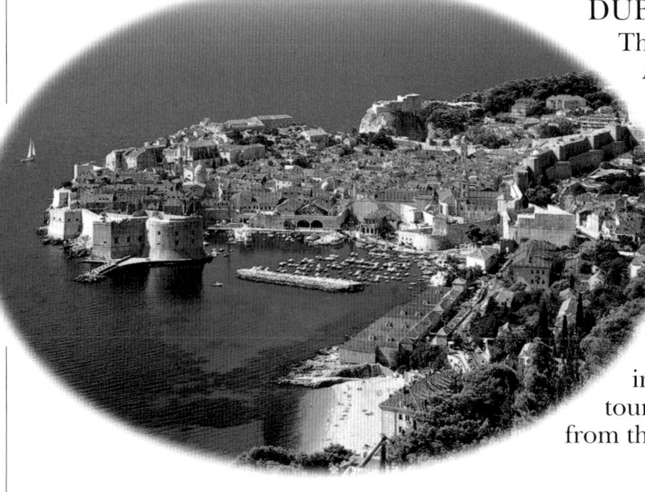

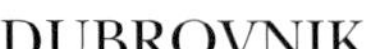

DUBROVNIK

The most picturesque city on the Adriatic coast, Dubrovnik has a history which dates back 1,000 years. With its steep and twisting narrow streets, ancient city walls and historic fortifications, Dubrovnik was once one of Croatia's main tourist attractions. In 1991, this beautiful city came under fire as a result of Croatia's independence struggle. The tourist industry has now recovered from the effects of civil war.

ZAGREB
The Croatian capital is a major commercial centre. Vegetables and fruit produced by local farmers are sold in markets in the town's squares. Much of the city dates to the 19th century, although there are some medieval buildings dating from the 13th century. Zagreb is Croatia's main industrial centre, specializing in manufacturing, textiles and chemicals.

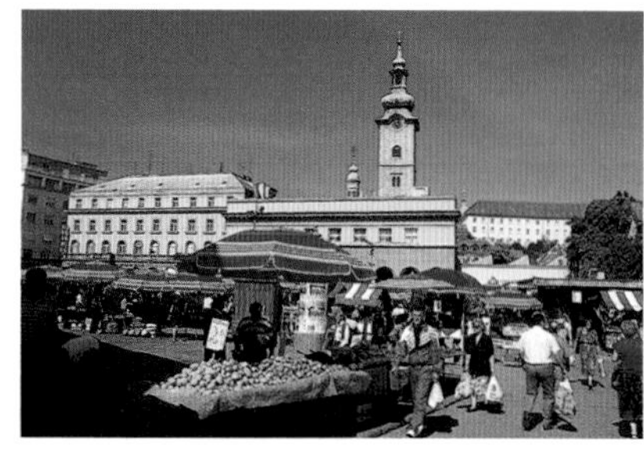

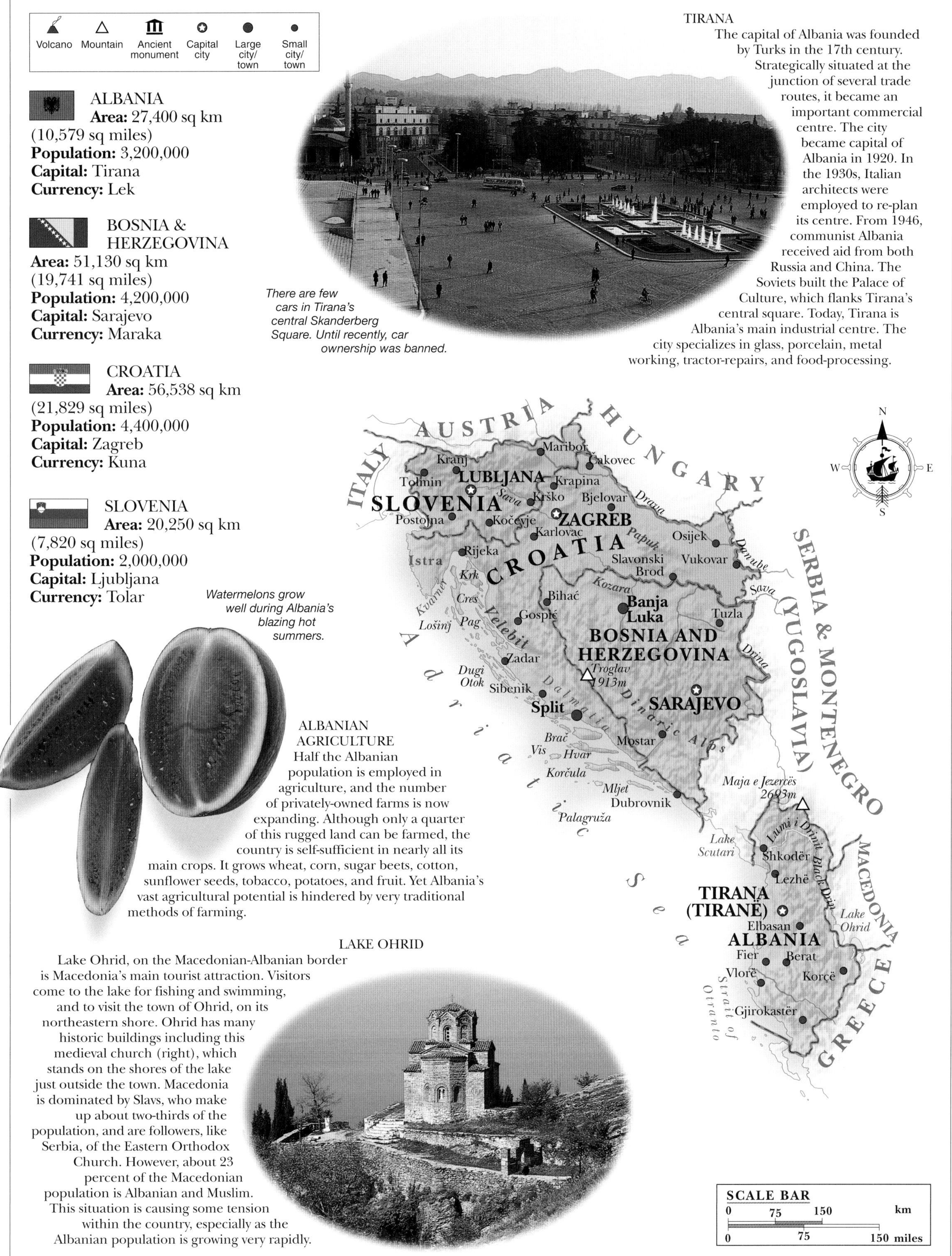

ALBANIA
Area: 27,400 sq km (10,579 sq miles)
Population: 3,200,000
Capital: Tirana
Currency: Lek

BOSNIA & HERZEGOVINA
Area: 51,130 sq km (19,741 sq miles)
Population: 4,200,000
Capital: Sarajevo
Currency: Maraka

CROATIA
Area: 56,538 sq km (21,829 sq miles)
Population: 4,400,000
Capital: Zagreb
Currency: Kuna

SLOVENIA
Area: 20,250 sq km (7,820 sq miles)
Population: 2,000,000
Capital: Ljubljana
Currency: Tolar

TIRANA

The capital of Albania was founded by Turks in the 17th century. Strategically situated at the junction of several trade routes, it became an important commercial centre. The city became capital of Albania in 1920. In the 1930s, Italian architects were employed to re-plan its centre. From 1946, communist Albania received aid from both Russia and China. The Soviets built the Palace of Culture, which flanks Tirana's central square. Today, Tirana is Albania's main industrial centre. The city specializes in glass, porcelain, metal working, tractor-repairs, and food-processing.

There are few cars in Tirana's central Skanderberg Square. Until recently, car ownership was banned.

Watermelons grow well during Albania's blazing hot summers.

ALBANIAN AGRICULTURE

Half the Albanian population is employed in agriculture, and the number of privately-owned farms is now expanding. Although only a quarter of this rugged land can be farmed, the country is self-sufficient in nearly all its main crops. It grows wheat, corn, sugar beets, cotton, sunflower seeds, tobacco, potatoes, and fruit. Yet Albania's vast agricultural potential is hindered by very traditional methods of farming.

LAKE OHRID

Lake Ohrid, on the Macedonian-Albanian border is Macedonia's main tourist attraction. Visitors come to the lake for fishing and swimming, and to visit the town of Ohrid, on its northeastern shore. Ohrid has many historic buildings including this medieval church (right), which stands on the shores of the lake just outside the town. Macedonia is dominated by Slavs, who make up about two-thirds of the population, and are followers, like Serbia, of the Eastern Orthodox Church. However, about 23 percent of the Macedonian population is Albanian and Muslim. This situation is causing some tension within the country, especially as the Albanian population is growing very rapidly.

SOUTHERN AFRICA

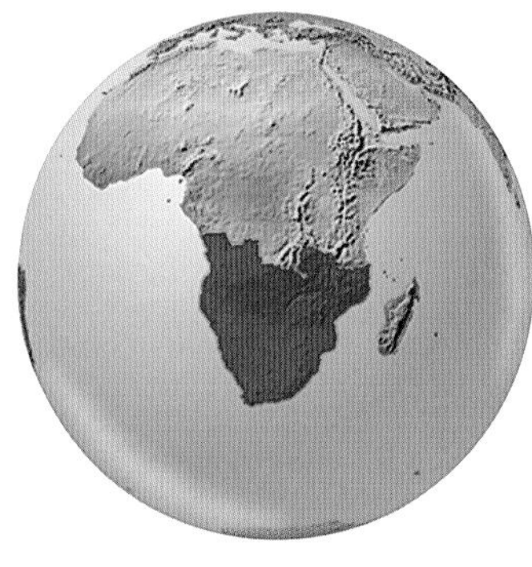

Bordered on the west by the Atlantic Ocean and on the east by the Indian Ocean, much of southern Africa lies within the tropics. The landscape includes the Namib and Kalahari Deserts. Madagascar, the fourth largest island in the world, lies to the east.

THE COUNTRIES OF SOUTHERN AFRICA are dominated by dry savannah and woodland, with humid subtropical forests in the north and, to the centre and west, the Kalahari and Namib Deserts. Traditionally, agriculture has been the mainstay of these countries' economies, but rich mineral deposits, in particular diamonds, uranium, copper and iron, are being discovered and exploited, especially in Namibia, Zambia, and Botswana. Economically, the region is dominated by South Africa, with its well-developed mining industries and large cities. Zimbabwe has reserves of coal, gold and nickel, but the country's economy has been brought close to collapse by drought and misgovernment. Both Angola and Mozambique, former Portuguese colonies, have been devastated by civil wars since independence and are only now beginning to re-build their shattered economies.

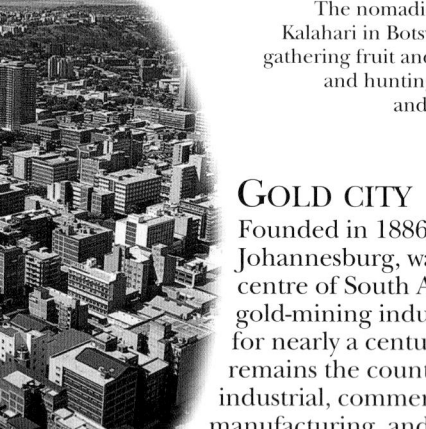

DESERT NOMADS
The nomadic San of the Kalahari in Botswana live by gathering fruit and vegetables and hunting springbok and wildebeest.

URANIUM WEALTH

The largest open pit uranium mine in the world is located at Rössing in the Namib Desert. The mine was opened in 1976 by a group of British, South Africa, French, and Canadian companies. As well as being the world's largest uranium producer, Namibia also has extensive reserves of tin, lead, zinc, copper, silver, and tungsten, and produces 30 per cent of the world's diamond output.

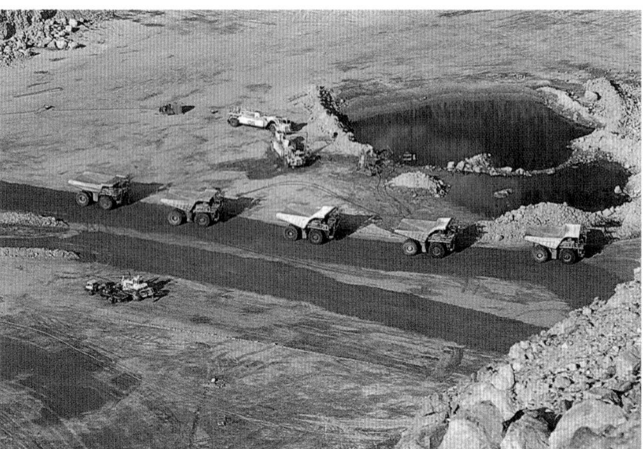

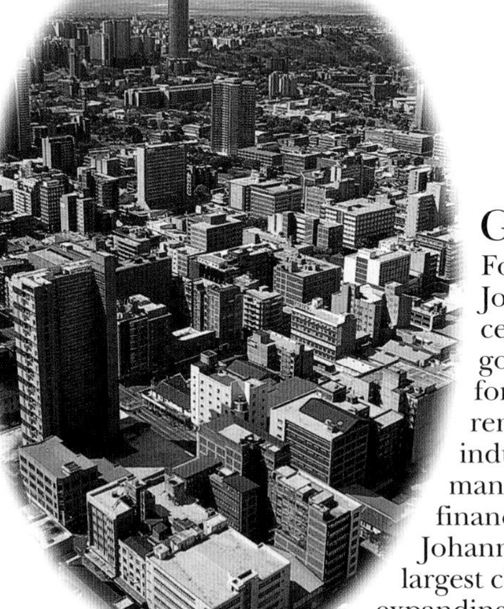

GOLD CITY

Founded in 1886, Johannesburg, was the centre of South Africa's gold-mining industry for nearly a century, and remains the country's chief industrial, commercial, manufacturing, and financial centre. Greater Johannesburg is one of Africa's largest cities, the heart of an expanding motorway system and the South African rail network.

VICTORIA FALLS

Located on the Zambezi River, on the border between Zimbabwe and Zambia, the Victoria Falls are 1,700 m (5,500 ft) at their widest point, and fall to a maximum depth of 108 m (354 ft) in the chasm below. The huge volume of plummeting water creates a mighty roar, known to locals as "the smoke that thunders", which can be heard 40 km (25 miles) away. From the chasm, the river carves a narrow gorge before plunging into a deep pool known as the Boiling Pot.

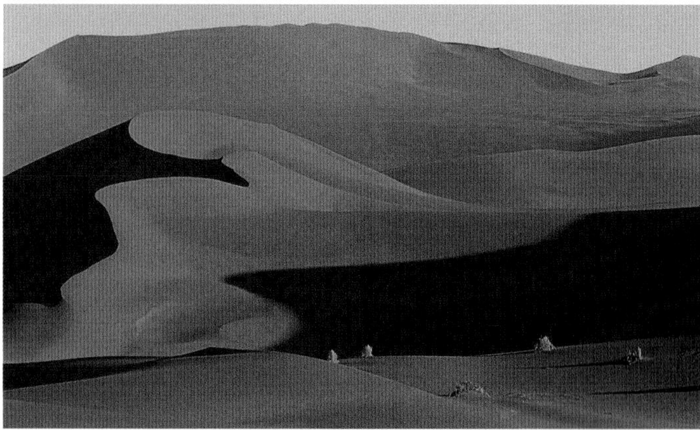

NAMIB DESERT
The Namib Desert extends up to 160 km (100 miles) inland along the coast of southwest Africa. Sand dunes can reach heights of 240 m (800 ft). Moisture from coastal fogs supports some vegetation.

Find out more

AFRICA
AFRICA, HISTORY OF
AFRICAN WILDLIFE
SOUTH AFRICA

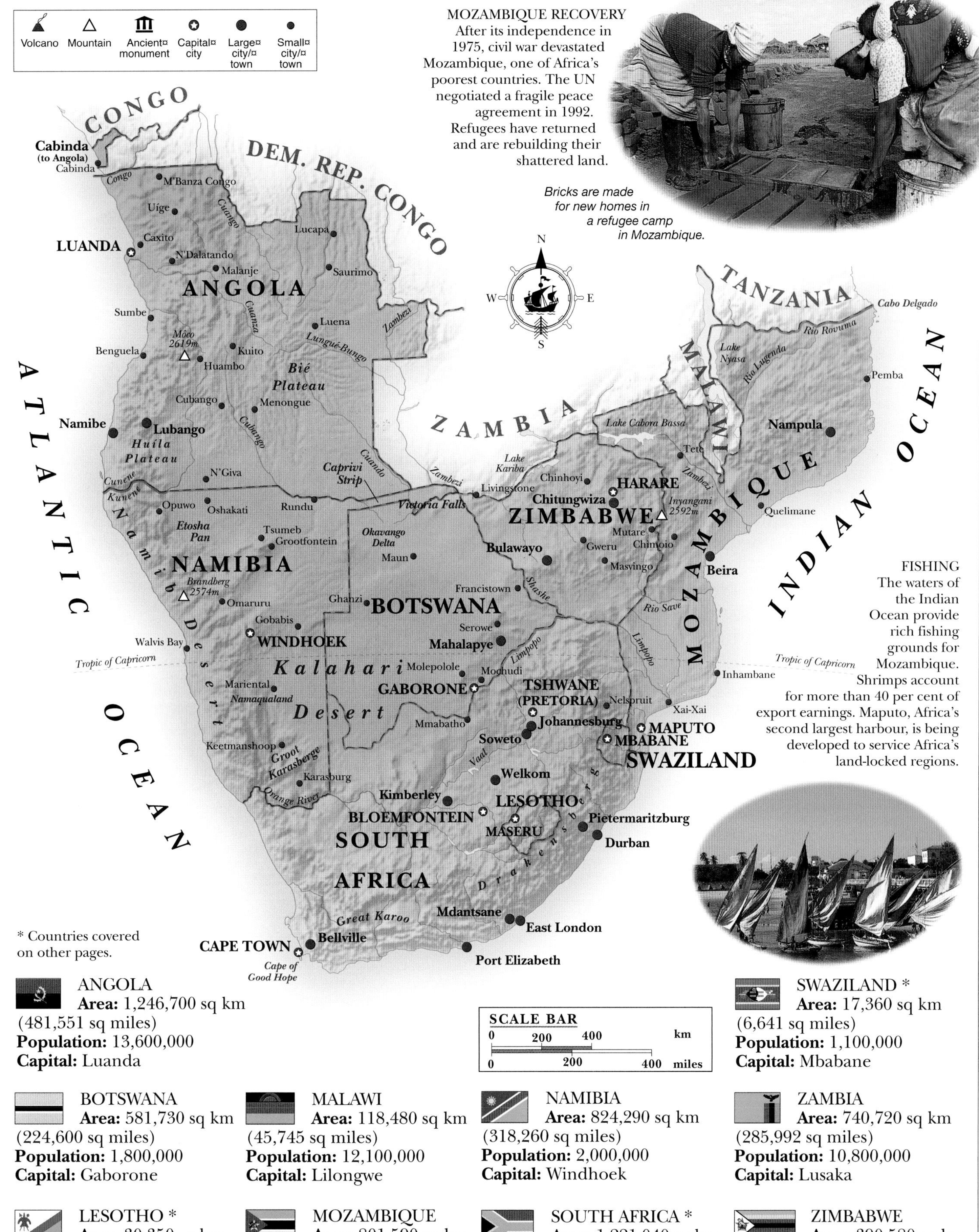

MOZAMBIQUE RECOVERY
After its independence in 1975, civil war devastated Mozambique, one of Africa's poorest countries. The UN negotiated a fragile peace agreement in 1992. Refugees have returned and are rebuilding their shattered land.

Bricks are made for new homes in a refugee camp in Mozambique.

FISHING
The waters of the Indian Ocean provide rich fishing grounds for Mozambique. Shrimps account for more than 40 per cent of export earnings. Maputo, Africa's second largest harbour, is being developed to service Africa's land-locked regions.

* Countries covered on other pages.

ANGOLA
Area: 1,246,700 sq km (481,551 sq miles)
Population: 13,600,000
Capital: Luanda

SWAZILAND *
Area: 17,360 sq km (6,641 sq miles)
Population: 1,100,000
Capital: Mbabane

BOTSWANA
Area: 581,730 sq km (224,600 sq miles)
Population: 1,800,000
Capital: Gaborone

MALAWI
Area: 118,480 sq km (45,745 sq miles)
Population: 12,100,000
Capital: Lilongwe

NAMIBIA
Area: 824,290 sq km (318,260 sq miles)
Population: 2,000,000
Capital: Windhoek

ZAMBIA
Area: 740,720 sq km (285,992 sq miles)
Population: 10,800,000
Capital: Lusaka

LESOTHO *
Area: 30,350 sq km (11,718 sq miles)
Population: 1,800,000
Capital: Maseru

MOZAMBIQUE
Area: 801,590 sq km (309,493 sq miles)
Population: 18,900,000
Capital: Maputo

SOUTH AFRICA *
Area: 1,221,040 sq km (471,443 sq miles)
Population: 45,000,000
Capital: Pretoria

ZIMBABWE
Area: 390,580 sq km (150,800 sq miles)
Population: 12,900,000
Capital: Harare

HISTORY OF THE

SOVIET UNION

IN 1922, A NEW NATION came into being. The Union of Soviet Socialist Republics, or the Soviet Union, was the new name for Communist Russia, led by Vladimir Lenin (1870-1924). The years following the 1917 Revolution were difficult. Civil war between Communists and anti-Communists had torn Russia apart. More than 20 million people had died. When Lenin died, Joseph Stalin took over as dictator. In a reign of terror, he eliminated all opposition to his rule. He started to transform the Soviet Union into a modern industrial state. The huge industrial effort made the Soviet Union strong. It survived German invasion in 1941, although World War II (1939-1945) cost the nation many lives. After 1945 the Soviet Union became a superpower, but it still had difficulty providing enough goods for its people. In 1985, Mikhail Gorbachev came to power. He introduced reforms and began a policy of openness with the West. In 1991, the Communist Party was declared illegal, and the Soviet Union broke up.

INDUSTRIALIZATION
Stalin introduced a series of Five-Year Plans to increase production of coal, steel, and power. The plans were successful for the country, but workers had little reward for their efforts and many were used as slave labour.

КОМСОМОЛ-УДАРНАЯ БРИГАДА ПЯТИЛЕТКИ

Posters showing muscular workers encouraged people to work hard.

This shows how collective farms were organized under Stalin. The collective included a school where children were educated, a factory, and a hospital. The collective had to send fixed deliveries of crops to the State.

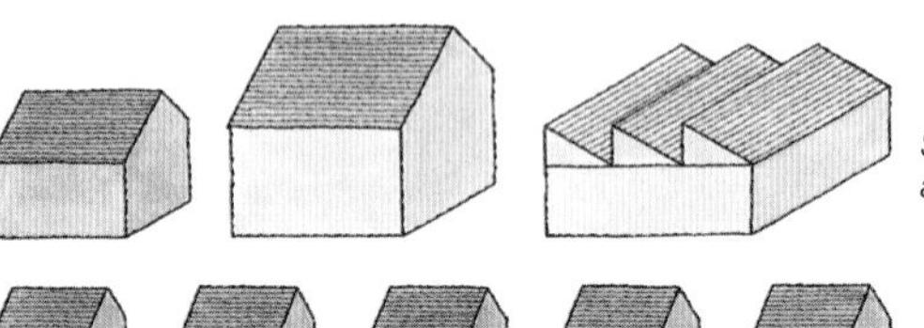

School, hospital, and factory

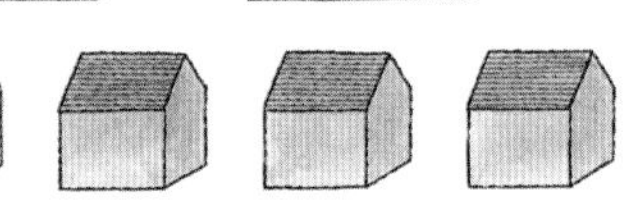

Workers' homes

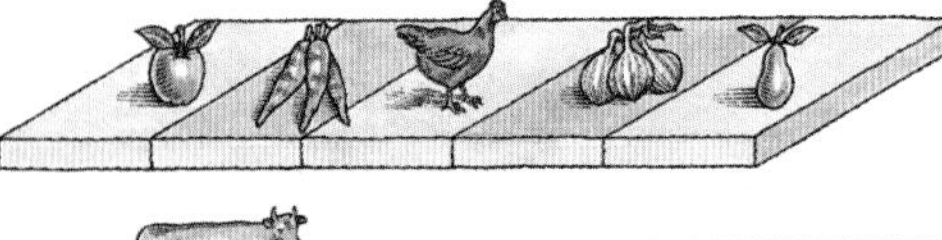

Private plots for fruit, vegetables, and poultry

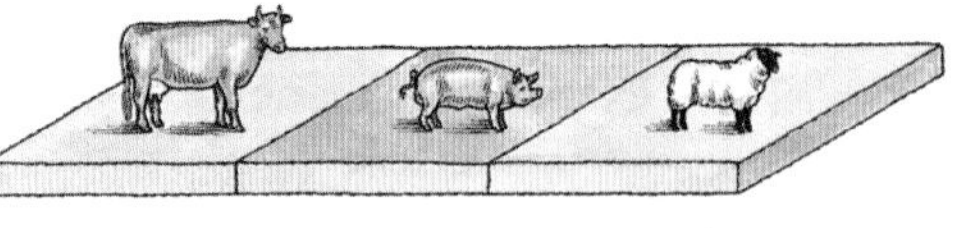

Grazing land for pigs, sheep, and cattle

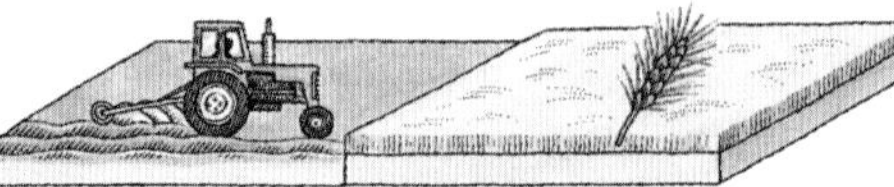

Land for growing crops

COLLECTIVE FARM
Stalin wanted to get rid of all the old-fashioned peasant farms and increase productivity. He reorganized the land into *kolkhozy* (giant collective farms), controlled by the government. The government took the land and livestock of millions of *kulaks* (richer peasants); those who protested were sent to work in prison labour camps. Most of the collectives' products were exported, or sent to the government to feed the city workers.

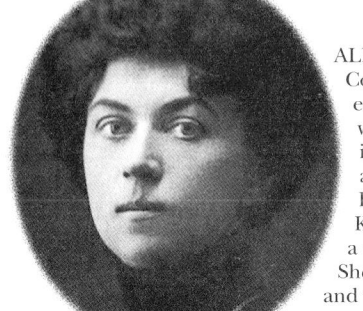

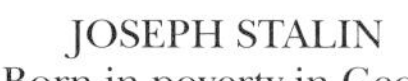

JOSEPH STALIN
Born in poverty in Georgia, southwestern Russia, Joseph Stalin (1879-1953) was a follower of Lenin. After Lenin's death, Stalin seized power and destroyed his opponents. He formed a secret police force to arrest, torture, and execute millions of suspected enemies. These ruthless "purges" enabled Stalin to remain unchallenged as Soviet leader until his death.

ALEXANDRA KOLLONTAI
Communism was supposed to introduce equality into Soviet society. However, while women worked alongside men in heavy industry, they were not allowed to hold real power. But a woman named Alexandra Kollontai (1872-1952) did become a member of Stalin's government. She made many important speeches and wrote several articles about peace and women's rights.

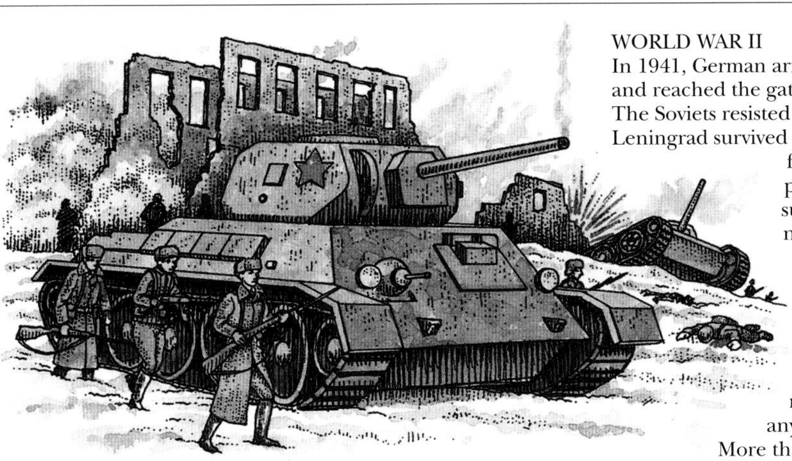

WORLD WAR II

In 1941, German armies invaded the Soviet Union and reached the gates of Moscow, the capital. The Soviets resisted heroically. Stalingrad and Leningrad survived long and bitter sieges. New factories in the east began to produce advanced weapons, such as the T-34 tank, in large numbers. In 1943, Soviet armoured forces, led by Marshal Zhukov, fought and won the largest tank battle ever. But the Soviets paid a high price for victory. They suffered more military casualties than any other country in the war. More than 20 million people died.

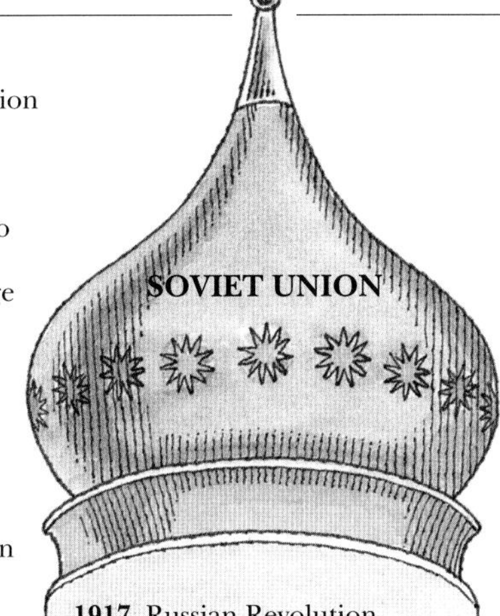

1917 Russian Revolution

1922 Soviet Union formed.

1924 Lenin dies and is replaced by Stalin.

1941-45 More than 20 million Soviets die in World War II.

1955 Warsaw Pact, an alliance of Communist states, created.

1962 Soviet Union builds missile bases on Cuba. US Navy blockades island. Soviet Union removes missiles.

1980 Soviet invasion of Afghanistan.

1988 Soviet troops withdraw from Afghanistan.

1991 Soviet Union breaks up as Lithuania, Latvia, and other republics declare their independence.

CHERNOBYL

In 1986 there was a major disaster at Chernobyl, near Kiev. A nuclear power plant exploded, killing at least 30 people and injuring hundreds more. Radioactive dust and smoke blew all over Europe and exposed thousands of people to contamination. Instead of keeping this disaster secret, the Soviets followed their new policy of *glasnost*, or openness, and warned the rest of the world of the danger.

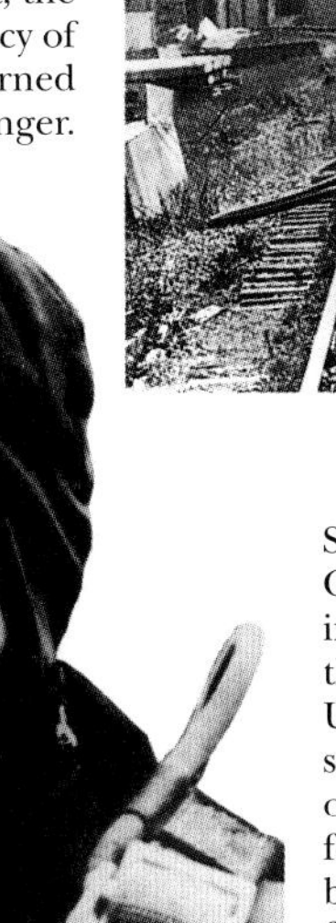

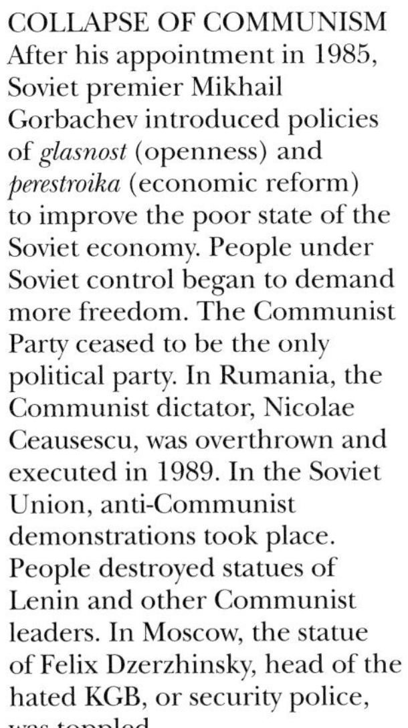

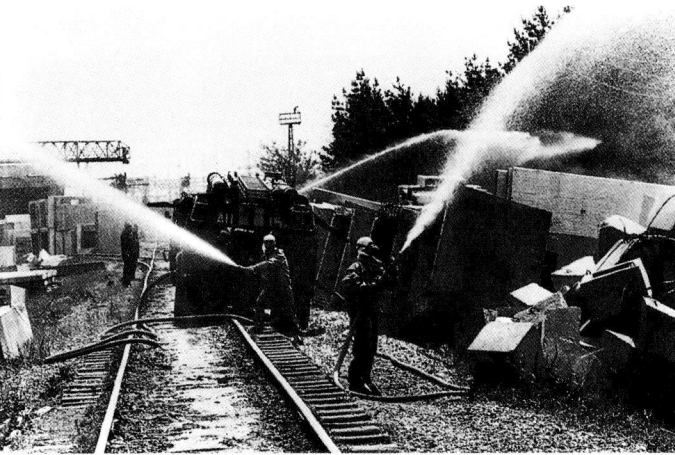

SPACE RACE

On 4 October 1957, the whole world listened in amazement to a strange beeping sound that came from space. The Soviet Union had launched the first satellite, called *Sputnik 1*, into orbit around Earth. It was followed four years later by Yuri Gagarin (left), the first human in space.

COLLAPSE OF COMMUNISM

After his appointment in 1985, Soviet premier Mikhail Gorbachev introduced policies of *glasnost* (openness) and *perestroika* (economic reform) to improve the poor state of the Soviet economy. People under Soviet control began to demand more freedom. The Communist Party ceased to be the only political party. In Rumania, the Communist dictator, Nicolae Ceausescu, was overthrown and executed in 1989. In the Soviet Union, anti-Communist demonstrations took place. People destroyed statues of Lenin and other Communist leaders. In Moscow, the statue of Felix Dzerzhinsky, head of the hated KGB, or security police, was toppled.

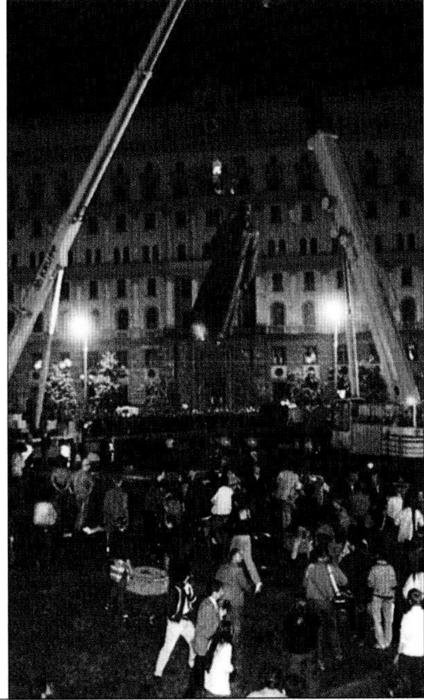

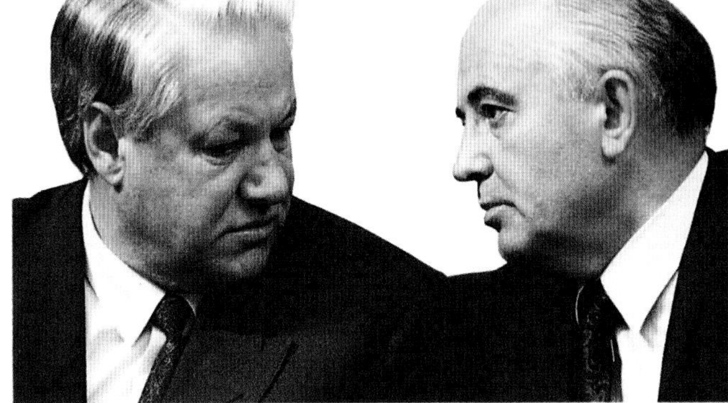

Gorbachev and Yeltsin

Throughout the late 1980s, Soviet people suffered from terrible economic hardship. Many thought that the changes brought about by Gorbachev's policy of *perestroika* were too slow. Mikhail Gorbachev (right) resigned in 1991. Boris Yeltsin (left) became the leader of the new Russian Federation. The Soviet Union broke up as the republics formed their own governments. Boris Yeltsin resigned in December 1999.

Find out more

Caucasus republics
Cold war
Communism
Russia, history of
Russian revolution
World war II

SPACE FLIGHT

SPACE SHUTTLE

A space shuttle is an aircraft that can make repeated flights into space. Since the *Columbia* disaster in 2003, when a shuttle broke up on re-entry to the Earth's atmosphere, the shuttle program has been restricted for safety reasons. A new type of spacecraft is currently being developed to replace the shuttle.

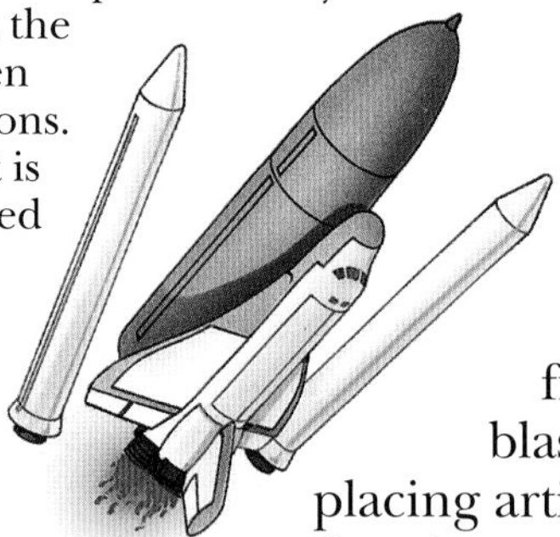

The booster rockets break away at a height of about 47 km (29 miles). They are recovered from the ocean and used again.

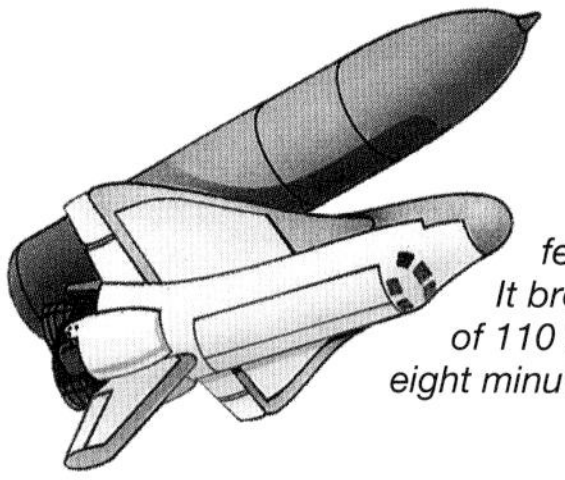

A large fuel tank feeds the main engines. It breaks away at a height of 110 km (70 miles), just eight minutes after launch.

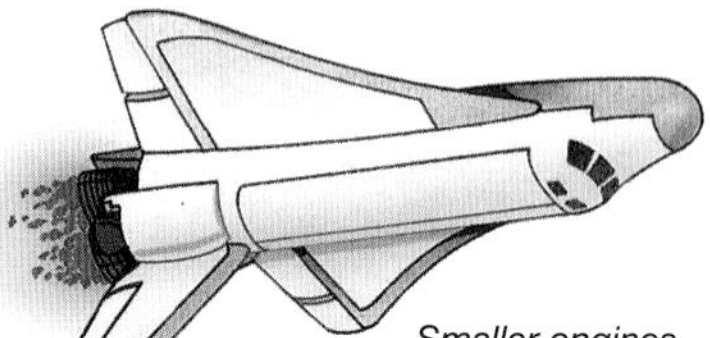

Smaller engines guide the shuttle into orbit.

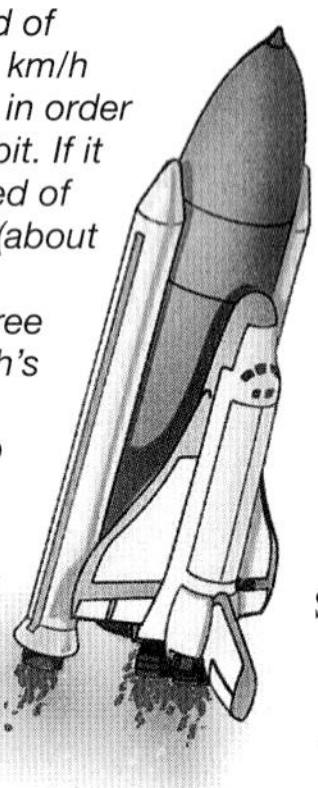

A spacecraft must reach a speed of about 28,000 km/h (17,500 mph) in order to get into orbit. If it attains a speed of 40,000 km/h (about 25,000 mph), it can break free from the Earth's gravity and travel out into space. This speed is called the Earth's escape velocity.

ONLY A FEW DECADES ago, stories about space flight were found only in science fiction books. Today, spacecraft blast off regularly from the Earth, placing artificial satellites in orbit around the planet and carrying space probes and astronauts into space. Space flight became a reality because of two inventions: the rocket engine, which is the only engine that can work in the vacuum of space; and the computer, which is needed to guide a spacecraft on its mission. Spacecraft have been used to do many jobs in space, including launching satellites that map the Earth and provide communication links between countries. However, the most exciting part of space flight is the exploration of space itself. Spacecraft have carried astronauts to the Moon. Although this dramatic journey took three days, it covered only a tiny speck of the universe. The real space explorers are *Voyager, Pioneer,* and other unmanned craft which travel many years through the solar system and beyond, photographing planets, moons, and other objects on their way.

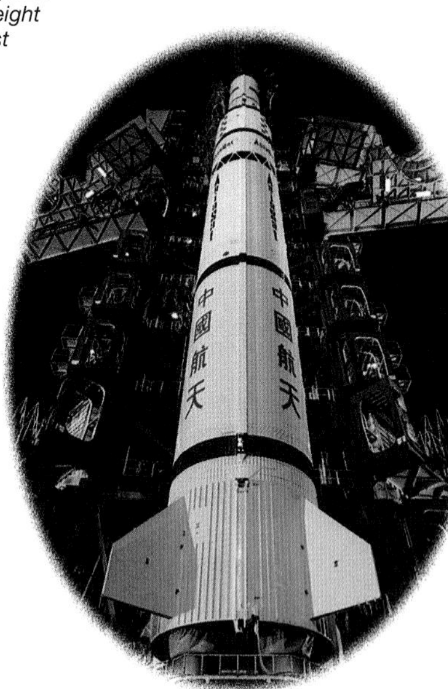

SPACE ROCKET

Spacecraft are carried into space by launch vehicles, or rockets. The launch rocket consists of several parts called stages, each with its own rocket engine. Each stage breaks away as it uses up its fuel, eventually leaving only the spacecraft to fly in space. Returning to the Earth, spacecraft use a small engine to slow them down until they fall out of orbit.

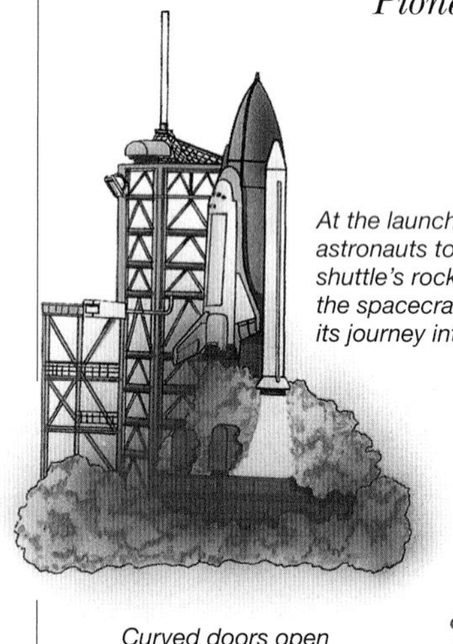

At the launch pad, a tall gantry enables astronauts to enter the shuttle. The shuttle's rocket engines fire, and the spacecraft lifts off to begin its journey into space.

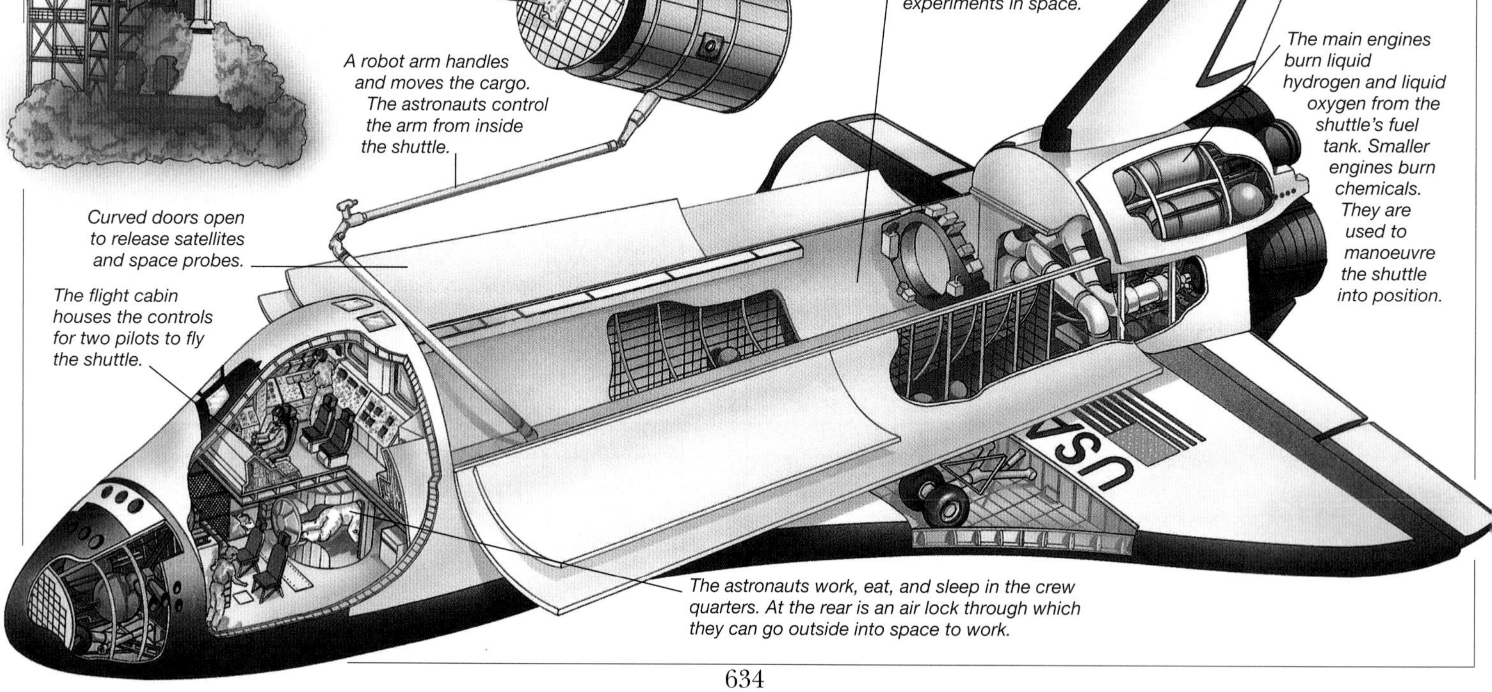

A robot arm handles and moves the cargo. The astronauts control the arm from inside the shuttle.

The payload bay holds the shuttle's cargo, which consists of satellites, space probes, and equipment for carrying out experiments in space.

The main engines burn liquid hydrogen and liquid oxygen from the shuttle's fuel tank. Smaller engines burn chemicals. They are used to manoeuvre the shuttle into position.

Curved doors open to release satellites and space probes.

The flight cabin houses the controls for two pilots to fly the shuttle.

The astronauts work, eat, and sleep in the crew quarters. At the rear is an air lock through which they can go outside into space to work.

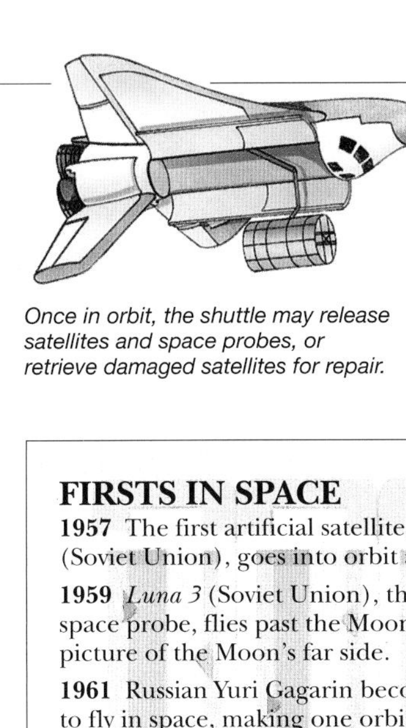

Once in orbit, the shuttle may release satellites and space probes, or retrieve damaged satellites for repair.

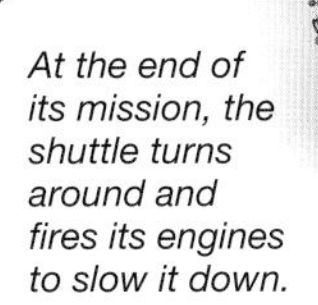

At the end of its mission, the shuttle turns around and fires its engines to slow it down.

Space probes

Space probes leave the Earth and travel out into space. They are equipped with cameras and all kinds of sensors that collect information about space and the planets, which is beamed back to Earth by radio.

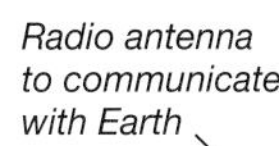

Once the shuttle is travelling slowly enough, it leaves its orbit and begins to descend towards Earth.

Radio antenna to communicate with Earth

Instruments for studying Jupiter's surface

Atmospheric entry probe

GALILEO
In 1995, the *Galileo* spacecraft entered orbit around Jupiter. It discovered that Jupiter's largest moon Ganymede has magnetism within the strong magnetism of Jupiter, a phenomenon not known anywhere else in the solar system.

FIRSTS IN SPACE

1957 The first artificial satellite, *Sputnik 1* (Soviet Union), goes into orbit around the Earth.

1959 *Luna 3* (Soviet Union), the first successful space probe, flies past the Moon and sends back the first picture of the Moon's far side.

1961 Russian Yuri Gagarin becomes the first person to fly in space, making one orbit of the Earth.

1962 *Mariner 2* (US), the first successful planetary space probe, flies past Venus.

1969 Neil Armstrong becomes the first person to walk on the Moon.

1971 The first space station, *Salyut 1* (Soviet Union), goes into orbit.

1981 US space shuttle *Columbia* makes its first test flight into space.

1986 European space probe *Giotto* sends back close-up pictures of the nucleus (centre) of Halley's Comet.

1995 *Discovery* (US) is the first shuttle mission to be flown by a female pilot, Eileen Collins.

2001 Businessman Dennis Tito becomes the first space tourist, aboard the Russian craft *Soyuz*.

When the shuttle enters the Earth's atmosphere, friction of the air makes the heat-proof underside of the shuttle glow red-hot.

A parachute lowered the entry probe into Jupiter's atmosphere.

The spacecraft released a probe containing instruments that measured conditions in Jupiter's atmosphere. They worked for only 75 minutes because Jupiter's gravity crushed the probe like an egg when it got close to the planet's surface.

Heat shield

The shuttle lands on the runway and rolls to a halt. After months of intensive checking, it is ready to fly again.

The shuttle glides down towards a runway, just like an ordinary aircraft.

INSIDE THE ISS
While on board the International Space Station (ISS), astronauts conduct experiments and repair equipment under weightless conditions. The space station is currently under construction, due to be completed in 2010.

Space station

People can make the longest space flights on board space stations – large spacecraft that spend several years in orbit around the Earth. Smaller spacecraft carry teams of astronauts to the space station, where they will live and work for weeks or months at a time. Supplies and relief crews come aboard in spacecraft that dock, or link up, with the space station.

Solar panels rotate to point at the Sun.

Thermal control panels regulate temperature.

Pressurized modules provide living quarters and laboratories.

Spacecraft dock at ports in positions like this one.

International Space Station

Radiators turn edge-on to the Sun to lose excess heat.

Remote sensing instruments look down on Earth.

Find out more
Astronauts
Comets and meteors
Gravity
Moon
Planets
Rockets and missiles
Satellites

Spain

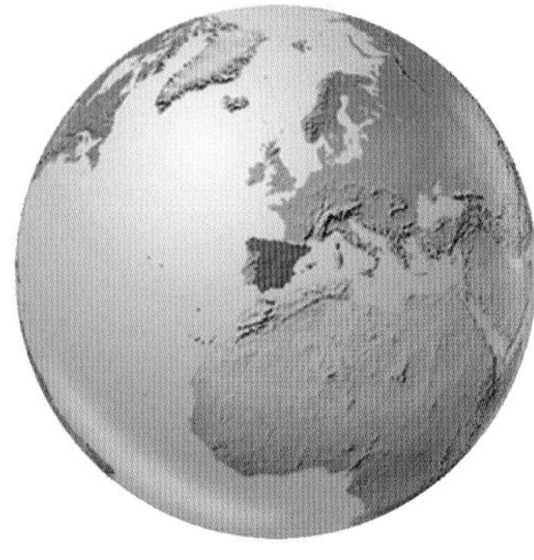

Spain is situated on the Iberian Peninsula in the southwest corner of Europe. France and the Bay of Biscay are to the north, the Mediterranean Sea to the east, the Strait of Gibraltar and Africa are to the south, and Portugal is to the west.

SPAIN SHARES THE IBERIAN PENINSULA with Portugal. It is the fourth largest country in Europe, and both its landscape and its people are varied. The centre of Spain is a hot, dry plateau with snowcapped mountain ranges to the north and south. The southern region of Spain contains Europe's only desert. The Spanish are divided into regional groups, each with their own language and culture. About 16 per cent are Catalan, Galicians make up seven per cent, and just two per cent are Basques. Most of the rest are Castilian Spanish. The country was torn apart by a vicious civil war from 1936-39, and right-wing dictators ruled Spain for much of the 20th century. However, in the mid-1970s the country formed democratic governments. This change allowed Spain to join the European Community, now known as the European Union (EU), in 1986 and to benefit from the higher standard of living in the rest of Europe. Once reliant on farming and fishing for its income, Spain has experienced economic growth since joining the EU. The economy is now dominated by tourism.

In many parts of Spain the donkey cart is still a common form of transport.

FLAMENCO

Flamenco music and dance was developed by gypsies in Andalucia, in the south of Spain. Flamenco songs deal with the entire range of human emotion, from despair to ecstasy. Dancers dress in traditional costume and are usually accompanied by guitars and their own hand-held percussion instrument called castanets. The men's steps are intricate, with toe and heel clicking; women's dancing depends on the grace of the hands and body, rather than on footwork.

Tourism

More than 60 million tourists from all over the world visit Spain. Tourism employs 10 per cent of the work-force and is a major source of income. Tourists come to enjoy the sun, as the climate is mild in the winter and hot in the summer. The country boasts fine beaches, and its old towns are full of interesting buildings and fine works of art.

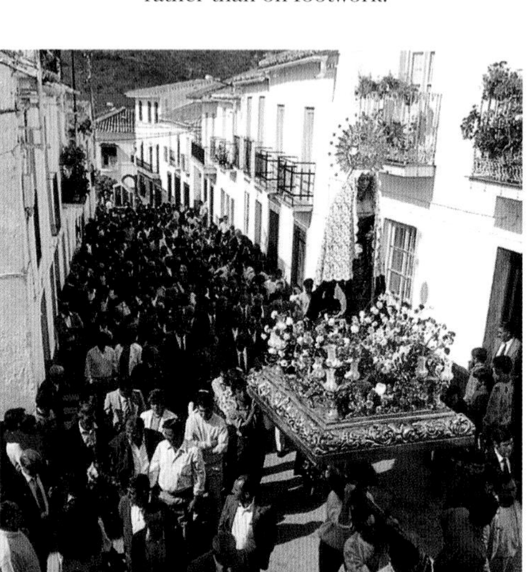

Religion

The Roman Catholic Church plays an important part in the lives of most Spanish people. Nearly everybody is a member of the church and attends mass on Sundays. The priest is an influential member of the community, and the church is a centre of local activities.

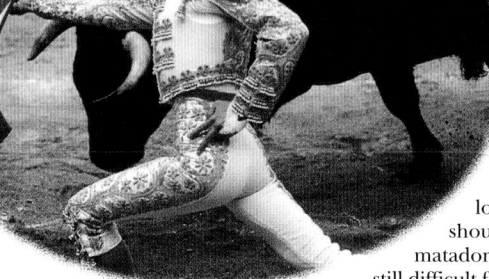

In Spain, bullfighting is a national sport. It is very popular, but many people consider it to be unnecessarily cruel.This bullfighter is shown wearing a typically elaborate costume.

BULLFIGHTING

In Spain, men fight with bulls to entertain crowds. The matador, or bullfighter, stands in the bullring and teases the bull into a rage by waving a red cape. When the bull charges, the matador sticks long, pointed barbs into the bull's shoulders. Once it is exhausted, the matador uses a sword to kill the bull. It is still difficult for women to break into the sport.

Old-fashioned horse drawn carriages ferry tourists around a number of Spanish cities. These carriages (left) are pictured in the Plaza de España, Seville.

King Juan Carlos

The Spanish Civil War of 1936-39 resulted in a dictatorship by General Franco. In 1975 Franco died and was succeeded by King Juan Carlos, grandson of the last Spanish king. Under his rule, Spain became a multi-party democracy, and attained membership of the EU.

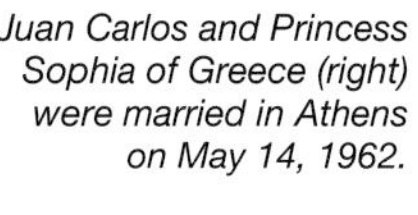

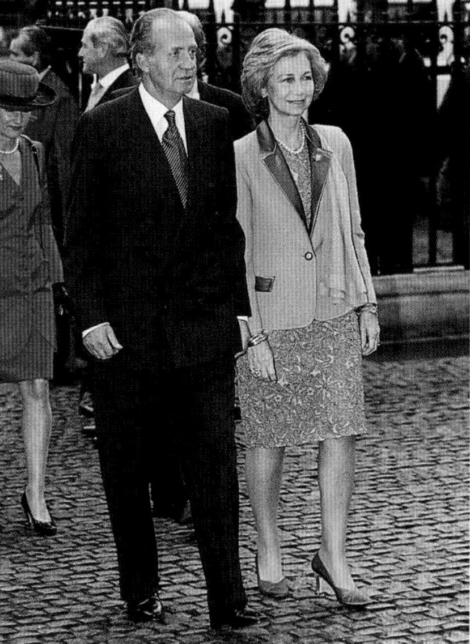

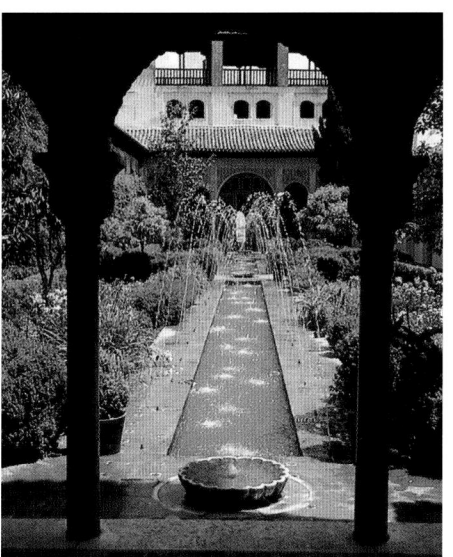

Juan Carlos and Princess Sophia of Greece (right) were married in Athens on May 14, 1962.

Seville

Seville is a major port as well as an important industrial, cultural, and tourist centre. With the discovery of the New World, Seville entered its greatest period of prosperity, being the chief port of trade with the new colonies until 1718 when it was superseded by Cádiz. The city is the capital of bullfighting in Spain and a centre of the Andalusian gypsies, famed for their songs and dances.

Regional dishes include salt-cured ham (above), Spanish omelette (left), and mussels in an onion and garlic sauce (below).

The splendid gardens and architecture of the Moorish palace in Granada

GRANADA

North African Muslims, known as the Moors, once ruled most of Spain. The town of Granada was the capital of their kingdom, and the Alhambra fortress overlooking the town enclosed a magnificent Moorish palace which remains to this day. The palace and its gardens (left) gradually fell into ruin after the Moors were defeated in 1492, but they have since been restored to their former glory.

REGIONAL FOOD

Spain boasts a variety of regional dishes, the most famous of which are paella and tapas. Paella is a classic dish from the Valencia region, where rice is grown. It consists of a variety of meat, fish, fresh vegetables, and saffron-flavoured rice. Tapas, sometimes known as pinchos, are small snacks that originated in Andalusia in the 19th century to accompany sherry. Stemming from a bartenders' practice of covering a glass with a saucer or tapa (cover) to keep out flies, the custom progressed to food being placed on a platter to accompany a drink. Tapas range from cold meats or cheeses to elaborately prepared hot dishes of seafood, meat, or vegetables. A tapa is a single serving, whereas a *ración* serves two or three.

The climax of Pamplona's (left) annual fiesta, Los Sanfermines, is when bulls stampede through the city.

SPANISH GUITAR

The guitar originated in spain in the 16th century. It plays a central role in flamenco, traditionally accompanying the singer. The flamenco guitar developed from the modern classical guitar, and evolved in Spain in the 19th century. Flamenco guitars have a lighter, shallower construction and a thickened plate below the soundhole, used to tap rhythms. Today, flamenco guitarists often perform solo.

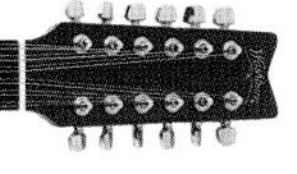

The classical guitar is Spain's national instrument.

Fiestas

More than 3,000 fiestas take place each year in Spain. On any day of the year there is a fiesta happening somewhere - usually more than one. Fiestas are a means for a village, town, or city to honour either its patron saint, the virgin mother, or the changing seasons. Fiestas can take the form of processions, bull-running (above), fireworks, re-enacted battles, some ancestral rite, or a mass pilgrimage to a rural shrine. Whatever the pretext, a fiesta is a chance for everybody to take a break from normal life and let off steam, with celebrations going on around the clock.

PAINTING

Many great artists lived and worked in Spain. Diego Velasquez (1599-1660) was famous for his pictures of the Spanish royal family. Several modern painters, including Pablo Picasso (1881-1973) and Salvador Dali (1904-89), were born in Spain.

Velasquez included himself as the painter in his picture The Maids of Honour.

INDUSTRY

Farming and fishing were once the basis of the Spanish economy. The country has now developed additional industries including textiles, metals, shipbuilding, car production, and tourism. Iron, coal, and other minerals are mined in the Cordillera Cantabrica in the north of Spain. In the 1980s, many foreign-owned electronics and high-tech industries began to locate in the country. Major agricultural products include cereals, olives, grapes for wine, and citrus fruits, especially oranges from around Seville.

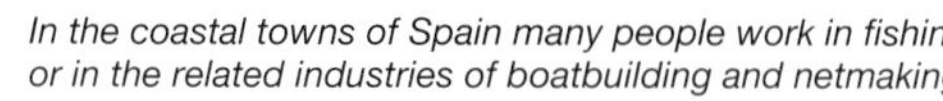

In the coastal towns of Spain many people work in fishing or in the related industries of boatbuilding and netmaking.

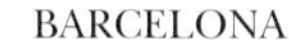

BARCELONA

The city of Barcelona lies on the Mediterranean coast of eastern Spain. It is the second largest city in the country (Madrid is the largest) and is a bustling port of almost two million people. Barcelona is the capital of the province of Catalonia. It lies at the heart of a large industrial area and was the site of the 1992 Olympic Games. Its people speak Catalan, a language that sounds similar to Spanish but has many differences. The city is renowned for its beautiful architecture and many historic buildings.

The cathedral of Sagrada Familia in Barcelona was designed by Antonio Gaudi and begun in 1882. It is still not finished today.

GIBRALTAR

Spain claims that Gibraltar, at its southern tip, is Spanish. However, since 1713 this rocky outcrop has been a British colony. Gibraltar is just 6.5 sq km (2.5 sq miles) in area. Most of the 28,000 inhabitants work in tourism.

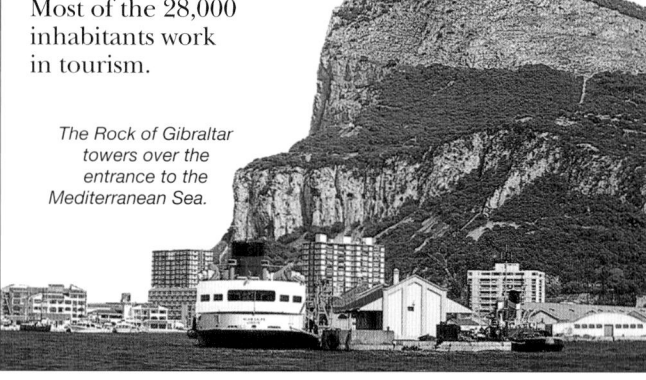

The Rock of Gibraltar towers over the entrance to the Mediterranean Sea.

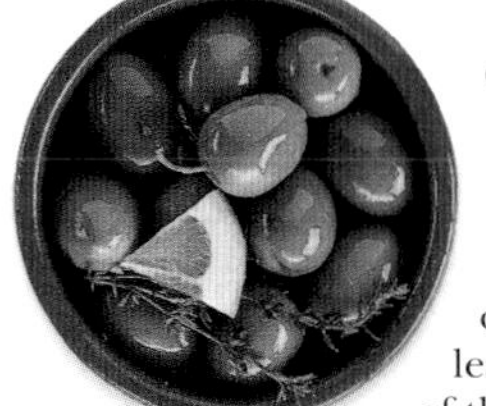

OLIVES

The deep fertile soils and warm climate of southern and eastern Spain are ideal for olive cultivation. The country is one of the world's leading olive producers. Most of the crop is made into olive oil.

Find out more

EUROPE, HISTORY OF
EUROPEAN UNION
PORTUGAL, HISTORY OF
SPAIN, HISTORY OF

Madrid

Spain's largest city, Madrid, lies at the centre of the country, surrounded by a broad plain. Madrid has been Spain's capital city since the 16th century. Recently it has become an important centre for commerce and industry. Madrid's main roads radiate out from the Plaza del Sol (left), which is positioned at the heart of the old city. The newer parts of the city lie to the east.

STATISTICS

Area: 499,440 sq km (192,834 sq miles)
Population: 41,100,000
Capital: Madrid
Languages: Spanish, Catalan, Galician, Basque
Religions: Roman Catholic
Currency: Euro
Main Occupations: Manufacturing, shipbuilding, fishing, agriculture
Main Exports: Textiles, chemicals, ships, cars, fish, fruit and vegetables
Main Imports: Oil, natural gas

POPULATION
In the first half of the 20th century, most of the Spanish population lived in villages or small towns, scattered around the country. Today, tourism and industry have drawn most of the population to the cities and the coastal areas.

CORDILLERA CANTABRICA
These rugged, forested mountains rise on Spain's Atlantic coast. They form the northern edge of the Meseta.

MESETA
Much of this vast plateau of ancient rock is covered with dry, dusty high plains. It has thin soils and is mainly used to graze sheep.

PYRENEES
These majestic mountains form a natural boundary with France.

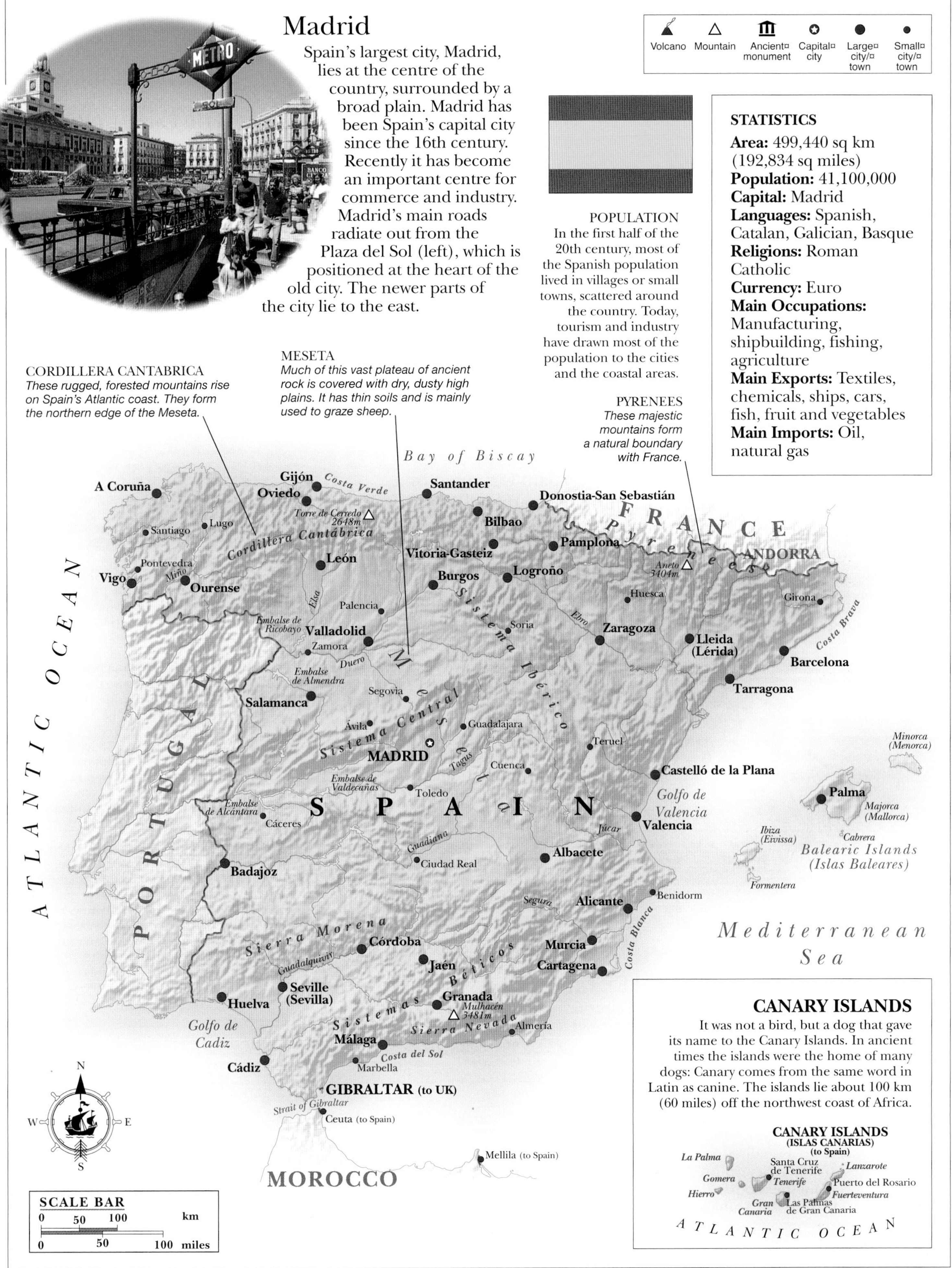

CANARY ISLANDS

It was not a bird, but a dog that gave its name to the Canary Islands. In ancient times the islands were the home of many dogs: Canary comes from the same word in Latin as canine. The islands lie about 100 km (60 miles) off the northwest coast of Africa.

HISTORY OF

SPAIN

BY 1550, SPAIN had become one of the greatest powers in Europe. It had explored other lands and set up a huge empire with colonies in Africa, the Americas, the Caribbean, and Asia. Its early story is one of visiting conquerors. First of all came Celts from the North. From about 1000 B.C., the Phoenicians, then the Carthaginians and Greeks, built trading colonies on the peninsula. The Romans, and then the Visigoths, a Germanic tribe, occupied the whole land. In A.D. 711 Muslim Moors from North Africa invaded Spain and Portugal. By the end of the 15th century Spain, together with Portugal, had driven out the Moors, but rivalry between the two countries developed when they competed in building up their empires overseas. In 1580, Spain invaded Portugal and held it for 60 years. After this, the Portuguese became determined to remain independent of Spanish rule. Spain fought against Portugal during the Napoleonic Wars with the French. More recently, Spain was ruled by a dictator until his death in 1975. Now it has a democratic government.

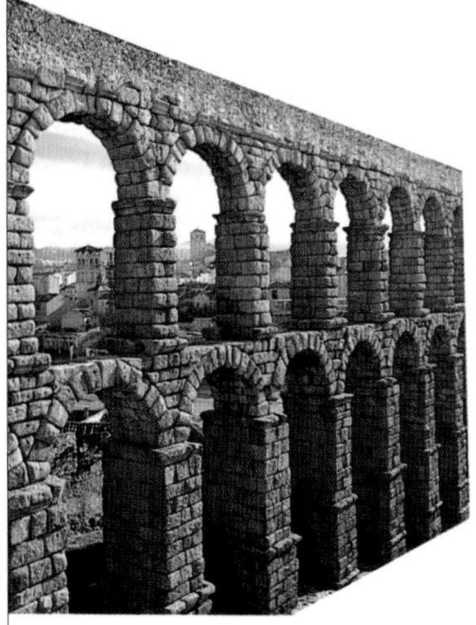

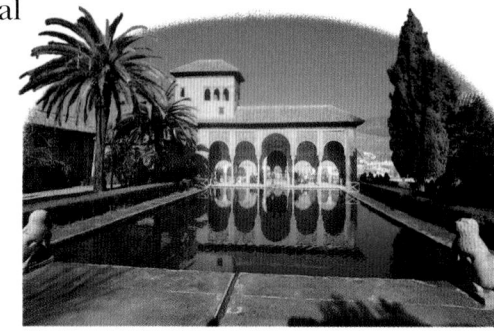

HISPANIA
In 201 B.C. the Romans conquered Spain. The Romans named the region Hispania and introduced Latin as the official language. They also built huge aqueducts (such as the one in Segovia, Spain, above) which carried water to cities. Several of Rome's greatest emperors, including Hadrian and Trajan, were born in Hispania.

ALHAMBRA
Begun in 1248, the Alhambra palace in Granada was the last stronghold of the Moors in Spain. The outer wall is made of red bricks, which gave the palace its name (*alhambra* is the Arabic word for red). It also has 13 towers. The Alhambra contains the finest examples of Moorish art in Europe.

SPANISH CONQUESTS
During the European age of discovery in the late 1400s, Spain, on the edge of the Atlantic, was in an ideal spot to send out explorers to the Americas. By the middle of the 16th century it had colonized the area from Mexico to Peru.

EL CID

During the Moorish occupation, the people of Castile in northern Spain emerged as champions of Christianity. Rodrigo Díaz de Vivar (1040-99) was a nobleman and soldier who heroically fought the Christian cause under King Sancho II of Castile. But when Sancho's brother Alfonso became king, he banished Rodrigo. Rodrigo quickly gathered a small army and fought the Moors. In 1094, he captured the city of Valencia from the Moors. He was given the title El Cid (from the Arabic word *sidi*, meaning "lord") and is one of Spain's national heroes. He died immensely wealthy, ruler of his own kingdom.

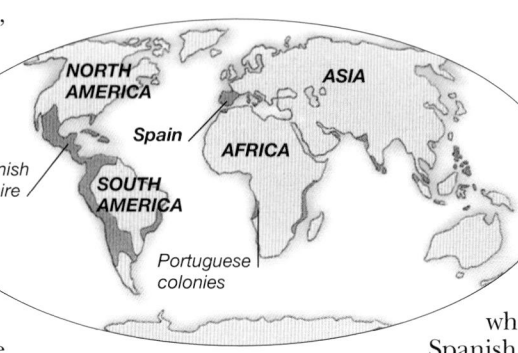

SPANISH EMPIRE

In the Treaty of Tordesillas the Pope divided the non-European world between Spain and Portugal, to avoid wars between them. In 1588, when Portugal was under Spanish rule, the Spanish Empire was at the height of its power.

The Spanish empire, 1588

Elaborately designed and inscribed with its history, this sword was surrendered by the French governor of a Spanish fortress during the Peninsular War.

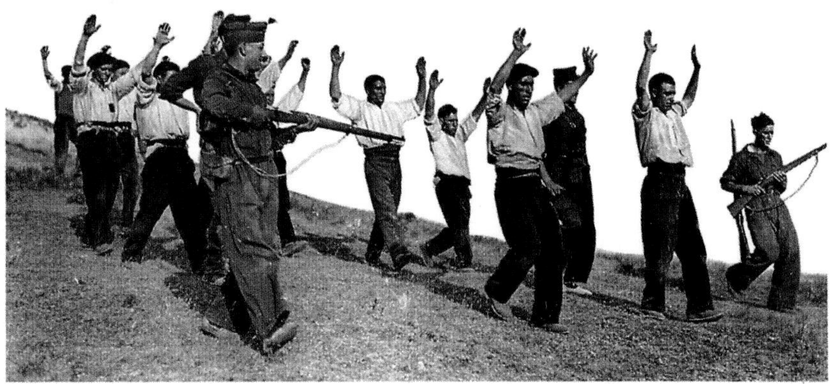

PENINSULAR WAR

In 1807, Spain agreed to support French Emperor Napoleon I in a war with Portugal. French troops defeated Portugal but occupied major Spanish cities in the process. In 1808, Napoleon overthrew the Spanish monarch and had his brother Joseph Bonaparte proclaimed king of Spain. The Spanish people rose in revolt and finally, by 1814, drove out the French. Spain calls it the Spanish War of Independence.

SPANISH CIVIL WAR

In February 1936, a left-wing (radical) Republican government was elected in Spain. Most of the Spanish army (right-wing and conservative) rebelled and tried to overthrow the government. Led by General Franco, the army fought bitterly with the Republicans for nearly three years. Mussolini sent Italian troops, and Hitler sent German troops to help the right-wing cause. Thousands of Spaniards died in this bloody civil war. In 1939, the Republican armies collapsed, and Franco emerged as dictator of Spain.

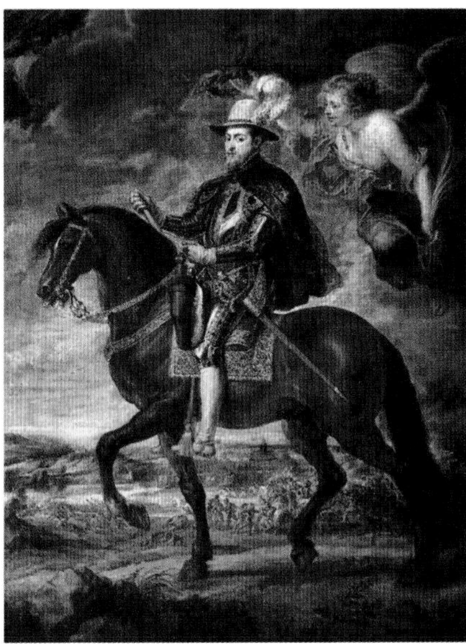

The policy of Philip II was to establish an absolute monarchy.

PHILIP II

King Philip II (1527-98) ruled Spain at the height of its power. Under him, Spanish art, writing, and fashions led Europe. He united Spain with Portugal and conquered the Philippines. He was involved in many wars; during a war against the English, the Spanish Armada (fleet) was destroyed. Poverty spread throughout Spain because of these wars, and after Philip died, Spanish power began to fail.

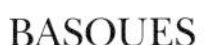

BASQUES

The Basque people have lived in the Pyrenees (mountains between France and Spain) for thousands of years. They have their own language, called Euskera. In the 1960s, the Spanish Basques demanded a separate, independent Basque state. Some Basques formed terrorist groups to fight against the Spanish government. The Basques now have their own parliament and some control over their government.

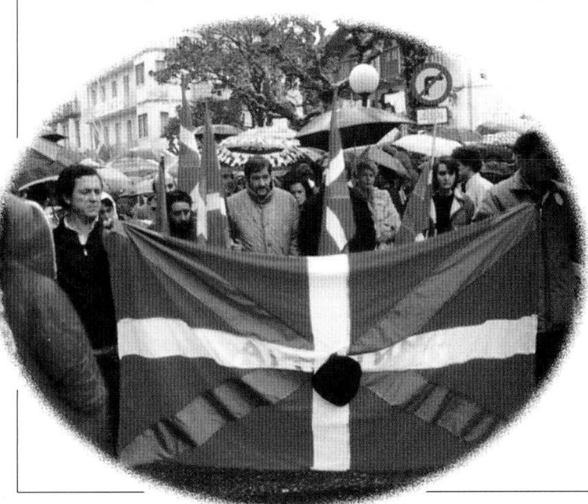

FRANCO

General Francisco Franco (1892-1975) had a successful army career before he became dictator of Spain. He kept Spain out of World War II (1939-45). After the war there was rapid economic growth, and the standard of living improved. But many people were unhappy with Franco's restrictions on personal freedom. Many Spaniards were arrested and executed by Franco's police for protesting and demanding more freedom.

SPAIN

800-200 B.C. Phoenicians, Carthaginians, and Greeks set up trading colonies along the coast of Spain.

201 B.C. Roman control begins.

711 A.D. Visigoths invade. Muslim Moors from North Africa conquer Spain.

1094 El Cid captures Valencia.

1385 Spaniards attempt invasion of Portugal but are defeated.

1494 Treaty of Tordesillas between Spain and Portugal carves out their empires.

1580 Philip II of Spain invades Portugal and unites the two countries.

1588 English navy defeats the Spanish Armada.

1640 Spain loses Portugal and all the Portuguese colonies. Decline of the Spanish empire begins.

1807 Peninsular War begins.

1898 Spanish war with United States over Cuba leads to the end of the Spanish empire.

1931 King Alfonso XIII of Spain flees the country. Spain becomes a republic.

1936-39 Spanish Civil War.

1939 General Franco becomes dictator of Spain.

1975 General Franco dies. Spain becomes a democracy.

1986 Spain joins the European Community (EC).

1992 Summer Olympic games held in Barcelona.

Find out more

COLUMBUS, CHRISTOPHER
HAPSBURGS
SOUTH AMERICA, HISTORY OF
SPAIN

SPIDERS AND SCORPIONS

FEW ANIMALS ARE MORE FEARED but less understood than spiders and scorpions. We often call these scurrying little creatures insects, but they really belong to the group of animals called arachnids, along with ticks and mites. Insects have six legs; spiders and other arachnids have eight legs. There are about 40,000 kinds of spiders and 1,400 kinds of scorpions. All are carnivores (meat eaters). Scorpions hunt down their prey and kill it with their pincers. If the prey is big, or struggles, the scorpion uses the sting in its tail. Many spiders capture insects by spinning a silken web. The silk of some webs is stronger than steel wire of the same thickness. Not all spiders spin webs, however; some catch their prey by dropping a net of silk onto it. A few spiders, such as the trap-door spider, rush out at their victim from a burrow. Some scorpions and several spiders are dangerous to humans, including the Australian funnel web spider and the Durango scorpion of Mexico.

WEB
Spiders make webs with a special silken thread from glands at the rear end of the body. Tubes called spinnerets squeeze out the thread like toothpaste. The silk hardens as the spider's legs pull it out.

GARDEN SPIDER

Thousands of spiders live in our houses and gardens, feeding on flies, gnats, and moths. The common garden spider spins a beautiful, complicated web called an orb web, often between the stems of plants. Some spiders lie in wait for their prey in the centre of the web; others hide nearby. Many orb-web spiders spin a new web almost every day.

SPIDERLINGS
Young spiders are called spiderlings. They hatch from eggs inside a silken cocoon and feed on stores of yolk in their bodies. After a few days, weeks, or months, depending on the weather, they cut their way out of the cocoon and begin to hunt for food.

The female black widow has a deadly bite.

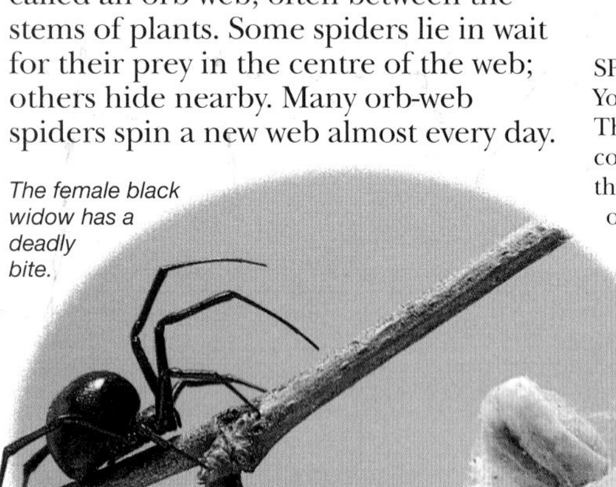

BLACK WIDOW
The female black widow spider is so named because it sometimes kills its mate. This spider is also one of the few spiders that can kill humans. The female black widow shown here is standing near its eggs, which are wrapped in a silken egg sac or cocoon.

TARANTULA
True tarantulas are shy spiders which live mainly in burrows. False tarantulas, such as the big spider shown here, include various large, hairy hunting spiders from North and South America. They are also called bird or monkey spiders. Their bite is painful to humans, but it is less poisonous than the bite of smaller spiders such as the black widow.

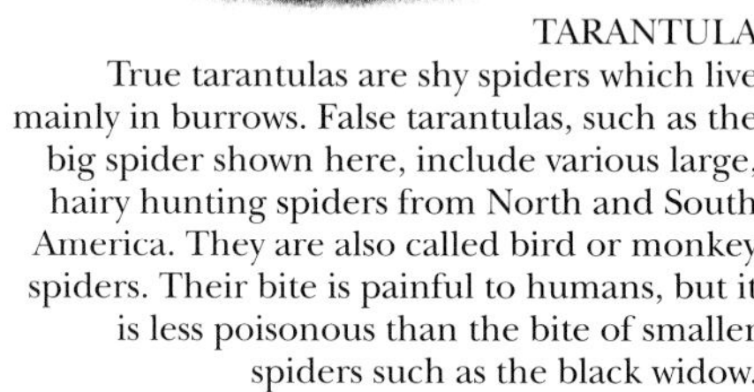

FOOD
Spiders eat animal prey. Their most common victims are insects, worms, sow bugs, and other spiders. The spider's venom subdues or paralyses the prey while the spider wraps it up in a silk bag to eat later.

YOUNG SCORPIONS
Scorpions are born fully formed. At first the female scorpion carries the young on its back, where they are well protected from predators. After the young have moulted (shed their skin) for the first time, they leave their mother to fend for themselves.

Mother carries the young on her back.

Imperial scorpion

The sting is connected to twin poison glands at the end of the tail.

Scorpion's large pincers are called pedipalps. They seize, crush, and tear the prey, then pass it to the jaws.

SCORPION

Scorpions live mainly in warm regions, lurking beneath rocks or in cracks or burrows. Most feed at night, ambushing or hunting down their prey. They feed mainly on insects and spiders. The scorpion uses the sting at the end of the tail in self-defence, as well as to subdue its prey.

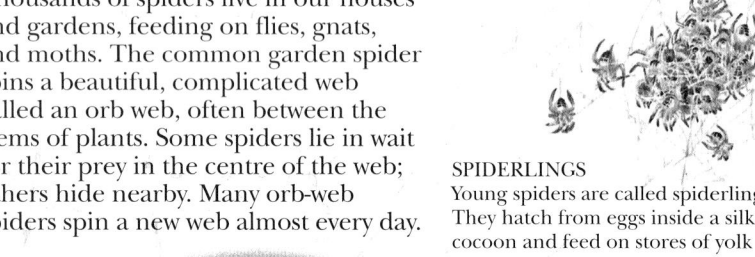

Find out more
ANIMALS
AUSTRALIAN WILDLIFE
DESERT WILDLIFE

SPIES AND ESPIONAGE

MATA HARI
The most notorious spy of World War I was a dancer who worked in Paris using the stage name Mata Hari. She was born in the Netherlands as Gertrude Margarete Zelle in 1876. Mata Hari was probably a double agent: she spied on the Germans for their enemies the French, but she also gave French secrets to the Germans. She was arrested by the French and executed in 1917.

Charmed by Mata Hari's beauty, military men gave her secret information.

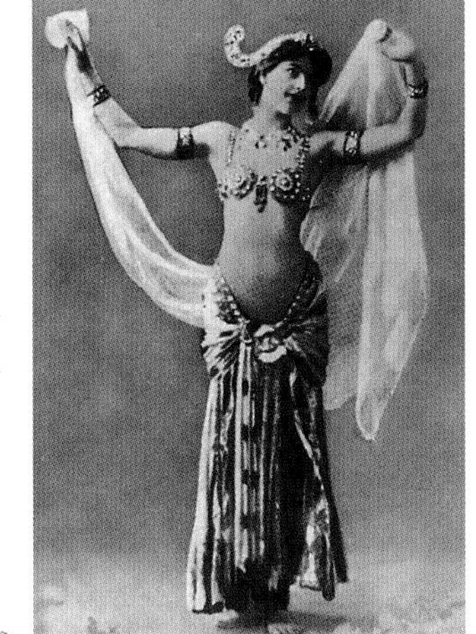

NATIONS AT WAR try hard to discover what their enemy will do next, so that they can mount a more secure defence or an effective attack. Secretly trying to discover the plans of an enemy or competitor is called spying, or espionage. The people who do it are called spies, and they have a difficult job. They often pretend to be working for one side while collecting information for the other. Their work is also dangerous: spies caught in wartime are executed.

Spying is an ancient trade, but it reached a peak during World War II (1939-45) and in the years that followed. Though the United States and the former Soviet Union were not at war, each feared attack from the other. So both sides used espionage to estimate the strength of the opponent's forces. Today, much spying is not military but industrial. By copying a competitor's plans, a manufacturer can make a similar product without the cost of research.

Undercover spies may seek low-paying work such as cleaning in offices where they know secrets are filed.

SECRET AGENTS

Spies may use false identities to hide their activities. They seem to lead regular lives but are secretly collecting information. These spies are called agents or secret agents. They may bribe people to steal secrets. Or they use blackmail: they find out damaging facts about someone who has access to secrets, then threaten to reveal these facts unless the victim becomes a spy.

Tiny bugs transmit signals that a spy can pick up a city block away.

Night-vision binoculars help spies see long distances in darkness.

Phone capsule transmitters broadcast telephone calls and are difficult to detect.

Even a cigarette pack is big enough to hide a tiny tape recorder.

Cameras hidden in watches enable spies to take photographs secretly.

Bug detectors disguised as pens give warning that a spy has hidden a bug in the room.

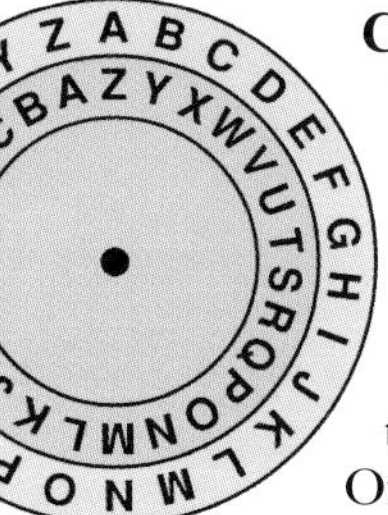

CODES

When spies send messages, they encode them – write them in code – to hide the meaning. The spy changes each letter for a different one, so that only someone else who knows the code can read the words. On this code disc, the letters of the message are marked in blue, and their coded form is in green. For example, C becomes X. HELP I AM TRAPPED would be SVOK R ZN GIZKKVW in code. This code is easy to break, or understand. But computer-generated codes are almost impossible to break.

SPY EQUIPMENT
Spies need special equipment so that they can watch and listen to people and send messages secretly. To hear private conversations, spies hide "bugs" – tiny microphones and radio transmitters – in their subjects' homes or offices. The spy tunes in a radio receiver to hear the signals transmitted by the bug. A spy can use a camera with a powerful magnifying lens to take embarrassing photographs with which to blackmail. Hacking into a computer to discover top-secret files of government and big business is a growing trend.

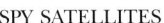

SPY SATELLITES
In 1961, the United States launched the first spy satellite. It had cameras pointed at the ground to photograph troop movements. Today, there are many spy satellites, and they are much more sophisticated. They can monitor radio signals and distinguish individual vehicles on the ground. Spying from space has greatly reduced the need for conventional spies.

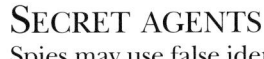

Find out more

LAW
POLICE
SATELLITES
WORLD WAR II

SPORTS

EVERYONE WHO takes part in a sport does so for his or her own individual reasons. Early-morning joggers feel good by keeping fit and trying to beat a personal best time. Backpackers enjoy the fresh air and like to learn outdoor survival skills. And in a sports competition, no experience can match the sensation of winning. Sports are games and activities that involve physical ability or skill. Competitive sports have fixed rules and are organized so that everyone has an equal opportunity to succeed.

Many of today's sports developed from activities that were necessary for survival, such as archery, running, and wrestling. Some sports, such as basketball and volleyball, are modern inventions. And as the equipment improves, the rules change to ensure that no competitor has an advantage. Sponsorship and television are now major influences on sports. Leading players become millionaires, and most popular events have huge international audiences.

Many ancient sports are still played today but some, such as foot-wrestling, have long been forgotten.

Officials make sure each game lasts the same time.

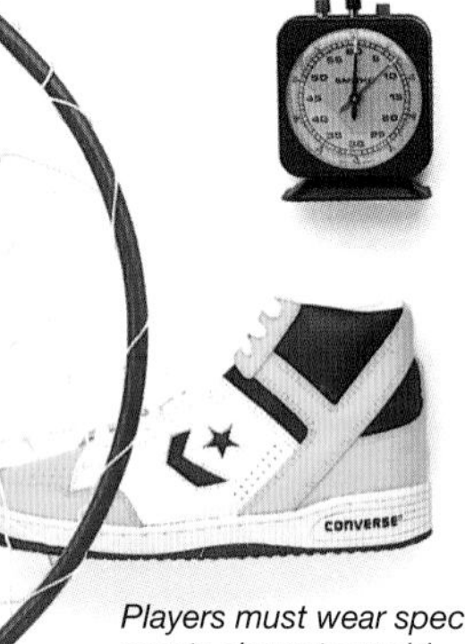

Players must wear special sports shoes to avoid slipping on the floor.

EQUIPMENT AND UNIFORMS

Uniforms are important in team sports. They help players and spectators quickly recognize fellow team members and tell them apart from the opposing side. Underneath the basic shirt and shorts or jersey and trousers, players wear protective gear, especially in games such as football and hockey. Shoes are designed to suit the playing surface – rubber-soled for a basketball court, for example, and cleated (spiked) for grass. Other equipment includes a standard ball and, for some sports, bats or rackets.

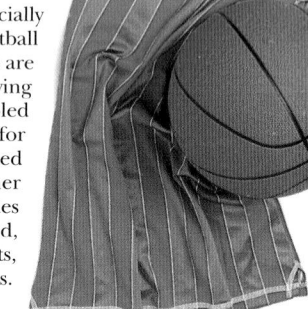

Basketball hand signals

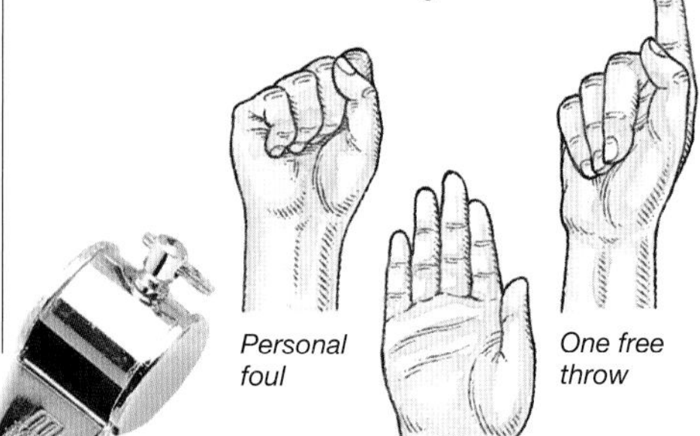

RULES

Each team sport has its own rules so that everyone taking part knows how to play the game. Referees, umpires, or other judges stand at the edge of the playing area and make sure that the players obey the rules. In some sports, they use a loud whistle to stop and start play. They also signal with their hands or with flags to let the players know their decisions.

TEAM SPORTS

In a team sport such as basketball, everybody must co-operate, or work together, in order to win. The stars in a team sport are usually the attacking players who score points or kick for a goal. However, if every player tried to be a star, there would be no one to play a defensive role and prevent the opposing team from scoring. So every player on the team has a special job, and each plays an equal part in a successful game.

FIELD

The rules of every team sport include standard sizes for the field or court, its markings, and other features such as goal posts. There may be more than one standard if the game is played by both adults and young people. For example, the dimensions of the free-throw lane and the backboard are different for high school, college, and professional basketball. The rules of some sports, such as baseball and soccer, give the largest and smallest sizes allowed for the playing area.

The ring of the basket stands 3 m (10 ft) above the floor.

Basketball court

COMPETITION

In individual competition, contestants compete alone. Some try to beat a record; some measure their performance against other contestants. Players compete "one-on-one" in sports such as fencing, judo, and tennis. Several contestants compete together in racing sports such as horse racing or the 100-metre dash. In some sports, such as alpine skiing and archery, contestants compete separately to record the best timing or scores. In other sports, such as diving or gymnastics, judges decide the scores.

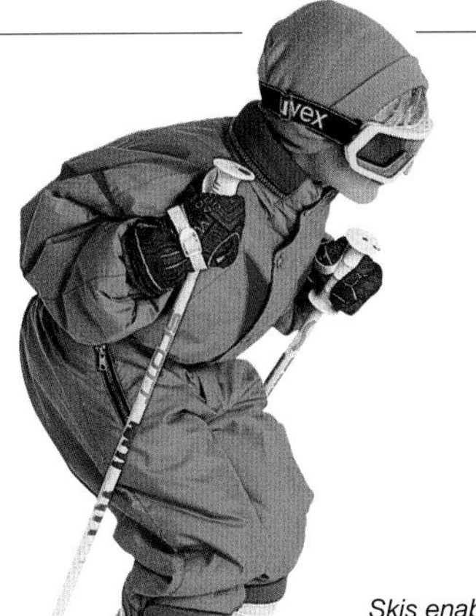

Skis enable the wearer to slide swiftly over snow.

GYMNASTICS

In classic gymnastics, contestants perform exercises on the floor and on pieces of apparatus. This apparatus includes a padded stand called a horse, wooden rings hanging from straps, and arrangements of bars. Men and women do different exercises, and each is excluded from certain events. For instance, only men compete on rings, and only women use the balance beam.

Men's rings

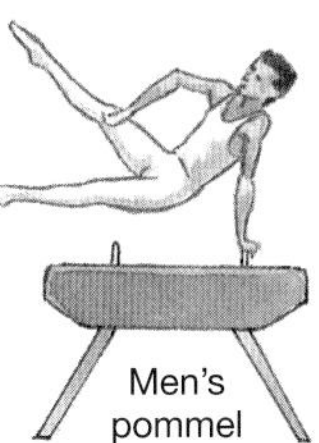

Men's pommel horse

Women's balance beam

Women's uneven parallel bars

Men's horse vault

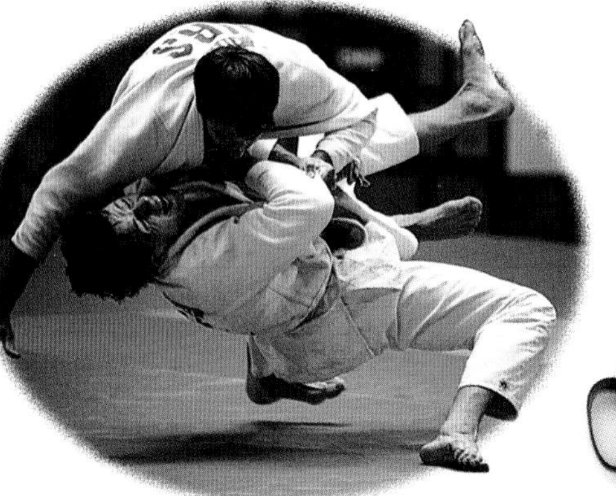

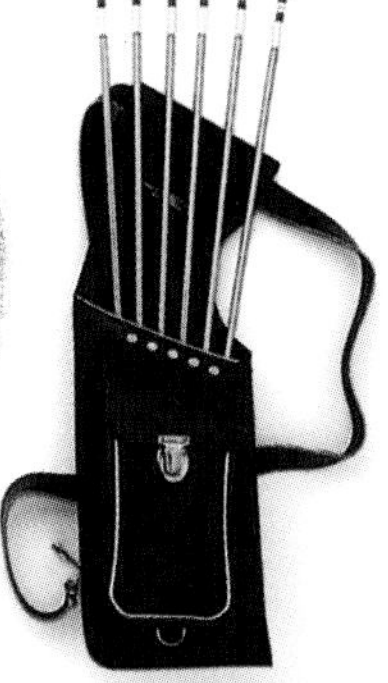

Archery target

TARGET SPORTS

Firing at targets began with archery, or bow-and-arrow practice, about 500 years ago. In modern archery, competitors shoot a series of arrows at a target from a range of distances. They score ten points for arrows that hit the centre, or bull, and get lower scores the closer the arrow is to the edge of the target. Another target sport is shooting, in which competitors fire rifles or pistols at targets.

COMBAT SPORTS

Modern combat sports originated in the fighting sports of Ancient Greece, although people wrestled for sport 15,000 years earlier. Various styles of unarmed combat evolved – boxing and wrestling in the West and jujitsu in the East. The martial arts, such as judo, karate, aikido, and tae kwon do, come from jujitsu.

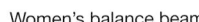

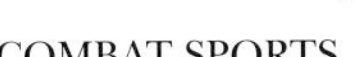

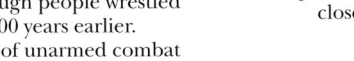

WHEEL SPORTS

Competitions on wheels include everything from roller-skating to Grand Prix automobile racing. Physical skill and fitness are most important in unpowered wheel sports such as skateboarding, cycling, and bicycle motocross.

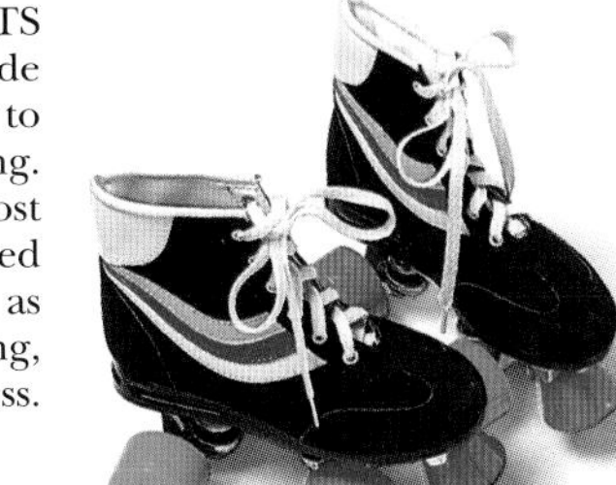

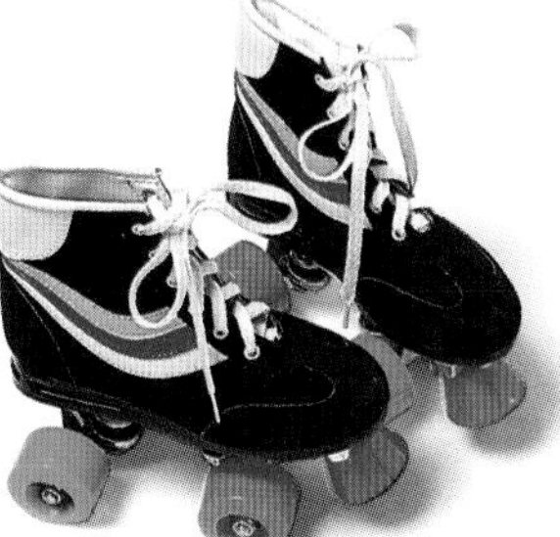

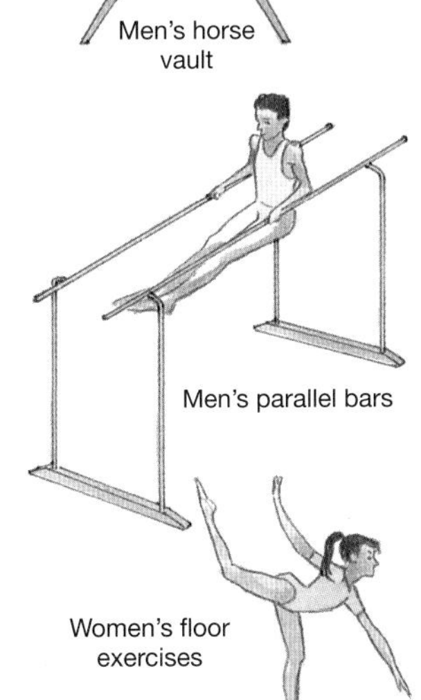

Men's parallel bars

Women's floor exercises

AIR SPORTS

Flying, gliding, and skydiving provide some of the greatest thrills in sport. Pilots race aeroplanes and, in aerobatics, perform manoeuvres. Glider, balloon, and hang glider pilots use warm air currents to move around without power. Skydiving parachutists "free fall" for thousands of metres, linking hands in formation before opening their parachutes to land safely.

In parasailing, a tow vehicle lifts the participant into the air with the aid of a special parachute.

ANIMAL SPORTS

Greyhounds, pigeons, camels, and sled dogs compete in races, but horse racing is the best-known animal sport. Horse racing takes place over jumps as well as on flat ground. In harness racing, the horse pulls its driver around a track in a two-wheeled "sulky", like the chariot of ancient times. Other horse sports include show jumping, eventing, dressage, and polo.

Find out more

ATHLETICS
BALL GAMES
CRICKET
FOOTBALL AND RUGBY
GAMES
OLYMPIC GAMES

STAMPS AND POSTAL SERVICES

MILLIONS OF LETTERS pass through the postal system each day. But even those posted to you from the other side of the world reach your home within only a few days. To accomplish this miracle, the postal system relies on a network of sorting offices. Every letter passes through several sorting processes at different offices. If you post a letter to a friend far away, workers from the post office first collect your letter from the postbox. Then they take it back to the sorting office and put it into a sack along with others destined for the same county or urban area. Vans, trains, or aeroplanes rush the sack to the correct destination, where more postal workers empty out the sack and sort the letters once more – this time by town, or by city district. Again, the post travels onwards to the local sorting office, then on to a neighbourhood office. There, postal workers sort the letters by street and by house before delivering them on foot or by van.

HILLTOP BEACONS
Fires carried messages long before there was a regular postal service. During the 16th century a chain of hilltop fires warned the British of the danger of a Spanish invasion. Watchers on each hilltop lit their beacon when they saw a flame on the horizon. The signal travelled from beacon to beacon faster than a messenger could ride on horseback.

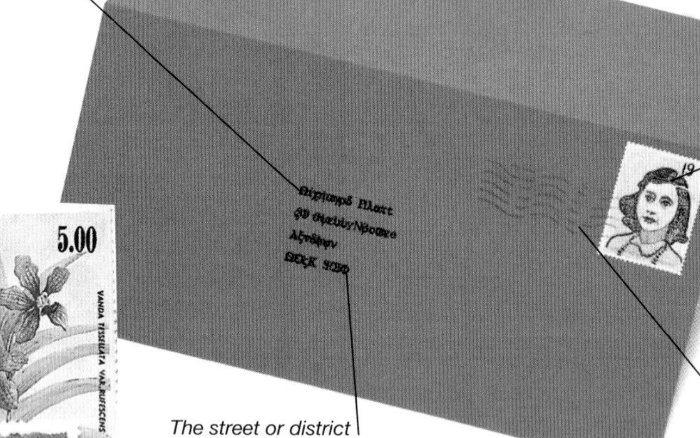

The name and address must be easy for the postal worker to read.

Stamps are always placed in the top right-hand corner.

Cancellation with a postmark means a stamp cannot be re-used.

The street or district address is shown in the form of a postcode.

The weight of mail and the speed of its delivery determine the price of postage.

Parcels and packages still need to be sorted by hand.

STAMPS

The first postage stamps appeared in Britain in 1840. They were prepaid; postage cost one penny regardless of how far the letter had to travel. In 1847 the United States also started producing stamps, and other countries soon followed. Today, every country produces stamps in a range of prices, often using the illustrations to commemorate national events and famous citizens.

SORTING SYSTEM
The use of machines has made the task of sorting mail much quicker and easier. Machines read and postmark the stamps so they cannot be used again. A keyboard operator translates the postal codes into a series of phosphor dots that can be sorted automatically. A modern sorting system can deal with 350,000 letters per hour.

PONY EXPRESS

In 1860 in the United States, the Pony Express company introduced a fast postal service between Missouri and California. Stagecoach post took six weeks, but the relays of riders employed by the Pony Express cut this to eight days, with each rider covering up to 120 km (75 miles) a day. There were 80 riders. One of them was 14-year-old William Cody, later famous as Buffalo Bill. The service was short-lived and was soon replaced by the telegraph.

Find out more

TRADE AND INDUSTRY
TRANSPORT, HISTORY OF

STARFISH AND SEA URCHINS

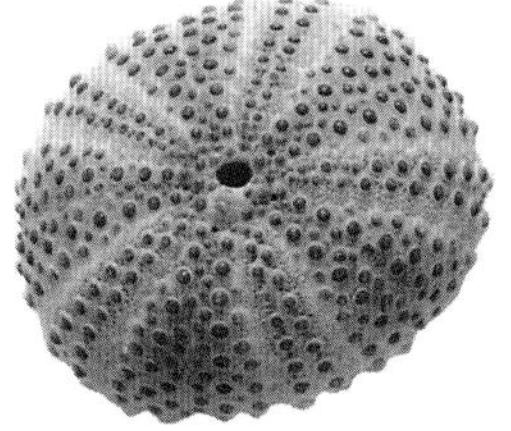

A sea urchin's shell is also known as a test. This one has lost all its spines.

THE SEABED PROVIDES HOMES for many spiny-skinned creatures including starfish, sea urchins, and brittle stars. Starfish range in size from 8 cm (3 in) to 1 m (3 ft) across, and have a central body from which five arms radiate outwards. The sea urchin looks like a starfish whose arms have curled upwards and joined at the top to make a ball shape. Sea urchins have a hard outer skeleton covered with long spines. Starfish usually have short spines, like little bumps on the skin. Sea urchins graze on tiny animals and plants from rocks and the seabed, and starfish feed on corals and shellfish. Both animals move using tubes inside the body which pump water in and out of hundreds of "tube feet". These tube feet lengthen and bend under the pressure of the water, propelling the creature along. Each tube foot has a sucker on the end. Using these suckers, a sea urchin can move up a vertical rock, and a starfish can prise open a shellfish and eat the flesh inside.

FEEDING
The common starfish uses its arms to force open shellfish, then turns its stomach inside out, onto the prey, to digest its flesh.

INSIDE A STARFISH
The central part of a starfish contains a stomach, with the mouth below and the anus above. Branches of the nerves, stomach, and water canals go into each arm.

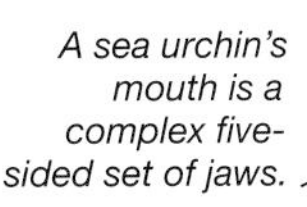

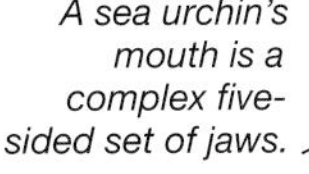

A sea urchin's mouth is a complex five-sided set of jaws.

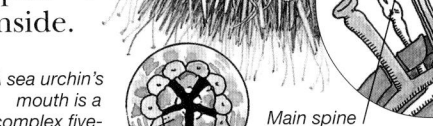

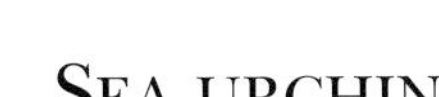

SEA POTATO
Sea urchins such as sea potatoes burrow in sand with their flattened spines. Their tube feet are shaped at the tips for passing food to the mouth. An extra long tube foot reaches the surface of the sand like a periscope, so that the sea urchin can breathe. There is another tube foot for passing out waste products.

SEA URCHIN

A sea urchin has long spines for defence, and between them wave the tube feet with suckers on the end. Some tube feet bear tiny pincers for clinging on to prey. These are called pedicellariae. In some urchins the pedicellariae are surrounded by venom sacs that are full of poison.

GROWING NEW ARMS
Most starfish can grow new body parts, particularly arms, if the old ones are broken or bitten off. This means they can leave an arm behind to escape from a predator. A new arm grows within a few weeks.

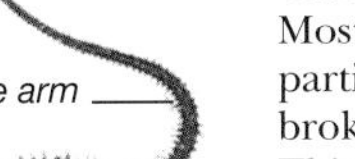

BRITTLE STAR
The brittle star shown here feeds by trapping food on its slimy mucus-covered arms. It pushes the food towards the mouth with its tube feet. This starfish moves by "rowing" with its arms, and is called a brittle star because its long, slim arms break off easily.

CROWN-OF-THORNS STARFISH
These large, prickly starfish eat living coral, and they have severely damaged many coral reefs, including Australia's Great Barrier Reef. Covered with razor-sharp poisonous spines, crown-of-thorns starfish attack coral reefs from Kenya to Tahiti.

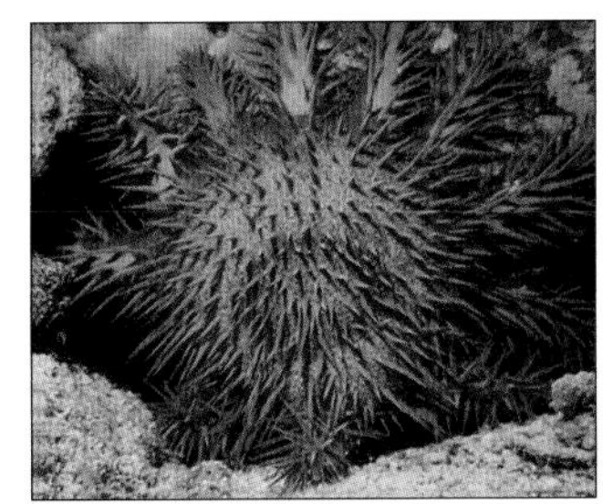

The crown-of-thorns has more than a dozen arms covered with poisonous spines.

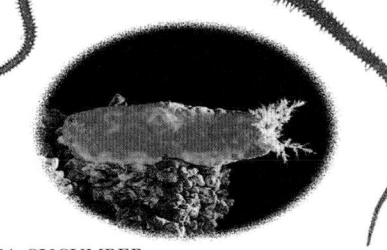

SEA CUCUMBER
This curious sea creature lies on its side looking like a cucumber. Feathery tentacles around the mouth gather tiny food particles from the water.

Find out more
ANIMALS
DEEP-SEA WILDLIFE
SEASHORE WILDLIFE

STARS

IF YOU LOOK UP AT THE SKY ON A CLEAR night, it is possible to see about 3,000 of the billions of stars in our galaxy. Although they appear as tiny dots, they are, like our closest star the Sun, huge, hot balls of gas, deep in space. Some stars are gigantic – if placed in the centre of our solar system, they would stretch beyond the Earth's orbit. Others are far smaller, about the size of our planet, and give off only faint light. Stars are unimaginably distant; so distant, in fact, that light from our nearest star (apart from the Sun) takes more than four years to reach us.

Ancient skywatchers noticed that stars seem to form patterns in the sky. They imagined that the shapes represented pictures called constellations. These constellations, such as the Great Bear, are still useful for learning the positions of the stars. Astronomers identify the brightest individual stars according to their constellation and with Greek letters such as alpha, beta, and gamma (which stand for A, B, and C). For instance, the second brightest star in the constellation of Centaurus (the Centaur) is called Beta Centauri.

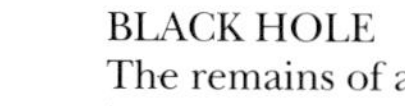

BLACK HOLE
The remains of a very massive star may collapse into a tiny volume, forming a black hole. The gravitational pull of a black hole is so strong that matter and radiation, such as light, cannot escape from it.

NEUTRON STAR
A supernova may leave a neutron star – a spinning ball with a mass greater than the Sun's, yet only about 16 km (10 miles) across. As a neutron star spins, it sends out a powerful beam of radiation.

SUPERNOVA
When a massive star dies, it collapses in less than one second. This is followed by a colossal explosion called a supernova. The explosion produces other substances which scatter through space in an expanding gas cloud.

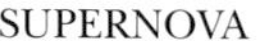

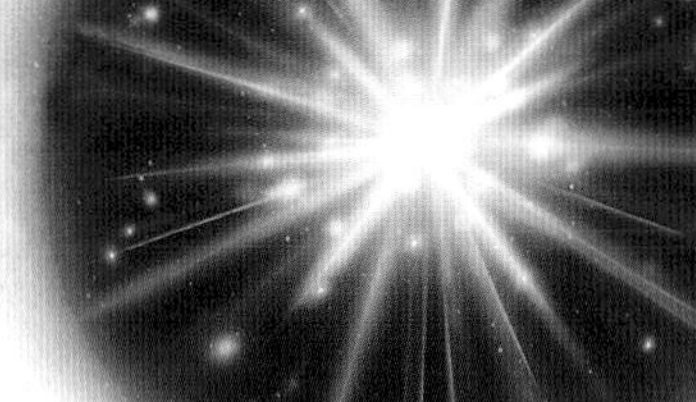

RED SUPERGIANT
Some dying stars grow into huge, cool stars called red supergiants, which can be up to 1,000 times the diameter of the Sun. A red supergiant contains many substances formed by nuclear reactions.

A group of growing stars in a cluster.
The gas and dust in a mini-globule pack closer together, and it spins faster and gets hotter. The mini-globule has become a protostar (a young star).
Death of a massive star
Temperature at centre of red supergiant is about 10 billion°C (18 billion°F).
Death of a star about the size of the Sun
The planetary nebula survives only for a few thousand years.
White dwarf

STAR STARTS TO SHINE
When the centre of the protostar reaches about 10 million°C (18 million°F), nuclear reactions begin which slowly change hydrogen into helium. The protostar begins to shine, and has become a true star.

NEBULA
Stars are born from great clouds of dust particles and hydrogen gas, called nebulae. The word nebula (plural nebulae) comes from the Latin for "mist".

BIRTH OF A STAR
Gravity pulls parts of a nebula into blobs called globules. These get smaller and spin faster, finally breaking up into a few hundred "mini-globules". Each of these will eventually become a star.

RED GIANT
As a sunlike star runs low in hydrogen, it swells into a cooler, larger star called a red giant. This will happen to our own Sun in about 5,000 million years.

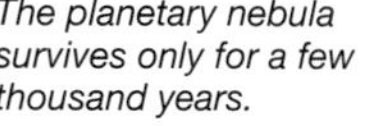

LIFE AND DEATH OF A STAR

Throughout the universe, new stars form and old stars die. The birthplaces of stars are clouds of gas and dust scattered through space. Stars the size of the Sun shine for about 10 billion years. The most massive stars (which contain 100 times as much matter as the Sun) shine very brightly, but live for a shorter time – only about 10 million years.

PLANETARY NEBULA
At the end of its life, a red giant blows off its outer layers of gas. These make a glowing shell called a planetary nebula, which eventually disperses. At the centre is a white dwarf, a tiny hot star that is the burned out core of the red giant. It will outlast the nebula by billions of years.

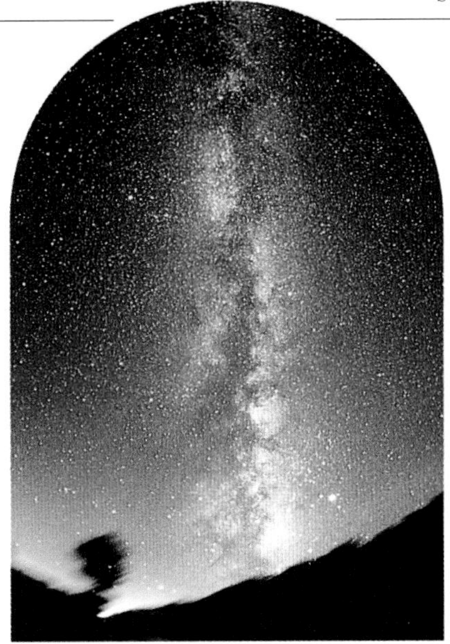

TWINKLING STARLIGHT
Nuclear reactions inside a star heat the star up from the centre, causing it to emit light and heat from its surface. A star appears to flicker or twinkle because its light passes through the Earth's atmosphere, which is a constantly shifting blanket of gases. Seen from a travelling spacecraft, stars shine steadily because there is no surrounding atmosphere to disturb the path of the light.

CONSTELLATIONS

Modern astronomers group stars into 88 constellations. Each has a Latin name, such as Ursa Major (the Great Bear) or Corona Australis (the Southern Crown). The "sun signs" of astrology have the same names as the 12 constellations of the zodiac – the band of sky along which the Sun and planets appear to pass during the course of a year.

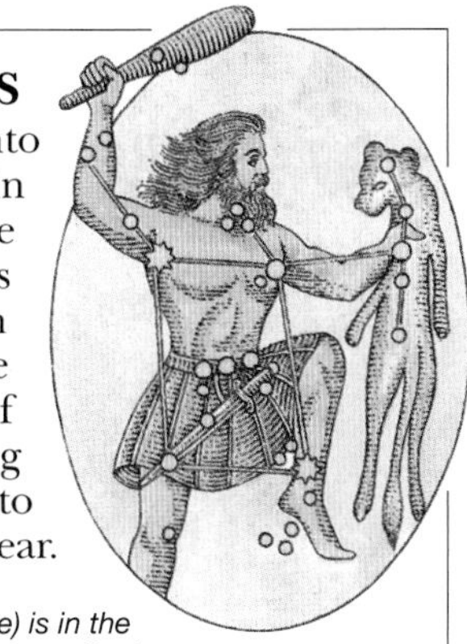

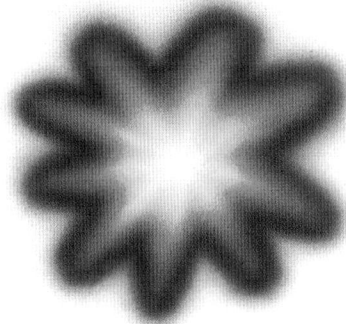

When the constellation of Orion (above) is in the night sky, it can be seen from anywhere on Earth.

WHITE DWARF
At the end of its life, a sunlike star shrinks to about the size of the Earth, forming a white dwarf. A white dwarf is intensely hot, but because it is so small it is very faint.

BLACK DWARF
After perhaps thousands of millions of years, a white dwarf will cool to become a dark, cold, black dwarf. However, no black dwarf has ever been observed because there may not yet have been enough time since the creation of our galaxy for one to appear.

PARALLAX

Astronomers use a technique called parallax to measure the distance of a star from the Earth. As the Earth moves around the Sun, the closest stars seem to move very slightly compared with stars further away. Astronomers measure the position of a star once, and then again six months later. From their measurements they can then calculate the distance of a star.

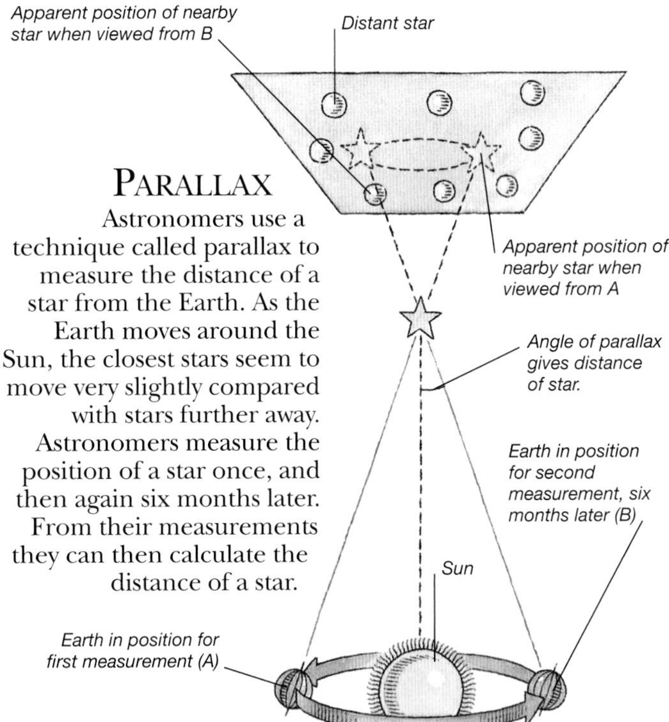

VARIABLE STARS

Many stars, called variable stars, appear to vary in brightness. Some stars constantly swell and shrink, becoming alternately fainter and brighter. Other variables are really two stars that circle each other and block off each other's light from time to time.

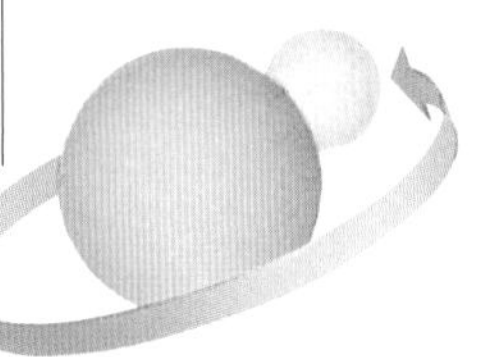

Double stars circle around each other. When one star is in front of the other, the brightness dims. When both stars can be seen, the brightness increases.

Some variable stars are produced by exploding stars. The explosion makes the star appear much brighter than usual for a period that can last from a few days to a few years.

STAR QUALITIES

The colour of a star's light corresponds to the surface temperature of the star: red stars are the coolest, blue stars are the hottest. A star's brightness (the amount of energy it gives out) is linked to its mass (the amount of material it contains): heavier stars are brighter than lighter stars. Astronomers can use the colour and brightness of the light emitted from a star to help calculate its size and distance from the Earth.

Neutron stars (pulsars) are the smallest stars. They have about the same mass as the Sun, but are only about 16 km (10 miles) in diameter.

White dwarfs are small stars at the end of their life; some are smaller than the Earth.

Yellow dwarfs, or medium-sized stars, are about the same size as the Sun.

Giants have diameters between 100 and 1,000 times larger than that of the Sun.

Supergiants are the largest stars, with diameters up to 1,000 times that of the Sun.

Find out more
ASTRONOMY
BLACK HOLES
GRAVITY
NAVIGATION
PLANETS
SUN
TELESCOPES
UNIVERSE

STATISTICS

THE WORD STATISTICS has two meanings. Firstly, statistics are actual data, or facts, that are given as numbers – for instance, how many children there are in a class, how often it rains every year, or how much money is raised through taxes. Secondly, statistics is the way in which statisticians, people who work with statistics, analyse or interpret numerical data in order to understand and use it. For instance, by analysing data such as annual rainfall, statisticians can work out averages and percentages, and forecast how much rain may fall in the future, which could be useful for farmers, or people planning holidays. Statistics is a science, and a branch of mathematics. Governments, industry, and planners of all kinds use statistics.

COLLECTING DATA
Before statistics can analysed, data must be collected. If statistics are about people, the data can be collected through interviews or by asking people to fill in questionnaires (written questions). People being questioned may belong to a particular group or may be chosen at random. They may answer in words or by ticking a box, but all answers must be converted into numerical data.

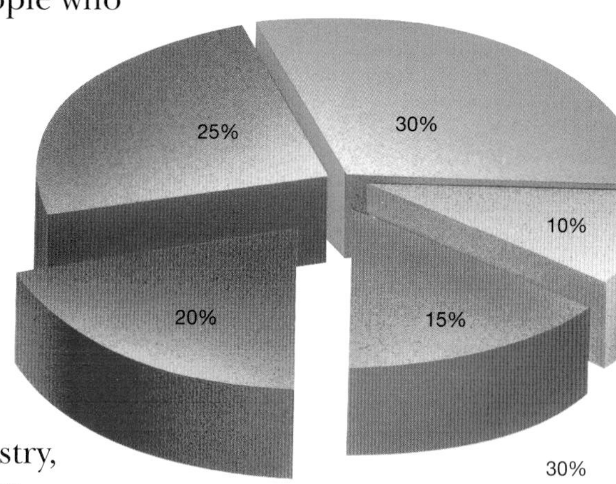

Pie chart

30%
25%
20%
15%
10%
Bar chart

PIE AND BAR CHARTS
Statistical information can be shown as tables of data, but these can be difficult to read. An easier way is to show the information on a pie chart or a bar chart. Pie charts look like pies with slices cut out. Bar charts show information as columns, or bars, of different heights.

CENSUS

One way of gathering statistical information about people is to hold a census. A census is an official survey or examination of a country's population carried out by its government. A census counts the number of people in the country, as well as asking about people's age, income, and gender. The first modern census was in the USA in 1790. The first British census was in 1801.

Some Victorian school-children were shown how to fill in a census form, because their parents could not read.

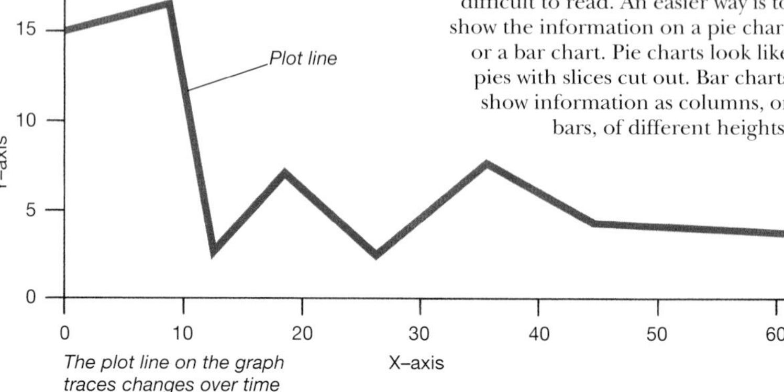

The plot line on the graph traces changes over time

GRAPHS
Like charts, graphs show statistical data in a way that is easy to understand. The vertical line, called the Y-axis, is marked to show one kind of information, for example numbers of things, people, or events. The horizontal line, or X-axis, is marked to show a different kind of information, for example, periods of time. The plot line shows at a glance what is happening.

AVERAGES

An average is a quantity that is typical of a certain group or set. It is not a guess; it is worked out mathematically by adding all the figures together and then dividing the total by the number of figures in the set. The average height of five people, for example, can be found by adding their heights together and then dividing the total by five.

The child in the centre represents the average height for this set of five children.

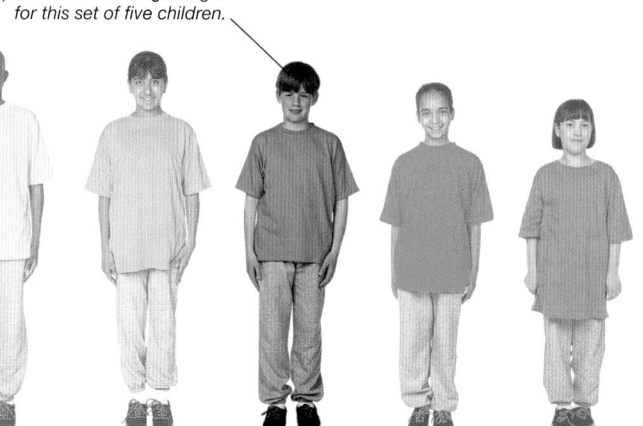

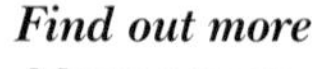

Find out more
MATHEMATICS
NUMBERS
SCIENCE

STATUE OF LIBERTY

ON A BRONZE PLAQUE inside the base of the Statue of Liberty are the words of a poem written by Emma Lazarus in 1883. Part of it reads: "Give me your tired, your poor,/ Your huddled masses yearning to breathe free./ The wretched refuse of your teeming shore./ Send these, the homeless, tempest-tost to me./ I lift my lamp beside the golden door!" The "masses" were the people fleeing poverty and oppression in Europe; the "golden door", the opportunity to start a new life in the United States. The French historian Edouard de Laboulaye planned the statue in 1865 to symbolize liberty and to commemorate the friendship of France with the United States. It was designed by Frédéric Auguste Bartholdi and built by Alexandre Gustave Eiffel, whose famous Eiffel Tower dominates the skyline of Paris.

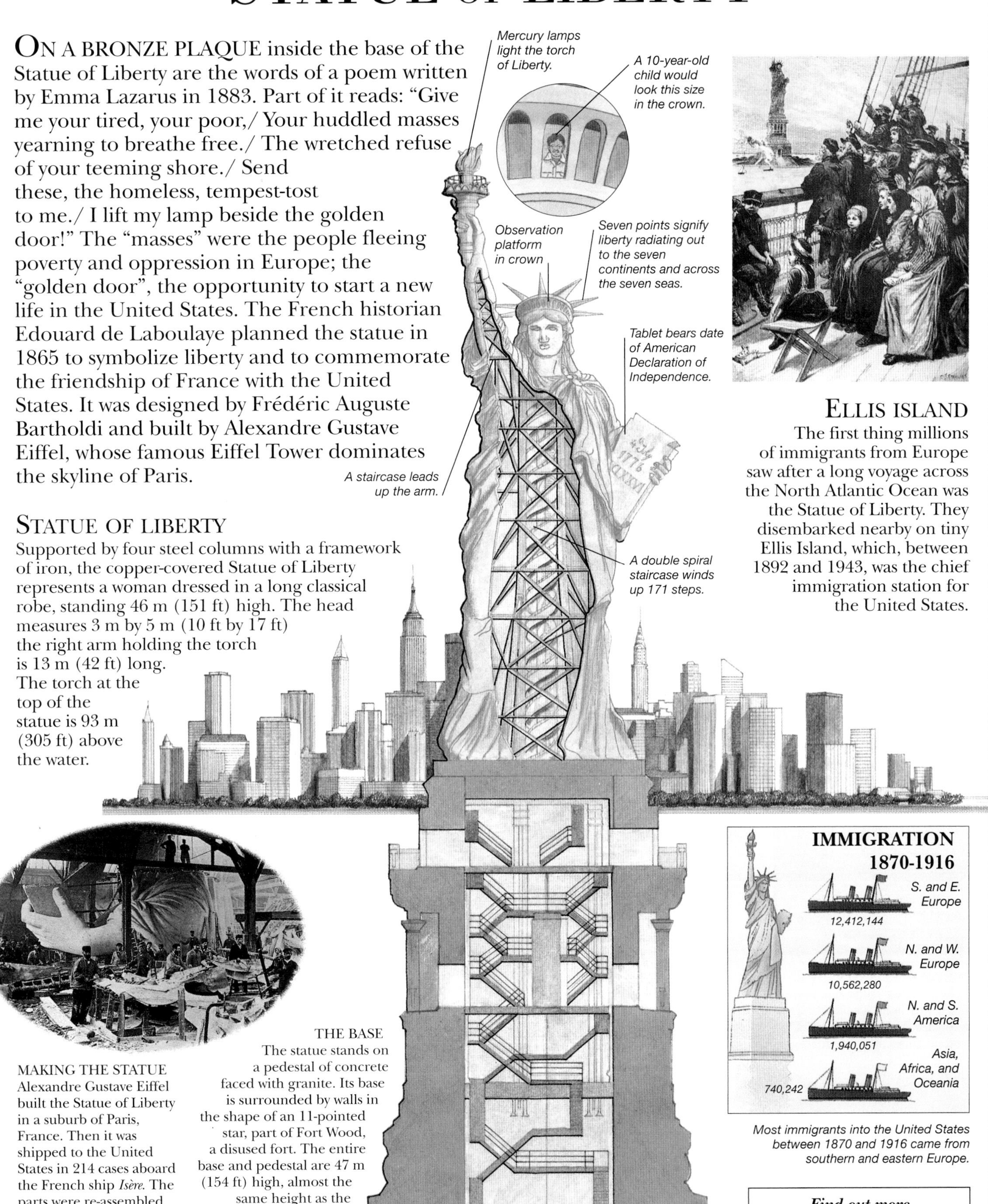

Mercury lamps light the torch of Liberty.
A 10-year-old child would look this size in the crown.
Observation platform in crown
Seven points signify liberty radiating out to the seven continents and across the seven seas.
Tablet bears date of American Declaration of Independence.
A staircase leads up the arm.
A double spiral staircase winds up 171 steps.
Visitors enter here and take a lift to the base of the statue.

STATUE OF LIBERTY

Supported by four steel columns with a framework of iron, the copper-covered Statue of Liberty represents a woman dressed in a long classical robe, standing 46 m (151 ft) high. The head measures 3 m by 5 m (10 ft by 17 ft) the right arm holding the torch is 13 m (42 ft) long. The torch at the top of the statue is 93 m (305 ft) above the water.

ELLIS ISLAND

The first thing millions of immigrants from Europe saw after a long voyage across the North Atlantic Ocean was the Statue of Liberty. They disembarked nearby on tiny Ellis Island, which, between 1892 and 1943, was the chief immigration station for the United States.

MAKING THE STATUE

Alexandre Gustave Eiffel built the Statue of Liberty in a suburb of Paris, France. Then it was shipped to the United States in 214 cases aboard the French ship *Isère*. The parts were re-assembled in New York.

THE BASE

The statue stands on a pedestal of concrete faced with granite. Its base is surrounded by walls in the shape of an 11-pointed star, part of Fort Wood, a disused fort. The entire base and pedestal are 47 m (154 ft) high, almost the same height as the statue itself.

IMMIGRATION 1870-1916

Region	Immigrants
S. and E. Europe	12,412,144
N. and W. Europe	10,562,280
N. and S. America	1,940,051
Asia, Africa, and Oceania	740,242

Most immigrants into the United States between 1870 and 1916 came from southern and eastern Europe.

Find out more

UNITED STATES OF AMERICA, history of

Stock exchange

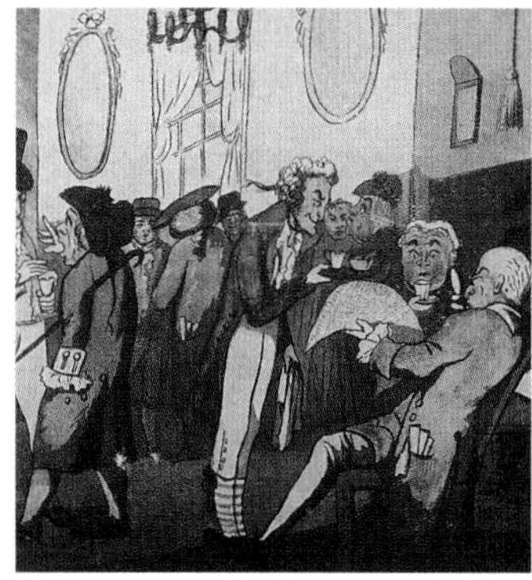

COFFEE HOUSE EXCHANGE
In 1760, Jonathan's Coffee House was the first home of what would become the modern London stock exchange. Brokers met there to buy and sell shares. In 1773, it changed its name to the Stock Exchange. The London Stock Exchange is now one of the biggest in the world.

A STOCK EXCHANGE IS A MARKET where stocks and shares are bought and sold. The public is not allowed into a stock exchange. Buying and selling is done by special traders called brokers. If ordinary people want to buy or sell shares, they have to pay brokers to do it for them. A stock or a share is a certificate to show that you have invested – paid for a part-ownership – in a company. Most companies sell shares to bring in money so they can expand their business. People buy shares because they can make money by waiting until the shares go up in value and then selling them. Sometimes this only takes a few hours. The first exchange in Europe was founded in 1531 in Antwerp, Belgium. In the USA, the New York Stock Exchange was set up in 1792 on Wall Street, where brokers originally met under a buttonwood tree. Today, the world's most important stock exchanges are in Tokyo, Hong Kong, London, and New York.

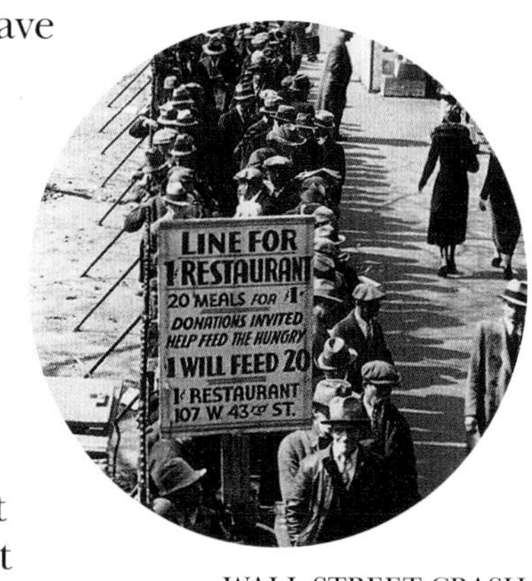

WALL STREET CRASH
In 1929, shares in many American companies fell in price all at once. The stock market could not work. This was known as the Wall Street Crash. Companies closed, and millions lost their jobs.

Share trading

In a traditional stock exchange, traders worked in areas called "pits". Each pit dealt in shares in a particular sort of company. Brokers outside the pits sent messages to those inside to buy or sell shares on instructions from their customers. Today, many exchanges, such as the one in London, buy and sell by telephone, e-mail, and computer.

Traders on the New York Stock Exchange buy and sell for their customers.

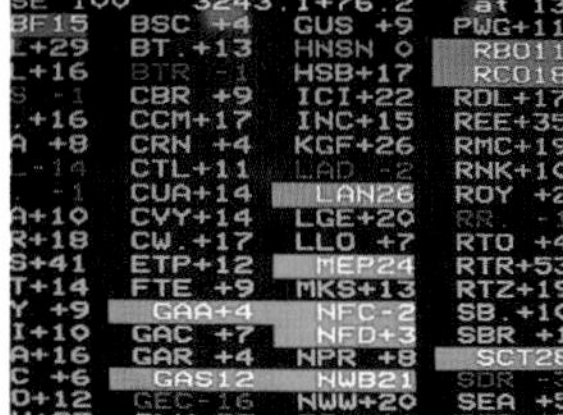

INDICATORS AND INDEXES
Inside a stock exchange, huge electronic boards called indicators show the prices of shares. To see how the market is doing at a glance, the share prices are added up and an average, called an index, is worked out. The index is given in points, not money. It can go up and down daily. Falling markets are called "bear" markets; rising markets are known as "bull" markets.

CHECKING INVESTMENTS
Information technology has made it quicker and easier for everybody to buy shares. Some people are given shares in the company they work for as part of their earnings. Anybody can find out how their shares are doing by looking at the lists of share prices published daily in financial newspapers.

Oranges for juice

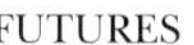

FUTURES
A future is a contract to buy shares in something for an agreed price at a set time in the future. For example, you buy "futures" in next year's harvest of coffee beans or oranges. If the price goes higher than the one you agreed, you make money because you still pay the agreed price; but if it goes lower, you lose money.

Coffee beans

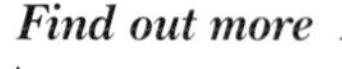

Find out more
ASIA, HISTORY OF
MONEY
SHOPS AND SHOPPING
TRADE AND INDUSTRY

Stone Age

More than two million years ago, stone was the most valuable raw material known to people. They made stone tools and weapons, usually from flint. These early people were called hominids, and were more apelike than us. They gradually learned to make specialized implements, such as knife blades. Stone Age people moved constantly, looking for hunting areas and setting up camps in small groups. A few groups lived in caves during the coldest seasons. They gathered fruits, berries, and roots, and hunted wild animals. By the start of the Mesolithic Age (Middle Stone Age; 10,000 years ago) many types of larger animals had died out. Mesolithic people, who were "modern people" (*Homo sapiens*) like us, used new stone-edged tools to fish and hunt deer and wild pigs. About 5,000 years ago some Neolithic (New Stone) Age people learned how to domesticate animals and grow crops. They settled on farms.

c. 2,500,000 B.C. Palaeolithic Age begins.

c. 2,000,000 B.C. Hominids make the first stone tools.

c. 1,500,000 B.C. First hand axe.

c. 125,000 B.C. Ice Age retreats; people return to Europe, hunt large animals.

c. 75,000 B.C. People use fire and bury their dead.

c. 20,000 B.C. Spear thrower invented. Also harpoon, bow and arrows, sewing, and cave painting.

c. 8300 B.C. Mesolithic Age.

c. 6500 B.C. Neolithic Age.

c. 3000 B.C. Metal tools and weapons replace stone.

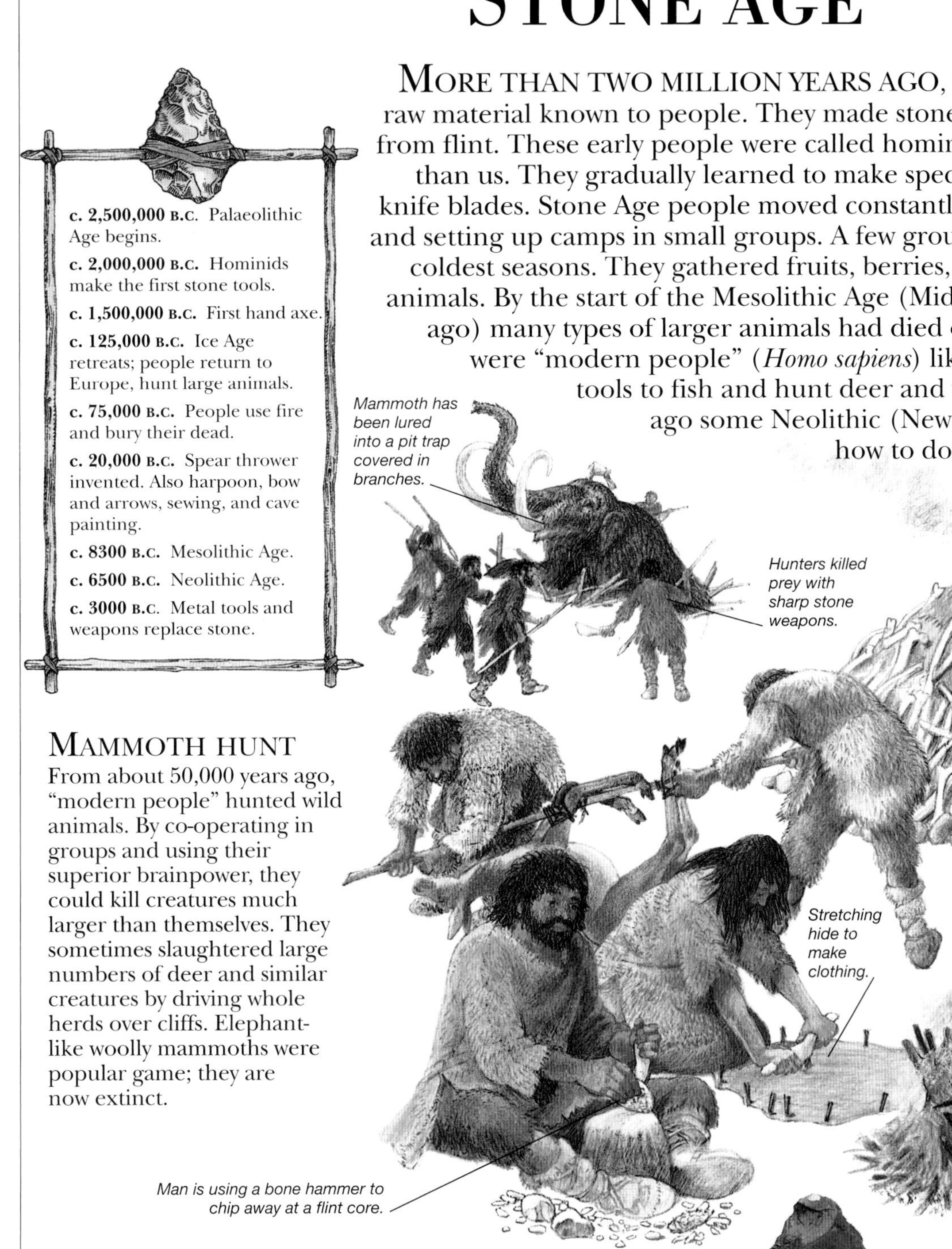

Mammoth has been lured into a pit trap covered in branches.
Hunters killed prey with sharp stone weapons.
Dwelling places made from animal hides and mammoth bones kept out the cold wind.
Woman cooks a hare on a spit over the fire.
Stretching hide to make clothing.
Man is using a bone hammer to chip away at a flint core.

Mammoth hunt

From about 50,000 years ago, "modern people" hunted wild animals. By co-operating in groups and using their superior brainpower, they could kill creatures much larger than themselves. They sometimes slaughtered large numbers of deer and similar creatures by driving whole herds over cliffs. Elephant-like woolly mammoths were popular game; they are now extinct.

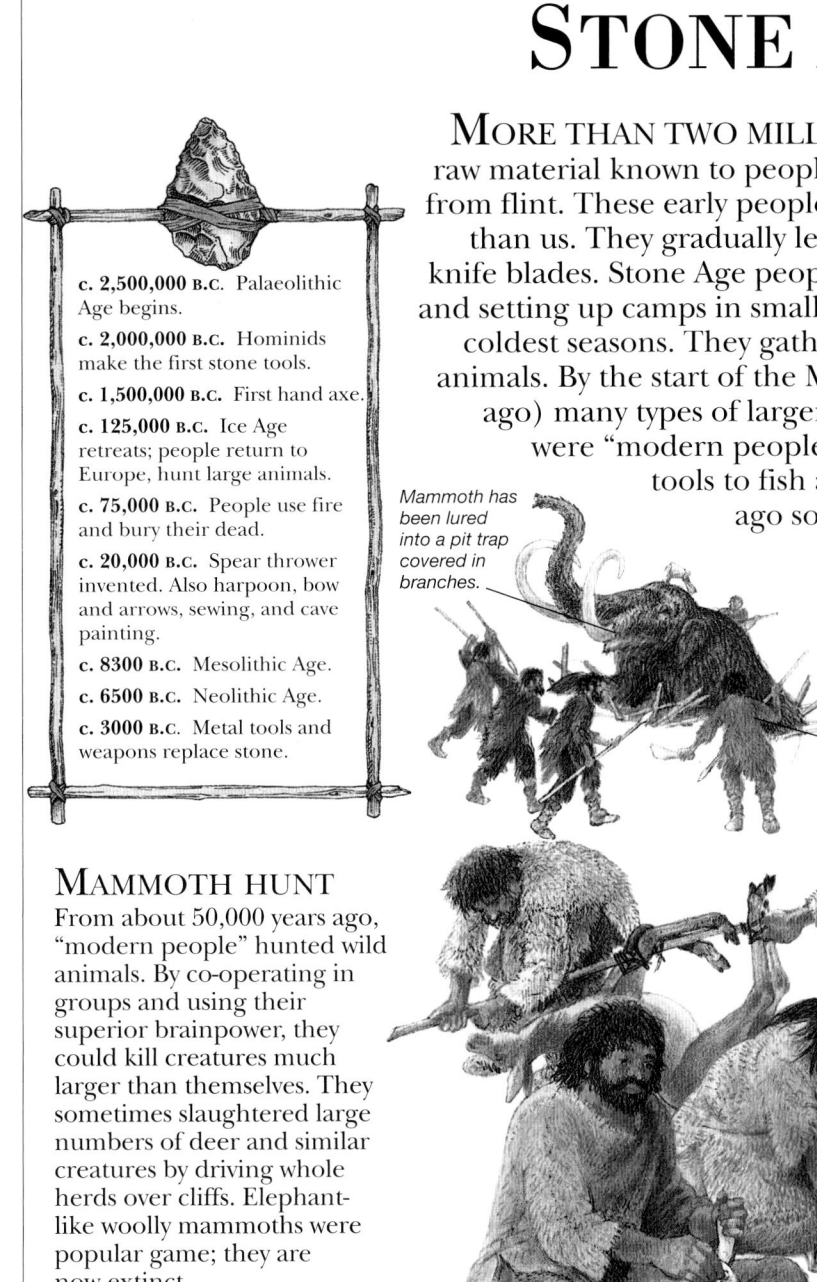

MAKING FLINT TOOLS AND WEAPONS

1 The first flint implements were crude. People used the sharp edge of a broken rock as a cutting tool.

2 Later tools were much better. The toolmaker prepared a flint core by skillful chipping.

3 Hitting the core with a bone hammer made flakes, each one a special tool.

HAND AXE

The hand axe was the first deliberately shaped tool made by humans. It was gripped at the rounded end and used to cut meat or dig roots. Popular for over a million years, it was used longer than any other tool.

This flint hand axe was found in a desert area near Thebes, Egypt.

Find out more

Archaeology
Britain, ancient
Evolution
Prehistoric peoples

STORMS

TORNADOES

The most violent storms are tornadoes, or whirlwinds. A twisting column of rising air forms beneath a thunder cloud, sometimes producing winds of 400 km/h (250 mph). The air pressure at the centre is very low, which can cause buildings to explode. A waterspout is a tornado over water, formed when water is sucked up into the funnel of air. Dust devils are tornadoes which have sucked up sand over the desert.

ABOUT 2,000 thunderstorms are raging throughout the world at this very moment, and lightning has struck about 500 times since you started reading this page. Storms have enormous power: the energy in a hurricane could illuminate more light bulbs than there are in the United States. A storm is basically a very strong wind. Severe storms such as thunderstorms, hurricanes, and tornadoes all contain their own strong wind system and blow along as a whole. Certain areas, such as the region around the Gulf of Mexico, are hit regularly by severe storms because of the local conditions. Storms can cause great damage because of the force of the wind and the devastating power of the rain, snow, sand, or dust which they carry along. One of the most destructive forces of a hurricane is a storm surge. The level of the sea rises because of a rapid drop in air pressure at the centre of the storm. This rise combines with the effect of the wind on the sea to create a huge wall of water which causes terrible damage if it hits the coast.

Severe storms build up as moist air, heated by warm land or sea, rises. Storm clouds develop as the rising air cools and rain forms. Air rushes in to replace the rising air, and strong winds begin to blow.

The base of the tornado is fairly narrow – about 1.5 km (1 mile) across.

The rising air spirals up the column, sucking up dirt and objects as heavy as trucks from the ground.

DESTRUCTION AND DEVASTATION
Winds of 320 km/h (200 mph) leave a trail of destruction (below) when the hurricane strikes the shore. The strongest winds are in a belt around the calm eye.

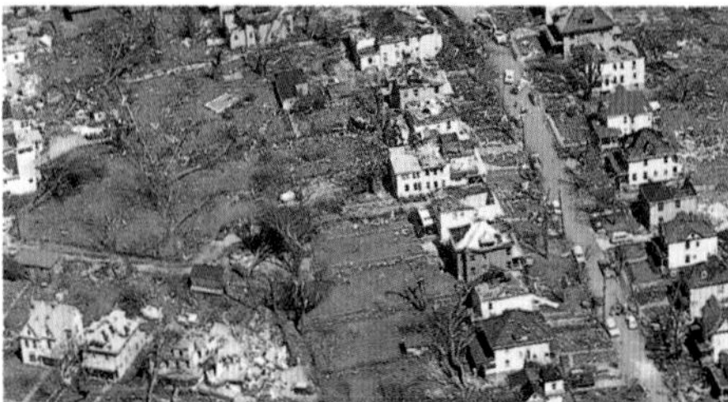

THUNDER AND LIGHTNING

Thunder clouds often form on hot, humid days. Strong air currents in the cloud cause raindrops and hailstones to collide, producing electric charges. Lightning flashes in giant sparks between the charges, and often leaps to the ground. A burst of heat from the flash makes the air nearby expand violently and produces a clap of thunder.

Negative charges in the bottom of the cloud attract positive charges in the ground. Eventually, a huge spark of lightning leaps from the cloud to the highest point on the ground.

Buildings are protected by lightning rods – strips of metal on the roof which attract the lightning and lead the electricity safely to the ground.

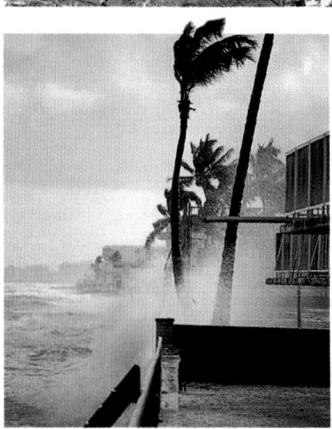

HURRICANES

When warm, moist air spirals upward above tropical oceans, it forms a hurricane – a violent storm which is also called a typhoon or a cyclone. The spin of the Earth causes the storm winds to circle around a calm centre called the eye. The eye usually moves along at about 25 km/h (15 mph). It can measure as much as 800 km (500 miles) across.

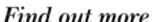

Find out more
CLIMATES
RAIN AND SNOW
WEATHER
WIND

STUARTS

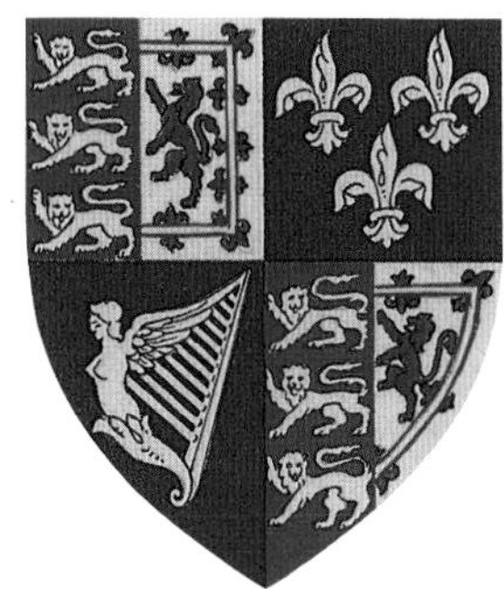

COAT OF ARMS
The Stuart coat of arms included the English and Scottish lions, the Irish harp, and the French fleur-de-lys.

IN 1603, THE LAST TUDOR MONARCH – Elizabeth I – died without leaving an heir. Her cousin, James Stuart, already James VI of Scotland, took over the English throne as well, becoming James I of England. The Stuarts united England and Scotland peacefully, but there were deep differences between King and Parliament over the power of the monarch. In 1642, these differences led to civil war. James I's son, Charles I, was executed, and England became a republic under Cromwell. In 1660, the Stuarts were restored (brought back to power) under Charles II. However, when his Catholic brother James II came to the throne in 1685, people resented his religion and his harsh laws. He was banished to Scotland and his son-in law, the Protestant William of Orange, became king. The last Stuart was Queen Anne, James II's second daughter.

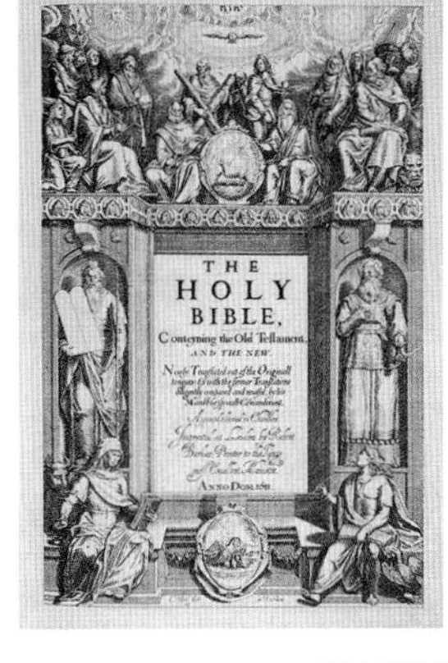

JAMES I
A vain man, James I believed God had made him ruler, and he ignored Parliament for much of his reign. Instead, he relied on the advice of favourites, and this weakened his government. However, James did achieve peace with Spain, England's old enemy. He also ordered an important new English translation of the Bible.

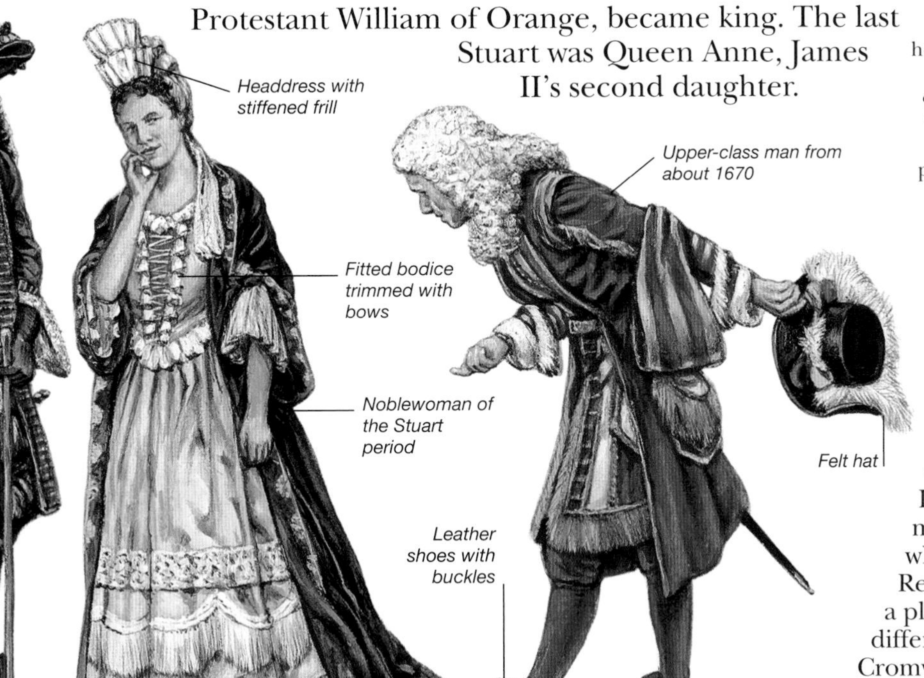

RESTORATION

After Oliver Cromwell's death, parliamentary leader George Monck (1608-70) negotiated with the exiled Charles II, and Britain became a monarchy again. During what historians call the Restoration, Charles II led a pleasure-seeking life, quite different to the Puritanism of Cromwell and his followers.

STUARTS

1603-25 Reign of James I.

1605 Gunpowder Plotters try to blow up parliament.

1625-49 Reign of Charles I.

1642-49 English Civil War.

1649-60 England becomes a republic.

1660 Monarchy restored.

1660-85 Reign of Charles II.

1666 Great Fire of London.

1685-88 Reign of James II.

1688 "Glorious Revolution" brings William of Orange to Britain.

1689-1702 Reign of William and Mary.

1702-14 Queen Anne rules, the last of the Stuart dynasty.

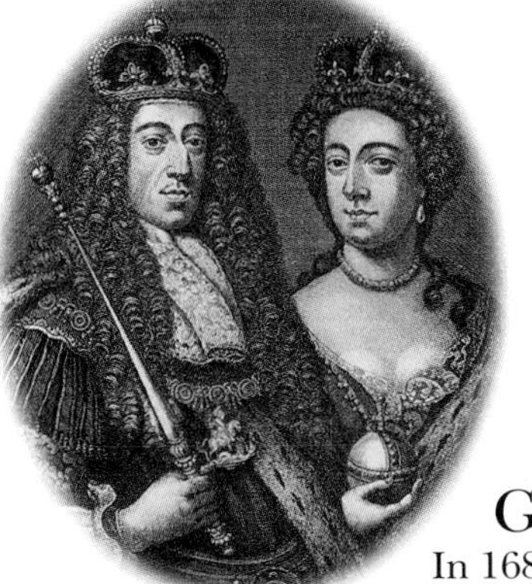

QUEEN ANNE
The last Stuart ruler was Queen Anne (1665-1714),She had a troubled life, and her reign was also difficult, as England waged a long war against France. However, British forces under John Churchill, Duke of Marlborough, gained victories which made England more powerful overseas. The decorative arts, such as furniture-making, flourished during Anne's reign.

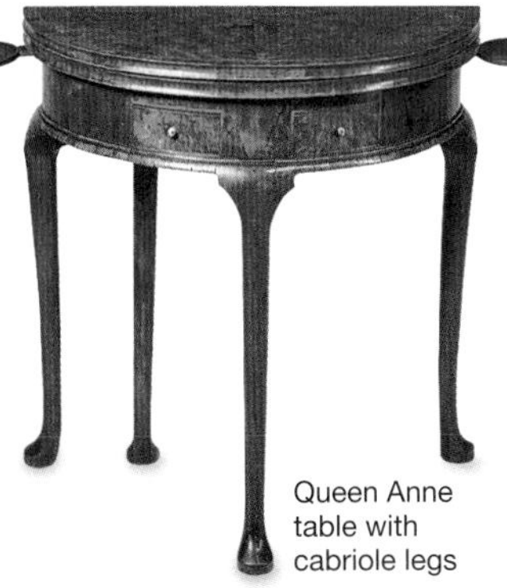

Queen Anne table with cabriole legs

GLORIOUS REVOLUTION

In 1688, British leaders opposed to James II's Catholicism, invited Protestant Dutch King William of Orange to rule Britain. William, who reigned jointly with his wife, Mary, agreed a Bill of Rights forbidding the introduction of laws or taxes without Parliament's approval. Known as the "Glorious Revolution", this marked the start of modern constitutional monarchy, by which Parliament has greater powers than the king or queen.

Find out more
ENGLISH CIVIL WAR
CROMWELL, OLIVER
FIRE OF LONDON
GUNPOWDER PLOT

SUBMARINES

THE GREAT POWER of a submarine lies in its ability to remain hidden. It can travel unseen beneath the waves, carrying its deadly cargo of missiles and torpedoes, and remain underwater for months at a time. However, the submarine had humble beginnings; legend states that during the siege of Tyre (Lebanon) in 332 B.C., Alexander the Great attacked the inhabitants from a submerged glass barrel. Aided by the invention of the electric motor for underwater propulsion and the torpedo for attacking ships, modern submarines developed into powerful weapons during the two world wars of the 20th century. Today's submarines are powered either by a combination of diesel and electric motors or by nuclear-powered engines. There are two main types: patrol submarines, which aim to seek and destroy ships and other submarines, and missile-carrying submarines. Small submarines called submersibles are used mainly for non-military purposes, such as marine research.

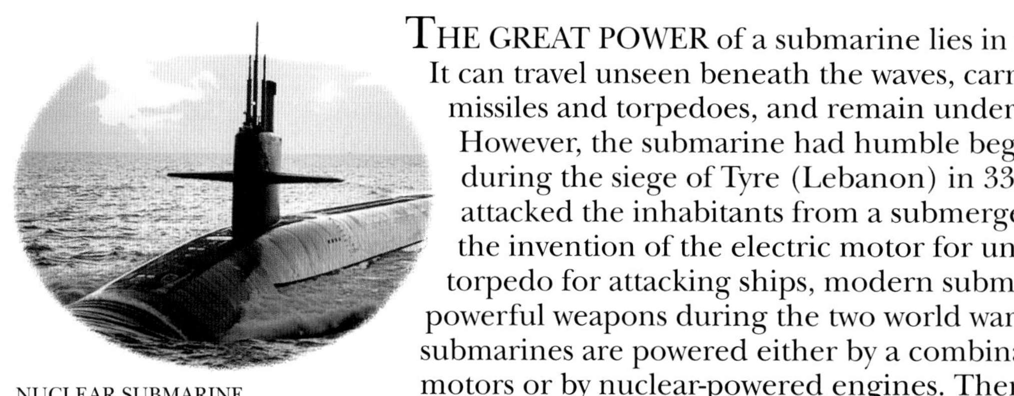

NUCLEAR SUBMARINE
The most powerful of all weapons is the nuclear missile-carrying submarine. Its nuclear-powered engines allow it to hide underwater almost indefinitely without coming up for air, and it carries sufficient nuclear missiles to destroy several large cities.

Periscope and communication antennas

Propeller drives the submarine through the water.

Diesel-electric engines are specially designed to make as little noise as possible.

The conning tower stands clear of the water when the submarine is on the surface.

Torpedoes ready for firing

Small movable wings called hydroplanes control the submarine's direction.

Tubes for launching torpedoes

Crew's living quarters are usually cramped. Some submarines carry a crew of more than 150.

Control room, from where the captain commands the submarine

HUNTER-KILLER SUBMARINE

A diesel engine powers this hunter-killer submarine when it travels on the surface, and an electric motor when it is underwater. Buoyancy tanks fill with water to submerge the submarine; to surface again, compressed air pushes the water out of the tanks.

TORPEDOES
Torpedoes are packed with explosives and have their own motors to propel them to their targets. They are launched by compressed air from tubes in the nose and rear of the submarine.

PERISCOPE
With a periscope, the captain can see what is on the surface while the submarine is submerged. A periscope is a hollow tube which extends from the conning tower. It contains an angled mirror at either end and a system of lenses which form an image of the object on the surface.

Anti-submarine helicopter trails active sonar system in the water.

The missile-carrying submarine will dive to escape its attackers.

Hunter-killer submarine uses active sonar to detect enemy submarine.

Submarine captain sees helicopter through periscope.

SONAR
Helicopters, ships, and hunter-killer submarines are equipped with sonar (sound navigation and ranging) for detecting submarines. Passive sonar consists of microphones, which pick up the sound of the submarine's engines. Active sonar sends out ultrasonic sound pulses which are too high-pitched to be heard but bounce off a hidden submarine and produce a distinctive echo.

Find out more
NAVIES
ROCKETS AND MISSILES
SHIPS AND BOATS
UNDERWATER EXPLORATION
WARSHIPS

SUMERIANS

THE WORLD'S FIRST CITIES were built on the banks of the Tigris and Euphrates rivers in what is now Iraq. About 5,000 years ago, the people of Sumer, the area of southern Iraq where the two rivers flow together, began to build what would become great, bustling cities. They made bricks from the riverside mud to build houses and massive temples. The Sumerians also developed one of the world's earliest writing systems, by making marks in soft tablets of clay, which they left in the sun to harden. Their earliest cities, such as Ur and Uruk, became famous all over the Middle East as Sumerian merchants travelled abroad trading food grown in the fertile local fields. The Sumerians flourished until about 2000 B.C., when desert tribes invaded.

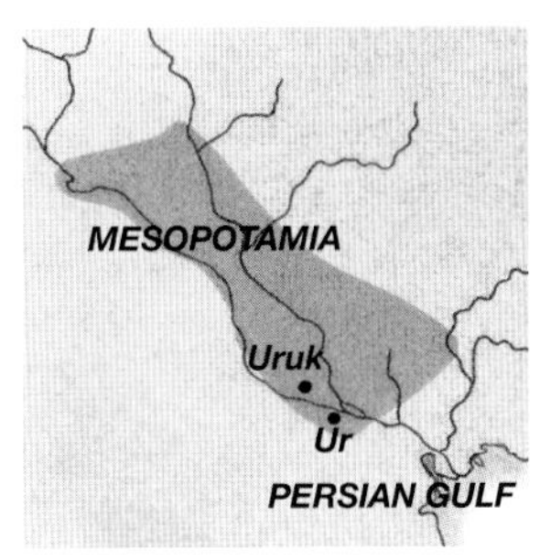

MESOPOTAMIA
The land between the Tigris and Euphrates rivers is known as Mesopotamia. The home of the Sumerians was in southern Mesopotamia and Ur was one of their greatest cities.

GILGAMESH
The Sumerians created the earliest written story that has survived to modern times. Written on clay tablets, the story tells of Gilgamesh, King of Uruk and the son of a goddess and a man. Gilgamesh begins as a cruel king, but be becomes a hero when he kills two fearsome monsters. Later, Gilgamesh visits the underworld to try to search for immortal life.

Cuneiform script consisted of wedge-shaped marks made with a reed writing-stylus.

ZIGGURAT
At the centre of each Sumerian city was a stepped tower called a ziggurat, topped by a temple. By building their ziggurats high, the Sumerians believed that they were reaching up to the heavens, so that each temple could become a home for one of Sumer's many gods and goddesses. Only priests were allowed to worship in the temples.

SUMER

The land between the two rivers was fertile but dry. Farmers dug canals to bring water to their fields, and found that this meant they could produce huge harvests – there was usually enough to sell. The Sumerians found other useful resources near the rivers. They used reeds for boat-building and simple houses, and clay for making bricks and pottery.

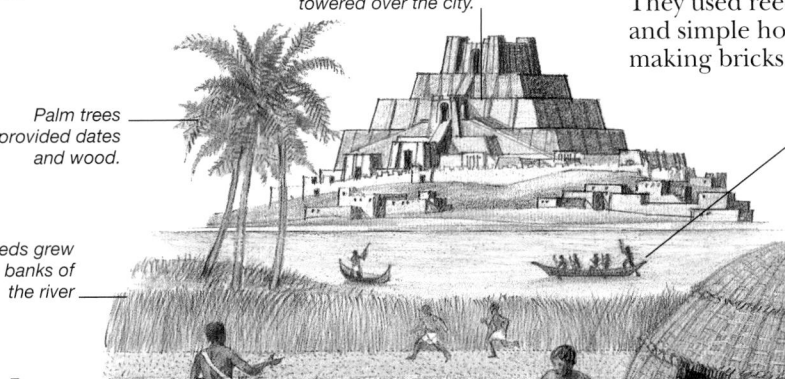

Mud-brick ziggurat towered over the city.

Palm trees provided dates and wood.

Sumerians travelled along the rivers in boats made from local reeds. Fishermen used similar boats.

Reed beds grew on the banks of the river

Farmers scattered seeds by hand.

Oxen pulled wooden ploughs.

Brickmakers poured soft mud into a mould.

Reed huts were common in southern Mesopotamia.

Bricks were left to bake dry in the hot sun.

Workers dug up clay to make bricks.

Neatly trimmed beard typical of Mesopotamian fashion.

SARGON
Originally the servant of a king of Kish, in Akkad, north of Sumer, Sargon rose to become Akkad's ruler. In around 2350 B.C., he conquered Sumer, Mesopotamia and the eastern territory of Elam. He made Mesopotamia into a united country for the first time. Sargon was a powerful king who protected merchants, and built up flourishing trade.

Find out more
ALPHABET
BRONZE AGE
WHEELS

SUN

THE NIGHT SKY is full of stars, so distant that they are mere points of light. The Sun is one of these stars, but we are closer to it than to any other star. Along with the other planets of the solar system, the Earth moves around the Sun, trapped in orbit by the force of gravity. The Sun sustains nearly all life on Earth with its light and heat. The Sun is a ball of glowing gases, roughly three-quarters hydrogen and one-quarter helium, along with traces of other elements. Within its hot, dense core, hydrogen particles crash together. This produces nuclear reactions that release enormous amounts of energy, keeping the core of the Sun very hot. The energy travels outwards and leaves the Sun's surface mainly as light, and infrared and ultraviolet radiation. Energy sources that humans use to provide power originate from the Sun. For example, coal is the remains of ancient plants, which trapped the Sun's energy.

STORY OF THE SUN
The Sun formed just under 5,000 million years ago from a cloud of hydrogen, helium, and dust, which contracted under its own gravity. The contraction heated the cloud until nuclear reactions began, converting hydrogen into helium. At this point the Sun began to shine steadily. It is believed that the Sun will continue to shine for another 5,000 million years before it runs out of hydrogen fuel and begins to die.

SOLAR FLARES
Huge explosions on the Sun's surface, called solar flares, fire streams of electrically charged particles into space.

CORONA AND SOLAR WIND
The corona is a thin atmosphere of gases that extends for millions of kilometres around the Sun. A blast of electrically charged particles, called the solar wind, blows out from the corona at a rate of millions of tonnes each second. The Earth is protected from these particles by its magnetic field, but they can damage spacecraft and satellites. Coronal Mass Ejections are sudden blasts of great clouds from the corona. These are thought to cause auroras – coloured lights in the sky above the Earth's poles – and magnetic storms.

Energy travels outwards in the form of heat and electromagnetic waves such as infrared, light, and radio waves.

Relatively cool and dark areas, called sunspots, form on the surface of the Sun. Sunspots develop in places where the Sun's magnetic field becomes particularly strong.

Great streamers of glowing hydrogen gas, called prominences, frequently soar up from the Sun. Prominences are often about 60,000 km (more than 37,000 miles) long.

Core extends to about 175,000 km (about 110,800 miles) from the Sun's centre.

The hot, glowing surface of the Sun is called the photosphere (sphere of light). It is about 400 km (250 miles) deep.

A glowing red layer of hydrogen gas called the chromosphere (sphere of colour) lies above the photosphere. The chromosphere is a few thousand kilometres deep.

Light from the Sun takes about eight minutes to reach the Earth.

The Sun's diameter is 109 times that of the Earth. More than 1,300,000 globes the size of the Earth could fit into the Sun.

Warning: Never look at the Sun, either directly or through dark glasses. The intense light could seriously damage your eyesight.

SOLAR ENERGY

Electronic devices called solar cells convert sunlight into electricity. Solar cells power satellites and produce electricity in experimental houses and cars. In 2003, the solar-powered *Nuna II* car (below) drove across Australia at an average speed of 96.8 km/h (60 mph).

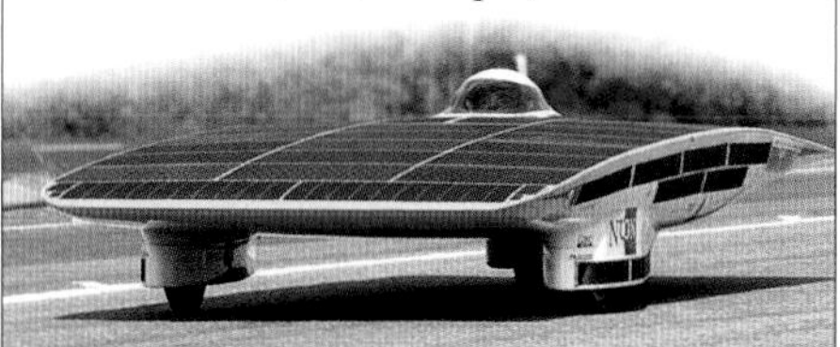

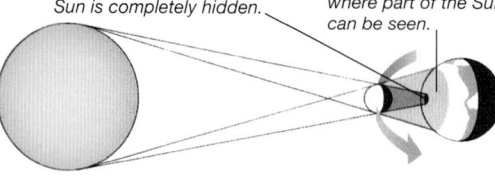

Umbra is the centre of the moon's shadow, where the Sun is completely hidden.

Penumbra is the outer part of the moon's shadow, where part of the Sun can be seen.

SOLAR ECLIPSES
When the moon passes between the Earth and the Sun, the Sun is hidden. This is called a solar eclipse. A total solar eclipse occurs at places on the Earth where the Sun appears to be completely hidden (although prominences, chromosphere, and corona can be seen). Elsewhere the eclipse is partial, and parts of the Sun can be seen.

SUN FACTS

Earth–Sun distance	149.6 million km (92.9 million miles)
Diameter at equator	1,392,000 km (864,950 miles)
Time to rotate once	25.4 days
Temperature at surface	5,500°C (10,000°F)
Temperature at centre	15,000,000°C (27,000,000°F)

Find out more
ASTRONOMY
ENERGY
STARS

Swimming

From crowds on a beach to bathers by a pool, most people enjoy swimming. It is one of the most popular sports for people of all ages. Swimming – using your arms and legs to move through water – exercises every part of the body, encouraging health and fitness. It is also an important international sport. Competitive swimmers need to be very strong and fit. They train for hours, swimming huge distances every week. For swimmers such as these, an Olympic gold medal is the ultimate goal. But almost anyone can learn to swim, whether using a fast-moving crawl, slower breaststroke, or even a doggy paddle. Learning to swim well is an important safety measure, and it can save lives.

CAPTAIN WEBB
On 25 August, 1875, Captain Matthew Webb became the first person to swim across the English Channel. It took him 22 hours to cross between England and France. Long-distance swimming needs stamina. Swimmers cover themselves with grease for insulation against the cold water.

Fun and safety

Swimming is fun, whether on holiday at the seaside, or at the local pool or leisure centre. But knowing how to swim properly also makes other water sports such as canoeing, boating, surfing, and water skiing much safer.

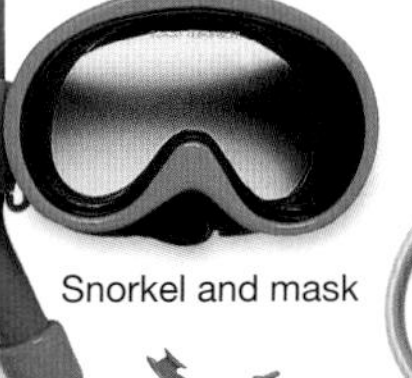
Snorkel and mask

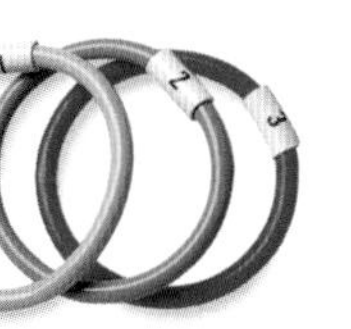
Dive weights

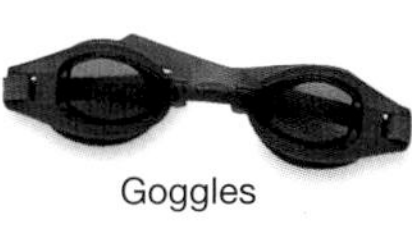
Goggles

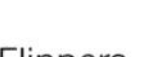
Flippers

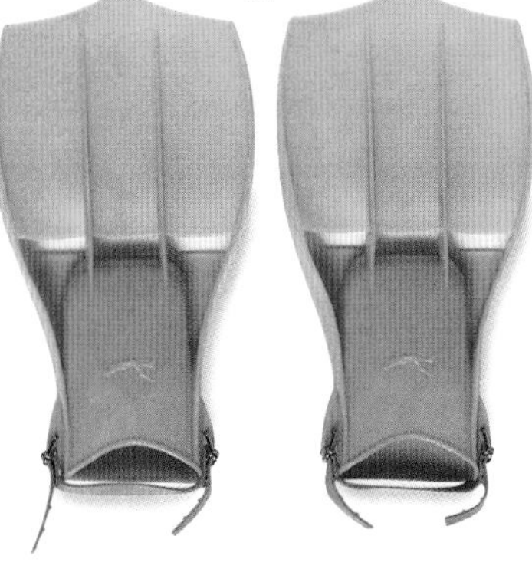

EQUIPMENT
Using a mask and snorkel, a swimmer can see and breathe underwater; the top of the snorkel sticks above the surface of the water. Goggles protect the eyes and allow swimmers to see what is going on without their eyes stinging. Flippers are like the fins of fish, and make swimming easier. Diving weights make it easy to stay underwater.

Swimming strokes

There are four main strokes, or methods of swimming: freestyle, or crawl, backstroke, butterfly, and breaststroke. Crawl is the fastest. Swimmers kick up and down, bringing their arms forward out of the water. For backstroke, swimmers lie on their backs. Butterfly involves using arms and legs together, pulling the body forward. In breaststroke, swimmers pull their hands sidewise, and kick like a frog.

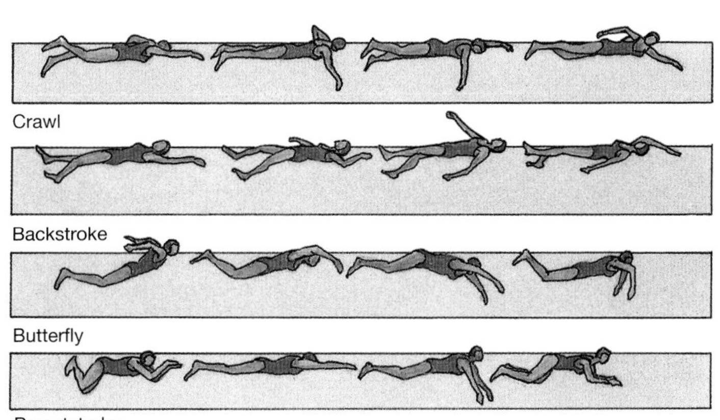

MAKING A TURN
Swimmers save time by doing somersault, or tumble, turns when they finish a length. Just before the end of the pool the swimmer takes a breath, swivels underwater and pushes off from the wall with their feet. A good turn can mean the difference between winning and losing.

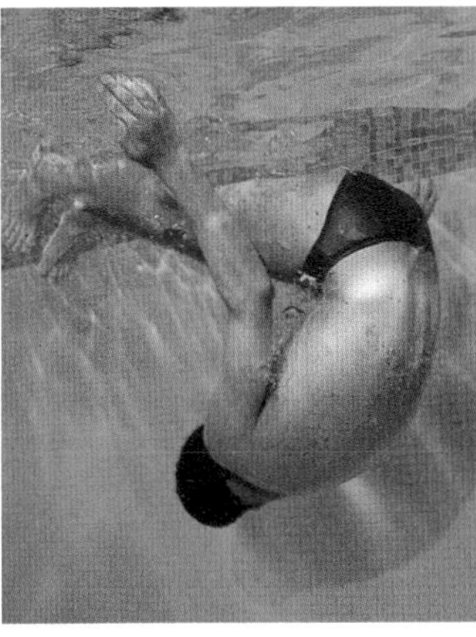

Find out more
Health and fitness
Sports
Water sports

SWITZERLAND

Switzerland is a land-locked country at the heart of Europe. The Alps create a major barrier to the south. To the north the Jura Mountains form its border with France. Lake Geneva, on the French border, is formed by the Rhône river.

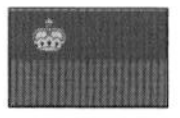

LIECHTENSTEIN
Area: 160 sq km (62 sq miles)
Population: 33,100
Capital: Vaduz
Languages: German, Alemannish dialect, Italian
Religions: Roman Catholic, Protestant
Currency: Swiss franc

SWITZERLAND
Area: 41,290 sq km (15,940 sq miles)
Population: 7,200,000
Capital: Bern
Languages: German, Swiss-German, French, Italian, Romansch
Religions: Roman Catholic, Protestant, Muslim, non-religious
Currency: Swiss franc

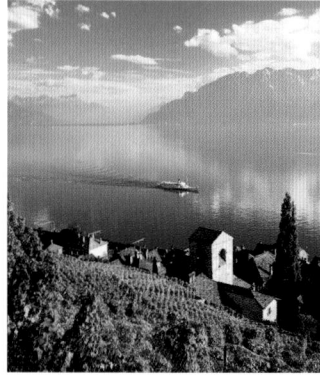

LAKE GENEVA
Picturesque villages line the shores of Europe's largest Alpine lake, especially to the north, where the soil is fertile. Geneva, at the southwest of the lake, is a major banking and insurance centre. Many international organizations, such as the Red Cross, are based in the city.

A LAND OF HIGH MOUNTAINS and isolated valleys, the 26 provinces (cantons) of Switzerland have been a united confederation since 1291. With access to the north via the Rhine river and control of the Alpine passes to the south, Switzerland has dominated Europe's north-south trade routes for many centuries. The country lacks natural resources, but has become a wealthy financial, banking and commercial centre, with a worldwide reputation for precision engineering, especially watch-making. Although mountains cover nearly three-quarters of the land, dairy farming is very important, and the Swiss export a wide range of cheeses and milk chocolate. Liechtenstein, a tiny mountainous country on Switzerland's eastern border, is also an important financial and manufacturing centre.

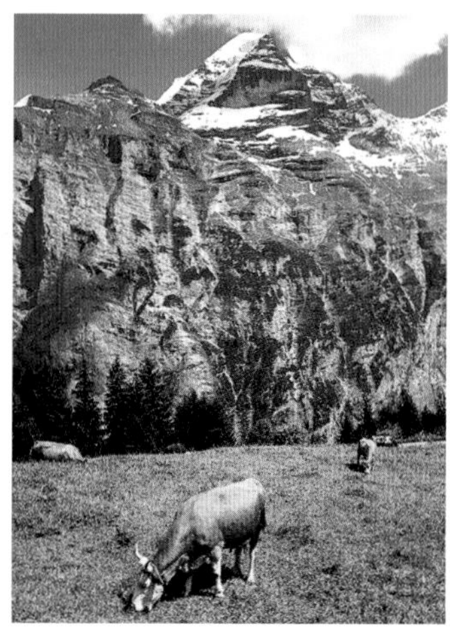

ALPINE PASTURES
Most Alpine villages are clustered at the base of mountain slopes and in valley plains. These locations provide fertile soil, adequate water and temperate weather. Vines can even be grown on south-facing slopes. Swiss dairy farmers keep their cattle in the valleys during the winter. In summer they are taken up to lush, green Alpine meadows to graze.

WINTER SPORTS

Over 100 million visitors a year come to the Swiss Alps to enjoy climbing, hiking and winter sports. Alpine skiing has been included in the Olympic Games since 1936. Mountain resorts, with chair lifts, ski runs, and ski instructors, cater for winter visitors. But tourism is having a dangerous impact. Trees are cleared to make way for ski runs. Without these natural barriers, there is a much greater risk of avalanches.

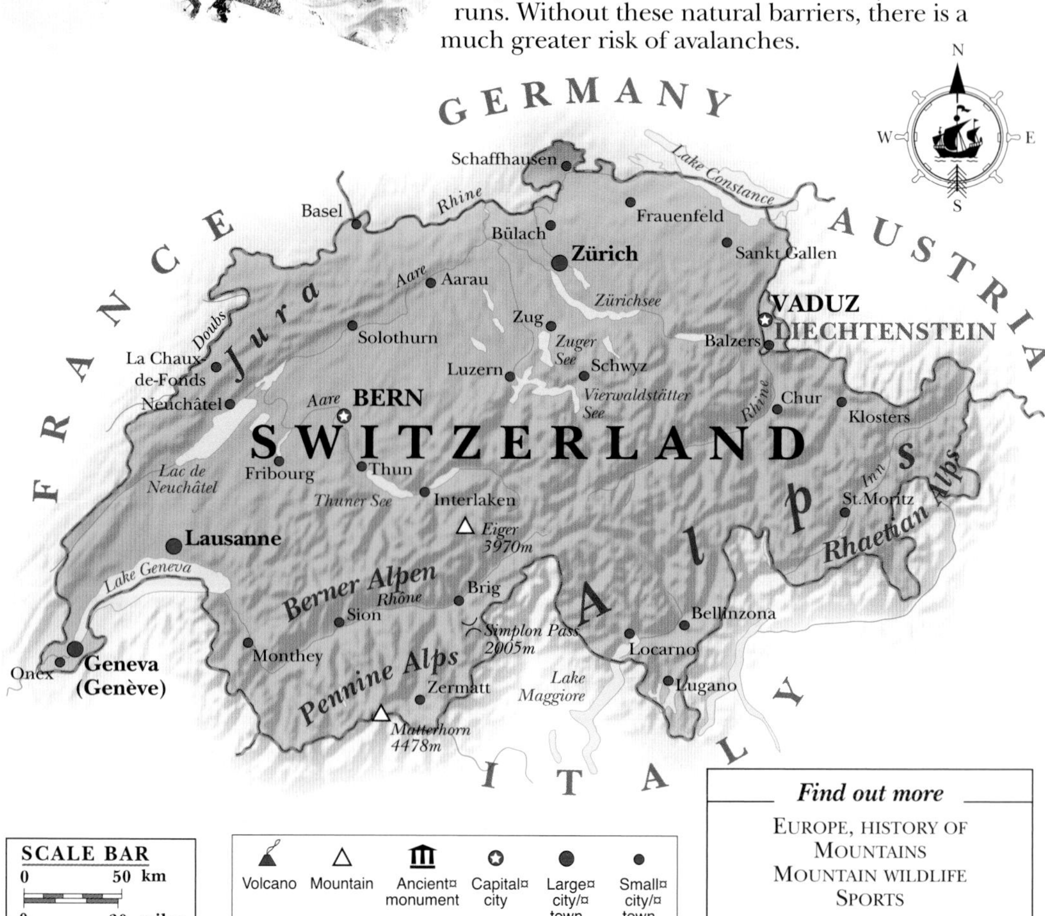

Find out more
EUROPE, HISTORY OF
MOUNTAINS
MOUNTAIN WILDLIFE
SPORTS

TANKS

MILLIONS OF YEARS AGO, nature equipped animals such as turtles with a shell of armour to protect them from enemies. Early in the 20th century, armies adopted the same idea in battle. The result was the tank – a steel monster that lumbered over the battlefields of World War I (1914-18), destroying enemy defences and machine-gun positions. Tanks have now developed into sophisticated weapons that combine fire power, protection, and mobility. Each tank is fitted with a powerful gun which is guided by computers and a laser rangefinder to ensure pinpoint accuracy. Hardened-steel armour, which may be up to 11 cm (4.3 in) thick, protects the crew. Tanks can manoeuvre their way over terrain that would stop any other vehicle, including water, and some light tanks can travel at speeds of more than 80 km/h (50 mph).

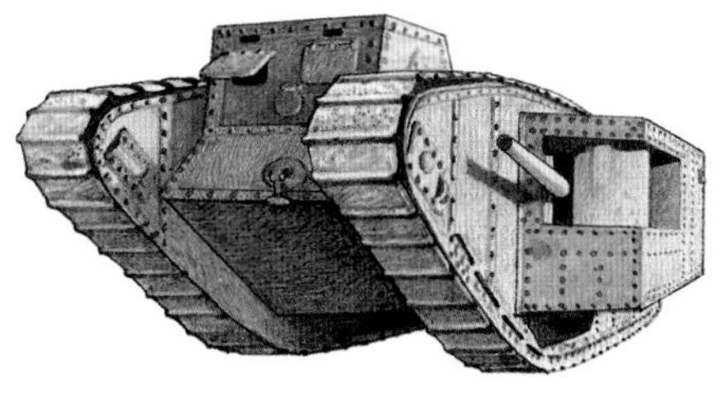

THE EARLY TANK
In 1916, the British Mark I became the first tank to be used in battle. Its strange shape allowed it to cross the wide trenches, mud, and barbed wire of the battlefield. Over the next 30 years, tanks evolved into advanced fighting machines. Recent developments are concerned with improving weaponry, speed, and the armour of tanks.

MAIN BATTLE TANK

The German-built *Leopard 2* battle tank is one of the most powerful tanks in the world. It can travel at 72 km/h (45 mph) despite its weight of 55 tonnes (54 tons), which is equivalent to more than 30 small family saloon cars. It is armed with a main gun and two machine guns and carries a crew of four.

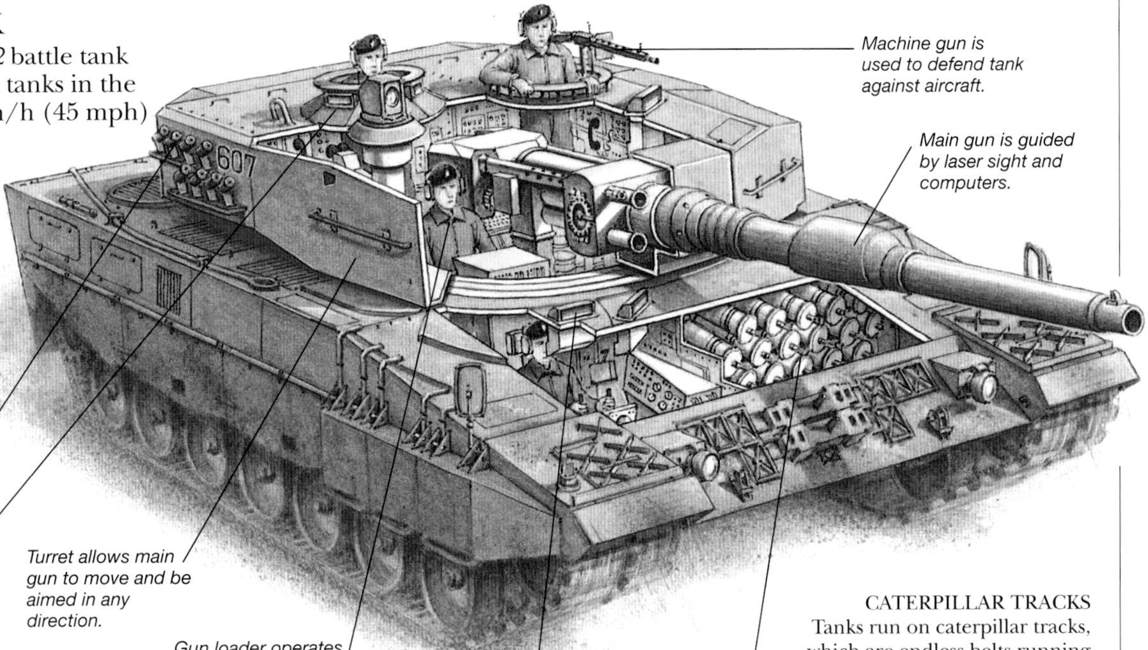

Machine gun is used to defend tank against aircraft.

Main gun is guided by laser sight and computers.

Smoke dischargers produce huge cloud of smoke to hide the tank if it is under attack.

Commander's cupola with periscopes that give all-round vision.

Turret allows main gun to move and be aimed in any direction.

Gun loader operates main gun and radio communications.

Ammunition store with shells for main gun.

Periscope allows driver to see out from inside the hull of the tank.

CATERPILLAR TRACKS
Tanks run on caterpillar tracks, which are endless belts running over several wheels. To turn the tank, the driver makes the tracks on either side of the tank run at different speeds.

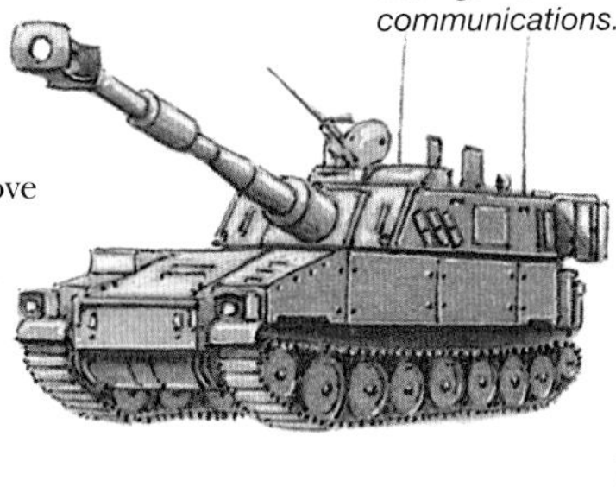

SELF-PROPELLED GUN
Because mobile artillery weapons are mounted on a tanklike vehicle, they can move rapidly into new positions.

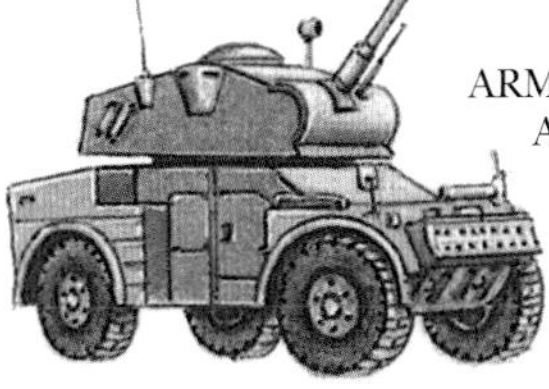

M1 Abrams

120mm cannon fires rocket-shaped projectiles to penetrate enemy tanks and explode.

ARMOURED CAR
Armoured cars are perfect for reconnaissance (scouting) missions and patrols because they are small and fast.

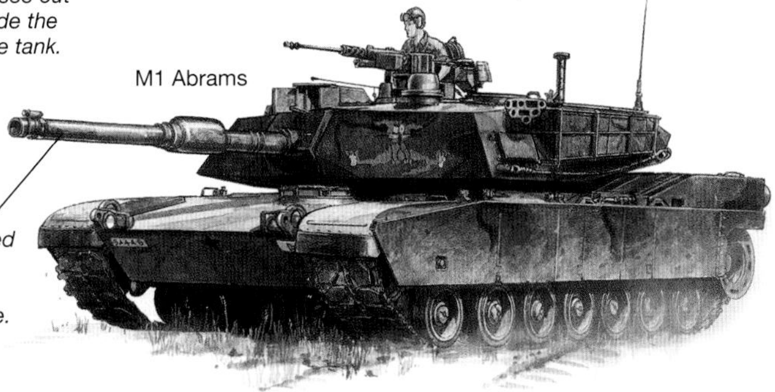

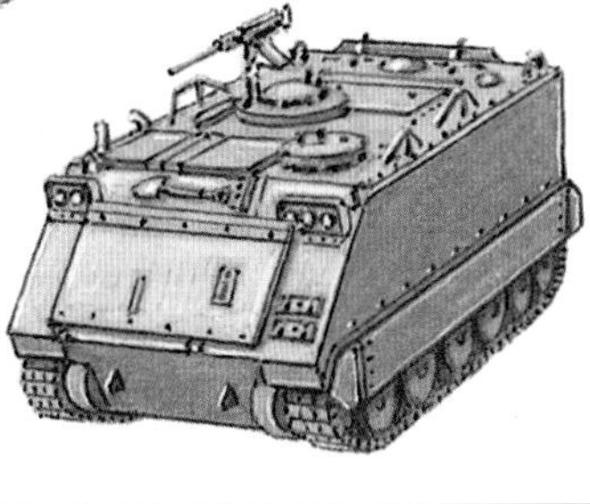

US ABRAMS

The M1 Abrams took 10 years to develop and was used by the US Army during the 1980s and 1990s. It has a more comfortable cabin and stronger armour than older tanks. It uses lasers to calculate the distance to a target. During the Gulf War in 1991 it destroyed more than 2,000 enemy tanks without any US losses.

PERSONNEL CARRIER
Soldiers travel into battle inside an armoured personnel carrier. It transports them on water and on land, propelled by its caterpillar tracks.

Find out more

ARMIES
GUNS
WEAPONS
WORLD WAR I
WORLD WAR II

TECHNOLOGY

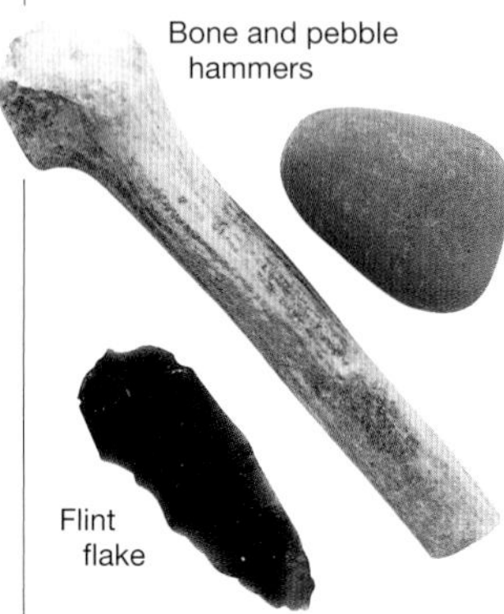

EARLY TECHNOLOGY
Humans living during the Stone Age developed a variety of tools for everyday purposes. They used rounded pebbles and bones as hammers to form cutting tools from a strong stone called flint. Flint was chipped and flaked to produce a sharp cutting edge like a blade.

THE INVENTION OF STONE TOOLS more than two million years ago marked the beginning of technology. For the first time in history, people found that cutting or chopping was easier to do with tools than with bare hands. Technology is the way in which people use the ideas of science to build machinery and make tasks easier. Although technology began in prehistoric times, it advanced rapidly during and after the Industrial Revolution, beginning in the 18th century. Since that time technology has dramatically changed our world. It has given us fast, safe transport, materials such as plastics, increased worldwide communications, and many useful daily appliances. Perhaps the greatest benefits of technology are in modern medicine, which has improved our health and lengthened our lives. Advances in technology have been mainly beneficial to humans and our lifestyle. However, increased technology has a negative side, too – it has produced weapons with the power to cause death and destruction. Technology and development have caused many environmental problems such as ozone depletion, and is often dependent on non-renewable resources, such as oil, which has a limited life. Governments and other organizations are now trying to use new technology to find solutions to these problems.

Threshing machines help farmers separate the heads from the stalks of rice plants. Previously, this job had to be done by hand.

COMPUTERS

The development of computers has been one of the most important recent advances in technology. The invention of the microchip (right) changed the emphasis of producing goods from mechanical to electronic. This meant that many tasks which had previously been done manually were now automated. Computers perform many different tasks and are used in banking, architecture, manufacturing, and a range of other businesses. Computers also aid new technology, because they can help develop new machines.

Microchips lie at the heart of a computer. These tiny devices store and process huge amounts of information at high speed.

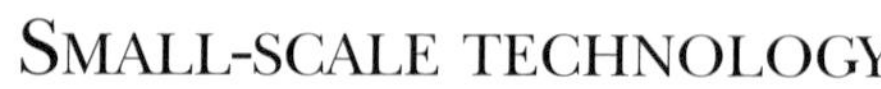

SMALL-SCALE TECHNOLOGY

People in poorer countries cannot afford to buy the technological goods that are common in richer parts of the world such as North America and Europe. Their primary concern is feeding and housing their families, and they tend to use smaller, simpler machines, such as windmills that drive pumps for irrigation.

Synthetic clothing materials are lightweight, machine-washable, and allow ease of movement.

The cyclist's helmet is made from plastic and polystyrene. It has an aerodynamic shape to increase the speed of the cyclist.

Disabled members of the community can participate in more activities because of advanced technology, such as this specially designed tricycle.

Wheel technology, developed in 3500 B.C, revolutionized machines and modes of transportation.

LIFESTYLE
In the western world, technology has generally made daily life easier. Washing machines, cars, and cash machines all make daily tasks more convenient, providing more time for leisure, hobbies, and sports. People also now have the time and means to travel to other countries to experience different cultures and environments.

MEDICAL TECHNOLOGY

Inventions such as x-ray machines and brain scanners help doctors to detect and treat illness. Doctors can transplant organs, implant tiny electronic pacemakers to keep a heart beating, and repair damaged tissue with plastic surgery. Medical technology, such as glasses, contact lenses, or hearing aids, also helps to improve the daily lives of many people affected by impaired vision or hearing. Prosthetic (artificial) limbs are also being improved and now allow their users more movement and flexibility.

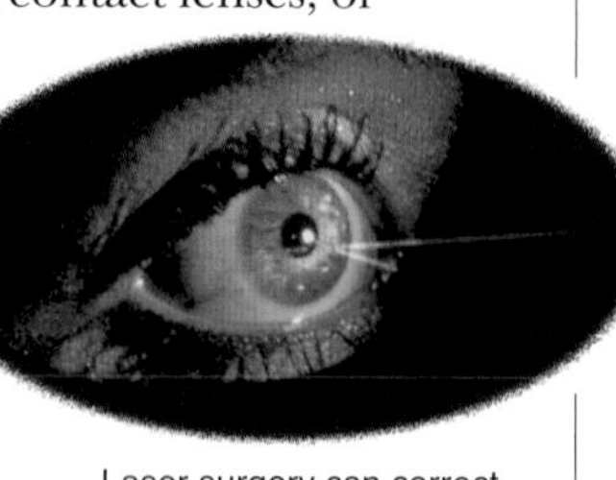

Laser surgery can correct many eye defects without needing to cut the eye.

MILITARY TECHNOLOGY

The military uses technology to develop new weapons and navigation methods. Many machines built for the military also benefit civilians, such as the jet engine and radar, which are vital to modern airliners.

COMMUNICATIONS

Today, people across the globe communicate instantly. Speech, pictures, and text are turned into signals that are transmitted via wires, radio waves, or satellite to telephones, faxes, radios, computers, and televisions almost anywhere.

FOOD TECHNOLOGY

Every aspect of food and its production has been affected by technology, from growing and harvesting, to preserving and distribution. There is now a larger variety of food available due to international influences and transportation technology.

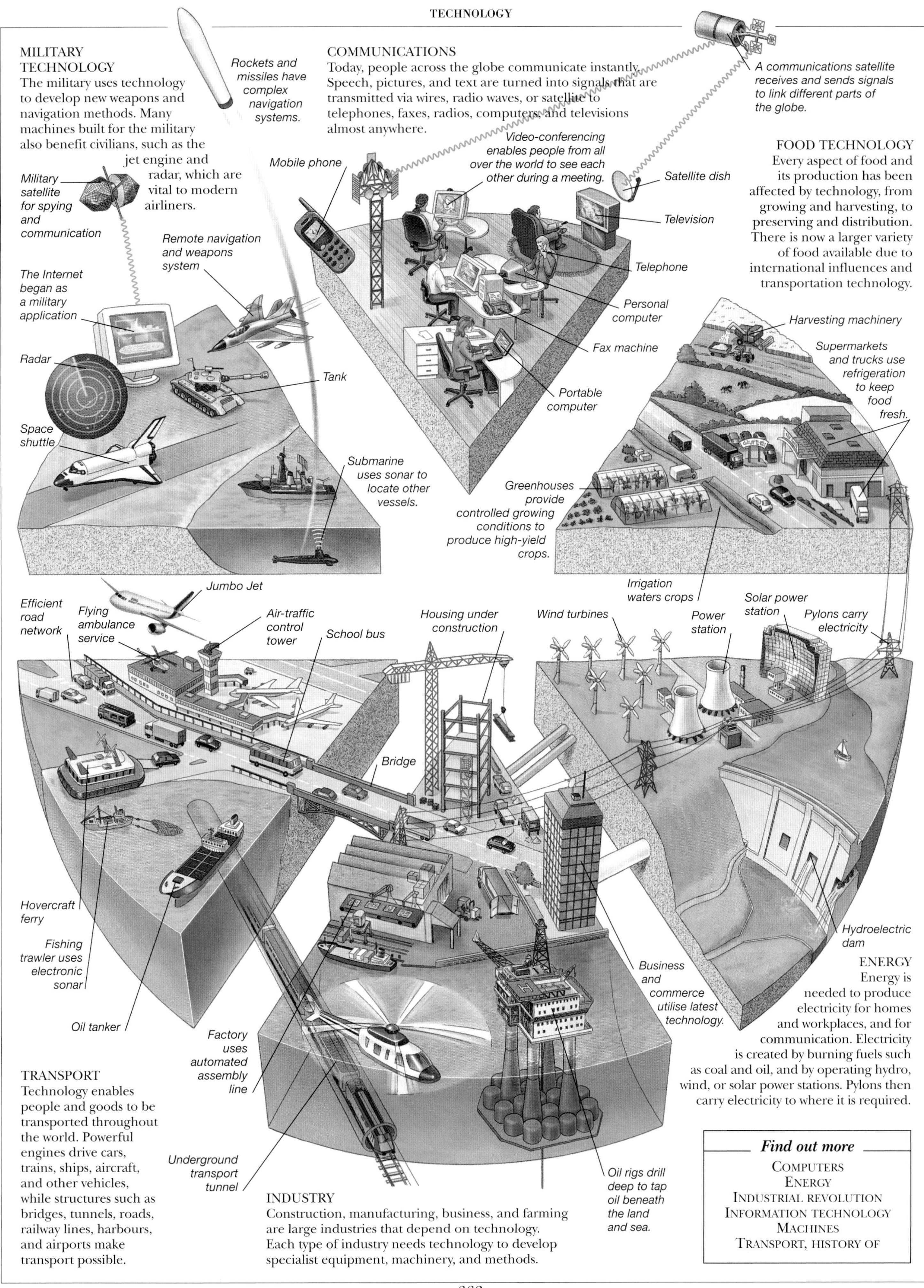

ENERGY

Energy is needed to produce electricity for homes and workplaces, and for communication. Electricity is created by burning fuels such as coal and oil, and by operating hydro, wind, or solar power stations. Pylons then carry electricity to where it is required.

TRANSPORT

Technology enables people and goods to be transported throughout the world. Powerful engines drive cars, trains, ships, aircraft, and other vehicles, while structures such as bridges, tunnels, roads, railway lines, harbours, and airports make transport possible.

INDUSTRY

Construction, manufacturing, business, and farming are large industries that depend on technology. Each type of industry needs technology to develop specialist equipment, machinery, and methods.

Find out more

COMPUTERS
ENERGY
INDUSTRIAL REVOLUTION
INFORMATION TECHNOLOGY
MACHINES
TRANSPORT, HISTORY OF

TEETH

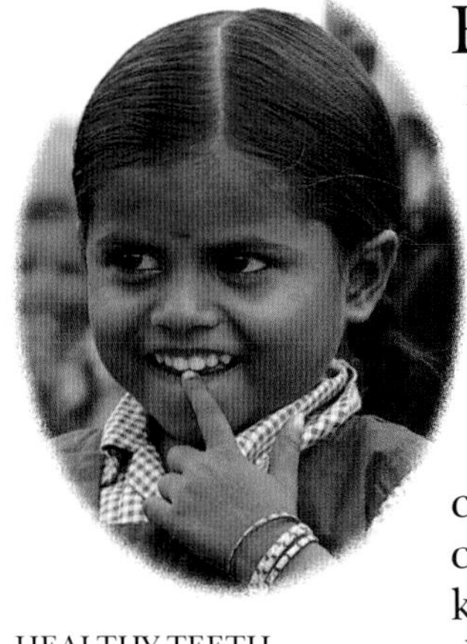

HEALTHY TEETH
It is important to take care of your teeth to keep them healthy. Teeth should be cleaned with a toothbrush and toothpaste after every meal. Dental floss should be used regularly. Sugary foods are damaging to teeth and cause tooth decay.

EVERY TIME WE EAT we use our teeth – to bite, chew, crunch, and grind food. Teeth enable us to break up food properly so that our bodies can digest it and turn it into energy. A tooth has three main parts – the crown of the tooth, which shows above the gum; the neck, which shows at gum level; and the root, which is hidden in the jawbone. The root of the tooth is fixed securely in the jaw by a substance called cementum. A tooth has three layers – creamy white enamel on the outside (the hardest substance in the body); a layer of dentine beneath; and the pulp cavity in the centre. The pulp contains many nerves, which connect to the jawbone. There are four main kinds of teeth; each kind is shaped for a different job. Chisel-like incisors at the front of the mouth cut and slice food; longer, pointed canines tear and rip food; and flat, broad premolars and molars crush and grind it. During our lives, we have two sets of teeth – milk teeth as children, and a second set of teeth as adults.

Enamel
Pulp cavity
Dentine
Gum
Root
Blood vessels
Cementum
Jawbone
Nerve

Cross-section of a molar

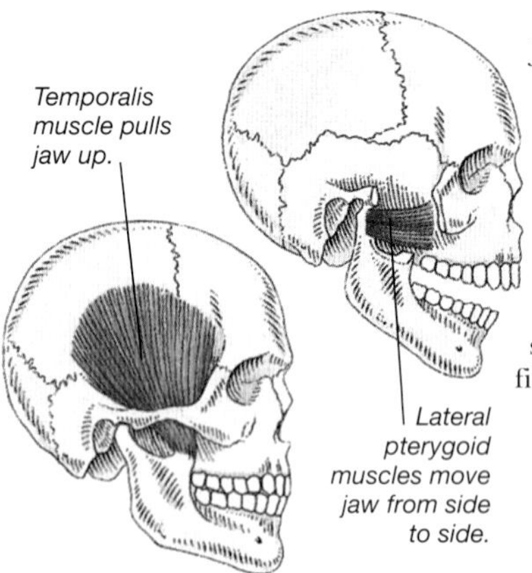

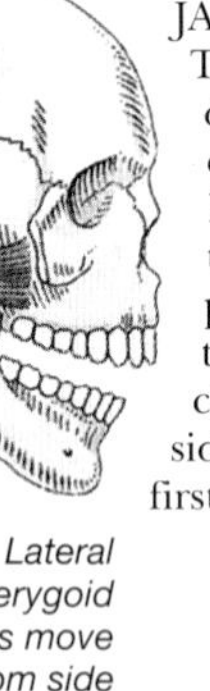

JAWS
The upper jaw is fixed to the skull and does not move. Powerful muscles in the cheeks and the side of the head pull the lower jaw up towards the upper jaw, so that the teeth come together with great pressure for biting. Other muscles pull the lower jaw sideways, so that we can chew with both up-and-down and side-to-side movements. Teeth are an important first step in the process of digesting food.

STRUCTURE OF A TOOTH

Teeth have one, two (like this molar), three, or occasionally four roots, which anchor them securely in the jawbone and withstand the pressure of biting and chewing. Blood vessels which carry nutrients and oxygen, and nerves which transmit sensation, pass out through tiny holes in the base of each root.

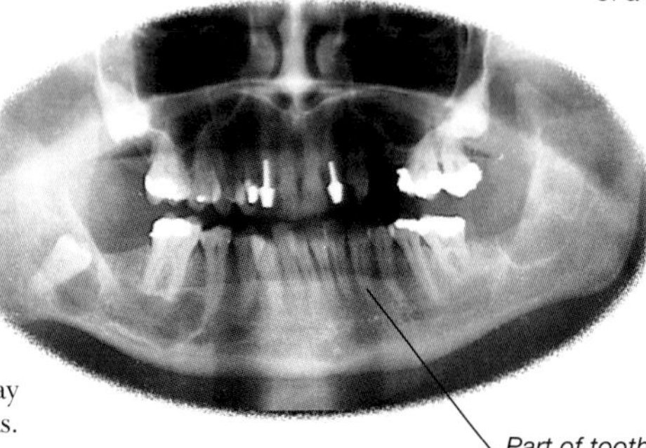

DENTISTS
Dentists use X-rays (right) to see the roots of teeth and to identify any cavities. In the past, dentists extracted decaying teeth, but now only the affected parts are removed and the hole is filled with hard artificial materials. The white areas on this X-ray are fillings and two crowns on posts.

MILK TEETH AND ADULT TEETH

Children have 20 milk teeth which gradually fall out and are replaced by a second set of permanent adult teeth. Adults have 32 teeth in total. Each jaw has 4 incisors, 2 canines, 4 premolars, and 6 molars (2 of which are wisdom teeth). Wisdom teeth grow when a person is about 20, although some may never push through the gum.

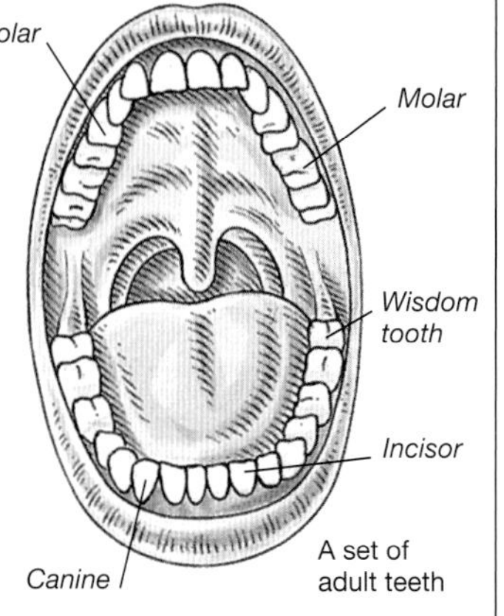

A set of adult teeth

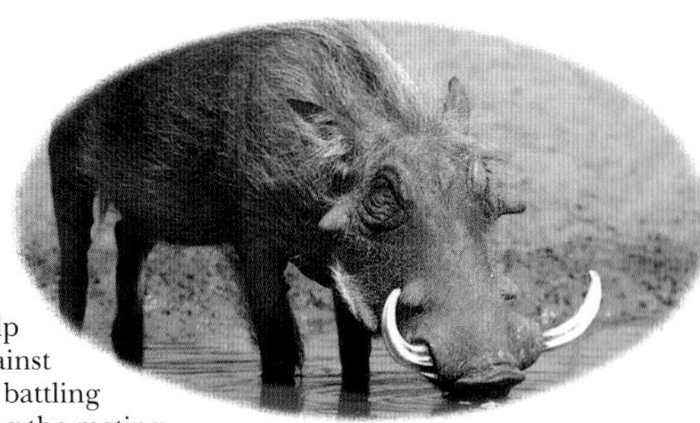

TUSKS
Animals use their teeth for more than just eating food. Large teeth help to defend against enemies, or when battling with rivals during the mating season. The warthog's tusks shown here are huge canine teeth – like the tusks of an elephant. Tusks are used to frighten off predators and, sometimes, to dig up food.

Find out more
FOOD AND DIGESTION
HUMAN BODY
SKELETONS

TELEPHONES

WITH THE PUSH of a few buttons on the telephone, it is possible to talk to someone nearly anywhere else in the world. By making instant communication possible, the telephone has done more to "shrink" the world than almost any other invention. A telephone signal can take several forms on its journey. Beneath the city streets it travels in the form of electric currents in cables, or as light waves in thin glass fibres. Telephone signals also travel as radio waves when they beam down to other countries via satellites, or when they carry messages to and from mobile phones. Many electronic devices "talk" to each other by sending signals via telephone links. Computers exchange information and programmes with one another, and fax machines use telephone lines to send copies of pictures and text to other fax machines across the world within seconds.

Earpiece

A loudspeaker, called the receiver, contains a thin metal disc that vibrates, converting electric signals into sound waves.

Silicon chip

Electronic circuits generate signals corresponding to each button as it is pressed. They also amplify (boost) incoming electric signals and send them to the receiver.

Microphone

Soundwaves of the user's voice strike a microphone called the transmitter, creating an electrical signal that is sent down the telephone cable.

TELEPHONE HANDSET
A small direct (one-way) electric current flows in the wires connected to a telephone handset. Signals representing sounds such as callers' voices, computer data, and fax messages consist of rapid variations in the strength of this current.

The electric cable connects to the telephone network, allowing access all over the world.

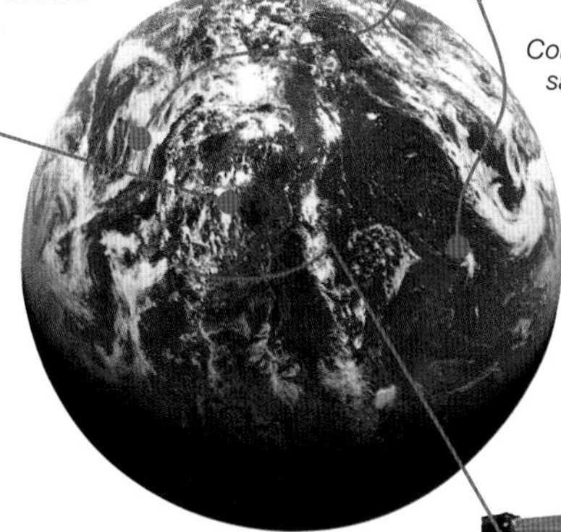

Communication satellites orbit the Earth at such a height and speed that they remain stationary over the same part of the globe all the time. They receive telephone signals from one country on Earth, boost the signals, then beam them back down to another country.

TELEPHONE NETWORK

Computer-controlled telephone exchanges make the connections needed to link two telephones. When a person dials a telephone number, automatic switches at the local exchange link the telephone lines directly. International calls travel along undersea cables or, in the form of radio waves, by way of satellites.

Fibre-optic cables use light waves to carry thousands of phone calls at one time.

Words and pictures printed by a fax machine have jagged edges because they are made up of thousands of dots.

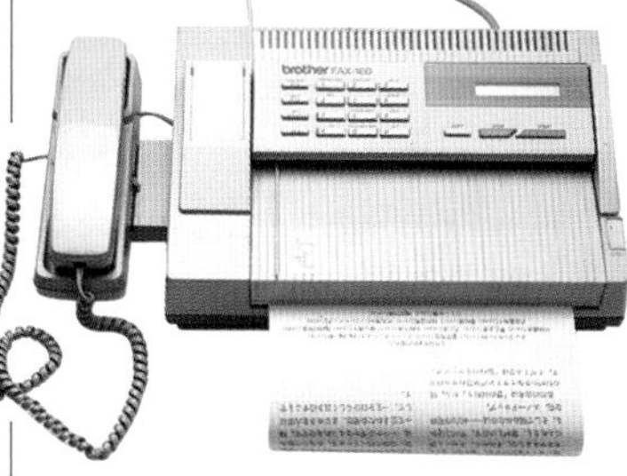

FAX
A facsimile, or fax, machine scans a picture or a written page, measuring its brightness at thousands of individual points. The machine then sends signals along the telephone wire, each representing the brightness at one point. A printer inside the receiving fax machine prints a dot wherever the original picture is dark, making a copy.

ALEXANDER GRAHAM BELL

The inventor of the telephone was a Scottish-American teacher named Alexander Graham Bell (1847-1922). In 1875, Bell was experimenting with early telegraph systems. For this he used vibrating steel strips called reeds. He found that when a reed at one end of the line vibrated, a reed at the other end gave out a sound. In 1876, Bell patented the world's first practical telephone.

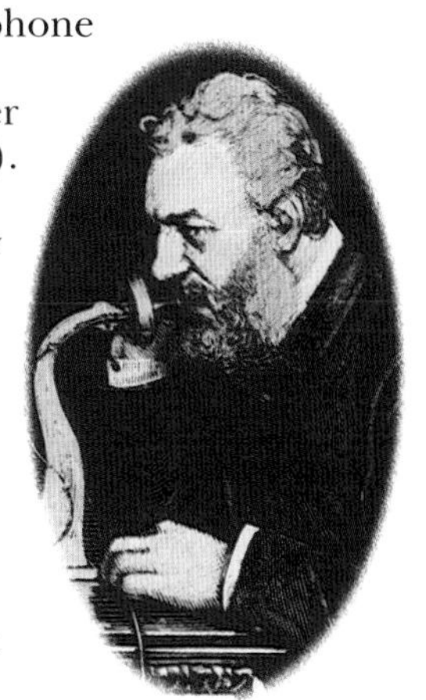

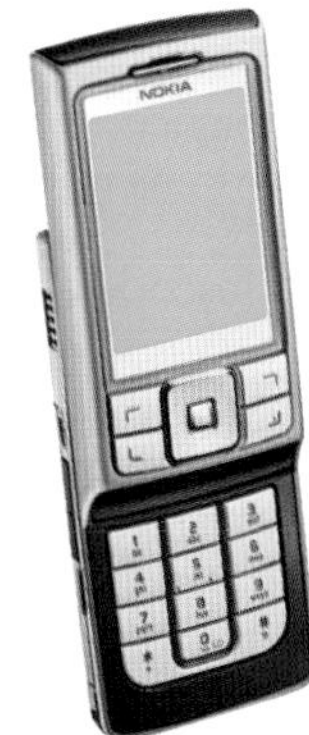

PORTABLE PHONES
A cordless telephone has a built-in radio transmitter and receiver. It communicates with a unit connected to a telephone line in a home. Mobile phones (left) work with the aid of powerful relay stations such as cellular exchanges. Mobile phones are becoming increasingly versatile. Many now also function as cameras and can connect to the Internet.

Find out more

INTERNET
RADIO
SATELLITES
TECHNOLOGY

TELESCOPES

FROM FAR AWAY, a person looks like a tiny dot. But with a telescope, you can see a clear, bright image that reveals all the details of that person's face. Large modern telescopes make it possible to see incredibly distant objects. The Hale telescope on Mount Palomar, California, United States, can detect objects in space called quasars, which are about 30,000 million billion km (20,000 million billion miles) from the Earth. Less powerful telescopes are important too: they are valuable tools for mapmakers, sailors, and bird watchers. Telescopes have helped scientists make some of the greatest discoveries about the universe. In 1609, the Italian scientist Galileo first turned a telescope to the skies. His observations led him to suggest that the Earth moved around the Sun and was not the centre of the universe, as people believed at that time. Since then astronomers have used telescopes to probe into the farthest reaches of our solar system and beyond, discovering new stars and planets.

OPERA GLASSES
Opera glasses are the simplest kind of binoculars. They consist of two small telescopes placed side by side.

Eyepiece lenses are adjustable to match the strength of each eye.

Prisms "fold up" the light inside the binoculars, which magnifies objects as much as a long telescope.

A prism is a triangular-shaped piece of glass.

BINOCULARS
Binoculars are more complex than opera glasses. They contain a system of lenses and prisms that makes them powerful yet small in size.

When the Hale telescope was first built, the observer sat inside the telescope itself to view the stars. Today, there is an electronic detector placed there instead.

Doors of observatory slide open to give telescope a view of the stars.

Light enters the front of the telescope.

REFLECTING TELESCOPE

Most astronomers use reflecting telescopes, which are the best telescopes for picking up the faint light from distant stars. A large curved mirror catches the light and concentrates it to form an image. A smaller mirror then carries the image to a lens called the eyepiece. A camera or electronic light detector is often fitted to the eyepiece of astronomical telescopes.

Concave mirror is curved inward to focus the light. This mirror is called the objective mirror because it forms an image of a distant object.

The mountings allow the telescope to turn in order to follow the stars as the Earth moves.

The mirror is made as large as possible to collect the maximum amount of light and distinguish fine details. The objective mirror on the Hale telescope (above) is 5.8 m (16.6 ft) wide and weighs 20 tonnes (20 tons).

RADIO TELESCOPES

Stars and other objects in space give out invisible radio waves as well as light. Astronomers study the universe with radio telescopes, which are large dish-shaped antennas that pick up radio waves from space. Radio astronomy has led to the discovery of dying stars and distant galaxies that would not have been seen from their light alone.

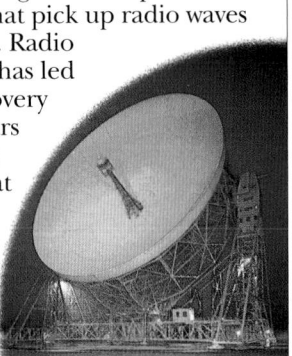

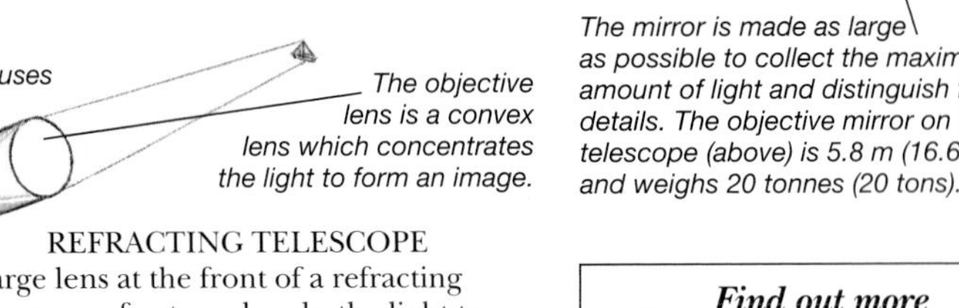

The eyepiece lens focuses the image into the observer's eye.

The objective lens is a convex lens which concentrates the light to form an image.

The middle lens turns the image the right way up.

REFRACTING TELESCOPE
A large lens at the front of a refracting telescope refracts, or bends, the light to form an image of a distant object. The eyepiece lens is at the back. Some refractors have a third lens in the middle. Without this lens, the telescope would produce an upside-down image.

Find out more
ASTRONOMY
LIGHT
MICROSCOPES
SCIENCE, HISTORY OF

TELEVISION AND VIDEO

SINCE ITS INVENTION early in the 20th century, television has become one of the world's most important sources of opinion, information, and entertainment. Television gives us the best seats in the theatre, at a rock concert, or at the Olympic Games. It also beams us pictures of war and disaster, the conquering of space, and other world events as they happen. Television programmes are actually electronic signals sent out as radio waves by way of satellites and underground cables. A television set converts the signals into sound and pictures. People can watch pre-recorded films and record broadcast programmes to play at a later time using a videocassette recorder (VCR), optical discs (DVDs), or a personal video recorder (PVR). Lightweight video cameras can also be used to make home movies. Closed-circuit (nonbroadcast) television cameras are used to guard shops and offices, monitor traffic conditions, and survey crowds at sports events.

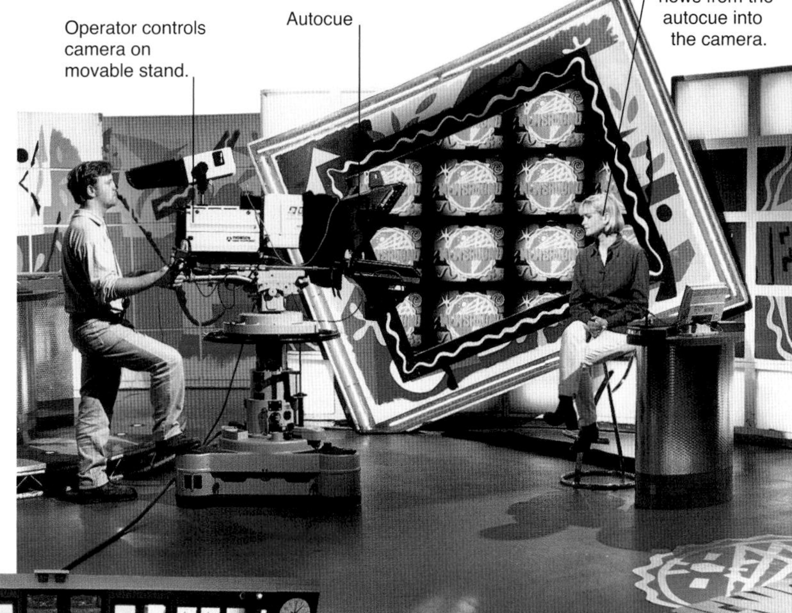

Operator controls camera on movable stand.

Presenter reads the news from the autocue into the camera.

TELEVISION STUDIO

Within the space of a few hours, a studio might be used for a game show, a play, a variety show, and a panel discussion, so studio sets have to be changed very rapidly. Presenters and people working behind the cameras receive instructions from the control room via headphones. Most programmes are recorded, sometimes months before they are broadcast.

CONTROL ROOM

The director and vision mixer sit in the control room (shown above) in front of a bank of screens showing pictures from several sources, such as from cameras at various angles in the studio and at outside broadcast locations, from videotape machines, and from satellites. Other screens show still photographs, captions, and titles. The vision mixer is instructed by the director which image to broadcast on screen and for how long. Sound is also mixed in at the same time. The producer has overall control of the final programme.

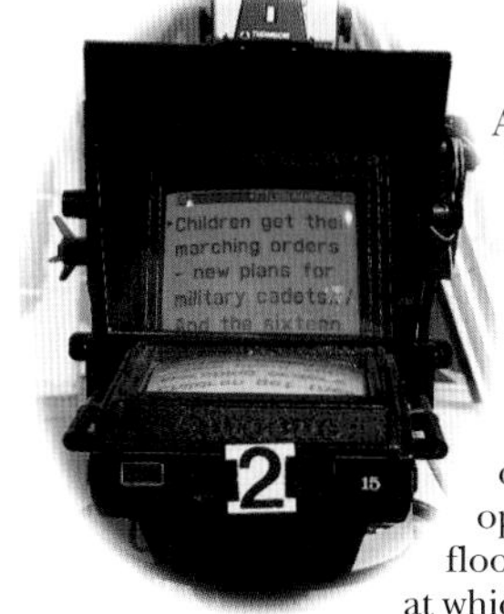

Children got the
marching orders
- new plans for
military cadets

AUTOCUE

The presenter reads the script from an autocue. The words are displayed on a monitor screen and reflected in a two-way mirror in front of the camera lens. An operator on the studio floor controls the speed at which the words move.

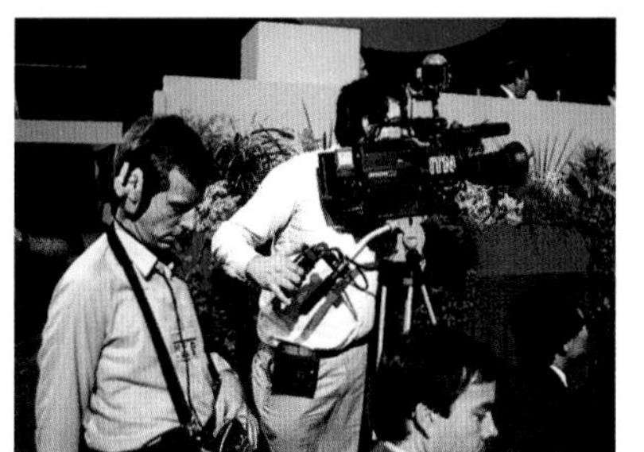

OUTSIDE BROADCAST

Outside broadcast teams use portable cameras when mobility is important, as in a news report, and large, fixed cameras for events such as football games. The pictures are recorded on videotape or beamed back to the studio via a mobile dish antenna.

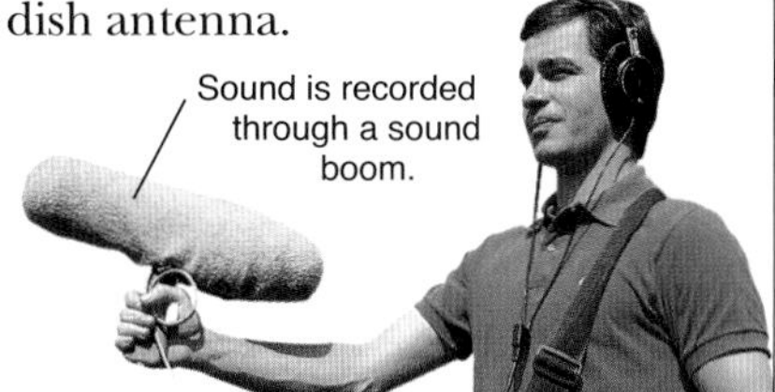

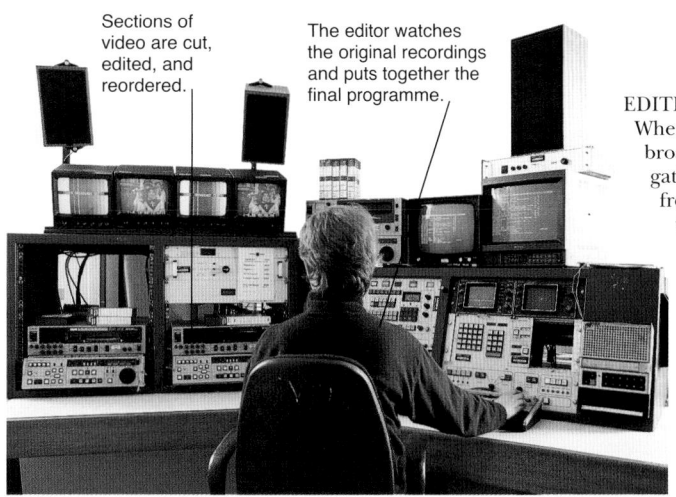

Sound is recorded through a sound boom.

Sections of video are cut, edited, and reordered.
The editor watches the original recordings and puts together the final programme.

EDITING SUITE

When a programme is not broadcast live, an editor gathers all the video recorded from each camera and selects the best sections and edits them together in the right order. This is done in an editing suite (left) with specialist equipment. Editing allows filming to be done out of sequence, and from many different angles. Smooth editing can be crucial to the flow and final cut of a programme.

Television receiver

A television receiver (or TV set) picks up signals broadcast by television stations and converts them to moving pictures using a picture tube. Images appear to move because 25-30 pictures appear each second. Beams of electrons (tiny charged particles from atoms) sweep across the inside surface of a colour screen, hitting dots of chemicals called phosphors. The electrons cause the dots to glow red, green, or blue, depending on the phosphor, and combine to reproduce every colour in the picture.

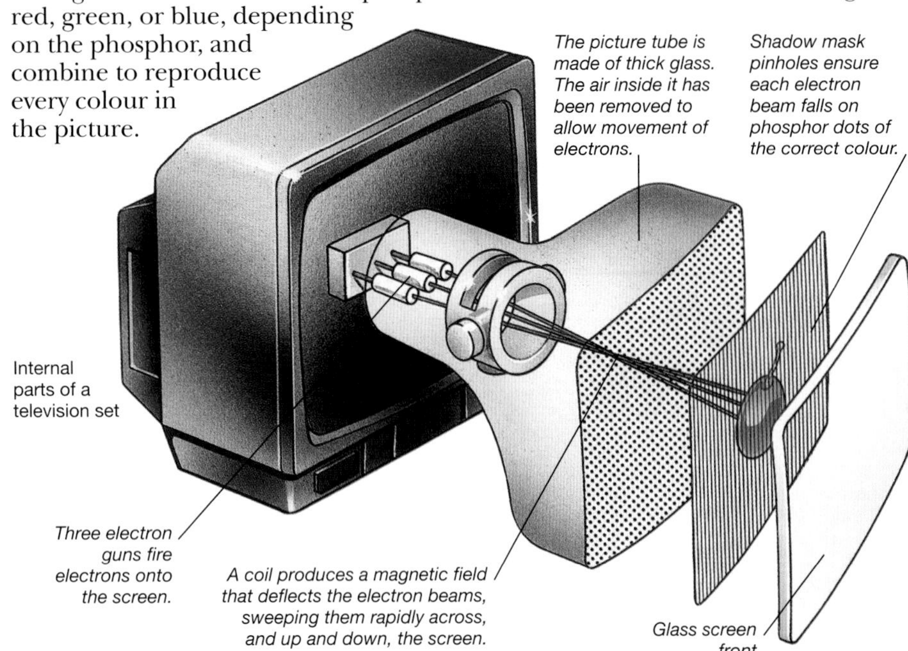

The picture tube is made of thick glass. The air inside it has been removed to allow movement of electrons.

Shadow mask pinholes ensure each electron beam falls on phosphor dots of the correct colour.

Internal parts of a television set

Three electron guns fire electrons onto the screen.

A coil produces a magnetic field that deflects the electron beams, sweeping them rapidly across, and up and down, the screen.

Glass screen front

NEW TECHNOLOGIES

Today's widescreen TV sets increasingly have flat plasma screens or liquid crystal displays instead of bulky picture tubes. Videocassette tapes are being replaced by optical discs (DVDs), which are like high-density music CDs, and by personal video recorders (PVRs), which work in the same way as computer hard disc drives. Movies and TV shows can now be downloaded from the Internet, too. Digital broadcasting uses binary code to carry TV signals with better quality sound and pictures. And with interactive television, viewers can select what to watch and when from a wide range of options.

Hand-held television

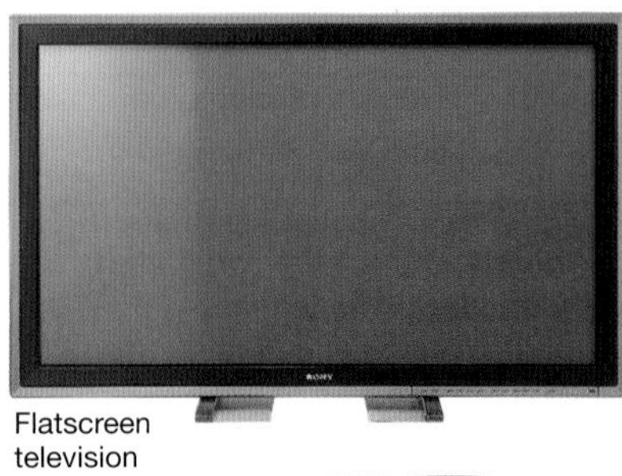

Flatscreen television

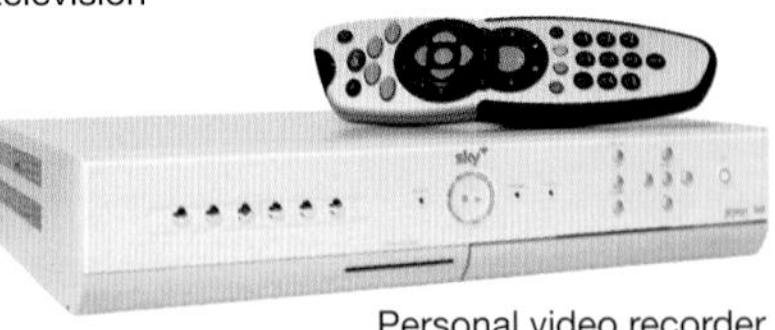

Personal video recorder

TELEVISION TRANSMISSION

Television signals can reach a viewer by several routes. Usually, transmitters broadcast television signals directly to homes as ultrahigh frequency (UHF) radio waves. Alternatively, the signals are sent up to a satellite, which transmits them over a larger region. Individual homes receive the satellite broadcast via dish antennas (right). In other cases, a ground station picks up the signals and sends them out along cables.

Satellite television sends signals from the TV station to homes via a satellite.

Television station

House aerial picks up UHF signals.

Cable television

Cable feeds the signal into the house to the receiver.

The horn collects concentrated incoming waves

Camcorder

INVENTION

In 1926, Scottish engineer John Logie Baird (1888-1946) gave the first public demonstration of television. At about the same time, the Russian American engineer Vladimir Zworykin (1889-1982) invented the electronic camera tube, which was more sophisticated than Baird's system and is the basis of today's television sets. In 1956 the U.S. company Ampex first produced videotape; videocassette recorders appeared in 1969, produced by Sony of Japan.

Video cameras

Today's video cameras or "camcorders" are tiny in comparison with the giant studio cameras used in the early days of TV. They fit easily in the palm of one hand. Most are now digital and record high-quality video sequences – including stereo sound as well – in the form of binary code stored on magnetic tape, optical DVD discs, memory cards, or a hard disc drive built into the camera.

Find out more

Cameras
Electronics
Information technology
Radio
Sound recording

TEXTILES

SPINNING, WEAVING, AND KNITTING turn a mass of short fibres into something much more useful: a textile. We are surrounded by decorative textiles; most clothing is made from them. Textiles keep us warm because they trap air within their mesh of threads. The air acts as an insulator, preventing body heat from escaping. But textiles do much more than keep out the cold. Tightly woven artificial fibres are flexible but tough, so they are ideal for making knapsacks, sails, and parachutes. The loose-weave loops of natural fibres in a towel have a great thirst for water, drying us quickly after a bath. Some special textiles are as strong as armour; Kevlar fabric, for instance, can stop a bullet.

Textiles date back to the taming and breeding of animals about 12,000 years ago. The people of Mesopotamia (now Iraq) rolled sheep wool into a loose yarn for weaving clothes. Plant fibres such as cotton came later, and synthetic fibres have been available only since the invention of nylon in 1938.

SPINNING WHEEL
Spinning thread by twisting fibres between the fingers is hard work. The pedal-powered spinning wheel made the process quicker and easier.

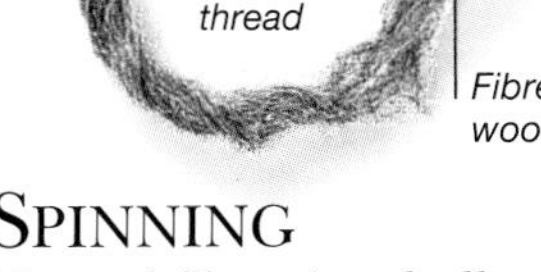

SOURCES OF TEXTILES

Natural fibres for textiles come from cotton bolls, flax (for linen), fleece (for wool), and silk cocoons. Synthetic fibres, such as nylon, are made of chemicals that are mostly produced from crude oil.

SPINNING

Natural fibres in a boll or fleece are tangled together. Spinning machines separate the fibres. They then twist natural or synthetic fibres together so the fibres firmly grip each other and form a strong thread.

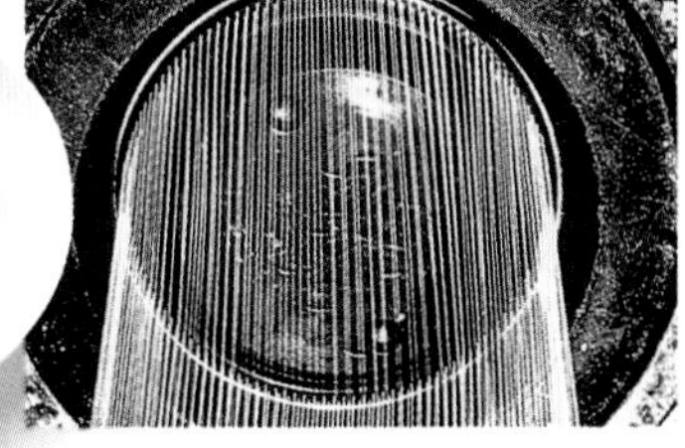

SYNTHETIC FIBRES
Squeezing a liquid called a polymer through tiny holes makes synthetic fibres. The polymer sets as it emerges.

WEAVING AND KNITTING

Looms are machines that crisscross long threads to make woven textiles. Knitting by hand requires just a pair of needles, but a machine does the job more quickly. Pressing unspun fibres together produces a thick textile called felt that is often used for hats.

Weaving passes threads over and under each other.

Knitting forms tiny loops of thread that interlock.

FINISHING TEXTILES

Many textiles are printed with beautiful patterns. Batik (above) uses wax or other materials to make a pattern by restricting where the dye penetrates the fabric. Special treatments make textiles fluffy or waterproof, or stop them from shrinking or wrinkling.

CARPET MAKING

A carpet loom weaves strong threads of wool, cotton, or synthetic fibres onto a mesh backing to make a carpet. The threads may also be knotted together or formed into loops. Cutting the loops turns the tufts of fibres into a carpet pile.

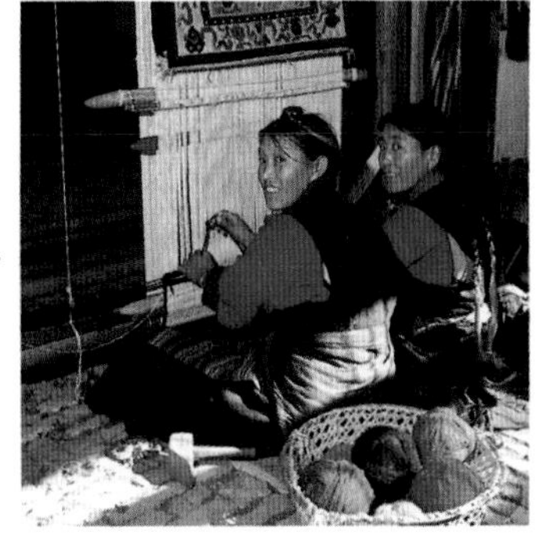

Find out more
BUTTERFLIES AND MOTHS
CLOTHES
INDUSTRIAL REVOLUTION
PLASTICS

THEATRE

AT THE HEART OF ALL THEATRE lies the excitement of watching a live performance. Bringing a play to life involves many people. The words of the dramatist, or playwright, the ideas of the director, and the actors' skill combine to make an audience believe that what is happening on the stage – the drama – is real. Early theatre grew out of religious festivals held in Greece in honour of the god Dionysus, and included singing and dancing as well as acting. The different forms of theatre that emerged in India, China, and Japan also had religious origins. In medieval Europe people watched "miracle plays", which were based on religious stories. Later, dramatists began to write about all aspects of life, and companies of actors performed their plays in permanent theatres. Theatre changes to suit the demands of each new age for fantasy, spectacle, or serious drama.

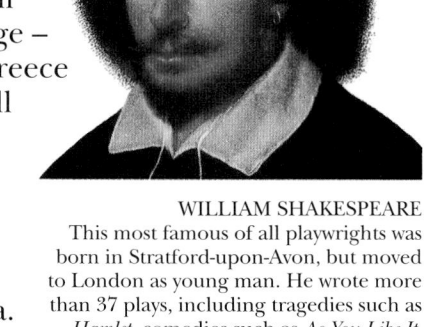

WILLIAM SHAKESPEARE
This most famous of all playwrights was born in Stratford-upon-Avon, but moved to London as young man. He wrote more than 37 plays, including tragedies such as *Hamlet*, comedies such as *As You Like It*, and history plays such as *Henry V*. He died in 1616 at the age of 52.

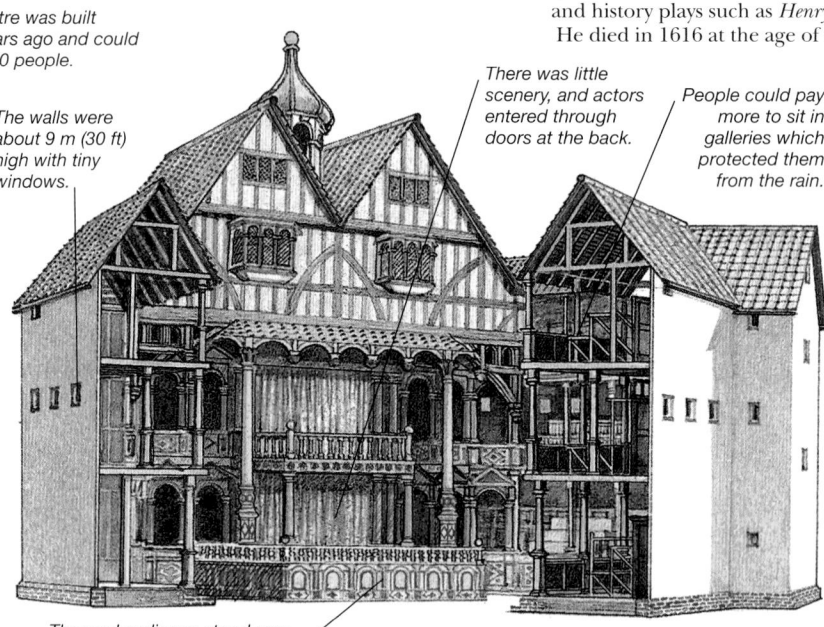

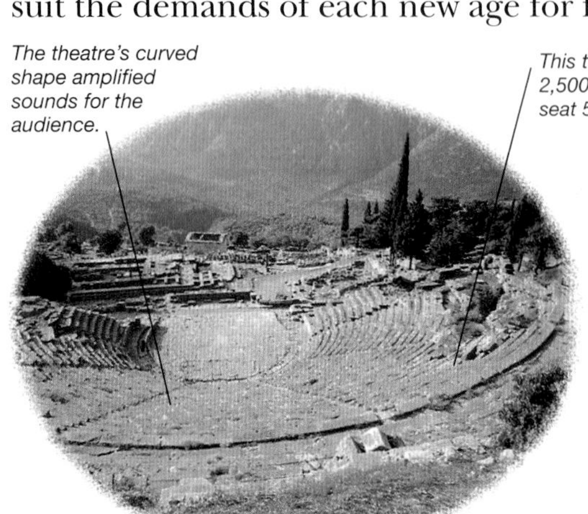
The theatre's curved shape amplified sounds for the audience.
This theatre was built 2,500 years ago and could seat 5,000 people.

OPEN-AIR THEATRE
Ancient Greek theatre made use of landscapes like this one at Delphi. Actors wore exaggerated masks so that characters could be recognized from afar.

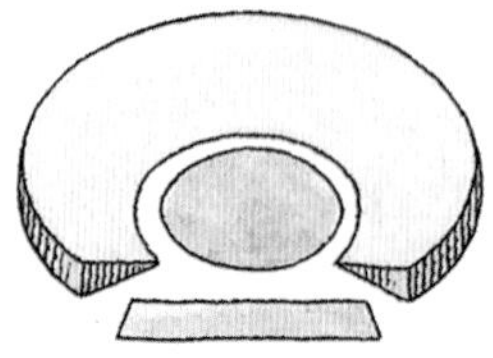

GREEK THEATRE
The audience sat in a semicircle of steplike seats. There was a circular orchestra – a space for dancing and singing – and a low stage for actors.

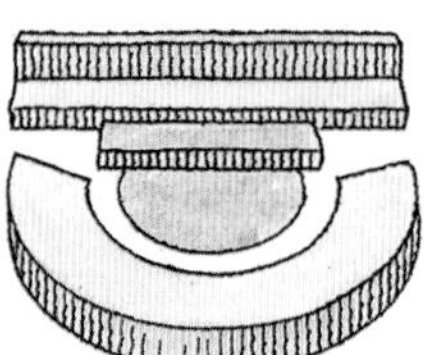

ROMAN THEATRE
Based on Greek theatres, the Roman theatre was usually open to the sky and enclosed on three sides. A permanent wooden roof sheltered the raised stage.

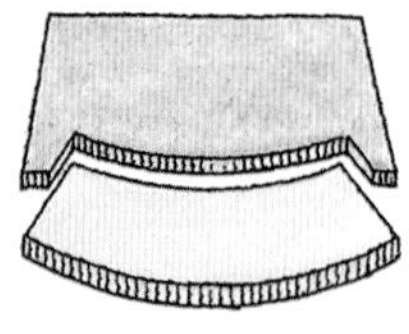

THE OPEN STAGE
Some modern theatres have an open stage without a curtain. The actors can address the audience more directly, as if holding a conversation.

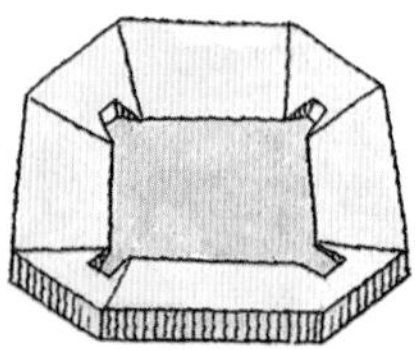

THEATRE-IN-THE-ROUND
Here the audience surrounds the cast on all four sides, bringing everyone close together. The actors enter through aisles between the seats.

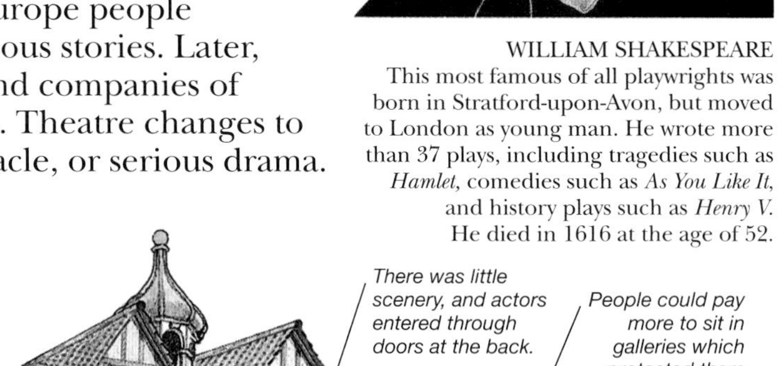

The walls were about 9 m (30 ft) high with tiny windows.
There was little scenery, and actors entered through doors at the back.
People could pay more to sit in galleries which protected them from the rain.
The yard audience stood very close to the actors on stage.

GLOBE PLAYHOUSE

Shakespeare was an actor and a writer at this famous theatre on the south bank of the River Thames in London. There was room for more than 2,000 people in the round wooden building. The audience stood in the open yard or sat in the enclosed gallery to watch a performance. In 1995, the Globe was rebuilt at a nearby site in London.

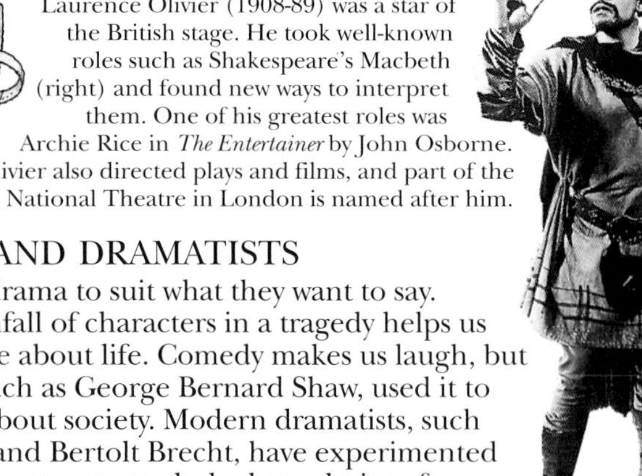

LAURENCE OLIVIER
Laurence Olivier (1908-89) was a star of the British stage. He took well-known roles such as Shakespeare's Macbeth (right) and found new ways to interpret them. One of his greatest roles was Archie Rice in *The Entertainer* by John Osborne. Olivier also directed plays and films, and part of the Royal National Theatre in London is named after him.

DRAMA AND DRAMATISTS

Playwrights adapt drama to suit what they want to say. Watching the downfall of characters in a tragedy helps us to understand more about life. Comedy makes us laugh, but some dramatists, such as George Bernard Shaw, used it to say serious things about society. Modern dramatists, such as Samuel Beckett and Bertolt Brecht, have experimented with words and characters to push the boundaries of drama even further.

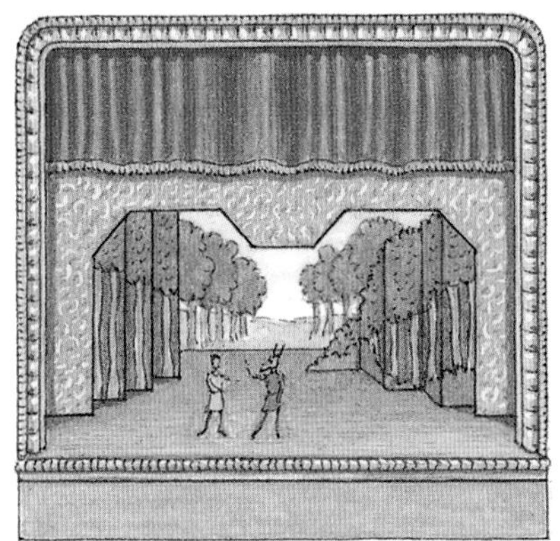

THE PICTURE FRAME
Clever use of scenery and a sloping stage helps to change the audience's view through the proscenium arch (the frame of the stage) and makes the stage look deeper.

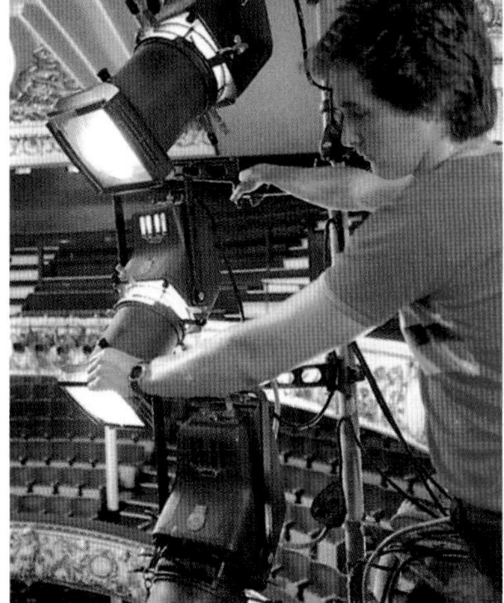

PROFILE-SPOT
Stagehands control this light from the rear of the upper circle. They use the strong beam to pick out and follow an actor in a pool of brilliant light.

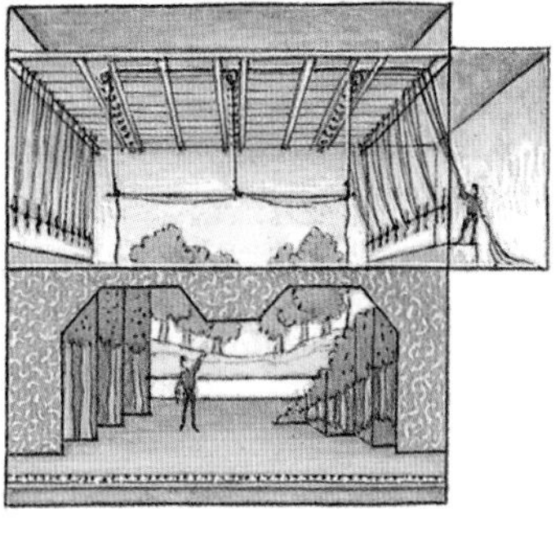

UP IN THE FLIES
High above the stage there is "fly" space in which scenery and equipment hang. A system of pulleys makes it possible to lower scenery.

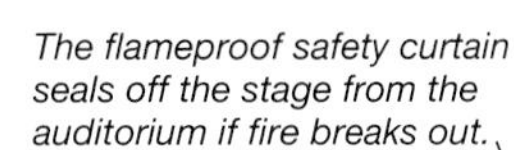

Lowering the curtain, or tabs, hides the stage while stagehands change scenery.

The flameproof safety curtain seals off the stage from the auditorium if fire breaks out.

Some of the actors share a dressing room where they put on makeup and change into costume.

Fly ropes raise and lower the lights as they are needed.

Loudspeaker announcements warn the actors to get ready to make their entrance.

Actors who play the lead roles may have a dressing room to themselves.

The wardrobe department makes the costumes and stores them until needed.

Scenery and props wait in the wings for rapid scene changes.

By raising or angling the stage slightly the designer can change the audience's view.

Musicians may sit in an orchestra pit below the front of the stage.

The elevator can lift an actor or prop onto the stage in a split second.

Most traditional theatres have a "picture frame" stage – the play takes place under a proscenium arch.

The busy carpentry department builds the sets. Props, such as furniture, are stored here when not in use.

Actors enter and leave the theatre by the stage door.

From the lighting control board or console, the operator can dim or brighten any light in the theatre. A lighting change can alter the mood of a play in seconds.

SOUND EFFECTS
Sound effects must happen at exactly the right moment. If an actor falls down before the sound of a gunshot, the whole scene is ruined. The sound operator listens and watches carefully for each cue.

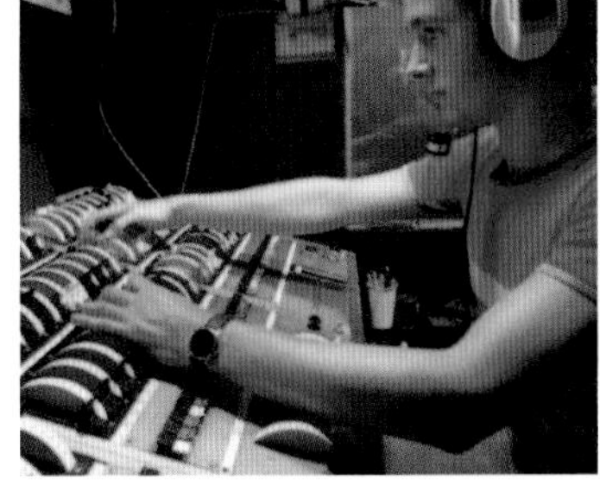

Find out more
Ballet
Literature
Music
Opera and singing
Shakespeare, William

TIME

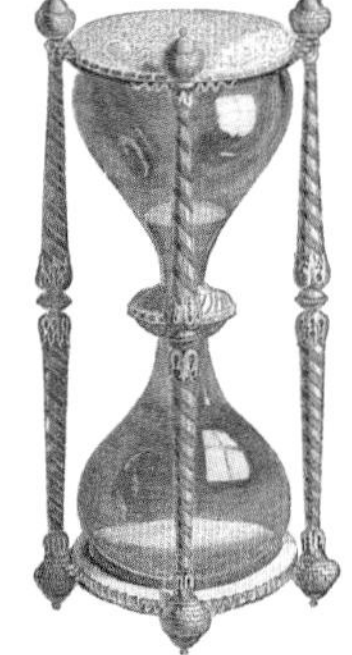

HOURGLASS
Sand draining through an hourglass shows the passing of time. It takes one hour for the sand to run from the top to the bottom bulb.

HOUR FOLLOWS HOUR as time passes. Time always flows steadily in the same direction. Behind us in time lies the past, which we know. Ahead lies the future, which we cannot know. We cannot change time, but we can measure it. People first measured time in days and nights, which they could easily see and count. They also measured time in months, by watching the phases of the Moon, and in years, by watching the cycle of the seasons. Today, we have clocks and watches that can measure time in fractions of a second.

In 1905, German physicist Albert Einstein proposed the scientific theory of relativity. This says that time is not constant, but that it would pass more slowly if you could travel very fast (near the speed of light), or in strong fields of gravity. Scientists believe that time may even come to a stop in black holes deep in space.

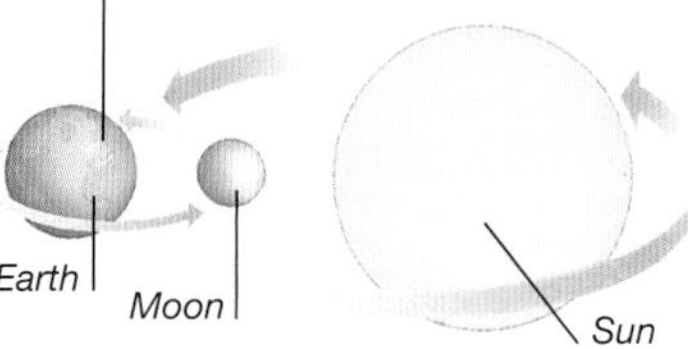

In reality, the Earth is 400 times further away from the Sun than it is from the Moon.

YEARS AND MONTHS
A year is based on the time the Earth takes to go once around the Sun, which is 365.26 days. Months vary from 28 to 31 days. They were originally based on the time the Moon takes to go around the Earth, which is 27.3 days.

The International Date Line is at 180 degrees longitude.

3 p.m. in Moscow, Russian Federation

INTERNATIONAL DATE LINE
The western side of the International Date Line is one day ahead of the eastern side. When you cross the line, the date changes.

12 noon in London, Britain

TIME ZONES
The world is divided into 24 regions, called time zones, each with a different time of day. This was done to avoid having several time differences within one area, and to ensure that all countries have noon during the middle of the day.

2 p.m. in Cairo, Egypt

7 a.m. in New York City, USA

The Earth spins counterclockwise.

UNIVERSAL TIME
The time at the prime meridian is used as a standard time known as Universal Time (UT) or Greenwich Mean Time (GMT).

The prime meridian is at 0 degrees longitude.

UNITS OF TIME

One full day and night is the time in which the Earth spins once. This is divided into 24 hours: each hour contains 60 minutes, and each minute contains 60 seconds. The Babylonians fixed these units about 5,000 years ago, using 24 and 60 because they divide easily by 2, 3, and 4.

9 a.m. in Rio de Janeiro, Brazil

DAYS AND NIGHTS
The Sun lights up one half of the Earth, where it is day. The other half, away from the Sun, is dark, and there it is night. Days and nights come and go because the Earth spins once every 24 hours. But the day and night may last different lengths of time because the Earth is tilted at an angle to the Sun.

Twice a year the Sun is directly overhead at 12 noon.

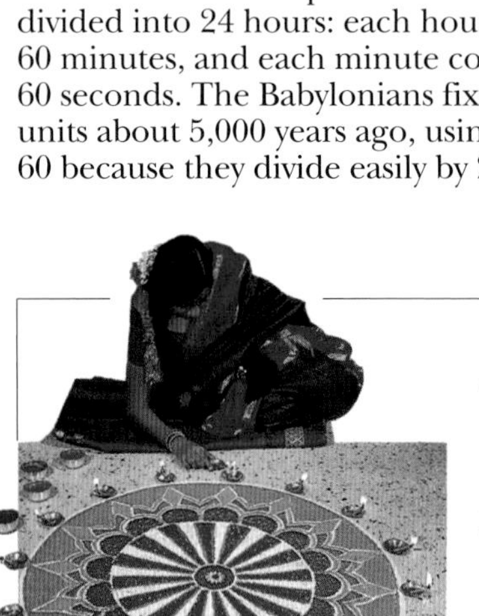

The Hindu calendar is based on lunar months. Diwali, the Festival of Lights, marks the start of the new year, which falls in October or November.

CALENDARS

The date is fixed by the calendar, which contains 12 months with a total of 365 days. Every fourth year is a leap year which has one extra day, February 29. Leap years are years that divide by four, such as 2008 and 2012. The calendar contains leap years because the Earth takes slightly longer than 365 days to go once around the Sun. Prehistoric peoples may have used monuments such as Stonehenge, in southern England (below), to measure the Sun's position and find the exact length of the year.

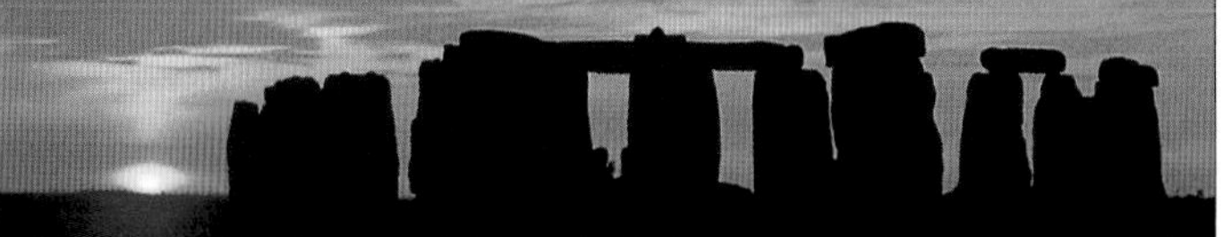

Find out more

CLOCKS AND WATCHES
EARTH
EINSTEIN, ALBERT
PHYSICS
SCIENCE
STARS
UNIVERSE

TOURISM AND TRAVEL

IT USED TO BE VERY UNUSUAL for people to travel far from their homes. It took weeks to do trips that today take hours in a car, and months or years to reach destinations that are now a few hours flight away. Religious pilgrimages were one of the few reasons why people made journeys. In the 17th and 18th centuries, only the rich could afford to travel. With the arrival of trains, and later buses, in the 19th century, journeys became cheaper and tourism – travel for pleasure – began. Today, cheap air travel has made holidays abroad available to many people. A huge industry, including travel agencies, package holiday companies and airlines, has grown up to serve the tourist trade, which is now an important part of the world's economy.

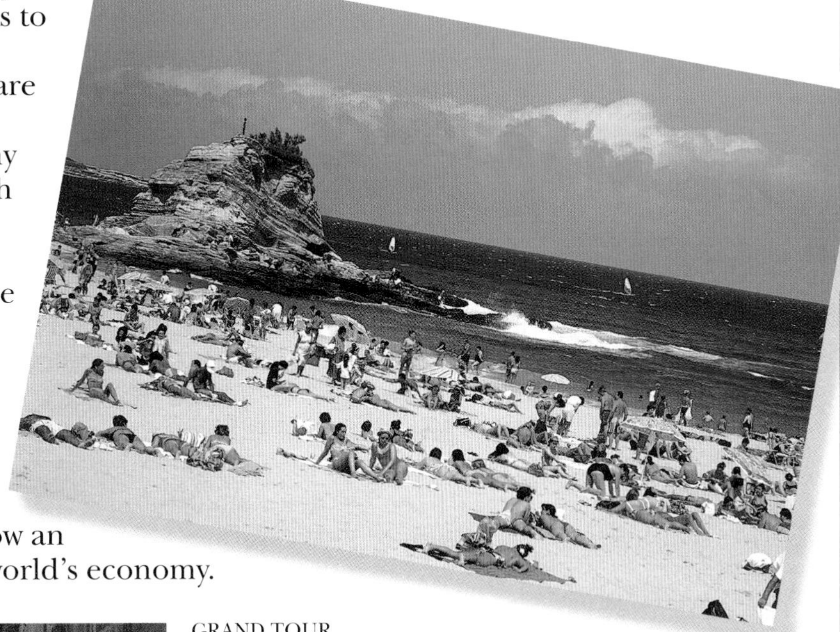

Cockle shell

PILGRIMS
Since ancient times, people all over the world have made pilgrimages – journeys to holy places – to pray for help and spiritual guidance. In medieval Europe, pilgrims who travelled to the shrine of St. James at Santiago de Compostela in Spain brought back a cockle shell to show that they had made the journey.

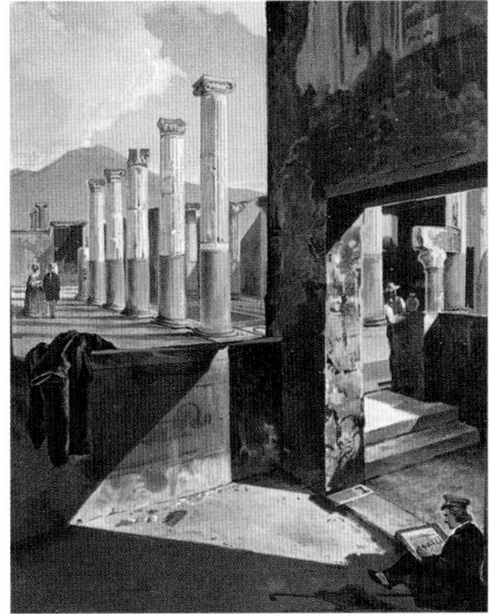

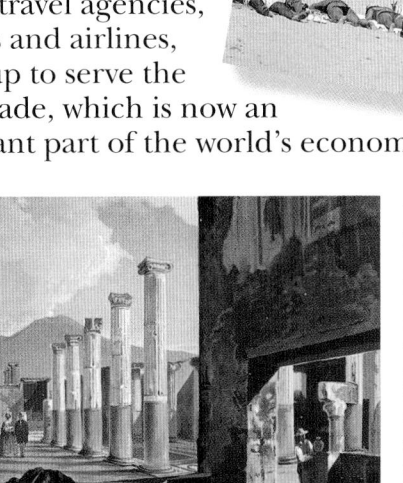

GRAND TOUR
A trip around Europe became fashionable among the British aristocracy in the 18th century, when it was considered a desirable way to complete a young person's education. The travellers would spend weeks, or possibly months, in cities such as Rome and Vienna, often staying with relatives or friends. Only the very rich could afford to do a Grand Tour.

PACKAGE HOLIDAYS

Travel agencies and holiday companies put together flights, hotels and meals to create all-inclusive holiday packages for tourists. Spain, Greece, and other places that have hot weather and sandy beaches, have built lots of hotels for tourists from colder countries such as Britain. Package holidays are a huge business that provides millions of jobs.

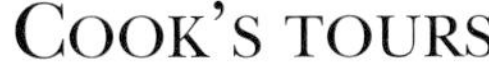

COOK'S TOURS

The first person to make a successful business from organizing excursions and travel groups was Thomas Cook (1808-92) in the late 1800s. He brought holidays to the middle classes by making them affordable, and created the modern holiday business. The travel agency named after him is part of a worldwide business.

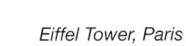

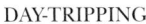

Snowboards are a challenging way to enjoy the ski slopes.

OUTDOOR HOLIDAYS
Some people want to be lazy on holiday, while others prefer to be active. Many tourists choose to go on adventure holidays, which focus on sports such as scuba diving and windsurfing. Skiing is also very popular and has become a big business. In recent years, many young people have decided to go backpacking – travelling to less-discovered places, away from the tourist crowds.

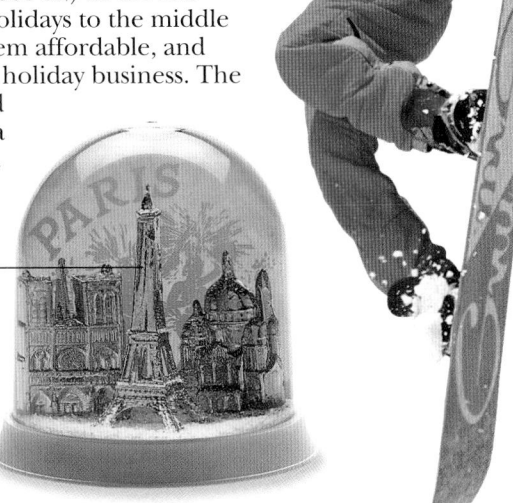

Eiffel Tower, Paris tourist attraction

DAY-TRIPPING
The development of the railways and buses made travel quicker as well as cheaper. Day trips were now possible for ordinary people. The souvenir industry grew up, making small ornaments and items for trippers to take back to their friends and family as gifts, or to remind them of the places they had visited.

Find out more
SPORTS
TRANSPORT, HISTORY OF
WATER SPORTS

Toys

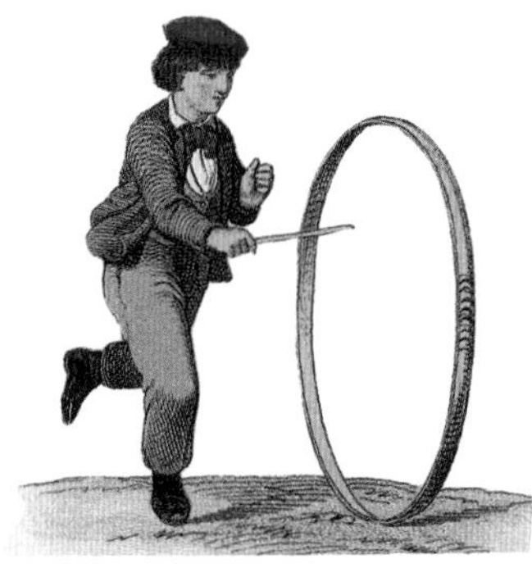

HOOPS
With a little imagination everyday objects can become toys. A stick becomes a hobby-horse, an old box a doll's bed. For centuries, children of many lands have used wooden wheels or rings from barrels as hoops. They can be rolled along, thrown in the air, or whirled around the body.

ALTHOUGH THE MAIN purpose of a toy is fun or amusement, toys have other functions too. Some toys prepare children for the activities of adult life. For example, hobby-horses helped children learn about horse-riding long before they were old enough to sit in the saddle. Similarly, today's toy cars can teach driving skills. In the Middle Ages toys such as tops and rattles were popular, but in later centuries only rich families could afford the elaborate toys that became fashionable. In strict families the only toys allowed on Sunday were those associated with the Bible, such as a model of Noah's Ark. Today, there are more toys than ever before. Children have a vast choice of mass-produced playthings, but there is still a demand for simple homemade toys like those that amused Ancient Egyptian children.

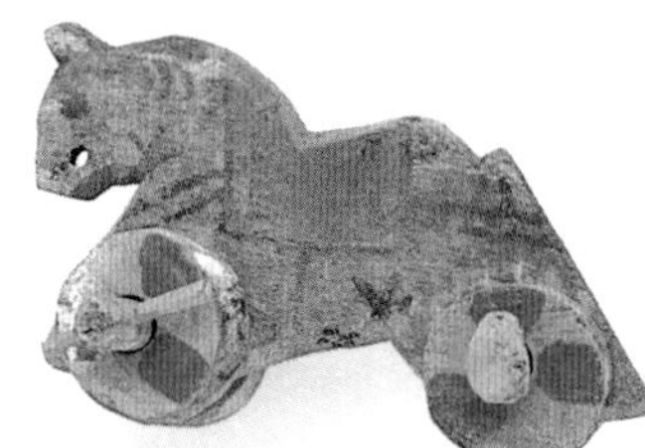

ANCIENT TOYS
Baked clay horses were found in Egypt that are almost 2,500 years old. Archaeologists in Rhodes, Greece, discovered animal toys which were even older. These ancient toys give us an idea of how children played long ago.

Dolls

Dolls were among the first toys. They have been made from rags, wax, wood, and paper. During the last century dolls were beautifully dressed and had fragile china heads. Modern dolls are much sturdier and some are able to walk, talk, and eat.

The ball is a universal toy and is found in every society.

Blocks can be used for games of counting, balancing, and building.

ELECTRONIC TOYS
Battery-powered games test a player's mental agility and speed of reflexes. The computer brains inside are tiny, so even complex games are small enough to fit in a pocket.

TEDDY BEARS

On a hunting trip in 1902, United States President Theodore "Teddy" Roosevelt refused to kill a bear cub. Soon after this was reported in the newspapers, a shopkeeper began to sell cuddly toys called "teddy bears". In Europe, a German company called Steiff made similar bears with movable arms and legs. This favourite toy now comes in all colours and sizes, but the basic shape remains the same.

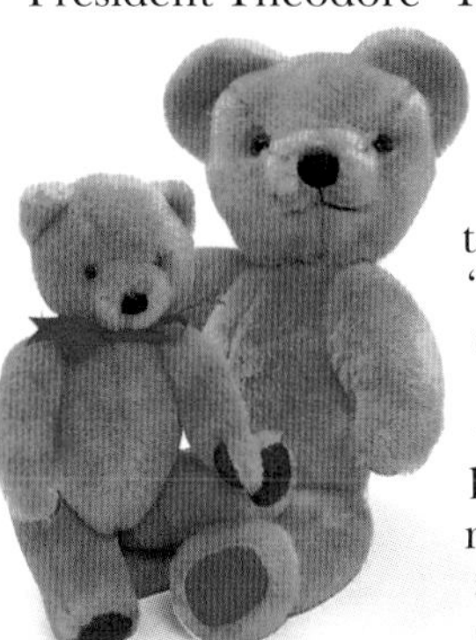

TOY CARS
Both children and adults enjoy and collect model cars. Some toy cars move in any direction by remote control.

CONSTRUCTION TOYS
Construction toys such as Lego® really challenge building skills and imagination. Sections of various sizes fit together to create model forts, castles, and spacecraft.

Find out more
GAMES
PUPPETS
PUZZLES

TRADE AND INDUSTRY

WITHOUT TRADE AND INDUSTRY, people would have to create everything they needed to live. If you wanted a loaf of bread you would have to grow wheat, grind the wheat to make flour, mix the dough, and bake it in an oven. You would also need to build the mill and make the oven! Industry organizes the production of bread, so that just a few farmers, millers, and bakers can make bread for everyone. Similarly, industry supplies us with most other essential and luxury goods, from fresh water to cars. Trade is the process of buying and selling. Trade gets the products from the people who make them to the people who need them. And through trade, manufacturers can buy the raw materials they need to supply their factories and keep production going. Together, the trade and industry of a nation are sometimes called the economy.

SILK ROAD
Trade between different regions and peoples goes back to ancient times. The Silk Road was one of the earliest and most famous trade routes. Traders led horses and camels along this route between 300 B.C. and A.D. 1600, carrying silk from China to Europe.

India exports cotton textiles to Europe.

India exports tea to the Russian Federation.

India imports cars from Japan.

India imports oil from the Middle East.

India exports rice to Australia.

Imports

Exports

INTERNATIONAL TRADE

Goods move around the world by sea, land, and air. This international trade takes materials such as oil from the countries that have a surplus to those that have no or insufficient oil deposits. International trade is also necessary because goods do not always fetch a high price in the country where they are made. For example, many clothes are made by hand in countries where wages are low. But the clothes are sold in another country where people are richer and can pay a high price. Money earned this way helps less rich countries for their imports.

IMPORTS AND EXPORTS

Goods that are traded internationally are called imports and exports. Goods that one country sells to another are called exports; imports are goods that a country buys from another. In most nations, private businesses control imports and exports. But in others, the government imposes strict controls on what can be bought and sold.

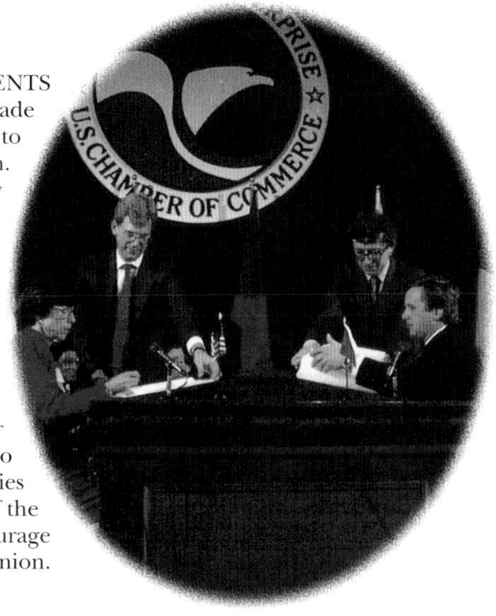

TRADE AGREEMENTS
Some countries sign trade agreements in order to control trade between them. The agreement may simply fix the price at which the two countries buy and sell certain goods, such as tea and wheat. The European Union (EU) has a complicated network of trade agreements which allow free exchange of goods between member countries. The EU also restricts trade with countries that are not members of the Union. This helps encourage industry within the Union.

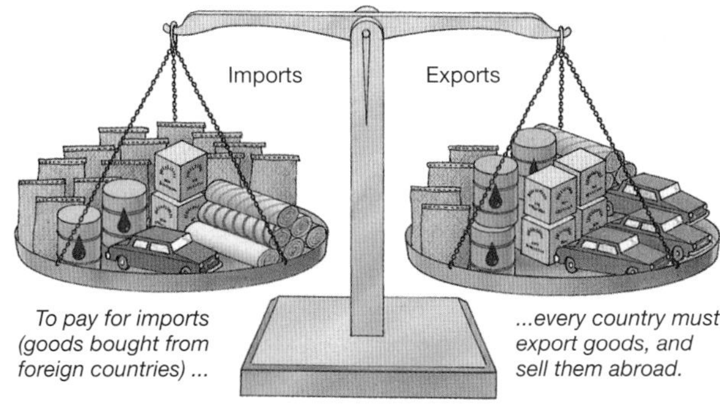

Imports
Exports
To pay for imports (goods bought from foreign countries) ...
...every country must export goods, and sell them abroad.

BALANCE OF PAYMENTS
Each country pays for imports with the money it earns by selling goods in other countries. This balance between imports and exports is called the balance of trade, or the balance of payments. Countries that do not export enough must borrow money from abroad to pay for imports.

FACTORIES

Some industry takes place in people's homes, but workers in factories make most of the products that we buy. In a factory each person has a small task in the manufacturing process. He or she may operate a large machine or assemble something by hand. No one person makes an entire product. This process of mass production makes manufacturing cheaper and quicker. Most factories are owned by large companies; a few factories are owned by governments or by the people who work in them.

SUPPLY AND DEMAND

Companies set up factories to produce goods that they think people will want to buy. They sell the goods at a price that allows the company to make a profit. As long as there is a demand for the goods, the factory will continue to supply them. When fewer people buy the goods that the factory makes, prices drop to try to attract buyers, and workers in the factory may lose their jobs.

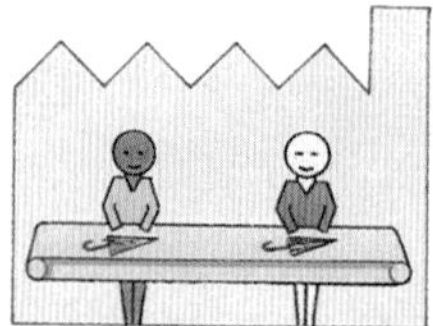

A factory starts by making a small number of umbrellas.

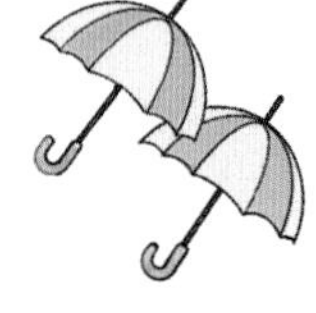

Shops put a few umbrellas on sale at a high price.

Many people need umbrellas and buy them, increasing demand.

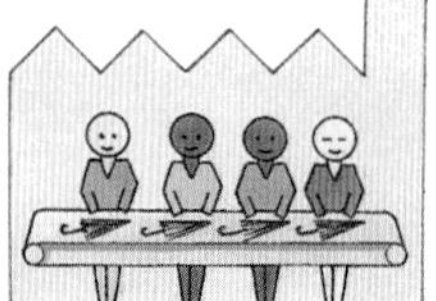

The factory employs more people to make more umbrellas.

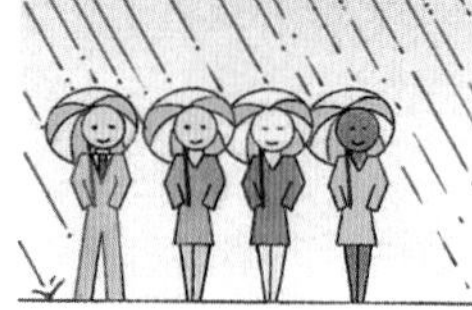

When everyone has an umbrella, demand for umbrellas falls.

Prices drop, and the factory needs fewer umbrella workers.

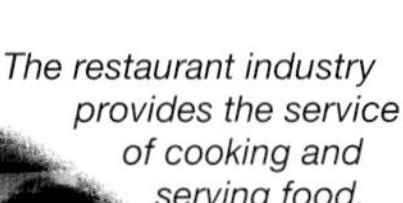

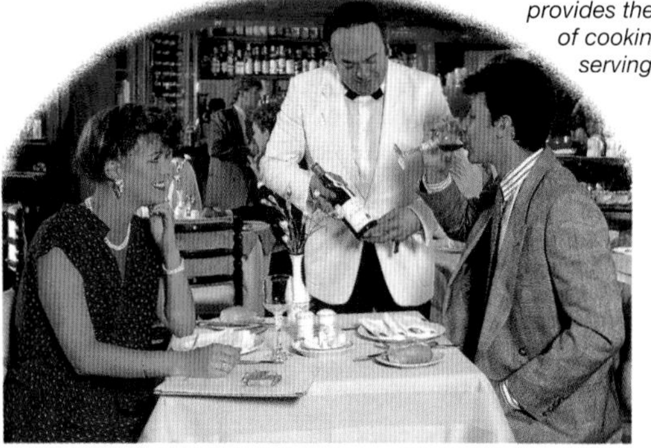

The restaurant industry provides the service of cooking and serving food.

SERVICE INDUSTRIES

Not all industries make objects for sale. Some industries provide a service in return for money. A garage, for instance, might charge a fee to adjust a car so that it runs more efficiently. People pay for this service rather than do the work themselves.

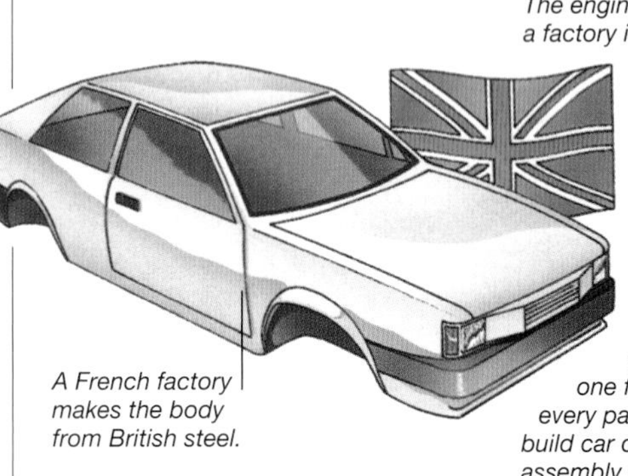

A French factory makes the body from British steel.

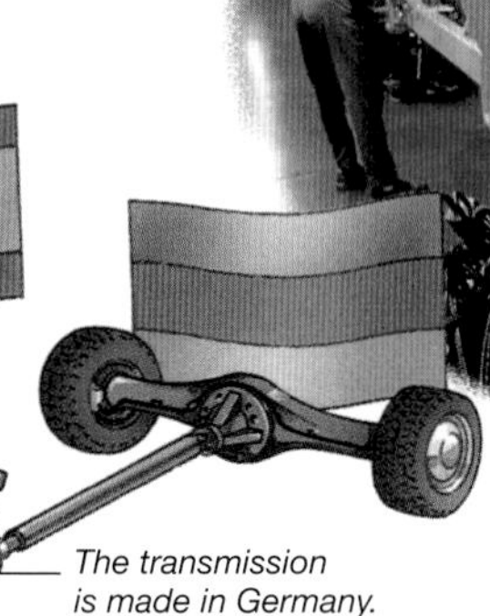

The engine comes from a factory in Spain.

The transmission is made in Germany.

A modern car is so complex that one factory cannot make every part. So, many factories build car components, and an assembly plant builds the vehicle.

Final assembly of the car may take place in Spain.

MANUFACTURING

The basic form of industry is manufacturing. This means working on materials to manufacture, or make, a finished product. Almost everything we use is the product of manufacturing, and most manufacturing takes place in large factories. However, craftsworkers manufacture goods alone or in small groups. Some goods go through many stages of manufacturing. For example, workers making cars assemble manufactured components or parts which, in turn, have been made in many other factories, often in other countries.

TRADE UNIONS

During the 19th century, workers began to form trade unions in order to obtain better pay and conditions for its members. If a union cannot achieve its aims, its members may go on strike – stop work – until their demands are met.

The successful strike of women workers in a London match factory in 1888 encouraged other workers to join unions.

Find out more

ADVERTISING
DEPRESSION OF THE 1930S
FACTORIES
INDUSTRIAL REVOLUTION
MONEY
SHOPS AND SHOPPING

TRAINS

WHEN THE FIRST RAILWAYS were built more than 150 years ago, many people said they were the most wonderful of all inventions. Others said the snorting, smoking steam engines were like ugly, metal monsters. Trains and railways certainly changed our world. Not only did embankments and cuttings alter the landscape, but also, for the first time, people and goods could be carried long distances in vast quantities – and at speeds undreamed of. Railways also allowed cities to grow more than ever before. Today, large networks of railways stretch through many countries. If the tracks of the world's main rail routes were laid end to end, they would circle the Earth more than 116 times. Trains are an efficient method of transport. They use less fuel and produce less pollution than cars and trucks because they carry large cargoes in a single journey. Because of the damage road vehicles do to our environment, many people believe trains are the best form of transport for the future.

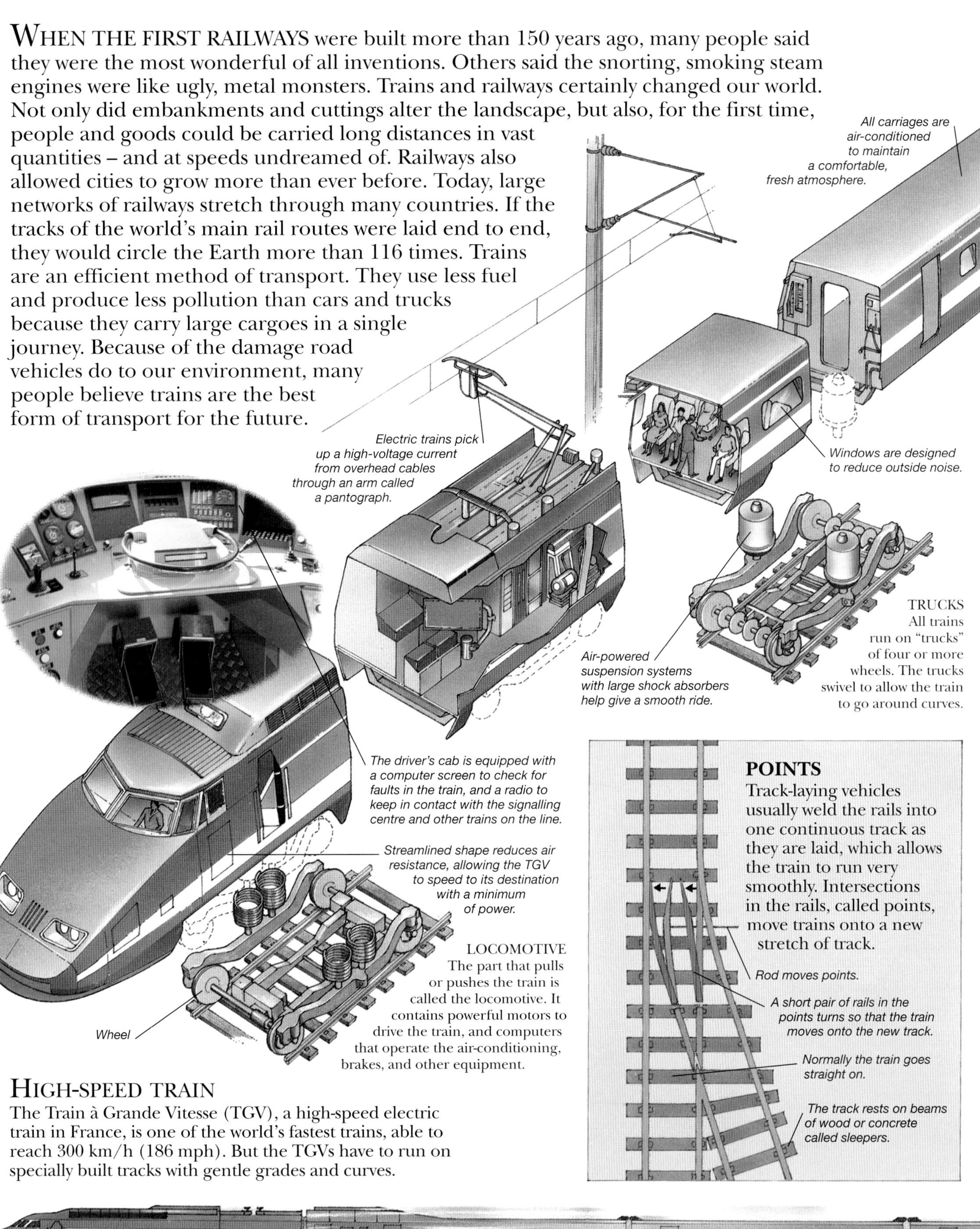

All carriages are air-conditioned to maintain a comfortable, fresh atmosphere.
Electric trains pick up a high-voltage current from overhead cables through an arm called a pantograph.
Windows are designed to reduce outside noise.
Air-powered suspension systems with large shock absorbers help give a smooth ride.
The driver's cab is equipped with a computer screen to check for faults in the train, and a radio to keep in contact with the signalling centre and other trains on the line.
Streamlined shape reduces air resistance, allowing the TGV to speed to its destination with a minimum of power.
Wheel
Rod moves points.
A short pair of rails in the points turns so that the train moves onto the new track.
Normally the train goes straight on.
The track rests on beams of wood or concrete called sleepers.

TRUCKS
All trains run on "trucks" of four or more wheels. The trucks swivel to allow the train to go around curves.

LOCOMOTIVE
The part that pulls or pushes the train is called the locomotive. It contains powerful motors to drive the train, and computers that operate the air-conditioning, brakes, and other equipment.

POINTS
Track-laying vehicles usually weld the rails into one continuous track as they are laid, which allows the train to run very smoothly. Intersections in the rails, called points, move trains onto a new stretch of track.

HIGH-SPEED TRAIN

The Train à Grande Vitesse (TGV), a high-speed electric train in France, is one of the world's fastest trains, able to reach 300 km/h (186 mph). But the TGVs have to run on specially built tracks with gentle grades and curves.

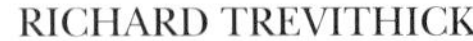

RICHARD TREVITHICK

In 1804, a steam locomotive (right) built by Englishman Richard Trevithick ran on rails for the first time. Trevithick thought that steam power had a future, and bet that his steam engine could haul 9 tonnes (9 tons) of iron 15 km (9.5 miles) along a mine railway in Wales. Trevithick won his bet; the engine carried not only the iron but also 70 cheering coal miners who climbed aboard.

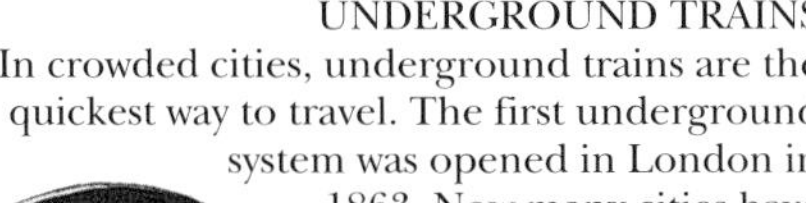

UNDERGROUND TRAINS

In crowded cities, underground trains are the quickest way to travel. The first underground system was opened in London in 1863. Now many cities have their own network. The Metro in Paris is one of the most efficient underground systems in the world.

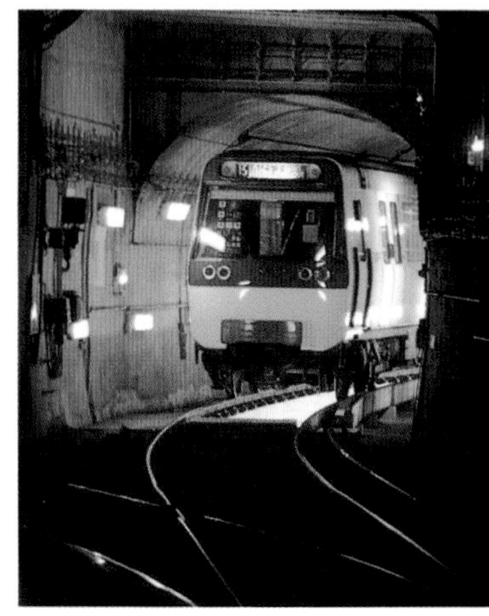

The Rocket, built by English engineer George Stephenson in 1829, was a new design that heralded the age of the passenger train.

STEAM RAILWAYS

Railways date back 4,000 years to the Babylonians, who pushed carts along grooves. But the age of railways really began in the early 1800s when steam engines first ran on rails. In 1825, the first passenger line opened in England; 30 years later, vast railway systems stretched across Europe and North America. By the 1890s, steam engines could reach speeds of more than 160 km/h (100 mph).

A front truck was introduced on early American locomotives to give a smoother ride around curves.

During the mid-1800s, England's railway system developed into a large network.

Engines could reach 200 km/h (126 mph) by the 1930s – the peak of the steam age.

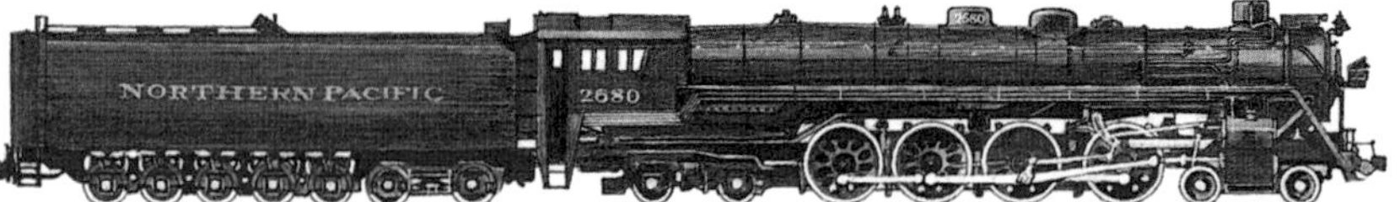

Steam locomotives of the1930s were very sophisticated compared to the first engines.

SIGNALS AND SAFETY

Trackside signals tell the driver how fast to go and when to stop. In the past, signals were mechanical arms worked by levers in the signal box. Nowadays they are usually sets of coloured lights controlled by computers that monitor the position of every train.

MAGLEVS AND MONORAILS

One day we may be whisked along silently at speeds of 480 km/h (300 mph) on trains that glide a small distance above special tracks, held up by magnetic force – which is why they are called Maglevs (for magnetic levitation). Some countries, such as Japan, already have Maglev lines. Other new designs include monorail trains, which are electric trains that run on, or are suspended from, a single rail.

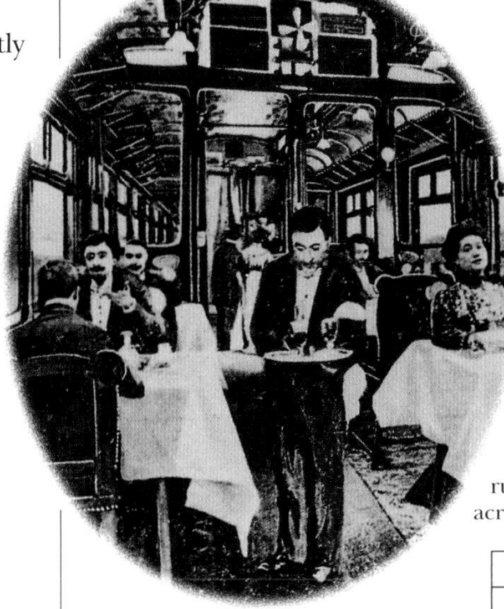

ORIENT EXPRESS

Some trains have become famous for their speed, some for their luxury, and others for the length of their route. From 1883, the *Orient Express*, for example, provided a first-class service from Paris to Constantinople (Istanbul), Turkey. It still travels part of this route today. The world's longest train route is the *Trans-Siberian Express*, which runs 9,438 km (5,864 miles) across Siberia.

Find out more

BUSES
ENGINES
TOURISM AND TRAVEL
TRANSPORT, HISTORY OF

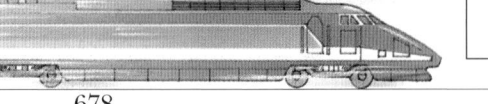

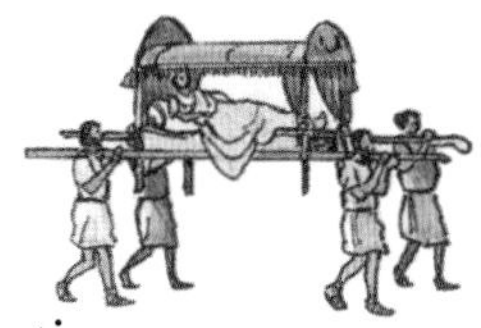

HISTORY OF
TRANSPORT

WE LIVE IN AN AGE when people can fly across the Atlantic Ocean in less than three hours. Straight roads link city to city across the world. Yet 7,000 years ago the only way that people could get from one place to another was by walking. In around 5,000 B.C. people began to use donkeys and oxen as pack animals, instead of carrying their goods on their backs or heads. Then, 1,500 years later, the first wheeled vehicles developed in Mesopotamia. From around A.D. 1500, deep-sea sailing ships developed rapidly as Europeans began to make great ocean voyages to explore the rest of the world. During the 1700s, steam power marked another milestone in transport. Steam engines were soon moving ships and trains faster than anyone had imagined. During the next century the first cars took to the road and the first flying machines took to the air.

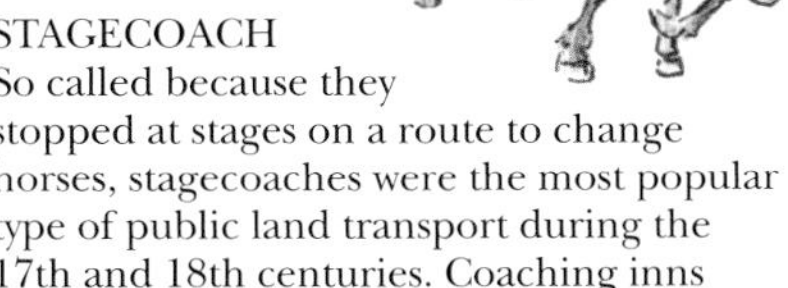

STAGECOACH
So called because they stopped at stages on a route to change horses, stagecoaches were the most popular type of public land transport during the 17th and 18th centuries. Coaching inns sprung up along popular stagecoach routes.

Railways began to appear in the United States in the 1820s. Trains could carry more goods and people than any other kind of transport.

LAND TRAVEL

Land travel is the most common kind of transport. It all began with walking. Two thousand years ago the Romans built a network of superb roads over which people travelled by foot or by horse-drawn cart. It was only in the 1800s that steam power took the place of horse power. Steam locomotives provided cheap long-distance travel for ordinary people. In the early years of this century, engine-powered cars, trucks, and buses were developed.

CARS
Cars are now the most popular form of private transport. They were invented towards the end of the 19th century.

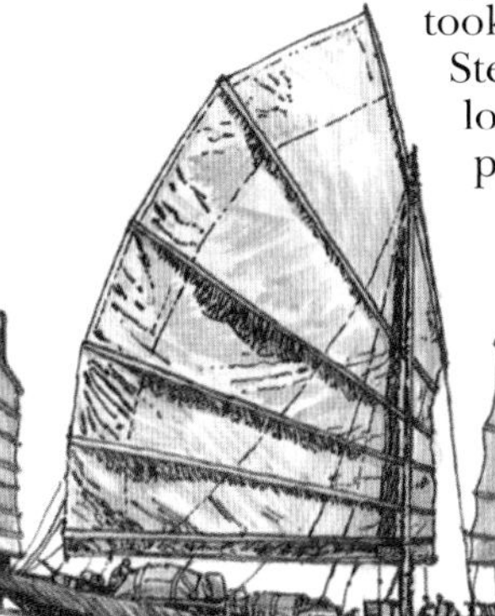

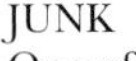

JUNK
One of the world's strongest sailing ships, the junk has been used in Asia for thousands of years. Mainly a trading vessel, it has large, highly efficient sails made of linen or matting.

BARGE
A barge is a sturdy boat which transports cargo, such as coal, from place to place along canals and rivers.

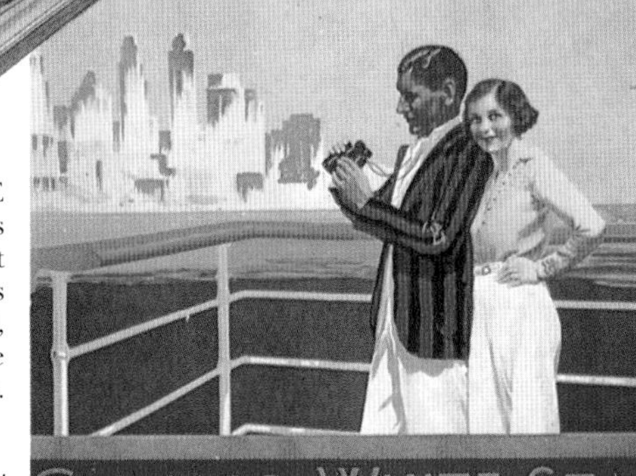

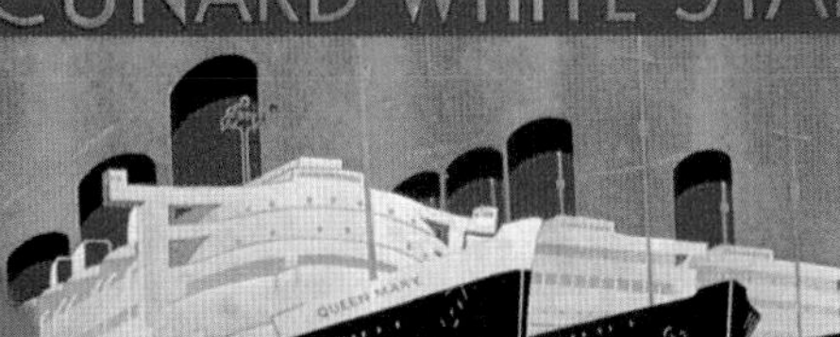

Ocean liners (below) are used as floating hotels. They take passengers on cruises and call at different resorts along the way.

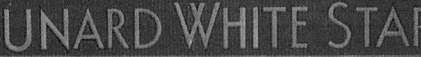

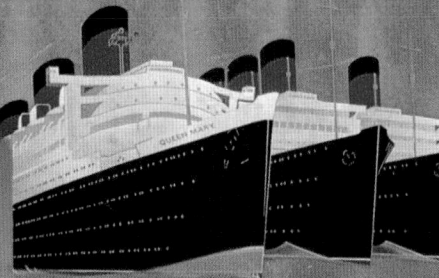

SEA TRAVEL

Floating logs led to the first watercraft, the simple raft. In around 3500 B.C. the Sumerians and the Egyptians made fishing boats out of reeds from the riverbank. They also built watertight wooden ships with oars and a sail, for seagoing voyages. In the 19th century, steel replaced wood, and steam engines gradually took over from sails. Today's engine-powered ships can carry huge loads of cargo at speeds never reached under sail.

AIR TRAVEL

In 1783 the Frenchmen Pilâtre de Rozier and the Marquis d'Arlandes made the first human flight in a hot air balloon. Then, in 1903, to everyone's amazement, brothers Orville and Wilbur Wright built and flew the first powered plane near Kitty Hawk, North Carolina, U.S.A. Aircraft developed rapidly in the two world wars that followed. In 1918, the U.S. Post Office began the first airmail service. Today, it is hard to imagine a world without aircraft.

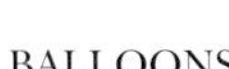

BALLOONS

Long before aeroplanes were invented, people flew in balloons – bags filled with hot air or a lighter-than-air gas. In 1783, the Montgolfier brothers of France built the first balloon to lift humans into the air. Balloons were used by the French emperor Napoleon as flying lookout posts, and later, baloons were used during the Civil War and World War I. Today, ballooning is a popular sport.

In the early days of flying, airline companies used colourful posters to encourage people to fly with them.

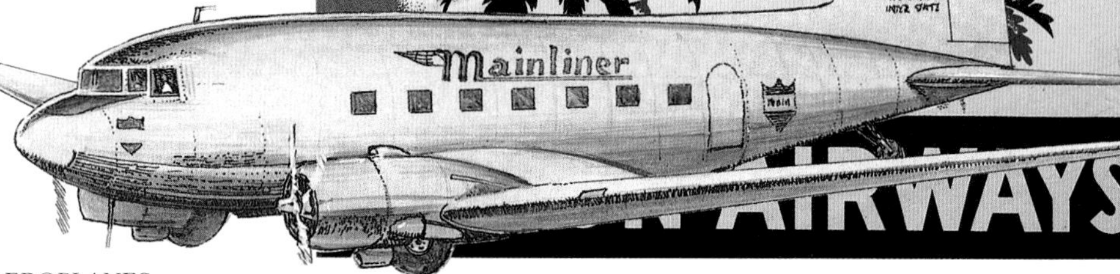

AEROPLANES

Today, millions of people depend on aeroplanes for both business and pleasure. But the golden age of aeroplane development occurred only 80 years ago, when daring pilots took great risks in testing aeroplanes and flying long distances. Jet-powered passenger aeroplanes appeared in the 1950s. A supersonic airliner, *Concorde*, was in service from 1976 to 2003. At 2,500 km/h (1,550 mph), it travelled faster than the speed of sound.

The *Apollo II* spacecraft

SPACE TRAVEL

Not content with the sky, humans wanted to explore space and distant planets as well. In 1957, the Soviets fired the first satellite, *Sputnik,* into orbit (a path around the Earth). In 1968, the United States sent the first manned craft around the Moon. Then, in 1969, astronaut Neil Armstrong became the first person to walk on the Moon.

POLLUTION-FREE TRANSPORT

Many of today's forms of powered transport pollute the environment because their engines send out dangerous gases. Cars, in particular, upset the natural balance of the atmosphere. Lead-free petrol helps reduce the amount of poison which cars release into the air. The transport systems that cause the least pollution are those using natural power, such as wind. On land, people can help preserve our planet by walking, bicycling, or using animals to pull wheeled vehicles. At sea, large loads can be moved in sailing ships powered only by the wind.

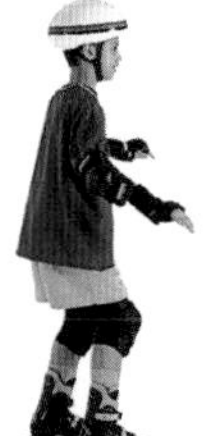
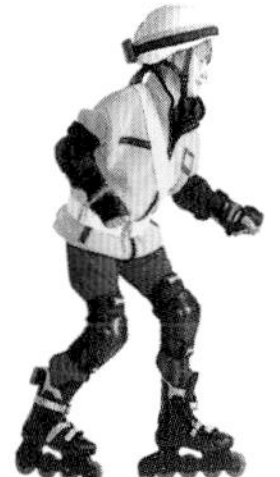
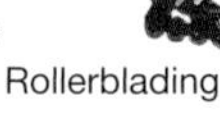

Rollerblading

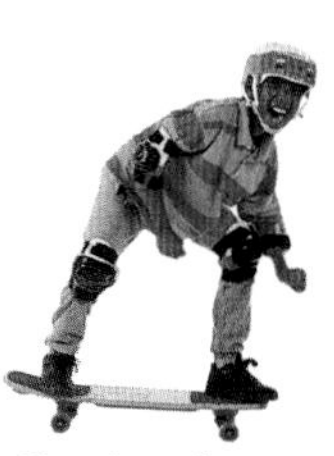

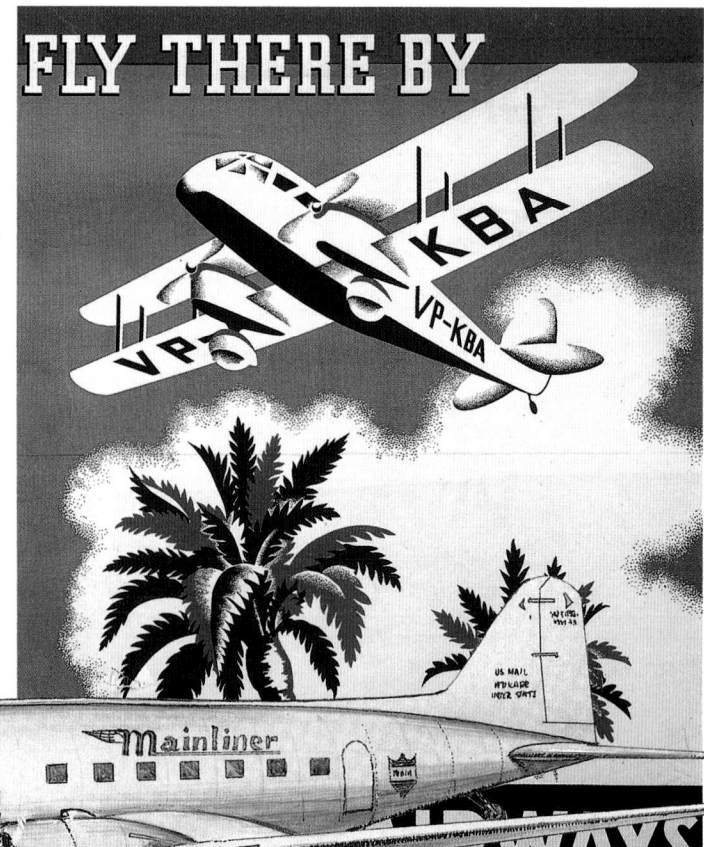

Skateboarding

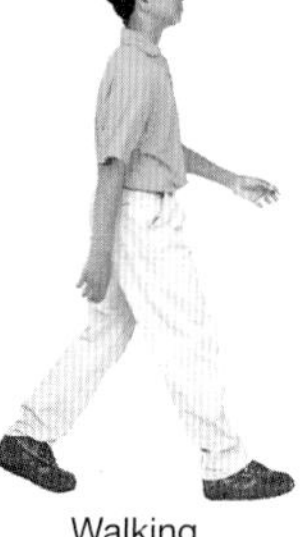
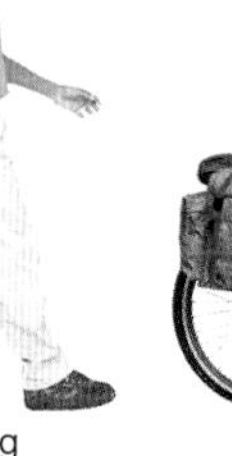

Walking

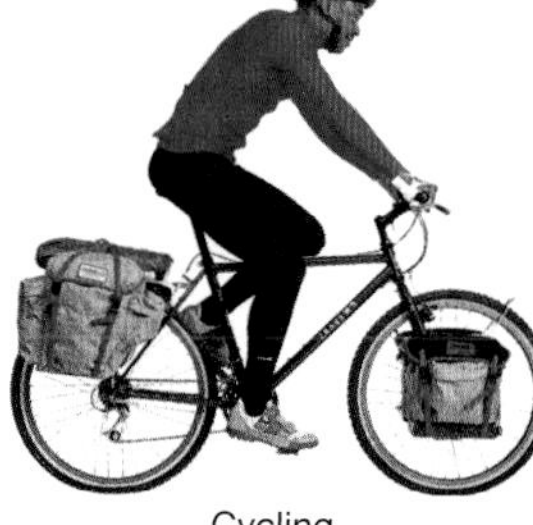

Cycling

Find out more

AIRCRAFT
BALLOONS AND AIRSHIPS
CARS
SHIPS AND BOATS
TRAINS

TREES

Giant sequoia trees are the largest living things – more than 84 m (270 ft) high, and 2,000 tonnes (1,970 tons) in weight; an elephant weighs about 5 tonnes (5 tons).

WITHOUT PLANTS such as trees there could be no life on Earth. Trees take in carbon dioxide from the air and give off oxygen by the process of photosynthesis, so maintaining the balance of the atmosphere. Tree roots stabilize the soil so it is not washed away by the rain, and their leaves give off vast amounts of water vapour, which affects the balance of the world's weather. Forests cover about 39 million sq km (15 million sq miles) of the planet's surface. Trees vary greatly in size, from towering redwoods to dwarf snow willows, that are only a few centimetres high. They supply food for millions of creatures, and produce wood to make buildings, furniture – even the pages of this book.

Leaves

English oak tree in spring and autumn

Buds

Oak bark

Acorns are the fruits of the oak tree; they develop from the pollinated female flowers during autumn.

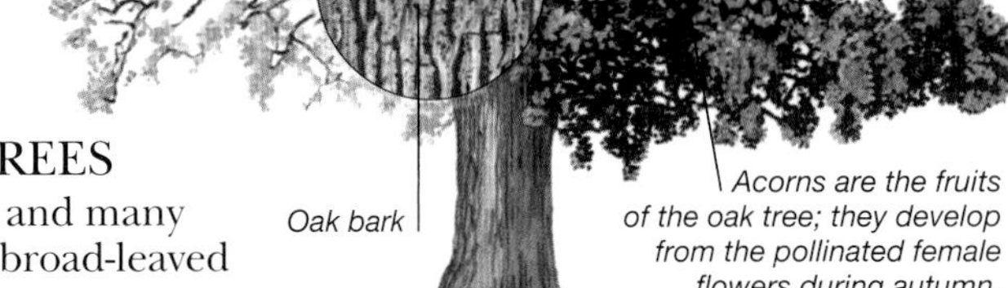

The roots of a deciduous tree may reach out sideways to the same distance as the tree's height.

CONIFEROUS TREES

Pines, firs, cedars, and redwoods are called coniferous trees, or conifers, because they grow their seeds in hard, woody cones. The long, narrow leaves, called needles, stay on the tree all winter. These trees are also called evergreens, because they stay green all year.

CONES

Each tree has its own type of cone, which develops from the fertilized female flowers.

Larch cone

Scots pine needles grow in pairs.

Pine cone

Arolla pine needles

Conifer roots usually spread out sideways.

Sitka spruce cone turns brown as it ripens.

NEEDLES

Every conifer has distinctively shaped needles that grow in a certain pattern. Sitka spruce needles are long and sharp.

Needle

Sitka spruce is an evergreen coniferous tree often seen in forest plantations.

BROAD-LEAVED TREES

Oaks, beeches, willows, and many other trees are called broad-leaved because their leaves are broad and flat, unlike the sharp needles on coniferous trees. Some broad-leaved trees are also called deciduous, because their leaves die and drop off in autumn.

LEAVES

Broad-leaved trees can be recognized by the shape of their leaves and the pattern in which the leaves grow on the twigs. In winter, you can identify a bare tree by its bark, buds, and overall shape.

Leaves of the holly tree are spiky.

Japanese maple leaves have deep notches.

The gingko tree has fan-shaped leaves.

Sweet chestnut leaves have a jagged edge.

Rowan or mountain ash trees have compound leaves.

GROWTH

All trees grow from small seeds inside their fruit. Each seed contains a food store and a tiny embryo tree. The seed begins to grow when the temperature and moisture of the soil are suitable. A young tree is called a sapling.

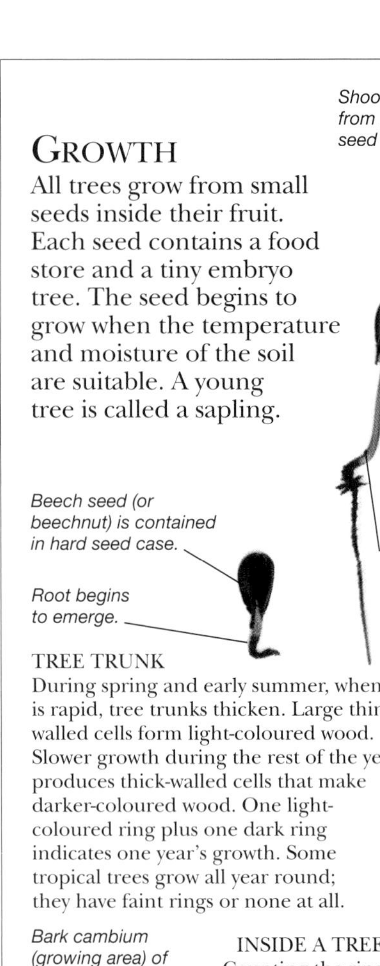

Shoot grows from between seed leaves.
First true leaves develop and seed case falls away.
Seed case splits.
Beech seed (or beechnut) is contained in hard seed case.
Root and stem of seedling grow longer.
Root begins to emerge.

SEASONAL GROWTH

In temperate regions, where there are definite seasons each year, trees grow during spring and summer. Growth occurs mainly at the ends of the tree, the tips of the branches, and the roots. The twigs lengthen, and flowers and leaves appear from the buds. Root tips grow longer and push their way through the soil. The roots and branches thicken, as does the tree trunk, so that the tree's girth, or waistband, also increases in size.

New leaves develop each spring.

Twig tips grow.

Trunk and branches thicken.

Roots become fatter.

Root tips lengthen.

TREE TRUNK

During spring and early summer, when growth is rapid, tree trunks thicken. Large thin-walled cells form light-coloured wood. Slower growth during the rest of the year produces thick-walled cells that make darker-coloured wood. One light-coloured ring plus one dark ring indicates one year's growth. Some tropical trees grow all year round; they have faint rings or none at all.

INSIDE A TREE

Counting the rings on a section of trunk can tell us the age of a tree. This is a section of a very old giant sequoia tree.

A.D. 1800 Washington, D.C., becomes U.S. capital.

A.D. 1400 Joan of Arc burned at the stake.

A.D. 800 Charlemagne crowned emperor.

Native Americans used the smooth bark of birch trees to make canoes.

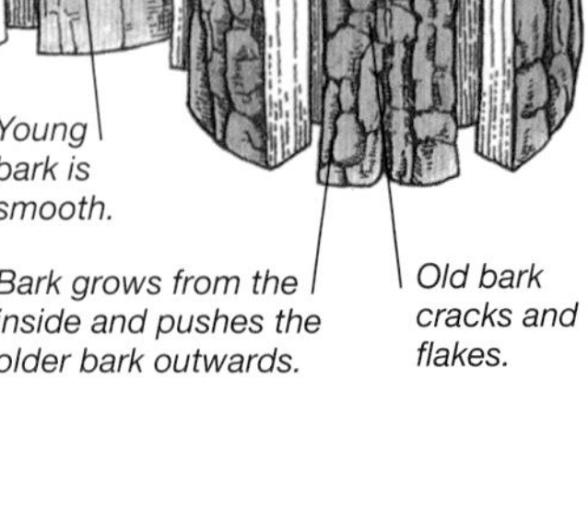

Bark cambium (growing area) of young tree
Young bark is smooth.
Bark grows from the inside and pushes the older bark outwards.
Old bark cracks and flakes.

BARK

The tree's bark is its skin. It shields the living wood within, stops it from drying out, and protects it from extreme cold and heat. Bark prevents damage from moulds, but some animals, such as deer and beavers, eat the bark, and a few wood-boring beetles can tunnel through. A tree with no leaves can be identified by the colour and texture of its bark.

The rough bark of the cork tree is stripped off every eight to 10 years; it is used to make bottle stoppers and floor tiles.

Coconut palm tree

PALM TREES

The 2,700 kinds of palm tree are found in warm Mediterranean and tropical regions. These tall, straight trees provide many products, including palm oils, dates, and coconuts from the coconut palm.

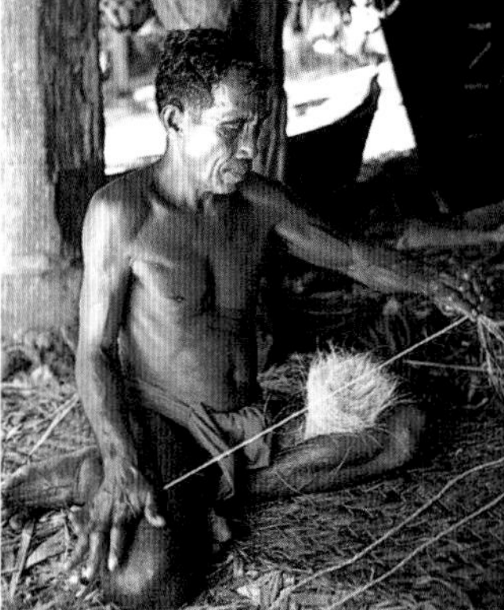

The outer husk of the coconut is used to make coconut matting (above). Coconuts are a valuable source of milk, edible fats, and animal food.

WOOD

Each year we use thousands of tonnes of wood for building, as fuel for cooking and heating, and to make tools, furniture, and paper. As the world's population grows, vast areas of forest are cut down, particularly in South America, where much of the tropical rain forest has been destroyed.

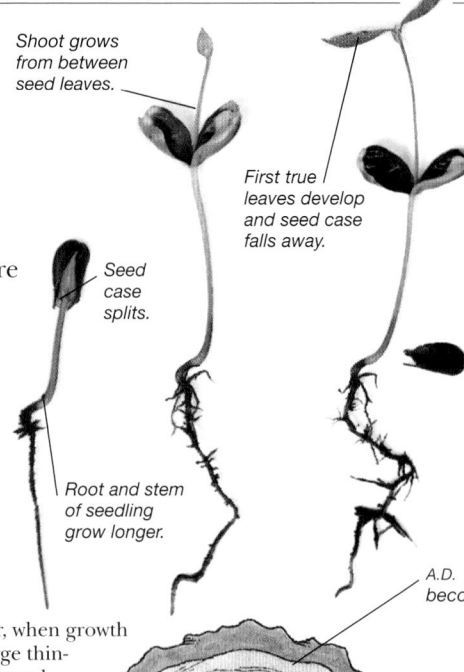

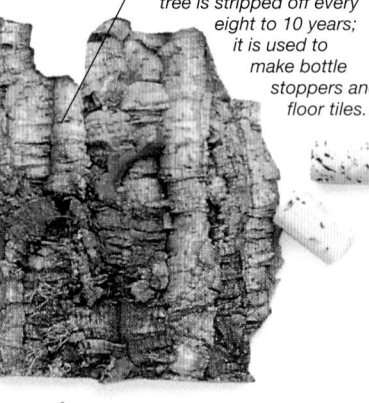

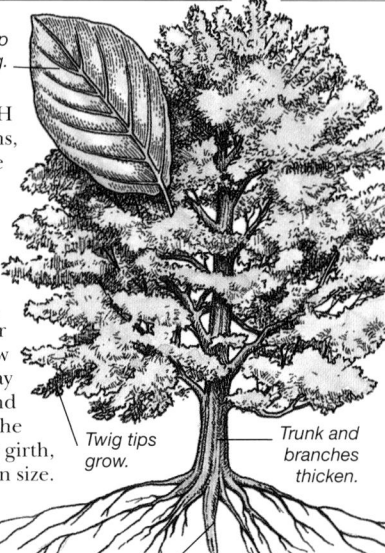

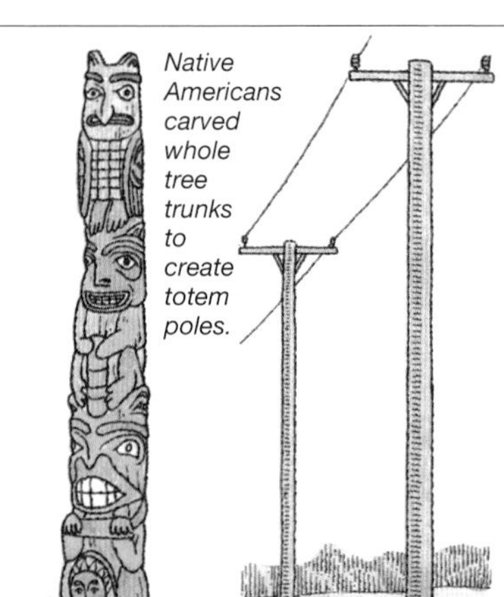

Whole tree trunks are used to make telephone poles.

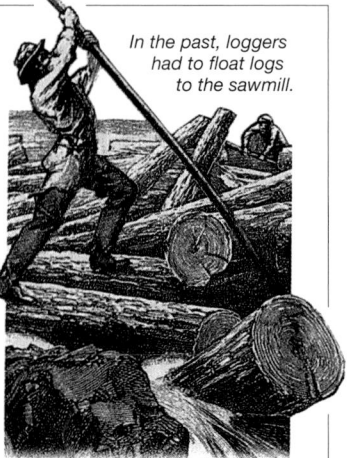

In the past, loggers had to float logs to the sawmill.

Find out more

FOREST WILDLIFE
FRUITS AND SEEDS
PLANTS
SOIL

TRUCKS AND LORRIES

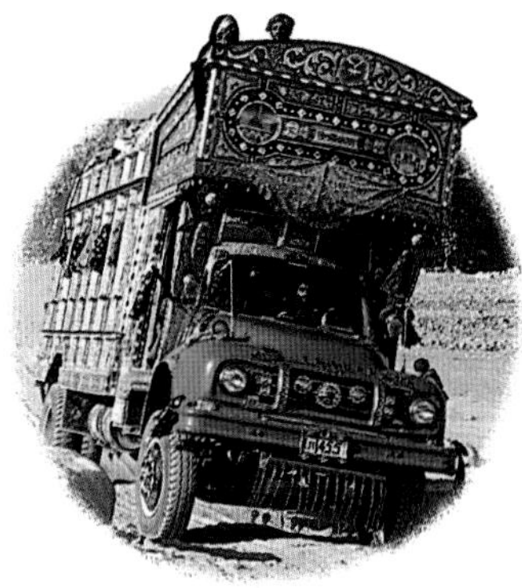

FROM THE SMALLEST VAN to the largest juggernaut that towers over all other traffic, trucks and lorries play a vital role in our lives. They are powerful, rugged vehicles designed to carry goods of all kinds. They transport food to shops, raw materials to factories, fuel to power stations, and much more. In many countries, trucks and lorries now carry all but the bulkiest goods. Trains can carry larger loads, but they are restricted to railway networks. A lorry or truck can pick up and deliver goods from door to door. It can be specially built to carry nearly any kind of load – big or small, heavy or light, liquid or solid, and it can reach remote places far from the nearest railway. For the icy settlements of Finland, the desert towns of the Middle East, and many starving people in countries such as Ethiopia, trucks are an essential lifeline.

ROUGH-ROAD LORRIES
Trucks and lorries are often the only way to get goods in and out of rugged mountain regions. But to survive the rough tracks, the trucks have to be tough and reliable. They also need big wheels to give plenty of ground clearance.

The air deflector, a specially shaped metal flap, helps air flow smoothly over the tractor and trailer and cuts down on fuel consumption.

Long-distance lorry drivers spend many hours on the road, so the cab is made as comfortable as possible. Many cabs contain a bed for overnight stops.

The turbo-charged diesel engine is very powerful, because it must pull heavy loads. Some lorries have up to 20 forward and 10 reverse gears, allowing them to cope with all kinds of road conditions.

Cab tips forward to make the engine easier to work on.

Triple wheels spread the load over a bigger road area.

Trailer pivots on a special joint. When necessary, hydraulic rams lift the trailer for disconnection.

ARTICULATED LORRIES
Most large, modern lorries are articulated, or jointed. The load is pulled along on a separate trailer behind a tractor unit containing the engine and the driver's cab. Because an articulated lorry bends, it is much more manoeuvrable than a rigid one. Articulated lorries have different kinds of trailers that are built to carry a wide range of loads, such as food, wood, oil, and animals.

SPECIAL VEHICLES
There are several kinds of lorries and trucks that are designed for special purposes. Many carry particularly large or heavy loads, such as this quarry truck (below), or the huge trailer that carries the space shuttle to its launch pad.

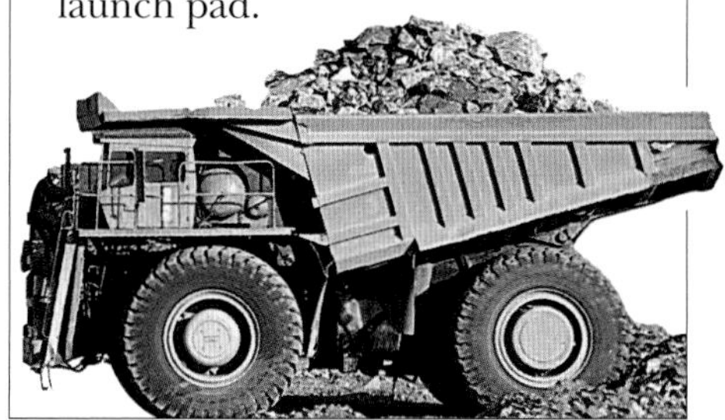

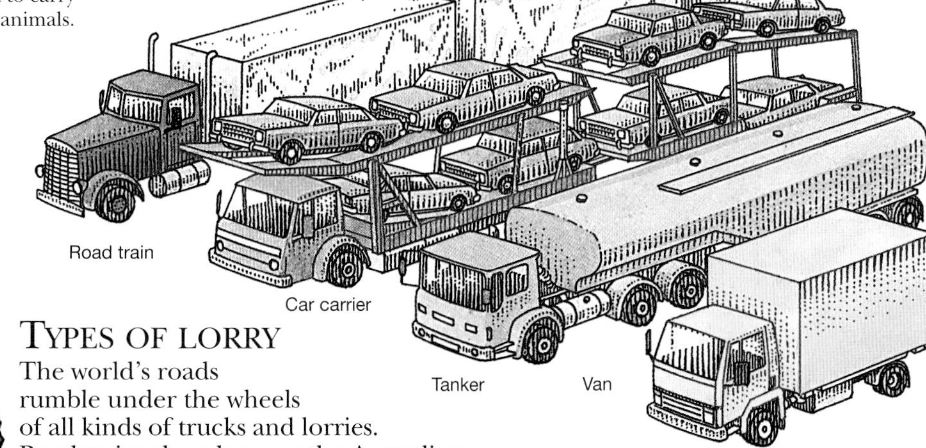

TYPES OF LORRY

The world's roads rumble under the wheels of all kinds of trucks and lorries. Road trains thunder over the Australian plains hauling two, or even three, trailers to keep costs low. Car carriers have trailers too, to take up to 18 cars. Tankers carry petrol, wine, milk, and even flour. Most common are vans, which are able to carry many small loads.

Find out more
BUSES
CARS
TRANSPORT, HISTORY OF

HARRIET TUBMAN

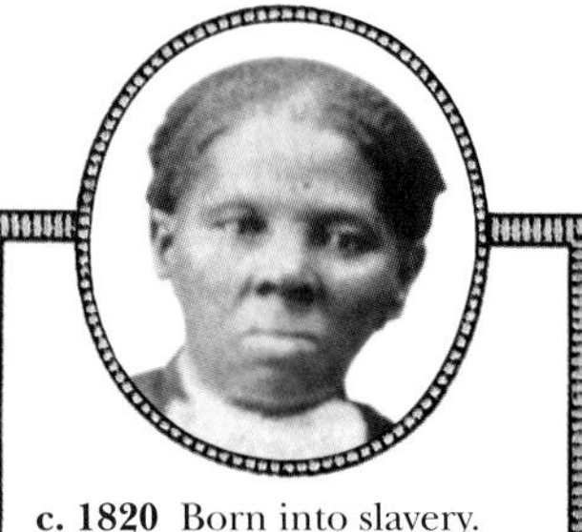

c. 1820 Born into slavery.

1849 Escapes from slavery via the Underground Railroad.

1850 Fugitive Slave Act makes it a crime to help runaway slaves. Tubman makes her first trip as a "conductor".

1850-61 Leads over 300 people to freedom.

1857 Leads her parents to freedom in Auburn, New York.

1861-65 Serves as nurse, scout, and spy for the Union Army.

1913 Dies.

BLACK AMERICANS OWE MUCH to the bravery and determination of Harriet Tubman. Between 1850 and 1861, she led more than 300 black American slaves to freedom on what was known as the "Underground Railroad". Her courageous work earned her the nickname "General Moses", after the Biblical figure Moses who led the Jews out of slavery in Egypt. Tubman was born into slavery and like many other slaves experienced brutal treatment at the hands of her white masters. In 1849, she escaped from a Maryland plantation and made her way to Philadelphia. She vowed to go back and rescue other slaves, and a year later, she returned to Maryland to help members of her family escape. In all, she made 19 journeys back to the South, risking capture, and possible death. During the American Civil War (1861-65), she worked for the Union Army in South Carolina. After slavery was abolished, she continued to fight for black rights, setting up schools for black children, and a home for elderly black Americans.

VALUABLE GANG OF YOUNG
NEGROES
By JOS. A. BEARD.
Will be sold at Auction,
ON WEDNESDAY, 25TH INST.
At 12 o'clock, at Banks' Arcade,
17 Valuable Young Negroes, Men and Women, Field Hands. Sold for no fault; with the best city guarantees.
Sale Positive
and without reserve!
TERMS CASH.
New Orleans, March 24, 1840.

SLAVES FOR SALE
Slaves had no rights. They were bought and sold as property. By law, they were not allowed to own anything, assemble in groups of more than five, or even learn to read and write.

UNDERGROUND RAILROAD

The "Underground Railroad" was not really a railway, but an elaborate network of escape routes that was described using railway terms. Runaway slaves, known as "freight" or "passengers", were helped to flee secretly at night. Guides called "conductors" led them from one "station", or stopping place, to the next. The escape routes stretched all the way from the states of the South to the North and Canada. During the day, helpers hid fugitives in barns and haylofts. Thousands of anti-slavery campaigners – both black and white, and many of them women – risked their lives to operate the "railroad".

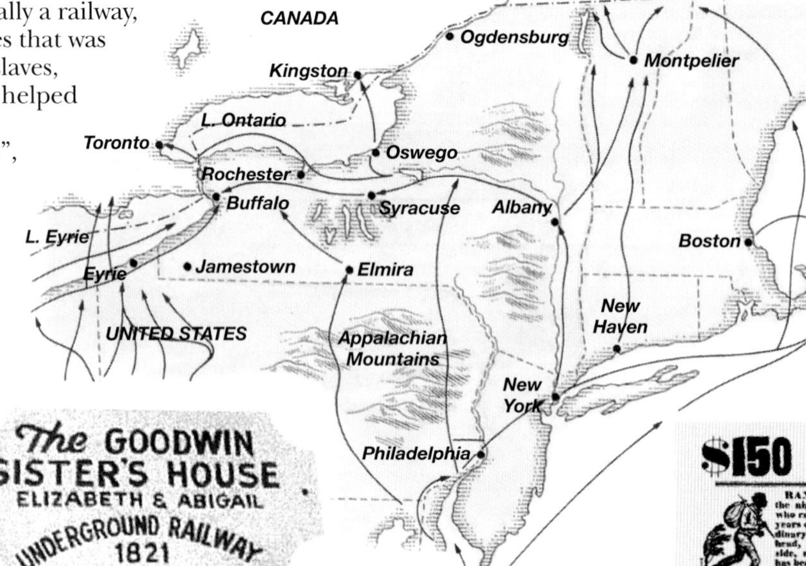

Map of Underground Railroad escape routes

STOPPING PLACE
Every 15–30 km (10–20 miles) along the route was a "station", or safe house, where the "passengers" could rest or hide in safety. This sign (right) commemorates a "station" of 1821.

$150 REWARD

RANAWAY from the subscriber, on the night of the 2d instant, a negro man, who calls himself *Henry May*, about 22 years old, 5 feet 6 or 8 inches high, ordinary color, rather chunky built, bushy head, and has it divided mostly on one side, and keeps it very nicely combed; has been raised in the house, and is a first rate dining-room servant, and was in a tavern in Louisville for 18 months. I expect he is now in Louisville trying to [illegible]

RUNAWAY SLAVES
Northern states banned slavery in the 1780s, but it remained legal in the South until 1865. Laws passed in 1793 and 1850 made it a crime to help runaway slaves.

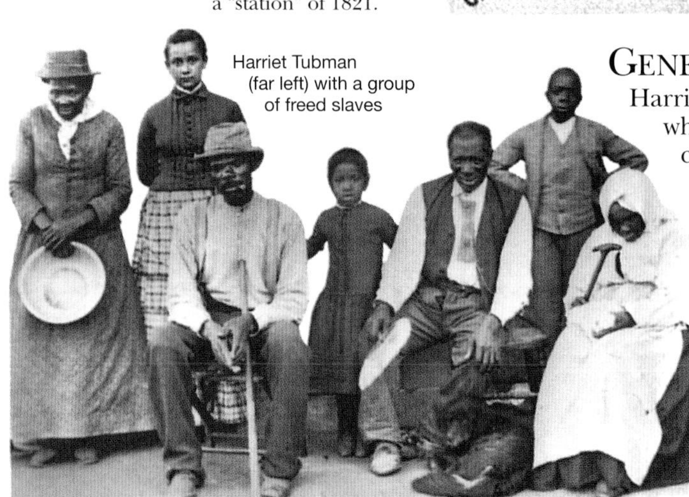

Harriet Tubman (far left) with a group of freed slaves

GENERAL MOSES

Harriet Tubman was a brave woman who believed that God gave her courage and strength. She was so successful a "conductor" that angry plantation owners offered a $40,000 reward for her capture. She travelled during winter, meeting runaway slaves about 15 km (10 miles) from their plantations and then leading them to safety. She escaped capture more than once, and never lost a slave on her escape missions.

Find out more

AMERICAN CIVIL WAR
HUMAN RIGHTS
KING, MARTIN LUTHER
SLAVERY
UNITED STATES, HISTORY OF

Tudors

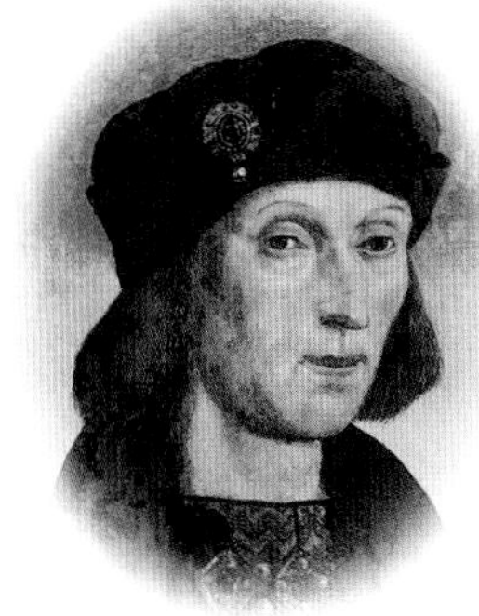

HENRY VII
The first Tudor king was Henry VII (r. 1485-1509). His name was Henry Tudor, and the dynasty (ruling house) took its name from him. A member of the House of Lancaster, he married Elizabeth of York to unite their two houses. He kept other noble families under control, banning their armies, and defeating two rivals to the throne.

THE TUDORS CAME TO the throne in 1485. Before that, there had been years of civil war between two rival ruling family groups, the House of York and the House of Lancaster. But during the Tudor period, which ended in 1603, England enjoyed a time of lasting peace. Rulers such as Henry VII, who united the warring houses, and Elizabeth I, improved the economy, making the country a richer place. It was also a golden age for the arts, with major poets, great playwrights, and fine composers creating important works. However, there were damaging disputes over religion, with the official faith of England changing repeatedly until Elizabeth I became queen. Under her, there was a lasting period of Protestantism.

THE TUDORS

1485 Battle of Bosworth: Henry Tudor defeats Richard III. He rules as Henry VII.

1497 Henry supports voyages to America by John and Sebastian Cabot.

1509-47 Henry VIII reigns.

1534 Henry VIII rebels against the pope and becomes head of the Church of England.

1547-53 Edward VI reigns.

1553-58 Reign of Mary I.

1554 Mary marries Philip of Spain, creating an alliance between the two countries.

1558-1603 Reign of Elizabeth I, last of the Tudors.

Daily life

In Tudor times, most people lived in the countryside, and there was much poverty. Many country people had a difficult life, working hard and earning little. A few made money farming sheep and exporting the wool to Europe. In the towns, merchants and craftworkers could make a good living. Some of their houses still survive.

Gaps between timbers filled in with wattle (thin strips of wood) and daub (mud or clay).

Framework made of strong oak timbers

Roof covered with baked clay tiles

Overhang, or "jetty", gave more room on the upper floor.

This house, belonging to a wealthy Tudor merchant, had two storeys. Its central hall reached up through both levels.

Fireplace had a brick chimney, to keep heat away from the timbers.

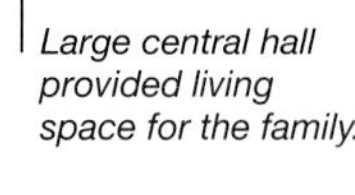

Large central hall provided living space for the family.

Mary Tudor

England was a Protestant country when Mary Tudor (r. 1553-58) became queen. Mary married Philip II of Spain, and made England Catholic again. She ordered that Protestants who refused to change their faith were to be burned at the stake, for which she earned the nickname "Bloody Mary".

Protestants being burned at the stake.

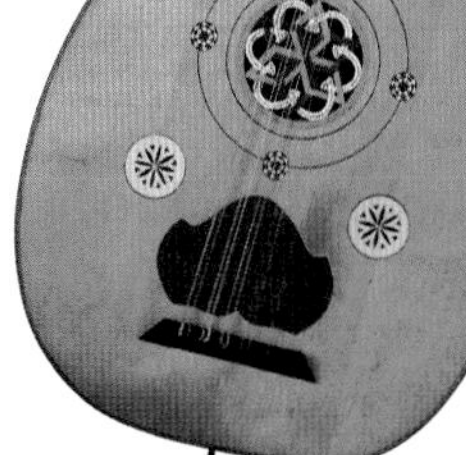

Lute

MUSIC AND ENTERTAINMENT
The Tudors enjoyed good food and drink, dancing, and music. Some of England's greatest composers lived during the Tudor period. They included Thomas Morley and John Dowland, who wrote songs and music for the lute, and Thomas Tallis and William Byrd, who composed choral music.

Find out more
ELIZABETH I
HENRY VIII
STUARTS

TUNNELS

A CITY HIDES MANY of its most important structures from view; some we never see at all. Among these are tunnels, and a city may be honeycombed with them. Beneath the streets run tunnels carrying trains, pedestrians, motor vehicles, sewage, water supplies from reservoirs, and even small rivers. These kinds of tunnels serve cities and towns. Other tunnels allow trains and motor vehicles to pass through hills and mountains and under rivers and seas. Canals, which must be level, sometimes have tunnels to take boats under hills. Mine systems have the deepest tunnels of all. People dug tunnels in ancient times, hacking out the rock with picks. On the island of Samos in Greece, a tunnel dug in about 525 B.C. can still be seen. It is 1 km (3,400 ft) long. The tunnel was started from both ends, and the teams of diggers met in the middle of the mountain. In medieval times, many palaces and forts had tunnels to serve as escape routes in case of seige.

RECORD TUNNELS
The St. Gotthard Road Tunnel in Switzerland (above) is one of the world's longest road tunnels. It is 16 km (10 miles) long. The longest rail tunnel is the Seikan Rail Tunnel in Japan. It has a length of 54 km (33.5 miles). At 169 km (105 miles), a water supply tunnel in New York State, USA, is the longest of all.

KINDS OF TUNNELS

Many city tunnels are "cut-and-cover" tunnels. Machines excavate a deep trench; a cover is then placed over it. Other tunnels are bored through rock or soil, and may go much deeper. Still others, designed for use under rivers, are made in sections on land and joined together on the river-bed.

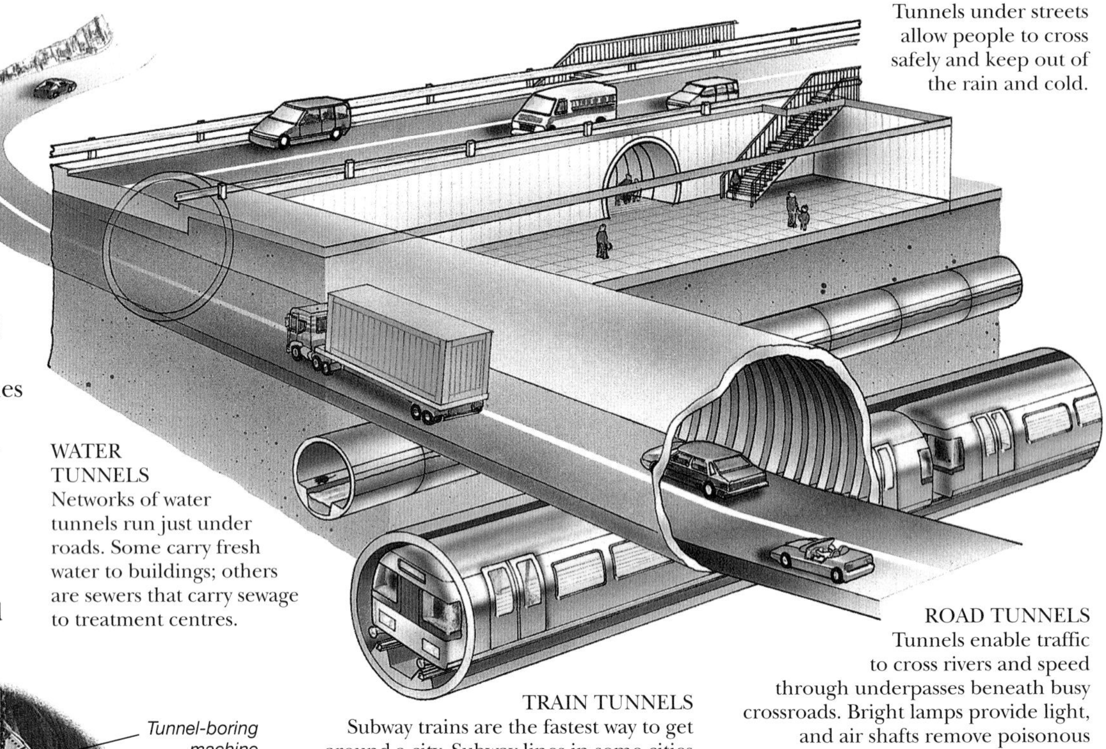

PEDESTRIAN TUNNELS
Tunnels under streets allow people to cross safely and keep out of the rain and cold.

WATER TUNNELS
Networks of water tunnels run just under roads. Some carry fresh water to buildings; others are sewers that carry sewage to treatment centres.

ROAD TUNNELS
Tunnels enable traffic to cross rivers and speed through underpasses beneath busy crossroads. Bright lamps provide light, and air shafts remove poisonous exhaust fumes from long tunnels.

TRAIN TUNNELS
Subway trains are the fastest way to get around a city. Subway lines in some cities travel under streets just below the roadway. In other cities train tunnels are very deep.

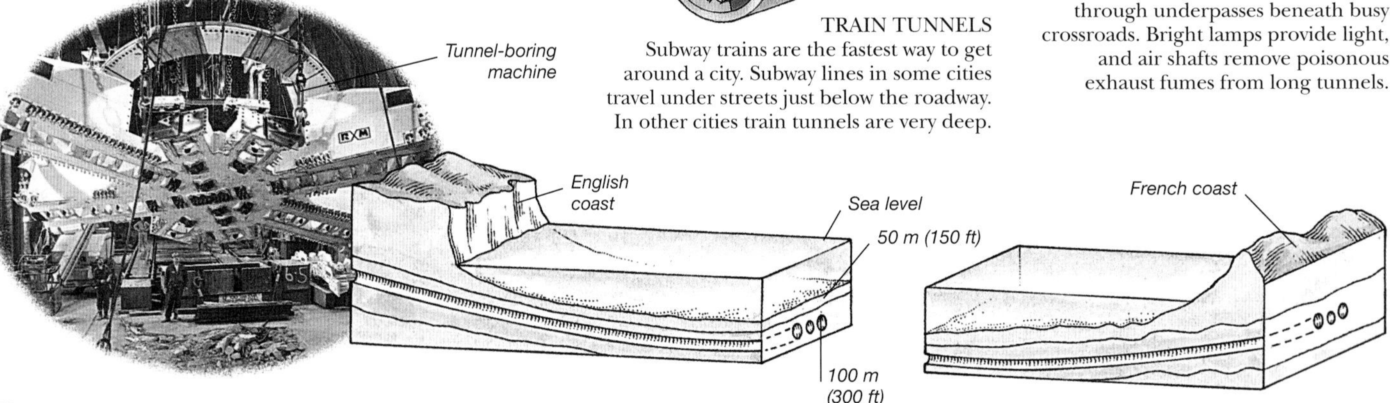

BORING A TUNNEL

Huge tunnelling machines, often guided by lasers and computers, bore tunnels through rock and soil. At the front of the machine is a round cutting head that digs out the rock or soil. Sections of tunnel lining are fitted behind the cutting head. The lining supports the roof, floor, and sides of the tunnel.

CHANNEL TUNNEL
In 1994 a rail link was opened under the English Channel between Britain and France. It is 50 km (31 miles) long, of which 38 km (23 miles) are under the sea. The link has three separate tunnels: two to carry the trains and one for emergency and maintenance work. Special trains have been designed to carry cars as well as passengers.

Find out more
CITIES
COAL
TRAINS
WATER

TURKEY

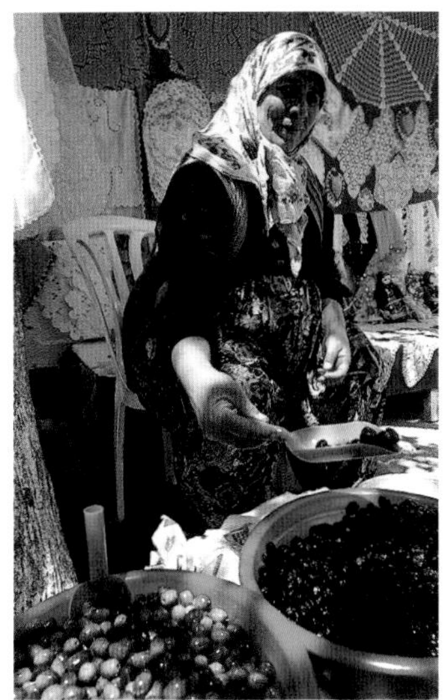

MARKET PRODUCE
Street markets are an important part of every Turkish town. Stalls sell a variety of produce, from olives, spices and vegetables to clothing and household goods. This woman is wearing traditional Turkish clothes – loose, baggy trousers and a printed headscarf – which are still widely worn, especially in the countryside.

TURKEY LIES in both Asia and Europe; today it is on the verge of becoming part of modern Europe, yet retains many elements of its Asian history. Western Turkey was an important part of both the Greek and Roman worlds. The invasion of Turkish nomads (Ottomans) from the east in the 15th century brought the Islamic religion and the nomadic culture of Central Asia. Turkey became a republic in 1923, and rapidly entered the 20th century. Islam is no longer the state religion, although it is widely practised. A wide range of manufacturing and textile industries have strengthened Turkey's growing economic links with Europe. With its warm climate and fertile soils, Turkey is able to produce all its own food – even in the arid southeast huge dams on the Euphrates river are used to water the land. The west and south coasts are visited by increasing numbers of tourists.

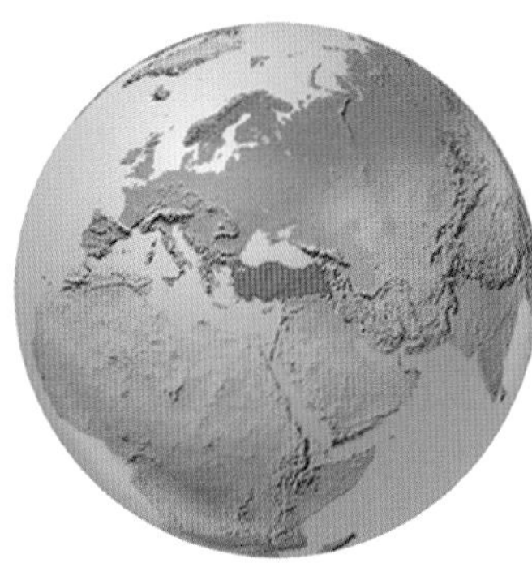

Turkey lies at the western edge of Asia, and extends into the south-eastern tip of Europe. It is bounded on three sides by the Black, Mediterranean and Aegean Seas.

Bodrum's St. Peter's castle (right) is a fine example of Crusader architecture.

ISTANBUL

Turkey's largest city and sea port straddles the continents of Europe and Asia, which are separated by the Bosporus Strait. Founded by Greeks in the 8th century B.C., later to become capital of the Eastern Roman Empire, Istanbul fell to the Ottoman Turks in 1453. The Ottomans beautified the capital with mosques, and built the sumptuous Topkapi Palace, the home of the sultan and his many wives. Today Istanbul is a sprawling, bustling city with a population of more than 6 million.

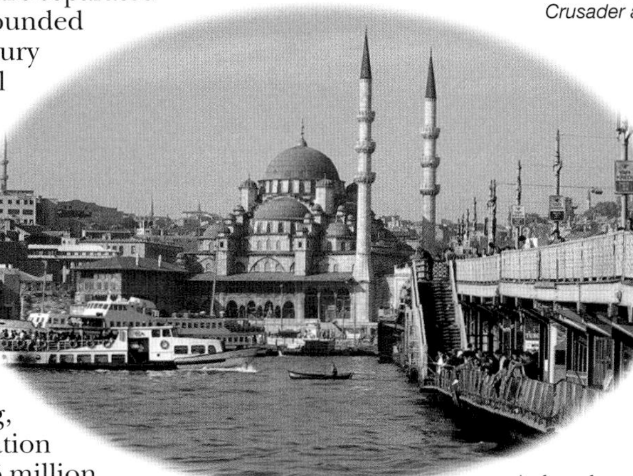

TURKISH TOURISM

Turkey's warm climate, beautiful coastline and rich history attract many tourists from northern Europe. Most of the tourists travel to the Aegean and Mediterranean coasts where picturesque harbours, such as Bodrum (above), are accessible to beautiful beaches. There are some worries that the fast pace of development is spoiling the landscape.

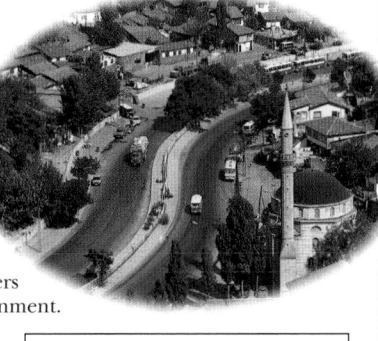

ANKARA
Ankara became capital of the new Turkish republic in 1923 – a break with the Ottoman past. Ankara's history dates back to the 2nd millennium B.C. It was an important Ottoman cultural and commercial centre, located on the main caravan routes. Today, the modern city centre is the headquarters of the government.

The Library of Celsus at Ephesus was built in the 2nd century A.D. for a Roman consul.

CLASSICAL RUINS
The Aegean coast was colonized by Greeks by the 7th century B.C., and western Turkey was an important part of the Greek, and subsequently, the Roman worlds. Many well preserved classical cities attract both archaeologists and tourists to Turkey. Ephesus was the home of the Temple of Artemis, one of the Seven Wonders of the ancient world.

Find out more
ASIA, HISTORY OF
GREECE, ANCIENT
OTTOMAN EMPIRE
ROMAN EMPIRE
WONDERS of the Ancient World

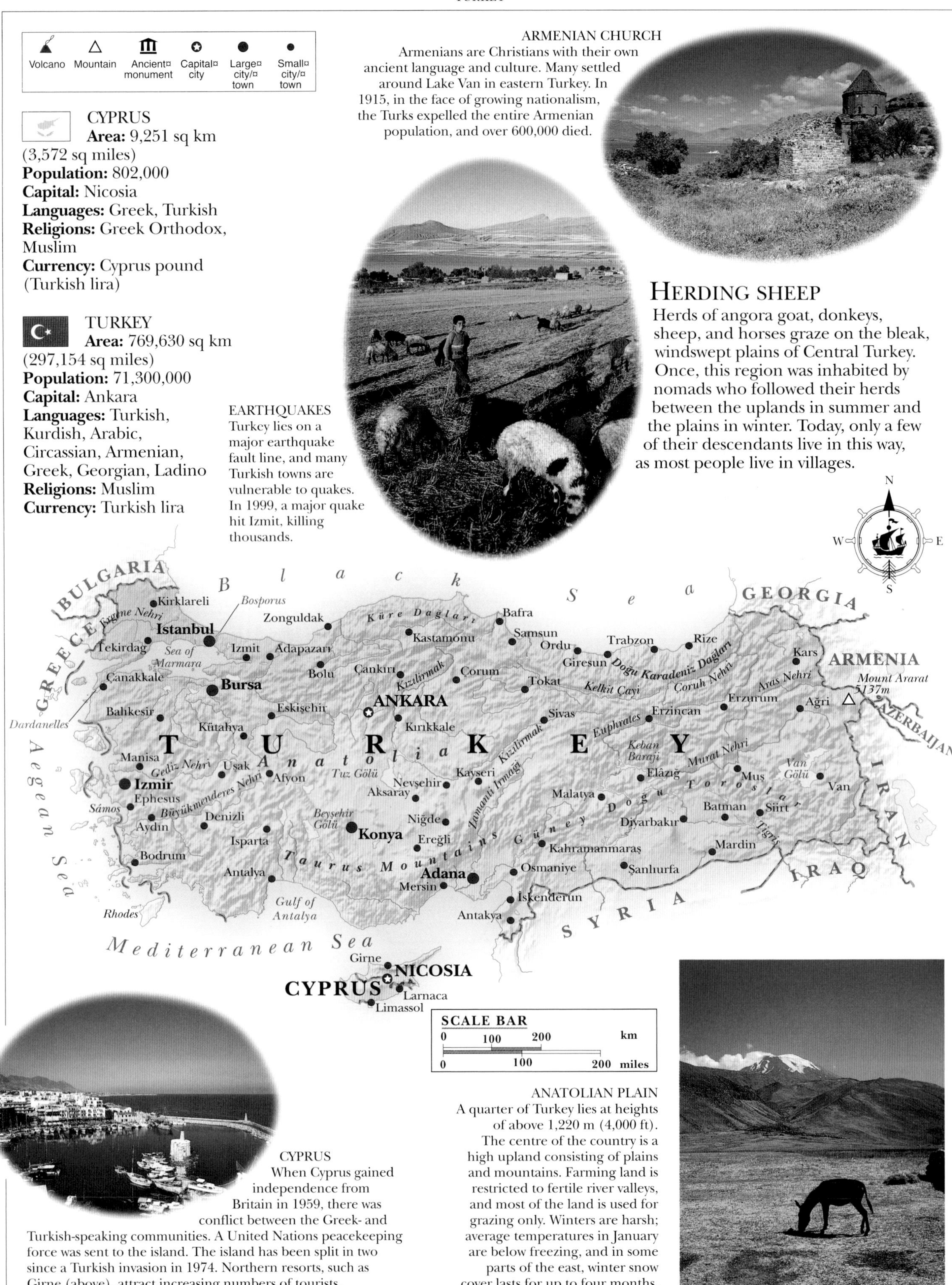

CYPRUS
Area: 9,251 sq km (3,572 sq miles)
Population: 802,000
Capital: Nicosia
Languages: Greek, Turkish
Religions: Greek Orthodox, Muslim
Currency: Cyprus pound (Turkish lira)

TURKEY
Area: 769,630 sq km (297,154 sq miles)
Population: 71,300,000
Capital: Ankara
Languages: Turkish, Kurdish, Arabic, Circassian, Armenian, Greek, Georgian, Ladino
Religions: Muslim
Currency: Turkish lira

ARMENIAN CHURCH
Armenians are Christians with their own ancient language and culture. Many settled around Lake Van in eastern Turkey. In 1915, in the face of growing nationalism, the Turks expelled the entire Armenian population, and over 600,000 died.

Herding sheep

Herds of angora goat, donkeys, sheep, and horses graze on the bleak, windswept plains of Central Turkey. Once, this region was inhabited by nomads who followed their herds between the uplands in summer and the plains in winter. Today, only a few of their descendants live in this way, as most people live in villages.

EARTHQUAKES
Turkey lies on a major earthquake fault line, and many Turkish towns are vulnerable to quakes. In 1999, a major quake hit Izmit, killing thousands.

CYPRUS
When Cyprus gained independence from Britain in 1959, there was conflict between the Greek- and Turkish-speaking communities. A United Nations peacekeeping force was sent to the island. The island has been split in two since a Turkish invasion in 1974. Northern resorts, such as Girne (above), attract increasing numbers of tourists.

ANATOLIAN PLAIN
A quarter of Turkey lies at heights of above 1,220 m (4,000 ft). The centre of the country is a high upland consisting of plains and mountains. Farming land is restricted to fertile river valleys, and most of the land is used for grazing only. Winters are harsh; average temperatures in January are below freezing, and in some parts of the east, winter snow cover lasts for up to four months.

UKRAINE

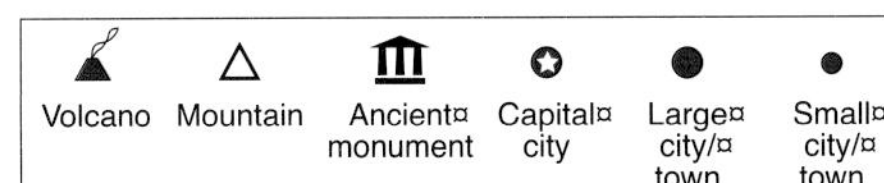

The Carpathian Mountains form Ukraine's western border. To the south lies the Black Sea. The Crimean peninsula extends into the Black Sea, forming the Sea of Azov to the east. Ukraine's flat steppes are bisected by the Dnieper river, which drains into the Black Sea.

UKRAINE HAS BEEN an independent republic since 1991, when the Soviet Union collapsed. The country is dominated by rolling flat grasslands, rich in fertile soils, and is crossed by major rivers such as the Dnieper, Donets, and Bug. The year-round warm climate and sandy beaches of the Crimean peninsula attract many tourists, especially from Russia and Germany. With its fertile land and mild climate, Ukraine is a major cereals producer, once called the "bread-basket" of the Soviet Union. In the east, the basin of the River Donets is rich in deposits of coal, iron ore, manganese, zinc, and mercury. It is the centre of a major industrial heartland. During the Soviet era, Ukraine was a major weapons producer; efforts are now being made to convert weapons factories for the manufacture of consumer goods. In 1986, a radiation leak at Chornobyl', one of Ukraine's nuclear power stations, caused panic in Europe. Much of the land around the plant is still contaminated and towns stand desolate and empty.

STATISTICS
Area: 603,700 sq km (223,090 sq miles)
Population: 47,700,000
Capital: Kiev
Languages: Ukrainian, Russian, Tatar
Religions: Ukrainian Orthodox, Roman Catholic, Protestant, Jewish
Currency: Hryvna
Main occupations: Agriculture, mining
Main exports: Coal, titanium, iron ore, manganese ore, steel
Main imports: Oil, natural gas

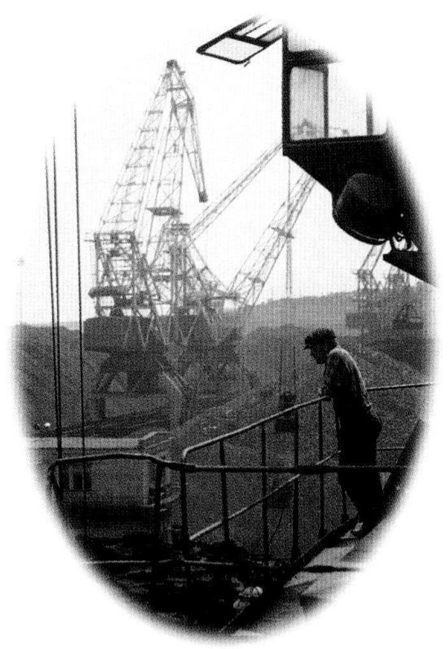

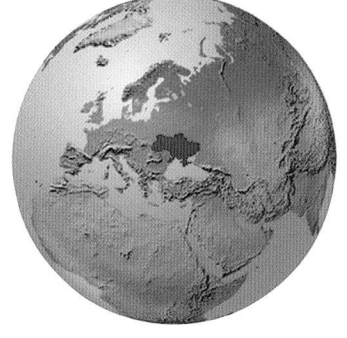

INDUSTRIAL HEARTLAND
Eastern Ukraine, with its rich reserves of iron, coal, gas, and oil, is a major centre of industry. Ukraine is one of the world's top steel producers, and large iron and steel works dominate the landscape. Ukraine also manufactures mining and transport equipment, trucks, cars, railway locomotives, ships, and turbines.

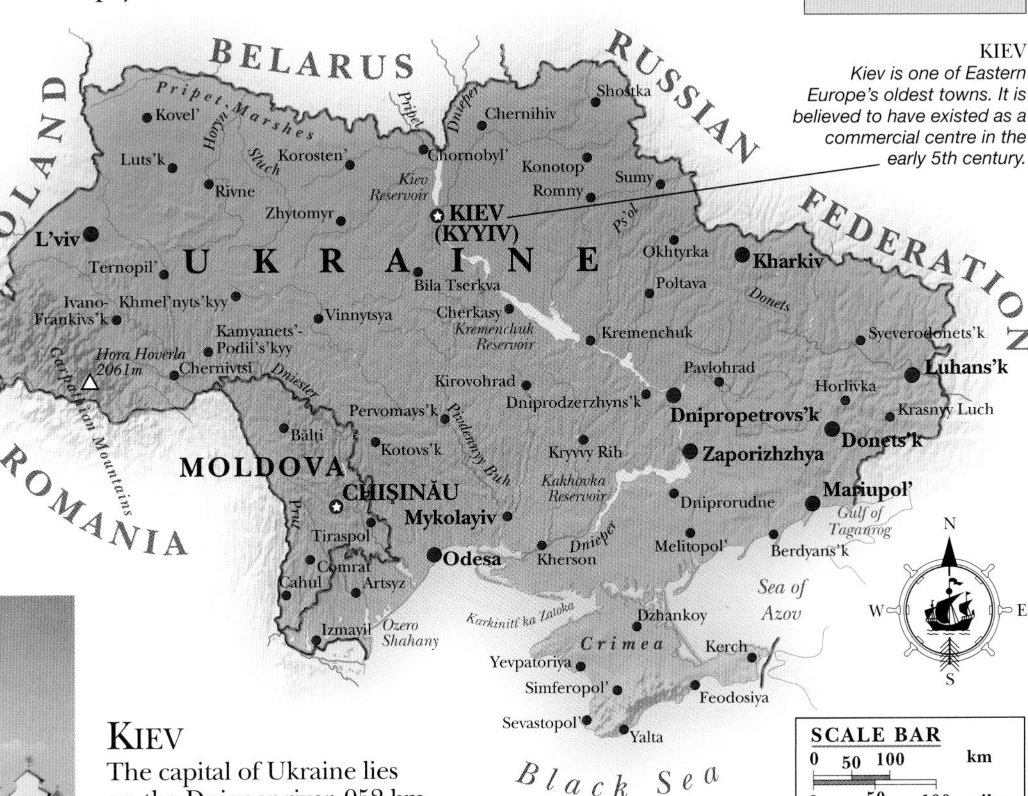

KIEV
Kiev is one of Eastern Europe's oldest towns. It is believed to have existed as a commercial centre in the early 5th century.

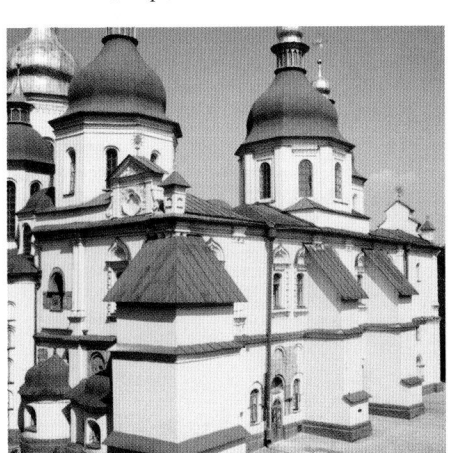

KIEV

The capital of Ukraine lies on the Dnieper river, 952 km (591 miles) from the river's mouth in the Black Sea. Kiev was founded in the 8th century as the capital of the state of Kievan Rus. The focus of the city is the ancient Upper Town where historic buildings still survive despite the damage done during World War II. The Church of Saint Sophia (left), founded in the 11th century, is a famous landmark of the Eastern Orthodox faith.

Find out more

EUROPE
EUROPE, HISTORY OF
IRON AND STEEL
NUCLEAR ENERGY
SOVIET UNION, HISTORY OF

UNDERWATER EXPLORATION

BENEATH THE WAVES lies another world waiting to be discovered. Divers go down to explore the edges of the underwater world. Only a few metres below the surface they can find fascinating sea creatures, beautifully coloured coral reefs, and strange rock formations. On the seabed lie wrecks of ships which may have sunk hundreds of years ago. They contain pots, coins, and other objects which show how people lived in ancient times. Divers also work in the sea. They service underwater structures, such as oil rigs, and study life on the seabed. But diving can be dangerous, and divers must follow strict safety rules.

The dark depths of the ocean lie beyond divers. Only submersibles, which are small submarines, can reach the ocean floor. There they have discovered previously unknown creatures and have studied undersea mountains and trenches that reveal the structure of the Earth.

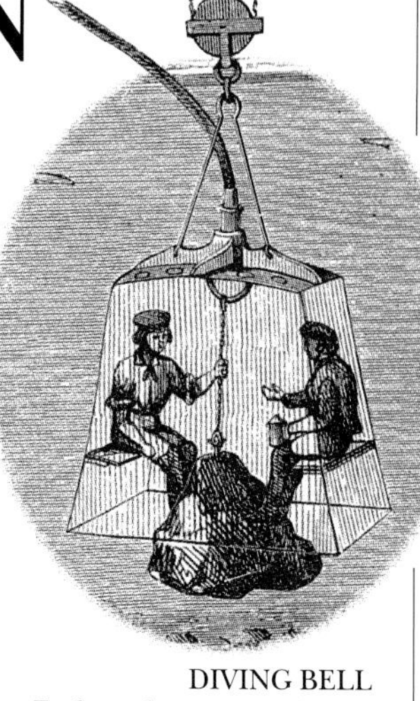

DIVING BELL
Early underwater explorers used diving bells – air-filled chambers that were lowered to the seabed.

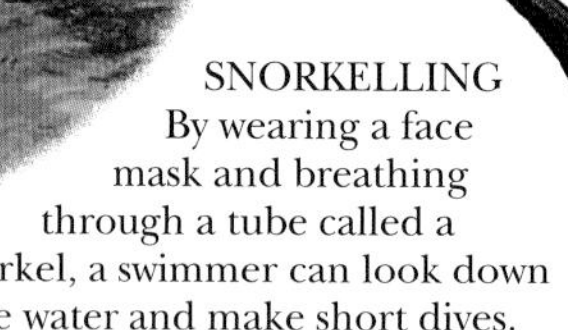

SNORKELLING
By wearing a face mask and breathing through a tube called a snorkel, a swimmer can look down into the water and make short dives.

SCUBA DIVING
Self-contained underwater breathing apparatus (scuba for short) enables divers to swim underwater for an hour or so. The safe maximum depth for scuba diving is 50 m (160 ft).

REACHING THE DEPTHS

People can dive simply by holding their breath and swimming down into the water. But such dives are short-lived and shallow. In order to dive deeper, divers carry air cylinders or receive air pumped through tubes from the surface. Divers using special equipment can reach a maximum depth of approximately 500 m (1,600 ft). Underwater vessels take people on the deepest dives.

SUBMERSIBLES
Teams of people dive to the ocean floor in submersibles, which sometimes go as deep as 6,000 m (20,000 ft). The submersible dives from, and returns to, a mother ship on the surface.

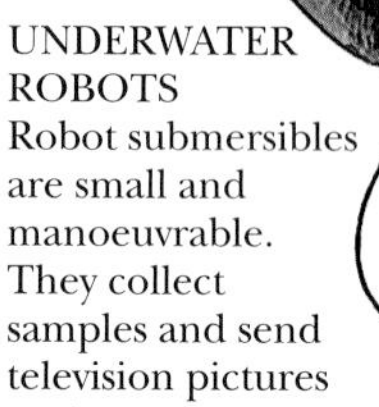

Mechanical arms take samples and grip tools.

UNDERWATER ROBOTS
Robot submersibles are small and manoeuvrable. They collect samples and send television pictures to the surface.

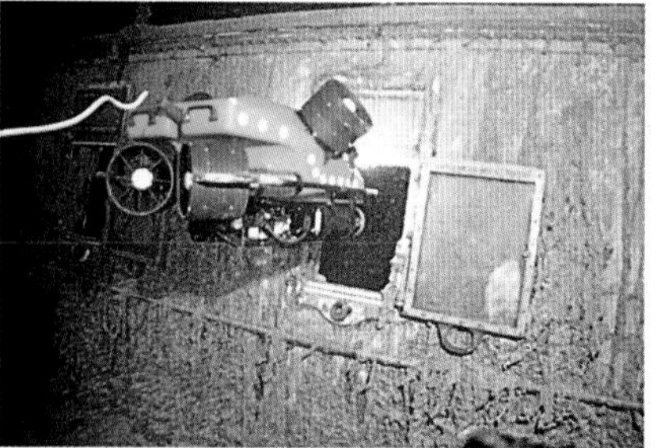

EXPLORING THE *TITANIC*
In 1986, the US submersible *Alvin* explored the wreck of the great ocean liner *Titanic*. The crew used a robot submersible, called *Jason Junior* (left), to inspect the hull and look inside the ship. The *Titanic*, which was thought to be unsinkable, struck an iceberg on its maiden voyage in 1912. It sank more than 3.2 km (2 miles) to the floor of the North Atlantic Ocean.

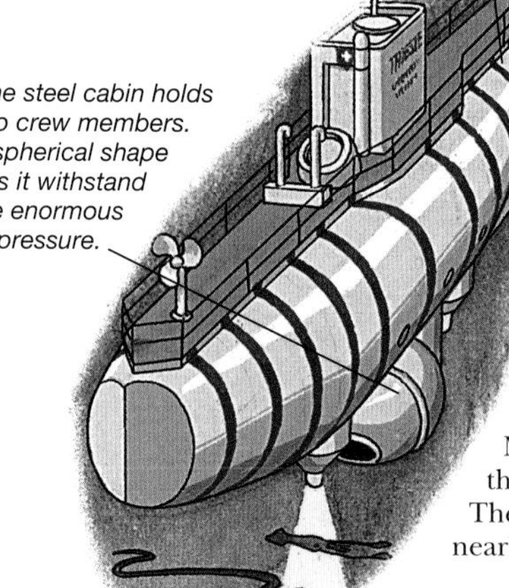

Float contains petrol which keeps bathyscaphe weightless in the water.
The steel cabin holds two crew members. Its spherical shape helps it withstand the enormous water pressure.

BATHYSCAPHES
Special deep-diving vessels called bathyscaphes can dive to the deepest seabed. In 1960 the bathyscaphe *Trieste* dived almost 11 km (7 miles) to reach the very deepest part of the ocean, the Marianas Trench in the Pacific Ocean. The descent took nearly five hours.

Scuba equipment

A diver needs several pieces of equipment to survive underwater. An aqualung provides air, and a wet suit keeps the diver warm. A buoyancy jacket may also be necessary, since divers tend to sink in the water as they dive deeper. The diver maintains a constant depth by blowing air into or expelling air from the jacket.

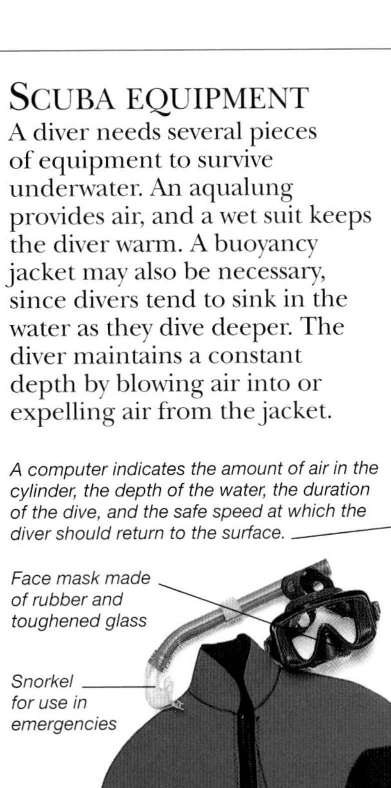
Mouthpiece for inflating buoyancy jacket in emergency
Mouthpiece and demand valve
Air from the aqualung inflates the buoyancy jacket. The emergency cylinder can be used if the main one fails, or the diver can blow into the mouthpiece.
A computer indicates the amount of air in the cylinder, the depth of the water, the duration of the dive, and the safe speed at which the diver should return to the surface.
Face mask made of rubber and toughened glass
Emergency air cylinder
Main air cylinder
Snorkel for use in emergencies
Compass for navigating underwater
Diaphragm moves in and out as diver inhales and exhales.
Lever opens and closes air inlet valve.
Tube from air cylinder
Air inlet valve
Air outlet valve opens when diver breathes out.
Knife
Weights on the belt cancel out the buoyancy of the diving suit and help the diver sink. The belt can be released in an emergency.
A film of water trapped between the rubber wet suit and the diver's body prevents heat from escaping and keeps the diver warm in cold water.
Scuba divers wear large fins, or flippers, to propel themselves through the water.

AQUALUNG

The diver breathes from an aqualung, which consists of an air cylinder, a pressure-reducing valve, and a tube that leads air to the mouthpiece. The cylinder contains air at high pressure. The diver can only breathe in air at the same pressure as the surrounding water. The demand valve on the mouthpiece automatically controls the air pressure so the diver can breathe in and out easily.

JACQUES COUSTEAU

Two Frenchmen, Jacques Cousteau (above) and Emile Gagnan, invented the aqualung in 1943. Later, Cousteau became a famous underwater explorer.

ATMOSPHERIC DIVING SUIT

Divers can reach greater depths, make longer dives, and avoid the dangers of the bends by using an atmospheric diving suit. This suit encloses the diver's body, and has its own air supply so the diver can breathe normally.

Buoyancy tank

Thrusters propel suit.

Hand-operated manipulators

DANGERS OF DIVING

Air contains nitrogen gas. Increasing pressure forces nitrogen into a scuba diver's blood as he or she dives deeper. Too much nitrogen is harmful, so the diver must not dive too deep or stay underwater too long. The diver must return slowly from a deep dive, or the nitrogen forms bubbles in the blood. This condition, called the bends, is very painful and can cause permanent injury.

The spherical cabin can be released from the Alvin to carry the crew back to the surface in an emergency.

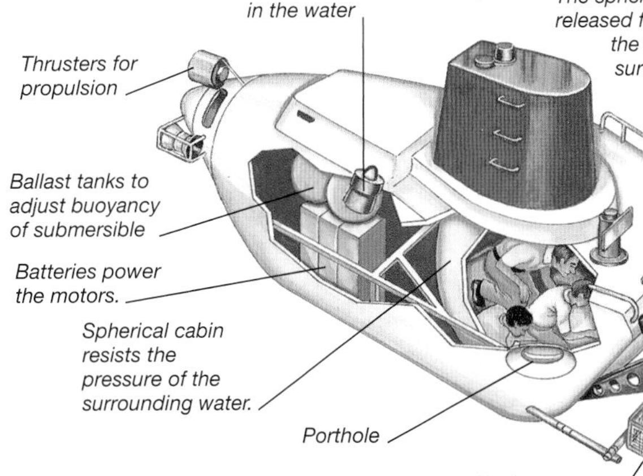
Thrusters for manoeuvring in the water
Thrusters for propulsion
Ballast tanks to adjust buoyancy of submersible
Batteries power the motors.
Spherical cabin resists the pressure of the surrounding water.
Porthole
Television camera
Twin-lens stereo camera
Manipulator arm
Equipment tray

UNDERWATER ARCHAEOLOGY

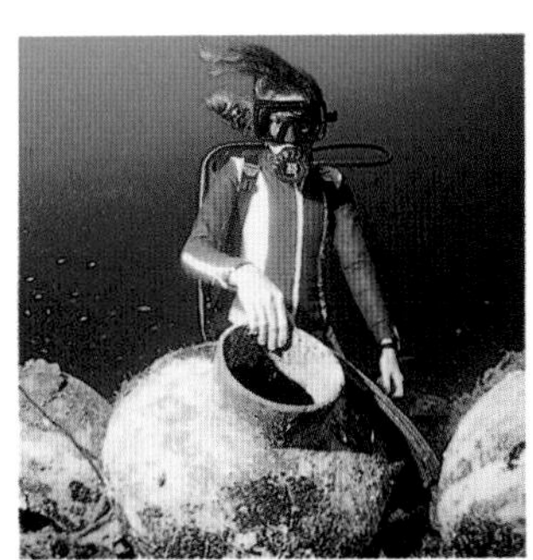

Ancient vessels often carried pottery containers called amphorae that were used to store wine or oil.

Divers are able to uncover the wrecks of old ships just as archaeologists on land dig up the remains of old buildings. They carefully recover objects from the shipwrecks, some of which contain treasure. A few ships have been raised to the surface and preserved.

THE *ALVIN* SUBMERSIBLE

Since it began service in 1964, *Alvin* has made more than 2,000 dives deep into the world's oceans. The submersible mainly undertakes scientific research. Three people – one pilot and two scientists – make dives of six to ten hours to a maximum depth of 4,000 m (13,000 ft).

Find out more

Deep-sea wildlife
Oceans and seas
Submarines

UNITED KINGDOM

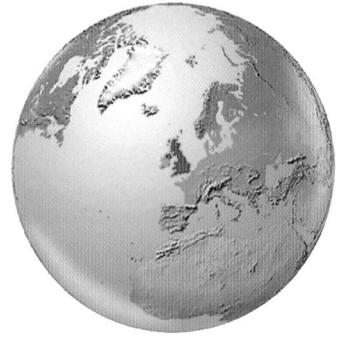

The United Kingdom is just off the northwest coast of Europe. To its east lies the North Sea. The Atlantic Ocean washes its northern and western coasts. The English Channel separates the country from mainland Europe.

THE UNITED KINGDOM of Great Britain and Northern Ireland was formed under the Act of Union of 1801. It is made up of England, Wales, and Scotland, which together form the island of Great Britain, and the province of Northern Ireland. In the late 1990s, the British government devolved power to regional governments by creating new parliaments in Northern Ireland, Scotland and Wales. The English countryside is famed for its gently sloping hills and rich farmland. Wales and Scotland are mostly wild and mountainous. Much of Northern Ireland is low-lying and marshy. In Wales and parts of Scotland, many of the people speak a language of their own. Britain is a multicultural country, for the English, Scots, Welsh, and Irish are all separate peoples. In the last 100 years refugees and immigrants from Europe, Africa, Asia, and the Caribbean have settled in Britain, bringing with them their own languages and religions. Britain once controlled a vast empire that stretched around the world. In recent years its economy has declined, but the discovery of oil in the North Sea has helped to make the country self-sufficient in energy.

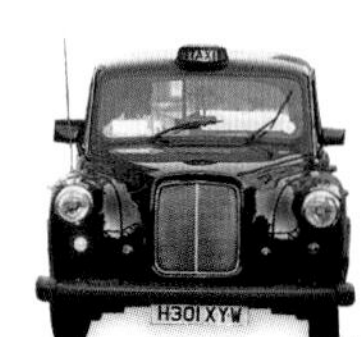

Distinctive red double-decker buses and black taxis ferry Londoners around their city.

LONDON

When the Roman armies invaded Britain almost 2,000 years ago, they built a fortified town called Londinium to safeguard the crossing over the River Thames. By 1100, the city of London had grown in size to become the capital of the entire country. Today, London is a huge city of almost 7 million people and is the political, financial, and cultural centre of Britain. Tourists come from all over the world to admire the historic buildings, particularly the Tower of London (left), an 11th-century fortress.

Cricket began in Britain, and is the country's national sport. Many villages have their own teams.

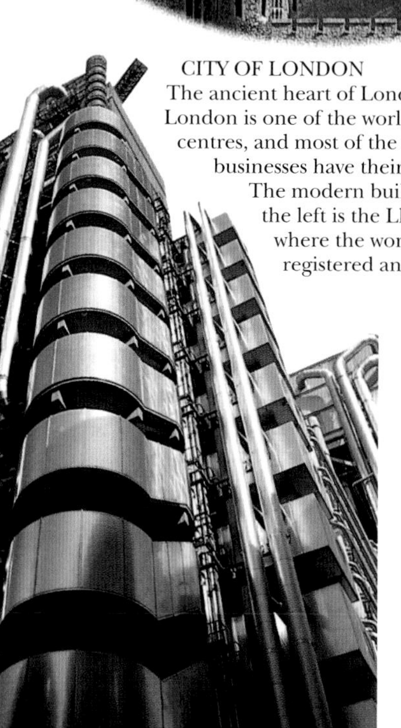

CITY OF LONDON

The ancient heart of London is called the City. London is one of the world's leading financial centres, and most of the nation's banks and businesses have their headquarters here. The modern building shown on the left is the Lloyd's Building, where the world's shipping is registered and insured.

ENGLAND

The biggest and most populated part of the United Kingdom is England. Many people live in large towns and cities, such as London, Birmingham, and Manchester. Parts of the southeast and the north are very crowded. The English countryside is varied, with rolling farmland in the south and east and hilly moors in the north and west. England is dotted with picturesque villages where old houses and shops are often grouped around a village green.

The rose is the national flower of England.

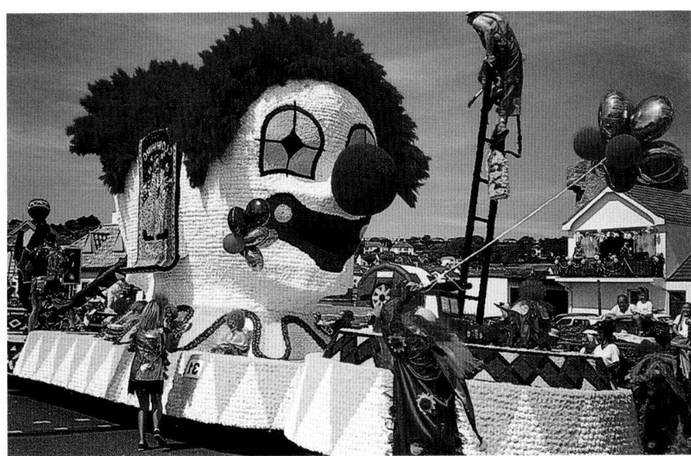

Thousands of colourful flowers are used to decorate floats for Jersey' s "Battle of the Flowers" festival.

JERSEY AND GUERNSEY

The Channel Islands of Jersey and Guernsey are closer to France than they are to Britain. The French coast is just 24 km (15 miles) away from Jersey, the largest island. Close to Jersey and Guernsey are some smaller islands that are also part of the Channel Islands group. All of the islands have a mild climate, so one of the principal occupations is the growing of vegetables. The warm weather and ample sunshine also attract holidaymakers, who in the summer months swell the islands' usual population of 156,000.

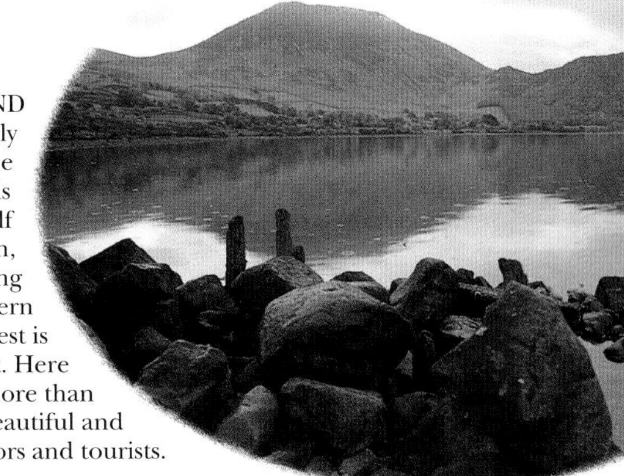

NORTHERN ENGLAND

The north of England has traditionally been the most heavily industrialized part of the United Kingdom. During the Industrial Revolution of the 19th century, factories and mills made goods for export to a British empire that covered half the world. Today the industrial cities of the north remain, but many of the factories stand empty because manufacturing is more profitable in other parts of the world. Northern England is also famous for its natural beauty; in the northwest is a rugged, mountainous region called the Lake District. Here deep lakes separate steep hills which rise to a height of more than 975 m (3,200 ft). The Lake District is beautiful and attracts many visitors and tourists.

"Mad Sunday" motor cyclist on the Isle of Man

ISLE OF MAN

The Isle of Man is part of the United Kingdom but enjoys a certain amount of independence. The Manx people, as islanders are called, have their own government, called the Tynwald, which makes many decisions about how the island is run. There is also a Manx language, though it is now used only for formal ceremonies. Manx independence has a long history, and between 1405 and 1765 the island was a kingdom separate from England.

FISHING INDUSTRY

The waters of the northeast Atlantic are among the world's richest fishing grounds. But EU regulations, designed to reduce catches and conserve fish stocks, are causing widespread discontent amongst fishermen.

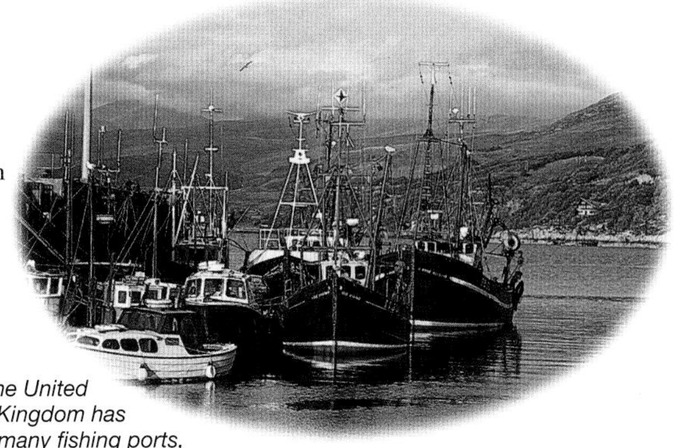

The United Kingdom has many fishing ports, like this one in Scotland.

PEOPLE

The United Kingdom is densely populated, with most of the people living in urban areas, particularly in the southeast of England. Almost 12 per cent of the total population of the country lives in London. The southeast is also the most prosperous area. Other parts of the country are less crowded. For example, the Highlands in Scotland have less inhabitants today than 200 years ago.

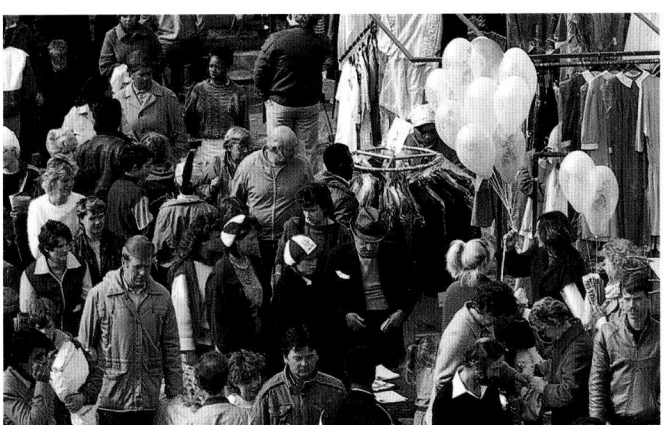

SHETLAND AND ORKNEY

To the northeast of Scotland, two groups of islands form Britain's most northerly outposts. Orkney and Shetland comprise about 170 islands in all, but only the larger islands are inhabited. The landscape is bleak and there are few trees. The land is too poor to make farming profitable, and the traditional local industry is fishing. The islands are also famous for their hand-knitted wool clothes: Fair Isle has given its name to a distinctive knitting pattern.

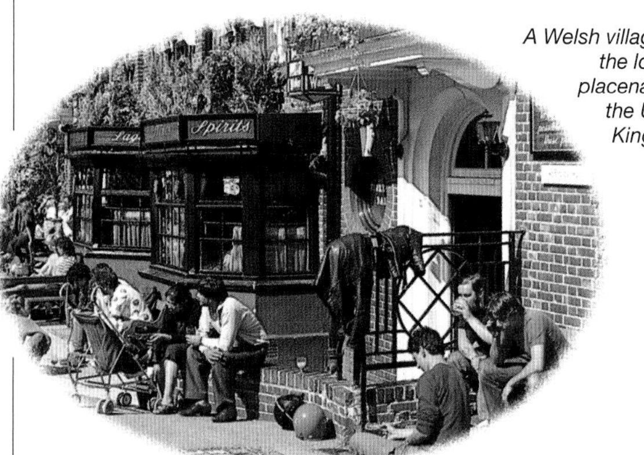

A Welsh village has the longest placename in the United Kingdom.

LLANFAIRPWLLGWYNGYLLGOGERYCHWYRN-DROBWLLLLANTYSILIOGOGOGOCH

Wales

Farming, forestry, and tourism are the most important occupations in the rural regions of Wales. Farms tend to be small and average 40 hectares (16 acres) in size. Farmers in the upland regions keep cattle and sheep. Wales was once one of the main coal-producing areas in the world. There were 630 collieries in the region in 1913. However, the coal industry declined in the years after the first World War. By 1990, a mere seven collieries remained open.

PUBLIC HOUSES
Public houses, more usually called pubs, developed from inns which offered travellers food, drink, and shelter. The pub played a part in British culture, too. In the *Canterbury Tales* by Geoffrey Chaucer (1340-1400), pilgrims on their way to Canterbury in southeast England rest at pubs and tell each other tales. Many of the plays of William Shakespeare (1564-1616) were performed in the yards of London pubs. Today the pub is a social centre where adults meet to discuss the events of the day. Pubs often entertain their customers with music or poetry, and many British rock bands began their careers playing in a pub.

The leek is the Welsh National emblem.

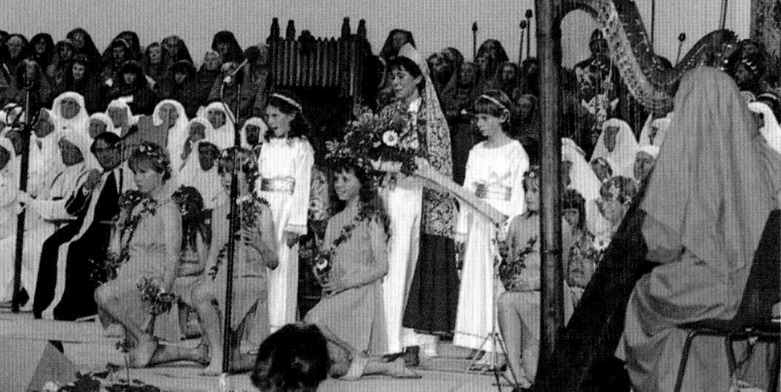

EISTEDDFOD
Every year a festival of poetry, music, and drama celebrates and promotes the Welsh language. This National Eisteddfod began in the 7th century. Today colourful choirs and orchestras compete for awards at the event.

By custom, the first son of the British king or queen becomes Prince of Wales, and wears a gold crown.

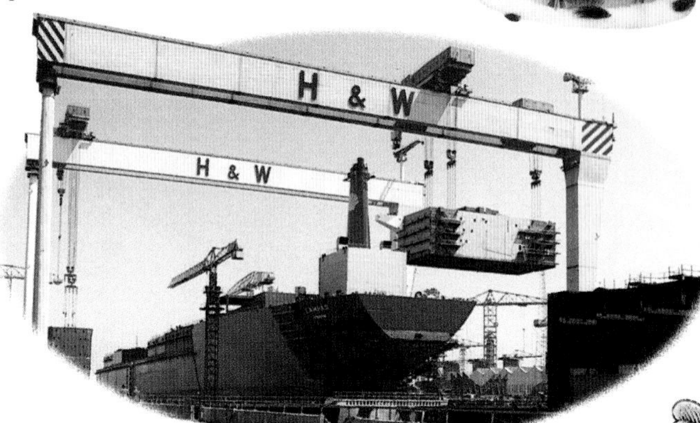

Scottish tourism

Tourism is an important source of income for Scotland. People are lured to the region by its beautifully wild Highland scenery. Scotland is steeped in history and visitors often take the opportunity to visit its many ancient castles. For centuries, Scotland was dominated by struggles between rival families, known as clans. Today one of the most popular tourist souvenirs is tartan – textiles woven in the colours of the clans.

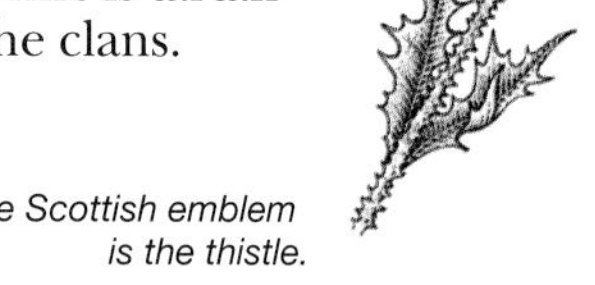

The Scottish emblem is the thistle.

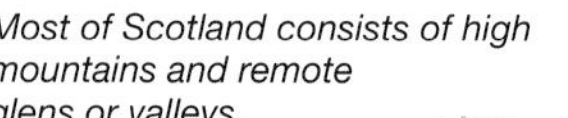

Most of Scotland consists of high mountains and remote glens or valleys.

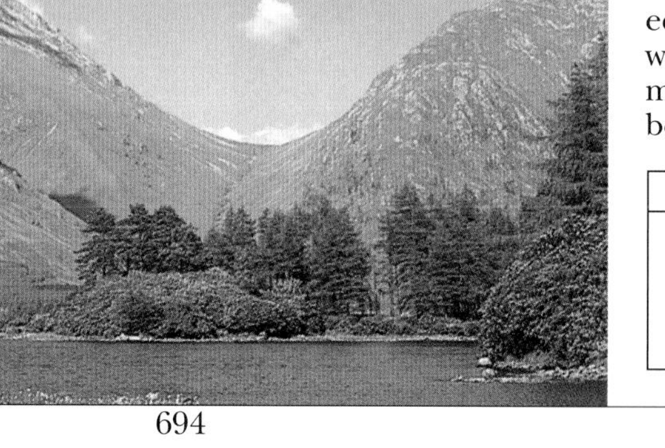

The Irish shamrock emblem

Northern Ireland

Prior to the the 1960s, the economy of Northern Ireland was based on manufacturing, engineering, shipbuilding, and textiles. Heavy industry was concentrated in Belfast where shipbuilding (above) was the largest employer. However, civil disorder after 1968 had a detrimental effect on the economy and, as across the whole of the UK, the manufacturing industry has been in decline.

Find out more

England
Northern Ireland
Scotland
Wales

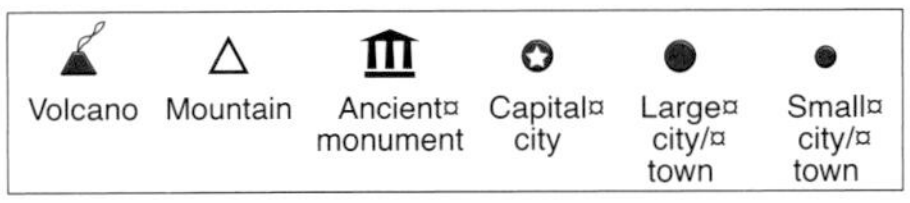

Volcano | Mountain | Ancient monument | Capital city | Large city/town | Small city/town

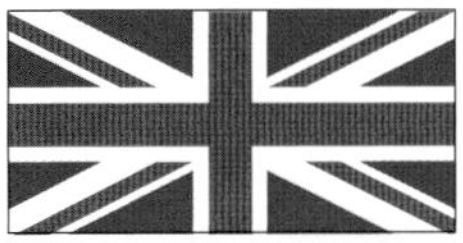

STATISTICS

Area: 244,880 sq km (94,550 sq miles)
Population: 59,800,000
Capital: London
Languages: English, Welsh, Scottish Gaelic, Irish Gaelic
Religions: Anglican, Roman Catholic, Presbyterian, Muslim, Methodist
Currency: Pound sterling
Main occupations: Finance, engineering, oil and gas production, manufacturing, agriculture
Main exports: Oil, natural gas, chemicals, electronics, cars, aircraft
Main imports: Machinery, fruit and vegetables, metals, raw materials

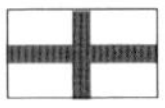

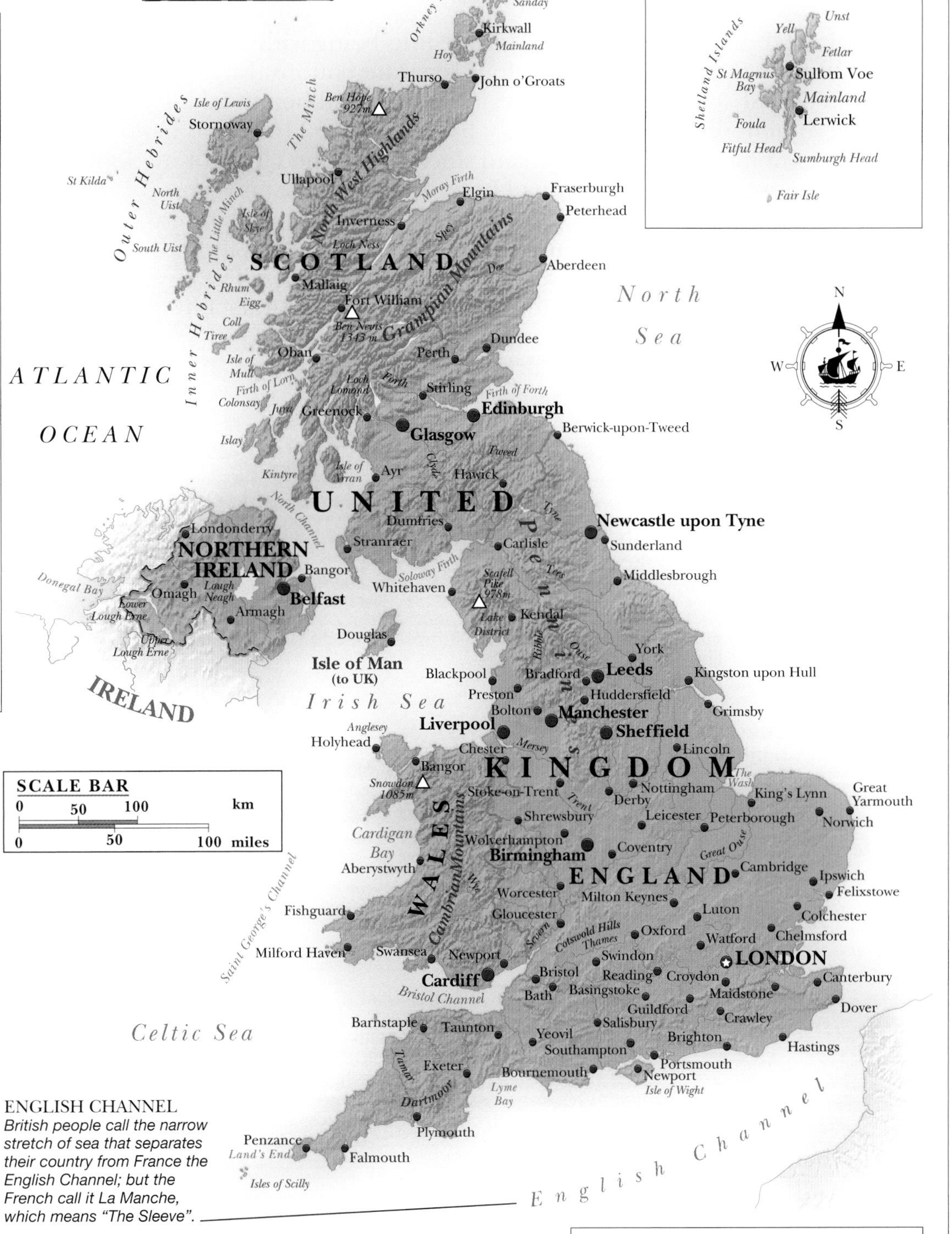

ENGLAND
Area: 130,423 sq km (50,356 sq miles)
Population: 50,093,800
Capital: London

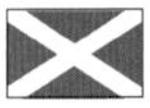

SCOTLAND
Area: 78,133 sq km (30,167 sq miles)
Population: 5,078,400
Capital: Edinburgh

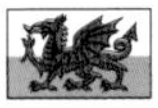

WALES
Area: 20,766 sq km (8,017 sq miles)
Population: 2,952,500
Capital: Cardiff

NORTHERN IRELAND (no official flag)
Area: 14,695 sq km (5,674 sq miles)
Population: 1,700,100
Capital: Belfast

SHETLAND ISLANDS
Unst
Yell
Fetlar
Shetland Islands
St Magnus Bay
Sullom Voe
Mainland
Lerwick
Foula
Fitful Head
Sumburgh Head
Fair Isle

Orkney Islands
Sanday
Kirkwall
Mainland
Hoy
Thurso
John o'Groats
Ben Hope 927m
Isle of Lewis
Stornoway
The Minch
North West Highlands
Outer Hebrides
St Kilda
North Uist
South Uist
The Little Minch
Isle of Skye
Ullapool
Moray Firth
Elgin
Fraserburgh
Peterhead
Inverness
Loch Ness
Spey
Grampian Mountains
Dee
Aberdeen
SCOTLAND
Mallaig
Rhum
Eigg
Inner Hebrides
Fort William
Ben Nevis 1343 m
Coll
Tiree
Isle of Mull
Oban
Firth of Lorn
Colonsay
Jura
Islay
Loch Lomond
Forth
Perth
Dundee
Stirling
Firth of Forth
Edinburgh
Greenock
Glasgow
Berwick-upon-Tweed
Tweed
Clyde
Kintyre
Isle of Arran
Ayr
Hawick
North Sea
ATLANTIC OCEAN
UNITED KINGDOM
North Channel
Londonderry
NORTHERN IRELAND
Donegal Bay
Lower Lough Erne
Upper Lough Erne
Omagh
Lough Neagh
Bangor
Belfast
Armagh
IRELAND
Dumfries
Stranraer
Tyne
Newcastle upon Tyne
Sunderland
Carlisle
Solway Firth
Pennines
Tees
Middlesbrough
Whitehaven
Scafell Pike 978m
Lake District
Kendal
Douglas
Isle of Man (to UK)
Irish Sea
Ribble
Ouse
York
Blackpool
Bradford
Leeds
Kingston upon Hull
Preston
Huddersfield
Bolton
Manchester
Grimsby
Liverpool
Sheffield
Anglesey
Holyhead
Chester
Mersey
Lincoln
Bangor
Snowdon 1085m
Stoke-on-Trent
Trent
Nottingham
Derby
The Wash
King's Lynn
Great Yarmouth
Norwich
Shrewsbury
Leicester
Peterborough
Cardigan Bay
Wolverhampton
Birmingham
Coventry
Great Ouse
Aberystwyth
WALES
Cambrian Mountains
Wye
ENGLAND
Cambridge
Ipswich
Felixstowe
Saint George's Channel
Fishguard
Worcester
Milton Keynes
Gloucester
Luton
Colchester
Severn
Cotswold Hills
Thames
Oxford
Watford
Chelmsford
Milford Haven
Swansea
Newport
Swindon
LONDON
Cardiff
Bristol
Reading
Croydon
Canterbury
Bristol Channel
Bath
Basingstoke
Maidstone
Guildford
Dover
Celtic Sea
Barnstaple
Taunton
Salisbury
Crawley
Yeovil
Brighton
Hastings
Southampton
Tamar
Exeter
Bournemouth
Portsmouth
Newport
Isle of Wight
Lyme Bay
Dartmoor
Plymouth
Penzance
Land's End
Falmouth
Isles of Scilly
English Channel

N
W
E
S

SCALE BAR
0 50 100 km
0 50 100 miles

ENGLISH CHANNEL
British people call the narrow stretch of sea that separates their country from France the English Channel; but the French call it La Manche, which means "The Sleeve".

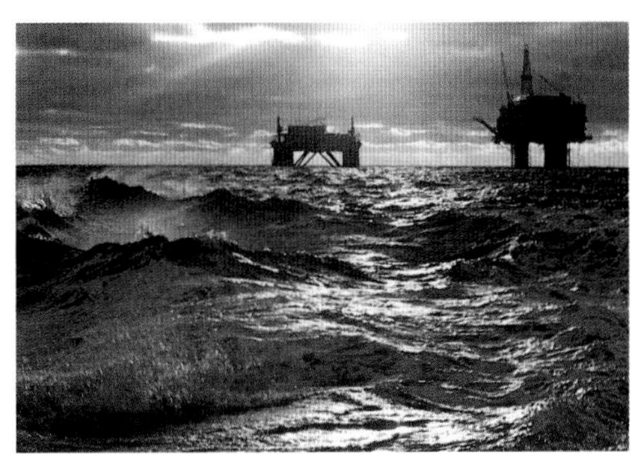

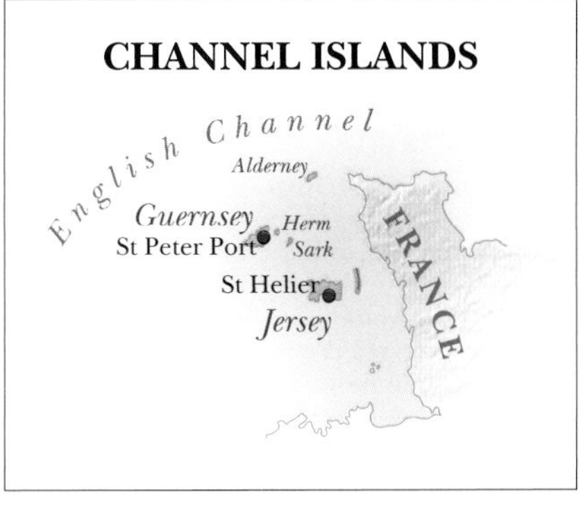

NORTH SEA OIL

The discovery of oil under the North Sea greatly benefitted the British economy from the 1980s. Construction and operation of the oil drilling platforms provided many jobs, and money from oil sales allowed the British government to cut taxes.

HISTORY OF THE

UNITED KINGDOM

IN 1801, THE UNITED KINGDOM came into being with the Act of Union. Before that there had been four separate nations: England, Wales, Scotland, and Ireland. However, England had begun taking over the government of Wales in the 1000s, Ireland in the 1100s, and had shared a joint monarchy with Scotland since 1603. The United Kingdom is a small country, but by 1850 it had become the richest and most powerful nation in the world, controlling the largest empire in history. Even today, the British Commonwealth of Nations includes more than 40 independent countries that were once British colonies. The United Kingdom has often been forced to fight long and bitter wars, but has survived and prospered because of its island position and its strong navy. The British system of laws and government by Parliament has become a model which many other nations have copied.

PALAEOLITHIC SETTLERS
A quarter of a million years ago, during mild conditions between two Ice Ages, people began to settle in Britain. They walked across the bridge of land which joined Britain to Europe at the time.

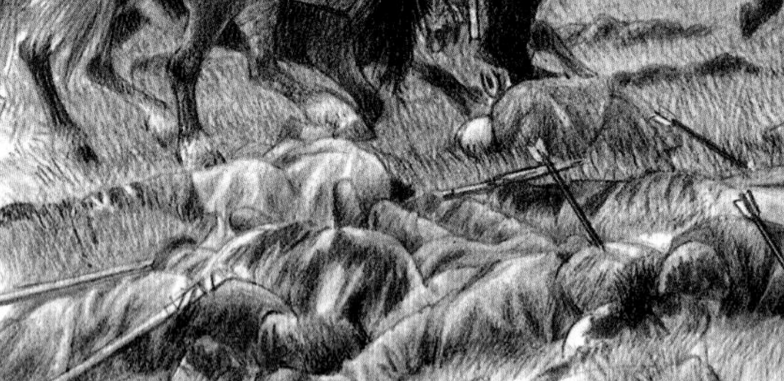

BATTLE OF HASTINGS

In 1066, a battle changed the course of English history. A Norman army led by William the Conqueror defeated an English king, Harold of Wessex, at Hastings, in southern England. William's descendants have ruled the country ever since. As king, he built castles in his new kingdom and gave land to powerful barons. They in turn give land to local lords for agreeing to fight for them. Peasants farmed the land of the local lord, and paid rent in produce and money. This system was called feudalism.

HENRY VIII
A truly multitalented king, Henry VIII was an expert at many things, from jousting and archery to lute-playing and languages. His impact on England was tremendous. In 1541, he forced the Irish Parliament to recognize him as king of Ireland. He also broke from the Roman Catholic Church, in order to divorce his wife, and became head of a new Church of England. Henry was an absolute ruler who executed anyone who displeased him, including two of his six wives.

MAGNA CARTA
The Magna Carta (Great Charter) of 1215 was an agreement between the king and the nobles of England. The charter promised that the king would not abuse his royal power to tax the nobles. This important moment in English history was the start of the belief that even kings must obey certain laws of the land.

UNITED KINGDOM

A.D. 43 Ancient Romans, under Claudius, invade Britain and make it part of their empire.

400 Romans leave Britain.

c. 500 Christian missionaries arrive in Britain and preach Christianity to the people.

c. 870 Viking conquest of Britain begins.

1066 Normans invade Britain.

1215 Magna Carta agreement between the king and the nobles of England.

1282 Edward I, king of England, conquers Wales.

1485 Battle of Bosworth. Henry VII becomes the first Tudor king.

1534 Parliament declares Henry VIII head of the Church of England.

1588 English navy defeats the Spanish Armada (fleet) sent by Philip II, king of Spain.

UNION FLAG
The flag of the United Kingdom is made up from the red crosses of St. George of England and St. Patrick of Ireland, plus the white St. Andrew's cross of Scotland, on a blue background. Wales has its own flag.

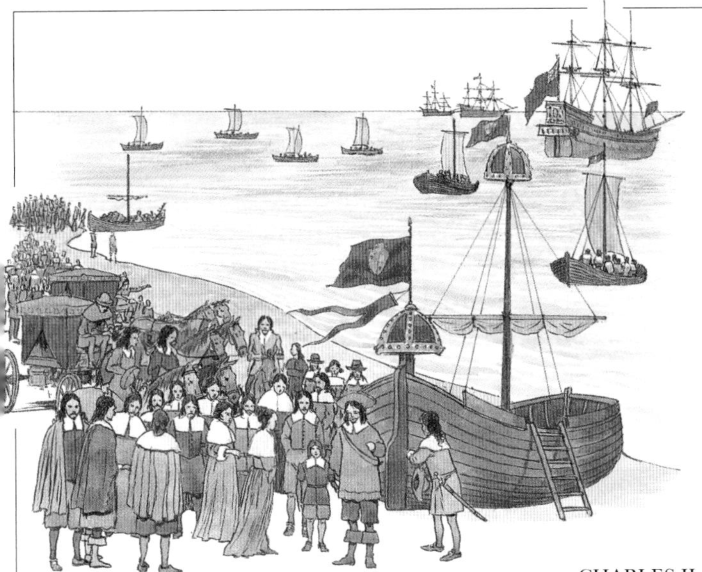

CHARLES II
The Parliamentary army defeated and executed King Charles I during the English Civil War (1642-51). For nine years Oliver Cromwell (1599-1658), a member of Parliament, and his army ruled the country as a republic. In 1660, Charles' son returned from travels abroad (above) and claimed the throne as King Charles II. The nation, weary of the republic, welcomed him.

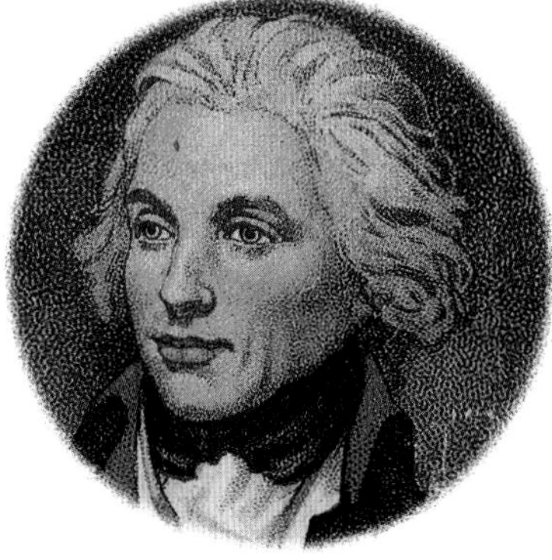

ADMIRAL NELSON

The most famous and daring commander of the British Royal Navy was Admiral Horatio Nelson (1758-1805), who defeated the Spanish and French at the Battle of Trafalgar. Before the battle he said "England expects every man to do his duty". Nelson was fatally wounded in the battle.

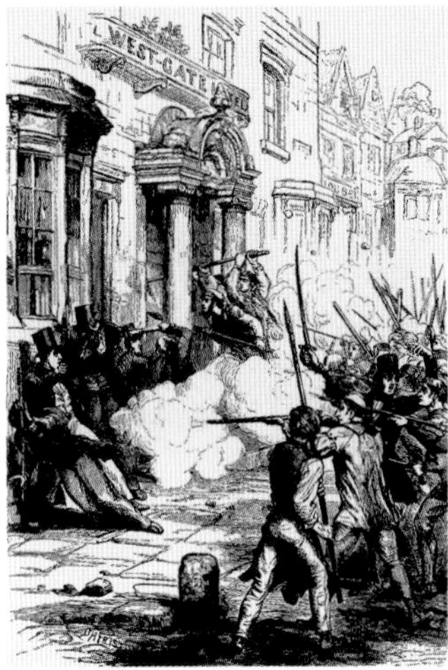

CHARTISTS
During the 19th century, British people fought for the right to vote. Groups such as the Chartists (1837-48) organized demonstrations demanding a fairer system with representation for all, a secret voting system, and regular elections. Above is a Chartist riot being crushed by the police.

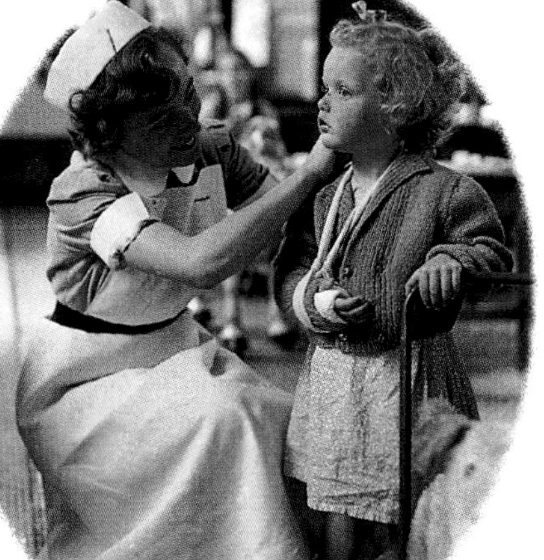

IMMIGRATION

The United Kingdom has become a multiracial and multicultural society, with immigration mainly from Commonwealth countries in the Caribbean, and from many of the Asian nations. This picture, taken in the 1960s, shows new arrivals from Jamaica receiving meals at a hostel set up to provide support for immigrants.

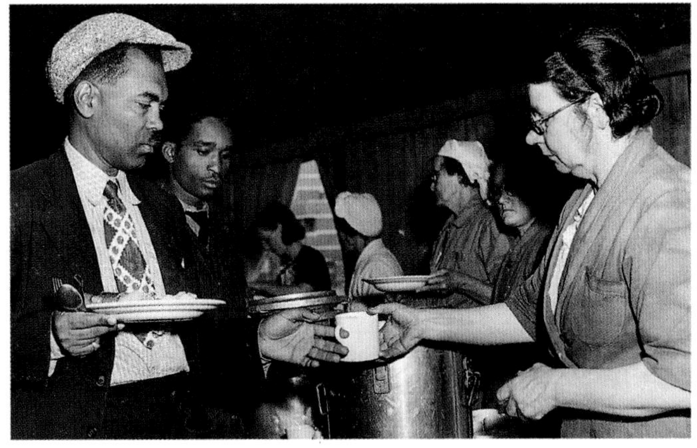

WELFARE STATE
In 1945, following the end of World War II, a Labour government came into power and introduced a welfare state. This put a number of private businesses under public control. It also provided welfare for people "from the cradle to the grave", including free medical treatment under the National Health Service.

NEW LABOUR

When the Labour Party achieved a landslide victory over the Conservatives in 1997, Tony Blair (left) became prime minister of the United Kingdom. Under Blair's leadership, the Party moved to the political centre, re-christening themselves "New Labour". Blair won two more elections, in 2001 and 2005, despite widespread opposition to his decision to take part in the American-led invasion of Iraq.

UNITED KINGDOM

1642-51 Civil War between the King and Parliament.

1660 Charles II becomes King of England.

1707 Act of Union unites England, Wales, and Scotland.

1801 Ireland united with Great Britain.

1900 Britain is the strongest, richest country in the world.

1914-18 Britain fights in World War I.

1931 Commonwealth of Nations is established.

1939-45 Britain fights in World War II.

1945 Welfare state introduced.

1973 Britain becomes a member of the European Union (EU).

1997 Scotland votes in favour of its own parliament.

Find out more

CIVIL WAR, ENGLISH
ELIZABETH I
INDUSTRIAL REVOLUTION
IRELAND, HISTORY OF
NORMANS
UNITED KINGDOM
VICTORIANS

REGIONAL HISTORY OF

UNITED KINGDOM

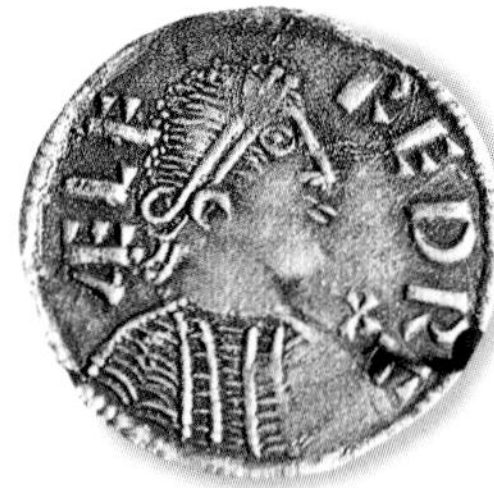

ALFRED THE GREAT
Known as the "Great", Alfred was the grandson of Ecgberht of Wessex (r. 829-39), the first person to unite England.

FOR MUCH OF ITS HISTORY, the United Kingdom has been anything but united. England, Wales, Scotland, and Ireland were all once separate countries and have often split into rival kingdoms themselves. Since the 1100s, England has tried to unite the countries of the British Isles under its rule. In 1171 England invaded Ireland, although it failed to win control; a century later, England conquered Wales. Until the 1600s, Scotland and England were deadly enemies. They were only united when a Scottish king inherited the English throne. The United Kingdom as we know it came into being in 1801, when the final Act of Union was passed between Ireland and the rest of the country, athough most of Ireland left the union in 1922. Today, the separate parts of the country are regaining control of their affairs from London.

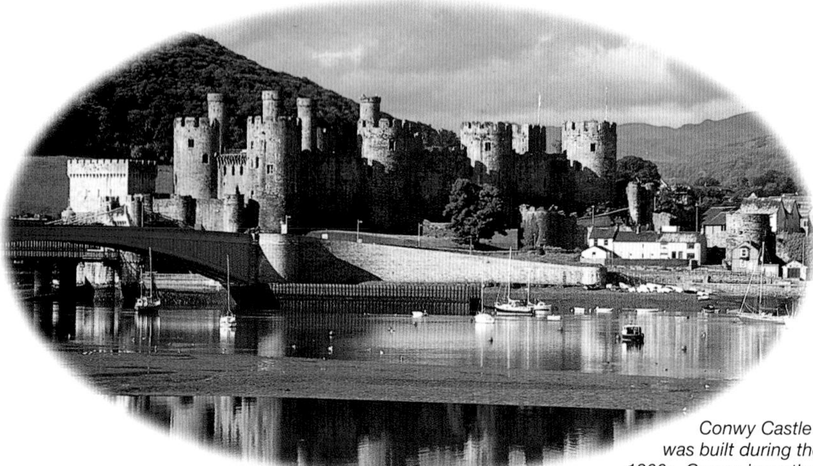

Conwy Castle was built during the 1200s. Conwy is on the north coast of Wales.

Melrose Abbey

INVASION OF WALES
In 1277, the English King Edward I demanded that the Welsh Prince Llywelyn Yr Ail accept him as the ultimate ruler of Wales. Llywelyn refused and so Edward invaded. After the death of Llywelyn in 1282, Wales became part of England. In order to keep control, Edward built 10 great stone castles throughout the principality.

SCOTLAND

The first true king of Scotland was Kenneth MacAlpin, who united the country north of the River Forth in 843. By 1018 the country was united within roughly its present borders. For the next 200 years Scottish kings fought a long series of border wars with England. They built many stone castles, as well as several abbeys, such as Melrose.

Robert the Bruce

Hero of Scottish independence, Robert the Bruce led 30,000 men to victory against an English army of 100,000 under King Edward II at the Battle of Bannockburn.

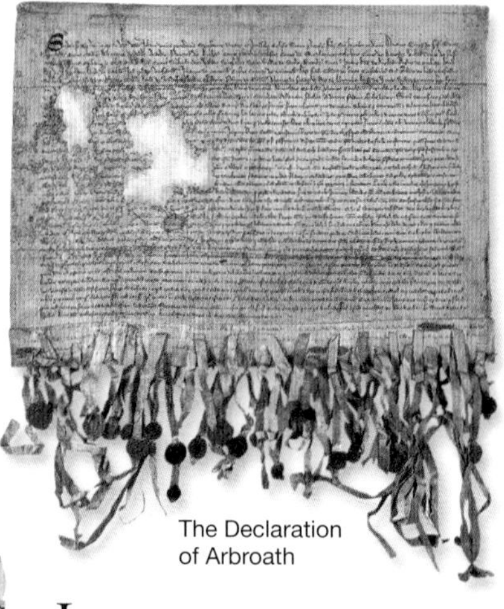

The Declaration of Arbroath

DECLARATION OF ARBROATH
After their victory at Bannockburn, the Scots expected the English to leave them alone. This did not happen, so in 1320 the Scottish lords and bishops met at Arbroath to draw up a petition to Pope John XXII, asking him to recognize Scottish independence. In 1328, the English finally recognized Scotland as an independent nation.

BANNOCKBURN
In 1290 Margaret, the young queen of Scotland, died without an heir. The Scottish lords asked Edward I of England to choose a successor, but in 1296 he took direct control of Scotland. William Wallace (c. 1274-1305) – Braveheart – rose in revolt against English rule but was excuted in 1305. Robert the Bruce (1274-1319) continued the fight, finally defeating the English army at Bannockburn in 1314.

INVASION OF IRELAND

In 1155, Pope Adrian IV authorized King Henry II to bring the Irish Church into line with the Catholic Church in Rome. Henry invaded in 1171, forcing the Irish bishops to submit to Rome at the Rock of Cashel. The invasion marked the start of English involvement in Ireland.

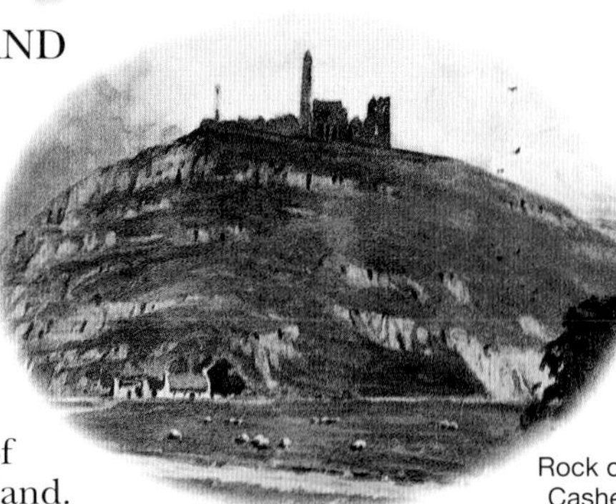

Rock of Cashel

UNION OF ENGLAND AND SCOTLAND

In 1603, Elizabeth I of England died. Her heir was her distant cousin, James VI of Scotland. He also took over the English throne as James I, so uniting the two countries. Scotland kept its own parliament, Church, and judicial system until 1707, when the Act of Union united the two parliaments in London. In 1999, Scotland once again had its own parliament.

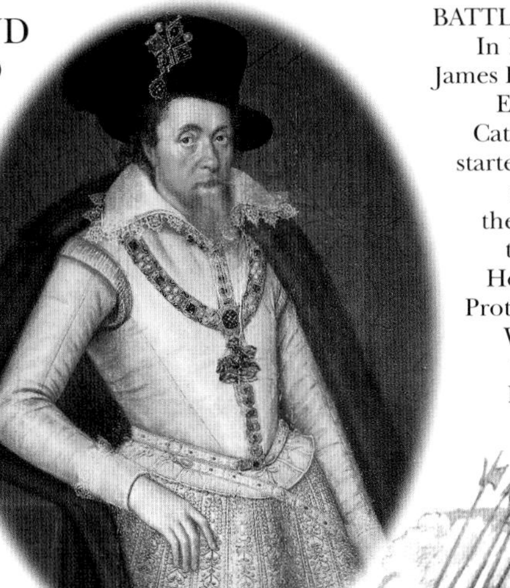

James I of England and VI of Scotland

BATTLE OF THE BOYNE

In 1688, Catholic King James II was forced off the English throne. Irish Catholics objected and started a rebellion. They asked James to lead them, and he brought troops from France. However, in 1620, the Protestant English King William III defeated the Catholics at the Battle of the Boyne.

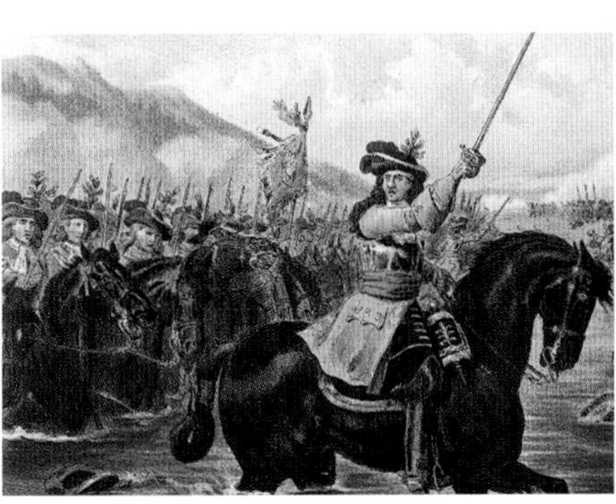

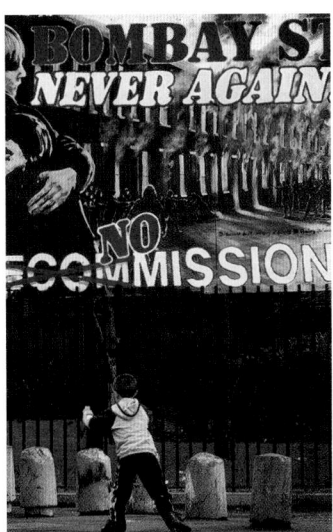

CULLODEN

After Queen Anne died in 1714, the British throne went to the German King George I. Many Scots believed that Catholic James Edward Stuart (1688-1766), son of James II, should be king. In 1715, they rose in revolt. The rebellion failed, but in 1745, the Scots tried again under Charles Edward Stuart (1720-88), known as Bonnie Prince Charlie. They were defeated at Culloden Moor in 1746.

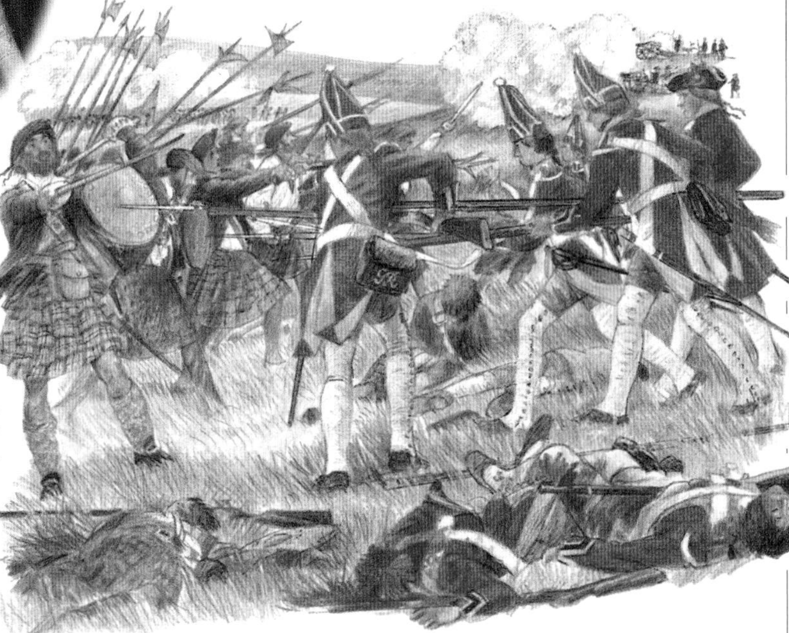

NORTHERN IRELAND

During the 19th century, Irish Catholics campaigned for Home Rule for Ireland. Northern Irish Protestants objected to this. In 1920-22 the British government divided Ireland, setting up separate states in northern and southern Ireland, each with its own parliament. Many Northern Irish Catholics, continue to campaign for a united Ireland free of British rule.

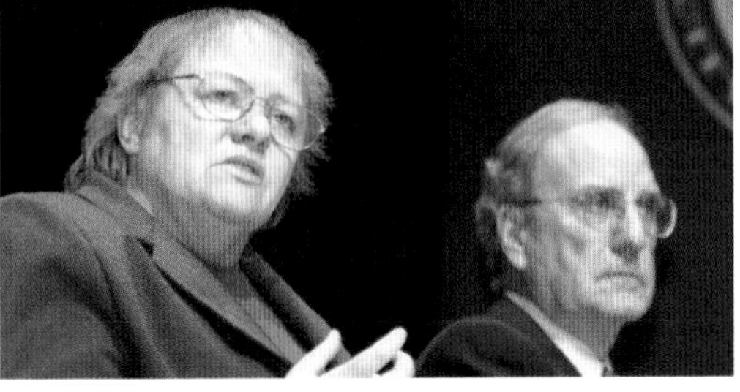

GOOD FRIDAY

In 1972 the Northern Ireland parliament was closed because it could not keep the peace between Protestants and Catholics. Eventually, US senator George Mitchell and the British minister Mo Mowlam worked out an agreement to share power between all political parties. It was signed on Good Friday, 10 April, 1998. However, there have been problems making power-sharing work.

DEVOLUTION

For some years, many people in Scotland and Wales have wanted devolution, the passing of power from England to their own parliaments. In 1998, the British government held a vote on devolution in both countries. A Scottish parliament and a Welsh Assemby were then set up. They both met for the first time in 1999.

Many football fans, such as this young Scot, paint their country's flag on their faces in support of their national team.

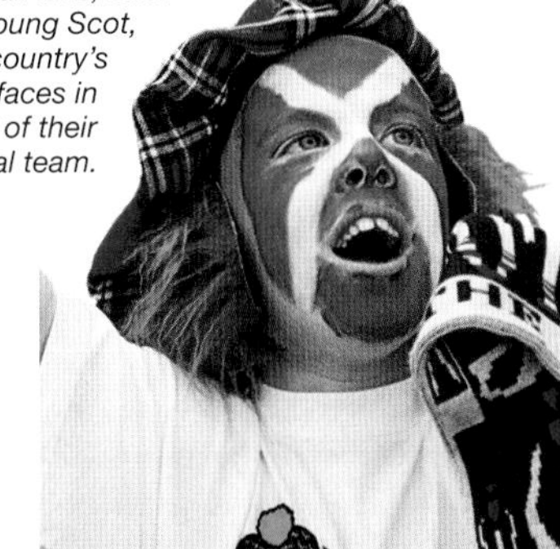

THE REGIONS OF THE UNITED KINGDOM

871-899 Alfred rules England.

1018 Malcolm II unites Scotland.

1171 Henry II invades Ireland.

1200s Wales united.

1277-84 England conquers Wales.

1296 Edward I of England rules Scotland.

1314 English defeated at Bannockburn and driven out of Scotland.

1320 Scottish lords draw up Declaration of Arbroath.

1536 Act of Union between England and Wales.

1603 Scottish and English crowns unite.

1690s Protestants take complete control of Ireland.

1707 Act of Union between Scotland and England.

1746 Scots defeated at Culloden.

1801 Act of Union between Britain and Ireland.

1920-22 Ireland divided into north and south.

1999 Scotland and Wales get devolved government.

Find out more

ENGLAND
NORTHERN IRELAND
SCOTLAND
WALES

UNITED NATIONS

IN 1945, AT THE END of World War II, the nations that opposed Germany, Italy, and Japan decided that such a war must never be repeated. They set up the United Nations, with the aim of preventing future conflicts, and drew up the United Nations Charter. The United Nations (UN) met for the first time in San Francisco in 1945. Today, 185 nations belong to the UN. The UN consists of six main organs: the General Assembly, the Security Council, the Secretariat, the Economic and Social Council, the Trusteeship Council, and the International Court of Justice. Each is concerned with world peace and social justice. The UN also has agencies which deal with global issues such as health. Each member nation of the UN has a seat in the General Assembly; 15 nations sit on the Security Council. The UN is not without problems. Its members often disagree, and it suffers financial difficulties.

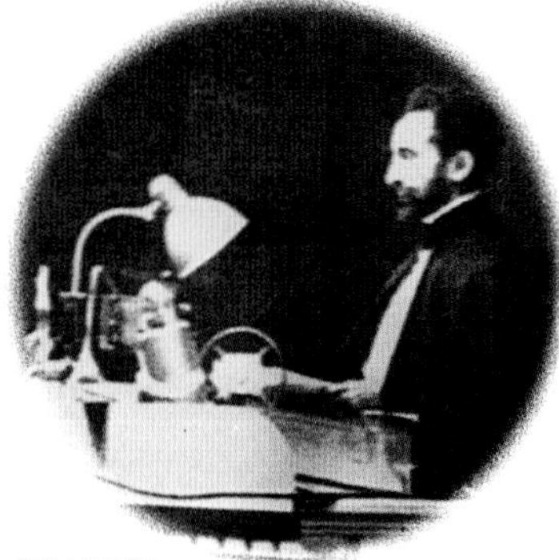

LEAGUE OF NATIONS
In 1919, the victors of World War I including Great Britain, founded the League of Nations to keep peace. But in 1935 the League failed to prevent Italy from invading Ethiopia. In 1946, the League's functions were transferred to the UN. Haile Selassie, emperor of Ethiopia, is seen addressing the League, above.

UNITED NATIONS
The headquarters of the UN in New York City, United States, is where the General Assembly and Security Council meet, as well as many of the specialist agencies of the organization. Politicians from every member nation come to New York to address the UN, and many international disputes and conflicts are settled here.

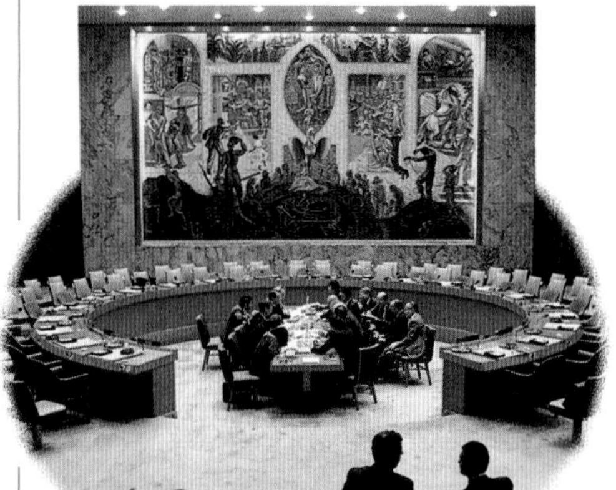

SECURITY COUNCIL

The aim of the Security Council is to maintain peace in the world. It investigates any event which might lead to fighting. The council has five permanent members – Britain, the United States, the Russian Federation, France, and China – and 10 members elected for two years each.

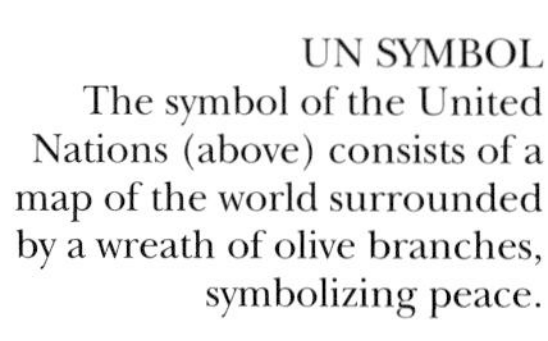

UN SYMBOL
The symbol of the United Nations (above) consists of a map of the world surrounded by a wreath of olive branches, symbolizing peace.

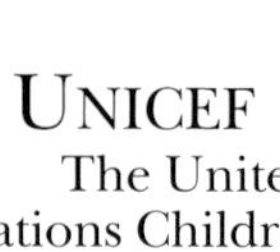

UNICEF

The United Nations Children's Fund (UNICEF) is one of the most successful agencies of the UN. UNICEF was originally founded to help child victims of World War II. The fund now provides education, health care, and medical help for children across the world, particularly in areas devastated by war or famine. Much of its work takes place in the poorer countries of Africa and Asia.

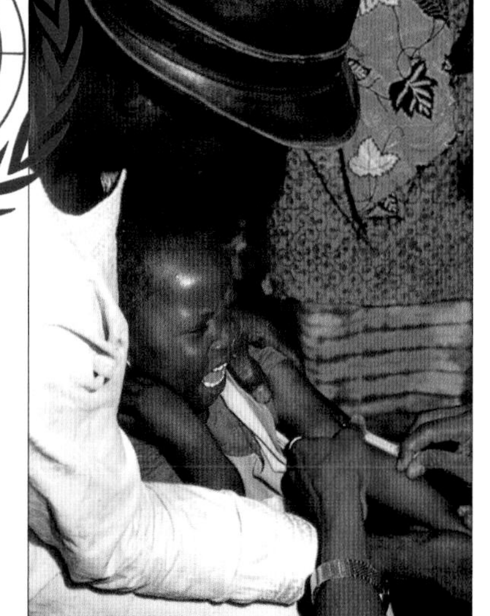

Children in underdeveloped countries are immunized against disease, thanks to UNICEF.

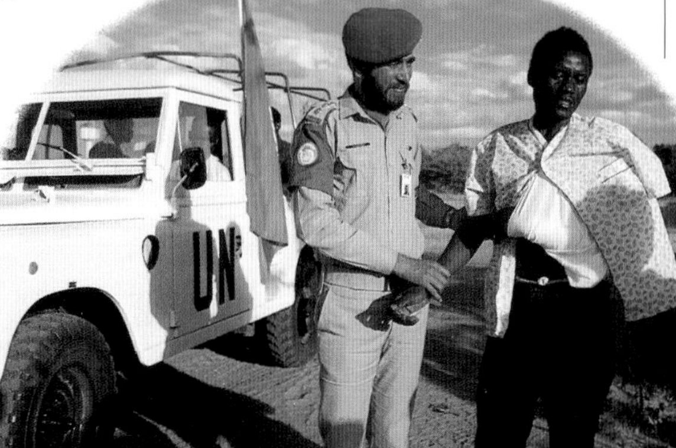

PEACEKEEPING
The UN is sometimes called on to send a peacekeeping force to a country in order to prevent war. In 1989, a UN force was sent to Namibia, southern Africa, to supervise the elections that led to Namibia's independence. More recently, UN forces were sent to Ethiopia, in eastern Africa, to uphold a peace agreement with neighbouring Eritrea.

Find out more
ARMIES
GOVERNMENTS AND POLITICS
WORLD WAR I
WORLD WAR II

UNITED STATES OF AMERICA

ON THE FLAG OF the United States, 50 identical stars represent the country's 50 states. But the states themselves could not be more different. If the stars showed their areas, the largest, for Alaska, would be nearly 500 times bigger than the star for the smallest state, Rhode Island. If the stars showed population, Alaska's star would be the smallest, and the star for California, which has the most people, would be 60 times larger. The states vary in other ways, too. The Rocky Mountains in the western states reach more than 4,400 m (14,400 ft) in height, but flat plains extend for hundreds of kilometres across the country's centre. At Barrow, Alaska, the most northerly town, the average temperature is just -13°C (9°F), yet in Arizona temperatures have reached 57°C (134°F). Since 1945, the USA has played a leading role in world affairs. The nation is the most powerful in the Western world. American finance, culture, and politics have spread outward from the United States. Products made in the United States are available in every country. Decisions made by American politicians affect the lives of many people throughout the world.

The United States covers much of the continent of North America. It reaches from the Atlantic to the Pacific oceans and from the Mexican border to Canada. The nation covers a total of 9.37 million sq km (3.68 million sq miles).

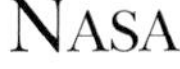

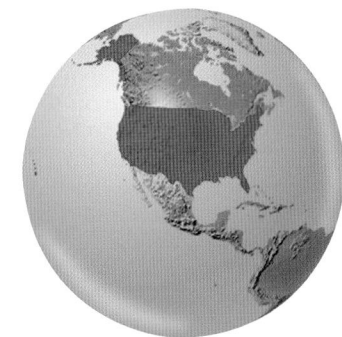

NASA

The United States is a world leader in technology, particularly in space research. The National Aeronautics and Space Administration (NASA) spends millions of dollars every year on satellites and spacecraft. In 1969, Neil Armstrong, commander of NASA's *Apollo 11*, became the first man to walk on the moon. One of NASA's recent successes is the space shuttle, a reusable spacecraft.

Operatives monitor data in a NASA space shuttle control centre.

STATE AND FEDERAL GOVERNMENT
The United States is a democracy and has a written constitution which sets out how government works. State governments, which meet in the state capital, have the authority to make laws affecting their own residents. The states were once nearly self-governing, but today the federal, or national, government has more power. It makes decisions on foreign policy and can pass laws which affect the entire country.

NEW YORK CITY

At the mouth of the Hudson River on the east coast of the United States is New York City, the country's biggest city. It is also one of the oldest. New York was founded in the 1620s and is now an urban area with 8 million people. The city is the financial heart of the nation and houses the offices of many large companies and dozens of theatres, museums, and parks. Skyscrapers more than 300 m (1,000 ft) tall dominate the city centre, Manhattan.

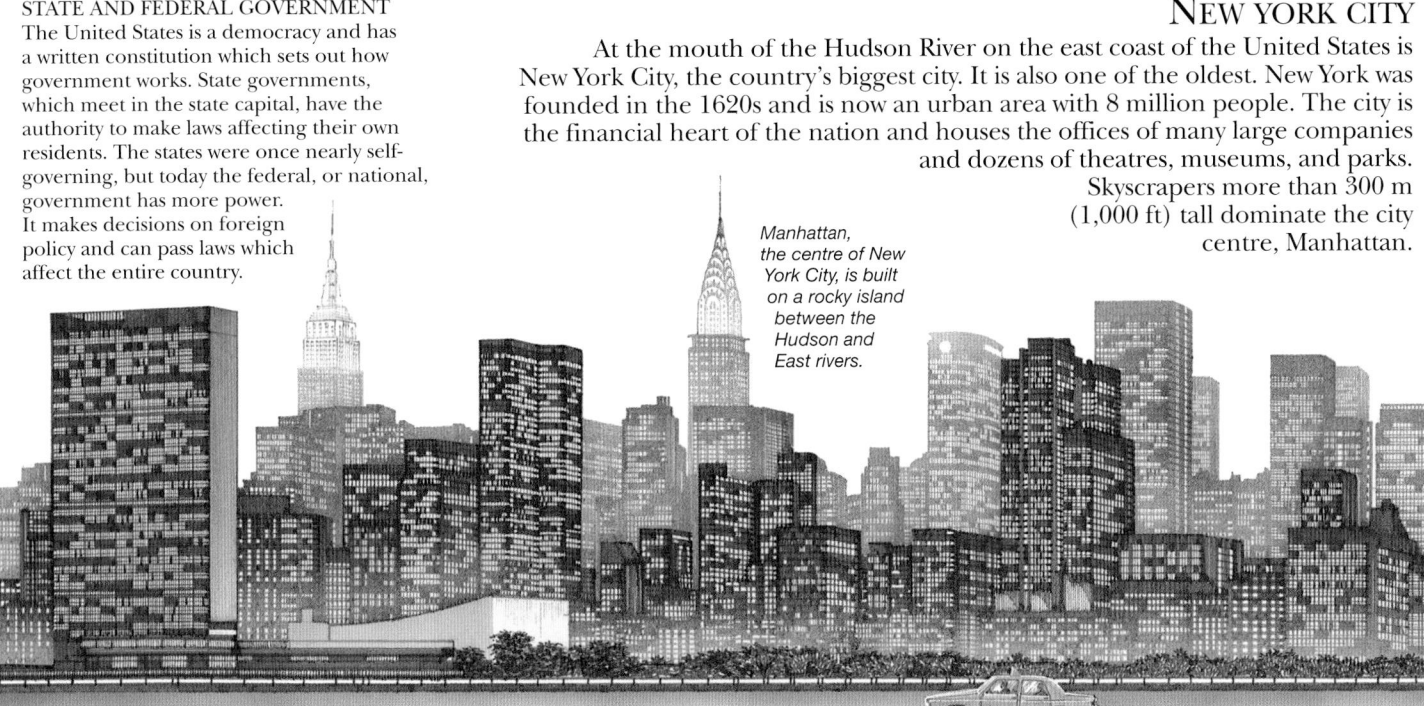

Manhattan, the centre of New York City, is built on a rocky island between the Hudson and East rivers.

HAWAII AND ALASKA

Hawaii, a group of tropical islands in the Pacific Ocean, became the fiftieth US state in 1959. The islands produce pineapples, sugar, and coffee. Polynesians first settled Hawaii in the 700s, and many native Polynesians still live here. Alaska lies outside the United States, too, separated from the other states by Canada.

The Sugar Train *on the Hawaiian island of Maui*

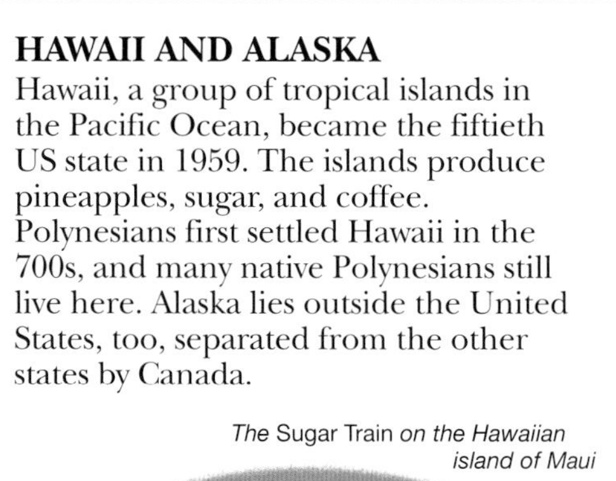

CALIFORNIA

In 1848 gold, was discovered in California, and many people rushed to the region to prospect for it. California is still the state with the most inhabitants. Nearly 36 million people live there. Most of the state has a mild, sunny climate and produces vast amounts of fruit. Many towns in California have become resorts. Modern industries have started up in California; the so-called Silicon Valley, for example, is a centre for the computer business.

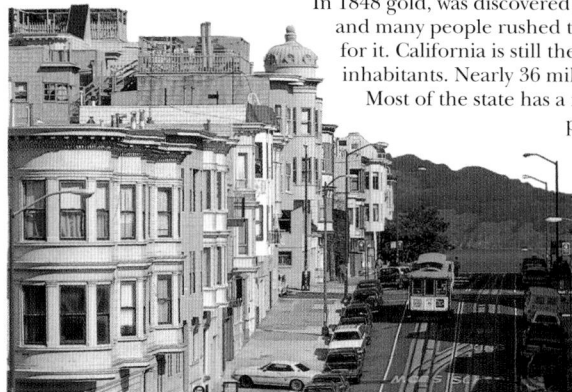

Cable cars still carry passengers up some of the 43 hills on which the city of San Francisco, California, is built.

AMERICAN PEOPLE

Native Americans, the original Americans, now make up only a small part of the total population of 295 million. Most people are the descendants of settlers from overseas and speak English. They live in the same neighbourhoods and mingle in everyday life. Their cultures have also mingled, producing a new form of English different from that spoken in England. Some groups, such as the Chinese and the Italians, also keep their own traditions and language alive in small, urban communities.

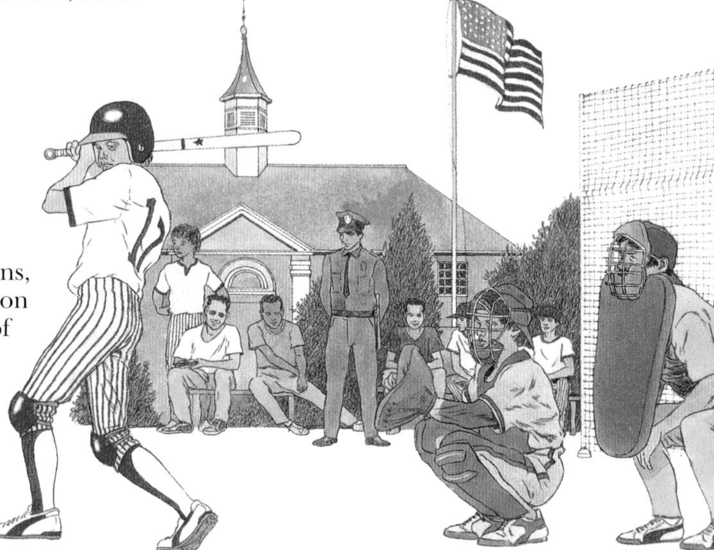

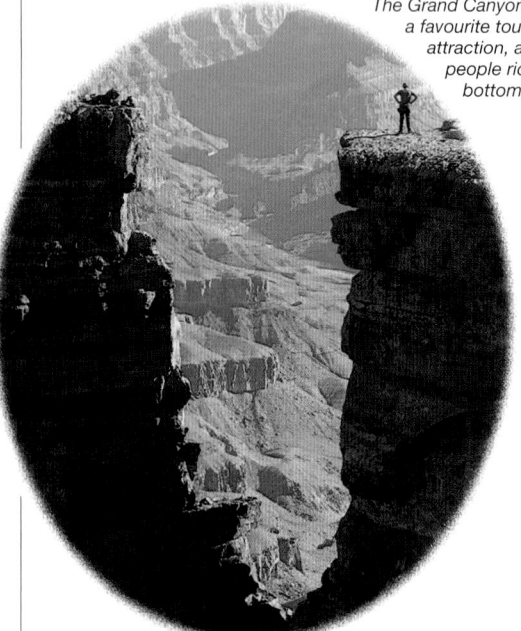

BASEBALL

Baseball is the USA's top sport, and was first played between two organized teams in 1846.

The Grand Canyon is a favourite tourist attraction, and many people ride to the bottom on mules.

HOLLYWOOD

Hollywood, in Los Angeles,was founded in 1887 as a community for Christians. Today, it is the centre of America's film industry. Many movie studios are based here, and actors, actresses and other celebrities live and work nearby. The area is a big tourist attraction. Visitors come to spot the stars and to take photos of the Hollywood sign (right) in the Hollywood Hills.

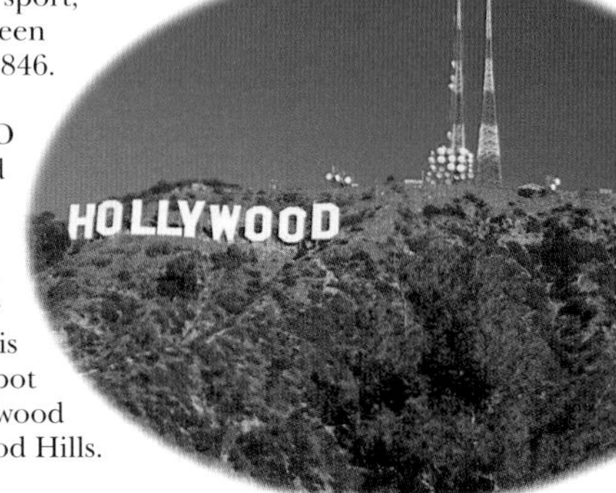

BLUES

During the 17th, 18th, and 19th centuries thousands of Africans were brought to America as slaves. Slavery was outlawed in 1865, and since then black writers, artists, and musicians have made their mark on American culture. The popular music known as blues originated among slaves in the southern states of America.

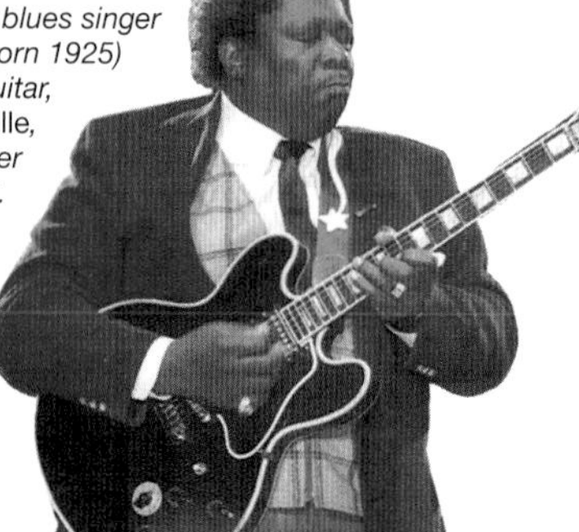

Famous blues singer B.B. King (born 1925) has played his guitar, named Lucille, *in concerts all over the world.*

GRAND CANYON

There are many natural wonders in the United States; one of the most impressive is the Grand Canyon in Arizona. The Colorado River took thousands of years to cut the canyon by natural erosion through solid rock. It is 29 km (18 miles) wide in places and more than 1,800 m (6,000 ft) deep.

Find out more

GOVERNMENT AND POLITICS
KING, MARTIN LUTHER
NATIVE AMERICANS
ROOSEVELT, FRANKLIN

SEAT OF GOVERNMENT

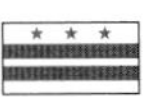
DISTRICT OF COLUMBIA
Area: 159 sq km (61sq miles)
Population: 553,500
Capital: Washington

STATES, with date of admission to Union

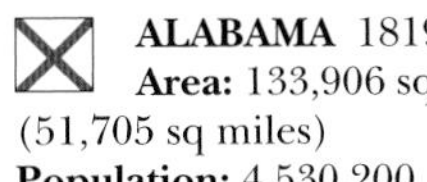
ALABAMA 1819
Area: 133,906 sq km (51,705 sq miles)
Population: 4,530,200
Capital: Montgomery

ALASKA 1959
Area: 1,530,572 sq km (591,000 sq miles)
Population: 655,400
Capital: Juneau

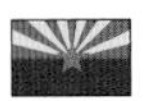
ARIZONA 1912
Area: 295,237 sq km (114,000 sq miles)
Population: 5,743,800
Capital: Phoenix

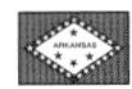
ARKANSAS 1836
Area: 137,744 sq km (53,187 sq miles)
Population: 2,752,600
Capital: Little Rock

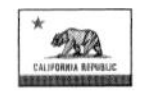
CALIFORNIA 1850
Area: 411,017 sq km (158,706 sq miles)
Population: 35,893,800
Capital: Sacramento

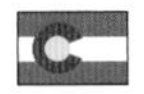
COLORADO 1876
Area: 269,575 sq km (104,091 sq miles)
Population: 4,601,400
Capital: Denver

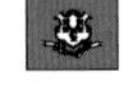
CONNECTICUT 1788
Area: 12,996 sq km (5,018 sq miles)
Population: 3,503,600
Capital: Hartford

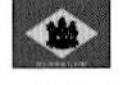
DELAWARE 1787
Area: 5,296 sq km (2,045 sq miles)
Population: 830,400
Capital: Dover

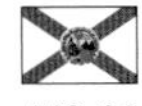
FLORIDA 1845
Area: 151,928 sq km (58,664 sq miles)
Population: 17,397,200
Capital: Tallahassee

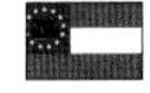
GEORGIA 1788
Area: 152,565 sq km (58,910 sq miles)
Population: 8,829,400
Capital: Atlanta

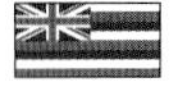
HAWAII 1959
Area: 16,759 sq km (6,471 sq miles)
Population: 1,262,800
Capital: Honolulu

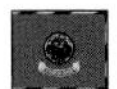
IDAHO 1890
Area: 216,414 sq km (83,564 sq miles)
Population: 1,393,300
Capital: Boise

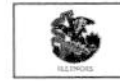
ILLINOIS 1818
Area: 145,922 sq km (56,345 sq miles)
Population: 12,713,600
Capital: Springfield

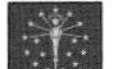
INDIANA 1816
Area: 93,712 sq km (36,185 sq miles)
Population: 6,237,600
Capital: Indianapolis

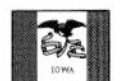
IOWA 1846
Area: 145,740 sq km (56,275 sq miles)
Population: 2,954,500
Capital: Des Moines

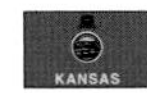
KANSAS 1861
Area: 213,081 sq km (82,277 sq miles)
Population: 2,735,500
Capital: Topeka

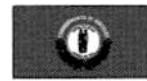
KENTUCKY 1792
Area: 104,654 sq km (40,410 sq miles)
Population: 4,145,900
Capital: Frankfort

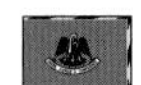
LOUISIANA 1812
Area: 123,678 sq km (47,752 sq miles)
Population: 4,515,800
Capital: Baton Rouge

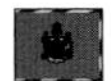
MAINE 1820
Area: 86,150 sq km (33,265 sq miles)
Population: 1,317,300
Capital: Augusta

MARYLAND 1788
Area: 27,089 sq km (10,460 sq miles)
Population: 5,558,000
Capital: Annapolis

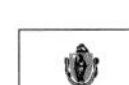
MASSACHUSETTS 1788
Area: 21,454 sq km (8,284 sq miles)
Population: 6,416,500
Capital: Boston

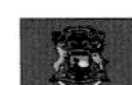
MICHIGAN 1837
Area: 151,573 sq km (58,527 sq miles)
Population: 10,112,600
Capital: Lansing

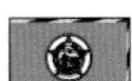
MINNESOTA 1858
Area: 218,584 sq km (84,402 sq miles)
Population: 5,101,000
Capital: St. Paul

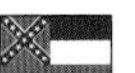
MISSISSIPPI 1817
Area: 123,505 sq km (47,689 sq miles)
Population: 2,903,000
Capital: Jackson

MISSOURI 1821
Area: 180,501 sq km (69,697 sq miles)
Population: 5,754,600
Capital: Jefferson City

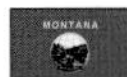
MONTANA 1889
Area: 380,820 sq km (147,046 sq miles)
Population: 926,900
Capital: Helena

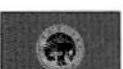
NEBRASKA 1867
Area: 200,334 sq km (77,355 sq miles)
Population: 1,747,200
Capital: Lincoln

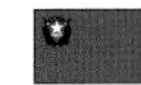
NEVADA 1864
Area: 286,331 sq km (110,561 sq miles)
Population: 2,334,800
Capital: Carson City

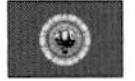
NEW HAMPSHIRE 1788
Area: 24,031 sq km (9,279 sq miles)
Population: 1,299,500
Capital: Concord

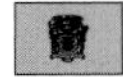
NEW JERSEY 1787
Area: 20,167 sq km (7,787 sq miles)
Population: 8,698,900
Capital: Trenton

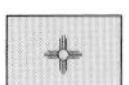
NEW MEXICO 1912
Area: 314,902 sq km (121,593 sq miles)
Population: 1,903,300
Capital: Santa Fe

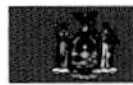
NEW YORK 1788
Area: 127,180 sq km (49,108 sq miles)
Population: 19,227,000
Capital: Albany

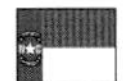
NORTH CAROLINA 1789
Area: 136,402 sq km (52,669 sq miles)
Population: 8,541,200
Capital: Raleigh

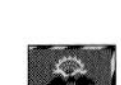
NORTH DAKOTA 1889
Area: 183,104 sq km (70,702 sq miles)
Population: 634,400
Capital: Bismarck

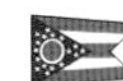
OHIO 1803
Area: 107,036 sq km (41,330 sq miles)
Population: 11,459,000
Capital: Columbus

OKLAHOMA 1907
Area: 181,076 sq km (69,919 sq miles)
Population: 3,523,600
Capital: Oklahoma City

OREGON 1859
Area: 251,400 sq km (97,073 sq miles)
Population: 3,594,600
Capital: Salem

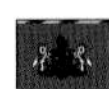
PENNSYLVANIA 1787
Area: 117,339 sq km (45,308 sq miles)
Population: 12,406,300
Capital: Harrisburg

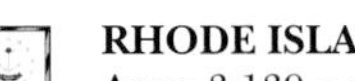

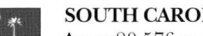
RHODE ISLAND 1790
Area: 3,139 sq km (1,212 sq miles)
Population: 1,080,600
Capital: Providence

SOUTH CAROLINA 1788
Area: 80,576 sq km (31,113 sq miles)
Population: 4,198,000
Capital: Columbia

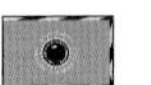
SOUTH DAKOTA 1889
Area: 199,715 sq km (77,116 sq miles)
Population: 770,900
Capital: Pierre

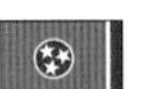
TENNESSEE 1796
Area: 109,145 sq km (42,144 sq miles)
Population: 5,901,000
Capital: Nashville

TEXAS 1845
Area: 690,977 sq km (266,807 sq miles)
Population: 22,490,000
Capital: Austin

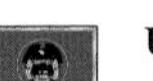
UTAH 1896
Area: 219,871 sq km (84,899 sq miles)
Population: 2,389,000
Capital: Salt Lake City

VERMONT 1791
Area: 24,898 sq km (9,614 sq miles)
Population: 621,400
Capital: Montpelier

VIRGINIA 1788
Area: 105,578 sq km (40,767 sq miles)
Population: 7,459,800
Capital: Richmond

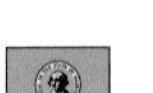
WASHINGTON 1889
Area: 176,466 sq km (68,139 sq miles)
Population: 6,203,800
Capital: Olympia

WEST VIRGINIA 1863
Area: 62,756 sq km (24,232 sq miles)
Population: 1,815,400
Capital: Charleston

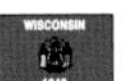
WISCONSIN 1848
Area: 145,425 sq km (56,153 sq miles)
Population: 5,509,000
Capital: Madison

WYOMING 1890
Area: 253,306 sq km (97,809 sq miles)
Population: 506,500
Capital: Cheyenne

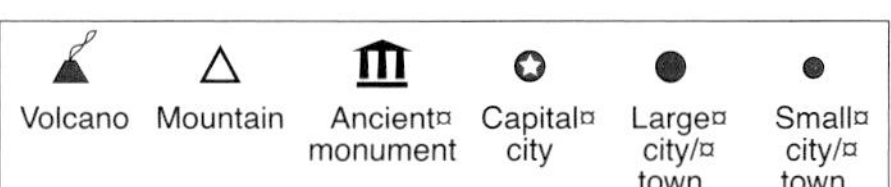

STATISTICS

Area: 9,372,610 sq km (3,681,760 sq miles)
Population: 295,734,000
Capital: Washington, DC
Languages: English, Spanish, Italian, German, French, Polish, Chinese, Tagalog, Greek
Religions: Protestant, Roman Catholic, Jewish, non-religious
Currency: US dollar
Main occupations: Research, manufacturing, agriculture
Main exports: Energy, raw materials, food, electronics, cars, coal
Main imports: Oil

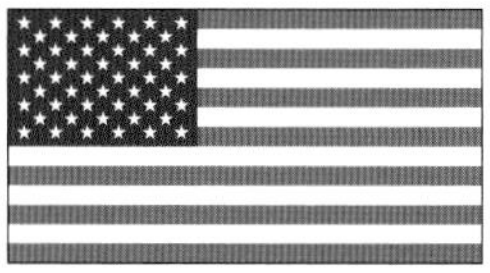

MIDWEST

The United States is the world's largest exporter of wheat and produces nearly half of the corn on Earth. This enormous quantity of food is grown on the open plains that cover the Midwest between the Mississippi River and the Rockies. Grain farming is highly mechanized, with giant machines operating in fields hundreds of hectares in size. The United States also produces one quarter of the world's oranges, one seventh of the world's nuts, and half of the world's soya beans.

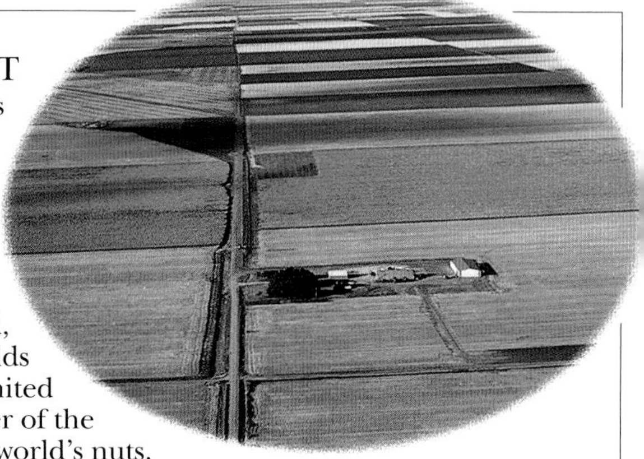

The seemingly endless wheat fields of the Midwest

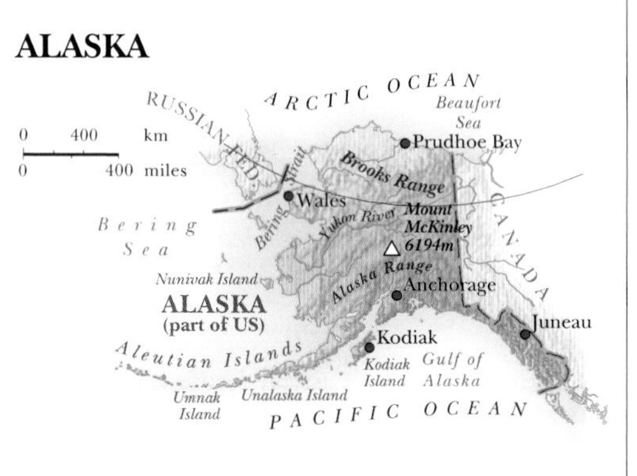

INDUSTRY

Most of the industries in the United States are the largest and most profitable of their type in the world. America has abundant mineral deposits, raw materials, and energy sources. The most economically important industries in the US include car manufacturing, food processing, textile and clothing manufacture, and the computer industry. "Silicon Valley" in California is a world centre for micro-electronics. New York is the nation's financial capital while Washington has an important aerospace industry.

BORDER
The border between Canada and the USA is the world's longest land border between any two countries.

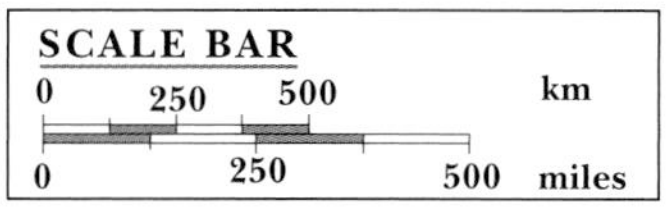

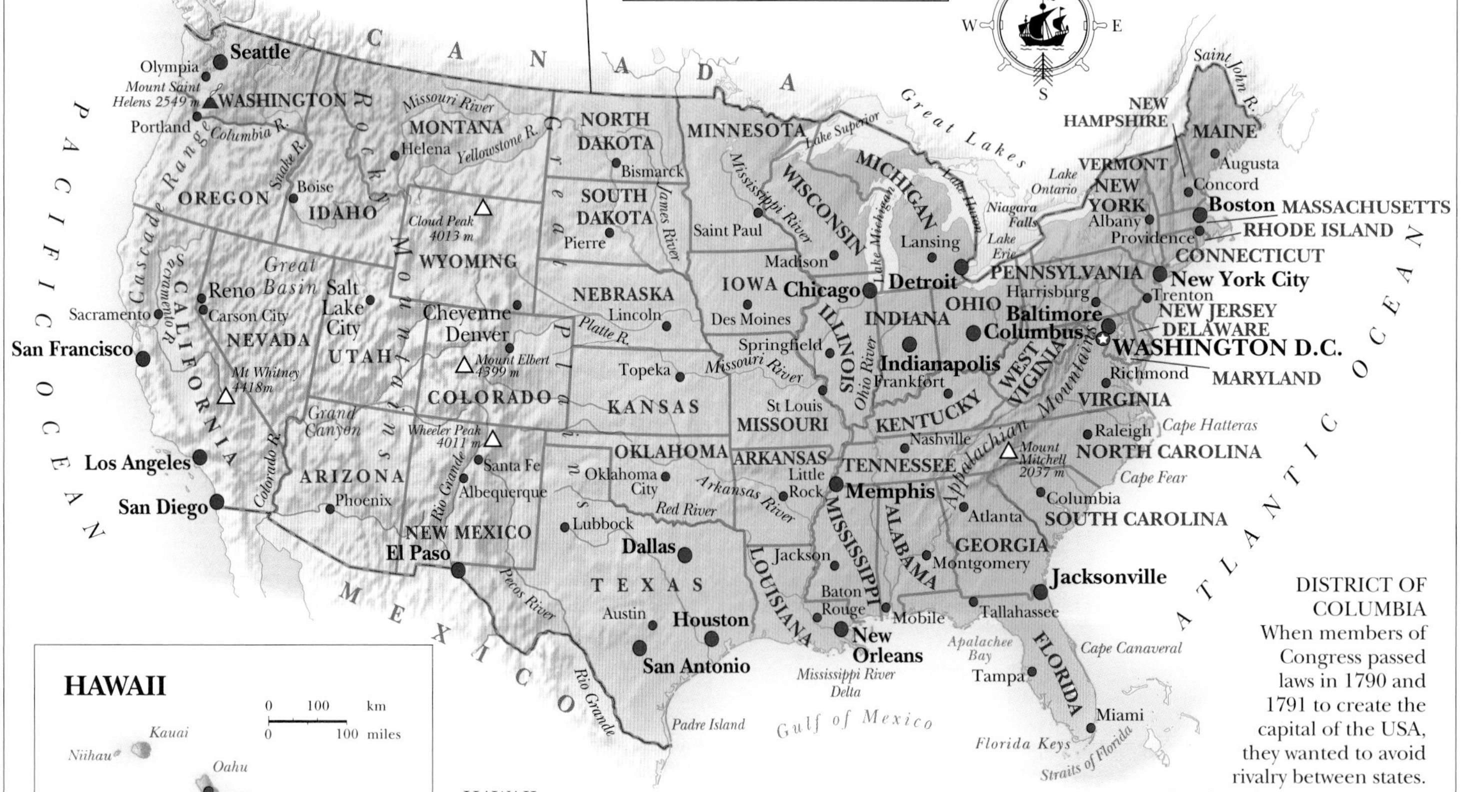

HAWAII

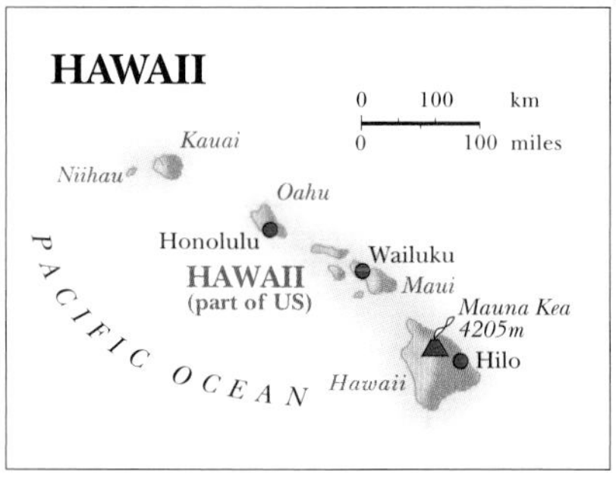

HAWAII
Hawaii is the only state that is not on the North American mainland. The eight main islands of the group are some 3,380 km (2,100 miles) southwest of San Francisco. Although most of the population lives on the island of Oahu, Hawaii itself is the biggest island.

DISTRICT OF COLUMBIA
When members of Congress passed laws in 1790 and 1791 to create the capital of the USA, they wanted to avoid rivalry between states. So when George Washington chose the site for the capital city that bears his name, the region was created as a special district, called the District of Columbia (D.C.). However, D.C. is not a state, and although the people who live there take part in Congressional elections, their delegate in the House of Representatives cannot vote.

HISTORY OF THE
UNITED STATES

TODAY, THE UNITED STATES OF AMERICA is the most powerful nation on Earth. Yet, just 230 years ago the United States was a new and vulnerable nation. It occupied a narrow strip of land on the Atlantic coast of North America and had a population of only about four million people. Beyond its borders lay vast areas of unclaimed land. Throughout the 19th century, American settlers pushed the frontier westwards across that land, fighting the Native Americans for control. At the same time, millions of immigrants from Europe were arriving on the East Coast. By 1900, the nation's farms and factories were producing more than any other country. That wealth and power led to its involvement in international affairs and drew it into two world wars. But the country continued to prosper. Since 1945 the system of individual enterprise that inspired the founders of the United States has made its people among the world's richest. American business, influence, and culture have spread to every other nation in the world.

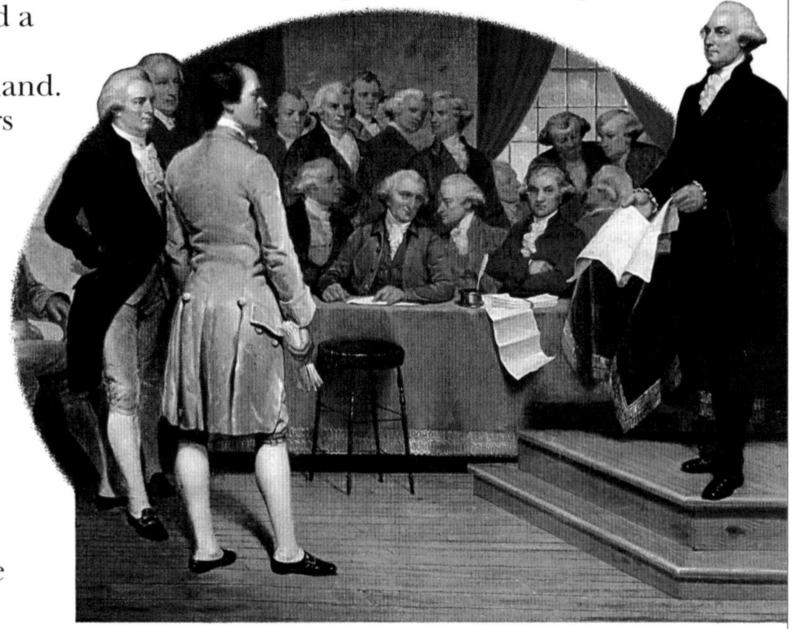

FOUNDING FATHERS
The United States originally consisted of 13 states, each with its own customs and history. In 1787 George Washington and other leaders, sometimes called the Founding Fathers, drew up the United states Constitution, a document that established a strong central government. The Constitution, which also safeguards the rights of the states and those of their people, has been in force since 1789.

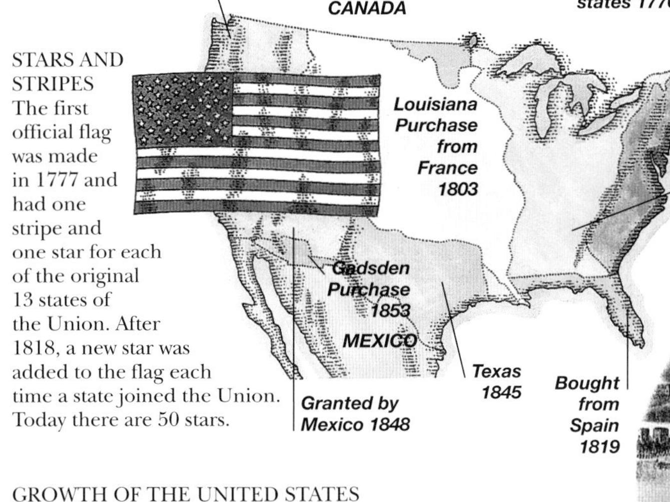

STARS AND STRIPES
The first official flag was made in 1777 and had one stripe and one star for each of the original 13 states of the Union. After 1818, a new star was added to the flag each time a state joined the Union. Today there are 50 stars.

GROWTH OF THE UNITED STATES
The 13 original colonies on the East Coast gained their independence from Britain in 1783, and acquired all the land as far west as the Mississippi River. In 1803 the vast area of Louisiana was bought from France, and by 1848 the United States had reached the Pacific Ocean.

FALL OF THE SOUTH

The Civil War ended in 1865, leaving the South in ruinous poverty. The hatred and bitterness caused by the war lasted for many years as the central government took temporary control of the defeated southern states.

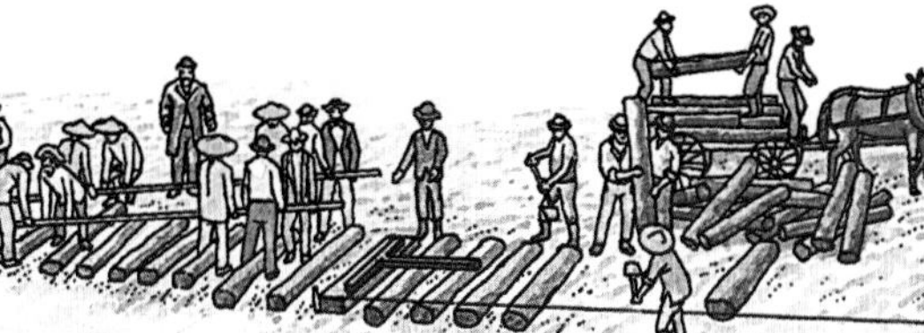

SPREAD OF THE RAILWAY
In 1860 there were more than 48,000 km (30,000 miles) of railways in the eastern United States, but almost none had been built west of the Mississippi River. On 10 May 1869, the first continental railway was completed, and the two coasts of America were joined for the first time. A ceremony was held at Promontory Point in Utah to mark the occasion. The growth of the national railway network helped unify the country.

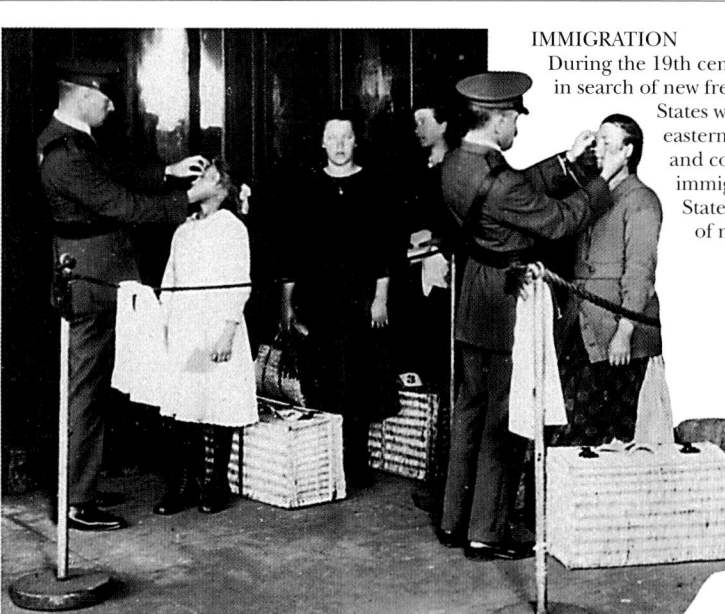

Immigrants arriving in the United States were examined at a reception centre on Ellis Island, New York.

IMMIGRATION

During the 19th century many Europeans crossed the Atlantic in search of new freedoms and opportunities. The United States welcomed Irish people escaping famine, eastern European Jews fleeing persecution, and countless others. By 1890, half a million immigrants were arriving each year in the United States. As a result, the country became a mixture of many different cultures and religions.

INDUSTRY

The United States offered an endless supply of raw materials to 19th-century industrialists, who soon took advantage of these resources. Manufacturers such as Ransom Olds pioneered mass production of cars and many other goods. In the Olds Motor Works, cars moved along a production line, with workers at intervals each performing a single task. This technique made assembly faster, and Henry Ford and other manufacturers quickly adopted it.

THE UNITED STATES AT WAR

Until the United States entered World War I in 1917, its armed forces had rarely fought overseas. After the war ended the United States tried once again to stay out of conflicts abroad. But in 1941 the Japanese attacked Pearl Harbor naval base in Hawaii, bringing the U.S. into World War II. Since 1945, the U.S. has fought in several overseas wars, notably in Korea (1950-53) and Vietnam (1961-73).

The Iwo Jima monument in Arlington National Cemetery is a memorial to Americans who died in World War II. It shows Marines raising the flag on Iwo Jima Island in the Pacific. Many US soldiers died in the battle for the island.

UNITED STATES

1783 The 13 colonies win their freedom from Britain.

1787 Constitution is drafted.

1789 George Washington becomes the first president.

1790-1800 A new capital, Washington, D.C., is built on the Potomac River.

1803 Louisiana Purchase doubles size of the country.

1845 Texas joins the Union.

1848 US defeats Mexico and acquires California and other territories.

1861-65 Civil War ends slavery

1869 First transcontinental railroad is completed.

1917-1918 US fights in World War I.

1929 Economic depression.

1941 United States enters World War II.

1963 President Kennedy assassinated.

1969 Neil Armstrong walks on the moon.

1991 US leads United Nations forces against Iraq in the Gulf War.

2001 Islamic terrorists destroy the World Trade Center.

2003 US invades Iraq.

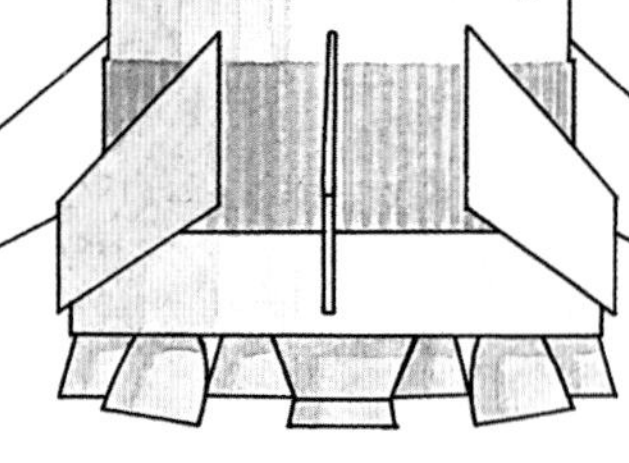

JOHN F. KENNEDY

In 1960, John F. Kennedy (1917-63) became the youngest man ever elected president. In 1961, Kennedy approved the invasion of Communist Cuba by US-backed Cuban exiles. The invasion, at the Bay of Pigs, was a disaster, and Kennedy was severely criticized. In 1962 the Soviets stationed nuclear missiles on the island. For one week, nuclear war seemed unavoidable, but Kennedy persuaded the Soviet Union to remove the missiles and averted the war. Kennedy's presidency ended tragically on 22 November 1963, when he was assassinated during a visit to Dallas, Texas, United States, after serving for exactly 1,000 days in office.

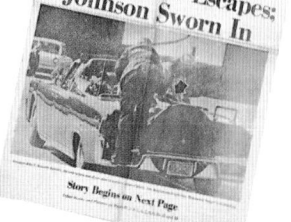

CHICAGO DAILY NEWS

PRESIDENT IS KILLED

Texas Sniper Escapes; Johnson Sworn In

Story Begins on Next Page

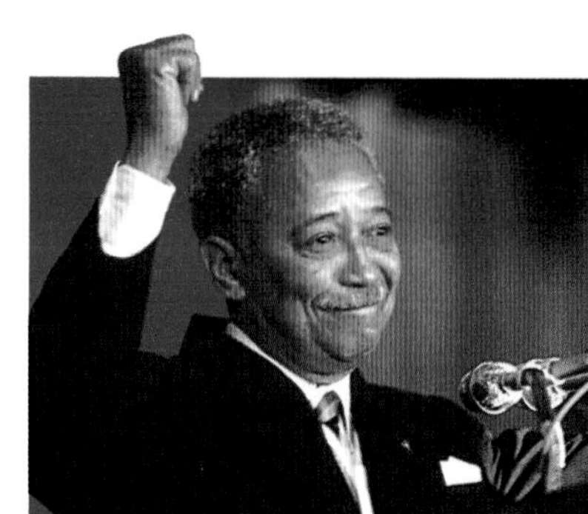

EQUAL OPPORTUNITIES

Since 1789, the US Constitution has guaranteed every citizen equal rights. In reality, many minority groups are only now starting to achieve equality. The photograph above shows David Dinkins, New York City's first black mayor.

Find out more

AMERICAN CIVIL WAR
AMERICAN REVOLUTION
EMIGRATION AND IMMIGRATION
KENNEDY, JOHN F.
NUCLEAR AGE
PILGRIMS
UNITED STATES OF AMERICA
WASHINGTON, GEORGE

UNIVERSE

THE VAST EXPANSE OF SPACE that we call the universe contains everything there is. It includes the Sun, the planets, the Milky Way galaxy, and all other galaxies too. The universe is continually growing, and each part is gradually moving further away from every other part. We know about the universe by using powerful telescopes to study light, radio waves, x-rays, and other radiations that reach Earth from space. Light travels nearly 9.5 billion km (6 billion miles) in a year. We call this distance a light-year. The light from a distant star that you can see through a telescope may have travelled thousands of years to reach us. Most scientists believe that the universe was created by a massive explosive event that happened billions of years ago. This idea is called the Big Bang theory. Many scientists now believe that visible matter makes up only 7% of the universe and that the rest is dark matter and dark energy.

Milky Way has a halo of stars and gas.

MILKY WAY
The Sun is just one of 100 billion stars in the large spiral galaxy we call the Milky Way. Like most other spiral galaxies, the Milky Way has curved arms of stars radiating from a globe-shaped centre. The Milky Way is 100,000 light-years across, and the Sun is 30,000 light-years from its centre.

GALAXIES

Galaxies, which contain gas, dust, and billions of stars, belong to one of three main groups – elliptical, irregular, or spiral. Most galaxies are elliptical, ranging from sphere shapes to egg shapes. A few galaxies are irregular. Others, such as the Milky Way, are spirals. The universe consists of billions of galaxies of all types.

Pieces of paper represent clusters of galaxies.

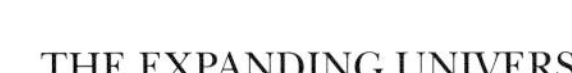

Balloon expands in the same way that the universe is expanding.

GALAXY CLUSTERS
Most galaxies belong to groups called clusters, which may contain thousands of galaxies of all types. These clusters form "walls" with great voids in between, so that the universe is like a foam.

In this image the galaxies are yellow and red, and the blue haloes around them represent dark matter.

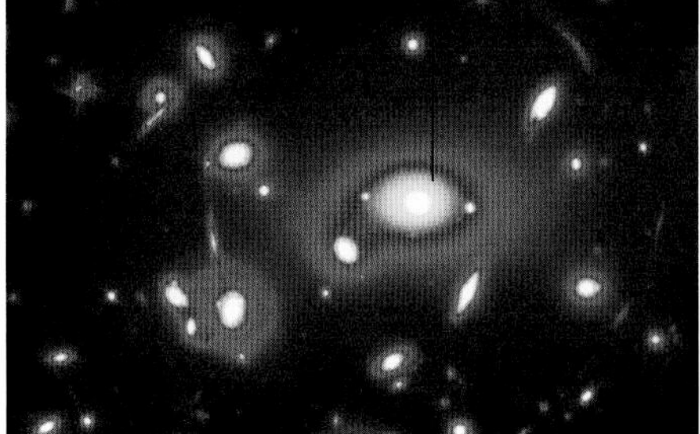

THE INVISIBLE UNIVERSE
When scientists estimate the mass of a galaxy cluster, the figure usually turns out to be much more than the mass of the visible galaxies alone. The extra, invisible matter is called dark matter, and no-one knows what it is. Dark matter and ordinary matter together account for only 30% of the universe. Scientists call the remaining 70% dark energy. Dark energy is like a force that acts against gravity and pushes the galaxies apart. It is causing the expansion of the universe to speed up.

THE EXPANDING UNIVERSE
You can get an idea of how the universe is expanding by imagining several small pieces of paper glued onto a balloon. Each piece represents a cluster of galaxies. As you blow up the balloon, all the paper pieces move further away from one another. In the same way, galaxy clusters are moving further away from one another. The further a cluster is, the faster it travels away from us.

LOOKING BACK IN TIME
If you look through a telescope you can see galaxies millions of light-years away. You are not seeing them as they are now but as they were long ago, when their light first set out on its journey – so in a sense, you are looking into the past.

Dinosaurs lived on Earth 65–215 million years ago.

Galaxy is 100 million light-years away. Light left this galaxy when the dinosaurs lived on Earth.

Find out more

BIG BANG
BLACK HOLES
COMETS AND METEORS
EARTH
LIGHT
MOON
PLANETS
STARS
SUN
TELESCOPES

VETERINARIANS

UNLIKE HUMANS, ANIMALS cannot explain where the pain is when they are ill. This makes healing sick animals particularly difficult. It is the job of the veterinarian. Veterinarians are doctors who study the care and healing of animals. Originally, they treated horses and farm animals. Today, veterinarians look after household pets, too. They carry out regular health checks on farm animals and help with delivering lambs and calves. Some veterinarians treat zoo animals, and some are animal dentists. If an animal is very sick or in great pain, a veterinarian may have to put it down (kill it painlessly) to relieve its suffering. The first veterinary schools opened in Europe in the 18th century. Today, veterinarians study for five years or more to learn the skills they need.

FARRIERS
Before there were vets, farriers (blacksmiths) treated horses and other farm animals such as cattle, using traditional folk remedies.

Vets often use the same instruments as doctors, such as stethoscopes.

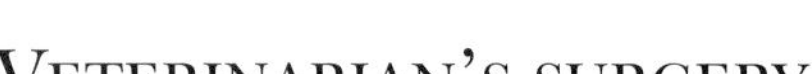

VETERINARIAN'S SURGERY

Many different animals go to the veterinarian's surgery for treatment. To avoid fights and prevent the spread of infection, dogs must be kept on a lead and cats should stay in baskets. The veterinarian examines the animal and asks the owner what the signs of the illness are. The veterinarian may need to give medicine or injections, take x-rays, or operate.

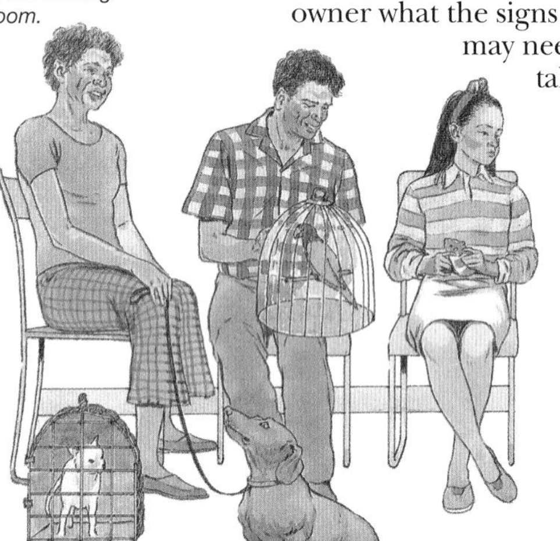

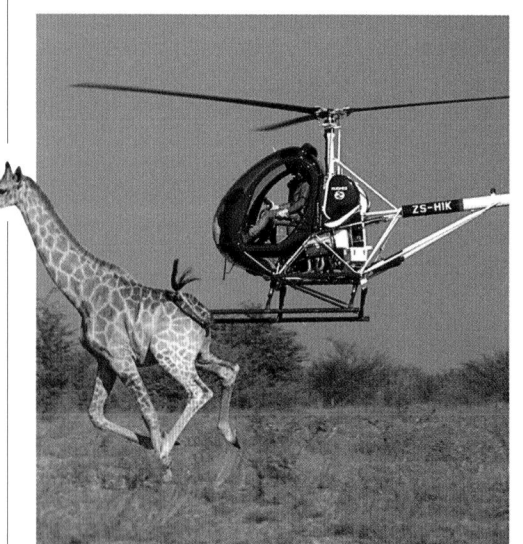

People wait with their pets in the waiting room.

Inoculating chickens prevents one diseased bird from infecting the whole flock.

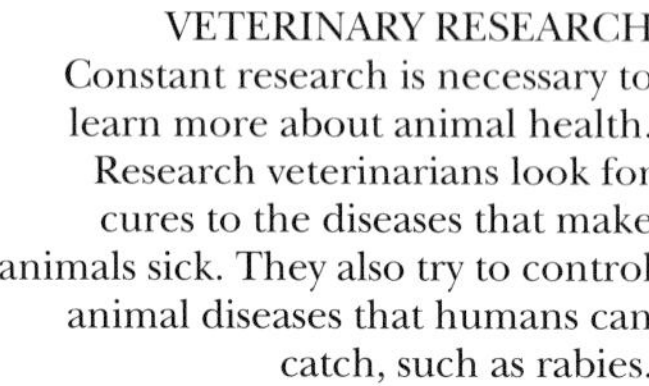

VETERINARY RESEARCH
Constant research is necessary to learn more about animal health. Research veterinarians look for cures to the diseases that make animals sick. They also try to control animal diseases that humans can catch, such as rabies.

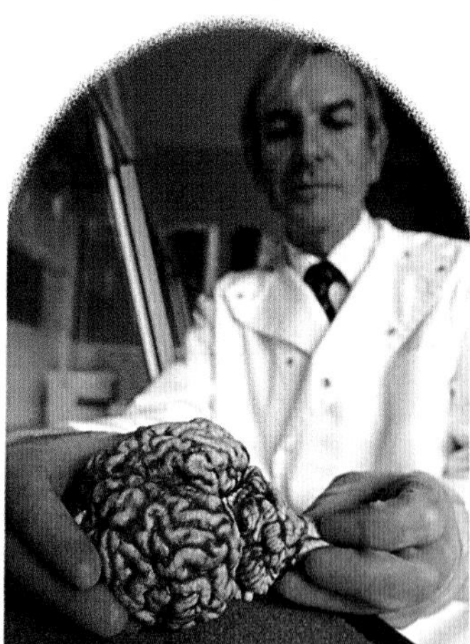

Vets sometimes have to use helicopters to locate and treat animals that range over wide areas.

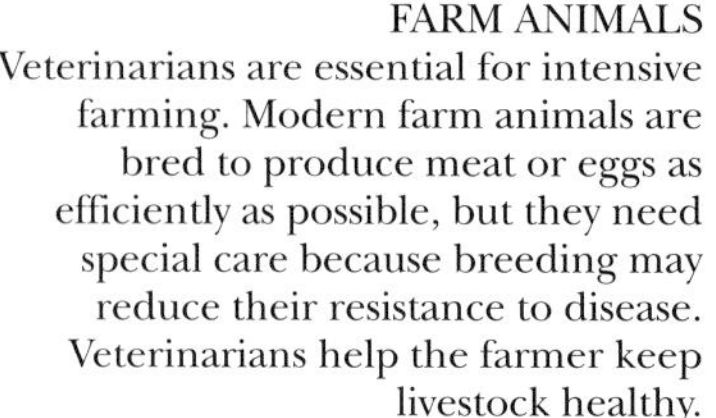

FARM ANIMALS
Veterinarians are essential for intensive farming. Modern farm animals are bred to produce meat or eggs as efficiently as possible, but they need special care because breeding may reduce their resistance to disease. Veterinarians help the farmer keep livestock healthy.

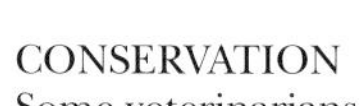

CONSERVATION
Some veterinarians are involved in wildlife conservation and treating wild animals. Large or ferocious animals, such as lions and giraffes, may have to be given a calming drug before the veterinarian can handle them. The drug eventually wears off, and does not harm the animal.

Find out more
CONSERVATION and endangered species
FARMING
PETS

QUEEN

VICTORIA

IN 1837, A YOUNG WOMAN called Victoria became Queen of Britain. She was only 18, but was determined to rule wisely and well. She reigned for 64 years, longer than any other British monarch. During her rule, Britain went through huge social, economic, and political changes, becoming the world's first industrial nation and creating a vast empire. Parliament made political decisions and governed the country, but Victoria involved herself closely in state affairs. Her dignified appearance and family life came to symbolize that period of British history, so historians call her reign the Victorian Age.

1819 Born at Kensington Palace, London.

1837 Becomes Queen after the death of her uncle, William IV.

1838 Coronation at Westminster Abbey, London.

1840 Marries her German cousin, Prince Albert.

1861 Albert dies; Victoria retires from public life.

1897 Diamond Jubilee: Victoria celebrates 60 years on the throne.

1901 Dies, aged 81.

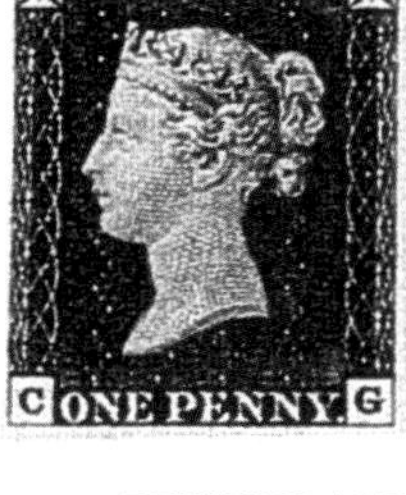

PENNY BLACK
Issued in 1840, the Penny Black was the first postage stamp. Victoria's head was printed on it.

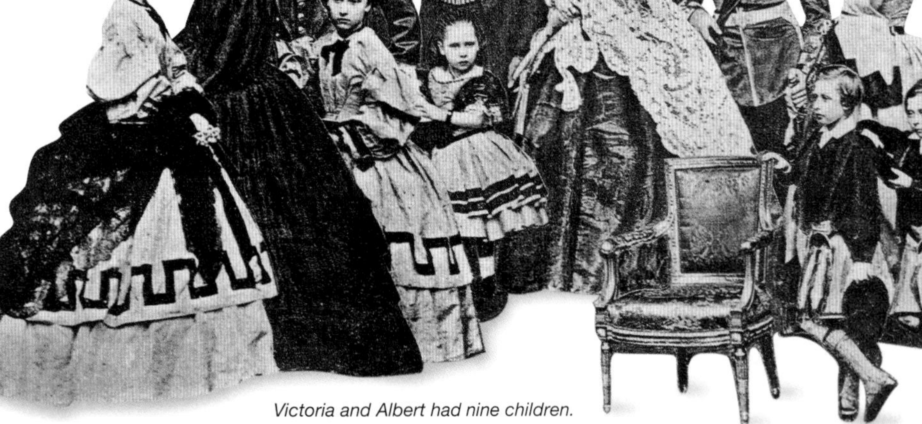

Through her children's marriages, Victoria was related to every major European royal family.

Victoria and Albert had nine children.

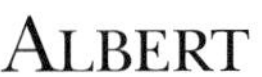

ALBERT

When Victoria was 20 she married her German cousin, Prince Albert. She adored him, and he advised her on political matters. He was also enthusiastic about education and industrial progress. Albert, who introduced the decorated Christmas tree into Britain,was a devoted father.

BENJAMIN DISRAELI
Politicians advised Victoria on political matters. During her long reign, there were 10 prime ministers. A great favourite was Benjamin Disraeli, prime minister in 1868, and from 1874-80. Victoria was interested in the British Empire, and it was Disraeli who brought India directly under British rule. In 1876, Disraeli persuaded Parliament to make Victoria "Empress of India".

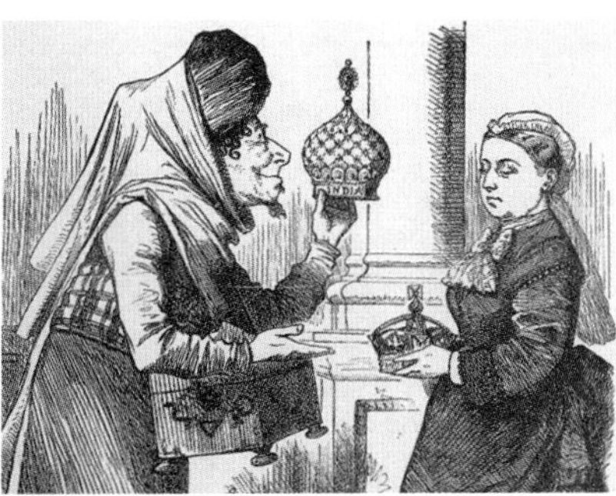

BALMORAL
Victoria and Albert created a much-loved family home at Balmoral in the Scottish Highlands, which is used by the royal family today. In 1861, Albert died of typhoid and Victoria was grief-stricken. She went into deep mourning and retired from public duties, spending time at Balmoral in the company of a household servant, John Brown. Her absence from public life made the British people angry, and for some years she was very unpopular.

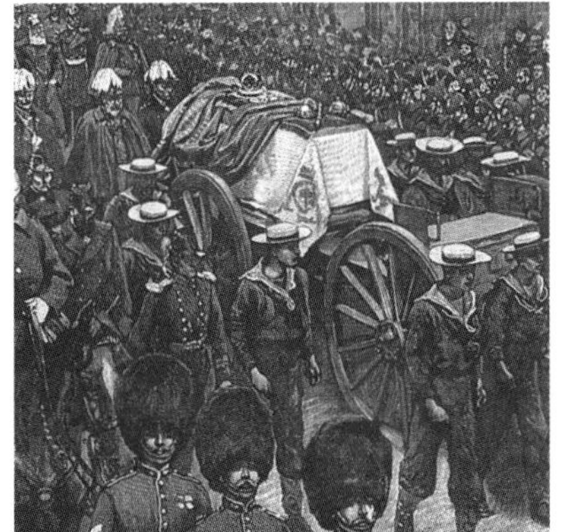

DEATH OF THE MONARCH
During the last 25 years of her reign, Victoria involved herself in matters such as housing for the poor, and her popularity soared. When she died in the first year of the 20th century, thousands of people lined London's streets to watch her funeral procession.

Find out more
BRITISH EMPIRE
INDUSTRIAL REVOLUTION
UNITED KINGDOM, HISTORY OF
VICTORIANS

VICTORIANS

UNDER THE RULE OF QUEEN VICTORIA, the British people enjoyed a long period of prosperity. Profits gained from the Empire overseas, as well as from industrial improvements at home, allowed a large, educated middle-class to develop. Great advances were made in the arts and sciences. In the cities, department stores were opened for the convenience of those with cash to spend. Domestic servants were employed in many homes, although vast numbers of people remained poor and lived in slums. Public transport, police forces, clean water supplies, and sewage treatment were introduced to ease conditions in the new towns. Like Victoria, middle-class people set high moral standards, and devised programmes to "improve" the lives of the poor. The Victorians thought themselves the most advanced society in the world.

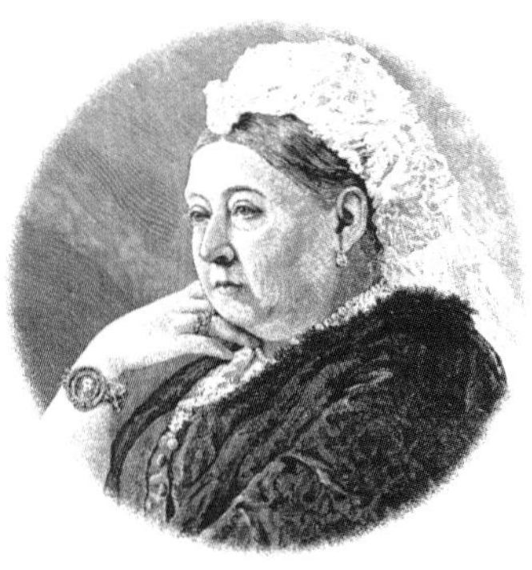

QUEEN VICTORIA
Victoria (1819-1901) is best remembered dressed all in black and in mourning for her husband Albert, who died in 1861. Queen Victoria had great dignity and was highly respected by her subjects.

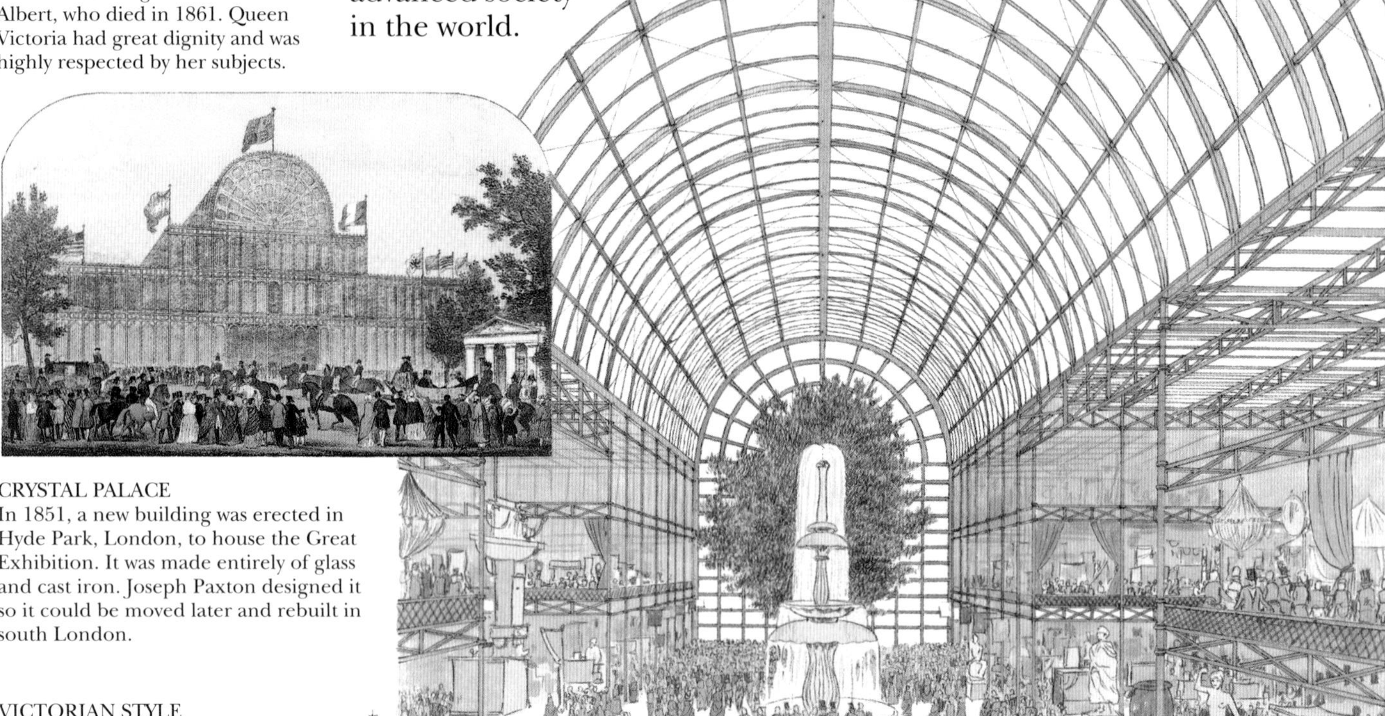

CRYSTAL PALACE
In 1851, a new building was erected in Hyde Park, London, to house the Great Exhibition. It was made entirely of glass and cast iron. Joseph Paxton designed it so it could be moved later and rebuilt in south London.

VICTORIAN STYLE
Victorians loved elaborate decoration. Almost all Victorian objects, from lamp posts to teaspoons were covered in carvings, patterns, and other ornamentation. Large houses and public buildings, such as St. Pancras station, London (right), were built in the style of ancient castles, cathedrals, and palaces.

St. Pancras station

THE GREAT EXHIBITION

In 1851, Prince Albert organized the first international exhibition in Britain. More than 6 million people visited the Crystal Palace (above) to celebrate the industrial age. The 14,000 exhibits included a 24-ton lump of coal, a railway engine, the Koh-i-noor diamond from India, and a stuffed elephant.

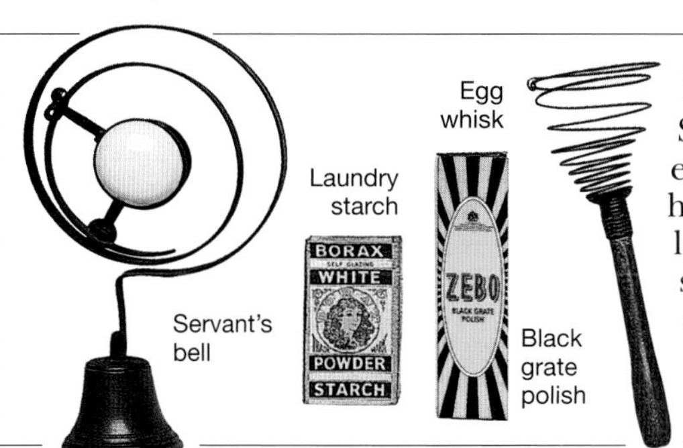

DOMESTIC LIFE

Servants were a feature of every upper- and middle-class household. Maids worked long hours for little or no pay, sometimes only for board and lodging. In 1871, more than $^{1}/_{3}$ of British women aged 12-20 were "in service".

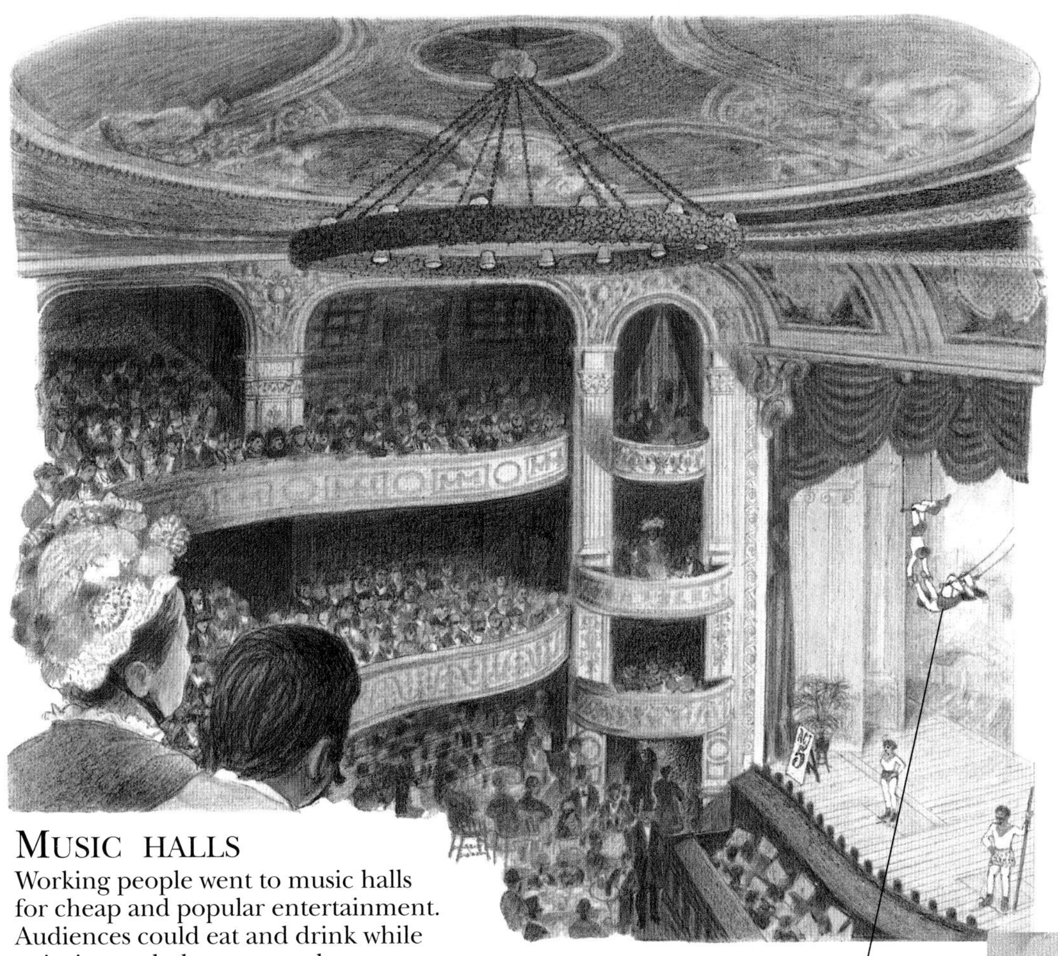

Music halls

Working people went to music halls for cheap and popular entertainment. Audiences could eat and drink while enjoying melodramas, acrobats, comedians, and singers. Sentimental songs were especially popular.

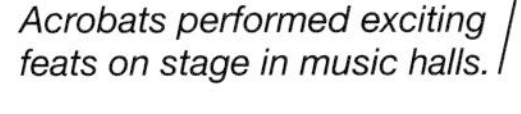

Acrobats performed exciting feats on stage in music halls.

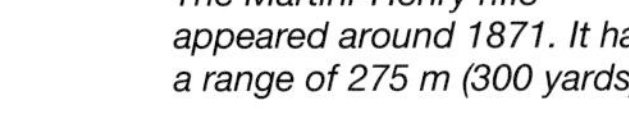

The Martini-Henry rifle appeared around 1871. It had a range of 275 m (300 yards).

The Gatling gun fired bullets at a rate of 1,000 rounds per minute.

Empire building

During Victoria's reign, there were dozens of small-scale wars as the various European nations carved out empires in Africa and Asia. The people who already lived in these places stood little chance against trained troops equipped with rifles and automatic guns.

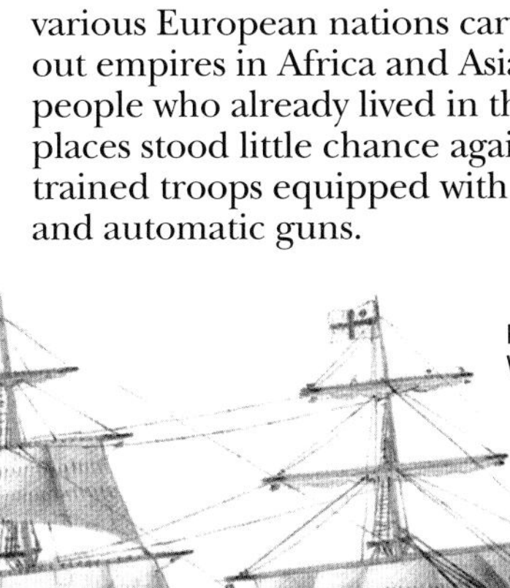

HMS Warrior

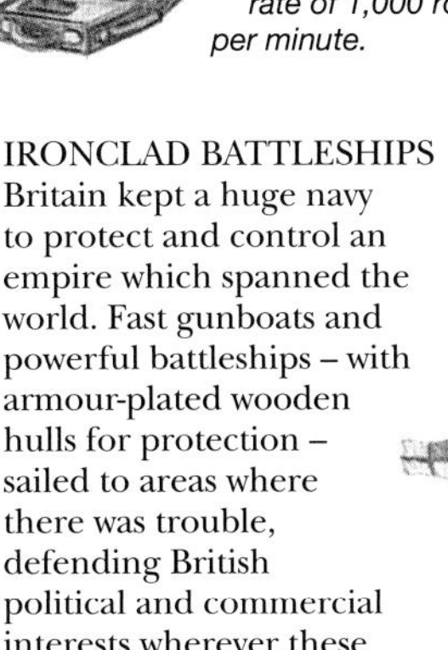

IRONCLAD BATTLESHIPS
Britain kept a huge navy to protect and control an empire which spanned the world. Fast gunboats and powerful battleships – with armour-plated wooden hulls for protection – sailed to areas where there was trouble, defending British political and commercial interests wherever these were threatened.

VICTORIANS

1837 Victoria becomes queen.

1842 Mines Act prevents women and children from working underground in mines.

1851 Great Exhibition held in London.

1863 First underground railway (the Metropolitan Line) opens, London.

1864 Factory Act bans children under eight years old from factory work.

1881 First electric street lighting is installed.

1884 Married Women's Property Act gives married women legal ownership of their property.

1891 Primary education in state schools made free.

1901 Queen Victoria dies.

SOCIAL REFORM
In Victorian times, a new industrial era resulted in a wealthy middle class. However, it also created a vast working class who often suffered terrible living and working conditions. Some boys worked as chimney sweeps in wealthy homes (above). Their plight was publicized by Charles Kingsley's novel *Water Babies*, and reformers such as Lord Shaftesbury campaigned for new labour laws.

Find out more

BRITISH EMPIRE
INDUSTRIAL REVOLUTION
TRANSPORT, HISTORY OF
UNITED KINGDOM, HISTORY OF

VIETNAM WAR

VIETNAM WAR

1859 France begins to colonize Vietnam.

1954 Vietnamese defeat French.

1956 Viet Cong lead rebellion against South Vietnamese government.

1961 United States sends advisers to train South Vietnamese army.

1964 Gulf of Tongkin clash between North Vietnamese and US naval craft leads to war.

1965 United States begins bombing of North; first US combat troops arrive in South.

1968 Tet (Vietnamese New Year) offensive by Viet Cong

1968 American troops massacre My Lai villagers.

1968 Antiwar protests in the US

1973 Cease-fire signed in Paris; American troops leave Vietnam.

1975 Vietnam reunited under Communist control.

BETWEEN 1956 AND 1975 Vietnam was the scene of one of the most destructive wars in modern history. In 1954, Vietnam defeated French colonial forces and was divided into two countries – a Communist North and a non-Communist South Vietnam. The Viet Cong (Vietnamese Communists) rebelled against the South Vietnamese government and, helped by North Vietnam under Ho Chi Minh, fought to reunite the country. This brought in the United States, which believed that if Vietnam fell to the Communists, nearby countries would fall too. During the 1960s the United States poured troops and money into Vietnam, but found itself in an undeclared war it could not win. Despite intensive bombing and the latest military technology, the Viet Cong were better equipped and trained for jungle warfare. Casualties in Vietnam were appalling, and strong opposition to the war developed in the United States. A cease-fire was negotiated, and in 1973 all American troops were withdrawn. Two years later North Vietnam captured Saigon, capital of South Vietnam, and Vietnam was united as a Communist country.

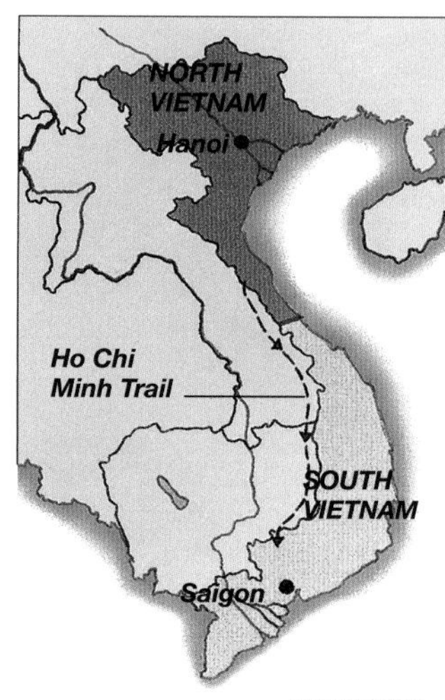

VIETNAM
Vietnam is in Southeast Asia. The war was fought in the jungles of South Vietnam and in the skies above North Vietnam. Viet Cong fighters received supplies from the North along the Ho Chi Minh trail. At the end of the war, the country was reunited with its capital at Hanoi. Saigon, the southern capital, was renamed Ho Chi Minh City.

TROOPS
The first American military personnel arrived in Vietnam during 1961 to advise the South Vietnamese government. By 1969 there were about 550,000 American troops in Vietnam.

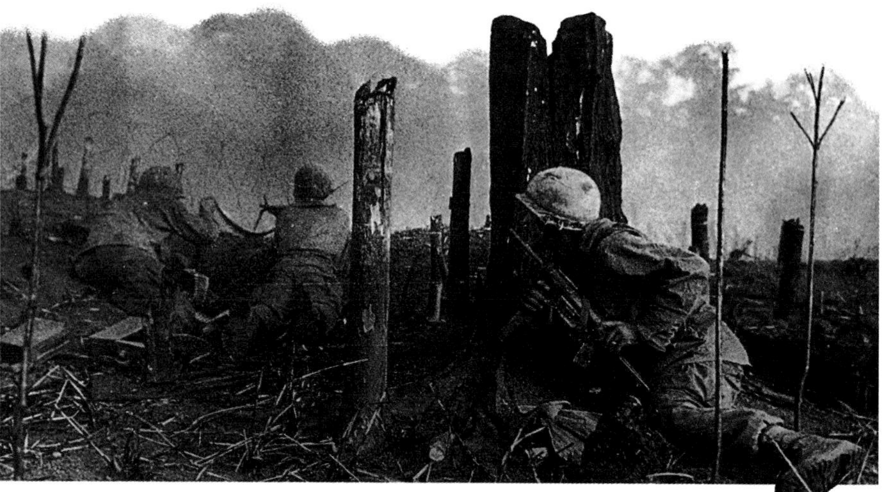

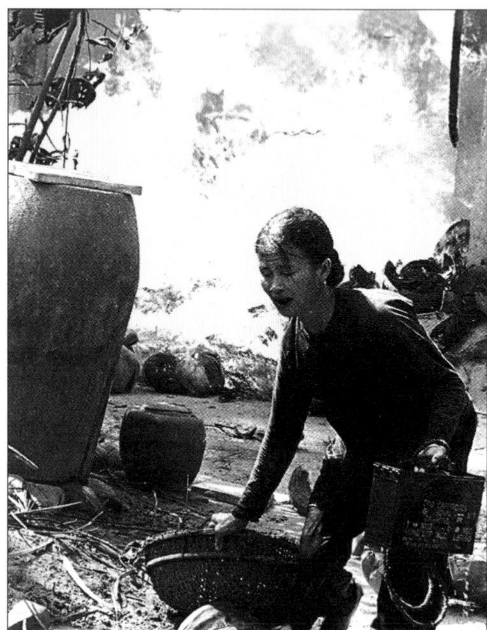

DESTRUCTION
The lengthy fighting had a terrible effect on the people of Vietnam. Their fields were destroyed, their forests stripped of leaves, and their houses blown up, leaving them refugees. Thousands were killed, injured, or maimed.

COSTS

It is unlikely that the exact cost of the Vietnam war will ever be known, but in terms of lives lost, money spent, and bombs dropped, it was enormous. Both sides suffered huge casualties and emerged with seriously damaged economies.

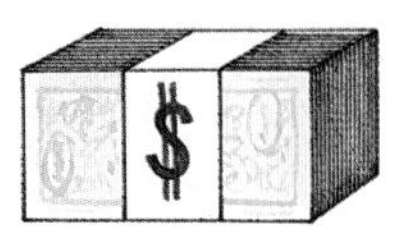

The United States spent $150 billion on the war; there are no figures for what North Vietnam spent.

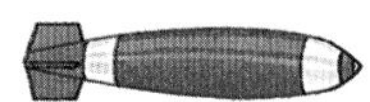

Four times as many bombs were dropped by the American Air Force on Vietnam than were dropped by British and American bombers on Germany during the whole of World War II.

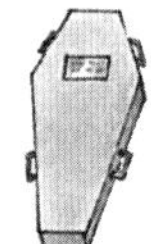

More than one million South Vietnamese and between 500,000 and one million North Vietnamese died in the war; over 58,000 American soldiers and nurses lost their lives.

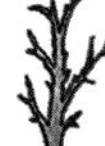

The US Air Force bombed the jungle with chemicals to strip the leaves off the trees. Much of Vietnam is still deforested today.

Find out more

SOUTHEAST ASIA, history of
UNITED STATES, HISTORY OF

VIKINGS

BETWEEN THE 8TH AND 12TH CENTURIES A.D., fierce warriors called Vikings terrorized the people of Europe. They came from Norway, Sweden, and Denmark, where the weather was cold and the soil was poor, to look for loot. At first they made lightning raids on coastal villages and isolated farms. They stole horses and food, captured prisoners for slaves, and robbed churches of their gold and silver. Later they conquered and settled in parts of England, France, Germany, Italy, and Russia. The Vikings were the finest shipbuilders of the time, and their swift, light boats could travel far from their homelands. They settled in Iceland and Greenland and were the first Europeans to reach North America. Although they are chiefly remembered for their conquests, most Nordic people lived peacefully in small settlements and worked as farmers, merchants, and craftsworkers.

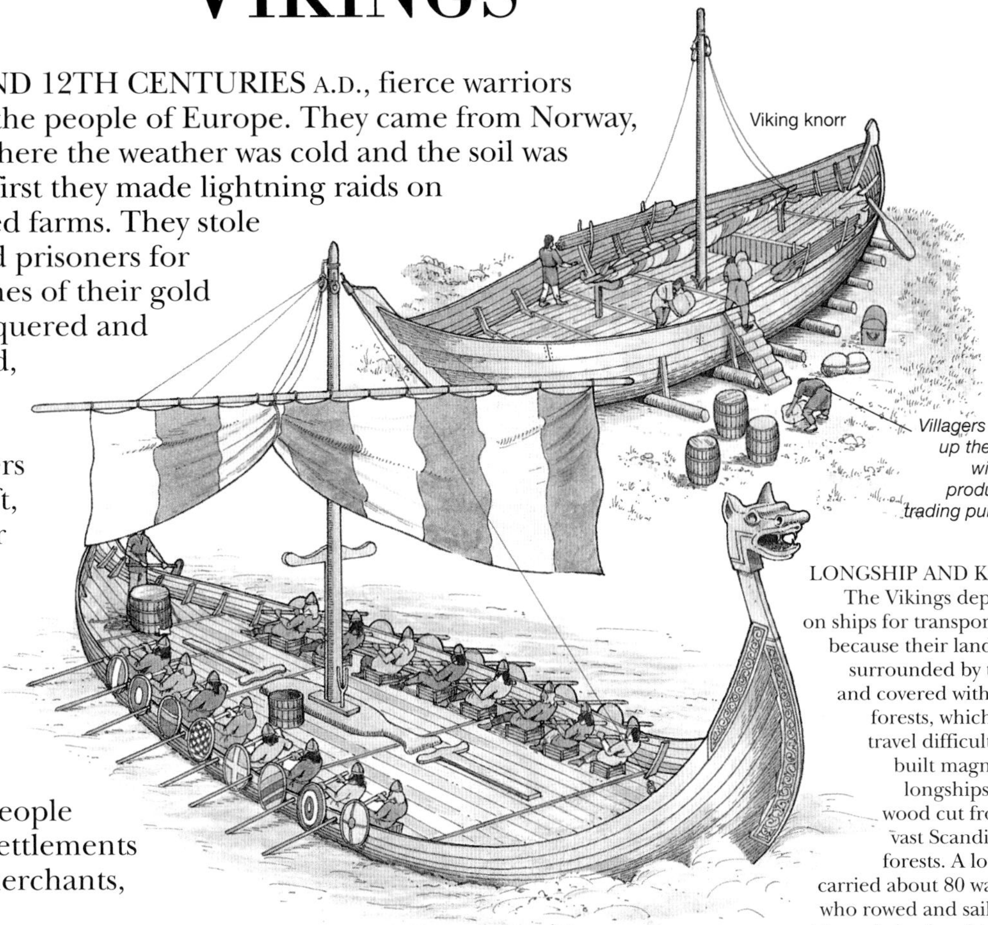

Viking knorr

Villagers loaded up the knorrs with farm produce, for trading purposes.

Viking longship

LONGSHIP AND KNORR
The Vikings depended on ships for transportation, because their lands were surrounded by the sea and covered with dense forests, which made travel difficult. They built magnificent longships out of wood cut from the vast Scandinavian forests. A longship carried about 80 warriors, who rowed and sailed the ship and also fought battles when they reached land. The Vikings also built smaller ships called knorrs, which they used for trading and transporting goods.

WARRIORS

Viking warriors usually fought with swords and battle axes, although some used spears, and bows and arrows. They carried wooden shields, and some wore armour made of layers of thick animal hides. Viking chieftains often wore metal helmets and chainmail armour.

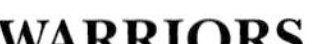

Swedish helmet (7th century)

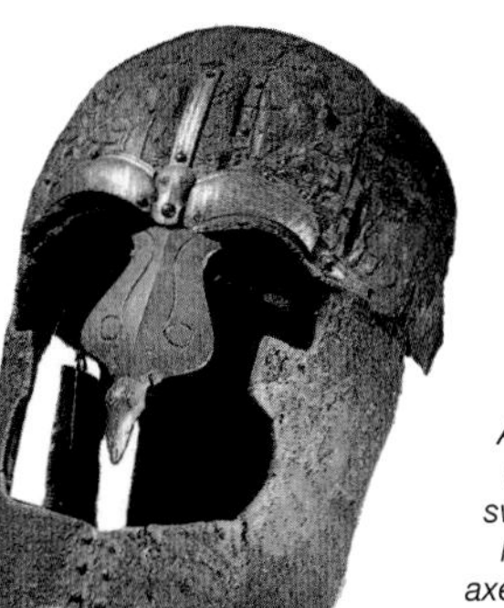

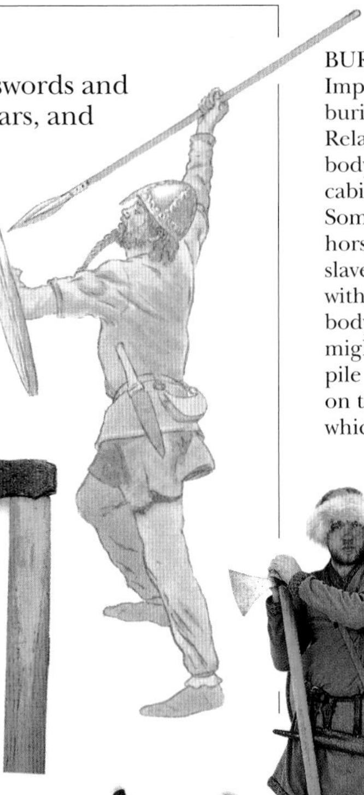

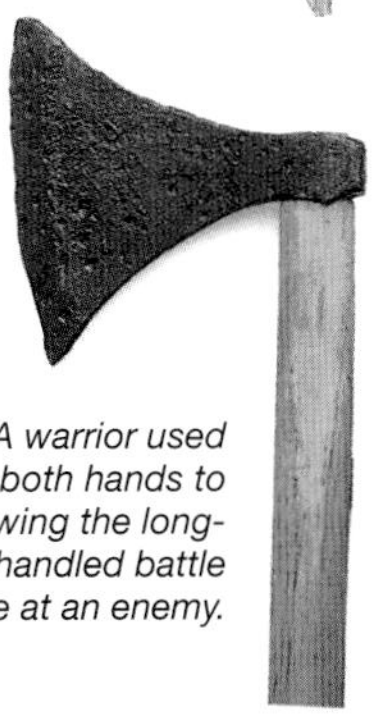

A warrior used both hands to swing the long-handled battle axe at an enemy.

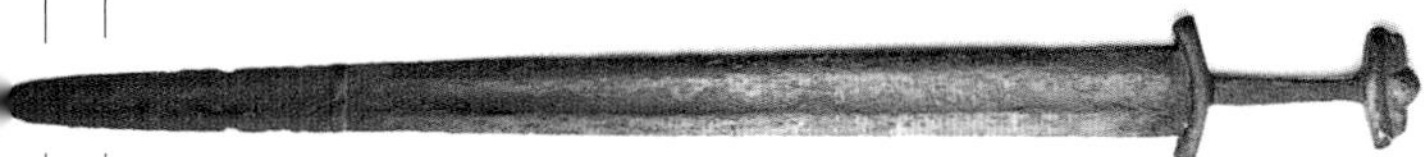

The sword was a Viking's most important weapon.

BURIALS
Important Vikings were buried with their ships. Relatives placed the body in a wooden cabin on the deck. Sometimes, dogs, horses, cattle, and slaves were buried with their owners. The body of a great warrior might be burned on a pile of wood or placed on the deck of a longship which was then set alight.

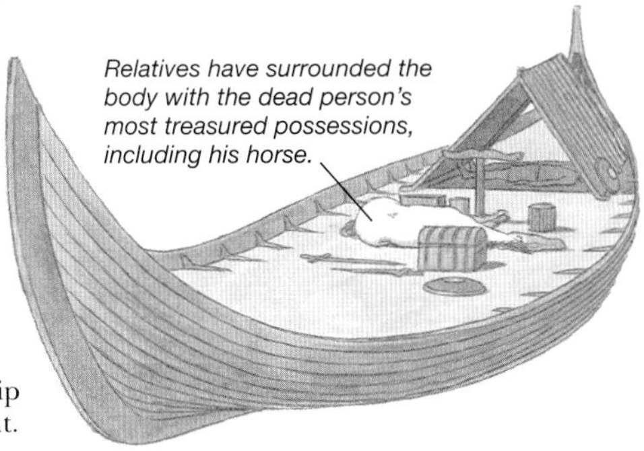

Relatives have surrounded the body with the dead person's most treasured possessions, including his horse.

VIKING FAMILIES

Some Vikings lived in bustling trading towns, such as York, England. But most lived in isolated farming settlements. Everything the family needed had to be made or grown on the farm. Viking women had more rights than many other European women of the time. For instance, they were allowed to get divorced if they wished.

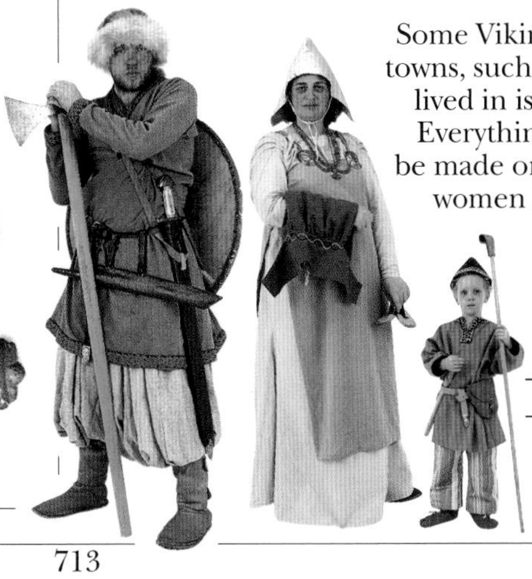

Find out more
NORMANS
SCANDINAVIA, HISTORY OF

VOLCANOES

LIVING IN THE SHADOW of a volcano can be a source of constant fear. An active volcano can erupt with little warning: smoke and hot ash billow from the crater at the volcano's summit, and red-hot lava flows down the slopes, setting fire to everything in its path. Volcanoes are caused by the movement of vast slabs of rock, called plates, in the Earth's surface. When the plates collide or spread apart, molten rock from deep underground is forced to the surface, at or near the place where the plates meet. There are about 850 active volcanoes in the world. Most lie in a belt called the Ring of Fire, which surrounds the Pacific Ocean. Volcanoes also occur in the ocean, where they form underwater mountains or islands, such as Hawaii.

Cloud of ash and gas pours out from crater.

Red-hot lava flows down side of volcano.

Earth's crust is formed of layers of different kinds of rock. Close to the centre of the Earth, the intense heat melts the rock.

Magma rises up the main pipe and branch pipes. If thick, slow-flowing lava blocks the main pipe, the volcano may explode.

Magma chamber forms deep underground.

Volcano builds up with layers of ash and solidified lava.

VOLCANIC ERUPTIONS

A volcano lies over a deep chamber of red-hot, molten rock, called magma. Pressure from hot gases forces the magma up to the surface. The molten rock, now called lava, melts a hole through the rock above and flows out. Layers of lava and volcanic ash cool and solidify, building up a cone-shaped mountain with a central pipe through which lava flows. Most volcanoes do not erupt continuously. Between eruptions, active volcanoes are called dormant. Extinct volcanoes are those that are no longer active.

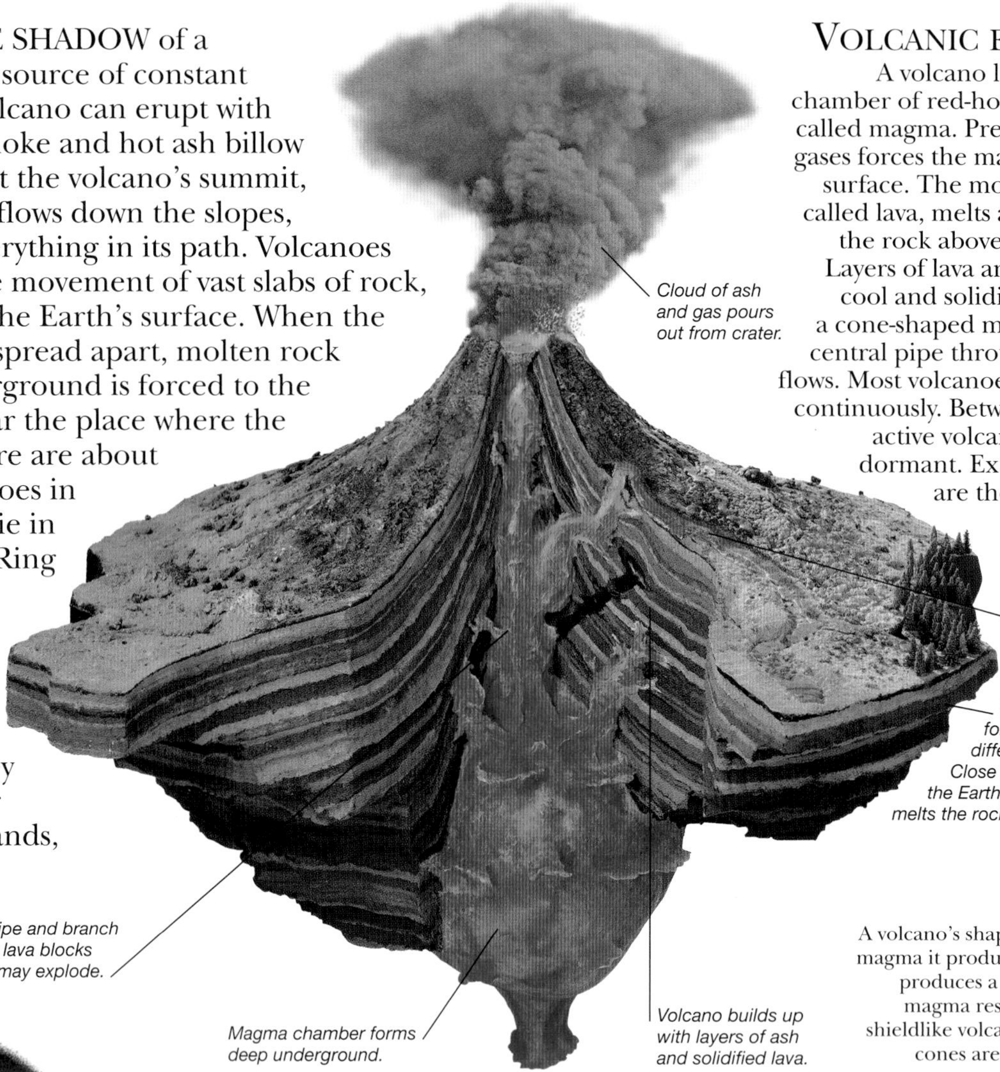

MAGMA

A volcano's shape depends on the magma it produces. Thick magma produces a steep cone; runny magma results in a flattened, shieldlike volcano. Some volcano cones are made only of ash.

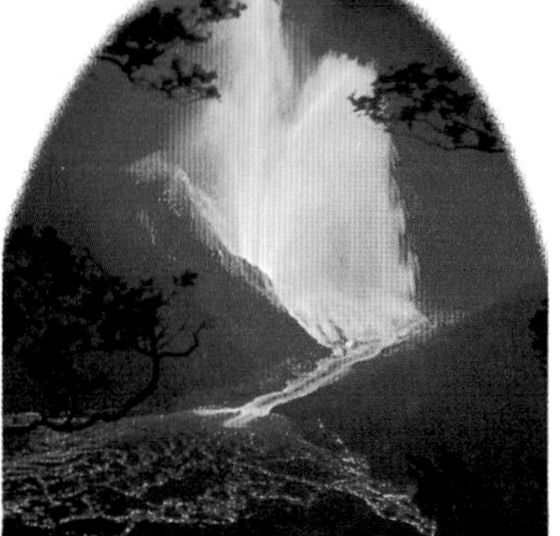

LAVA

Molten rock which has escaped to the Earth's surface is called lava. A bubbling lake of molten rock fills the crater of the volcano, and fountains of fiery lava leap high into the air. Glowing streams of lava pour out of the crater and flow down the sides of the volcano like rivers of fire. The lava has a temperature of about 1,100°C (2,000°F), which is hot enough to melt steel.

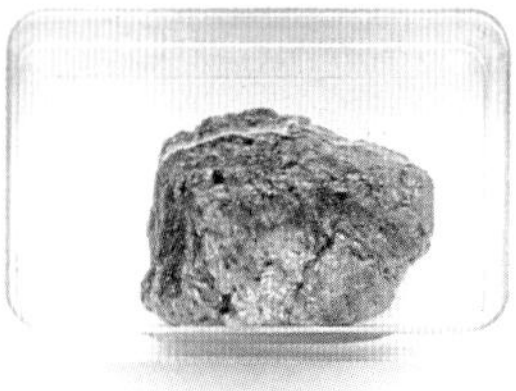

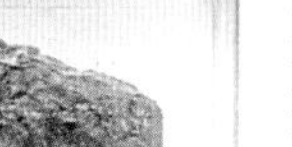

PUMICE

Lava containing bubbles of gas hardens to form a rock called pumice, which is peppered with tiny holes. The holes make pumice very light; it is the only rock that can float in water.

POMPEII

In A.D. 79, Mount Vesuvius in Italy erupted, burying the Roman city of Pompeii and its inhabitants in a deep layer of hot ash. Archaeologists have now uncovered Pompeii, much of which is well preserved. The bodies of victims left hollows in the ash; the plaster cast below is made from such a hollow and shows the last moments of one victim. Vesuvius last erupted in 1944. It could erupt again at any time. One of the greatest of all volcanic disasters occurred when the island of Krakatoa, Indonesia, exploded in 1883.

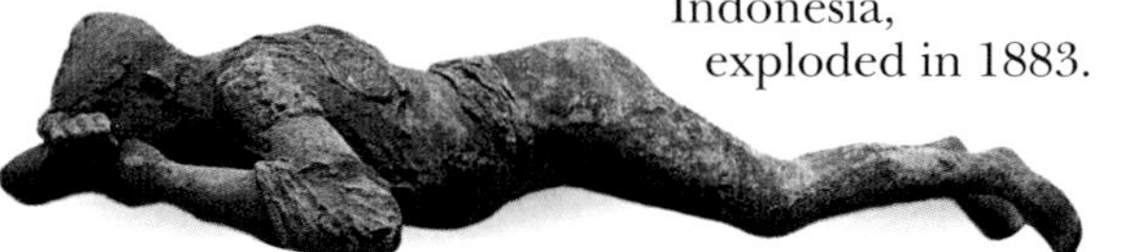

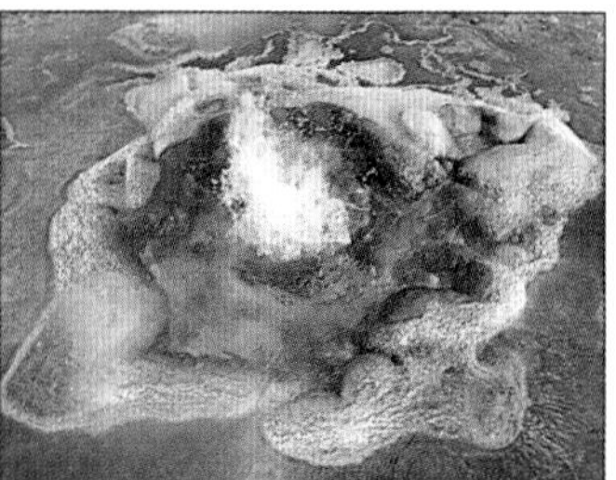

GEYSERS

A jet of boiling water which suddenly shoots up from the ground is called a geyser. Hot rock deep below the surface heats water in an underground chamber so that it boils. Steam forces the water out in a jet. When the chamber refills and heats up, the geyser blows again.

Find out more

CONTINENTS
EARTHQUAKES
GEOLOGY
MOUNTAINS
ROCKS AND MINERALS

WALES

WELSH DRAGON
The Welsh flag carries a red dragon, the national symbol of Wales.

FROM THE WILDS OF ITS NORTHERN mountains to the industrial valleys of the south, Wales covers an area of 20,761 sq km (8,014 sq miles). It has a population of 2.9 million and is the smallest country in the United Kingdom. Wales has been under English control since the late 13th century, although in 1999 a Welsh Assembly was introduced, giving Wales limited self-government. Until recently, coal mining was a major industry, particularly in the south, but by the 1990s most mines had closed, causing widespread unemployment. Sheep and cattle farming have remained economically important. Wales has a strong national identity, with its own language and a long tradition of music and song. Welsh choirs are famous worldwide.

Wales lies on a peninsula (land jutting into the sea) in the western British Isles. It is bordered by England on its eastern border and the Irish Sea to the west.

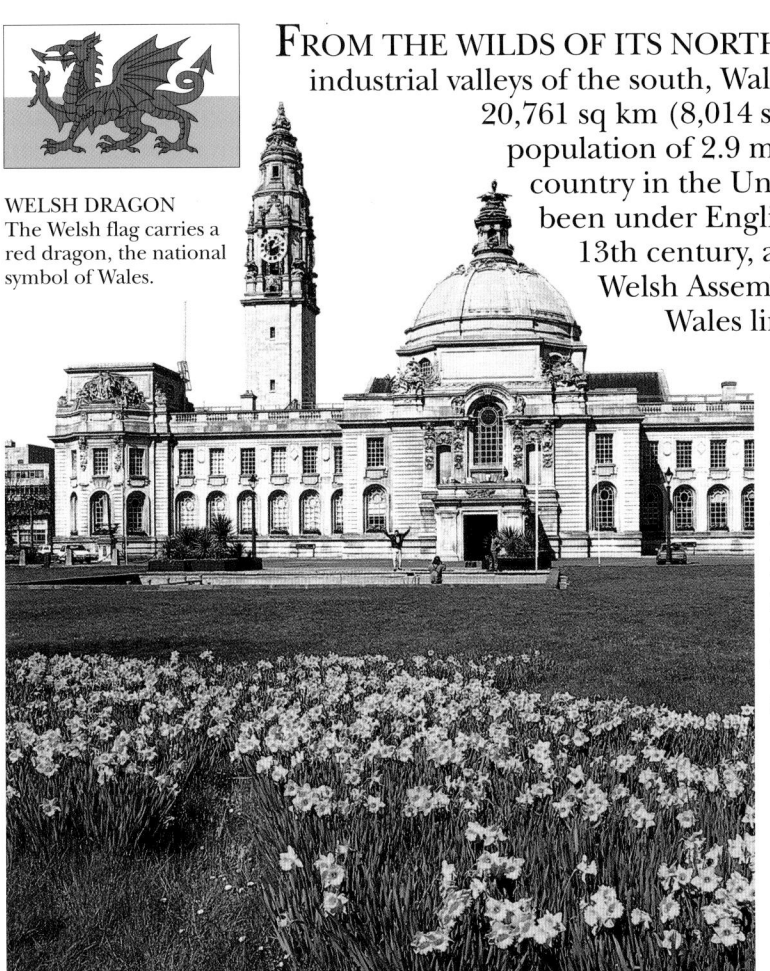

CARDIFF

Located on the south coast of Wales, Cardiff is the country's capital and the largest city. It is also the headquarters of the new Welsh Assembly. For many years Cardiff was a major port, exporting coal from the valleys in the south. The port has declined, but the city is still an administrative and business centre.

WELSH COUNTRYSIDE
Much of Wales is extremely beautiful, particularly around St. David's Bay on the Pembrokeshire coast in the west. Welsh landscape is varied. Snowdonia, in the north of the country, has spectacular mountain scenery, and is a national park. Green hills cover mid-Wales.The southeast is industrial.

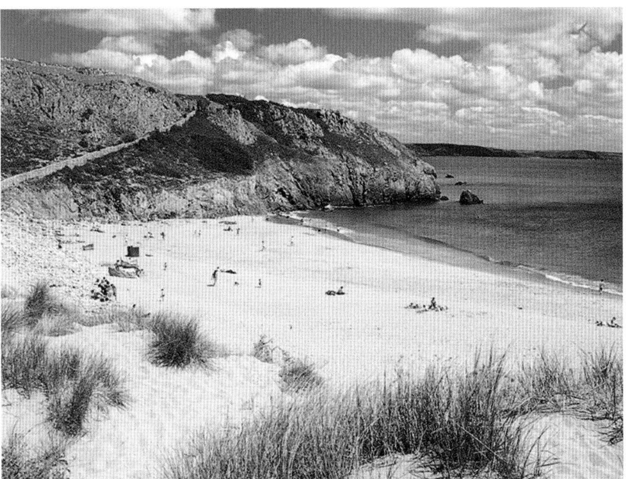

PRINCE OF WALES
Edward I of England conquered Wales in 1284, but told the Welsh he would find them a prince who had never spoken English. He then held up his baby son as Prince of Wales at Caernarfon (Caernarvon) Castle. The title passes to the heir to the British throne. Today, Prince Charles is the Prince of Wales.

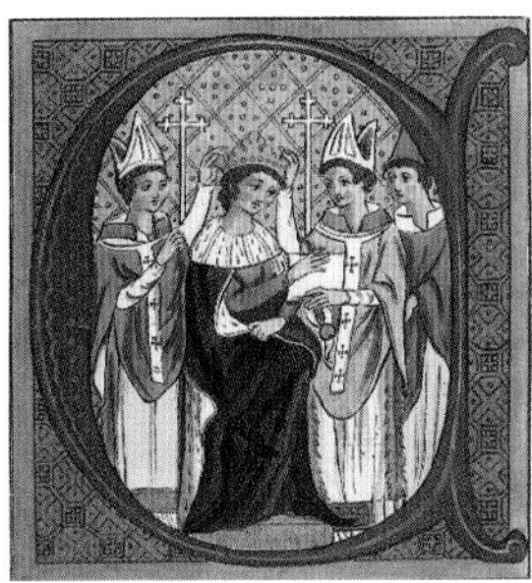

RUGBY
The national sport of Wales is Rugby Union. The game plays an important part in daily life and Welsh teams play at national and international level. The Millennium Stadium in Cardiff is the world's finest.

Neil Jenkins, Welsh rugby star

KEEP WALES TIDY
PLEASE TAKE YOUR LITTER HOME
EWCH Â'CH SBWRIEL GYDA CHI
CADWCH GYMRU'N DACLUS
MAX PENALTY £1000 COSB UCHAF

WELSH LANGUAGE
Wales is bilingual, that is two languages – Welsh and English – are officially recognized. Road signs are in Welsh and English, and many people in the north speak Welsh as a first language. Teaching Welsh in schools has revived interest in traditional Welsh culture. Poets, speakers, and choirs compete at traditional festivals called *eisteddfods*.

Find out more
FOOTBALL AND RUGBY
UNITED KINGDOM
UNITED KINGDOM, HISTORY OF

WARSHIPS

IN A MODERN NAVY, there are several different types of warships, each designed to carry out a special function. The largest warship is the aircraft carrier, which is like a floating runway about 300 m (more than 1,000 ft) long that acts as a base for up to 100 aircraft. Battleships are heavily armoured warships equipped with powerful guns that can fire shells over distances of about 30 km (20 miles). Other warships include destroyers for protecting fleets of ships; frigates, which are usually armed with missiles; mine-sweepers for clearing mines; and small coastal protection vessels. The role of the warship has changed with the invention of nuclear arms. One of its most important functions is the ability to locate and attack missile-carrying submarines. Thus, warships increasingly rely on advanced electronic equipment to detect their targets, and are armed with an array of guided missiles and guns.

FRIGATE

A frigate is a light, fast, medium-sized warship, which is particularly useful for escorting other ships. Frigates carry equipment for seeking submarines, anti-ship missiles for defence against other warships, and an array of anti-aircraft weapons.

Cross-section of British-built Type 22 frigate

Anti-aircraft missiles

Radar for detecting enemy aircraft

Main living quarters for crew of about 250

Captain commands the ship from the bridge.

Ship's helicopter, used for reconnaissance (scouting), transport, rescue work, and anti-submarine warfare

Anti-aircraft missiles with a range of about 5 km (3 miles)

Hull made of aluminium, which is lighter than steel and makes the frigate faster and more manoeuvrable

Twin gas-turbine engines capable of producing a top speed of 55 km/h (35 mph) with a range of about 8,300 km (5,200 miles)

Control room, from where all weapons are fired and guided

Anti-ship missiles, for use against enemy warships up to 32 km (20 miles) away

The first modern battleship was the British Navy Dreadnought, *which was introduced in 1906. The* Dreadnought *was armed with heavy guns and protected by thick steel armour.*

MODERN WARSHIPS

Many warships now carry missiles as well as guns. Warships have various types of missile. Some are used as a defence against aircraft. Other types of missile can attack enemy warships, which may be so distant that they are visible only on a radar screen.

HISTORY OF WARSHIPS

The first true warships were the galleys of Ancient Greece and Rome which used oars and sails for propulsion. Major leaps forward came with the invention of the cannon, steam power, and the use of steel in shipbuilding. During World War I (1914-18) and World War II (1939-45) warships developed into huge, heavily armed battleships, the forerunners of today's warship.

The heavily armed galleon was developed by the Spanish in the early 15th century and used in their voyages of conquest in the Americas and Asia.

During the 9th century, Viking warriors used longships to travel from their homelands in Scandinavia to conquer countries of northern Europe.

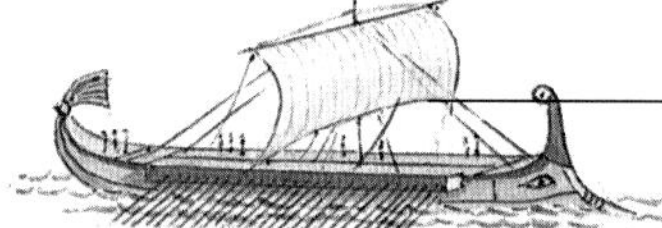

The trireme, or Roman galley, of 200 B.C. had three banks of oars. The pointed beak at the prow (front) of the ship allowed it to ram enemy vessels.

Find out more

NAVIES
ROCKETS AND MISSILES
SUBMARINES
WEAPONS
WORLD WAR I
WORLD WAR II

GEORGE
WASHINGTON

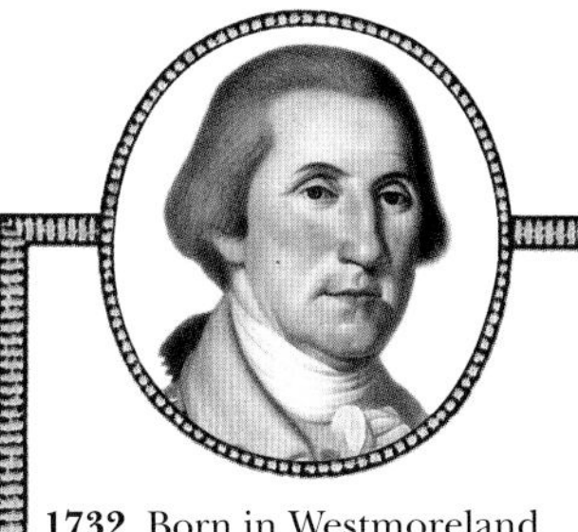

1732 Born in Westmoreland, Virginia.

1759-74 Member of the Virginia parliament

1775-81 Leads Continental forces in the Revolution.

1787 Helps draft the Constitution of the United States of America.

1789 Chosen as first president of the United States.

1793 Elected to second term as president.

1797 Retires as president.

1799 Dies at Mount Vernon.

"THE FATHER OF HIS COUNTRY" was a nickname that George Washington earned many times over. First, he led the American forces to victory against the British in the Revolution, then he served the American people again as the first president of the United States. As a military leader, he was capable and strong-willed. Even when the British seemed set to win the war, Washington did not give up hope and continued to encourage the American troops. As president, he was an energetic leader who used his prestige to unite the new nation. Yet, despite his many personal strengths, Washington was an unlikely figure to lead a revolution. He was born into a wealthy family and trained as a surveyor before serving in the local militia. He could have had a brilliant military career, but at the age of 27 he returned to farming in Virginia. He did the same at the end of the Revolution, and only went back to national politics in 1787 because he felt the country needed his help once more.

VICTORY AT TRENTON

On Christmas night, 1776, George Washington led his troops across the icy Delaware River and attacked the British in Trenton, New Jersey, before they had time to prepare themselves for battle. The surprise attack did much to increase American morale at the start of the Revolution.

Troops had to break the ice in order to make their way across the river.

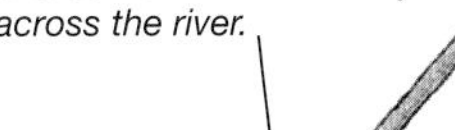

CONTINENTAL CONGRESS

In 1774, the 13 British colonies in North America set up a Continental Congress to protest against unfair British rule. George Washington was one of the delegates from Virginia. Although the Congress favoured reaching an agreement with Britain, fighting broke out between the two sides in 1775. The Congress raised an army under Washington and on 4 July 1776, issued the Declaration of Independence. Peace was declared in 1781 and the Congress became the national government of the newly formed United States of America. In 1789 it was abolished and a new government structure was established.

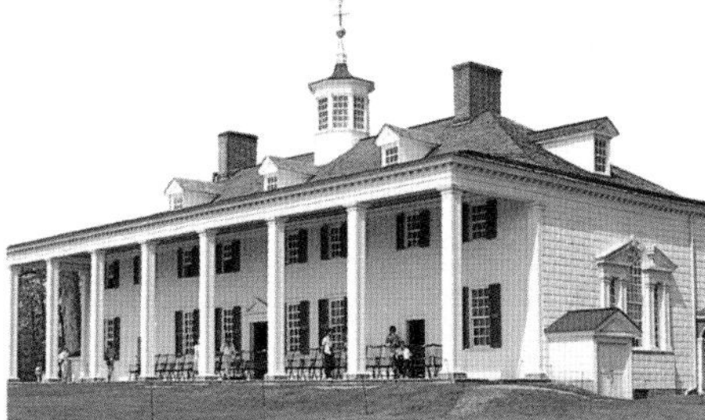

MOUNT VERNON
Built in 1743, Mount Vernon was the home of George Washington for more than 50 years. The wooden house overlooks the Potomac River near Alexandria, Virginia, and is now a museum dedicated to Washington.

Find out more

AMERICAN REVOLUTION
UNITED STATES OF AMERICA, history of

WATER

WE ARE SURROUNDED by water. More than 70 per cent of the Earth's surface is covered by vast oceans and seas. In addition, 10 per cent of the land – an area the size of South America – is covered by water in the form of ice. However, little new water is ever made on Earth. The rain that falls from the sky has fallen billions of times before, and will fall billions of times again. It runs down the land to the sea, evaporates (changes into vapour) into the clouds, and falls again as rain in an endless cycle. Water has a huge effect on our planet and its inhabitants. All plants and animals need water to survive; life itself began in the Earth's prehistoric seas. Seas and rivers shape the land over thousands of years, cutting cliffs and canyons; icy glaciers dig out huge valleys. Water is also essential to people in homes and factories and on farms.

The force of surface tension holds water molecules together so that they form small, roughly spherical drops.

SURFACE TENSION
The surface of water seems to be like an elastic skin. You can see this if you watch tiny insects such as water striders walking on water – their feet make hollows in the surface of the water, but the insects do not sink. This "skin" effect is called surface tension. It is caused by the attraction of water molecules to each other. Surface tension has another important effect: it causes water to form drops.

Molecules at the surface have other molecules pulling on them only from below. This means there is a force pulling on this top layer of molecules, keeping them under tension like a stretched elastic band.

In the body of the liquid, each water molecule is surrounded by others, so the forces on them balance out.

WATER FOR LIFE
All plants and animals, including humans, are made largely of water and depend on water for life. For instance, more than two thirds of the human body is water. To replace water lost by urinating, sweating, and breathing, we must drink water every day to stay healthy. No one can survive more than four days without water.

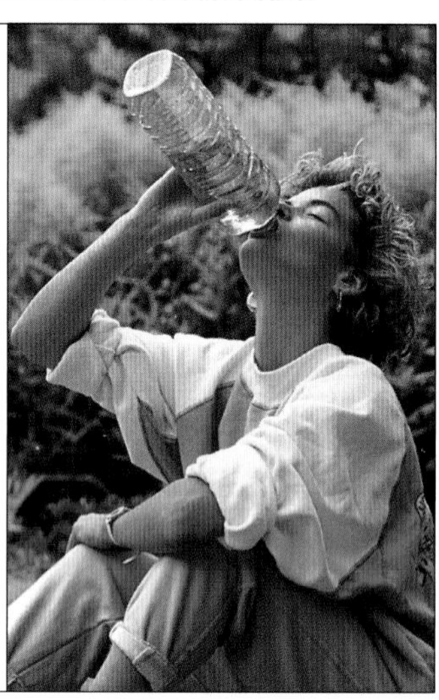

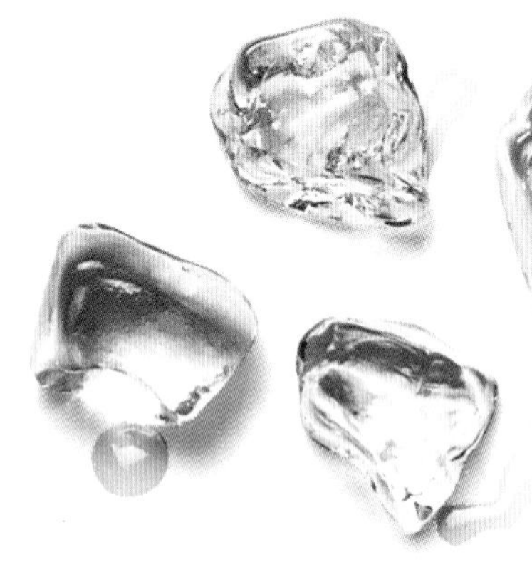

ICE
Water freezes when the temperature drops below 0°C (32°F). Water expands, or takes up more space, as it freezes. Water pipes sometimes burst in very cold winters as the water inside freezes and expands.

STATES OF WATER

Pure water is a compound of two common elements, hydrogen and oxygen. In each water molecule there are two hydrogen atoms and one oxygen atom; scientists represent this by writing H_2O. Water is usually in a liquid state, but it can also be a solid or a gas. If left standing, water slowly evaporates and turns into water vapour, an invisible gas. When water is cooled down enough, it freezes solid and turns to ice.

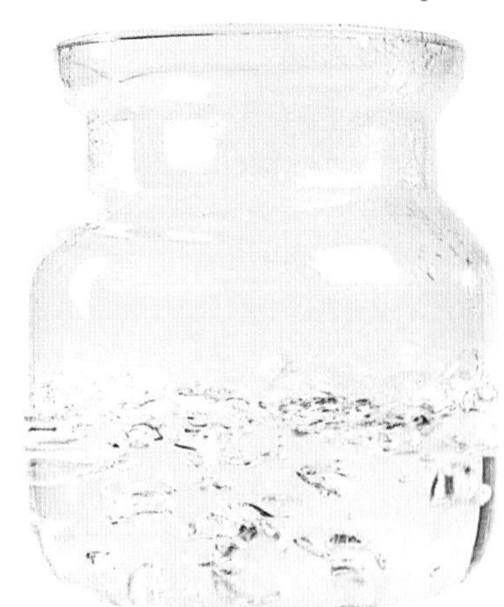

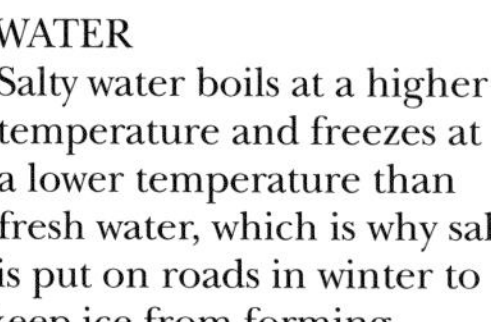

WATER
Salty water boils at a higher temperature and freezes at a lower temperature than fresh water, which is why salt is put on roads in winter to keep ice from forming.

WATER VAPOUR
Water boils at 100°C (212°F). At this temperature it evaporates so rapidly that water vapour forms bubbles in the liquid. Water vapour is invisible; visible clouds of steam are not water vapour but are tiny droplets of water formed when the hot vapour hits cold air.

Water tank stores clean water.

Water falls as rain and is collected in lakes and artificial reservoirs.

Water is cleaned in a treatment plant.

Once the water is treated, it is pumped up into a high tank, ready to be used.

With the water high above the ground, the tap can be opened and the water runs out.

WATER TREATMENT

Water in a reservoir is usually not fit to drink. It must pass through a treatment centre which removes germs and other harmful substances. Chlorine gas is often dissolved into the water to kill bacteria and viruses. In addition, the water is stored in huge basins so that pieces of dirt sink to the bottom; filters made of stones and sand remove any remaining particles.

Water can provide an unlimited supply of power, unlike the underground resources such as coal and gas.

SOLUTIONS

Pure water is rarely found in nature because water dissolves other substances to form mixtures called solutions. For example, sea water is salty because there are many minerals dissolved in it. Water solutions are vital to life; blood plasma, for instance, is a water solution.

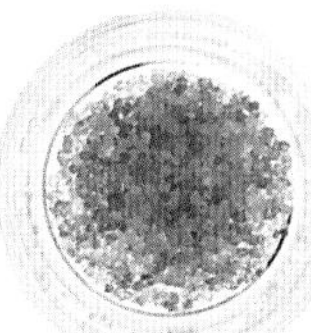

Sugar dissolves in water, making a sweet-tasting sugar solution.

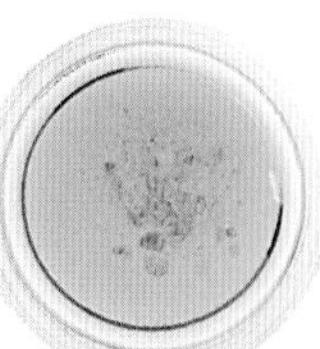

The sugar disappears when it is completely dissolved.

HYDROELECTRIC POWER

People have used water as a source of power for more than 2,000 years. Today, water is used to produce electricity in hydroelectric (water-driven) power stations. Hydroelectric power stations are often built inside dams. Water from a huge lake behind the dam flows down pipes. The moving water spins turbines which drive generators and produce electricity. Hydroelectric power produces electricity without causing pollution or using scarce resources.

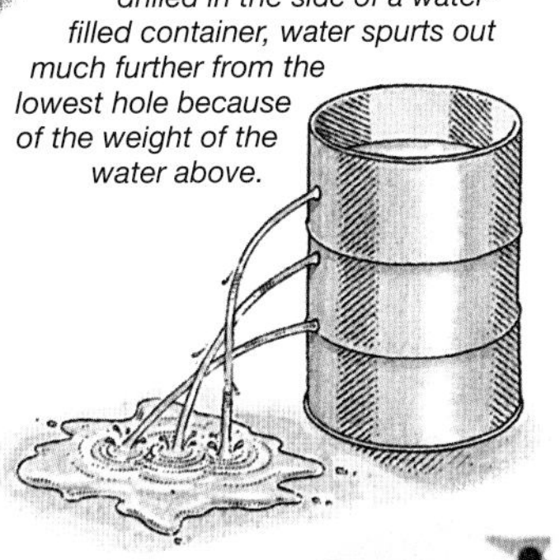

If three identical holes are drilled in the side of a water-filled container, water spurts out much further from the lowest hole because of the weight of the water above.

WATER PRESSURE

Water rushes out of a tap because it is under pressure; that is, it is pushed from behind. Pressure is produced by pumps that force water along using pistons or blades like those on a ship's propeller. Water pressure is also created by the sheer weight of water above. The deeper the water, the greater the pressure. If you dive into a pool, you can feel the water pressure pushing on your eardrums.

POLLUTION AND DROUGHT

In many places, such as East Africa, there is insufficient rain and constant drought. Plants cannot grow, and people and animals must fight a constant battle for survival. Fresh, clean water can also be difficult to obtain even in places with lots of rain. This is because waste from cities and factories pollutes the water, making it unsafe to drink.

Fire fighters connect their hoses to fire engines which contain powerful pumps. The pumps increase the pressure so that the water can reach flames high up in buildings.

Deep underground water stores exist below the surface of the Earth. After a drought, these stores dry out; it may take years for them to be refilled.

Find out more

ELECTRICITY
HEAT
LAKES
OCEANS AND SEAS
RAIN AND SNOW
RIVERS

WATER SPORTS

SPLASHING AROUND IN WATER – whether swimming, diving, surfing, or just floating on your back – is one of the most enjoyable ways of relaxing and keeping fit. Water sports are fun for people of all ages: even babies can learn to swim. And for the elderly or the physically handicapped, swimming provides a gentle yet vigorous way to exercise. Swimming became popular for fitness and recreation with ancient peoples in Egypt, Greece, and then Rome. Swimming races began in the 19th century and were included in the first Olympics, in 1896. Like swimming, surfing and water-skiing take place on the surface of the water. Scuba divers, however, dive deep below the waves. They can stay under water for an hour or more by breathing air from cylinders on their backs. Snorkellers swim to a depth of about 9 m (30 ft) with just a face mask, flippers, and a snorkel, or breathing tube.

Diver twists in mid-air

Straightening out as he descends

The body should enter the water straight, with legs, arms, and hands extended.

DIVING

In diving competitions, judges award points for technique as each competitor performs a series of dives. More difficult dives win higher points. Divers leap from a platform at 10 m (33 ft) above the water, and from a springboard at 3 m (10 ft).

There are three types of competitive water-skiing: slalom, jumping, and trick-skiing.

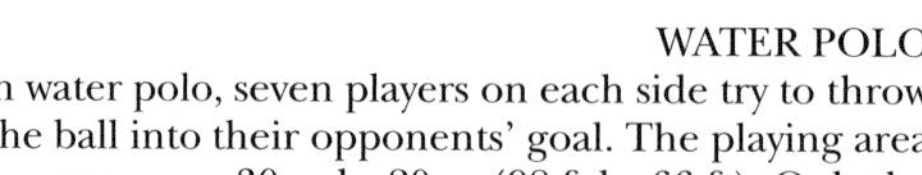

WATER POLO

In water polo, seven players on each side try to throw the ball into their opponents' goal. The playing area measures 30 m by 20 m (98 ft by 66 ft). Only the goalkeeper may hold the ball with both hands.

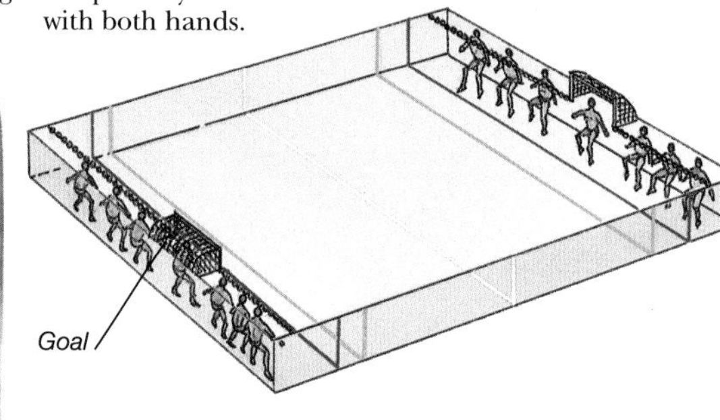

WATER-SKIING

A fast powerboat tows water-skiers along at the end of a rope. Skiers can cross from side to side behind the boat, and can jump through the air by skiing up a ramp in the water.

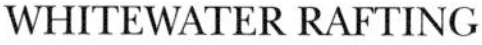

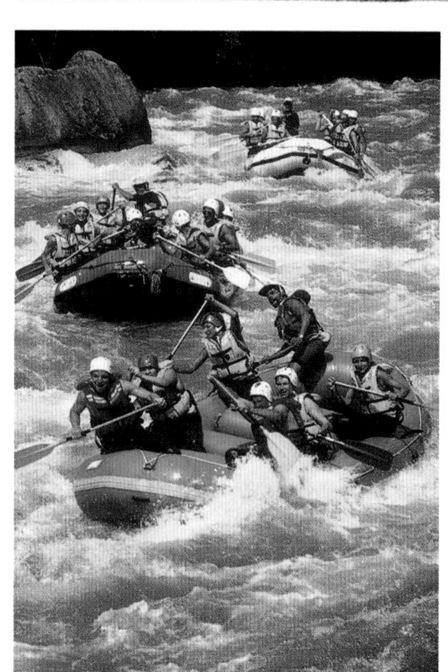

WHITEWATER RAFTING

Rowing in turbulent waters (or rapids) is a dangerous and thrilling sport because it takes extraordinary skill and agility to go over the water without tipping over. It has taken its name from the white foam that tips the waves of fast-flowing water. Whitewater rafts have to be light in order to stay afloat and navigate between rocks and sharp turns in the river, and are therefore made of inflated rubber.

WINDSURFING

Windsurfing, or sailboarding, began as a leisure activity in the 1960s and became a competitive Olympic event in 1984. The windsurfer balances the craft by holding on to a boom fixed around the sail. A daggerboard, or fin, on the underside of the board keeps the board upright in the water. There are several kinds of competition in the sport. These include racing around buoys, slalom races, and performing tricks that require great balance.

Sail by which the board is steered

Surfer balances the craft.

Board on which surfer stands

Find out more

SAILING AND BOATING
SPORTS
SWIMMING
UNDERWATER EXPLORATION

WEAPONS

PREHISTORIC HUNTERS LEARNED that they could kill their prey more quickly and safely with a stone knife than with their bare hands. This crude weapon later became refined into the dagger and the sword. Both are members of a group of weapons we now call side arms. However, an even less dangerous way to hunt was to use missile weapons. By throwing rocks or spears, early hunters could disable wild beasts and human enemies alike from a distance of 10 paces or more. Simple changes to a missile weapon made it much more effective: with slingshots or bows and arrows, hunters could hit smaller, more distant targets. Since these early times, better technology has greatly increased the range and accuracy of weapons. Seven centuries ago the invention of gunpowder made possible much more powerful weapons. Gunpowder launched bullets and cannonballs much faster than an arrow could fly. Muskets and cannons were thus more deadly than bows, and quickly came to dominate the battlefield. Modern developments have increased both power and range still farther. Today, nuclear weapons can destroy in seconds a whole city on the other side of the world.

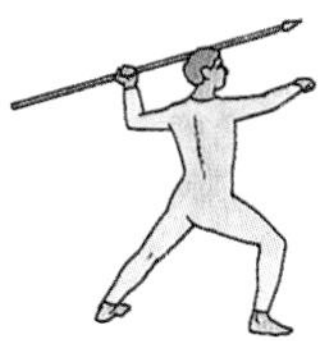
Spears could be thrown or used for stabbing.

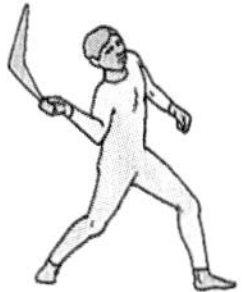
Boomerangs return to the thrower if they miss their target.

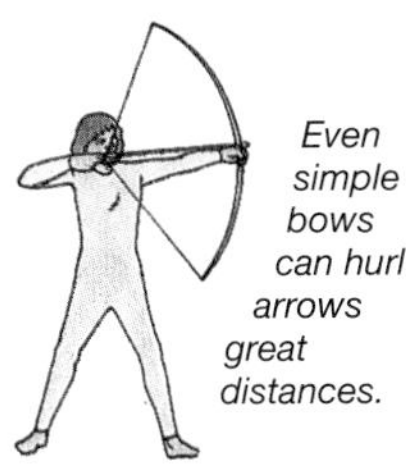
Even simple bows can hurl arrows great distances.

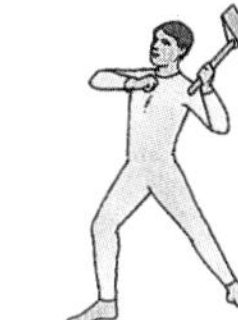
Some fighting axes were made to be thrown.

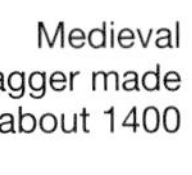
Medieval dagger made about 1400

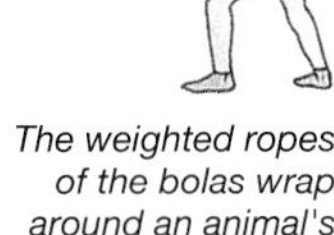
The weighted ropes of the bolas wrap around an animal's legs and trip it up.

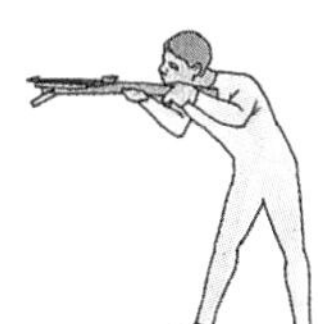
Powerful crossbows were even more deadly and accurate than simple bows.

SWORDS

Armed with swords, warriors could inflict injuries at a greater distance than with daggers or knives. The earliest swords were made in about 1500 B.C., when bronze working first developed. Later swords were made of iron and steel. Many different types evolved. Some were for thrusting, others for cutting. Today pistols have replaced swords in close combat, but the sword still has a role to play. It is used as a symbol of power in military ceremonies, in courts of law, and in governments.

SAMURAI DAGGER
Very high-quality steel was used for Samurai weapons such as this dagger. It took craftsworkers many hours to produce them.

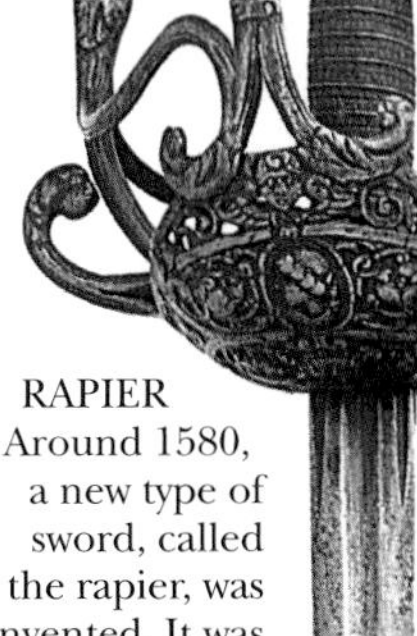
RAPIER
Around 1580, a new type of sword, called the rapier, was invented. It was long and thin and was used for thrusting.

BRONZE AGE SWORD
Shaping the sword so that it was wider near the end of the blade made it more effective as a slashing weapon. The handle of this Bronze Age sword would have been wrapped in leather for comfort.

SAMURAI WARRIORS

Swordfighting and archery were the two most important skills of the Samurai warriors of Japan. These warriors first appeared in the 12th century as private armies of landowners. They became very powerful, and the shogun, head of all the Samurai warlords, controlled Japan for the next seven centuries.

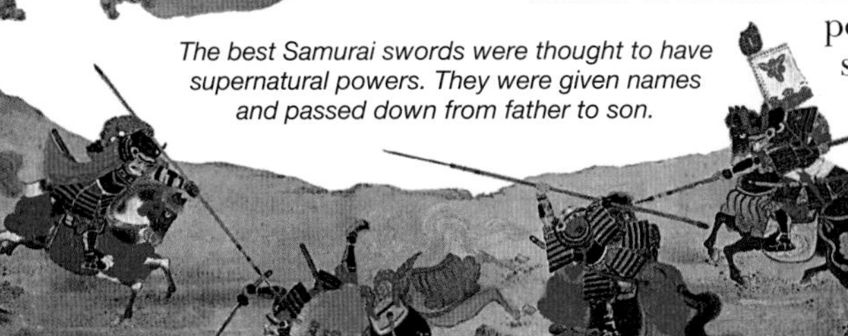
The best Samurai swords were thought to have supernatural powers. They were given names and passed down from father to son.

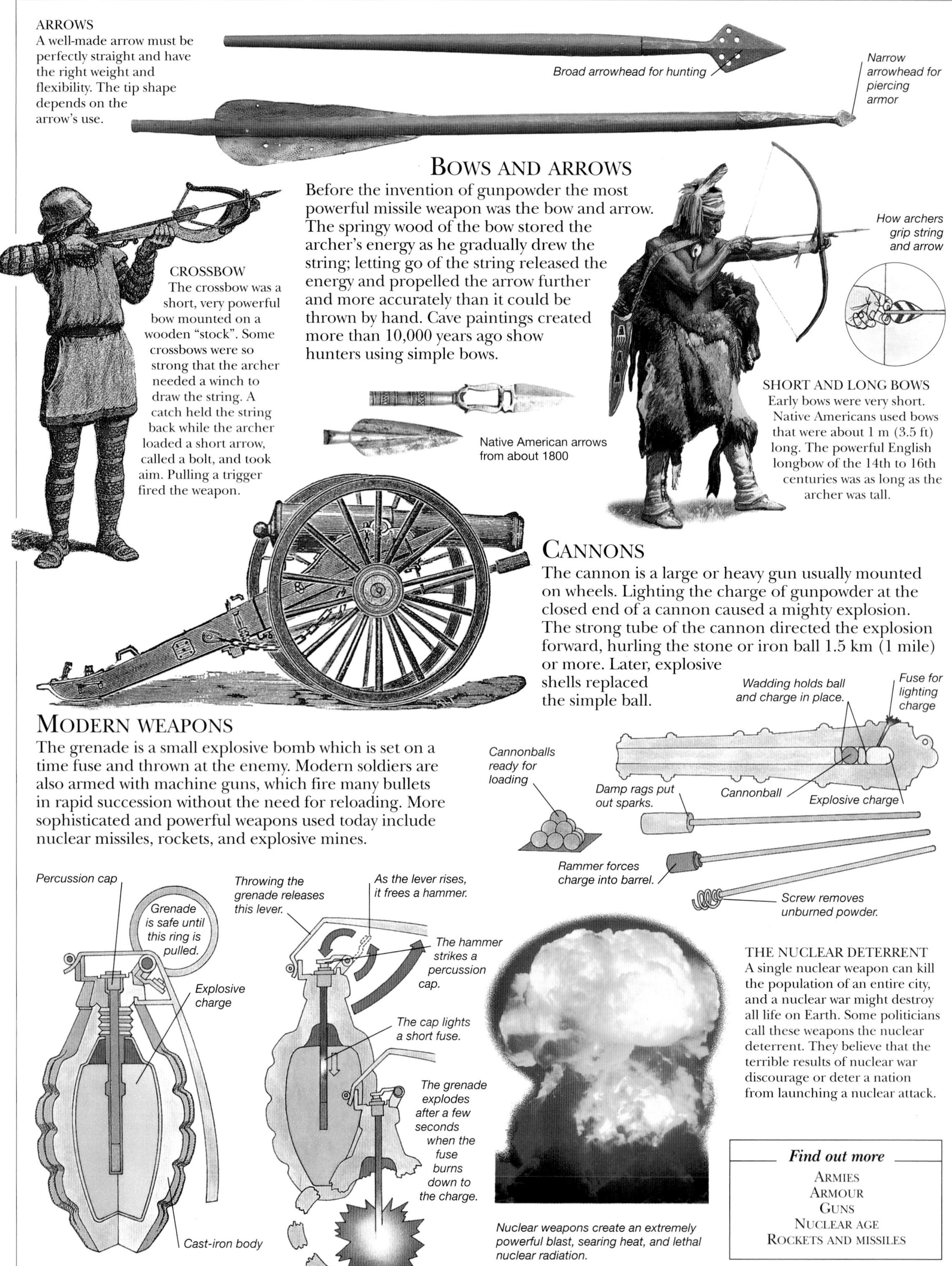
Broad arrowhead for hunting
Narrow arrowhead for piercing armor
How archers grip string and arrow
Native American arrows from about 1800
Wadding holds ball and charge in place.
Fuse for lighting charge
Cannonballs ready for loading
Damp rags put out sparks.
Cannonball
Explosive charge
Rammer forces charge into barrel.
Screw removes unburned powder.
Percussion cap
Grenade is safe until this ring is pulled.
Explosive charge
Cast-iron body
Throwing the grenade releases this lever.
As the lever rises, it frees a hammer.
The hammer strikes a percussion cap.
The cap lights a short fuse.
The grenade explodes after a few seconds when the fuse burns down to the charge.

ARROWS
A well-made arrow must be perfectly straight and have the right weight and flexibility. The tip shape depends on the arrow's use.

Bows and arrows

Before the invention of gunpowder the most powerful missile weapon was the bow and arrow. The springy wood of the bow stored the archer's energy as he gradually drew the string; letting go of the string released the energy and propelled the arrow further and more accurately than it could be thrown by hand. Cave paintings created more than 10,000 years ago show hunters using simple bows.

CROSSBOW
The crossbow was a short, very powerful bow mounted on a wooden "stock". Some crossbows were so strong that the archer needed a winch to draw the string. A catch held the string back while the archer loaded a short arrow, called a bolt, and took aim. Pulling a trigger fired the weapon.

SHORT AND LONG BOWS
Early bows were very short. Native Americans used bows that were about 1 m (3.5 ft) long. The powerful English longbow of the 14th to 16th centuries was as long as the archer was tall.

Cannons

The cannon is a large or heavy gun usually mounted on wheels. Lighting the charge of gunpowder at the closed end of a cannon caused a mighty explosion. The strong tube of the cannon directed the explosion forward, hurling the stone or iron ball 1.5 km (1 mile) or more. Later, explosive shells replaced the simple ball.

Modern weapons

The grenade is a small explosive bomb which is set on a time fuse and thrown at the enemy. Modern soldiers are also armed with machine guns, which fire many bullets in rapid succession without the need for reloading. More sophisticated and powerful weapons used today include nuclear missiles, rockets, and explosive mines.

Nuclear weapons create an extremely powerful blast, searing heat, and lethal nuclear radiation.

THE NUCLEAR DETERRENT
A single nuclear weapon can kill the population of an entire city, and a nuclear war might destroy all life on Earth. Some politicians call these weapons the nuclear deterrent. They believe that the terrible results of nuclear war discourage or deter a nation from launching a nuclear attack.

Find out more
Armies
Armour
Guns
Nuclear age
Rockets and missiles

WEASELS
STOATS, AND MARTENS

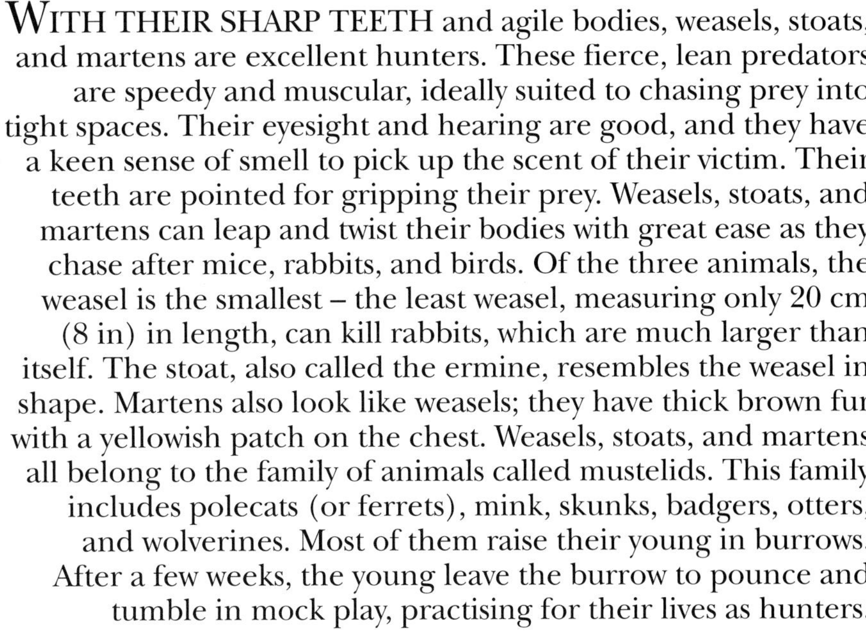

WITH THEIR SHARP TEETH and agile bodies, weasels, stoats, and martens are excellent hunters. These fierce, lean predators are speedy and muscular, ideally suited to chasing prey into tight spaces. Their eyesight and hearing are good, and they have a keen sense of smell to pick up the scent of their victim. Their teeth are pointed for gripping their prey. Weasels, stoats, and martens can leap and twist their bodies with great ease as they chase after mice, rabbits, and birds. Of the three animals, the weasel is the smallest – the least weasel, measuring only 20 cm (8 in) in length, can kill rabbits, which are much larger than itself. The stoat, also called the ermine, resembles the weasel in shape. Martens also look like weasels; they have thick brown fur with a yellowish patch on the chest. Weasels, stoats, and martens all belong to the family of animals called mustelids. This family includes polecats (or ferrets), mink, skunks, badgers, otters, and wolverines. Most of them raise their young in burrows. After a few weeks, the young leave the burrow to pounce and tumble in mock play, practising for their lives as hunters.

MARTEN

Although it hunts mainly on the ground, the pine marten is a skilful climber. It is so nimble in the treetops that it can easily catch a squirrel. Pine martens hunt beetles, mice, birds' eggs and chicks, and also eat berries.

STOAT

During the spring and summer months, stoats are brown like weasels. In winter, however, their coats change colour to white, and this coat is known as ermine. In the coldest parts of northern Europe, North America, and Asia the stoat's white fur provides good camouflage as the animal hunts rabbits, lemmings, and mice in the snow. Like other members of the weasel family, stoats steal birds' eggs and raid chicken coops in search of eggs.

MINK

With their partly webbed feet and supple bodies measuring 40 to 50 cm (16 to 20 in) in length, mink are expert swimmers and divers. They live on the banks of rivers and lakes, where they feed on water birds, water voles, and fish. Many mink have been killed for their beautiful fur, and in some areas they are bred for this purpose.

Mink

POLECAT

The polecat is also called the ferret. There are three kinds – the European polecat, the steppe polecat, and the black-footed ferret from North America. Black-footed ferrets are on the official list of endangered species. They are threatened because their main source of food – the prairie dog – has been greatly reduced in numbers.

Markings on face enable ferrets to recognize one another.

Lithe, muscular body

Sharp claws for digging and for catching prey

Black-footed ferret

COMMON WEASEL

With its long, thin body and short legs, the European common weasel can dart into a rabbit burrow or rat tunnel to grab its prey. Weasels are so long and slender and flexible that they can easily perform a U-turn in a rabbit burrow. Weasels are fierce hunters, ripping a mouse or vole apart within seconds in a flurry of teeth and claws.

The weasel sniffs around a tunnel entrance in search of prey such as young rabbits.

Common weasel

When it finds a victim such as a rabbit, the weasel gives it a fatal bite to the back of the neck.

Find out more

ANIMALS
BADGERS AND SKUNKS
CONSERVATION and endangered species
MAMMALS
RABBITS AND HARES

WEATHER

The air over the Sahara Desert is so stable and dry that rain seldom falls.

Clouds hang over the hot and rainy tropics of Central Africa.

Swirls of cloud mark patterns of winds.

Snow and ice cover the cold Antarctic continent.

WEATHER DESCRIBES CONDITIONS, such as rain, wind, and sunshine, that occur during a short period of time in a particular place; climate is the overall pattern of weather in a region. From one moment to the next the weather can change. A warm, sunny day can be overtaken by a violent storm. Dark clouds form, high winds blow, and rain lashes the ground, yet it may be only a few minutes before the sunny weather returns. However, in some parts of the world, such as the tropics, the weather barely changes for months at a time. There it is always hot, and heavy rains fall.

Meteorologists are scientists who measure and forecast the weather. They do this by studying clouds, winds, and the temperature and pressure of the Earth's atmosphere. But despite the use of satellites, computers, and other technology in weather forecasting, weather remains a force of nature that is hard to predict.

WORLD WEATHER
The Sun is the driving force for the world's weather. The heat of the Sun's rays produces wind and evaporates water from the seas, which later forms clouds and rain. The direct heat above the equator makes the weather hot, while the poles, which get less of the Sun's heat, are cold and cloudy.

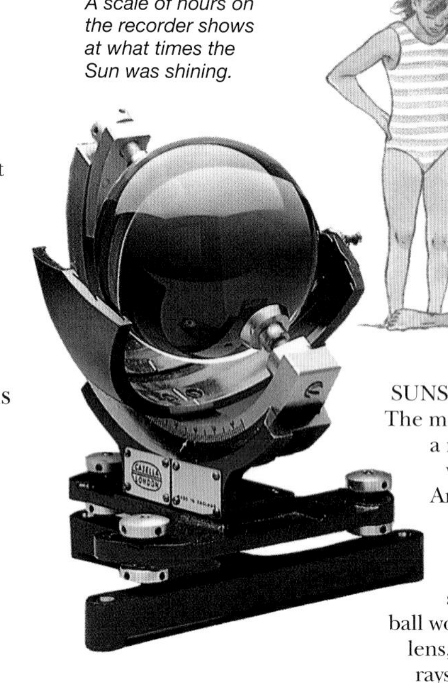

A scale of hours on the recorder shows at what times the Sun was shining.

SUNSHINE RECORDER
The more direct sunshine a region receives, the warmer it becomes. An instrument called a sunshine recorder measures daily hours of sunshine. The glass ball works like a powerful lens, focusing the Sun's rays, which leave a line of burn marks on a piece of cardboard.

MEASURING THE WEATHER

Several thousand weather stations on land, ships, and aircraft measure weather conditions around the world. The stations contain instruments that record temperature, rainfall, the speed and direction of wind, air pressure, and humidity (the amount of water vapour in the air). Balloons called radiosondes carry instruments to take measurements high in the air. Weather satellites in space send back pictures of the clouds.

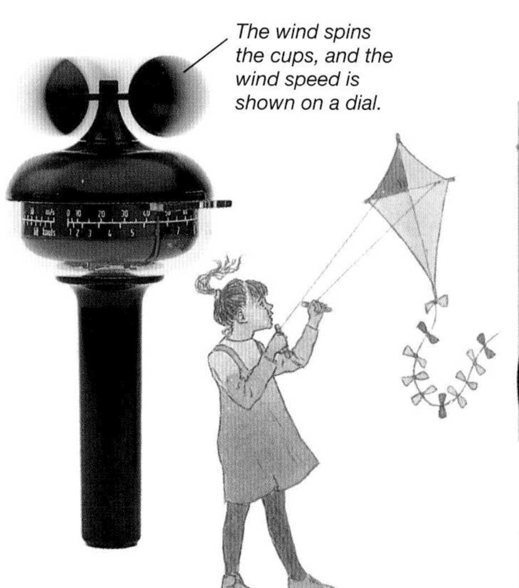

The wind spins the cups, and the wind speed is shown on a dial.

ANEMOMETER
The Sun's heat produces winds – moving currents of air that flow over the Earth's surface. Meteorologists use anemometers to measure wind speed, which shows the rate of approaching weather.

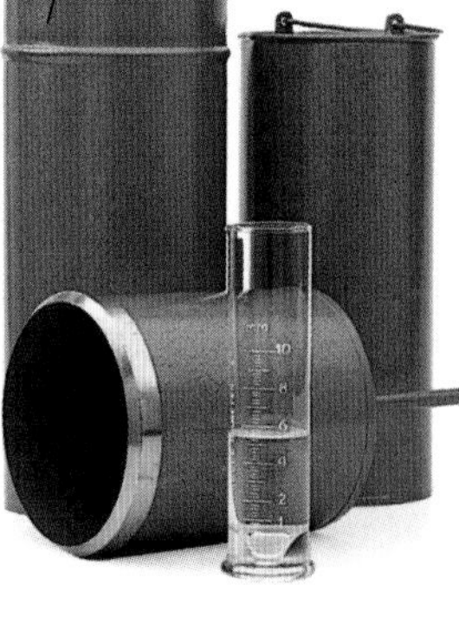

Rain pours through a funnel into a container. After every 24 hours the collected water is poured into a measuring cylinder that gives a reading of the day's total rainfall.

RAIN GAUGE
Droplets of water and tiny ice crystals group together to form clouds, and water falls from the skies as rain and snow. Meteorologists measure rainfall, which is the depth of water that would occur if the rain did not drain away.

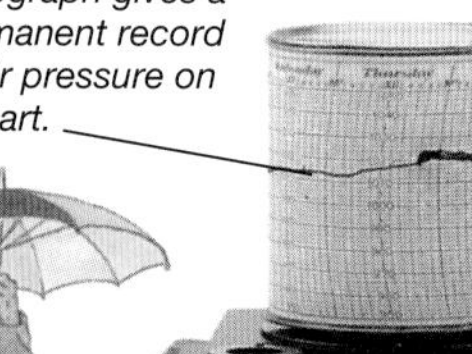

Barograph gives a permanent record of air pressure on a chart.

BAROGRAPH

A barograph measures air pressure. This is important in weather forecasting because high pressure often brings settled weather; low pressure brings wind and rain.

Clouds

Low-lying clouds at the top of a hill cause the air to become cold, foggy, and damp. This is because the clouds contain many tiny droplets of water. Clouds form in air that is rising. The air contains invisible water vapour. As the air ascends, it becomes cooler. Colder air cannot hold so much vapour, and some vapour turns to tiny droplets or freezes to ice crystals, forming a cloud. Slow-rising air produces sheets of cloud. Air that is ascending quickly forms clumps of cloud.

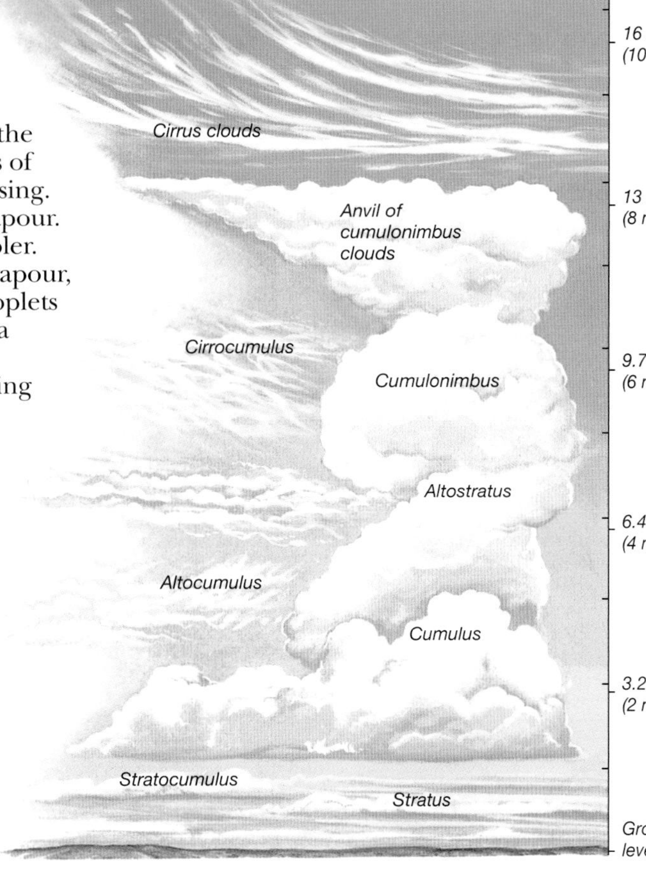

CLOUD FORMATION
There are three main kinds of clouds, that form at different heights in the air. Feathery cirrus clouds float highest of all. Midway to low are fluffy cumulus clouds. Sheets of stratus clouds often lie low in the sky; grey stratus bears rain. Cumulonimbus cloud, a type of cumulus cloud, towers in the sky and often brings thunderstorms.

CIRRUS CLOUDS
Cirrus clouds form high in the sky so they contain only ice crystals. Cirrocumulus (above) and cirrostratus also form at high altitudes.

CUMULUS CLOUDS
Separate masses of cloud are called cumulus clouds. Altocumulus is medium-high patchy cloud, and low stratocumulus contains low, dense clumps of cloud.

Air masses and fronts

Huge bodies of air, called air masses, form over land and sea. Air masses containing warm, cold, moist, or dry air bring different kinds of weather as they are carried by the wind. A front is where two air masses meet. The weather changes when a front arrives.

WARM FRONT
Long spells of rain occur as warm air rises above cold air before the front arrives on the ground.

Warm, moist air mass

Cold, moist air mass

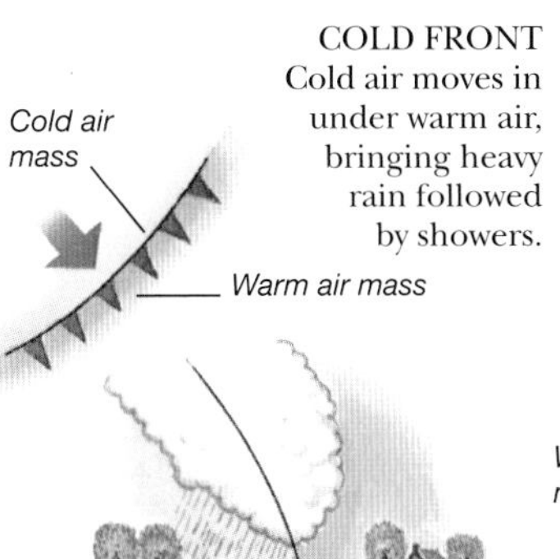

COLD FRONT
Cold air moves in under warm air, bringing heavy rain followed by showers.

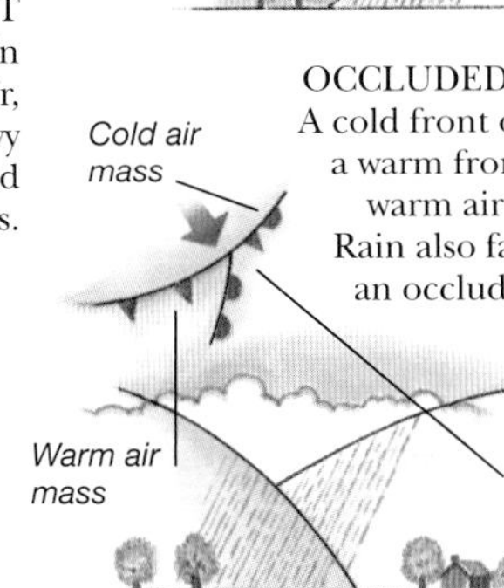

OCCLUDED FRONT
A cold front overtakes a warm front, lifting warm air above it. Rain also falls along an occluded front.

Weather forecasting

The weather centres in different countries receive measurements of weather conditions from satellites and observers around the world. They use this data to forecast the weather that lies ahead. Supercomputers do the many difficult calculations involved and draw charts of the weather to come. Forecasters use the charts to predict the weather for the next few days, producing weather reports for television, newspapers, shipping, and aircraft.

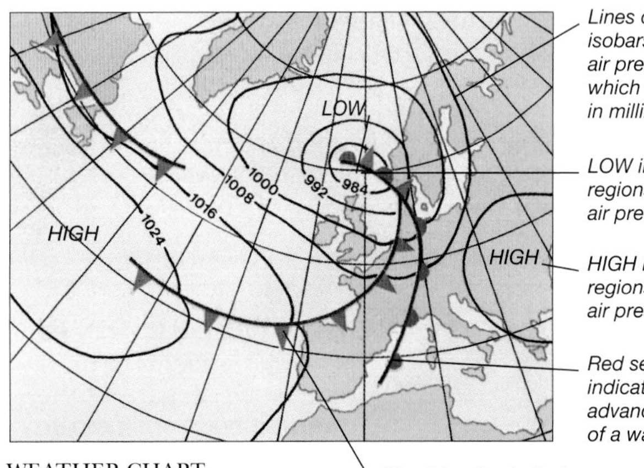

WEATHER CHART
A weather forecaster predicts the day's weather using a chart showing air pressure and fronts over a large region. Lines called isobars connect regions with the same atmospheric pressure. Tight loops of isobars of decreasing pressure show a low, where it is windy and possibly rainy. Isobars of rising pressure indicate a high, which gives settled weather.

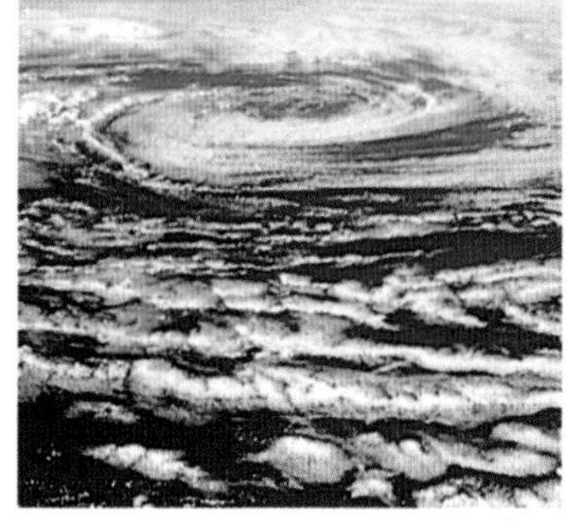

HIGHS AND LOWS
The pressure of the air varies from time to time and from place to place. Regions of low pressure are called cyclones or lows. The air rises and cools, bringing clouds and rain. An anticyclone, or high, is a region of high pressure. The air descends and warms, bringing clear, dry weather. Winds circle around highs and lows, as can be seen in this satellite picture of a cyclonic storm.

Find out more

Atmosphere
Climates
Earth
Rain and snow
Storms
Wind

WEIGHTS AND MEASURES

HOW FAR AWAY is the moon? How deep are the oceans? How tall are you? How hot is it on Mars? It is possible to measure all of these things and many more. Every day we need to make measurements. In cooking, for example, a recipe requires the correct weight of each ingredient, and once mixed, the ingredients have to be cooked at a certain temperature. We make measurements using measuring instruments. For example, a thermometer measures temperature, a ruler measures distance, and a clock measures time. All measurements are based on a system of units. Time, for example, is measured in units of minutes and seconds; length is measured in metres or feet. Precise measurements are very important in science and medicine. Scientists have extremely accurate measuring instruments to determine everything from the tiny distance between atoms in a piece of metal, to the temperature of a distant planet, such as Neptune.

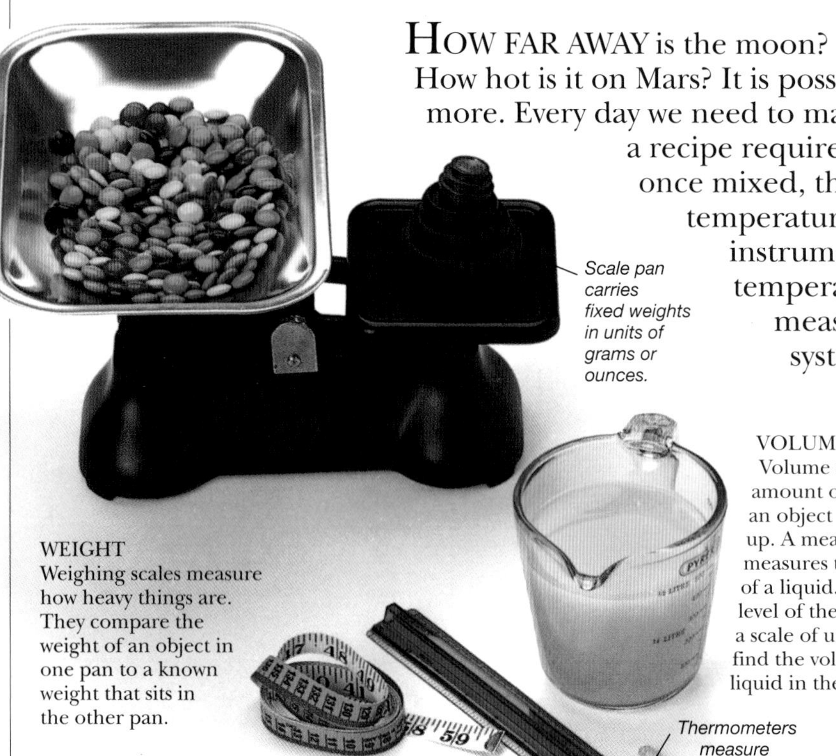

Scale pan carries fixed weights in units of grams or ounces.

WEIGHT
Weighing scales measure how heavy things are. They compare the weight of an object in one pan to a known weight that sits in the other pan.

VOLUME
Volume measures the amount of space that an object or liquid takes up. A measuring jug measures the volume of a liquid. By reading the level of the liquid against a scale of units, you can find the volume of the liquid in the jug.

Thermometers measure temperature.

LENGTH AND AREA
Tape measures and rulers indicate length. They can also be used to calculate area, which indicates, for example, the amount of land a football field takes up or the amount of material needed to make a coat.

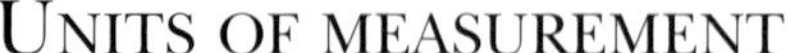

We can also measure things that we cannot see. This digital meter measures the strength of an electric current in amperes (A).

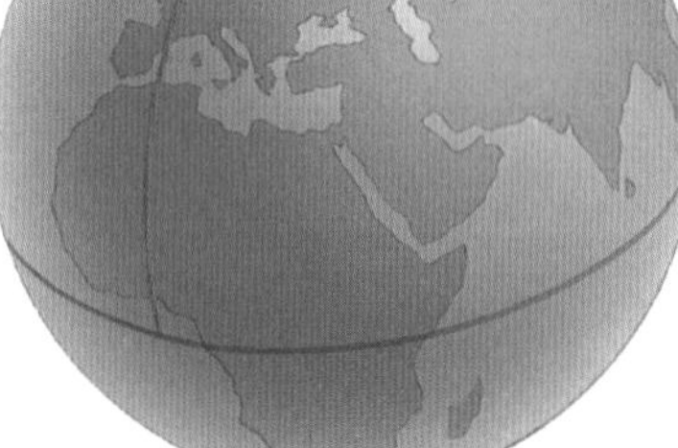

UNITS OF MEASUREMENT

When you measure something, such as height, you compare the quantity you are measuring to a fixed unit such as a metre or a foot. Scientists have set these units with great precision, so that if you measure your height with two different rulers, you will get the same answer. The metre, for example, is defined (set) by the distance travelled by light in a specific time. This gives a very precise measure of length.

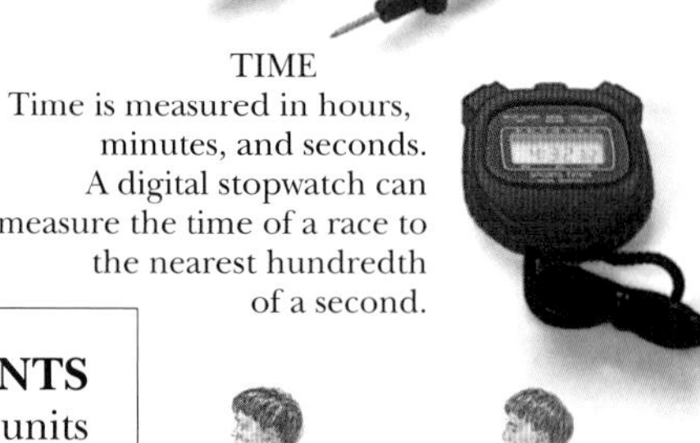

TIME
Time is measured in hours, minutes, and seconds. A digital stopwatch can measure the time of a race to the nearest hundredth of a second.

METRIC SYSTEM
A system of measurement defines fixed units for quantities such as weight and time. Most countries use the metric system, which was developed in France about 200 years ago. Then the metre was fixed as the 10 millionth part of the distance between the North Pole and the equator. The metre is now fixed using the speed of light.

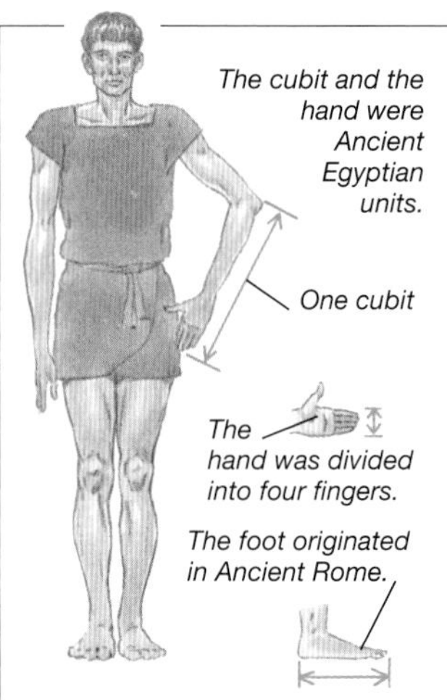

The cubit and the hand were Ancient Egyptian units.

One cubit

The hand was divided into four fingers.

The foot originated in Ancient Rome.

BODY MEASUREMENTS

The earliest systems of units were based on parts of the human body, such as the hands or feet. Both the Ancient Egyptians (about 3000 B.C.) and the Romans (from about 800 B.C.) used units of this kind. However, body measurements present a problem. They always give different answers because they depend on the size of the person making the measurement.

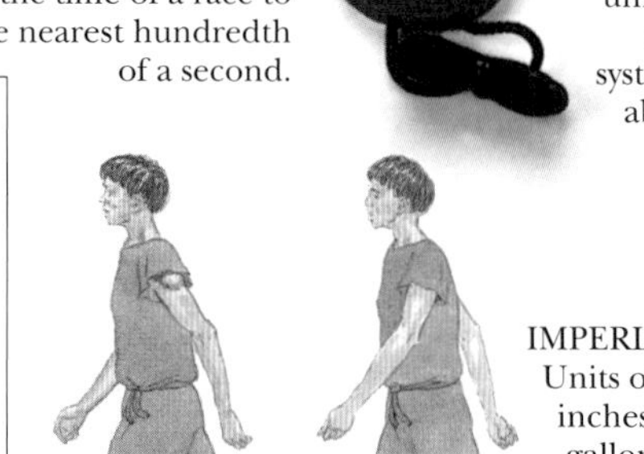

Many imperial units were first used in Ancient Rome. The mile was 1,000 paces, each pace being two steps. The word mile comes from the word for 1,000 in Latin.

IMPERIAL SYSTEM
Units of the imperial system include inches and feet for length, pints and gallons for volume, and pounds and tons for weight. The imperial system is used mainly in the United States.

Find out more

CLOCKS AND WATCHES
EGYPT, ANCIENT
MATHEMATICS
ROMAN EMPIRE

WEST AFRICA

THE VARIED CLIMATES, landscapes, and resources of the countries of West Africa have attracted both traders and colonizers. Arabs operated trading caravans across the Sahara Desert, while the Europeans sought both West African slaves and gold. Today, most of the countries in this region are desperately poor, their problems made worse by corrupt governments, debt, and occasional civil wars. The vast majority of people live by farming. Coffee, cocoa, and oil palms are all cultivated in the humid tropical lowlands of the west and south, while cattle, sheep, and goats are herded by the nomads of the Sahel. Vast reserves of oil have been found in the Niger Delta and off Ivory Coast, and there is mineral wealth in both Mauritania and Sierra Leone, but these resources are still not having an impact on most peoples' daily lives.

PLANTAINS
Plantains are members of the banana family. They are cooked and mashed to make a staple food in many parts of tropical West Africa.

FISHING IN MAURITANIA
Two-thirds of Mauritania is covered by the Sahara Desert. Only one per cent of the land, the area drained by the Senegal River, can be cultivated. However, Mauritania has some of the richest fishing grounds in the world. Many other nations fish there. Catches are sold through the state fishing company, and fishing provides over half of Mauritania's export earnings.

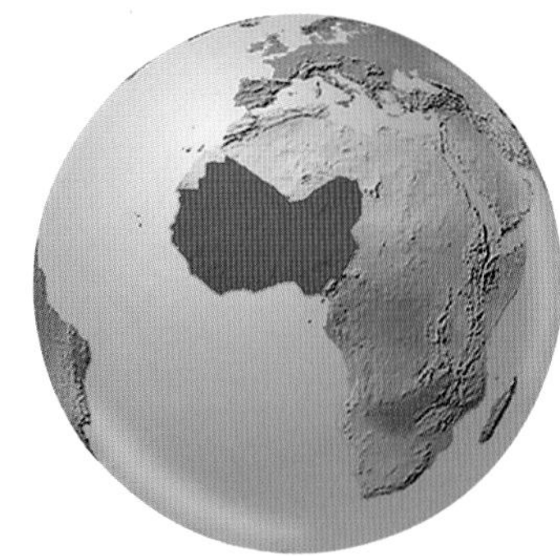

Most of the countries of this region border the Atlantic Ocean. The northern countries lie on the fringes of the Sahara Desert and the Sahel, a vast area of semi-desert. The tropical rainforests of the west and south are irrigated by three major rivers – the Niger, Volta, and Senegal.

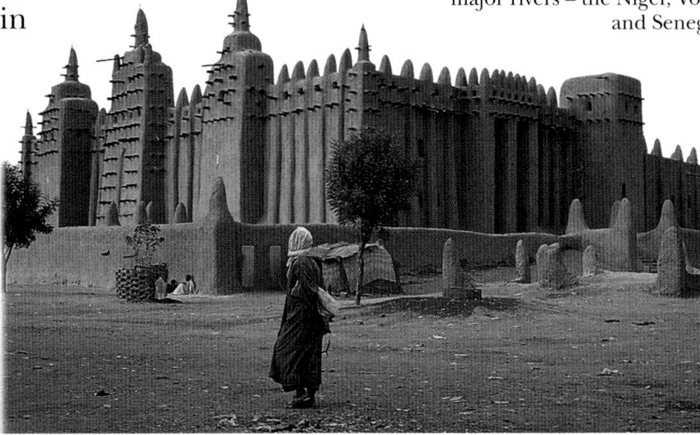

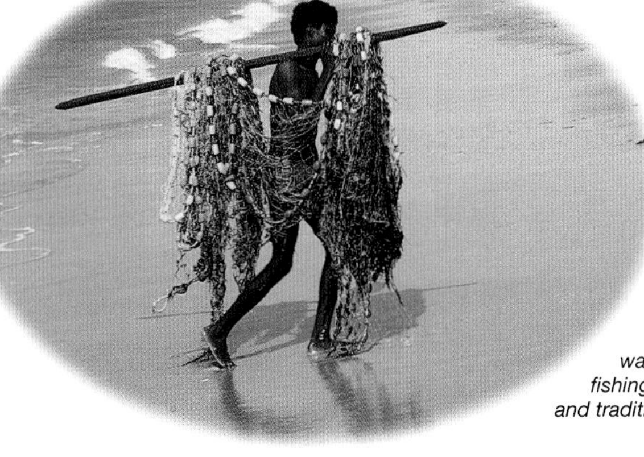

A Mauritanian fisherman uses a pole to carry his nets to the water's edge. Local fishing is small-scale and traditional.

ISLAM

Many of the countries of West Africa are Islamic. The religion was spread by Arab traders, who controlled the great caravan trading routes across the Sahara from the 8th century. The rulers of the West African kingdoms adopted Islam from the 13th century. The Grand Mosque at Djenne, in Mali, is the largest mud-brick building in the world. It dates to the 14th century, but requires constant rebuilding.

SAHARA DESERT
The Sahara is spreading south, turning much of Mauritania, Mali, and Niger into desert. In Mauritania, 75 per cent of grazing land has been lost in the past 25 years. Drought, cutting down trees for fuel, and over-grazing are all contributing to this process. When soil has no roots to cling to, the wind blows it away. Windbreaks of trees and shrubs are being planted in order to halt the desert's advance.

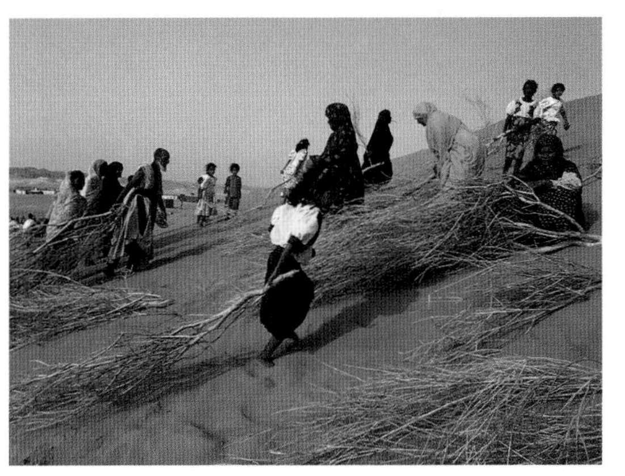

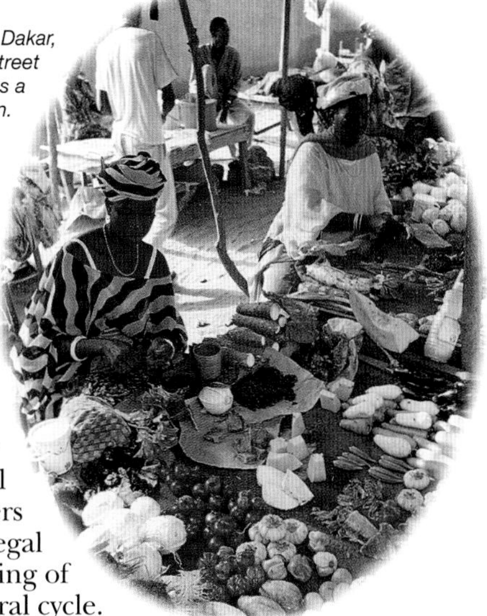

The streets of Senegal's capital, Dakar, are lined with market stalls and street sellers. This busy, expanding port has a population of more than one million.

FARMING

Throughout West Africa, most people live by small-scale farming. In Senegal, the main crops that are grown for export include groundnuts, cotton, and sugar-cane. Rice, millet, and sorghum are staple foods. Many farmers travel regularly into local towns, or even Dakar, the capital city, to sell their excess produce. Most farmers rely on the flooding of the Senegal river to water their land. The damming of the river is disrupting this natural cycle.

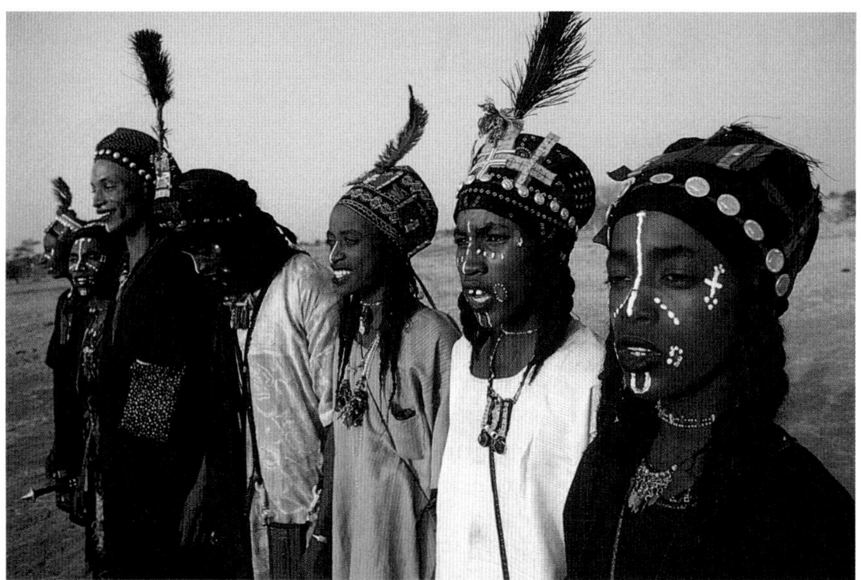

The Wodaabe are nomadic cattle herders, who only come into towns for trading and festivals.

The main dye used in this cloth is indigo, a blue colour produced by pulping the leaves of the indigo vine.

NIGERIAN TEXTILES
The Yoruba and Hausa are the main ethnic groups in Nigeria. The Hausa are found in the north of the country, the traditionally city-dwelling Yoruba in the southwest. Both groups produce patterned textiles, hand-dyed using natural plant extracts.

Wodaabe people

The nomadic Wodaabe people graze their herds along the Nigerian-Niger borderlands. Every year they hold a beauty contest, where the men compete for wives. Under the careful scrutiny of the women, they parade themselves in make-up which emphasizes their eyes and teeth.

Downtown Lagos

Lagos is Nigeria's largest city, chief port, and until 1991, the country's capital. It developed as a major Portuguese slave centre until it fell under British control in 1861. The city sprawls across the islands and sandbars of Lagos lagoon, linked by a series of bridges. Most of the population is concentrated on Lagos Island. The southwest of the island, with its striking high-rise skyline, is the commercial, financial, and educational centre of the city. Lagos is Nigeria's transport hub; it is served by a major international airport, and is also the country's main outlet for exports. Lagos suffers from growing slums, traffic congestion, and overcrowding. Pollution is also a major problem.

BAMBUKU HEAD
In many parts of West Africa, traditional beliefs are still very much alive. Ancestors are worshiped, or called upon to cure sickness and help people in difficulties. Spirits are worshiped at rituals and ceremonies. In eastern Nigeria, the fierce expression on this Bambuku head is used to frighten away evil spirits. It is left in a small shelter at the entrance to the village.

NIGERIAN OIL

Since the 1970s, Nigeria has become dependent on its vast oil reserves in the Niger Delta. It is the tenth largest producer in the world, and oil accounts for 90 per cent of its exports. The Nigerian government has become over-dependent on oil; the country was once a major exporter of tropical fruits, but agriculture has declined. When world oil prices declined in the 1980s, Nigeria was forced to rely on financial assistance from the World Bank. There are also growing concerns about the pollution problems caused by the oil industry in the Niger Delta. Protesters have attacked Shell, one of the main companies operating in Nigeria.

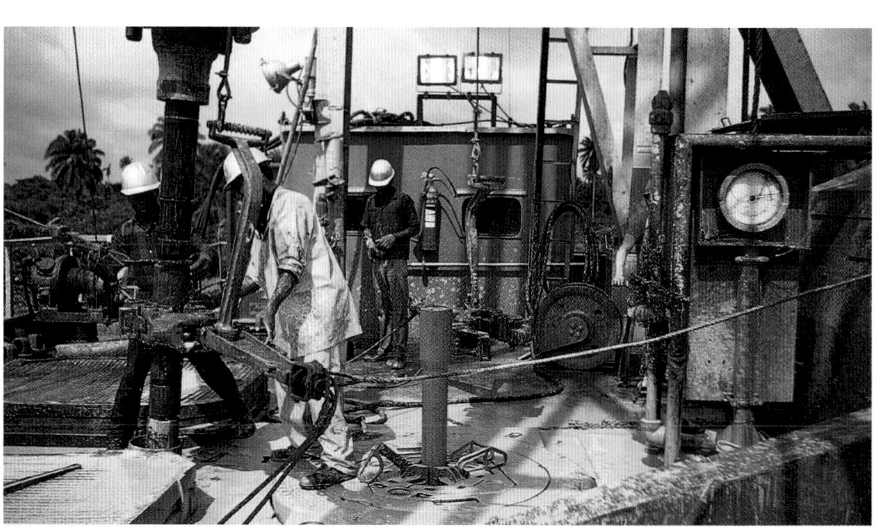

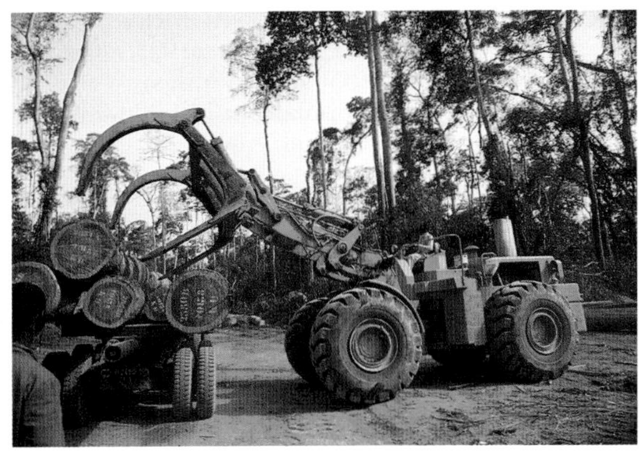

The use of modern equipment (left) in the logging industry in Ivory Coast is speeding up the process of deforestation.

AFRICAN GOLD

The gold of West Africa is found underground, or as a fine dust, obtained by sifting soil in shallow river beds. In the 19th century, African gold produced great wealth for European traders. In Asante, Ghana, goldsmiths were a privileged class. They created this magnificent head, taken as loot by the British in 1874.

LOGGING IN IVORY COAST

The tropical rain forests in the moist, humid interior of Ivory Coast have suffered considerable damage. Many trees have been cut down in order to grow more profitable cocoa trees which thrive in the tropical conditions. Cocoa beans are transported to factories along the coast where they are made into cocoa butter, an ingredient in chocolates and some cosmetics. Exports are sent through the port of Abidjan, once the capital and now West Africa's main port.

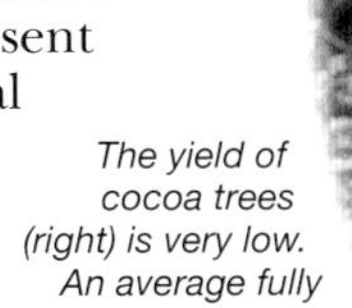

The yield of cocoa trees (right) is very low. An average fully grown tree bears only 20 cocoa pods.

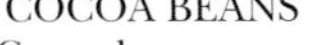

COCOA BEANS

Cocoa beans were first discovered by the Aztec peoples of Mexico. They used the seeds to make a drink called *chocolatl*, which was exported to Europe by Spanish and Portuguese colonists, where it became an instant success. West Africa now produces over half the world's supply of cocoa beans. Seeds are sun-dried, fermented, roasted, and ground to make cocoa butter.

TOURISM IN GAMBIA

Gambia is a narrow country, clinging to the banks of the Gambia River, and almost entirely surrounded by Senegal. Most people live off the land, but increasing numbers are moving to the coast. Here, sandy beaches and mild winters are attracting many visitors from northern Europe. Tourism is Gambia's fastest-growing industry.

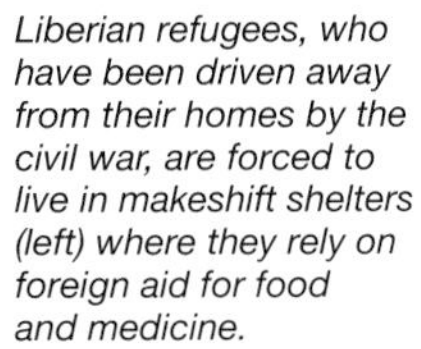

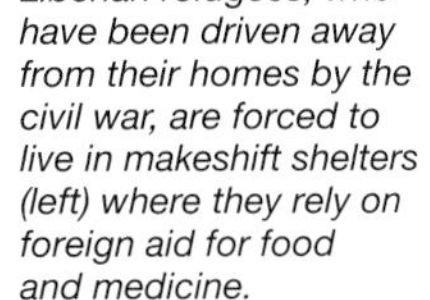

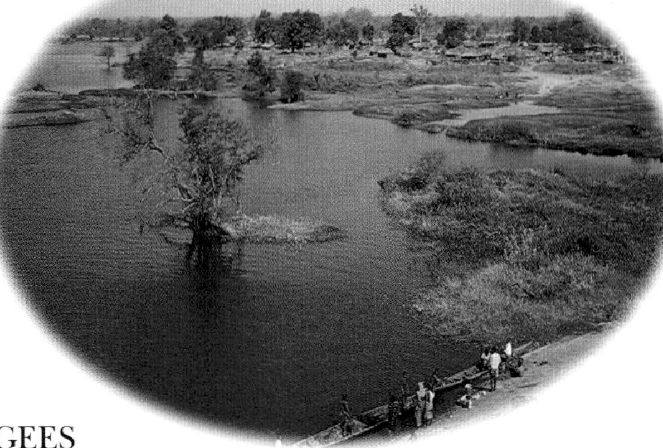

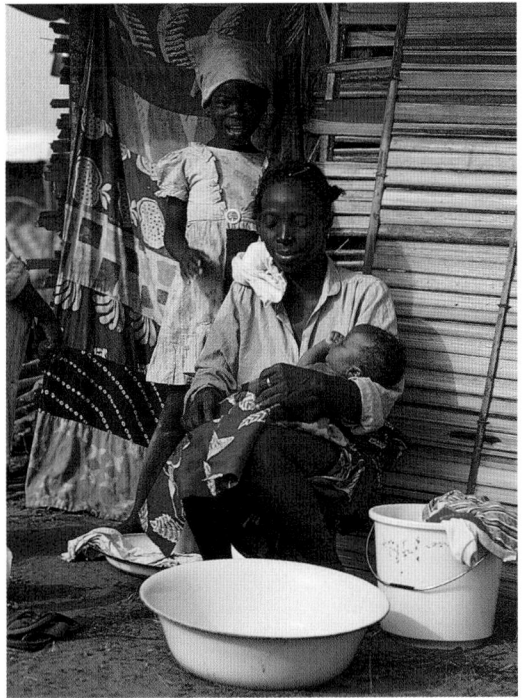

Liberian refugees, who have been driven away from their homes by the civil war, are forced to live in makeshift shelters (left) where they rely on foreign aid for food and medicine.

LIBERIAN REFUGEES

Liberia has never been colonized, making it the oldest independent republic in Africa. It was founded by the USA in the 1820s as a refuge for Africans who had been freed from slavery. The name Liberia means "freed land". Descendants of the American slaves mixed uneasily with the majority native population. For many years, Liberia was a devastated war zone, the result of violent conflict between the country's ethnic groups, which include the Kpelle, Bassa, and Kru peoples. Homeless victims of the fighting were forced to live in vast refugee camps, where disease and food shortages were common. In 2003, UN peacekeepers entered the country, and the armed groups have now largely been disbanded.

LAKE VOLTA

One of the largest man-made lakes in the world, Lake Volta was formed by the building of the Askosombo Dam on Ghana's Volta River in 1965. Some 78,000 people, living in 740 villages, were resettled when the dam was built. The lake is a major fishing ground, and also supplies water for farmers. The hydroelectric dam generates most of Ghana's power.

Find out more

AFRICA
AFRICA, HISTORY OF
AFRICAN WILDLIFE
DESERTS
VOLCANOES

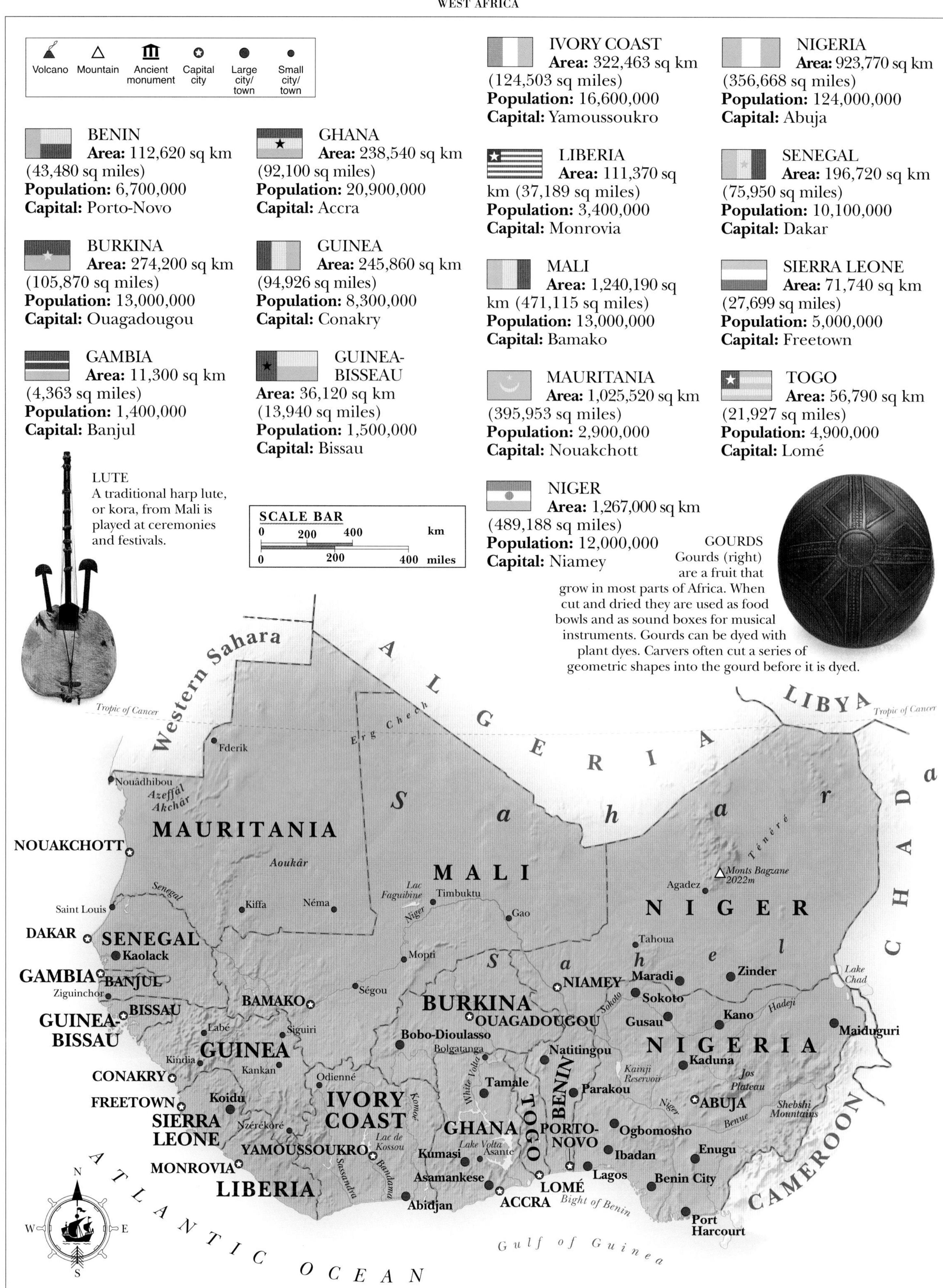

LUTE
A traditional harp lute, or kora, from Mali is played at ceremonies and festivals.

GOURDS
Gourds (right) are a fruit that grow in most parts of Africa. When cut and dried they are used as food bowls and as sound boxes for musical instruments. Gourds can be dyed with plant dyes. Carvers often cut a series of geometric shapes into the gourd before it is dyed.

WHALES AND DOLPHINS

TEN MILLION YEARS before humans first lived on Earth, whales were swimming in the oceans. Whales are among the most intelligent of all creatures. They are also the largest living animals, and among the gentlest and most graceful. Whales, dolphins, and porpoises make up a fascinating group of mammals. They are warm-blooded, but unlike seals, they have no fur; a thick layer of fatty blubber under the skin keeps them warm. The whale group is divided into those with teeth (toothed whales) and those without teeth (baleen whales). There are dozens of different toothed whales, including the friendly bottle-nosed dolphin and the ferocious killer whale, which eats almost anything in the sea. Toothless or baleen whales include the humpback and blue whales, which feed by sieving small sea creatures, such as krill, into their mouths. Since all whales and dolphins breathe air, they must swim to the surface of the water regularly. Whales and dolphins swim by moving their tails up and down; fish move their tails from side to side. Whales have suffered greatly from hunting by humans, and 21 kinds are on the official lists of endangered species. Today, whaling is not allowed, in the hope that the population of whales will increase.

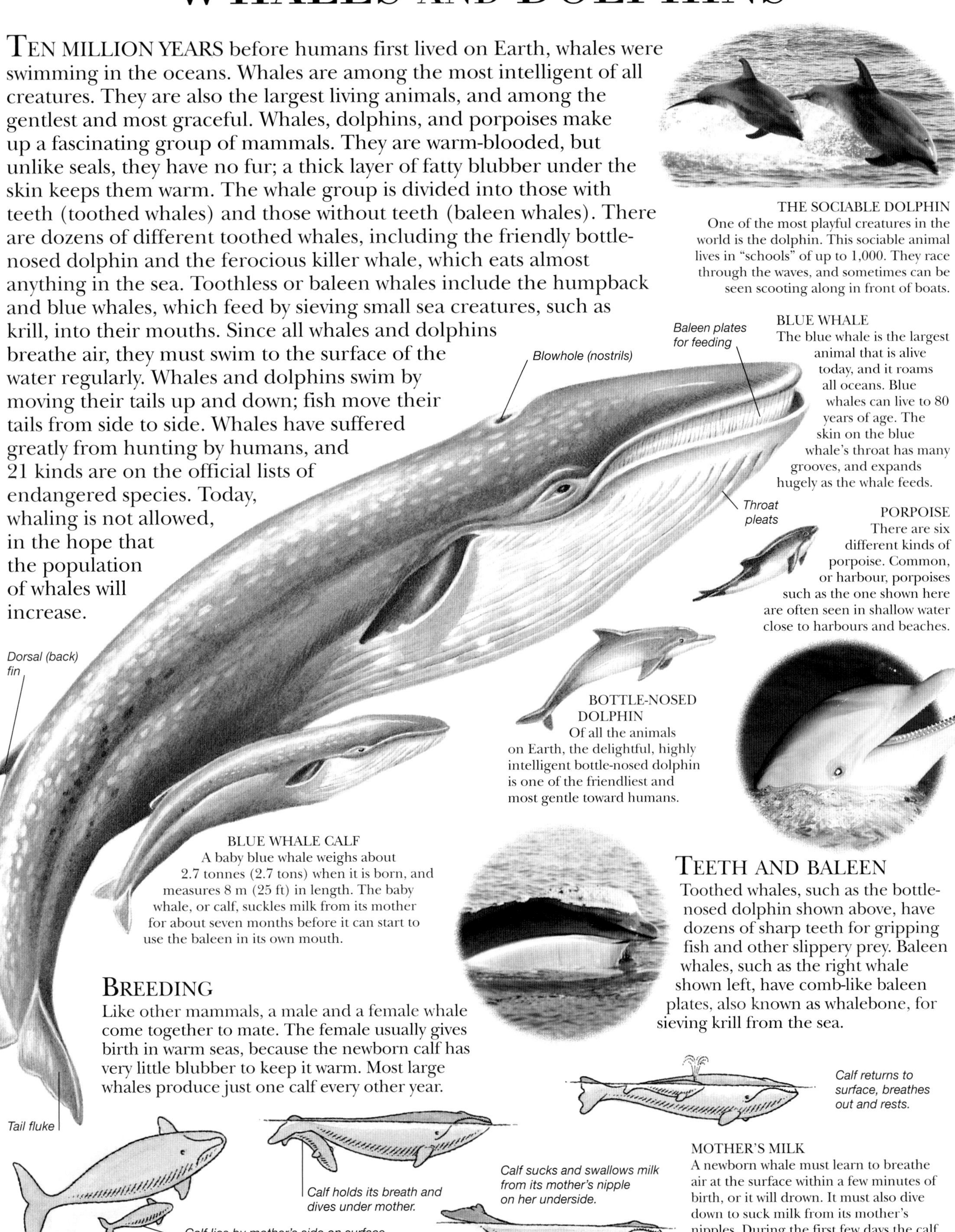
Baleen plates for feeding
Blowhole (nostrils)
Throat pleats
Dorsal (back) fin
Tail fluke
Calf returns to surface, breathes out and rests.
Calf holds its breath and dives under mother.
Calf sucks and swallows milk from its mother's nipple on her underside.
Calf lies by mother's side on surface of water and breathes in air.

THE SOCIABLE DOLPHIN
One of the most playful creatures in the world is the dolphin. This sociable animal lives in "schools" of up to 1,000. They race through the waves, and sometimes can be seen scooting along in front of boats.

BLUE WHALE
The blue whale is the largest animal that is alive today, and it roams all oceans. Blue whales can live to 80 years of age. The skin on the blue whale's throat has many grooves, and expands hugely as the whale feeds.

PORPOISE
There are six different kinds of porpoise. Common, or harbour, porpoises such as the one shown here are often seen in shallow water close to harbours and beaches.

BOTTLE-NOSED DOLPHIN
Of all the animals on Earth, the delightful, highly intelligent bottle-nosed dolphin is one of the friendliest and most gentle toward humans.

BLUE WHALE CALF
A baby blue whale weighs about 2.7 tonnes (2.7 tons) when it is born, and measures 8 m (25 ft) in length. The baby whale, or calf, suckles milk from its mother for about seven months before it can start to use the baleen in its own mouth.

TEETH AND BALEEN

Toothed whales, such as the bottle-nosed dolphin shown above, have dozens of sharp teeth for gripping fish and other slippery prey. Baleen whales, such as the right whale shown left, have comb-like baleen plates, also known as whalebone, for sieving krill from the sea.

BREEDING

Like other mammals, a male and a female whale come together to mate. The female usually gives birth in warm seas, because the newborn calf has very little blubber to keep it warm. Most large whales produce just one calf every other year.

MOTHER'S MILK
A newborn whale must learn to breathe air at the surface within a few minutes of birth, or it will drown. It must also dive down to suck milk from its mother's nipples. During the first few days the calf learns how to suckle, then surface for air.

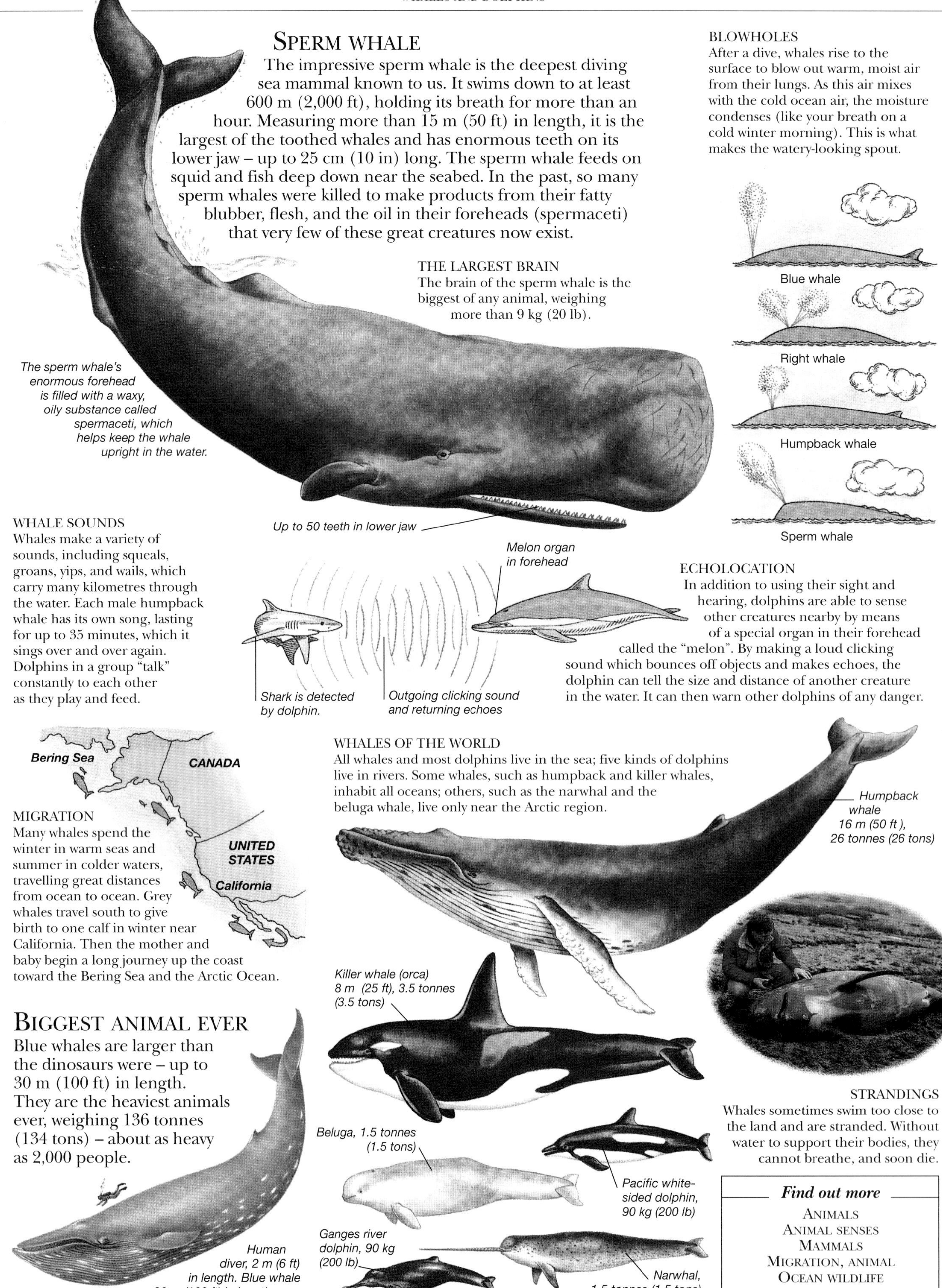

Sperm whale

The impressive sperm whale is the deepest diving sea mammal known to us. It swims down to at least 600 m (2,000 ft), holding its breath for more than an hour. Measuring more than 15 m (50 ft) in length, it is the largest of the toothed whales and has enormous teeth on its lower jaw – up to 25 cm (10 in) long. The sperm whale feeds on squid and fish deep down near the seabed. In the past, so many sperm whales were killed to make products from their fatty blubber, flesh, and the oil in their foreheads (spermaceti) that very few of these great creatures now exist.

The largest brain

The brain of the sperm whale is the biggest of any animal, weighing more than 9 kg (20 lb).

The sperm whale's enormous forehead is filled with a waxy, oily substance called spermaceti, which helps keep the whale upright in the water.

Up to 50 teeth in lower jaw

Blowholes

After a dive, whales rise to the surface to blow out warm, moist air from their lungs. As this air mixes with the cold ocean air, the moisture condenses (like your breath on a cold winter morning). This is what makes the watery-looking spout.

Whale sounds

Whales make a variety of sounds, including squeals, groans, yips, and wails, which carry many kilometres through the water. Each male humpback whale has its own song, lasting for up to 35 minutes, which it sings over and over again. Dolphins in a group "talk" constantly to each other as they play and feed.

Echolocation

In addition to using their sight and hearing, dolphins are able to sense other creatures nearby by means of a special organ in their forehead called the "melon". By making a loud clicking sound which bounces off objects and makes echoes, the dolphin can tell the size and distance of another creature in the water. It can then warn other dolphins of any danger.

Migration

Many whales spend the winter in warm seas and summer in colder waters, travelling great distances from ocean to ocean. Grey whales travel south to give birth to one calf in winter near California. Then the mother and baby begin a long journey up the coast toward the Bering Sea and the Arctic Ocean.

Whales of the world

All whales and most dolphins live in the sea; five kinds of dolphins live in rivers. Some whales, such as humpback and killer whales, inhabit all oceans; others, such as the narwhal and the beluga whale, live only near the Arctic region.

Humpback whale 16 m (50 ft), 26 tonnes (26 tons)

Killer whale (orca) 8 m (25 ft), 3.5 tonnes (3.5 tons)

Beluga, 1.5 tonnes (1.5 tons)

Pacific white-sided dolphin, 90 kg (200 lb)

Ganges river dolphin, 90 kg (200 lb)

Narwhal, 1.5 tonnes (1.5 tons)

Biggest animal ever

Blue whales are larger than the dinosaurs were – up to 30 m (100 ft) in length. They are the heaviest animals ever, weighing 136 tonnes (134 tons) – about as heavy as 2,000 people.

Human diver, 2 m (6 ft) in length. Blue whale 30 m (100 ft) in length.

Strandings

Whales sometimes swim too close to the land and are stranded. Without water to support their bodies, they cannot breathe, and soon die.

Find out more

Animals
Animal senses
Mammals
Migration, animal
Ocean wildlife

WHEELS

SOMETIMES THE SIMPLEST INVENTIONS are the most important. Although no one is sure exactly who invented the first wheel, the earliest records go back to about 5,500 years ago. The wheel has made possible a whole range of machines, from photocopiers to jet engines, that we take for granted today. Wheels have a unique characteristic – they are circular, without corners, enabling them to roll or spin evenly. This allows almost all forms of land transportation – bicycles, cars, trains, and trams – to roll smoothly along roads, rails, and rough ground. In addition, the circular motion of a wheel means that it can transmit power continuously from an engine. Many more inventions are based on wheels. The crane, for example, relies on pulleys (grooved wheels around which a rope is passed), which reduce the effort needed to lift heavy weights; gears multiply or reduce the speed and force of a wheel and are essential in countless other machines.

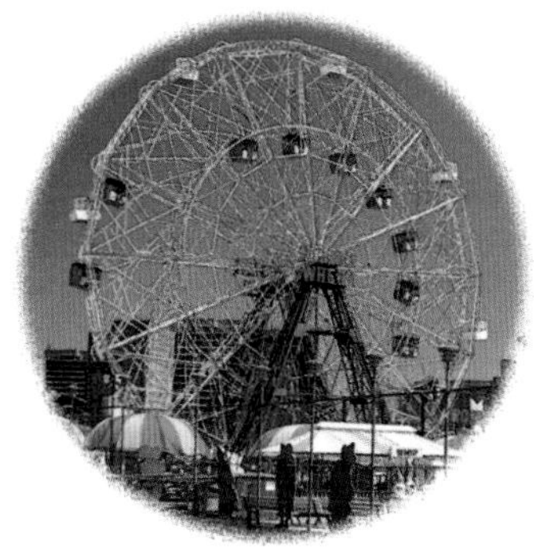

AXLE AND BEARINGS
A wheel spins on a shaft called an axle. Wheels often have ball bearings – several small steel balls that run between the axle and the wheel, allowing it to turn smoothly. Without bearings, the great weight of a Ferris wheel (above) would squeeze the wheel against the axle and prevent it from turning.

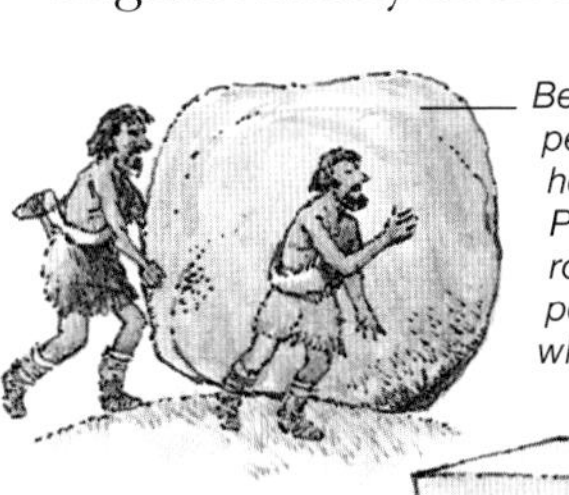

Before wheels were invented, people had to push or drag heavy loads over the ground. Perhaps watching a smooth rock roll down a hill gave people the idea of using wheels for transport.

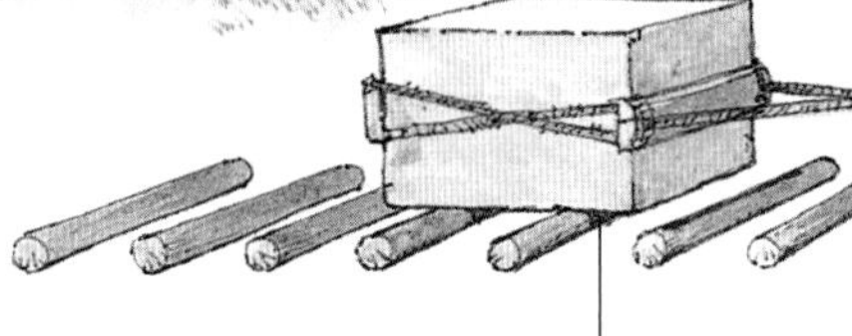

About 4,500 years ago, the Ancient Egyptians built great triangular pyramids as tombs and temples. Gangs of workers dragged huge blocks of stone with the aid of log-rollers.

INVENTING THE WHEEL

The first recorded use of a wheel dates back to around 3500 B.C. This was the potter's wheel, a simple turntable used in southwest Asia by Mesopotamian pottery workers to make smooth, round clay pots. About 300 years later, the Mesopotamians fitted wheels to a cart, and the age of wheeled transportation began.

The first vehicle wheels used for carts were solid wood. They were made of two or three planks of wood fixed together and cut into a circle. They first appeared in about 3200 B.C.

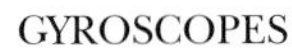

GYROSCOPES
A gyroscope is a rotating wheel mounted on a frame. When the wheel spins, its momentum makes it balance like a spinning top. Once a gyroscope is spinning, it always tries to point in the same direction. Aircraft, ships, and missiles use gyroscopes to navigate, or direct themselves, to their destinations.

Wheels with spokes developed in about 2000 B.C. Spoked wheels are lighter and faster than solid wheels and were fitted to war chariots.

Bibendum, the famous symbol of the French tire company Michelin

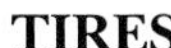

Wheels held together by wire spokes appeared in about 1800. They are very light and strong, and were first used for cars, bicycles, and early airplanes. In the 1950s, metal wheels replaced wire wheels on cars.

The gear wheels are connected by teeth that interlock (fit exactly) into each other. Their mutual positions decide how the force changes.

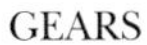

TIRES

Car and bicycle wheels have rubber tires filled with air. They give a comfortable ride and all, except those of racing cars, have a tread (a pattern of ridges) to help them grip the road. Scottish engineer Robert W. Thomson invented the first air-filled tire in 1845.

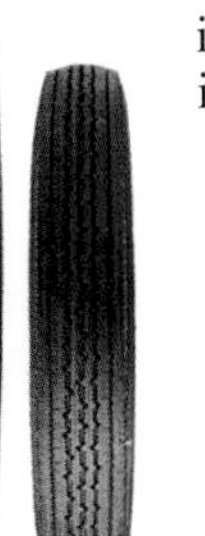

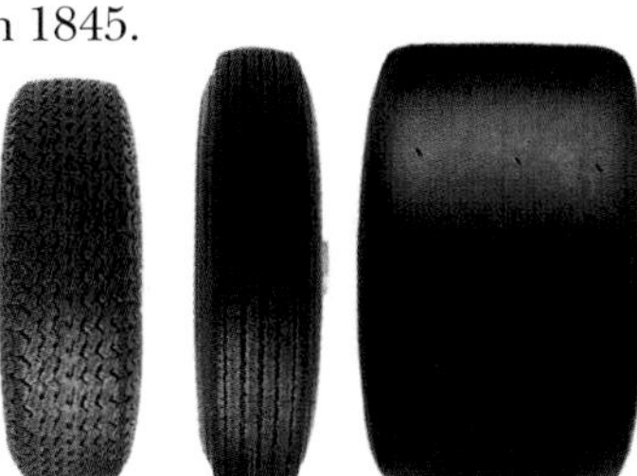

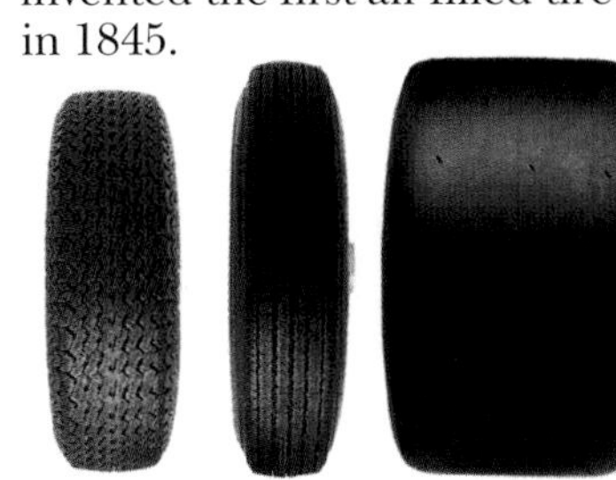

GEARS
Sets of interlocking toothed wheels are called gears. Gears transfer movement in machines and change the speed and force of wheels. For example, a large gear wheel makes a small gear wheel rotate faster, but the faster moving wheel produces less force. Gears can also change the direction of the motion.

Find out more
BICYCLES AND MOTORCYCLES
CARS
TRANSPORT, HISTORY OF

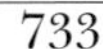

WIND

AS A GENTLE BREEZE or a powerful hurricane, wind blows constantly around the world. Winds are belts of moving air that flow from one area to another, driven by the Sun's heat. Warm air is lighter than cold air, so warm air rises as it is heated by the Sun, and cold air flows in to take its place. This sets up a circular current of air which produces winds. Light, warm air exerts less pressure on the Earth than cold air, creating an area of low pressure toward which cold air flows. Similarly, cold air sinks and produces an area of high pressure from which air flows outward. The greater the difference in pressure between two areas, the stronger the winds. Weather forecasters use the Beaufort scale to measure the speed of wind. It runs from 0 to 12: for example, force 2 is a light breeze; force 12 is a hurricane. The size and shape of areas of land and water affect local winds, which are often given special names, such as the chinook in North America and the sirocco in Italy.

WIND DIRECTION
A wind is often named according to the direction from which it is coming. For example, a wind which comes from the west is called a westerly. Windsocks (above) and vanes are used to show wind direction.

At the equator, the Sun's heat warms the air. In this area, the air rises, causing a belt of calm air called the doldrums.

Horse latitudes
Path of air
Doldrums

When the air has risen very high, it cools and sinks back to the Earth in the horse latitudes.

Doldrums
Path of air
Horse latitudes

Polar easterlies

The westerlies are warm winds which blow away from the horse latitudes in the direction of the poles.

Westerlies

Horse latitudes

NE trade winds

The trade winds flow from the horse latitudes toward the equator.

Equator

In between the westerlies and the trade winds is an area of calm called the horse latitudes. The name may refer to the many horses that died on ships that were becalmed in this region.

SE trade winds

Horse latitudes

Westerlies

The polar easterlies are cold winds which blow away from the poles.

WORLD WINDS

Besides local and seasonal winds, there are certain winds that always blow. These are called prevailing winds. There are three main belts of prevailing winds on each side of the equator. They are called the trade winds, the westerlies, and the polar easterlies. The direction they blow in is affected by the spin of the Earth. They are angled toward the left in the southern hemisphere and toward the right in the northern hemisphere.

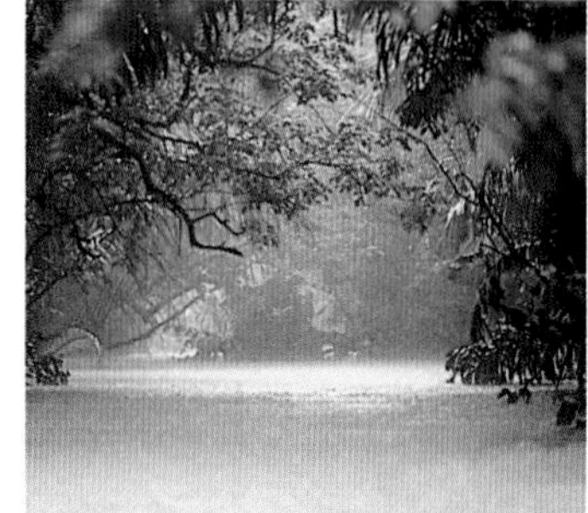

MONSOONS

Seasonal winds that blow in a particular direction are called monsoons. For example, during the summer in southern Asia, the wind blows from the Indian Ocean toward the land, bringing heavy rains. In winter, the wind blows in the opposite direction, from the Himalayas toward the ocean.

WIND TURBINES

The earliest ships used wind power to carry them across the sea. Wind also powers machines. Windmills were used in Iran as long ago as the 7th century for raising water from rivers, and later for grinding corn. Today huge windmills, or wind turbines, can produce electricity; a large wind turbine can supply enough electricity for a small town. Wind turbines cause no pollution but they are large and noisy and take up huge areas of land.

A wind farm in the United States uses 300 wind turbines to produce electricity.

Find out more

CLIMATES
ENERGY
STORMS
WEATHER

WOMEN'S RIGHTS

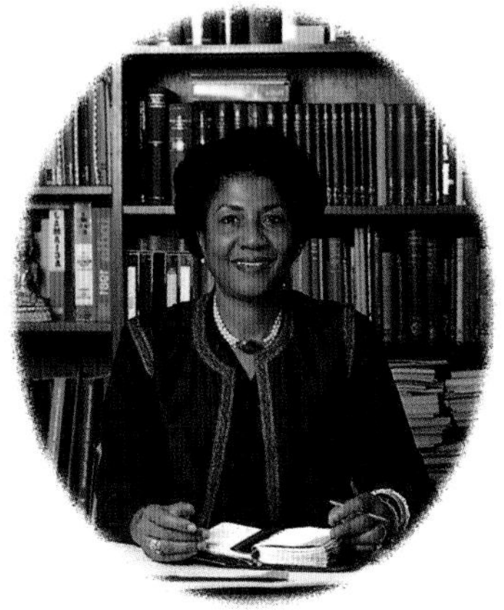

WORKING WOMEN
In the United States about 43 per cent of workers are women. But few hold important positions, and most earn less than men doing the same jobs.

UP UNTIL TWO HUNDRED YEARS AGO women had few rights. They were not allowed to vote, and were considered the property of their fathers or husbands. By the middle of the 19th century, women were demanding equality with men. They wanted suffrage – the right to vote in elections – and an equal chance to work and be educated. They demanded the right to have their own possessions, to divorce their husbands, and to keep their children after divorce. The fight for women's rights was also called feminism, and involved many dedicated women. The first organized demand for the vote occurred in the United States in 1848. By the 1920s, women had won some battles, particularly for the vote and greater education. In the 1960s, women renewed their call for equal rights. This new wave of protest was named the women's liberation movement. It led to the passage of laws in many countries to stop discrimination against women.

WOMEN'S RIGHTS

1792 Mary Wollstonecraft publishes *A Vindication of the Rights of Woman.*

1848 First Women's Rights Conference, USA calls for voting rights for women.

1893 New Zealand is first country to grant voting rights to women.

1903 Emmeline Pankhurst launches Women's Social Political Union in Britain.

1918 British women over 30 earn voting rights.

1920 The United States grants vote to women over 30.

1960 World's first woman prime minister in Sri Lanka.

1963 US Federal Equal Pay Act outlaws paying women less than men for the same job.

1970 First Women's Liberation Conference, UK.

1970 Equal Pay Act, Britain.

1979 United Nations approves Convention on the Elimination of All Forms of Discrimination Against Women.

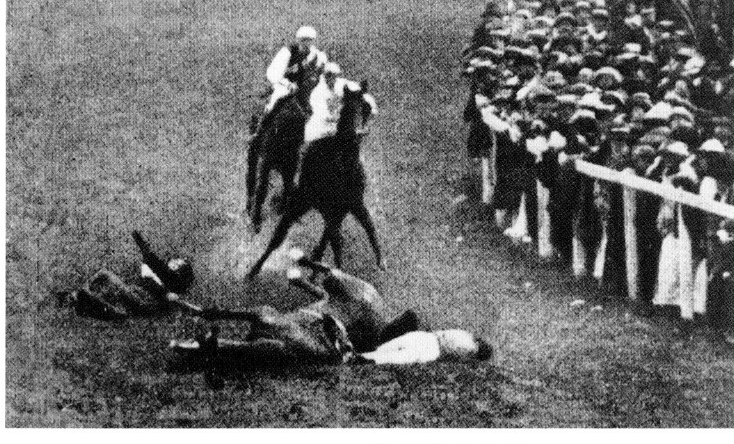

EMILY DAVISON
In 1913 British suffragette Emily Davison leaped under the king's horse at a race and died. Her protest drew attention to the Votes for Women campaign.

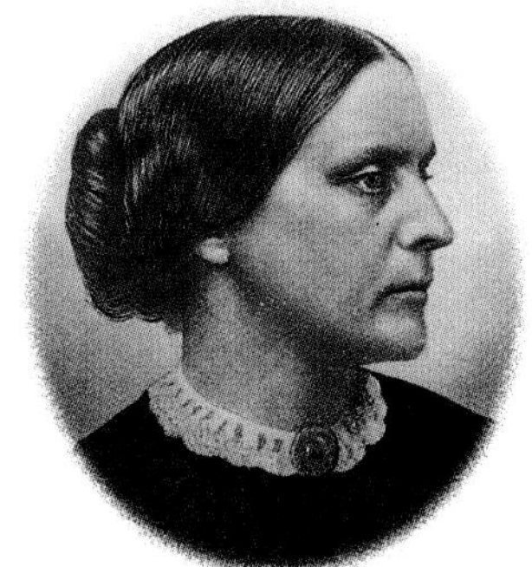

SUSAN B. ANTHONY
One of the leaders of the suffrage movement in the United States, Susan B. Anthony (1820-1906) helped launch *Revolution,* the first feminist newspaper.

ON HER THEIR LIVES DEPEND
WOMEN MUNITION WORKERS
Enrol at once

WOMEN AT WAR
During World War I (1914-18), women in Britain worked to keep factories going while the men fought. They proved that women were just as capable as men. In 1918, British women over 30 got voting rights. Two years later, all American women also gained the vote.

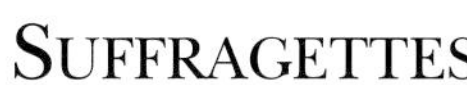

SUFFRAGETTES

In 1905, a British newspaper used the word suffragette to insult women who were fighting for the vote. However, the suffragettes themselves were delighted. People have used the name ever since. Many suffragettes broke the law and went to prison for their beliefs. Women who used peaceful means to obtain the vote were called suffragists.

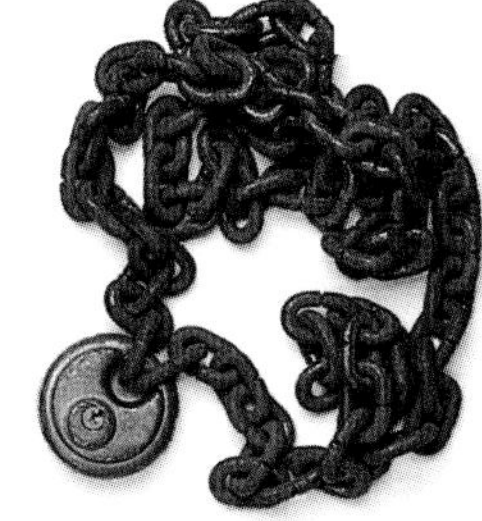

Suffragettes publicized their campaign by chaining themselves to the railings of famous buildings.

FORCE FEEDING
In 1909, suffragettes in prison refused to eat. Warders fed them by pouring food down tubes that they forced through the women's noses and into their stomachs. It was painful and seriously injured some women. Force-feeding ended in 1913.

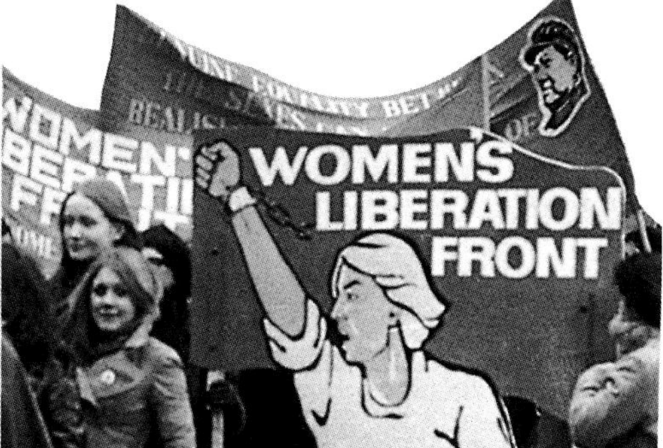

WOMEN'S LIBERATION MOVEMENT
During the late 1960s and 1970s, the women's liberation movement fought for further improvements in women's rights. Women everywhere demonstrated for equal pay, better health care, and an end to pornography and violence against women.

Find out more
DEMOCRACY
LAW
PANKHURST FAMILY
SCHOOLS

WONDERS
OF THE ANCIENT WORLD

PYRAMIDS
Three pyramids were built at Giza, Egypt, in about 2600 B.C. as tombs for three Egyptian kings. The largest, made from more than two million huge blocks of limestone, stands 147 m (482 ft) high.

TWO THOUSAND YEARS AGO Ancient Greek and Roman tourists visited the world's great landmarks just as we do today. Ancient "travel agents" compiled lists of amazing things that travellers should see. These "wonders" were outstanding examples of human artistic or engineering achievement. The seven most commonly listed monuments to human endeavour are called the Seven Wonders of the Ancient World. They all had qualities that made them stand out from the rest. Some were the most beautiful statues, others the largest structures of the day. Of the seven wonders, only one, the Great Pyramids, can still be seen today. The Hanging Gardens, the Temple of Artemis, the Statue of Zeus, the Mausoleum, the Colossus, and the Lighthouse at Pharos have all vanished or are in ruins.

HANGING GARDENS
In 605 B.C. Nebuchadnezzar II, king of Babylon, built the Hanging Gardens in his kingdom. He planted many exotic plants on a brick terrace 23 m (75 ft) above the ground. Machines worked by slaves watered the plants.

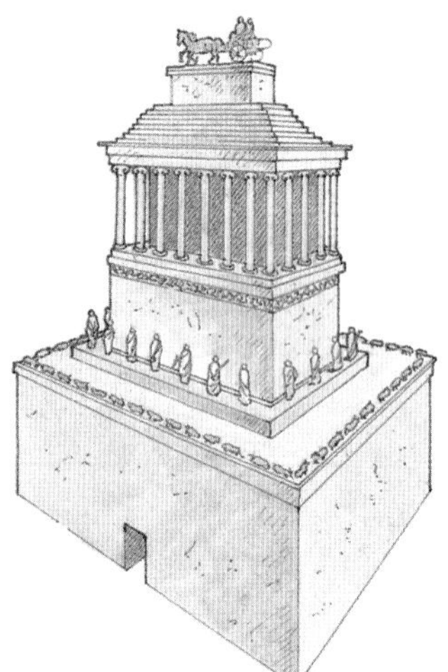

MAUSOLEUM
The Mausoleum at Halicarnassus (in modern Turkey) was a huge marble tomb built for Mausolus, a rich governor. It stood 41 m (135 ft) high, with a base supporting 36 columns, under a stepped pyramid. An earthquake destroyed most of the mausoleum.

LIGHTHOUSE
The Greek architect Sostratos designed the world's first lighthouse. It was built around 304 B.C. on the island of Pharos, Alexandria, Egypt. It stood about 134 m (440 ft) high. A fire burned at the top to mark the harbour entrance.

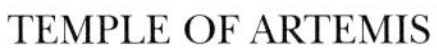

TEMPLE OF ARTEMIS
This, the largest temple of its day, was dedicated to Artemis, goddess of the moon and hunting. Built almost entirely of marble by the Greeks at Ephesus (in modern Turkey), it burned down in 356 B.C., leaving only a few broken statues.

COLOSSUS
The bronze statue of the sun god Helios towered 37 m (120 ft) over the harbour entrance on the island of Rhodes in the Aegean Sea. Built in 292 B.C., it was about the same size as the Statue of Liberty in New York.

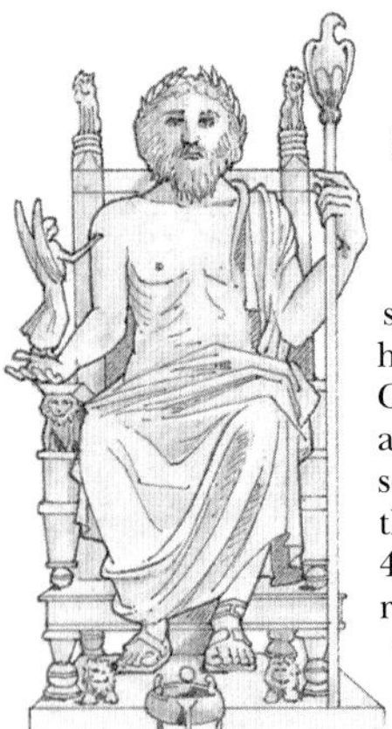

ZEUS
The great Statue of Zeus, king of the Greek gods, stood 12 m (40 ft) high at Olympia, Greece. Phidias, a famous Greek sculptor, created the statue in about 435 B.C. The god's robes and ornaments were made of gold, and the skin was of ivory.

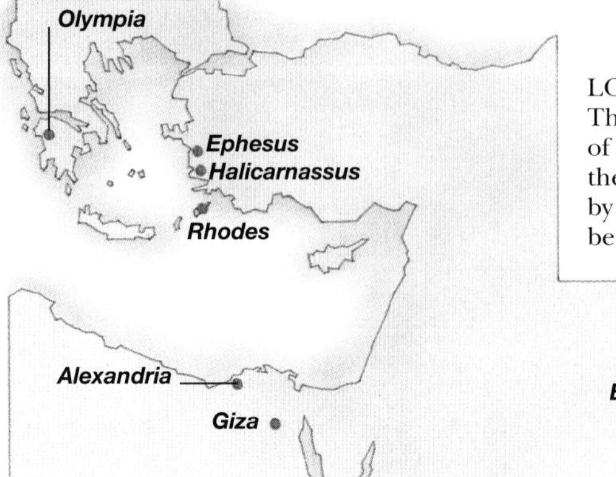

LOCATION OF THE WONDERS
The map shows the location of the Seven Wonders of the Ancient World. Travellers visited many of them by ship. Most of the wonders were destroyed by earthquakes or fire, but some remains can still be seen in the British Museum in London, England.

Find out more
ALEXANDER THE GREAT
BABYLONIANS
EGYPT, ANCIENT

WORLD WAR I

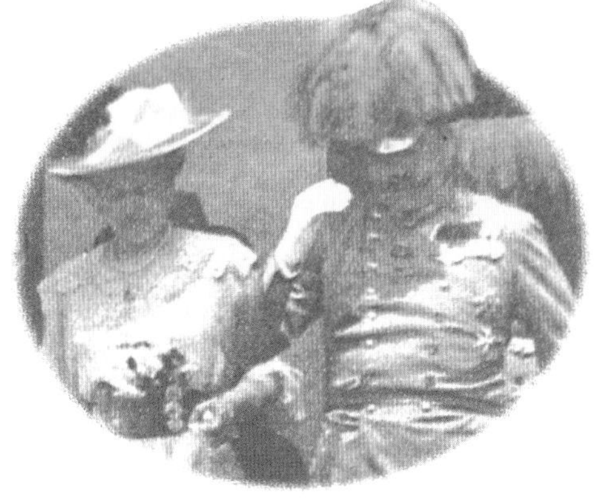

ARCHDUKE FERDINAND
On 28 June 1914, a Serbian terrorist shot Franz Ferdinand, heir to the throne of Austria and Hungary. Germany encouraged Austria to retaliate, or fight back, by declaring war on Serbia. A month after the assassination, World War I had begun.

BETWEEN 1914 AND 1918, a terrible war engulfed Europe. The war was called the First World War, or the Great War, because it affected almost every country in the world. It began because of the rivalry between several powerful European countries. Fighting started when the empire of Austria and Hungary declared war on Serbia. Soon, other countries joined the war. They formed two main groups: the Allies, composed of Britain, France, Italy, Russia, and the United States, versus the Central Powers – Germany, Austria-Hungary, and Turkey. In the beginning everyone thought the war would be short and glorious. Young men rushed to join the armies and navies. But it soon became clear that none of the opposing armies was strong enough to win a clear victory. Thousands of troops died, fighting to gain just a few hundred feet of the battlefield. In the end, the war, which some called the "war to end all wars", had achieved nothing. Within a few years a worse war broke out in Europe.

Allied countries are green, Central Powers are pink, and neutral countries are shown in beige.

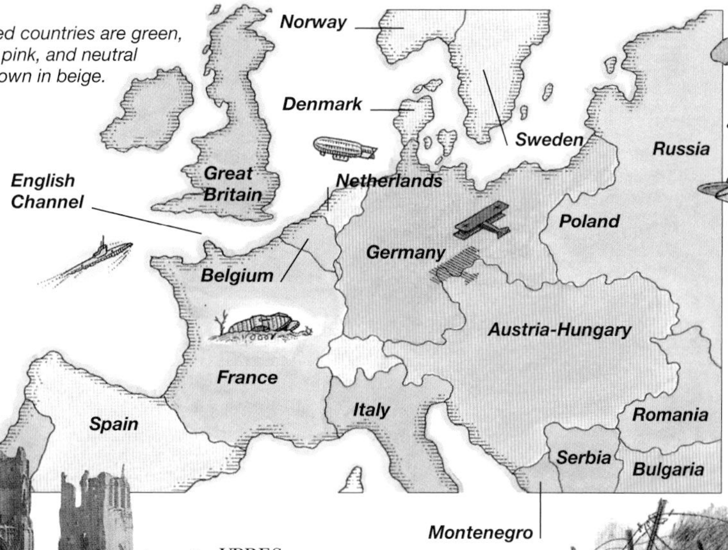

Norway
Denmark
Sweden
Russia
English Channel
Great Britain
Netherlands
Poland
Belgium
Germany
Austria-Hungary
France
Italy
Romania
Spain
Serbia
Bulgaria
Montenegro

COUNTRIES AT WAR
The war involved nearly 30 countries – more countries than any previous war. There was fighting in the Middle East, Africa, and the Pacific. However, most of the war was fought in Europe. The western front in northern France was a line of trenches that stretched from Switzerland to the English Channel. Soldiers on the eastern front fought in what is now Poland. Fighting took place on land, at sea, and in the air.

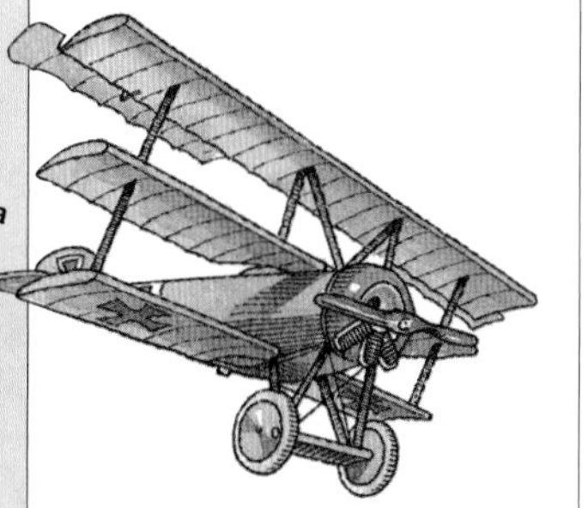

RED BARON
World War I was the first war in which airplanes were used for fighting. Germany's Manfred von Richthofen (the Red Baron) became one of the first air aces.

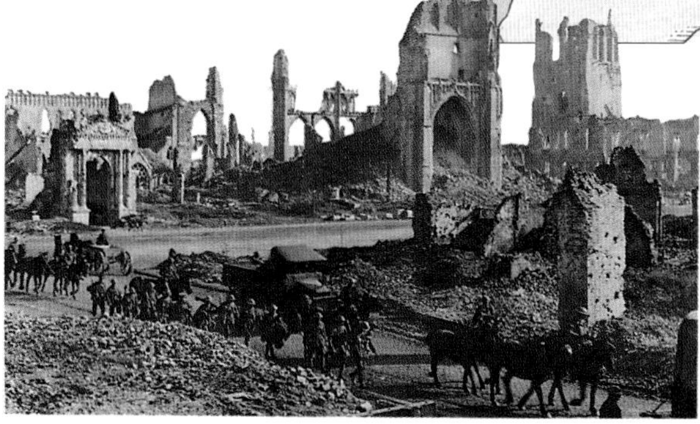

YPRES
The Belgian city of Ypres was a battleground several times during World War I. It was here that the Germans first used poison gas on the western front. By 1918 the town was devastated (left).

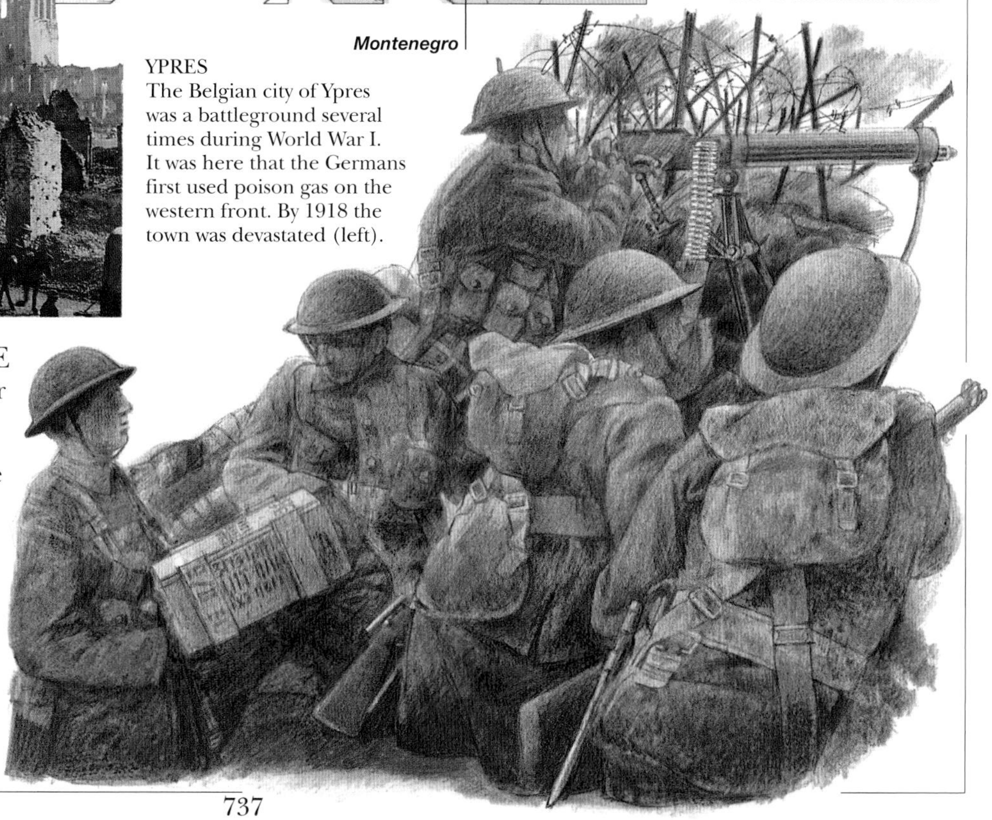

TRENCH WARFARE

The armies advanced as far they could, then dug trenches for shelter. Life in the trenches was miserable. Soldiers were often up to their knees in mud. Lice and rats added to their discomfort. When soldiers left the trenches to advance further, the enemy killed them by the millions with machine guns. Each side also had artillery – guns that fired huge shells – which killed many more and churned up the battlefield into a sea of mud.

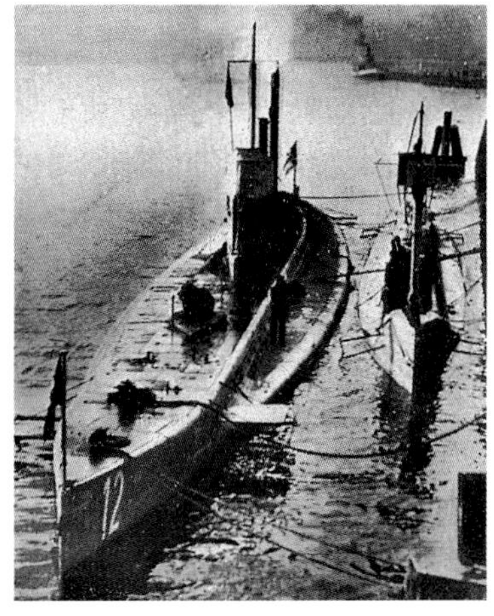

U-BOATS
German submarines called underwater boats, or U-boats, sank many cargo ships in the Atlantic, causing food shortages in Britain.

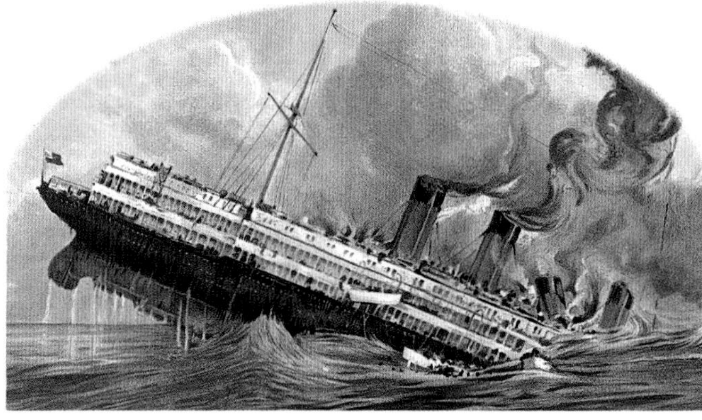

LUSITANIA
On 7 May 1915, a German U-boat torpedoed the British passenger liner *Lusitania.* More than 100 American passengers drowned, some of whom were very rich and famous. This angered many Americans and turned them against Germany. The sinking helped to bring the United States into the war on the Allied side.

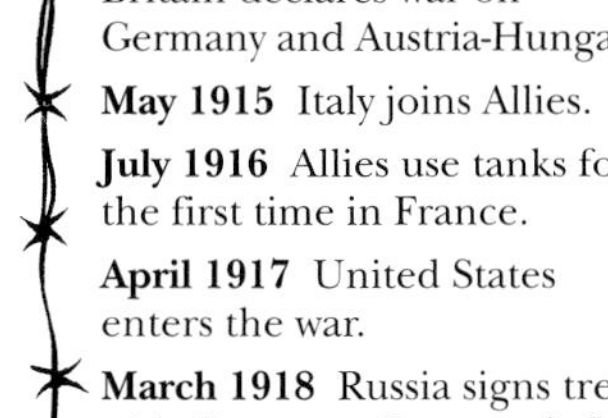

WORLD WAR I

June 1914 Assassination of Archduke Franz Ferdinand

July 1914 Austria-Hungary declares war on Serbia.

August 1914 Germany declares war on Russia and France and invades Belgium. Britain declares war on Germany and Austria-Hungary.

May 1915 Italy joins Allies.

July 1916 Allies use tanks for the first time in France.

April 1917 United States enters the war.

March 1918 Russia signs treaty with Germany. Germany's final huge attack at Marne fails.

September 1918 Allies begin their final attack.

November 1918 Germany signs armistice, ending the war.

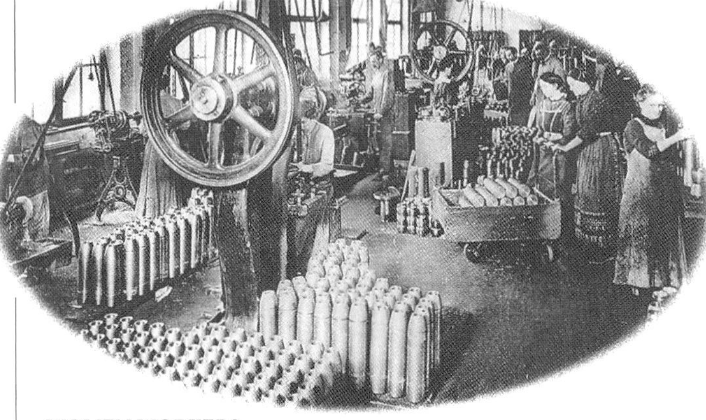

WOMEN WORKERS
As thousands of men went off to war, women took over their jobs in the factories. Most women worked long hours, and many had dangerous jobs, such as making ammunition. Their efforts disproved the old idea that women were inferior to men, and eventually led to women gaining the right to vote. But when the troops returned after the war, there was massive unemployment, and women lost their jobs.

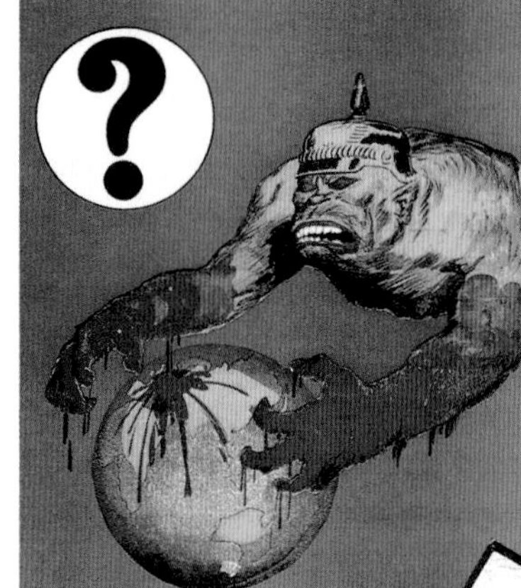

PROPAGANDA
Wartime posters and newspapers aimed to persuade people that the enemy was evil and that war must go on. The message of this propaganda, or government-controlled news, was that everyone should help by fighting, working, raising money, and making sacrifices. The poster (left) shows a frightening image of Germany with its hands on Europe.

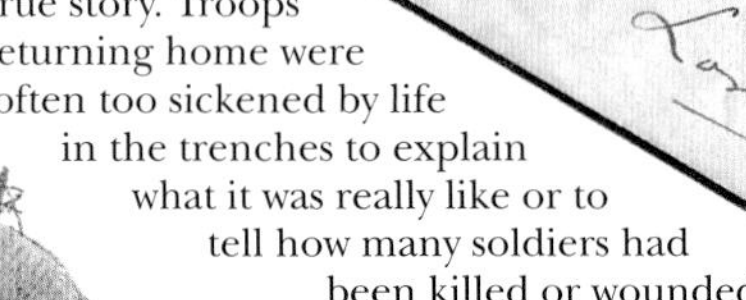

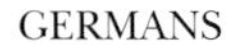

COMMUNICATION
People at home had little idea of the real conditions of the war. Officers read mail from soldiers and censored, or cut out, information that told the true story. Troops returning home were often too sickened by life in the trenches to explain what it was really like or to tell how many soldiers had been killed or wounded.

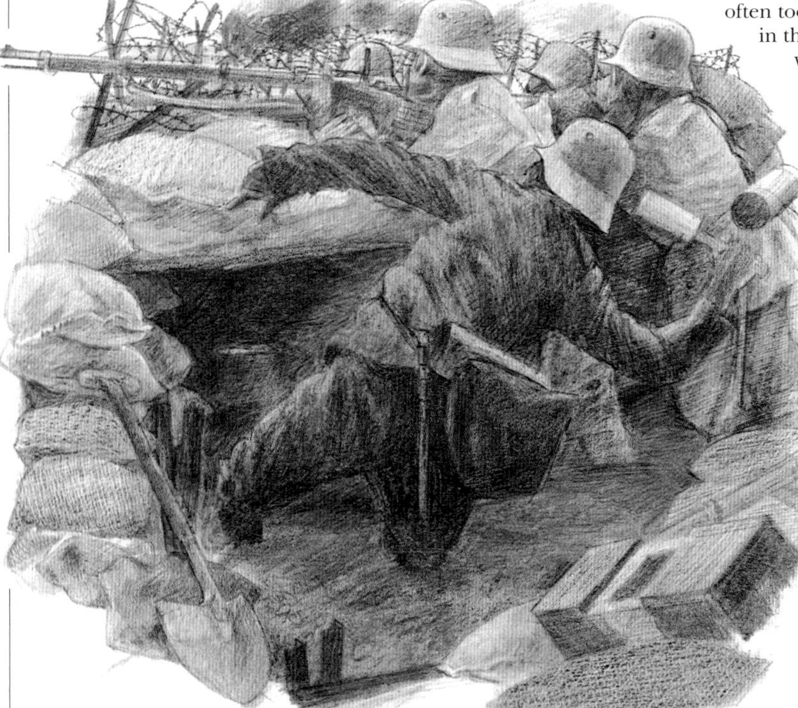

GERMANS
Until 1918, it looked as if Germany and her allies might win. But they were outnumbered, and when the British navy blocked the ports and cut off supplies of food and vital war materials, the German people rioted. They demanded food and peace, and the Kaiser – the German emperor – gave up his throne. Germany then made a peace treaty called the Treaty of Versailles with the Allied forces. The Germans lost much land and took the blame for starting the war.

DEATH TOLL
Germany and Russia each lost nearly two million soldiers in the war. Britain lost nearly one million. In all, 10 million died.

Find out more

DEPRESSION OF THE 1930S
WOMEN'S RIGHTS
WORLD WAR II

WORLD WAR II

IN 1939, GERMAN TANKS and bombers attacked Poland, and the bloodiest war in history began. Like World War I, World War II was a global war and was fought on the ground, in the air, and at sea. The war was a result of the rise to power of the German National Socialist or Nazi party, led by Adolf Hitler. The Nazis wanted to wipe out the memory of defeat in World War I. Within a year, German armies, with help from Italy, had occupied much of Europe. Only Britain opposed them. In 1941, Hitler invaded the Soviet Union. But the Soviet people fought hard and millions died. In the Pacific, the Japanese formed an alliance, called the Axis, with Germany and Italy. Japanese warplanes bombed the American naval base at Pearl Harbour, in Hawaii. This brought the United States into the war, and they joined the Soviet Union and Britain to form the Allies. By June 1945, Allied forces had defeated the Nazis in Europe; Japan surrendered in August. When the war ended, 45 million people had died and much of Europe was in ruins. Two new "superpowers" – the Soviet Union and the United States – began to dominate world politics.

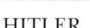

HITLER
In 1933, Adolf Hitler came to power in Germany as leader of the Nazi party. The Nazis were fascists: they were against Communism and believed in strong national government. The Nazis ruthlessly crushed anyone who opposed them. They enslaved and murdered Jews, gypsies, and other minorities, whom they blamed for all of Germany's problems, from defeat in World War I to unemployment and inflation.

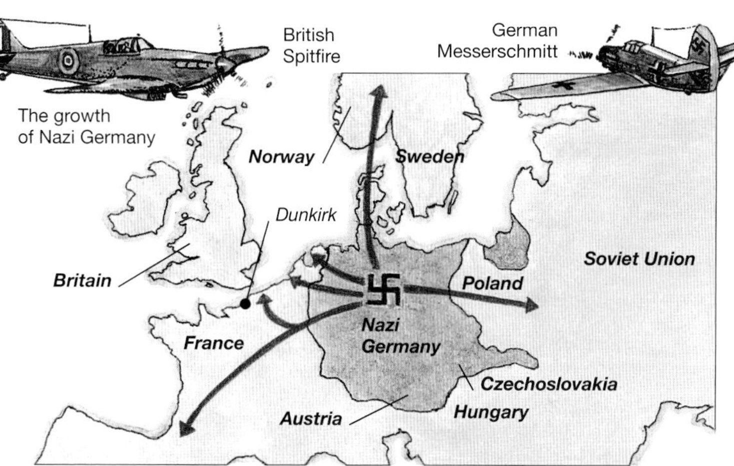

INVASION
In 1938, Hitler took control of Austria and parts of Czechoslovakia. Britain and France did not oppose him, and he went on to invade Poland. Britain and France then declared war on Germany. German troops smashed into France in 1940, sweeping aside the armies of Britain and France. Fleets of fishing boats and pleasure steamers from the southern coast of England helped the Royal Navy to rescue the retreating Allied soldiers from the beaches at Dunkirk, on the coast of France.

BLITZ

Between August and October 1940, the British Royal Air Force fought the Luftwaffe – the German air force – in the Battle of Britain, and finally won. Without control of the skies, Hitler could not invade Britain. His bombers began to bomb British cities during the night. This "blitzkrieg" or blitz, killed 40,000 people, mostly civilians.

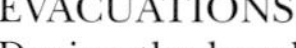

EVACUATIONS
During the bombing of major cities, such as London, thousands of British children were evacuated to country towns and villages where they were much safer.

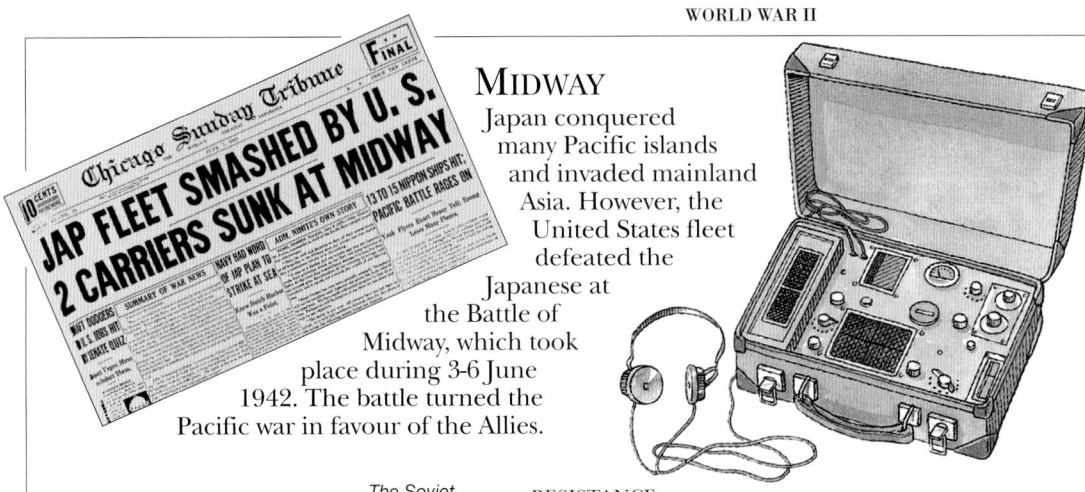

Chicago Sunday Tribune
FINAL
JAP FLEET SMASHED BY U. S.
2 CARRIERS SUNK AT MIDWAY
13 TO 15 NIPPON SHIPS HIT;
PACIFIC BATTLE RAGES ON
SUMMARY OF WAR NEWS
NAVY HAD WORD OF JAP PLAN TO STRIKE AT SEA
ADM. NIMITZ'S OWN STORY

MIDWAY

Japan conquered many Pacific islands and invaded mainland Asia. However, the United States fleet defeated the Japanese at the Battle of Midway, which took place during 3-6 June 1942. The battle turned the Pacific war in favour of the Allies.

RESISTANCE
Many people in Europe hated the Nazi occupation of their countries. So they formed secret resistance movements to spy on and fight the enemy. They used hidden radios (above) to work behind the battle lines. Resistance workers risked torture and death if they were discovered.

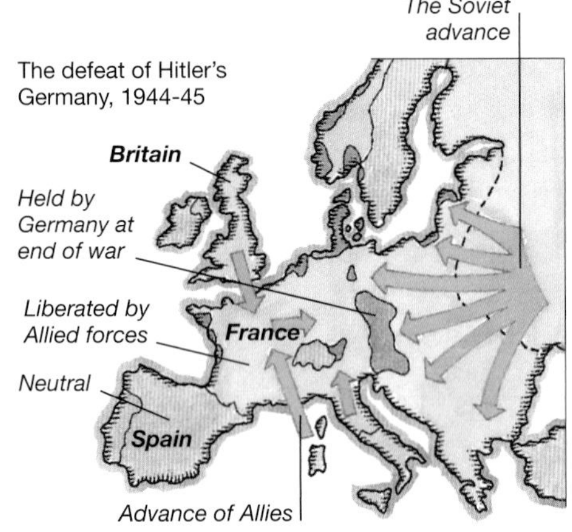

The Soviet advance
The defeat of Hitler's Germany, 1944-45

Neutral
Spain
Advance of Allies

PEACE IN EUROPE
By the spring of 1945, the Allies had recaptured most of occupied Europe and began to cross the Rhine River into Germany. In the east, the Soviet army swept toward Berlin, Germany's capital. Crushed between these two powerful forces, the German armies surrendered. Hitler committed suicide, and the biggest and most expensive war in human history ended.

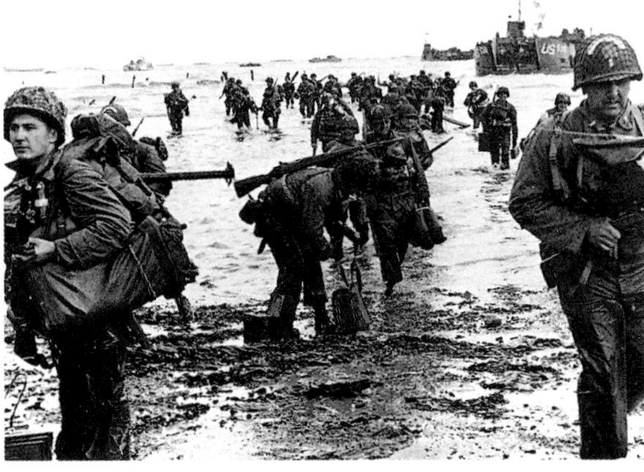

D-DAY
In June 1944, Allied troops invaded occupied Europe in the greatest seaborne landing ever mounted. Invasion day was code-named D-day. The D stood for deliverance. After a bitter struggle, and aided by resistance fighters, the Allied forces broke through, and the German soldiers retreated or were taken as prisoners.

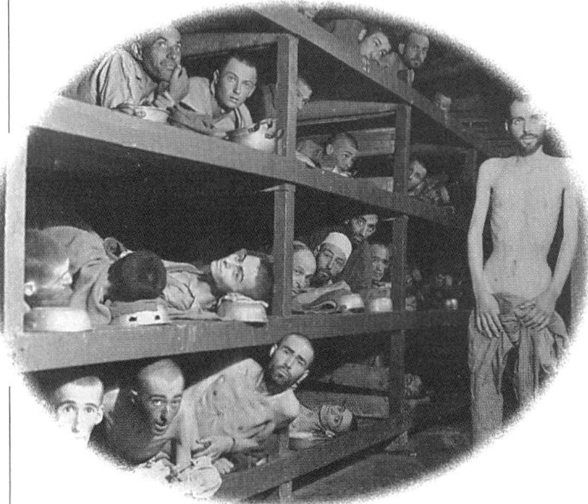

CONCENTRATION CAMP

After Germany surrendered, Allied troops discovered horrifying concentration (prison) camps throughout Europe, where the Nazis had imprisoned up to 26 million people they considered "undesirable", including millions of Jews. The prisoners were starved and tortured, and many were eventually gassed to death.

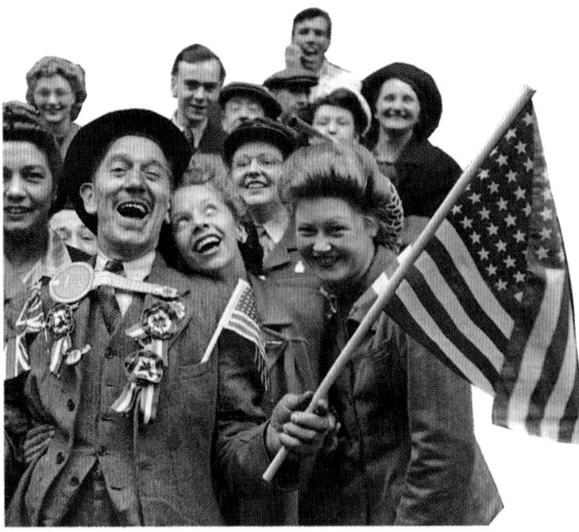

VE DAY
On May 8, 1945, the Allies celebrated VE (Victory in Europe) Day. However, there were still another three months of bitter fighting in the Pacific. In August 1945, US planes dropped two atom bombs on Japan, destroying the cities of Hiroshima and Nagasaki. This was done to force Japan to surrender quickly and so save Allied lives that would be lost if the Allies invaded Japan. Within a few weeks the Japanese surrendered and the war ended.

WORLD WAR II

1 September 1939 Germany invades Poland. Britain and France declare war on Germany two days later.

April 1940 Germany invades Denmark and Norway.

May 1940 Germany invades Belgium, the Netherlands, and France.

June 1940 Germans enter Paris, and France signs an armistice (peace agreement) with Germany.

April 1941 Germany invades Greece and Yugoslavia.

June 1941 Germany invades the Soviet Union.

September 1941 Siege of Leningrad (Soviet Union) begins; lasts over two and a half years.

December 7, 1941 Japanese planes attack Pearl Harbor. The United States, Britain, and Canada declare war on Japan.

February 1942 Japanese capture many Pacific islands.

August 1942 German attack on Stalingrad (Soviet Union) begins.

November 1942 Under General Montgomery the British defeat Germany, led by Rommel, at El Alamein, Egypt. Allied troops land in French North Africa to fight Germany and Italy.

January 1943 German armies besieged in Stalingrad surrender.

May 1943 German armies in North Africa surrender to the Allies.

July 1943 Allies invade Sicily.

September 1943 Allied forces land in Italy. Italy surrenders.

June 1944 Allied forces land in Normandy, north-west France, in the D-day invasion.

May 1945 German forces surrender; war in Europe ends.

August 1945 Allies drop atomic bombs on Japan.

September 2, 1945 Japan signs an unconditional surrender, ending World War II.

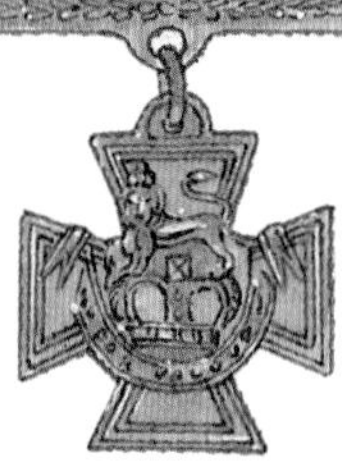

Find out more

Held by Germany at end of war
Liberated by Allied forces

CHURCHILL, SIR WINSTON
HOLOCAUST
NUCLEAR AGE
ROOSEVELT, FRANKLIN DELANO
WORLD WAR I

WORMS

WE DESCRIBE MANY long, slender, soft, legless creatures as worms. There are thousands of different kinds, ranging from the tiny hookworm to the much larger bootlace worm. The word worm is a fairly general term, and there are a number of distinct groups. Annelids, or segmented worms, include leeches, earthworms, and ragworms. Nematodes, or roundworms, have long tubelike bodies without segments. There are at least 12,000 kinds of roundworms. Some, including hookworms, cause serious diseases in humans such as river blindness and elephantiasis. Flatworms, or playhelminths, make up a third group. There are more than 17,500 kinds, and they include the parasitic flukes and tapeworms that infest sheep, pigs, and other animals.

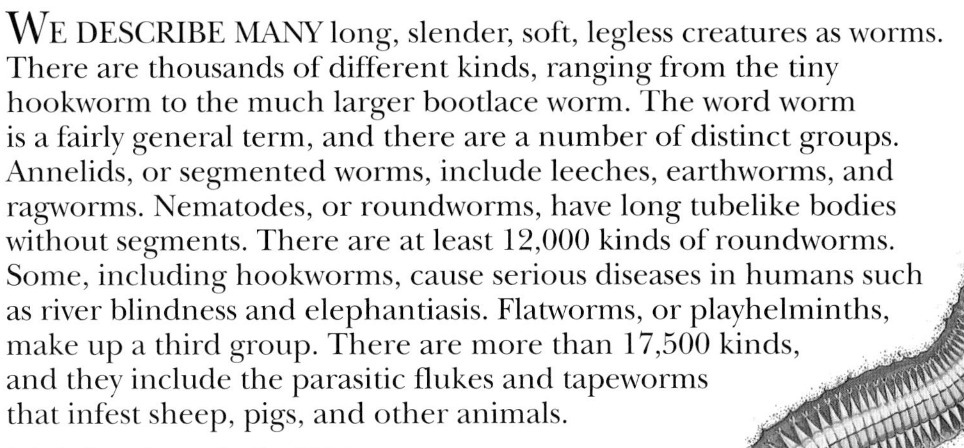

Ragworm lives in sand and under rocks.

Undigested sand comes out of the worm's rear end and forms a worm cast on the surface.

Lugworm eats sand at head end.

SEASHORE WORMS
Ragworms are active predators that seize prey such as smaller worms. Their name comes from the flaps along the body that make the animal look like a strip of torn rag. Large ragworms can bite through human skin and draw blood. Lugworms live in U-shaped burrows under the surface of the sand, eating the sand and mud and digesting the nutrients in them.

Entire body may be more than 9 m (30 ft) long.

Proglottis (single segment)

Scolex (pin-sized head) has hooks.

TAPEWORM
These long worms are parasitic; they live in the digestive systems of animals such as cats and dogs. A cat, for example, becomes infected when it eats a mouse that has eaten a plant coated with tapeworm eggs. The eggs hatch into larvae inside the mouse, then develop into tapeworms once inside the cat. When waste matter passes out of the cat, tapeworm eggs also pass out.

Tapeworm grows in segments. These segments grow from the head in a long, widening ribbon. Each segment contains a full set of reproductive organs.

POND WORMS
Even a small pond contains many worms, such as leeches and bloodworms. Leeches have 33 body segments. They suck the blood or fluids of other animals, including mammals and fish. The leech can swim by flapping its body, which has a sucker at each end. Bloodworms, or tubifex worms, show deep red blood through their thin skin.

Worm's tiny bristles grip the soil particles.

Intestine

Upper main blood vessel

Hearts

Mouth

Reproductive organs

Main nerve

INSIDE AN EARTHWORM
Although earthworms are annelids, with a body divided into many similar segments, not all the segments are the same. A digestive tube runs along the worm's body. The main nerves come together at the head end of the body to form a simple brain. The blood vessels in the worm's body sometimes form five pairs of hearts.

Tubifex (bloodworm)

Hirudo (Medicinal leech)

Fat part of body is called the saddle.

EARTHWORM

There are more than 3,000 kinds of earthworm. These long-bodied animals are responsible for the health of the soil. As the earthworms push their way along, they take in soil at the head end, digesting nutrients in the soil particles. The undigested remains that come out at the rear end form a worm cast. By burrowing in the earth, worms mix the soil layers, and their burrows allow air and water to soak downward, generally increasing the fertility of the soil.

BLOODWORM TAILS
Pond-dwelling bloodworms, or tubifex worms, wave their rear ends in the water to gather oxygen. Their heads are buried in the mud, taking in nutrients.

Find out more
ANIMALS
MEDICINE, HISTORY OF
SOIL

WRITERS AND POETS

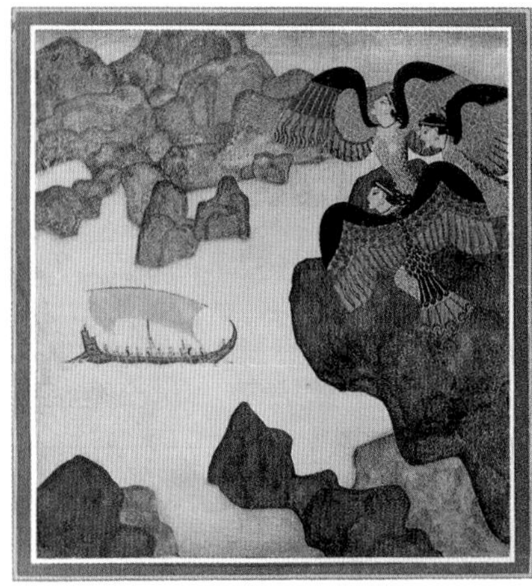

A READER'S IMAGINATION can be excited by the way in which writers and poets use words. Writers create fantasy worlds for readers to explore. Historical novelists and science fiction writers transport us back to the past or into the distant future. Others writers, such as journalists, write in a way that creates a lifelike picture of real events they have experienced. And poets arrange words into patterns or rhymes that bring pleasure just by their sound or their shape on the page. A writer is anyone who expresses facts, ideas, thoughts, or opinions in words. Most writers hope or expect that their work will be published – printed in books or magazines and read by thousands of people. But some writers, including diarists such as the Englishman Samuel Pepys (1633-1703), write for their own pleasure. They do not always expect their work to be published. Poets are people who write in verse, or poetry. Poets make sure the lines of their poems form a regular pattern, so that, unlike prose, or ordinary writing, the poem has a rhythmic sound.

HOMER
One of the world's first writers was the Ancient Greek poet Homer, who lived about 2,700 years ago. He wrote long epic verses called *The Iliad* and *The Odyssey*. In *The Odyssey* the beautiful singing of the bird-like sirens lured sailors to the island where the sirens lived.

WRITING
Even a short novel has more than 50,000 words, so writing can be hard work. To make it easier, most writers organize their work carefully. Writing methods are quite individual. Although many authors use word processors, pen and paper are still popular writer's tools. American Raymond Chandler (1888-1959), who wrote detective novels, had a favourite way of writing throughout his working life.

Like any author, Chandler would have used maps to check his hero's movements around Los Angeles, the setting for many of his novels.

Chandler typed the first draft, or version, of his books on yellow paper. He used half-size sheets because he made changes by retyping, not by changing words with a pen. Retyping a whole sheet would have taken longer.

Books such as J. S. Hatcher's Textbook of Pistols *gave Chandler the accurate information he needed to make his stories seem lifelike and real.*

Chandler's secretary typed a clean version of the finished draft on white paper.

Chandler smoked a pipe and drank coffee as he worked. At times he also drank a lot of alcohol

ANNE FRANK
During World War II, the German Nazi government persecuted millions of European Jews. To escape, Anne Frank (born 1929) and her Jewish family hid in a secret attic in a Netherlands office. The diary that Anne wrote while in hiding was later published. It is a deeply moving and tragic account of her ordeal. Anne died in a prison camp in 1945.

MANUSCRIPT
A writer's original typed or handwritten version of a work is called a manuscript. The publisher writes instructions to the printer on the manuscript, and may also make changes and revisions to improve the writing. For example, F. Scott Fitzgerald (1896-1940) was bad at spelling, and his publisher corrected these errors.

The manuscript for this page, with the publisher's corrections

CHAUCER

Geoffrey Chaucer (c.1340-1400) was an English government official. He wrote poems in English at a time when most English writers were writing in French and Latin. Chaucer began his most famous work, the *Canterbury Tales*, in about 1386. It is a collection of stories told by pilgrims travelling from London to Canterbury. The stories tell us much about 14th-century life and are often very amusing.

HARRIET BEECHER STOWE

Uncle Tom's Cabin is a powerful anti-slavery novel written by Harriet Beecher Stowe (1811-96) in 1852. It became extremely popular all over the world, even in the southern states of America, where owning a copy was illegal at the time.

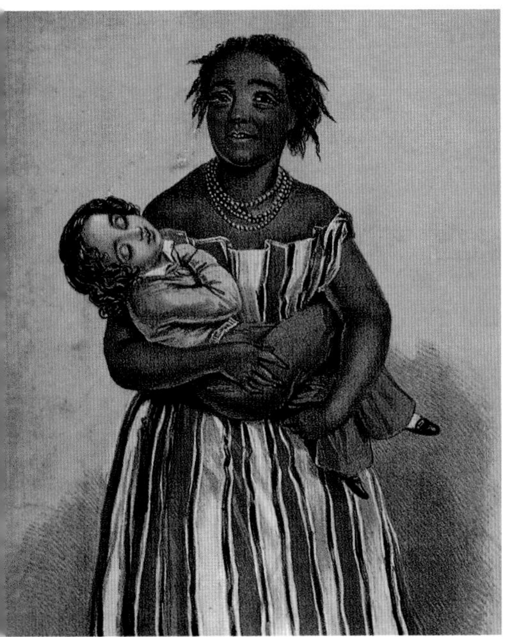

DICKENS

Some of the greatest novels in the English language are the work of Charles Dickens (1812-70). He wrote colourful and exciting novels, such as *Oliver Twist*, *Nicholas Nickleby*, and *David Copperfield*, which also drew attention to the poverty and social injustices of 19th-century England.

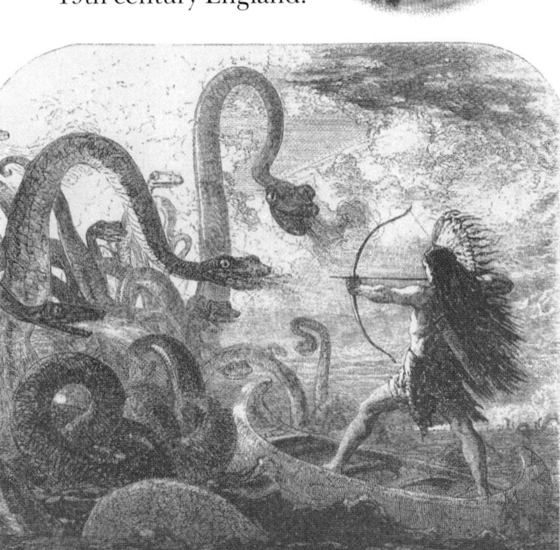

LONGFELLOW

During his lifetime, Henry Wadsworth Longfellow (1807-82) was the most popular poet in the United States. His *Song of Hiawatha*, which was published in 1855, sold more than a million copies while Longfellow was still alive. The poem tells the story of a Native American tribe before America was colonized by Europeans. Longfellow wrote on many subjects and in many styles, but he is best remembered for his romantic "picture poems" about American life.

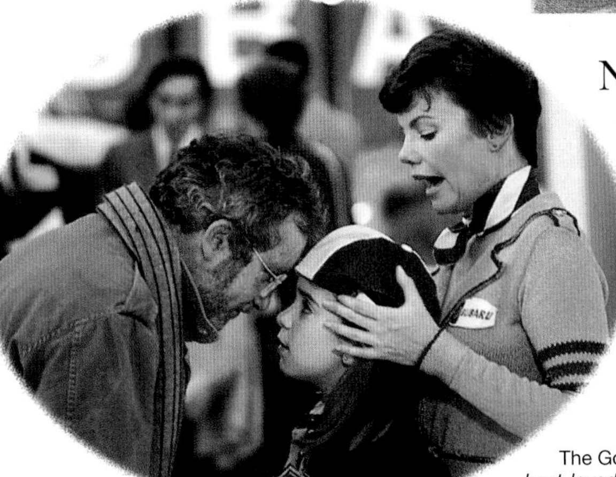

The Goodbye Girl, one of Neil Simon's best-loved films, is set in New York.

NEIL SIMON

Playwright Neil Simon was born in New York City on 4 July 1927. He has written more than 25 plays and musicals, many of which have been made into films. Most of his plays deal with aspects of ordinary American life. However, the writer's insight and sense of humour ensure that his plays appeal to people of all nationalities.

LITERARY FILE

c. 2300 B.C. Ancient Egyptian writers create the world's first literature, the *Book of the Dead.*

c. 600 B.C. Greek poet Sappho writes early lyric poetry (poetry with music).

c. 500 B.C. Greek poet Aeschylus (525-456 B.C.) writes the earliest dramas.

c. A.D.100 Greek writer Plutarch (A.D. 46-120) writes *The Parallel Lives*, the first biography.

1420 Zeami Motokiyo (1363-1443), the greatest writer of Japanese Noh dramas, writes *Shikadosho* (Book of the Way of the Highest Flower).

1740-42 Englishman Samuel Richardson (1689-1761) writes one of the first English novels, *Pamela, or, Virtue Rewarded.*

1765 Horace Walpole (1717-97), an Englishman, writes a ghost story, *The Castle of Otranto.*

1819-20 American Washington Irving (1783-1859) publishes one of the first books of short stories, which includes *The Legend of Sleepy Hollow* and *Rip Van Winkle.*

1841 American writer Edgar Allan Poe (1809-49) publishes *The Murders in the Rue Morgue*, the first detective story.

1847 English novelist Charlotte Brontë writes *Jane Eyre* under the false name Currer Bell, because it is still unacceptable for "respectable" women to write fiction.

1864 Jules Verne (1828-1905), a Frenchman, writes the first science fiction story, *Journey to the Center of the Earth.*

1956 The performance of *Waiting for Godot* by Irish-French dramatist Samuel Beckett (1906-89) opens the way for modern drama.

1993 American novelist Toni Morrison (born 1931), author of *Song of Solomon* and *Beloved*, becomes the first black American to win the Nobel Prize for Literature.

Find out more

BOOKS
BYRON, LORD
DICKENS, CHARLES
LITERATURE
POETRY
SLAVERY

X-RAYS

TO THE EARLY pioneers of medicine, the thought of looking through the body of a living person would probably have seemed like magic. But today it is routine for doctors and dentists to take pictures of their patients' bones and teeth with an x-ray camera. X-rays are invisible waves, like light or radio waves. They can travel through soft materials just as light passes through glass. For example, x-rays can travel through flesh and skin. But hard materials such as bone and metal stop x-rays, so bone and metal show up as a shadow on an x-ray picture. X-rays have many uses: scientists use them to probe into the molecular structure of materials such as plastics, and engineers make x-ray scans of aircraft to find cracks that could cause mechanical failure. In addition, the Sun, stars, and other objects in space produce x-rays naturally.

WILHELM ROENTGEN
The German scientist Wilhelm Roentgen (1845-1923) discovered x-rays in 1895. Roentgen did not understand what these rays were, so he named them x-rays.

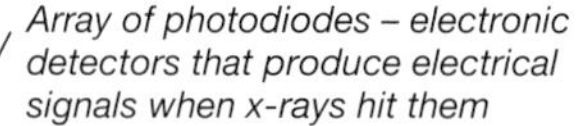

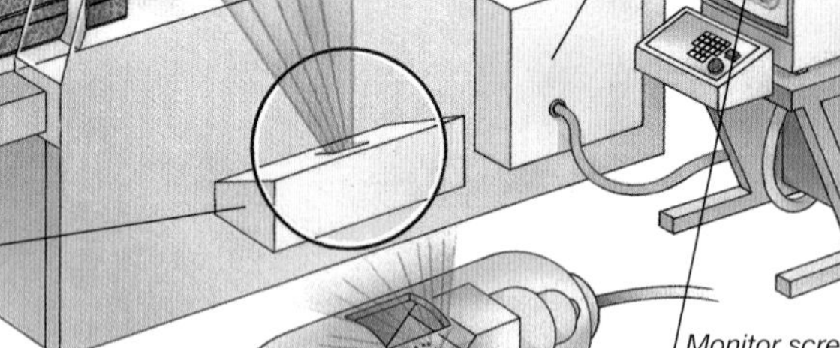

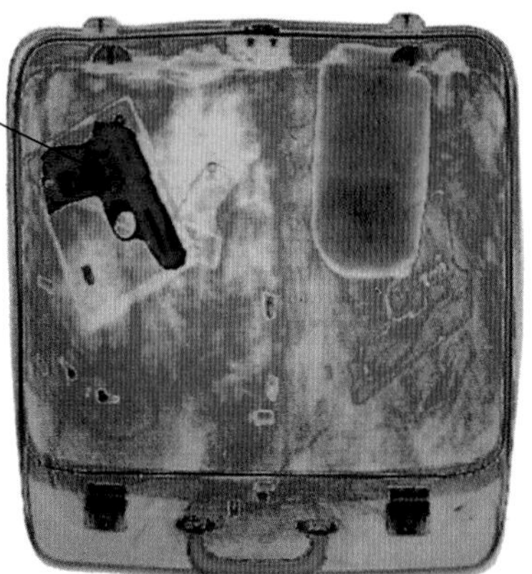

Scanner is lined with lead to prevent x-rays from escaping.

Computer receives electrical signals from the photodiodes and converts them into an image of the case.

Monitor screen displays contents of case to security guards.

A metal object such as a pistol does not allow x-rays to pass through it, so the pistol shows up on screen.

BAGGAGE SCANNER

Airports have x-ray scanners (left) to check baggage for weapons and other dangerous objects. An x-ray tube produces a beam of x-rays, and a conveyor belt carries each suitcase into the path of the beam. Electronic detectors pick up the x-rays once they have passed through the case. A computer uses signals from the detectors to build up a picture of the contents of the case.

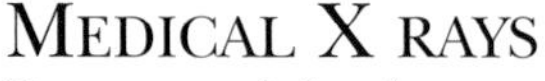

As the electrons crash into the target, atoms of the metal produce the x-ray beam.
A strong electric current heats a wire. The energy from the electric current knocks some electrons out of the atoms in the wire.
A powerful electric field pulls electrons at high speed toward the metal target.

X-RAY TUBE
Like a light bulb, an x-ray tube is filled with an inert (non-reacting) gas, but produces x-rays instead of light.

MEDICAL X RAYS

Doctors and dentists use x-ray machines to look inside their patients' bodies without using surgery. The machine makes an x-ray picture on a piece of photographic film. The photograph is a negative, and bones show up in white. Large doses of x-rays are harmful, so x-ray examinations must be carefully controlled as a precaution.

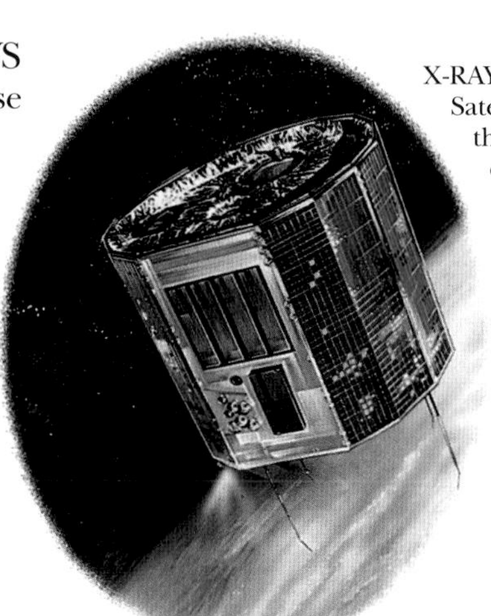

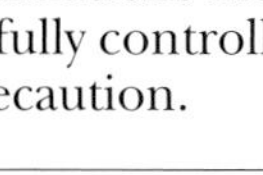

X-RAYS IN SPACE
Satellites containing x-ray telescopes orbit the Earth. The telescopes detect x-rays coming from the Sun and stars, and from objects such as black holes. The satellites send x-ray pictures back to Earth. Astronomers use these pictures to discover and understand more of the universe.

Find out more
AIRPORTS
ATOMS AND MOLECULES
DOCTORS
MEDICINE, HISTORY OF
STARS

ZOOS

PEOPLE BEGAN TO KEEP animals in zoological gardens, or zoos, more than 3,000 years ago, when rulers in China established a huge zoo, called the Gardens of Intelligence. Today, most cities have a zoo, wildlife park, or aquarium, which provide a chance to observe and study hundreds of different animals. However, many people do not agree on the value of zoos. Zoo supporters say that zoos give people the opportunity to be close to animals, which they would never otherwise experience; zoos help us appreciate the wonder of the natural world; and zoo staff carry out scientific research and important conservation work, such as breeding rare species. Zoo critics believe that it is wrong to keep animals in captivity; the creatures behave unnaturally, and in poorly run zoos they suffer because of stress, unsuitable food, dirty conditions, and disease.

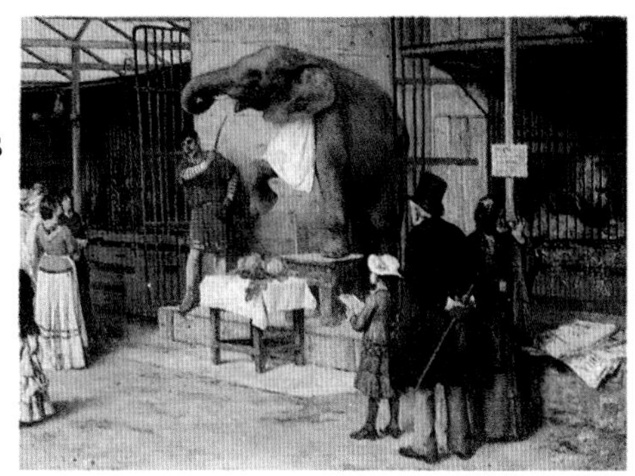

EARLY ZOOS
In early zoos, animals such as elephants were taught to perform for the visitors, as shown in this picture. Animals are no longer trained to perform for the public. The purpose of a zoo is to enable people to see how wild animals behave in their natural surroundings. The ideal solution is to save wild areas, with their animals and plants, and allow people to visit these, but this is not always possible.

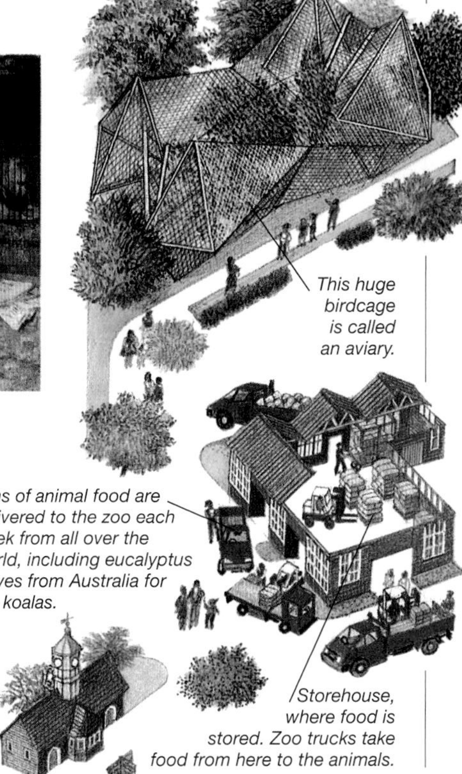

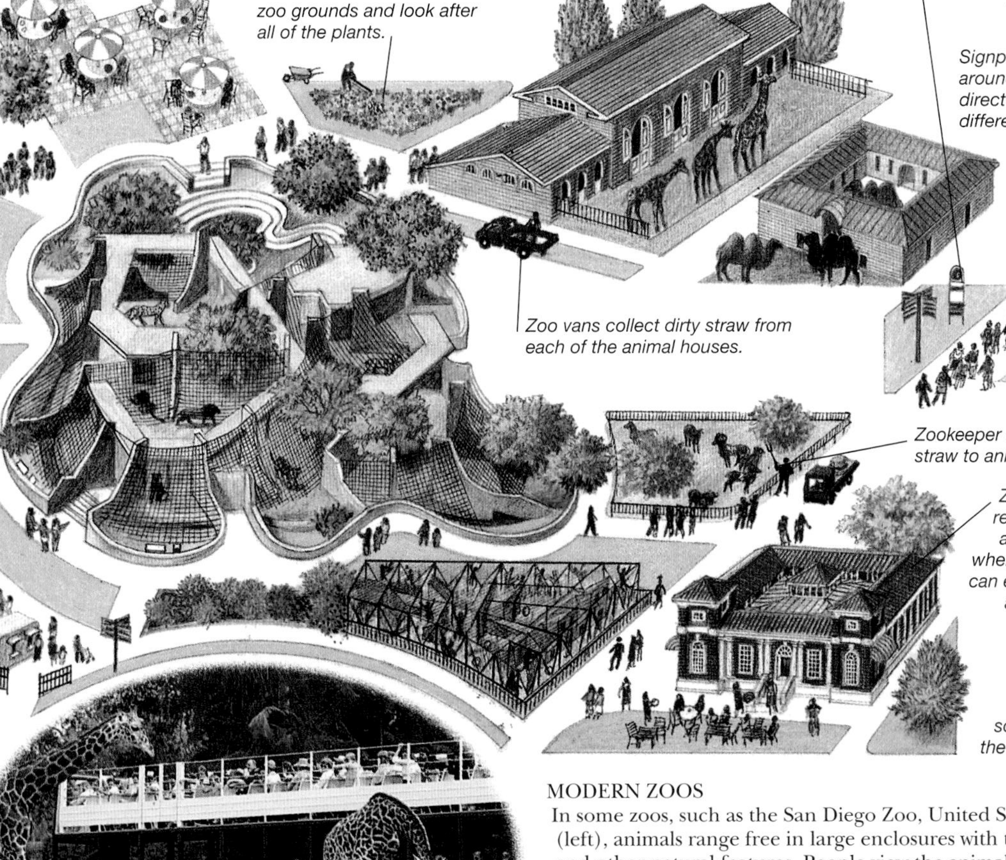

This huge birdcage is called an aviary.
Tons of animal food are delivered to the zoo each week from all over the world, including eucalyptus leaves from Australia for the koalas.
Storehouse, where food is stored. Zoo trucks take food from here to the animals.

Display boards and guide books full of information provide education.
Gardeners take care of the zoo grounds and look after all of the plants.
Signposts around the zoo direct visitors to different areas.
Thousands of school-children visit zoos each year with their teachers.
Zoo vans collect dirty straw from each of the animal houses.
Zookeeper delivering straw to animals
Zoos have restaurants and cafés, where visitors can eat, drink, and relax.
Visitors can buy souvenirs in the zoo shop.

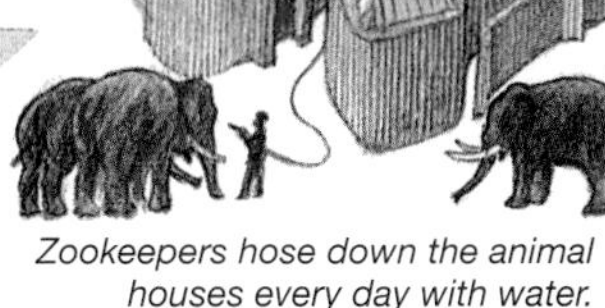

Zookeepers hose down the animal houses every day with water.

MODERN ZOOS
In some zoos, such as the San Diego Zoo, United States, (left), animals range free in large enclosures with trees and other natural features. People view the animals through glass panels rather than iron bars. You can even see the animals from an open-topped bus. In most countries, inspectors can arrive unannounced to check the welfare of the creatures. A few zoos still treat their captives badly, and organizations such as Zoo Check work toward ensuring better conditions in zoos.

HOW ZOOS ARE RUN
A zoo employs zookeepers to look after the animals, zoologists (scientists who study animals), veterinarians, accountants, architects, cooks, gardeners, builders, and many other people. The zoo manager must keep all of these people organized because there are many jobs to do, such as ordering the correct food for each animal and running the souvenir shop and the restaurants. Visitors have to pay an entrance fee toward the upkeep of the zoo, but most zoos also need government funds.

Find out more
ANIMALS
CONSERVATION and endangered species

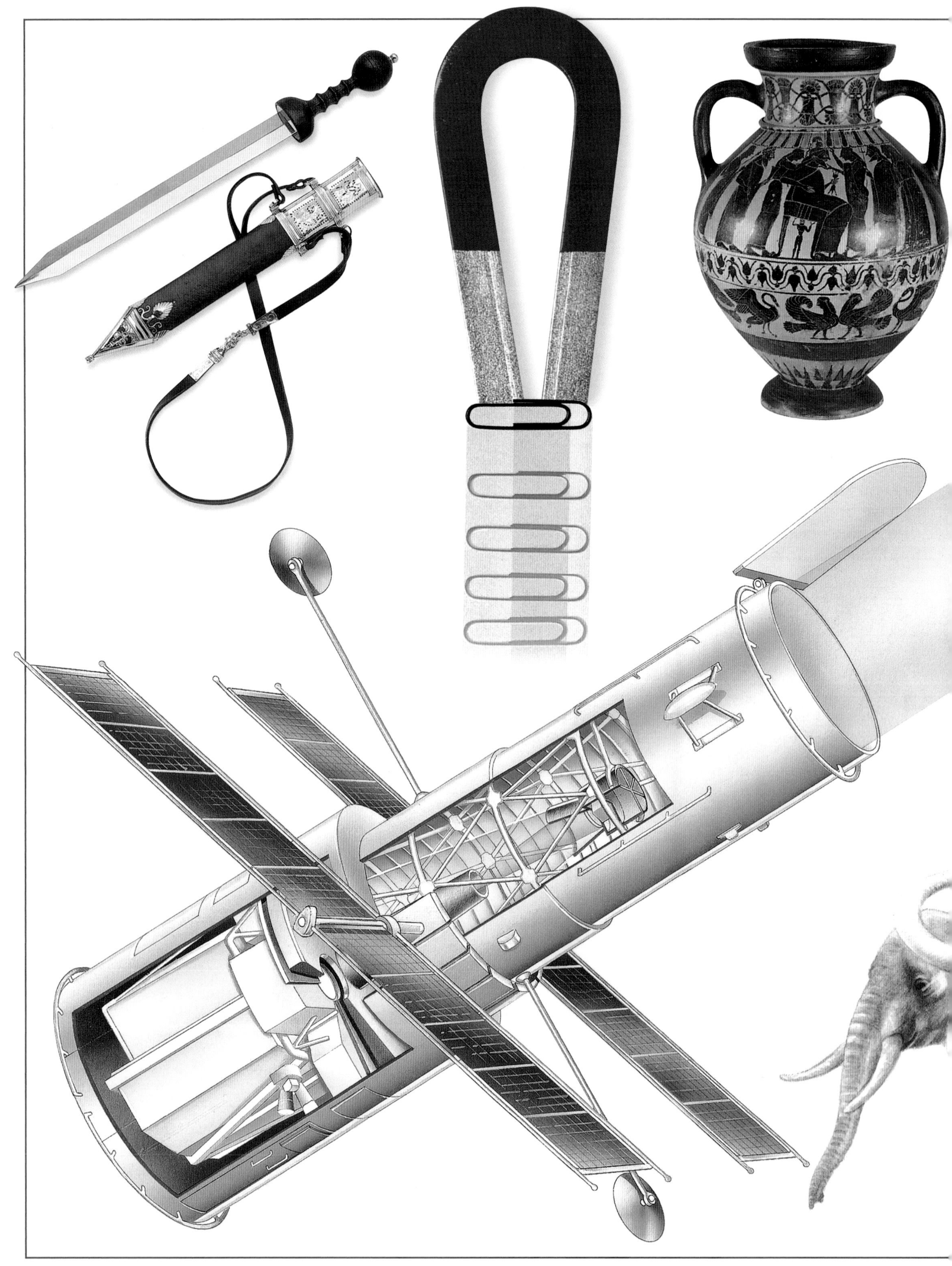

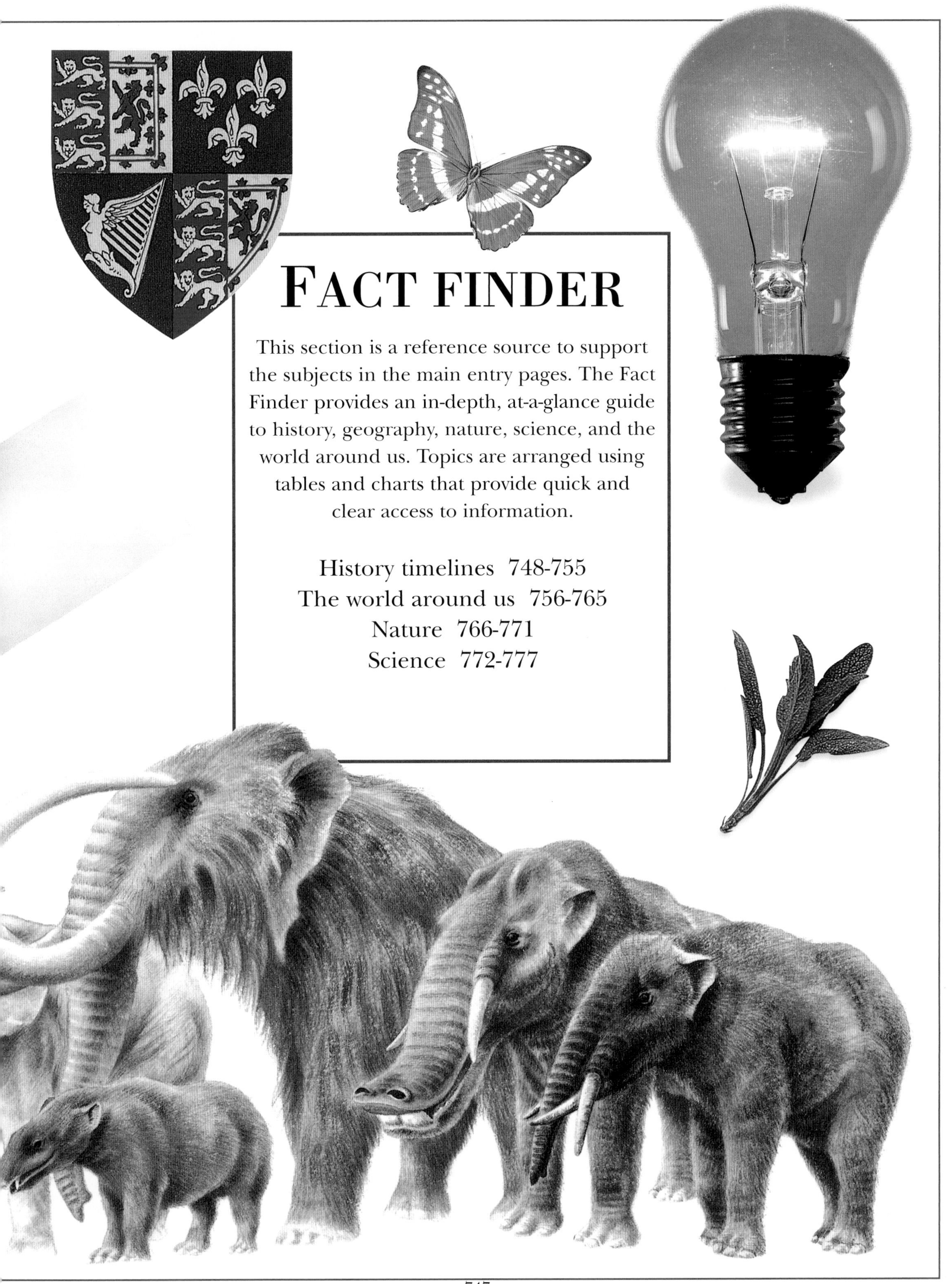

FACT FINDER

This section is a reference source to support the subjects in the main entry pages. The Fact Finder provides an in-depth, at-a-glance guide to history, geography, nature, science, and the world around us. Topics are arranged using tables and charts that provide quick and clear access to information.

B.C.	7000	6000	5000	4000	3000	2000
AFRICA	c. 7000 Fishing starts in the Sahara, North Africa		c. 5000 Farming begins in Egypt	c. 3200 The earliest hieroglyphic script, Egypt	c. 2650 Pyramid building begins in Egypt	
AMERICAS	c. 7000 Earliest crops grown in Mexico		c. 5000 Maize first cultivated in Mexico	c. 3500 Llama first used as pack animal, Peru		c. 1100 Olmec culture, San Lor
ASIA	c. 7000 Farming begins in western Asia		c. 5000 Stone Age settlements appear in China	c. 3100 Bronze casting starts in the Middle East	c. 2300 Sumer civilization reaches its height	c. 2000 Sumeria rule ends
EUROPE	c. 6500 Cereal farming begins in Southeast Europe	c. 6000 Copper and gold metalworking starts	c. 4500 Vinca copper culture begins in Yugoslavia		c. 3000 Bronze Age begins in Crete	c. 2000 Minoan civilization, Crete
OCEANIA	Oceania remains in Stone Age until A.D. 1770.					

AFRICA

1,500,000 B.C. – 2500 B.C. EARLIEST PEOPLES

1,500,000 B.C.
Our direct ancestors, *Homo erectus*, inhabit Africa and move outwards to Middle East and the rest of the world.

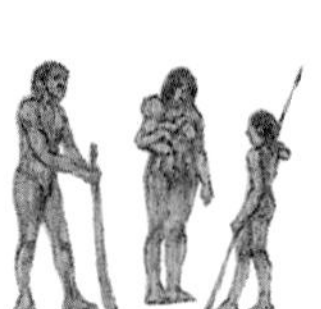

c. 7000 B.C.
People begin to herd cattle in the Sahara.

c. 3000 B.C.
Egyptians develop hieroglyphic writing.

c. 2600 B.C.
Construction of the Great Pyramid at Giza, Egypt.

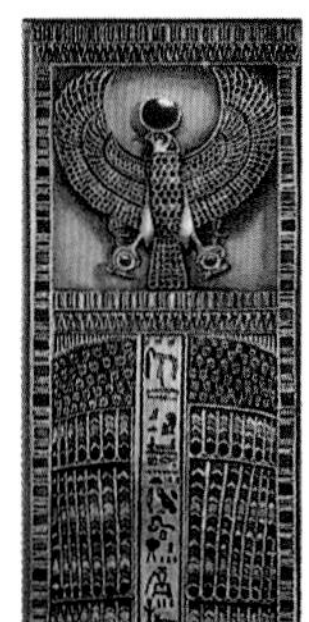

2500 B.C. – A.D. 1400 GREAT CIVILIZATIONS

c. 1503 B.C.
Hatshepsut, woman pharaoh (ruler) of Egypt, begins her reign.

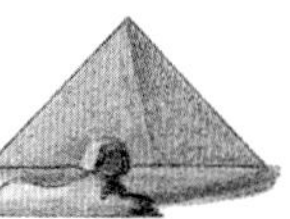

900 B.C.
Kingdom of Meroë established. Towns, temples, and pyramids are built, all showing influence of Egypt.

814 B.C.
Phoenicians found the city of Carthage in North Africa. Phoenician industries include dyeing, metal-working, glass-working, pottery, and carving.

c. 671 B.C.
Assyrians conquer Egypt.They are great builders, and decorate their palaces with big stone reliefs.

500 B.C.
Nok culture begins in Nigeria. People produce terracotta sculptures.

332 B.C.
Alexander the Great conquers Egypt.

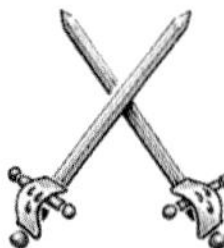

c. 290 B.C.
World's greatest library founded in Alexandria, Egypt.

100 B.C.
Camel arrives in the Sahara from Arabia.

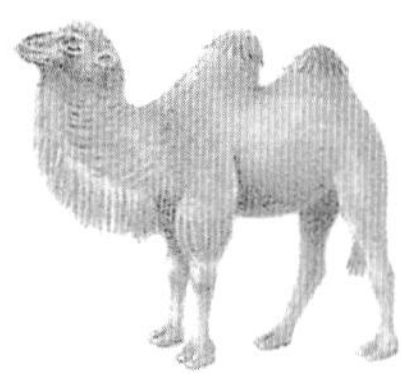

A.D. 100
Civilization of Aksum begins in Ethiopia. It trades at sea and exports ivory.

A.D. 641
Islamic Arabs occupy Egypt; they begin a conquest of North Africa.

A.D. 971
The world's first university is founded in Cairo, Egypt.

c. 1300
West African kingdom of Benin excels in casting realistic figures in bronze.

1400 – 1900 EUROPEAN IMPACT AND THE SLAVE TRADE

1430
Great Zimbabwe is built and trades gold to Muslims on the East African coast.

1488
The Portuguese navigator Bartholomeu Diaz rounds the Cape of Good Hope.

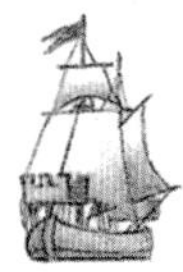

1510
The first African slaves are shipped to the Caribbean.

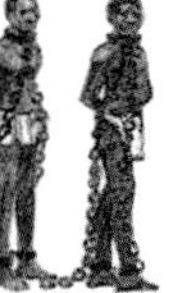

1652
Boers – Dutch settlers – set up a colony in Cape of Good Hope.

1787
The British establish a colony in Sierra Leone, West Africa.

1795
The British acquire the Cape of Good Hope from Dutch.

1822
United States sets up Liberia, West Africa, as a home for freed slaves.

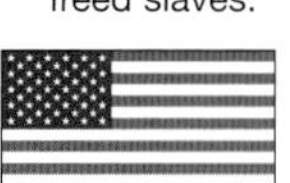

1835-37
Boers trek north from the Cape to escape British rule.

1899-1902
Boer War is fought between the Boers and the British. Treaty makes Boer republics British colonies.

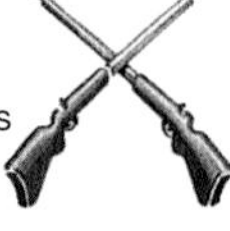

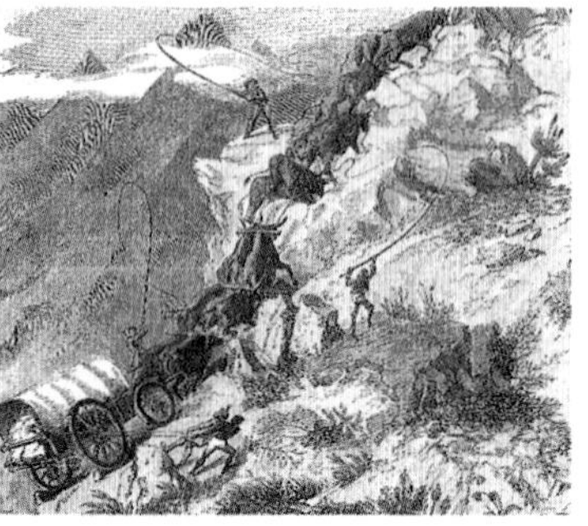

1900 – 2000 INDEPENDENCE AND THE MODERN WORLD

1910
Union of South Africa is created.

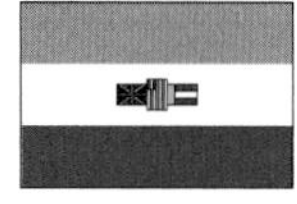

1914-1918
World War I: German colonies in Africa conquered by British and French.

1935
Italy conquers Ethiopia; leads to end of League of Nations.

1949
Apartheid (separation of races) begins in South Africa.

1954
Gamal Abdel Nasser becomes premier of Egypt.

1957
Ghana becomes independent; it is the first African state to gain independence.

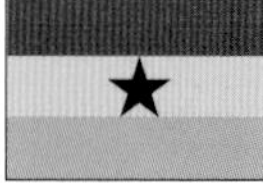

1962
Algeria wins independence from France.

1963
Organization of African Unity (OAU) is founded.

1964
ANC leader Nelson Mandela is jailed for life.

1965
Rhodesia declares independence from Britain.

1967-70
Civil war fought in Nigeria.

1975
Moroccans begin occupation of the Spanish Sahara.

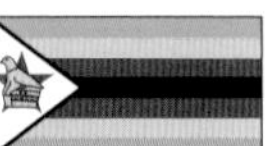

1980
Rhodesia becomes independent and is renamed Zimbabwe.

1984
Ten-year drought leads to appalling famine in Ethiopia, Sudan, and Chad.

1989
Namibia, the last colony in Africa, becomes independent from South Africa.

1993
Eritrea becomes independent.

1994
Nelson Mandela, released in 1990, becomes president of South Africa.

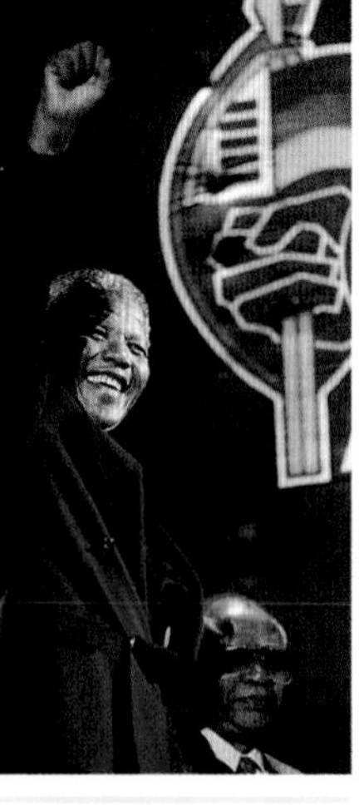

00	500	A.D. 100	400	500	600	800
00 Ironworking begins Africa	c. 400 Copper smelting begins in Mauritania	238 Revolt in Africa begins against Roman rule	c. 400 Use of iron spreads through eastern Africa	c. 500 Rise of the Ghanaian Empire, West Africa		
00 Oaxaca culture ws stronger, Mexico	c. 200 Beginning of early Mayan period	c. 100 Moche civilization begins on Peruvian coast		c. 500 Thule people move into Alaska	c. 600 Height of Mayan civilization	
-529 Reign of Cyrus the at, Persia	c. 250 Arsaces I founds the Parthian kingdom, Persia	c. 224 Parthian rule ends in Persian Empire	c. 400 Gupta Empire stretches across India	c. 500 The figure zero is introduced in India	634 Arab Empire begins	
000 Early Iron Age ins in Italy	431 Great Peloponnesian War	116-117 Roman Empire is at its greatest extent		527-565 Reign of Justinian, Byzantine emperor	787 Vikings make their first raids on the coasts of Britain	c. 800 First castles built
	c. 500 Aboriginal culture develops	c. 300 Beginning of early eastern Polynesian culture		c. 500 Polynesians navigate eastwards	c. 700 First Polynesians settle in the Cook Islands	

AMERICAS

40,000 – 2000 B.C. EARLIEST PEOPLES

c. 40,000 B.C.
The first peoples arrive in the Americas from Siberia across the Bering Strait.

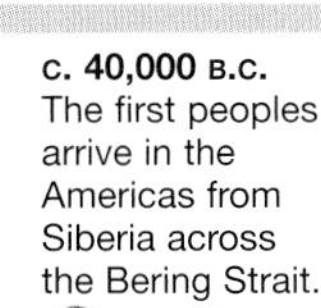

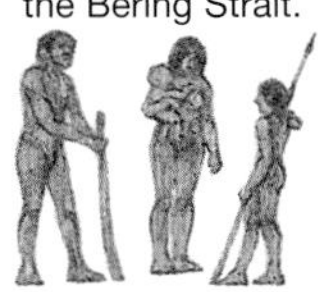

c. 15,000 B.C.
Cave art produced in what is now Brazil.

c. 6500 B.C.
Farming begins in the Peruvian Andes, South America.

c. 3200 B.C.
Pottery begins to be made in Ecuador, and Colombia, South America.

2000 B.C. – A.D. 1450 EMPIRES AND CIVILIZATIONS

2000 B.C.
The Mayan culture begins in Central America. Farmers begin to settle in villages.

c. 1150 B.C.
Olmec people in Mexico, North America, develop a picture-writing and number system that spreads through continent.

c. 300 B.C.
Mayan culture develops. Large political and religious centres are built, such as Palenque.

c. A.D. 300
Hopewell Indians build burial mounds and trade in North America.

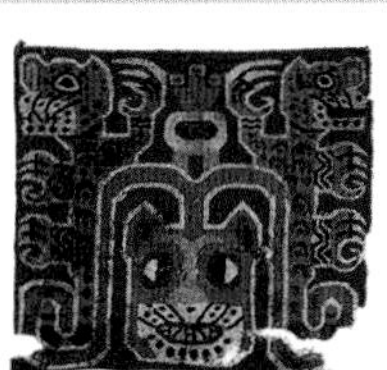

c. A.D. 700
People weave tapestries in Peru, South America. Cotton and wool tapestry, above, shows jaguars.

c. A.D. 900
Toltecs conquer the Mayans and create an empire in Central America.

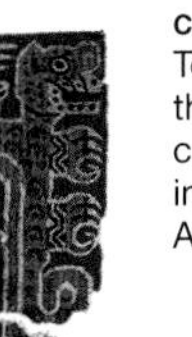

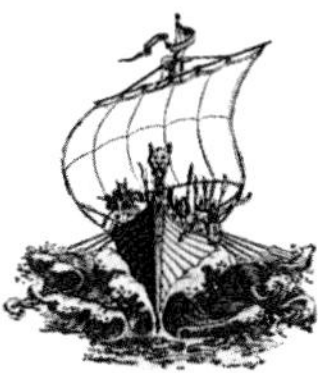

c. A.D. 1000
Vikings from Europe arrive in North America.

1450 – 1750 EUROPEAN CONQUEST AND TRADE

1492
Italian explorer Christopher Columbus reaches the Caribbean and claims islands for Spain; other Europeans follow with horses and guns, seeking treasure.

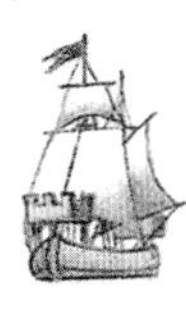

1494
Treaty of Tordesillas divides the Americas between Spain and Portugal.

1499
Amerigo Vespucci explores the Amazon, South America; gives his name to the American continent.

c. 1510
First African slaves are taken to the Caribbean.

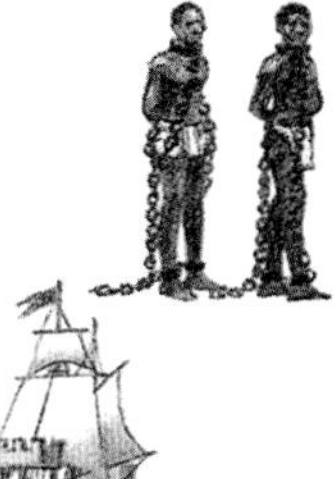

1519
Hernando Cortés, a Spanish Conquistador, conquers Mexico; the Aztec Empire, under emperor Montezuma, ends.

1620
Mayflower ship arrives in New England, North America, carrying Puritan refugees from Britain (the Pilgrims).

1636
The first university in the future US, Harvard College, is founded.

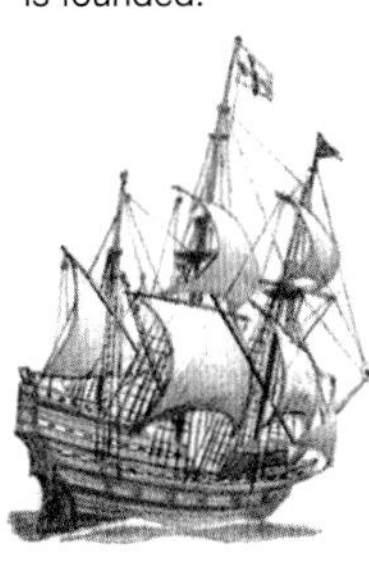

1750 – 1900 THE NEW NATIONS

1783
Birth of Simón Bolívar, liberator of South America.

1776
America issues Declaration of Independence.

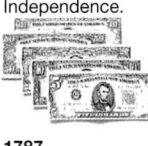

1787
Dollar currency is introduced into America.

1791
Slave revolt in Haiti, led by Toussaint L'Ouverture against the French.

1803
Louisiana Purchase: US buys land from France, doubling the size of the country.

1861-65
American Civil War.

1849
Gold rush begins in California.

1852
Elisha Otis invents the elevator.

1861-65
Civil War fought in United States. Slaves are freed.

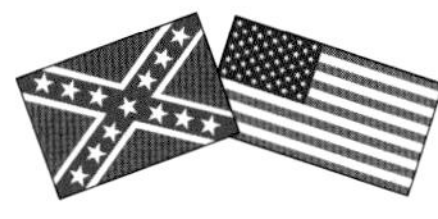

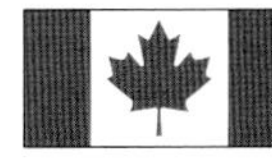

1867
Canada becomes independent.

1869
Railway crosses United States from coast to coast.

1876
Battle of the Little Bighorn between Indians and white troops.

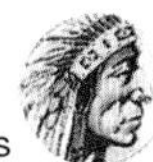

1877
Thomas Edison invents the phonograph.

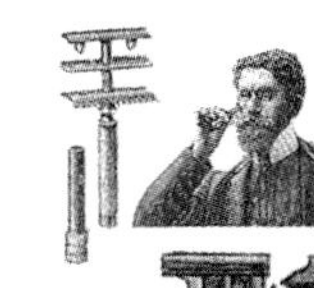

1895
King C. Gillette invents the safety razor, with a convenient disposable blade.

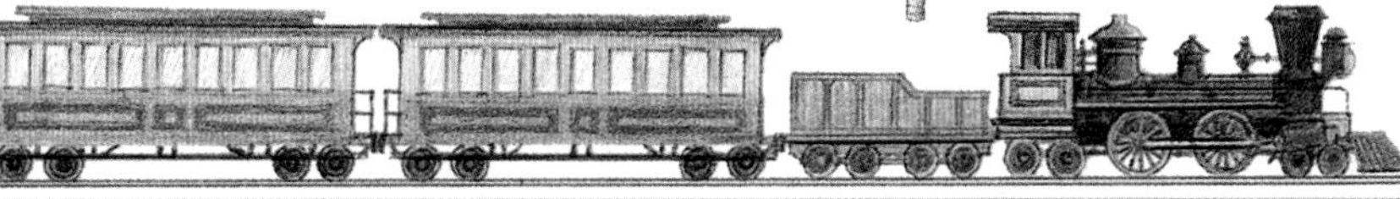

1900 – 2000 THE MODERN WORLD

1903
Wright brothers make first powered flight.

1908
Henry Ford produces Model T Ford car.

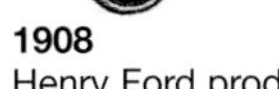

1913
Hollywood becomes centre of film industry.

1917
United States enters World War I, following rupture in diplomatic relations with Germany.

1920
Boom years: jazz age follows World War I (1914-18).

1929
The Wall Street crash: the US Stock Exchange collapses; start of Depression of 1930s.

1941
United States enters World War II.

1945
United Nations begins, San Francisco.

1958
Silicon chip developed by Texas Instruments Co.

1959
Ernesto "Che" Guevara helps Fidel Castro overthrow Cuban government.

1969
Apollo 11 takes US astronauts to the Moon. Neil Armstrong is the first man to walk on the Moon.

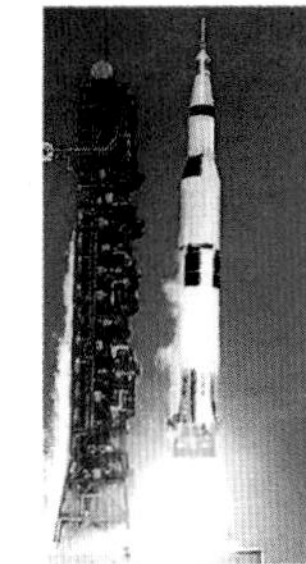

1987
Intermediate-Range Nuclear Forces (INF) Treaty signed with Soviet Union.

1991
Gulf War.

2001
Islamic terrorists destroy the Twin Towers of the World Trade Center in New York City.

A.D.	900	950	1000	1050	1100	1150
AFRICA		969 Cairo is built and becomes capital of Egypt	c. 1000 Kingdoms of Takrur and Gao flourish in West Africa		c. 1100 Ghana Empire in West Africa declines	1173 Saladin bec Sultan of Egypt
AMERICAS	c. 900 Mayan power in northern Mexico starts to fade		c. 1000 Farmers in Peru grow sweetcorn and potatoes		c. 1100 Rise of Incas, farmers led by warrior chiefs, in Peru	c. 1150 End of Hopewell culture
ASIA	906-906 Tang Dynasty, China collapses after years of war	969 China is reunified under the Song Dynasty	c. 1000 Chinese perfect the art of making gunpowder	c. 1090 Mechanical clock, driven by water, built in China	1099 Crusaders capture Jerusalem, Palestine	
EUROPE	911 Rollo, a Viking chief, settles in Normandy, France	962 Otto the Great is crowned Holy Roman Emperor	c. 986 Viking Eric the Red sets up colony in Greenland	1066 Normans conquer England, Battle of Hastings	1132-35. The first Gothic church is built in Paris	1171-72 Henry II invades Ireland
OCEANIA	c. 900 First settlers reach South Island, New Zealand		c. 1000 Maori people settle in New Zealand		c. 1100 Organized societies form in Hawaiian Islands	c. 1150 Maoris settle in river are

ASIA

800,000 B.C. – 1500 B.C. EARLIEST CIVILIZATIONS

800,000 B.C.
First humans arrive in Asia from Africa.

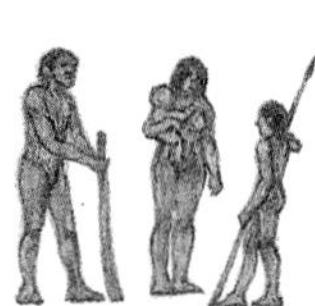

c. 9000 B.C.
Palestinian sheep are the world's first domesticated animals identified so far.

c. 8350 B.C.
Jericho, the world's first known walled city, is founded. It consists of mud brick houses behind a strong wall.

c. 3500 B.C.
The Sumerians invent the wheel.

c. 3250 B.C.
The Sumerians develop picture writing and build the world's first cities. They also grow barley, bake bread, and make beer. Sumerian picture writing was called cuneiform, and was scratched onto clay tablets.

c. 2698 B.C.
Legendary Chinese emperor Shen Nung writes Chinese "Canon of Herbs" with over 252 plant descriptions.

c. 2500 B.C.
Indus Valley civilization, based on agriculture, in India.

c. 1750 B.C.
Hammurabi establishes the Babylonian Empire.

1500 B.C. – A.D. 1500 EMPIRES AND RELIGIONS

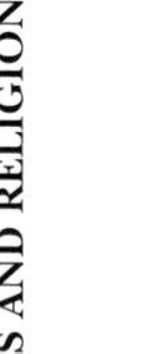

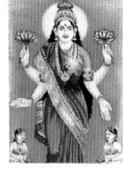

c. 1500 B.C.
Hindu religion begins to be established in India.

c. 1200 B.C.
Beginning of Judaism, Palestine.

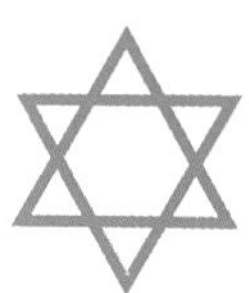

650s B.C.
World's first coins are produced in the Near East.

c. 600 B.C.
Chinese philosopher Lao-tzu develops philosophy of Taoism.

c. 563 B.C.
Birth of Siddhartha Gautama, the Buddha, founder of Buddhism, India.

551 B.C.
Birth of Confucius, founder of a philosophical system in China.

200s B.C.
Great Wall of China is built to keep out invaders.

c. A.D. 30
Jesus Christ is executed; Christianity is born in Judea.

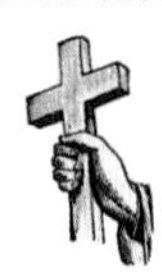

c. A.D. 100
Paper is invented in China.

A.D. 606
First examinations for entry to public offices in China.

A.D. 632
Death of Muhammad, the Prophet. Spread of Islamic religion, led by caliphs (successors).

A.D. 868
World's first printed book, Diamond Sutra, in China

c. A.D. 1000
The Chinese perfect their invention of gunpowder.

A.D. 1206
Mongols begin conquest of Asia.

1259
Kublai Khan becomes Mongol ruler of China; sets up Yuan dynasty, which lasts 1279-1368.

1290
Ottomans (Turkish Muslims) rise to power.

1333
China suffers drought, famine, floods, and plague. Five million people die.

1421
Peking (now Beijing) becomes capital of China.

1453
Ottomans capture Constantinople, ending the Byzantine Empire.

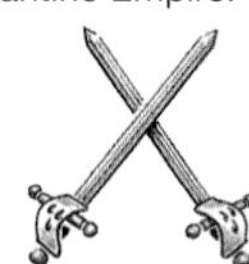

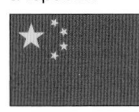

1498
Portuguese navigator Vasco da Gama reaches India, via Africa.

1500 – 1900 TRADE AND CONQUEST

1556
Akbar the Great, the greatest of the Mogul rulers, comes to power, India.

1600
English East India trading company is founded.

1639
Japan closed to foreigners.

1648
Taj Mahal is built in India by emperor Shah Jahan as a tomb for his favourite wife, Mumtaz Mahal.

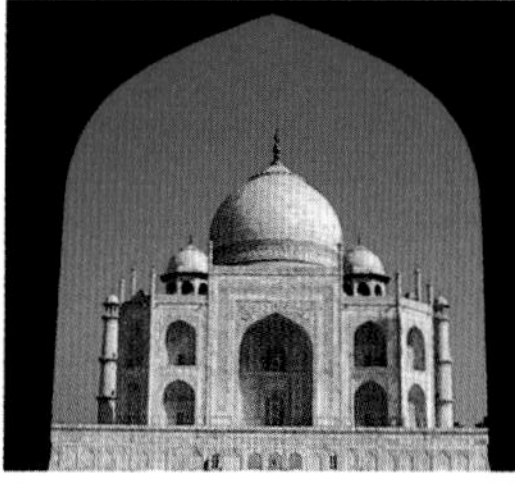

1649
Russians conquer Siberia and reach the Pacific Ocean.

1857
Outbreak of Indian Mutiny against British rule. Put down by British a year later.

1900 – 2000 THE MODERN WORLD

1911
China becomes a republic.

1918
Ottoman Empire collapses.

1920
Mahatma Gandhi begins campaign for Indian independence.

1921
Mao Zedong and Li Ta-chao found the Chinese Communist Party in Beijing.

1926
Hirohito becomes the emperor of Japan.

1934
Communists in China, led by Mao Zedong, begin Long March through the mountains of China to Yenan, where they set up government.

1941
Japanese attack US fleet at Pearl Harbor, Hawaii.

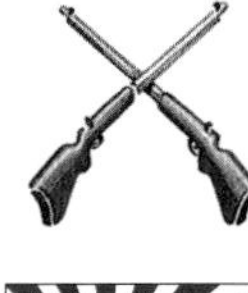

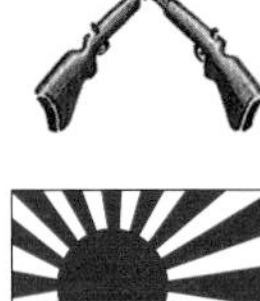

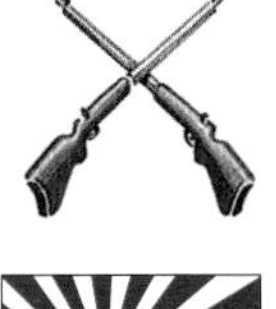

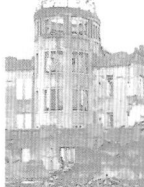

1945
World's first atomic bombs are dropped on Japan.

1947
India and Pakistan independent.

1947
Partition of Palestine into Arab and Jewish states leads to fighting between Arabs and Jews in Palestine.

1948
Jewish state of Israel founded.

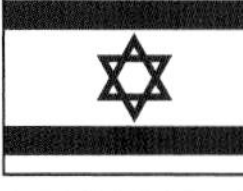

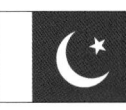

1966
Mao Zedong starts Cultural Revolution in China.

1967
Six-Day War between Arabs and Israelis.

1980-1989
War between Iran and Iraq.

1989
Pro-democracy movement in Beijing is crushed by military force.

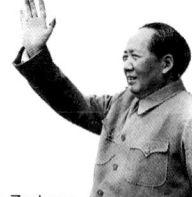

Mao Zedong

1990-1991
Gulf War. Iraq invades Kuwait. UN intervenes.

2003
US and British forces invade Iraq.

2004
Tsunami around the Indian Ocean kills 300,000 people.

200	1250	1300	1350	1400	1450	1500
200-30 King of Ethiopia churches cut from rock	c. 1250 Kanem kingdom breaks up into rival factions	1348 Egypt devastated by plague, called the Black Death		c.1400 Gold trade thrives in Kingdom of Great Zimbabwe	c. 1450 Songhai Empire reaches its greatest height	
200 Incas in Peru centre ınd settlement of Cuzco	c. 1250 Chimu people expand their empire in Peru	c. 1300 Incas expand their empire in the central Andes		c. 1400 Inca Empire flourishes in South America	1519 Conquistadors destroy Aztec and Inca Empires	
5 Ghengis Khan founds ıgol Empire	c. 1254 Explorer, Marco Polo, born in Venice	c. 1300 Osman founds Ottoman Dynasty in Turkey	1368 Mongols are driven out of China		c. 1450 Portuguese set up trading posts in Indian Ocean – Christianity spreads in Asia	
5 English King John seals gna Carta	1282-84 Edward I of England conquers Wales	1337 Start of 100 Years' War between England and France	1370 Chaucer writes his first book, *Book of the Duchess*	c. 1400 Renaissance of art and learning begins		
	c. 1250 Valley irrigation schemes in Hawaiian islands	c. 1300 Huge stone statues are built on Easter Island	c. 1350 Maoris flourish in North Island, New Zealand		c. 1450 Advanced societies develop in Polynesian islands	

EUROPE

1,000,000 B.C. – A.D. 450 EARLY PEOPLES AND THE ANCIENT WORLD

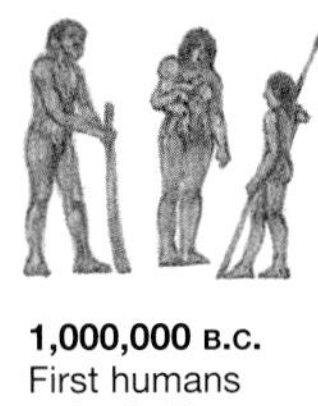

1,000,000 B.C.
First humans arrive in Europe.

6500 B.C.
People begin farming in Greece and the Balkans.

c. 1900 B.C.
Civilization of Mycenae develops in Greece. The Mycenaeans build splendid, rich palaces.

c. 1500 B.C.
Linear B script, used to write an early version of the Greek language, develops in Crete.

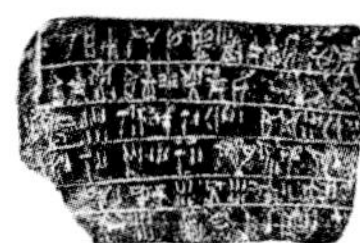

c. 1250 B.C.
Trojan War between Greeks of Mycenae and the Trojans. According to legend, after a 10-year siege the Greeks entered Troy hidden inside a huge wooden horse, and destroyed the city.

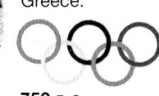

c. 753 B.C.
Rome founded by the legendary brothers Romulus and Remus.

776 B.C.
First Olympic Games held in Greece.

750 B.C.
Homer composes the *Iliad*, an epic poem describing the Trojan War.

c. 500 B.C
Celts occupy much of Europe.

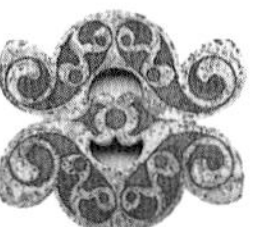

146 B.C.
Romans conquer Greece.

44 B.C.
Julius Caesar is assassinated.

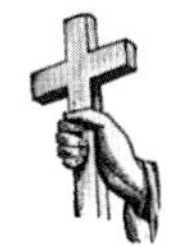

A.D. 391
Christianity becomes the official religion of the Roman Empire.

A.D. 450 – 1450 RELIGION AND THE MIDDLE AGES

A.D. 500
Barbarian tribes overrun much of western Europe.

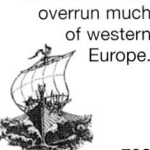

793
Vikings raid northern Europe.

1096
First Crusade leaves England for Palestine.

c. 1150
One of the first European universities is founded in Paris.

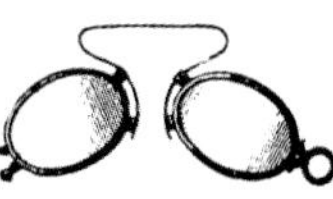

1290
Reading glasses are invented in Italy.

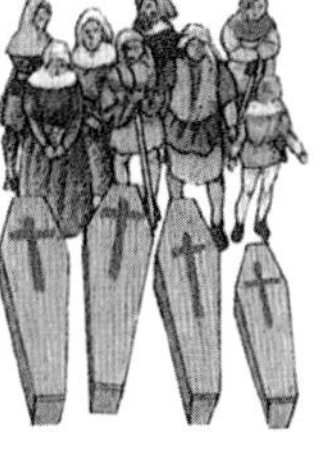

1348
Bubonic plague, called the Black Death, kills one-third of the population of Europe.

1454
The German Johann Gutenberg publishes the Gutenberg Bible, the first printed book in Europe. It was printed with movable copper type.

1450 – 1780 EXPLORATION AND SCIENCE

1453
Ottoman Turks capture Constantinople; end of Byzantine Empire.

1516
Hapsburg Empire expands under Charles V of Spain.

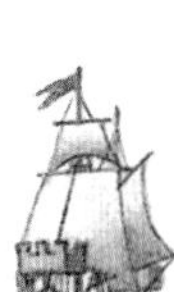

1517
German Martin Luther pins a list of complaints about Roman Catholic Church practices on a church door in Wittenberg; Reformation begins.

1519-1521
Portuguese Ferdinand Magellan leads the first voyage around the world.

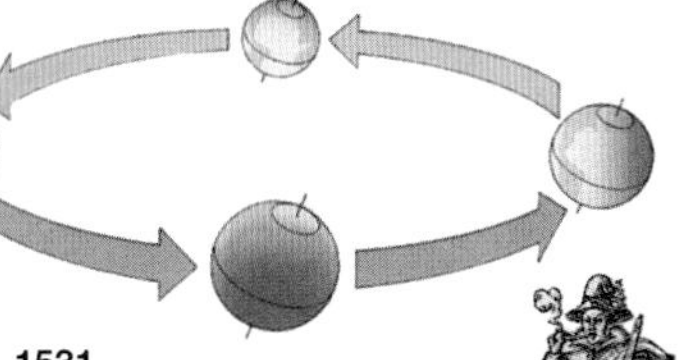

1531
Polish astronomer Copernicus suggests that Earth revolves around the Sun.

1555
Tobacco taken to Europe from the Americas.

1603
Union of Scotland and England.

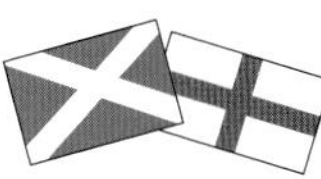

1628
William Harvey, English doctor, discovers circulation of blood.

1665
English scientist Isaac Newton discovers laws of gravity.

1682
Peter the Great becomes czar of Russia.

1683
Ottoman Turks fail in their siege of Vienna.

1690
William III of England defeats the exiled Catholic James II and his Irish supporters at the Battle of the Boyne, Ireland.

1710
Russia conquers Swedish provinces in the Baltic.

1760 – 2000 REVOLUTION AND THE MODERN WORLD

1789
French Revolution breaks out.

1805
British Admiral Nelson defeats French in the sea battle of Trafalgar.

1825
First passenger railway, Britain

1840
First postage stamp, the Penny Black, is issued in Britain.

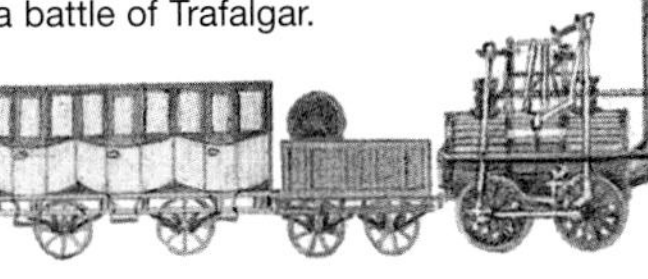

1846
Potato famine in Ireland.

1848
Karl Marx and Friedrich Engels write *Communist Manifesto*.

1859
Charles Darwin publishes theory of evolution.

1876
Alexander Graham Bell invents telephone.

1895
Italian Guglielmo Marconi invents the radio.

1902
Polish scientist Marie Curie and her French husband, Pierre, discover radium, a chemical element to treat cancer.

1914
World War I begins.

1917
Russian Revolution breaks out.

1922
The Irish Free State is formed.

1930s
Economic depression in Europe.

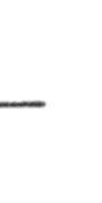

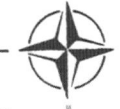

1939
German scientists discover that energy can be released by splitting uranium atoms into two.

1939
World War II begins.

1949
North Atlantic Treaty Organization (NATO) formed.

1957
European Union is formed.

1957
Soviets launch first space satellite.

1961
Berlin Wall built.

1990
East and West Germany unite.

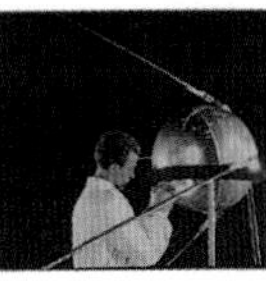

1991
Soviet Union collapses.

1992
Civil war breaks out in Bosnia.

1999
NATO forces attack Serbia in defence of Kosovan Muslims.

2002
Euro introduced.

A.D.	1550	1600	1650	1700	1725	1750
AFRICA	c. 1500 Songhai Empire expands in West Africa	c. 1600 Ivory trade expands in Kalonga kingdom	1652 Dutch found Cape Town in South Africa		c. 1740 The Lunda create prosperous new kingdom	1755 The first ou of smallpox, Cape
AMERICAS		c. 1608 Quebec in Canada founded by France		c. 1700 North American colonies begin to prosper	1727 First discovery of diamonds in Brazil	1776 US Declarat Independence, Ju
ASIA		c. 1619 Dutch control spice trade in Indonesian islands	c. 1620 Japan restricts contact with rest of world	1709 Death of shogun Tsunayoshi of Japan	1722-35 Siberian-Mongolian border defined	
EUROPE	1558-1603 Reign of Elizabeth I of England	1618-48 30 Years War involves all Europe but Britain	1652-54 First Dutch war with England	1707 Act of Union unites England and Scotland		1789 Outbreak of French Revolution
OCEANIA		1642-44 Abel Tasman founds Tasmania	c. 1680 Civil war starts on Easter Island	c. 1700 First contact between Tahitians and Europeans		1768-71 Captain C first voyage to Pac

OCEANIA

50,000 B.C. – A.D. 1600 FIRST SETTLERS

c. 40,000 B.C.
Aboriginal people arrive in Australia from Southeast Asia.

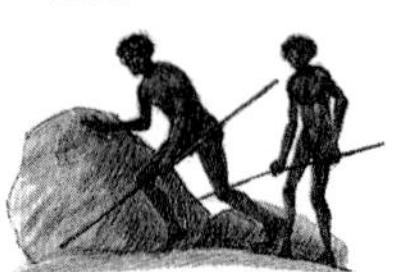

c. 2000 B.C.
People arrive in New Guinea.

c. 1300 B.C.
People reach Fiji, Tonga.

c. A.D. 300
People reach Polynesia.

c. A.D. 950
Polynesians, later known as Maori people, settle in New Zealand and the Pacific islands.

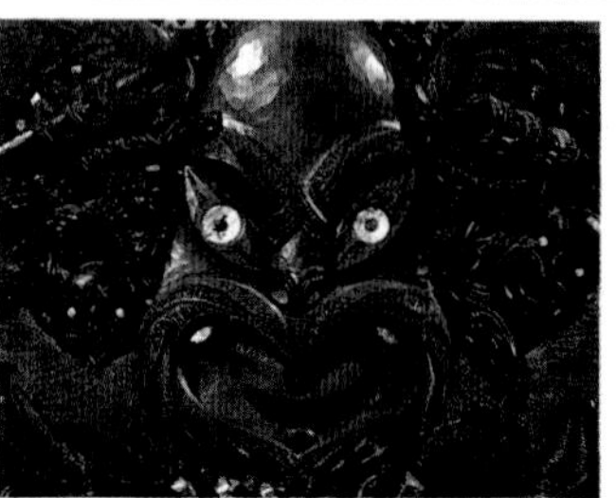

1600 – 1850 CONQUEST AND COLONIZATION

1606
Dutch navigator Willem Jansz visits Australia.

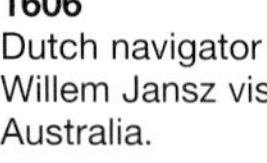

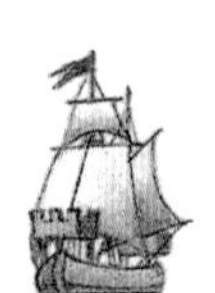

1642
Dutch navigator Abel Tasman sails around Australia to New Zealand.

1770
English navigator Captain Cook claims Australia for Britain. He discovers species of animals and plants not yet heard of in Europe.

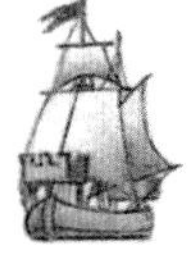

1788
First British convicts are transported from British prisons to Botany Bay, site of the first European settlement, Australia.

1826
English settlers and Aboriginals fight in the "Black War" in Tasmania.

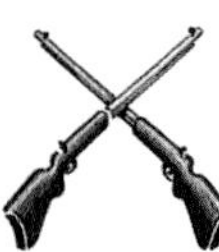

1840
In the Treaty of Waitangi, Maori chiefs in New Zealand give sovereignty over New Zealand to Britain. New Zealand becomes British colony.

1851
Gold rush, Victoria, Australia. Settlers arrive from Europe.

1850 – 2000 THE MODERN WORLD

1860
Burke and Wills are the first people to cross Australia from coast to coast. Both die of starvation on the journey back in 1861.

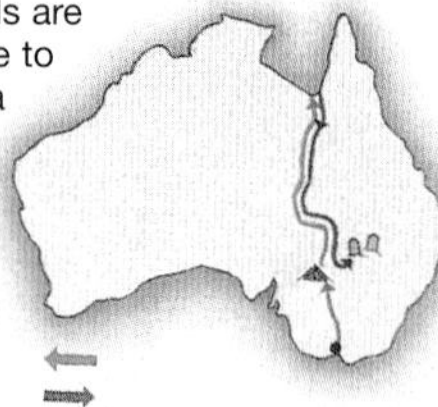

1893
New Zealand women gain the vote.

1901
Australia gains independence from Britain; Commonwealth of Australia is proclaimed.

1907
New Zealand gains independence from Britain.

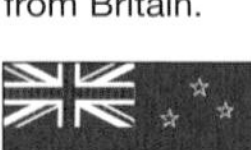

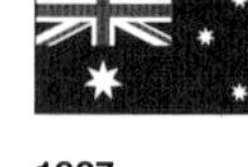

1927
Canberra becomes the capital city of Australia.

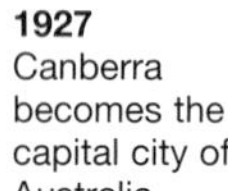

1941-42
Japan invades the Pacific islands.

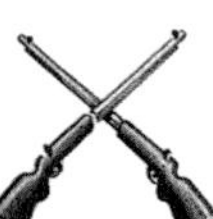

1945
Assisted passages to Australia for Europeans. Two million people emigrate.

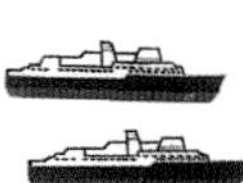

1950s
Nuclear testing carried out in the Pacific islands.

1951
ANZUS defence treaty between Australia, New Zealand, and the United States.

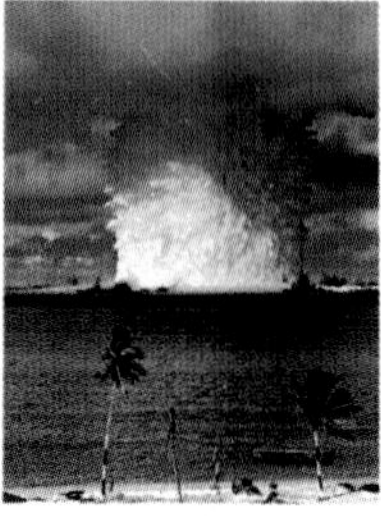

1985
South Pacific Forum treaty – Pacific is a nuclear-free zone.

1993
Australia passes Native Title Bill to confirm the Aboriginal right to claim back land.

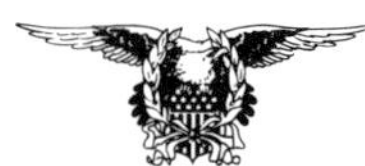

PRESIDENTS OF THE UNITED STATES

GEORGE WASHINGTON (1732-1799) Term of office: **1789-1797**

JOHN ADAMS (1735-1826) Term of office: **1797-1801**

THOMAS JEFFERSON (1743-1826) Term of office: **1801-1809**

JAMES MADISON (1751-1836) Term of office: **1809-1817**

JAMES MONROE (1758-1831) Term of office: **1817-1825**

JOHN QUINCY ADAMS (1767-1848) Term of office: **1825-1829**

ANDREW JACKSON (1767-1845) Term of office: 1829-1837

MARTIN VAN BUREN (1782-1862) Term of office: **1837-1841**

W.H. HARRISON (1773-1841) Term of office: **Mar.-Apr. 1841**

JOHN TYLER (1790-1862) Term of office: **1841-1845**

JAMES K. POLK (1795-1849) Term of office: **1845-1849**

ZACHARY TAYLOR (1784-1850) Term of office: **1849-1850**

MILLARD FILLMORE (1800-1874) Term of office: **1850-1853**

FRANKLIN PIERCE (1804-1869) Term of office: **1853-1857**

JAMES BUCHANAN (1791-1868) Term of office: **1857-1861**

ABRAHAM LINCOLN (1809-1865) Term of office: **1861-1865**

ANDREW JOHNSON (1808-1875) Term of office: **1865-1869**

ULYSSES S. GRANT (1822-1885) Term of office: **1869-1877**

RUTHERFORD B. HAYES (1822-1893) Term of office: **1877-1881**

JAMES A. GARFIELD (1831-1881) Term of office: **Mar.-Sept. 1881**

CHESTER A. ARTHUR (1830-1886) Term of office: **1881-1885**

GROVER CLEVELAND (1837-1908) Term of office: **1885-1889**

BENJAMIN HARRISON (1833-1901) Term of office: **1889-1893**

GROVER CLEVELAND (1837-1908) Term of office: **1893-1897**

WILLIAM MCKINLEY (1843-1901) Term of office: **1897-1901**

THEODORE ROOSEVELT (1858-1919) Term of office: **1901-1909**

WILLIAM H. TAFT (1857-1930) Term of office: **1909-1913**

WOODROW WILSON (1856-1924) Term of office: **1913-1921**

WARREN G. HARDING (1865-1923) Term of office: **1921-1923**

CALVIN COOLIDGE (1872-1933) Term of office: **1923-1929**

HERBERT HOOVER (1874-1964) Term of office: **1929-1933**

FRANKLIN D. ROOSEVELT (1882-1945) Term of office: **1933-1945**

HARRY S. TRUMAN (1884-1972) Term of office: **1945-1953**

DWIGHT EISENHOWER (1890-1969) Term of office: **1953-1961**

JOHN F. KENNEDY (1917-1963) Term of office: **1961-1963**

LYNDON B. JOHNSON (1908-1973) Term of office: **1963-1969**

RICHARD NIXON (1913-1994) Term of office: **1969-1974**

GERALD R. FORD (BORN 1913) Term of office: **1974-1977**

JIMMY CARTER (BORN 1924) Term of office: **1977-1981**

RONALD REAGAN (1911-2004) Term of office: **1981-1989**

GEORGE BUSH (BORN 1924) Term of office: **1989-1993**

BILL CLINTON (BORN 1946) Term of office: **1993 to 2001**

GEORGE W. BUSH (BORN 1946) Term of office: **2001 to date**

800	1825	1850	1900	1925	1950	1990
	1825 Egyptians found the city of Khartoum in Sudan	1897 Slavery banned in Zanzibar	1902 End of second Boer War in South Africa	1930 White women given vote in South Africa	1958-60 Independence for Zaire, Nigeria, Somalia	
01 Thomas Jefferson comes third US president	1849 California Gold Rush begins	1861-65 Civil War between southern and northern states		1929 US Stock Exchange crashes	1963 US president John F. Kennedy assassinated	
19 Stamford Raffles unds Singapore		1851 Thailand is open to foreign trade	1905 Japan becomes world power after defeat of Russia		1965-73 Vietnam War	
04 Napoleon becomes nperor of the French	1837 Victoria becomes Queen, United Kingdom		1914-18 World War I	1939-1945 World War II	1961 Berlin Wall divides East and West Germany	
10 Kamehameha I comes king of Hawaii	1840 British and Maoris sign Treaty of Waitangi	1860-70 Second Maoris War in New Zealand	1907 New Zealand becomes a dominion	1927 Canberra becomes federal capital of Australia	1970 Tonga and Fiji gain independence from Britain	

KINGS AND QUEENS OF GREAT BRITAIN

RULERS OF ENGLAND

	REIGNED
Saxon line	
EGBERT	827-839
ETHELWULF	839-858
ETHELBALD	858-860
ETHELBERT	860-865
ETHELRED I	865-871
ALFRED THE GREAT	871-899
EDWARD THE ELDER	899-924
ATHELSTAN	924-939
EDMUND	939-946
EDRED	946-955
EDWY	955-959
EDGAR	959-975
EDWARD THE MARTYR	975-978
ETHELRED THE UNREADY	978-1016
EDMUND IRONSIDE	1016
Danish line	
CANUTE (CNUT)	1016-1035
HAROLD I HAREFOOT	1035-1040
HARDECANUTE	1040-1042
Saxon line	
EDWARD THE CONFESSOR	1042-1066
HAROLD II (GODWINSON)	1066
House of Normandy	
WILLIAM I (THE CONQUEROR)	1066-1087
WILLIAM II	1087-1100
HENRY I	1100-1135
STEPHEN	1135-1154
House of Plantagenet	
HENRY II	1154-1189
RICHARD I	1189-1199
JOHN	1199-1216
HENRY III	1216-1272
EDWARD I	1272-1307
EDWARD II	1307-1327
EDWARD III	1327-1377
RICHARD II	1377-1399
House of Lancaster	
HENRY IV	1399-1413
HENRY V	1413-1422
HENRY VI	1422-1461
(also)	1470-1471
House of York	
EDWARD IV	1461-1470
(also)	1471-1483
EDWARD V	1483
RICHARD III	1483-1485
House of Tudor	
HENRY VII	1485-1509
HENRY VIII	1509-1547
EDWARD VI	1547-1553
MARY I	1553-1558
ELIZABETH I	1558-1603

MONARCHS OF SCOTLAND

MALCOLM II	1005-1034
DUNCAN I	1034-1040
MACBETH	1040-1057
MALCOLM III	1057-1093
DONALD BANE	1093-1094
DUNCAN II	1094
DONALD BANE	1094-1097
EDGAR	1097-1107
ALEXANDER I	1107-1124
DAVID I	1124-1153
MALCOLM IV	1153-1165
WILLIAM THE LION	1165-1214
ALEXANDER II	1214-1249
ALEXANDER III	1249-1286
MARGARET OF NORWAY	1286-1290
JOHN DE BALIOL	1292-1296
ROBERT I (BRUCE)	1306-1329
DAVID II	1329-1371
House of Stuart	
ROBERT II	1371-1390
ROBERT III	1390-1406
JAMES I	1406-1437
JAMES II	1437-1460
JAMES III	1460-1488
JAMES IV	1488-1513
JAMES V	1513-1542
MARY	1542-1567
JAMES VI *(became James I of England)*	1567-1625

MONARCHS OF GREAT BRITAIN

House of Stuart	
JAMES I	1603-1625
CHARLES I	1625-1649
Commonwealth	1649-1660
CHARLES II	1660-1685
JAMES II	1685-1688
WILLIAM III	1689-1702
MARY II	1689-1694
ANNE	1702-1714
House of Hanover	
GEORGE I	1714-1727
GEORGE II	1727-1760
GEORGE III	1760-1820
GEORGE IV	1820-1830
WILLIAM IV	1830-1837
VICTORIA	1837-1901
House of Saxe-Coburg-Gotha	
EDWARD VII	1901-1910
House of Windsor	
GEORGE V	1910-1936
EDWARD VIII	1936
GEORGE VI	1936-1952
ELIZABETH II	1952 to date

PRIME MINISTERS OF GREAT BRITAIN

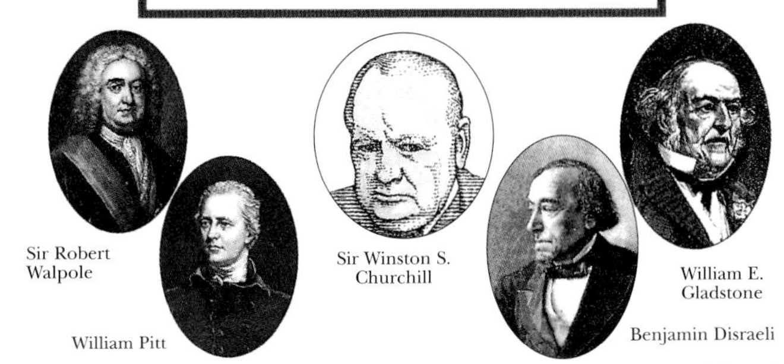
Sir Robert Walpole

William Pitt

Sir Winston S. Churchill

Benjamin Disraeli

William E. Gladstone

PRIME MINISTER	TERM OF OFFICE
SIR ROBERT WALPOLE	1721-1742
EARL OF WILMINGTON	1742-1743
HENRY PELHAM	1743-1754
DUKE OF NEWCASTLE	1754-1756
DUKE OF DEVONSHIRE	1756-1757
DUKE OF NEWCASTLE	1757-1762
EARLE OF BUTE	1762-1763
GEORGE GRENVILLE	1763-1765
MARQUESS OF ROCKINGHAM	1765-1766
WILLIAM PITT (EARL OF CHATHAM)	1766-1767
DUKE OF GRAFTON	1767-1770
LORD NORTH	1770-1782
MARQUESS OF ROCKINGHAM	1782
EARL OF SHELBORNE	1782-1783
DUKE OF PORTLAND	1783
WILLIAM PITT (THE YOUNGER)	1783-1801
HENRY ADDINGTON	1801-1804
WILLIAM PITT	1804-1806
BARON GRENVILLE	1806-1807
DUKE OF PORTLAND	1807-1809
SPENCER PERCEVAL	1809-1812
EARL OF LIVERPOOL	1812-1827
GEORGE CANNING	1827
VISCOUNT GODERICH	1827-1828
DUKE OF WELLINGTON	1828-1830
EARL GREY	1830-1834
VISCOUNT MELBOURNE	1834
DUKE OF WELLINGTON	1834
SIR ROBERT PEEL	1834-1835
VISCOUNT MELBOURNE	1835-1841
SIR ROBERT PEEL	1841-1846
LORD JOHN RUSSELL	1846-1852
EARL OF DERBY	1852
EARL OF ABERDEEN	1852-1855
VISCOUNT PALMERSTON	1855-1858
EARL OF DERBY	1858-1859
VISCOUNT PALMERSTON	1859-1865
EARL RUSSELL	1865-1866
EARL OF DERBY	1866-1868
BENJAMIN DISRAELI	1868
WILLIAM E. GLADSTONE	1868-1874
BENJAMIN DISRAELI	1874-1880
WILLIAM E. GLADSTONE	1880-1885
MARQUESS OF SALISBURY	1885-1886
WILLIAM E. GLADSTONE	1886
MARQUESS OF SALISBURY	1886-1892
WILLIAM E. GLADSTONE	1892-1894
EARL OF ROSEBERY	1894-1895
MARQUESS OF SALISBURY	1895-1902
ARTHUR J. BALFOUR	1902-1905
SIR HENRY CAMPBELL-BANNERMAN	1905-1908
HERBERT HENRY ASQUITH	1908-1915
HERBERT HENRY ASQUITH	1915-1916
DAVID LLOYD GEORGE	1916-1922
ANDREW BONAR LAW	1922-1923
STANLEY BALDWIN	1923-1924
J. RAMSAY MACDONALD	1924
STANLEY BALDWIN	1924-1929
J. RAMSAY MACDONALD	1929-1931
J. RAMSAY MACDONALD	1931-1935
STANLEY BALDWIN	1935-1937
NEVILLE CHAMBERLAIN	1937-1940
WINSTON S. CHURCHILL	1940-1945
CLEMENT R. ATTLEE	1945-1951
SIR WINSTON S. CHURCHILL	1951-1955
SIR ANTHONY EDEN	1955-1957
HAROLD MACMILLAN	1957-1963
SIR ALEC DOUGLAS-HOME	1963-1964
HAROLD WILSON	1964-1970
EDWARD HEATH	1970-1974
HAROLD WILSON	1974-1976
JAMES CALLAGHAN	1976-1979
MARGARET THATCHER	1979-1990
JOHN MAJOR	1990-1997
TONY BLAIR	1997 to date

B.C.	7000	3500	1000	A.D. 100	250	500
ENGLAND		Stonehenge under construction c. 2950-2500.	Iron Age begins c. 800.	London founded c. A.D. 50.	Angles, Jutes, and Saxons arrive in England from 400s.	*Beowulf* is written down c. 700.
SCOTLAND	Prehistoric peoples arrive from Ireland c. 6000.	Neolithic village built at Skara Brae c.3000.		Picts dominate Scotland A.D. 100s-800s.		St Columba founded Iona, 563.
N. IRELAND		Bronze Age begins c.2200.	Celts invade c. 600.		St. Patrick's mission to Ireland c. 432.	
WALES			Celts from central Europe occupy Wales c. 400.	Wales becomes part of Roman Empire A.D. 50-60.		

UNITED KINGDOM

350000 B.C. – 500 B.C. EARLIEST CIVILIZATIONS

350000 B.C. Swanscombe Man, early form of human lives near River Thames.

8000 B.C. Early Britons begin settling in Great Britain.

6000 B.C. First settlers reach Ireland from Scotland.

2950-2500 B.C. Ancient Britons build Stonehenge, huge stone circle, on Salisbury Plain, England.

c. 800 B.C. Iron Age begins in Britain.

500 B.C. Celts begin settling in the British Isles.They are skilled metalworkers.

55 B.C. Julius Caesar makes first expedition to Britain.

100 B.C. – 999 A.D. ROMANS AND SAXONS

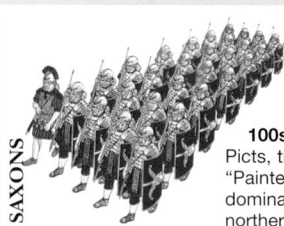

43 B.C.-A.D. 411 Romans occupy Great Britain.

100s-800s Picts, the "Painted People", dominate northern Scotland.

128 Romans build Hadrian's Wall to keep the Picts out of England.

300s Irish tribes called Scots begin settling in western Scotland.

400s Angles, Saxons, and Jutes begin settling in England.

800s Vikings invade from Denmark.

878 Battle of Edington: Alfred defeats the Danes.

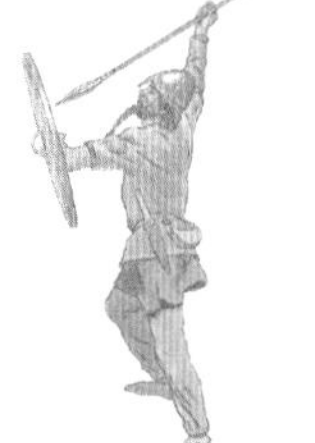

959 Edgar becomes the first king of a united England.

1000 – 1199 NORMAN BRITAIN

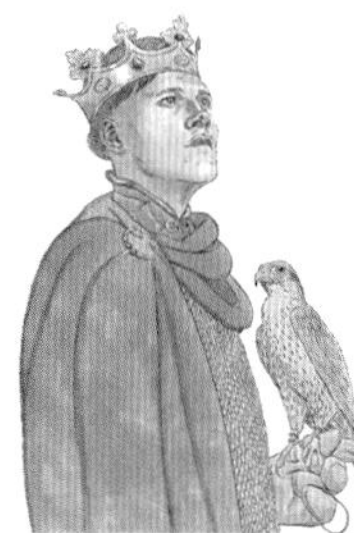

1066 Duke William of Normandy begins the conquest of England and becomes king as William I.

1085 Work begins on the Domesday Book, a record of English lands and possessions.

1169 Normans from England begin trying to conquer Ireland.

1173-89 Scotland becomes a state but is dependent on England.

1200 – 1399 WARS AND REBELLIONS

1215 England's barons force King John to agree to Magna Carta – the Great Charter.

1282 Edward I of England conquers Wales and kills its ruler, Prince Llwelyn.

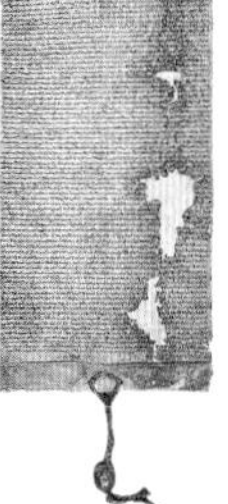

1314 Robert Bruce defeats the English at Bannockburn and becomes king of independent Scotland.

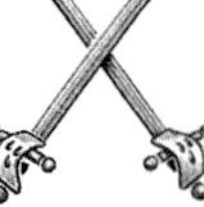

1320 Declaration of Arbroath demands Scottish independence.

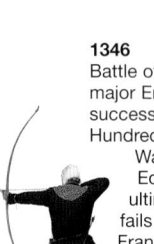

1346 Battle of Créçy: major English success in Hundred Years War; but Edward III ultimately fails to take France.

1371 Robert II becomes the first Stuart king of Scotland.

1381 Wat Tyler leads Peasants' Revolt against an unfair poll tax.

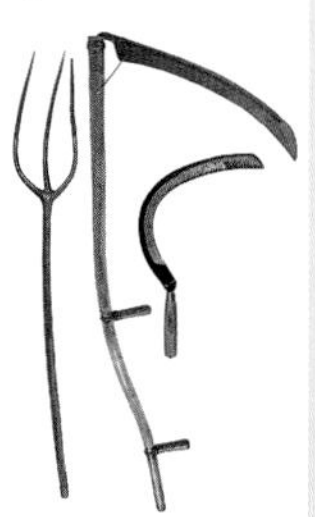

1400 – 1599 TUDORS AND REFORMATION

1400-10 Welsh prince Owain Glyn Dwr leads revolt against the English.

1455-85 Wars of the Roses: two royal families fight for the English throne.

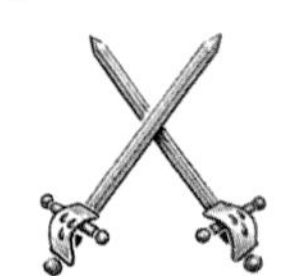

1485 Battle of Bosworth. Henry Tudor, last Lancastrian prince, becomes king as Henry VII.

1534 English Reformation: Henry VIII of England breaks with Rome and becomes head of the Church of England.

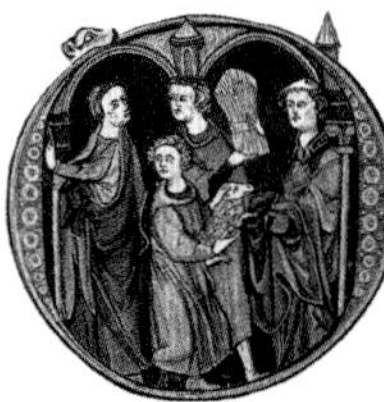

1536 Act of Union unites Wales and England.

1553 Mary II of England tries to restore Roman Catholicism; 300 Protestants burned at the stake.

1558-1603 Elizabeth I rules England; period of prosperity. The arts flourish.

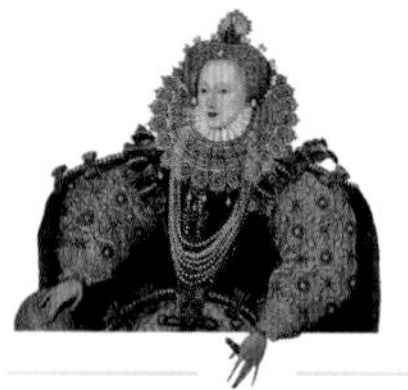

1564 Elizabethan playwright William Shakespeare is born.

1567 The English execute Mary, Queen of Scots for plotting against Elizabeth I of England.

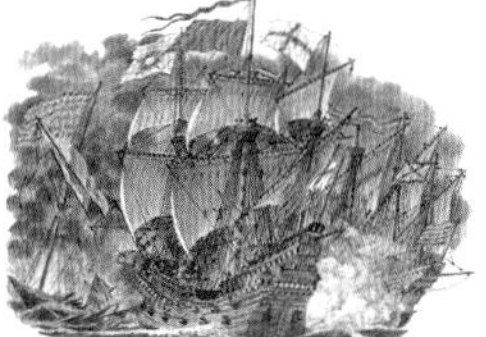

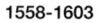

1588 English navy defeats the Spanish Armada, sent against England by Philip II, King of Spain.

1600 – 1799 STUARTS AND CIVIL WAR

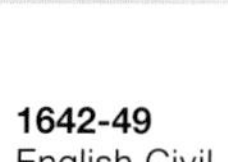

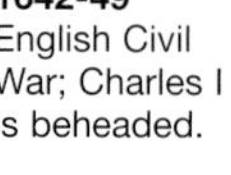

1603 Elizabeth I dies; her nephew James VI of Scotland becomes king of England as James I.

1605 Gunpowder Plot to blow up the Houses of Parliament. Plot fails, and leaders, including Guy Fawkes, are executed.

1607 First British overseas colony established at Jamestown, North America.

1642-49 English Civil War; Charles I is beheaded.

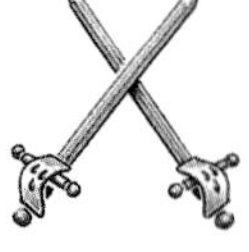

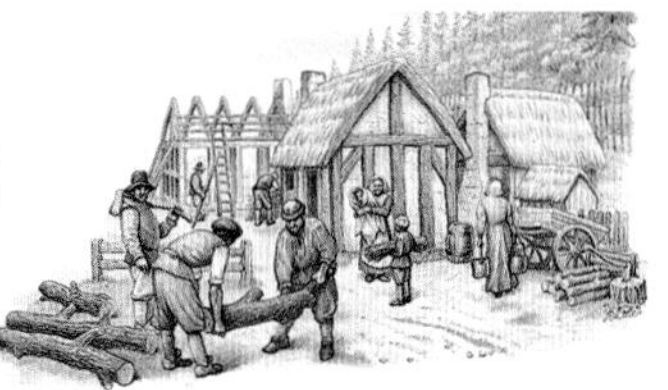

50	1000	1400	1600	1800	1900	2000
king invasions begin 795.	Norman conquest, 1066.	Black Death kills about 30% of population, 1348-49.	Act of Union between England and Scotland, 1707.	Great Exhibition held in London 1851.		Millennium Dome
nneth MacAlpine unites ts and Scots c.843.	Battle of Bannockburn, 1314; Scots defeat English.	Battle of Flodden, 1513, Scots defeated by English.	Jacobite rebellions during 1700s.		Scotland regains own parliament, 1999.	
	Brian Boru defeats Vikings at Battle of Clontarf, 1014.		Battle of Boyne, 1690, leads to Protestant domination.	Act of Union unites Ireland with England, 1800.	Good Friday Agreement, 1998.	
odri Mawr of Gwyndd 44-78) unites Wales.	Wales conquered by England, 1282.	Welsh uprisings against English until 1500.		Miners and other trade unionists active, 1800s.	First Plaid Cymru (Welsh Nationalist) MP elected, 1966.	

UNITED KINGDOM

1653-58
Puritan leader Oliver Cromwell rules England as dictator.

1660
The Restoration: Charles II becomes king of England.

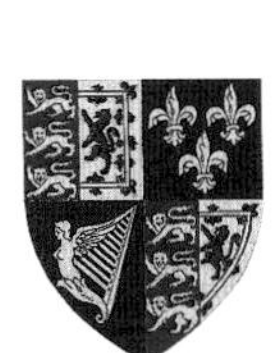

1666
Great Fire, following a bubonic plague epidemic, destroys most of London.

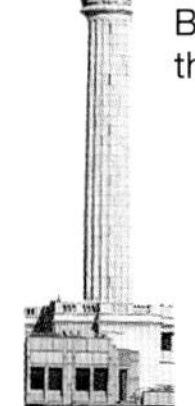

1688
Glorious Revolution brings William of Orange to British throne.

1700 – 1799 INDUSTRIAL REVOLUTION

1714-1837
German princes of the House of Hanover rule Great Britain.

1715
Robert Walpole becomes Britain's first prime minister.

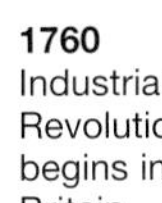

1715-46
Jacobite (Stuart) rebellions in Scotland.

Jacobites finally defeated at Culloden Moor; Scottish clans abolished.

1760
Industrial Revolution begins in Britain.

1783
Britain loses its North American colonies after American Revolutionary War.

1788
First British convicts sent to Australia.

1799-1815
Britain fights a long war against Napoleon I of France.

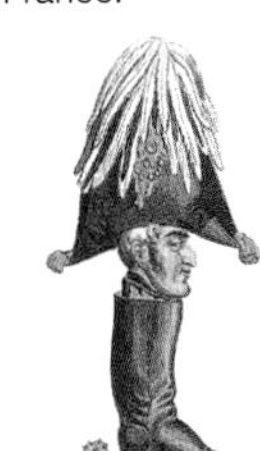

1800 – 1899 THE AGE OF EMPIRE

1800
Ireland is annexed, forming the United Kingdom of Great Britain and Ireland.

1832
First Reform Act gives the vote to middle-class, property-owning men.

1837-1901
Reign of Queen Victoria, the "Victorian Age"; the British Empire expands.

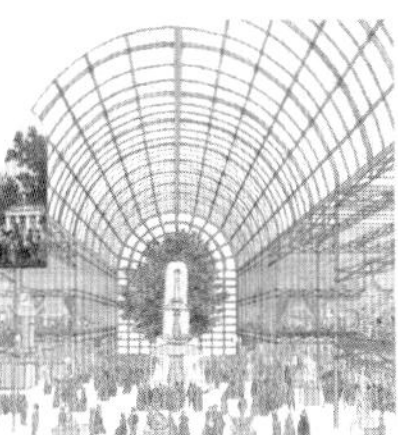

1851
Great Exhibition is held in London in the Crystal Palace.

1853-56
Florence Nightingale reforms nursing during the Crimean War.

1870
Forster's Education Act: introduces state education for children up to age 13.

1899-1902
Anglo-Boer War: Britain defeats Dutch colonists in South Africa.

1900 – 1950 MODERN WORLD

1903
Pankhursts found the Women's Social and Political Union (WSPU).

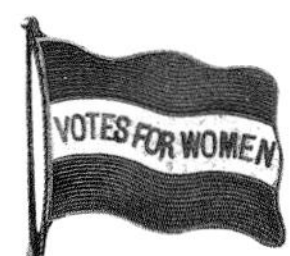

1914-18
World War I; Britain and the Allies fight Germany and Austro-Hungarian Empire.

1916
Easter Rebellion in Ireland fails.

1918
British women over 30 gain the vote.

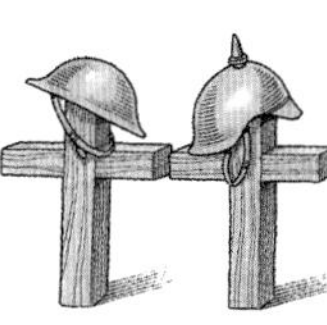

1919
Irish Republican army (IRA) is formed to fight for Irish independence.

1921
Ireland is partitioned: 26 southern counties form a dominion; six northern counties remain in the UK. There is civil war in southern Ireland and in 1922 the Irish Free State is formed.

1925
Plaid Cymru, the Welsh nationalist party, is founded.

1928
Universal suffrage: men and women over the age of 21 can vote.

1931
British Commonwealth of Nations formed.

1939-45
World War II.

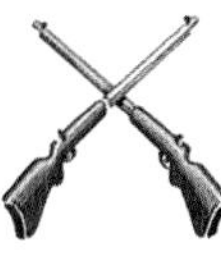

1945
Welfare State established; leads to National Health Service in 1948.

1948
Empire Windrush brings 510 Jamaicans to Britain.

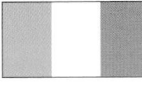

1949
Southern Ireland becomes an independent republic.

1950 – 2000 INTO THE NEW MILLENNIUM

1951
Festival of Britain.

1953
Elizabeth II becomes Queen.

1969
IRA begins campaign of civil disobedience against the British in Northern Ireland.

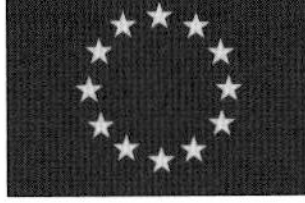

1973
United Kingdom joins the Common Market (now the European Union).

1976
Race Relations Commission set up to work for an end to racial discrimination in Britain.

1979
Margaret Thatcher becomes the UK's first woman prime minister.

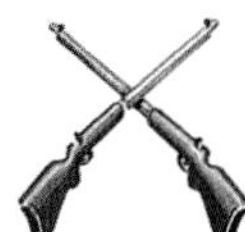

1982
Falklands War; Britain goes to war with Argentina over possession of the Falkland Islands (Malvinas).

1988
Education Act: introduces national curriculum into Britain.

1985
Live Aid, British rock concert, raises money for Ethiopia, and is broadcast worldwide.

1994
Channel Tunnel opens, linking England with Europe.

1997
Diana, Princess of Wales killed in car crash.

1998
Good Friday Agreement in Northern Ireland; IRA promises ceasefire.

1999
UK parliament agrees to abolish voting rights of hereditary peers as a first step to reforming the House of Lords.

1999
Devolution: Scotland regains own parliament; Wales gets National Assembly.

1999/2000
Millennium Dome opens in Greenwich, London to celebrate the arrival of the year 2000. Thousands attend the opening party.

2005
Tony Blair, prime minister since 1997, wins third consecutive general election victory for the Labour Party.

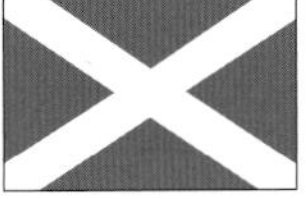

THE WORLD

SINCE TIME BEGAN, world population has risen and fallen as health and food supplies have changed. The number of people alive at any one time rose when there was plenty of food, and fell when famine or disease struck. Until about 800 A.D., the population of the world stayed below 200 million. But since then it has risen dramatically. The rise was greatest in the 20th century; by the year 2020, experts predict that there will be more than 8.5 billion people living. The population graph below charts the world's rising population since 1500, and includes a forecast.

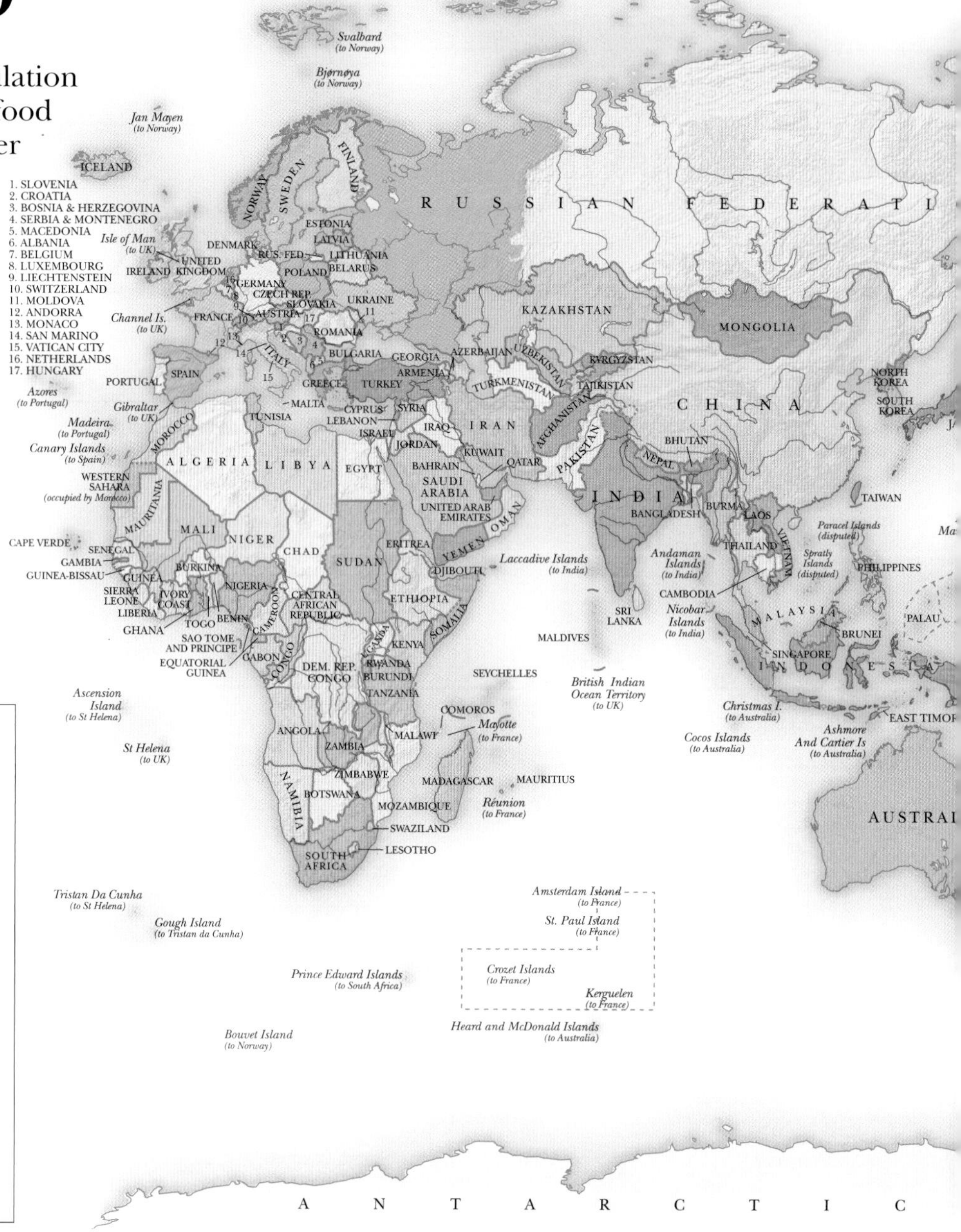

1. SLOVENIA
2. CROATIA
3. BOSNIA & HERZEGOVINA
4. SERBIA & MONTENEGRO
5. MACEDONIA
6. ALBANIA
7. BELGIUM
8. LUXEMBOURG
9. LIECHTENSTEIN
10. SWITZERLAND
11. MOLDOVA
12. ANDORRA
13. MONACO
14. SAN MARINO
15. VATICAN CITY
16. NETHERLANDS
17. HUNGARY

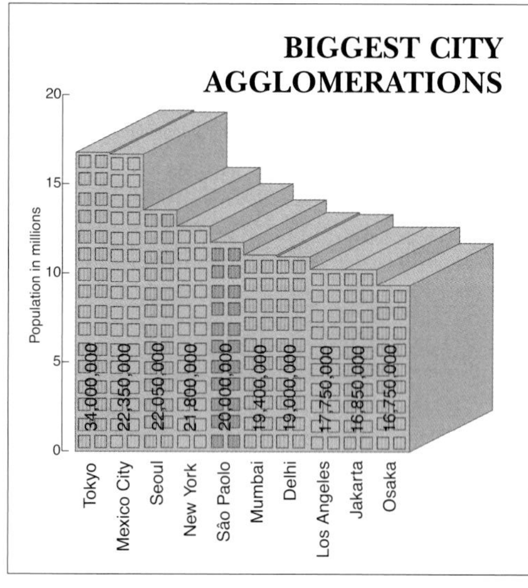

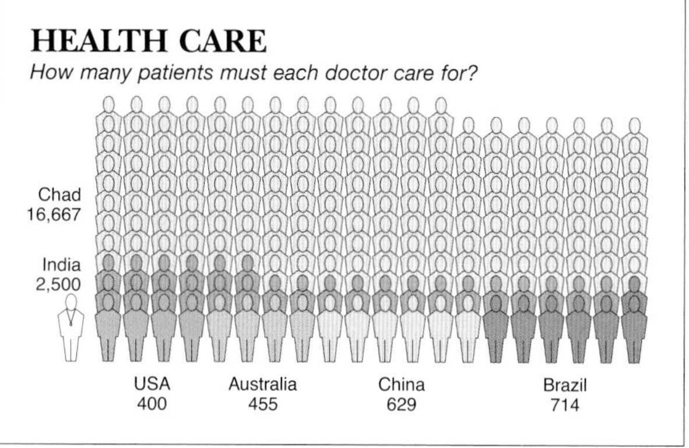

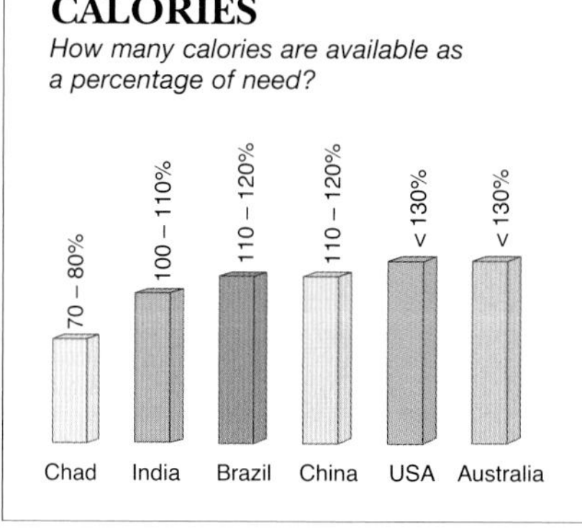

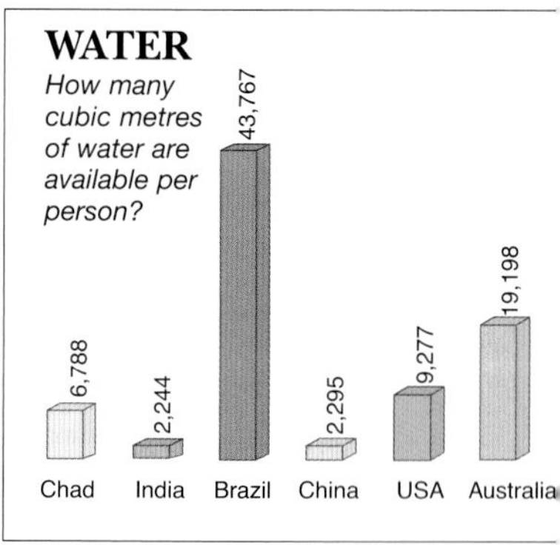

WORLD POPULATION GROWTH SINCE 1500

One figure represents 500 million people

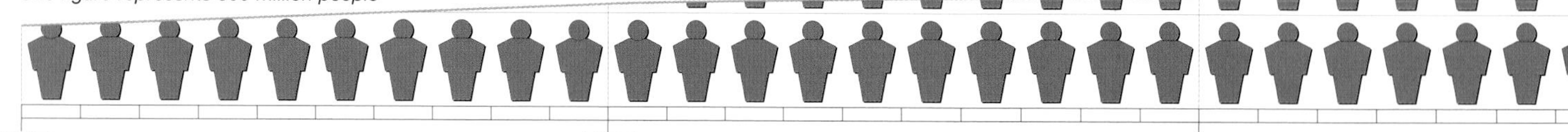

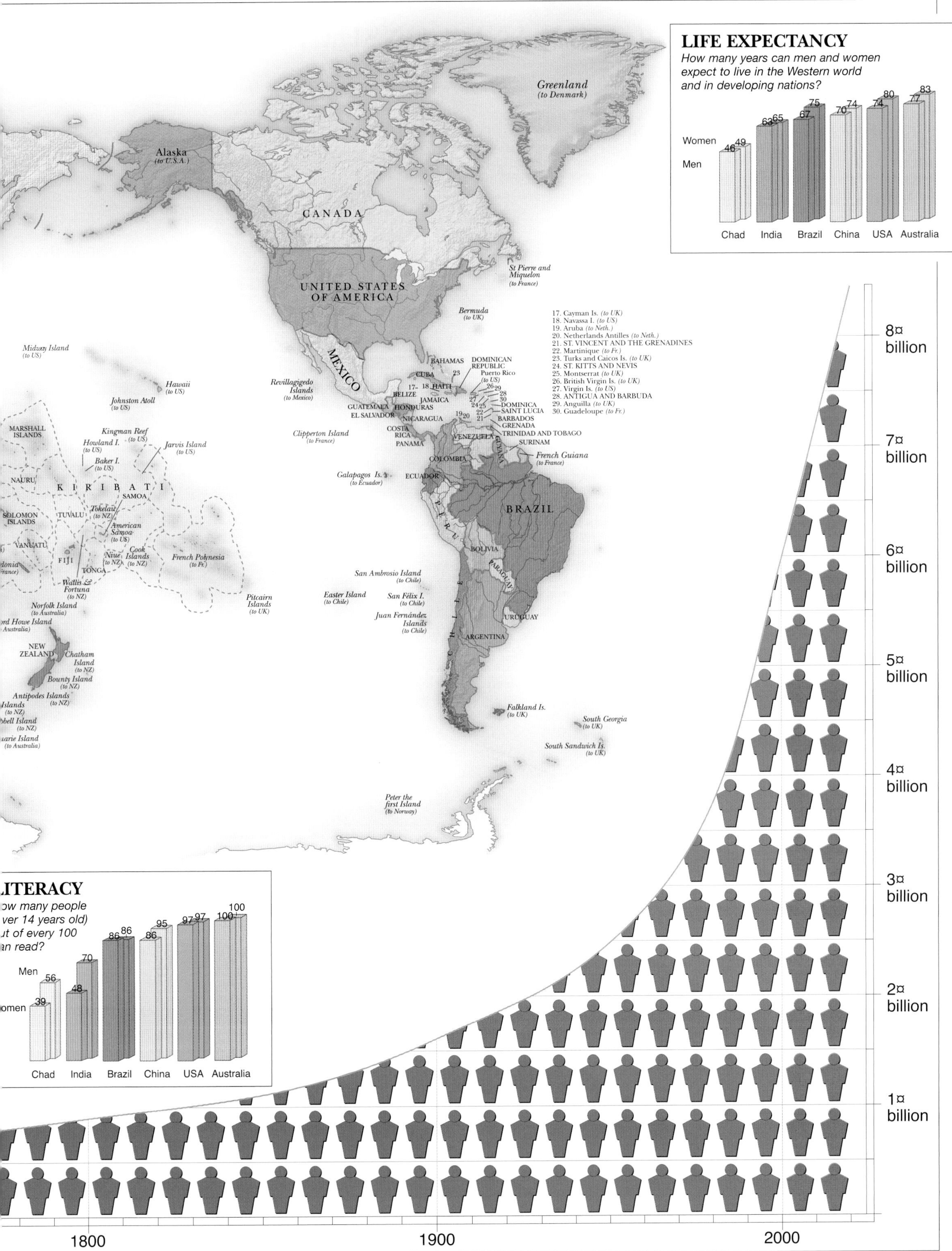
LIFE EXPECTANCY
How many years can men and women expect to live in the Western world and in developing nations?
Women
Men
46 49
63 65
67 75
70 74
74 80
77 83
Chad
India
Brazil
China
USA
Australia
Greenland
(to Denmark)
Alaska
(to U.S.A.)
CANADA
UNITED STATES OF AMERICA
St Pierre and Miquelon
(to France)
Bermuda
(to UK)
17. Cayman Is. (to UK)
18. Navassa I. (to US)
19. Aruba (to Neth.)
20. Netherlands Antilles (to Neth.)
21. ST. VINCENT AND THE GRENADINES
22. Martinique (to Fr.)
23. Turks and Caicos Is. (to UK)
24. ST. KITTS AND NEVIS
25. Montserrat (to UK)
26. British Virgin Is. (to UK)
27. Virgin Is. (to US)
28. ANTIGUA AND BARBUDA
29. Anguilla (to UK)
30. Guadeloupe (to Fr.)
Midway Island
(to US)
Hawaii
(to US)
Johnston Atoll
(to US)
Revillagigedo Islands
(to Mexico)
MEXICO
BAHAMAS
CUBA
HAITI
DOMINICAN REPUBLIC
Puerto Rico
(to US)
BELIZE
JAMAICA
GUATEMALA
HONDURAS
EL SALVADOR
NICARAGUA
COSTA RICA
PANAMA
DOMINICA
SAINT LUCIA
BARBADOS
GRENADA
TRINIDAD AND TOBAGO
SURINAM
French Guiana
(to France)
VENEZUELA
GUYANA
COLOMBIA
ECUADOR
Clipperton Island
(to France)
Galapagos Is.
(to Ecuador)
MARSHALL ISLANDS
Kingman Reef
(to US)
Howland I.
(to US)
Jarvis Island
(to US)
Baker I.
(to US)
NAURU
KIRIBATI
SAMOA
SOLOMON ISLANDS
TUVALU
Tokelau
(to NZ)
American Samoa
(to US)
VANUATU
FIJI
Niue
(to NZ)
Cook Islands
(to NZ)
French Polynesia
(to Fr.)
TONGA
Wallis & Fortuna
(to NZ)
Norfolk Island
(to Australia)
Pitcairn Islands
(to UK)
BRAZIL
PERU
BOLIVIA
PARAGUAY
San Ambrosio Island
(to Chile)
Easter Island
(to Chile)
San Félix I.
(to Chile)
Juan Fernández Islands
(to Chile)
CHILE
URUGUAY
ARGENTINA
NEW ZEALAND
Chatham Island
(to NZ)
Bounty Island
(to NZ)
Antipodes Islands
(to NZ)
Falkland Is.
(to UK)
South Georgia
(to UK)
South Sandwich Is.
(to UK)
Peter the first Island
(to Norway)
LITERACY
How many people over 14 years old out of every 100 can read?
Men
Women
39 56
48 70
86 86
86 95
97 97
100 100
Chad
India
Brazil
China
USA
Australia
8 billion
7 billion
6 billion
5 billion
4 billion
3 billion
2 billion
1 billion
1800
1900
2000

Energy production and consumption

Fossil fuels – oil, coal and gas – still supply most of the world's energy, but they are rapidly being used up. Most of the fossil fuels come from countries in the Middle East. Although each year new reserves of oil and natural gas are found, no-one knows how long these reserves will last. Because people in the developed countries have so many cars and electrical appliances, they use far more energy than people in the less-developed countries. The USA alone uses 25 per cent of the world's energy, but only has five per cent of its population. Nuclear power is being used in increasing amounts, but there are concerns about its safety and the nuclear waste it produces. The use of alternative sources of energy, such as wave power, solar power, and wind power, is also increasing, but still only supplies a tiny fraction of the energy the world needs.

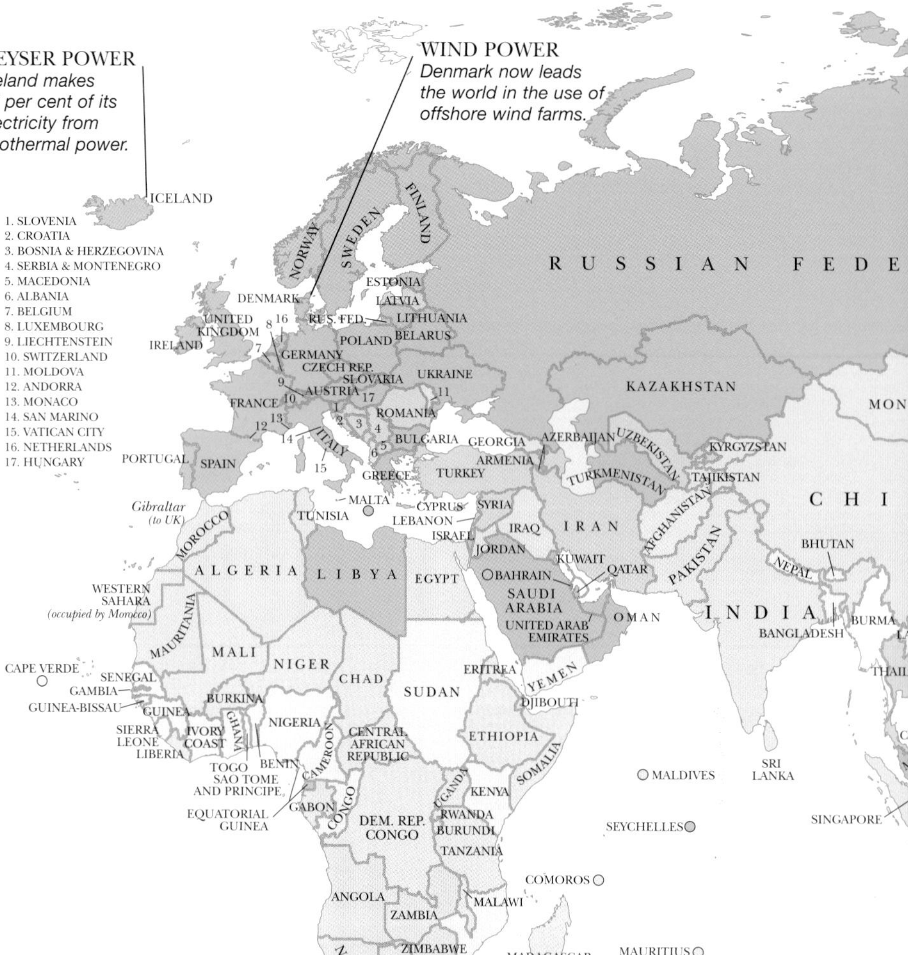

ENERGY CONSUMPTION (Kilograms of coal equivalent per person a year)

- more than 10,000¤
- 5000 – 10,000¤
- 1000 – 5000¤
- 100 – 1000¤
- less than 100¤
- no data

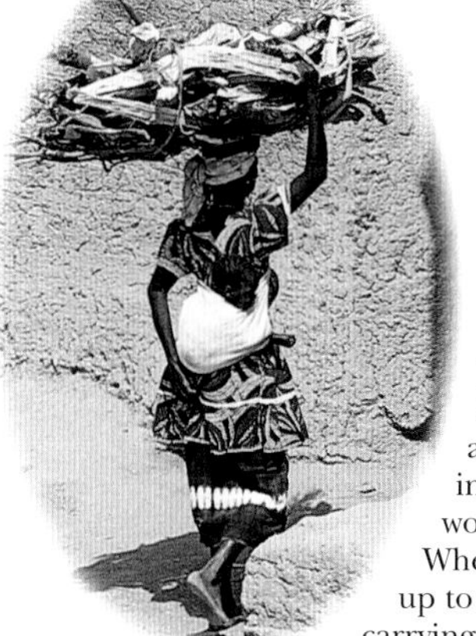

WOOD POWER
In the villages of Africa, Brazil, and India the burning of wood is the main source of energy. But as the forests are cut down, firewood becomes increasingly hard to find. Collecting wood is traditionally women's work. Where wood is scarce, women can spend up to four hours a day searching for it and carrying it long distances back to their villages.

Oil

Modern industrial economies greatly depend on oil to drive their machines and factories. To feed the global appetite for oil, almost nine million tonnes of oil are produced each day. Saudi Arabia is the world's largest oil producer; the USA is the largest consumer. Countries that produce more oil than they need export it to countries that have no oil reserves. The crude oil is either shipped in huge oil tankers, or piped. Since the 1960s, oil spills have been a major environmental problem, polluting the oceans and destroying wildlife.

World exporters of energy

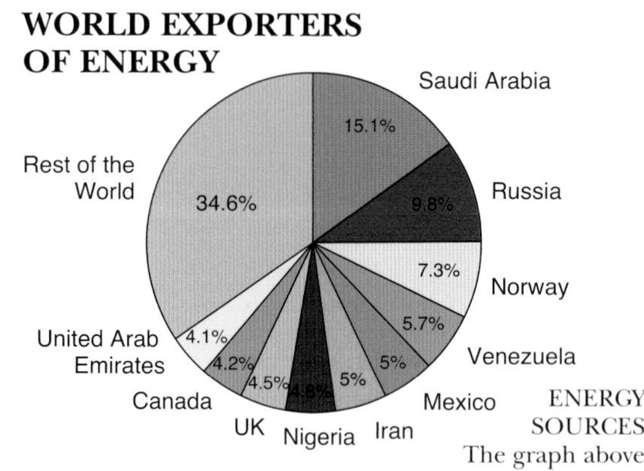

ENERGY SOURCES
The graph above shows that only ten countries provide almost two thirds the world's fossil fuels – oil, coal, and gas. Burning these fuels is the major cause of global warming, whereas hydro-electric power is a cheap and renewable energy source.

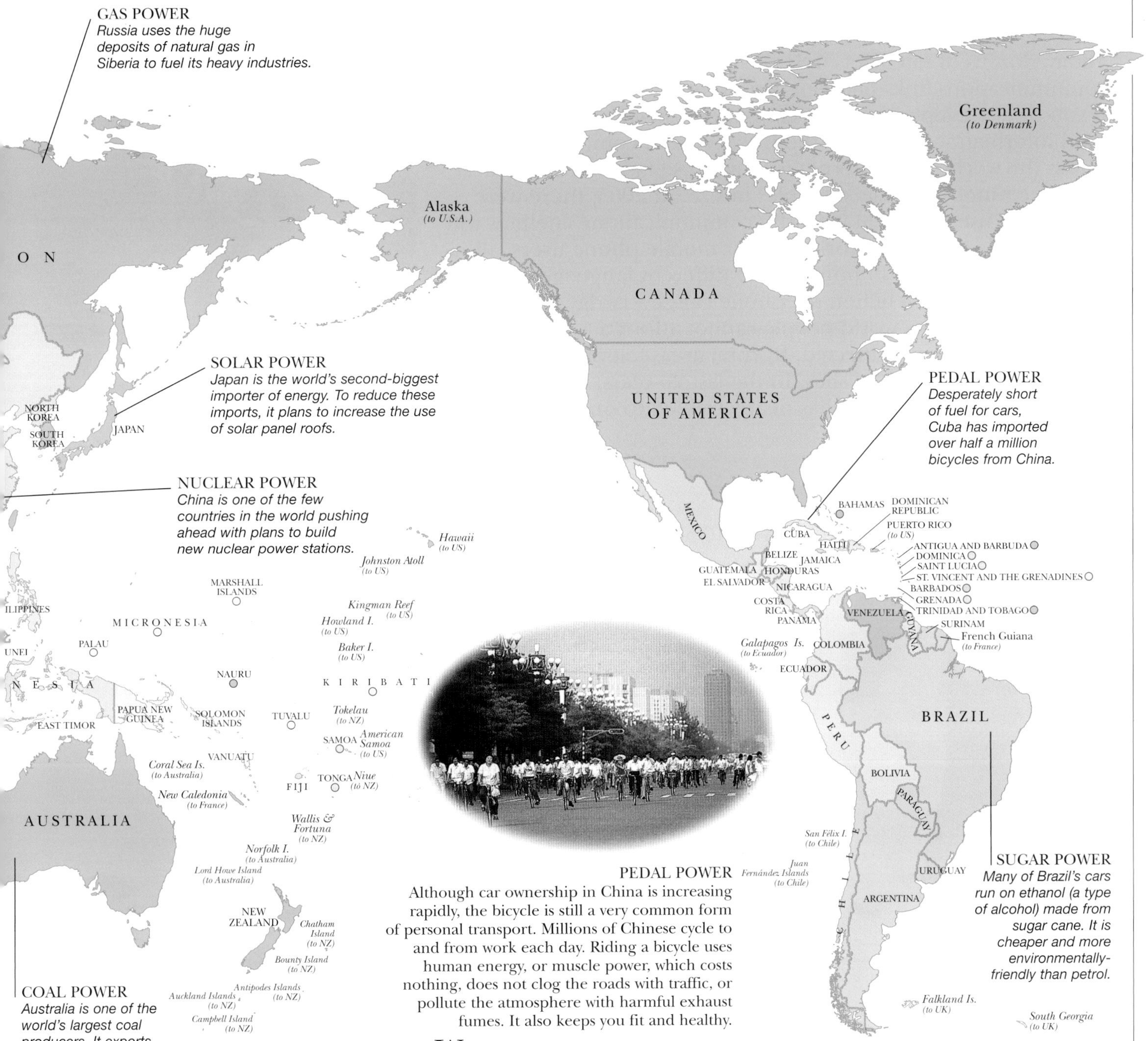

GAS POWER
Russia uses the huge deposits of natural gas in Siberia to fuel its heavy industries.

SOLAR POWER
Japan is the world's second-biggest importer of energy. To reduce these imports, it plans to increase the use of solar panel roofs.

NUCLEAR POWER
China is one of the few countries in the world pushing ahead with plans to build new nuclear power stations.

PEDAL POWER
Desperately short of fuel for cars, Cuba has imported over half a million bicycles from China.

PEDAL POWER
Although car ownership in China is increasing rapidly, the bicycle is still a very common form of personal transport. Millions of Chinese cycle to and from work each day. Riding a bicycle uses human energy, or muscle power, which costs nothing, does not clog the roads with traffic, or pollute the atmosphere with harmful exhaust fumes. It also keeps you fit and healthy.

SUGAR POWER
Many of Brazil's cars run on ethanol (a type of alcohol) made from sugar cane. It is cheaper and more environmentally-friendly than petrol.

COAL POWER
Australia is one of the world's largest coal producers. It exports millions of tonnes each year, much of it to Japan.

WASTE

The richer and more developed a country is, the more waste it produces. Every day people in the USA dump tonnes of paper, newspapers, disposable babies' nappies, aluminium cans, clothing, and car tyres. Getting rid of these mountains of waste is a major world problem. Recycling rubbish helps; of the 520,000 tonnes of rubbish produced by the USA every day, 20 per cent is recycled. Germany has the best record for recycling waste. In some cities in the less-developed world, the poor make a living by picking through rubbish dumps and selling what they find to recycling centres.

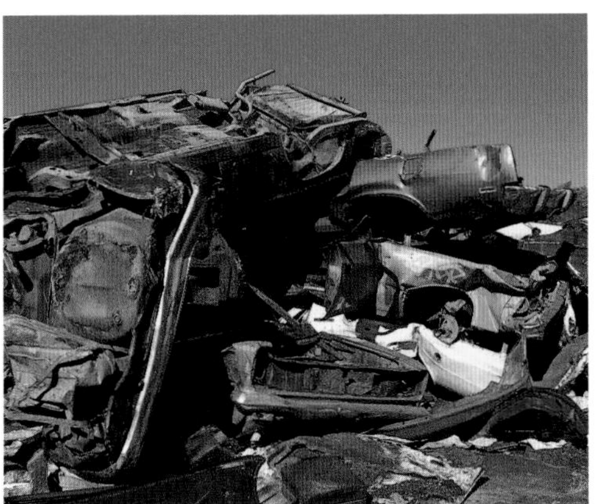

USED CARS
Every day, hundreds of thousands of vehicles roll off the world's production lines. By the year 2025, there will be an estimated one billion cars on the world's roads. The USA and Japan manufacture more cars each year than any other country in the world. But every day in the USA some 32,000 tonnes of used cars are put on the scrap-heap. The exhaust from cars pollutes the air. In many of the world's major cities, the very act of breathing is a health hazard.

Find out more

ENERGY
COAL
GAS
NUCLEAR ENERGY
OIL
POLLUTION
TRADE AND INDUSTRY

Global communications

Today, dozens of satellites circle the globe, providing communications links between various points on Earth. If you have a telephone and a computer, you can receive and send information, log on to the Internet, and communicate across the world. The Internet is growing so fast that every three years the number of users doubles in size. In 2005, there were 900 millon users. Special low-orbit communications satellites will soon provide reception worldwide for mobile phone users, all talking to each other in hundreds of different languages. Americans make 1.3 billion telephone calls every day. However, in some parts of the world people cannot afford a telephone, or it takes years to get connected. In rural areas television images can be received via satellite dishes. In the last 20 years, the number of television sets in the world has nearly trebled to one billion.

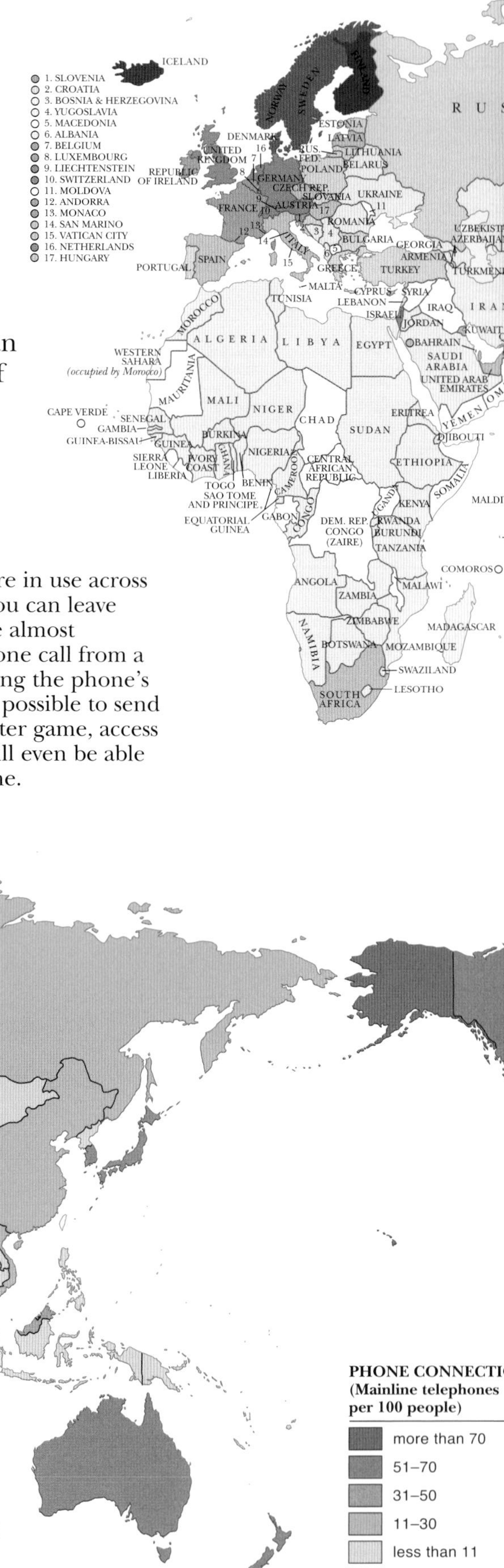

Mobile phones

Every day, around two billion mobile phones are in use across the world. With your phone in your pocket, you can leave home and still be able to telephone someone almost anywhere on the planet. You can make a phone call from a bus or call home from a holiday abroad. Using the phone's super-large high-resolution screen, it is now possible to send and receive e-mails and faxes, play a computer game, access the Internet, or listen to music. Soon you will even be able to watch your favourite television programme.

SWEDEN
In the year 2003, with 73.6 telephones per 100 people, Sweden had the highest proportion of telephones in the world.

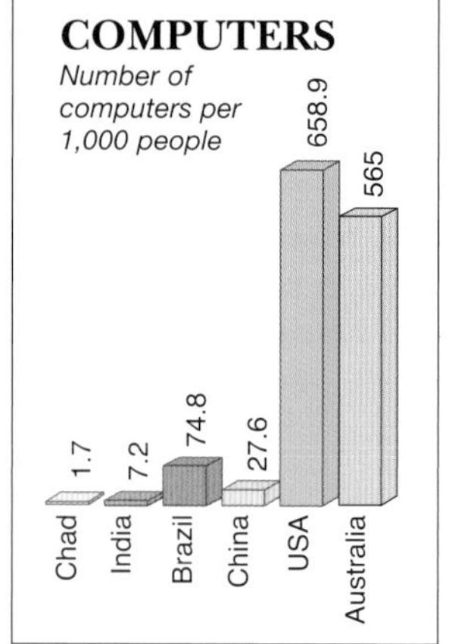

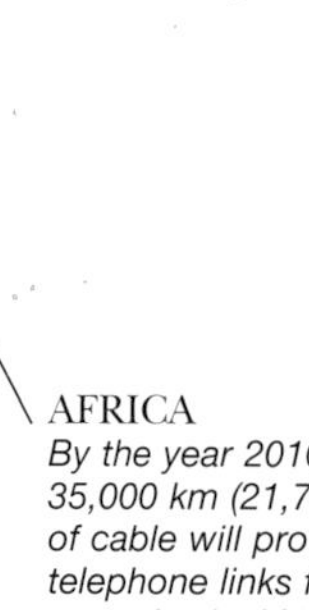

AFRICA
By the year 2010, 35,000 km (21,749 miles) of cable will provide telephone links for 41 countries in Africa.

PHONE CONNECTIONS
(Mainline telephones per 100 people)

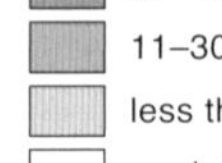

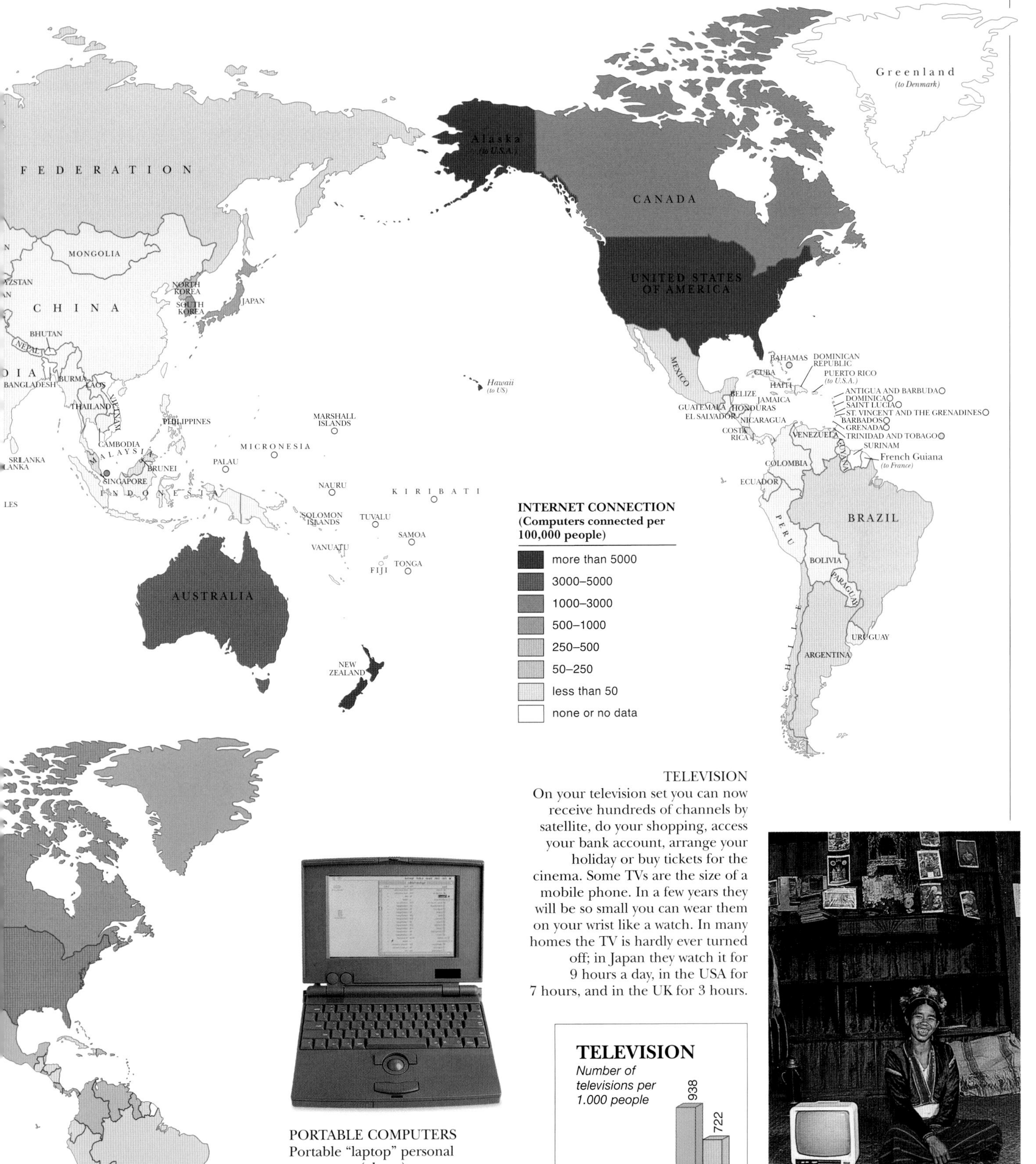

TELEVISION
On your television set you can now receive hundreds of channels by satellite, do your shopping, access your bank account, arrange your holiday or buy tickets for the cinema. Some TVs are the size of a mobile phone. In a few years they will be so small you can wear them on your wrist like a watch. In many homes the TV is hardly ever turned off; in Japan they watch it for 9 hours a day, in the USA for 7 hours, and in the UK for 3 hours.

PORTABLE COMPUTERS
Portable "laptop" personal computers (above) are now so small and light that they can be used while flying over the Atlantic Ocean as easily as in the office or in your home. You can sit on the beach and send a letter to a friend by tapping it out on the keyboard as an email, or you can send a voice message by talking into the computer.

Find out more

Computers
Internet
Satellites
Telephones
Television and video

UK COUNTIES

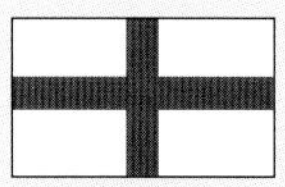

ENGLAND

COUNTY	COUNTY TOWN	AREA SQ KM (SQ MILES)
Bedfordshire	Bedford	1,192 (460)
Buckinghamshire	Aylesbury	1,565 (604)
Cambridgeshire	Cambridge	3,410 (1,316)
Cheshire	Chester	2,320 (896)
Cornwall	Truro	3,550 (1,370)
Cumbria	Carlisle	6,810 (2,629)
Derbyshire	Matlock	2,550 (984)
Devon	Exeter	6,720 (2,594)
Dorset	Dorchester	2,541 (981)
Durham	Durham	2,232 (862)
East Sussex	Lewes	1,725 (666)
Essex	Chelmsford	3,670 (1,417)
Gloucestershire	Gloucester	2,640 (1,019)
Hampshire	Winchester	3,679 (1,420)
Hertfordshire	Hertford	1,630 (629)
Kent	Maidstone	3,730 (1,440)
Lancashire	Preston	3,040 (1,173)
Leicestershire	Leicester	2,084 (804)
Lincolnshire	Lincoln	5,890 (2,274)
Norfolk	Norwich	5,360 (2,069)
Northamptonshire	Northampton	2,370 (915)
Northumberland	Morpeth	5,030 (1,942)
North Yorkshire	Northallerton	8,037 (3,102)
Nottinghamshire	Nottingham	2,160 (834)
Oxfordshire	Oxford	2,610 (1,007)
Shropshire	Shrewsbury	3,490 (1,347)
Somerset	Taunton	3,460 (1,336)
Staffordshire	Stafford	2,623 (1,012)
Suffolk	Ipswich	3,800 (1,467)
Surrey	Kingston upon Thames	1,660 (641)
Warwickshire	Warwick	1,980 (764)
West Sussex	Chichester	2,020 (780)
Wiltshire	Trowbridge	3,255 (1,256)
Worcestershire	Worcester	1,640 (1,020)

NORTHERN IRELAND

COUNTY	CO. TOWN	AREA SQ KM (SQ MILES)
Antrim	Belfast	2,845 (1,098)
Armagh	Armagh	1,265 (488)
Down	Downpatrick	2,460 (950)
Fermanagh	Enniskillen	1,850 (714)
Londonderry	Londonderry	2,075 (801)
Tyrone	Omagh	3,265 (1,260)

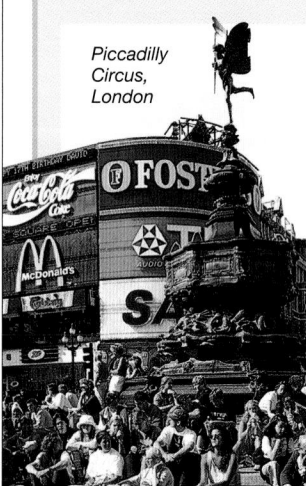

Piccadilly Circus, London

TOP TEN CITIES

CITY	POPULATION (URBAN AREA)
London	7,926,000
Birmingham	2,360,000
Manchester	2,337,000
Glasgow	1,648,000
Leeds	1,581,000
Newcastle upon Tyne	797,000
Liverpool	780,000
Sheffield	673,000
Nottingham	631,000
Bristol	568,000

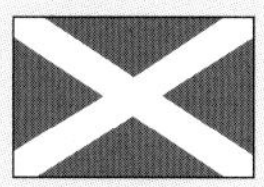

SCOTLAND

COUNTY	CO. TOWN	AREA SQ KM (SQ MILES)
Aberdeen City	Aberdeen	184 (71)
Aberdeenshire	Aberdeen	6,289 (2,428)
Angus	Forfar	2,184 (843)
Argyll and Bute	Lochgilphead	4,001 (1,545)
Clackmannanshire	Alloa	161 (62)
Dumfries and Galloway	Dumfries	6,394 (2,468)
Dundee City	Dundee	65 (25)
East Ayrshire	Kilmarnock	1,271 (491)
East Dunbartonshire	Glasgow	202 (78)
East Lothian	Haddington	681 (263)
East Renfrewshire	Giffnock	172 (66)
Edinburgh City	Edinburgh	261 (101)
Eilean Siar/Western Isles	Stornoway	2,900 (1,120)
Falkirk	Falkirk	294 (114)
Fife	Glenrothes	1,340 (517)
Glasgow City	Glasgow	177 (68)
Highland	Inverness	25,304 (9,767)
Inverclyde	Greenock	157 (60)
Midlothian	Dalkeith	355 (137)
Moray	Elgin	2,217 (856)
North Ayrshire	Irvine	878 (339)
North Lanarkshire	Motherwell	466 (180)
Orkney Islands	Kirkwall	970 (375)
Perth and Kinross	Perth	5,328 (2,058)
Renfrewshire	Paisley	261 (101)
Scottish Borders	Newtown St. Boswells	4,712 (1,819)
Shetland Islands	Lerwick	1,400 (541)
South Ayrshire	Ayr	1,202 (464)
South Lanarkshire	Hamilton	1,776 (686)
Stirling	Stirling	2,195 (848)
West Dunbartonshire	Dumbarton	155 (60)
West Lothian	Livingston	2,900 (1,120)

WALES

COUNTY	CO. TOWN	AREA SQ KM (SQ MILES)
Anglesey	Llangefai	720 (278)
Blaenau Gwent	Ebbw Vale	109 (42)
Bridgend	Bridgend	40 (15)
Caerphilly	Hengoed	270 (104)
Cardiff	Cardiff	139 (54)
Carmarthenshire	Carmarthen	2,390 (923)
Ceredigion	Aberaeron	1,793 (692)
Conwy	Conwy	1,107 (427)
Denbighshire	Ruthin	844 (326)
Flintshire	Mold	437 (167)
Gwynedd	Caernarfon	2,546 (983)
Merthyr Tydfil	Merthyr Tydfil	111 (43)
Monmouthshire	Cwmbran	851 (328)
Neath Port Talbot	Port Talbot	442 (171)
Newport	Newport	190 (73)
Pembrokeshire	Haverfordwest	1,588 (613)
Powys	Llandridnod Wells	5,179 (1,999)
Rhondda Cynon Taff	Clydach Vale	440 (170)
Swansea	Swansea	377 (156)
Torfaen	Pontypool	98 (38)
Vale of Glamorgan	Barry	337 (130)
Wrexham	Wrexham	500 (193)

UK GEOGRAPHY

HIGHEST MOUNTAIN PEAKS, BY COUNTRY

Scotland	Ben Nevis	1,392 m (4,406 ft)
Wales	Snowdon	1,085 m (3,560 ft)
England	Scafell Pike	978 m (3,210 ft)
N. Ireland	Slieve Donard	852 m (2,796 ft)

LARGEST LAKES, BY COUNTRY

England	Windermere	14.7 sq km (5.7 sq miles)
Wales	Llyn Tegid (Lake Bala)	4.38 sq km (1.7 sq miles)
Scotland	Loch Lomond	71.2 sq km (27.5 sq miles)
N. Ireland	Lough Neagh	381.73 sq km (147.4 sq miles)

TOP TEN RIVERS, BY LENGTH

NAME	LOCATION	LENGTH
Severn	Wales/England	354 km (220 miles)
Thames	England	346 km (215 miles)
Trent/Humber	England	297 km (185 miles)
Aire/Ouse	England	259 km (169 miles)
Great Ouse	England	230 km (143 miles)
Wye	Wales/England	215 km (135 miles)
Tay	Scotland	188 km (117 miles)
Clyde	Scotland	158 km (99 miles)
Spey	Scotland	158 km (98 miles)
Tweed	Scotland/England	155 km (97 miles)

UK STRUCTURES

NOTABLE TUNNELS AND BRIDGES

TUNNEL	ROUTE	LENGTH
Channel Tunnel	Cheriton-Calais	49.94 km (31.22 miles)
Northern Line	Finchley-Morden	27.84 km (17.4 miles)
Severn Rail	Bristol-Newport	7.00 km (4.38 miles)
Mersey Road	Liverpool-Birkenhead	3.42 km (2.38 miles)

BRIDGE	TYPE	LENGTH
Severn Bridge 2	Suspension	5,150 m (16,896 ft)
Tay Bridge	Multiple span	3,220 m (10,564 ft)
Humber Bridge	Suspension	2,220 m (7,282 ft)
Forth Rail Bridge	Cantilever	521 m (1,709 ft)
London Bridge	Multiple arch	275 m (902 ft)
Tower Bridge	Bascule	83 m (272 ft)
Ironbridge	World's first iron bridge	183 m (600 ft)

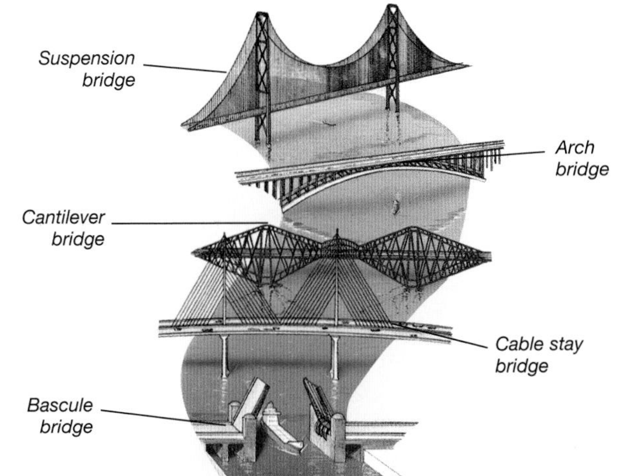

UK LIFESTYLE

TOP TEN NEWSPAPERS

TITLE AND DATE OF FOUNDING	DAILY CIRCULATION (2005)
1 *The Sun* (1964)	3,653,168
2 *Daily Mail* (1896)	2,359,003
3 *Mirror* (1903)	2,248,111
4 *Daily Telegraph* (1855)	915,711
5 *Express* (1900)	898,396
6 *Daily Star* (1978)	863,083
7 *The Times* (1785)	684,695
8 *Financial Times* (1888)	431,287
9 *The Guardian* (1821)	372,562
10 *The Independent* (1986)	263,043

FOOD FACTS

- On average, British people eat 16 g of hamburger per person per week
- On average, British people eat 4 g of apple per person per week
- On average, British people eat 12 g of pizza per person per week
- On average, British people eat 73 g of chips per person per week
- On average, British people eat 17 g of sweets and chocolate per person per week

PETS

PET	PERCENTAGE OF PET-OWNING HOUSEHOLDS
Dog	23.4%
Cat	21.4%
Goldfish	9.3%
Rabbit	3.9%
Hamster	3.2%

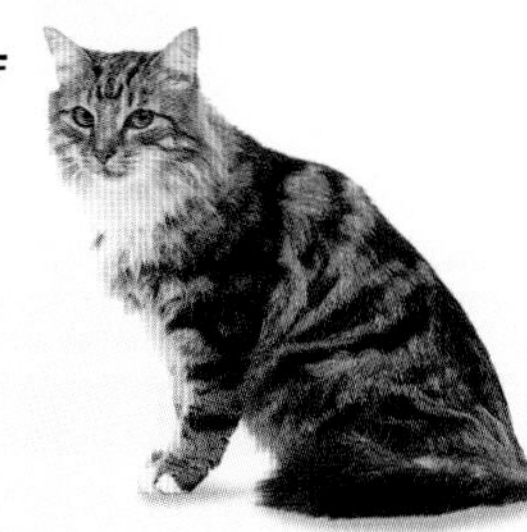

Over half of all households in the UK contain a pet. Dogs and cats are the most popular.

UK COMMEMORATIVE DAYS

Burns Night	25 January
St. David's Day	1 March
Commonwealth Day	13 March
St. Patrick's Day	17 March
St. George's Day	23 April
Queen's Official Birthday	17 June
Orangeman's Day	12 July
Guy Fawkes Night	5 November
Remembrance Day	11 November
St. Andrew's Day	30 November

TOP TEN FOOTBALL TEAMS*

CLUB	AVERAGE ATTENDANCE
Manchester United	67,641
Newcastle United	51,440
Manchester City	46,834
Liverpool	42,677
Chelsea	41,234
Everton	38,837
Arsenal	38,079
Leeds United	36,666
Aston Villa	36,622
Tottenham Hotspur	34,876

*Average attendance 2003–04

OLYMPIC GAMES

The categories for the Games are reviewed frequently. Some of the most popular events are listed below.

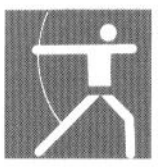
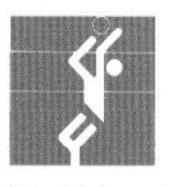

Archery
Athletics
Badminton
Baseball

Field hockey
Judo
Pentathlon
Rowing

Basketball
Boxing
Canoeing
Cycling

Shooting
Swimming
Tennis
Volleyball

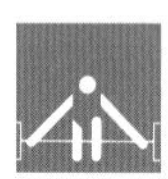

Equestrian sports
Football
Gymnastics

Water polo
Weightlifting
Wrestling
Yachting

SUMMER GAMES HISTORY

SITE	YEAR
Athens	1896
Paris	1900
St. Louis	1904
London	1908
Stockholm	1912
Antwerp	1920
Paris	1924
Amsterdam	1928
Los Angeles	1932
Berlin	1936
London	1948
Helsinki	1952
Melbourne	1956
Rome	1960
Tokyo	1964
Mexico City	1968
Munich	1972
Montreal	1976
Moscow	1980
Los Angeles	1984
Seoul	1988
Barcelona	1992
Atlanta	1996
Sydney	2000
Athens	2004
Beijing	2008

INTERNATIONAL ORGANIZATIONS

Listed below are some of the major international organizations that work towards co-operation between their member countries. The subjects that each are concerned with range from financial matters and trade, to peace, education, and crime.

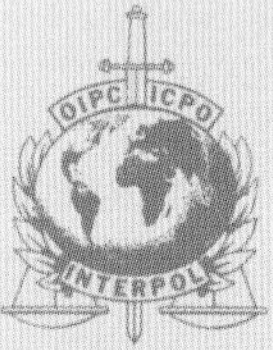

INTERPOL
International Criminal Police Organization
Est. 1994
182 member states
www.interpol.com

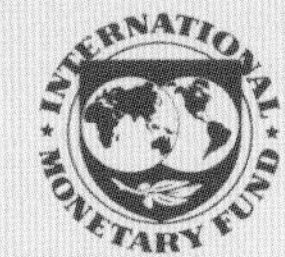
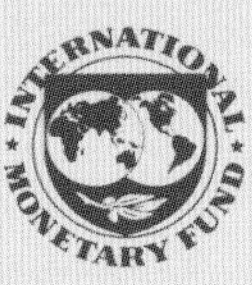

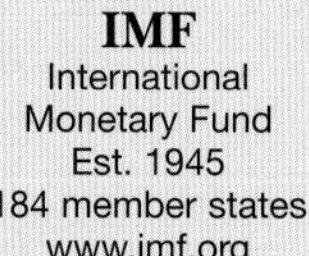

IMF
International Monetary Fund
Est. 1945
184 member states
www.imf.org

UNESCO
United Nations Educational, Scientific, and Cultural Organization
Est. 1945
191 member states
www.unesco.org

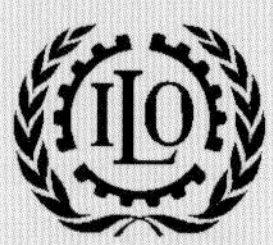

ILO
International Labour Organization
Est. 1919
www.ilo.org

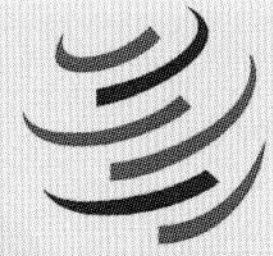

WTO
World Trade Organization
Est. 1995
148 member states
www.wto.org

COMPOSERS

The list below gives the birth and death dates of some major composers, and the country in which they were born, together with one of their most famous works.

Vivaldi, Antonio
1675-1741 Italy
The Four Seasons

Bach, Johann Sebastian
1685-1750 Germany
St. Matthew Passion

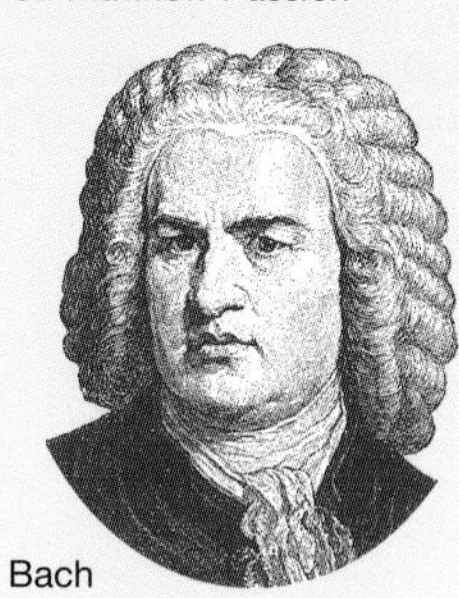

Bach

Handel, George F.
1685-1759 Germany
Messiah

Haydn, Franz Joseph
1732-1809 Austria
The Creation

Mozart, Wolfgang
1756-91 Austria
The Magic Flute

Beethoven, Ludwig van
1770-1827 Germany
Symphony No. 9 "Choral"

Chopin, Frédéric
1810-49 Poland
Piano Études

Verdi, Giuseppe
1813-1901 Italy
La Traviata

Brahms, Johannes
1833-97 Germany
Hungarian Dances

Tchaikovsky, Peter I.
1840-93 Russia
The Nutcracker

Puccini, Giacomo
1858-1924 Italy
Madame Butterfly

Mahler, Gustav
1860-1911 Czech Republic
Resurrection Symphony

Debussy, Claude
1862-1918 France
La Mer

Strauss, Richard
1864-1949 Germany
Der Rosenkavalier

Rachmaninov, Sergei
1873-1943 Russia
Piano Concerto No. 3

Ravel, Maurice
1875-1937 France
Bolero

Stravinsky, Igor
1882-1971 Russia
The Rite of Spring

Prokofiev, Sergei
1891-1953 Russia
Love for Three Oranges

Gershwin, George
1898-1937 USA
Rhapsody in Blue

Copland, Aaron
1900-90 USA
Appalachian Spring

Bernstein, Leonard
1918-90 USA
West Side Story

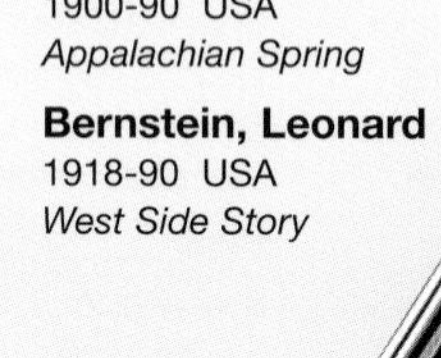
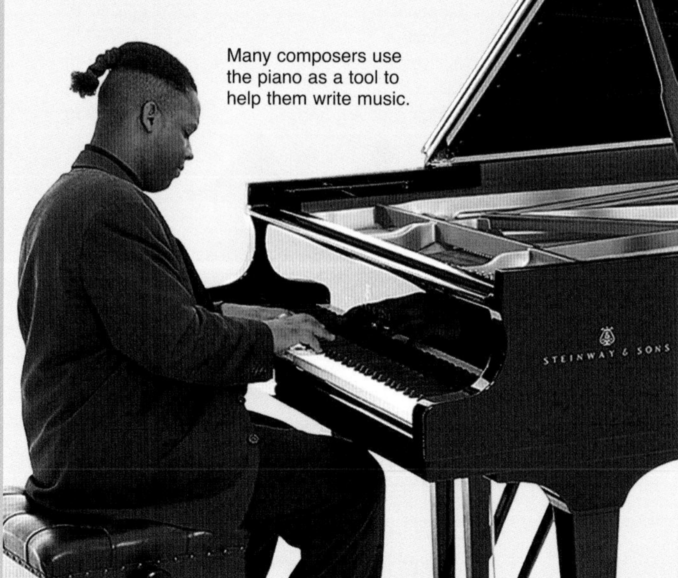

Many composers use the piano as a tool to help them write music.

ARTISTS

The list of artists below gives their birth and death dates, the country in which they were born, and one of their most famous works.

Da Vinci, Leonardo
1452-1519 Italy
Mona Lisa

Dürer, Albrecht
1471-1528 Germany
The Great Piece of Turf

Michelangelo
1475-1564 Italy
David

Raphael
1483-1520 Italy
Sistine Madonna

Rubens, Peter Paul
1577-1640 Belgium
Self-Portrait

Rembrandt van Rijn
1606-69 Holland
The Night Watch

Goya, Francisco
1746-1828 Spain
The Gypsies

Hokusai
1760-1849 Japan
The Wave

Degas, Edgar
1834-1917 France
Dancers on a Stage

Cézanne, Paul
1839-1906 France
The Card Players

Rodin, Auguste
1840-1917 France
The Burghers of Calais

Monet, Claude
1840-1926 France
Water Lilies

Renoir, Pierre-Auguste
1841-1919 France
Le Jugement de Paris

Cassatt, Mary
1845-1926 USA
Morning Toilette

Gauguin, Paul
1848-1903 France
The Yellow Christ

Van Gogh, Vincent
1853-90 Holland
Sunflowers

Toulouse-Lautrec
1864-1901 France
At the Moulin Rouge

Matisse, Henri
1869-1954 France
The Dance

Picasso, Pablo
1881-1973 Spain
Guernica

O'Keeffe, Georgia
1887-1986 USA
Pelvis Series

Rothko, Mark
1903-70 Russia
Yellow Band

Dalí, Salvador
1904-89 Spain
Persistence of Memory

Kahlo, Frida
1907-54 Mexico
The Wounded Deer

Pollock, Jackson
1912-56 USA
Full Fathom Five

Warhol, Andy
1928-87 USA
Campbell's Soup Cans

Riley, Bridget
1931- UK
Colour Moves

Hockney, David
1937- UK
A Bigger Splash

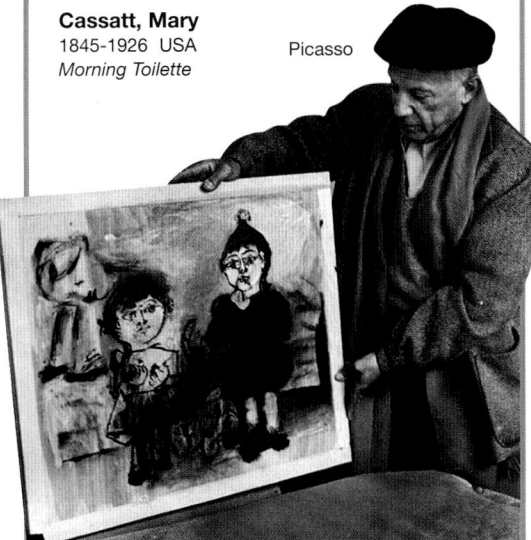

Picasso

WRITERS

The list of adults' and children's writers below gives the birth and death dates of each, the country in which they were born, and one of their most famous works.

Chaucer, Geoffrey
1340-1400 England
The Canterbury Tales

Cervantes, Miguel de
1547-1616 Spain
Don Quixote

Shakespeare, William
1564-1616 England
Romeo and Juliet

Swift, Jonathan
1667-1745 UK
Gulliver's Travels

Voltaire
1694-1778 France
Candide

Wordsworth, William
1770-1850 UK
The Daffodils

Austen, Jane
1775-1817 UK
Pride and Prejudice

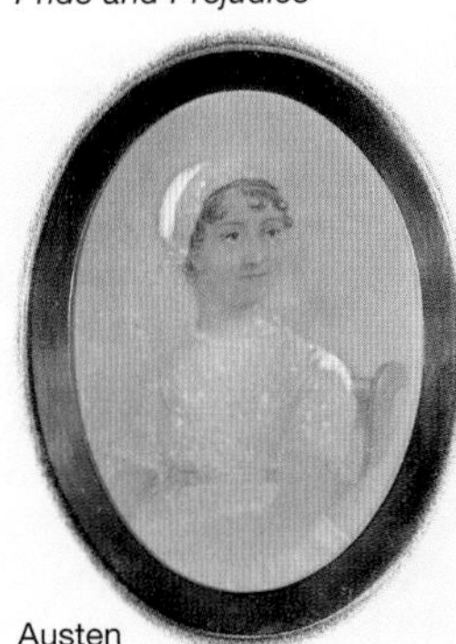

Austen

Byron, Lord
1788-1824 UK
Don Juan

Poe, Edgar Allan
1809-49 USA
The Raven

Dickens, Charles
1812-70 UK
Oliver Twist

Dostoevsky, Fyodor
1821-81 Russia
Crime and Punishment

Ibsen, Henrik
1828-1906 Norway
Hedda Gabler

Dickinson, Emily
1830-86 USA
Letters of Emily Dickinson

Stevenson, Robert Louis
1850-94 Scotland
Treasure Island

Chekhov, Anton
1860-1904 Russia
The Cherry Orchard

Colette
1873-1954 France
Chéri

Frost, Robert
1874-1963 USA
The Road Not Taken

Joyce, James
1882-1941 Ireland
Ulysses

Lawrence, D.H.
1885-1930 UK
The Rainbow

Eliot, T.S.
1888-1965 UK
The Wasteland

Faulkner, William
1897-1962 USA
Absalom, Absalom!

Hemingway, Ernest
1899-1961 USA
For Whom the Bell Tolls

Morrison, Toni
1931- USA
Beloved

Plath, Sylvia
1932-63 USA
The Bell Jar

Lovelace, Earl
1935- Trinidad
The Dragon Can't Dance

Allende, Isabel
1942- Chile
The House of Spirits

Walker, Alice
1944- USA
The Color Purple

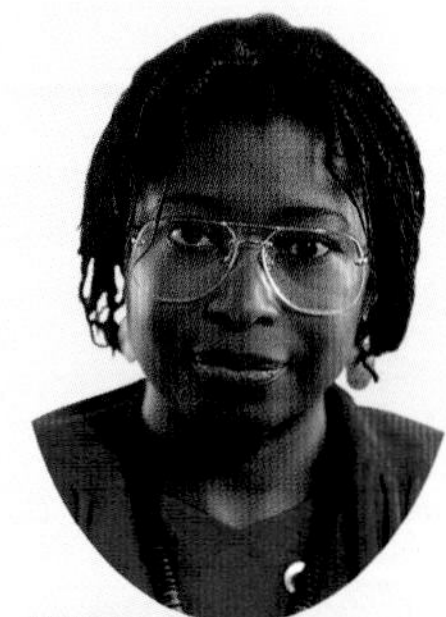

Walker

Seth, Vikram
1952- India
A Suitable Boy

Okri, Ben
1959- Nigeria
The Famished Road

CHILDREN'S WRITERS

Andersen, Hans Christian
1805-75 Denmark
The Snow Queen

Carroll, Lewis
1832-98 UK
Alice in Wonderland

Twain, Mark
1835-1910 US
The Adventures of Tom Sawyer

Baum, L. Frank
1856-1919 US
The Wonderful Wizard of Oz

White, E.B.
1899-1985 US
Charlotte's Web

Kipling, Rudyard
1865-1936 UK
The Jungle Book

Potter, Beatrix
1866-1943 UK
The Tale of Peter Rabbit

Seuss, Dr.
1904-91 US
The Cat in the Hat

Dahl, Roald
1916-90 UK
Willy Wonka and the Chocolate Factory

Rowling, J.K.
1965- UK
Harry Potter

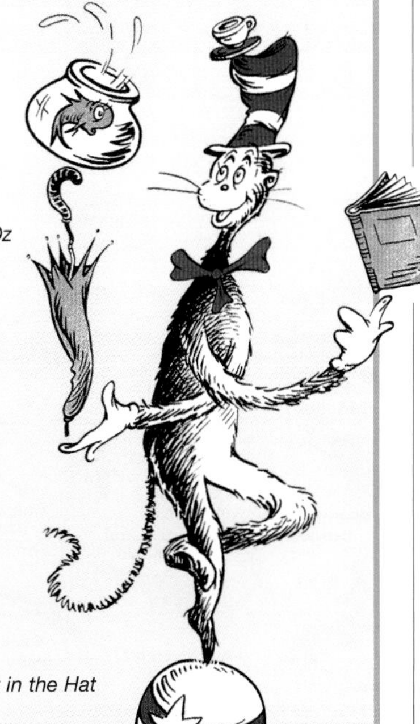

The Cat in the Hat

CLASSIFYING LIVING THINGS

SCIENTISTS CLASSIFY living things (organisms) into groups called kingdoms. This chart shows the five main kingdoms and typical organisms that belong to each one. Within a kingdom, organisms are divided into groups called phyla (singular, phylum). Scientists divide phyla into subphyla, and again into classes. Classes are divided into orders, then into suborders. Orders and their suborders are divided into families, then into genera (singular, genus), and finally into species.

MONERANS

The moneran kingdom includes simple organisms such as bacteria, which live in the air, on land, and in water. There are at least 4,000 species of monerans.

PROTOCTISTS

The protoctist kingdom includes simple organisms such as amoebas, which live mainly in water. There are about 50,000 species of protoctists.

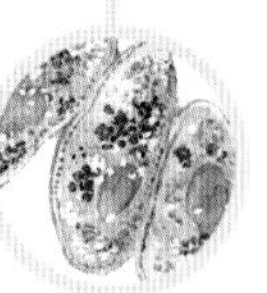

Bacteria
About 2,000 species

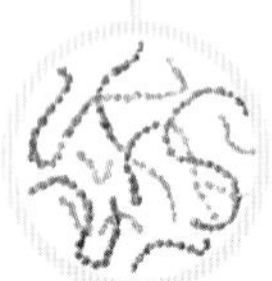

Blue-green algae
About 2,000 species

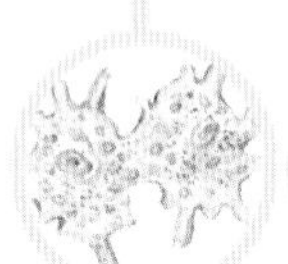

Amoebas
10,000 species

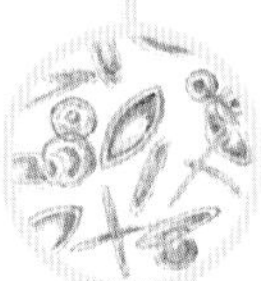

Diatoms
2,000 species

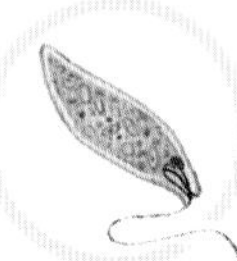

Euglenas
10,000 species

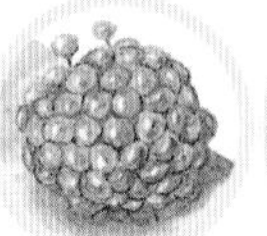

Slime moulds
5,000 species

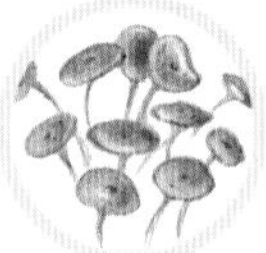

Green Algae
6,000 species

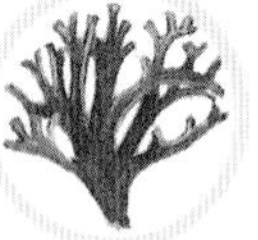

Red Algae
4,000 species

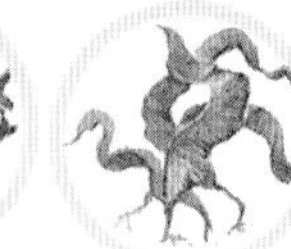

Brown Algae
2,000 species

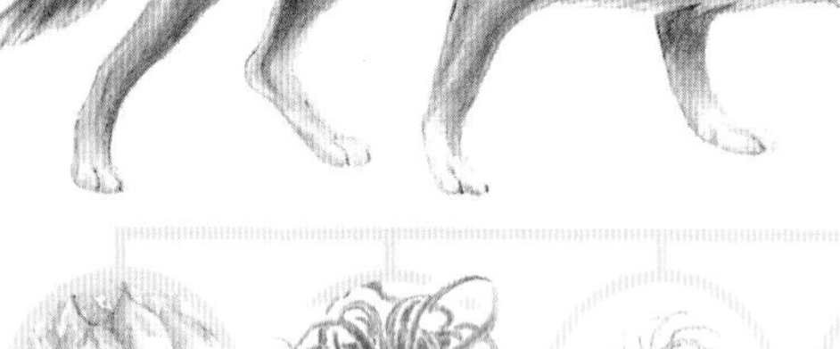

ANIMALS

The animal kingdom includes organisms which are able to move around, and survive by eating other animals or plants. There may be more than 10 million species in the animal kingdom.

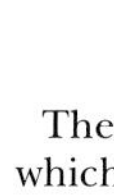

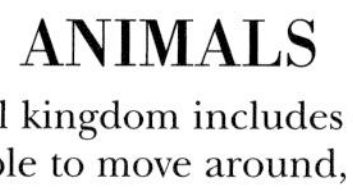

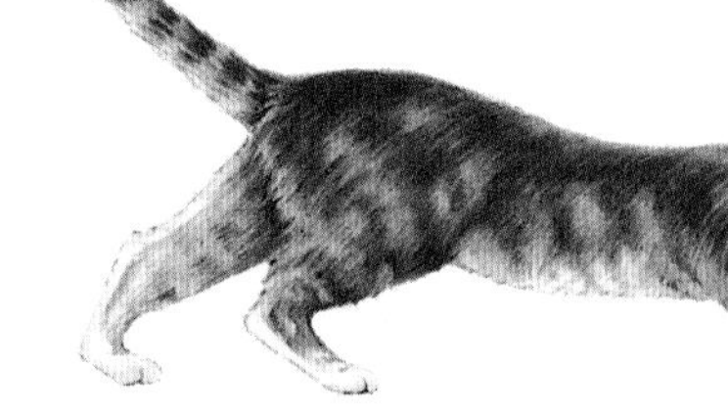

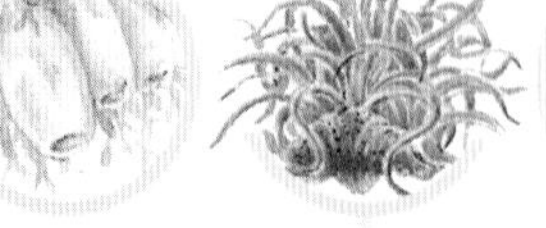

Sponges
5,000 species

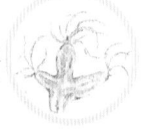

Coelenterates
9,400 species

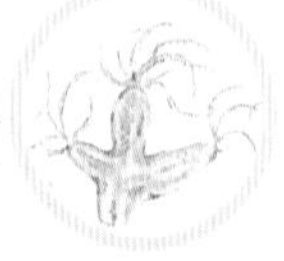

Bryozoans
4,000 species

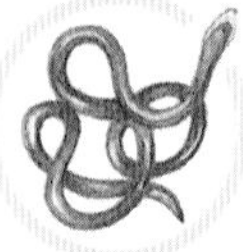

Small phyla
5,500 species

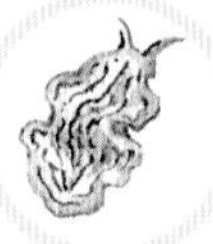

Flatworms
10,000 species

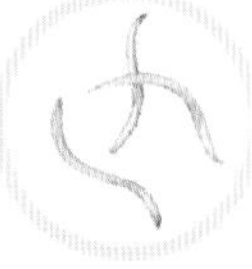

Nematode worms
12,000 species

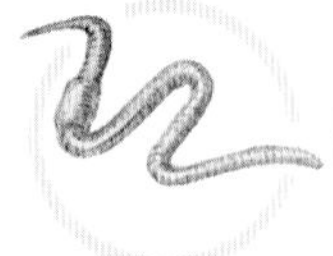

True worms
12,000 species

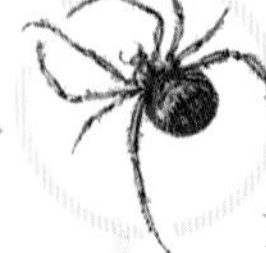

Arthropods
More than 1 million species

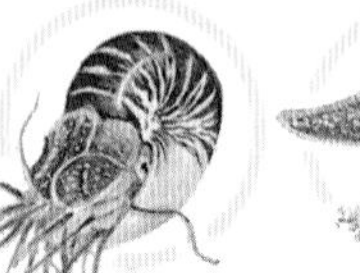

Mollusks
40,000 species

Echinoderm
6,000 speci

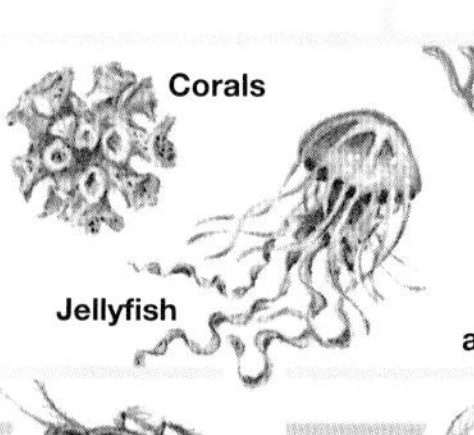

Ctenophores (comb jellies)
Velvet worms
Ribbon worms
Lamp shells

Flukes
Free-living flatworms
Tapeworms

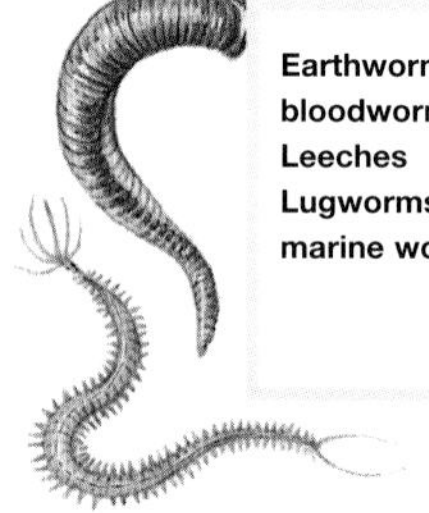

Earthworms and bloodworms
Leeches
Lugworms and other marine worms

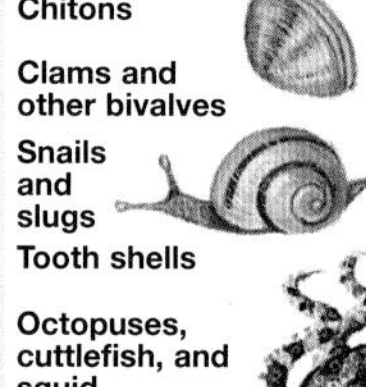

Brittle stars
Sea urchins
Sea cucumbers
Starfish
Sea lilies and feather stars

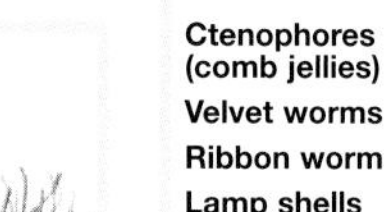

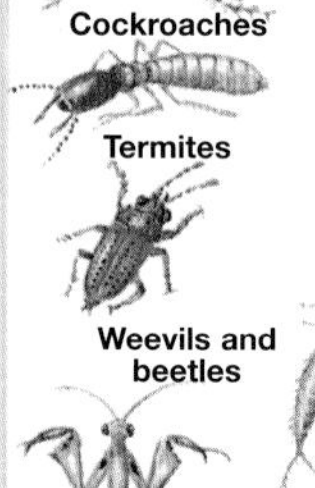

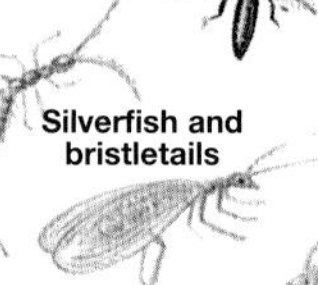

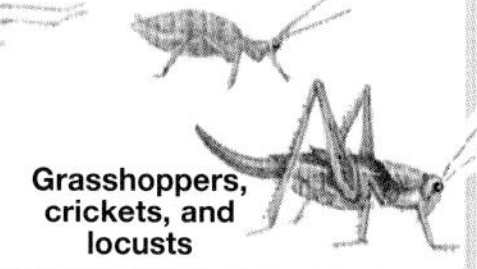

Millipedes
7,000 species

Centipedes
1,700 species

Insects
More than 1 million species

Crustaceans
40,000 species

Barnacles
Crabs and prawns
Fish lice
Sand hoppers
Water fleas
Woodlice

Arachnids
70,000 specie

Spiders
Scorpions
Daddy-longle
Mites and tic
King crabs

FUNGI

The fungi kingdom includes mushrooms, toadstools, and moulds, which are neither plants nor animals. There are more than 100,000 species of fungi.

PLANTS

The plant kingdom contains living organisms which can produce their own food using sunlight. Unlike animals, plants cannot move around freely. There are at least 400,000 species in the plant kingdom.

HOW TO USE THE CHART

These colours are a guide to the main plant and animal groupings. You can see at a glance which groups each organism belongs to.

Kingdom	Class
Phylum	Subclass
Subphylum	Order

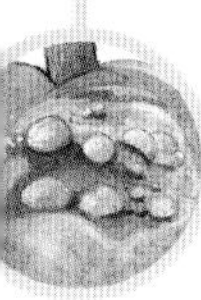

gomycetes
55 species

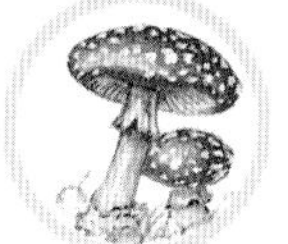

True fungi
About 100,000 species

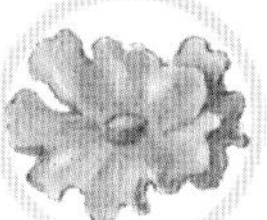

Mosses and liverworts
25,000 species

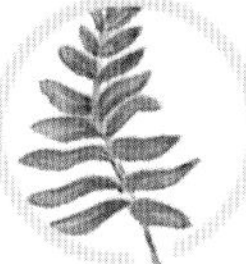

Ferns
12,000 species

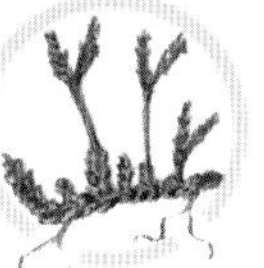

Club mosses
400 species

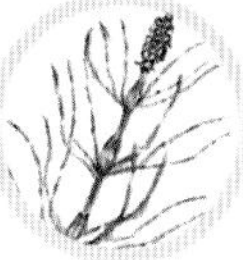

Horsetails
35 species

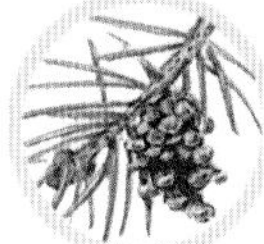

Conifers
500 species

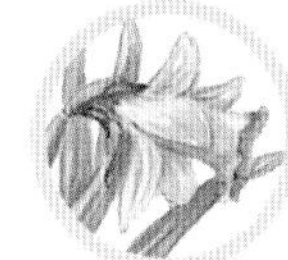

Flowering plants
at least 300,000 species

MONOCOTYLEDONS

A group of 55,000 species with one pair of seed leaves (cotyledons) when they germinate – food for the embryo plant.

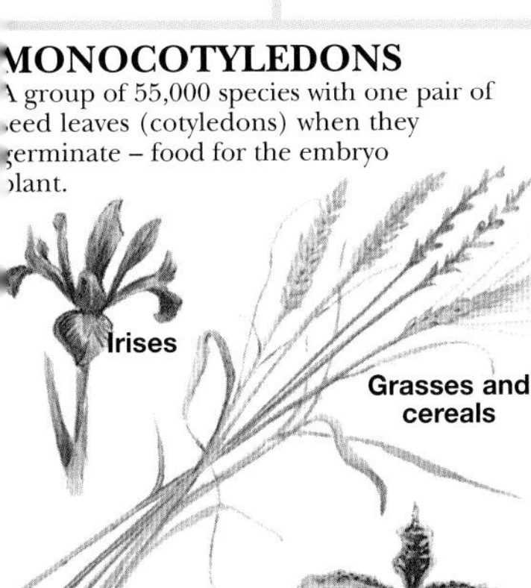

DICOTYLEDONS

A group of 250,000 species, these plants have two pairs of seed leaves (cotyledons) when they germinate.

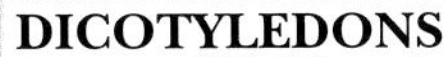

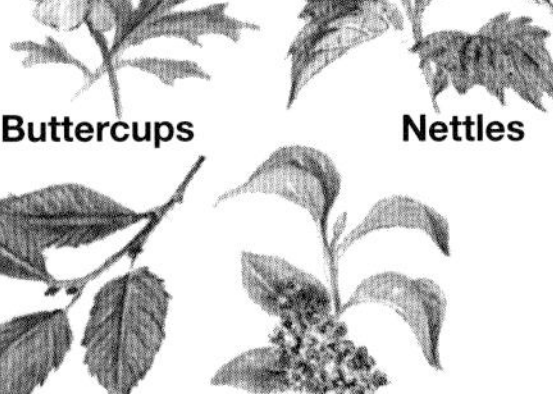

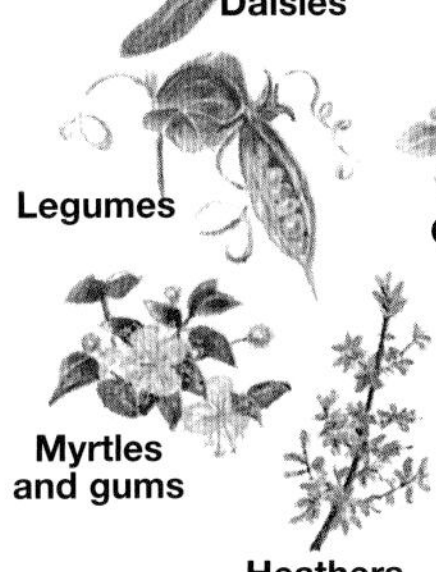

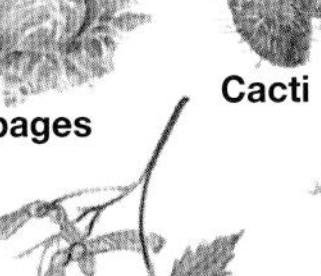

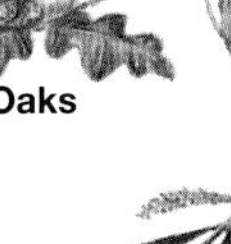

Daisies, Primroses, Roses, Teas, Poppies, Buttercups, Nettles, Legumes, Cabbages, Cacti, Oaks, Parsleys and carrots

Chordates
44,000 species

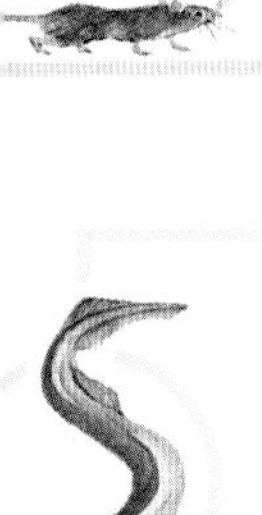

Jawless fish
60 species

Sharks and rays
700 species

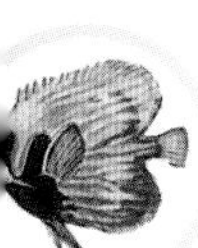

Bony fish
,000 species

- wfins, garfish
- stlemouths, viperfish, dragonfish
- ps, catfish, characins, hatchetfish
- elacanth, birchir, lungfish
- d, anglers, clingfish
- phant fish, featherbacks
- s, tarpons
- rings, anchovies
- ternfish, lancetfish
- ch, barracudas, sea horses,
- ordfish
- e, salmon, trout
- ersides, ricefish, flying fish
- rgeons, paddlefish

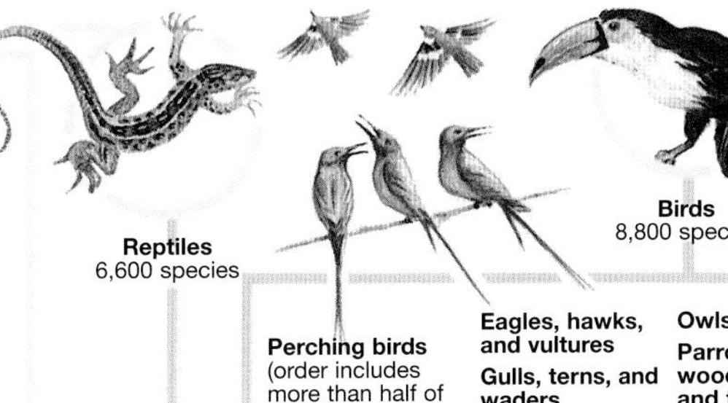

Reptiles
6,600 species

Birds
8,800 species

- **Perching birds** (order includes more than half of all kinds of birds, such as crows and thrushes)
- **Albatrosses and petrels**
- **Cranes and coots**
- **Cuckoos and roadrunners**
- **Ducks, geese, and swans**
- **Eagles, hawks, and vultures**
- **Gulls, terns, and waders**
- **Herons, storks, and flamingos**
- **Kingfishers, bee-eaters, and hornbills**
- **Nightjars, swifts, and hummingbirds**
- **Ostriches, emus, and kiwis**
- **Owls**
- **Parrots, woodpeckers, and toucans**
- **Pelicans, gannets, and cormorants**
- **Penguins**
- **Pheasants, turkeys, and jungle fowl**
- **Pigeons, doves, and sand grouse**

Amphibians
3,100 species

- **Newts and salamanders**
- **Legless amphibians (caecilians)**
- **Frogs and toads**

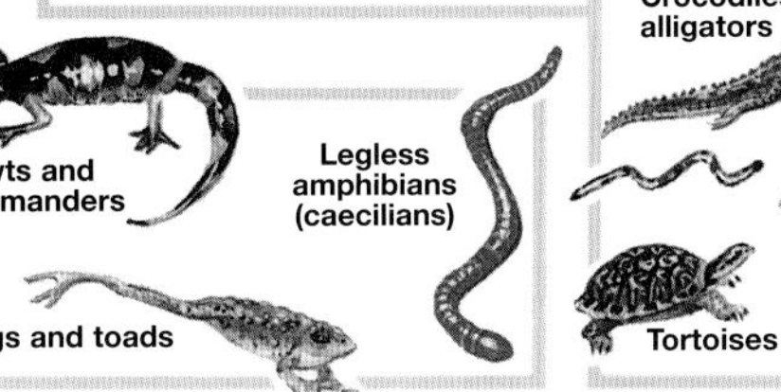

- **Crocodiles and alligators**
- **Lizards and snakes**
- **Tuatara**
- **Tortoises and turtles**

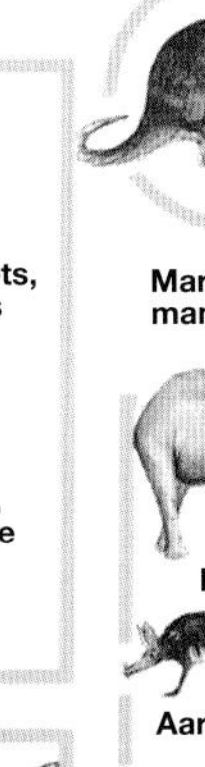

Mammals
4,070 species

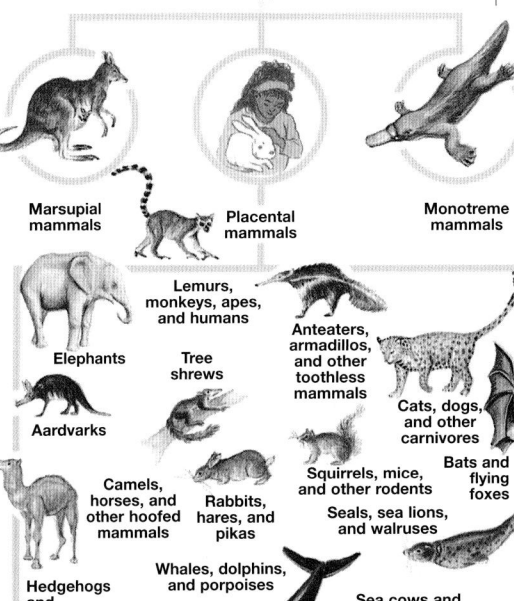

WILDLIFE FACTS

Here are dozens of useful facts about all kinds of plants and animals.

PLANT AND ANIMAL LIFESPANS

The chart below shows you how long wild plants and animals live. The ages given are the maximum average lifespans.

HOW TO USE THE CHA
The colours in this key indicate nine main groups to which each plant or animal belongs.

SEVERAL HOURS	SEVERAL DAYS	SEVERAL WEEKS	SEVERAL MONTHS	1-5 YEARS	5-15 YEARS	15-30 YEARS	30-45 YEARS	45-60 YEARS	60-80 YEARS	80- YE
Some bacteria 20 minutes	**Morning glory flower** 1 day	**Fruit fly** 2 weeks	**Footprint carp** 8 months	**Common poppy** 1 year	**Common starfish** 6 years	**Pitcher plant** 20 years	**Jewel beetle** 35 years	**Blue whale** 45 years	**Alligator** 61 years	**A ane** 80
Mayfly (adult) 12 hours	**Fairy ring mushroom** 5 days	**Common housefly** 3 weeks	**Common field speedwell** 6 months	**Monarch butterfly** 1-2 years	**Red fox** 8 years	**Fruit bat** 25 years	**Canary** 34 years	**Orangutan** 50 years	**Blue macaw** 64 years	**Eu** 80
Some kinds of fungi 18 hours	**Water flea** 7 days	**Skipper butterfly** 3 weeks	**Bedbug** 6 months	**Wild parsnip** 2 years	**Badger** 15 years	**Goldfish** 30 years	**Brown bear** 40 years	**Green turtle** 50 years	**Andean condor** 70 years	**L stu** 81
		Shepherd's purse 6 weeks	**Black widow spider** 3-9 months	**Common shrew** 3 years	**Queen ant** 15 years	**Komodo dragon** 30 years	**Common boa** 40 years	**Royal albatross** 53 years	**Elephant** 75 years	**K w** 90

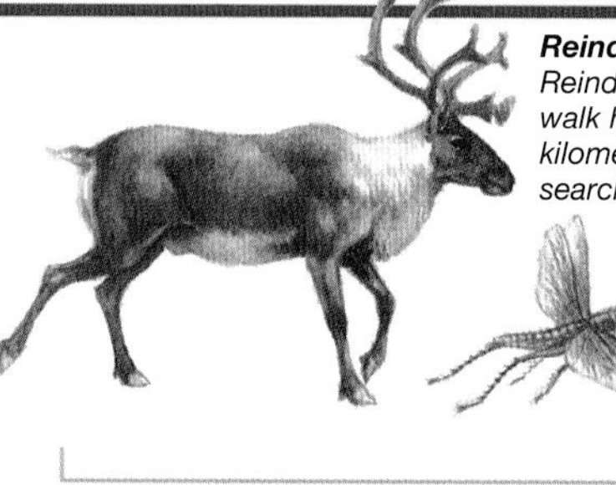

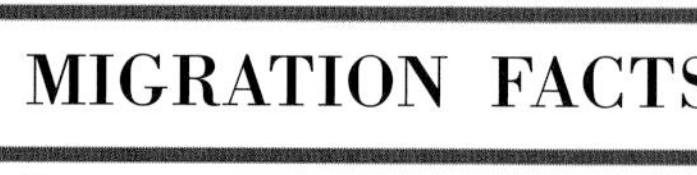

MIGRATION FACTS

Many animals migrate great distances once, a often twice, a year to fi fresh pasture, a place t breed, or to escape ha winters. Here are some animals that migrate – by land, sea, or air.

Reindeer *Reindeer (caribou) walk hundreds of kilometres each year in search of fresh pasture.*

Locust *Swarms of desert locusts migrate more than 3,000 km (2,000 miles) in less than 2 months.*

Fur seal *The Northern fur seal makes a journey of 3,000 km (2,000 miles) and back again each year.*

European swallow *This swallow flies about 11,000 km (7,000 miles) from Northern Europe to South Africa and back again each year.*

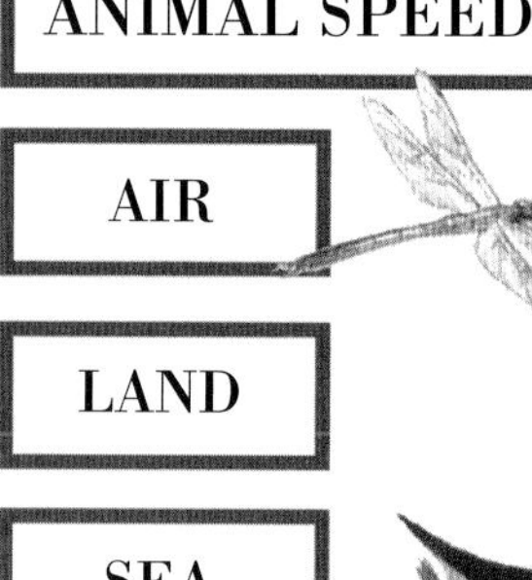

ANIMAL SPEEDS

AIR

Dragonfly *58 km/h (36 mph)*

Frigate bird *153 km/h (95 mph)*

Spine-tailed swift *170 km/h (106 mph) – fastest level flier*

Racing pigeon *177 km/h (110 mph)*

LAND

Brown hare *25 km/h (16 mph)*

Ostrich *72 km/h (45 mph) – fastest bird on land*

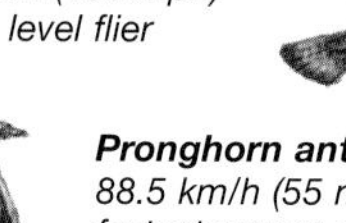

Pronghorn antelope *88.5 km/h (55 mph) – fastest runner over long distances*

Cheetah *96.5 km/h (60 m fastest runner c short distance*

SEA

Gentoo penguin *27 km/h (17 mph) – fastest bird in water*

Killer whale *55.5 km/h (34.5 mph)*

Marlin *80 km/h (50 mph)*

Sailfish *109 km/h (68 m fastest fish*

AMMALS	FISH	FUNGI
BIRDS	ARTHROPODS	PLANTS
EPTILES, HIBIANS	OTHER INVERTEBRATES	SIMPLE ORGANISMS

00-1,000 YEARS	OVER 1,000 YEARS
uatara 1 years	English oak 1,500 years
Tortoise 20 years	Yew 3,500 years
European beech 00 years	Giant sequoia 6,000 years
nderosa pine 0 years	Creosote bush 11,000 years

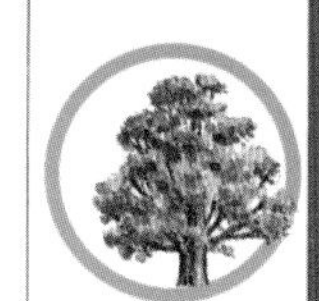
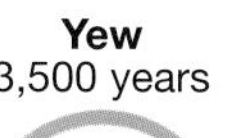
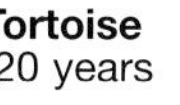
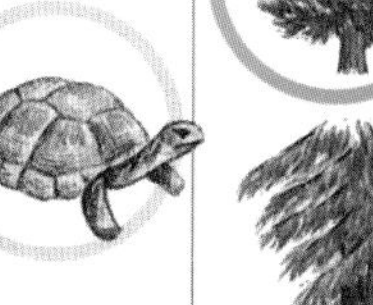
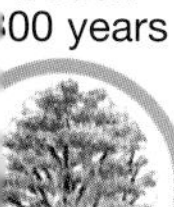
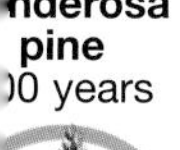
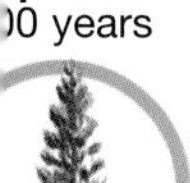
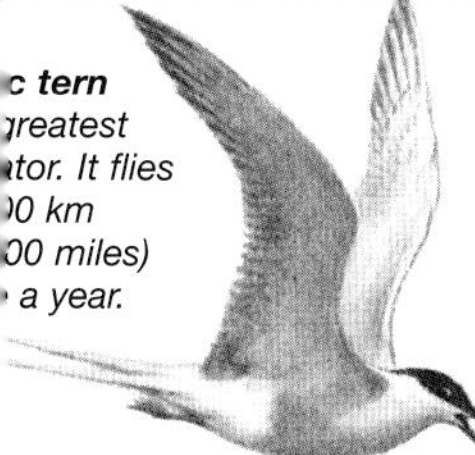

c tern
greatest
tor. It flies
0 km
00 miles)
a year.

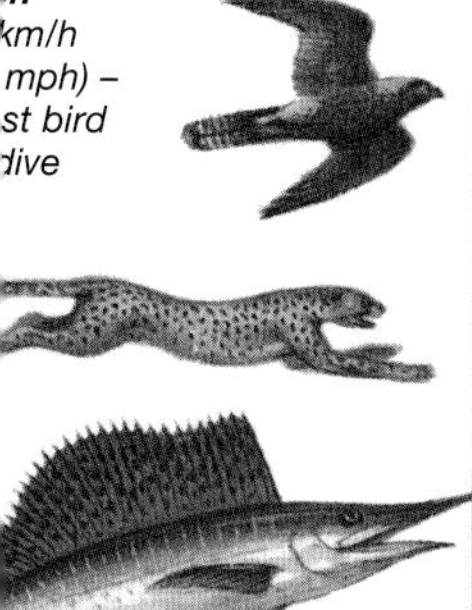

grine
n
km/h
mph) –
st bird
dive

PLANT AND ANIMAL RECORDS

This chart gives you information about plant and animal sizes. It is divided into groups, such as mammals, fish, and birds.

HOW TO USE THE CHART
The colours in this key indicate the different habitats of each of the plants and animals on this page.

LAND
AIR
WATER

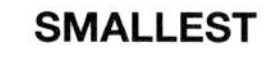
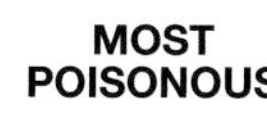

MAIN GROUP	BIGGEST		SMALLEST		LONGEST	TALLEST	MOST POISONOUS
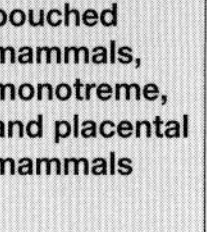 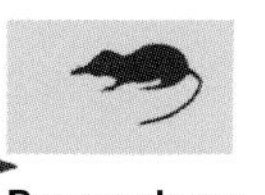 **MAMMALS** including pouched mammals, monotreme, and placental mammals	**African elephant** 3.2 m (10 ft 6 in) high; weighs 5.2 tonnes (5.1 tons).	**Blue whale** 30 m (100 ft) long; weighs 120 tonnes (118 tons).	**Pygmy shrew** This shrew is 40 mm (1.6 in) long and weighs 1.5 g (0.05 oz).	**Bumblebee bat** 15 cm (6 in) long; weighs 1.5 g (0.05 oz).	**Finback whale** The longest mammal after the blue whale is 25 m (85 ft) long.	**Giraffe** The giraffe is 5.2 m (17 ft) high and weighs 1.2 tonnes (1.2 tons).	**Some moles and shrews can give a bite that contains poisonous saliva (spit).**
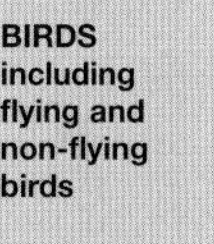  **BIRDS** including flying and non-flying birds	**Kori bustard** The biggest flying bird, weighing 18 kg (40 lb).	**Ostrich** The ostrich is the biggest of all birds, weighing 130 kg (280 lb).	**Bee hummingbird** 57 mm (2.2 in) long; weighs 1.6 g (0.06 oz).	**Hummingbirds use so much energy that they eat half their weight in food each day.**	**Phoenix red jungle fowl** This bird has tail feathers 10 m (33 ft) long.	**The ostrich is the tallest bird on Earth, measuring 2.4 m (8 ft) in height.**	**The only poisonous birds are the Hooded Pitohui and the Ifrita, both from Papua, New Guinea.**
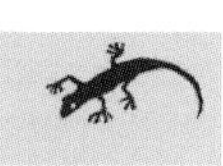 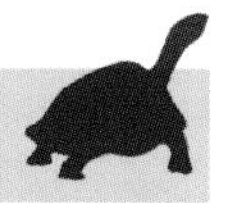 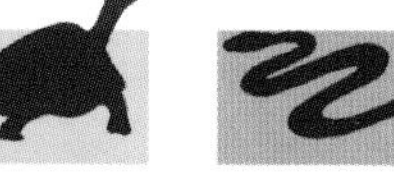 **REPTILES** such as snakes **AMPHIBIANS** such as frogs and newts	**Chinese giant salamander** Biggest amphibian, 1.8 m (6 ft) long; weighs 0.91 tonnes (0.89 tons).	**Saltwater crocodile** Biggest reptile, 5 m (18 ft) long; weighs 1 tonne (0.98 tons).	**Gecko** Some geckos are only 1.8 cm (0.7 in) long.	**Cuban arrow-poison frog** 1 cm (0.5 in) long.	**Reticulated python** 10 m (33 ft) long.	**Giant tortoise** This tortoise is 1.2 m (4 ft) high.	**Black-headed sea snake** The black-headed sea snake is the most poisonous of all reptiles.
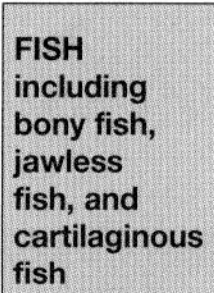 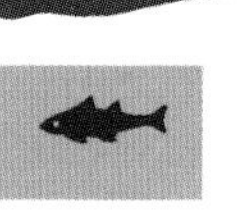 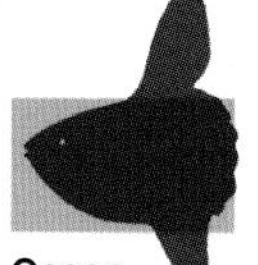 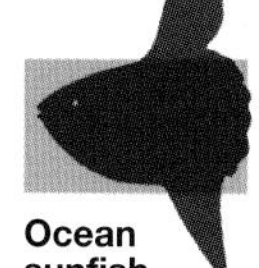 **FISH** including bony fish, jawless fish, and cartilaginous fish	**Whale shark** This is 18 m (60 ft) long and weighs 40 tonnes (39 tons).		**Dwarf pygmy gobi** This is 2.03 cm (0.8 in) long and weighs 5 mg (0.00018 oz).	**Some of the smallest fish eggs are those of the ling, which lays millions during its lifetime.**	**Oarfish** 14 m (46 ft) long.	**Ocean sunfish** 4.3 m (14 ft) high; 3 m (10 ft) long; weighs 2.2 tonnes (2.1 tons).	**Stonefish horrida** A stonefish that has spines to inject its victim with venom.
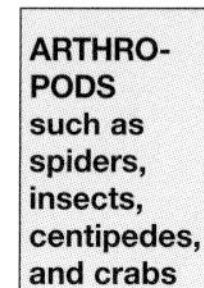 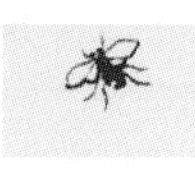 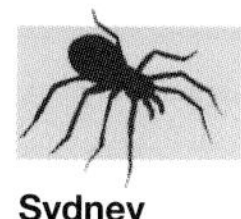 **ARTHROPODS** such as spiders, insects, centipedes, and crabs	**Goliath beetle** The heaviest insect, weighing 100 g (3.5 oz), is 110 mm (4.3 in) long.	**Japanese spider crab** The biggest crustacean, 3.5 m (11 ft) across.	**Fairy fly** The fairy fly is the smallest insect, only 0.02 mm (0.0008 in) long when adult.	**Alonella water flea** The smallest crustacean is only 0.25 mm (0.0098 in) long.	**Giant stick insect** Biggest insect 38 cm (15 in) long.		**Sydney funnel-web spider** This spider has a deadly poisonous bite.
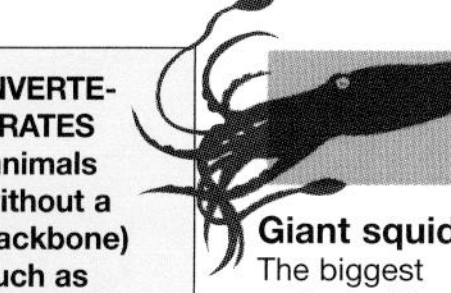 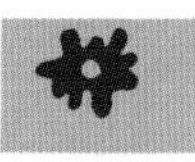 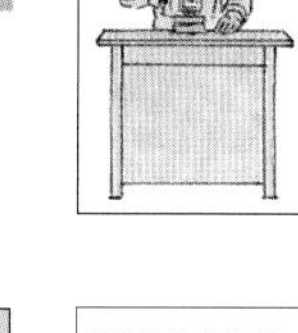 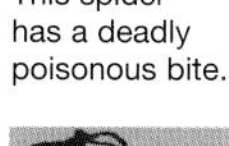 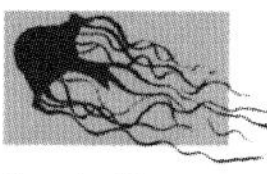 **INVERTEBRATES** (animals without a backbone) such as mollusks	**Giant squid** The biggest mollusk, this squid is 17.4 m (57 ft) long.	**African giant snail** The largest land mollusk, weighing 907 g (2 lb).	**Amoebas** These are too small to be seen with the naked eye.		**African giant earthworm** The longest segmented worm is 6.7 m (22 ft) long.	**Arctic giant jellyfish** The longest coelenterate; 36 m (120 ft) tentacles.	**Australian sea wasp** This sea wasp has the most painful sting of all animals.
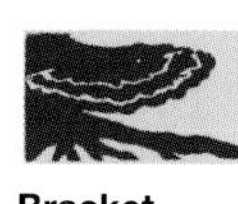 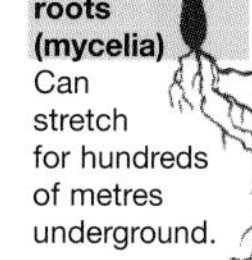 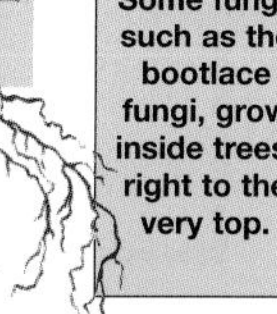 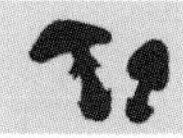 **FUNGI** such as mushrooms, toadstools, moulds, and yeasts	**Bracket fungus** This fungus can be several metres across.	**American giant puffball** A large fungus, this generally measures 194 cm (76 in) across.	**All fungi produce microscopic spores. Bracket fungi make 30 million a day.**	**WARNING! DO NOT TOUCH WILD FUNGI. MANY ARE EXTREMELY POISONOUS.**	**Fungi roots (mycelia)** Can stretch for hundreds of metres underground.	**Some fungi, such as the bootlace fungi, grow inside trees, right to the very top.**	**Death cup** The death cup is the most poisonous of all the fungi.
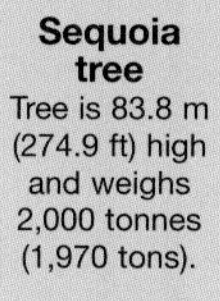 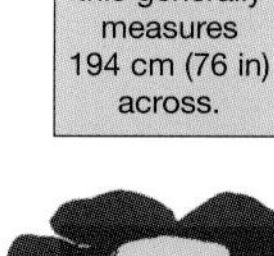 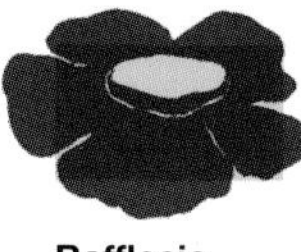 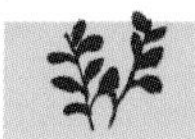 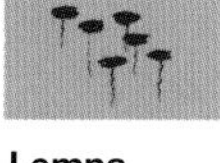 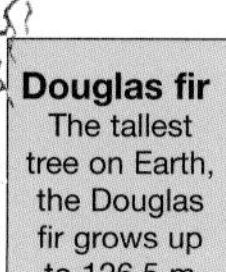  **PLANTS,** such as trees, flowering plants, and grasses	**Sequoia tree** Tree is 83.8 m (274.9 ft) high and weighs 2,000 tonnes (1,970 tons).	**Rafflesia** This is the largest of all flowering plants.	**Dwarf snow willow** A few centimetres long, this is the smallest land plant.	**Lemna aquatic duckweed** Only 0.6 mm (1/42 in) long.	**Pacific giant kelp seaweed** The longest seaweed, measuring 60 m (200 ft).	**Douglas fir** The tallest tree on Earth, the Douglas fir grows up to 126.5 m (415 ft) high.	**Deadly nightshade** This is one of the most poisonous of all plants.

THREATS TO WILDLIFE

The main threat to wildlife is loss of habitat, with pollution another damaging factor. Some animals are also hunted, or must compete with people for food. Rare plants are removed from the wild by collectors.

North America
Africa
Asia
South America
Australia
Rain forests 100 years ago

North America
Africa
Asia
South America
Austr
Rain forests today

These two maps show areas of the world covered by rain forests 100 years ago and today. You can see how the forests are being destroyed.

POLLUTION PYRAMID
This picture and the key (right) show how a small amount of chemical pesticide sprayed onto plants becomes concentrated in the bodies of the animals that feed on each other up the food chain.

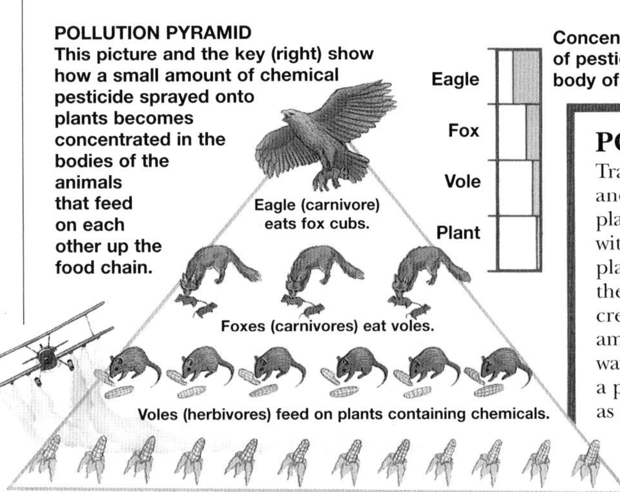

Farmer sprays chemical pesticide onto each plant in a field.

POLLUTION

Traffic fumes, oil slicks, acid rain, litter, and chemicals threaten the lives of plants and animals. When we spray crops with chemicals, a residue is left on the plant. If an animal feeds on these crops, the chemical enters its body. As each creature is eaten by another, certain amounts of the chemical work their way up the food chain. This is called a pollution pyramid. Many animals die as a result of chemical crop spraying.

ATMOSPHERIC WASTE (ACID RAIN)

Woodland plants
Forest trees
Beavers
Fish

DUMPING WASTE AT SEA

Seals
Fish
Penguins

PESTICIDES (CHEMICAL SPRAYS)

Butterflies
Ladybirds

COMPETING WITH HUMANS

All kinds of sea creatures, including seals and dolphins, are at risk from humans because they feed on the fish that humans want. Many dolphins die each year because they become caught up in fishing nets. Other sea creatures die because they cannot get enough food.

Dolphins
Seals
Porpoises

HABITAT LOSS

Only 100 years ago, large areas of the world were covered by forests, where millions of species of plants and animals lived. Today forests are much smaller due to people burning the forests and cutting down the trees for farmland and housing. All sorts of unusual animals and plants now have nowhere to live. Today many species are rare, and scientists believe that huge numbers are already extinct.

RAIN FOREST DESTRUCTION (DEFORESTATION)

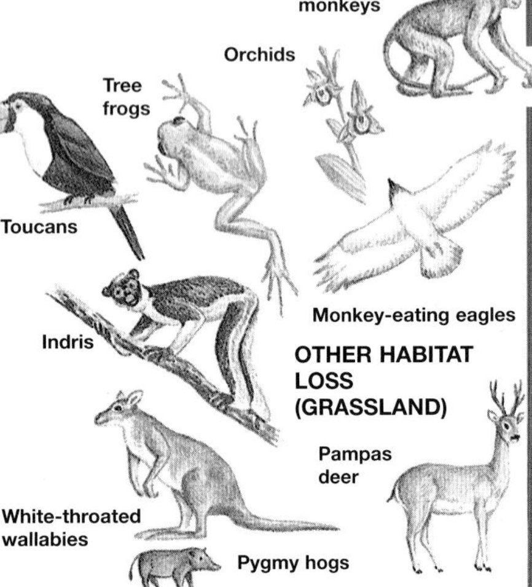

RATE OF EXTINCTION

Many species of animals have died out since the Earth formed. This is often due to habitat loss, and the exploitation of animals for profit. In recent years, many more species have become extinct and, if this continues at the current rate, 50,000 species will die out each year. This graph shows some of the animals which have become extinct in the past few hundred years. It also shows those that are in danger of extinction today.

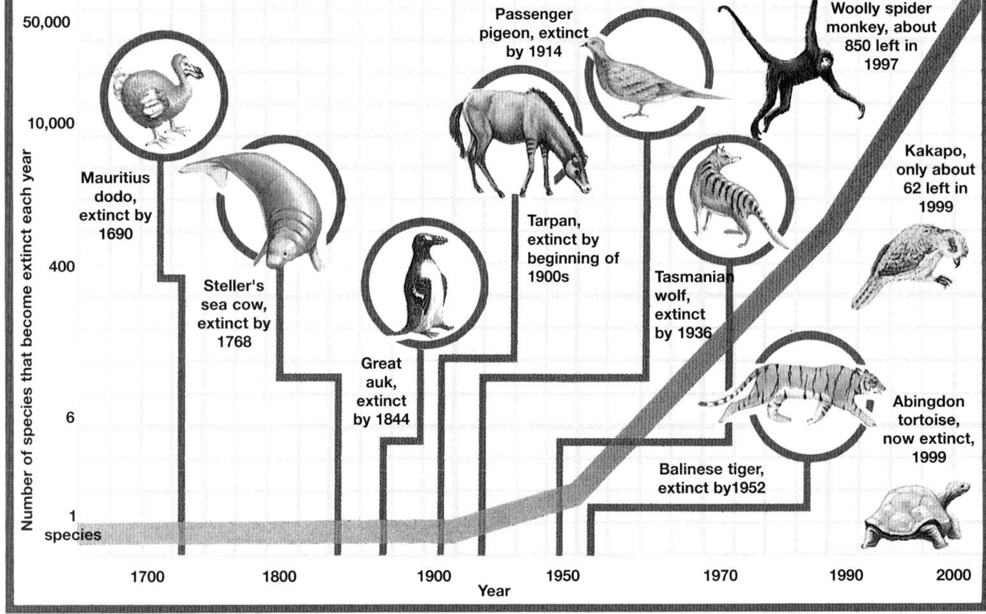

HUNTING AND COLLECTING

Many plants and animals are on the verge of extinction because people have hunted them for centuries for fur, horns, meat, and skin. Today it is illegal to hunt many species of animals, including big cats, rhinoceroses, and whales. It is also illegal to dig up plants from the wild in many areas.

Butter
Polar bears

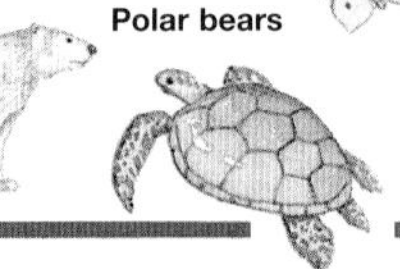

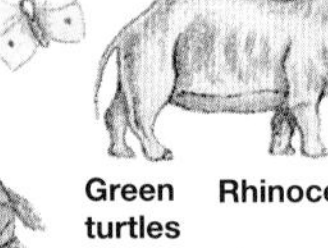

CONSERVATION ACTION

WORLD WILDLIFE ORGANIZATIONS

There are many organizations around the world concerned with the protection of wildlife, working to stop the trade in animal products – and to save animals and plants from extinction. Some of the best-known international organizations and their contact details are listed below.

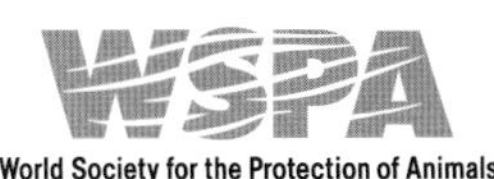

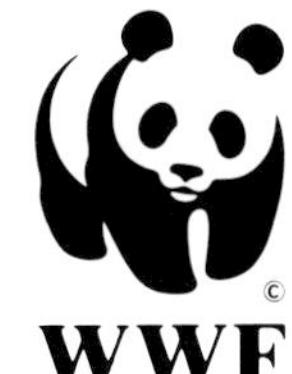

FRIENDS *of the* earth
for the planet for people

GREENPEACE

WORLD SOCIETY FOR THE PROTECTION OF ANIMALS
89 Albert Embankment
London
SE1 7TP
England
020 7587 5000
www.wspa.org.uk

Seeks to relieve the suffering of all animal life throughout the world

WORLD WIDE FUND FOR NATURE (WWF U.K.)
Panda House
Weyside Park
Godalming
Surrey
GU7 1XR
England
01483 426 444
www.wwf-uk.org

Protects all kinds of wildlife

FRIENDS OF THE EARTH
26-28 Underwood Street
London
W1 7JQ
England
020 7490 1555
www.foe.co.uk

Committed to the preservation and sensible use of the environment

INTERNATIONAL FUND FOR ANIMAL WELFARE (IFAW)
87-90 Albert Embankment
London
SE1 7UD
England
020 7587 6700
www.ifaw.org

Aims to ensure the kind treatment of all animals

GREENPEACE
Canonbury Villas
London
N1 2PN
England
020 7865 8100
www.greenpeace.org.uk

Works as a pressure group against damage to the natural world

NATIONAL WILDLIFE PARKS AND RESERVES

In many parts of the world wildlife parks and reserves help endangered animals and plants survive in their natural habitats. This chart lists some of the parks and wildlife reserves around the world. The information tells you how large these wildlife areas are, when they were set up, and the animals and plants they seek to protect.

SALONGA RESERVE, DEM. REP. CONGO, AFRICA
Forest habitat
36,417 sq km
(14,115 sq miles)
The biggest wildlife reserve in Africa

African elephants, pygmy chimps

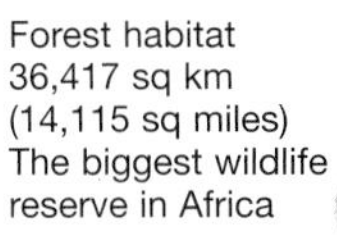
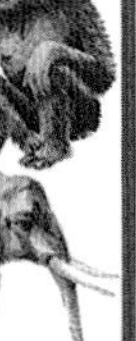

GREENLAND NATIONAL PARK, SCANDINAVIA
Tundra habitat
700,000 sq km
(270,271 sq miles)
The world's largest park

Polar bears, seals, walruses

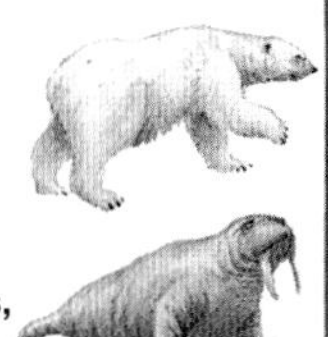

FIORDLAND NATIONAL PARK, NEW ZEALAND
Mountain and island habitat
10,232 sq km
(3,950 sq miles)

Sea birds, seals

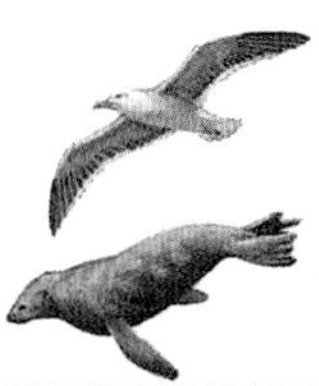

EVERGLADES NATIONAL PARK, FLORIDA
Swamp habitat
5,661sq km
(2,185 sq miles)

Alligators, West Indian manatee

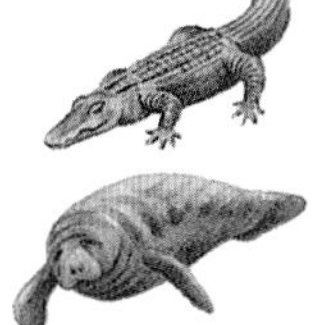

KUSHIRO PARK, HOKKAIDO, JAPAN
Wetland marsh habitat
200 sq km
(77 sq miles)

Japanese red-crowned crane

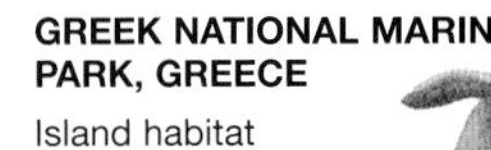

GREEK NATIONAL MARINE PARK, GREECE
Island habitat

Mediterranean monk seal

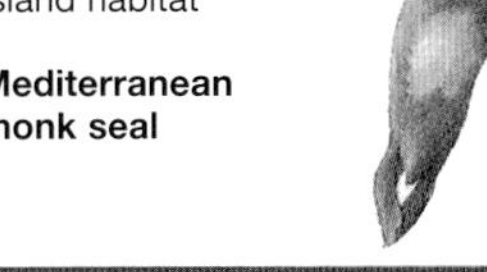

GALAPAGOS ISLANDS, SOUTH AMERICA
Island habitat
6,912 sq km
(2,668 sq miles)

Giant tortoise, finches, marine iguana

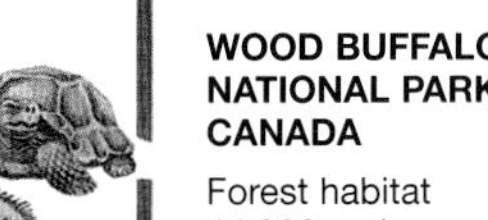

WOOD BUFFALO NATIONAL PARK, CANADA
Forest habitat
44,900 sq km
(17,335 sq miles)

Buffalo, lynx, reindeer

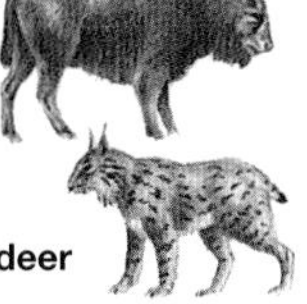

YELLOWSTONE PARK, NORTH AMERICA
Mountain habitat
8,945 sq km
(3,467 sq miles)

Bighorn sheep, moose

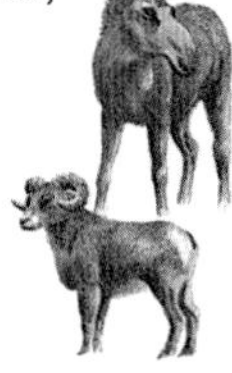

SNOWDONIA NATIONAL PARK, WALES
Mountain habitat
2,188 sq km
(845 sq miles)

Mountain plants, kite, merlin, peregrine falcon

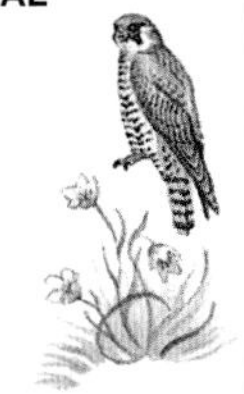

GREAT BARRIER REEF, CAIRNS SECTION, AUSTRALIA
Sea habitat
36,000 sq km
(13,899 sq miles)

Corals, jellyfish, and other sea creatures

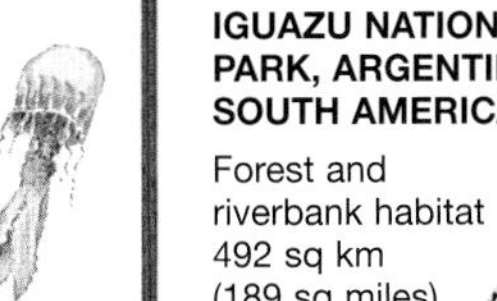

IGUAZU NATIONAL PARK, ARGENTINA, SOUTH AMERICA
Forest and riverbank habitat
492 sq km
(189 sq miles)

Caiman, jaguar

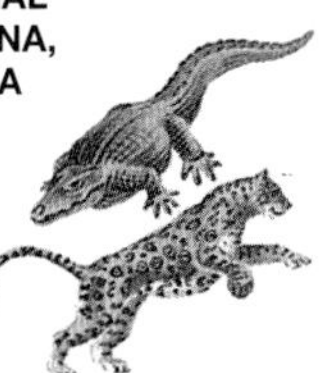

TAI NATIONAL PARK, IVORY COAST, AFRICA
Moist forest habitat
3,300 sq km
(1,274 sq miles)

Many rare trees

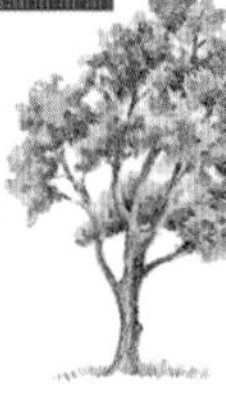

ULURU NATIONAL PARK, AUSTRALIA
Desert habitat
132,490 sq km
(51,671 sq miles)

Desert plants, thorny devil

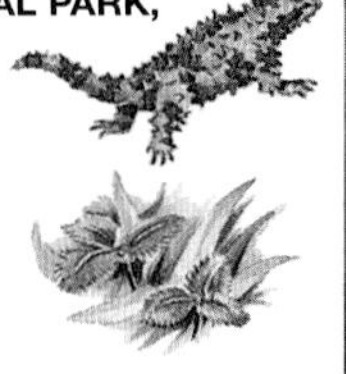

ROYAL CHIAWAN SANCTUARY, NEPAL, ASIA
Forest habitat
932 sq km
(359 sq miles)

Rhinoceros, tigers

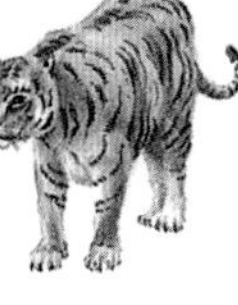

PYRENEES OCCIDENTALES PARK, FRANCE
Mountain habitat
457 sq km
(176 sq miles)

Bears, chamois

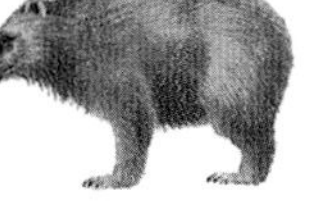

STAR MAPS

ABOUT 6,000 STARS are visible from Earth without using a telescope – roughly 3,000 in the northern sky and 3,000 in the southern sky. Constellations, or groups of stars, are visible depending on the season, the time of night, and which hemisphere you are in. Clarity is also affected by city lights, which light up the sky and make stars harder to see. These star maps show the main stars visible from the Northern and Southern Hemispheres.

NORTHERN HEMISPHERE

The size of the stars on the maps represents their brightness as seen from Earth. The larger the dot, the brighter the star.

Ursa Minor, also called the Little Bear

As the Earth spins on its axis, so the stars appear to move across the sky. This means you will need to rotate these star maps so that they match up with the night sky.

LUNAR PROBES

LUNA 1 (USSR)
Launched January 2, 1959. First probe to successfully fly past the Moon.

LUNA 3 (USSR)
Launched October 4, 1959. Took first photographs of the far side of the Moon.

RANGER 7 (US)
Launched July 28, 1964. Took first close-up photographs of the lunar surface.

Ranger 7

APOLLO 11 (US)
Launched July 16, 1969. First spacecraft to carry people to the Moon. On July 20, 1969, Neil Armstrong and Edwin Aldrin landed on the Moon.

Apollo 11 lunar module

SMART-1 (EUROPE)
Launched September 27, 2003. Used new technology, in the form of solar-powered ion thrusters.

SOLAR PROBES

YOHKOH (JAPAN)
Launched August 30, 1991. Studied x-rays from the Sun.

SOHO (EUROPE/US)
Launched December 2, 1995. Monitors changes on the Sun and solar radiation.

THE SOLAR SYSTEM

Planet	Diameter at equator		Average distance from Sun (millions of)		Mass	Volume	Surface temperature	
	km	miles	km	miles	(Earth = 1)	(Earth = 1)	°C	°F
Mercury	4,879	3,033	57.9	36.0	0.055	0.056	+350	+662
Venus	12,104	7,523	108.2	67.2	0.86	0.82	+480	+896
Earth	12,756	7,928	149.6	93	1	1	+22	+72
Mars	6,794	4,222	227.9	141.5	0.107	0.15	-23	-9
Jupiter	142,884	88,784	778.3	483.3	318	1,319	-150	-238
Saturn	120,536	74,914	1,427	886.1	95	744	-180	-292
Uranus	51,118	31,770	2,871	1,783	15	67	-214	-353
Neptune	50,538	31,410	4,497	2,793	17	57	-220	-364
Pluto	2,360	1,519	5,914	3,666	0.002	0.01	-230	-382

In the Northern Hemisphere (left), locate Polaris (the North Star) and the constellation Ursa Major. From there use the map to locate other constellations.

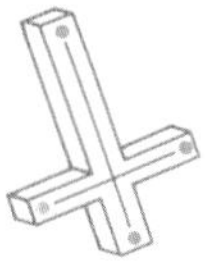

SOUTHERN HEMISPHERE

Crux, also called the Southern Cross

In the Southern Hemisphere, locate the constellation Crux (left) – it is small but very bright; from there you can find your way around the stars in the southern sky.

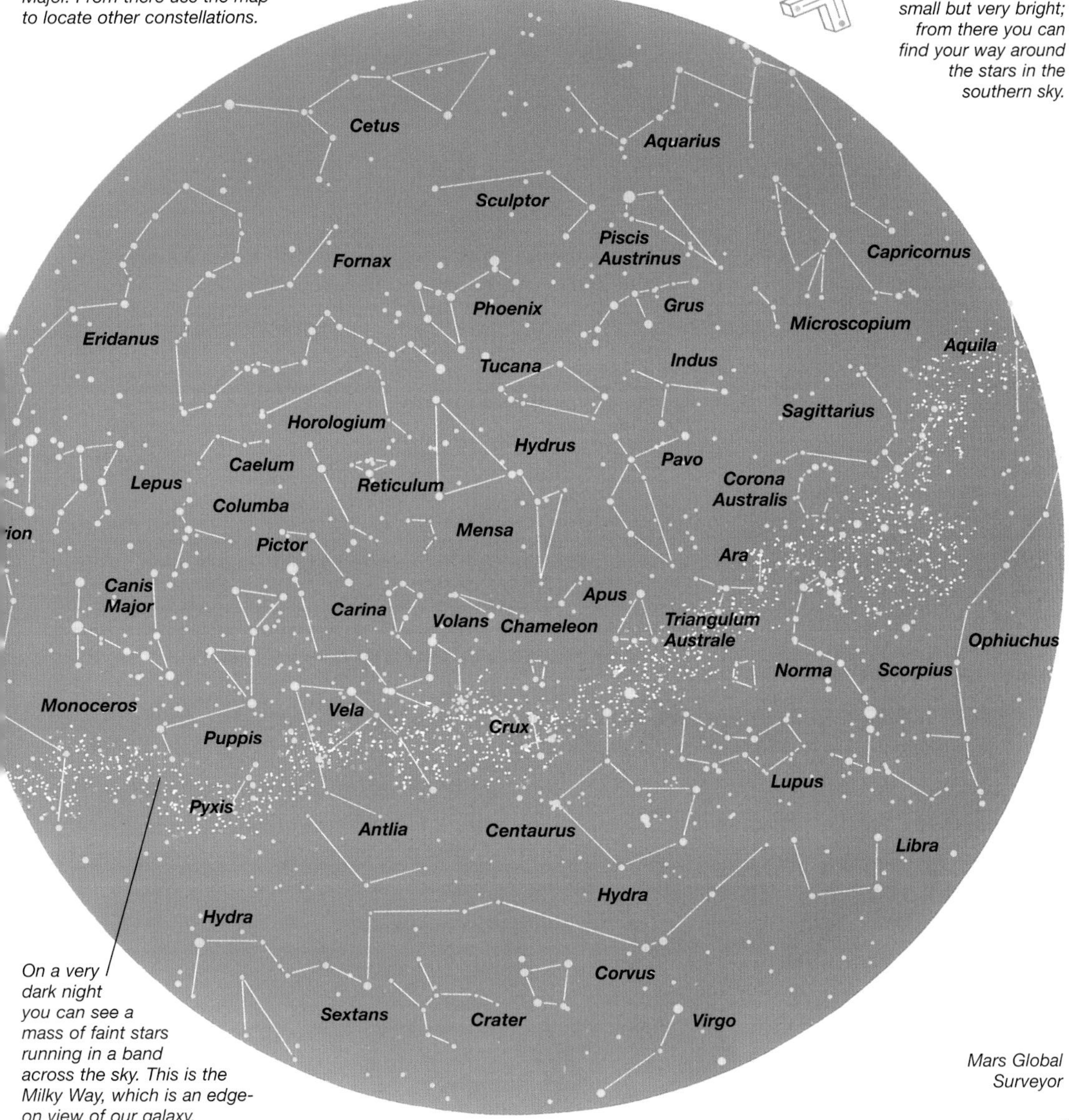

Cetus
Aquarius
Sculptor
Piscis Austrinus
Fornax
Capricornus
Phoenix
Grus
Microscopium
Eridanus
Aquila
Tucana
Indus
Sagittarius
Horologium
Hydrus
Caelum
Pavo
Corona Australis
Lepus
Reticulum
Columba
Orion
Mensa
Pictor
Ara
Canis Major
Apus
Carina
Volans
Chameleon
Triangulum Australe
Ophiuchus
Norma
Scorpius
Monoceros
Vela
Crux
Puppis
Lupus
Pyxis
Antlia
Centaurus
Libra
Hydra
Hydra
Corvus
Sextans
Crater
Virgo

On a very dark night you can see a mass of faint stars running in a band across the sky. This is the Milky Way, which is an edge-on view of our galaxy.

Surface gravity (Earth = 1)	Time taken to orbit Sun	Time taken to spin once on axis	Orbital velocity per second km	miles	Number of moons
0.38	87.97 days	58.65 days	47.9	29.7	0
0.9	224.7 days	243.16 days	35	21.8	0
1	365.26 days	23 hr 56 min 4 sec	29.8	18.5	1
0.38	779.9 days	24 hr 37 min 23 sec	24.1	15	2
2.64	11.86 years	9 hr 50 min 30 sec	13.1	8.1	63
1.16	29.46 years	10 hr 39 min	9.6	6	47
0.93	84.01 years	17 hr 14 min	6.8	4.2	27
1.2	164.8 years	16 hr 3 min	5.4	3.4	13
0.05	247.7 years	6 days 9 hr	4.7	2.9	1

PLANETARY PROBES

These are some of the most important space probes launched to date.

VOYAGER (US)
Two probes, *Voyager 1* and *2*, were launched in 1977. Between them they explored much of the solar system, including Jupiter, Saturn, Uranus, and Neptune.

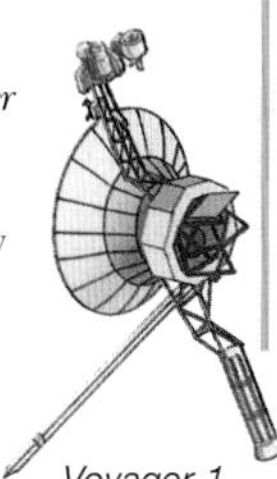

Voyager 1

MAGELLAN (US)
Launched May 4, 1989. Collected information about Venus's gravity field and used radar to map its surface.

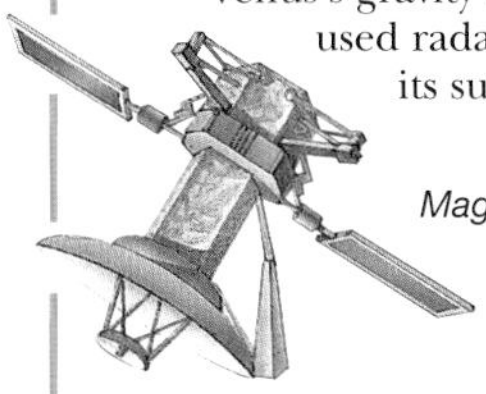

Magellan

GALILEO (US)
Launched October 18, 1989. Probe launched from the space shuttle *Atlantis*, which entered Jupiter's atmosphere on December 7, 1995. First probe to measure the atmosphere of the solar system's largest planet.

NEAR SHOEMAKER (US)
Launched February 17, 1996. The first spacecraft to orbit an asteroid, it studied 433 Eros, a near-Earth asteroid.

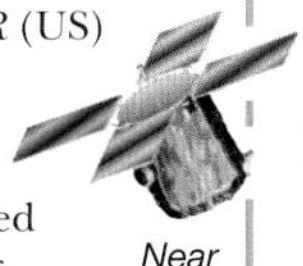

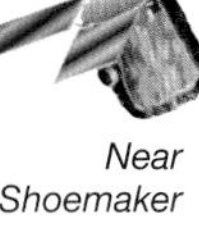

Near Shoemaker

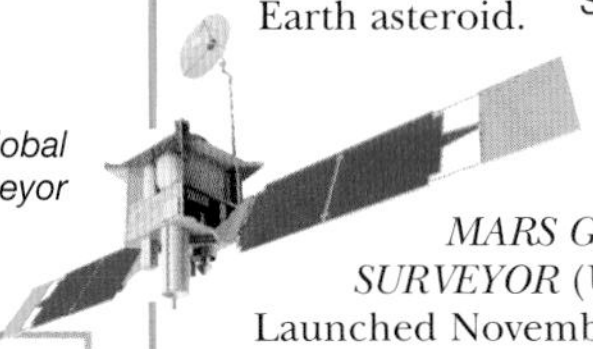

Mars Global Surveyor

MARS GLOBAL SURVEYOR (US)
Launched November 7, 1996. Orbited Mars and sent back pictures and data.

CASSINI (US)
Launched October 6, 1997. Mission to learn about Saturn and its moon Titan.

MARS EXPLORATION ROVERS (US)
Launched June 10 and July 7, 2003. Two unmanned rovers, *Spirit* and *Opportunity*, landed on different sides of Mars in 2004. They carried out scientific experiments on rocks found there and transmitted the information back to Earth.

DEEP IMPACT (US)
Launched January 12, 2005. Mission to learn about comet Tempel 1. Released first probe to impact on a comet's nucleus.

WORLD'S GREATEST OCEANS AND SEAS

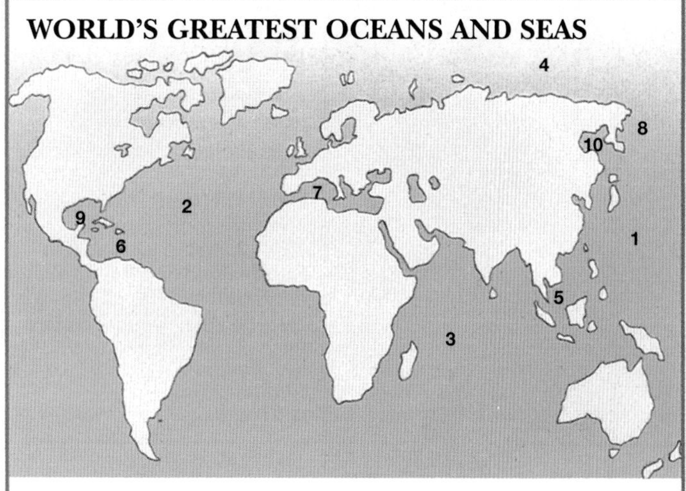

1 Pacific Ocean
166,240,000 sq km (64,185,629 sq miles)

2 Atlantic Ocean
86,560,000 sq km (33,421,006 sq miles)

3 Indian Ocean
73,430,000 sq km (28,351,484 sq miles)

4 Arctic Ocean
13,230,000 sq km (5,108,132 sq miles)

5 South China Sea
2,974,600 sq km (1,148,499 sq miles)

6 Caribbean Sea
2,753,000 sq km (1,062,939 sq miles)

7 Mediterranean Sea
2,510,000 sq km (969,116 sq miles)

8 Bering Sea
2,261,000 sq km (872,977 sq miles)

9 Gulf of Mexico
1,542,985 sq km (595,749 sq miles)

10 Sea of Okhotsk
1,527,570 sq km (589,788 sq miles)

WORLD'S GREATEST DESERTS

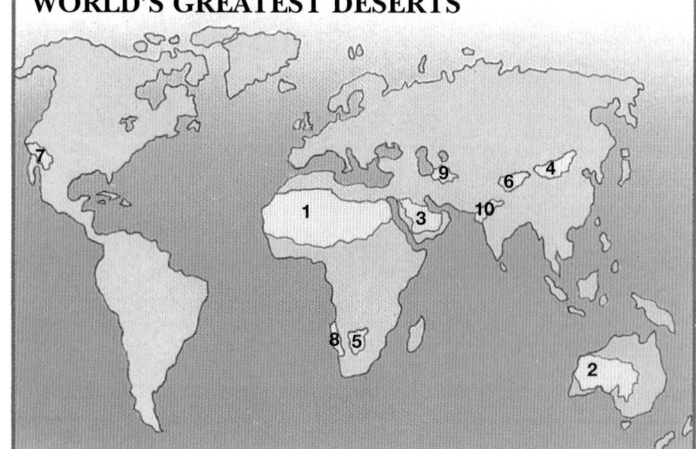

1 Sahara Desert (North Africa)
9,000,000 sq km (3,500,000 sq miles)

2 Australian Desert
3,800,000 sq km (1,470,000 sq miles)

3 Arabian Desert (Southwest Asia)
1,300,000 sq km (502,000 sq miles)

4 Gobi Desert (Central Asia)
1,040,000 sq km (401,500 sq miles)

5 Kalahari Desert (Southern Africa)
520,000 sq km (201,000 sq miles)

6 Takla Makan Desert (West China)
327,000 sq km (125,000 sq miles)

7 Sonoran Makan Desert (USA/Mexico)
310,000 sq km (120,000 sq miles)

8 Namib Desert (Southwest Africa)
310,000 sq km (120,000 sq miles)

9 Kara Kum (Turkmenistan)
270,000 sq km (105,000 sq miles)

10 Thar Desert (India and Pakistan)
260,000 sq km (100,000 sq miles)

WORLD'S LARGEST ISLANDS

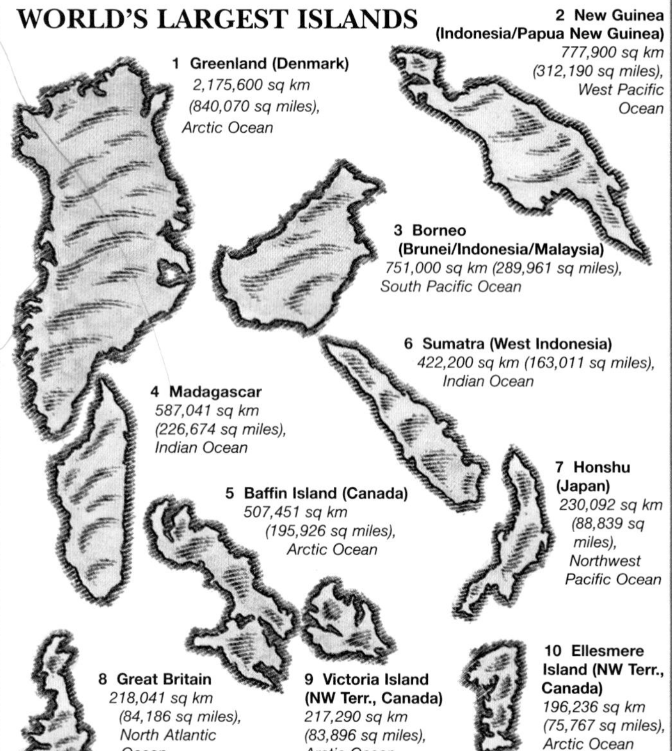

WEATHER RECORDS

Greatest Snowfall
31.1 m (102 ft), Paradise, Mt. Rainier, Washington State, USA, 19 February 1971 to 18 February 1972

Greatest Rainfall
In a 24-hour period 1.9 m (6.1 ft), Cilaos, Réunion, Indian Ocean, 15-16 March 1952

Driest Place / Longest Drought
Annual average of nil in the Atacama Desert, near Calama, Chile. 400 years of drought also in Atacama Desert, 1571-1971

Highest Surface Wind Speed
371 km/h (231 mph), Mt. Washington (1,916 m/6,288 ft), New Hampshire, USA, 12 April 1934

Maximum Sunshine
97% (more than 4,300 hours), Eastern Sahara Desert, North Africa

Minimum Sunshine
Nil, for average winter stretches of 182 days, North Pole

Highest Shade Temperature
58°C (136.4°F), al'Azizyah, Libya (111 m/367 ft), 13 Sept 1922

Hottest Place
Annual average of 34.4°C (94°F), Dallol, Ethiopia, 1960-66

Coldest Place
Average of -56.6°C (-70°F), Plateau Station, Antarctica

Most Rainy Days
Annual average of 350 days, Mt. Waialeale 1,569 m (5,148 ft), Kauai, Hawaii

Windiest Place
Gales can reach 320 km/h (200 mph), Commonwealth Bay, George V Coast, Antarctica

WORLD'S MAJOR MOUNTAINS

All of the world's highest mountains lie in the Himalayas, South Asia.

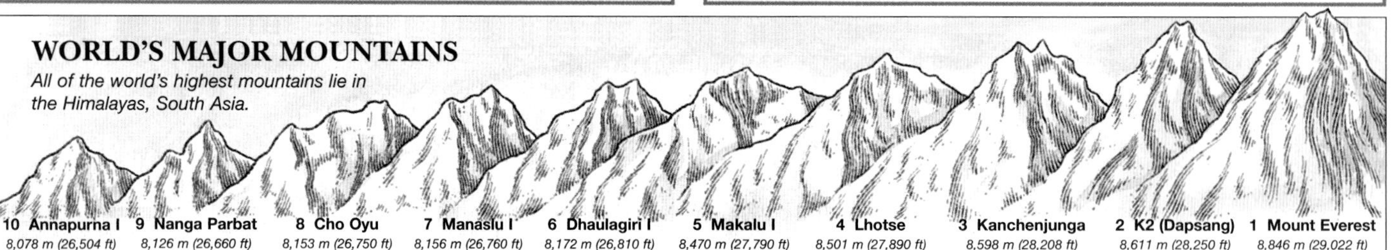

EARTHQUAKES

There are two different scales for measuring earthquakes: the Richter scale and the Modified Mercalli scale.

RICHTER SCALE

The Richter scale measures the strength of an earthquake at its source. It is a logarithmic scale, which means that each time the magnitude increases by one unit, the ground moves 10 times more and the earthquake releases about 30 times as much energy. The scale below gives an indication of the probable effects of earthquakes of particular magnitudes.

Magnitude	Probable effects
1	Detectable only by instruments.
2-2.5	Can just be felt by people.
4-5	May cause slight damage.
6	Fairly destructive.
7	A major earthquake.
8-9	A very destructive earthquake.

MODIFIED MERCALLI SCALE

The Modified Mercalli scale measures how much an earthquake shakes the ground at a particular place. This is called the felt intensity. The scale below gives a list of descriptions of earthquake effects.

Intensity	Probable effects
1	Not felt by people.
2	May be felt by some people on upper floors.
3	Detected indoors. Hanging objects may swing.
4	Hanging objects swing. Doors and windows rattle.
5	Felt outdoors by most people. Small objects moved or disturbed.
6	Felt by everyone. Furniture moves. Trees and bushes shake.
7	Difficult for people to stand. Buildings damaged, loose bricks fall.
8	Major damage to buildings. Branches of trees break.
9	General panic. Large cracks form in the ground. Some buildings collapse.
10	Large landslides occur. Many buildings are destroyed.
11	Major ground disturbances. Railway lines buckle.
12	Damage is almost total. Large objects thrown into the air.

BEAUFORT SCALE OF WIND SPEED

Force	Description	Average Speed km/h	Average Speed mph
0	Calm	Less than 1	Less than 1
1	Light air	1-5	1-3
2	Light breeze	6-11	4-7
3	Gentle breeze	12-19	8-12
4	Moderate breeze	20-29	13-18
5	Fresh breeze	30-39	19-24
6	Strong breeze	40-50	25-31
7	Moderate gale	51-61	32-38
8	Fresh gale	62-74	39-46
9	Strong gale	75-87	47-54
10	Whole gale	88-101	55-63
11	Storm	102-117	64-73
12	Hurricane	Above 119	Above 74

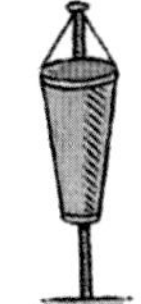
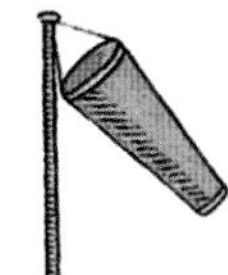
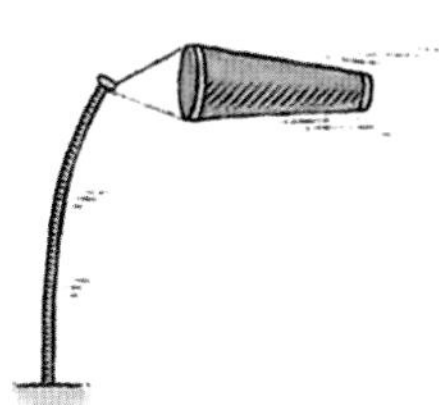

TALLEST STRUCTURES

Towers (including those supported by guy ropes)

		Metres	Feet	Built
1	KTHI-TV Tower, North Dakota, USA	629	2,064	1963
2	CN Tower, Toronto, Canada	553	1,815	1975

Habitable Buildings

		Metres	Feet	Built
1	Taipei 101, Taipei, Taiwan	509	1,671	2003
2	Petronas Towers, Kuala Lumpur, Malaysia	452	1,482	1997
3	Sears Towers, Chicago, Illinois, USA	443	1,454	1974
4	Jin Mao Tower, Shanghai, China	421	1,380	1998
5	Two International Finance Centre, Hong Kong	415	1,362	2003
6	CITIC Plaza, Guangzhou, China	391	1,283	1997
7	Shun Hing Square, Shenzhen, China	384	1,260	1996
8	Empire State Building, New York, USA	381	1,250	1931
9	Central Plaza, Hong Kong	374	1,227	1992
10	Bank of China Tower, Hong Kong	367	1,205	1990

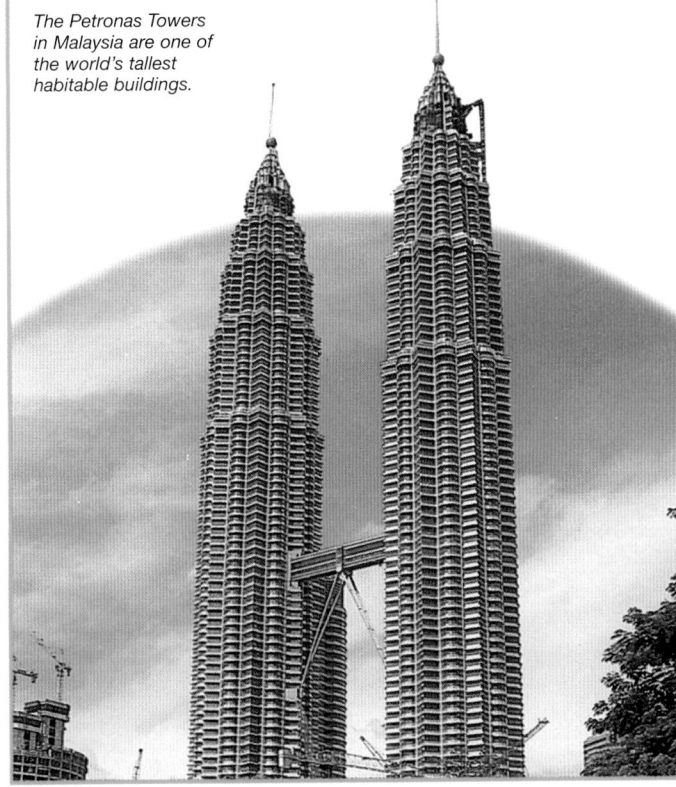

The Petronas Towers in Malaysia are one of the world's tallest habitable buildings.

LONGEST BRIDGES

The figures given below show the top ten longest bridges in the world. The measurements relate to the length of the central span of each bridge. All the bridges listed are suspension bridges.

1 Akashi-Kaikyo
1,780 m (5,839 ft), Honshu-Shikoku, Japan, completed 1997
2 Great Belt East
1,624 m (5,328 ft), Denmark, completed 1998
3 Humber Estuary
1,410 m (4,626 ft), Humber, UK, completed 1980
4 Jiangyin
1,385 m (4,544 ft), China, completed 1999
5 Tsing Ma
1,377 m (4,518 ft), Hong Kong, completed 1997
6 Verrazano-Narrows
1,298 m (4,260 ft), New York City, USA, completed 1964
7 Golden Gate
1,280 m (4,200 ft), San Francisco, USA, completed 1937
8 Höga Kusten
1,200 m (3,937 ft), Sweden, completed 1997
9 Mackinac Straits
1,158 m (3,800 ft), Michigan, USA, completed 1957
10 Minami Bisan-Seto
1,100 m (3,608 ft), Japan, completed 1988

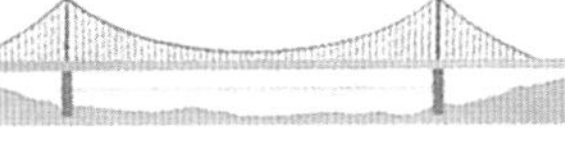

LONGEST RAIL SYSTEMS

The list below provides the measurements of the ten longest rail systems in the world, and where they are.

1 USA
240,000 km (149,129 miles)
2 Russia
154,000 km (95,691 miles)
3 Canada
70,176 km (43,605 miles)
4 India
62,462 km (38,812 miles)
5 China
58,399 km (36,287 miles)
6 Germany
43,966 km (27,319 miles)
7 Australia
38,563 km (23,962 miles)
8 Argentina
37,910 km (23,556 miles)
9 France
33,891 km (21,059 miles)
10 Brazil
27,418 km (17,037 miles)

The total length of all world rail systems is estimated to be 1,201,337 km (746,476 miles).

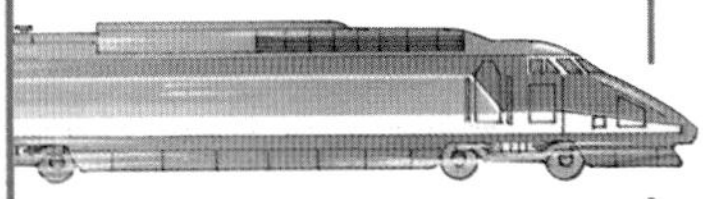

Many geographical statistics are approximate because of factors such as seasonal changes and the method of measurement.

AREA AND VOLUME

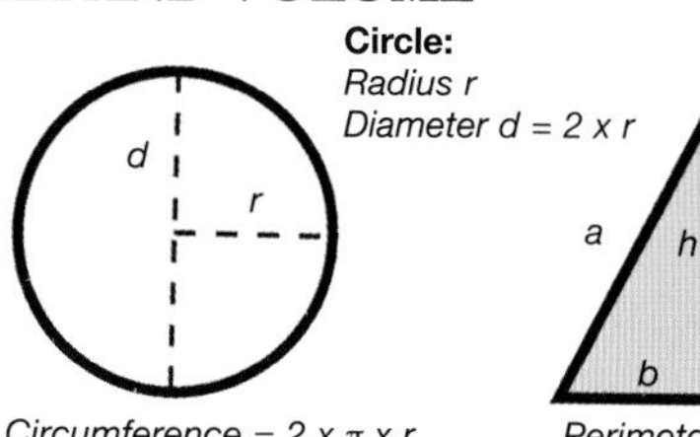

Circle:
Radius r
Diameter d = 2 x r

Circumference $= 2 \times \pi \times r$
Area $= \pi \times r^2$ $(\pi = 3.1416)$

Triangle:
Height h
Sides a, b, c

Perimeter $= a + b + c$
Area $= \frac{1}{2} \times b \times h$

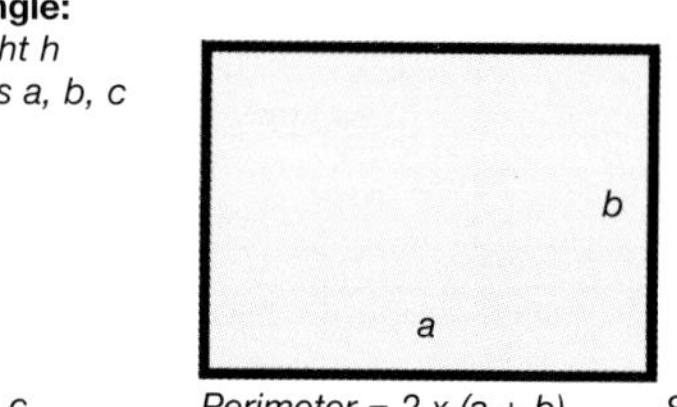
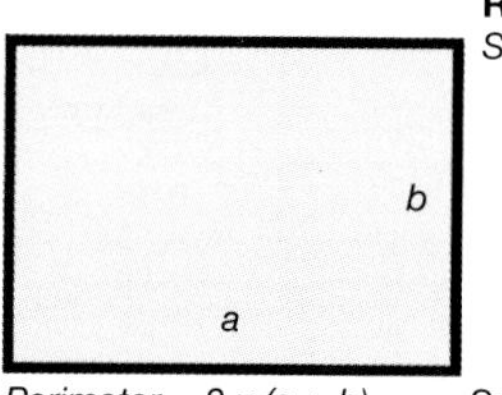

Rectangle:
Sides a, b

Perimeter $= 2 \times (a + b)$
Area $= a \times b$

Cylinder:
Height h
Radius r

Surface area $= 2 \times \pi \times r \times h$ *(excluding ends)*
Volume $= \pi \times r^2 \times h$

Cone:
Height h
Radius r
Side l

Surface area $= \pi \times r \times l$ *(excl*
Volume $= \frac{1}{3} \times \pi \times r^2 \times l$

UNITS OF MEASUREMENT

METRIC UNIT	EQUIVALENT	IMPERIAL UNIT	EQUIVALENT
Length		**Length**	
1 centimetre (cm)	10 millimetres (mm)	1 foot (ft)	12 inches (in)
1 metre (m)	100 centimetres (cm)	1 yard (yd)	3 feet
1 kilometre (km)	1,000 metres	1 mile	1,760 yards
Mass		**Mass**	
1 kilogram (kg)	1,000 grams (g)	1 pound (lb)	16 ounces (oz)
1 tonne (t)	1,000 kilograms	1 ton	2,240 pounds
Area			
1 square centimetre (cm^2)	100 square millimetres (mm^2)	1 square foot (ft^2)	144 square inches (in^2)
1 square metre (m^2)	10,000 square centimetres	1 square yard (yd^2)	9 square feet
1 hectare	10,000 square metres	1 acre	4,840 square yards
1 square kilometre (km^2)	1 million square metres	1 square mile	640 acres
Volume			
1 cubic centimetre (cc)	1 millilitre (ml)	1 pint	34.68 cubic inches (in^3)
1 litre (l)	1,000 millilitres	1 quart	2 pints
1 cubic metre (m^3)	1,000 litres	1 gallon	4 quarts

METRIC-IMPERIAL CONVERSION

Metric units into imperial units

To convert	*into*	*multiply*
Length		
Centimetres	inches	0.39
Metres	feet	3.28
Kilometres	miles	0.62
Area		
Square cm	square inches	0.16
Square metres	square feet	10.76
Hectares	acres	2.47
Square km	square miles	0.39
Volume		
Cubic cm	cubic inches	0.061
Litres	pints	1.76
Litres	gallons	0.22
Mass		
Grams	ounces	0.04
Kilograms	pounds	2.21
Tonnes	tons	0.98

BINARY SYSTEM

The binary number system is used in computers to represent numbers and letters. The binary system uses only two symbols – 0 and 1 – which represent "On" and "Off" in computer circuits.

Decimal	Binary
1	1
2	10
3	11
4	100
5	101
6	110
7	111
8	1000
9	1001
10	1010
11	1011
12	1100

MATHEMATICAL SYMBOLS

+	plus
–	minus
±	plus or minus
x	multiplication (times)
÷	divided by
=	equal to
≠	not equal to
≈	approximately equal to
>	greater than
<	less than
≥	greater than or equal to
≤	less than or equal to
%	per cent
√	square root
π	pi (3.1416)
°	degree
'	minute, foot
"	second, inch

PERIODIC TABLE

The periodic table classifies chemical elements in order of atomic number (the number of protons in each atom of the element). The elements are arranged in horizontal rows, called periods, and vertical columns, called groups. In this way, elements with similar chemical properties (such as the alkali metals) lie in the same vertical group.

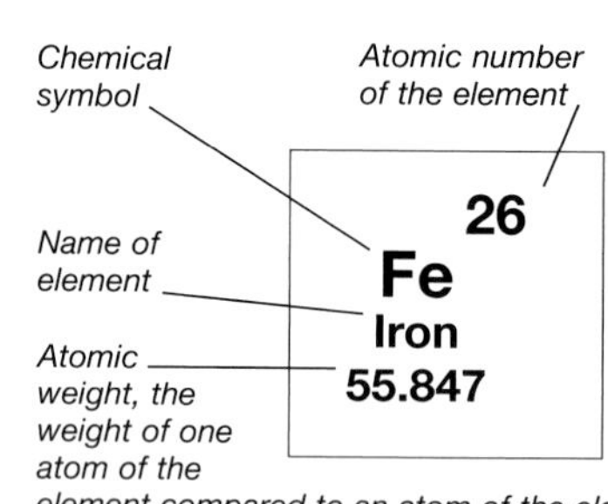

1 H Hydrogen 1.008								
3 Li Lithium 6.941	4 Be Beryllium 9.012							
11 Na Sodium 22.990	12 Mg Magnesium 24.305							
19 K Potassium 39.098	20 Ca Calcium 40.08	21 Sc Scandium 44.956	22 Ti Titanium 47.90	23 V Vanadium 50.941	24 Cr Chromium 51.996	25 Mn Manganese 54.938	26 Fe Iron 55.847	Co Coba 58.93
37 Rb Rubidium 85.468	38 Sr Strontium 87.62	39 Y Yttrium 88.906	40 Zr Zirconium 91.22	41 Nb Niobium 92.906	42 Mo Molybdenum 95.94	43 Tc Technetium (97)	44 Ru Ruthenium 101.07	Rh Rhodi 102.9
55 Cs Caesium 132.910	56 Ba Barium 137.34		72 Hf Hafnium 178.49	73 Ta Tantalum 180.948	74 W Tungsten 183.85	75 Re Rhenium 186.207	76 Os Osmium 190.2	Ir Iridiu 192.2
87 Fr Francium (223)	88 Ra Radium 226.025		104 Unq Unnilquadium (260)	105 Unp Unnilpentium (262)	106 Unh Unnilhexium (263)	107 Uns Unnilseptium (262)	108 Uno Unniloctium (265)	1 Une Unnilenr (266)

57 La Lanthanum 138.906	58 Ce Cerium 140.12	59 Pr Praseodymium 140.908	60 Nd Neodymium 144.24	61 Pm Promethium (145)	62 Sm Samarium 150.4	63 Eu Europium 151.96	Gd Gadolini 157.2
89 Ac Actinium (227)	90 Th Thorium 232.038	91 Pa Protactinium 231.036	92 U Uranium 238.029	93 Np Neptunium 237.048	94 Pu Plutonium (244)	95 Am Americium (243)	Cm Curiu (247)

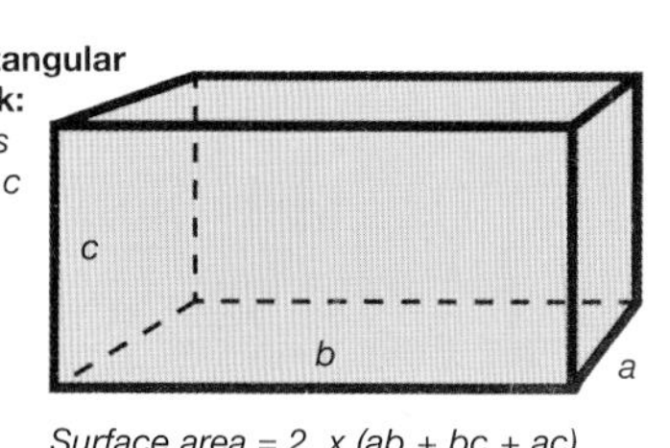

Surface area = 2 x (ab + bc + ac)
Volume = a x b x c

erial units into metric units

onvert	into	multiply by
gth		
es	centimetres	2.54
	metres	0.30
s	kilometres	1.61
a		
are inches	square cm	6.45
are feet	square metres	0.09
s	hectares	0.41
are miles	square km	2.59
me		
ic inches	cubic cm	16.39
s	litres	0.57
ons	litres	4.55
s		
ces	grams	28.35
nds	kilograms	0.45
	tonnes	1.02

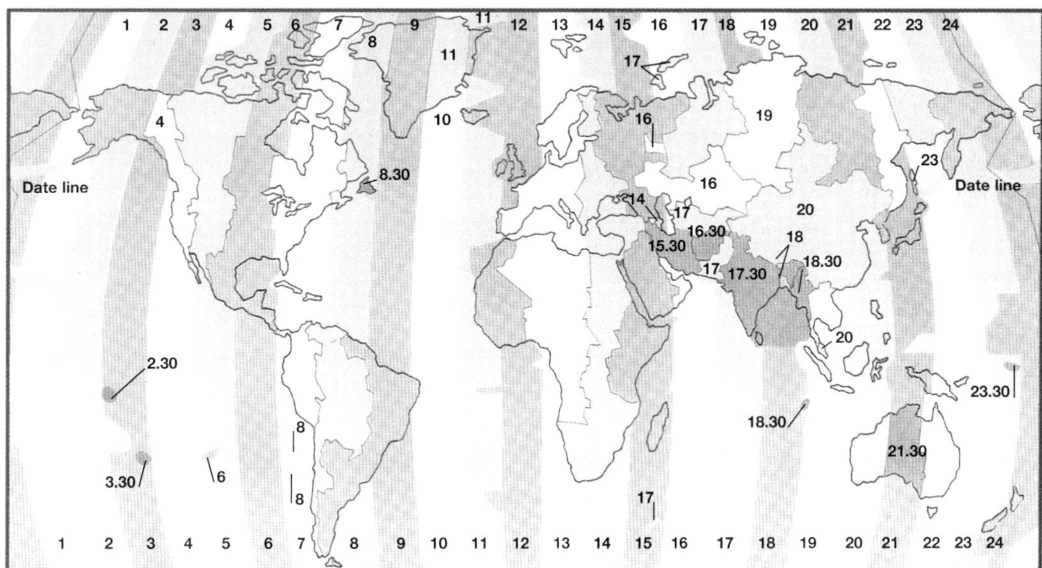

TIME ZONES

As Earth spins, the Sun appears to rise and set. However, while the Sun is rising at one place on the globe, it is setting at another. For instance, when it is 5 A.M. in New York, it is 8 P.M. in Australia. To take account of this, the Earth is divided into a series of time zones, starting from the Date line. Clocks are set to a different time in each zone, calculated to ensure that in every part of the world, the time is about 12 noon during the middle of the day, and midnight during the middle of the night.

Alkali metals · *Alkaline earth metals* · *Transition metals* · *Other metals* · *Nonmetals* · *Noble gases* · *Lanthanide series* · *Actinide series*

								2 **He** Helium 4.003
			5 **B** Boron 10.81	6 **C** Carbon 12.011	7 **N** Nitrogen 14.007	8 **O** Oxygen 15.999	9 **F** Fluorine 18.998	10 **Ne** Neon 20.179
			13 **Al** Aluminium 26.982	14 **Si** Silicon 28.086	15 **P** Phosphorus 30.974	16 **S** Sulphur 32.06	17 **Cl** Chlorine 35.453	18 **Ar** Argon 39.948
28 **Ni** ickel 8.70	29 **Cu** Copper 63.546	30 **Zn** Zinc 65.38	31 **Ga** Gallium 69.72	32 **Ge** Germanium 72.59	33 **As** Arsenic 74.922	34 **Se** Selenium 78.96	35 **Br** Bromine 79.904	36 **Kr** Krypton 83.80
46 **Pd** ladium 06.4	47 **Ag** Silver 107.868	48 **Cd** Cadmium 112.40	49 **In** Indium 114.82	50 **Sn** Tin 118.69	51 **Sb** Antimony 121.75	52 **Te** Tellurium 127.60	53 **I** Iodine 126.905	54 **Xe** Xenon 131.30
78 **Pt** tinum 95.09	79 **Au** Gold 196.967	80 **Hg** Mercury 200.59	81 **Tl** Thallium 204.37	82 **Pb** Lead 207.2	83 **Bi** Bismuth 208.98	84 **Po** Polonium (209)	85 **At** Astatine (210)	86 **Rn** Radon (222)

New elements are sometimes discovered, but it takes time for them to be officially recognized and named.

65 **Tb** rbium 8.925	66 **Dy** Dysprosium 162.50	67 **Ho** Holmium 164.930	68 **Er** Erbium 167.26	69 **Tm** Thulium 168.934	70 **Yb** Ytterbium 173.04	71 **Lu** Lutetium 174.97
97 **Bk** kelium 247)	98 **Cf** Californium (251)	99 **Es** Einsteinium (254)	100 **Fm** Fermium (257)	101 **Md** Mendelevium (258)	102 **No** Nobelium (255)	103 **Lr** Lawrencium (260)

TEMPERATURE SCALES

To convert from Celsius to Fahrenheit:

°F = °C x 9/5 + 32

To convert from Fahrenheit to Celsius:

°C = (°F – 32) x 5/9

Celsius/°C: 100, 90, 80, 70, 60, 50, 40, 30, 20, 10, 0, -10, -20

Fahrenheit/°F: 210, 200, 190, 180, 170, 160, 150, 140, 130, 120, 110, 100, 90, 80, 70, 60, 50, 40, 30, 20, 10, 0

INDEX

Page numbers in **bold** type have most information in them. Numbers in *italics* refer to pages in the Fact Finder.

A

D · E

F · G

H · I · J

K · L · M

N · O · P

Q · R

S · T

U · V · W

X · Y · Z

GAZETTEER

A

Abu Dhabi United Arab Emirates **435**
Abuja Nigeria **730**
Acapulco Mexico **428**
Accra Ghana **730**
Addis Ababa Ethiopia **215**
Adelaide Australia **68**
Aden Yemen **435**
Adriatic Sea *sea* Mediterranean Sea **364**
Aegean Sea *sea* Mediterranean Sea **309**
Afghanistan *country* C Asia **141**
Africa *continent* **17**
Alabama *state* USA **704**
Alaska *state* USA **704**
Albania *country* SE Europe **629**
Alberta *province* Canada **120**
Alexandria Egypt **473**
Algeria *country* N Africa **473**
Algiers Algeria **473**
Alicante Spain **639**
Alice Springs Australia **68**
Alps *mountains* C Europe **238**
Amazon *river* Brazil/Peru **100**
Amazon Basin *basin* South America **100**
American Samoa *dependency* Pacific Ocean **499**
Amman Jordan **435**
Amsterdam Netherlands **403**
Andes *mountains* S America **617**
Andorra *country* SW Europe **278**
Andorra la Vella Andorra **278**
Angola *country* SW Africa **631**
Anguilla *dependency* West Indies **123**
Ankara Turkey **688**
Antananarivo Madagascar **344**
Antarctica *continent* Antarctica **38**
Antigua and Barbuda *country* West Indies **123**
Antwerp Belgium **403**
Appennines *mountains* Italy/San Marino **364**
Arabian Peninsula *peninsula* SW Asia **434**
Arabian Sea *sea* Indian Ocean **53**
Arctic Ocean *ocean* **45**
Argentina *country* S South America **47**
Arizona *state* USA **704**
Arkansas *state* USA **704**
Armenia *country* SW Asia **132**
Aruba *dependency* West Indies **123**
Ascension Island *dependency* Atlantic Ocean **62**
Ashgabat Turkmenistan **141**
Ashmore and Cartier Islands *dependency* Indian Ocean **344**
Asia *Continent* **53**
Asmara Eritrea **215**
Astana Kazakhstan **53**
Asunción Paraguay **617**
Atacama Desert *desert* Chile **617**
Athens Greece **309**
Atlantic Ocean *Ocean* **62**
Atlas Mountains *mountains* N Africa **473**
Auckland New Zealand **468**
Australia *country* Oceania **68**
Australian Capital Territory *territory* Australia **68**
Austria *country* W Europe **73**
Ayers Rock *see* Uluru
Azerbaijan *country* SE Asia **132**

B

Baffin Bay *bay* Atlantic Ocean **120**
Baghdad Iraq **435**
Bahamas *country* West Indies **123**
Bahrain *country* SW Asia **435**
Baku Azerbaijan **132**
Balearic Islands *islands* Spain **639**
Baltic Sea *sea* Atlantic Ocean **238**
Bamako Mali **730**
Bandar Seri Begawan Brunei **623**
Bangalore India **340**
Bangkok Thailand **623**
Bangladesh *country* S Asia **340**
Bangui Central African Republic **137**
Banjul Gambia **730**
Barbados *country* West Indies **123**
Barcelona Spain **639**
Basel Switzerland **660**
Basseterre Saint Kitts and Nevis **123**
Bavarian Alps *mountains* Austria/Germany **73**
Beijing China **147**
Beirut Lebanon **435**
Belarus *country* E Europe **80**
Belfast UK **695**
Belgium *country* NW Europe **403**
Belgrade Serbia and Montenegro **627**
Belize *country* Central America **139**
Belmopan Belize **139**
Belo Horizonte Brazil **100**
Ben Nevis *mountain* UK **695**
Bengal, Bay of *bay* Indian Ocean **340**
Benin *country* W Africa **730**
Bering Strait *strait* Russian Federation/USA **704**
Berlin Germany **296**
Bermuda *dependency* Atlantic Ocean **62**
Bern Switzerland **660**
Berner Alpen *mountains* Switzerland **660**
Bethlehem West Bank **361**
Bhutan *country* S Asia **340**
Birmingham UK **695**
Biscay, Bay of *bay* Atlantic Ocean **639**
Bishkek Kyrgyzstan **141**
Bissau Guinea-Bissau **730**
Black Forest *physical region* Germany **296**
Black Sea *sea* Atlantic Ocean **238**
Blackpool UK **695**
Blanc, Mont *mountain* France/Italy **364**
Bloemfontein South Africa **612**
Bogotá Colombia **162**
Bohemian Forest *mountains* C Europe **296**
Bolivia *country* W South America **617**
Bombay *see* Mumbai
Bonn Germany **296**
Bordeaux France **278**
Borneo *island* SE Asia **623**
Bosnia and Herzegovina *country* SE Europe **629**
Boston USA **704**
Botswana *country* S Africa **631**
Bouvet Island *dependency* Atlantic Ocean **62**
Brahmaputra *river* S Asia **147**
Brasília Brazil **100**
Bratislava Slovakia **238**
Brazil *country* C South America **100**
Brazzaville Congo **137**
Bridgetown Barbados **123**
Brisbane Australia **68**
Bristol Channel *inlet* UK **695**
British Columbia *province* Canada **120**
British Indian Ocean Territory *dependency* Indian Ocean **344**
British Virgin Islands *dependency* West Indies **123**
Bruges Belgium **403**
Brunei *country* SE Asia **623**
Brussels Belgium **403**
Bucharest Romania **627**
Budapest Hungary **238**
Buenos Aires Argentina **47**
Bujumbura Burundi **215**
Bulgaria *country* SE Europe **627**
Burkina *country* W Africa **730**
Burma *country* SE Asia **623**
Burundi *country* C Africa **215**

C

Cabinda *province* Angola **137**
Cádiz Spain **639**
Cairo Egypt **473**
Calais France **278**
Calcutta *see* Kolkata
Calgary Canada **120**
California *state* USA **704**
California, Gulf of *gulf* Pacific Ocean **428**
Cambodia *country* SE Asia **623**
Cameroon *country* W Africa **137**
Canada *country* N North America **120**
Canary Islands *islands* Spain **639**
Canberra Australia **68**
Cape Town South Africa **612**
Cape Verde *country* Atlantic Ocean **62**
Caracas Venezuela **617**
Cardiff UK **695**
Cardigan Bay *bay* Atlantic Ocean **695**
Caribbean Sea *sea* Atlantic Ocean **477**
Cartagena Colombia **162**
Casablanca Morocco **473**
Castries Saint Lucia **123**
Cayenne French Guiana **617**
Cayman Islands *dependency* West Indies **123**
Central African Republic *country* C Africa **137**
Central America *geopolitical region* **139**
Chad *country* C Africa **137**
Channel Islands *islands* W Europe **695**
Chennai India **340**
Chicago USA **704**
Chile *country* SW South America **617**
China *country* E Asia **147**
Chisinau Moldova **689**
Christchurch New Zealand **468**
Christmas Island *dependency* Indian Ocean **344**
Cocos Islands *dependency* Indian Ocean **344**
Cologne Germany **296**
Colombia *country* N South America **162**
Colombo Sri Lanka **340**
Colorado *state* USA **704**
Comoros *country* Indian Ocean **344**
Conakry Guinea **730**
Congo *country* C Africa **137**
Congo Basin *basin* C Africa **137**
Congo, Democratic Republic of *country* C Africa **137**
Connecticut *state* USA **704**
Cook Islands *dependency* Pacific Ocean **499**
Copenhagen Denmark **579**
Corfu *island* Greece **309**
Cork Ireland **356**
Corsica *island* France **278**
Costa Rica *country* Central America **139**
Crete *island* Greece **309**
Crimea *peninsula* Ukraine **689**
Croatia *country* SE Europe **629**
Cuba *country* West Indies **123**
Cyprus *country* Mediterranean Sea **53**
Czech Republic *country* C Europe **238**

D

Dakar Senegal **730**
Dallas USA **704**
Damascus Syria **435**
Danube *river* C Europe **296, 627**
Darwin Australia **68**
Dead Sea *salt lake* Israel/Jordan **361**
Delaware *state* USA **704**
Delhi India **340**
Denmark *country* N Europe **579**
Detroit USA **704**
Dhaka Bangladesh **340**
Dijon France **278**
Dili East Timor **623**
Dingle Bay *bay* Atlantic Ocean **356**
Djibouti *country* E Africa **215**
Djibouti Djibouti **215**
Dodecanese *islands* Greece **309**
Dodoma Tanzania **215**
Doha Qatar **435**
Dominica *country* West Indies **123**
Dominican Republic *country* West Indies **123**
Donegal Bay *bay* Atlantic Ocean **356**
Dordogne *river* France **278**
Douro *river* Portugal/Spain **532**
Dubai United Arab Emirates **435**
Dublin Ireland **356**
Durban South Africa **612**
Dushanbe Tajikistan **141**
Düsseldorf Germany **296**

E

East Timor *country* SE Asia **623**
Ecuador *country* NW South America **617**
Edinburgh UK **695**
Egypt *country* NE Africa **473**
Eiger *mountain* Switzerland **660**
El Salvador *country* Central America **139**
Elburz Mountains *mountains* Iran **354**
England *national region* UK **695**
English Channel *channel* France/United Kingdom **238**
Equatorial Guinea *country* C Africa **137**
Erie, Lake *lake* Canada/USA **704**
Eritrea *country* E Africa **215**
Estonia *country* NE Europe **80**
Ethiopia *country* E Africa **215**
Etna, Monte *volcano* Italy **364**
Euphrates *river* SW Asia **688**
Europe *Continent* **238**
Everest, Mount *mountain* China/Nepal **340**

F

Faeroe Islands *dependency* NW Europe **579**
Falkland Islands *dependency* Atlantic Ocean **47**
Fiji *country* Pacific Ocean **499**
Finland *country* N Europe **579**
Florence Italy **364**
Florida *state* USA **704**
Florida Keys *islands* USA **704**
France *country* W Europe **278**
Frankfurt am Main Germany **296**
Freetown Sierra Leone **730**
French Guiana *dependency* N South America **617**
French Polynesia *dependency* Pacific Ocean **499**

G

Gabon *country* C Africa **137**
Gaborone Botswana **631**
Galilee, Sea of *lake* Israel **361**
Galway Bay *bay* Atlantic Ocean **356**
Gambia *country* W Africa **730**
Ganges *river* S Asia **340**
Garda, Lago di *lake* Italy **364**
Garonne *river* France **278**
Gaza Strip *disputed region* Gaza Strip **361**
Geneva Switzerland **660**
Geneva, Lake *lake* France/Switzerland **660**
Genoa Italy **364**
Georgetown Guyana **617**
Georgia *country* SW Asia **132**
Georgia *state* USA **704**
Germany *country* N Europe **296**
Ghana *country* W Africa **730**
Gibraltar *dependency* **639**
Glasgow UK **695**
Gothenburg Sweden **579**
Grampian Mountains *mountains* UK **695**
Gran Chaco *lowland plain* South America **47**
Grand Canyon *canyon* USA **704**
Great Barrier Reef *reef* Australia **68**
Great Bear Lake *lake* Canada **120**
Great Lakes *lakes* Canada/USA **704**
Great Wall of China *Ancient monument* China **147**
Great Plains *plains* Canada/USA **120**
Great Rift Valley *depression* Asia/Africa **215**
Great Slave Lake *lake* Canada **120**
Greater Antilles *islands* West Indies **123**
Greece *country* SE Europe **309**
Greenland *dependency* NE North America **579**
Grenada *country* West Indies **123**
Grenoble France **278**
Guadeloupe *dependency* West Indies **123**
Guam *dependency* Pacific Ocean **499**
Guatemala *country* Central America **139**
Guatemala City Guatemala **139**
Guernsey *island* Channel Islands **695**
Guinea *country* W Africa **730**
Guinea-Bissau *country* W Africa **730**
Gulf, The *gulf* SW Asia **435**
Guyana *country* N South America **617**

H

Haifa Israel **361**
Haiti *country* West Indies **123**
Halifax Canada **120**
Hamburg Germany **296**
Hamilton New Zealand **468**
Hanoi Vietnam **623**
Hanover Germany **296**
Harare Zimbabwe **631**
Havana Cuba **123**
Hawaii *state* USA **704**
Hebrides *islands* UK **695**
Hebron Israel **361**
Helsinki Finland **579**
Himalayas *mountains* S Asia **340**
Hindu Kush *mountains* Afghanistan/Pakistan **141**
Hiroshima Japan **369**
Hô Chi Minh Vietnam **623**
Hobart Australia **68**
Hokkaido *island* Japan **369**
Honduras *country* Central America **139**
Hong Kong *former UK dependency* China **147**
Honshu *island* Japan **369**
Houston USA **704**
Hudson Bay *bay* Atlantic Ocean **120**
Hungary *country* C Europe **238**

I·J

Ibiza *island* Spain **639**
Iceland *country* NW Europe **579**
Idaho *state* USA **704**
Illinois *state* USA **704**
India *country* S Asia **340**
Indian Ocean *ocean* **344**
Indiana *state* USA **704**
Indianapolis USA **704**
Indonesia *country* SE Asia **623**
Indus *river* S Asia **340**
Innsbruck Austria **73**
Iowa *state* USA **704**
Iran *country* SW Asia **354**
Iranian Plateau *plateau* Iran **354**
Iraq *country* SW Asia **435**
Ireland *country* NW Europe **356**
Irian Jaya *province* Indonesia **623**
Irish Sea *sea* Atlantic Ocean **356**
Islamabad Pakistan **340**
Isle of Man *dependency* NW Europe **695**
Israel *country* SW Asia **361**
Istanbul Turkey **688**
Italy *country* S Europe **364**
Ivory Coast *country* W Africa **730**
Jakarta Indonesia **623**
Jamaica *country* West Indies **123**
Japan *country* E Asia **344**
Java *island* Indonesia **623**
Jersey *island* Channel Islands **695**
Jerusalem Israel **361**
Johannesburg South Africa **612**
Jordan *country* SW Asia **435**
Jutland *peninsula* Denmark **579**

K·L

K2 *mountain* China/Pakistan **340**
Kabul Afghanistan **141**
Kalahari Desert *desert* S Africa **631**
Kamchatka *peninsula* Russian Federation **571**
Kampala Uganda **215**
Kansas *state* USA **704**
Kathmandu Nepal **340**
Kazakhstan *country* C Asia **53**
Kentucky *state* USA **704**
Kenya *country* E Africa **215**
Khartoum Sudan **215**
Khyber Pass *pass* Afghanistan/Pakistan **340**
Kiev Ukraine **689**
Kigali Rwanda **215**
Kilimanjaro *volcano* Tanzania **215**
Killarney Ireland **356**
Kingston Jamaica **123**
Kingstown Saint Vincent and the Grenadines **123**
Kinshasa Congo, Dem. Rep. of **137**
Kiribati *country* Pacific Ocean **499**
Kisangani Congo, Dem. Rep. of **137**
Kobe Japan **369**
Kolkata India **340**
Kosovo Serbia and Montenegro **628**
Kuala Lumpur Malaysia **623**
Kuwait *country* SW Asia **435**
Kuwait Kuwait **435**
Kyoto Japan **369**
Kyrgyzstan *country* C Asia **141**
Kyushu *island* Japan **369**
La Paz Bolivia **617**
Laâyoune Western Sahara **473**
Lahore Pakistan **340**
Land's End *headland* UK **695**
Laos *country* SE Asia **623**
Latvia *country* NE Europe **80**
Lausanne Switzerland **660**
Le Havre France **278**
Lebanon *country* SW Asia **435**
Leeds UK **695**
Leeward Islands *islands* West Indies **123**
Lesbos *island* Greece **309**
Lesotho *country* S Africa **612**
Lesser Antilles *islands* West Indies **123**
Liberia *country* W Africa **730**
Libreville Gabon **137**
Libya *country* N Africa **473**
Libyan Desert *desert* N Africa **17**
Liechtenstein *country* C Europe **238**
Liffey *river* Ireland **356**
Lille France **278**
Lilongwe Malawi **17**
Lima Peru **617**
Limoges France **278**
Lisbon Portugal **532**
Lithuania *country* NE Europe **80**
Liverpool UK **695**
Ljubljana Slovenia **629**
Llanos *physical region* Colombia/Venezuela **617**
Loire *river* France **278**
Lomé Togo **730**
London UK **695**
Los Angeles USA **704**
Louisiana *state* USA **704**
Luanda Angola **631**
Lusaka Zambia **17**
Luxembourg *country* NW Europe **403**
Luxembourg Luxembourg **403**
Lyon France **278**

M

Maastricht Netherlands **403**
Macedonia *country* SE Europe **627**
Madagascar *country* Indian Ocean **344**
Madras *see* Chennai
Madrid Spain **639**
Maine *state* USA **704**
Majorca *island* Spain **639**
Malabo Equatorial Guinea **137**
Málaga Spain **639**
Malawi *country* S Africa **17**
Malaysia *country* SE Asia **623**
Maldives *country* Indian Ocean **344**
Male Maldives **344**
Mali *country* W Africa **730**
Malta *country* S Europe **364**
Managua Nicaragua **139**
Manama Bahrain **435**
Manchester UK **695**
Manila Philippines **623**
Manitoba *province* Canada **120**
Maputo Mozambique **631**
Marrakech Morocco **473**
Marseille France **278**
Marshall Islands *country* Pacific Ocean **499**
Martinique *dependency* West Indies **123**
Maryland *state* USA **704**
Maseru Lesotho **612**
Massachusetts *state* USA **704**
Massif Central *plateau* France **278**
Matterhorn *mountain* Italy/Switzerland **660**
Mauritania *country* W Africa **730**
Mauritius *country* Indian Ocean **344**
Mayotte *dependency* Indian Ocean **344**
Mbabane Swaziland **612**
Mediterranean Sea *sea* Atlantic Ocean **238**
Mekong *river* SE Asia **147**
Melbourne Australia **68**
Memphis USA **704**
Mexico *country* Central America **428**
Mexico City Mexico **428**
Mexico, Gulf of *gulf* Atlantic Ocean **477**
Michigan *state* USA **704**
Micronesia *country* Pacific Ocean **499**
Midway Islands *dependency* Pacific Ocean **499**
Milan Italy **364**
Minnesota *state* USA **704**
Minorca *island* Spain **639**
Minsk Belarus **80**
Mississippi *state* USA **704**
Mississippi River *river* USA **704**
Missouri *state* USA **704**
Mogadishu Somalia **215**
Moldova *country* SE Europe **689**
Mombasa Kenya **215**
Monaco *country* W Europe **278**
Mongolia *country* E Asia **53**
Monrovia Liberia **730**
Montana *state* USA **704**
Montevideo Uruguay **617**
Montréal Canada **120**
Montserrat *dependency* West Indies **123**
Morocco *country* N Africa **473**
Moroni Comoros **344**
Moscow Russian Federation **571**
Mozambique *country* S Africa **631**
Mumbai India **340**
Munich Germany **296**
Muscat Oman **435**
Myanmar *see* Burma

N

Nagasaki Japan **369**
Nairobi Kenya **215**
Namib Desert *desert* Namibia **631**
Namibia *country* S Africa **631**
Naples Italy **364**
Nassau Bahamas **123**
Nauru *country* Pacific Ocean **499**
Navassa Island *dependency* West Indies **123**
Nazareth Israel **361**
Ndjamena Chad **137**
Nebraska *state* USA **704**
Negev *desert* Israel **361**
Nepal *country* S Asia **340**
Netherlands *country* NW Europe **403**
Nevada *state* USA **704**
New Brunswick *province* Canada **120**
New Caledonia *dependency* Pacific Ocean **499**
New Delhi India **340**
New Hampshire *state* USA **704**
New Jersey *state* USA **704**
New Mexico *state* USA **704**
New Orleans USA **704**
New South Wales *state* Australia **68**
New York USA **704**
New York *state* USA **704**
New Zealand *country* Oceania **468**
Newcastle upon Tyne UK **695**
Newfoundland *province* Canada **120**
Niagara Falls *waterfall* Canada/USA **120, 704**
Niamey Niger **730**
Nicaragua *country* Central America **139**
Nice France **278**
Nicosia Cyprus **53**
Niger *country* W Africa **730**
Niger *river* W Africa **730**
Nigeria *country* W Africa **730**
Nile *river* N Africa **17**
Niue *dependency* Pacific Ocean **499**
North America *Continent* **477**
North Carolina *state* USA **704**
North Dakota *state* USA **704**
North European Plain *plain* N Europe **238**
North Geomagnetic Pole *pole* **45**
North Island *island* New Zealand **468**
North Korea *country* Asia **380**
North Pole *pole* **45**
North Sea *sea* Atlantic Ocean **238**
Northern Ireland *political division* UK **695**

Northern Mariana Islands *dependency* Pacific Ocean **499**
Northern Territory *territory* Australia **68**
Northwest Territories *territory* Canada **120**
Norway *country* N Europe **579**
Nouakchott Mauritania **730**
Nova Scotia *province* Canada **120**
Nubian Desert *desert* Sudan **215**
Nunavut *province* Canada **120**
Nuremberg Germany **296**
Nyasa, Lake *lake* E Africa **631**

O · P

Ob' *river* Russian Federation **571**
Ohio *state* USA **704**
Oklahoma *state* USA **704**
Oklahoma City USA **704**
Oman *country* SW Asia **435**
Ontario *province* Canada **120**
Oporto Portugal **532**
Oregon *state* USA **704**
Orléans France **278**
Osaka Japan **369**
Oslo Norway **579**
Ottawa Canada **120**
Ouagadougou Burkina **730**
Pacific Ocean *ocean* **499**
Pakistan *country* S Asia **340**
Palau *country* Pacific Ocean **499**
Palma Spain **639**
Pampas *plain* Argentina **47**
Panama *country* Central America **139**
Panama Canal *shipping canal* Panama **139**
Panama City Panama **139**
Papua New Guinea *country* Pacific Ocean **499**
Paraguay *country* C South America **617**
Paramaribo Surinam **617**
Paris France **278**
Patagonia *semi arid region* Argentina/Chile **47**
Peloponnese Greece **309**
Pennsylvania *state* USA **704**
Perth Australia **68**
Peru *country* W South America **617**
Philippines *country* SE Asia **623**
Phnom Penh Cambodia **623**
Pindus Mountains *mountains* Greece **309**
Pitcairn Islands *dependency* Pacific Ocean **499**
Plenty, Bay of *bay* Pacific Ocean **468**
Poland *country* C Europe **238**
Port Louis Mauritius **344**
Port-au-Prince Haiti **123**
Port-of-Spain Trinidad and Tobago **123**
Porto-Novo Benin **730**
Portugal *country* SW Europe **532**
Prague Czech Republic **238**
Praia Cape Verde **62**
Pretoria South Africa **612**
Puerto Rico *dependency* West Indies **123**
Pyongyang North Korea **380**
Pyrenees *mountains* France/Spain **639**

Q · R

Qatar *country* SW Asia **435**
Québec Canada **120**
Québec *province* Canada **120**
Queensland *state* Australia **68**
Quito Ecuador **617**
Riga Latvia **80**
Rabat Morocco **473**
Rangoon Burma **623**
Red Sea *sea* Indian Ocean **17**
Réunion *dependency* Indian Ocean **344**
Reykjavík Iceland **579**
Rhine *river* W Europe **296**
Rhode Island *state* USA **704**
Rhodes *island* Greece **309**
Rhône *river* France/Switzerland **278**
Rio de Janeiro Brazil **100**
Riyadh Saudi Arabia **435**
Rocky Mountains *mountains* Canada/USA **477**
Romania *country* SE Europe **627**
Rome Italy **364**
Roseau Dominica **123**
Rotterdam Netherlands **403**
Rouen France **278**
Ruhr *river* Germany **296**
Russian Federation *country* Asia/Europe **571**
Rwanda *country* C Africa **215**
Ryukyu Islands *islands* Japan **369**

S

Sahara *desert* N Africa **17**
Sahel *physical region* C Africa **17**
Saint Helena *dependency* Atlantic Ocean **62**
Saint Helens, Mount *volcano* USA **704**
Saint Kitts and Nevis *country* West Indies **123**
Saint Lucia *country* West Indies **123**
Saint Petersburg Russian Federation **571**
Saint Vincent and the Grenadines *country* West Indies **123**
Salonica Greece **309**
Salvador Brazil **100**
Salzburg Austria **73**
Samoa *country* Pacific Ocean **499**
San Diego USA **704**
San Francisco USA **704**
San José Costa Rica **139**
San Marino *country* S Europe **364**
San Salvador El Salvador **139**
Santiago Chile **617**
Santo Domingo Dominican Republic **123**
São Paulo Brazil **100**
São Tomé São Tomé and Príncipe **137**
São Tomé and Príncipe *country* Atlantic Ocean **137**
Sarajevo Bosnia and Herzegovina **629**
Sardinia *island* Italy **364**
Saskatchewan *province* Canada **120**
Saudi Arabia *country* SW Asia **435**
Scafell Pike *mountain* UK **695**
Scotland *national region* UK **695**
Seattle USA **704**
Seine *river* France **278**
Senegal *country* W Africa **730**
Seoul South Korea **380**
Serbia and Montenegro SE Europe **627**
Serengeti Plain *plain* Tanzania **215**
Seville Spain **639**
Seychelles *country* Indian Ocean **344**
Shannon *river* Ireland **356**
Sheffield UK **695**
Shetland Islands *islands* UK **695**
Shikoku *island* Japan **369**
Siberia *physical region* Russian Federation **571**
Sicily *island* Italy **364**
Sierra Leone *country* W Africa **730**
Singapore *country* SE Asia **623**
Skopje Macedonia **627**
Slovakia *country* C Europe **238**
Slovenia *country* SE Europe **629**
Snowdon *mountain* UK **695**
Sofia Bulgaria **627**
Solomon Islands *country* Pacific Ocean **499**
Somalia *country* E Africa **215**
South Africa *country* S Africa **612**
South America *Continent* **617**
South Australia *state* Australia **68**
South Carolina *state* USA **704**
South Dakota *state* USA **704**
South Geomagnetic Pole *pole* Antarctica **38**
South Georgia *dependency* Atlantic Ocean **62**
South Island *island* New Zealand **468**
South Korea *country* E Asia **379**
South Pole *pole* Antarctica **38**
South Sandwich Islands *dependency* Atlantic Ocean **62**
Spain *country* SW Europe **639**
Sri Lanka *country* S Asia **340**
St George's Grenada **123**
St John's Antigua and Barbuda **123**
Stockholm Sweden **579**
Strasbourg France **278**
Stuttgart Germany **296**
Sucre Bolivia **617**
Sudan *country* N Africa **215**
Sumatra *island* Indonesia **623**
Superior, Lake *lake* Canada/USA **704**
Surinam *country* N South America **617**
Swansea UK **695**
Swaziland *country* S Africa **612**
Sweden *country* N Europe **579**
Switzerland *country* C Europe **660**
Sydney Australia **68**
Syria *country* SW Asia **435**

T

T'bilisi Georgia **132**
Tagus *river* Portugal/Spain **531**
Taipei Taiwan **147**
Taiwan *country* E Asia **147**
Tajikistan *country* C Asia **141**
Takla Makan Desert *desert* China **147**
Tallinn Estonia **80**
Tanzania *country* E Africa **215**
Tashkent Uzbekistan **141**
Tasmania *state* Australia **68**
Taurus Mountains *mountains* Turkey **688**
Tegucigalpa Honduras **139**
Tehran Iran **354**
Tel Aviv-Yafo Israel **361**
Tennessee *state* USA **704**
Texas *state* USA **704**
Thailand *country* SE Asia **623**
Thames *river* UK **695**
Thar Desert *desert* India/Pakistan **340**
The Hague Netherlands **403**
Thimphu Bhutan **340**
Tibet *autonomous region* China **147**
Timor *island* Indonesia **623**
Tirana Albania **629**
Tisza *river* SE Europe **627**
Togo *country* W Africa **730**
Tokelau *dependency* Pacific Ocean **499**
Tokyo Japan **369**
Tonga *country* Pacific Ocean **499**
Toronto Canada **120**
Toulouse France **278**
Transylvanian Alps *mountains* Romania **627**
Trieste Italy **364**
Trinidad and Tobago *country* West Indies **123**
Tripoli Libya **473**
Tristan da Cunha *dependency* Atlantic Ocean **62**
Tunis Tunisia **473**
Tunisia *country* N Africa **473**
Turin Italy **364**
Turkey *country* SW Asia **688**
Turkmenistan *country* C Asia **141**
Turks and Caicos Islands *dependency* West Indies **123**
Tuvalu *country* Pacific Ocean **499**
Tuz, Lake *lake* Turkey **688**

U · V

Uganda *country* E Africa **215**
Ukraine *country* SE Europe **689**
Ulan Bator Mongolia **53**
Uluru *rocky outcrop* Australia **68**
United Arab Emirates *country* SW Asia **435**
United Kingdom *country* NW Europe **695**
United States of America *country* North America **704**
Ural Mountains *mountains* Kazakhstan/Russian Federation **571**
Uruguay *country* E South America **617**
Utah *state* USA **704**
Uzbekistan *country* C Asia **141**
Vaduz Liechtenstein **238**
Valletta Malta **364**
Van, Lake *salt lake* Turkey **688**
Vancouver Canada **120**
Vanuatu *country* Pacific Ocean **499**
Vatican City *country* S Europe **364**
Venezuela *country* N South America **617**
Venice Italy **364**
Vermont *state* USA **704**
Victoria Seychelles **344**
Victoria *state* Australia **68**
Victoria Falls *waterfall* Zambia/Zimbabwe **631**
Victoria, Lake *lake* E Africa **215**
Vienna Austria **73**
Vientiane Laos **623**
Vietnam *country* SE Asia **623**
Vilnius Lithuania **80**
Virgin Islands (US) *dependency* West Indies **123**
Virginia *state* USA **704**
Vladivostok Russian Federation **571**
Volta, Lake *reservoir* Ghana **730**

W

Wake Island *dependency* Pacific Ocean **499**
Wales *national region* UK **695**
Wallis and Futuna *dependency* Pacific Ocean **499**
Warsaw Poland **238**
Washington *state* USA **704**
Washington DC USA **704**
Waterford Ireland **356**
Wellington New Zealand **468**
West Bank *disputed region* West Bank **361**
West Virginia *state* USA **704**
Western Australia *state* Australia **68**
Western Dvina *river* E Europe **80**
Wexford Ireland **356**
Wicklow Mountains *mountains* Ireland **356**
Wien Austria **73**
Windhoek Namibia **631**
Winnipeg Canada **120**
Wisconsin *state* USA **704**
Wyoming *state* USA **704**

Y · Z

Yangtse *river* China **147**
Yaoundé Cameroon **137**
Yellow River *river* China **147**
Yellowknife Canada **120**
Yemen *country* SW Asia **435**
Yenisey *river* Mongolia/Russian Federation **571**
Yerevan Armenia **132**
Yokohama Japan **369**
Yukon Territory *territory* Canada **120**
Zagreb Croatia **628**
Zagros Mountains *mountains* Iran **354**
Zaire *see* Congo, Democratic Republic of
Zambia *country* S Africa **17**
Zanzibar *island* Tanzania **215**
Zimbabwe *country* S Africa **631**
Zurich Switzerland **660**

ACKNOWLEDGEMENTS

Contributors Simon Adams, Neil Ardley, Norman Barrett, Gerard Cheshire, Judy Clark, Chris Cooper, Margaret Crowther, John Farndon, Will Fowler, Adrian Gilbert, Barbara Gilgallon, Peter Lafferty, Margaret Lincoln, Caroline Lucas, Antony Mason, Rupert Matthews, Dan McCausland, Steve Parker, Steve Peak, Theodore Rowland-Entwistle, Sue Seddon, Marilyn Tolhurst, Marcus Weeks, Philip Wilkinson, Frances Williams, Tim Wood, Elizabeth Wyse
Additional editorial assistance from Sam Atkinson, Jane Birdsell, Lynn Bresler, Azza Brown, Liza Bruml, Caroline Chapman, Claire Gillard, Carl Gombrich, Samantha Gray, Sudhanshu Gupta, Prita Maitra, Caroline Murrell, Pallavi Narain, Connie Novis, Louise Pritchard, Ranjana Saklani, Jill Somerscales
Additional design assistance from Sukanto Bhattacharjya, Tina Borg, Duncan Brown, Darren Holt, Shuka Jain, Ruth Jones, Sabyasachi Kundu, Clare Watson, Simon Yeomans
Illustration Coordinator Ted Kinsey
Picture Research Maureen Cowdroy, Diane LeGrand, Samantha Nunn, Deborah Pownall, Louise Thomas, Bridget Tily, Emma Wood
Cartographers Pam Alford, Tony Chambers, Ed Merritt, Rob Stokes, Peter Winfield
DTP Harish Aggarwal, Georgia Bryer, Siu Chan, Nomazwe Madonko, Pankaj Sharma, Claudia Shill
Photography Stephen Oliver
Index Hilary Bird, Sylvia Potter
Gazetter Sylvia Potter
Additional Production Chris Avgherinos

ADVISORS AND CONSULTANTS

Chemistry and Physics
Ian M. Kennedy BSc
Jeff Odell BSc, MSc, PhD
David Glover

Culture and Society
Iris Barry
Margaret Cowan
John Denny B.Mus.Hons
Dr. Peter Drewett BSc, PhD, FSA, MIFA
Dr. Jamal, Islamic Cultural Centre
Miles Smith-Morris
Brian Williams BA
The Buddhist Society

Earth Resources
April Arden Dip.M
Hedda Bird BSc
Conservation Papers Ltd.
Peter Nolan, British Gas Plc
Stephen Webster BSc, M. Phil
Earth Conservation Data Centre

Earth Sciences
Erica Brissenden
Alan Heward PhD
Keith Lye BA, FRGS
Rodney Miskin MIPR, MAIE
Shell UK Ltd.
Christine Woodward
The Geological Museum, London
Meteorological Office

Engineering
Karen Barratt
Jim Lloyd, Otis Plc
Alban Wincott
Mark Woodward MSc, DICC.Eng

History
Reg Grant
Dr. Anne Millard BA, Dip Ed, PhD
Ray Smith
The Indian High Commission
Campaign for Nuclear Disarmament

Medicine and the Human Body
Dr. Sue Davidson
Dr. T. Kramer MB, BS, MRCS, LRCP
Dr. Frances Williams MB, BChir, MRCP

Music
Simon Wales BA, MBA,
London Symphony Orchestra

Natural History
Kim Bryan
Wendy Ladd and the staff of the Natural History Museum
London Zoo

Space Science
NASA
Neil MacIntyre MA, PhD, FRGS
Dr. Jacqueline Mitton
John Randall BSc, PGCE
Christian Ripley BSc, MSc
Carole Stott BA, FRAS

Sport
Brian Aldred
David Barber
Lance Cone
John Jelley BA
International Olympic Committee

Technology
Alan Buckingham
Jeremy Hazzard BISC
Paul Macarthy BSc, MSc
Cosson Electronics Ltd.
Robert Stone BSc, MSc, C. Psychol, AFBsF, M.ErgS,
Advanced Robotic Research Ltd.
Stuart Wickes B. Eng

Transport
Doug Lloyd, Westland Helicopters
John Pimlott BA, PhD
Tony Robinson
Wing Commander Spilsbury, RAF
M. J. Whitty GI Sore.E

In addition, Dorling Kindersley would like to thank the following people and organizations for their assistance in the production of this book:

Liz Abrahams, BBC; Alan Baker; All England Tennis Club; Alvis Ltd.; Amateur Swimming Assoc.; Apple UK Ltd.; Ariane Space Ltd.; David Atwill, Hampshire Constabulary; Pamela Barron; Beech Aircraft Corp; Beaufort Air Sea Equipment; Bike UK Ltd.; BMW; Boeing Aircraft Corporation; BP Ltd.; British Amateur Athletics Assoc.; British Amateur Gymnastics Assoc.; British Antarctic Survey; British Canoe Union; British Coal Ltd.; British Forging Industry Assoc.; British Foundry Assoc.; British Gas Ltd.; British Museum; British Paper and Board Federation; British Parachuting Assoc.; British Post Office; British Ski Federation; British Steel; British Sub-Aqua Club; British Telecom International Ltd.; Paul Bush; Michelle Byam; Karen Caftledine, Courtauld Fibres; Martin Christopher, VAG Group; Citroen; CNHMS; Colourscan, Singapore; "Coca-Cola" and "Coke" are registered trade marks which identify the same products of The Coca-Cola Company; Commander Richard Compton-Hall; Lyn Constable-Maxwell; Cottrell & Co Ltd.; Geoffrey Court; Sarah Crouch, Black & Decker Ltd.; F. Darton and Co. Ltd.; Department of Energy, Energy Conservation Support Unit; Adrian Dixon; DRG Paper Ltd.; Patrick Duffy, IBA Museum; Earth Observation Data Centre; Electronic Arts; Embassy of Japan, Transport Department; Esso Plc; Eurotunnel Ltd.; Ford UK Ltd.; Sub Officer Jack Goble, London Fire Brigade; Julia Golding; Brian Gordon; Paul Greenwood, Pentax Cameras Ltd.; Patrick and Betty Gunzi; Hamleys, Regent Street, London; Helmets Ltd.; Jim Henson Productions Ltd.; Alan Heward, Shell UK Ltd.; cartoon frames taken from "Spider in the Bath", reproduced by permission from HIBBERT RALPH ENTERTAINMENT © and SILVEYJEX PARTNERSHIP ©; Hoover Ltd.; Horniman Museum; House of Vanheems Ltd.; IAL security products; ICI Ltd.; Ilford Ltd.; Imperial War Museum; Institute of Metals; Institution of Civil Engineers; Janes Publications Ltd.; Nina Kara; Jonathan Kettle, Haymarket Publishing; Julia Kisch, Thorn EMI Ltd.; Kite Shop, London; Sarah Kramer; Krauss-Maffei GMBH; Lambda Photometrics Ltd.; Sandy Law; Richard Lawson Ltd.; Leica GmbH; Leyland Daf Ltd.; London Transport Museum; London Weather Centre; The Lord Mayor of Westminster's New Year Parade; Lyndon-Dykes of London; Joan MacDonnell, Sovereign Oil and Gas Ltd.; Neil MacIntyre; Marconi Electronic Devices Ltd., Lincoln; Paul McCarthy, Cosser Electronics Ltd.; McDonnell Douglas Aircraft Corporation; Philip Mead; Mercedes; The Meteorological Office, London; Ruth Milner, Comark Ltd.; A. Mondadori Editore, Verona; Mysteries New Age Centre, London; National Army Museum; National Grid Company Ltd.; National Physical Laboratory; National Remote Sensing Centre, Farnborough; Nautilus Ltd.; Newcastle Hindu Temple; Helene Oakley; Olympus Ltd.; The Ordinance Survey; Osel Ltd.; Otis PLC; Gary Palmer, Marantz Ltd.; Personal Protection Products; Pilkington Glass Ltd.; Pioneer Ltd.; Philips Ltd.; Porter Nash Medical; Powell Cotton Museum; John Reedman Associates; Renaissance Musée du Louvre; Robertson Research Ltd.; Tony Robinson; Rockware Glass Ltd.; Rod Argent Music; Rolls Royce Ltd.; Liz Rosney; Royal Aircraft Establishment; Royal Astronomical Society, London; Royal Military Academy, Sandhurst; SNCF; Andrew Saphir; Malcolm Saunders, Simon Gloucester Saro Ltd.; Seagate Ltd.; Sedgewick Museum; Shell UK Ltd.; Skyship International Ltd.; Dennis Slay, Wessex Consultants Ltd.; Amanda Smith, Zanussi Ltd.; Ross Smith, Winchcombe Folk Police Museum; Sony Ltd.; Rachael Spaulding, McDonald's Restaurant Ltd.; Stanfords Map Shop, London; Steelcasting Research and Trade Assoc.; Stollmont Theatres Ltd.; Swatch Watches Ltd.; Tallahassee Car Museum; Texaco Ltd.; The Theatre Museum, Covent Garden, London; Toyota; Trafalgar House, Building and Civil Engineering; Trevor Hyde; Wastewatch; Jim Webb; Westland Helicopters Ltd.; Westminster Cathedral; Malcolm Willingale, V Ships, Monaco; Wiggins Teape Ltd.; Howard Wong, Covent Garden Records, London; Woods Hole Oceanographic Institute; Yarrow Shipbuilders Ltd.; The YHA Shop, London.

PICTURE SOURCES

The publisher would like to thank the following for their kind permission to reproduce their photographs:

Abbreviations: a = above, b = below, c = centre, f = far, l = left, r = right, t = top.

A

Architectural Association: Joe Kerr 445cl.
Action Plus: Glyn Kirk 179tl, 715bl; Richard Francis 88tl, 314bl.
Airship Industries: 79crb.
AKG London: 326bc, 550bl; Michael Teller 326c.
Alamy Images: Keith Dannemiller 440bl; Images Etc Ltd 320tr;Tom Tracy Photography 202br.
Album: 254t.
Bryan And Cherry Alexander Photography: 412bc.
Max Alexander: 468br.
Alvis Ltd: 559br.
Allsport: 100cl; Ben Bradford 122cl; Howard Boylan 694cl; Shaun Botterill 467bl.
Amtrak: 230br.
Ancient Art & Architecture Collection: 27cl, 102bl, 112tl, 347tl, 387tl, 387bc; Charles Tait 102tr; N.P.Stevens 221tr; Ronald Sheridan 102cr, 197tl, 310cla, 347bl, 357tl, 372crb, 438tr, 438bc, 505bl, 551ca, 657tl, 698tl, 698bl.
Animal Photography: Sally Anne Thompson 509bl.
Animals Unlimited: Patty Cutts 509cr.
Ardea London Ltd: 176tr; Francies Gohier 174bc.
The Art Archive: 112cl, 142bc, 181bl, 240cl, 240bl, 373cr, 414bl, 459tr, 459crb, 502bc; bib Arts Decoratifs Paris 673c; Chateau Malmaison 241cla.
Ashmolean Museum, Oxford: 27tr, 220bc.
Catherine Ashmore: 77c.
Associated Press Ap: 238cr, 375crb, 625cl, 633crb.
Australian Tourist Commission: 65bl.
National Archaelogical Museum: 106cl.
Neil Audley: 59bl.
Australian Overseas Information Services, London: 12bc, 70bl.
Axiom: Chris Bradley 472c; Chris Caldicott 472cl, 473tr, 549br.

B

Barnaby's Picture Library: 672bl.
N.S. Barrett: 269tr.
Beech Aircraft Corporation: 521clb, 521bc.
Belkin.com: 170fcrb.
Walter Bibikow: 558bl.
Bite Communications Ltd.: 352cl, 352c.
BMW: 230cb.
The Boeing Company: 22ca, 24c.
D. C. Brandt, Joyce and Partners: 42cb, 43clb.
Bridgeman Art Library, London / New York: *Catherine, Mulatte of the Bradeo* portrait by A. Durer, 1521 87br; *Greeks under Seige* by Eugene Delacroix 112br, 167tl, 227tr, 251cla; *King James I of England* by Paul Van Somer 312cla, 323clb, 400br, 407tl, 409tl, 409cl; *William Morris*, photographic portrait by Hollyer, 1884 445tl, 501bc; *Henry Wrothesley 3rd Earl Southampton* 593cl; *Sir Francis Bacon* bust by Roubillac 593cr, 604tr, 655br, 745tr; Archivo de la Catedral *Oviedo Alfonso III* c838-910 533tl; Ashmolean Museum Oxford Chinese Stirrup 6th-7th century bronze 327tr; *Belvoir Castle Henry VIII* by Hans Holbein younger 323tr; Berger Collection, Denver Art Museum *Oliver Cromwell* c1649 181tr; Bibliotheque Nationale, Paris 500c; Bonhams *Samuel Pepys* portait by John Riley 256tr; Bristol City Museum Art Gallery *Bristol Harbour* 1785, by Nicholas Pocock 604tl; British Library 31bc, St. Cuthbert from Bede 12th century 32clb, Queen Mary Psalter, bailiff berating peasants 508bc; British Museum 28cb, Benin sword 87bc; British Museum London, *Nineveh Epic of Gilgaresh* (clay tablet 7th Century BC) 657tl; British Museum, London 64cb, 297tl, 421cl, 500tl; Cairo Museum/Giraudon 41clb; Chateau de Versailles 366c; Chester Beatty Library & Gallery of Art 370bc; Christies, London 18bl, 535tr, 573bl, 721bl; City of Bristol Museum Art Gallery 372tl; Dept. of the Environment 754cra; Eton College, Windsor 421cr; Fabbir 114cb; Fine Art Society *Seige at Droghedon* 1641 181bc; Forbes Magazine Collection 458crb; Galleria Degli Uffizi 699tl; Galleria dell Accademia Firenze 551bl; Hertford Cathedral 415tl; Hever Castle 323crb; Lambeth Palace Library collection, burning of Thomas Cranmer from the *Foxe's Book of Martyrs* 1563 (woodcut), 685bl; Lauros Girandon Musée de la Ville de Paris, Carvaralet 404tr; *Leeds Museum and Gallery Kirkstall Abbey* by George Alexander 323bl; Liberty and Co. London 1972 Bauhaus fabric by Collier and Campbell for Liberty 195br; Louvre, Paris 280tc, 310bc, 547bc; Mallett & Sons Antiquities, London 285cl; Mozart Museum, Salzburg, Austria, *Mozart and his sister Maria-Anna*, ivory by Eusebius Johann Alphen 73c; Musée Conde, Chantilly 279bc; Musée d'Orsay, Paris (© DACS) 501cr; Musée des Beaux Arts, Tourcoing, Giraudon 207br; National Army Museum, London 342tc; National Maritime Museum, Greenwich 463tr; National Portrait Gallery 227tl; New Zealand High Commission, London 468cl; Oriental Museum, Durham University 522tl; *Henry VIII,* portait, Philip Mould 323tl; Phillips Fine Art Auctioneers 685tl; Prado, Madrid 459tl, 637tr, 641cl; Private Collection, Chariot, Qin Dynasty 148tr, *The Charge of the Light Brigade* 397tr, Sherlock Holmes 397crb, 400br, 705cr; Queenland Art Gallery, Brisbane 12tl; Rafael Valls Gallery, London 181cl; Richard Philip 31br; Roy Miles Gallery *Lord Byron* by Sir William Allan 112bc; Roy Miles Gallery, London 365bc; Royal Albert Memorial Museum *Olandah Equiano* portrait 1780's 604bc; Sante Maria delle Grazie, Milano 372bl; *Self Portrait with Gloves*, 1498 (panel) by Albrecht Durer, Prado, Madrid, Spain 295tr; *Snow White and the Seven Dwarves*, c.1912 (block print), English School. Stapleton Collection, UK. 295b; Staaliche Museen zu Berlin 134bc; T.U.C. London 346cb; Tate Gallery, London 75bc; Victoria & Albert Museum, London 341bl; Wallace Collection, London, *Oliver Cromwell* (portrait) 181tl; Wilberforce House Museum, Hull *The Kneeling Slave* 18th century, England (painting) 604cl; William Morris Gallery, Walthamstow 377br.
Paul Brierly: 610bl.
British Film Institute: Stills, Posters and Designs 254tr.
British Library, London: 32tl, 93cra, 93crb, 95tl, 106bl, 424bl, 424bc, 439bl, 469clb; Stuart 655tr.
British Museum, London: 74cl, 106br, 292tr, 419bc; British Museum 32bc, 292tr; Museum of Mankind 419tl.
British Airways Archive Museum Collection: 320cra, 680tr.
British Steel: 359cl, 359crb.
Britstock-ifa: 312bc.
British Tourist Authority: 692bl.

C

Camera Press: 90br, 105cb.
Casio: 668tr.
Coca-Cola Company: 13tr, 13cr.
Bruce Coleman Ltd: 97crb, 138cr, 144cr, 146tl, 176bl, 176br, 182cl, 207cl, 209bl, 210tl, 226clb, 277cl, 284bc, 328tr, 359clb, 378cl, 454cr, 465cl, 478cra, 498bc, 498bcr, 520crb, 582c, 588tl, 589tc, 589crb, 589bl, 590cra, 598bl, 647br, 669bc, 670cl, 682br, 702bl, 706bc, 723cl; Jack Dermid 592tl; A.J. Deane 337br; Alain Compost 267tl, 492tr, 539bl, 669crb; Bernol Thies 592cla; Bob and Clara Calhoun 83clb; Brian and Cherry Alexander 577tr; Brian Coates 92bl, 177bl, 498bcl; C. B. Frith 493bc; C.B. & D.W. Frith 107c; C.B. Frith 201tl, 201tl, 329tr; Charles Henneghein 156bc, 382tr, 636bl; Charlie Ott 541cl; Chris Hollerbeck 287bl, 702tl; Colin Moyneux 671tc; David C. Houston 339bl; David Davies 557bc; David Hughes 591tl; Dieter & Mary Plage 734crb, 454cl; Douglas Pike 15cl; Dr. Echart Pott 391bc, 528bl; Dr. Frieder Sanct 431c; E. Breeze-Jones 496tl; Eric Crichton 265cb; Erwin and Peggy Bauer 255bl; Fitz Prenzel 63bl; Frans Lanting 462crb; Fransisco Erize 590bc; Fritz Penzel 234clb, 491tr; G. D. Plage 328cl, 393cl, 208tl, 329c; G. Zienter 115crb; Gene A. Ahrens 701tl; Gerald Cubitt 50bc, 173cr, 248clb, 300tl, 325bc, 343c, 411bl, 504tl; H. Rivarola 85cl, 86cl; Hans Reinhardt 130tr, 237bl; 411cb; Hans Richard 224tr; Herbert Kranawetter 279cl; Inigo Everson 525tc, 525cr; Jane Burton 36bc, 217bc, 307cl, 428bc, 452crb, 556tl; Jaroslav Poncar 719cla; Jeff Foott 36c, 590cb; Jeff Simon 382clb; Jen and Des Bartlett 392tr; Joe Van Wormer 525bl; John Markhom 93clb; John Shaw 211c, 214cl, 435clb, 545br; John Topham 277tr; John Wallis 493bl; Jonathan T. Wright 370cl; Jonathan Wright 484tl, 597tr; Joseph Van Werner 493br; Keith Gunner 447cl; Kim Taylor 135bl, 225bc, 243cl, 452cra, 608cl, 736tl; L.C. Marigo 218br, 249ca, 331br, 534bc; Lee Lyon 76cr; Leonard Lee Rue III 479clb, 664br; Liz Marigo 285cb; M. Timothy O' Keefe 555tr; Marquez 416tl; Michael Fogden 192tr, 512br; Michael Freeman 151br, 325clb, 456bc; Michael Klinec 157tr, 160bl; Michel Viard 452tl; N.A.S.A. 210cr, 216tl, 444bl; Neville Fox-Davies 446clb; Norbert Rosig 237tr; Norbert Schwertz 714crb; Norman Myers 14br, 443bl, 528tr; Norman Owen Tomalin 35tr, 60tl, 442crb, 557cra, 700cra; Norman Plyers 393tr; Norman R. Lightfort 321c; R. Campbell 274crb; R.I.M. Campbell 41ca, 41cl; Robert Perron 512cr; Rod Williams 111bc, 443cl; Ron Cartnell 392br; Stephen J. Krasemann 84tr, 479tl; Udo Hirsch 336cl; Vatican Museums and Galleries, Rome 500clb; Walter Lankinen 382cl, 324cb, 324bl, 63bc; Werner Stoy 210c, 714clb.
Collections: Bill Wells 483bc; Brian Keen 694cr; Brian Shuel 355cr, 356bl, 386tc; Gena Davies 715cla; Geoff Howard 386crb; John Callan 527br; John Miller 386bl; Nigel Hawkins 232bl; Richard Davies 219c; Sandra Lousada 694br; Select 480bc; Yuri Lewinski 32cr.
Collection Viollet: 373tl.
Colorific!: Eric Sampers 451bl; Joe McNally/Wheeler Pics 300cra; Roger de la Harpe 630tr.
Columbia Pictures: 185bl.
Thomas Cook Archive: 673bl.
Corbis UK Ltd.: Archivo Iconografico S.A. 689bl; Dean Conger 140b, 570b, 689cl; Earl and Nasima Kowall 141br; John Noble 44b; Lawrence Manning 531crb; Michael St Maur Sheil 402bc; Nik Wheeler 638br; Stephanie Maze 578tc; Frederic Larson/San Francisco Chronicle 212clb; Walt Disney Pictures/Pixar Animation/Bureau L.A.Collections 127br; Ariel Skelley 352crb; Tom Wagner 349tl.
H.M. Customs & Excise: 25bl.

D

James Davis Travel Photography: 61cr, 401cl, 531b, 687bl, 688br.
Duncan Brown: 568tr, 568c, 568br.
Douglas Dickens: 624cr.
Dickens House Museum: 197tr, 197bl.
C.M. Dixon: 341tl.
DK Images: NASA 635bl.
Dominic Photography: Zoe Dominic 593bl.
Zoe Dominic: 491c, 491br.
Courtesy of **Dyson:** 195bc.

E

Earth Satellite Corporation: 415crb.
Empics Ltd: 270cr, 490tr; 305198 270cr; Andy Heading 720cl, 720bl; Tony Marshall 270tl.
The English Heritage Photo Library: Down House 186bl; Jonathan Bailey, Down House 186tl.
T. Malcolm English: 322bc.
Environmental Images: 247bc; Graham Burns 583c; Steve Morgan 303ca; Toby Adamson 290bl.
European Space Agency: 59cra, 531cra.
European Parliament Photolibrary: 239cl, 239bl.
Mary Evans Picture Library: 19tl, 19tr, 23br, 25crb, 40tr, 41bc, 64tr, 64bl, 70tl, 70cl, 77cr, 79tl, 79cl, 82tl, 88tr, 101cr, 113clb, 121crb, 124cl, 127cr, 134tl, 148bl, 149clb, 150c, 153tr, 157tl, 157cl, 171cr, 171bl, 171br, 183cr, 183bl, 183bl, 185tl, 186bc, 190tr, 190cl, 202tr, 206tr, 207cl, 211bv, 218bl, 219tl, 219tc, 224bl, 231cb, 233tr, 233cb, 233bl, 242tl, 244ce, 245cla, 247tr, 251clb, 252tl, 256tl, 260tr, 268tl, 279br, 280cla, 281tl, 290tc, 291bl, 297br, 298tl, 298tc, 298ca, 301tl, 301br, 302tl, 311clb, 312tr, 312cra, 313tl, 315bl, 330tl, 331tl, 346tl, 346clb, 346bc, 357cb, 366tl, 366tc, 371cl, 372bc, 373bc, 386tl, 391cl, 400tl, 404tc, 404cl, 418bl, 421bl, 421br, 422cb, 422bc, 430clb, 439crb, 439bc, 457clb, 457bl, 458bl, 461tr, 464cra, 470bl, 488tl,

490c, 492bl, 494bc, 495clb, 503tr, 506bl, 508clb, 512tr, 512clb, 520cr, 520cr, 526tl, 533bl, 538bc, 543tr, 543bc, 545tr, 546tr, 550br, 572bl, 573c, 573bc, 574tr, 574cb, 580tl, 580tr, 581cl, 581bl, 582cl, 585ca, 585bc, 586tl, 586ca, 598c, 598bc, 600cra, 603clb, 604cr, 604bl, 610tc, 619cl, 641crb, 641t, 644tr, 652tl, 665bc, 666tl, 669tl, 670tr, 672tl, 674tl, 675tr, 676bl, 678cr, 678cr, 682cr, 682bc, 690tr, 698cra, 698br, 699tr, 706tl, 708tl, 709ca, 709crb, 709bl, 710tl, 710cl, 710cl, 711cr, 715br, 722tr, 735c, 738tl, 738tc, 738cla, 739ca, 742tl, 743tc, 743ca, 743cl, 743cb, 744tr; 522cra; Bruce Castle Museum 495bl; Explorer 168cla, 168cl, 281cl; Illustrazione 241tr; ILN 650cl; Spencer 508tr.
Eye Ubiquitous: David Cumming 401tl; David Foreman 688bl; Helen A. Lisher 694tl; Mike Southern 61tl; P. Maurice 688tc; Tim Durham 531cb.

F

Family Life Picture Library: Angela Hampton 348c, 352br.
FLPA – Images of Nature: 589cl, 654clb; Dick Jones 135bc; Roger Wilmshurst 45ctr; W.S. Clark 476tl.
Michael & Patricia Fogden: 266cr.
Werner Forman Archive: 56tr, 457bc, 565tr, 713bl; British Museum 56clb; Metropolitan Museum of Art, New York 285tr; Mr & Mrs C.D. Wertheim 371cr.
Ford Motor Company Ltd: 21cl, 247cl.
Format Photographers: Jacky Chapman 124tr, 583cra; Karen Robinson 228cl; Mo Wilson 303tl; Sasha Lefreund 303cl.
Fortean Picture Library: Allen Kennedy 240tl.
French Railways: 677cl.
John Frost Historical Newspapers: 740tl.

G

General Motors Corporation: 658bl.
Geoscience Features: 133bc, 212bl, 291tr, 509crb.
German National Tourist Office: 294b.
Getty Images: 561bl; AFP 433bc; 2005 Dave M. Benett 561c; Iconica 513br; Photographer's Choice 475br; Stone 119cr, 512cr; Taxi 517br.
Photographie Giraudon: 424ca, 459bc; Lauros 458cl.
Google: 352bl.
Greenpeace Inc: 172tl.

H

Sonia Halliday Photographs: 113bc, 240cr, 277b, 378cra, 494tl; James Wellard 251tc; R.H.C. Birch 310tr.
Hampshire County Constabulary: 526cra.
David Hamilton: 692cl.
Robert Harding Picture Library: 14tl, 15br, 17tr, 37bc, 46cr, 46bc, 59cr, 120tc, 139tc, 145tl, 145cr, 148cb, 148cb, 148bc, 148bc, 162cl, 276cl, 276b, 354bl, 354br, 363bl, 370tl, 432cr, 467br, 467t, 472br, 473br, 474tr, 588tr, 588clb, 611cr, 616tr, 620tr, 622cl, 728cl, 729cl; Adam Woolfit 627bc, 628tr; C. Bowman 476cr; David Hughes 239bc; F.J. Jackson 44cl; Frans Lanting 145c; Fraser Hall 611bc; G. P. Corrigan 43tl; G. Renner 38tc; G.Boutin 472bl; G.M. Wilkins 612tc; G.R. Richardson 293bl; Gavin Hellier 73br, 611ct; Goldstrand 627cr; J.K.Thorne 466bl; James Strachan 140tr; Jeff Greenberg 80cl; Jeremy Lightfoot 309c; J.H.C. Wilson 339cl; Julia Thorne 532bl; Michael Jenner 368br, 434b; Mitsuaki Iwago 38tr; Paul van Riel 364br; Phil Robinson 626br; R. Ashworth 354tl; R. Cundy 476ct; Rob Cousins 120cr; Robert Cundy 611clb; Robert Francis 67cl; Robert Frerck/Odyssey 476cl; Roy Rainford 474bl; T. van Goubergen 402tc; T. Waltham 477tr; Thierry Borridon 275bl; Victor Engelbert 729cr; Weisbecker 338cr.
Henson Association Inc.: 539cr, 539cb.
Frames taken from "Spider in the Bath". Reproduced by permission from **Ralph Entertainment © and Silveryjex Partnership:** 127t.
Hewlett Packard: 170br.
Kaii Higashiyama: 501tr.
The Historical Society of Pennyslvania: 717bl.
David Hoffman: 527crb.
© Michael Holford: 75tl, 75clb, 142c, 152crb, 341br, 509cb, 511cr, 516br; British Library 164cr; British Museum 453tr.
Holt Studios International: Duncan Smith 250bl; Richard Anthony 662cr.
Houses & Interiors: Nick Huggins 196clb.
Hulton Getty: 27tl, 55tr, 70cb, 89tl, 94tr, 103cl, 103cr, 103cb, 103bl, 104tl, 104tr, 112tr, 153tl, 153bl, 161tl, 161bl, 166bc, 191bc, 197crb, 222tl, 222tr, 228bc, 231tr, 239 tl, 251bc, 292tl, 326tr, 342cl, 342c, 357clb, 366cl, 371cb, 391tl, 506cl, 506CB, 506crb, 523tl, 544tr, 567tl, 586crb, 586bl, 613cb, 625clb, 633cl, 655bc, 659tl, 735bc, 737clb, 739bl, 740c, 740clb, 740cb, 742bl; A.C. Michael 409bl; Bettmann Archive 42cl, 161cr, 515bc; Bettmann/UPI 101crb; Douglas Miller 228cr; Ernst Haas 222c; Keystone 124br; Keystone, Max Schneider, Zurich 613clb; MPI Archives 652tr; Val Doone 527tl.
Jacqui Hurst: Robert Aberman 433br.
Hutchison Library: 46cl, 54tl, 54br, 55br, 98cl, 99tr, 99ctl, 136cr, 149bc, 162bl, 166bl, 339c, 343cl, 344tr, 361br, 505tr, 583tl, 607c, 614cl, 615tr, 616tl, 727cl, 729bl; Anna Tully 202bl; B. Regent 511bc, 729tl; Bernard Green 607tl; Bernard Regent 136bl, 136bc; Carlos Freste 337bc; Christina Dodwell 343bl; Christine Pemberton 55tl; Crispin Hughes 213bl, 628tc, 727cr, 729ctr; Eric Lawrie 615tl; F. Greene 55c; Felix Greene 13br, 414cr; H.R. Dorig 421tl, 618crb; Jeremy Horner 54crb, 145cl; John Downman 477br; John G. Egan 629cr; Juliet Highey 338tl; Kerstin Rodseps 735tl; Leslie Woodhead 728tl; M. Friend 626cl; M. Jeliffe 137tr; Mary Jeliffe 472tr; Maurice Harvey 570clb; Melanie Friend 629b; N. Durrell McKenna 147tr; Nick Hadfield 583bl; Nick Haslam 80tr, 80bl, 570cr, 627tr; Nigel Sitwell 99cr; P. Moszynski 206cr; P.E. Parker 708br; Philip Wolmuth 228crb; R. Ian Lloyd 379bc; Richard Howe 98br; Robert Aberman 687br; Robert Francis 54cra; Sarah Erinngton 17c, 137bc, 144br, 201bc, 201bc, 213tl, 249bl, 250tl, 631br, 728br; Timothy Beddow 213c; Titus Moser 141tr; Trevor Page 132bl, 140cl; V. Ivleva 140cr; Vanessa S. Boeye 54bl.

I

I.A.L. Security Products: 744cr.
I.C.I.: 669cb.
Illustrated London News Picture Library: 342bl, 679br.
Image Bank: 51tr, 53br, 67tl, 67br, 74crb, 78cr, 118c, 118bc, 119c, 122tr, 122bl, 122br, 139br, 146cr, 146bl, 160cl, 171tr, 184bl, 254bc, 271tl, 278bl, 287bc, 300bc, 330bc, 361tl, 361bl, 368bl, 433cl, 441bc, 441bc, 450tl, 499cr, 575bc, 614cl, 614b, 617cl, 617br, 620bc, 640tl, 644tl, 654bl, 656tl, 664tl, 676tl, 678tr, 679bc, 720cl, 720br; Alan Beeker 679ca; Alex Hamilton 407bc; Andrea Pistolesi 563tl; Anne der Vaeren 152tl; Anthony A. Broccaccio 257cl; Ben Rose 512c; Bernard van Berg 278tr; Brett Frooner 260bc; Brian McNeely 690cla; Colin Molyneux 319tl; 269bl; David Hiser 382ca; David Martin 407tr; David W. Hamilton 129tc, 702tr; Don Klumpp 432b, 434tr; Dr. J. Gebhardt 261cb; Eric L. Wheeler 115cb; Erik Leigh 464crb; Francis Hildago 336bc; Francisco Ontanon 637bl; Frank Roiter 75crb; Fulvio Roiter 308bc; G. A. Wilton 199tr; G. Gundberg 578br; G. Rontmeester 695bc; Gary Gladstone 676tl; Georgina Bowater 294t; Gianalberto Cigolini 151tl; Giulliano Colliva 118bl; Guido Alberto Rossi 720cl, 636bc, 119cr, 362cl, 637br; Harold. Sand 426cr, 704tr; Hank Delespinesse 644cl; Isy-Schwart 252cl; J. Bronsseau 108crb; J. Bryson 116bl; Jean Pierre Pienchat 545bl; Joe Azzara 733tr; John P. Keely 720br; Joseph B. Brignolo 433tr, 530crb, 683bl; Kay Charmost 218cl; Kaz Mori 210cl; Kodansha Images 596tr; Lou Jones 609bc; Luis Castaneda 238bl; M. Melford 425bc; Marc Solomon 271br; Marvin E. Newman 577cl; Michael Melford 543cla; Michael Salas 69tr; Milan Skarya 25crb; P. & G. Bower 129tr; Paul Kleuenz 620cr; Peter Thomann 160cl; Robert Holland 497crb; Robert Phillips 530bl; Ronald R. Johnson 636cr, 367tl; Sah Zarember 674cl; Stan Drexter 152bl; Steve Dunwell 440bl; Steve Niedorf 202br, 420ca; Stockphotos 410cr; Thomas R. Rampy 85crb; Toyotumi Mori 368c; Trevor Wood 694tr; Ulli Seer 510tl.
Impact Photos: Caroline Penn 385bc.
Imperial War Museum: 48tl, 104cla, 735clb, 738c.
Innes Photo Library: Ivor Innes 101cl, 101clb; John Blackburn 101bl.
Intercity: 230crb.

J

Lou Janitz: 608tl.
JET Joint Undertaking: 482tl.

K

Katz Pictures: Resnick 652c.
Royal Borough of Kensington and Chelsea Public Library: 219cl.
Barnabas Kindersley: 368tl, 368clb, 368crt; 144bl.
David King Collection: 166tr.
Kobal Collection: 65br, 197c, 253cra, 254bl, 335cb, 339tl, 454bc, 559tr, 743bl.
Courtesy of **Kodak:** 513tr.

L

Lada: 571bl.
Leitz: 293br.
Link Picture Library: 413cb; Greg English 413br; Orde Eliason 413cl, 413bl; Philip Schelder 613bc.
London Features International: 456crb.
Lotus Cars Ltd: 300cb.
Lupe Cunha: 316cl, 330clb, 420ce. **Ann Lyons:** 646tr.

M

Magnum: 633bc.
Mander & Mitchenson: 154cl, 154cr, 154cb.
Mansell/Time Inc: 167br.
Mansell Collection: 40bc, 70cr, 114cl, 580bl, 737tl.
Marconi Electronic Devises: Bruce Stone 385cr.
Marshall Cavendish: Osel Group 691cr.
McDonald's Restaurants Ltd: 600c.
Mercedes Benz: 125clb.
The Metropolitan Museum of Art: Rogers Fund 1904 373clb.
Michelin: 733clb.
William Morris Gallery: 445tr, 445bl, 445bc.
Museum Of London: 40br, 181crb, 256bc.

N

N.A.S.A.: 57cl, 63cr, 165c, 444cb, 497bl, 531c, 559bl, 645cr, 680cl, 680br, 724tl, 725bl, 707clb; Finlay Holiday Films 300cr; N.A.S.A 94c.
The National Archives of Scotland: 698cb.
National Gallery, London: 501tl, 502tl, 502bl, 503tl, 503cl, 551tl.
National Trust Photographic Library: Andrew Butler 409bc; Ian Shaw 460bc; Jennie Woodstock 460c; Martin Trelawny 715c.
National Maritime Museum, London: 175tl, 240bc, 463tl, 494bl; James Stevenson 145br, 292clb.
National Portrait Gallery, London: 112cr, 502cl, 709tl; Brnte, Patrick Branwell, 1817-1848 397ca.
The Natural History Museum, London: 39tl, 274cr.
Network Photographers Ltd.: 138br, 526crb; Gideon Mendel 413tl, 413cr; Goldwater 48bc; Jenny Matthews 219bl; Louise Gubb 413tc; Peter Jordan 527c.
Peter Newark's Pictures: 29cl, 29cr, 153cr, 159c, 191c, 191br, 391tr, 461crb, 461bc, 462tl, 462cl, 495br, 516bc, 603bc, 618br, 646bc, 651tr.
N.H.P.A.: 47cl, 68tr, 99bc, 615br, 616br; Anthony Bannister 135tl; Bill Wood 555tc; Brian and Cherry Alexander 44tr, 44c, 474cl; Daryl Balfour 215tr; J. H. Carmichael 486cra; Jerry Sauvanet 273tl; John Shaw 476b; Manfred Danegger 448tr; Martin Harvey 621br; Phillipa Scot 399cla; Roger Tidney 194tl; Stephen Dalton 82c; Stephen Krasemann 214t; Willima S. Pakon 416c.
New Millennium Experience Company: 437tc, 437c, 437bc.
Nobel Foundation: 581crb.
Nokia: 170cb, 665br.
Novosti (London): 569br, 572tl, 574bl, 632tr, 632crb, 632bc; Vladimir Vyatkin 570bl.

O

Olympic Co-ordination Authority: 490tr.
Open University: 219bc.
Ordnance Survey © Crown Copyright: 415c.
Christine Osborne: 12cl, 50bl, 420tl, 588cr, 683tl.
OSF/photolibrary.com: 72crb.
Oxford Scientific Films: 605bc, 606bc, 615bl; Animals Animals, M. Austerman 556bl, Fran Allen 328cr; Fran Allen 329cr; B.G. Murray/JR Garth Scenes 545c; David Fox 208cl; Edward Panker 20tr; Fritz

Penzel 72bc; G.I. Bernard 262bc, 544crb; J.A.L. Cooke 39bc, 305cr, 351tl; JAL Cooke 605clb; John Paling 36clb; Kathie Atkinson 71tr, 411tl; Kim Westerskov 188tc; Lawrence Gould 259cl; Michael Fogden 72cl; Pam & Willy Kemp 217tl; Raymond Blythe 86tl; Ronald Toms 734bl; Stan Osolinksi 180c; Sue Trainer 289bc.
Courtesy of **Otis' Elevators:** 234bc.

P

Palace of Versailles: 400cra. **Panasonic:** 116cl.
Panos Pictures: 46bl, 727br; Alain le Garsmeur 759cr; Alfredo Cadeno 99bl; B. Klass 340b; Caroline Penn 617bl, 761br; Chris Stowers 627c; Dermot Tatlow 549bc; Dominic Harcourt-Webster 213cr; Fred Hoogervorst 758cl; Giacomo Pirozzi 612 ctr; 15tr, 136tr, 136cl; Gregory Wrona 132tl; Heidi Bradner 627bl; Howard Davies 629tl; Jean-Leo Dugast 621tc; Jeremy Hartley 727br; John Miles 99cl; Liba Taylor 214bl; Maya Kardum 158cl; N. Durrell Mc Kenna 630c; Neil Cooper 631tr; Pietro Cenini 213br; Trgve Bolstad 630cl.
PA News Photo Library: 301bl.
Patankar, Aditya: 457ct.
Philips Scientific: 430crb, 430bc.
Photofusion: Sam Tanner 470br.
Pickthall Picture Library: Barry Pickthall 575tl.
Pictor International: 301cr, 309cl, 309cr, 362cr, 363tr, 401tr, 401b, 475br, 531tr, 531cr, 578bl, 626tr, 626c, 627tl, 638tl, 692tr.
Picture Mate: 116cr.
Planet Earth Pictures: 45bl, 594bl, 612br, 691tr, 691bl, 745bl; Adam Jones 474cr, 475cl; Anup Shah 214br, 621tl; Brian and Cherry Alexander 44cr; Christin Petron 41cr; David Phillips 446bc; Doug Perrine 475tl; Gary Bell 68c; John Downer 630bl; Jonathan Scott 214cr, 708bl; Joyce Photographics 37cr; Mary Clay 475cr; Paul Cooper 260crb; Peter David 187tr, 187bcl; Peter Lillie 630br; Tom Walker 338bl, 474br; Warren Williams 482ca; William Smithey 188c.
Richard Platt: 79bc, 224bc, 408crb, 415cl.
Popperfoto: 19cl, 19c, 55cb, 105bc, 149crb, 151bl, 153cl, 153br, 241tc, 241cl, 241cb, 280bl, 280bc, 298cl, 305bc, 375bl, 447tr, 484bl, 490br, 501clb, 533bc, 567bl, 567br, 586c, 619cb, 619bl, 643t, 700tl, 712cl, 712cr; Bilderberg 699br; David Crosling, Reuters 104crb; Dmitri Messinis 241cb; Dylan Martinez, Reuters 104cb; Michael Stephens, Reuters 312bl; Reuters 222bc, 302ca, 699cl.
Post Office Picture Library: 646cb.
Powerstock Photolibrary / Zefa: 105tl, 232ca, 247crb, 332tl, 374bl, 451cr, 520tr, 598cr, 676cr, 762bl; 451bc; D.H. Teuffen 40tl; Geoff Kalt 609tr; Hales 672bc; Ingo Seiff 125tl; R.G. Everts 148br; S. Palmer 744bl; K. Scholz 148cr; T.Schneider 142tl; Transglobe 404bc.
Press Association Picture Library: 699bc.
Public Record Office Picture Library: 471cb.

Q

© **QA Photos Ltd.:** Eurotunnel 686bl.
Quadrant Picture Library: Mark Wagner 232crb.

R

Redferns: Charlyn Zlotnik 560bl; David Redfern 561tl; Des Willie 560tl; Elliot Landy 561tr; Glenn A. Baker Archives 560cb; Kieran Doherty 561c; Michael Ochs 560crb; Mick Hutson 480cr, 561bl; Patrick Ford 561cr; S&G 560br; Simon Ritter 560tc; Steve Grillett 454tl.
Reuters: 658bl.
Rex Features: 51tl, 61br, 105bc, 159cl, 235tla, 235tlb, 296t, 316cl, 397tl, 414tl, 468bc, 473bl, 522bc; Chat 386cb; David Pratt 141bl; Fotex 578tl; J. Sutton-Hibbert 290c; James Fraser 303cr; Julian Makey 303bc; Richard Gardner 386cl; Sipa 124bc, 758bl; Steve Wood 638tr; Times 652cl; Wheeler 229tl; LXL 560tl.
Bridget Riley: 503crb.
Ann Ronan Picture Library: 165bc, 251c, 423tl.
Cliff Rosney: 702bc. **Rover Group:** 235cr.
The Royal Collection (© 1999 Her Majesty Queen Elizabeth II): 167tr, 387crb.
The Royal Mint (Crown copyright): 440tl.

S

Saatchi Gallery: 503bl.
Scala: 500br, 585crb; Museo Nazionale Athenai 106cb.
Science & Society Picture Library: 451cl; Science Museum 105c, 105bl.
Science Photo Library: 518br, 647bl, 666bl, 678bl; Alan Hart-Davies 319br; Alexander Isiaras 482clb, 662br; Alta Greenberg 701cr; Astrida Hans Frieder Michler 662c; Chris Bjornberg 201bl; Chris Butler 518br; CNRI 198bc, 201cl, 201cr; David Parker 542cl; David Parker 600 Group 559c; David Parker/Max Planck/ Institut for Aeronomie 165c; David Wintraub 477tl; Dr Fred Espenak 649tl, 418cl; Dr. Gerald Schatten 316br; Dr. Jeremy Burgess 431tl, 431bl; Dr. T. E. Thompson 202c; Earth Satellite Corp. 576ca; Earth Satellite Corporation 475cl; Eric Grave 430c; E.W. Space Agency 517bcl; Frank Espanak 59cra; Hubert Raguet 760cl; Ian Boddy 316cr; I.B.M. 430br; Jane Stevenson 552tl; Jim Stevenson 114tl; John Bavosi 198bl; John Mead 759bl; John Sanford 165bl, 444tl; Johns Hopkins University Applied Physics Laboratory 773cr; Julian Baum 773crb; Ken Briggs 229bl; Lawrence Migoale 201bl; M.I. Walker 431cl; Michael Dohrn 21cb, 286tr; N.A.S.A. 59cl, 384br, 517bl, 517bc, 518bc, 518 bl, 518bcl, 518bcr, 529tl, 571tr, 744bc; N.I.B.S.C. 318bl; N.R.A.O. 59v; Pasieka 201crb; Philippe Plailly 420cb; Philippe Reilly 384bl; Professor Harold Edgerton 512cra; Proffessor R. Gehz 59ca; R.E. Litchfield 431bc; Royal Greenwich Observatory 157bc; Simon Fraser 156tr, 523bl; Smithsonian Institute 59tc; St. Mary's Hospital Medical School 422c; Takeshi Takahara 678bl; Tim Malyon 384tr; Tom McHugh 331bl; U.S. Navy 722bc; US Geological Survey 517br; W. Crouch & R.Ellis/NASA 707cb; William Curtsinger 37tr; Yves Bauken 349cb.
National Museum of Scotland: Mayan bowl 419crb.
Scottish Highland Photolibrary: R. Weir 587cra.
Shakespeare Globe Trust: 593tr. **Shell UK:** 489bc.
Ronald Sheridan: 471t. **Silkeborg Museum:** 41tl.
SKR Photos: LFI 453bl. **Sky TV:** 668crb.
South American Pictures: 619cra; Tony Morrison 74bc.
Spectrum Colour Library: 184br; E. Hughes 693cl.
Frank Spooner Pictures: 15cr, 17bl, 121bl, 276tr, 367bc, 675bl; Bartholomew Liaison 190cr; Blanche 481bc; Chip Hines 190bc, 298bc; Eric Bouver 19bc; Eric Bouvet/Gamma 625cb; G. Nel Figaro 469cl; Gamma 145tr, 161bc, 357bc, 379tl, 433bl, 562cr; Gamma/V. Shone 212tr; Jacques Graf 514crb; John Chiason 49br; K. Kristen 481ca; Kahu Karita 371bl; L. Novovitch-Liaison 706bc; Manaud/Figaro 581cb; Nickelsberg/Gamma 313bl; Novosti/Gamma 633ca; Pierre Perin/Gamma 641bl.
Sporting Pictures (UK) Ltd: 88cr, 269cr, 277tl, 362bl, 490cl, 497tl, 588bc, 645cl.
Still Pictures: 529c; Edward Parker 529clb; Harmut Schwartzbach 247bl; Mark Edwards 529br.
The Stock Market: 374cb; Zefa 553br.
Tony Stone Images: 62tr, 96tr, 98bl, 100br, 237br, 343br, 349tr, 349cla, 349cl, 349bl, 403bl, 466bc, 587cl, 587crb, 621bl, 676cl; Bob Thompson 476tr; Demetrio Carrasco 548cra; Donald Nausbaum 100tc; Donovan Reese 105cr; Doug Armand 295tl; Gary Yeowell 687tl; Glen Allison 474c; Hugh Sitton 363bc, 687c; James Balog 660c; John Beatty 45tl, 61cl; John Callahan 344cr; John Lamb 275br; Jon Gray 676cl; Manfred Mehlig 73bl, 660bl; Martin Puddy 343tr; Michael Busselle 232clb; Nigel Hillier 687cr; Nigel Snowdon 67tr; Peter Cade 659tr; Ragnar Sigurdsson 61bc; Randy Wells 475tc; Robert Everts 626bl; Rohan 402bl; Seigfreid Layda 295c; Shaun Egan 363tl; Stephen Studd 660tr; Stuart Westmoreland 65cr; Tom Parker 693bl; Tom Walker 45tc.
Superstock Ltd.: 673cr.
Survival Anglia Photo Library: 173cl, 173c; Jeff Foott 173crb.
Don Sutton: 480cla, 480bl; DS17633 480br.
Syndication International: 651bl.

T

Tass News Agency: 299clb, 635cl.
© **Tate Gallery, London:** 445cr, 503ca.
Ron & Valerie Taylor: 488clb.
Telegraph Colour Library: 542cr, 584cl; Bavania/Bild Agentur 652crb; Jason Childs 65cl.
Thames & Hudson Ltd: *The Complete Architecture Works* 155bc.
Louise Thomas: 621cr.
Topham Picturepoint: 375cl, 481tl, 481cl, 643b, 667bl, 668bl, 697cb, 739tl; Image Works, Lee Snider 451tr.
Toy Brokers Ltd: 602tr.
Toyota (GB) PLC: 230bl.
Art Directors & TRIP: B. Vikander 688tr; G. Spenceley 629cl.

U

Unicef: 700bc.
United Nations: 700cl.
Reproduced by permission of United Feature Syndicate Inc.: 127cl.
University of Manchester: Barri Jones, Department of Archaeology 41tr.

V

V&A Picture Library: 148br, 149tl, 195crb.
La Vie Du Rail: 678.
View Pictures: Dennis Gilbert 326br.
Virginia Museum of Fine Arts: gift of Col. & Mrs Edgar W. Garbisch 705tr.

W

National Museum of Wales: 693cra.
The Wallace Collection: 501c.
John Walmsley Photo Library: 90tr, 527tc, 549ca, 715bc.
John Watney: 355c.
Reg Wilson: 77cl, 168, 491tr.
Winchester City Council: 27crb.
Windsor Castle Royal Library (by permission HM The Queen): 205br.
Harland and Wolf: 693cr.
Alexander Wolf/Herge Verlag: 127bc.
Woods Hole Oceangraphic Instititution: 690bl.

X

Xinhua News agency: 634tl.

Y

Jerry Young: 263bl.

Z

Zefa Picture Library: 48cl, 53bl, 67bl, 109bl, 117cl, 123c, 133tl, 139cr, 146bc, 148br, 235bc, 280tl, 294cr, 294bl, 315bc, 356t, 360bc, 362tr, 363c, 427cr, 427bl, 466cl, 485cl, 548bc, 570tl, 622cr, 638cl, 640cra, 654c, 676cr, 693tl, 694bl, 708cb, 716cr, 717br, 718c, 719crb; Abril 557c; B. Croxford 433cr; B. Keppelmeyer 276cr; Colin Kaket 340tr; Damm 279tl, 433tl, 622bc; Dr. David Conker 93bl; Dr. R. Lorenz 505tl; Fritz 469bc; G. Hunter 119bl; Groebel 569cr; H. Grathwohl 427tr; Heilman 249tl, 250bc; Helbig 83tr; J. Zittenzieher 338br; K. Goebel 220tl, 295cr, 432cl; K. Keith 639tl; K. Scholz 15tl; K. Schotz 438crb; Kim Heebig 192crb; Klaus Hackenburg 686tl; Knight & Hunt Photo 192bc; Kohler 294cl; Leidmann 339tr; Messershmidt 155tr; O. Langrand 299bc; Orion Press 107tr; Praedel 578cr; R.G. Everts 299crb; Scholz 148cr; Starfoto 338cl; UWS 393cr; W. Benser 338c; W. Deuter 261cr; W. F. Davidson 150tl; W. Mole 453br; W.F. Davidson 714bc; Werner H. Muller 151cr.

Additional thanks to: Max Alexander; Peter Anderson; Tony Barton Collection; Geoff Brightling; Jane Burton; Peter Chadwick; Joe Cornish; Andy Crawford; Geoff Dann; Tom Dobbie, Philip Dowell; Niel Fletcher; Bob Gathany; Frank Greenaway; Steve Gorton; Alan Hill; Chas Howson; Colin Keates; Barnabas Kindersley; Dave King; Bob Langrish; Liz McAulay; Andrew McRobb; Ray Moller; Tracey Morgan; Stephen Oliver; Susannah Price; Rob Reichenfeld; Tim Ridley; Kim Sayer; Karl Shone; Steve Shott; Clive Streeter; Harry Taylor; Kim Taylor; Wallace Collection; Matthew Ward; Francesca Yorke, Jerry Young.

Every effort has been made to trace the copyright holders and we apologise in advance for any unintentional omissions. We would be pleased to insert the appropriate acknowledgments in any subsequent edition of the publication.

ILLUSTRATION CREDITS

Abbreviations: a = above, b = below, c = centre, l = left, r = right, t = top.

A

Graham Allen: 442
David Ashby: 24bl; 125cl, tl, tr; 256c; 313t; 346; 538; 458cl; 603c; 683b; 705; 706r; 633tl; 603cr; 749
Graham Austen/Garden Studios: 189tl, bl

B

Stephen Biesty: 22; 23; 125cr; 128; 129; 322t; 656c; 661; 666; 671c; 671tl; 716; 749
Rick Blakely/Studio Art and Illustration: 223cl; 320; 384; 406c; 430; 444; 463c; 542t; 562c; 576tl; 596c; 597t, c; 610; 634; 635b, l; 676; 744; 772bl; 773r
Peter Bull Art Studio: 108tl, cr, bl; 116tr; 231bc; 299c; 292tr; 347c, bc; 483cl, cr; 544bl; 691br; 725
Christopher Butzer: 385c; 387c

C

Julia Cobbold: 133; 376b; 447c; 528; 557; 692br; 693tr
Stephen Conlin: 25c; 42t; 43c; 152; 155; 196bc; 280c; 431cr; 439; 551c; 701b
John Crawford-Fraser: 185cr; 457cr; 491; 539cr

D

William Donahue: 113c; 365; 438; 565c, bl; 624t; 677; 713t; 736
Richard Draper: 59
Keith Duran/Linden Artists: 507bl

E

Angelika Elsebach: 33t, c; 34c; 39; 82; 86; 204cr; 243; 248; 249; 272 except tl; 273; 283cl, br; 284; 304bl; 351; 393tl, c, b; 412; 416; 589; 605; 608; 642; 681tl; 723; 731c
Angelika Elsebach/David Moore: 681tr, bl
Gill Elsebury: 193; 194; 282; 305; 465; 606

G

L.R. Galante: 26cl; 56cr; 179cr; 245bc; 315cl; 332c, cr; 333c; 335c; 400cr; 502c; 508c
Tony Gibbons: 596b; 597b

H

Nick Hall: 210; 211c; 535; 536; 663
Nicholas Hewetson: 12cr; 14c; 15bl; 21t; 24cr; 25bc; 40c, bc; 48r; 50r; 51; 57t, b; 74t; 75cl; 107; 118tr, bl, cr; 122cr; 138tr; 144cl, tr; 119tl; 159b; 166cl; 168; 175c, br; 190bl; 200cr; 202cl; 218; 220; 221b, tl; 353 tl, bl; 252; 254tl; 257; 275c; 277c; 286t; 294; 297c; 301tr; 308bl; 310c; 311cl; 315tl, cl; 316; 319b; 325; 336; 337c; 355br; 367b; 370; 371; 372tr; 373; 374; 376tl, cl; 389bl; 394; 400br; 408bl; 414tr; 422tl; 428cr; 429b; 441; 454tr; 455; 463b; 468tl, cr; 469tl; 471cl, cr; 490; 494cl, br; 495; 498; 523c, cr; 526; 534; 537tr, b; 541br; 550c; 555cl; 559cl; 564b; 567cr; 569; 573c; 575cr; 577tl, br; 580; 722tl, tr; 609bc; 614cl; 615; 618; 619; 620cl; 624b; 625r; 636cl; 641tl; 643cl; 645; 651c; 697tl; 702; 707cr, bl; 708cl; 710; 713bl; 724; 726bl, br; 735tr
Trevor Hill: 313b
Adam Hook/ Linden Artists: 31cl; 32c; 56cr; 186c; 461c; 506cr; 613cl; 655cl

J

Kevin Jones Associates: 482

K

Aziz Khan: 26cr; 27cr; 31tr, cr, bl; 55l; 87tr, bl; 104c, bl; 124bl; 164tr; 171cr; 183cl; 186bl; 209c; 219tr; 228bl; 232tr; 239cr; 239br; 241br; 245cr; 290br; 303bl; 326bl; 335tr, bl; 347tr; 397b; 403cr; 404br; 419tr; 458cr; 460br; 480tr; 515tl; 533br; 549bc; 561cl; 587tr; 603c; 613tr; 650cr; 655tl, bl; 657tr; 685tr; 699bl; 715tr
Steven Kirk: 200tl; 554; 555tl, b

L

Jason Lewis: 88; 148; 160; 231tl; 285; 322r; 331; 461tc
Richard Lewis: 24cl; 165; 211t; 229; 271; 319c; 514; 543; 559bl; 576tr; 609tc, bl; 654t; 658; 675; 751cl
Ruth Lindsay: 71; 72; 85; 110; 115; 131; 203cr; 265tl; 266; 306; 307; 324; 329; 350; 398br; 399; 428l; 448 except cl; 510; 732bl; 748
Chen Ling: 748; 749; 750; 751
Mick Loates/Linden Artists: 35; 36b; 76b; 83; 84r; 172; 173; 182t; 187; 188; 207bl, br; 216; 242; 380; 381; 392; 488; 517; 518; 590t; 771

M

Kathleen McDougall: 506tl
Janos Marffy: 463cr
Coral Mula: 478; 653tl, bl

P

Brian Poole: 84b
Warren Poppiti: 522c

Q

Sebastian Quigley/Linden Artists: 180; 184t, bl; 300bl; 425; 447b; 521cr; 686c; 768b

R

Eric Robson/Garden Studios: 20c, bl; 556; 591; 592
Jackie Rose: 377l, b; 378r, b
Clifford Rosney: 750cl
Simon Roulstone: 89c, bl, bc; 94tl, cl;125c; 157c, cr; 169c; 222cl; 224tl, cr, c; 230tl; 231cl; 234cl, cr, tr; 291c; 319cr; 352tr; 359c; 464bl; 538c; 543c; 558c; 663

S

Sergio: 97; 209; 246; 318; 332cl, bl; 405; 450; 552; 553
Rodney Shackell: 26c; 42b; 43b; 56br; 90cl; 143; 225; 245c (insets); 353tr; 260cl; 261r; 286bl; 297bl; 304c; 310b; 337bl; 311bc; 406tc; 407br; 500; 501; 504b; 505tl; 511tr; 549; 585; 586tc; 603tl; 649tr; 692bl; 693ct, cb, cr; 753tc
Eric Shields: 377c
Rob Shone: 21bl, cr; 29; 37bl; 150; 151; 174br; 192c; 267cr; 279tr; 280r; 288br; 382; 389r, cl; 390; 457r; 497; 537tl, cr; 545; 563c; 564cr; 566t, cl; 654br; 669; 691; 712; 721; 722
Francesco Spadoni: 183tl, bc, br; 441cl; 515tc, cr, bl
Francesco Spadoni/Lorenzo Cecchi: 164cl, tr, bl, br
Clive Spong/Linden Artists: 287; 598tl; 690
Mark Stacey: 27bl; 102cl; 103tr, br; 114cr; 142cr; 171cl; 382cl; 391cr; 419c; 593c; 685c

T

Eric Thomas: 18cr; 19br; 30; 69; 70bl; 81c; 91bl, br; 93; 121tr, cl, bc; 125tc; 134; 233cl; 196t; 227bl; 235cl; 237; 281; 293c; 321tl, cr; 341; 342tr; 355tr, cl; 357c; 358; 360; 366b; 403c; 423r; 424; 452; 455; 459tr, cl; 403cl; 511c; 516; 547tl, cl; 572; 574; 625t; 636tr; 640c; 653c; 670bl; 678tl, cl; 696cr; 711; 717c; 737br; 738bl; 745; 748; 749; 750; 751; 751c, cr; 752tl

V

François Vincent: 635tr

W

Richard Ward/Precision: 18tr; 20tl; 57c; 63t; 64t; 70tl; 71tl; 75tr; 79c; 81cr; 113tl; 142br; 156; 161c; 163; 166cr; 174t, bl; 187cr; 192bl; 212c, cr, b; 217; 245t; 262bl; 272tl; 275tl; 291; 308t; 342br; 461bl; 462bl; 372cl; 393b (maps); 406br; 407tl, bl; 410bl; 414c; 415bc; 435; 436; 448cl; 479tl; 481; 484; 485; 509bcl, bl; 524tl; 542b; 573tl; 651br; 656b; 672; 683cr; 707t, c; 718tc; 733br; 734; 752cr, bc; 770tl, bl, tr; 772t, br; 773l; 774t; 775r; 777
Craig Warwick/Linden Artists: 489
Phil Weare: 519l; 607bl; 741
David Webb/Linden Artists: 36t; 91bc; 135; 177c; 176; 207c; 226; 258bl, tl; 262tc, tr, bc, br; 263bl; 321c, b; 411br; 478; 479b; 482; 486; 524b; 525; 541tr, bl; 732t, bc; 768t; 770br
Ann Winterbotham: 117br; 208br; 258r; 446c; 493tr; 594; 647tr
Gerald Wood: 56bl; 60; 78c; 109; 250; 253; 254br; 255; 260cr; 269br; 330; 509tlc; 530; 644br; 668bc; 680tl, cr; 679; 686b; 720; 733c; 739
John Woodcock: 14cr; 28cb; 63c; 79b; 92tl, c; 178; 182br; 201; 206b; 207t, cr; 208tr; 223c; 259bl; 298; 311r; 315tr, br; 328; 345b; 357br; 366r; 410tl, c, cr; 420l; 422br; 431cr; 459bl; 471bc; 493tl, cl; 494tr; 519cr; 551r; 565br; 573r; 575bl; 576bl; 581tr; 586r; 590bl; 595cl, bl; 641r; 644bl; 647cl; 649cr; 670cl; 670bc; 682; 696b; 697b; 700; 632; 633tr; 719; 731b; 732cl, tr, c; 737c, cr; 738tr, br; 740; 743; 769; 770 (insets); 774b; 775t, l
Dan Wright: 130; 262c; 443; 767br; 770bl

JACKET CREDITS

Abbreviations: FC = front cover, BC = back cover, a = above, b = below, c = centre, l = left, r = right, t = top.

Pekka Parviainen/Science Photo Library: FC al.
Corbis © Renee Lynn/Corbis: FC br.
Corbis © Bettmann/Corbis: FC cl.
ESA, NASA, and P. Anders (Göttingen University Galazy Evolution Group, Germany): BC cl.

treatment channels. Each tube ends in a fragile plastic catheter which is inserted into the appropriately numbered applicator and secured by a coupling device. The unit has a supply of compressed air and it is air pressure that the system uses to transfer the sources from the safe within the unit to the applicators along the connecting tubes. Operation of the unit is initiated from a remote-control unit situated outside the protected treatment area. Together these components form the basis of the remote-controlled afterloading system (Blake, 1991).

The selectron provides an accurate and safe method of radiotherapy treatment for cancers of the cervix, uterus and upper part of the vagina.

The advantages of the selectron system are threehold:

1. Remote afterloading eliminates contact with radioactive material and protects personnel.
2. It allows highly accurate dosimetry.
3. The activity of the caesium-137 sources is such (up to 40 microCurie (mCi) that treatment times for patients are considerably shorter than for conventional techniques.

While the selectron has been used predominantly for the treatment of gynaecological cancers, features of its design render it potentially useful for treating a number of other tumours such as cancers of the oesophagus, bladder or colon.

Patients have hollow, lightweight stainless steel applicators positioned in the operating theatre under a general anaesthetic. These are usually modified Fletcher-type applicators consisting of a uterine tube and two vaginal ovoids held in place with a proflavine-soaked vaginal packing. However, several other applicators are available. Accurate positioning of the applicators is confirmed by taking X-rays with dummy sources *in situ* and the optimum source configuration is selected, taking account of individual anatomical variations.

The selectron is programmed by the physicist. For each treatment channel being used, active source pellets are interspersed with inactive stainless steel space pellets to achieve the desired dose distribution. The treatment time required to reach the prescribed dose is also entered. With a six-channel selection unit it is possible to treat two patients with Fletcher-type applicators simultaneously. The radiotherapist is responsible for connecting the transfer tubes to the applicators. The transfer tubes are led over a bed bracket which supports the weight of the tubes and prevents traction being applied to the applicators in the patient. If the wrong catheter is connected to the applicator, the system will fail to operate.

Operating the selectron

Treatment is commenced by activation of the remote control unit when all staff have left the treatment area. While treatment is in progress it can be interrupted and restarted from the remote control unit by pressing the stop and start buttons. The display panel indicates which channels are being used for treatment and which are unused with red and green lights respectively. The time of the longest treatment is displayed in decimal hours and a telephone intercom system allows for communication with the patient without the need to interrupt treatment.

Interrupting the treatment by pressing the green stop button results in the sources being withdrawn into the selectron unit and stops the timer. This allows nursing staff to enter the treatment area in safety and give routine or specific care to the patient. Pressing the red start button transfers the sources back into the applicators and restarts the timer. The red lights demonstrate that the channels are operating again satisfactory.

The system has built-in safety features. In the event of a failure in the system, treatment usually stops automatically. An audible and visual alarm at the remote control unit alerts staff to a problem and indicates whether this is a fault related to the air or power supply, the pellets or the timer. There is an optional nurse station display unit with a similar alarm indicator which also emits an audible signal when treatment has been interrupted. This helps to prevent treatment being inadvertently left interrupted for long periods.

A record of any break in treatment is shown on the print-out from the unit itself, together with any programming or system fault. These appear as an error code and can be identified by reference to the selectron users' manual.

At the end of the treatment time, all sources will be withdrawn automatically from the applicators back into the selectron unit. When two patients are being treated simultaneously termination of the treatment of one patient may be some time before that of the other. This means the timer will register the longer treatment time but the channels used for the first patient will have changed from red to green.

Additional safety features include a door switch facility to retract sources immediately if the door to the treatment area is opened when treatment is in progress, and/or Geiger dose rate meters visible when entering the treatment area and approaching the patient, which indicate when there are radioactive sources either in the patient or in the connecting tubes.

Preparation of the patient

This is similar to that required before other gynaecological intracavitary techniques. Information given should include explanation that the patient will be connected to the selectron unit via the flexible plastic tubes and that these will restrict turning in bed. Patients should also be prepared for the various mechanical noises that the system makes, especially when the sources are being transferred in and out of the applicators. Some patients find the prospect of treatment alarming and may prefer to receive regular sedation for the duration of the treatment.

References and further reading

Amersham International Ltd (1978) *Interstitial Therapy Using Iridium-192*. Amersham International Ltd.

Amersham International Ltd (1981) *Radioisotope Sources for Brachytherapy*. Amersham International Ltd.

Baker, J. (1979) Implants and applications. In Scan-technology in nursing – radiotherapy (Ed. by R. Tiffany), *Nursing Times*, 148, Suppl. pt. 10, 37–40.

Blake, P. R. (1991) Radiotherapy and chemotherapy in the treatment of gynaecologic cancer. In *Textbook of Gynaecology* (Ed. by R. Varma). Edward Arnold, London.

Dean, E. M. *et al.* (1988) Gynaecological treatments using the selectron remote afterloading system. *British Journal of Radiology*, 61(731), 1053–7.

Department of Health and Social Security (1985) *The Ionising Radiations Regulations Schedule 1*. HMSO, London.

Hodt, H. J. *et al.* (1952) A gun for interstitial implantation of radioactive gold grains. *British Journal of Radiology*, 25, 419–21.

Holmes (1988) *Radiotherapy. The Lisa Sainsbury Foundation Series*. Austen Cornish, London.

Hussey, K. (1985) Demystifying the care of patients with radioactive implants. *American Journal of Nursing*, 85, 789–92.

Lambert, J. E. & Blake, P. R. (1992) *A Guide to Gynaecology Oncology*. Oxford University Press, London.

Nucletron Engineering (1981) *Selectron Users' Manual*, Nucletron Engineering, Chester.

Paine, C. H. (1972) Modern afterloading methods for interstitial radiotherapy. *Clinical Radiology*, 23, 263–72.

Pierquin, B. *et al.* (1978) The Paris system in interstitial radiation therapy. *Acta Radiologica: Oncology, Radiation, Physics, Biology*, 17(1), 33–48.

Royal Marsden Hospital (1968) *Rules for the Protection of Nursing Staff Exposed to Ionising Radiation* (rev. edn). The Royal Marsden Hospital, London.

Royal Marsden Hospital (1978) *Physics Manual Protocol*. The Royal Marsden Hospital, London.

Shell, J. & Carter, J. (1987) The gynaecological implant patient. *Seminars in Oncology Nursing* 3(1), 54–66.

Shepherd, J. H. & Monagham, J. M. (1990) *Clinical Gynaecological Oncology*, 2nd edn. Blackwell Scientific Publications, Oxford.

Tiffany, R. (1979) *Cancer Nursing – Radiotherapy*. Faber & Faber, London.

Welby-Allen, M. (1982) Selectron treatment in gynaecology. *Nursing Times*, 78(46), 1948–50.

GUIDELINES: CARE OF PATIENTS WITH INSERTIONS OF SEALED RADIOACTIVE SOURCES

Action	Rationale
1. When transferring patients from theatre to ward, the nurse and porter should remain at the head and foot of the bed and at least 120 cm from the centre of the bed in the event of any delay in the transfer. If the source is intra-oral, the nurse should stand at the foot of the bed.	To minimize the risk of exposure to radiation.
2. A yellow radiation hazard board should accompany the patient back from theatre. This must remain at the bottom of the bed or outside the cubicle until the source is removed.	To warn everybody that the patient has a radioactive source.
3. Nursing staff must calculate the time allowed with the patient in any 24-hour period. This time should be written on the yellow hazard notice on the bed or cubicle door.	To minimize exposure to radiation.
4. A Geiger counter should be available on the ward.	To monitor radioactivity if a dislodged source is suspected, e.g. in the bed linen.
5. One nurse should be delegated responsibility for	To minimize the risk of overexposure to radiation.

Action	Rationale
the nursing care of the patient. The time spent with the patient should be shared between all of the staff on duty, and time spent in nursing procedures must be kept to a minimum.	
6. Every nurse must wear a radiation badge above the level of the lead shield.	To record the extent of exposure to radiation.
7. All bed linen and waste materials removed from the patient area should be monitored before being removed from the ward.	To prevent loss of an accidentally dislodged source.
8. If a source becomes dislodged, use the long-handled forceps to put the source into a lead pot. Care should be taken not to damage the source. It must never be handled directly with the fingers.	To minimize the dose of radiation received.
9. Visitors must remain at least 120 cm away from the patient. The visit should not last longer than the time shown on the warning notice. No children or pregnant women are allowed to visit.	To minimize the risk of overexposure to radiation.

GUIDELINES: CARE OF PATIENTS WITH INTRA-ORAL SOURCES

Preparation of the patient

Dental assessment of the patient is usually carried out before oral brachytherapy so that caries, mouth infections and dental extractions may be dealt with in case of the oral blood supply being impaired by the treatment. The patient is usually admitted 24 hours before the implant, during which time the nature of the procedure and the implications of having a radioactive source should be explained to the patient. Ideally, the patient should be nursed in a cubicle or in a bed away from other patients to reduce the amount of radiation exposure to other people.

Action	Rationale
1. Encourage frequent mouth care. The patient should void the solution into a bowl and not into a handbasin.	To reduce the risk of infection. To prevent the loss of a dislodged source.
2. Provide a soft, puréed or liquid diet.	To reduce the risk of the patient biting into the source or tongue. Eating is often difficult when implants are present.
3. Avoid spicy and/or hot foods. Discourage the patient from smoking and/or drinking alcohol.	To prevent exacerbation of local reaction or soreness.
4. Encourage ingestion of carbonated drinks.	To alleviate dryness.
5. Provide crushed ice for the patient to suck and/or soluble aspirin as a mouthwash.	To minimize oral pain and discomfort.
6. Give steroids as prescribed.	To prevent and/or minimize swelling.
7. Provide writing equipment for the patient.	To reduce the need for oral communication. This is liable to increase soreness and alter the distribution of the sources.
8. Provide paper tissues and a bowl for saliva.	The patient may have difficulty in swallowing due to soreness and oedema.

Guidelines: Care of patients with intra-oral sources

Action	Rationale
9. The sources should be checked at regular intervals, e.g. at the beginning of a span of duty.	To make sure that the sources have not become dislodged.
10. The patient must be confined to the cubicle or the space around the bed. Washing is carried out in the bed area, but the general toilet facilities should be used, provided that the patient remains at a distance from other people.	To minimize the risk of radiation exposure to other people on the ward.

Discharge of the patient

The patient is usually discharged the day after the removal of the implant. The patient should be warned about the brisk local reaction which may be experienced due to rapid cell breakdown induced by the radiation. In order to minimize the risk of infection or soreness, the patient should be taught how to care for the treated area, e.g. frequent oral toilet.

GUIDELINES: CARE OF PATIENTS WITH GYNAECOLOGICAL SOURCES

Preparation of the patient

The patient is usually admitted 12 to 48 hours before the procedure so that any pre-anaesthetic investigations may be performed. An enema or suppositories are usually given to reduce the chance of the patient having a bowel action while the sources are in place, which could dislodge the sources. Some patients, however, have diarrhoea on admission due to previous radiotherapy and will need regular medication, such as codeine phosphate, both before and during the application of the sources. It is arguable whether the vulval area needs to be shaved. The patient should be bathed before any premedication is administered. A full explanation should be given to the patient along with information about the implications of having a radioactive source inside her.

Action	Rationale
1. The patient must remain in bed in a recumbent or semi-recumbent position while the applicators or implants are in place.	To prevent the applicators becoming dislodged or changing their position with relation to the internal organs.
2. Rolling from side to side is permitted and should be encouraged if the patient is at risk of developing a pressure sore.	To promote comfort and to relieve prolonged pressure on any one area.
3. On return from theatre, the sanitary towel should be checked for discharge.	
Disposable pants may be worn.	To secure the position of the sanitary towel.
Check that the catheter is correctly positioned to allow drainage.	To ensure that urine is draining freely.
4. Observe for any blood or other discharge from the vagina. Check the temperature and pulse every two hours.	To monitor haemorrhage, shock and other postoperative complications.
5. Administer prescribed analgesics, antiemetics and antidiarrhoeal agents.	For the patient's comfort.

Action	Rationale
6. Encourage fluid intake as soon as the patient is allowed to drink. If the source is to be in for longer than 24 hours:	
(a) Encourage a fluid intake of 50 to 100% a day over and above the patient's normal intake.	To ensure adequate hydration. To reduce the risk of urinary tract infection.
(b) A low-residue diet may be taken.	To prevent the stimulation of a bowel action.

GUIDELINES: REMOVAL OF GYNAECOLOGICAL CAESIUM

The removal of applicators is usually performed by nursing staff. Only nurses holding a certificate of competence, or nurses supervised by a suitably qualified nurse, should perform this procedure.

Equipment

1. Sterile gynaecological pack containing large receiver, green towel, paper towel, long dissecting forceps, sanitary towel, cotton wool balls.
2. Equipment for the administration of Entonox.
3. Solutions of choice for swabbing, e.g. normal saline.
4. Sterile gloves.
5. Sterile scissors or stitch cutter.
6. Clean draw sheet.
7. Geiger counter.

Procedure

Action	Rationale
1. Explain the procedure to the patient.	To obtain the patient's consent and co-operation.
2. Check the date and time for removal on the form that was received from the physics department when sources were inserted.	The accurate timing of the removal is essential for the administration of the correct therapeutic dose of radiation.
3. Check that any pre-removal drugs (e.g. sedatives, analgesics) have been administered.	
4. Check, with another nurse, the exact time of removal and the number of applicators.	To reduce the risk of error.
5. Ensure that:	
(a) The lead shield is suitably positioned beside the patient.	To shield the nurse from exposure to radiation.
(b) The lead pot is also suitably positioned with the lid removed.	So that sources can be placed in the pot immediately after removal.
6. Begin the administration of Entonox at least two minutes before commencing the procedure.	To allow time for the effects of the gas to be felt. (For further information on Entonox administration, see Chapter 15.)
7. Prepare a trolley, put on gloves and open the pack before going to the bedside.	This is a clinically clean, not an aseptic procedure. To reduce the time spent in close proximity to the source.
8. Working from behind the lead shield, assist the patient into the dorsal position with knees apart. Remove the sanitary towel.	To obtain access to the sources.
9. Remove any sutures, if present. Remove the vaginal packing.	

Guidelines: Removal of gynaecological caesium

Action	Rationale
10. Remove the caesium sources in reverse order of insertion. Contact the radiotherapist immediately if difficulty is encountered in removing a source. Place the removed sources in a lead pot immediately and cover with the lid.	To contain radioactivity.
11. Remove the lead pot to a designated area, e.g. an isotope sluice or safe. Ensure that the lid of the pot or the sluice door is locked.	To remove the radioactive source from the ward area. To prevent unauthorized access to the source.
12. Monitor the patient's level of radioactivity.	To ensure that no sources remain inside the patient.
13. Remove the urinary catheter.	
14. Swab the vulva and perineal area with a solution such as normal saline. Ensure that the patient has a clean sanitary towel in position and is made comfortable.	To promote patient hygiene and comfort.
15. Monitor the bed linen, paper bags, vaginal packing and other waste material. (Two nurses should monitor the patient independently.)	To ensure that no source has been lost or remains inside the patient.
16. The patient should remain in bed until the physics department staff are satisfied that all sources are accounted for.	To ensure that all sources have been accounted for before the patient moves around.
17. Remove the radiation warning notice.	

NURSING CARE PLAN

Problem	Cause	Suggested action
Patient has a bowel action.		Inform the radiotherapist.
Patient removes caesium source herself.	Confusion, e.g. post-anaesthetic.	Using long-handled forceps place the source in the lead container or safe. Inform the radiotherapist and the physics department.
Pyrexia.	Pelvic cellulitis or abscess. Reaction to the proflavine pack. Urinary infection. Physiological reaction to the breakdown of the tumour. Chest infection. Peritonitis due to perforation of the uterus.	If the patient's temperature remains over 37.5°C for two consecutive readings, inform the radiotherapist. The caesium may have to be removed if the pyrexia persists.

GUIDELINES: CARING FOR THE PATIENT WITH GOLD-198 GRAINS

Preparation of the patient

The patient is usually admitted at least one day before treatment: Patients should be nursed ideally in a single room but, more importantly, in a bed away from the main thoroughfare.

Gold grains are implanted permanently into the tissue and therefore the patient must agree to stay in hospital until the physics staff state that the radioactivity is at a legally permissible level for discharge.

Breast and lymph node implantation

Action	Rationale
1. The dressing to be left securely in position unless special instructions are given by the radiotherapist.	Sources may become detached, dressings will prevent them from becoming lost.
2. If dressing becomes dislodged leave it at the bedside, preferably in a lead pot and inform the physics staff.	If sources have become detached and are in the dressings physics staff will take the necessary action.
3. If there is any possibility that the sources have become detached inform physics department staff immediately and do not remove anything from the room.	It is important that the source is not lost as this could result in contamination of the environment. The patient's total dose will be altered and the medical staff will need to be informed.

Lung implantation

Action	Rationale
1. Check all sputum and drainage from the chest with the Geiger counter. If no radioactivity is found the sputum and drainage may be disposed of in the usual way unless special instructions are given by the physics department or radiotherapy staff.	To check for radioactivity in case any gold grains are coughed up or expelled in the drainage.
2. If radioactivity is detected, inform physics department staff immediately. Save the sputum or drainage for them to deal with.	To prevent contamination of the hospital environment.

Bladder and prostate implantation

Action	Rationale
1. Check all urine with the Geiger counter. If no radioactivity is found the urine may be disposed of in the usual way.	To check for radioactivity in case any gold grains are expelled in the urine.
2. If radioactivity is detected inform physics staff immediately and save urine for them to deal with.	To prevent contamination of the hospital environment.
3. Leave suspect urine in a safe place at the bedside, e.g. under the bed.	To prevent accidental disposal.

GUIDELINES: CARE OF PATIENTS WITH BREAST SOURCES

Preparation of the patient

The patient will usually be admitted for local excision of the breast tumour and an axillary clearance. Drains are inserted and these are usually removed before the iridium wire sources are loaded 24 to 48 hours after surgery. When the sources are loaded, the patient should be nursed in a bed away from other patients.

Action	Rationale
1. Any dressing is left undisturbed for the duration of treatment.	To minimize the time spent in proximity to the patient.
2. The patient is confined to the cubicle or the space around the bed. Washing is carried out at the bed area. If general toilet facilities have to be used the patient must remain at a distance from other people.	To minimize the risk of radiation to other people on the ward.
3. Administer prescribed analgesia as required throughout the treatment period and before removal.	For the patient's comfort.

Discharge of the patient

The patient should normally be discharged the day after the removal of the implant. The patient should be warned about the brisk local reaction which she may experience due to the rapid cell breakdown induced by the radiation. In order the minimize the risk of infection or soreness, the patient should be taught how to care for the treated area.

GUIDELINES: CARE OF PATIENTS UNDERGOING SELECTRON TREATMENT

Action	Rationale
1. Nurse the patient on a pressure-relieving mattress or with a foam wedge under her buttocks.	To promote comfort and to relieve backache since rolling is not permitted.
2. Ensure the plastic transfer tubes are supported securely in the bed bracket, leaving slight slack.	To enable the patient to change position slightly without putting traction on the applicators.
3. Limit the frequency and duration of interruption to treatment. Visitors are discouraged unless the patient is markedly distressed.	To prevent unnecessary prolongation of treatment time.
4. Unless otherwise indicated by the patient's physical or psychological mental condition, check two-hourly:	
(a) Temperature, pulse and vaginal loss.	To monitor for haemorrhage, shock or other postoperative complications.
(b) Contents of catheter drainage bag.	To ensure urine is draining freely.
(c) Assist patient to adjust her position.	To promote comfort and relieve prolonged pressure on any one area.
5. Administer prescribed analgesics, antiemetics, antidiarrhoeal and sedative agents as appropriate and evaluate effect.	To promote the patient's comfort and wellbeing.

Action	Rationale
6. Encourage fluid intake as soon as the patient is able to drink.	To ensure adequate hydration and reduce the risk of urinary tract infection.
7. If the patient wishes to eat, a light, low-residue diet may be taken.	To prevent stimulation of a bowel action.

GUIDELINES: REMOVAL OF SELECTRON APPLICATORS

If two patients are being treated simultaneously, removal of the applicators may be delayed until both patients have finished treatment, depending on the individual treatment times.

Equipment

As for removal of other gynaecological applicators see 'Guidelines: Removal of gynaecological caesium', above, (items 1–7) plus:

8. Rubber caps for the applicators.

Procedure

Action	Rationale
1. Check treatment has been terminated by: (a) Ensuring the appropriate channel lights are green. If the other patient's treatment is continuing, interrupt treatment. (b) Ensure time display on the selectron unit reads zero for the appropriate channels. (c) Ensure the print-out indicates treatment has stopped for those channels.	The applicators should be removed only on completion of treatment.
2. Record the finish time on the patient's dosimetry sheet.	This is kept as a record in the patient's notes.
3. Check that the close-circuit television camera is not focused on the patient.	To ensure privacy.
4. Explain the procedure to the patient.	To obtain patient's consent and co-operation.
5. Ensure any pre-removal drugs have been administered.	To allow analgesic or sedative to be felt.
6. Assist the patient into a comfortable position with her knees apart.	To allow access to the applicators.
7. Uncouple the plastic transfer tubes by rotating the black coupling anticlockwise in the direction of the arrow and very carefully store the tubes on the plastic supporting mantle attached to the selectron unit.	To prevent the plastic catheter becoming damaged or kinked.
8. Place rubber caps on the ends of the applicators.	To ensure no fluid or debris is allowed to enter the applicator tubes.
9. Commence administration of Entonox (see Chapter 15) at least two minutes before removal of the applicators.	To allow the effect of the gas to be felt.
10. Prepare the equipment and put on gloves.	The procedure is clinically clean and not aseptic.

Guidelines: Removal of selectron applicators

Action	Rationale
11. Remove the vulval dressing pads, any sutures and vaginal packing.	These must be removed before the applicators can be eased out.
12. Dismantle the applicators by loosening the screws holding them togeter.	To promote ease of removal.
Remove the uterine tube first, ensuring it is taken out complete with its small white flange, followed by the ovoids.	To prevent the flange being left in the patient's vagina.
13. Remove the catheter, swab the vulval area and ensure the patient has a clean sanitary pad and a fresh draw sheet.	To promote cleanliness and patient comfort.
14. The patient can then be assisted into a comfortable position and is permitted up to have a bath.	The patient is reassured that the procedure has been completed, that she is no longer radioactive and can resume normal activities.

Applicators are retained carefully for cleaning in accordance with local policies.
Remaining treatment can then be given to the second patient.

NURSING CARE PLAN

See also 'Nursing care plan' for conventional gynaecological sources, above.

Problem	Cause	Suggested action
Patient removes the applicators herself.	Confusion, e.g. post-anaesthetic.	Interrupt treatment. Deposit applicators and attached tubing in the lead pot. Inform radiotherapist and physicist. Restart treatment if two patients are being treated.
Applicator is partially dislodged.	Patient may have moved too much or too vigorously.	Interrupt treatment. Inform physicist and radiotherapist. The applicator may have to be removed as above.
Alarm sounding at nurse station.	Treatment has been interrupted and inadvertently left off.	Check patient is unattended and recommence treatment.
Sources are not transferred to the applicators.	Incorrect coupling or loose connection.	Check print-out to identify which channel is at fault. Tighten appropriate coupling device.
Alarm activated at remote control unit.	Failure in the system.	Check the error code on the print-out with the selectron users' manual. Rectify as indicated in the manual or seek technical assistance from the physics department.
Pellets stuck in the applicator or transfer tubing.	A damaged or kinked catheter.	Inform the physics department. Withdraw the plastic catheter

using long-handled forceps and deposit in the protected container until technical assistance can be provided. Reassure the patient.

36

Specimen Collection

Definition

Specimen collection is the collection of a required amount of tissue or fluid for laboratory examination.

Indications

Specimen collection is required when microbiological, biochemical or other laboratory investigations are indicated. Nursing staff should be able to identify the need for microbiological investigations and, if appropriate, initiate the taking of specimens. Specimen collection is often a first crucial step in investigations that define the nature of the disease and determine diagnosis and the mode of treatment.

REFERENCE MATERIAL

General principles

Successful laboratory diagnosis depends on the collection of specimens at the appropriate time, using the correct technique and equipment and transporting them to the designated laboratory safely without delay. For this to be achieved, good liaison is essential between medical, nursing, portering and laboratory staff. The nurse's role is:

1. To identify the need and importance for microbiological investigation.
2. To initiate, if appropriate, the taking of a swab or specimen, e.g. during wound dressing it is usually the nurse who identifies signs of infection.
3. To know the appropriate investigation to be taken so as to avoid indiscriminate specimen collection which wastes time and money.
4. To collect the desired material in the correct container.
5. To arrange prompt delivery to the laboratory.

Collection of specimens

The greater the quantity of material sent for laboratory examination, the greater the chance of isolating a causative organism. Anaerobic and other fastidious micro-organisms particularly are more likely to survive. It is, therefore, preferable to send a few millimetres of pus aspirated with a sterile syringe than to send a swab. Specimens are readily contaminated by poor technique. Cultures taken from such specimens often result in confusing or misleading results.

Specimens should always be collected in sterile containers with close-fitting lids. Swabs should never be removed from their sterile containers until everything is ready for taking the sample.

Ideally, samples should be collected before beginning any treatment, e.g. antibiotics or antiseptics. If the patient is receiving such treatment at the same time the specimen is collected, the laboratory staff must be informed. Both antibiotics and antiseptics may destroy organisms that are, in fact, active in the patient and will affect the outcome of the laboratory test. Specimens should also be obtained using safe technique and practices (Hart, 1991). For example, gloves should always be worn when handling all body fluids.

Documentation

Requests for microbiological investigations must include the following information:

1. Patient's name, ward and/or department.
2. Hospital number.
3. Date collected.
4. Time collected.
5. Diagnosis.
6. Relevant signs and symptoms.
7. Relevant history, e.g. recent foreign travel.
8. Any antimicrobial drug being taken by the patient.
9. Type of specimen.
10. Consultant's name.
11. Name of the doctor who ordered the investigation, as it may be necessary to telephone the result before the typed report is dispatched.

Without full information, it is impossible to examine a specimen adequately or to report it accurately.

Transportation of specimens

Guidelines are now available on the labelling, transport and reception of specimens (Health Services Advisory Committee, 1986). The sooner a specimen arrives in the laboratory, the greater is the chance of organisms present surviving and being identified. Delays will cause changes that may radically alter the result. The laboratory count of bacteria in a delayed specimen could be out of all proportion to that of the specimen when it was collected.

If specimens cannot be sent to a laboratory immediately, they should be stored as follows:

1. Blood culture samples in a 37°C incubator.
2. All other specimens in a specimen refrigerator at a temperature of 4°C.

In diagnostic pathology it is likely that at any given time there will be a number of specimens that present a risk of infection. Every health authority, therefore, must ensure that medical, nursing, phlebotomy, laboratory, portering and any other staff involved in handling specimens are trained to do so. Specimen containers must be sufficiently robust and must not leak when used. They must also be closed securely and any accidental spillage cleaned immediately. Ideally, all specimens should be placed in a double self-sealing bag with one compartment containing the request form and the other the specimen. Specimens should be transported to the laboratory in washable baskets or trays.

It is the responsibility of the person who requests and takes specimens that are known to be infectious to ensure that both the form and the container are labelled with biohazard labels.

Types of investigation

Bacterial

A wide range of methods is available for obtaining cultures and identifying organisms from a specimen or swab. To employ all these tests would be time consuming and costly. Testing, therefore, tends to be selective. It is at this stage that the laboratory request form plays a particularly important part. A faecal specimen, for example, from a patient with diarrhoea who also has a recent history of foreign travel, would be investigated for organisms not normally looked for in faecal specimens from patients without such a history.

The majority of specimens undergo microscopic investigation. This is valuable as an early indication of the causative organisms in an infection. The specimen is often cultured for 24 to 48 hours longer in the case of blood cultures. This is followed by antibiotic sensitivity testing on any pathogenic organisms that are isolated. Normally this takes a further 24 hours.

Viral

Three types of technique are available for the diagnosis of viral infections:

1. Electron microscopy.
2. Culture.
3. Serology.

For culture specimens the use of viral transport media and speed of delivery to the laboratory are important as viruses do not survive well outside the body. With good liaison, the nursing personnel should obtain the specimen when the laboratory staff have the transport ready to take it to the virus laboratories. If delays occur, the specimen should be refrigerated at a temperature of 4°C.

The time at which specimens are collected for viral investigations is important. Many viral illnesses have a prodromal phase during which the multiplication and shedding of the virus are at a peak and the patient is most infectious.

Serological

Serological testing for the presence of antigens and antibodies is used when it is not possible to isolate the organism from the patient's tissue easily. By demonstrating serum antibodies to suspected organisms it is inferred that the patient is, or has been, infected with the organism. A single test is inadequate as if the titres are raised it is impossible to determine whether this is due to past or present infection. Two tests need to be carried out, both of which involve the collection of 10 ml of blood once at the beginning of the illness and again 10 to 14 days later. If a rising titre level is demonstrated it suggests the patient's infection is current.

Mycosis

Although many pathogenic fungi will grow on ordinary becteriological culture media, they grow better and with less risk of bacterial overgrowth on special mycological media. Alternatively, they may be demonstrated in skin and nail scraping. The presence of fungi in clinical specimens is difficult to interpret as *Candida albicans*, for example, is commonly present in the upper respiratory, alimentary and female genital tract and on the skin of healthy people.

Mycobacteriological

For further information, please refer to the procedure on tuberculosis (see Chapter 4).

Protozoa

Most protozoa do not cause disease but those that do, e.g. malaria, make a formidable contribution to human illness (Akinola, 1984). Laboratory investigations depend on direct microscopy which necessitates specimens being delivered to the laboratory as quickly as possible.

Blood

For information on the collection of blood see the procedure on venepuncture (Chapter 44).

Quantitative analysis of drugs in blood

Therapeutic drug monitoring by blood analysis can provide valuable objective information to guide clinicians in achieving optional treatment with selected therapeutic agents.

With drugs that possess a narrow therapeutic range in serum, as with the aminoglycoside antibiotics (Barza *et al.*, 1978), if the serum levels are too low the patient is jeopardized by the probable lack of efficacy. However, if the serum concentration is excessive, the patient may suffer serious toxicity. In the case of gentamicin, exposure to high serum levels for a prolonged period may cause renal impairment or ototoxicity (Cipolle, 1981). However, when the serum levels are within the normal range, the incidence of dose-related side-effects is minimal in most patients (Koch-Weser, 1972).

In order to correctly individualize drug dosage, and then to monitor the drug effectively, the doctor needs to be familiar with the metabolic processes and relationships between a drug dose and drug concentration in biological fluids (Greenblatt *et al.*, 1975). This is affected by many factors, such as route of administration (Riegelman, 1973) and age (Rane, 1976). Disease processes, for example liver (Blaschke, 1977) and renal disease (Peters, 1978), will also affect metabolism and excretion of the drug.

Drug monitoring is time consuming and costly. However, it is important to evalute the cost of the test in the light of the information it yields, in providing optimal patient care and the cost it might be avoiding, for example, damage to the ear.

Analysis involves laboratory testing of blood serum. Although this knowledge can be gained from random sampling, most benefit will be obtained by the correct timing of sample collection. This will provide a direct relationship to drug administration, and therefore give the correct interpretation of the serum concentration results.

Ideally, a trough sample just before the next scheduled dose, plus a peak level at a set time following the administration of the drug, will provide the most useful information.

In the procedure guidelines below two examples of drug analysis have been discussed; the laboratory will supply specific times for blood sampling for other drugs.

References and further reading

Akinola, J. (1984) Malaria. *Nursing Times*, 80(38), 40–3.

Ayton, M. (1982) Microbiological investigations. *Nursing*, 2(8), 26–9, 232.

Barza, M. *et al.* (1978) Why monitor serum levels of gentamicin? *Clin. Pharmacokinetics*, 3, 202–15.

Blaschke, T. F. (1977) Protein binding and kinetics of drugs in liver disease. *Clin. Pharmacokinetics*, 2, 32–44.

Cipolle, R. J. *et al.* (1981) Therapeutic use and serum concentration monitoring. In *Individualizing Drug Therapy: Practical Applications of Drug Monitoring* (Ed. by W. J. Taylor & A. L. Finn). Gross, Townsend & Frank, New York.

Greenblatt, D. J. *et al.* (1975) Clinical pharmacokinetics. *New England Journal of Medicine*, 293, 964–70.

Hargiss, C. O. & Larson, E. (1981) How to collect specimens and evaluate results. *American Journal of Nursing*, 81, 2166–74.

Hart, S. (1991) Blood and body fluid precautions. *Nursing Standard*, 5, 25–7.

Health Services Advisory Committee (1986) *Safety in Health Services Laboratories: The Labelling, Transport and Reception of Specimens*. HMSO, London.

Koch-Weser, R. J. (1972) Serum drug concentration as therapeutic guides. *New England Journal of Medicine*, 287, 227–31.

Parker, M. J. (1982) *Microbiology for Nurses*, 6th edn. Baillière Tindall, London.

Peters, U. *et al.* (1978) Digoxin metabolism in patients. *Archives of Internal Medicine*, 138, 1074–6.

Rane, A. *et al.* (1976) Clinical pharmacokinetics in infants and children. *Clin. Pharmacokinetics*, 1, 2–24.

Reigelman, S. (1973) Effects to route of administration on drug disposition. *J. Pharmacokin. Biopharm.*, 1, 419–34.

Smith, A. L. (1985) *Principles of Microbiology*, 10th edn. C. V. Mosby, St Louis.

Wilson, M. E. & Mizer, H. E. (1969) *Microbiology in Nursing Practice*. Macmillan, London.

GUIDELINES: SPECIMEN COLLECTION

Procedure

Action	Rationale
1. Explain the procedure to the patient and ensure privacy while the procedure is being carried out.	To obtain the patient's consent and co-operation.
2. Wash hands using bactericidal soap and water or bactericidal alcohol hand rub.	Hand washing greatly reduces the risk of infection transfer.
3. Place specimens and swabs in the appropriate, correctly labelled containers.	To ensure that only organisms for investigation are preserved.
4. Dispatch specimens promptly to the laboratory with the completed request form.	To ensure the best possible conditions for any laboratory examinations.

Eye swab

Action	Rationale
1. Using either a plastic loop or a cotton wool-covered wooden stick, hold the swab parallel to the cornea and gently rub the conjunctiva in the lower eyelid.	To ensure that a swab of the correct site is taken. To avoid contamination by touching the eyelid.
2. If possible, smear the conjunctival swab on an agar plate at the bedside.	Eye swabs are often unsatisfactory because of the action of tears, which contain the enzyme lysozyme which acts as an antiseptic. Conjunctival scrapings are preferable. This procedure is usually performed by medical staff.

Nose swab

Action	Rationale
1. Moisten the swab beforehand with sterile water.	To prevent discomfort to the patient. The healthy nose is virtually dry and a dry swab may cause discomfort.
2. Move the swab from the anterior nares and direct it upwards into the tip of the nose (Figure 36.1).	To swab the correct site and to obtain the required sample.
3. Gently rotate the swab.	

Perinasal swab (for whooping cough)

Action	Rationale
1. Using a special soft-wire mounted swab, pass it along the floor of the nasal cavity to the posterior wall of the nasopharynx (see Figure 36.1).	To minimize trauma to nasal tissue. To obtain a swab from the correct site.
2. Rotate the swab gently.	

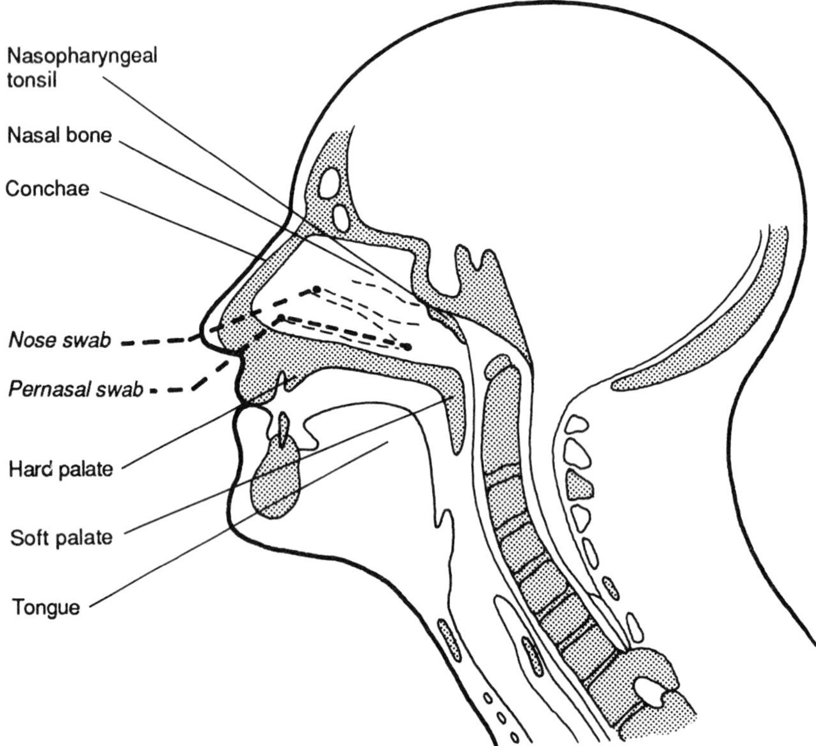

Figure 36.1 Area to be swabbed when sampling the nose.

Guidelines: Specimen collection

Sputum

Action	Rationale
1. Use a specimen container that is free from organisms of respiratory origin. This need not, therefore, be a sterile container.	Sputum is never free from organisms since material originating in the bronchi and alveoli has to pass through the pharynx and mouth, areas that have a normal commensal population of bacteria.
2. Care should be taken to ensure that the material sent for investigation is sputum, not saliva.	
3. Encourage patients who have difficulty producing sputum to cough deeply first thing in the morning. Alternatively, a physiotherapist should be called to assist.	To facilitate expectoration.
4. Send any sputum specimen to the laboratory immediately.	The bacterial population alters rapidly and rapid dispatch should ensure accurate results.

Throat swab

Action	Rationale
1. Ask the patient to sit in such a position that he/	To ensure maximum visibility of the area to be

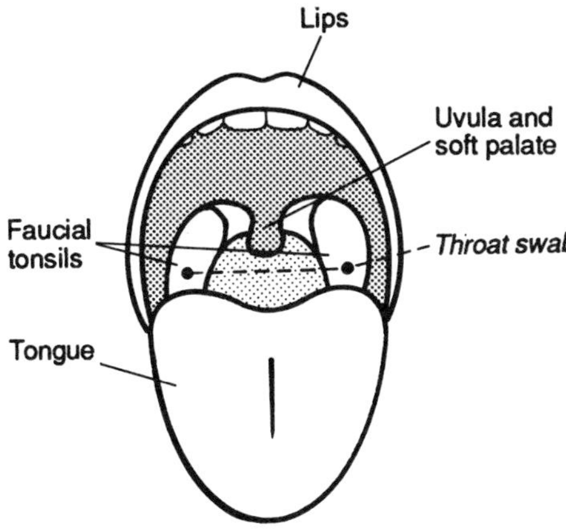

Figure 36.2 Area to be swabbed when sampling the throat.

she is facing a strong light source. Depress the patient's tongue with a spatula.

swabbed. The procedure is one that is likely to cause the patient to gag and the tongue will move to the roof of the mouth, contaminating the specimen.

2. Quickly, but gently, rub the swab over the prescribed area, usually the onsillar fossa or any area with a lesion or visible exudate (Figure 36.2).

To obtain the required sample.

3. Avoid touching any other area of the mouth or tongue with the swab.

To prevent contamination by other organisms.

Ear swab

Action	Rationale
1. No antibiotics or other chemotherapeutic agents should have been used in the aural region three hours before taking the swab.	To prevent contamination from other organisms. To prevent collection of traces of such therapeutic agents.
2. Place the swab into the outer ear as shown in Figure 36.3. Rotate the swab gently.	To avoid trauma to the ear. To collect any secretions.

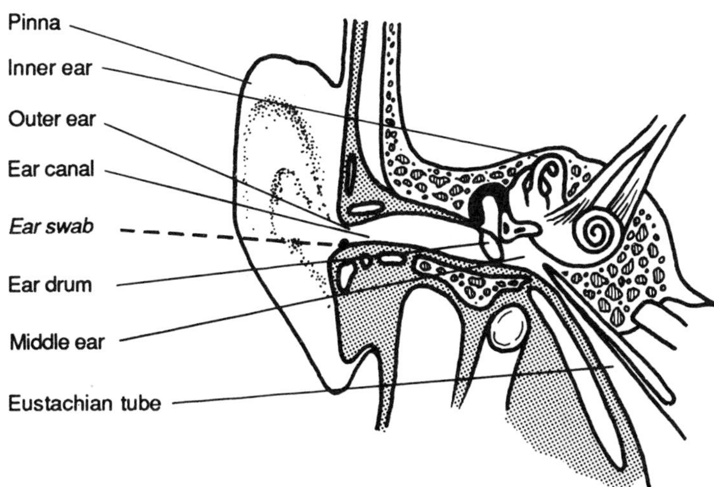

Figure 36.3 Area to be swabbed when sampling the outer ear.

Guidelines: Specimen collection

Wound swab

Action	Rationale
1. Take any swabs required before dressing procedure begins.	To prevent collection of any therapeutic agents that may be employed in the dressing procedure.
2. Rotate the swab gently.	To collect samples. It is preferable to send samples of purulent discharge to swabs.

Note: The use of disposable gloves is recommended in the following procedures in order to prevent cross-infection.

Vaginal swab

Action	Rationale
1. Introduce a speculum into the vagina to separate the vaginal walls. Take the swab as high as possible in the vaginal vault.	To ensure maximum visibility of the area to be swabbed. To ensure that the swab is taken from the best site. If infection by Trichomonas species is suspected, a charcoal-impregnated swab is recommended as this organism survives longer in this medium.

Penile swab

Action	Rationale
1. Retract prepuce.	To obtain maximum visibility of area to be swabbed.
2. Rotate swab gently in the urethral meatus.	To collect any secretions.

Rectal swab

Action	Rationale
1. Pass the swab, with care, through the anus into the rectum.	To avoid trauma. To ensure a rectal and not an anal sample is obtained.
2. Rotate gently.	
3. In patients suspected of suffering from threadworms, take the swab from the perianal region.	Threadworms lay their ova on the perianal skin.

Faeces

Action	Rationale
1. Ask the patient to defaecate into a clinically clean bedpan.	To avoid unnecessary contamination from other organisms.
2. Scoop enough material to fill a third of the specimen container using a spatula or a spoon, often incorporated in the specimen container.	To obtain a usable amount of specimen. To prevent contamination.
3. Examine the specimen for such features as	To monitor any fluctuations and trends.

colour, consistency and odour, and record your observations.

4. Segments of tapeworm are seen easily in faeces and any such segments should be sent to the laboratory for identification.

Unless the head is dislodged, the tapeworm will continue to grow. Laboratory confirmation of the presence of the head is essential.

5. Patients suspected of suffering from amoebic dysentery should have any stool specimens dispatched to the laboratory immediately.

The parasite causing amoebic dysentery exists in a free-living nonmotile cyst. *Both* are characteristic in their fresh state but are difficult to identify when dead.

Urine

Action	Rationale
1. Specimens of urine should be collected as soon as possible after the patient wakens in the morning and at the same time each morning if more than one specimen is required.	The bladder will be full as urine has accumulated overnight. If specimens are taken at other times, the urine may be diluted. All specimens will be comparable if taken at the same time each morning.
2. Dispatch all specimens to the laboratory as soon after collection as possible.	Urine specimens should be examined within two hours of collection or 24 hours if kept refrigerated at a temperature of 4°C. At room temperature overgrowth will occur and lead to misinterpretation. The cellular elements of urine break up quickly. Boric acid is sometimes used in specimen containers as a urine preservative.

Midstream specimen of urine: male

Action	Rationale
1. Retract the prepuce and clean the skin surrounding the urethral meatus with soap and water, saline or a solution that does not contain a disinfectant.	To prevent other organisms contaminating the specimen. Disinfectants may irritate or be painful to the urethral mucous membrane.
2. Ask the patient to direct the first and last part of his stream into a urinal or toilet but to collect the middle part of his stream into a sterile container.	To avoid contamination of the specimen with organisms normally present on the skin.

Midstream specimen of urine: female

Action	Rationale
1. Clean the urethral meatus with soap and water, saline or a solution that does not contain a disinfectant.	To prevent other organisms contaminating the specimen. Disinfectants may irritate or be painful to the urethral mucous membrane.
2. (a) Use a separate wool swab for each swab. (b) Swab from the front to the back.	To prevent cross-infection. To prevent perianal contamination.
3. Ask the patient to micturate into a bedpan or toilet. Place a sterile receiver or a wide-mouthed container under the stream and remove before the stream ceases.	To avoid contamination of the specimen with organisms normally present on the skin.
4. Transfer the specimen into a sterile container.	

Guidelines: Specimen collection

Specimen of urine from an ileal conduit

For further information see the relevant section in the procedure on stoma care (Chapter 37).

Catheter specimen of urine

For further information see the relevant section in the procedure on urinary catheterization (Chapter 43).

24-Hour urine collection

Action	Rationale
1. Request the patient to void the bladder at the time appointed to begin this procedure. Discard this specimen.	To ensure the urine collected is that produced in the 24 hours stated.
2. All urine passed in the next 24 hours is collected in a large specimen bottle. The final specimen is collected at exactly the same time the bladder was voided 24 hours earlier.	Body chemistry alters constantly. A 24-hour collection will accommodate all the variables within a representative period.
3. Care must be taken to ensure the patient understands the procedure in order to eliminate the risk of an incomplete collection.	A 24-hour collection will not be obtained if one sample is lost and the results will be invalid.

Semen

Action	Rationale
1. Sexual intercourse should not have taken place for three to four days before the specimen is collected.	To ensure the sperm count will be at maximum levels. It takes between three and four days for the sperm count to return to normal after ejaculation.
2. A fresh masturbated specimen must be collected in a sterile container and delivered to the laboratory within two hours of the collection of the specimen.	Sperm will die if there is a delay in testing. Specimens must not be collected in a condom as sperm die when in contact with materials such as rubber.

Cervical scrape

Action	Rationale
1. The ideal time for smear testing is mid-cycle.	To allow for accuracy of results as the cervix is usually free of contamination from menstrual flow at this time.
2. The menses should be avoided.	This is less uncomfortable for the patient.
3. The smear must be taken before a vaginal examination is carried out.	To ensure normal tissue samples are obtained.
4. Label the ground glass end of the slide with the patient's name.	To ensure patient identification.
5. Expose the cervix by using a dry speculum or one moistened with warm tap water.	To ensure maximum visibility. Greasy lubricants inhibit specimen collection.

6. Using the bilobed end of the cervical spatula, scrape firmly but gently around the squamocolumnar junction of the cervix. If the os is splayed open or scarred, a wider sweep with the broad end of the spatula may be necessary.	To obtain a usable amount of specimen.
7. Smear both sides of the spatula evenly on the slide with one stroke from each side of the spatula.	To ensure complete specimens.
8. Fix immediately.	To preserve the specimen and ensure accurate results.
9. Allow the fixing agents to dry for 20 minutes.	Dry specimens are less likely to be damaged.
10. Place the slides in a transport container.	To safeguard delicate glass slides.
11. Send, with a completed cervical cytology request form, to the appropriate laboratory.	

GUIDELINES: ANALYSIS OF DRUG LEVELS IN BLOOD

Procedure

Gentamicin levels

Action	Rationale
1. Following venepuncture guidelines (see Chapter 44), withdraw 10 ml blood to obtain specimen for clotted sample to provide trough serum using a new needle or winged infusion device. Blood specimen container to be clearly labelled 'pre-gentamicin administration blood'.	To obtain a blood sample safely via an intravenous device that is not contaminated by previous administration of gentamicin residue, which could provide an inaccurate result.
2. Administer intravenous gentamicin (following administration of drugs by direct injection, bolus, or push; see Guidelines, Chapter 21) via patient's established cannula.	To continue with patient's prescribed drug regime.
3. 20 minutes after administration of gentamicin withdraw 10 ml blood to obtain specimen for clotted sample to provide peak level serum either using the needle from which the pre-gentamicin administration blood was withdrawn or a new device. Blood specimen container to be clearly labelled 'post-gentamicin administration blood'.	Time gap allows for even distribution of gentamicin thorough the blood and for peak blood levels to be achieved.
4. Rarely but occasionally when only poor and limited venous access is available, the blood specimens may have to be obtained from the patient's existing device.	The possibility of these specimens being contaminated with residue drug is high.
The device must be flushed thoroughly before taking the blood sample.	Contamination can be reduced by thorough flushing of the line.
The blood specimen container and request care must be labelled to indicate this deviation from the usual procedure.	The clinician interpreting the result will be aware of the method of obtaining the blood specimen.

Guidelines: Analysis of drug levels in blood

Vancomycin levels

Action	Rationale
1. Following venepuncture guidelines (see Chapter 44), withdraw 10 ml blood to obtain specimen for clotted sample to provide trough serum using a new needle or winged infusion device. Blood specimen container must be clearly labelled 'pre-vancomycin administration blood'.	To obtain a blood sample safely via an intravenous device that is not contaminated by previous administration of vancomycin, which could provide an inaccurate result.
2. Administer vancomycin intravenously (following administration of drugs by continuous infusion guidelines, Chapter 21) via patient's established cannula.	To continue with patient's prescribed drug regime.
3. Two hours after completion of administration of vancomycin, withdraw 10 mls blood to obtain specimen for clotted sample to provide peak level serum.	Time span allows for even distribution of vancomycin throughout the blood and for peak blood levels to be achieved.
4. Blood specimen container to be clearly labelled 'post-vancomycin administration blood'.	

37

Stoma Care

Definition

'Stoma' is a word of Greek origin meaning 'mouth' or 'opening'. A bowel or urinary stoma is usually created on the abdominal wall as a diversionary procedure because the urinary or colonic tract beyond the position of the stoma is no longer viable.

Indications

Stoma care is required for the following purposes:

1. To collect urine or faeces in an appropriate appliance.
2. To achieve and maintain patient comfort and security.
3. To maintain good skin and stoma hygiene.

REFERENCE MATERIAL

Types of stoma

Colostomy

In a colostomy the stoma may be formed from any section of the large bowel, e.g. 'end' or 'terminal' sigmoid colostomy (usually permanent, Figure 37.1).

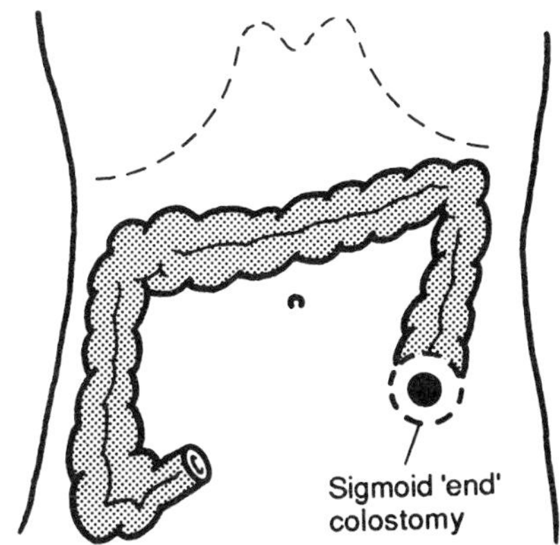

Figure 37.1 Sigmoid 'end' colostomy.

A temporary (usually transverse) colostomy may be raised to divert the faecal output, thus allowing healing of an anastamosis further along the colon. With a defunctioning loop colostomy, a rod or bridge may be used to maintain a hold on the abdominal surface. Such a rod or bridge is removed seven to ten days after insertion (Figure 37.2). The term 'defunctioning' is used to indicate that the bowel distal to the stoma is being rested.

Ileostomy

In an ileostomy the ileum is brought out onto the abdominal wall (Figure 37.2), as when, for example, the large colon is affected by inflammatory disease. Many patients with ulcerative colitis are offered a Park's pouch and therefore do not have to have a permanent stoma. For this operation a colectomy is performed and the terminal ileum is made into a reservoir (pouch) and brought down and attached to the anus. A temporary ileostomy allows the pouch to heal (Nemer & Rolstad, 1985).

Ileal loop, ileal conduit or urostomy

The performance of such operations (when the bladder is removed or diseased), requires the ureters to be transplanted from the bladder into a length, approximately 15 cm, of ileum which has been isolated, along with its mesentery, from the remainder of the small bowel. One end of the ileum, with the resected ureters, remains inside the abdomen, while the other is brought out on to the abdominal wall and everted to form a slightly protruding stoma (Figure 37.3).

Other types of urinary diversion

Other types of urinary diversion include ureterostomy, a procedure that brings the ureters out onto the abdominal wall together (one stoma) or separately (two stomas). It may be possible for some patients with bladder disease to have a continent pouch or 'new' bladder formed internally. One example of this is the Mitrofanoff technique (Horn, 1991; Gelister, 1991).

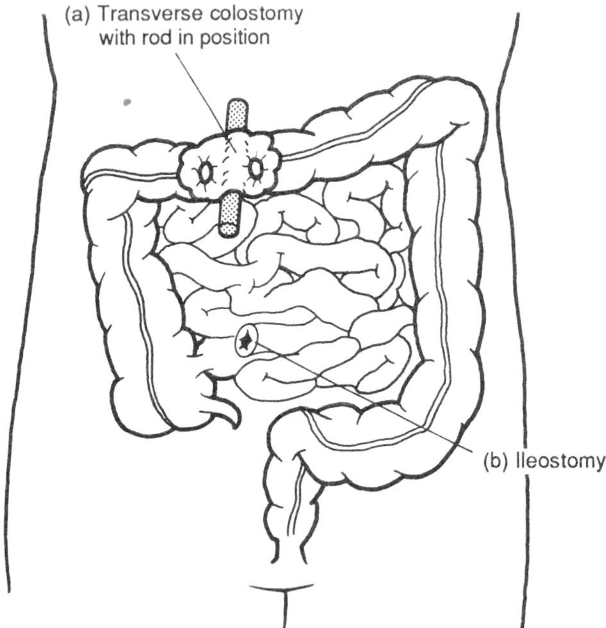

Figure 37.2 (a) Traverse colostomy and (b) ileostomy.

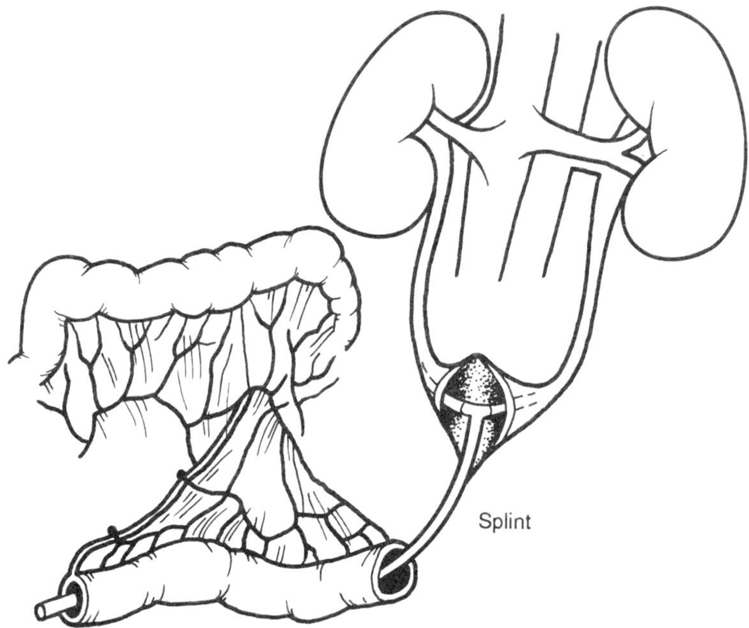

Figure 37.3 Urostomy.

For further information on these continent urinary diversions, see Chapter 10.

Indications for bowel stoma

1. Cancer of the bowel.
2. Cancer of the pelvis.
3. Trauma.
4. Neurological damage.
5. Congenital disorders.
6. Ulcerative colitis.
7. Crohn's disease.
8. Diverticular disease.

9. Familial polyposis coli.
10. Intractable incontinence.

Indications for urinary stoma

1. Cancer of the bladder.
2. Cancer of the pelvis.
3. Trauma.
4. Congential disorders.
5. Neurological damage.
6. Intractable incontinence.

Pre-operative preparation for stoma surgery

Physical preparation of the patient will vary according to the type of operation and the policies of individual surgeons and hospitals. This will involve the usual preparation for anaesthesia, preparation of the area of the body involved and of the bowel. Other specific procedures may also be included.

Psychological preparation of the individual facing stoma surgery should begin as soon as surgery has been considered, preferably by utilizing the skills of a trained stoma care nurse. Boore (1978) and Hayward (1978) have illustrated the importance of pre-operative information and explanation in reducing postoperative physical and psychological stress. The aims of presenting such information are as follows:

1. To help the individual with a stoma to return to their previous place in society whenever possible.
2. To help in the process of adapting to a changed body image (Price, 1990; Salter, 1988).
3. To reduce anxiety. The patient's perception of life with a stoma may have a positive or detrimental influence on rehabilitation. There may be myths and wrong information to dispel, and the patient's awareness of the experiences of another ostomist to discuss.
4. To explain that the presence of a stoma need not adversely affect any previous quality of life such as hobbies, work, social life or any other interests, although the underlying disease might.
5. To prepare the patient for the appearance and likely behaviour pattern of the stoma.
6. To reassure patients that they will be able to manage an appliance whatever the environment.
7. To assure patients that they will be supported fully while in hospital and will not be discharged until they are confident about the stoma's care and that continuing support will be available in the community.

Such pre-operative education has been shown to increase co-operation and trust and reduce anxiety, the length of time the patient remains in hospital and the amount of postoperative analgesia required. It should be borne in mind that any information given should be relevant to the patient's needs. Family and/or close friends may also be involved, when appropriate, on agreement with the patient.

Diet

All patients should be encouraged to eat a wide variety of foods.

Colostomy

Certain foods, e.g. large portions of fruit and vegetables (onions, sprouts, cabbage, etc.) may cause diarrhoea or excess flatus. It is suggested that rather than eliminate these items from the diet, the foods identified should be tried again in smaller portions. No food item affects everyone in the same way and it is best for the individual to experiment. It might be preferable to reduce the portion and prepare for the consequences. Beer may cause excess flatus. Other forms of alcohol will affect the ostomist as they do everyone else.

Ileostomy

Certain foods will cause excess flatus. Pulses, dried fruit, peanuts and coconut are digested slowly and so they will need to masticated well before swallowing.

If these foods are taken in excess and not masticated well they could swell in the gut and cause a 'bolus' obstruction. Some foods, e.g. tomato skins or pips, may pass into the appliance unaltered.

Urostomy

There are no dietary restrictions. It must be stressed, however, that an adequate fluid intake must be maintained to minimize the risk of urinary infection. Approximately 1.5 litres (or 12 cups per day) is the recommended minimum. The slow return of both a normal appetite and bowel function is a common feature following this operation (due to bowel handling in surgery) and it gives cause for much anxiety. The patient should be warned of this and advised to take small, light meals supplemented by nutritious drinks. Normal appetite may not return for two or three months after the operation.

Fear of malodour

This is a common fear for patients with bowel stomas, often based on hearsay or experience with other ostomists in hospital or the community. Appliances are odour free when fitted correctly. Flatus may be released via charcoal filters and deodorizers are available. The individual must be reassured, however, that any problems that occur postoperatively will be investigated, with a good possibility of them being solved by such means as the use of alternative appliances.

Sex and the ostomist

The possibility of sexual impairment for both men and women after stoma surgery depends on the nature of the operation and ensuing damage to the nerves and tissues involved. Impairment may be permanent or temporary. In the latter case, resolution of the difficulty may take anything up to two years. Pre- and postoperative counselling should be offered for both patient and partner. In cases of male impotence, surgical intervention, such as insertion of penile implants, may be appropriate if impairment becomes permanent. Papaverine injections (not to be confused with papaveretum) to induce an erection may be used, with the patient being taught to self-administer the injections (Brindley, 1986).

Useful references of the psychological and sexual aspects can be found in Devlin and Plant (1979), Davies (1990) and MacDonald (1982).

Female patients may experience narrowing or shortening of the vagina and require the use of a lubricant. Pre- and postoperative counselling to help acceptance of a change in the patient's body image is of paramount importance (Salter, 1988).

Personnel who may be expected to provide information

1. Medical staff.
2. Stoma care nurse.
3. Nursing staff on ward.
4. Primary health care team.
5. Another suitable ostomist. 'Visitors' are trained by the voluntary associations and, ideally, should be of similar age, sex and background to the patient.

Useful aids

1. Information booklets.
2. Samples of the various appliances.
3. Diagrams.

These aids are valuable to reinforce and clarify the verbal information.

Pre-operative assessment

It is important to determine whether a patient will be able to manage a stoma by assessing the following:

1. Eyesight.
2. Manual dexterity.
3. The presence of other debilitating diseases, e.g. Parkinson's disease or arthritis.
4. Mental state.

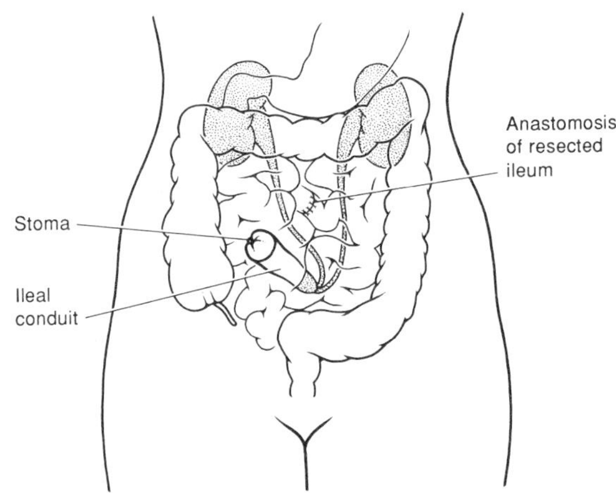

Figure 37.4 Position of stoma.

5. Loss of an upper limb.
6. Skin conditions.
7. Abnormal contours, e.g. the changes that occur with spina bifida.

Siting of the stoma is one of the most important preoperative tasks to be carried out by the doctor, stoma care nurse or experienced ward nurse (Figures 37.4 and 37.5). This minimizes future difficulties such as interference by the stoma with clothes, or skin problems caused by leakage of the appliance due to a badly sited stoma (e.g. on the waistline or in a body crease). When siting the stoma, consideration should be given to the following:

1. A flat area of the skin to facilitate safe adhesion of the appliance.
2. Avoidance of body prominences such as hips, ribs or pendulous breasts.
3. Avoidance of skin creases, especially in the region of the groin or the umbilicus, to avoid urine or faecal matter tracking along the skin creases.
4. Avoidance of scars.
5. Avoidance of wasitline or belt areas.
6. Maintenance of the stoma within the rectus sheath, as this reduces the risk of herniation later. The muscle may be identified by asking the patient to lie flat then to raise the head. The muscle may also be palpated and easily felt when the patient coughs.
7. Ideally, the patient should be able to see the stoma site.

The patient must be observed while lying, sitting in a comfortable chair, with the abdominal muscles relaxed, and standing. Consideration must be given to any bending of lifting involved with the patient's work

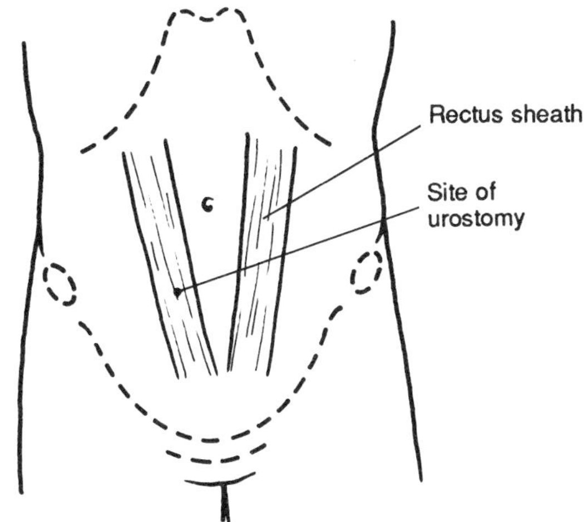

Figure 37.5 Site of urostomy.

and any other activities in which the patient partakes. Account must also be taken of any weight gain or loss in the postoperative period.

Post-operative period

Control of stoma action

Ileal loop

Urine will dribble from the stoma every 20 to 30 seconds. The output may be slightly less after periods of reduced fluid intake, e.g. at night. An appliance has to be worn at all times.

Ileostomy

Once the stoma starts to act a few days after surgery, the fluid output normally 500 to 800 ml every 24 hours, becomes of a porridge consistency once a normal intake of food is routine. The effluent contains enzymes that will excoriate the skin if contact is allowed. While the effluent cannot be controlled, the ostomist may find that the stoma is more active after main meals.

Colostomy

Due to its position, faecal matter from a transverse colostomy will be unformed. Patients with a sigmoid colostomy may find that wholemeal foods assist in producing a formed stool once or twice daily.

Medications that reduce peristaltic action, e.g. codeine phosphate, may also be used to control diarrhoea. The only means of controlling a sigmoid colostomy, however, is by regular irrigation or by use of a conseal plug system. This method must be taught under supervision to suitable ostomists.

Irrigation

Irrigation is a method of controlling the output of a colostomy by means of washing out the stoma with warm tap water (with the use of a coned irrigation set), every 24 to 48 hours.

The advantage of successful colostomy irrigation is that there is no stool leakage between irrigations (De-Hong, 1991).

Postoperative stages

Stage I

In theatre an appropriately sized skin-protective wafer should be applied around the stoma, followed by a drainable, transparent appliance, which should be left on for approximately five days. For the first 48 hours postoperatively, observe stoma colour (pink and healthy appearance ensures a good blood supply), size and stoma output (bearing in mind that it may take a few days for a bowel stoma to act). The drainable appliance should always be emptied frequently, gas should be allowed to escape and the appliance should not be allowed to get more than half full with effluent.

Immediately postoperatively patients would not be expected to perform their own stoma care but would be encouraged to observe the nurse caring for them and may discuss it with the nurse. Viewing the stoma may be difficult for the patient, who may be very aware of other people's reaction to it.

Stage II

As the patient's condition improves, a demonstration change of the appliance will be given with full explanation of the principles of stoma care. This will be followed by further opportunities to discuss any problems or raise new queries. Provided the patient agrees, it is useful to involve the patient's partner or close friends or relatives at this stage. Their acceptance of the stoma may encourage the patient and help to restore the patient's self-esteem. In the following days patients will be encouraged to participate in and gradually assume responsibility for their own stoma care. They may now be ready to discuss appliances and choose the one that they wish to use at home. Preparation for discharge will be discussed.

Stage III

Ideally, the patient should now be independent, eating a normal diet, be ready for discharge and should be confident in stoma care.

The family or close friends should be closely

involved during all stages. They are also likely to require support and information so that they are in a position to help the ostomist. Acceptance of the stoma is a gradual process and, on discharge from hospital, patients may only be beginning to adapt to life with a stoma.

Specific discharge plans

Follow-up support

The patient is discharged with adequate supplies until a prescription is obtained from the general practitioner. Written reminders are provided of how to care for the stoma, how to obtain supplies of appliances, and any other information that may be required. The patient should have details of non-medical stoma clinics, details about the relevant agencies and information about voluntary associations. Arrangements should also have been made for a home visit from the stoma care nurse and/or the community nurse.

Obtaining supplies

All National Health Service patients with a permanent stoma are entitled to free prescriptions for their stoma care products, and should complete the relevant forms for exemption from payment. Appliances can then be obtained from the local chemist, a free home delivery service or directly from the appropriate manufacturers.

Stoma appliances and accessories

Many of the appliances now available are very similar in style, colour and efficiency and often there is very little to choose between them when the time comes for the ostomist to decide what to wear.

The aim of good stoma care is to return patients to their place in society. One of the ways in which this can be achieved is to provide them with a safe, reliable, appliance. This means that there must be no fear of leakage or odour and the appliance should be comfortable, unobtrusive and easy to handle. The ostomist should also be allowed a choice of bag from a selection of appropriate appliances. It is also necessary to ensure that there are no problems with the stoma or peristomal skin.

Appliances

Choosing the right size of appliances

Bags are labelled according to the size of the opening that fits around the stoma. To keep the skin unblemished, it must be protected from the stoma output. The size chosen, therefore, should be one that fits snugly around the stoma to within 0.5 cm of the stoma edge. This narrow edge of skin is left exposed to prevent any of the adhesives, some of which are more rigid than others, rubbing against the stoma. The appliances usually come with measuring guides to allow for correct choice of size. During the first weeks the oedematous stoma will reduce in size and the bags or flange of the two-piece type appliances will have to be changed accordingly.

Types of appliance

Although some people whose stomas were created several years ago are wearing non-disposable rubber bags, most appliances used today are made of a specially designed laminate composed of three types of plastic. This should ensure that the appliances are:

1. Leak proof.
2. Odourproof.
3. Unobtrusive.
4. Noiseless.
5. Disposable.

The appliances differ slightly according to the stoma for which they are meant. All types, however, fall within one of two broad categories:

1. One-piece. This comprises a bag with an adhesive wafer that fits around the stoma. When the bag is renewed, the adhesive is removed from the skin. Its advantage is that is easy to handle, e.g. by an ostomist suffering from arthritis.
2. Two-piece. This comprises a flange for the skin that fits around the stoma and a bag that clips on to the flange. It can be used with sore and sensitive skin as when bags are removed from the flange, the skin is left undisturbed. However, the patient must have the dexterity to clip the bag securely onto the flange.

Drainable bags

1. Bowel stoma bags.
   Suitable for: ileostomy, transverse colostomy.
   Stoma output: fluid to semiformed (volume is too great for closed bags).
   Use: emptied frequently, taking care to rinse outlet afterwards; may be left on for up to three days.
   Additional features: flatus filters are absent in some as the fluid would obstruct the charcoal, rendering it useless, or will leak through the small opening; the outlet may have a separate clip or fixed 'roll-up' closure.
   Colour: clear, white, pink/beige.
2. Urinary stoma bags.
   Suitable for: urostomy.

Stoma output: urine.
Use: emptied frequently via a fixed tap; may be left on for up to three days.
Additional features: may be used with large collecting bag and tubing for night drainage.
Colour: clear or white.

3. Closed bags.
Suitable for: sigmoid colostomy.
Stoma output: a formed stool.
Use: changed once or twice a day.
Additional features: some have incorporated flatus filters that allow the release of flatus through charcoal patches that absorb the odour.
Colour: clear, white or pink/beige.

Some may be fitted with protective adhesive especially for sensitive skin and may now have a cotton-weave backing to prevent perspiration and to prevent the plastic from sticking to the skin.

Accessories

The specific products in this section have been mentioned as examples of what aids are available and reference to them is not necessarily intended as a recommedation.

Solutions for skin and stoma cleaning

Mild soap and water, or water only, are sufficient. Detergents, disinfectants and antiseptics cause dryness and irritation and should not be used. The stoma is not a wound or a lesion and should be regarded as a resited urethra or anus.

Skin barriers

1. Creams.
Unless made specifically for use on peristomal skin, these should not be used, as the residual surface film of grease prevents adherence of the appliance. Creams usually have a smoothing and moisturizing effect.
Use: for sensitive skin, as a protective measure.
Method: use sparingly; massage gently into the skin until completely absorbed; excess grease may be wiped off with a soft tissue.
Example: Chiron barrier cream (aluminium chlorohydrate 2% in an emulsified base).
Precaution: not to be used on broken or sore skin.
2. Skin gels/sealants.
Use: act as a film on the skin, first to prevent irritation and, second, to give protection as it is removed with the adhesive of the bag, thus preventing removal of the stratum corneum of the skin.
Method: use sparingly; pat onto the skin gently; dries quickly.
Example: Skin Gel, Skin Prep.
Precaution: should not be used on broken skin as they contain alcohol and cause stinging.
3. Protective wafers.
Use: these are hypo-allergenic and are designed to cover and protect skin, and allow healing if the skin is sore or broken. May be useful in cases of skin reaction or allergy to the adhesive or an appliance.
Method: the wafers may be cut with the aid of a template (pattern) to the required shape and fitted on to the skin. The appliances are then attached to the wafer. The rim of the wafer should not press against the stoma but should fit to 0.5 cm around it.
Examples: Stomahesive or Comfeel type of wafers. (Stomahesive is composed of gelatin, pectin, sodium carboxymethycellulose, and polyisobutylene; it adheres painlessly to normal, erythematous, moist or broken skin; it is available in three sizes.)
Precautions: allergy may occur, but rarely.
4. Protective rings.
Use: protective rings are used to provide skin protection around the stoma; they will protect a smaller area than the wafers mentioned above. They are also useful to fill in 'dips' or 'gulleys' in the skin.
Method: like the wafers, they have an adhesive side and may be applied directly to the skin. They form an integral part of some of the appliances.
Precautions: as for protective wafers above.
5. Pastes.
Use: useful to fill in crevices and 'gulleys' in the skin to provide a smooth surface for an appliance.
Examples: Stomahesive paste, Karaya gum paste and Orobase paste.
Method: *Stomahesive* – either leave for 60 seconds after applying to the skin, when the surface will be dry, making the paste easier to mould into the skin contour, or apply with a spatula, or wet the finger first to prevent the paste sticking and mould the paste immediately. Will sting on raw areas as it contains alcohol. Apply a little Orahesive powder to these areas first. *Orobase* – similar to Stomahesive in composition but with the addition of liquid paraffin. For protection of raw areas. Does not contain alcohol so will not cause local irritation.
6. Powders.
Use: for protection of sore or raw areas without impeding adhesion of the appliance.
Method: sprinkle on affected areas.
Examples: Orahesive powder.

Adhesive preparations

1. Sprays.
   Use: only required when appliance does not adhere well to the skin, e.g. due to leakage problems, difficult stoma site or with abdominal fistulae.
   Method: spray on appliance, not on the skin. Follow specific instructions on packaging. Removal should not be difficult.
   Examples: Dow Corning Adhesive.
   Precaution: the individual products differ considerably in the method of application and it is recommended that the user consults the manufacturer's instructions.
2. Lotions.
   Use: as above.
   Method: pat gently onto skin. The individual products differ considerably in their method of application and it is recommended that the user consults the manufacturer's instructions.
   Examples: Saltair solution.

Deodorants

1. Aerosols.
   Use: absorb odour.
   Method: one or two puffs into the air before emptying or removal of appliance.
   Examples: Atmacol, Oziom, Limone.
2. Drops and powders.
   Use: for deodorizing bag contents.
   Method: one drop into appliance.
   Examples: Nilodor (drops).
   Precaution: beware of over enthusiastic use which may result in a strong and distinctive odour that will become associated with stoma care.
3. Flatus filters (charcoal filled) usually incorporated into the bag.
   Use: to allow gradul release of flatus from the bag while allowing absorption of odour by the charcoal. The charcoal may only be effective for between six and 12 hours, depending on brand of filter.
   Precaution: use of flatus filters is not advised when the stoma effluent is very fluid as the charcoal may become moist and the air outlet blocked.

Useful addresses

1. Association of Spina Bifida and Hydrocephalus, Tavistock House North, Tavistock Square, London SW1V 1PS (Tel: 071-388 1382/5).
2. British Colostomy Association, 13–15 Station Road, Reading, Berkshire RG1 1LG (Tel: 0734 391537).
3. Ileostomy Association of Great Britain and Ireland, Amblehurst House, Black Scotch Lane, Mansfield, Nottingham NG18 4PF (Tel: 0623 28099).
4. Urostomy Association, 'Buckland', Beaumont Park, Danbury, Essex CM3 4DE (Tel: 024-541 4294).

References and further reading

Bailey, A. J. (1977) Nursing the patient with a colostomy. *Nursing Times*, 73, 382–5.

Boore, J. R. P. (1978) *A Prescription for Recovery: the Effects of Preoperative Preparation of Surgical Patients on Postoperative Stress, Recovery and Infection*. Royal College of Nursing, London.

Breckman, B. (1981) *Stoma Care*. Beaconsfield Publishers, Beaconsfield.

Brindley, G. (1986) Pilot experiments on the actions of drugs injected into the human corpus cavernosum penis. *British Journal of Pharmacology*, 87, 495–500.

Broadwell, D. C. & Jackson, B. S. (1982) *Principles of Ostomy Care*. C. V. Mosby, St Louis.

Brooke, B. N. *et al.* (1982) *Stomas*. W. B. Saunders,

Cassel, P. (1980) Management of ulcerative colitis.

Coloplast (undated) *Back on Your Feet Again*, Coloplast.

Davies, K. (1990) Impotence after surgery. *Nursing*, 4(18), 13–26.

De-Hong, Y. (1991) An assessment of colostomy irrigation. *Ostomy International*, 11(2), *Nursing* (1st series),, no. 17, pp. 727–9.

Devlin, H. B. & Plant, J. (1979) Sexual function – an aspect of stoma care. *British Journal of Sexual Medicine*, 1(6), 33–4, 37; 2(6), 22, 24, 26.

Gelister, J. F. & Woodhouse, C. R. (1991) Role of Continent Suprapubic Diversion in Pelvic Cancer. *British Journal of Urology*, 68, 376–9.

Gray, A. (1980) A new lease of life. *Nursing Times*, 76, 1616–20.

Hayward J. (1978) *Information – A Prescription Against Pain*. Royal College of Nursing, London.

Horn, S. (1991) Nursing patients with a continent urinary diversion. *Nursing Standard*, 4(21), 24–6.

MacDonald, L. (1982) Problems of the colostomy population. *Stoma Care News*, Vol. 1, p. 45, in *Nursing Mirror* (1983) Clinical Forum 8: Stoma Care, *Nursing Mirror*, Vol. 157, no. 11, Supplement.

Nemer, E. & Rolstad, B. (1985) The role of the ileo–anal reservoir in patients with ulcerative colitis and familial polyposis. *Journal of Enterostomal Therapy*, 12(3), 74–83.

Price, B. (1990) *Body Image Nursing: Concepts and Care*. Prentice Hall, New York.

Salter, M. (1988) *Body Image – The Nurse's Role*. Scutari Press, London.

Squibb Surgicare (undated) *Understanding Colostomy*. Squibb Surgicare.

Squibb Surgicare (undated) *Understanding Ileostomy*. Squibb Surgicare.

Squibb Surgicare (undated) *Understanding Urostomy*. Squibb Surgicare.

Turner, A. G. (1979) Urinary diversion. *Journal of Community Nursing*, 2(10), 20–1, 28.

Whitethread, M. (1981) Ostomists: a world of difference. *Journal of Community Nursing*, 5(2), 4–5, 10.

GUIDELINES: STOMA CARE

These procedural guidelines contain the basic information needed for changing a stoma appliance. Modifications may be made according to the following factors:

1. The place of change, i.e. bathroom, bedside, availability of sink, etc.
2. The person changing the appliance, i.e. nurse or patient.
3. Type of appliance used, e.g. one- or two-piece, closed or drainable.
4. Any accessories used, e.g. flatus filters, hypo-allergenic tape, barrier creams, etc.

Equipment

1. Clean tray holding:
   (a) Tissues.
   (b) New appliances.
   (c) Disposal bags for used appliances and tissues.
   (d) Relevant accessories, e.g. flatus filters, tape, etc.
2. Bowl of warm water.
3. Soap.
4. Jug for contents of appliance.
5. Gloves. (It is now common practice and, in many cases, hospital policy, to wear gloves when dealing with blood and body fluids. Thus they should be worn for cleaning stomas. It is recognized that it could be difficult to attach an appliance with gloves *in situ* (due to the adhesive), but once the stoma has been cleaned of excreta and blood, the gloves may be removed to apply the bag.) This practice should be explained to the patient so that they do not feel it is just because they have a stoma that gloves are worn.

Procedure

Action	Rationale
1. Inform the patient of the proposed activity.	To obtain the patient's consent and co-operation.
2. Explain the procedure.	To familiarize the patient with the procedure.
3. Ensure that the patient is lying in a suitable and comfortable position where the patient will be able to watch the procedure, if well enough.	To allow good access to the stoma for cleaning and for secure application of the stoma bag. The patient will become familiar with the stoma and will also learn much about the care of the stoma by observation of the nurse.
4. Use a small protective pad to protect the patient's clothing from drips if the effluent is fluid and apply gloves for nurse's protection.	Prevents the necessity of renewing clothing or bedclothes and demoralization of the patient due to any soiling.
5. If the bag is of the drainable type, empty the contents into a jug before removing the bag.	For ease of handling the appliance and prevention of spillage.
6. Remove the appliance. Peel the adhesive off the skin with one hand while exerting gentle pressure on the skin with the other.	To reduce trauma to the skin. Erythema as a result of removing the appliance is normal and quickly settles.
7. Remove excess faeces or mucus from the stoma with a damp tissue.	So that the stoma and surrounding skin are clearly visible.
8. Examine the skin and stoma for soreness, ulceration or other unusual phenomena. If the skin is unblemished and the stoma is a healthy red colour, proceed.	For the prevention of complications or the treatment of existing problems.
9. Wash the skin and stoma gently until they are clean.	To promote cleanliness and prevent skin excoriation.

Guidelines: Stoma care

Action	Rationale
10. Dry the skin and stoma gently but thoroughly.	The appliance will attach more securely to dry skin.
11. Apply a clean appliance.	
12. Dispose of soiled tissues and the used bag. Rinse the bag through in the sluice with water, wrap it in a disposable bag and place it in an appropriate plastic bin. At home the bag should be emptied into the toilet; a closed bag may be cut at the lower end, then rinsed using a jug or by holding it under the flushing water. Wrap the bag in newspaper, tie it in a plastic bag and dispose of it in a rubbish bag.	Faecal material in waste bags is a potential source of infection. Excreta should be disposed of down the sluice.
13. Wash hands thoroughly using bactericidal soap and water or bactericidal alcohol hand rub.	To prevent spread of infection by contaminated hands.

GUIDELINES: COLLECTION OF A SPECIMEN OF URINE FROM AN ILEAL CONDUIT OR UROSTOMY

Equipment

1. Sterile dressing pack.
2. Soft catheter – tracheal type, not larger than 12 or 14 gauge.
3. Disposable plastic apron.
4. Universal specimen container.
5. Skin-cleansing solution.
6. Alcohol-based hand wash solution.
7. Clean stoma appliance.

Procedure

Action	Rationale
1. Explain the procedure to the patient.	To gain the patient's consent and co-operation.
2. Ensure that the patient is in a comfortable position, e.g. sitting up, supported by pillows, and that the stoma is easily accessible.	
3. Screen the bed, then wash hands using bactericidal soap and water or bactericidal alcohol hand rub. Then dry them.	For the patient's privacy and to reduce the risk of cross-infection. Curtains are drawn at this stage so that dust and airborne organisms disturbed by the curtains do not settle on the sterile trolley.
4. Prepare the trolley and take it to the patient's bedside.	
5. Put on a disposable plastic apron.	To prevent cross-infection.
6. Remove the sterile dressing pack, catheter and receiver from their outer wrappings. Place them on the top shelf of the trolley.	

7. Remove the appliance from the stoma and cover the stoma with a clean topical swab.	To absorb spillage from the stoma.
8. Clean hands with a bactericidal alcohol hand rub, and put on clean disposable gloves before opening the sterile field on the trolley.	To reduce the risk of introducing infection into the stoma during the procedure.
9. Remove the non-linting gauze with forceps, check and discard it. Arrange a towel to absorb spillage from the stoma.	To keep the areas as clean as possible and to protect the patient and the bedclothes from spilled urine.
10. Clean around the stoma with water or saline, from the centre outwards.	Good cleansing of the area reduces the risk of introduction of surface pathogens into the ileal loop.
11. Insert the catheter tip gently to a depth of 2.5 to 5 cm only and wait for urine to drain through. Collect the sample in the specimen container. The recommended volume is 3 to 5 ml.	Gentle handling reduces the risk of ileal perforation and is more comfortable for the patient.
12. Remove the catheter and seal in the specimen container. Remove gloves and attend to stoma care and apply a pouch as usual. Make the patient comfortable.	
13. Dispose of equipment.	
14. Wash and dry hands.	To prevent cross-infection.
15. Check that the specimen is labelled correctly and dispatch it to the laboratory with the appropriate forms.	

NURSING CARE PLAN

Problem	Cause	Suggested action
Leakage of urine or faeces.	Ill-fitting appliance.	The opening of the appliance should fit snugly around the stoma.
	Skin creases or 'gulleys' preventing correct application of adhesive.	Build up indented areas and fill in gulleys to create a smooth surface e.g. using paste.
	Infrequent emptying of drainable bag leading to stress on adhesion.	Drainable bags should be emptied frequently, e.g two to three hourly if necessary.
Sore skin.	Leakage.	As above.
	Skin reaction to adhesive.	Change the make of appliance or apply a protective square between skin and adhesive. Anti-inflammatory agents may be required for very severe reactions.
	Poor hygiene.	Improve the technique of nurses or patient.
Odour.	Ill-fitting appliance; lack of seal	Fit the appliance with care.

Nursing care plan

Problem	Cause	Suggested action
	between skin and adhesive.	Consider a change of the type of appliance.
	Poor hygiene.	Improve the technique of nurses or patient.
	Poor technique, e.g. when emptying drainable bag.	Empty the bag, then rinse the end with water to ensure that it is clean before closing.

Urostomy specimen

Problem	Cause	Suggested action
Stoma specimen of urine contaminated.	Contaminants introduced during specimen collection.	Take a repeat speciment, observing aseptic procedure and cleaning the stoma well.
Ileum perforated during specimen collection.	Catheter too hard or inserted too roughly.	Report to a doctor immediately.
Difficulty passing catheter into conduit.	Small degree of retraction of ileum.	Apply gentle pressure to the area around the stoma to make it protrude.
	Unpredictable direction of ileum.	Gently insert your little (gloved) finger into the stoma to determine the direction of the conduit. Insert the catheter tip along this line.

38

Syringe Drivers

Definition

A syringe driver is a portable battery-operated infusion pump weighing approximately 175 g (including the battery) and measuring 165 mm by 53 mm by 23 mm.

Indications

The syringe driver is used to deliver drugs at a predetermined rate via the appropriate parenteral route. Typical applications include its use in pain control, cytotoxic chemotherapy, coronary care and neonatal care; for the administration of heparin and insulin, and treatment of thalassaemia.

REFERENCE MATERIAL

The syringe driver was developed in 1979 by Dr Martin Wright for use in treating thalassaemia with infusions of desferrioxamine (Wright & Callam, 1979).

Since its first introduction, the syringe driver has proved to be effective in the treatment of chronic pain in advanced cancer for patients requiring regular opioid treatment who are unable to tolerate oral or rectal medications (Dickson *et al.*, 1984; Russell, 1979). More recently, management of certain cancers with continuous intravenous infusions of cytotoxic chemotherapy via the subclavian vein using the portable syringe driver is becoming more common (Adams *et al.*, 1987; Greidanus *et al.*, 1987). Advantages of this technique include reduced toxicity and adverse effects while allowing longer term exposure to anti-cancer therapy (Lokich, 1983). The patients are able to continue to be ambulant and frequently treatment continues in the community. Where appropriate, patients are educated in reloading and caring for the syringe driver, thus maintaining independence with minimal input from the primary health care team. The details in this chapter concentrate on the clinical application of the syringe driver in the administration of subcutaneous drugs to patients unable to tolerate oral or rectal preparations. The following principles, however, remain valid when using this technique in other areas.

There are a growing number of syringe drivers on the market – the Graseby Medical MS16A series (Figure 38.1) is typical of one of these and will be used as the example throughout. Users of other types of syringe driver should always check the instruction manual for details.

The MS series syringe drivers may be used with most sizes and makes of plastic syringe. The different types of syringe driver allow drug administration on an hourly rate (for example, Graseby Medical, type MS16A) or on a daily rate (Graseby Medical type MS26). The wide variety of barrel sizes of syringes means that when calculating the delivery rate of the drug, it is necessary to calibrate in millimetres, i.e. the distance the syringe plunger has to travel. The Graseby Medical MS16A pump is calibrated in millimetres per hour (the MS 26 is calibrated in millimetres per day).

Indications for use

Careful selection of patients who may benefit from continuous subcutaneous infusion of drugs must be undertaken and the use of a syringe driver should not be viewed as a convenient alternative to oral or rectal medication. It should be used only for an indicated clinical condition, e.g. dysphagia, intractable nausea or vomiting, intestinal obstruction, local disease, or intractable pain unrelieved by oral or intermittent injections.

Advantages in the use of the syringe driver

1. Avoids the necessity of intermittent injections.
2. Mixtures of drugs may be administered (see 'Drug stability and compatability', below).
3. Infusion timing is accurate, which is particularly advantageous in the community.
4. The device is lightweight and compact allowing mobility and independence.

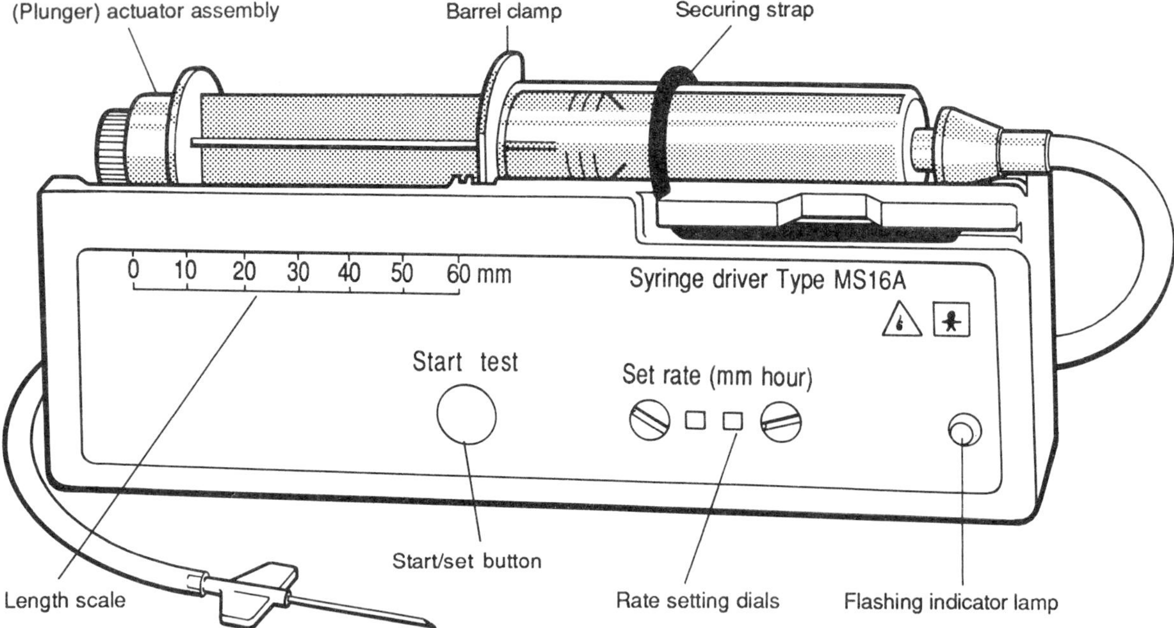

Figure 38.1 Graseby Medical MS16A syringe driver.

5. Rate can be increased and bolus doses given (see 'Additional notes' at end of chapter).
6. Simple calculations of dosage are required over a 12- or 24-hour period.

Disadvantages in the use of the syringe driver

1. Patient may become psychologically dependent on the device. (Radstone & Crowther, 1989)
2. Inflammation or infection may occur at the site of the cannula insertion.
3. Rate calculation can be confusing for the novice, particularly if the patient's dose requirements alter (see 'Additional notes', below).
4. The alarm system of some syringe drivers, e.g. the Graseby, operates only if the plunger is obstructed. It does not alert the nurse if the flow is too rapid or if the skin site has perished.

Skin site selection for subcutaneous infusion

The best sites to use for continuous infusion of drugs are the lateral aspects of the upper arms and thighs, the abdomen, the anterior chest below the clavicle and, occasionally, the back (Nicholson, 1986). Areas which should not be used for cannula placement are:

1. Lymphoedematous limbs. The rate of absorption from a skin site would be adversely affected. A cannula breaches skin integrity thus increasing the risk of infection in a limb which is already susceptible.
2. Sites over bony prominences: the amount of subcutaneous tissue will be diminished, impairing the rate of drug absorption.
3. Previously irradiated skin area. Radiotherapy can cause sclerosis of small blood vessels, thus reducing skin perfusion (Tiffany, 1988).
4. Sites near a joint: excessive movement may cause cannula displacement and patient discomfort.

Care of the skin site

The infusion site should be renewed when there is evidence of inflammation (erythema or reddening) or poor absorption (a hard subcutaneous swelling). The time taken for this to occur can vary from hours to over three weeks, dependent on the patient, and the drug(s) being infused (Brenneis *et al.*, 1987; Bruera *et al.*, 1987; Coyle *et al.*, 1986; Nicholson, 1986; Regnard & Newbury, 1983). There would appear to be a relationship between the concentration of drug(s) being infused, and the duration of a skin site (Nicholson, 1986). In one study, the average frequency of needle resiting was 5.1 days for patients receiving 7.5 to 30 mg of diamorphine per 24 hours, but only 2.4 days for those receiving 1000 to 2000 mg per 24 hours (Nicholson, 1986).

Another study noted no statistically significant relationship between duration of skin site and sex and age of patients, type or dose of narcotic, rate of infusion, or triceps skinfold measurement (Brenneis *et al.*, 1987). Clearly, further research into the factors influencing skin site survival is required.

If skin sites break down rapidly, suggestions include:

1. Further dilute the drug infused.
2. Change the infusion device.
3. Use a different site cleanser.
4. Where appropriate *and prescribed*, a glyceryl trinitrate transdermal patch may be placed above the entry site. Additional care must be taken that this is not contraindicated (see 'Additional notes', below).
5. Change the site dressing.

Drug stability and compatibility

In the context of single drug infusions, instability is not a clinically significant problem. The drug simply has to be:

1. Available in injectable form.
2. Suitable for subcutaneous administration.
3. Stable in solution for the duration of the infusion (usually 12 to 48 hours).

For example, diamorphine hydrochloride is stable, in solution, for up to two weeks (Jones & Hanks, 1986).

Problems of drug instability and incompatibility arise when higher drug concentrations and combinations of two or more drugs, are used. In addition, exposure of drug solutions to direct light and increased storage temperatures (up to 32°C) may exacerbate the problem.

Where drug combinations (commonly an analgesic and an antiemetic are used), further criteria must be met:

1. The drugs must be compatible with each other.
2. The diluents must be compatible with each other.
3. Each drug must be compatible with the diluent(s) of the other drug(s) in the combination.

Studies by Allwood (1984) and later work by Regnard and Davies (1986) have examined the stability and compatibility of analgesic/anti-emetic combinations. Regnard and Davies (1986) make the following recommendations:

1. Protect the syringe from direct light whenever possible.
2. Visual inspection of drug solutions should be made daily, and the syringe discarded if signs of crystallization, precipitation or discoloration occur.
3. Avoid high concentrations of drugs if used in combination.
4. Avoid mixing more than two drugs in one syringe.
5. Do not infuse antiemetics for more than 24 hours, particularly if part of a combination of drugs.

However, it remains the responsibility of each individual practitioner to ensure that the drug(s) prescribed are suitable for continuous subcutaneous infusion, and are stable under these conditions. If in any doubt, seek advice from an appropriate professional.

References and further reading

Adams, P. S. *et al.* (1987) Pharmaceutical aspects of home infusion therapy for cancer patients. *The Pharmaceutical Journal*, 238, 476–8.

Allwood, M. C. (1984) Diamorphine mixed with antiemetic drugs in plastic syringes. *British Journal of Pharmaceutical Practice*, 6, 88–90.

Auty, B. & Protheroe, D. T. (1986) Syringe pumps: a review. *British Journal of Parenteral Therapy*, 7, 72–7.

Badger, C. & Regnard, C. (1986) Pumping in pain relief. *Nursing Times*, 82, 52–4.

Baines, M. (1981) Drug control of common symptoms. *World Medicine*, 7(4), 47–59.

Beswick D. T. (1987) Use of syringe driver in terminal care. *The Pharmaceutical Journal*, 239, 656–8.

Brenneis, C. *et al.* (1987) Local toxicity during the subcutaneous infusion of narcotics (SCIN). *Cancer Nursing*, 10(4) 172–6.

Bruera, E. *et al.* (1987) Continuous SC infusion of narcotics using a portable disposable device in patients with advanced cancer. *Cancer Treatment Reports*, 71(6), 635–7.

Cox, P. & Potter, M. (1984) Controlling pain. *Journal of District Nursing*, 3(4), 4–3, 9.

Coyle, N. *et al.* (1986) Continuous subcutaneous infusions of opiates in cancer patients with pain. *Oncology Nursing Forum*, 13(4), 53–7.

Cunningham, D. (1989) Cytotoxic drugs for gastric and colorectal cancer. *British Medical Journal*, 299, 1479–80.

Dover, S. B. (1987) Syringe driver in terminal care. *British Medical Journal*, 294, 553–5.

Greidanus, J. *et al.* (1987) Evaluation of a totally implanted venous access part and portable pump in a continuous chemotherapy infusion schedule on an outpatient basis. *Eur. J. Cancer Clin. Oncol*, 23(11), 1653–7.

Hanks, G. W. *et al.* (1987) Diamorphine stability and pharmacodynamics. *Anaesthesia*, 42, 664–73.

Hawkett, S. & Nicholson, R. (1987) Syringe drivers (drug

administration for the terminally ill in the community). *Journal of District Nursing*, 5(8), 4–6.

Hoskin, P. *et al.* (1988) Syringe drivers. *Anaesthesia*, 43, 708.

Hoskin, P. *et al.* (1988) Sterile abscess formation by continuous subcutaneous infusion of diamorphine. *British Medical Journal*, 296, 1605.

Jones, V. A. & Hanks, G. W. (1986) New portable infusion pump for prolonged administration of opioid analgesics in patients with advanced cancer. *British Medical Journal*, 292, 1496.

Jones, V. A. *et al.* (1985) Solubility of diamorphine. *The Pharmaceutical Journal*, 235, 426.

Jones, V. A. *et al.* (1987) Diamorphine stability in aqueous solution for subcutaneous injection. Proceedings of the BPS, 17 to 19 December. *British Journal of Clinical Pharmacology*, 23, 651.

Latham, J. (1987) Syringe drivers in pain control. *The Professional Nurse*, 2(7), 207–9.

Ledger, T. (1986) Administering heparin with syringe pumps. *The Professional Nurse*, 1(7), 176–7.

Leggett, A. (1990) Looking at infusion devices (advantages and disadvantages of syringe pumps and drivers). *Nursing Standard*, 4(18), 29–31.

Lokich, J. J. (1983) Cancer chemotherapy by constant infusion. *Hospital Practice*, 18(11), 50C-50Q.

Nicholson, H. (1986) The success of the syringe driver. *Nursing Times* 82, 49–51.

Oliver, D. J. (1988) Syringe drivers in palliative care: a review. *Palliative Medicine*, 2, 21–26.

Oliver, D. J. & Sykes, C (1988) Histopathological study of subcutaneous drug infusion sites in patients dying with cancer. *The Lancet*, 1, 478.

Radstone, D. J. & Crowther, A. G. O. (1989) The appropriate use of syringe drivers. In *The Edinburgh Symposium on Pain Control and Medical Education* (Ed. by Twycross). Royal Society of Medicine, London.

Regnard, C. F. & Davies, A. (1986) *A Guide to Symptom Relief in Advanced Cancer*. Haigh & Hochland, Manchester.

Regnard, C. & Newbury, A. (1983) Pain and the portable syringe pump. *Nursing Times*, 79, 25–8.

Regnard, C. *et al.* (1968) Anti-emetic/diamorphine mixture compatibility in infusion pumps. *British Journal of Pharmaceutical Practice*, 8, 218–20.

Russell, P. S. B. (1979) Analgesia in terminal malignant disease. *British Medical Journal*, Vol 1 (6177) 1561.

Storey, P. *et al.* (1990) Subcutaneous infusions for control of cancer symptoms. *Journal of Pain and Symptoms Management*, 5(1), 33–41.

Tiffany, R. (Ed.) (1988) *Oncology for Nurses and Health Care Professionals, Vol. I. Pathology, Diagnosis and Treatment*, 2nd edn. Harper & Row, London.

Twycross, R. G. & Lack, S. A. (1984) *Therapeutics in Terminal Cancer*, Pitman, London.

Vere, D. W. (1978) Pharmacology of morphine drugs used in terminal care. In *Topics in Therapeutics* (Ed. by D. W. Vere). Pitman Medical, London.

Weston, A. (1989) Graseby syringe driver (brief research project). *Nursing Times and Nursing Mirror*, 85, 60–61.

Wright, B. M. & Callam, K. (1979) Slow drug infusions using a portable syringe driver. *British Medical Journal*, 2, 582.

GUIDELINES: SUBCUTANEOUS ADMINISTRATION OF DRUGS USING A SYRINGE DRIVER (E.G. GRASEBY MEDICAL MS16A)

Equipment

1. Syringe driver MS16A.
2. Battery (PP3 size, 9 volt alkaline).
3. Winged infusion set (for example, Vygan microflex PVC infusion set tube 100 cm, 0.5 mm G25)
4. Luer lock syringe of suitable size (5 ml or larger).
5. Swab saturated with isopropyl alcohol 70%.
6. Transparent adhesive dressing.
7. Drugs and diluent.
8. Needle (to draw up drug).
9. Drug additive label.
10. Patient's prescription.

Calculating the rate setting for administration of drugs using a syringe driver (e.g. Graseby Medical MS16A) over a 12-hour period

1. Measure stroke length in millimetres. The stroke length is the *length* of fluid to be infused, i.e. the distance the plunger has to travel (irrespective of the number of millilitres) (see Figure 38.2).
2. Check the delivery time (previously prescribed) in hours.
3. Calculate:

$$\frac{\text{Stroke length (mm)}}{\text{Delivery time (hr)}} = \text{Rate setting}$$

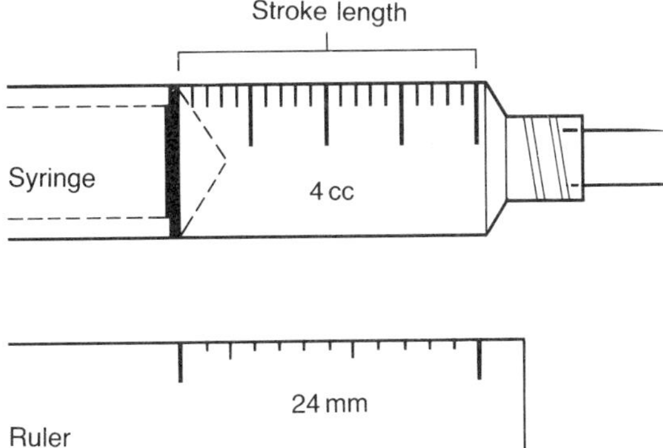

Figure 38.2 Measuring the stroke length.

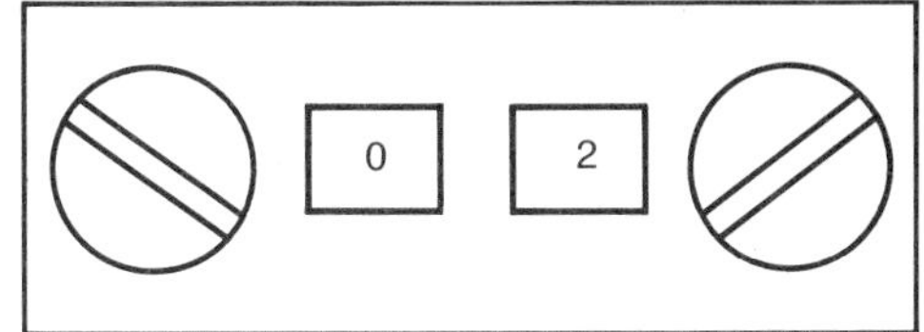

Figure 38.3 Setting the rate.

Example:
Stroke length = 24 mm
Delivery time = 12 hr
Rate setting = 2 mm/hr
Set rate using screwdriver provided.
If the set rate is a single figure, e.g. 2, this must be preceded by 0 (Figure 38.3).
See instruction booklets provided with individual syringe pumps.

GUIDELINES: PREPARATION OF THE SYRINGE FOR 12-HOUR DRUG ADMINISTRATION USING GRASEBY MEDICAL MS16A SYRINGE DRIVER

Action	Rationale
1. Calculate dosage of drugs and minimum volume of diluent required over 12 hours (use at least 1 ml diluent per 250 mg diamorphine hydrochloride injection).	This is more comfortable for the patient. Smaller volumes reduce the risk of inflammation at infusion site.
2. Draw up drugs with diluent, withdrawing the plunger until the stroke length corresponds with a number divisible by 12, e.g. 24, 36 or 48 hours.	Ensures accuracy as the infusion rate can only be set in whole numbers.
3. Establish the rate setting of the pump and check (or where appropriate educate the patient to check) the rate four- to six-hourly.	Ensures drug is given over the prescribed time period.

GUIDELINES: PRIMING THE INFUSION SET

Action	Rational
1. Using previously prepared syringe, connect a 100 cm winged infusion set.	Adding further diluent to syringe reduces the potency and therefore the effect of drug to be infused. This length of tubing allows patient greater freedom of movement.
2. Gently depress the plunger until the infusion tubing is filled up to the needle end.	This removes extraneous air from the system.

Guidelines: Priming the infusion set

Action	Rationale
3. Having previously calculated the rate setting, allow time for speedier first infusion rate.	Ensures patient receives drugs immediately and accuratelly. (Usually priming the line reduces delivery time by approximately half an hour.) Do not alter previously calculated rate setting despite volume reduction in barrel of syringe.

GUIDELINES: INSERTING THE WINGED INFUSION SET

Action	Rationale
1. Explain the procedure to the patient.	To obtain the patient's consent and co-operation.
2. Assist the patient into a comfortable position.	
3. Expose the chosen site for infusion (see skin site selection under 'Reference material', above).	
4. Clean the chosen site with a swab saturated with 70% isopropyl alcohol. Wait until the alcohol evaporates.	To reduce the number of pathogens introduced into the skin by the needle at the time of the insertion. Reduces pain on insertion which may be caused by introducing alcohol.
5. Grasp the skin firmly.	To elevate the subcutaneous tissue.
6. Insert the infusion needle into the skin at an angle of 45° and release the grasped skin.	Shallower positioning than 45° may shorten the life of the infusion site.
7. Tape the infusion wings firmly to the skin using transparent adhesive dressing (see 'Care of the skin site' under 'Reference material', above).	Transparent dressing allows observation of the infusion site and maintains the correct position of the needle.
8. Connect the syringe to the syringe driver (see instructions below).	To ensure the syringe is connected correctly to the syringe driver.
9. Record, in the appropriate documents, that the infusion has been commenced.	To comply with local drug administration policies.

Connecting the syringe to the syringe driver

1. Place the syringe on the syringe driver along the grooved lines, with barrel clamp firmly in position.
2. Secure in place with rubber strap.
3. Slide the actuator assembly along the lead screw by pressing white release button as shown in Figure 38.4, until it rests against the end of the plunger.
4. Secure plunger with additional safety clamp (Figure 38.5).
5. Press start/test button to commence infusion. The indicator light should flash to indicate functioning syringe pump.

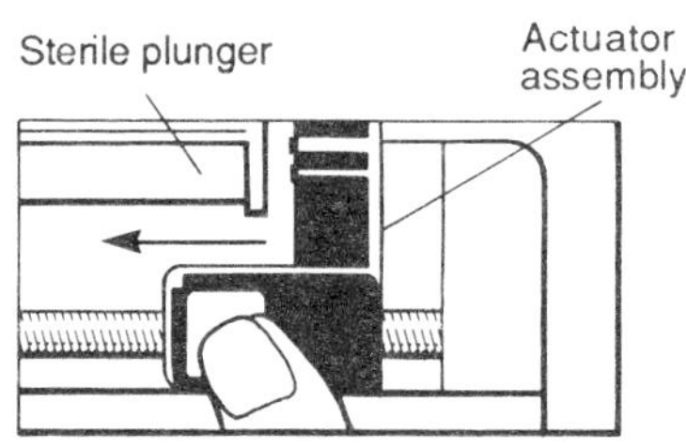

Figure 38.4 Connecting the syringe to the syringe driver.

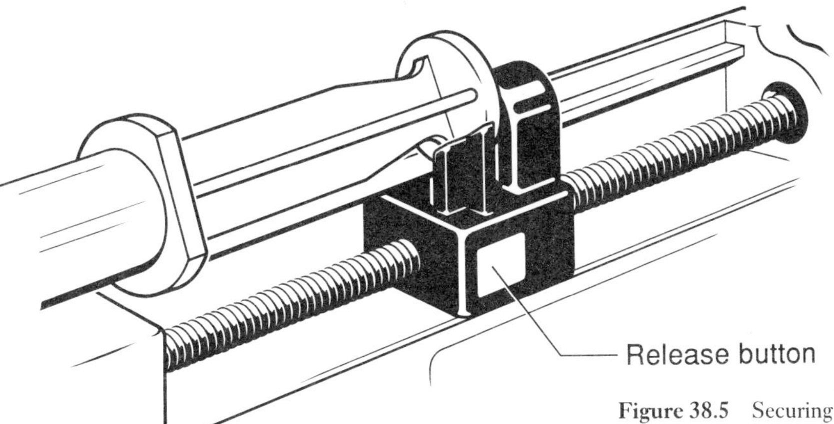

Figure 38.5 Securing the plunger with additional safety clamp.

Additional notes

1. Different manufacturers of syringes have different barrel sizes, i.e. 4 ml in a 10 ml syringe made by one company may yield a different stroke length to 4 ml in a 10 ml syringe made by another.
2. If more than one drug is to be administered, for example, analgesic and antiemetic, it is important not to increase the rate of the syringe driver to yield more pain relief, as this will increase the antiemetic dose.
3. If 'breakthrough' analgesia is required, it is preferable to administer the equivalent of a four-hourly dose as a separate extra statim subcutaneous injection. Bolus pushes using the boost button is not recommended, for the following reasons.
   (a) Those outlined in point 2 above.
   (b) A 'boost' push yields only 0.2 mm of extra analgesia.
   (c) Pain assessment is more difficult and evaluation of pain control is hindered.
   (d) Inaccuracies of infusion time may occur as a result.
4. Glyceryl trinitrate patches are to be positioned above the entry site. The pharmacological basis is that vasodilation will enhance site integrity, although this theory requires further research. This information is based on anecdotal evidence of two patients with whom site breakdown was greatly decreased with use of a glyceryl trinitrate patch.

39

Tracheostomy Care

The care of patients with a tracheostomy varies from one hospital to another. The changing of a tracheostomy tube will usually be undertaken by a doctor or a trained nurse who has been instructed in this procedure. It is important, however, that nurses are aware of the procedures and basic principles and know how to respond in an emergency situation.

Definition

A tracheostome is an artificial opening made into the trachea through the neck (Figure 39.1a) (Stell & Moran, 1978).

Indications

Tracheostomy may be carried out:

1. To provide and maintain a patent airway.
2. To enable the removal of tracheobronchial secretions.

A tracheostomy may be performed as a temporary, permanent or emergency procedure (Stell & Moran, 1978).

General care of tracheostomy patients

1. When caring for a tracheostomy patient the following should always be at the bedside or accessible if the patient is self-caring or ambulant.
   (a) Humidified oxygen with tracheostomy mask.
   (b) Suction machine with a selection of suction catheters.
   (c) Covered bowl of sodium bicarbonate (one teaspoon to 500 ml sterile water) to clear suction tubing of secretions when suctioning has been performed.
   (d) Clean disposable gloves.
   (e) Two cuffed tracheostomy tubes, one the same size as the patient is wearing, the other a size smaller, in the event of an emergency tracheostomy tube change.
   (f) One 10 ml syringe to inflate cuff on tracheostomy tube.
   (g) One clamp to ensure that air stays in cuff.
   (h) Tracheal dilators, in the event of tracheostomy tube falling out or being removed and inability to insert another tube. Tracheal dilators can be used to keep stomal opening patent until medical assistance arrives.
2. Tracheostomy tube changes are mostly dependent on the type of secretions the patient has, for example, a patient with copious, tenacious secretions will need a daily tube change, sometimes twice a day, as this will be the only way of ensuring that the stoma and tube are free from any accumulation of secretions. If the patient has minimal secretions then the necessity to change the tube decreases until some patients need to have their tube changed only weekly.

Sometimes if the patient has a wound area up to the stoma edge, the tracheostomy tube has to be removed to gain access for cleaning the wound and observing its general status.

The tracheostomy dressing can be renewed without removing the tube and this should be done daily or twice a day to ensure that any secretions are cleared, and do not lay wet against the skin and cause any excoriation.

REFERENCE MATERIAL

Types of tracheostomy

Temporary

A temporary tracheostomy (see Figure 39.1b) is performed for patients as an elective procedure, e.g. at the time of major surgery.

Permanent

A permanent tracheostomy is the creation of a tracheostome following a total laryngectomy (see Figure 39.1c). The top three tracheal cartilages are brought to the surface of the skin and sutured to the neck wall to form a stoma. The 'end' tracheostome is

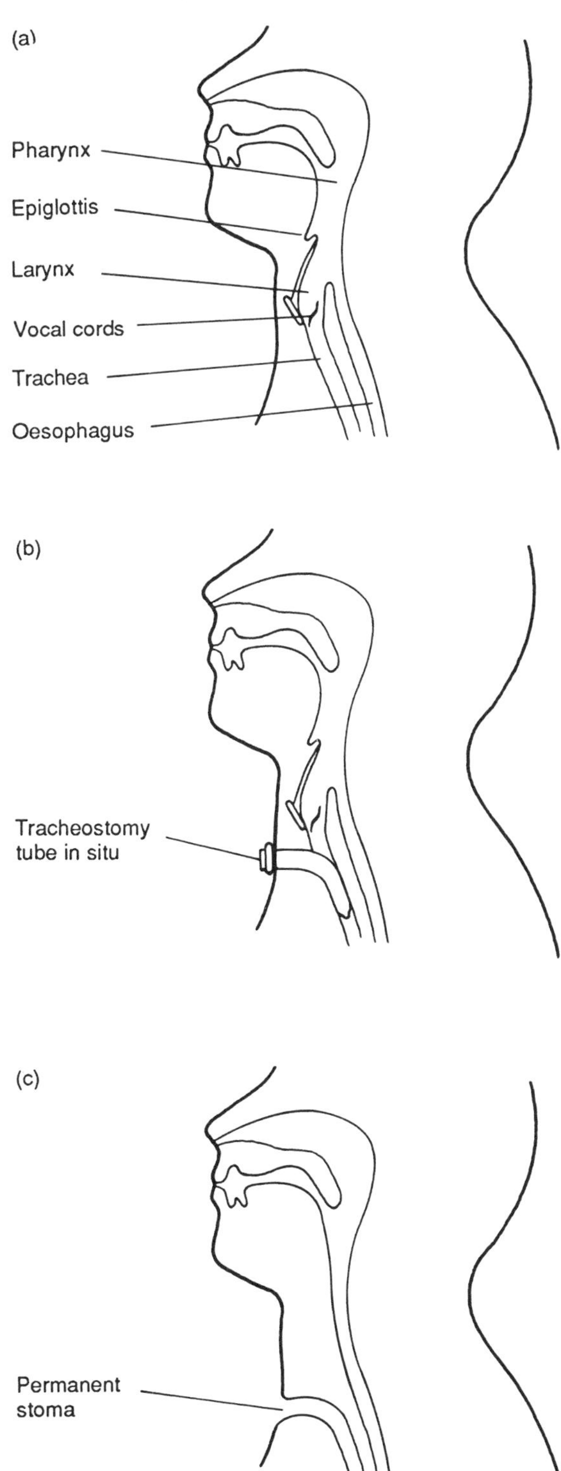

Figure 39.1 (a) Anatomy of the head and neck. (b) Temporary tracheostomy. (c) Permanent tracheostomy (total laryngectomy).

permanent and the rigidity of the tracheal cartilage keeps the stoma open. The patient will breathe through this stoma for the remainder of his/her life. As a result, there is no connection between the nasal passages and the trachea.

Emergency
A tracheostomy may be performed as an emergency procedure when a patient has an obstructed airway. Among the more common conditions causing obstruction are trauma to the airway or neck, poisoning, infections or neoplasms.

Types of tubes

Experience has shown that the choice of tracheostomy tube depends on the type of operation performed; the patient's ability to tolerate the tube depends on various external factors. A selection of tubes is listed below.

Portex cuffed tracheostomy tube
This is a disposable plastic tracheostomy tube with an introducer and inflatable cuff to give an airtight seal (Figure 39.2a). The cuff prevents blood from reaching the lungs and the seal facilitates ventilation at the time of surgery.

It is an anaesthetic tube which is usually in site for 24 to 48 hours. Depending on the patient's condition, the portex tube will be removed and the stoma left exposed, or a more suitable sturdier tube will be inserted, such as a Shiley tracheostomy tube.

Portex uncuffed tracheostomy tube
This is a disposable plastic tracheostomy tube (Figure 39.2b) used, for example, during radiotherapy to the neck area when a metal tube would cause tissue reaction.

Shiley plain tracheostomy tube (Figure 39.3a)
This is plastic tube with an introducer and two inner tubes. One inner tube has an extension at its upper aspect. This facilitates connection to other equipment, e.g. nebulizers and speaking valves.

This tube is usually used for the following reasons:

1. To keep the tracheostomy tract patent if the patient is going to have further surgery.
2. In place of a metal tracheostomy tube if the patient is going to have radiotherapy to the neck area when a metal tube would cause tissue reaction.
3. For a laryngectomy patient who has a benign or malignant stenosis of the trachea and requires a longer tube than the regular length laryngectomy tube to keep the stenosis patent.

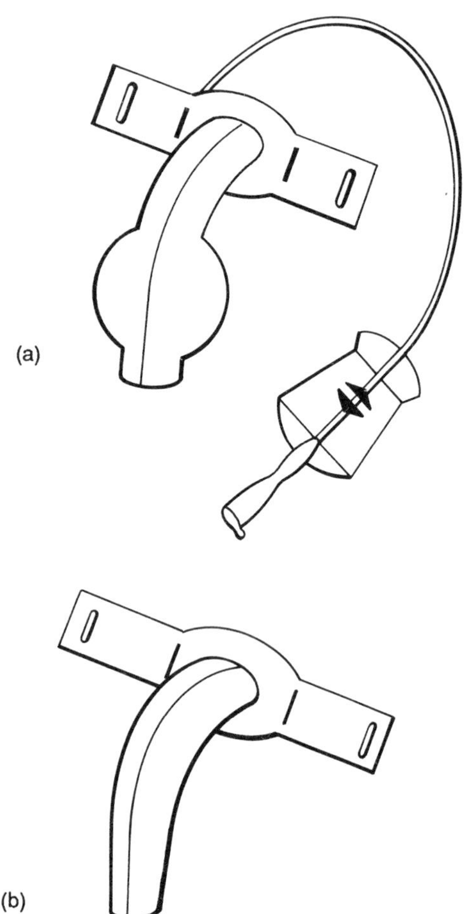

Figure 39.2 Tubes for temporary tracheostomies. (a) Portex cuffed tube. (b) Portex uncuffed tube.

4. As a weaning method. For example, the patient could occlude the tube with a cap for certain periods of time to get used to breathing normally again, until the cap can be worn for a full uninterrupted 24 hours, breathing comfortably via the oral airway.

Alternatively, the cuffless tube can be used to assist with maintaining a patent airway while the patient is learning to swallow without aspirating food.

These weaning methods can also be used with the Shiley plain fenestrated tube, and the cuffed fenestrated tube.

Shiley cuffed tracheostomy tube (Figure 39.3b)
This is a plastic tube with an introducer and two inner tubes. One inner tube has an extension at its upper aspect to facilitate connection to other equipment. The outer tube has an inflatable cuff to give an airtight seal. The cuff prevents secretions from reaching the lungs. The seal facilitates ventilation.

Shiley plain fenestrated tube (Figure 39.3c)
This is a plastic tube with an introducer and two inner tubes. One inner tube has an extension at its upper end to facilitate connection to other apparatus. The outer tube has a fenestration in the middle of the cannula. This is to encourage the passage of air and secretions into the oral and nasal passage. It is useful when attempting to encourage a return to normal function following long-term use of a temporary tracheostomy.

Shiley cuffed fenestrated tube (Figure 39.3d)
This is a plastic tube with an introducer and two inner tubes. One inner tube has an extension at its upper aspect to facilitate connection to other apparatus. The outer tube has a fenestration in the middle of the cannula, again to encourage a return to normal function. The outer tube also has an inflatable cuff to give an airtight seal. The cuff prevents secretions from reaching the lungs. This tube is useful for patients with swallowing problems but who are starting to return to normal function.

Jackson's silver tracheostomy tube
This is a silver tube with an introducer and inner tube (Figure 39.4a). The inner tube is locked in position by a small catch on the outer tube and may be removed and cleaned as necessary without disturbing the outer tube.

Negus's silver tracheostomy tube
This is a silver tracheostomy tube with an introducer and a choice of inner tubes, with and without speaking valves (Figure 39.4b). The outer tube does not have a safety catch, consequently the inner tube may be coughed out inadvertently.

Rusch speaking valve
This is a plastic device with a two-way valve which fits onto the extended aspects of the Shiley inner tube (Figure 39.5a). When breathing, the valve stays open but when the patient attempts to speak the valve closes, thus redirecting air up through the normal air passages and allowing the production of voice.

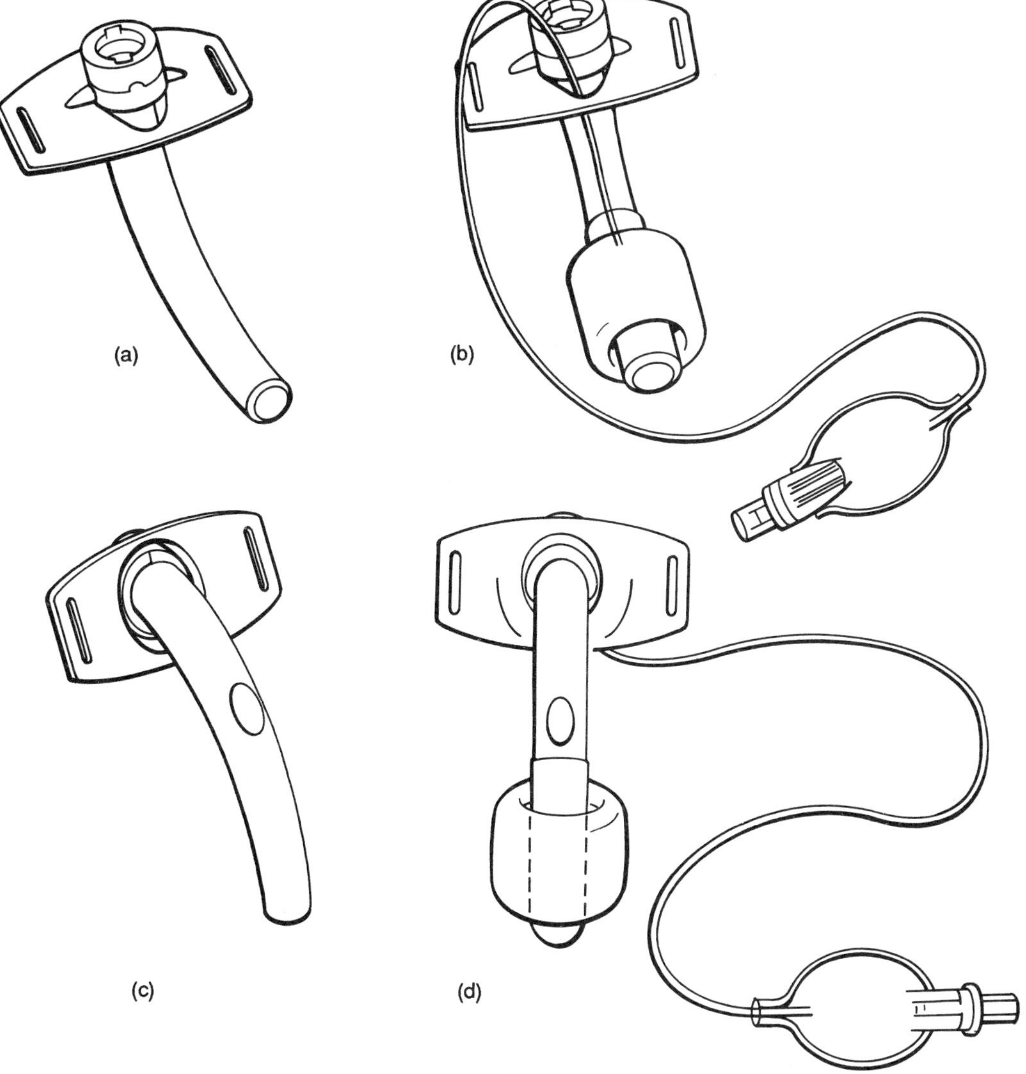

Figure 39.3 Shiley's tracheostomy tubes. (a) Shiley plain tube. (b) Shiley cuffed tube. (c) Shiley plain fenestrated tube. (d) Shiley cuffed fenestrated tube.

Shiley decannulation plug

This is a plastic inner tube with a red blind and or a small red plastic plug (Figure 39.5b) which fits in the tracheostomy tube. It should be used when encouraging patients to breath via normal air passages before removal of the tracheostomy tube.

It is not advisable to leave the red decannulation plug in a fenestrated tube for periods longer than two or three hours at a time due to the risk of granulation tissue forming in the fenestration. For longer periods the red, blind-ended decannulation inner tube should be used.

Colledge silver laryngectomy tube

This is a silver laryngectomy tube with an introducer (Figure 39.6a). It is an old-fashioned tube, often worn by laryngectomy patients who dislike their stoma being exposed.

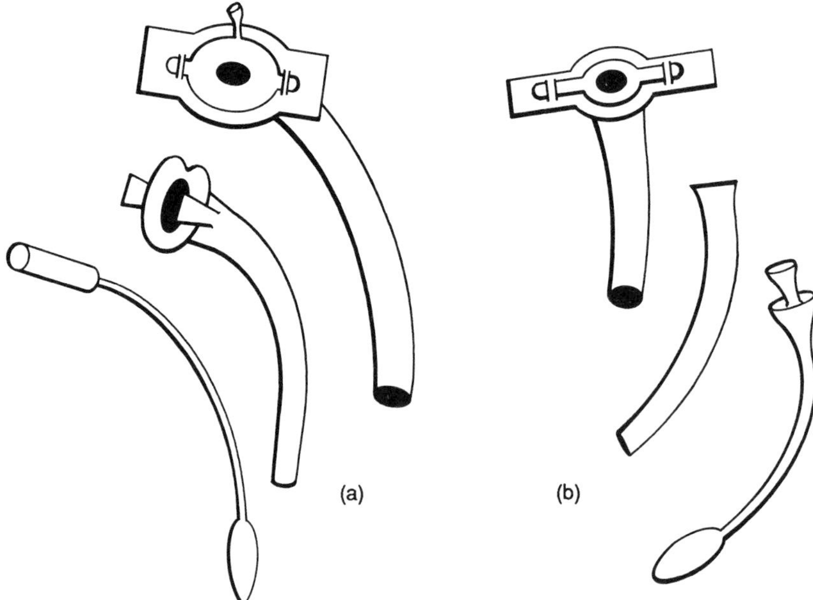

Figure 39.4 (a) Jackson's silver tube. (b) Negus's silver tube.

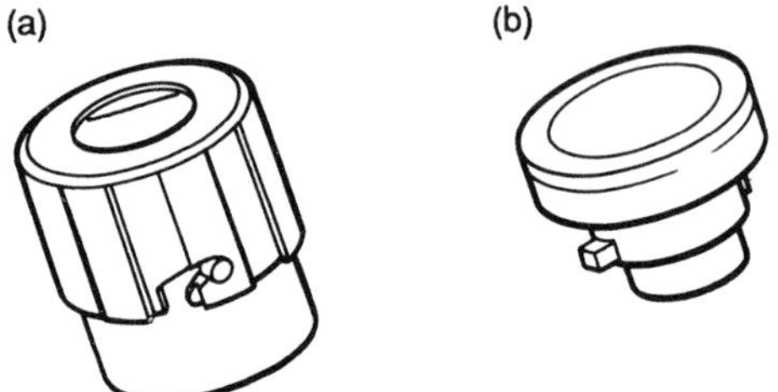

Figure 39.5 (a) Rusch speaking valve. (b) Shiley decannulation plug.

Shiley laryngectomy tube
This is a plastic tube with an introducer and inner tube (Figure 39.6b). The inner tube may be removed and cleaned frequently without disturbing the outer tube. It is sometimes worn postoperatively while the stoma is healing to help facilitate a good shaped stoma.

Shaw's silver laryngectomy tube
This is a silver laryngectomy tube with an introducer and an inner tube beyond both lower and upper aspects of the outer tube (Figure 39.6c). Thus pressure dressings may be secured without occluding the stoma. The lower extension of the tube ensures that crusting does not occur when the tube is changed regularly. The silver catch on the outer tube keeps the inner tube in position.

Stoma button
This is a soft Silastic 'button' (Figure 39.6d). It may be used in place of a laryngectomy tube. It is very light and comfortable to wear and is the appliance of choice when the patient has a blom singer speaking valve *in situ*.

References and further reading

Ballantyne, J. C. *et al.* (1978) *Otolaryngology*, 3rd edn. John Wright, Bristol.

Cox, S. & Jones, G. (1980) Head and neck nursing care. In *Cancer Nursing: Surgical* (Ed. by R. Tiffany). Faber & Faber, London.

Davis, J. (1980) Surgical treatment – preparation of the patient. I By the nurse. In *Laryngectomy, Rehabilitation Seminars* (Ed. by Poole (1978) Abindon (1980)) pp. 67–72. National Society for Cancer Relief.

Edels, Y. (1983) *Laryngectomy – Diagnosis to Rehabilitation*. Croom Helm, London.

Freud, R. H. (1979) *Principles of Head and Neck Surgery*. Appleton Century Crofts, New York.

Harris, R. B. & Hyman, R. B. (1983) Clean vs sterile tracheostomy care and level of pulmonary infection. *Nursing Research*, 33(2), 80–5.

Iveson-Iveson, J. (1981) Students' forum. Tracheostomy.

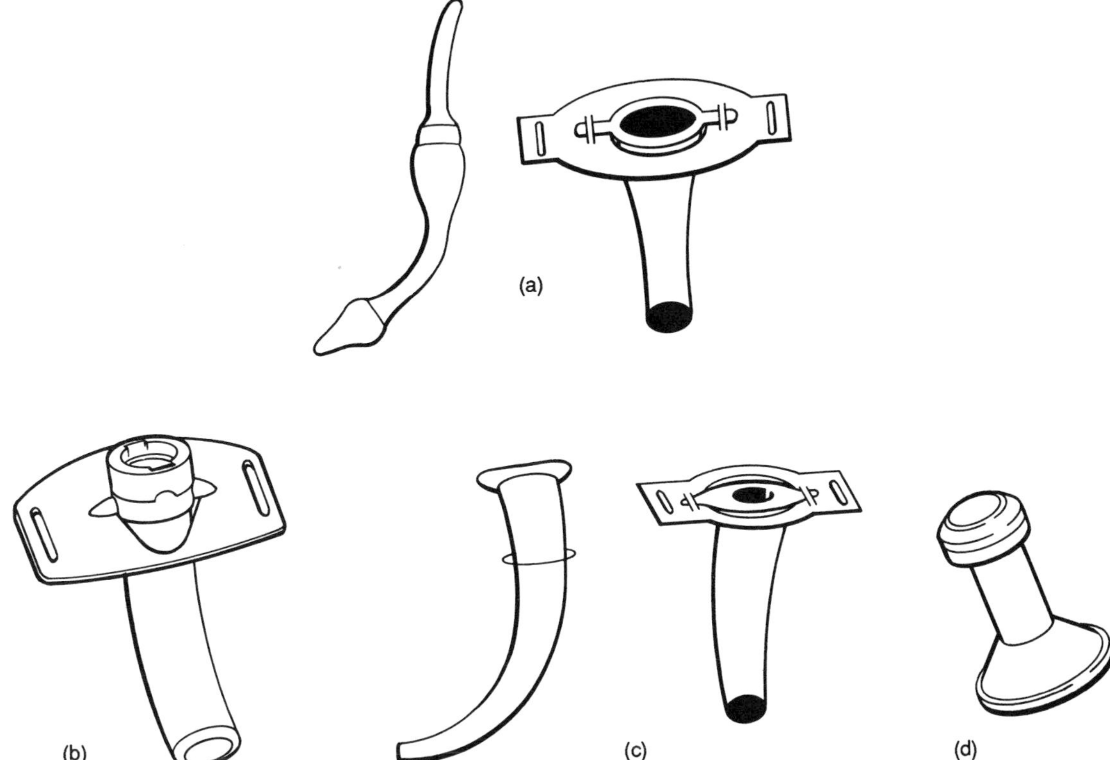

Figure 39.6 Tubes for permanent tracheostomies. (a) Colledge silver tube. (b) Shiley laryngectomy tube. (c) Shaw's laryngectomy tube. (d) Stoma button.

Nursing Mirror, 153(4), 30–1.

McKelvie, P. L. (1980) Surgical aspects of laryngectomy. In *Laryngectomy Rehabilitation Seminars* (Ed. by Poole (1978), Abindon (1980)) pp. 80–1. National Society for Cancer Relief.

McMinn, R. M. H. *et al.* (1981) *A Colour Atlas of Head and Neck Anatomy*. Wolfe Medical, London.

Moore, G. V. & Stafford, N. (1987) *Aids to Ear, Nose and Throat*. Churchill Livingstone, Edinburgh.

Nursing (US) (1976) Up to date survey of tracheal tubes. *Nursing* (US), 5(11), 66–72.

Serra, A. *et al.* (1986) *Ear, Nose and Throat Nursing*. Blackwell Scientific Publications, Oxford.

Stell, P. M. & Moran, A. G. D. (1978) *Head and Neck Surgery*. Heinemann Medical Books, London.

Thurston-Hookway, F. & Seddon, S. (1989) Care after laryngectomy. *Ear, Nose and Throat*, 3(35).

Tiffany, R. (1979) *Cancer Nursing: Surgical*. Faber & Feber, London.

Turner, A. L. (1988) *Nose, Throat and Ear*, 10th ed (Ed. by A. G. D. Moran). J. Wright, Bristol.

GUIDELINES: CHANGING A TRACHEOSTOMY DRESSING

Equipment

1. Sterile dressing pack.
2. Tracheostomy dressing or a keyhole dressing.
3. Cleaning solution, such as saline.
4. Tracheostomy tape.
5. Bactericidal alcohol hand rub.

Guidelines: Changing a tracheostomy dressing

Procedure

Action	Rationale
1. Explain the procedure to the patient.	To obtain the patient's consent and co-operation.
2. Screen the bed or cubicle.	To ensure the patient's privacy.
3. Wash hands using bactericidal soap and water or bactericidal alcohol hand rub, and prepare the dressing tray or trolley.	To reduce the risk of infection.
4. Perform the procedure using aseptic technique.	To prevent infection.
5. Remove the soiled dressing around the tube and clean around stoma with saline.	To avoid discomfort to the patient. To remove secretion and crusts.
6. Replace with a tracheostomy dressing or a comfortable keyhole dressing.	To ensure the patient's comfort. To avoid pressure from the tube.
7. Renew tracheostomy tapes.	To secure the tube.

GUIDELINES: SUCTION AND TRACHEOSTOMY PATIENTS

The aim of suction is to maintain an airway and to prevent the formation of crusts. The frequency of suction varies with individual patients, according to their needs.

Equipment

1. Suction machine (wall source or portable).
2. Areo-flow sterile suction catheters (assorted sizes; see notes below).
3. Disposable gloves.
4. Jug of sodium bicarbonate solution (one teaspoon in 500 ml water).
5. ENT spray containing sterile normal saline.
6. Disposable plastic apron.
7. Bactericidal alcohol hand rub.

Note: it is advisable to use the right size of catheter for the lumen of the tracheostomy tube; a 10FG catheter is appropriate for a 27 to 30FG tube, a 12FG catheter for a 33 to 36FG tube, a 14FG catheter for a 39FG tube.

Procedure

Action	Rationale
1. Instruct the patient to use the spray every two hours or more frequently if secretions are tenacious, i.e. two or three sprays directly into the tracheostomy.	Suction will not be achieved if the secretions become too tenacious or dry. Regular spraying minimizes this occurrence.
2. Suctioning should be taught if the patient is able to perform his/her own suction. Otherwise inform the patient what is to be done.	To obtain the patient's co-operation. The procedure is unpleasant and can be frightening for the patient. Reassurance is vital. Self-control of the patient's

suction is preferable if the patient is able to manage it.

3. Wash hands with bactericidal soap and water or bactericidal alcohol hand wash, and put on a disposable plastic apron.	To reduce the risk of cross-infection. Most patients cough directly onto the nurse's clothes after spraying or suction; standing to one side minimzies this risk.
4. Checking that the suction machine is set to the appropriate level.	Sputum which is more tenacious requires more powerful suction.
5. Open the end of the suction catheter pack and use the pack to attach the catheter to the suction tubing. Keep the rest of the catheter in the sterile packet.	To reduce the risk of transferring infection from hands to the catheter and to keep the catheter as clean as possible.
6. Put on disposable gloves and withdraw the catheter from the sleeve.	Gloves minimize the risk of infection transfer to the catheter or from the sputum to the nurse's hands.
7. Introduce the catheter to about one-third of its length and apply suction by placing the thumb over the suction port control.	Gentleness is essential; damage to the tacheal mucosa can lead to trauma and respiratory infection. The catheter should go no further than the carina to prevent trauma. The catheter is inserted with the suction turned off so as not to irritate mucous membrane.
8. Withdraw the catheter gently with a rotating motion. Do not suction the patient for more than 15 seconds at a time.	To remove secretions from around the mucous membranes. Prolonged suction will result in infection if the mucous membranes are traumatized, and the patient may experience a choking sensation.
9. Wrap catheter around gloved hand then pull back glove over soiled catheter, thus containing catheter in glove, then discard.	Catheters are used only once to reduce the risk of introducing infection.
10. Rinse the connection by dipping its end in the jug of sodium bicarbonate solution with the suction turned on to clear secretions into the receptacle.	To loosen secretions which have adhered to the inside of the tube.
11. If the patient required further suction, repeat the above actions using new gloves and a new catheter.	
12. Repeat the suction until the airway is clear.	

HUMIDIFICATION

Definition

Humidification may be defined as increasing the moisture content of air. In health, inspired air is filtered, warmed and moistened by the ciliated lining, and mucus is produced in the upper respiratory pathways. Because the upper respiratory pathways are bypassed in patients with a tracheostomy, they need artificial humidification to ensure that these pathways remain moist.

GUIDELINES: HUMIDIFICATION

Procedure

Immediate postoperative care, i.e. the first 24 to 48 hours

Action	Rationale
1. Fill a suitable nebulizer with sterile water and attach it to the oxygen supply. Set the oxygen rate at four litres per minute at 40%. Give a constant supply of humidified oxygen for 24 to 48 hours.	Constant humidification is required while new stoma adapts to the outside environment (especially for laryngectomy patients). Humidification also prevents the formation of crusts which are liable to obstruct the airway.
2. Spray saline into the trachea as necessary, using a spray or a syringe.	To loosen secretions prior to suction and to stimulate the cough reflex.
3. For patients in cubicles, a room humidifier may be placed at the bedside.	

Subsequent care

Action	Rationale
1. Give humidified oxygen as required. Usually, patients need about 10 to 15 minutes of humidification every four hours. This may be adapted according to the patient's needs, e.g. throughout the night, according to time.	Patients begin to adapt to breathing through their tracheostomy after the first 24 to 48 hours. Some humidification is required according to individual needs and to prevent crust formation in the airway.
2. If the patient does not require oxygen, blow humidifiers may be used.	These provide humidified air without the need for an oxygen supply.
3. Teach the patient to keep the tracheostomy moist by using a spray containing normal saline, before suctioning.	To loosen secretions and to prevent crust formation. To prevent contamination. Normal saline is supplied in small bottles which, if not used within 24 hours, should be changed. If a spray is used, this should be washed and dried each day and resterilized once the patient is discharged.
4. Provide bibs, such as Buchanan bibs or Romet, for patients.	To protect the airway.

GUIDELINES: CHANGING A TRACHEOSTOMY TUBE

Equipment

1. Sterile dressing pack.
2. Tracheostomy dressing or a keyhole dressing.
3. Tracheostomy tape.
4. Cleaning solution, such as normal saline.
5. Barrier cream.
6. Lubricating jelly.
7. Disposable plastic apron.
8. Bactericidal alcohol hand rub.

Procedure

Action	Rationale
1. Explain the procedure to the patient.	To obtain patient's consent and co-operation.
2. Wash hands using bactericidal soap and water or bactericidial alcohol hand rub, and prepare a dressing trolley.	
3. Screen the patient's bed.	To ensure the patient's privacy.
4. Perform the procedure using clean technique.	To prevent contamination.
5. Assist the patient to sit in an upright position, supported by pillows with the neck extended.	To ensure the patient's comfort and to maintain a patent airway. If the neck is not extended, skin folds may occlude the tracheostomy when the tube is removed.
6. Remove the dressing pack from its outer wrappings and open the tracheostomy dressing.	Technique should be clean to reduce the risk of cross-infection.
7. Put on a disposable plastic apron.	
8. Clean hands with bactericidal alcohol hand rub.	
9. Put on clean disposable plastic gloves.	To prevent infection.
10. Prepare the tracheostomy tube as outlined in steps 11 to 14.	So that the tube is ready for immediate insertion when required.
11. Thread on piece of tape through the slits in the flanges so that the tape passes behind the flange next to the stoma.	The tape is kept behind the flange to prevent it occluding the passage of air into the tracheostomy tube.
12. Put the tracheostomy dressing around the tube.	To prevent abrasion of the patient's skin by the tube.
13. Lubricate the tube sparingly with a lubricating jelly.	To facilitate insertion.
14. Remove the soiled tube from the patient's neck while asking the patient to breathe out.	Conscious expiration relaxes the patient and reduces the risk of coughing. Coughing can result in unwanted closure of the tracheostome.
15. Clean around the stoma with normal saline and dry gently. Apply barrier cream with topical swabs. (An aqueous cream may be used if the patient is having the site irradiated.)	To remove superficial organisms and crusts. Skin should not be left moist as this provides an ideal medium for the growth of micro-organisms.
16. Insert a clean tube with introducer in place, using an 'up and over' action.	Introduction of the tube is less traumatic if directed along the contour of the trachea.
17. Remove the introducer immediately.	The patient cannot breathe while the introducer is in place.
18. Place the inner tube in position.	The inner tube may be changed several times when the outer tube is in position, thus minimizing the risk

Guidelines: Changing a tracheostomy tube

Action	Rationale
	of trauma to trachea and stoma. The quantity of secretions present will determine the frequency with which the inner tube is changed.
19. Tie the tape securely at the side of the neck.	To secure the tube. Place the tie in an accessible place, at the same time ensuring that it will not cause discomfort to the patient.
20. Remove gloves and ask the patient to breathe out onto the palm of your hand.	Flow of air will be felt if the tube is in the correct position.
21. Ensure that the patient is comfortable.	
22. Clear away the trolley and equipment.	
23. Scrub the soiled tube with a brush under cold running water. If the tube is very soiled then use sodium bicarbonate to remove debris. The tube must be rinsed thoroughly and stored dry at the patient's bedside.	To remove debris that may occlude the tube and/or become a source of infection.

Note: plastic tubes should not be soaked in solutions as there is a danger that the material may absorb the solution which could then cause irritation of the trachea.

NURSING CARE PLAN

Problem	Cause	Suggested action
Profuse tracheal secretions.	Local reaction to tracheostomy tube.	Suction frequently, e.g. every one to two hours.
Lumen of tracheostomy tube occluded.	Tenacious mucus in tube.	Spray frequently with normal saline e.g. every one to three hours, and suction. Change the inner tube regularly, e.g. one- to three-hourly.
	Dried blood and mucus in the tube, especially in the postoperative period.	Provide humidified air. (For further information, see 'Guidelines: Humidification', above.)
Tracheostomy tube dislodged accidentally.	Tapes not secured adequately.	Put in a spare tube. This should be clean and ready at the bedside. *Note*: tracheal dilators must be kept at the bedside of patients with tracheostomies.
Unable to insert clean tracheostomy tube.	Unpredicated shape or angle of stoma.	Remain calm since an outward appearance of distress may cause the patient to panic and lose confidence. Lubricate the tube well and attempt to reinsert at various angles.

	Tracheal stenosis due to patient coughing, very anxious or because the tube has been left out too long.	Insert a smaller-size tracheostomy tube. If insertion still proves difficult, do not leave the patient but ask for a tube to be brought to the bed. Keep the tracheostomy patent with tracheal dilators if stenosis is pronounced until the tube is reinserted.
Tracheal bleeding following or during change of the tube.	Trauma due to suction or to the tube being changed. Presence of tumour. Granulation tissue forming in fenestration of tube.	Change the tube as planned if bleeding is minimal. For profuse bleeding, insert a cuffed tube and inflate. Inform the doctor. Suction the patient to remove the blood from the trachea.
Infected sputum.	Nature of surgery and condition of patient often predispose to infection.	Encourage the patient to cough up secretions and/or suction regularly. Change the tube and clean the stoma area frequently, e.g. four-hourly. Protect permanent stomas with a bib or gauze. Following result of sputum specimen, commence appropriate antibiotics as needed.

40

Traction

Definition

Traction may be defined as treatment in which two or more forces, or resultants of forces, are applied to distract involved parts of an injured or diseased portion of the body (Nutt, 1983).

The two forces involved are traction and counter traction. Traction is a process whereby a force is exerted on a part or parts of the body. Counter traction is a process whereby a force is exerted that opposes the direct pull of the traction. This is essential in order to overcome muscle spasm and to prevent the patient from being dragged towards the traction pull (Figure 40.1) (Heywood Jones, 1990).

Indications

Traction will control the movement of an injured part, thereby enabling bone and soft tissue to heal.

It can be used in a variety of conditions as a method of treatment. Its uses include:

1. Relieving pain and/or muscle spasm.
2. Restoring and maintaining alignment of bone following fracture.
3. Gradually correcting deformities due to contracted soft tissue.
4. Resting a diseased or inflamed joint while maintaining it in a tractional position.
5. As pre-operative measure before internal fixation.
6. As a postoperative measure to maintain the desired position.

(From Osborne & Di Giacomo, 1987; Brunner & Suddarth, 1989).

REFERENCE MATERIAL

Types of traction

The two main categories into which traction is divided are:

1. Manual.
2. Mechanical.

Manual traction

Manual traction is accomplished by an individual exerting a pulling force on another's extremity or joint by using the former's hands. This type of traction can be used to reduce fractures while mechanical traction is being adjusted or during the application of a cast. It should not be attempted by a novice. Its main use is as a primary form of traction within an accident and emergency department.

Mechanical traction

Mechanical traction uses mechanical devices and is further classified depending on the nature of attachment and the nature of the pulling force. Attachment may be to either:

1. Skin.
2. Skeleton.

The pulling force may be exerted by a variety of systems of weights and pulleys, examples of which are given here.

1. *Sliding or balanced traction.*
   Here weights and pulleys are used to apply and direct the pull of the traction. The counter traction is exerted by the weight of the patient's body, aided by gravity when the bed is tilted away from the pull of the traction (Figure 40.2).
2. *Fixed traction.*
   This is traction between two fixed points. Weights and pulleys are used to elevate the limb, not to create the pull. The patient is attached to traction apparatus at one point and the affected part is pulled away from the point of fixation by extensions and cords which are tied to the traction apparatus. The fixation point is the counter traction and the pulling extensions are the traction. This type of traction has the advantage of requiring a small degree of force. It is frequently used to reduce or eliminate muscle spasm. An example of this type of traction would be the application of a Thomas'

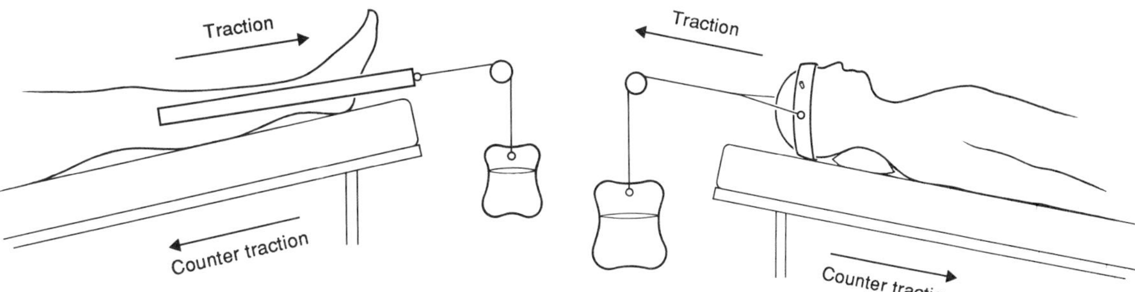

Figure 40.1 Traction and counter traction forces.

Figure 40.2 Balanced skeletal traction.

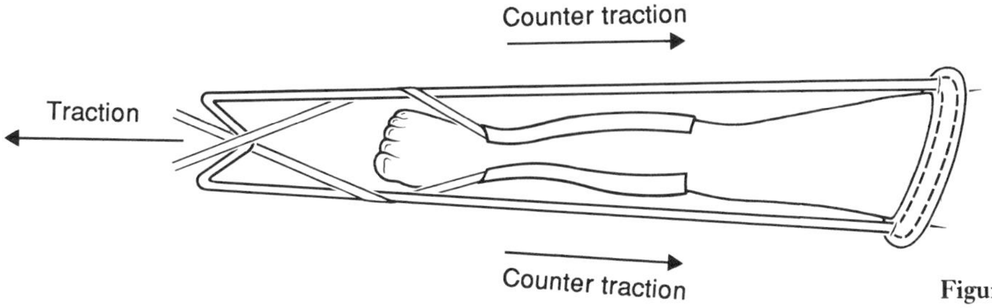

Figure 40.3 Fixed skin traction.

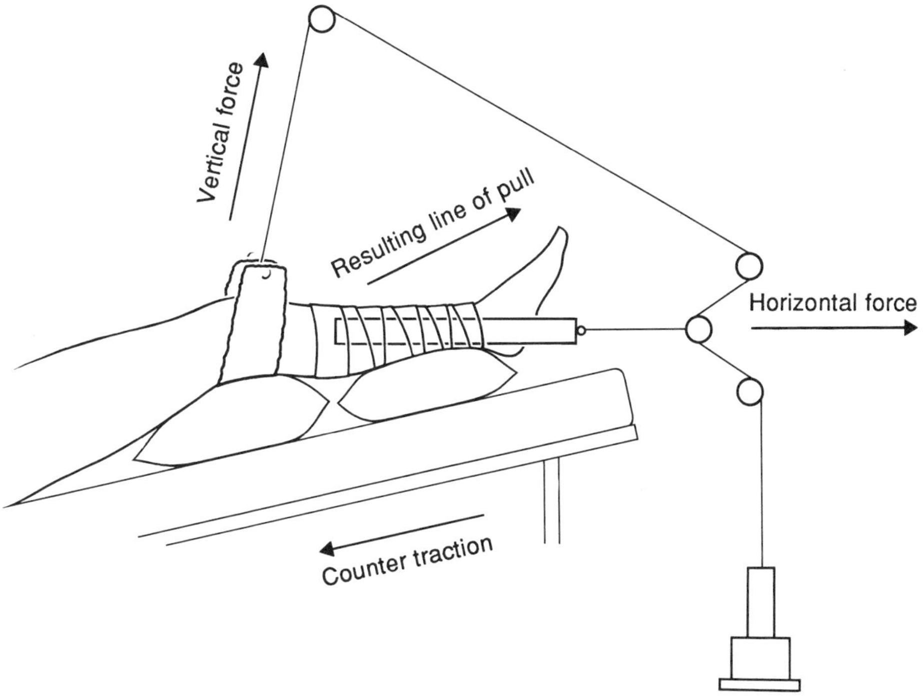

Figure 40.4 Hamilton-Russell traction, combining balanced traction with suspension.

splint to a leg using skin extensions tied to the end of the splint (Taylor, 1987) (Figure 40.3).

3. *Weight and pulley.*
A pulley is a wheel with a grooved edge suspended on an axle around which it rotates in a framework or block. A pulley block is a grouping of two or three pulleys on a single common axle in a frame. This type of traction may be a simple system using a single pulley to alter the direction of the force so that weights can be suspended conveniently, or a compound system using a number of pulleys in combination to increase the efficiency of the force applied as well as altering the direction. In all weighted traction the weights must hang freely and not touch the side of the bed or the floor (Figure 40.4).

SKIN TRACTION

Skin traction can be applied in a variety of ways. Extensions, slings or splints can be applied to the limbs; belts, halters and slings can be used for the spine or pelvis. Traction on the skin transmits traction to the musculoskeletal structures.

Skin is susceptible to damage from large traction forces applied for more than a few days. Therefore its use is limited to conditions where a relatively light or intermittent pull is required. Weights with a direct pull on skin do not generally exceed 3.6 kg since this can lead to skin necrosis (Cassels, 1983a).

Application of skin traction

The application of skin traction is generally contra-indicated in the presence of an existing skin condition, e.g. wounds, sores, abrasions, where the skin is thin and friable, where there is circulatory impairment or loss of normal skin sensation (Morris *et al.*, 1988a).

The application of skin traction may be painful. To minimize the patient's pain, the following principles should be adhered to:

1. Skill and gentleness are required when handling the affected part.
2. Manual traction must be maintained.
3. The traction should be applied with speed and dexterity.
4. The skin extension to which the traction will be attached should be applied on both sides of the limb, leaving a strip of skin free in order to prevent a constrictive tourniquet effect; when applied to a fractured limb the extension should not extend above the fracture site or traction will be exerted at the wrong site (Taylor, 1987).

There are two different types of skin extension:

1. Adhesive.
2. Non-adhesive.

Non-adhesive extensions are used on fragile skin. They are usually commercially available and consist of soft-vented foam rubber attached to a traction cord and weight, held in place by bandages. The weight applied is usually limited to 3.2 kg because the grip is less secure than that obtained by adhesive skin extensions (Taylor, 1987).

Adhesive skin extensions are used on intact skin in good condition. They are commercially available and consist of 'non-stretch' Elastoplast with padding to protect bony prominences. They are attached in a similar way but are more secure.

Most self-adhesive skin traction kits contain zinc oxide. A disadvantage of these is that some patients develop a reaction in the form of contact dermatitis. Hypo-allergenic kits are available and it is worth checking with the patient for previous allergies before application (Taylor, 1987).

References and further reading

Brunner, L. & Suddarth, D. (1989) *The Lippincott Manual of Medical–Surgical Nursing*, 2nd edn, Harper & Row, London.

Cassels, C. (1983a) Fundamentals of long bone traction – Part II. *Critical Care Update*, 10(4), 26–31.

Cassels, C. (1983b) Fundamentals of long bone traction – Part III. *Critical Care Update*, 10(5), 38–9.

Heywood Jones, I. (1990) Making sense of traction. *Nursing Times*, 86(23), 39–41.

Howard, M. & Corbo Pelia, S. (1982) Psychological after-effects of halo traction. *American Journal of Nursing*, 82, 1839–43.

Jones-Walton, P. (1988) Effects of pin care on pin reactions in adults with extremity fracture treated with skeletal traction. *Orthopaedic Nursing*, 7(4), 29–33.

Morris, L. *et al.* (1988a) Special care for skeletal traction. *Nursing Times*, 86(23), 24–9.

Morris, L. *et al.* (1988b) Nursing the patient in traction. *Registered Nurse*, January, S1, 26–31.

Nutt, R. (1983) Orthopaedic traction and the physical therapist. *Clinical Management*, 3(2), 21–4.

Osborne, L. & Di Giacomo, I. (1987) Traction: a review with nursing diagnoses and interventions. *Orthopaedic Nursing*, 6(4), 13–19.

Powell, M. (1986) *Orthopaedic Nursing and Rehabilitation*, 9th edn. Churchill Livingstone, Edinburgh.

Quain, M. & Tecklin, J. S. (1985) Lumbar traction: its effect on respiration. *Physical Therapy*, 65(9), 1343–6.

Smith, C. (1984) Nursing the patient in traction. *Nursing Times*, 80, 36–9.

Stewart, J. D. M. & Hallet, J. P. (1983) *Traction and Orthopaedic Appliances*, 2nd edn. Churchill Livingstone, Edinburgh.

Taylor, I. (1987) *Ward Manual of Orthopaedic Traction.* Churchill Livingstone, Edinburgh.

GUIDELINES: SKIN TRACTION

There are different types of skin traction, and different mechanical devices may be used to apply traction. This section is intended to give an overview. If in doubt about any procedure, a more exhaustive orthopaedic text should be consulted (Powell, 1986; Stewart & Hallet, 1983; Taylor, 1987).

Procedure

Adhesive

Action	Rationale
1. Explain the procedure to the patient.	To obtain the patient's consent and co-operation.
2. Ensure privacy for the patient while carrying out the procedure.	Maintains patient dignity.
3. Ensure that the affected part is clean and the skin intact.	To prevent infection from developing.
4. Shave any limb covered by thick, tough hairs.	To ensure that adhesive sticks to the skin and not to the hairs. The part affected will be sore if the traction is applied to the hair follicles only.
5. If possible, leave the ankle joint free.	To allow full plantar flexion and dorsiflexion in the foot in order to prevent stiffness and deformity.
6. If the lower limb is for traction, apply pieces of felt or latex foam to the malleoli and other bony prominences.	To protect them from friction. To prevent the development of pressure ulcers.
7. Leave the patellae and the knee 10 to 15° off full flexion.	To prevent limb deformity and joint stiffness.
8. The limb may be painted or sprayed with tincture of benzoin compound (Taylor, 1987).	To reduce moisture through perspiration. To increase the adhesive quality of the material used. To act as a barrier to the adhesive in the event of the patient developing contact dermatitis.
9. Apply the extension strapping and bandage without folds or creases.	To prevent discomfort. To prevent skin deterioration under the strapping.
10. Ensure that the part affected is in the correct anatomical position, e.g. feet and patellae pointing upwards when patient is in the supine position.	To prevent limb deformity.
11. Check the temperature and colour of the extremity affected as required, together with the degree of sensation and movement.	To ensure that the tension of strapping is correct, and that circulation and nerve pathways to the extremity are not being compromised.

Non-adhesive

As above, but omit steps 4 and 8.

Guidelines: Skin traction

Removing skin traction

Care must be taken to avoid skin damage during removal of adhesive extensions. Peeling the edges back slowly while pulling the skin taut is less damaging than trying to remove the adhesive quickly. Analgesia may be required. Adhesive solvents should be used where necessary. Manual traction should be maintained unless treatment is to be discontinued.

SKELETAL TRACTION

Skeletal traction is applied directly to bone by means of pins, wires or traction screws. It affords a greater degree of comfort than skin traction and is the preferred method when traction is required over long periods. More weight can be applied as this is a direct pull on bone (Taylor, 1987). It is important to note that skeletal traction is not applied directly to broken bone but to a bone on the other side of the joint, e.g. with a fractured femur the pin is applied through the tibia, not the femur.

It is used to overcome the powerful pull of muscles in the management of fractures of the lower limbs, pelvis and cervical spine. Weights of up to 18 kg can be used, depending on the fracture and the density of the bone at the site of insertion (Taylor, 1987). Skeletal traction can be applied to the skull, the proximal end of the ulna, the distal end of the femur, the proximal and distal ends of the tibia and the calcaneus (Morris *et al.*, 1988b). Lighter weights can be used instead of skin traction when the latter is contraindicated.

The insertion of skeletal traction is a surgical procedure performed under strict aseptic conditions. It is important that subsequent dealings with entry sites are also performed using aseptic techniques.

Complications

Preventing pin tract infections is a major priority. Infection at the insertion site can spread easily to bone and lead to osteomyelitis (Morris, 1988a). A predisposing factor to pin site infection apart from poor insertion technique is loosening of the pin or wire causing movement between the pin and surrounding tissues. Use of a threaded pin may prevent this.

Jones-Walton (1988) reviewed the effects of pin care on infectious pin reactions. Results showed that consistent application of routine pin care with hydrogen peroxide did not prevent pin reactions in those subjects with external fixators. Findings also suggested that factors such as fracture type, kind of traction and length of time pins were present may have had an impact on pin reaction development (sample size, 12). It is interesting to note that the three patients who did not receive pin care remained reaction free.

Other complications which can occur with skeletal traction include:

1 Traction on a pin or bending of the pin can result in local tissue damage such as necrosis, or tearing of the skin. This can be relieved by a surgeon incising the skin locally to allow for this slight amount of pin migration. The skin will usually heal behind the pin (Cassels, 1983b).
2. Pins improperly placed or placed in osteoporotic bone can actually pull out of the bone and create a new small fracture. Thus, observing for this is an essential part of nursing care. Improper placement can also lead to damage of surrounding tissues (Cassels, 1983b)
3. Over-pull and distraction of bone fragments are more likely to occur with the use of skeletal traction, rather than with skin traction due to the fact that heavier weights can be tolerated. Over-distraction will lead to delayed healing (Taylor, 1987).
4. Taylor (1987) reports that neurovascular damage can result from the use of heavy traction forces. It is important that neurovascular status of the injured and treated limb is established and evaluated at regular intervals so that later observations can highlight any progressive dysfunction. Taylor suggests that, as a general guideline, checks should be carried out hourly for 24 hours following the initial injury, surgery, application of cast, splint or traction. If there is no evidence of neurovascular compromise after this, the checks should be carried out four-hourly and should include evaluation of:
   (a) *Circulation.*
   Assessment of circulatory status involves monitoring colour, temperature, capillary refill in nail beds, and pulses. This should be compared to the unaffected limb.

(b) *Movement*.
This assessment involves the ability to contract muscle groups below the level of injury. Inability to do so may indicate compromised nerve function.

(c) *Sensation*.
Changes in sensation can also indicate compromised nerve function or compromised circulation.

Quain and Tecklin (1985) undertook a study to examine the effects of lumbar traction on respiration using 30 healthy volunteers. They found that application of lumbar traction significantly reduced inspiratory vital capacity and tidal volume. They suggested that when lumbar traction is used for patients who have respiratory disease, the patients should be observed closely for signs of respiratory distress during the first few treatments.

Removing skeletal traction

Skeletal traction should not be discontinued except under medical orders or in an emergency situation (e.g. cardiac arrest). Premature discontinuation can lead to muscle spasm and displacement of bone at fracture site causing delayed healing (Morris *et al.*, 1988a).

Removing skeletal traction pins

Removal technique will depend on the type of pin used, for example, a Denham pin will need to be unscrewed until the threaded section is free of the bone, whereas a Steinmann's pin is simply pulled out. Analgesia will be necessary. Skeletal traction is generally removed on the ward, using aseptic technique.

Taylor (1987) suggests that scarring at pin removal sites can be minimized by firmly pinching the pin tract at time of removal so that the adhesion of skin to deeper tissue is broken, giving a better cosmetic result.

GENERAL PRINCIPLES FOR THE CARE OF PATIENTS ON TRACTION

Maintenance of effective traction therapy

Care of apparatus (from Brunner & Suddarth, 1989; Smith, 1984)

1. Traction apparatus should be checked at regular intervals to ensure that the direction of the pull is correct; the cords are unobstructed; that weights are in proper position; and that the patient is comfortable.
2. Cords on pulleys should be freely movable. The cord should not have any frays or knots.
3. The traction must be continuous to be effective unless prescribed as intermittent, as with pelvic traction.
4. Weights should be of the correct prescription and should always hang freely and never rest on the floor, bed or chair.
5. The angle of elevation of the bed should not be altered as this affects the force of traction.
6. With *fixed* traction, the patient may not be turned without disrupting the line of the pull.
7. With *balanced* traction, the patient may be elevated, turned slightly and moved as desired.
8. A bed cradle should be used to prevent the pressure of the bedclothes interfering with the traction forces.

Care of the patient

A patient may be receiving traction therapy for prolonged periods of time. Thus, general complications associated with prolonged bedrest may occur, particularly in elderly, frail, immobilized patients. These include deep vein thrombosis and/or pulmonary embolism, chest infection, pressure sores, urinary stasis and constipation. (See Chapter 7, Bowel Care; Chapter 46, Wound Management (including pressure ulcers)). Nursing intervention should be aimed at preventing these complications.

Scant literature is available on the psychological effects of prolonged traction on patients and/or nurses. Howard and Corbo Pelia (1982) Offer an assessment of a patient who underwent halo traction.

NURSING CARE PLAN

Problem	Cause	Suggested action
Irritation or burning of skin under skin extensions.	Allergic reaction to skin extensions.	Inform appropriate personnel. Remove supporting material if appropriate. Use non-adhesive skin extensions.
Inadequate traction and potential skin excoriation.	Slipping skin extensions.	Reapply.
Pressure ulcers over bony prominences.	Inadequate padding of vulnerable areas.	Provide adequate padding; ensure bandages are not too tight.
Nerve palsy.	Leg rolled into lateral rotation compressing common peroneal nerve against supporting slings.	Check alignment of leg regularly. Assess patient's ability to dorsiflex the ankle. Check sensation.
Paraesthesia or coldness of affected part.	Supporting material bound too tightly.	Re-bandage.
Joint irritation or displacement of bone at fracture site.	Insufficient traction.	Ensure sufficient traction.
Delayed union or non-union of fracture.	Over-distraction at fracture site.	Inform appropriate personnel. Realign.
Pin slipping from side to side, carrying an area of non-sterile pin into the bone or tissue.	Pin is loose. Perhaps an area of necrotic or osteoporotic bone around the pin.	Report to medical staff.
Joint stiffness or muscle wasting.	Poor positioning and prolonged inactivity.	Report to medical staff and physiotherapist. Liaise about exercises.
Low-grade osteomyelitis.	Infection at site of entry.	Inform appropriate personnel. Ensure strict aseptic technique when attending to lesion.

41

Transfusion of Blood and Blood Products

Definition

A transfusion consists of the administration of whole blood or any of its components to correct or treat a clinical abnormality.

Indications

The range of products currently available, those most widely used, indications for their use and recommendations for administration are listed in Table 41.1.

REFERENCE MATERIAL

There are several problems or potential problems associated with the administration of blood or its components which can be classified as either immediate reactions or long-term complications.

Immediate reactions to blood transfusion

Fever

There are several causes of the development of the fever:

Pyrogenic reaction

This is probably the most common cause of fever. Pyrogens are the breakdown material from bacteria in the blood before sterilization (Davies & Brozovic, 1990).

The normal sequence seen is a rise in the patient's temperature without the signs and symptoms of shock, followed by the pyrexia subsiding when the transfusion is slowed. It is not thought to be a serious complication.

White cell antibody and platelet antibody reaction

Just as red blood cells have genetically transmitted antigens on their surface membrane from which the blood group is determined, so too have white cells. White cell antigens are more complex and are mainly linked with the human leucocyte antigen (HLA) system.

If a patient receives a number of transfusions he/she may develop antibodies against the foreign antigens. If transfusions containing white cells with similar antigens are then administered, the patient's previously manufactured antibodies will react against these (Huws & Brozovic, 1990).

White cell antibody reactions tend to be more severe than a pyrogenic reaction, showing signs and symptoms of chill and high fever. Platelet antibody reaction is very similar to white cell antibody reactions.

Both problems are normally associated with multiple transfusions but in the case of multigravida women the same reaction may occur on their first transfusion.

Foreign protein antibody reaction

This problem is very rarely seen and is associated with the development of antibodies to proteins present in the plasma of the transfused blood.

Infection

Infection can be bacterial growth in the transfusion product or it can be inadvertently introduced during cannulation or connection of giving set and transfusion bag.

Usually there is a brief period of the patient feeling hot, often associated with chest and abdominal pain, then the patient becomes severely shocked with a fall in blood pressure and a subnormal temperature. Later a pyrexia occurs (Watson & Royle, 1987).

Allergic reactions

These are often caused by the development of anti-immunoglobulin A (IgA) antibodies in the patient's plasma reacting against IgA protein in the transfused blood.

The reaction may be mild where the pyrexia is minimal with a rash soon appearing, or severe with

Table 41.1 Blood and products used for transfusion

Type	*Description*	*Indications*	*Cross-matching*	*Shelf life*	*Average infusion time*	*Technique*	*Special considerations*
Whole blood	Complete unadulterated blood, approx. 520 ml including anticoagulant	To restore blood volume lost due to massive, acute haemorrhage whatever the cause	ABO and Rh	28–35 days at 4–6°C (dependent on anticoagulant)	2–4 hours/unit	Give via a blood administration set	The prescription of whole blood will depend on a medical assessment of the patient's circulating blood volume
*Plasma reduced blood (packed red blood cells)	Whole blood minus approx. 200 ml plasma, and anticoagulant; haematocrit 60–65%	To correct red blood cell deficiency and improve oxygen-carrying capacity of the blood	ABO and Rh	21 days at 4–6°C	2–4 hours/unit	As above	–
Red cells in optimal additive solutions	Red cells minus all plasma: 100 ml fluid used as replacement to give optimal red cell preservation; haematocrit 60–65%	As above	ABO and Rh	35 days at 4–6°C	1–2 hours/unit	As above	An example of a replacement solution is saline/adenine/ glucose/mannitol
*Concentrated red cells	Plasma removed to produce a haematocrit of 70% plus	To correct anaemias when expansion of blood volume will not be tolerated	ABO and Rh	21 days at 4–6°C	1–2 hours/unit	As above	Availability varies
*Washed red blood cells	Red cells centrifuged free of plasma and resuspended in saline	To increase red cell mass and prevent tissue antigen formation in: 1. Immunosuppressed patients 2. Patients with previous transfusion reactions	ABO and Rh	Use within 12 hours or preferably immediately	1–2 hours/unit	As above	–

Frozen red blood cells	1. Cells from normal healthy donor with very rare blood group	To treat transplant patients or patients with atypical antibodies which react with almost the entire population	ABO and Rh	Stored frozen cells: 3 years. Use within 12 hours of thawing	2–3 hours/unit	As above	Available from a few centres. Freezing process and recovery are time consuming and expensive
	2. Patient's own cells taken in anticipation of later illness (autologous blood transfusion)	To increase safety of tranfusion therapy					
Leucocyte-poor blood	Red cells from which accompanying leucocytes have been removed	To prevent further reactions in patients who have had febrile attacks when receiving whole or plasma reduced blood	ABO and Rh	4–6°C. Time stated on pack. Usually within 12 hours of preparation, preferably immediately	2–3 hours/unit	As above	Frozen red cells may be used as an alternative
*White blood cells (leucocyte concentrate)	Mainly granulocytes obtained by leucophoresis or by 'creaming off' the buffy layers from packs of fresh blood	To treat patients with life-threatening granulocytopaenia, e.g. due to chemotherapy	ABO and HLA (human leucocyte group A antigen)	24 hours after collection. Stored at 5°C	60–90 minutes/unit	Administer via a blood administration set. Usually 1 unit only	White blood cell infusion *induces* fever, may cause hypertension, rigors and confusion. Treat symptoms and reassure patient. Preparation may be irradiated to prevent initiation of graft versus heart (GVH) disease in bone marrow transplant patients. Do not give to patients receiving amphotericin B

Table 41.1 *Continued*

Type	*Description*	*Indications*	*Cross-matching*	*Shelf life*	*Average infusion time*	*Technique*	*Special considerations*
*Platelets	Platelet sediment from platelet-rich plasma, resuspended in 40–60 ml plasma	To treat thrombocyto-paenia due to 1. Decreased production 2. Increased destruction 3. Functionally abnormal platelets 4. Dilutional problems following massive transfusions	Preferred but not essential	Up to 5 days after collection at 22°C, with continuous gentle agitation; best within 6 hours	20–30 minutes/unit	Administration using a component set is preferred. Flush the line with 100 ml normal saline after the infusion to ensure full dose is delivered. Do not use micro-aggregate filters	General guide to use: 1. Count less than 10×10^9/litre 2. Count 10–20 × 10^9/litre with haemorrhage 3. Count 20–50 × 10^9/litre or on chemotherapy may need platelets Prophylactic use in the absence of haemorrhage is controversial
Plasma: fresh or fresh, frozen (FFP)	Citrated plasma separated from whole blood. All coagulation factors preserved for several months	To treat a clotting factor deficiency, when specific concentrates are unavailable or precise deficiency is unknown, e.g. DIC	ABO compatibility; Rh preferred	Fresh: within 6 hours after collection. FFP: 12 months at −25°C. Use immediately after thawing	15–45 minutes/unit (approx. 200 ml)	Administer rapidly via a blood administration set	500 ml of FFP should be transfused after 8 units of blood (when massive transfusions given) to prevent dilutional hypocoagulability
Albumin 4.5% (plasma protein fraction)	Solution of selected proteins from pooled plasma in a buffered, stabilized saline diluent. Usually 400-ml bottle	To treat hypovolaemic shock or hypoproteinaemia due to burns, trauma, surgery or infection	Unnecessary	5 years at 2°C, 3 years at 25°C; store in the dark	30–60 minutes/unit	Administer via a blood administration set	Heated at 60°C for 10 hours to inactivate hepatitis virus. The solution should be crystal clear with no deposits

Salt poor human albumin 20%	Heat treated, aqueous chemically processed fraction of pooled plasma	To treat hypovolaemic shock or hypoproteinaemia due to burns, trauma, surgery or infection. To maintain appropriate electrolyte balance	Unnecessary	5 years at 2°C, 3 years at 25°C; store in the dark	30–60 minutes/unit	Administer via a blood administration set undiluted or diluted with saline or 5% glucose solution. Slower administration is advised if a cardiac disorder is present to avoid gross fluid shift	Heated at 60°C for 10 hours to inactivate hepatitis virus. The solution should be crystal clear with no deposits
Factor VIII (cryoprecipitates, dried anti-haemophilic globulin concentrates)	Cold-insoluble portion of plasma recovered from FFP – amount of factor VIII varies. Potency in freeze-dried concentrates can be assayed more reliably	To control bleeding disorders due to lack of factor VIII or fibrinogen, e.g. haemophilia, Von Willebrand's disease	ABO compatibility between donor plasma and recipient's red blood cells	Cryoprecipitates at −30°C for 1 year. Use immediately after thawing. Freeze-dried concentrates at +4°C. Reconstitute at room temperature and use immediately	15–30 minutes via infusion, 10–15 minutes via intravenous push	Administer rapidly via syringe or component set. Flush each unit with saline to obtain maximum dose	Heat treated 80°C for 72 hours to eliminate risk of hepatitis or HIV contamination, as multiple donors and imported preparation; limited availability
Dried factor IX concentrate	Preparation contains factor IX, prothrombin and factor X. Some may contain factor VII	To correct bleeding disorders due to lack of these factors, e.g. Christmas disease	Unnecessary	Refer to individual expiry dates	15–30 minutes	Administer via a blood administration set. Dose varies	As above. Limited availability

* Most commonly used blood products.

the development of oedema around the eyes and/or around the larynx with accompanying dyspnoea. A severe attack warrants urgent treatment.

It is essential to determine the exact nature and probable cause of fever as treatment, and the urgency with which it is implemented, may vary considerably.

Blood group antibodies

If a patient's blood contains blood group antibodies then haemolysis of the transfused blood can occur. This happens when blood is not cross-matched before transfusion or if blood is required urgently and certain antibodies are not detected in the cross-matching technique used in an emergency.

Occasionally, the reaction is such that the only sign of incompatibility is no increase in the patient's haemoglobin post-transfusion (Pritchard & David, 1988). However, the patient may experience a feeling of heat along the vein, flushing of the face and pain in the lumbar area and chest. Shock then follows with a fall in blood pressure. Urine output falls and the patient may become anuric and renal failure may develop (Pritchard & David, 1988).

Due to the rapid destruction of transfused red cells and the thromboplastin substances released from them, intravascular coagulation occurs, clotting factors are used up and the patient may develop a haemorrhagic diathesis. Therefore if the transfusion is being performed for a bleeding episode, the condition could be worsened (Pritchard & David, 1988).

Citrate and potassium intoxication

Due to the method used to prevent blood to be transfused form clotting, i.e. the use of acid citrate dextrose (ACD) or citrate phosphate dextrose (CPD) during storage, some potassium is passed from the red cells into the plasma. If blood is then transfused in large quantities or if the patient has hepatic or renal disease, the citrate and potassium levels in the patient's blood may become toxic and could lead to heart damage.

Long-term complications of blood transfusion

These are associated with the bacterial, parasitic and viral diseases that can be transmitted via a blood transfusion.

Bacterial infections

Bacterial infections of blood are now rare due to good collection methods. When they do occur they can rapidly be fatal, therefore as soon as it is suspected that a contaminated unit is being transfused, it should be stopped and blood samples from the patient and the unit of blood sent to the blood bank and microbiology department for investigation.

Reactions to contaminated blood usually develop quickly and include chills, rigors, fever, nausea, vomiting, pain and hypotension (Barbara *et al.*, 1990a).

The two bacterial diseases that have in the past been spread via blood transfusion are brucellosis and syphilis. Today, donors with a history of brucellosis are not accepted. *Treponema pallidum*, the cause of syphilis, can only be transmitted by fresh blood and platelets as it is inactivated by refrigeration for 72 hours. Screening for the *Treponema pallidum* antibody is mandatory. In very rare instances, both these bacterial infections have been reported post-transfusion.

Parasitic infections

Of the parasitic infections transmittable by blood, malaria is the most important. This organism is restricted to red blood cells, but may contaminate components such as platelets. Prevention depends on careful questioning of donors about foreign travel, and postponement of donation by those who have recently visited areas in which the disease is endemic (Hewitt *et al.*, 1990).

Occasional transmission still occurs in the United Kingdom despite the careful taking of histories. Of 18 374 cases of malaria in Britain, reported to the Malaria Reference Laboratory, between 1977 and 1986, only four were caused by blood transfusion (Barbara *et al.*, 1990b).

Viral infections

Most of transfusion-transmitted infections are caused by viruses and include:

1. Hepatitis B delta agent.
2. Hepatitis A (rarely).
3. Hepatitis non-A non-B (and possibly other hepatitis viruses).
4. HIV I and II (human immunodeficiency virus).
5. Cytomegalovirus.
6. Epstein-Barr virus.
7. HTLV I and II (human T-cell leukaemia virus).

The safety of blood relies on self-exclusion by potential donors who are at risk of contracting viruses that are transmissible by blood transfusion (Barbara *et al.*, 1990b). A survey in Glasgow for the regional health board showed that a third of people interviewed, incorrectly believed that they could be infected with HIV by giving blood (*AIDS Newsletter*, 1991).

Hepatitis B

Screening for hepatitis B surface antigen (HBsAg) is

mandatory. In the United Kingdom, hepatitis B virus is detected in 1 in 1000 donors or less because donors at risk of having HIV and hepatitis B are now excluding themselves (Barbara *et al.*, 1990b). Non-A and non-B hepatitis has now been shown usually to be due to a virus which has been called hepatitis C.

In the future the likely classification of viruses causing viral hepatitis is as follows (Barbara *et al.*, 1990b):

1. Hepatitis A virus – infectious hepatitis.
2. Hepatitis B virus – serum hepatitis.
3. Hepatitis C virus – principal } agents of non-A non-B hepatitis
4. Hepatitis ? virus – less common } agents of non-A non-B hepatitis
5. Hepatitis D virus – delta agent.
6. Hepatitis E virus – enteric or epidemic.

Human immunodeficiency virus (HIV I)

Before mandatory screening in 1985, HIV had been transmitted by most blood products including red cells, platelets, fresh frozen plasma and factor VIII and factor IX concentrates. Consequently, a large number of haemophiliacs were infected with HIV, as were a smaller number of people receiving the other blood products. The prevalence is now 1 in 70 000 of United Kingdom donors, and the risk of infection being transmitted by blood components is 1 in 3 000 000 units transfused in the United Kingdom. The virus can be inactivated in plasma products such as factor VIII and factor IX with heat at 80°C for 72 hours and chemicals, but red cells and platelets cannot be treated by these methods (Barbara & Contreras, 1986a, b).

Cytomegalovirus (CMV)

Screening of donors for cytomegalovirus is only necessary for neonates and immunosuppressed recipients who remain CMV-negative. Products are supplied for these two groups, as CMV infections, especially pneumonitis, can cause significant morbidity and mortality.

Future tests for blood donations

1. Antibody to human T cell leukaemia virus (HTLV 1), which is now mandatory in the United States.
2. HIV antigen and antibody to hepatitis C are being considered currently as mandatory tests in the United Kingdom in the future.

Concern by patients receiving blood transfusion has been noted (Kaberry, 1991). However, if a blood transfusion is essential and advisable, then today's small risk from infection is worthwhile.

Table 41.2 The ABO method of blood grouping

Blood group	*Approximate frequency % in the UK*	*Antigen present on cells*	*ISO antibodies present in serum*
O	46.5	Neither A nor B	Anti-A and anti-B
A	42.0	A	Anti-B
B	8.5	B	Anti-A
AB	3.0	A and B	Neither anti-A nor anti-B

Blood grouping and Rh factor

It is important that blood for transfusion is matched with the blood of the recipient to prevent a haemolytic reaction which could be life threatening. There follows a brief review of the blood group classification.

The most commonly used blood grouping system, the ABO method, was discovered in 1901 and is based on antigens on the red cells and antibodies in the serum (Table 41.2).

In 1940 the rhesus system was discovered. It is an antigen found on the red cell and because of the ease with which the antibody against it is built up in the blood, people without the antigen (Rh negative) need to be transfused with Rh-negative blood. If antibodies have developed and the patient is again transfused with Rh-positive blood, then the patient will react against it.

A similar problem of antibody formation can occur during pregnancy when the mother is Rh negative and the baby is Rh positive. The mother can develop Rh antibodies due to contact with the baby's blood during delivery. The risk of incompatibility and subsequent reaction can be minimized by following the procedures detailed in the 'Nursing care plan' (below).

Blood groups in bone marrow transplantation

The human lymphocyte antigen (HLA) is used to determine compatibility for organ transplantation, including bone marrow. Unfortunately, because ABO blood groups and HLA tissue types are determined genetically independently, it is not uncommon to find a well-matched HLA bone marrow donor who is ABO-incompatible with the recipient.

Major transfusion reactions can be avoided by red cell and/or plasma depleting the donor marrow in the laboratory before re-infusion. Very occasionally, if the recipient has a very high titre of anti-A or anti-B lytic antibody and the marrow donor is blood group A, B or AB, then plasmapheresis of the recipient is performed to lower the titre of this antibody to safe limits. This is necessary because it is not possible to remove all the red cells from the donor marrow and those remaining may cause a major transfusion reaction in this situation.

Delivery of blood and blood products

Inline blood filters

Filters are used to remove micro-aggregates and leucocytes present in the blood to be transfused.

Micro-aggregate filters

Micro-aggregate or micro-particle filters are used mainly to filter out red cell debris, platelets, white blood cells and fibrin strands that have clumped together. The number and size is variable and dependent on two main factors:

1. The storage time: in general the older the blood the more micro-aggregates it contains.
2. The anticoagulant used to prevent the blood from clotting.

The size of the particles can vary between 10 and 200 microns.

There are two main problems for the patient associated with the transfusion of micro-aggregates:

1. Pulmonary micro-emboli.
2. Non-haemolytic fevers.

These problems are more commonly associated with large transfusions of six units and above, and the use of blood stored for a long time. The filter compartment of commonly used blood administration sets will only remove particles of 170 to 200 microns and above.

Three types of filter are available:

1. Screen or surface filters, which effectively sieve the blood. The size of the particle removed will depend on the pore size on the surface. These filters tend to become more efficient the more blood flows through them. They remove particles of 40 micron or above.
2. Depth filters: these work by absorbing the particles into the layers of fibre. They tend to be effective for the removal of smaller particles but their efficiency diminishes as the number of units used increases. They also tend to slow the rate at which blood can be administered. These filters remove particles of 10 to 20 microns or above.
3. Combination filters, which consist of a surface filter above and a depth filter below.

As previously stated, the use of additional inline blood filters is not indicated for the majority of transfusions, and is contraindicated with certain components such as platelets.

Leucocyte depletion filters

The main problem for the patient associated with the transfusion of leucocytes is sensitization due to white cells or HLA antigens. Leucocyte depletion filters may be used prospectively for patients who are to undergo many transfusions, e.g. the transplant patient. There are specific filters designed for use in red cells and platelet transfusions, and it is important that the correct type is used.

Blood warmers

The warming of blood and blood products is not recommended as it is of limited benefit and is potentially dangerous. The use of blood warmers is indicated when:

1. Massive, rapid transfusion could result in cooling of cardiac tissue, causing dysfunction.
2. Frozen plasma or other components are prescribed and must be thawed before administration.
3. Transfusion is required by patients with potent cold agglutinins.
4. Exchange transfusion is indicated in the newborn.

Both waterbaths and dry heat blood warmers are available. Whatever device is chosen, the temperature should be maintained below 38°C, as warming in excess of this can cause haemolysis of red cells and can denature proteins.

The optimum effectiveness of dry heat blood warmers is reached when the rate of delivery to the patient is 150 to 160 ml per minute. This means that their use is restricted, and because of the greater flexibility of water baths these are more frequently used.

Wherever there is water, there is the risk of bacterial contamination of blood products, particularly with Pseudomonas. For the patient this could result a fatal systemic infection. Therefore, certain safety measures must be adhered to:

1. Waterbaths must be cleaned before and after use with disinfectant.
2. They must be stored dry and empty.
3. When needed, they should be refilled with sterile water.
4. A protective overbag should be considered for the blood produce to be thawed, to prevent entry of contaminants through microscopic punctures or breaks in the seal.

5. The blood warmer should be drained after each use.
6. The blood product should be used immediately after it has been thawed.

All devices should be serviced at regular intervals.

References and further reading

AIDS Newsletter (1991) *Survey Findings Transmission*, April, p. 2. Abbott Diagnostics Division.

Barbara, J. A. J. *et al.* (1990a) Infectious complications of blood transfusion bacteria and parasites. In *ABC of Transfusions* (Ed. by M. Contreras), pp. 45–8. British Medical Journal Publications, London.

Barbara, J. A. J. *et al.* (1990b) Infectious complications of blood transfusions viruses. In *ABC of Transfusions* (Ed. by M. Contreras), pp. 42–9, 45–52. British Medical Journal Publications, London.

Barbara, J. & Contreras, M. (1986a) Bacterial and parasitic diseases transmitted by blood transfusion. *Hospital Update*, 12, 629–31.

Barbara, J. & Contreras, M. (1986b) Viral diseases transmitted by blood transfusion. *Hospital Update*, 12, 697–708.

Brozovic, B. (1986) Blood and blood products: availability and indications. *Hospital Update*, 12, 445–58.

Canadian Red Cross Society Blood Transfusion Service (1982) *Clinical Guide to Transfusion*. Canadian Red Cross Society, Toronto, Canada.

Davies, S. & Brozovic, M. (1990) Transfusion of red cells. In *ABC of Transfusions* (Ed. by M. Contreras), pp. 9–24. British Medical Journal Publications, London.

Department of Health and Social Security, National Blood Transfusion Service, Scottish National Blood Transfusion Service (1984) *Notes on Transfusion*. DHSS, London.

Editorial (1985) Warming of blood and blood products. *Canadian Intravenous Nurses Association Journal*, 1(2), 5.

Hewitt, P. E. *et al.* (1990) The blood donor and tests on donor blood. In *ABC of Transfusions* (Ed. by M. Contreras), pp. 1–4. British Medical Journal Publications, London.

Huws, J. & Brozovic, B. (1990) Platelet and granulocyte transfusions. In *ABC of Transfusions* (Ed. by M. Contreras), pp. 14–17. British Medical Journal Publications, London.

Kaberry, S. (1991) Blood simple. *Nursing Times*, 87(2), 56.

Lloyd, G. M. & Marshall, L. (1986) Blood microaggregates: their role in transfusion reactions. *Intensive Care World*, 3(4), 119–22.

Lowe, G. D. (1981) Filtration in IV therapy: blood filters. *British Journal of Intravenous Therapy*, 2(6), 24–38.

Pritchard, A. P. & David, J. A. (1988) *The Royal Marsden Hospital Manual of Clinical Nursing Procedures*, 2nd edn. Harper & Row, London.

Smith, D. S. (1987) The appropriate use of diagnostic services: a guide to blood transfusion practice. *Health Trends*, 19, 12–16.

Swaffield, L. (1987) Circulating the blood. *Nursing Times*, 83(11), 16–17.

Watson & Royal (1987) Blood transfusion. In *Watson's Medical–Surgical Nursing and Related Physiology*, 3rd edn, p. 293. Ballière Tindall, Eastbourne.

Webster, A. (1987) Banking your own blood. *Nursing Times*, 83(31), 36–7.

NURSING CARE PLAN

The problems identified in this section are those associated specifically with blood or blood produce transfusion. Common problems associated with delivery of these substances are similar to those encountered in intravenous administration of any therapy and reference should be made to Chapter 21, Intravenous Management.

Examples of problems frequently encountered are:

1. The infusion slows or stops shortly after commencing the unit of blood. The most likely cause for this is venous spasm due to a cold solution being infused. The preventive or corrective measure would be to apply a warm compress to soothe and dilate the vein and increase blood flow.
2. The infusion slows or stops due to occlusion of the cannula. Maintenance of continuous flow is important here. If this problem is recognized early, then flushing the cannula gently with normal saline may resolve this. However, if some minutes have elapsed it may be necessary to prime a new administration set with normal saline to re-establish flow as clotting may have occurred in the tubing. Keeping the patient warm and relaxed will also increase the peripheral circulation and prevent problems.

Potential problem	Cause	Preventive measure	Suggested action
Elevated temperature after the commencement of a unit of blood with temperature falling if the blood is slowed.	Pyrogenic reaction.	Observation of the patient's temperature, pulse and blood pressure during the transfusion dependent on patient's condition and especially	Slow blood transfusion rate. Inform medical staff.

Nursing Care Plan

Potential problem	Cause	Preventive measure	Suggested action
		at the start of each unit. If patient has had multiple transfusions or experienced this type of reaction previously, ensure 'cover' of hydrocortisone and chlorpheniramine is written up and administered before commencement of therapy.	
A high temperature associated with fever and rigor during a transfusion.	White cell antibody reaction.	Observation as above.	Stop transfusion. Change giving set and commence normal saline slowly to keep vein open. Inform medical staff.
Slightly elevated temperature with associated rash, may be severe with oedema round the eyes and larynx and shortness of breath.	Allergic reaction to protein in the plasma.	Observation as above. Ensure patient is aware of symptoms to report, e.g. appearance of a rash or breathlessness. Close observation of patient for swollen eyes and signs of breathlessness.	If mild, slow the rate of transfusion. Inform medical staff. If severe, stop transfusion. Change giving set and commence normal saline to keep vein open, or hepflush cannula Lie patient flat, treat as for shock. Inform medical staff.
Patient complains of feeling hot with chest and abdominal pain. Fall in blood pressure, patient's temperature subnormal at first and later rising to a pyrexia.	Infection introduced either from bacteria in the blood or during the cannulation or connection set changes.	Adhere to strict aseptic technique when handling the blood bags and intravenous line. Use blood within 30 minutes of removal from refrigerator. Regular observations, as above. Adhere to recommended delivery time for each unit of blood; discard if hanging for eight hours.	Stop transfusion. Change giving set and commence normal saline slowly to keep vein open. Inform medical staff and institute prescribed treatment, e.g. steroids, antibiotics. Return remaining blood for examination by the bacteriology department.
Patient complaining of feeling a hot flush along the vein, facial flushing and lumbar pain. The patient may become shocked with a fall in the blood pressure and the urine output may fall.	Blood not cross-matched. Urgent cross-match completed and blood not fully compatible. Blood administered to wrong patient. Cross-matched blood sample wrongly labelled	Ensure blood cross-matching forms are completed correctly. If taking blood sample, check carefully that the name and number on the form matches the patient. Ensure that a unit	Stop transfusion. Change giving set and commence normal saline to keep vein open. Lay patient flat and treat as for shock. Inform medical staff.

	or taken from wrong patient.	is checked against the cross-match form for blood group, patient's name, patient's number, ward, Rh factor, unit number of blood, when blood taken, and expiry date. Begin transfusion slowly and observe the patient carefully at the start of each unit.

Note: tranfusion risks associated with administration of massive amounts of blood include:

1. Abnormal bleeding tendencies.
2. Hypocalacaemia.
3. Risk of development of adult respiratory distress syndrome.
4. Potassium intoxication.
5. Elevated blood ammonia level.
6. Haemosiderosis.
7. Hypothermia.

Massive transfusion refers to quantities in excess of six units and specific texts should be consulted in these circumstances.

42

The Unconscious Patient

Definition

In coma an individual's awareness, as well as those responses essential to comfort and self-preservation, no longer operate (Wong *et al.*, 1984)

Complete care of the unconscious patient presents a special challenge to the nurse because the patient is totally dependent on the nurse's skills – for his/her comfort needs and indeed for his/her life. This inability to respond must spur efforts to include the patient and the family or close friends in re-orientation programmes, by using stimuli associated with the patient's previous physiological and social experiences.

Indications

The normal reflexes protecting the conscious person are lost and their protective function is assumed by the nurse until the patient can function to maximum potential. In order to do so it would be necessary to:

1. Establish and maintain a clear airway.
2. Assess the level of consciousness (see Chapter 28, Neurological Observations).
3. Record and evaluate vital signs.
4. Maintain fluid and electrolyte balance.
5. Carry out nursing care as appropriate to the patient's condition.
6. Involve relatives and/or friends in care from the beginning.

REFERENCE MATERIAL

Causes of unconsciousness

Causes of unconsciousness are many and may dictate the length of the coma period. Some patients may recover spontaneously, e.g. after a seizure, while others remain unconscious until their death. This chapter deals mainly with the patient who is unconscious for some time and not with the anaesthetized and post-anaesthetic patient whose coma is controlled. The following list of causes of unconsciousness is not exhaustive, nor can it indicate the outcome of the comatosed state.

Poisons and drugs

1. Alcohol.
2. General anaesthetics.
3. Overdose of drugs, including solvents.
4. Gases, e.g. carbon monoxide.
5. Heavy metals, e.g. lead poisoning.

Vascular causes

1. Post-cardiac arrest.
2. Ischaemia.
3. Hypertensive encephalopathy.
4. Haemorrhage – intracerebral or subarachnoid.
5. Sudden reduction in circulating blood volume.

Infections

1. Septicaemia
2. Viruses, e.g. herpes, encephalitis, HIV.
3. Meningitis.
4. Protozoan infections, e.g. malaria.
5. Fungal, e.g. aspergillosis.

Seizures

1. Idiopathic or post-traumatic epilepsy.
2. Eclampsia.
3. Metabolic disorders.

Other causes

1. Neoplasm, primary, e.g. astrocytoma, or secondary tumour from other body primary, e.g. lung.
2. Trauma, e.g. head injury or trauma resulting in hyper/hypothermia, dehydration.
3. Liver, renal, cardiac or lung failure.
4. Tetany.
5. Metabolic causes, e.g. diabetic coma, myxoedema.
6. Degenerative diseases, e.g. multiple sclerosis.

Recording the level of consciousness

There are many methods of assessing and recording a patient's level of consciousness. One of the most commonly used in the United Kingdom is the Glasgow Coma Scale (Allan, 1986; Jennett & Teasdale, 1974). An extensive description of this scale can be found in

Allan (1986). Terms such as 'semiconscious' should be avoided since they mean different things to different people and can be misleading. It is more appropriate to describe the patient in terms of the responsiveness to environmental stimuli (Mangiardi, 1990).

Attitudes of nurses

Leon and Snyder (1980) explored the psychosocial problems in caring for head-injured patients and concluded that, in general, nurses accepted unconscious patients and were challenged by them. The phase of management appears to affect the attitude of the nursing staff, e.g. critical care, post-emergent care and continuing care. Bell (1986) discusses the hopelessness, guilt, ambivalence, frustration and depression felt by nurses in some situations. The involvement of families and friends of the patient may lead the nurse to experience professional, moral and ethical problems, depending on the likely outcome of the coma and the length of the comatosed state.

All nurses must recognize that 'it is difficult to provide constant and continuous excellent care to the comatosed (head-injured) patient when the professional rewards are minimal' (Flaherty, 1982). Peer support in units or wards caring for the unconscious patient is vital, particularly perhaps where the patient is a child, or the patient is brain dead (Pallis, 1983; Rudy, 1982). The needs of the patient's family and friends must also be addressed by the nursing staff. Grieving is a natural and necessary process for family and friends of the terminally ill or long-term unconscious patient, and they must be supported through and prepared for the eventual outcome (Allan, 1988; Penson, 1988).

References and further reading

Allan, D. (1986) Nursing the unconscious patient. *The Professional Nurse*, October, 2(1), 15–17.

Allan, D. (1988) The ethics of brain death. *The Professional Nurse*, May, 3(8), 295–8.

Bell, T. N. (1986) Nurses' attitudes in caring for comatose head-injured patients. *Journal of Neurological Nursing*, 18(5), 279–89.

De Young, S. (1987) Coma recovery program. *Rehabilitation Nursing*, May/June, 12(3), 121–4.

Flaherty, M. (1982) Care of the comatose: complex problems faced alone. *Nursing Management*, 13(10), 44–6.

Gooch, J. (1985) Mouth care. *The Professional Nurse*, 1(3), 77–9.

Jennett, B. & Teasdale, G. (1974) Assessment of coma and impaired consciousness. A practical scale. *Lancet*, 2, 81–3.

Leon, M. & Snyder (1980) The psychosocial aspects of the care of long-term comatose patients. *Journal of Neurosurgical Nursing*, 11(4), 235–7.

Mangiardi, J. R. (1990) Initial management of head injury. *Topics in Emergency Medicine*, 11(4), 11–23.

Nikas, D. (1983) Altered states of consciousness. Part I. *Focus and Critical Care*, 10(5), 10–14; Part II – December, 10(6), 10–13; Part III – February (1984), 11(1), 54–8.

Pallis, C. (1983) *ABC of Brain Stem Death*. British Medical Association, London.

Penson, J. (1988) The needs of the terminally ill patient's family. *The Professional Nurse*, 3(5), 153–5.

Podurgiel, M. (1990) The unconscious experience: a pilot study. *Journal of Neuroscience Nursing*, 22(1), 52–3.

Rudy, E. (1982) Brain death. *Dimensions of Critical Care Nursing*, 1(3), 178.

Scherer, P. (1986) Assessment: the logic of coma. *American Journal of Nursing*, 86(5), 542–9.

Taylor, S. J. (1988) A guide to nasogastric feeding. *The Professional Nurse*, 3(11), 439–43.

Taylor, S. J. (1989) Preventing complications in internal feeding. *The Professional Nurse*, 4(5), 247–9.

Taylor, S. J. (1989) A guide to internal feeding. *The Professional Nurse*, 4(4), 195–8.

Wong, J. *et al.* (1984) Care of the unconscious patient: a problem-orientated approach. *Journal of Neurosurgical Nursing*, 16(3), 148–50.

GUIDELINES: CARE OF THE UNCONSCIOUS PATIENT

Equipment

At the bedside:

1. Airway (of correct size).
2. Suction.
3. Oxygen.
4. Intravenous infusion equipment.
5. Personal hygiene equipment:
   (a) Eye toilet pack.
   (b) Oral toilet pack.
   (c) Catheter care pack.

6 Cot sides (if the patient is restless or likely to become so).

Guidelines: Care of the unconscious patient

7 Observation charts:
  (a) Neurological.
  (b) Intake and output.
8 Feeding equipment (as necessary).

Easy access to:
1. Ambu-bag with valve and mask; or intubation (and tracheostomy) equipment.
2. Neurological observation, tray, thermometer and sphygmomanometer.

Procedure

Action	**Rationale**
1. The room or ward area should be warm and well lit, and adequately ventilated with easy access to the patient.	To facilitate rapid assessment of the patient at a glance, e.g.: (a) colour of skin – cherry red after carbon monoxide poisoning, frost in uraemia, yellow in hepatic failure, blue in cyanosis. (b) Smell – alcohol; 'toasted almonds' after cyanide poisoning, the sickly sweet smell of diabetic ketoacdosis (Mangiardi, 1990).
2. Nurse the patient in a bed with a firm base, a detachable bed head (and cot sides as needed).	To failitate cardiac massage and intubation if required. (To prevent self-injury to the restless patient.)
3. Insert a bed cradle, if required.	To allow unhampered limb movements. To enhance vision of limbs if leg is in plaster or on traction (as in multiple injuries).
4. Place patient in lateral or semiprone position (if condition allows).	To prevent occlusion of airway by tongue falling back against the pharyngeal wall. To encourage drainage of respiratory secretions, and prevent pooling of same in throat.

Note: if a patient's injuries or other conditions prevent him/her from being nursed from side to side or prone, then a nurse should be in attendance at all times while there is an airway hazard.

5. Pass nasogastric tube.	To empty gastric contents regularly. Paralytic ileus occurs frequently in the unconscious patient and this may lead to aspiration of stomach contents.
6. Place the limbs as follows (Figure 42.1):	
(a) Head: put the patient's head on a pillow. (b) Trunk: keep the spine straight and place pillows at the patient's back for support.	To promote comfort and maintain proper alignment of the body.
(c) Upper limb: bring the uppermost arm forward in front of the patient. Bend the elbow slightly, but keep the wrist extended. Support the arm on a pillow and bring the bottom arm alongside the face with the palm facing upwards.	To prevent oedema by inappropriate pressure on venous flow.
(d) Lower limbs: flex the uppermost leg and bring it forward. Support it on pillows.	To prevent internal rotation of the hip.
Keep the lower leg extended straight and in line with the spine. Make sure the patient's uppermost leg does not rest on the lower leg.	To avoid pressure ulcers.

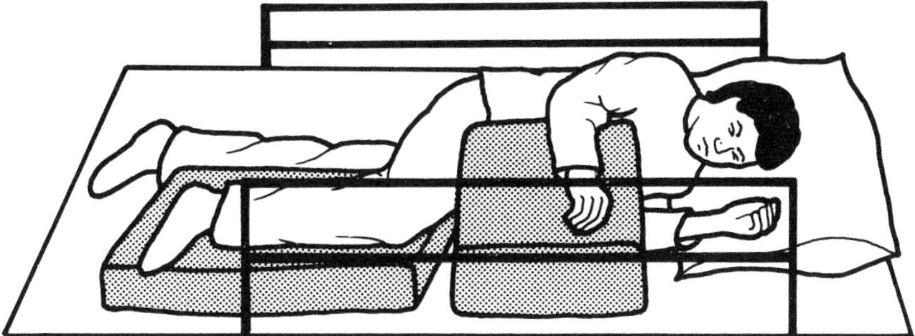

Figure 42.1 Positioning the unconscious patient.

(e) Consult with physiotherapist and anaesthetist about positioning exercises to enhance pulmonary function.

To effect optimal respiratory function and gaseous exchange.

(f) Institute passive physiotherapy exercises and observe colour, temperature and pulses of limbs.

To prevent deep vein thrombosis formation; to recognize early signs of limb deformity (Palmer & Wyness, 1988).

(g) Apply anti-embolism stockings as ordered.

To aid venous return to the heart.

7. Remove:
(a) All dental prostheses and note caps, loose teeth, bleeding gums etc.
(b) Clean patient's nostrils.
(c) Insert an airway (either oral or nasal) as appropriate.

To obtain and maintain clear airway.

8. Perform neurological assessment as frequently as physician or patient's condition dictates.

To note changes in condition and act on changes as appropriate.

9. (a) Administer intravenous fluids as prescribed and record.

To maintain electrolyte and fluid balance.

(b) Strict asepsis must be maintained when carrying out proceedings involving puncture site of cannula or sterile ends of intravenous infusion sets.

To prevent infections – local or systemic.

10. Maintain feeding regime either by nasogastric tube
– by fine bore continuous tube feeding
– by central venous catheter (see Chapter 9)

To maintain metabolic stasis.
To prevent weight loss (Goodinson, 1987; Taylor, 1988; Taylor, 1989).

11. Call the patient by preferred name. Introduce yourself, explain each procedure before starting; talk to patient; tell patient date, time, etc.

Hearing often remains intact in the unconscious patient.
To prevent sensory deprivation.

12. Touch the patient gently and describe boundaries and environment, e.g. place patient's hand on the bedside, blankets, locker and explain what each item is, describe the room.

Through touch, individuals establish (and maintain) their body boundaries and relationships with others, and their environment. Being denied opportunities to touch can impair physiological, psychological and social development (Podurgiel, 1990; de Young, 1987).

13. Give the patient daily baths (or as required).

To ensure patient's skin is kept clean, dry and supple (Gooch, 1989).

Guidelines: Care of the unconscious patient

Action	Rationale
14. Carry out eye care (see procedure on eye care, Chapter 18).	The blink reflex is absent during unconsciousness (or the patient's eyes may be open all the time). This may lead to corneal drying, irritation and ulceration (see Chapter 18).
15. Carry out mouth care (see procedure on mouth care, Chapter 27).	To maintain a clean, moist mouth, to prevent the accumulation of oral and postnasal secretions and to prevent the development of mouth infections (Gooch, 1985).
16. Observe the patient for signs of bladder distension (or urinary bypass of catheter; see Chapter 43, Urinary Catheterization).	To prevent urinary complication. In males an external sheath may be used and catheterization may be used and catheterization may become necessary. In females, catheterization may be immediately necessary.
(a) Read catheter information carefully.	To prevent over-distending the balloon and damaging urethra.
(b) Perform regular catheter care.	To prevent infection.
17. Carry out bowel care.	To prevent constipation and/or diarrhoea.
18. Change the patient's position every two hours or as dictated by condition.	To relieve pressure areas. To prevent respiratory complications by allowing for postural drainage, and for each side of the chest to receive a period free of compression by body weight when it can expand fully.
19. Keep relatives and friends informed of changes in the patient's condition and involve them in caring for the patient as appropriate.	To help family and friends adjust to the situation and (depending on prognosis) facilitate 'anticipatory grief' (Penson, 1988).

NURSING CARE PLAN

Problem	Cause	Suggested action
Restlessness and/or confusion.	A degree of restlessness may indicate that the patient is regaining consciousness. During this time there may be a clouding of consciousness with confusion, aggression, unco-operative behaviour and disorientation. Restlessness may also indicate brain damage, cerebral anoxia (when there is a partially obstructed airway), a full bladder or bowel pain or discomfort.	Ascertain, where possible, the cause of the discomfort and rectify as appropriate. Summon help if the patient becomes aggressive or violent. Ensure the patient does not inflict self-injury, e.g. place cot sides in position on the bed.
Seizures	An unconscious patient is a potential candidate for seizures.	Maintain a clear airway. Protect the patient from self-injury. Observe the patient during the

		seizure and record observations on a seizure chart. Administer prescribed drugs.
Cerebrospinal fluid leakage through nose or ears.	May be indicative of base of skull fracture, or some dural damage.	Place sterile swab against nose and ears and collect fluid. Test drainage for sugar (it will be positive if CSF is present). Inform medical staff.
Vomiting.	The unconscious patient is prone to paralytic ileus, or medulla oblongata may be involved.	Maintain a clear airway. Keep stomach empty until ileus resolves.
Distended bladder.	See Chapter 43, Urinary Catheterization, for problems associated with catheterization.	
Inability to maintain own nutritional intake.	See Chapter 14, Enteral Tube Feeding and Nutritional Assessment, for problems associated with this type of nutrition.	

43

Urinary Catheterization

Definition

Urinary catheterization is the insertion of a special tube into the bladder, using aseptic technique, for the purpose of evacuating or instilling fluids.

Indications

Male

In the male, urinary catheterization may be carried out for the following reasons:

1. To empty the contents of the bladder, e.g. before or after abdominal, pelvic or rectal surgery and before certain investigations.
2. To determine residual urine.
3. To allow irrigation of the bladder.
4. To bypass an obstruction.
5. To relieve retention of urine.
6. To introduce cytotoxic drugs in the treatment of papillary bladder carcinomas.
7. To enable bladder function tests to be performed.
8. To measure urinary output accurately, e.g. when a patient is in shock, undergoing bone marrow transplanation or receiving high-dose chemotherapy.
9. To relieve incontinence when no other means is practicable.

Female

In the female, urinary catheterization may be carried out for the nine reasons listed above and for two further reasons:

10. To empty the bladder before childbirth, if thought necessary.
11. To avoid complications during intracavitary insertion of radioactive caesium.

REFERENCE MATERIAL

Common sites of cross-infection

The common sites of cross-infection of a catheterized patient are as illustrated in Figure 43.1.

Types of material used for catheters

Latex

Latex is a purified form of rubber and is the softest material from which catheters are made. It has a smooth surface and has a tendency to attract crust formation. Latex can also produce urethral irritation and should be used only for short-term catheterization.

Teflon-coated latex

Teflon-coated latex was produced to reduce urethral reaction. It is appropriate for short-or medium-term catheterization.

Silicone-coated or all-silicone

Silicone is a very soft, inert material ideal for long-term drainage. This type of catheter is more expensive than those mentioned above and must be reserved for patients who require catheterization for two or more weeks.

Hydrogel catheters

This is a relatively new group of catheters. They are made of an inner core of latex, which has a hydrophilic polymer coating making them more compatible with the urethral mucosa, and thus reducing irritation. Manufacturers claim that the catheters can resist encrustation and bacterial colonization.

Catheter selection

Selection of catheter type, size and design is important if catheterization is to be effective. Careful consideration of the features required, i.e. shaft length, balloons size and materials used in manufacture, will assist the best selection. Five or 10 ml fill volume balloons should be used in the majority of cases. Preferably, 30 ml fill volume balloons should be used for patients following urological surgery.

Types of catheters

Types of catheters are listed in Table 43.1, together with their applications.

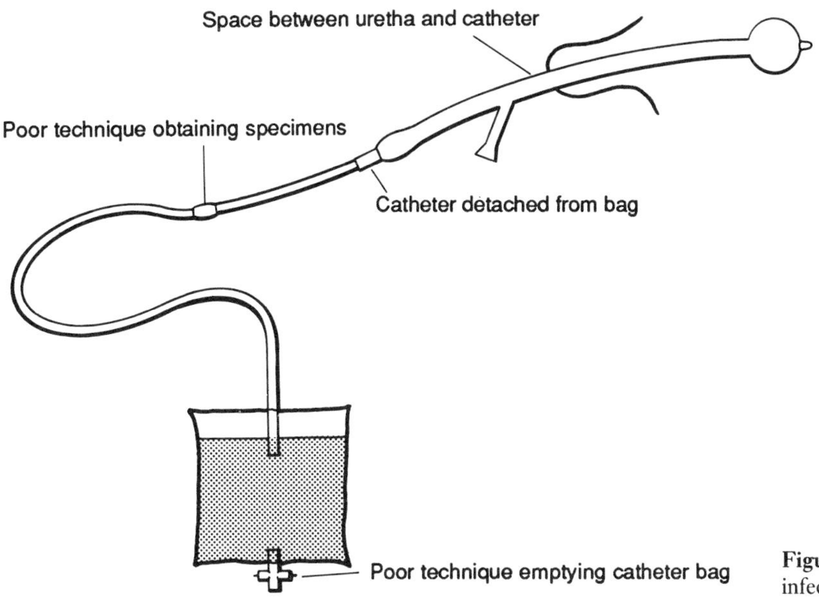

Figure 43.1 Common sites of cross-infection in a catheterized patient.

Table 43.1 Types of catheter

Catheter type	*Material*	*Uses*
Foley two-way	Latex	The usual choice when short-term indwelling catheterization is indicated. If Teflon coated, may remain in position for one month
Foley three-way	Latex	For those procedures where there is a need to irrigate the bladder or instil solutions into it. Potential infection is avoided by decreasing the need to break the closed system of drainage
Red rubber	Rubber	Use Foley latex or plastic intermittent types. Obtain sterile specimen from an ileal conduit. Rubber is extremely irritating to urethral mucosa
Silastic	Silicone	Long-term indwelling catheterization with an approximate lifespan of three months.
Intermittent	PVC and other plastics	To empty bladder or continent urinary reservoir intermittently (cannot be used for continuous drainage) and to dilate urethral stricture

Catheter size

Catheter size is measured in French gauge; 1 FG indicates an external tube diameter of the catheter of 0.66 mm.

Leg drainage bag

An active patient with a permanent urinary catheter in position should be instructed in the use of a leg drainage bag as this will allow the resumption of a full range of normal activities. Such patient education should begin several days before discharge so that any problems may be identified while the patient is still in hospital. If the patient has any physical or mental disabilities, a responsible relative or close friend should be taught the required catheter care before the patient is discharged.

Leg drainage bags have a limited capacity (350 to 750 ml). For night-time drainage, connection of a larger capacity bag to the outlet portal of the leg bag allows effective drainage without interruption of the closed system.

Intermittent self-catheterization (ISC)

This is not a new technique, although it has become noticeably more popular in recent years.

This procedure involves the episodic introduction of a catheter into the bladder to remove urine. After this the catheter is removed, leaving the patient catheter-free between catheterizations. The patient should perform the catheterization as often as necessary to prevent incontinence or to prevent prolonged retention of urine (usually four or five times a day) (Seth, 1987).

Patients suitable for intermittent self-catheterization include:

1. Those who can comprehend the technique.
2. Those with a reasonable degree of manual dexterity.
3. Those who are highly motivated.
4. Those who have a willing partner to perform the technique (i.e. if agreeable to both).
5. Those who can position themselves to attain reasonable access to the urethra (especially females) (Seth, 1987).

In 1970, Lasides, in the United States, found that patients using a clean rather than a sterile technique did not encounter problematic urinary tract infection. The catheters used for intermittent self-catheterization are technically described as semi-disposable, i.e. they are designed to be washed and re-used for a limited period only, usually one week.

They should always be rinsed in running water and properly dried after use; between uses they should be kept in a container such as a plastic envelope (Simcare booklet).

References and further reading

Bard Ltd (1984) *Guidelines for the Management of the Catheterized Patient*. Bard Ltd.

Bard Ltd (1987) *You, Your Patients, and Urinary Catheters*. Bard Ltd.

Bielski, M. (1980) Preventing infection in the catheterized patient. *Nursing Clinics of North America*, 15, 703–13.

Blannin, J. P. & Hobden, J. (1980) The catheter of choice. *Nursing Times*, 76, 2092–3.

Brunner, L. S. & Suddarth, D. S. (1986) *The Lippincott Manual of Nursing Practice*, 4th edn. J. B. Lippincott, Philadelphia.

Chilman, A. M. & Thomas, M. (1987) *Understanding Nursing Care*, 3rd edn. Churchill Livingstone, Edinburgh.

Crow, R. *et al.* (1988) Indwelling catheterization and related nursing practice. *Journal of Advanced Nursing*, 13(4), 489–95.

Crummey, V. (1989) Ignorance can hurt. *Nursing Times and Nursing Mirror*, 85, 67–8, 70.

Gupta, J. (1988) Effectiveness of different methods: effectiveness of three methods of periurethral hygiene in urinary catheterized surgical female patients. *Nursing Journal of India*, 79(10), 257–8, 280.

Heenan, A. (1990) Indications for long-term catheterization. *Nursing Times*, 86, 70–1.

Lowthian, P. (1989) Preventing trauma (in patients with indwelling catheters). *Nursing Times and Nursing Mirror*, 85, 73–5.

MacSweeney, P. (1989) Self-catheterization – a solution for some incontinent people. *The Professional Nurse*, 4(8), 399–401.

Mulhall, A. (1990) Bacteria, biofilm and bladder catheters. *Nursing Times*, 86, 57.

Oliver, H. (1988) Continence supplement. The treatment of choice. *Nursing Times and Nursing Mirror*, 84, 70.

Phipps, W. J. *et al.* (1986) *Medical-Surgical Nursing: Concepts and Clinical Practice*, 3rd edn. C. V. Mosby, St Louis.

Seth, C. (1987) Catheters ring the changes. *Nursing Times and Nursing Mirror*, 84, *Community Outlook*, 12, 14.

Sibley, L. (1988) Confidence with incontinence. *Nursing Times and Nursing Mirror*, 84, 42–3.

Simcare (undated) *Intermittent Self-Catheterization – A Guide For Patients' Families*. Simcare, Lancing.

Stickler, D. J. & Chawla, J. C. (1987) The role of antiseptics in the management of patients with long-term indwelling bladder catheters. *Journal of Hospital Infection*, 10(3), 219–28.

Wright, E. (1988) Catheter care: the risk of infection. *The Professional Nurse*, 3(12), 487–8, 490.

Wright, E. (1988) Minimising the risks of UTI. *The Professional Nurse*, 4(2), 63–4, 66–7.

GUIDELINES: URINARY CATHETERIZATION

Equipment

1. Sterile catheterization pack containing gallipots, receiver, non-linting material, disposable towels, disposable dissecting forceps.
2. Disposable pad.
3. Sterile gloves.
4. Selection of appropriate catheters.
5. Sterile anaesthetic lubricating jelly.
6. Universal specimen container.
7. Normal saline or antiseptic solution.
8. Alcohol-based hand wash solution.
9. Gate clip.
10. Hypo-allergenic tape.
11. Scissors.

12. Sterile water.
13. Syringe and needle.
14. Disposable plastic apron.
15. Drainage bag and stand or holder.

Procedure

Male

Action	Rationale
1. Explain the procedure to the patient.	To obtain the patient's consent and co-operation.
2. (a) Screen the bed.	To ensure patient's privacy. To allow dust and airborne organisms to settle before the field is exposed.
(b) Assist the patient to get into the supine position with the legs extended. (c) Do not expose the patient at this stage of the procedure.	
3. Wash hands using bactericidal soap and water or bactericidal alcohol hand rub.	
4. Put on a disposable plastic apron.	
5. Prepare the trolley, placing all equipment required on the bottom shelf.	
6. Take the trolley to the patient's bedside, disturbing screens as little as possible.	To minimize airborne contamination.
7. Remove cover that is maintaining the patient's privacy and position a disposable pad under his buttocks and thighs.	To ensure urine does not leak onto bedclothes.
8. Open the outer cover of the catheterization pack and slide the pack onto the top shelf of the trolley.	
9. Using an aseptic technique, open the supplementary packs.	The bladder is a sterile organ.
10. Clean hands with an alcohol-based hand wash solution.	Hands may have become contaminated by handling the outer packs.
11. Put on sterile gloves.	
12. Place sterile towels across the patient's thighs and under buttocks.	
13. Apply the nozzle to the tube of anaesthetic lubricating jelly.	
14. Wrap a sterile topical swab around the penis. Retract the foreskin, if necessary, and clean the glans penis with normal saline or an antiseptic solution.	

Guidelines: Urinary catheterization

Action	Rationale
15. Insert the nozzle of the lubricating jelly into the urethra. Squeeze the gel into the urethra, remove the nozzle and discard the tube. Massage the gel along the urethra.	Adequate lubrication helps to prevent urethral trauma. Use of a local anaesthetic minimizes the discomfort experienced by the patient.
16. Grasp the shaft of the penis, raising it until it is almost totally extended Maintain grasp of penis until the procedure is finished.	This manoeuvre straightens the penile urethra and facilitates catheterization. Maintaining a grasp of the penis prevents contamination and retraction of the penis.
17. Place the receiver containing the catheter between the patient's legs. Insert the catheter for 15 to 25 cm until urine flows.	The male urethra is approximately 18 cm long.
18. If resistance is felt at the external sphincter, increase the traction on the penis slightly and apply steady, gentle pressure on the catheter. Ask the patient to strain gently as if passing urine.	Some resistance may be due to spasm of the external sphincter.
19. Either remove the catheter gently when urinary flow ceases, or:	
(a) When urine begins to flow, advance the catheter almost to its bifurcation.	Advancing the catheter ensures that it is correctly positioned in the bladder.
(b) Inflate the balloon according to the manufacturer's direction, having ensured that the catheter is draining properly beforehand.	Inadvertent inflation of the balloon in the urethra causes pain and urethral trauma.
(c) Withdraw the catheter slightly and attach it to the drainage system.	
(d) Tape the catheter laterally to the thigh or on the abdomen.	This smoothes out the urethral curve and eliminates pressure on the penoscrotal junction which can lead to the formation of a fistula.
(e) Ensure that the catheter is not taut on the skin.	This allows room for movement should spontaneous erection occur.
20. Ensure that the glans penis is clean and then reduce or reposition the foreskin.	Retraction and constriction of the foreskin behind the glans penis (paraphimosis) may occur if this is not done.
21. Make the patient comfortable. Ensure that the area is dry.	If the area is left wet or moist, secondary infection and skin irritation may occur.
22. Measure the amount of urine.	
23. Take a urine specimen for laboratory examination, if required.	For further information, see the procedure on collection of a catheter specimen of urine, below.
24. Dispose of equipment in a yellow clinical waste bag and seal the bag before moving the trolley.	To prevent environmental contamination.
25. Draw back the curtains.	
26. Record information in any relevant documents.	

Female

Action	Rationale
1. Explain the procedure to the patient.	To obtain the patient's consent and co-operation.
2. (a) Screen the bed.	To ensure patient's privacy. To allow dust and airborne organisms to settle before the sterile field is exposed.
(b) Assist the patient to get into the supine position with knees bent, hips flexed and feet resting about 60 cm apart. (c) Do not expose the patient at this stage of the procedure.	
3. Ensure that a good light source is available.	To enable the genital area to be seen clearly.
4. Wash hands using bactericidal soap and water or bactericidal alcohol hand rub.	
5. Put on a disposable apron.	
6. Prepare the trolley, placing all equipment required on the bottom shelf, including female length catheters.	To reduce length of exposed catheter and provide extra patient comfort.
7. Take the trolley to the patient's bedside, disturbing screens as little as possible.	To minimize airborne contamination.
8. Remove cover that is maintaining the patient's privacy and position a disposable pad under the patient's buttocks.	To ensure urine does not leak onto bedclothes.
9. Open the outer cover of the catheterization pack and slide the pack on the top shelf of the trolley.	
10. Using an aseptic technique, open supplementary packs.	Catheterization requires the same aseptic precautions as a surgical procedure.
11. Clean hands with an alcohol-based hand rub.	Hands may have become contaminated by handling of outer packs, etc.
12. Put on sterile gloves.	
13. Place sterile towels across the patient's thighs.	
14. Separate the labia minora so that the urethral meatus is seen. Using non-linting gauze swabs, one hand should be used to maintain labial separation until catheterization is completed.	This manoeuvre helps to prevent labial contamination of the catheter and provides better access to the urethral orifice.
15. Clean around the urethral orifice with normal saline or an antiseptic solution, using single downward strokes. Forceps should be used to handle the cleaning swabs.	Inadequate preparation of the urethral orifice is a major cause of infection following catheterization.
16. Dry the area well before proceeding.	

Guidelines: Urinary catheterization

Action	**Rationale**
17. Lubricate the catheter with sterile anaesthetic lubricating jelly.	Lubricating the catheter reduces friction and trauma to the urethral mucosa. Use of a local anaesthetic minimizes the patient's discomfort.
18. Place the catheter, in the receiver, between the patient's legs.	
19. Introduce the tip of the catheter into the urethral orifice in an upward and backward direction. Advance the catheter until 5 to 6 cm have been inserted.	The direction of insertion and the length of catheter inserted should bear relation to the anatomical structure of the area.
20. Either remove the catheter gently when urinary flow ceases, or:	
(a) Advance the catheter 6 to 8 cm.	This prevents the balloon from becoming trapped in the urethra.
(b) Inflate the balloon according to the manufacturer's directions, having ensured that the catheter is draining adequately.	Inadvertent inflation of the balloon within the urethra is painful and causes urethral trauma.
(c) Withdraw the catheter slightly and connect it to the drainage system.	
(d) Tape the catheter and drainage system to the thigh.	This prevents traction and tension on the bladder and friction in the urethra.
21. Make the patient comfortable and ensure that the area is dry.	If the area is left wet or moist, secondary infection and skin irritation may occur.
22. Measure the amount of urine.	
23. Take a urine specimen for laboratory examination if required.	For further information, see the procedure on collection of a catheter specimen of urine (below).
24. Dispose of equipment in a disposable plastic bag and seal the bag before moving the trolley.	To prevent environmental contamination.
25. Draw back the curtains.	
26. Record information in any relevant documents.	

Note: when the bladder is very distended a gate clip should be applied to the drainage bag tubing to regulate the flow rate after 500 ml of urine have been drained. This prevents shock due to sudden reduction in intra-abdominal pressure. However, the catheter should not be left clamped because this allows bacteria, if present, to multiply above the clamp, increasing the risk of ascending infection.

An alternative way of preventing sudden emptying of the bladder on catheterization in the patient with a long history of urinary outflow obstruction would be to place the urinary collection bag at the height of the patient's bladder. This allows urine drainage to be gradual and controlled. However, once emptying has occurred, the bag should be placed below the level of the bladder to pevent pooling and potential ascending bacterial contamination.

GUIDELINES: INTERMITTENT SELF-CATHETERIZATION

Equipment

1. Mirror (for female anatomy).
2. Appropriately sized catheters for male/female patients.

3. Lubricating gel.
4. Clean container (e.g. plastic envelope) for catheter.

Procedure

Female

Action	Rationale
1. Wash hands using bactericidal soap and water or bactericidal alcohol hand rub, and dry them.	
2. Assist patient to adopt a comfortable position depending on mobility.	For patient's comfort.
3. Spread the labia and wash the genitalia from front to back with soap and water, then dry and insert the catheter, using lubricant if necessary.	To prevent introducing infection. For ease of insertion.
4. Drain the urine into a toilet or suitable container.	
5. Remove the catheter when flow has ceased.	
6. If catheter is to be re-used, wash through with tap water. Allow to drain and dry. Store in dry container.	To remove urine.
7. Wash hands.	To reduce the risk of infection.

Male

Action	Rationale
1. Wash hands using bactericidal soap and water or bactericidal alcohol hand rub.	To prevent infection.
2. Stand in front of a toilet or a low bench with a suitable container if it is easier.	To catch urine.
3. Clean glans penis with plain water. If the foreskin covers the penis it will need to be held back during the procedure.	To prevent infection.
4. Hold penis with left hand (if right handed), three forefingers underneath and the thumb on top. The penis should be held straight out. Coat the end of the catheter with lubricating gel.	To prevent trauma to the penis-scrotal junction, also gives easier observation of procedure.
5. Pass the catheter gently with the right hand; it can be felt as it passes the fingers holding the penis. There will be a change of feeling as the catheter passes through the prostrate gland and into the bladder. It may be a little sore on the first few occasions only. If there is resistance do not continue; withdraw the catheter and contact a nurse or doctor.	 The prostrate gland surrounds the urethra just below the neck of the bladder and consists of much firmer tissue. Can enlarge and cause obstruction, especially in older men.

Guidelines: Intermittent self-catheterization

Action	Rationale
6. Urine will drain as soon as the catheter enters the bladder, so have the end positioned over the toilet or a suitable container.	To keep the area clean.
7. Withdraw catheter slowly so that all the urine is drained. The catheter will slide out easily.	To prevent stasis of residual urine.
8. Wash catheter through if it is reusable and store in a clean container.	To prevent infection.
9. Wash hands and dry them.	To prevent infection.
10. A mirror to stand in front of is helpful for patients with a large abdomen.	For ease of observation.
11. Beware of patient having a vasovagal attack.	This is caused by the vagal nerve being stimulated so that the heart slows down, leading to a syncope faint. If it happens, lie the patient down in the recovery position. Inform doctors.

GUIDELINES: COLLECTION OF A CATHETER SPECIMEN OF URINE

Equipment

1. Swab saturated with isopropyl alcohol 70%.
2. Gate clip.
3. Sterile syringe and needle.
4. Universal specimen container.

Procedure

Action	Rationale
1. Explain the procedure to the patient.	To obtain the patient's consent and co-operation.
2. Screen the bed.	To ensure the patient's privacy.
3. Only if there is no urine in the tubing, clamp the tubing below the rubber cuff until sufficient urine collects. (An access point is now available on catheter bags.)	To obtain an adequate urine sample.
4. Wash hands using bactericidal soap and water or bactericidal alcohol hand rub.	
5. Clean the rubber cuff or access point with a swab saturated with isopropyl alchohol 70%.	To prevent cross-infection.
6. Using a sterile syringe and needle, aspirate the required amount of urine from the rubber cuff or access point (Figure 43.2).	The rubber cuff is specially designed to occlude the puncture hole when the needle is withdrawn. If the catheter bag or tubing is punctured it causes leakage of urine and aspiration of air inwards, carrying organisms with it. Specimens collected from the catheter bag may give false results due to organisms proliferating there.

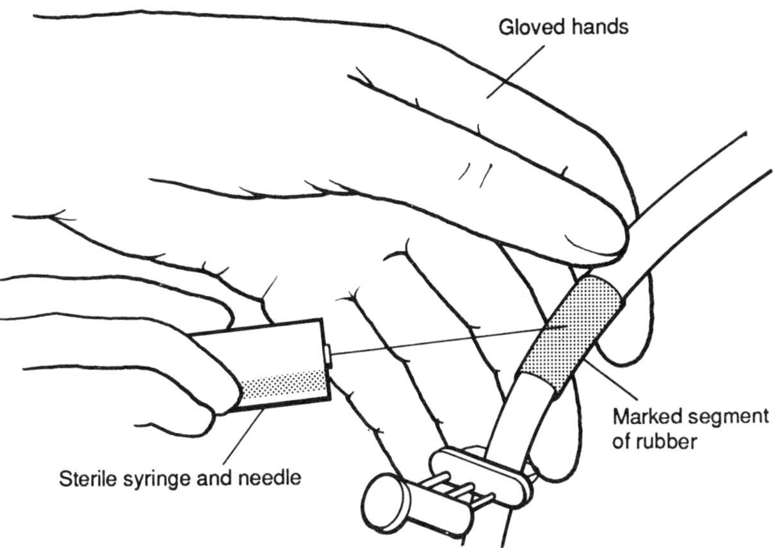

Figure 43.2 Taking a specimen.

7. Place the specimen in a sterile container.	
8. Wash and dry hands.	
9. Unclamp if necessary.	To allow drainage to continue.
10. Make the patient comfortable.	
11. Label the container and dispatch it to the laboratory as soon as possible after sample is taken to allow more accurate results from culture, with the completed request form.	

GUIDELINES: EMPTYING A CATHETER BAG

Equipment

1. Swabs saturated with isopropyl alcohol 70%.
2. Clean jug.
3. Disposable gloves.

Procedure

Action	Rationale
1. Explain the procedure to the patient.	To obtain the patient's consent and co-operation.
2. Wash hands using bactericidal soap and water or bactericidal alcohol hand rub, and put on disposable gloves.	To prevent cross-infection.
3. Clean the outlet valve with a swab saturated with isopropyl alcohol 70%.	
4. Allow the urine to drain into the appropriate jug.	

Guidelines: Emptying a catheter bag

Action	Rationale
5. Close the outlet valve and clean it again with a new alcohol-saturated swab.	To prevent cross-infection.
6. Cover the jug and dispose of contents in the sluice, having noted the amount of urine if this is requested for fluid balance records.	To prevent environmental contamination.
7. Heat-disinfect the jug after each use or return the jug for sterilization.	To prevent cross-infection.
8. Wash hands.	

GUIDELINES: REMOVING A CATHETER

Equipment

1. Dressing pack containing sterile towel, gallipot, foam swab or non-linting gauze.
2. Disposable gloves.
3. Needle and syringe for urine specimen, specimen container.
4. Syringe for deflating balloon.
5. Chlorhexidine solution to clean gloves.

Procedure

Action	Rationale
1. Catheter usually removed early in the morning.	So that any retention problems can be dealt with during the day.
2. Explain procedure to patients and inform them of post-catheter symptoms, i.e. urgency, frequency and discomfort. Symptoms should resolve over the following 24 to 48 hours. If not, further investigation may be needed.	So that patient knows what to expect, and can plan daily activity.
Encourage patient to exercise and to drink two to three litres of fluid per day.	For adequate flushing of bladder, especially to dilute and expel debris and infected urine, if present.
3. Wearing gloves, use saline to clean the meatus and catheter, always swabbing away from the urethral opening.	To prevent infection.
In women, never scrub from the perineum/vagina towards the urethra.	To help reduce the risk of bateria from the vagina and perineum contaminating the urethra.
4. Clean/change gloves. Take a catheter specimen of urine using specimen port hole. Curve catheter tubing so that the urine sample is taken from the top of the curve.	To assess if post-catheter antibiotic therapy is needed.
The catheter should not be clamped for this.	In case the catheter is left clamped for an excessive period of time, allowing bacteria to accumulate, and thus increasing the risk of infection.
5. Clean/change gloves.	
Release leg support.	For easier removal of catheter.
6. Having checked volume of water in balloon (see	To know how much water is in the balloon.

patient documentation), use syringe to deflate balloon.	
7. Ask patient to breathe in and then out; as patient exhales, gently – but quickly – remove catheter. Male patients should be warned of discomfort as the deflated balloon passes through the prostate gland.	To relax pelvic floor muscles.
8. Clean meatus, tidy away equipment, and offer the patient a cup of tea.	

NURSING CARE PLAN

With the catheter in place

Problem	Cause	Suggested action
Urinary tract infection introduced during catheterization.	Faulty aseptic technique. Inadequate urethral cleansing. Contamination of catheter tip.	Inform a doctor. Obtain a catheter specimen of urine.
Urinary tract infection introduced via the drainage system.	Faulty handling of equipment. Breaking the closed system. Raising the drainage bag above bladder level.	Inform a doctor. Obtain a catheter specimen of urine.
No drainage of urine.	Incorrect identification of external urinary meatus (female patients).	Check that catheter has been sited correctly.
	Blockage of catheter.	In the female, leave the catheter in position to act as a guide, re-identify the urethra and recatheterize the patient. Remove the inappropriately sited catheter.
	Empty bladder.	When changing the catheter, clamp the catheter 30 minutes before the procedure. On insertion of the new catheter, urine will drain.
Urethral mucosal trauma.	Incorrect size of catheter. Procedure not carried out correctly or skilfully. Movement of the catheter in the urethra.	Recatheterize the patient using the correct size of catheter. Check the strapping and reapply as necessary.
	Creation of false passage as a result of too rapid insertion of catheter.	Nurse may need to remove the catheter and wait for the urethral mucosa to heal.
Inability to tolerate indwelling catheter.	Urethral mucosal irritation.	Nurse may need to remove the catheter and seek an alternative means of urine drainage.
	Psychological trauma.	Explain the need for and functioning of the catheter.
	Unstable bladder. Radiation cystitis.	

Nursing care plan

Problem	**Cause**	**Suggested action**
Inadequate drainage of urine.	Incorrect placement of a catheter.	Resite the catheter.
	Kinked drainage tubing.	Inspect the system and straighten any kinks.
	Blocked tubing, e.g. pus, urates, phosphates, blood clots.	If a three-way catheter, such as Foley's, is in place, irrigate it. If an ordinary catheter is in use, milk the tubing in an attempt to dislodge the debris; then replace it with a three-way catheter.
Fistula formation.	Pressure on the penoscrotal angle.	Ensure that correct strapping is used.
Penile pain on erection.	Not allowing enough length of catheter to accommodate penile erection.	Ensure that an adequate length is available to accommodate penile erection.
Paraphimosis.	Failure to retract foreskin after catheterization or catheter toilet.	Always retract the foreskin.
Formation of crusts around the urtheral meatus.	Infection involving urea-splitting organisms that cause deposits of salts to form around the catheter.	Correct catheter toilet.
Leakage of urine around catheter.	Incorrect size of catheter.	Replace with the correct size, usually 2Ch sizes smaller.
	Incorrect balloon size.	Select catheter with 10-ml fill volume balloon.
	Bladder hyper-irritability.	Use double-balloon catheter. As a last resort bladder hyper-irritability can be reduced by giving diazepam or anticholinergic drugs.
Unable to deflate balloon.	Valve expansion. Valve displacement.	1. Check the non-return valve on the inflation/deflation channel. If jammed, use a syringe and needle to aspirate by means of the inflation arm above the valve.
	Channel obstruction.	2. Obstruction by a foreign body can sometimes be relieved by the introduction of a guidewire through the inflation channel. 3. Inject 3.5 ml of dilute ether solution (diluted 50/50 with sterile water or normal saline) into the inflation arm. 4. Alternatively, the balloon can be punctured suprapubically using a needle under ultrasound visualization. 5. Following catheter removal

		the balloon should be inspected to ensure it has not disintegrated leaving fragments in the bladder. *Note*: steps 2 to 4 should be attempted by or under the directions of a urologist. The patient may require cytoscopy following balloon deflation to remove any balloon fragments and to wash the bladder out.

After removal of the catheter

Problem	**Cause**	**Suggested action**
Dysuria.	Inflammation of the urethral mucosa.	Ensure a fluid intake of two to three litres per day. Advise the patient that dysuria is common but will usually be resolved once micturition has occurred at least three times. Inform medical staff it the problem persists.
Retention of urine.	May be psychological.	Encourage the patient to increase fluid intake. Offer the patient a warm bath. Inform medical staff if the problem persists.
Urinary tract infection.		Encourage a fluid intake of two to three litres a day. Collect a specimen of urine. Inform medical staff if the problem persists. Administer prescribed antibiotics.

44

Venepuncture

Definition
Venepuncture is the term used for the procedure of entering a vein with a needle.

Indications
Venepuncture is carried out for two reasons:

1. To obtain a blood sample for diagnostic purposes.
2. To monitor levels of blood components.

REFERENCE MATERIAL
Venepuncture is a routine procedure that is increasingly being performed by nursing staff. In order to do this safely the nurse must have a basic knowledge of the following:

1. The relevant anatomy and physiology.
2. The criteria for choosing both the vein and device to use.
3. The potential problems which may be encountered.
4. The correct disposal of equipment.

Certain principles, such as adherence to an aseptic technique, must be applied throughout. The circulation is a closed sterile system and a venepuncture, however quickly completed, is a breach of this system providing a method of entry for bacteria.

The nurse must be aware of the physical and psychological comfort of the patient. He/she must appreciate the value of adequate explanation and simple measures to prevent haematoma formation – a complication of venepuncture, not a natural consequence of it.

Anatomy and physiology
The superficial veins of the upper limb are most commonly chosen for venepuncture. These veins are numerous and accessible, ensuring that the procedure can be performed safely and with minimum discomfort. Occasionally, the veins of a lower limb may be utilized. This should be avoided if possible as blood flow in this region is diminished and the risk of ensuing complications is higher.

Criteria for choosing a site for venepuncture

Condition and accessibility of the peripheral veins
Veins may be tortuous, sclerosed, fibrosed or thrombosed, inflamed or fragile and unable to accommodate the device to be used. If the patient complains of pain or soreness over a particular site, this should be avoided, as should areas that are bruised. Veins adjacent to foci of infection must not be considered.

Preference is given to a vessel which is unused, easily detected by inspection and/or palpation, patent and healthy. These veins feel soft, bouncy and will refill when depressed.

Anatomical considerations
The venous anatomy of each individual differs, but care must always be taken to avoid adjacent structures, e.g. arteries and nerves. Accidental puncture of an artery may cause painful spasm and could result in prolonged bleeding. If a nerve is touched, this can result in severe pain and the attempted venepuncture at this site should be stopped.

Palpation is of value in distinguishing structures clinically, e.g. arteries and tendons, due to the presence of a pulse or resistance, and detecting deeper veins.

Use of veins which cross joints or bony prominences and those with little skin or subcutaneous cover, e.g. the inner aspect of the wrist, will subject the patient to more discomfort.

The sites of choice (Figure 44.1) are branches of:

1. The basilic vein.
2. The cephalic vein.
3. The median cubital vein in the antecubital fossa.

These are sizeable veins capable of providing copious and repeated blood specimens. The brachial artery and median nerve are in close proximity and must not be damaged.

The choice of vein, however, must be that which is

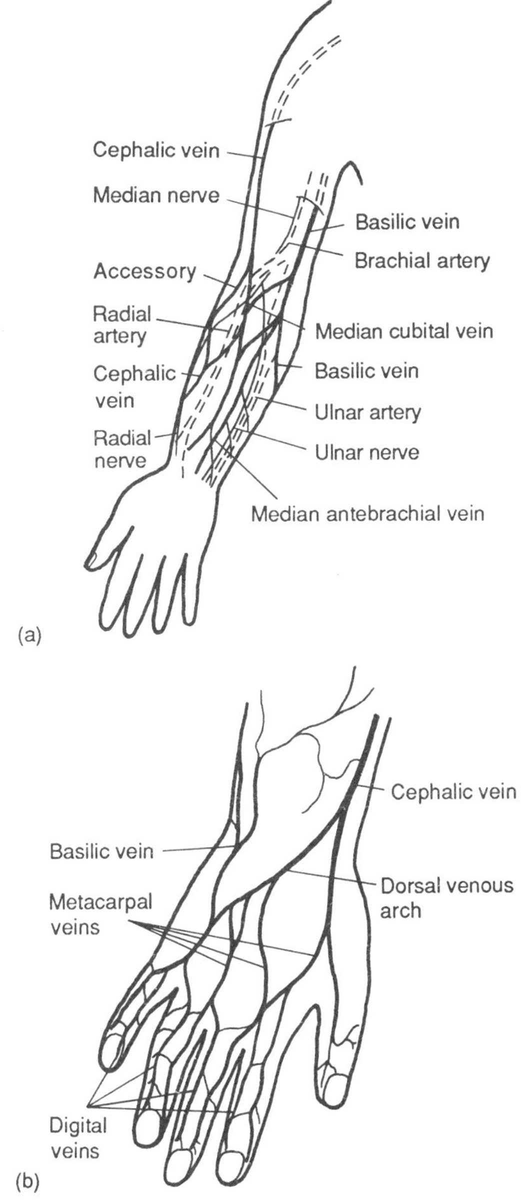

Figure 44.1 (a) Superficial veins of the forearm. (b) Superficial veins of the dorsal aspect of the hand.

best for the individual patient. When using other sites it is advisable to avoid junctions within the venous network. Another feature in veins is the presence of valves. These are folds of the endothelium present in larger vessels to prevent a backflow of blood to the extremity. If detected, a puncture should be performed above the valve in order to facilitate collection of the sample.

Clinical status of the patient

Injury or disease may prevent the use of a limb for venepuncture. Amputation, fracture and cerebrovascular accident are good examples of conditions that affect venous access. Use of a limb may be contraindicated because of an operation on one side of the body, e.g. mastectomy. Impairment of lymphatic drainage can influence venous flow regardless of whether there is obvious lymphoedema. An oedematous limb should be avoided as there is danger of stasis predisposing to such complications as phlebitis and cellulitis. Positioning of the patient may dictate the site of venepuncture.

Physiological factors

The tunica media, the middle layer of the vein wall, is composed of muscle fibres capable of constricting or dilating in response to stimuli from the vasomotor centre in the medulla via the sympathetic nerves. The nurse must be aware of the factors which can influence venous dilation. These are:

1. Anxiety.
2. Temperature.
3. Mechanical or chemical irritation.
4. The clinical state of the patient, e.g. hypovolaemia due to dehydration.

Anxiety may be reduced by presenting a confident manner together with an adequate explanation of the procedure. Careful preparation and an unhurried approach will help to relax the patient and the veins.

The temperature of the environment will influence venous dilation. If the patient is cold, no veins may be evident on first inspection. Application of heat, e.g. in the form of a hot compress or soaking the arm in hot water will increase the size and visibility of the veins, thus increasing the likelihood of a successful first attempt. Ointment or patches containing small amounts of glyceryl trinitrate have been used to cause local vasodilatation to aid venepuncture. (Gunawardene and Davenport, 1989; Hecker *et al.*, 1983).

Venepuncture may cause the vein to collapse or go into a spasm. This will produce discomfort and a reduction in blood flow. Good technique will reduce the likelihood of this and stroking the vein or applying heat will help resolve it.

Good technical skill also prevents trauma to the tunica intima, the lining of the vein. Roughening of the smooth endothelium encourages the process of thrombus formation.

Choice of device

The intravenous devices commonly used to perform a venepuncture for blood sampling are a straight steel

Table 44.1 The choice of intravenous device

Device	*Gauge*	*Advantages*	*Disadvantages*	*Use*
Needle	21	Cheap. Easy to use with large veins	Rigid. Difficult to manipulate with smaller veins in less conventional sites. May cause more discomfort	Large, accessible veins in the antecubital fossa. When small quantities of blood are to be drawn
Winged infusion device	21	Flexible due to small needle shaft. Easy to manipulate and insert at any site. Causes less discomfort	More expensive than steel needles	Veins in sites other than the antecubital fossa. When quantities of blood greater than 20 ml are required from any site
	23	As above	As above, plus there can be damage to cells which can cause inaccurate measurements	Small veins in more painful sites, e.g. inner aspect of the wrist, especially if measurements are related to plasma and not cellular components

needle and a steel winged infusion device. The optimum gauge to use is 21 swg (standard wire gauge). This enables blood to be withdrawn at a reasonable speed without undue discomfort to the patient or possible damage to the blood cells.

The nurse must choose the device dependent on the condition and accessibility of the individual patient's veins (see Table 44.1).

Given the concern about possible contamination by blood, a number of new systems of collection are now available commercially. The equipment available will depend on local policy.

Skin preparation

Asepsis is vital when performing a venepuncture as the skin is breached and an alien device is introduced into a sterile circulatory system. The two major sources of microbial contamination are:

1. Cross-infection from practitioner to patient.
2. Skin flora of the patient.

Good hand washing and drying techniques are essential on the part of the nurse; gloves should be changed between patients.

To remove the risk presented by the patient's skin flora, firm and prolonged rubbing with an alcohol-based solution, such as chlorhexidine 70% in spirit, is advised. This cleaning should continue for at least 30 seconds, although some authors state a minimum of one minute or longer. The area that has been cleaned should then be allowed to dry to facilitate coagulation of the organisms, thus ensuring disinfection. The skin must not be touched or the vein repalpated before puncture.

Skin cleansing is a controversial subject and it is acknowledged that a cursory wipe with an alcohol swab does more harm than no cleaning at all as it disturbs the skin flora. Good cleaning techniques in a hospital environment, where transient pathogens abound, are of value in controlling infection (Plumer, 1987).

Safety of the practitioner

With the increase over the past few years of blood-borne viruses, it is no longer appropriate to protect staff only when a disease is suspected or identified. Adherence to universal safe technique and practice is necessary, thus protecting staff from any potential blood spills. Good quality gloves should be worn at all times. Vacutainer systems should be used whenever possible, thus reducing further the risk of blood spillage. Used needles should always be discarded directly into an approved sharps container, without being re-sheathed. The specimens of patients with known or suspected disease should be double-bagged in clear polythene bags with a biohazard label attached. Only the required amount of blood should be drawn.

The accompanying request forms should be kept separately from the specimen to avoid contamination. All other non-sharp disposables should be placed in a universal yellow clinical waste bag.

There is no substitute for good technique. It must always be remembered that although gloves will protect practitioners from unexpected spillage, they will not prevent a needle stick injury if practice is not safe. Thus practitioners must always work carefully when performing this procedure.

Summary

In order to perform a safe and successful venepuncture, it is important that the practitioner (a) considers carefully the choice of vein and device, and (b) applies the principles of asepsis, and adheres to and understands safe technique and practices.

Supervision by an experienced member of staff is essential when the nurse begins to practise venepuncture.

References and further reading

Dyson, A. & Bogod, D. (1987) Minimizing bruising in the antecubital fossa after venepuncture. *British Medical Journal*, 294, 1659.

Gunawardene, R. D. & Davenport, H. T. (1989) Local application of EMLA and glyceryl trinitrate ointment before venepuncture. *Anaesthesia*, 45, 52–4.

Hecker, J. F. *et al.* (1983) Nitroglycerine ointment as an aid to venepuncture. *Lancet*, 12 February, 332–3.

Johnston-Early, A. *et al.* (1981) Venepuncture and problem veins. *American Journal of Nursing*, September, 1636–40.

Plumer, A. L. (1987) *Principles and Practice of Intravenous Therapy*, 4th edn. Little, Brown & Co., Boston, USA.

Sager, D. & Bomar, S. (1988) *Intravenous Medications*. J. B. Lippcncott, Philadelphia.

Sim, A. J. (1988) Intravenous therapy and HIV infection. *Intensive Therapy & Clinical Monitoring*, July/August, 140–5.

White, J. *et al.* (1970) Skin disinfection. *Johns Hopkins Medical Journal*, 126, 169–70.

Yuan, R. T. W. & Cohen, M. D. (1987) Lateral antebrachial cutaneous nerve injury as a complication of phlebotomy. *Journal of Canadian Intravenous Nurses Association*, 3(3), 16–17.

GUIDELINES: VENEPUNCTURE

Equipment

1. Clinically clean tray or receiver.
2. Tourniquet or sphygmomanometer and cuff.
3. Syringe(s) of appropriate size.
4. 21 swg needle or 21 swg winged infusion device.
5. Swab saturated with isopropyl alcohol 70%.
6. Sterile cotton wool balls.
7. Sterile adhesive plaster or hypo-allergenic tape.
8. Labelled blood specimen bottle(s).
9. Specimen requisition forms.
10. Gloves.
11. Plastic apron (optional).

Alternatively, there are a number of vacuum systems available that can be used for taking blood samples. These are simple to use and cost-effective. The manufacturer's instructions should be followed carefully if one of these systems is to be used and the following items will replace syringes, needles and specimen bottles:

1. 21G multiple sample needle *or* 21G winged infusion device and multiple sample Luer adaptor.
2. Plastic shell to hold specimen tubes.
3. Appropriate vacuumed specimen tubes, labelled.

Procedure

Action	Rationale
1. Approach the patient in a confident manner and explain the procedure to the patient.	To obtain the patient's consent and co-operation.
2. Allow the patient to ask questions and discuss any problems which have arisen previously.	A relaxed patient will have relaxed veins.
3. Assemble the equipment necessary for venepuncture.	To ensure that time is not wasted and that the procedure goes smoothly without any unnecessary interruptions.
4. Carefully wash hands using bactericidal soap and water or bactericidal alcohol hand rub, and dry, before commencement.	To minimize the risk of infection.

Guidelines: Venepuncture

Action	**Rationale**
5. Check hands for any visibly broken skin, and cover with a waterproof dressing.	To minimize the risk of contamination, by blood, to the practitioner.
6. Check all packaging before opening and preparing the equipment on the chosen clinically clean receptacle.	To maintain asepsis throughout and check that no equipment is damaged.
7. Take all the requirements to the patient, exhibiting a competent manner.	To put the patient at ease.
8. In both an inpatient and an outpatient situation, lighting, ventilation, privacy and positioning must be checked.	To ensure that both patient and operator are comfortable and that adequate light is available to illuminate this procedure.
9. Consult the patient as to any preferences and problems that may have been experienced at previous venepunctures.	To involve the patient in the treatment. To acquaint the nurse fully with the patient's previous venous history. To identify any changes in clinical status which may influence vein choice, e.g. mastectomy.
10. Support the chosen limb.	To ensure the patient's comfort.
11. (a) Apply a tourniquet to the upper arm on the chosen side, making sure it does not obstruct arterial flow. The position of the tourniquet may be varied, e.g. if a vein in the hand is to be used is may be placed on the forearm. A sphygmomanometer cuff may be used as an alternative.	To dilate the veins by obstructing the venous return.
(b) The arm may be placed in a dependent position. The patient may assist by clenching and unclenching the fist.	To increase the prominence of the veins.
(c) The veins may be tapped lightly.	
(d) If all these measures are unsuccessful, remove the tourniquet and apply moist heat, e.g. a hot compress, soak limb in hot water or, with medical prescription, apply glyceryl trinitrate ointment/patch.	To promote blood flow and therefore distend the veins.
12. Select the vein using the afore-mentioned criteria.	
13. Select the device, based on vein size, site, etc.	
14. Wash hands with bactericidal soap and water or bactericidal alcohol hand rub.	To maintain asepsis.
15. Put on gloves.	To adhere to universal safe standards.
16. Clean the patient's skin carefully for at least 30 seconds using an appropriate preparation and allow to dry. Do not repalpate the vein or touch the skin.	To maintain asepsis.
17. Inspect the device carefully.	To detect faulty equipment, e.g. bent or barbed needles. If these are present, discard them.

Action	Rationale
18. Anchor the vein by applying manual traction on the skin a few centimetres below the proposed insertion site.	To immobilize the vein. To provide countertension, which will facilitate a smoother needle entry.
19. Insert the needle smoothly at an angle of approximately 30°. The shaft of a straight needle may be bent slightly at the hub to enable the entry to be as flush with the skin as possible.	To ensure a successful, pain-free venepuncture.
20. Level off the needle as soon as a flashback of blood is seen in the tubing of a winged infusion device or when puncture of the vein wall is felt. If you are using a needle and syringe, pull the plunger back slightly prior to venepuncture and a flashback of blood will be seen in the barrel on vein entry.	
21. Advance the needle approximately 1 mm into the vein, if possible.	To stabilize the device within the vein and prevent it becoming dislodged during venepuncture.
22. Do not exert any pressure on the needle.	To prevent a through puncture occurring.
23. Withdraw the required amount of blood using a vacutainer system or syringes.	
24. Release the tourniquet. In some instances this may be requested at the beginning of sampling as inaccurate measurements may be caused by haemostasis, e.g. blood calcium levels.	To decrease the pressure within the vein.
25. Withdraw a small amount of blood into the syringe.	To reduce the amount of static blood in the vein and therefore the likelihood of leakage.
26. Pick up a sterile wool ball and place it over the puncture point.	
27. Remove the needle.	
28. Apply digital pressure directly over the puncture point.	To stop leakage and haematoma formation.
29. Do not apply pressure until the needle has been fully removed.	To prevent pain on removal.
30. Pressure should be applied until the bleeding has ceased, approximately one minute. Longer may required if current disease or treatment interferes with clotting mechanisms.	To prevent leakage or haematoma formation. To preserve vein by preventing leakage or haematoma formation.
The patient may apply pressure with the finger but should be discouraged from bending the arm if a vein in the antecubital fossa is used.	To prevent leakage and haematoma formation.
31. Where a syringe has been used, transfer the blood to appropriate specimen bottles as soon as possible, making sure that the correct quantity is placed in each container.	To prevent clotting in the syringe. To ensure that an adequate amount is available for each test.
32. Mix well if the bottle contains a chemical to prevent clotting or aid accurate measurements.	To ensure that the blood is correctly presented to the laboratory and that the patient does not have to have a repeat specimen taken.

Guidelines: Venepuncture

Action	Rationale
33. Label the bottles with the relevant details.	To ensure that the specimens from the right patient are delivered to the laboratory, the requested tests are performed and the results returned to the correct patient's records.
34. Inspect the puncture point before applying a dressing.	To check that the puncture point has sealed.
35. Ascertain whether the patient is allergic to adhesive plaster.	To prevent an allergic skin reaction.
36. Apply an adhesive plaster or alternative dressing.	To cover the puncture and prevent leakage or introduction of bacteria until healing is complete.
37. Ensure that the patient is comfortable.	To ascertain whether patient wishes to rest before leaving (if an outpatient) or whether any other measures need to be taken.
38. Discard waste, making sure it is placed in the correct containers, e.g. 'sharps' into a designed receptacle.	To ensure safe disposal and avoid laceration or other injury of staff. To prevent re-use of equipment.
39. Follow hospital procedure for collection and transportation of specimens to the laboratory.	To make sure that specimens reach their intended destination.
40. Remove gloves and discard.	

NURSING CARE PLAN

Problem	Cause	Suggested action
Excessive pain.	Anxiety, fear, low pain tolerance.	Confident, unhurried approach. Use all methods, including heat, to dilate veins. Use of local anaesthetic cream. Avoid hesitancy and skin 'tickling'. Consider use of winged infusion device.
	Frequently used vein.	Avoid this site, if possible, otherwise proceed as above.
	Nerve touched.	Remove the needle immediately and proceed to a different site.
Very anxious patient.	Previous trauma. Needle phobia.	Confident unhurried approach. Make sure the patient is comfortable, perhaps reclining/ lying down. Use all methods, including heat, to dilate veins. Consider use of winged infusion device.
Limited venous access.	Repeated use, e.g. prolonged cytotoxic therapy. Phlebitis.	Confident, unhurried approach. Use all methods including heat to dilate veins. Use a winged

		infusion device of 21G or 23G. Only proceed if sure of a successful first attempt. Consider referral to a more experienced colleague.
	Bruising due to: 1. Fragile veins in the elderly; 2. Anticoagulant therapy or low platelet levels.	As above plus apply tourniquet gently or do not use. Ensure adequate pressure to puncture site to prevent further damage.
	Peripheral shutdown.	Use all methods to dilate veins as listed. A sphygmomanometer and cuff may enable more effective restriction of the venous return. Work quickly if the patient is in a collapsed state. Pull blood back into the veins by massaging above the venepuncture site.
Infection.	Poor aseptic technique.	Practise good hand washing and skin cleansing and take particular care with immune-compromised patients.

Practical problems

Problem	**Cause**	**Suggested action**
Missed vein.	Inadequate anchoring. Wrong positioning. Poor lighting. Less than 100% concentration.	Withdraw the needle almost to the bevel and manoeuvre gently to realign needle and vein. Readvance, but if it becomes painful, remove. Better preparation next time.
Spurt of blood on entry.	Bevel tip of needle entering vein before entire bevel is under the skin, due to vein being very superficial.	Ignore. Reassure the patient if a small blood blister develops.
Blood flow stops.	Overshooting vein or advancing needle while withdrawing blood.	Gently ease needle back and continue.
	Vein collapse due to contact with valve or vein wall.	Manoeuvre gently. Release and retighten tourniquet and continue.
	Poor blood flow.	As above and massage above the needle tip to pull blood into vein.
Haematoma.	Perforation of opposite wall of vein.	Insert needle at correct angle and stop when a flashback is seen in syringe or tubing of winged fashion infusion device. Do not advance needle during taking of sample.
	Forgetting to remove tourniquet before removing needle.	Remember next time.
	Inadequate pressure on puncture site.	Press. Supervise the patient doing the same.

Nursing care plan

Problem	Cause	Suggested action
Hardening of the veins due to scarring and thrombosis.	Prolonged use of one site.	Alternate venepuncture sites to prevent this. Do not use hard veins as this is often not successful and will cause the patient pain.
Mechanical problems.	Faulty equipment, e.g. bent needle tips, cracked syringes.	Check carefully before use and discard.
Transmittable diseases.	Viruses pose the major risk, causing hepatitis B, cytomegalovirus, acquired immune deficiency syndrome.	All blood should be handled with care and caution used when handling specimens of infection, e.g. Australia antigen-positive people. Gloves should be worn when taking blood and handling samples. Hospital policy should be strictly observed.
Needle inoculation.	Lack of caution. Overfilling of 'sharps' containers.	Dispose of equipment safety to prevent inoculation. If it does occur, follow accident procedure and report the incident immediately. An injection of hepatitis B immunoglobulin may be required.

45

Violence: Prevention and Management

The problem of violence within public service organizations has become a matter of increasing concern to all those who work in the health service (Poyner & Warne, 1983). Incidents range from threats and abuse to permanently disabling injuries and, rarely, loss of life. This procedure is confined to the manifestation and management of violence in the hospital setting.

Definition

Stuart and Sundeen (1987) define violence as 'an act of destructive aggression which may involve injury to the self, assaulting people or objects in the environment'.

Robinson (1983) defines aggression as 'an assertive force which may be expressed through attitude or behaviour and is usually directed to external objects, though it may be turned inward, as reflected in self-destructive behaviour'. She states that 'aggression is a healthy force which sometimes needs to be channelled'.

Indications

Management of violence is necessary:

1. When a patient makes a physical attack on another person.
2. When a patient becomes disturbed to the extent that his/her behaviour is considered a threat to his/her own safety or to the safety of others.

REFERENCE MATERIAL

Principles

The following principles underlie the management of violent patients:

1. Restraint is always therapeutic, never punitive. As far as possible the therapeutic regime should be maintained.
2. The risk of physical injury should be minimized. Any restraint applied must be of a degree appropriate to the actual danger or resistance shown by the patient. This is particularly important with children and the elderly.
3. The agreed procedure for the nursing care of violent patients should be adhered to.

Theories of violence

Mechanisms which may combine to explain or produce a violent act are reviewed by Harrington (1972) and Gunn (1973). Generally, theories of violence may be classified as biological (Gray, 1971; Lorenz, 1966; Montague, 1979), psychological (Dollard & Miller, 1961; Freud, 1955) or sociocultural (Bandura & Walters, 1963; Gelles, 1972; Wertham, 1968). Violence may be viewed as a behaviour influenced by various factors including personality, environment and social culture. Each perspective may add to the development of a body of knowledge about the problem of violence in the hospital setting.

Agitation and aggression preceding violent behaviour have been identified particularly among elderly confused patients, and nursing interventions such as feeding, dressing and bathing represented the most common antecedents (Campbell *et al.*, 1989).

Physiological considerations

Under certain circumstances patients may have little or no ability to exercise control over their aggression. In these instances aggression may be related to pathological physiology. Internal stressors may include endocrine imbalance as in hyperthyroidism, hypoglycaemia, convulsive disorders, dementia, and brain tumours. The effects of alcohol and drug abuse should also be considered. Preventive measures may not be appropriate and the policy for the management of violence should be adhered to.

HIV involvement with the nervous system has been recognized (Royal College of Nursing, 1986). Fifty to 60% of AIDS patients are estimated to develop neurological complications, and 60 to 70% of patients contract HIV encephalopathy. Symptoms include memory and concentration impairment and, less frequently, organic psychosis with agitation, inappropriate behaviour and/or hallucinations (McArthur *et al.*, 1988). Although there have been no reported cases of violent incidents in hospitals involving patients with HIV or AIDS, the general principles for the management of such patients who become violent are no different to those for the management of other violent patients.

The care of violent patients or visitors

Among the guidelines recommended by the Royal College of Nursing and the National Council for Nurses of the United Kingdom (1972) for the care of violent patients, are the following:

1. Prevention of violence is the goal.
2. Physical confrontations should be avoided.
3. All hospital personnel within the vicinity of the violent incident are expected to render assistance.
4. Staff should receive instruction and guidance in the management of violence.
5. Staff should be aware of and control their own emotions.
6. The attitude of staff should be calm, non-critical and non-domineering.

There will be occasions when, for a variety of reasons, a patient or visitor will threaten violence or actually become violent. In these situations it is essential for the nurse to apply confidently the appropriate skills in order to manage the incident. Leiba (1980) isolates four aspects that need to be considered in the management of violence in the hospital setting:

1. Organization of the ward, department, etc.
2. Prevention.
3. Management.
4. Follow-up.

Organization

The way in which staff are deployed influences the likelihood and outcome of any violent incident. There must be adequate staff to deal with the violence and there must be a hospital policy for the management of violence. All hospital personnel should know what to do and how to do it. Teaching sessions on the management of violence should be held on a regular basis so that staff benefit from controlled practice of the required techniques for avoiding and containing violence. Topics may include alternatives to violent behaviour, appropriate expression of emotions or stress reduction techniques (Green, 1989). It is helpful if there is a team in the hospital that can be called if an emergency occurs. Teamwork is essential and the leader must be seen to be confident in making the necessary decisions. It is the responsibility of individual members of staff to state whether they have a physical disability, such as back injury or pregnancy, which would render them incapable of performing procedures.

Prevention

Identify high-risk patients, examples of whom may be those with physiological conditions as previously discussed or patients with a previous history of violent behaviour. A multidisciplinary approach may be helpful in establishing this. Violent incidents may be spontaneous, without apparent provocation, for example, with a patient suffering from a psychotic illness or cerebral lesions which affect behaviour. However, there may be signs of warning which would alert staff to a potentially violent situation and give opportunity for prevention of violence.

Signs may include increased motor agitation, verbal content, change in voice tone and volume, clenched fists or sudden cessation of activity (Smith, 1987). Megargee (1966) suggests that violent behaviour is part of a continuum of behaviour which also includes anger, frustration and aggression. Novaco (1976) attributes positive and therapeutic functions to be controlled expression of anger.

Stuart and Sundeen (1983) see violence as the culmination of an escalating process, where anger and aggression are considered as precursors to violence. They suggest that preventive therapeutic interventions can be used to intercept this process, thus deferring a potentially violent situation. Ritter (1989) suggests prevention of violence requires:

1. Detailed individual assessment of patients.
2. Close co-operation between multidisciplinary team members.
3. Attention to the methods of communication used by the patient.
4. Clearly defined systems for decision-making which allows the patient a degree of control.

Environmental measures can be taken to reduce aggression. Lighting, noise levels, furnishings and routine can be taken into consideration, while simple solutions such as providing information can alleviate frustration in waiting areas (Shuttleworth, 1989).

Knowledge of the propensities of individual patients will enable a nurse to recognize many of the signs of impending violence, thus allowing steps to be taken to help patients find alternative outlets for their aggressive feelings.

Management

Once violence has occurred, the following may

be regarded as among the important management decisions that need to be implemented:

1. All medical and nursing personnel must be involved immediately, the former because medication may be required as part of the management of the situation.
2. Some nurses must be delegated to attend to the needs of the remaining patients, to telephone for help and to prepare any required medication.
3. If immobilization is needed, the agreed policy for restraining a patient must be implemented.

Follow-up

Following the incident, staff should be given an opportunity to discuss their feelings about the patient, other members of staff involved and the way the incident was managed. This should happen as soon as possible after the incident has resolved and with as many of the staff concerned as possible. Some staff view incident-reporting as admission of failure, especially if violence is rare in the area in which they work (Drummond *et al.*, 1989), therefore de-briefing becomes particularly relevant.

Staff injured as a result of their involvement in the incident may be entitled to industrial injuries benefits or a payment under the criminal injuries compensation scheme, and will need to be informed of their rights. All documentation required by law or hospital policy should be completed and forwarded to the appropriate departments. If restraints have been used, how and by whom they were applied should be documented. Specific written records will aid recall if it is required, perhaps years later (Navis, 1987).

Summary

Violent incidents often arise from a patient feeling vulnerable. Attack may become the preferred means of defence. The manner in which a patient is approached may be crucial in determining whether the patient will feel secure enough to cease the behaviour or continue to feel threatened, perhaps leading on to violent behaviour. The need for physical restraint should be seen as the application of the appropriate technique in a particular situation and not as a failure of other methods. Protection against any administrative or legal problems lies in following the appropriate guidelines and applying them in good faith and with due restraint.

References and further reading

Bandura, A. & Walters, R. (1963) *Social Learning and Personality Development*. Holt, Rinehart & Winston, New York.

Bethlem Royal and Maudsley Hospital (1976) *Guidelines for the Nursing Management of Violence*. Bethlem Royal and Maudsley Hospital, London.

Blackburn, R. (1970) *Personality Types Among Abnormal Homicides. Special Hospitals Research Report No. 1*. Broadmoor Hospital, Special Hospitals Research Unit.

Campbell, B. *et al.* (1989) A high-risk occupation? *Nursing Times*, 85(13), 37–9.

Dollard, J. & Miller, N. E. (1961) *Frustration and Aggression*. Yale University Press, New Haven.

Drummond, D. J. *et al.* (1989) Hospital violence reduction among high-risk patients. *Journal of the American Medical Association*, 261(17), 2531–4.

Freud, S. (1955) *The Complete Psychological Works of Sigmund Freud, Vol. 18*. Hogarth Press, London.

Gelles, R. J. (1972) *The Violent Home*. Sage, Beverly Hills and London.

Gray, J. A. (1971) Sex differences in emotional behaviour in mammals including man: endocrine basis. *Acta Psychologica*, 35, 29–44.

Green, E. (1989) Patient care guidelines: management of violent behavior. *Journal of Emergency Nursing*, 15(6), 523–8.

Gunn, J. (1973) *Violence*. David & Charles, Newton Abbot.

Harrington, J. A. (1972) Violence: a clinical viewpoint. *British Medical Journal*, 1, 228–31.

Leiba, P. A. (1980) Management of violent patients. *Nursing Times*, Occasional Papers, 76(23), 101–4.

Lorenz, K. (1966) *On Aggression*. Harcourt, Brace & World, New York.

McArthur, J. H. *et al.* (1988) Human immunodeficiency virus and the nervous system. *Nursing Clinics of North America*, 23(4), 823–41.

Megargee, E. I. (1966) Under-controlled and over-controlled personality types in extreme antisocial aggression. *Psychological Monograph*, 80, 1–29.

Montague, M. C. (1979) Physiology of aggressive behaviour. *Journal of Neurosurgical Nursing*, 11, 10–15.

Navis, E. S. (1987) Controlling violent patients before they control you. *Nursing*, 17(9), 52–4.

Novaco, R. W. (1976) The functions and regulation of the arousal of anger. *American Journal of Psychiatry*, 133, 1124.

Poyner, B. & Warne, C. (1983) *Violence to Staff: A Basis for Assessment and Prevention*. Tavistock Institute of Human Relations, Health and Safety Commission, London.

Ritter, S. (1989) *The Bethlem Royal and Maudsley Hospitals Manual of Clinical Psychiatric Nursing Principles and Procedures*. Harper & Row, London.

Robinson, L. (1983) *Psychiatric Nursing as a Human Experience*. W. B. Saunders, Philadelphia.

Royal College of Nursing and the National Council for Nurses of the United Kingdom (1972) *The Care of the Violent Patient. Report of the Liaison Committee*. Royal College of Nursing, London.

Royal College of Nursing (1986) *Nursing Guidelines on the Management of Patients in Hospitals and the Community Suffering from AIDS*. Royal College of Nursing, London.

Royal College of Psychiatrists and Royal College of Nursing (1979) *Principles of Good Medical and Nursing Practice in the*

Management of Acts of Violence in Hospitals. Royal College of Psychiatrists/Royal College of Nursing, London.

Shuttleworth, A. (1989) Violence: is enough being done to protect you? *The Professional Nurse*, 4(5), 227–8.

Smith, D. (1987) Preventing violence in nursing. *New Zealand Nursing Journal*, 80(12), 18–19.

Stuart, G. W. & Sundeen, S. J. (1987) *Principles and Practice of Psychiatric Nursing*, 3rd edn. C. V. Mosby, St Louis.

Surrey Area Health Authority (1979) *Guidelines to Staff on the Management of Violent or Potentially Violent Patients*. Surrey Area Health Authority.

Wertham, D. J. (1968) *A Sign For Cain*. Hale, New York.

Video material

Nursing Management of Violence (1977), produced by the South East Thames Regional Health Authority.

GUIDELINES: PREVENTION AND MANAGEMENT OF VIOLENCE

Procedure

Prevention of violence

Action	Rationale
1. (a) It is important that the nurse makes other staff aware of a potentially violent situation and does not enter it unobserved. (b) Try not to encroach upon the patient's personal space. Keep at arm's length. (c) If possible ask other patients to leave the area. (d) Ensure that there is a clear exit from the situation. (e) Avoid cornering the patient. (f) Observe the area around the patient for potential weapons. (g) Try to appear confident, calm and relaxed. Do not fold your arms, maintain and open posture. Move slowly, showing that you have nothing in your hands.	To maintain a safe environment.
2. Talk quietly and clearly to the patient. Do not argue.	The nurse may be able to gauge the patient's level of frustration and give an opportunity of expressing anger verbally by initiating conversation.
3. Adopt an attentive expression.	Smiling could be interpreted as mockery. Frowning could be interpreted as anger.
4. Address the patient by name and name yourself.	To help orientate the patient and demonstrate respect.

Management of violence

General principles

Action	Rationale
1. Call for assistance by shouting or using any signalling system.	It is easier to manage the situation with two or more people.
2. Ask another patient to summon help when appropriate.	
3. Continue to hold on to the patient once immobilized.	To contain the violence.

4. Consider carefully the accessories you wear. Be aware of the length of your fingernails and the way long hair is dressed. Pens, badges and other items should be removed beforehand.	To minimize the risk of physical injury to patients.

Personal attack

Action	Rationale
1. Shout to the patient: 'Stop!'	A sharp command may bring the patient back to the reality of the situation.
2. Call for assistance.	
3. Sound any signalling alarm.	
4. If the above fails, either: (a) Stay close to the patient. (b) Grasp the patient's arm at elbow level and pull towards you. (c) Change your grip quickly and encircle patient with your arms. (d) Continue pulling the patient towards you. (e) Quickly get behind the patient. (f) Push the patient towards the nearest wall. (g) Retain your grip and lean against the patient, pressing the patient to the wall (Figure 45.1).	Immobilize the patient by pressing his/her body against the wall.
5. Or: (a) Move to one side. (b) Place your nearest leg behind the patient. (c) Keep your foot firmly on the ground. (d) Push the patient over your leg (Figure 45.2). (e) Lower the patient and yourself to the floor, turning the patient at the same time so that the patient's face is towards the floor.	Immobilize the patient by holding him/her face downwards on the floor.

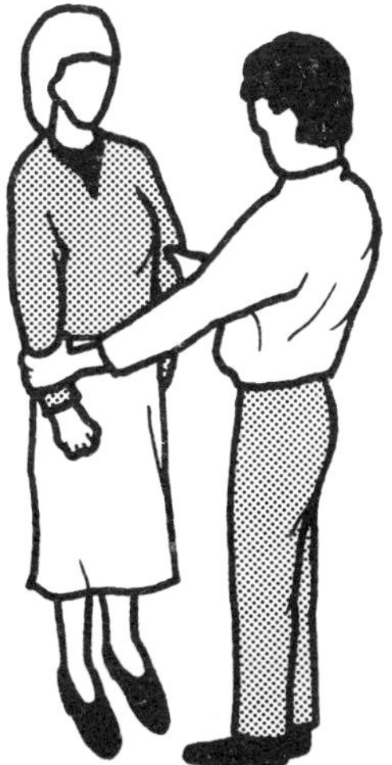
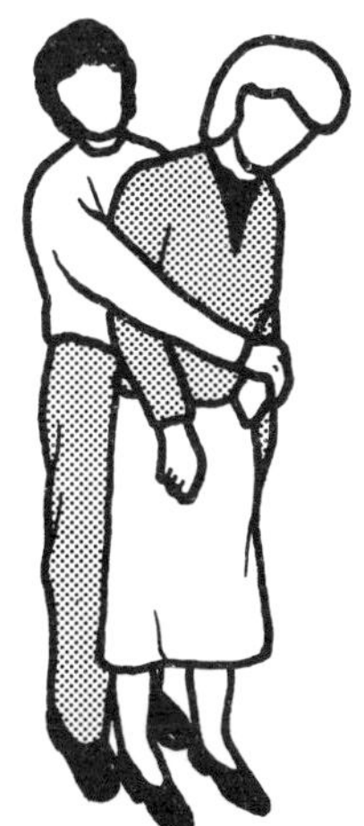

Figure 45.1 Managing the violent patient

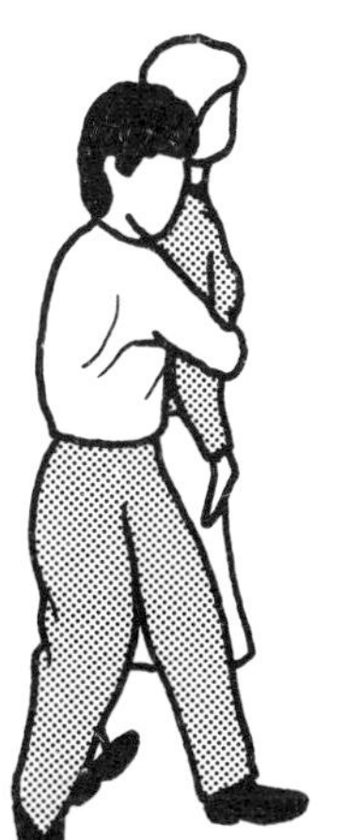
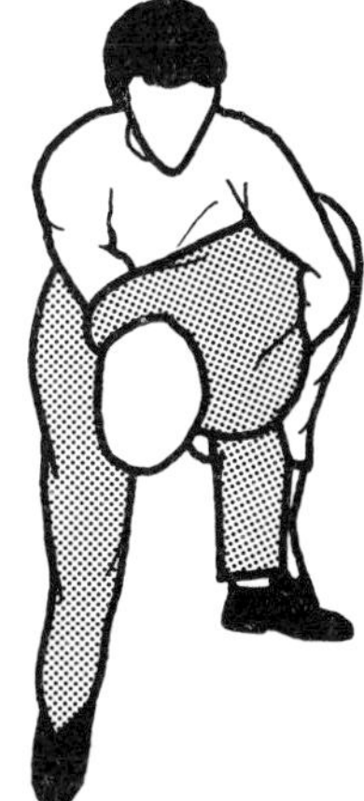

Figure 45.2 Managing the violent patient – a personal attack from behind.

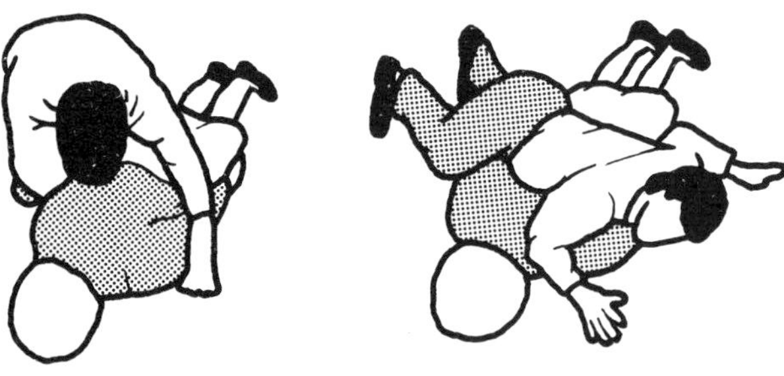

Figure 45.3 Managing the violent patient – a personal attack from behind.

Guidelines: Prevention and management of violence

Action	**Rationale**
(f) Lie across the patient's trunk (Figure 45.3).	
(g) Wrap the patient in a blanket if possible.	To restrict the use of limbs even further and to minimize the risk of physical injury to patient and staff.

Attempted choking

Action	**Rationale**
1. With patient in front of you:	
(a) Bend sharply forward from the waist (Figure 45.4).	To break the patient's grip.
(b) Cross your wrists in front of you and move back.	In case the patient brings the knees up.
(c) Carry out the procedure for personal attack outlined above.	
2. With patient behind you:	
(a) Grasp the little fingers on each of the patient's hands (Figure 45.5).	To break the patient's grip.

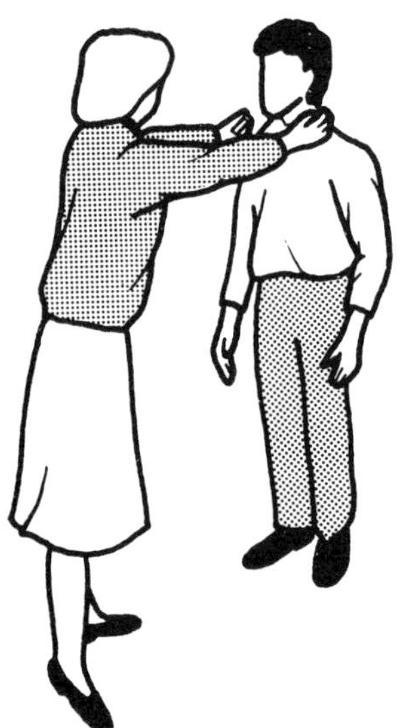

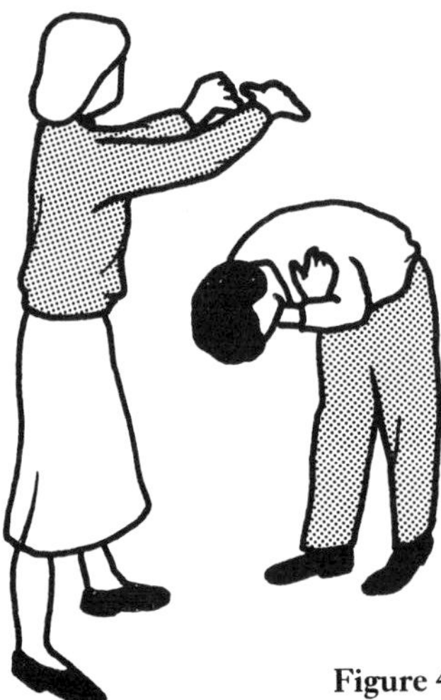

Figure 45.4 Managing the violent patient – attempted choking by a patient in front.

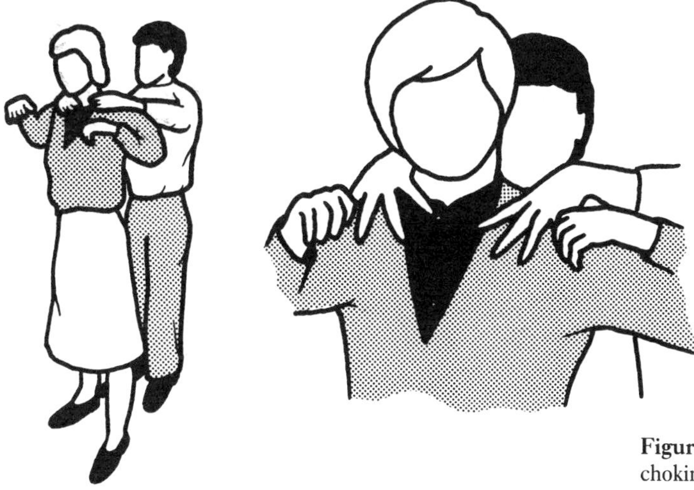

Figure 45.5 Managing the violent patient – attempted choking by a patient from behind.

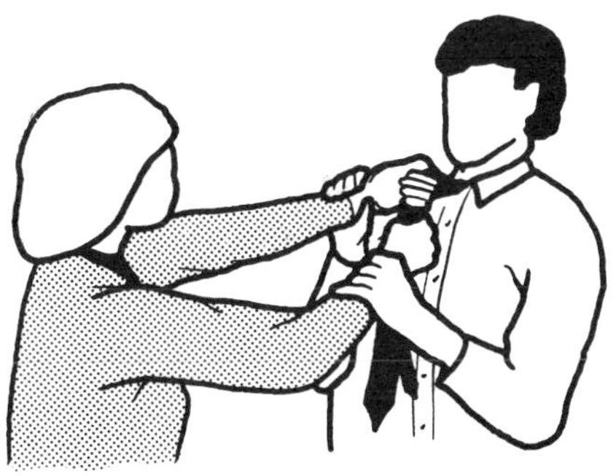

Figure 45.6 Countering tie and hair pulling.

(b) Pull the patient's arms forward, holding the patient close to you.
(c) Call for help.

Hair and tie pulling

Action	**Rationale**
1. Grasp the patient's wrists pulling the hands towards you (Figure 45.6).	To release the pressure on the hair or item of clothing being pulled.
2. Maintain this position.	
3. Call for help.	

Biting

Action	**Rationale**
1. Grasp attacker's hair and hold head still.	To minimize personal injury.
2. If possible, apply firm pressure to the back of the patient's head.	To release grip of patient's jaw.

Guidelines: Prevention and management of violence

Action	Rationale
3. Call for help.	
4. If blood is drawn through the biting the same emergency measures should be taken as those for a needlestick injury, regardless of the patient's HIV or hepatitis B status (see Chapter 4).	

Attack with objects

Action	Rationale
1. Back away from the situation.	To minimize the risk of physical injury.
2. Keep the patient in front of you.	
3. Call for help.	
4. If trapped, call for help and sound any signalling system.	
5. Use a chair or similar object as a shield.	To protect oneself.
6. Keep to the middle of the room.	
7. Defend yourself if attacked (Figure 45.7).	

Blunt objects

Action

1. Close in quickly.

2. Grasp object.

3. Hold on tightly.

4. Call for help.

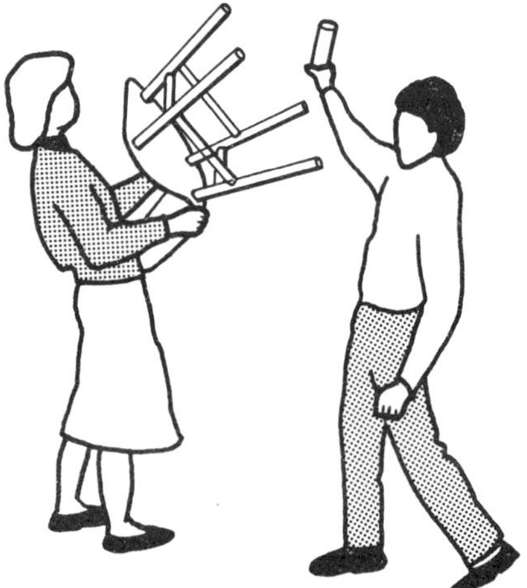

Figure 45.7 Countering an attack with an object.

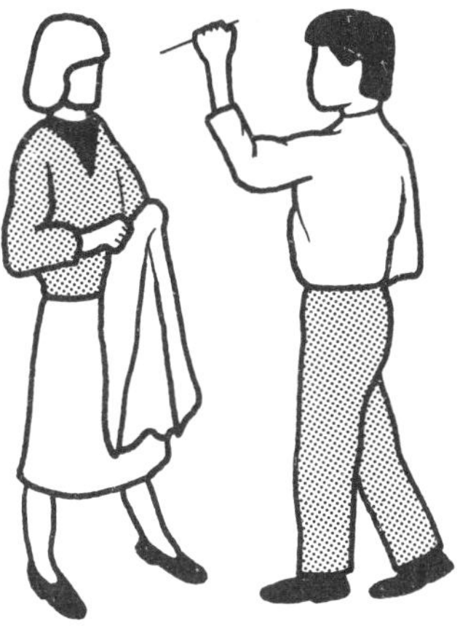
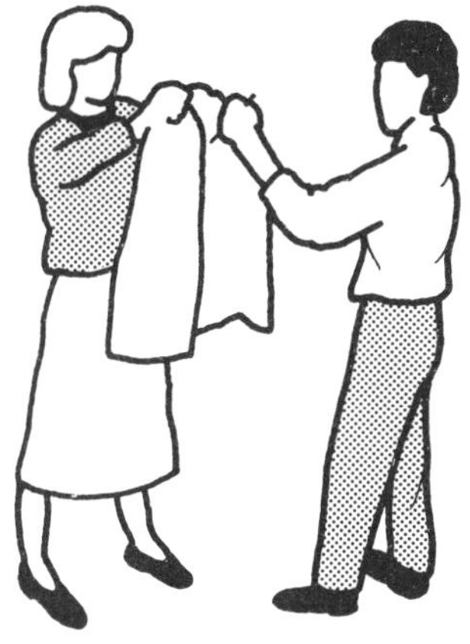
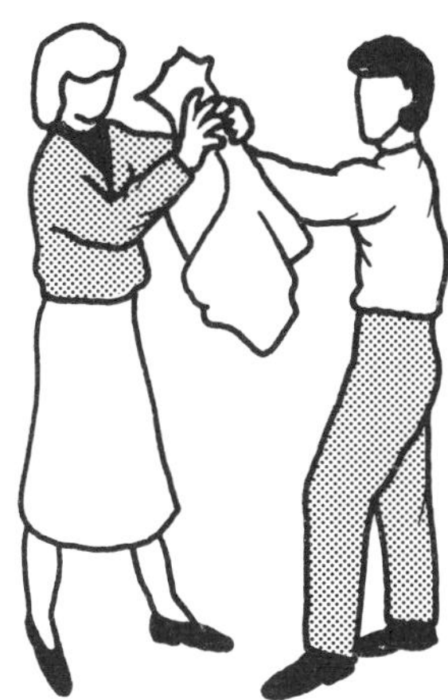

Figure 45.8 Countering an attack with a sharp object.

Sharp objects

Action

1. Pick up any piece of clothing or materials, the larger and thicker the better.
2. Use the material to absorb the impact of any blow.
3. Smother the weapon if possible with the material (Figure 45.8).
4. Call for help.

Threat with firearms

Action	Rationale
1. Do as the patient demands.	This is a life-threatening situation.

Management of personnel involved

Action	Rationale
1. The ward manager should assess whether or not there are enough staff, and inform the senior nurse if more are needed.	In order to contain the violence.
2. When help arrives, the staff should be organized. The manager should identify himself/herself as leader and should give a brief history of the patient and an account of the circumstances and events leading up to the incident.	Staff anxiety will need to be calmed.
3. A doctor, preferably the patient's own, should be called and must come immediately. A nurse should be allocated to draw up medication, and give injections if required.	Medication may be required in the management of the patient.

Guidelines: Prevention and management of violence

Action	**Rationale**
4. To restrain the patient, clear instructions should be given. The manager should indicate when the patient is to be restrained and co-ordinate staff during the procedure. Any disagreements between staff about decisions should not be voiced in front of the patient.	All staff must know the overall plan for restraint.
5. Specific staff should be allocated to be with the other patients, who should then be led away from the area where the patient is to be restrained.	Violent incidents are distressing and may trigger off more violence.
6. Each person should know which part of the patient's body is to be held, and from where to approach the patient.	To achieve full immobilization of the patient.
7. Allocate one member of staff, preferably someone the patient knows, to talk to the patient throughout the procedure.	To inform the patient about what is happening and why.
8. The first team member should help the nurse who is immobilizing the patient. They may need to disarm such patients and get them to the floor as quickly as possible in the face-downwards position if this has not already been achieved. This member of staff should lie across the patient's trunk.	
9. Two other nurses should each restrain a patient's leg.	
10. A further person should restrain the patient's head and shoulders and turn the patient's head to one side.	To ensure that the patient's airway is maintained.
11. Try to minimize discomfort. Reduce the amount of weight on the patient; use only what is necessary.	The procedure is not a punitive one.
12. As the patient calms down, the manager should indicate when restraint can be reduced. This should be done gradually, e.g. release one wrist slowly.	The patient may still be likely to strike.
13. The manager should withdraw staff from the patient gradually.	Restraint must be of a degree of appropriate to the actual resistance shown by the patient.
14. Some staff should stay with the patient.	To observe mood and behaviour.
15. Attend to any patients and staff injured during the incident. Inform such people of their legal rights.	To comply with legal obligations and hospital policy.
16. Record details of any violent incidents in the appropriate documents.	To comply with legal obligations and hospital policy.

17. The entire team should discuss the incident.	To ventilate feelings. Violent incidents are to be regarded as learning situations.

46

Wound Management

Definition of a wound

A wound can be defined as a cut or break in continuity of an organ or tissue caused by an external agent, such as injury or surgery (Cape & Dobson, 1977; *Dictionary of Nursing*, 1990), or a loss of continuity of the skin. Soft tissue, muscle and bone may or may not be involved (Milward, 1988). The first definition allows for tissue damage that occurs without a break in the skin, for example, 'bruising'. The second definition includes the premise that a wound involves a break in skin, which is often the assumption made by health care professionals and lay people.

Wounds are traditionally divided into four categories. These are:

1. Contusion (bruise).
2. Abrasion (graze).
3. Laceration (tear).
4. Incision (cut).

Puncture wounds may now also be incorporated into these groupings (Wingate & Wingate, 1988). Different causes of wounds include:

1. External, e.g. burns (chemical, electrical, fire); hypoxia; mechanical; micro-organisms; radiation; temperature extremes.
2. Internal, e.g. circulatory (venous, arterial, lymphatic); systematic (autoimmune, endocrine, haematological, neuropathies); local (infective, neoplastic) (Allen, 1988; David, 1986; Lawrence & Groves, 1988).

REFERENCE MATERIAL

Classification of wounds

Wounds can be classified in different ways depending on the information required and action to be taken on the data.

Classifications can be utilized to assess which treatment is most appropriate. These classifications most usefully contain an appraisal of the amount of tissue loss (Westaby, 1985). An example of such a system is that developed by the National Pressure Ulcer Advisory Panel (1989) which combines several of the most commonly used systems. There are four categories which begin with no tissue loss – 'non-blanchable erythema of intact skin' (stage one), and progress to 'full thickness skin loss with extensive destruction, tissue necrosis or damage to muscle, bone, or supporting structures' (stage four). The Panel also suggests that additional descriptions of these wounds, such as surface size, would assist in evaluation (National Pressure Ulcer Advisory Panel, 1989). Other grading of pressure ulcers has been determined using a five-point scale (Dealey, 1988).

Further classifications that might prove valuable for assessment of treatment entail whether the wound is clean or infected or dry or wet. The following categories are described as worthwhile when considering the application of disinfectants to wounds:

1. Dry, clean surgical wounds.
2. Wet, oozing, clean surgical wounds.
3. Open, contaminated wounds or lesions (Gustafsson, 1988).

A similar but more sophisticated system concerns both differing wounds and the various stages they pass through as they heal. This classification is designed for selection of a dressing:

1. Black and necrotic – covered with a hard, dry layer of skin.
2. Sloughy/necrotic – covered or filled with a soft yellow slough.
3. Clean and granulating with a significant amount of tissue loss.
4. Epithelializing (*The Dressing Times*, 1989 March)

In addition, surgical wounds can be identified as one of four types. These are: clean; clean contaminated; contaminated; or dirty. This is dependent on the infection encountered (Cruse & Foord, 1980).

Some classifications consider the origin of the

wound. For example: surgical trauma, accidental trauma or ulceration caused by pressure or vascular insufficiency (Turner, 1983); or intentional wounds and accidental wounds (Milward, 1988).

Although these classifications give an indication of the aetiology of the wound, from which some evaluation may be made of its likely nature, they are unsuitable for assessing relevant treatment. When treatment is deliberated, the most appropriate classifications will include those that consider both the degree of tissue loss and whether or not the wound is infected (Turner, 1983; Westaby, 1985).

Wound healing

Wound healing is the process by which tissues damaged or destroyed by injury or disease are restored to normal function (Cape & Dobson, 1977; Wingate & Wingate, 1988).

> Wound healing is only one aspect of the body's response to injury and the whole person, not just the visible injury, must be treated.
>
> (Torrance, 1985)

The latter statement reflects a holistic perspective and is, therefore, more appropriate as a framework for planning nursing care.

Healing may occur by first, second or third intention. Healing by first intention involves the union of the edges of a clean, incised wound under aseptic conditions without visible granulations (Cape & Dobson, 1977; *Dictionary of Nursing*, 1990).

Healing by second intention signifies the process of contraction and epithelialization. The wound edges are separated and the cavity is gradually filled with granulation tissue from the bottom and the sides (Winter, 1972). Epithelial tissue grows over the granulations and forms fibrous tissue which contracts to form a scar (Cape & Dobson, 1977; *Dictionary of Nursing*, 1990; Westaby, 1985).

Healing by third intention occurs when the wound ulcerates and granulations are slow to form (*Dictionary of Nursing*, 1990).

Phases of wound healing

Wound healing is a complex series of physiological events which occur in a predictable sequence (Messer, 1989). Generally, the mechanism is described in three or four stages. These are:

1. The inflammatory phase.
2. The destructive phase.
3. The proliferative or reconstructive phase or fibroplasia.
4. The remodelling phase or maturation phase (Cooper, 1990; Jackson & Rovee, 1988; Johnson, 1988a; Messer, 1989; Torrance, 1985; Westaby, 1985).

These stages overlap to an extent but will be discussed individually to enhance clarity (see also Table 46.1). Contraction and epithelialization are also necessary to the wound healing process but are not usually included in the above stages. These will be considered separately.

Inflammatory stage (0–3 days)

Vasoconstriction occurs within a few seconds of tissue damage. This lasts approximately five to ten minutes. During this time injured blood vessels bleed into the cavity and leucocytes arrive and marginate along the vessel walls. Platelets adhere to vessel walls and edges and are stabilized by a network of fibrin to form a clot. Bleeding ceases when the blood vessels thrombose. In the absence of noradrenaline (broken down by extracellular enzymes from damaged cells), and with the release of histamine, vasodilation begins. The liberation of histamine also increases the permeability of the capillary walls, and plasma proteins, leucocytes, antibodies and electrolytes exude into the surrounding tissues. The wound becomes red, swollen and hot.

Polymorphonuclear leucocytes and macrophages are chemotactically attracted to the wound to defend against infection and begin the process of repair. The macrophage is also known as the 'director cell' of wound healing. If the number and function of macrophages is reduced, as may occur in disease, e.g. diabetes (Tooke *et al.*, 1988), healing is seriously affected.

Destructive stage (2–5 days)

Polymorphonuclear leucocytes and macrophages combine to destroy and ingest bacteria, debris and devitalized tissue. This involves a great deal of cellular activity which requires up to 20 times the normal resting rate of oxygen of phagocytic cells. Patients with hypoxic wounds are, therefore, more susceptible to wound infection.

The degradation of unwanted material causes an increased osmolarity within the area resulting in further swelling by osmosis. This may increase pressure in restricted parts of the body thus precipitating ischaemia.

Proliferative stage (3–24 days)

Macrophages produce factors which are chemotactic to fibroblasts and angioblasts. The macrophage secretes a fibroblast-stimulating factor which in the presence of a growth factor released by the dead platelets causes the fibroplast to migrate into the wound soon after damage has occurred.

The fibroblasts are activated to divide and produce collagen by processes initiated by the macrophages. This develops a network of poorly organized collagen which increases the strength of the wound. Newly synthesized collagen creates a 'healing ridge' below an intact suture line, thus giving an indication of how wound healing is progressing. This mechanism is dependent on the presence of iron, vitamin C and oxygen. Therefore, appropriate levels of nutrition and oxygenation during this phase of wound healing are particularly necessary.

Angioblasts are required to form new blood vessels which grow into the wound under conditions of a hypoxic tissue gradient (Knighton *et al.* 1981). The vessels branch and join other vessels forming loops. The fragile capillary loops are held within a framework of collagen. This complex is known as granulation tissue. Granulation tissue can grow into wound dressings such as gauze. On removal of the dressing any adhered delicate granulation tissue is also destroyed.

There is an acceleration of the inflammatory and proliferative phases in moist conditions compared to dry conditions (Dyson *et al.*, 1988).

Remodelling phase (24 days onwards)

In this stage the collagen is reorganized so the fibres are enlarged and oriented along the lines of tension in the wound (right angles to the wound margin). This occurs via a process of lysis and resynthesis. Intermolecular cross-linking aids to increase the tensile strength of the wound. Maximum strength (about 80 per cent) is reached in approximately three months, although the scar never achieves the same strength as the original tissue. (From: Cooper, 1990; David, 1986; Jackson & Rovee, 1988; Johnson, 1988; Messer, 1989; Pritchard & David, 1988; Torrance, 1985; Westaby, 1985; Winter, 1972)

Contraction

If the wound is clean and granulating, myofibroblasts round the edge of the wound contract in unison. This can reduce significantly the size of the wound and the area that the new tissue must cover. When the edges first contract (about four days from injury) the wound becomes larger but after three or four days the wound area begins to decrease, leaving a scar in approximately three weeks. The position of the wound is relevant to the success of healing by contracture. If the skin is attached to nearby structures this may result in its distortion and limitation of movement. However, wounds on the abdomen and breasts may close with a small amount of scarring (David, 1986; Johnson, 1988a; Messer, 1989; Torrance, 1985; Westaby, 1985).

Oxygen-treated burns have been found to increase contraction significantly and healing of the wound in animals. However, this was accompanied by thicker scar formation which could prove detrimental for aesthetic and rehabilitative reasons (Kaufman & Alexander, 1988).

Epithelialization

Epithelial cells will migrate across healthy granulation tissue only by 'leap-frogging' over each other and will burrow under contaminated debris and unwanted material. Splinters, dirt and sutures may be 'worked out' of the wound (David, 1986; Torrance, 1985; Westaby, 1985; Winter, 1972). Epidermal cells also secrete an enzyme which separates the scab from the underlying tissue. Dissolving the eschar requires nearly 50 per cent of the cell's metabolic energy (Johnson, 1988a; Messer, 1989). Sources of epithelial cells include hair follicles, sweat glands and the perimeter of the wound (Johnson, 1988a; Torrance, 1985). As the epithelial cells migrate they begin to differentiate and cannot divide (Torrance, 1985). The ability of the epithelium to cover the wound surface is limited to approximately two centimetres. This means the process of contraction is of vital importance to healing in normal wounds (Messer, 1989).

Epithelialization (migration, mitosis and differentiation) is best achieved in moist conditions (Rovee *et al.*, 1972). Covering the wound in a polythene film accelerates epithelialization probably because hydration is maintained, while blowing air over wounds causes a deeper scab than normal to form and epidermal repair is delayed (Winter, 1972).

Raising oxygen tension in fluid in the wound has also been found to increase epidermal migration. This suggests that in normal wound healing the availability of oxygen may be the limiting factor (Winter, 1972). The epidermal migration under different types of films is perhaps directly related to their oxygen permeabilities (Winter, 1972). Oxygen breathing by man was not found to increase the partial pressure of oxygen in intact skin, while vasodilation produced by warming the body or limb did raise the oxygen tension (Silver, 1972). (Different results have been demonstrated in experiments involving animals (Knighton *et al.*, 1981)). This suggests that warming rather than giving oxygen may be of more clinical use, although this was probably not the limiting factor in the healthy subjects studied. Another trial is necessary in hypoxic patients.

Topical acidification and application of growth factors have also been found to increase epidermal regeneration, and may prove to be of use therapeutically (Brown *et al.*, 1989; Kaufman *et al.*, 1985; Jackson & Rovee, 1988).

Only by understanding the different stages of wound healing will the health carer be able to provide the appropriate treatment to produce the optimum wound environment.

Factors affecting wound healing

The rate of healing of a wound varies depending on the general health of the individual, the location of the wound, the degree of the damage (David, 1986) and the treatment applied.

Factors which may delay healing include systemic variables such as disease, poor nutritional state and infection. Other influences involve the local microenvironment of the wound including temperature, pH, humidity, air gas composition (Dyson *et al.*, 1988; Kaufman and Berger, 1988; Kaufman & Hirshowitz, 1982; Rovee *et al.*, 1982), oxygen tension (Kaufman & Alexander, 1988; Silver, 1972), blood supply, inflammation, etc. Whether this influence is positive or negative may depend on the stage of wound healing that has been reached. Other important considerations are external variables such as continuing trauma – possibly caused by treatment, the presence of foreign bodies etc.

It is necessary when treating a wound to appraise all potential detrimental factors and minimize them, where possible, in order to provide the optimum systemic, local and external conditions for healing. Wound care begins with the care of the patient.

Factors known to affect wound healing are listed in Table 46.1.

Promotion of wound healing

General care of the patient

Promotion of wound healing concerns optimizing the local, internal and external environments. This includes the control of disease or underlying pathology, reduction of external risk factors such as infection and maintaining an ideal microclimate for healing in the wound (see Table 46.1). Many factors need to be considered when assessing a patient with a wound.

Where possible, health care should be aimed at preventing wounding, for example, prevention of

Table 46.1 Factors that may delay wound healing

Disease, disorders and syndromes	Addisons' disease; anaemia; arteriosclerosis; auto-immune disorders; Buerger's disease; diabetes; cardiopulmonary disease; Crohn's disease; Cushing's syndrome; hepatic failure; hypovolaemia; hypoxia; immune disorders; infection; inflammatory bowel disease; jaundice; leucopenia; malignancy; protein loosing enteropathy; Raynaud's disease; renal failure; respiratory conditions; rheumatoid arthritis; thyroid deficiency; uraemia; vascular diseases; venous stasis
Drugs	Alcohol; antimicrobials; cytotoxics; immunosuppressives; nicotine; non-steroidal anti-inflammatories; penicillamine and penicillin; steroids
Poor nutritional state	Anaemia; malnutrition; mineral deificiency (particularly zinc); protein deficiency; vitamin deficiency (particularly A and C)
Micro-environment of wound	Blood supply; gas composition; humidity; infection; inflammation; high pH; low temperature; oxygen tension
Other	Aetiology of wound; age; fibrous ring round open wound; foreign body in wound; obesity; radiation; stress; suture materials; suture technique; trauma/mechanical stress; treatment (including use of antiseptics and/or linting materials)

Note: some conditions may affect the healing process via several mechanisms. (From: Cooper, 1990; David, 1986; Deas *et al.*, 1986; Dyson *et al.*, 1988; Kaufman & Hirshowitz, 1982; Kaufman & Alexander, 1988; Kaufman & Berger, 1988; Kaufman *et al.*, 1985; Lycarotti & Leaper, 1989; Messer, 1989; Rovee *et al.*, 1982; Silver, 1972; Tubman Papantonio, 1988a; and Westaby, 1985.)

pressure ulcers by regular turning and adequate nutrition. In addition, hydrocolloid dressings have been found to be effective in preventing pressure ulcers in 'at risk' patients (Johnson, 1989).

The psychological care of the patient is important to ensure acceptance of the wound and reduction in stress. It is also imperative to assess and treat pain. Apart from the obvious unpleasantness for the patient, this will also lead to stress which will then delay wound healing.

Attention must be given to adequate nutrition of the patient since this is necessary for wound healing (Roberts, 1988). A dietitian's assessment is advisable. Patients are considered 'at risk' for wound healing if they have lost 20 per cent or more of their body weight within the previous six months or 10 per cent in the previous two months (Messer, 1989).

Protein or calorie malnutrition are possible in patients with chronic or acute malabsorption. This includes diabetes, Crohn's disease, alcohol abuse, gastrointestinal surgery, liver disease and long-term steroid therapy. Malignancy, major trauma, fever, inflammatory disease, smoking, drug use, stress and iatrogenic starvation are associated with deficient intake or high energy demands (Messer, 1989).

Patients at risk of inadequate vitamin A levels include those with severe diabetes and rheumatoid arthritis (Messer, 1989). Vitamin A supplementation in these patients has been found to improve wound healing and should be considered as a supplement in steroid-dependent patients for at least five days post-wounding (Messer, 1989). This may be related to the fact that vitamin A is a potent immune stimulant which, when administered topically or orally, will reverse much of the steroid suppression of wound healing. However, it is not as effective in reversing the effects of non-steroidal anti-inflammatory drugs (Cohen & Cohen, 1973; Ehrlich *et al.*, 1973; Hunt and Dunphy, 1979; Hunt *et al.*, 1969).

Patients with sepsis and those having undergone major trauma are also at risk of depletion of vitamin A. Supplementation of vitamin A should be contemplated for these groups. In addition, losses of vitamin C and zinc may occur under these conditions (Messer, 1989).

In the absence of any malabsorption aetiology, the provision of adequate nutrition by diet or supplement is the easiest and often the cheapest method of ensuring the patient is nourished (Roberts, 1988).

The majority of chronic non-healing wounds are hypoxic wounds (Messer, 1989). The major conditions that predispose to this are diabetes, venous stasis, vascular insufficiency, cardiopulmonary disease, irradiation, oedema, hypovolaemia and smoking (Messer, 1989). It is possible that hyperbaric oxygen therapy may be helpful for healing wounds in these patients. This involves the patient breathing 100% oxygen while in a chamber where the pressure is elevated above atmospheric pressure, and enables the amount of oxygen in solution to be increased. This has been used to successfully treat chronic unhealed wounds (Barr *et al.*, 1990).

However, it is not always possible to overcome the deleterious effects of smoking with hyperbaric oxygen therapy while the patient continues to smoke (Messer, 1989). It is, therefore, important to educate the patient and assist them in this aspect of their care by helping them to reduce or stop smoking.

Drugs that may delay wound healing should be reduced or withdrawn where therapeutically possible. This includes penicillamine which prevents collagen cross-linking (Messer, 1989).

Other factors that require consideration are: the necessity to maintain adequate fluid replacement post-operatively or post-trauma to prevent hypovolaemia (Messer, 1989); containing and removing infection (both local and systemic); use of measures to assist healing (for example, using mattresses which can reduce the healing time of sores (Andrews & Balai, 1989), etc.

Physical and psychological rehabilitation may be necessary if the result of wounding and wound healing are debilitating and disfiguring and adjustment to changes in body image are necessary. This includes physiotherapy, counselling and occupational therapy.

Care of the microscopic wound environment

A considerable percentage of nurses' time is spent carrying out dressing procedures. Although research has examined wound physiology (Ayton, 1985; Johnson, 1984; Leaper, 1986; Torrance, 1985; Turner *et al.*, 1986; Westaby, 1985; Winter, 1971) and wound dressings (Ayton, 1986; Draper, 1985; Harkiss, 1985a and b; Johnson 1984), there is little that appraises different dressing packs and procedures.

Packs and procedures should be designed for safety, comfort and ease and speed of use. Opinion and research indicates that forceps (especially those made of plastic) are clumsy, can cause pain and damage and are difficult to use (Mallett, 1988; Wells 1984). Gloves are a more suitable alternative and, in addition, should assist in reducing the risk of cross-infection.

Cotton wool or gauze used in cleaning can leave fibres in the wound. This may stimulate foreign body reaction and lengthen the inflammatory phase. Not only will this act as a focus for infection and damage new epidermis, but it will also retard wound healing

(Johnson, 1984; Turner 1979; Winter, 1971 and 1972). Medical foam or low-linting material may be used instead. Appropriate use of hydrotherapy via a whirlpool, shower or a water or normal saline stream can be utilized to remove debris or for debridement (Gogia *et al.*, 1988; Jeter & Tintle, 1988; Trelstad & Osmundson, 1989; Zederfeldt *et al.*, 1980).

Introduction of a less complicated wound dressing procedure and new pack containing medical foam and gloves instead of cotton wool and forceps was evaluated in one London hospital. This demonstrated that it was not only quicker to use but also that nurses preferred the new pack to the original pack (Mallett, 1988).

The implications of research suggest that traditional packs are likely to be detrimental to the patient and are also more difficult to use by the health care professional. Study of new packs and procedures indicate that foam and gloves may be suitable subsitutes. Further research in this area is necessary.

Evaluation of the wound

The wound should be evaluated each time a dressing is applied or if it gives rise for concern. The aim of evaluating the wound is to assess healing and to establish which treatment will best provide the ideal environment for healing. The different classifications of wounds that relate to tissue loss and regeneration and absence or presence of infection may be of assistance in this process.

Table 46.2 Assessment of wounds

Factor	*Variables*
General	Aetiology; location; presence of haematoma, seroma, oedema; amount of necrosis; open/closed; number of times requires dressing per unit time
Pain	Amount; at change of dressing; only when traumatized; intermittent; continuous; time of day; type of pain (e.g. sharp, stabbing, dull, etc.)
Stage of healing	Original tissue loss; amount of granulation and epithelial tissue; area/volume/depth of wound; temperature; sensation; inflammation
Drainage	Colour; consistency; nature/type; volume over time; odour
Area surrounding wound	Colour; oedema; erythema; sensation; turgor; other skin conditions
Infection	Amount of pus; pain; temperature; positive swab culture; inflammation

Factors that should be appraised include the underlying pathology of the wound. For example, if an ulcer is present on the leg, is it venous, arterial, lymphatic, malignant, etc? In addition, the surface area or volume of the wound should be measured. This can be carried out using a number of methods (see Fincham Gee, 1990), and is necessary to ascertain the rate of healing. The amount and type of drainage is also important, both in traumatic and surgical wounds.

A list of variables that require regular assessment are shown in Table 46.2.

Principles of cleaning the wound

The aim of wound cleansing is to help create the optimum local condition for wound healing by removal of excess debris, exudate, foreign and necrotic material, toxic components, the food source of potential infecting micro-organisms, bacteria and other micro-organisms (Gustafsson, 1988; Jeter & Tintle, 1988; Morison, 1989; Turner *et al.*, 1986; Wells, 1984). Debridment is necessary to remove necrotic tissue which provides the ideal environment for bacterial growth and can hinder the healing process (Jackson & Rovee, 1988).

If the wound is clean and little exudate is present, repeated cleansing is contraindicated since it may damage new tissue, decrease the temperature of the wound unnecessarily and remove exudate (Morison, 1989). A fall in the temperature of the wound of 12°C is possible if the procedure is prolonged or the lotions are cold. This can take three hours or longer to return to normal warmth, during which time the cellular activity is reduced and therefore the healing process slowed (Stronge, 1984).

Sodium chloride (0.9%) used at body temperature is the safest and best cleansing solution for non-contaminated wounds (Ferguson, 1988; Jeter & Tintle, 1988; Morgan, 1990; Tubman Papantonio, 1988b). Although sodium chloride has no antiseptic properties it dilutes bacteria and is non-toxic to tissue (Morgan, 1990).

A number of other solutions have been used traditionally to clean wounds, some of which need to be used with caution (see Table 46.3). An example of this is povidine-iodine. This is sometimes used in a weak aqueous solution (1%) as an antiseptic. However, solutions of 5% povidine-iodine, have been found to reduce blood flow in granulation tissue (Brennan & Leaper, 1985).

Some compounds used to clean wounds have documented deleterious effects on tissue or have been

Table 46.3 Suitability of products used on wounds

Suitable	Sodium chloride (0.9%) (safe, non-irritant and non-toxic)
Not ideal, use with caution	Chlorhexidine – antiseptic (can cause sensitization and irritation; do not use alcoholic solutions)
	Hydrogen peroxide – antiseptic (use on dirty, infected, necrotic wounds only; do not use on large or deep wounds as may cause air embolism; may be caustic to skin and wound)
	Metronidazole – antibacterial (anaerobes only) (can cause nausea, neuropathy if used systemically)
	Povidone-iodine (1 %) antiseptic (do not use alcoholic solution; rarely causes skin reactions; some sources suggest that it should not be used on severe or extensive burns; if non-toxic goitre is present; or in pregnancy; or on lactating women)
Not suitable	Boric acid – bacteriocidal (toxic to tissues, fatal poisoning)
	Cetrimide – antibacterial and antifungal (toxic to wound tissue and causes skin hypersensitivity)
	Gentian violet – astringent, antiseptic (carcinogenic; is sometimes used on excoriating radiotherapy burns)
	Mercurochrome – weak bacteriostatic agent (toxic to tissue)
	Sodium hypochlorite – antiseptic (powerful oxidizing agent which is toxic to tissue)

(From: Bloomfield & Sizer, 1985; Brennan & Leaper, 1985; Deas *et al.*, 1986; Farrow & Toth, 1991; Johnson, 1988a; Morgan, 1990; Morison, 1989; *Nurses' Drug Alert*, 1987; Thorp *et al.*, 1987; Valdes-Dapena & Arey, 1962.)

found to have detrimental effects in mammals. These include the much discussed sodium hypochlorite which is found in several wound cleansing solutions (see Table 46.3). Eusol is a particularly well known solution containing sodium hypochlorite. Debate about its use has continued for a number of years. Many clinicians and researchers have recommended that it should not be used (Ferguson, 1988; Johnson, 1988b; Morgan, 1990; Spanswick *et al.*, 1990) or not be used routinely (Morison, 1989). In view of the mounting evidence against sodium hypochlorite (Bloomfield & Sizer, 1985; Brennan and Leaper, 1985; Deas *et al.*, 1986; Thorp *et al.*, 1987) and the availability of a range of alternatives, the use of sodium hypochlorite is not recommended in this manual except for short term use in exceptional circumstances, such as in recent war wounds and some patients' wounds in accident and emergency departments. Its use should be defined only by the clinical specialist.

Principles of dressing the wound

It is not possible or appropriate to describe here which dressing is most suitable for which types of wound, as each wound needs to be assessed individually. An ideal wound dressing may be described in general terms as follows:

> A material which, when applied to the surface of a wound, provides and maintains an environment in which healing can take place at the maximum rate.
> (Turner *et al.*, 1986)

More specifically, to provide such an environment the dressing must be capable of fulfilling the following functions:

1. To remove excess exudate and toxic components.
2. To maintain a high humidity at the wound–dressing interface.
3. To allow gaseous exchange.
4. To provide thermal insulation.
5. To be impermeable to bacteria.
6. To be free from particulate or toxic components.
7. To allow change without trauma (Turner, 1985).

In addition, the dressing should minimize pain, odour and bleeding and be comfortable and acceptable to the patient.

Occlusive dressings achieve many of these criteria. They affect the wound and healing in several ways. Occlusive dressings have the ability to maintain hydration and prevent the formation of an eschar. This leads to a more rapid epithelial migration. The lag phase before epithelial cell proliferation and the time for epidermal differentiation is reduced. Wound contraction occurs more quickly and there is a decrease in some signs of inflammation (redness, oedema) as well as pain. Dermal repair is also accelerated (Dyson *et al.*, 1988; Rovee *et al.*, 1972; Jackson & Rovee, 1988; Winter & Hewitt, 1990).

Protocols have been developed which suggest different types of treatment depending on whether the wound is clean, infected or necrotic or shallow or deep (Johnson, 1988d). Dry dressings do not afford

Table 46.4 Dressing groups

Dressing	*Advantages*	*Disadvantages*
Polymeric films	Only suitable for shallow wounds; prophylactic use against pressure sores; retention dressings; cool the surface of the wound; allow passage of water vapour; allow monitoring of wound	Possibility of adhesive trauma on removal; cool the surface of the wound
Dextranomers	Form stiff hydrophillic paste; useful in the treatment of infected wound cavities	Require retaining dressing
Hydrogels	Suitable light to medium exudating wounds; reduce pain; cool the wound surface; desloughing abilities; allow monitoring of wound; carrier for medicants; good permeability gas profile; low trauma at change; non-allergenic; non-sensitizing; easy to use	Cool the surface of the wound; some hydrogels cannot be used on infected wounds. Please refer to manufacturers' recommendations with regard to particular products.
Hydrocolloids	Provides a moist wound environment suitable for assisting debridment of wound; swelling of hydrocolloid increases pressure on the base of the wound, *may* aid healthy granulation; pain relief; waterproof; provide thermal insulation; most provide a barrier to micro-organisms; low trauma at change; non-allergenic; non-sensitizing; easy to use	May release degradation products into the wound; strong odour produced as dressing interacts with exudate; some hydrocolloids cannot be used on infected wounds. Please refer to manufacturers' recommendations with regard to particular products.
Alginates	Suitable for heavily exudating wounds; highly absorbent; can be used on infected wounds; useful for sinus and fissure drainage; hydrophillic gel formed in the presence of sodium ions provides a moist wound environment; sodium chloride (0.9%) can be used to flush away some alginates; fibres trapped in the wound are biodegradable; some alginates are haemostatic in action; odour remission	Cannot be used on wounds that are not exudating or exudating lightly; cannot be used on wounds with hard necrotic tissue; sometimes a mild burning occurs on application
Polyurethane foams	Suitable for use with open, exudating wounds; provide high thermal insulation; left *in situ* for long time	May be difficult to use in wounds with deep tracks

(From: Dealey, 1989; Fraser & Gilchrist, 1983; Gilchrist & Martin, 1983; Goren, 1989; Johnson, 1988c; Lawrence, 1985; Margolin *et al.*, 1990; Mertz *et al.*, 1985; Morgan, 1990; Piper, 1989; Pottle, 1987.)

most of the criteria for an ideal dressing and should not be used as a primary contact layer (Dealey, 1991). Care should be taken with wounds that are difficult shapes to treat. These include long, narrow cavities which require a dressing that can be comfortably inserted into the space but removed easily without leaving any fibres behind (Bale, 1991) and without trauma. (See Table 46.4 for details of groups of dressings.)

Other treatments

Other treatments for wounds include the possibility of topical acidification (Kaufman *et al.*, 1985) and active treatment using growth factors or autologous platelet derived factors (Jackson & Rovee, 1988). Some suggest the use of yoghurt and buttermilk, but this has not yet been evaluated sufficiently (Ivetic & Lyne, 1990).

Small, full-thickness skin loss can be repaired easily using skin grafts (Westaby, 1985). Where possible, it is preferable to use autografts. However, if donor sites are limited, homografts can be utilized. Muscle, tendon and bone may also be used to replace lost tissue (Pritchard & David, 1988).

PARTICULAR WOUNDS: LEG ULCERATION

REFERENCE MATERIAL

> Ulceration of the skin of the lower limb has been an affliction of the human race since the time of Hippocrates. It is almost certainly the price we pay for having emerged from the ocean and learnt to stand erect
>
> (Burnand, 1990)

Prevalence and cost

Approximately 1% of the general population are affected by leg ulceration during their lifetime (Callam *et al.*, 1985). Ulceration is often recurrent (Callam *et al.*, 1987b), persistent (Dale & Gibson, 1986a), and affects more women than men (Anning, 1954, Dale & Gibson, 1986a; Callam *et al.*, 1987b; Ryan, 1987).

The annual cost of treatment to the National Health Service of leg ulceration is between £300 million and £600 million per annum (Thomas, 1990). Leg ulceration treated by community nurses was estimated to use over £400 000 of resources in Paddington and North Kensington Health District (PNK) in 1988 (Mallett & Charles, 1989); much of this is borne by the cost of the district nursing service (Callam *et al.*, 1987b).

Aetiology

The most common predisposing factors to leg ulceration are venous and arterial disease.

Venous disease

Venous disease has been found to be prevalent in 70% to 95% of cases (Callam *et al.*, 1987b; Fangrell, 1979; Perkins, 1989; Williamson, 1988). Venous hypertension precipitating micro-oedema is probably the main cause of venous leg ulcers (Fangrell, 1979; Ryan, 1985b). This, in turn, can lead to lymphatic damage with resulting lymphoedema, fibrosis or liposclerosis (Robinson, 1988; Ryan, 1988a).

The reason that more women than men are prone to leg ulceration is due to the presence of varicose veins and episodes of deep vein thrombosis associated with pregnancy, which can lead to venous damage and ulceration in the affected leg (Dale & Gibson, 1986a; Knight, 1990; Ryan, 1987). Only 12% of women with varicose veins had never been pregnant, compared to 57% who had four or more pregnancies (Henry & Corless, 1989). In addition, further research indicates that multiple pregnancies enlarge the gonadal veins leading to vulvar, inner and posterior thigh and leg varicosities which do not follow the saphenous system. Symptoms are pain and heaviness in the thigh and legs and lateral aspects of the leg and foot (Lechter *et al.*, 1987). Venous pathology is also related to the menstrual cycle, when the level of circulating oestrogens are at their lowest (Marcelon *et al.*, 1988).

Warming can induce venous dilation resulting in decreased venous return and 'heavy legs' (Marcelon & Vanhoutte, 1988), and disorders relating to chronic venous insufficiency appear especially when the ambient temperature is high (Boccalon & Ginestet, 1988).

Venous ulcers are often described as occurring in the area around or on the medial malleolus, shallow and extensive and on the left leg (Callam *et al.*, 1987b; Falanga & Eaglstein, 1986; Matthews, 1986; Ryan, 1987; Swanwick & MacLellan, 1988; Thomas, 1988a; Williamson, 1988). This may be associated to iliocaval syndrome which occurs when the left common iliac vein is compressed by the common iliac artery (Ryan, 1987; Taheri *et al.*, 1987). These findings were not supported by the Paddington and North Kensington Health District survey, which suggested that significantly more ulcers were found on the anterolateral aspect of the lower leg. Ulceration was also statistically more likely to be on the right leg (Mallett & Charles, 1990). A larger, more recent survey has not strengthened either claim (Mallett and Charles, unpublished data).

Venous ulcers develop gradually and produce intermittent pain (Dale & Gibson, 1986a; Thomas, 1988a). Data from a survey in Parkside Health District do not support this (Mallett & Charles, unpublished data).

Arterial disease

Between 4% and 30% of patients with leg ulceration have been reported to have arterial insufficiency. This proportion increases with age to 50% in the very elderly (Callam *et al.*, 1987a and b; Matthews, 1986; Perkins, 1989; Williamson, 1988). Women are also more prone to arterial ulceration than men (Knight, 1990), although some research contradicts this (Callam *et al.*, 1987a).

Arterial ulcers are deep and 'punched out' (Dale & Gibson, 1986b; Mani *et al.*, 1988; Perkins, 1989; Williamson, 1988), and found on the feet or the anterior or lateral aspect of the ankle (Thomas, 1988a). These ulcers develop rapidly and give continuous or persistent pain, especially at night (Dale & Gibson, 1986c; Perkins, 1989; Thomas, 1988a). This is not supported by recent research (Mallett & Charles, unpublished data).

Other predisposing and aggravating factors

Rheumatoid arthritis causes vasculitis which can lead to small, painful, 'punched out' ulcers (Williamson, 1988). In addition, treatment with steroids leads to thinning of the skin and susceptibility to trauma.

Diabetes is also associated with vasculitis and neuropathy, and has been found to be five times more common in patients with leg ulceration (Callam *et al.*, 1987b).

Diastolic hypertension can led to (usually) painful bilateral ischaemic ulceration, known as 'Martorell's ulcer' (Alberdi, 1988).

Blood disease, such as sickle cell anaemia or thalassaemia, can cause haematological ulcers (Hallows, 1987; Williamson, 1988).

Obesity, immobilization and dependency of the lower limb, limitation of ankle joint and poor gait due to ulceration (the latter both leading to an inadequately functioning calf muscle pump) can aggravate ulceration and contribute to its persistence (Callam *et al.*, 1987b).

Treatment

It is imperative to distinguish between ulcers of varying pathologies as the management and treatment are very different. Assessment must be carried out to elicit which of the three vascular systems (arterial, venous and/or lymphatic) are diseased to provide the most appropriate care (Ryan, 1988a). Understanding and systematic management of the underlying disease, as well as topical wound care are necessary for a therapeutic approach (Falanga & Eaglstein, 1986). However, nurses and doctors may use the above factors associated with leg ulceration to appraise pathology. The problem arises when health care professionals are confronted with such concepts as 'shallow and extensive', 'develop rapidly' etc. Evaluation of the underlying pathology of ulceration must be underpinned where possible by definable and sound criteria.

Venous and lymphatic disease can be treated by improving the function of the calf muscle pump by graduated compression (Blair *et al.*, 1988b; Callam *et al.*, 1987b; Dale & Gibson, 1987; Dale and Gibson, 1990; Evans, 1988; Smith, 1988; Thompson, 1990). This has been found to be more important than certain types of dressing (Blair *et al.*, 1988a). Compression bandaging is detrimental to those with arterial insufficiency. Surgery may be necessary in these cases to increase the perfusion of the tissues, although it should be noted that arterial surgery can also lead to a decrease in the venous return time (Struckmann, 1988).

As with all wound care, it is important that nutritional requirements (especially vitamin A, vitamin C and zinc) are met and pain control is adequate (Cherry & Ryan, 1987; Hallows, 1987; Ryan, 1988a; Thomas, 1988b).

PRESSURE ULCERS OR DECUBITUS ULCERS

Definition

The terms 'decubitus ulcer' or 'pressure ulcer or sore' are used to describe any area of damage to the skin or underlying tissues caused by direct pressure or shearing forces. The extent of this damage can range from persistent erythema to necrotic ulceration involving muscle, tendon and bone.

REFERENCE MATERIAL

Aetiology of pressure ulcers

There are three major factors which have been identified as being significant contributory factors in the development of pressure ulcers. These are:

1. Pressure. The blood pressure at the arterial end of the capillaries is approximately 30 mm Hg, while at the venous end this drops to 10 mm Hg (the average mean capillary pressure equals about 17 mm Hg (Guyton, 1984)). Any external pressures exceeding this will cause capillary obstruction. Tissues that are dependant on these capillaries are deprived of their blood supply. Eventually, the ischaemic tissues will die (David, 1986; Department of Infection Control, Memorial Hospital, 1989; Johnson, 1989; Waterlow, 1988; Wyngaarden & Smith, 1988). However, research has demonstrated that with constant pressure, even in denigrated tissues, a critical period of one to two hours exists before pathological changes occur (Kosiak, 1958, 1976).
2. Shearing. This may occur when the patient slips down the bed or is dragged up the bed. As the skeleton moves over the underlying tissue the micro-circulation is destroyed and the tissue dies of anoxia. In more serious cases lymphatic vessels and muscle fibres may also become torn, resulting in a deep pressure ulcer (Department of Infection Control, Memorial Hospital, 1989; Johnson, 1989;

Waterlow pressure sore prevention/treatment policy
Ring scores in table, add total. Several scores per category can be used.

Build/weight for height	★	**Skin type visual risk areas**	★	**Sex Age**	★	**Special risks**	★
Average	0	Healthy	0	Male	1	**Tissue malnutrition**	★
Above average	1	Tissue paper	1	Female	2	e.g.: Terminal cachexia	8
Obese	2	Dry	1	14–49	1	Cardiac failure	5
Below average	3	Oedematous	1	50–64	2	Peripheral vascular disease	5
Continence	★	Clammy (temp. ↑)	1	65–74	3	Anaemia	2
Complete/catheterized	0	Discoloured	2	75–80	4	Smoking	1
Occasion. incont.	1	Broken/spot	3	81+	5	**Neurological deficit**	★
Cath./incontinent of faeces	2	**Mobility**	★	**Appetite**	★	e.g.: Diabetes, multiple sclerosis, CVA	
Doubly incont.	3	Fully	0	Average	0	Motor/sensory	
		Restless/fidgety	1	Poor	1	Paraplegia	4–6
		Apathetic	2	Nasogastric tube/fluids only	2	**Major surgery/trauma**	★
		Restricted	3	Nil by mouth/anorexic	3	Orthopaedic – below waist, spinal	5
		Inert/traction	4			On table >2 hours	5
		Chairbound	5			**Medication**	★
						Cytotoxics	4
						High-dose steroids	
						Anti-inflammatory	

Score	10+ At risk	15+ High risk	20+ Very high risk

Obtainable from: Newtons, Curland, Taunton TA3 5SG

Figure 46.1 The Waterlow Scale (with permission).

REMEMBER: TISSUE DAMAGE OFTEN STARTS PRIOR TO ADMISSION, IN CASUALTY. A SEATED PATIENT IS ALSO AT RISK

ASSESSMENT: (See Over) IF THE PATIENT FALLS INTO ANY OF THE RISK CATEGORIES THEN PREVENTATIVE NURSING IS REQUIRED.
A COMBINATION OF GOOD NURSING TECHNIQUES AND PREVENTATIVE AIDS WILL DEFINITELY BE NECESSARY.

PREVENTION:

PREVENTATIVE AIDS:

Special mattress/bed:	10+ Overlays or specialist foam matresses 15+ Alternating pressure overlays, mattresses and bed systems. 20+ Bed Systems: Fluidised, bead, low air loss and alternating pressure mattresses. Note: Preventative aids cover a wide spectrum of specialist features. Efficacy in the 20+ area should be judged on the basis of independent evidence.
Cushions:	No patient should sit in a wheelchair without some form of cushioning. If nothing else is available – use the patient's own pillow. 10+ 4″ Foam cushion. 15+ Specialist Gell and/or foam cushion 20+ Cushion capable of adjustment to suit individual patient.
Bed Clothing:	Avoid plastic draw sheets, inco pads and tightly tucked in sheets/sheet covers, especially when using Specialist bed and mattress overlay systems. Duvet – plus vapour permeable cover

NURSING CARE:

General:	Frequent changes of position, lying or sitting. Use of pillows?
Pain	Appropriate pain control
Nutrition	High Protein, vitamins, minerals
Patient Handling:	Correct Lifting technique Hoists Monkey Pole Transfer devices
Patient Comfort Aids:	Real sheepskins Bed cradle
Operating Table/ Theatre/A&E Trolley	4″ cover plus adequate protection
Skin Care:	General Hygiene, NO rubbing. Correct lifting and positioning. Cover with an appropriate dressing.

IF TREATMENT IS REQUIRED, FIRST REMOVE PRESSURE

WOUND CLASSIFICATION

BLANCHING HYPERAEMIA	Stage I	Is wound RED?	YES Semi-permeable film hydrocolloid sheet
NON-BLANCHING HYPERAEMIA	Stage II	Is wound Red, clean but not healed?	YES Hydrocolloid, alginate, hydrogel, Silastic Foam (deep)
ULCERATION PROGRESSES	Stage III	Is wound YELLOW/ infected/inflamed?	YES Alginate, hydrogel, hydrocolloid
ULCERATION EXTENDS	Stage IV	Infected?	YES Alginate ribbon or rope, non adherent topical antimicrobial dressing, polysaccharide paste
INFECTIVE NECROSIS	Stage V	Is wound BLACK/ Necrotic?	YES Debride-surgical excision, hydrocolloid, hydrogel, enzymatic treatment

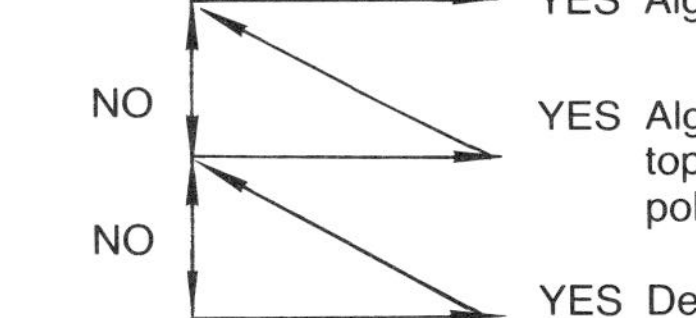

Figure 46.1 Continued

Pritchard & David, 1988; Waterlow, 1988; Wyngaarden & Smith, 1988).
3. Friction. This is a component of shearing which causes stripping of the stratum corneum, leading to superficial ulceration (Johnson, 1989; Waterlow, 1988; Wyngaarden & Smith, 1988).

The most likely sites for pressure ulcer development are:

1. Sacral area.
2. Coccygeal area.
3. Ischial tuberosities.
4. Greater trochanters (Wyngaarden & Smith, 1988).

Indentification of at-risk patients

Many predisposing factors are involved in the development of pressure ulcers:

1. Immunosuppression (Pritchard & David, 1988).
2. Immobility (National Pressure Ulcer Advisory Panel, 1989; Waterlow, 1988).
3. Moisture (Wyngaarden & Smith, 1988).
4. Inactivity (National Pressure Ulcer Advisory Panel, 1989).
5. Faecal and urinary incontinence (Department of Infection Control, Memorial Hospital, 1989; National Pressure Ulcer Advisory Panel, 1989; Waterlow, 1988).
6. Decreased level of consciousness (Department of Infection Control, Memorial Hospital, 1989; National Pressure Ulcer Advisory Panel, 1989).
7. Infection (Waterlow, 1988).
8. Circulatory diseases (for example, peripheral vascular disease, cardiac disease) (Barton, 1977; Department of Infection Control, Memorial Hospital, 1989).
9. Personal hygiene (Waterlow, 1988).
10. Neurological diseases (for example, multiple sclerosis) (Department of Infection Control, Memorial Hospital, 1989; Waterlow, 1988).
11. Weight distribution (Waterlow, 1988).
12. Treatment regimes (Waterlow, 1988).
13. Malnutrition/nutritional status (Department of Infection Control, Memorial Hospital, 1989; Waterlow, 1988).
14. Drugs which affect mobility (for example, sedatives) (Department of Infection Control, Memorial Hospital, 1989; Waterlow, 1988).
15. Anaemia (Waterlow, 1988).
16. Malignancy (Waterlow, 1988).
17. Patient-handling methods (Department of Infection Control, Memorial Hospital, 1989; Waterlow, 1988).
18. Shortage of nursing staff where patients require regular positioning (Department of Infection Control, Memorial Hospital, 1989).
19. Design of beds, mattresses, chairs and wheelchairs (Department of Infection Control, Memorial Hospital, 1989).
20. Advanced age (National Pressure Ulcer Advisory Panel, 1989).
21. Fracture (National Pressure Ulcer Advisory Panel, 1989).
22. Chronic systemic illness (National Pressure Ulcer Advisory Panel, 1989).

A patient's risk of developing a pressure ulcer should be assessed either on admission to hospital or in the community when they first come into contact with health services. Norton *et al.* (1985) and Waterlow (1991) have produced 'at risk' scales which are shown in Table 46.5 and Figure 46.1. In Norton's scale, patients with scores of 14 or below are considered to run the greatest risk of developing pressure ulcers. Patients with scores of 14 to 18 are not considered to be at risk, but they will require reassessment immediately any change in their condition is observed. Scores of 18 to 20 indicate patients at minimal risk. Waterlow's scale defines patients with a score of 11 to 15 being 'at risk', 16 to 20 as 'high risk' and over 20 as 'very high risk' (Figure 46.1, © Waterlow, 1992). A recent study comparing the use of the Norton and Waterlow scales showed that 22 (75.7%) of the patients who were predicted as being 'at risk' on admission using Waterlow's scale (a score of 10 and over), developed pressure ulcers, compared to 18 (62%) of patients using a score of 16 or less on the Norton scale. The author concluded that the Waterlow scale was more accurate at predicting the ulcer formation (Smith, 1989). Further research in

Table 46.5 The Norton Scale (Norton, 1975)

Physical condition	*Score*	*Mental condition*	*Score*	*Activity*	*Score*	*Mobility*	*Score*	*Incontinent*	*Score*
Good	4	Alert	4	Ambulant	4	Full	4	Not	4
Fair	3	Apathetic	3	Walk/help	3	Slightly limited	3	Occasionally	3
Poor	2	Confused	2	Chairbound	2	Very limited	2	Usually/urine	2
Very bad	1	Stuporous	1	Bedfast	1	Immobile	1	Doubly	1

Table 46.6 Pressure sore grades (David *et al.*, 1983)

Grade	*Description*
1	(a) Where the skin is likely to break down (red, black and blistered areas) (b) Healed areas still covered by a scab
2	Superficial break in the skin
3	Destruction of the skin without cavity (full skin thickness)
4	Destruction of the skin with cavity (involving underlying tissues)

this area with a larger sample of patients is required.

Grades of pressure ulcers

If a pressure ulcer develops then classification of the wound will assist in determining the most appropriate treatment (see 'Reference material', above). There are, however, grading systems that have been produced specifically for use with pressure ulcers, such as that by David *et al.* (1983) (Table 46.6), or the National Pressure Ulcer Advisory Panel (1989). These are valuable in describing the state of the ulcer and the most pertinent care required by the patient.

Treatment of pressure ulcers

Treatment of pressure ulcers is the same as for any other wound. The aetiology and underlying or related pathology, as well as the wound itself, must be assessed in order to provide the most appropriate treatment. Care should be aimed at relief of pressure, the minimization of symptoms from predisposing factors and the provision of the ideal micro-environment for wound healing.

The most effective treatment for and prevention of pressure ulcers includes frequent turning or moving the patient (for example, at least every two hours), keeping the skin clean and using an air or foam mattress (Andrews & Balai, 1989; David, 1986; Wyngaarden & Smith, 1988). Of prime consideration in nursing care is the positioning and regular repositioning of the patient (Pritchard & David, 1988).

The affected area should not be rubbed as this causes maceration and degeneration of the subcutaneous tissues, especially in elderly patients (Dyson, 1978).

Devices used for relief of pressure

The most effective way of preventing pressure ulcers or facilitating healing is to minimize the pressure in the affected area(s). Usually it is sufficient for the patient to be nursed on alternating aspects of the body surface, provided they are repositioned regularly. Sometimes this is inappropriate or impossible due to individual patients' circumstances, for example, surgical intervention, body deformities, etc. (Pritchard & David, 1988).

A wide variety of devices are available to help relieve pressure over susceptible areas. These devices

Table 46.7 A selection of mechanical methods for relieving pressure

Aid	*Use*	*Advantages*	*Disadvantages*
Sheepskin	Low risk patients. Norton score 14 or above. Good for under heels	Warm and comfortable. Machine washable. Decreases friction	Does *not* relieve pressure. Hardens and matts with washing. Needs to be changed frequently. *Not recommended* for regularly incontinent patients
Heel and elbow pads: sheepskin, foam, silicone	Norton scale 14 or less or patients on prolonged bedrest	Reduce friction and shearing over the elbow and heel	Often have inadequate methods of keeping them on. Become hardened by washing
Silicone-filled mattress pad	Norton scale 14 or less or patients on prolonged bedrest, able to move spontaneously	Relieves pressure by distributing it over a greater area. Comfortable. Machine (industrial) washable. Acceptable in community settings as well as in hospital. Can be used for incontinent patients. Relatively cheap purchase price	If the patient is very incontinent of urine, even if the plastic side is uppermost, there is seepage into the core material. Stitching comes undone after several launderings. Reduces self-motivated movements in very debilitated patients

Table 46.7 *Continued*

Aid	*Use*	*Advantages*	*Disadvantages*
Roho air-filled mattress	Norton scale 10–14, high to medium risk. To wear off pressure equalizing beds	Interlinked air cells transfer air with movement. Patient can be nursed sitting or recumbent. Non-mechanical. Washable	Can be punctured and is expensive to repair. Often incorrectly inflated
Alternating pressure beds (Pegasus, ripple, Alphabed)	Medium risk, 12–14 Norton scale	Mechanical alteration of pressure. Reduce the frequency of (but not need for) repositioning. Available on hire at short notice	Older types prone to breakdown. Must be checked and maintained. May increase pressures in very thin patients. Punctures possible
Mechanaid netbed	Moderate risk patients. Norton score 14 or less	Fits any bed. Easy to assemble and dismantle. Easy to store. No servicing, maintenance or laundry difficulties. Patients can be repositioned by one nurse. Appears to encourage relaxation and sleep. Can be lowered on to the bed surface when a firm base is required	Patients do not always like it. Wedge of pillows needed to sit patient up. Patients may lose heat. Reduces self-motivated movement. Not always easy for patients to communicate with people sitting by bed
Water bed	Moderate risk, Norton score 12–16	Spreads pressure. Is warm and comfortable. Available on hire at short notice	Patient is supported on the skin of the water sac thus reducing the pressure-relieving properties. Difficult to get the patient in and out
Water flotation bed	Moderate to high risk patients. Norton score 14 or less	Equalizes pressure and weight. Heated	Expensive to buy, run and maintain. Makes some patients feel 'sea-sick'. Reduces self-motivated movement. Heavy to move. If not filled correctly can create more pressure than conventional bed. Not to be confused with water trough above
Fluidized air bed	High risk patients, Norton score 10 or less or indicated because of medical condition	As near to levitation as possible. Warm, sterile air produces a beneficial environment for healing wounds. One nurse can manage even very heavy or debilitated patients on his/her own. Can be used for incontinent patients or those with heavy wound exudate	Expensive to hire, run and in old buildings maintain. Need to reinforce floors before it can be installed. Minimizes self-motivation. Can be difficult for the patient to get in and out of bed even with help. Available on hire basis only
Low air loss bed	High risk patient, Norton score 10 or less. Orientated and immobile patients	Pressure-equalizing properties equal to the fluidized air bed. Patient can be nursed in any position including prone. (Patient can control position.) Mobilization easy	Expensive to buy but can be hired. Nurses need education in the use of the equipment

(From: Pritchard and David, 1988.)

differ in function and complexity, and choice must be based on meeting the patient's individual need (Table 46.7) (Pritchard & David, 1988).

References and further reading

Alberdi, J. M. Z. (1988) Hypertensive ulcer: Martorell's ulcer. *Phlebology*, 3, 139–42.

Allen, S. (1988) Ulcers: treating the cause. *Nursing Times*, 84(51), 62–3.

Andrews, J. & Balai, R. (1989) The prevention and treatment of pressure sores by use of pressure distributing mattresses. *Care – Science and Practice*, 7(3), 72–6.

Anning, S. T. (1954) *Leg Ulcers, their Cause and Treatment*. Churchill, London cited in *The Management of Leg Ulcers* (1987), 2nd edn (Ed. by T. J. Ryan). Oxford University Press, Oxford.

Ayton, A. (1985) Wounds that won't heal: wound care. *Community Outlook*, November 16–19.

Bale, S. (1991) A holistic approach and the ideal dressing. *The Professional Nurse*, 6(6), 316–23.

Barr, P. O. *et al.* (1990) Hyperbaric oxygen and problem wounds. *Care – Science and Practice*, 8(1), 3–6.

Barton, A. A. (1988) Prevention of pressure sores. *Nursing Times*, 73, 1593–5.

Blair, S. D. *et al.* (1988a) Do dressings influence the healing of chronic venous ulcers? *Phlebology*, 3, 129–34.

Blair, S. D. *et al.* (1988b) Sustained compression and healing of chronic leg ulcers. *British Medical Journal*, 297(6657), 1159–61.

Bloomfield, S. F. & Sizer, T. J. (1985) Eusol BPC and other hypochlorite formulations used in hospitals. *The Pharmaceutical Journal*, 3 August, 153–7.

Boccalon, H. & Ginestet, M. C. (1988) Influence of temperature variations on venous return: clinical observations. *Phlebology*, 3, Supplement 1, 47–9.

Brennan, S. S. & Leaper, D. J. (1985) The effect of antiseptics on the healing wound: a study using the rabbit ear chamber. *British Journal of Surgery*, 72, 780–2.

Brown, G. L. *et al.* (1989) Enhancement of wound healing by topical treatment with epidermal growth factor. *The New England Journal of Medicine*, 321(2), 76–9.

Burnand, K. G. (1990) Aetiology of venous ulceration. *British Journal of Surgery*, 77, 483–4.

Callam, M. J. *et al.* (1985) Chronic ulceration of the leg: extent of the problem and provision of care. *British Medical Journal*, 290, 1855–6.

Callam, M. J. *et al.* (1987a) Arterial disease in chronic leg ulceration: an underestimated hazard? Lothian and Forth Valley Leg Ulcer Study. *British Medical Journal*, 294, 929–31.

Callam, M. J. *et al.* (1987b) *Lothian and Forth Valley Leg Ulcer Study*. Buccleuch Printers Limited, Hawick.

Cape, B. F. & Dobson, P. (eds) (1978) *Baillière's Nurses' Dictionary*, 18th edn. Baillière Tindall, London.

Cherry, G. W. & Ryan, T. J. (1987) *Blueprint for the Treatment of Leg Ulcers and the Prevention of Recurrence*. Squibb Surgicare, Hounslow.

Cohen, B. E. & Cohen, I. K. (1973) Vitamin A: adjuvant and steroid antagonist in the immune response. *Journal of Immunology*, 3(5), 1376–1380, quoted in Messer, M. S. (1989) Wound care. *Critical Care Nursing Quarterly*, 11(4), 17–27.

Cooper, D. M. (1990) Optimizing wound healing. *Nursing Clinics of North America*, 25(1), 165–80.

Cox, B. D. *et al.* (1987) *The Health and Lifestyle Survey*, Health Promotion Trust, London.

Cruse, P. J. E. & Foord, R. (1980) The epidemiology of wound infection. *Surgical Clinics of North America*, 60(1), 27–40, quoted in Pritchard, A. P. & David, J. A. (eds) (1988) *The Royal Marsden Hospital Manual of Clinical Nursing Procedures*, 2nd edn. Harper & Row, London.

Cunliffe, W. J. (1990) Eusol – to use or not to use? *Dermatology in Practice* 8(2), 5–7.

Dale, J. J. & Gibson, B. (1986a) Leg ulcers: a disease affecting all ages. *The Professional Nurse*, 1(8), 213–16.

Dale, J. J. & Gibson, B. (1986b) Leg ulcers: the nursing assessment. *The Professional Nurse*, 1(9), 236–8.

Dale, J. J. & Gibson, B. (1986c) The treatment of leg ulcers. *The Professional Nurse*, 1(12), 321–4.

Dale, J. J. & Gibson, B. (1987) Compression bandaging for venous ulcers. *The Professional Nurse*, 2(7), 211–14.

Dale, J. J. & Gibson, B. (1990) Back-up for the venous pump. *The Professional Nurse*, 5(9), 481–6.

David, J. A. (1983) Normal physiology from injury to repair. *Nursing*, 2(11), 296–7.

David, J. A. (1986) *Wound Management: A Comprehensive Guide to Dressing and Healing*. Martin Dunitz, London.

David, J. A. (1987) Beds. *Nursing*, 3(13), 503–5.

David, J. A. (1990) Recent venous ulcer treatments. *Nursing Standard*, 4(23), 24–6.

David, J. A. *et al.* (1983) *An Investigation of the Current Methods Used in Nursing For the Care of Patients With Established Pressure Sores*. Nursing Practice Research Unit, University of Surrey.

Dealey, C. (1988) The role of the tissue viability nurse. Supplement, *Nursing Standard*, 2(51), 4–5.

Dealey, C. (1989) Management of cavity wounds. *Nursing*, 3(39), 25–7.

Dealey, C. (1991) Criteria for wound healing. *Nursing*, 4(29), 20–1.

Deas, J. *et al.* (1986) The toxicity of commonly used antiseptics on fibroblasts in tissue culture. *Phlebology*, 1, 205–9.

Department of Infection Control, Memorial Hospital (1989) *Blueprint for the Prevention and Management of Pressure Sores*. Convatec Limited, England.

Dictionary of Nursing. Oxford Reference (1990) Consultant editor, P. Wainwright; general editors, R. Fergusson *et al.* Oxford University Press, Oxford.

Draper, J. (1985) Make the dressing fit the wound. *Nursing Times*, 81(41), 32–5.

Dyson, R. (1978) Bed sores – the injuries hospital staff inflict on patients. *Nursing Mirror*, 146(24), 30–2.

Dyson, M. *et al.* (1988) Comparison of the effects of moist and dry conditions on dermal repair. *The Journal of Investigative Dermatology*, 91(5), 434–9.

Ehrlich, H. P. *et al.* (1973) The effects of vitamin A and

glucocorticoids upon inflammation and collagen synthesis. *Annals of Surgery*, 2, 222–7, quoted in Messer, M. S. (1989) Wound care. *Critical Care Nursing Quarterly*, 11(4), 17–27.

Evans, P. (1988) Venous disorders of the leg. *Nursing Times*, 84(49), 46–7.

Fader, R. C. *et al.* (1983) Sodium hypochlorite decontamination of split-thickness cadaveric skin infected with bacteria and yeast with subsequent isolation and growth of basal cells to confluency in tissue culture. *Antimicrobial Agents and Chemotherapy*, 24(2), 181–5.

Falanga, V. & Eaglstein, W. (1986) A therapeutic approach to venous ulcers. *Journal of American Academy of Dermatology*, 14(5), 777–84.

Fangrell, B. (1979) Local microcirculaton in chronic venous incompetence and leg ulcers. *Vascular Surgery*, 13(4), 217–25.

Farrow, S. & Toth, B. (1991) The place of Eusol in wound management. *Nursing Standard*, 5(22), 25–7.

Ferguson, A. (1988) Best performer. *Nursing Times*, 84(14), 52–5.

Fincham Gee, C. (1990) Measuring the wound size. *Nursing*, 4(2), 34–5.

Florey, C. du V. (1982) Diabetes mellitus (Chapter 25). In *Epidemiology of Diseases* (Ed. by D. L. Miller & R. D. T. Farmer). Blackwell Scientific Publications, Oxford.

Forrest, R. D. (1980) The treatment of pressure sores. *Journal of International Medical Research*, 8, 430–5.

Fraser, R. & Gilchrist, T. (1983) Sorbsan calcium alginate fibre dressings in footcare. *Biomaterials*, 4, 222–4.

General Household Survey, 1986 (1989) HMSO, London, pp. 290–3.

Gilchrist, B. (1989) The treatment of leg ulcers with occlusive hydrocolloid dressings: a microbiological study, Chapter 6. In *Directions in Nursing Research*, (Ed. by J. Wilson-Barnett & S. Robinson). Scutari Press, London, pp. 51–8.

Gilchrist, T. & Martin, A. M. (1983) Wound treatment with Sorbsan – an alginate fibre dressing. *Biomaterials*, 4, 317–20.

Gogia, P. P. *et al.* (1988) Wound management with whirlpool and infrared cold laser treatment. *Physical Therapy*, 68(8), 1239–42.

Goren, D. (1989) Use of omniderm in treatment of low-degree pressure sores in terminally ill cancer patients. *Cancer Nursing*, 12(3), 165–9.

Gould, D. (1984) Clinical forum. *Nursing Mirror*, 159(16), pp. iii–vi.

Griffin, T. (ed.) (1989) *Social Trends 19. Central Statistical Office*. HMSO, London.

Gustafsson, G. (1988) Guidelines for the application of disinfectants in wound care. *Nursing RSA Verpleging*, 3(11/12), 8–9.

Guttman, L. (1976) The prevention and treatment of pressure sores. In *Bed Sore Biomechnics* (Ed. by R. M. Kenedi *et al.*). Macmillan, London.

Guyton, A. C. (1984) *Physiology of the Human Body*, 6th edn. CBS College Publishing, USA.

Hallows, L. (1987) Leg ulcers. An underlying problem. *Community Outlook*, September, 6–14.

Harkiss, K. J. (ed.) (1971) *Surgical Dressings and Wound Healing*. Bradford University Press, Bradford.

Harkiss, K. J. (1985a) Leg ulcers: cheaper in the long run. *Community Outlook*, August, 19–28.

Harkiss, K. J. (1985b) Wound management: cost analysis of dressing materials used in venous leg ulcers. *Pharmaceutical Journal*, 31 August, 268–9.

Henry, M. & Corless, C. (1989) The incidence of varicose veins in Ireland. *Phlebology*, 41, 133–7.

Holmes, S. (1990) Good food for long life. *The Professional Nurse*, 6(1), 43–6.

Hunt, T. K. & Dunphy, J. E. (1979) *Fundamentals of Wound Management*. Appleton-Century-Crofts, New York. Quoted in Messer, M. S. (1989) Wound care. *Critical Care Nursing Quarterly*, 11(4), 17–27.

Hunt, T. K. *et al.* (1969) Effect of vitamin A on reversing the inhibitory effect of cortisone on healing of open wounds in animals and man. *Annals of Surgery*, 170, 633–41. Quoted in Messer, M. S. (1989) Wound care. *Critical Care Nursing Quarterly*, 11(4), 17–27.

Husian, T. (1953) An experimental study of some pressure effects on tissues, with reference to the bed-sore problems. *Journal of Pathology and Bacteriology*, 66, 347–58.

Ivetic, O. & Lyne, P. A. (1990) Fungating and ulcerating malignant lesions: a review of the literature. *Journal of Advanced Nursing*, 15, 83–8.

Jackson, D. S. & Rovee, D. T. (1988) Current concepts in wound healing: research and theory. *Journal of Enterostomal Therapy*, 15(3), 133–7.

Jeter, K. F. & Tintle, T. (1988) Principles of wound cleaning and wound care. *Journal of Home Health Care Practice*, 1, 43–7.

Johnson, A. (1984) Towards rapid tissue healing. *Nursing Times*, 80(48), 39–43.

Johnson, A. (1988a) Natural healing processes: an essential update. *The Professional Nurse*, 3, 149–52.

Johnson, A. (1988b) The case against the use of hypochlorites in the treatment of open wounds. *Care – Science and Practice*, 6(3), 86–8.

Johnson, A. (1988c) Modern wound care products. *The Professional Nurse*, 3, 392–8.

Johnson, A. (1988d) Standard protocols for treating open wounds. *The Professional Nurse*, 3(12), 498–501.

Johnson, A. (1989) Granuflex wafers as a prophylactic pressure sore dressing. *Care – Science and Practice*, 7(2), 55–8.

Kaufman, T. & Alexander, J. W. (1988) Topical oxygen treatment promoted healing and enhanced scar formation of experimental full-thickness burns. In *Beyond Occlusion: Wound Care Proceedings. Royal Society of Medicine International Congress and Symposium Series* (Ed. by T. J. Ryan, 1988b), pp. 61–6. Royal Society of Medicine, London.

Kaufman, T. & Berger (1988) Topical pH and burn wound healing: a review. In *Beyond Occlusion: Wound Care Proceedings. Royal Society of Medicine International Congress and Symposium Series* (Ed. by T. J. Ryan, 1988b), pp. 55–60. Royal Society of Medicine, London.

Kaufman, T. *et al.* (1985) Topical acidification promotes healing of experimental deep partial thickness skin burns: a randomized double-blind preliminary study. *Burns*, 12, 84–90.

Kaufman, T. & Hirshowitz, B. (1982) The influence of various microclimate conditions on the burn wound: a review. *Burns*, 9, 84–90.

Knight, A. (1990) The skin clinic. *Modern Medicine*, 35(8), 608–8.

Knighton, D. R. *et al.* (1981) Regulation of wound healing angiogenesis. Effect of oxygen gradients and inspired oxygen concentration. *Surgery*, 90(2), 262–70.

Kosiak, M. (1958) Evaluation of pressure as a factor in the production of ischial ulcers. *Archives of Physical Medicine and Rehabilitation*, 40, 62–9.

Kosiak, M. (1976) A mechanical resting surface: its effect on pressure distribution. *Archives of Physical Medicine and Rehabilitation*, 57, 481–3.

Lawrence, J. D. (1985) The physical properties of a new hydrocolloid dressing. In *An Environment for Healing: The Role of Occlusion. Royal Society of Medicine International Congress and Symposium Series* (Ed. by T. J. Ryan, 1985), pp. 69–76. Royal Society of Medicine, London.

Lawrence, J. D. & Groves, A. R. (1988) *Blueprint for the Management of Minor Burns*. Squibb Surgicare, Hounslow.

Leaper, D. (1986) Antiseptics and their effects on healing tissue. *Nursing Times*, 82(22), 45–6.

Lechter, A. *et al.* (1987) Pelvic varices and gonadal veins. *Phlebology*, 2, 181–8.

Lycarotti, M. E. & Leaper, D. J. (1989) Measurement in wound healing. *Care – Science and Practice*, 7(3), 68–71.

Maibach, H. I. & Rovee, D. T. (1972) *Epidermal Wound Healing*. Year Book Medical Publishers, Chicago.

Mallett, J. (1988) Wound dressing made easier. *Senior Nurse*, 8(5), 31–3.

Mallett, J. & Charles, H. (1989) *Survey of Clients with Leg Ulceration Treated by District Nurses in Paddington and North Kensington*. Report produced for Paddington and North Kensington Health Authority.

Mallett, J. & Charles, H. (1990) Defining the leg ulcer problem. *Journal of District Nursing*, 9(1), 5–10.

Mani, R. *et al.* (1988) Non-invasive oxygen measurements: have they a role in ulcer investigations? In *Beyond Occulsion: Wound Care Procedings. Royal Society of Medicine International Congress and Symposium Series* (Ed. by T. J. Ryan, 1988b). Royal Society of Medicine, London.

Marcelon, G. & Vanhoutte, P. M. (1988) Venotonic effect of ruscus under variable temperature conditions *in vitro*. *Phlebology*, 3, Supplement 1, 51–4.

Marcelon, G. *et al.* (1988) Oestrogens impregnation and ruscus action on the human vein *in vitro*, depending on preliminary results. *Phlebology*, 3, Supplement 1, 83–5.

Margolin *et al.* (1990) Management of radiation-induced moist skin desquamation using hydrocolliod dressing. *Cancer Nursing*, 13(2), 71–80.

Martindale, W. (1982) *The Extra Pharmcopoeia*, 28th edn. The Pharmaceutical Press, London.

Masi, A. T. & Medsger, T. A. (1979) Epidemiology of the rheumatic diseases. *In Arthritis and Allied Conditions* (Ed. by D. J. McCarty), pp. 11–35. Lea & Febiger, Philadelphia. Quoted in Walker, J. M. *et al.* (1989) The nursing management of pain in the community: a theoretical framework. *Journal of Advanced Nursing*, 14, 240–7.

Matthews, R. N. (1986) Leg ulcers. *Surgery*, 1(33), 790–5.

Mertz, P. M. *et al.* (1985) Occlusive wound dressings to prevent bacterial invasion and wound infection. *Journal of the American Academy of Dermatology*, 12(4), 662–8.

Messer, M. S. (1989) Wound care. *Critical Care Nursing Quarterly*, 11(4), 17–27.

Miller, D. L. & Farmer, R. D. T. (Eds) (1982) *Epidemiology of Diseases*. Blackwell Scientific Publications, Oxford.

Milward, P. (1988) The healing process. Educational Leaflet Supplement to *Care – Science and Practice*, 6(3).

Morgan, D. A. (1990) *Formulary of Wound Management Products. A Guide for Health Care Staff*, 4th edn. Britcare Ltd, UK.

Morison, M. J. (1989) Wound cleansing – which solution? *The Professional Nurse*, 4, 220–5.

National Pressure Ulcer Advisory Panel (1989) Pressure ulcers: incidence, economics and risk assessment. *Care – Science and Practice*, 7(4), 96–9.

Nicholls, R. (1989) Leg ulcers: collecting the facts. *Nursing Standard*, Special Supplement, 6 pp. 12–13 December.

Nicholls, R. (1990) Leg ulcers: a study in the community. *Nursing Standard*, Special Supplement, 7 pp. 4–6 April.

Norton, D. *et al.* (1985) *An Investigation of Geriatric Nursing Problems in Hospital*. Churchill Livingstone, Edinburgh.

Nurses' Drug Alert (1987) *Avoid Use of Hydrogen Peroxide and Povidine-Iodine in Open Wounds*. M. J. Powers, Publishers, New Jersey.

Official Population Census Statistics (1983) *Midyear Population* Estimates for Parkside Health District. HMSO, London.

Pattie, A. H. & Gilleard, C. J. (1979) *Manual of the Clifton Assessment Procedures of the Elderly (CAPE)*. Hodder & Stoughton, Great Britain.

Perkins, P. (1989) A clinic to cope with leg ulcers. *MIMS Magazine*, April, pp. 73–4.

Piper, S. M. (1989) Effective use of occlusive dressings. *The Professional Nurse*, 4(8), 402–4.

Pottle, B. (1987) Trial of a dressing for non-healing ulcers. *Nursing Times*, 83(12), 54–8.

Pritchard, A. P. & David, J. A. (Eds) (1988) *The Royal Marsden Manual of Clinical Nursing Procedures*, 2nd edn. Harper & Row, London.

Raiman, J. (1986) Pain relief – a two-way process. *Nursing Times*, 82(15), 24–8.

Roberts, G. (1988) Nutrition and wound healing. Supplement to *Nursing Standard*, 2(51), 8–12.

Robinson, B. (1988) Aetiology and treatment of leg ulcers. Focus on wound healing. Supplement to *MIMS Magazine*, July, p. 23.

Rovee, D. T. *et al.* (1972) Effect of local wound environment on epidermal healing, Chapter 8. In *Epidermal Wound Healing*, (Ed. by H. I. Maibach & D. T. Rovee), pp. 159–81. Year Book Medical Publishers, Chicago.

Royal College of General Practitioners (1986) *Alcohol: A Balanced View*. Royal College of General Practitioners (Report from General Practice, 24), Exeter.

Ryan, T. J. (Ed) (1985a) *An Environment for Healing: The Role of Occlusion. Royal Society of Medicine, International Congress and Symposium Series*, pp. 5–14. Royal Society of Medicine, London.

Ryan, T. J. (1985b) Current management of leg ulcers. *Drugs*, 30(5), 461–8.

Ryan, T. J. (1987) *The Management of Leg Ulcers*, 2nd edn. Oxford University Press, Oxford.

Ryan, T. J. (1988a) Management of leg ulcers. *The Practitioner*, 232, 1014–21.

Ryan, T. J. (Ed) (1988b) *Beyond Occlusion: Wound Care Proceedings. Royal Society of Medicine, International Congress and Symposium Series.* Royal Society of Medicine, London.

Saunders, J. (1989) Toilet cleaner for wound care? *Community Outlook*, pp. 11–13. *Nursing Times*, 85(10).

Silver, I. A. (1972) Oxygen tension and epithelialization, Chapter 17. In *Epidermal Wound Healing* (Ed. by H. I. Maibach & D. T. Rovee), pp. 291–305. Year Book Medical Publishers, Chicago.

Smith, I. (1989) Waterlow/Norton scoring system – a ward view. *Care – Science and Practice*, 7(4), 93–5.

Smith, S. (1988) Doing the leg work. *Community Outlook*, pp. 17–18. *Nursing Times*, 84(33).

Spanswick, A. *et al.* (1990) Eusol – the final word. *The Professional Nurse*, 5(4), 211–14.

Stronge, J. L. (1984) Principles of wound care. Supplement, *Nursing*, 2(26), 7–10.

Struckmann, J. R. (1988) Venous muscle pump function following reconstructive arterial surgery. *Phlebology*, 3, 169–73.

Swanwick, T. & MacLellan, D. (1988) The treatment of venous ulceration. *Nursing*, 3(32), 40–3.

Taheri, S. A. *et al.* (1987) Iliocaval compression syndrome. *Phlebology*, 2, 173–9.

The Dressing Times (1988) 1(2). Welsh Centre for the Quality Control of Surgical Dressings, East Glamorgan Hospital, Glamorgan.

The Dressing Times (1989) 2(1). Welsh Centre for the Quality Control of Surgical Dressings, East Glamorgan Hospital, Glamorgan.

Thomas, L. (1988a) Treating leg ulcers. *Nursing Standard*, 2(18), 22–3.

Thomas, L. (1988b) Treating leg ulcers. *Nursing Standard*, 2(19), 28.

Thomas, S. (1990) Cost-effective management of leg ulcers. *Community Outlook*, pp. 21–2. *Nursing Times*, 86(11).

Thompson, J. (1990) Foot and leg care, *Community Outlook*, pp. 14–17. *Nursing Times*, 86(8).

Thorp, J. M. *et al.* (1987) Gross hypernatraemia associated with the use of antiseptic surgical packs. *Anaesthesia*, 42, 750–3.

Tomlinson, D. (1987) To clean or not to clean? *Journal of Infection Control/Nursing Times*, 83(9), 71–5.

Tooke, J. E. *et al.* (1988) Diabetes and wound healing: the skin response to injury, and white cell behaviour *in vivo* in diabetic patients. In *Beyond Occlusion: Wound Care Proceedings. Royal Society of Medicine International Congress and Symposium Series* (Ed. by T. J. Ryan, 1988b), pp. 71–4. Royal Society Medicine, London.

Torrance, C. (1985) Wound care in accident and emergency, pp. 1–3. Supplement, *Nursing*, 2(42).

Trelstad, A. & Osmundson, D. (1989) Water piks: wound cleansing alternative. *Plastic Surgical Nursing*, 9(3), 117–19.

Tubman Papantonio, C. (1988a) Holistic approach to healing: part I. *Home Healthcare Nurse*, 6(5), 31–4.

Tubman Papantonio, C. (1988b) Holistic approach to healing: part II. *Home Healthcare Nurse*, 6, 31–5.

Turner, T. D. (1979) Hospital usage of absorbant dressings. *The Pharmaceutical Journal*, May, 421–2.

Turner, T. D. (1983) A practical guide to absorbant dressings. Supplement, *Nursing*, 12.

Turner, T. D. (1985) Semiocclusive and occlusive dressings. In *An Environment for Healing: The Role of Occlusion. Royal Society of Medicine International Congress and Symposium Series* (Ed. by T. J. Ryan). Royal Society of Medicine, London.

Turner, T. D. *et al.* (1986) *Advances in Wound management Symposium Proceedings*, John Wiley, Cardiff. Quoted in *Blueprint for the Treatment of Leg Ulcers and the Prevention of Recurrence* (Ed. by G. W. Cherry & T. J. Ryan, 1987). Squibb Surgicare, Hounslow.

Valdes-Dapena, M. A. & Arey, J. B. (1962) Boric acid poisoning. *Journal of Pediatrics*, 61(4), 531–46.

Walker, J. M. *et al.* (1989) The nursing management of pain in the community: a theoretical framework. *Journal of Advanced Nursing*, 14, 240–7.

Waterlow, J. (1987) Calculating the risk. *Nursing Times*, 83(39), 58–60.

Waterlow, J. (1988) Prevention is cheaper than cure. *Nursing Times*, 84(25), 69–70.

Wells, R. J. (1984) Controversial issues in wound care. *Journal of Clinical Nursing*, Suppl., June, 10–11.

Westaby, S. (1985) *Wound Care.* Heinemann, London.

Williams, I. (1989) A company wraps up the bandage market with new deal for wounded. *The Guardian*, 13 March.

Williamson, D. (1988) Leg ulcers. Taking your time with leg ulcers. *Mims Magazine*, 1 May, 105–8.

Willington, F. L. (1977) The use of non-ionic detergents in sanitary cleansing: a report of a preliminary trial. *Journal of Advanced Nursing*, 3, 373–82.

Wilson-Barnett, J. & Robinson, S. (Eds) (1989) *Directions in Nursing Research*, Scutari Press, London.

Wingate, P. & Wingate, R. (1988) *The Penguin Medical Enclyopedia* 3rd edn. Pengiun Books, England.

Winter, A. & Hewitt, H. (1990) Testing a hydrocolloid. *Nursing Times*, 86(50), 59–62.

Winter, G. D. (1971) Healing of skin wounds and the influence of dressings on the repair process. In *Surgical Dressings and Wound Healing* (Ed. by K. J. Harkiss), pp. 46–50. Bradford University Press, Bradford.

Winter, G. D. (1972) Epidermal regeneration studied in the domestic pig, Chapter 4. In *Epidermal Wound Healing* (Ed. by H. I. Maibach & D. T. Rovee), pp. 71–112. Year Book Medical Publishers, Chicago.

Wood, P. H. N. (1977) In *Epidemiology of Diseases* (Ed. by D. L. Miller & R. D. T. Farmer, 1982). Blackwell Scientific Publications, Oxford.

Wyngaarden, J. B. & Smith, L. H. (1988) *Cecil Textbook of Medicine*, 18th edn. W. B. Saunders, Philadephia.

Zederfeldt, B. *et al.* (1980) *Wounds and Wound Healing.* Wolfe Medical Publications, New York.

GUIDELINES: CHANGING WOUND DRESSINGS

Equipment

1. As for 'Guidelines: Aseptic technique' (Chapter 3).
2. Cleansing fluid for irrigation (see Table 46.3).
3. Appropriate dressing (see Table 46.4).

Procedure

See procedure for 'Aseptic technique' (Chapter 3) up to and including step 10, then loosen the dressing.

Action	Rationale
11. Where appropriate, loosen the old dressing.	The dressing can then be lifted off without causing trauma.
12. Clean hands with a bactericidal alcohol hand rub.	Hands may become contaminated by handling outer packets, dressing, etc.
13. Using the forceps in the pack, arrange the sterile field with the handles of instruments in one corner or around the edge of the sterile field.	The time the wound is exposed should be kept to a minimum to reduce the risk of contamination.
Where appropriate, swab along the 'tear area' of lotion sachet with chlorhexidine gluconate 0.5% and isopropyl alcohol. Tear open sachet and pour lotion into gallipots or an indented plastic tray (see Table 46.3).	To minimize risk of contamination of lotion.
14. Remove dressing by placing a hand in the plastic bag, lifting the dressing off and inverting the plastic bag so that the dressing is now inside the bag. Thereafter use this as the 'dirty' bag.	To reduce the risk of cross infection.
15. Attach the bag with the dressing to the side of the trolley below the top shelf.	Contaminated material is below the level of the sterile field.
16. Assess the wound healing with reference to volume, amount of granulation tissue and epithelialization, signs of infection, underlying pathology etc (see Table 46.2). (Record assessment in relevant documentation at the end of the procedure.)	To evaluate wound care.
17. Put on gloves, touching only the inside wrist end.	To reduce the risk of infection to the wound and contamination of the nurse. Gloves provide greater sensitivity than forceps and are less likely to traumatize the wound or the patient's skin.
18. If necessary, gently clean the wound with a gloved hand using normal saline (unless another solution is indicated [see Table 46.3]) and non-linting material, such as foam. If appropriate, irrigate by flushing with water or normal saline.	To reduce the possibility of physical and chemical trauma to granulation and epithelial tissue.
19. Apply the dressing that is most suitable for the wound using the criteria for an ideal dressing (see Table 46.4).	To promote healing.

Guidelines: Changing wound dressings

Action	Rationale
20. Remove gloves and fasten with non-allergenic tape as required.	
21. Make sure the patient is comfortable and the dressing is secure.	A dressing may slip or feel uncomfortable as the patient changes position.

Continue with steps 15 to 18 from the procedure for 'Aseptic technique'.

GUIDELINES: REMOVAL OF SUTURES, CLIPS OR STAPLES

Equipment

1. As for 'Guidelines: Aseptic technique' (Chapter 3).
2. Sterile scissors, stitch cutter, Michel clip-removing forceps or staple remover.
3. Sterile adhesive sutures.

Procedure

Action	Rationale
1. Explain the procedure to the patient.	To obtain the patient's consent and co-operation.
2. Perform procedure using aseptic technique.	To prevent infection (for further information see procedure on aseptic technique, Chapter 3).
3. Clean the wound with an appropriate sterile solution such as normal saline (see Table 46.3).	To prevent infection.
For removal of sutures	
4. Lift knot of suture with metal forceps. Snip stitch close to the skin. Pull suture out gently (see Figure 46.2).	Plastic forceps tend to slip against nylon sutures. To prevent infection by drawing exposed suture through the tissue.
5. Use tips of scissors slightly open or the side of the stitch cutter to gently press the skin when the suture is being drawn out.	To minimize pain by counteracting the adhesion between the suture and surrounding tissue.
For removal of clips	
6. Squeeze wings of Kifa clips together with forceps to release from skin (see Figure 46.3). For Michel clips use special forceps under the clips to flatten the loop (see Figure 46.4).	To release clips atraumatically from the wound.

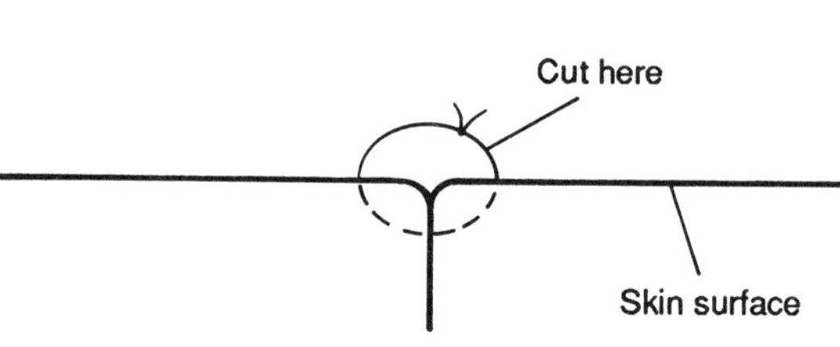

Figure 46.2 Suture removal.

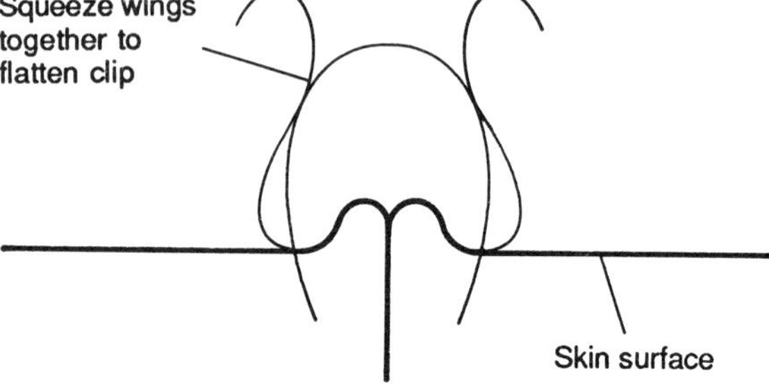

Figure 46.3 Kifa clip removal.

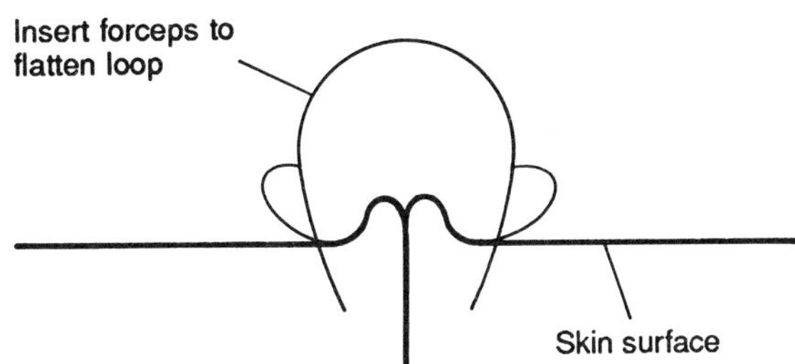

Figure 46.4 Michel clip removal.

Action	Rationale
7. If the wound gapes use adhesive sutures to oppose the wound edges.	To improve the cosmetic effect.
8. When necessary, cover the wound with an appropriate dressing (see Table 46.4).	To provide the best possible environment for wound healing to take place. To reduce the risk of infection. To prevent the suture line from rubbing against clothing.

For removal of staples

Action	Rationale
9. Slide the lower bar of the staple remover with the V-shaped groove under the staple at an angle of 90 degrees. Squeeze the handles of the staple removers together to open the staple. If the suture line is under tension, use free hand to gently squeeze the skin either side of the suture line.	To release the staple atraumatically from the wound. If the angle of the staple remover is not correct, the staple will not come out freely. To reduce tension of skin around suture line and lessen pain on removal of staple.
10. If the wound gapes use adhesive sutures to oppose the wound edges.	To improve the cosmetic effect.

For all suture lines

Action	Rationale
11. Record condition of suture line and surrounding skin (for example, amount of exudate, pus, inflammation, pain, etc., see Table 46.2).	To document care and enable evaluation of the wound.

GUIDELINES: DRAIN DRESSING (REDIVAC – CLOSED DRAINAGE SYSTEMS)

Equipment

1. As for 'Guidelines: Aseptic technique' (Chapter 3).
2. Keyhole dressing.
3. Sterile padded dressing.

Procedure

Action	Rationale
1. Explain the procedure to the patient.	To obtain the patient's consent and co-operation.
2. Perform procedure using aseptic technique.	To prevent infection (for further information on asepsis, see procedure on aseptic technique, Chapter 3).

Guidelines: Drain dressing

Action	Rationale
3. Clean the surrounding skin with an appropriate sterile solution such as normal saline (see Table 46.3).	To prevent infection.
4. Ensure that the skin suture holding the drain site in position is intact.	To prevent the drain from leaving the wound.
5. Cover the drain site with a keyhole dressing.	To protect the drain site, prevent infection entering the wound and absorb exudate.
6. Tape securely.	To ensure continuity of drainage.
7. Ensure that the drain is primed or that the suction pump is in working order.	

GUIDELINES: CHANGE OF VACUUM BOTTLE (REDIVAC – CLOSED DRAINAGE SYSTEMS)

Equipment

1. Sterile topical swab.
2. Artery forceps.
3. Sterile drainage bottle.

Procedure

Action	Rationale
1. Explain the procedure to the patient.	To obtain the patient's consent and co-operation.
2. Wash hands using bactericidal soap and water or bactericidal alcohol hand rub.	To minimize the risk of infection.
3. Clean the nozzle of wall suction apparatus with an appropriate antiseptic solution and prime a sterile vacuum bottle.	To ensure sterility and to prepare the bottle for attachment to the drainage tube.
4. Measure the contents of the bottle to be changed and record this in the appropriate documents.	To maintain an accurate record of drainage from the wound and enable evaluation of state of wound.
5. Clamp the tube with artery forceps and remove the bottle.	To prevent air and contamination entering the wound via the drain.
6. Put on clean gloves.	To prevent contamination from blood and body fluids.
7. Clean the end of the tube and attach it to the sterile bottle.	To maintain sterility.
8. Remove the artery forceps.	To re-establish the drainage system.
9. Ensure that the bottle is primed.	To ensure that drainage continues.
10. If the vacuum is constantly lost, take down the dressing and examine the entry site of the drain.	To ensure that the drain has not become dislodged.
11. If necessary, re-dress as drain dressing (above).	

GUIDELINES: REMOVAL OF DRAIN (REDIVAC – CLOSED DRAINAGE SYSTEMS, AND PENROSE, ETC. – OPEN DRAINAGE SYSTEMS)

Equipment

1. As for 'Guidelines: Aseptic technique' (see Chapter 3).
2. Sterile scissors or suture cutter.

Action	Rationale
1. Check the patient's operation notes.	To establish the number and site(s) of internal and external sutures.
2. Explain the procedure to the patient.	To obtain the patient's consent and co-operation.
3. If appropriate (Redivac and closed drainage systems) release vacuum.	To prevent pulling at wound tissue.
4. Perform the procedure using aseptic technique.	To minimize the risk of infection. (For further information on asepsis, see Chapter 3.)
5. Where the wound is covered with an occlusive dressing (e.g. following lumpectomy in the breast), lift and snip the dressing from around the drain. Do not remove it from the entire wound.	To prevent disturbing the incision or contaminating the wound.
6. Only clean the wound if necessary, using an appropriate sterile solution, such as normal saline (see Table 46.3).	To prevent infection.
7. Hold the knot of the suture with metal forceps and gently lift upwards.	Plastic forceps tend to slip against nylon sutures. To allow space for the scissors or stitch cutter to be placed underneath.
8. Cut the shortest end of the suture as close to the skin as possible.	To prevent infection by allowing the suture to be liberated from the drain without drawing the exposed part through tissue.
9. Remove drain gently. If there is resistance place free gloved hand against the tissue to oppose the tugging of the drain being removed. If the resistance is felt to be excessive Entonox may be required.	To minimize pain and reduce trauma.
10. Cover the drain site with a sterile dressing and tape securely.	To prevent infection entering the drain site.
11. Measure and record the contents of the drainage bottle in the appropriate documents.	To maintain an accurate record of drainage from wound and enable evaluation of state of wound.
12. If disposable drainage bottle is used, dispose of in yellow clinical waste bag.	To prevent environmental contamination. Yellow is the recognized colour for clinical waste.
13. If glass drainage bottle is used, empty contents into bedpan washer and send bottle to the central sterile supplies department for cleaning and sterilizing.	To prevent environmental contamination. To ensure reusable bottles are cleaned and sterilized before use.

GUIDELINES: SHORTENING OF DRAIN (PENROSE, ETC. OPEN DRAINAGE SYSTEMS)

Action	Rationale
1. Follow steps 1 to 8 above (removal of drain), i.e. to the stage where the suture has been cut.	
2. Using gloved hand, gently ease the drain out of wound to the length requested by surgeons. Usually 3 to 5 cm.	Allows healing to take place from base of wound.
3. Using gloved hand, place a sterile safety pin through the drain as close to the skin as possible, taking great care not to stab either the nurse or patient.	To prevent retraction into the wound and minimize the risk of cross-infection.
4. Cut same amount of tubing from distal end of drain as withdrawn from wound.	So there is a convenient length of tubing to drain into the bag. To ensure patient comfort.
5. Place a sterile, suitably sized drainage bag over the drain site.	To allow effluent to drain into the bag. To prevent excoriation of the skin. To contain any odour.
6. Check bag is secure and comfortable for the patient.	For patient comfort.
7. Record by how much the drainage tube was shortened.	To ensure the length remaining in the wound is known.

GUIDELINES: DRAINAGE DRESSING (PENROSE, PAUL'S TUBING, CORRUGATED AND NAUNTON MORGAN DRAINAGE SYSTEMS)

Equipment

1. As for 'Guidelines: Aseptic technique' (see Chapter 3).
2. Sterile padded dressings.
3. Stomahesive wafers.
4. Keyhole dressing.
5. Drainage stoma bag.

Procedure

Minimum drainage

Action	Rationale
1. Explain the procedure to the patient.	To obtain the patient's consent and co-operation.
2. Perform the procedure using aseptic technique.	To prevent infection. (For further information on asepsis, see Chapter 3.)
3. Clean the surrounding skin with an appropriate sterile solution.	To prevent infection.
4. Cut a hole slightly larger than the site in a stomahesive wafer and apply the wafer to the skin surrounding the drain.	To protect the skin from the drainage which may cause excoriation. The wafer should fit as close as possible without interrupting the flow of effluent.

5. Leave the stomahesive wafer in position until the drain is removed.	To continue to protect vulnerable skin.
6. Cover the drain site and the stomahesive wafer with a keyhole dressing and sterile dressing pad. Tape securely.	To absorb drainage. To prevent infection.
7. Change the dressing whenever it becomes soiled.	To prevent infection.
8. Describe the wound and type of drainage in appropriate documents and amend the care plan accordingly.	For accurate evaluation of progress of drainage.

Copious drainage

1. Follow steps 1 to 5 above, i.e. to the stage where the stomahesive wafer has been applied.	
2. Cover the drain with a clinically clean drainage stoma bag preferably with a woven back.	To allow effluent to drain into the bag. To reduce sweating and so aid patient comfort.
3. Ensure that the drain is enclosed by the aperture of the bag.	To prevent excoriation of surrounding skin. To contain any odour.
4. Where necessary, pad under the bag and secure with Netelast.	To prevent bag rubbing skin and to keep it secure.
5. Empty the contents of the bag regularly and record the amount in appropriate documents.	To prevent accumulated fluid from detaching the bag from the skin due to its weight. To maintain an accurate record of drainage.

GUIDELINES: PREVENTION OF PRESSURE ULCERS

Action	Rationale
1. Assess every patient on admission using a recognized scale, such as the Norton (Table 46.5) or Waterlow (Figure 46.1) Scale.	To identify the patient at risk from developing decubitus ulcers.
2. Reassess every patient on a regular basis and/or if there has been any deterioration or change in condition.	To provide appropriate data on which to base treatment.
3. Do not rub any area at risk.	Rubbing causes maceration and degeneration of subcutaneous tissues, especially in the elderly.
4. Wash areas at risk only if the patient is incontinent or sweating profusely. Use mild soap or a liquid detergent. Ensure that all detergent or soap is rinsed off and that the area is patted dry. Use moisturizer if the skin is very dry. Ask the patient what suits his/her skin.	To maintain skin integrity and prevent the formation of sores. Excessive use of soap can be harmful to the skin. Thorough gentle drying of the skin promotes comfort and discourages the growth of micro-organisms. Dry skin cracks allow entry of micro-organisms (Pritchard & David, 1988).
5. Use barrier creams only when indicated.	Barrier creams prevent damage to the epidermis. They are, however, occlusive and prevent moisture exchange from the skin (Pritchard & David, 1988).

Guidelines: Prevention of pressure ulcers

Action	Rationale
6. Educate the patient to shift position, to pull or push up regularly and to examine the vulnerable areas.	After discharge the patient may be self-caring and possibly still vulnerable to sores. To encourage the patient to participate in own care.
7. Initiate a mobility programme for the patient. Call on the physiotherapist or occupational therapist as appropriate.	To reduce further tissue damage and improve the circulation.
8. Where possible relieve the pressure over areas vulnerable to tissue breakdown. Use appropriate pressure relief devices (Table 46.7). If necessary, turn the patient at least two-hourly and record the position on the relevant charts.	To reduce pressure where possible. Use of inappropriate aids may increase pressure to vulnerable areas.
9. Have the patient recumbent whenever possible. Support with bead bags or pillows in bed. Reduce period spent sitting in chair if pelvic sores develop.	Avoid the use of bedrests as these increase shearing (Pritchard & David, 1988).

Index